Dr. Sarah Hobday
Belper Clinic

Dr. Sarah Hobday

Clinics in Developmental Medicine
DISEASES OF THE NERVOUS SYSTEM IN CHILDHOOD
2nd Edition

Clinics in Developmental Medicine

Diseases of the Nervous System in Childhood

2nd Edition

JEAN AICARDI
Institute of Child Health
London

with contributions from

MARTIN BAX
Charing Cross and Westminster Hospital
London

CHRISTOPHER GILLBERG
Department of Child and Adolescent Psychiatry
University of Göteborg

HÉLÈNE OGIER
Metabolic Investigation Unit
Hôpital Robert Debré
Paris

1998
Mac Keith Press

Distributed by 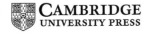 **CAMBRIDGE**
UNIVERSITY PRESS

© 1998 Mac Keith Press
High Holborn House, 52–54 High Holborn, London WC1V 6RL

Senior Editor: Martin C.O. Bax
Managing Editor: Michael Pountney

Editor: Pamela A. Davies
Sub Editor/Design: Pat Chappelle

Indexer: Jill Halliday
Cover/Title Design: Ninety Seven Plus Ltd

Set in Adobe Garamond and Avant Garde on QuarkXPress

First edition 1992

Second edition 1998
Reprinted 1999, with corrections and amendments

British Library Cataloguing-in-Publication data:
A catalogue record for this book is available from the British Library

ISBN: 1 898683 16 6

Printed by The Lavenham Press Ltd, Water Street, Lavenham, Suffolk

Mac Keith Press is supported by **Scope** (formerly The Spastics Society)

CONTENTS

PREFACE TO SECOND EDITION

The pace of progress both in medicine and in communication techniques has been so fast in the past few years that there are those who wonder whether books are still useful. They argue that new data are accumulating so rapidly that only computerized data bases and networks can permit users to keep abreast of current developments in basic and clinical sciences, and that books are irremediably condemned to be outdated even at the time of publication. However, immediate availability of such an overwhelming volume of information may be a mixed blessing as assessment of the quality and relevance is left to the judgement of each user, whereas books may be of some help in soliciting the most important data and giving an idea of their organization and significance, assuming that the author's choices are backed by a certain experience and provided they are not excessively biased. Moreover, books are more friendly companions than computers and are more easily accessible, even at the bedside.

Such considerations led my collaborators and myself to prepare a second edition of this book in an attempt to incorporate the major developments of the last six years, a long enough interval at the current pace of progress in child neurology. Major changes have been made in several chapters in addition to the general updating, but the overall outline of the preceding edition has in the main been kept, as has its resolute clinical orientation. Because the coverage of such a wide subject as the neurological diseases of childhood in a single volume is of necessity incomplete, an essential function of such a book is to serve as a key to access more detailed information in the literature. A special effort has therefore been made to include an extensive choice of references, especially recent ones. Obviously, the selection is biased by our special interests and cannot be expected to be completely representative.

I am grateful to the same small group of collaborators—and friends—who have once more generously given their work time and knowledge and punctually delivered their contributions in spite of their many pressing commitments.

JEAN AICARDI
London, November 1997

ACKNOWLEDGEMENTS

I wish to express my gratitude to Professor B. Neville who welcomed me into the Department of Neurosciences, Institute of Child Health and the Hospital for Sick Children, Great Ormond Street, London, and constantly supported me during the past six years, making possible the preparation of this second edition.

I thank Professors T. Billette de Villemeur and B. Lake, and Doctors S. Boyd, Kling Chong, M. Duchowny and F. Goutières for their contribution to the iconography.

My former secretary Brigitte Tricot achieved the impossible feat of typing and retyping the manuscript in addition to her other tasks and in spite of communication difficulties due to our different geographical locations.

Finally, I wish to express my thanks to Mac Keith Press—to Martin Bax, who prompted me to write this book, which I would never have done without his pressing persuasion, and especially to Pamela Davies and Pat Chappelle for their outstanding editorial help.

PREFACE TO FIRST EDITION*

Diseases of the nervous system in infancy and childhood have a profound impact on the life of patients and their families and are probably the most disruptive of all paediatric ailments. They constitute the matter of Child Neurology, a paediatric sub-specialty whose objectives are the diagnosis, management, alleviation and, if possible, cure of infants, children and adolescents with neurological illnesses.

Neurological diseases account for a significant proportion of the serious paediatric diseases, as between 15 and 20 per cent of hospitalized children have a neurological problem, either as their sole or as an associated complaint. However, many well-educated paediatricians not uncommonly feel uncomfortable and hesitant about what to do to children and what to tell the families of patients with neurological disorders.

This applies to common diseases and, not unexpectedly, even more to unusual ones. Yet, rare neurological disorders are collectively not uncommon. The frequency of the degenerative central nervous system (CNS) disorders as a whole is roughly equal to that of hemiplegic cerebral palsy (Hagberg, personal communication).

The aim of this book is to provide physicians with a sufficiently comprehensive description of neurological diseases of children to permit diagnostic orientation, prognosis and management, and to give access to a selection of references for further, more detailed information, as only limited coverage is compatible with available space.

Care has been taken to limit the references, except on specific points, to recent articles; relatively 'old' references, even when of historical interest, have been omitted, unless they were clearly basic or no or few articles on the particular topic had been recently published.

The book is resolutely clinically oriented, but when necessary some notions concerning pathogenesis and mechanisms are provided. It is meant for physicians with an interest in paediatric neurological disorders, whether paediatricians, neurologists, child neurologists or physicians dedicated to developmental medicine, and deals only with diseases of the nervous system (as indicated by its title). For this reason, I have deliberately not included a section on the neurological examination of infants and children at various ages or given data on maturation of the nervous system. Excellent books and monographs are available on these topics (Neligan and Prudham 1969; Touwen 1976, 1979; Prechtl 1977; Casaer 1979; Amiel-Tison and Grenier 1980, 1985; Dubowitz

and Dubowitz 1981; Saint-Anne Dargassies 1982; Baird and Gordon 1983; Bax and Whitmore 1987; Egan 1990) and the reader is referred to those works for detailed information. Obviously, this is not to detract from the value of the neurological examination. Child neurology is, and probably will remain, a clinical discipline. However spectacular future progress in imaging and in neurophysiological or other laboratory examinations might be, such techniques will remain of little value when applied indiscriminately without a previous careful clinical analysis.

I wish to formulate a few remarks, based on 30 years experience, on what could be termed the 'philosophy' of paediatric neurological examination. In the first place, the eminent importance of history-taking needs to be re-emphasized. It is not going to be superseded by any type of technical examination, especially if asked randomly or systematically. Indeed, medical diagnosis, especially in neuropaediatrics, remains an intellectual process, and the history of the disease—as well as that of the child from conception and that of her/his family—forms the initial and most important step of the diagnostic approach. This applies even more to paroxysmal disorders in which the essential part of the disease—the seizures—is generally known only through oral information from patients and/or caretakers. It is thus critical to get a correct description by listening to patients and by asking questions formulated in adequate words that are both intelligible to lay persons and not suggestive of the 'desired' response (Stephenson 1990); and it is illogical to expect that interictal examinations should indicate the nature of intermittent ictal events.

Neurological examination itself should be as complete as possible and largely guided by historical data. In children, and especially in infants or neonates, it cannot be conducted systematically as in adults. Attempts at 'adult-type' examination will lead to crying and fussing and will thus give only minimal information on the child's nervous system. Much of the examination should not require that the child be lying, as the lying position will often frighten the child by reminding her/him of previous unpleasant medical experience, and certainly gives a minimum of information on CNS functioning. After all, the vertical posture has been a major evolutionary acquisition and, since the time of *Homo erectus*, most human activities take place in the standing position. Therefore, children should be watched patiently in their spontaneous activity, and playing or otherwise interacting with the child is the best manner of assessing CNS function. It cannot be overemphasized that the major role of the CNS is to produce not just reflexes—necessary as these

*Abridged from the original version (published 1992), with some updating of references.

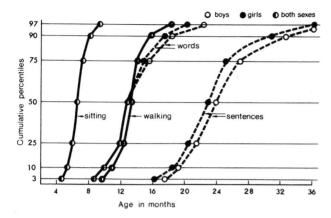

Cumulative percentile curves for four standard developmental milestones. (Neligan and Prudham 1969, reproduced by permission.)

may be—but above all complex and adaptive behaviours. I am always surprised to see physicians interrupt a child's complex spontaneous activity, which is highly informative about the state of the brain, to impose the systematic search of simple responses to non-physiological stimuli, the only merit of which is to be elicited by the doctor but which tell virtually nothing about CNS function! All too often, children are examined but not looked at. On the contrary, watching the child while playing with her/him or simply talking at the bedside to parents or medical students provides a continuous flow of information that runs from the patient to the physician, provided the latter is attentive and knows how to capture and interpret it.

Based on this information, a diagnostic hypothesis arises, in part subconsciously and in part through systematic reflection, and the rest of the examination can be used to look for signs that will vindicate or falsify the hypothesis. In many cases, only a few manoeuvres will be required. In difficult cases, an hypothesis may not emerge initially but will do so only after further reflection and/or repeat examination at another time and under different circumstances. In such cases, having the patient available for frequent re-examination, and not just the need for technical examinations, may be the major reason for demanding hospitalization.

The interpretation of the neurological examination of infants and children is rendered difficult by the necessity to take into account the qualitative aspects of the activity observed, which requires much more experience than to look at the results of relatively standardized tests, useful as these are. The qualitative approach to examination of CNS function in neonates and infants has been illustrated by the work of Brazelton and Nugent (1995), which takes into account such features as 'consolability', 'intensity of gaze' and 'directed attention' that remain highly dependent on the observer's judgement, even though quantification has been proposed.

Likewise, Ferrari *et al.* (1990) have shown that simple observation of the *quality* of the spontaneous movements of preterm infants is strongly correlated with the neurodevelopmental outcome and that normal movements are good predictors of a normal outcome.

In general, there is a tendency among paediatricans to underestimate the abilities of young infants, and this is due in part to excessive emphasis put on the more easily quantitated tonic and postural acquisitions.

A remarkable degree of variability exists among normal infants and children. This is clear in the timing of the main milestones of infancy and early childhood. The figure opposite illustrates this variability as well as the fact that the more complex the skill, the wider the age range when it may be acquired. Thus, children acquire the sitting position within a narrow period, whereas talking in sentences may appear at any time between 18 months and 3 years (Neligan and Prudham 1969). A good knowledge of the *variants of normal development* is therefore essential. Such variants have been well studied for certain skills, *e.g.* prewalking locomotor movements (Robson 1970,1984; Lundberg 1979). Some of the various modes, *e.g.* bottom shuffling, are often associated with late bipedal ambulation to the point that children exhibiting such movements are not infrequently referred to a child neurologist or submitted to useless investigations, which raises parental anxiety. Conversely, the hypotonia of the body axis and lower limbs that is associated with 'shuffling' and contrasts with the normal skill of fine manipulation (Hagberg and Lundberg 1969) may be responsible for delayed diagnosis of spastic diplegia (Robson and Mac Keith 1971). Other variants probably exist in several developmental fields and even in physical characteristics such as the size and time of closure of the fontanelles (Duc and Largo 1986). It is striking that some of the milestones that are culturally regarded as essential are in fact quite variable, whereas skills such as reaching for objects under visual control, whose importance is not culturally emphasized, may be acquired at a reasonably fixed date and may be more significant as predictors of CNS development. This is clearly the case for voluntary reaching, provided it is distinguished from movements such as grasping. In general, the best predictors of development are those skills that are more heavily loaded with intentionality and with cognitive or relational significance, rather than purely tonic or motor milestones.

Diseases of the Nervous System in Childhood, because of the experience—and limitations—of its writers, is mainly focused on child neurology in developed countries. A large part is applicable with minimal adjustment to Third World countries, and I believe that the clinical approach that I favour is particularly appropriate in countries where technical facilities may not be optimal or are lacking altogether. Although efforts have been made to mention at least some aspects of child neurology in developing countries, I am fully aware that important topics have not been covered. My hope is that, with those inevitable limitations, this book will be found useful by those involved in the care of children with neurological diseases throughout the world, as the bases of child neurology are universal.

JEAN AICARDI

REFERENCES

Amiel-Tison, C., Grenier, A. (1980) *Evaluation Neurologique du Nouveau-né et du Nourrisson.* Paris: Masson.

—— (1985) *La Surveillance Neurologique au Cours de la Première Année de la Vie.* Paris: Masson.

Baird, H.W., Gordon, E.C. (1983) *Neurological Evaluation of Infants and Children. Clinics in Developmental Medicine No. 84/85.* London: Spastics International Medical Publications.

Bax, M.C.O., Whitmore, K. (1987) 'The medical examination of children on entry to school. The results and use of neurodevelopmental assessment.' *Developmental Medicine and Child Neurology,* **29,** 40–55.

Brazelton, T.B., Nugent, J.K. (Eds.) (1995) *Neonatal Behavioral Assessment Scale, 3rd Edn. Clinics in Developmental Medicine No. 137.* London: Mac Keith Press.

Casaer, P. (1979) *Postural Behaviour in Newborn Infants. Clinics in Developmental Medicine No. 72.* London: Spastics International Medical Publications.

Dubowitz, L., Dubowitz, V. (1981) *The Neurological Assessment of the Preterm and Full-term Newborn Infant. Clinics in Developmental Medicine No. 79.* London: Spastics International Medical Publications

Duc, G., Largo, R.H. (1986) 'Anterior fontanel: size and closure in term and preterm infants.' *Pediatrics,* **78,** 904–908.

Egan, D.F. (1990) *Developmental Examination of Infants and Preschool Children. Clinics in Developmental Medicine No. 112.* London: Mac Keith Press.

Ferrari, F., Cioni, G., Prechtl, H.F.R. (1990) 'Qualitative changes of general movements in preterm infants with brain lesions.' *Early Human Development,* **23,** 193–232.

Hagberg, B., Lundberg, K. (1969) 'Dissociated motor development simulating cerebral palsy.' *Neuropädiatrie,* **1,** 187-199.

Lundberg, A. (1979) 'Dissociated motor development: developmental patterns, clinical characteristics, causal factors and outcome with special reference to late walking.' *Neuropediatrics,* **10,** 161–182.

Neligan, G., Prudham, D. (1969) 'Norms for four standard developmental milestones by sex, social class and place in family.' *Developmental Medicine and Child Neurology,* **11,** 413–422.

Prechtl, H. (1977) *The Neurological Examination of the Full-term Newborn Infant, 2nd Edn. Clinics in Developmental Medicine No. 68.* London: Spastics International Medical Publications.

Robson, P. (1970) 'Shuffling, hitching, scooting or sliding: some observations in otherwise normal children.' *Developmental Medicine and Child Neurology,* **12,** 608–617.

—— (1984) 'Prewalking locomotor movements and their use in predicting standing and walking.' *Child: Care, Health and Development,* **10,** 317–330.

—— Mac Keith, R. (1971) 'Shufflers with spastic diplegic cerebral palsy: a confusing clinical picture.' *Developmental Medicine and Child Neurology,* **13,** 651–659.

Saint-Anne Dargassies, S. (1982) *Le Développement Neuro-moteur et Psycho-affectif du Nourrisson.* Paris: Masson.

Stephenson, J.B.P. (1990) *Fits and Faints. Clinics in Developmental Medicine No. 109.* London: Mac Keith Press.

Touwen, B.C.L. (1976) *Neurological Development In Infancy. Clinics in Developmental Medicine No. 58.* London: Spastics International Medical Publications.

—— (1979) *The Examination of the Child with Minor Neurological Dysfunction. Clinics in Developmental Medicine No. 71.* London: Spastics International Medical Publications.

PART I

FETAL AND NEONATAL NEUROLOGY

1
FETAL NEUROLOGY

The nine months that elapse between conception and birth are crucial for the future life of a human being. A considerable number of pathological processes take place during this period, many unassociated with maternal disease or discomfort. An extreme example is the fact that two-thirds of twin pregnancies detected by routine ultrasonography at 10 weeks of gestation result in a singleton birth (Levi 1976). Similarly, a vast majority of fetuses with chromosomal abnormalities are aborted at an early stage (see Chapter 5). Conversely, some maternal disorders do not seem to affect the fetus, thus illustrating the fact that, although the mother and fetus form a functional unit, each partner keeps a fairly high degree of independence.

Although maternal disorders can often result in fetal or embryonic disease or death, their effect is variable depending on the cause of maternal illness and on the dates of occurrence of disease, at least for many conditions. The concept of timing of an insult is important (Chapter 3), as the effect on the fetus often depends more on the stage of development at the time of injury than on its specific nature. Thus, *Toxoplasma* or rubella virus infections produce significant brain damage only during the first trimester of pregnancy, even though, in the case of toxoplasmosis, infection of the fetus is much more common during the second half of gestation than earlier.

In many cases, infectious maternal disorders that may dangerously injure the fetus are clinically silent or difficult to recognize. Thus, screening of pregnant mothers for such disorders has become routine practice in some countries, in addition to neonatal screening for the detection of metabolic or other diseases (Chapter 9).

Due to the difficulty of studying the unborn fetus, our knowledge of antenatal diseases is much too limited. It is increasingly apparent, however, that the prenatal period, in a broad sense, is of extreme importance, especially with reference to later dysfunction of the nervous system. Around 70 per cent of conceptuses are eliminated, mostly very early in gestation, and postnatal and minor problems resulting from prenatal disturbances afflict nearly 10 per cent of those who survive embryonic and fetal life (Evrard *et al.* 1989). Possibly 25 per cent of conceptuses are affected by developmental prenatal disorders of the central nervous system (CNS), and these account for a high percentage of fetal losses (Williams and Caviness 1984, Freeman 1985). Even more importantly, prenatally acquired disorders threaten postnatal survival and function. It has been estimated that 40 per cent of infant deaths during the first year of life are rooted in prenatal developmental disturbances, and it is now accepted that a large majority of cases of cerebral palsy and severe mental retardation are of prenatal rather than of perinatal or postnatal origin (Freeman 1985, Nelson and Ellenberg 1986, Naeye and Peters 1987, Volpe 1995).

However, too strict a distinction between prenatal and peri/postnatal disorders is artificial. Many fetal or embryonic diseases are not recognizable before birth (*e.g.* encephalopathies without major dysmorphism of the brain) and others are responsible only for postnatal clinical manifestations (*e.g. Toxoplasma* or cytomegalovirus infections). Moreover, perinatal difficulties are much more common in infants who suffered adverse prenatal conditions such as growth retardation (Chiswick 1985, Levene *et al.* 1985) or in those born preterm (Papiernik *et al.* 1985). There is also evidence that problems with labour and the neonatal period occur more commonly in infants with pre-existing abnormalities, for example CNS malformations (Biale *et al.* 1985); and the neonatal problems associated with twin or multiple pregnancies are well-recognized (Larroche *et al.* 1990).

Fetal disorders, in a broad sense, include many metabolic diseases in which CNS pathology is recognizable from an early stage (Chapter 9), and the vast group of CNS malformations. These are described in Chapter 3, and only a few general remarks about their prenatal diagnosis and some of their causes are given here.

The past few years have witnessed a remarkable advance in our knowledge of the embryonic and fetal periods and their disorders due to the development of new techniques which, for the first time, have allowed direct or indirect access to the fetus, enabling us to watch its development and to observe and diagnose some of its diseases at the time of their occurrence or in their early stages. It has even become possible to diagnose some disorders, especially neurometabolic or chromosomal ones, during the first weeks of pregnancy, at a time when there is no recognizable pathology and long before complete formation of the CNS.

In many countries, societal changes have made it possible to consider the extreme consequence of early detection, as termination of pregnancy has become accepted by a large fraction of the population even though it still raises major ethical controversies. Fetal diagnosis also has generally consensual consequences, such as indications for induced labour or caesarian section in cases of fetal distress, and the selection of obstetrical method, timing of delivery and preparation for immediate specialized care for infants with prenatally recognized malformations or other severe disorders.

TABLE 1.1
Indications for prenatal diagnostic techniques*

General risk factors**
• Maternal age 35 years or over at time of expected delivery***

Specific risk factors
• Previous child with malformation or chromosomal abnormality
• Previous history of stilbirth or neonatal death
• Structural abnormality in mother or father (*e.g.* neural tube defect)
• Balanced chromosomal translocation in one parent
• Family history of inherited disease in first degree relatives
• Maternal diabetes mellitus, phenylketonuria, exposure to teratogens or some infectious diseases

Risk factors peculiar to certain ethnic groups
• Tay–Sachs disease (screening in Ashkenazi Jews of eastern European origin)
• Sickle cell disease (screening in African and Afro-American Blacks)
• Thalassaemia (screening in some Mediterranean and some Asian populations)

*Modified from D'Alton and DeCherney (1993).
**Mostly for chromosomal anomalies.
***Risk of Down syndrome increases significantly after 35 years. Other chromosomal abnormalities are also increasingly common and double or treble the overall risk.

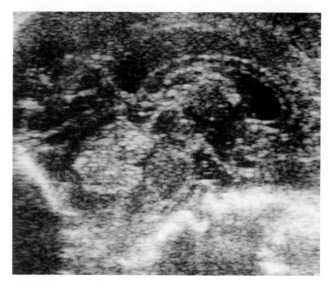

Fig. 1.1. Normal ultrasound scan of fetal head at 33 weeks gestation (sagittal cut, back of head is on left of picture). Note clear delineation of fourth ventricle, corpus callosum, septum pellucidum, cerebellum. (Courtesy Dr M-C. Aubry, Maternité Port Royal, Paris.)

OVERVIEW OF THE TECHNIQUES AND POSSIBILITIES OF FETAL NEUROLOGY

Techniques for investigation of the unborn fetus have progressed enormously over the past few years and are ever expanding. They permit not only morphological examination of the fetus but also evaluation of its growth and well-being, as well as the diagnosis of many metabolic and genetic conditions. The latter play an important role in the pathology of the fetus. The techniques of genetic diagnosis, their indications and limitations have been recently reviewed (American Academy of Pediatrics 1994).

INDICATIONS AND RISKS

Many available tests are invasive and should be used only on specific indications (D'Alton and DeCherney 1993, American Academy of Pediatrics 1994). Ultrasound examination on the other hand is innocuous and is routinely performed once or several times during pregnancy in most Western European countries, although in the USA it tends to be done only on specific indications. The risk factors that justify the practice of invasive investigations are shown in Table 1.1.

Amniocentesis is usually practised at 16 weeks gestational age, although earlier exploration is possible (Chard and Macintosh 1992). The fluid drawn is used for karyotyping and various biochemical investigations, the most common being alpha-fetoprotein and other tests of screening for trisomy 21 (Haddow *et al.* 1995; Chapter 5) and neural tube defects (Chapter 3). Miscarriage following the procedure is rare (0.3–1.5 per cent). Difficulties in diagnosis may be caused by maternal cell contamination and by mosaicism and chromosomal abnormalities confined to the placenta, but these are rare.

Chorionic villus sampling (CVS) may be undertaken from eight weeks onwards and allows chromosomal studies by direct

examination or by culture. The size of the samples also permits biochemical studies (d'Alton and DeCherney 1993). Possible errors are more frequent than with amniocentesis. Mosaicism may be found either as an artefact of culture (pseudo-mosaicism) or as a genuine difference between placenta and fetus. Abortion rate following CVS is about 0.8–1.0 per cent higher than with amniocentesis at 2–4 per cent (Chard and Macintosh 1992).

Fetal blood sampling can be performed under ultrasound guidance from 18 weeks onwards with a fetal loss rate of 1–2 per cent in experienced hands. It is useful to clarify ambiguous amniocentesis/CVS results, to perform rapid karyotyping, to diagnose fetal infections, and for the diagnosis of isoimmunization and of many haematological conditions.

Ultrasound examination aims at detecting structural abnormalities that might indicate termination or early intervention. It is often performed at 18–20 weeks and may be easily repeated (Fig. 1.1). Routine anomaly scans have a sensitivity of 58–83 per cent in the diagnosis of congenital malformations (Whittle 1991, Chard and Macintosh 1992, Ewigman *et al.* 1993, Couture *et al.* 1994), with a striking variation in the pick-up rate between various centres. Ultrasound examination is used for evaluation of fetal age and for assessment of intrauterine growth (using various measurements such as abdominal circumference, femur length and the like, thus allowing early diagnosis and surveillance of intrauterine growth retardation) and, especially, for cephalic growth. It is also a powerful tool in the antenatal diagnosis of many neurological fetal abnormalities (Aubry and Aubry 1986, Callen 1988). Table 1.2 indicates some of the most important conditions that can be diagnosed by fetal ultrasonography. The method requires considerable skill, and its reliability is highly dependent on the experience of the examiner and on the type of abnormality present. Thus, the diagnoses of anencephaly or of holoprosencephaly are easily made, but those of spina bifida, cysts of the posterior fossa or agenesis of the corpus callosum are more difficult and can be made only later in pregnancy. In routine practice, the sensitivity of sonography is not always satisfactory. A study from France indicated that only 75 per cent of major malformations were diagnosed (Macquart-Moulin *et al.* 1989). Moreover, diagnosis was often late: only 28 per cent of major malformations were detected on the first routine echography between 20 and 22 weeks, and 14 per cent had not yet been diagnosed at 32 weeks. Nonetheless, rapid progress in the reliability of the technique is being made. In a recent study from Finland (Saari-Kemppainen *et al.* 1990), 50 per cent of all major abnormalities were detected with a one-stage screening, and the neonatal mortality was cut from 9 to 4.5 per 1000 live births, largely because of termination.

BIOCHEMICAL, CYTOGENETIC AND MOLECULAR BIOLOGY

The *diagnosis of genetic conditions* and the *determination of biochemical abnormalities* (mostly enzymatic deficits) are possible by culturing fibroblasts obtained by *amniocentesis* or by *biopsy of chorionic villi*. In selected cases, biochemical examinations can be performed directly on fetal blood collected by cordocentesis under ultrasound control. The information obtained in this way is highly reliable, and well over 100 conditions can be so diagnosed (Winchester 1990). Problems may arise in some cases such as in compound heterozygotes or cases of pseudodeficiency of certain enzymes (Chapter 9). Other biochemical techniques such as enzyme assay or determination of long-chain fatty acids are possible with varying degrees of reliability.

The *techniques of DNA analysis* make possible the prenatal diagnosis of several genetic conditions for which no biochemical abnormality is known, either by detecting directly a mutant gene or, more commonly, by linkage study with restriction fragment length polymorphisms (RFLPs) or other DNA markers for a specific condition in a family. This requires that the family is informative, that a sufficient number of persons are examined and that adequate probes closely linked to the mutant gene are available (Antonarakis 1989, American Academy of Pediatrics

1994). Progress in this field is so rapid that keeping contact with a specialized centre has become necessary.

Other techniques such as fetal biopsy (of skin and even of liver and muscle) are only rarely used. Prenatal diagnosis by analysis of fetal cells in maternal blood is becoming feasible (Bianchi 1995).

Whenever possible, the use of several techniques makes antenatal diagnosis more precise and reliable. It is essential, however, that the limitations of available techniques are properly explained to couples and that they are made to understand that no method will completely ensure that the fetus will be normal, contrary to what many lay people are led to believe by sensational information in the media. This is all the more important as a majority of antenatal diagnoses are made by sonography, a technique that is highly dependent on the skill of examiners. Sixty per cent of all diagnoses in one study rested on sonography, 36 per cent on amniocentesis followed by chromosomal or biochemical study, and 4 per cent on DNA analysis (Macquart-Moulin *et al.* 1989).

TECHNIQUES FOR ASSESSMENT OF FETAL WELL-BEING AND DETECTION OF FETAL DISTRESS

Many of these techniques are mainly applicable towards the end of pregnancy and are especially useful for pregnancies in which abnormalities are present, for example maternal diabetes mellitus, maternal hypertension or fetal growth retardation. In such cases repeated assessment of the fetus is mandatory and obstetrical management will depend on its results (Schifrin 1989). Surveillance may variably include monitoring of fetal heart rate patterns (Biale *et al.* 1985) and of general and specific activities of the fetus such as gross body movements, sucking activity and the like (Rayburn 1989), and assessment of intrauterine environment including quantitative determination of amniotic fluid volume (Chamberlain *et al.* 1984). The fetal heart rate may be assessed at rest particularly during gross fetal movements (the nonstress test: Smith and Phelan 1989), or during induced contractions (the stress test: Phelan and Smith 1989). These various components can be combined to produce a fetal biophysical score (Brar and Platt 1989) that may represent the best evaluation of fetal well-being. Measurement of fetal pH is used near term and is discussed in Chapter 2. In special cases more elaborate techniques such as measurement of blood flow in umbilical vessels (Fitzgerald and Stuart 1989) or even in the fetal cephalic circulation (Wladimiroff *et al.* 1986) may become increasingly used in the future.

Assessment of fetal well-being in early or middle gestation may be important in high risk pregnancies, although the value of tests used remains controversial (Mohide and Enkin 1992). Study of the patterns of fetal movements (Rayburn 1989), eye movements (Birnholz 1989) and the development of fetal behaviour with individualization of different stages (Prechtl 1989) can give interesting information in this regard.

The whole question of fetal behaviour and well-being has been extensively reviewed by Hill and Volpe (1989).

INTRAUTERINE FETAL THERAPY

Direct intervention on the fetus has become possible over the past three decades. Fetal exchange transfusion was first performed in the early 1960s (review in Evans *et al.* 1989). Fetal surgery for hydrocephalus (Chapter 7) was first attempted in the early 1980s, but the results of shunt diversion between the lateral ventricle and the amniotic cavity have proved rather disappointing (Evans *et al.* 1989) and a moratorium on the technique has been accepted.

Other methods available for fetal intervention include vasocentesis, catheterization of the bladder, withdrawal of fluid from fetal body cavities, and some more complex surgical procedures (American Academy of Pediatrics 1994).

Biochemical therapy has been reviewed by Evans and Schulman (1989), and the possibilities of gene therapy are being actively explored.

INFECTIOUS EMBRYONIC AND FETAL DISEASES

The embryo becomes vulnerable to infectious agents when the primary germ layers have been established. Congenital malformations mainly occur with infections during the first and, occasionally, the second trimester. Later infections cause destructive changes. The response of the fetal brain to injury is altered. The inflammatory response which later often contributes to the damage produced by infectious agents is missing or less marked than later in life. A glial response with consequent scarring does not occur before 26–28 weeks gestational age (Barkovich *et al.* 1992). Calcification of necrotic areas may occur at the end of gestation. When present in a newborn baby or young infant, calcification constitutes a strong argument in favour of a clastic process and against a genetic condition. The results of fetal infections are very variable. At one extreme, they may cause abortion or stillbirth; at the other extreme the infection may be unapparent at birth and remain subclinical with purely serological evidence, or may be the origin of delayed complications, such as hearing loss, microcephaly, mental retardation or ocular lesions, which may become apparent only after several years.

Most embryonic and fetal infections are due to the action of viruses. Bacterial diseases are exceptional (Hori and Fischer 1982), though they may be underdiagnosed. Parasitic infestations are rare except for *Toxoplasma* (Lowichik and Siegel 1995). It is noteworthy that in humans many common maternal viral diseases either have no consistent effect on the fetus or result in abortion but do not produce fetal disease. In animals, however, a variety of viruses can induce cerebral malformations including neural tube defects, porencephaly and hydrocephalus (Volpe 1995). The latter has occasionally been reported in humans following maternal mumps infection (Johnson and Johnson 1972) and infection with human T-cell leukaemia virus type 1 (HTLV-1) (Tohyama *et al.* 1992).

Most fetal infections, with the exception of late bacterial disorders, are transmitted to the fetus via the placenta. The invading virus may be cytopathic for fetal cells or cause reduction or arrest of cell growth and multiplication. Certain viruses, especially that of rubella, produce damage of the endothelium of chorionic and fetal blood vessels. Indeed, visualization in the newborn infant of the lenticulostriate arteries as echogenic stripes in the basal ganglia is highly suggestive of fetal infection (Ben-Ami *et al.* 1990, Hughes *et al.* 1991), although this can occur in many circumstances (Govaert and de Vries 1997). Blood vessel damage, in turn, produces ischaemic brain lesions notably in the subependymal germinal matrix, with the frequent development of subependymal cysts (Rademaker *et al.* 1993). Destruction of the matrix may result in further cytoarchitectonic brain damage (Chapter 3). Once established, some viral infections can persist in the host for months or years.

The most important infections that affect the fetal brain include those caused by cytomegalovirus, rubella virus, herpes simplex virus, *Toxoplasma gondii*, *Treponema pallidum* and human immunodeficiency virus. Other causal agents are less common.

CYTOMEGALOVIRUS (CMV) INFECTION

CMV infection is the most common viral disease known to be transmitted *in utero* and to affect the central nervous system. CMV is ubiquitous and can be isolated from the urine of 1.0–1.4 per cent of asymptomatic newborn infants (Stagno 1990). Fewer than 10 per cent of infected infants are symptomatic at birth. Five to 15 per cent of asymptomatic infants are at risk of developing neurological complications within the first two years of life. The factors responsible for the development of clinically apparent infections are unclear. Maternal disease is transmitted to the fetus transplacentally. The seroconversion rate during pregnancy in susceptible women averages 2–2.5 per cent and is higher in women of low-income groups. Primary infection leads to transmission in only about 40 per cent of fetuses (Stagno *et al.* 1982). Only 11 per cent of infants thus infected have any type of clinical manifestation, and the risk of sequelae is 10 per cent. A prospective study of 35,000 newborn infants (Peckham and Logan 1988) found that clinical manifestations at birth were much rarer, only five infants showing symptoms during the neonatal period. However, 10 per cent of infected children had CMV-related problems by 3 years, most commonly sensorineural hearing loss that in some patients may be progressive (Souza and Bale 1995). Gestational age has no influence on the rate of transmission of the virus, but the risk of severe disease seems greater when infection is acquired during the first 4-24 weeks of pregnancy (Stagno and Whitley 1985a). Infection of two consecutive offspring is exceptional (Nigro *et al.* 1993). Most maternal infections are asymptomatic. Maternal immunity does not prevent virus reactivation, which occurs in 0.7–2.9 per cent of pregnancies, and spread of the virus. Studies of strains isolated repeatedly from mother and offspring by DNA analysis indicate reactivation of an identical latent virus rather than exogenous reinfection (Bale *et al.* 1989). In highly seropositive populations, a majority of intrauterine infections are due to reactivation. Congenital infections that result from recurrent infection are less likely to produce fetal damage than those due to primary infection (Fowler *et al.* 1992). Infection can also occur at birth, through contact with an infected

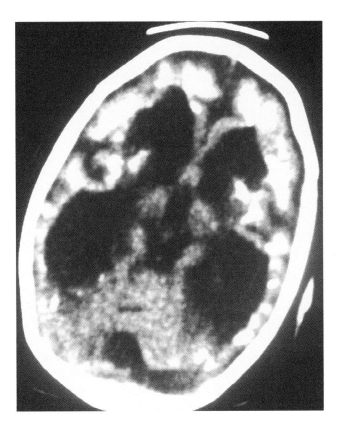

Fig. 1.2. Congenital cytomegalovirus infection. Extensive periventricular calcification. The brain parenchyma is markedly atrophic. The ventricles are considerably dilated with irregular contours. (Courtesy Dr Kling Chong, Great Ormond Street Hospital, London.)

cervix. Preterm infants have become infected following transfusions of unscreened blood.

It is therefore difficult to determine whether intrauterine infection has occurred, and routine serological screening of pregnant women is of limited value. Infection should always be suspected in women with a heterophil-negative mononucleosis-like syndrome. In such patients, fetal blood sampling (Daffos *et al.* 1984) can confirm infection of the fetus, but assessment of fetal disease remains impractical.

PATHOLOGY
The virus has an affinity for rapidly growing germinal cells of the lateral ventricles. Periventricular lesions are frequent, with necrosis and calcification. Aqueductal stenosis is not a feature. Cytomegalic inclusions are found in glial cells and occasionally in neurons.

A different type of cerebral CMV infection with widespread microglial nodular encephalitis of brainstem, cerebellum and cerebral hemispheres may occur in preterm infants and in immunodepressed patients (Friede 1989).

Cortical malformations, especially polymicrogyria, are frequently found in CMV infected infants (Hayward *et al.* 1991). They may be associated with other CNS malformations. Barkovich and Lindan (1994) studied nine children with abnormal gyral patterns ranging from agyria to less gross dysplasias.

Cerebellar atrophy, abnormalities of hippocampi and white matter changes were often associated. The mechanism of migration disorders is not clear, but haemodynamic consequences of infection may be an important factor and direct viral invasion does not seem to be essential (Marques-Dias *et al.* 1984).

CLINICAL MANIFESTATIONS
Clinical manifestations of CMV infection may appear during the neonatal period or early infancy. In the severe form that is observed in 1 per cent of infants, hepatomegaly, splenomegaly, intrauterine growth retardation, jaundice, microcephaly, intracranial calcification, pneumonitis and encephalitis are prominent. Such cases have a high mortality, particularly in preterm infants (Perlman and Argyle 1992), and survivors are usually microcephalic, mentally retarded and may have seizures and choroidoretinitis. Calcification, especially in the periventricular region, is suggestive of the diagnosis in infants with negative serology for toxoplasmosis (Fig. 1.2). A few cases of corneal opacities, optic atrophy and arthrogryposis are on record (Souza and Bale 1995).

A milder form is present in 5 per cent of infected neonates, with hepatosplenomegaly, jaundice and thrombocytopenia (Hanshaw *et al.* 1985, Boppano *et al.* 1992). Although no neurological abnormalities are noted in the neonatal period, almost half of these infants will later demonstrate mental retardation, microcephaly, seizures or deafness.

A majority of infants are asymptomatic at birth, but 5–15 per cent of them will develop sensorineural hearing loss which is bilateral in half the cases and may be progressive. It may be accompanied by apparently isolated microcephaly (Hanshaw *et al.* 1985), mental delay and learning difficulties (Williamson *et al.* 1982). However, in prospective studies, Conboy *et al.* (1986) and Pearl *et al.* (1986) found no difference between CMV infected infants asymptomatic at birth and controls. Images of migration abnormalities such as pachygyria or microgyria are suggestive when associated with calcification (Hayward *et al.* 1991, Barkovich and Lindan 1994). Hydrocephalus is only rarely present (Bale *et al.* 1985). Subependymal cysts may be recognized early by sonography (Beltinger and Saule 1988). Postnatal progression of congenital CMV disease, with development of multicystic encephalomalacia and hydranencephaly, has been observed (Bale *et al.* 1986). Cases of late intrauterine infection can produce microcephaly, ataxia and leukoencephalopathy (Steinlin *et al.* 1996). Riikonen and Donner (1980) suggested that steroid treatment of infantile spasms may induce reactivation of a latent CMV infection. A progressive course is rare in patients without immunosuppression (Koeda *et al.* 1993). Bale *et al.* (1990) found no correlation between the clinical features of the neonatal disease and neurodevelopmental outcome. Postnatal microcephaly and seizures were significantly associated with mental retardation.

DIAGNOSIS
The diagnosis of congenital CMV infection may be difficult to prove. The association of a compatible clinical picture and excretion of CMV in urine is reasonable proof, and certain signs, such as periventricular calcification, are highly suggestive. A few

cases of apparently genetic (recessive) disorders closely simulating CMV infection, with microcephaly, intracranial calcification, mental retardation, and even purpura and liver involvement in some, are on record (Burn *et al.* 1986, Hreidarsson *et al.* 1988, Reardon *et al.* 1994, Aalfs *et al.* 1995). Therefore, the diagnosis of CMV infection should not be firmly made when proof of infection is lacking. In CMV disease, periventricular calcification is usually associated in the perinatal period with areas of hypodensity of the white matter on CT scan. The CSF has a raised protein level often with oligoclonal banding and a high cell count (mononuclear). The virus has been occasionally isolated from the CSF. Intrauterine diagnosis is possible by viral assay on amniotic fluid, a culture technique that gives results in 24–48 hours (Grose *et al.* 1992) and possibly by polymerase chain reaction (Souza and Bale 1995).

Viruria is present in infected infants irrespective of the clinical picture and may persist for several years. Viruria alone is not sufficient to attribute clinical manifestations to congenital CMV disease. Griffiths *et al.* (1982) detected IgM-specific antibodies in 89 per cent of congenitally infected infants. However, a low titre of complement-fixing antibodies does not exclude the diagnosis.

TREATMENT
Treatment of symptomatic CMV infection by ganciclovir (Nigro *et al.* 1994) or foscarnet is effective, but brain damage is usually extensive by the time of birth. Prenatal administration of ganciclovir has not been evaluated.

PREVENTION
Prevention is not feasible at present. The risk of spread of CMV infection to child care personnel is not fully known, and female employees in their reproductive years should be informed of the potential risk, and strict hygienic measures enforced (Stagno and Whitley 1985a).

CONGENITAL RUBELLA
Congenital rubella can produce an embryopathy that frequently affects the CNS in addition to the heart and blood vessels. The frequency of congenital rubella following maternal infection is variably estimated between 40 and 80 per cent during the first 12 weeks of pregnancy, between 30 and 50 per cent during weeks 13–16 and between 0 and 25 per cent at the end of second trimester. Fetal infection after this is unusual, although there is an increase during the last month. After the 10th week, sequelae tend to be limited to a single organ, usually the organ of Corti. Severe malformations occur in a high proportion of fetuses infected before the 12th week. One third of those infected during the 13th to 16th weeks will have deafness alone (Miller *et al.* 1982). Deafness is often detected late and may develop after birth. Infants infected during the second trimester tend to demonstrate delayed mental development and disorders of communication. Intrauterine growth retardation is common. Fetal involvement following reinfection with rubella virus is exceptional (Cradock-Watson *et al.* 1985, Best *et al.* 1989). Intrauterine

TABLE 1.3
Clinical features of congenital rubella syndrome*

Clinical features	% of cases	
Congenital heart disease (patent ductus with or without stenosis of pulmonary arteries and atrial or ventricular septal defects)	52	
Bilateral or unilateral loss of hearing due to damage to the organ of Corti	52	
Cataracts, microphthalmos, retinopathy	40	
Psychomotor retardation (often associated with microcephaly)	40	
Severe		24
Mild		16

*Modified from Cooper and Krugman (1967).

infection has also been seen following immunization with rubella vaccine which should not be given in potentially pregnant women, even though such infection is rare (Philipps *et al.* 1970).

There is a high incidence of persistent chronic infection after fetal rubella, and the virus has been recovered from urine and throat washes of patients up to 12 months after birth. The infection may remain quiescent for as long as 13 months after birth and be activated by postnatal stress.

The *neuropathological abnormalities* of the rubella syndrome include meningoencephalitis, reduction of brain weight by about one quarter, probably as a result of inhibition of cell proliferation by the virus, and meningeal and brain lesions. There are extensive degenerative arterial changes with calcification and intimal proliferation, and infiltrates of mononucleated cells in the leptomeninges and perivascular spaces (Rorke 1973). Destruction of the periventricular germinal cells was ascribed to rubella infection by Shaw and Alvord (1974), and subependymal cysts have been observed by sonography in infants with the congenital rubella syndrome (Beltinger and Saule 1988). It is not established whether fetal rubella infection induces specific cerebral malformations (Friede 1989).

CLINICAL MANIFESTATIONS
The main features of the congenital rubella syndrome are shown in Table 1.3. Any combination of CNS, ear, heart and eye involvement is possible. In about 80 per cent of patients there are symptoms and signs of CNS involvement (Desmond *et al.* 1969). In almost three-quarters of such cases, irritability, lethargy, hypotonia and a bulging fontanelle are noted from birth. The CSF frequently shows increased protein and a mild pleocytosis, and it is often possible to isolate the virus from CSF. CSF abnormalities can present in asymptomatic infants. Many of these infants also have systemic manifestations in the neonatal period, including purpura, thrombocytopenia and jaundice.

In later infancy and childhood, opisthotonic attacks and marked developmental delay become apparent. Seizures occur in a minority of patients. Microcephaly is a common occurrence, and peripheral hearing loss is present in over 40 per cent of cases and may increase progressively; it can also develop months or even years after birth. Retarded language may also result from mental retardation. Autistic behaviour has been repeatedly recorded (Chess 1971). Cataracts may also appear at several weeks of age, and the virus can often be isolated from cataract material even after several years. Diffuse pigmentary disturbance of the retina is common, with alternating patchy areas of increased and decreased pigmentation. It does not affect vision but is a useful diagnostic marker. Intracranial calcification is rare.

A late-onset syndrome may be observed in infants infected *in utero* but with mild or no symptoms at birth. The syndrome has its onset at 4–6 months with diarrhoea, rashes, hepatosplenomegaly, thrombocytopenia and rapid neurological deterioration and is usually fatal (Tardieu *et al.* 1980).

DIAGNOSIS
The diagnosis can be made by finding an elevated level of IgM in the serum at birth and by identifying this IgM as specific rubella antibody. Isolation of the virus is also possible in tissue culture by coculture (Souza and Bale 1995).

PROGNOSIS
The prognosis of congenital rubella is severe. Most affected children are deaf and a significant proportion also have low visual acuity or blindness due to cataracts or choroidoretinitis. A rare complication of congenital rubella is *late progressive rubella panencephalitis* (Townsend *et al.* 1975; Chapter 11).

There is no effective treatment. The disorder has become rare since vaccination of prepubertal girls has become routine.

HERPES SIMPLEX VIRUS (HSV) INFECTIONS
Almost all cases of HSV infection in fetuses are with type 2 virus. They are much less common than CMV infection. Primary maternal infection with HSV appears to carry a significant risk to the fetus both in early pregnancy and at term. In the first 20 weeks of pregnancy, primary infection is associated with an increased frequency of spontaneous abortion and stillbirth (Robb *et al.* 1986). Severe brain abnormalities may occur. Hutto *et al.* (1987) found eight instances of choroidoretinitis, seven of microcephaly, five of hydranencephaly and two of microphthalmia in 13 neonates with HSV infection proved by viral isolation. Multicystic encephalomalacia has also ben reported (Smith *et al.* 1977). Recurrent infection is the most common form of infection during gestation (Stagno and Whitley 1985b). Often, infection is acquired during labour and vaginal delivery. Symptoms most commonly appear in the first week, but many occur in the ensuing three weeks of the neonatal period. Antepartum vaginal cultures for HSV do not reliably predict the risk of exposure to the virus and are not considered cost-effective (Libman *et al.* 1991, Gibbs and Mead 1992). The rate of transmission depends on the serological status of the mother and is higher for women with primary infection (Brown *et al.* 1991). New techniques for detection of HSV2-specific antibodies are being assessed (Gibbs and Mead 1992, Kulhanjian *et al.* 1992). Routine caesarean section for women with genital herpes infection is not justified. It is often recommended only if clinical lesions are present at onset of labour (Glaser and Dorfman 1991). Prophylactic administration of antiviral drugs (acyclovir) to clinically asymptomatic women excreting herpes virus at delivery or to their offspring is not now indicated (Stagno and Whitley 1985b)

CONGENITAL TOXOPLASMOSIS
Toxoplasma gondii is a protozoan parasite (coccidian) whose usual host is the cat and which exists in three forms: oocyst, trophozoite and cyst. Transmission of the acquired disease is by ingestion of tissue cysts or oocysts, and the prevalence of toxoplasmosis depends mostly on the meat-cooking habits in the community. The rate of seropositivity is 50–80 per cent in women of childbearing age in France as against about 30 per cent in the USA. Infection of the human fetus appears to occur transplacentally at or after the second month of gestation, from a maternal infection that is more commonly (85 per cent) subclinical than overt. Fetal infection in the first trimester is rare, but when it does occur it is more severe than later acquired disease. Infection is most common during the third trimester but then usually results in localized (ocular) disease or in subclinical infection. Fetal contamination is preceded by placental infection, and the organism has occasionally been identified in placental samples. Recurrent infection in two consecutive pregnancies has been rarely recorded (Garcia 1968). However, infection of the fetus by mothers with infections incurred before pregnancy does occur in immunodepressed subjects and even in some individuals with no detectable immunodeficiency (Desmonts *et al.* 1990, Remington and Desmonts 1990).

The cerebral lesions of toxoplasmosis include areas of necrosis with deposition of calcium salts, granular ependymitis that is often responsible for aqueductal stenosis and hydrocephalus, and granulomatous areas in the cortex and meninges. Parasites may be seen in recent lesions. Destructive lesions may be extensive and result in widespread cavitated necrosis that may amount to multicystic encephalomalacia or hydranencephaly (Altshuler 1973).

CLINICAL MANIFESTATIONS
The clinical manifestations of congenital toxoplasmosis depend on the time of fetal infection, and several clinical syndromes may be observed (Remington and Desmonts 1990, Gordon 1993).

The most classical presentation is the *severe neonatal form* with systemic signs that include hepatosplenomegaly, fever and purpura. Hydrocephalus is a major feature, although its frequency is now decreasing due to preventive measures. It is often unnoticed at birth because head circumference may not be increased. Prospective sonographic studies by Desmonts *et al.* (1985) indicated that ventricular dilatation existed *in utero* in six of nine cases diagnosed prenatally. Hydrocephalus is the result of aqueductal stenosis and is often associated with severe brain damage, mental retardation and epilepsy. *Choroidoretinitis* is the most frequent sign and is found in 76–85 per cent of cases. Cerebral calcification is also common. It may be disseminated or assume a periventricular disposition (Fig. 1.3). The *cerebrospinal fluid* (CSF) in severe forms is often xanthochromic

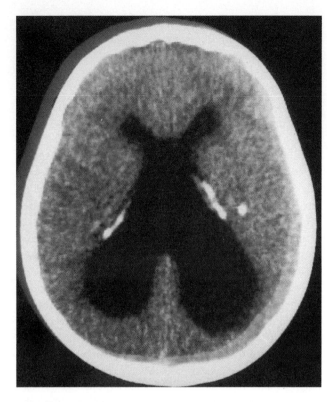

Fig. 1.3. Congenital toxoplasmosis: note dilatation of posterior horns of lateral ventricles and periventricular calcification.

with a high protein content and lymphocytosis. Oligoclonal bands are present in some cases. *Toxoplasma gondii* can be isolated from abnormal CSF, and an increased immune load of specific IgG in CSF can have diagnostic, prognostic and therapeutic significance (Couvreur *et al.* 1984).

A second syndrome of congenital toxoplasmosis is that of a less severe disease occurring in the first months of life. Choroidoretinitis is the most frequent feature in such cases. It can be isolated and can occur in a retina that was clinically intact during the first weeks of life. Nine out of ten cases of choroidoretinitis in infants and children are due to congenital toxoplasmosis. Microcephaly, intracranial calcification and various neurological symptoms and signs may accompany the choroidoretinitis or become evident later in life. The CSF is usually abnormal.

Subclinical infection is the most common form of congenital toxoplasmosis (Sever *et al.* 1988). Its diagnosis rests on systematic serologic surveillance of pregnancies which permits prenatal diagnosis and prospective follow-up of infected fetuses. Subclinical infection is the rule, with late contamination. It may remain asymptomatic or be complicated by the late appearance of choroidoretinitis, which has been found in between 28 and 85 per cent of patients prospectively followed up to adolescence (Couvreur and Desmonts 1988, Sever *et al.* 1988). Relapsing ocular involvement is not rare.

DIAGNOSIS

The diagnosis is usually made by tests measuring IgG- or IgM-specific antibody. The former include the dye and IFA tests, the latter the IgM-IFA and IgM-ELISA tests, the last of which is the most reliable. Low titres are found during the first months of life before significant infant synthesis of antibodies. Maternally transmitted IgG antibodies may persist beyond 6 months of age if originally present in high titres, but begin to decline by 5 years of age.

Prenatal diagnosis can be suspected when maternal infection occurs during early pregnancy, but fetal involvement is uncommon. Ninety-five per cent of fetuses do not become infected, as shown by blood cord sampling (Desmonts *et al.* 1985). Ultrasound examination allows some assessment of lesions in the pre- and postnatal periods, although in the latter, CT or MRI scan is more precise.

TREATMENT

Any form of congenital toxoplasmosis, even a subclinical one, should be treated in an attempt to prevent the development of new lesions or extension of established damage. Couvreur and Desmonts (1988) recommend three to five courses of pyrimethamine (0.5–1 mg/kg/d) with sulfadiazine (50 mg/kg/d), alternating with spiramycin for 1–2 months, during the first year of life. After one year of age, treatment does not seem worthwhile, unless relapses occur. These should be treated with one or two courses of pyrimethamine and sulfadiazine, followed by pyrimethamine with sulfadiazine for several months. One-year treatment is significantly better than one-month therapy. A majority of infants so treated have a normal IQ, and even 70 per cent of those with hydrocephalus have no severe cognitive defect (Roizen *et al.* 1995). Treatment should be monitored by serial blood counts. Bone marrow depression can be prevented by folinic acid, 5–10 mg/d orally or parenterally. The adjuvant use of steroids is debatable. Treatment appears to reduce the risk of secondary choroiditis. Neurosurgical treatment is indicated for active hydrocephalus (Chapter 7).

PREVENTION

Prevention is based on systematic serologic diagnosis of maternal infections and treatment of women who become positive during pregnancy. Such screening is not considered cost-effective in some countries with a low frequency of toxoplasmosis, and the balance of risks and benefits is indeed delicate (Hall 1992) and may vary from one country to another. Prompt treatment with spiramycin may reduce the rate of fetal infection for infected mothers, but no controlled trial is available. The drug has little effect on severe brain damage in first trimester infections, so termination may be considered in such cases. Daffos *et al.* (1988) have proposed that women with seroconversion during pregnancy should have fetal cord blood sampling with culture of fetal blood, serologic testing of fetal blood for IgM-specific antibodies, search for nonspecific biological signs of infection, and ultrasound of the brain. In 746 pregnancies, an antenatal diagnosis of fetal infection was made in 39 cases. Of the 15 cases in which pregnancy was continued (with treatment), 13 infants were clinically well and two had choroidoretinitis. Hohlfeld *et al.* (1989) followed 52 pregnancies with seroconversion. The mothers were treated with spiramycin alone (nine cases) or a combined regime of pyrimethamine, sulfadiazine and spiramycin (43 cases). Of the 54 live infants resulting from these pregnancies, 41 had serological evidence of toxoplasmosis, 12 had a benign clinical disorder and one a severe form. These authors concluded that treatment was effective. Recently, the polymerase chain reaction test has been used on amniotic fluid for the diagnosis of fetal infection and appears reliable (Hohlfeld *et al.* 1994). Prenatal blood sampling may rule out infection, and thus avoid termination, in up to 95 per cent of cases (Desmonts *et al.* 1985). According to Daffos *et al.* (1988), termination is only indicated when there is evidence of both fetal infection and an abnormal brain ultrasonogram. Avoiding undercooked meat and contact with cats is effective in preventing infection (Jeannel *et al.* 1990).

VARICELLA-ZOSTER VIRUS INFECTIONS

Varicella-zoster virus infections rarely occur during pregnancy. Transmission to the fetus occurs in around a quarter of cases, although in most cases no significant adverse consequence ensues (Stagno and Whitley 1985b, Paryani and Arvin 1986). Maternal infection before 20 weeks gestational age can result in miscarriage and, uncommonly, in an embryopathy. Perinatal infection may result in severe varicella in the infant (Michie *et al.* 1992). A syndrome of hypoplasia of the limbs, cicatricial skin lesions and ocular abnormalities has been identified in a few fetuses infected before 20 weeks gestation (Alkalay *et al.* 1987). Of 27 such infants, 14 were small for their gestational age, 11 had motor or sensory disturbances of the limbs, often in association with hypoplasia of the affected limb, 10 had choroidoretinitis and 10 had 'brain damage'. All 27 had unilateral cutaneous lesions ipsilateral to the affected limb and in a dermatomal distribution. Evidence of encephalitis was found in a few cases (Higa *et al.* 1987). Vocal cord paralysis may be the presenting manifestation (Randel *et al.* 1996). Some cases may be due to zoster. The risk of embryopathy is small. Pastuszak *et al.* (1994) found only four infants with defects among 106 pregnancies complicated by varicella during the first 20 weeks, and estimated the risk of encephalopathy in various series at 1.2–2.2 per cent. Prevention with specific immunoglobulin may be indicated in case of close contact within 72 hours (Prober *et al.* 1990, Enders *et al.* 1994). When varicella occurs during the last five days of pregnancy, preventive administration of specific gammaglobulins and of acyclovir to the infant has been advised (Haddad *et al.* 1987).

HUMAN IMMUNODEFICIENCY VIRUS (HIV)

INFECTION (see also Chapter 11)

HIV infection of mothers is transmitted to the fetus in approximately 15–20 per cent of cases in Western countries and approximately 30 per cent in Africa (European Collaborative Study 1991). Most mothers are seropositive but asymptomatic during pregnancy. There is evidence that HIV can be transmitted as early as 15 weeks gestation, but perinatal infection, especially during labour, seems to be predominant (Peckham and Gibb 1995), as suggested by the more frequent involvement of the first member of twin pairs because of longer exposure to contamination in the

birth canal (Duliège *et al.* 1995), by the higher infection rate of infants born to severely ill mothers, and by the possible prevention of contamination by perinatal zidovudine treatment (Connor *et al.* 1994). It also appears that a longer duration of membrane rupture is associated with more frequent contamination (Landesman *et al.* 1996). A significantly lower frequency of transmission is reported when membranes were ruptured less than four hours before birth (McCarthy 1996) and with caesarean section (European Collaborative Study 1994a), the latter probably because of intact membranes. Contamination by breast milk is possible.

Most infected neonates remain asymptomatic with positive serology for variable durations up to several years (Abrams *et al.* 1995). Only 1.6 per cent of infected neonates have symptoms in the neonatal period. In a series of 990 infants, 23 per cent had developed acquired immunodeficiency syndrome (AIDS) before age 1 year and 39 per cent by age 4 (European Collaborative Study 1994b). A bimodal progression of the disease has been found (Duliège *et al.* 1992, Blanche *et al.* 1994) in infants born to severely immunodepressed mothers with advanced disease, developing earlier disease and dying before 18 months of age. Such infants may have been infected *in utero* and/or have received a larger viral load (Blanche *et al.* 1994). Other infants remain asymptomatic for months or years. Preterm infants have more severe disease than those born at term (Abrams *et al.* 1995). The incidence of preterm delivery and low birthweight is increased. Most infected children develop milder disease between 2 and 5 years of age but some cases remaining asymptomatic at 12 years have been reported (Belman 1992). Those with severe forms (about 15–20 per cent) have progressive developmental deterioration and diffuse neurological signs, microcephaly and often calcification of the basal ganglia (Belman 1992). Less severely involved infants may have severe mental and motor involvement with a later onset (about 10–15 per cent) or mild signs such as clumsiness, slow progress in language and school failure (10 per cent). A small proportion present with spastic diplegia, so AIDS should be considered in cases presenting like cerebral palsy. Children over 5–6 years may show progressive dementia. Infants of HIV-positive mothers may be smaller at birth than uninfected controls but this seems to be related to the fact that they were born to drug-addicted women (Chapter 2). However, this may not apply in countries of high endemicity where growth retardation seems more common.

Diagnosis in the neonatal period is difficult. The techniques of diagnosis are discussed in Chapter 11 but diagnosis before 18 months to 2 years of age poses a special problem because of the passive transmission of antibodies of maternal origin.

OTHER VIRUSES

No consistent pattern of malformation or fetal disease has been found with infection caused by variola, influenza A and B, measles and hepatitis viruses or by entero- or adenoviruses. Cases of aqueductal stenosis following maternal mumps are on record (Johnson and Johnson 1972, Lahat *et al.* 1993). Hydrocephalus and extensive choroidoretinal scarring have also been observed following lymphocytic choriomeningitis in the second half of pregnancy. Wright *et al.* (1997) reported on 26 cases mimicking toxoplasmosis or CMV infection and suggested that the disease may be more common than suspected and should be looked for when serological reactions for toxoplasmosis or CMV are negative. Three infants born to mothers infected with parvovirus B19 had congenital arthrogryposis, polymicrogyria, infantile spasms and intracranial calcification (Conry *et al.* 1993). A few cases of meningoencephalitis or meningitis in infants of mothers with Western equine encephalitis and Venezuelan encephalitis have been reported (see Souza and Bale 1995). Infection with HTLV1 is probably transmitted congenitally in many cases but is rarely recognized as causing illness in the newborn baby. One case of hydrocephalus has been attributed to this agent (Tohyama *et al.* 1992). Hydrocephalus has also been reported as a complication of maternal infection with the lymphocytic choriomeningitis virus (Larsen *et al.* 1993).

CONGENITAL SYPHILIS
Infection by *Treponema pallidum* can be transmitted from mother to fetus at any time in pregnancy, usually between the fourth and seventh months. Twenty-five to 80 per cent of children of untreated mothers with syphilis become infected, and clinical signs of congenital neurosyphilis occur in 2–16 per cent of them (Weil and Levin 1995). Neurosyphilis can take either a meningovascular or a parenchymatous form. In both forms, the process begins in the meninges and diffuses along vessels into the cortex. Small veins and arteries are involved and infarction may result. Meningeal thickening and inflammatory perivascular exudates can result in hydrocephalus. With parenchymal disease, there is diffuse degeneration of the cerebrum and cerebellum with inflammatory infiltrates, microglial proliferation and presence of spirochaetes.

Active fetal infection may result in spontaneous abortion or stillbirth. In the liveborn infant its features include hepatosplenomegaly, chronic haemorrhagic rhinitis, osteochondritis (which is a classical cause of pseudoparalysis in the newborn infant) and interstitial keratitis. However, congenital syphilis may become manifest only between 3 and 14 weeks of age following an asymptomatic neonatal period (Dorfman and Glaser 1990).

During the first few months of life, syphilitic meningitis may be marked by irritability, vomiting, cranial nerve palsies and chronic hydrocephalus (Marcus 1982). The CSF contains an excess of protein, with oligoclonal banding, and of mononuclear cells.

Tertiary syphilis is now rare. Juvenile paresis only appears many years after birth, marked by progressive mental deterioration, disturbed behaviour, and often by spasticity and cerebellar signs. Optic atrophy and deafness may be present. Late 'stigmata' of syphilis such as Hutchinson teeth, saddle nose or sabre shins are seldom present. Tabes dorsalis is exceptional. There has been a marked recrudescence of congenital syphilis over the past decade (Rawstron *et al.* 1993) so that the possibility should always be kept in mind.

The diagnosis of congenital syphilis is serological. Serological testing during pregnancy can miss cases of late infection with transmission to the fetus. Serological tests should be repeated at delivery in both mother and infant to ensure the greatest chance of success. The VDRL (Venereal Disease Reference Laboratory) test has a specificity of 100 per cent but the sensitivity is only 27 per cent. The *T. pallidum* immobilization test and the fluorescent treponemal antibody absorption test (FTA-ABS) are more sensitive but do not distinguish between active and past syphilis. In early infancy, transmitted maternal antibodies can be responsible for positive tests in noninfected infants. Demonstration of IgM–FTA reactivity is specific for fetal infection (Müller *et al.* 1984). Demonstration of *T. pallidum* DNA by polymerase chain reaction test is more precise but not always easily available (Sánchez *et al.* 1993, Beeram *et al.* 1996). Although serology is the essential tool of diagnosis, other studies can be of value. X-ray films of the lower limbs were diagnostic in 20 of 59 asymptomatic children in one study (Dorfman and Glaser 1990). Full blood count and liver function tests are useful to assess the general consequences of the disease.

Treatment of neurosyphilis is with aqueous penicillin G, 30–60 mg (50,000–100,000 units) per kg body weight for 14 days. Benzathine penicillin G or aqueous procaine penicillin G may not achieve therapeutic levels with the same doses and are not recommended. Erythromycin and tetracycline (5–8 mg/kg/d every six hours for 10 days) may be used in the rare patient who does not tolerate penicillin but are less effective. Negative serological tests should be maintained by 2 years, and CSF should be reexamined one year after completion of treatment. Treatment of all mothers with positive serology is in order.

LYME DISEASE
Rare instances of maternal–fetal transmission of *Borrelia burgdorferi* infection with encephalitis (Weber *et al.* 1988) or multiple malformations have been reported (Schlesinger *et al.* 1985). Williams *et al.* (1988), however, could not find an association between the presence of cord blood antibodies and congenital malformations.

OTHER INFECTIONS
Congenital malaria is rare. Fever is usually present and clinical features are reminiscent of those of CMV disease (Souza and Bale 1995).

Congenital brucellosis (Al Eissa *et al.* 1992) is a rare occurrence in industrialized countries.

FETAL CIRCULATORY AND VASCULAR DISORDERS

Disturbances of blood supply to the brain, whether due to diseases of the vessels themselves or to haemodynamic failure from any origin, are a major cause of cerebral damage in the embryo and fetus and are probably responsible for a large part of the neurological disorders of infancy and childhood and for many cases of associated mental retardation. Some of the consequences of intrauterine circulatory and vascular disorders will be studied elsewhere in this book (Chapters 2, 3, 7, 8, 23). The present chapter is concerned exclusively with the acute stage of constitution of brain damage. It is not always possible to separate damage that

TABLE 1.4
Main causes of fetal encephalopathies of circulatory origin*

Lesions related to maternal pathological conditions
 Systemic diseases
  Maternal anaemia
  Toxaemia with hypertension
  Renal diseases
  Repeated seizures during second semester of pregnancy
  Severe hypoxia
 Maternal trauma
  Direct trauma to abdomen
  Maternal accidents
 Gas intoxication
  Carbon monoxide
  Butane

Lesions related to fetal conditions
 Twinning (especially with one macerated twin)
 Prenatal arterial occlusions
 Blood dyscrasias
  Haemolytic disease with or without incompatibility
  Thrombocytopenia (genetic, isoimmune or of infective origin)
 Nonimmune hydrops fetalis

Lesions related to placental or cord abnormalities
 Fetomaternal haemorrhage
 Chronic placental insufficiency with fetal distress
 Abruptio placentae
 Cord knotting

*Adapted from Larroche (1986).

occurs only prenatally from that incurred during the perinatal and immediate postnatal periods. Such a distinction is especially difficult in the case of circulatory disorders. However, as already indicated at the beginning of this chapter, considerable evidence including demonstration of prenatal brain lesions in neonates and stillborn fetuses (Scher *et al.* 1991, Cohen and Roessmann 1994, Lou *et al.* 1994) indicates that prenatal factors play a most important role in the genesis of CNS damage and impairment (Nelson and Ellenberg 1981, Freeman 1985).

CAUSES AND MECHANISMS OF FETAL CIRCULATORY DISORDERS

The main causes of circulatory disturbances in the fetus are shown in Table 1.4, but the exact cause is often impossible to determine for several reasons. The same cause may produce brain damage through different mechanisms. For example, infective fetal disorders can produce damage by direct effects of the virus on neurons or glial cells, but also indirectly by inducing circulatory failure which, in turn, will result in brain compromise (Marques-Dias *et al.* 1984).

Similar causes can produce different lesions depending on the date at which they act. However, prenatal circulatory disturbances, if severe enough, are capable of producing virtually any type of brain lesion, depending on the precise nature of the insult and, especially, on the gestational age at which they occur. Bilateral ligation of carotid arteries in fetal monkeys between 70 and 100 days of pregnancy produced hydranencephaly (Myers 1972). The same injury before the 70th day failed to induce cavitated lesions but resulted in an abnormal gyral pattern. It is likely that similar phenomena occur in humans. True porencephaly, which

is often termed 'schizencephaly', was thought to result from focal agenesis of the hemispheric mantle but probably results from destruction of the mantle as a consequence of a failing vascular supply and faulty reparation so that there is interference with neuronal migration (Chapter 3).

In humans, circulatory disturbances tend to involve more the periventricular white matter in preterm infants and the cortex and basal ganglia in term fetuses. However, the same lesion may be pre- or postnatal depending on the date of birth. Periventricular leukomalacia tends to occur between 26 and 35 weeks of gestation and may thus be prenatal in term infants. In preterm infants it is most often a perinatal event, most lesions not being present in the very first days of life, and it is associated with, and probably caused by, postnatal disturbances responsible for hypoxia or anoxia (Hagberg and Hagberg 1993, Krägeloh-Mann *et al.* 1995). However, damage to the white matter may be of prenatal origin in up to 30 per cent of cases (Murphy *et al.* 1995, 1996).

Prenatal and perinatal causes are often jointly responsible for the same lesions. Acute fetal hypoxia is a major cause of fetal brain damage. However, the fetal brain is capable of withstanding prolonged periods of hypoxia without damage. It is clear that prolonged intrauterine hypoxia–ischaemia considerably increases the likelihood of damage following an acute event that would otherwise have been tolerated. Gaffney *et al.* (1994) demonstrated in a case–control study the high frequency of adverse factors during delivery (*e.g.* abnormal cardiotachogram, meconium staining of the liquor) in infants whose brains showed at autopsy lesions of clear prenatal origin. Episodes of cardiac deceleration have been shown to precede acute hypoxic perinatal events that result in brain damage (Visser 1992), and the same is true of intrauterine disturbances of fetal haemodynamics such as partial abruptio placentae (Gibbs and Weindling 1994), intrapartum haemorrhage, eclampsia and intrauterine growth retardation (Weindling and Russell 1992). These conditions are associated with diminished uterine blood flow (Fitzgerald and Stuart 1989), which seems to be caused by increased placental resistance (Trudinger *et al.* 1985). Superimposed stress, *e.g.* at the time of labour, which would be insignificant in the case of a previously normal pregnancy, is then liable to produce damage. For this reason, careful monitoring of pregnancy by the techniques described earlier (p. 5) is important in such cases (Erkkola *et al.* 1984, Leveno *et al.* 1986, Luthy *et al.* 1987, Brar and Platt 1989, Low 1989, Schifrin 1989, Nelson *et al.* 1996; see also Chapter 2). Additional stress may occur even before labour, as acute reduction of uterine blood flow can be induced by pressure of the fetal head in the supine position and this can be alleviated simply by changing maternal posture. Moreover, examination of the placentae of infants with apparent birth hypoxia has shown the frequency of old infarctions and scars, thus indicating the role of prenatal factors (Scher *et al.* 1991, Altschuler 1993, Burke and Tannenberg 1995).

Several mechanisms (Table 1.4) can interfere with the blood supply to the fetal brain, either locally or diffusely, and produce more or less extensive damage.

Ischaemia can be the result of several causes. *Acute hypovolaemia* occurs with massive maternal haemorrhage as in placenta praevia. Less obvious but at times significant bleeding can occur as a result of large *fetomaternal transfusion* which may lead to fetal death (Boyce *et al.* 1994) or to massive cystic brain degeneration, which I have seen in three cases. It seems likely that *fetofetal transfusion* is one of the mechanisms that lead to brain destruction in the parabiotic twin syndrome, as suggested by the frequency of a low haemoglobin at birth in the surviving twin (Aicardi *et al.* 1972, Larroche *et al.* 1990). Another mechanism in this syndrome is disseminated intravascular coagulation in the surviving twin, induced by transfer through placental anastomoses of products with a thromboplastin action from the dead co-twin (Yoshioka *et al.* 1979, Schmitt 1984). This pattern of disseminated CNS lesions associated with multiple visceral infarcts has been repeatedly confirmed (Barth and van der Harten 1985, Szymonowicz *et al.* 1986). Although a similar pattern of brain disruption related to the fetofetal transfusion syndrome rarely occurs in dichorionic twins (Friede 1989), monochorionic twins are clearly at a much greater risk (Larroche *et al.* 1990, Weig *et al.* 1995). Jung *et al.* (1984) found that the ratio of monozygotic to dizygotic twins was 9:1 in cases of hydranencephaly–porencephaly, whereas in normal twins this ratio is 0.4:1, indicating a significant association with monozygotic twinning. Hughes and Miskin (1986) could follow by means of computed tomography the sequence from death of the co-twin to cyst formation in the survivor's brain. This syndrome is one of the causes of the excess mortality in multiple gestations. Acute vascular collapse generates identical brain damage.

Focal ischaemia with resulting infarction occurs mainly towards the end of pregnancy and may result from embolic migration of obscure origin or from general haemodynamic factors. Several cases of congenital hemiplegia due to localized infarcts of clear prenatal origin are on record (Ong *et al.* 1983, Mito *et al.* 1989). The diagnosis can sometimes be made prenatally by ultrasound or MRI (Amato *et al.* 1991). Other loci of prenatal infarcts have been reported (Bouza *et al.* 1994). An extreme example of CNS destruction of probable vascular origin with almost complete destruction of the brainstem was reported by Robinson *et al.* (1993).

Fetal hypoxia probably causes brain damage largely through its effect on cardiac function, and cardiac failure supervenes long before a direct effect of hypoxia on the brain is apparent (Myers 1972).

Acute vascular collapse also generates identical brain damage; it was probably the major factor in cases of hydranencephaly or multicystic encephalomalacia observed in a case of bee-sting anaphylaxis during pregnancy (Erasmus *et al.* 1982) and in a baby born to a mother involved in an aircraft accident (Fowler *et al.* 1971). The mechanisms of brain damage generated by accidents during pregnancy may include small placental detachment or uterine artery spasm due to catecholamine discharge. These may produce several types of damage, including periventricular leukomalacia and asymmetrical necrotic lesions. Cardiac failure causes poor peripheral perfusion with lactic acidosis and generates brain oedema that may prevent normal reflow and thus lead to diffuse or disseminated ischaemic damage. Such an intrauterine sequence

of events in the fetus has been observed following maternal carbon monoxide intoxication (Larroche 1986). Depending on the date of occurrence, the result may be polymicrogyria (Chapter 3) or necrosis of the white matter such as observed after carbon monoxide intoxication of experimental monkeys (Ginsberg and Myers 1972), in association with extensive cortical damage. Similar lesions have been produced by maternal intoxication with butane gas which is not toxic in itself but produces hypoxia by displacing air (Fernàndez *et al.* 1986).

Hypoxia is thus an example of the multifactorial nature of the mechanisms of fetal brain damage, the final common pathway being ischaemia. Hypoxia can also stimulate the excitatory glutamate receptors with resulting excitotoxic damage. A role for such a mechanism during pregnancy is suggestd by the fact that a much lower proportion of infants who later developed cerebral palsy were born to mothers who had received magnesium sulfate at the end of pregnancy for treatment of toxaemia or pre-eclampsia than to mothers who had not been so treated (Nelson and Grether 1995). Such an effect could be due to the prevention of excitotoxicity mediated through *N*-methyl-D-aspartate (NMDA) receptors that are blocked by magnesium (Marret *et al.* 1995).

Chronic fetal anaemia, such as occurs in haemolytic disease, haemoglobinopathies and parvovirus B19 infection, may cause cardiac failure resulting in immunological or nonimmunological hydrops and severe hypoxic–ischaemic brain damage. Massive fetomaternal haemorrhage (Boyce *et al.* 1994) and nonimmune hydrops fetalis (Laneri *et al.* 1994) are documented causes of prenatal hypoxic brain damage.

NEUROPATHOLOGY OF PRENATAL VASCULAR OR CIRCULATORY DISORDERS

Neuropathological lesions of prenatal origin cannot be entirely differentiated from perinatal or early postnatal ones (Chapters 2, 8). Malformations (Chapter 3) can also be a consequence of such disturbances. Here I will discuss primarily necrotic and cavitary lesions which are the hallmark of prenatal injury (Barth 1984). Lesions of the white matter are the most common and are usually incurred during the 26th to 35th weeks of gestation.

Periventricular leukomalacia is described in detail in Chapter 2 as it is most frequently seen in preterm infants as a postnatal event. However, some 10–25 per cent of occurrences may be of prenatal origin (Sinha *et al.* 1990). Iida *et al.* (1992) found prenatal leukomalacia in 20 per cent of stillborn fetuses and in 16.4 per cent of infants who died at <3 days of age. Cystic lesions were found by Bejar *et al.* (1988) in 13 of 127 preterm infants by day 3, and by Ellis *et al.* (1988) in 25 per cent of infants who died at <7 days (16 per cent of preterm and 48 per cent of term infants). Even higher figures were reported by Squier and Keeling (1991), who found such lesions in 15 of 39 stillborn babies and in 15 of 90 liveborn infants who died <7 days of age. Other investigators (Truwit *et al.* 1992, Krägeloh-Mann *et al.* 1995) have adduced evidence suggesting that many white matter lesions in older children are a late result of prenatal leukomalacia (Chapter 8). Lower figures were found by other groups, probably as a result of the different populations studied.

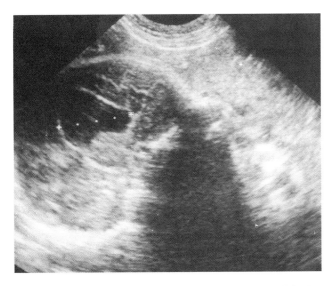

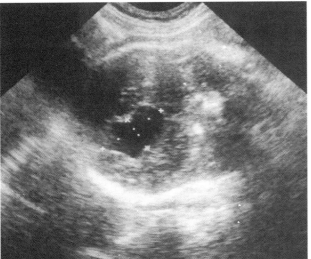

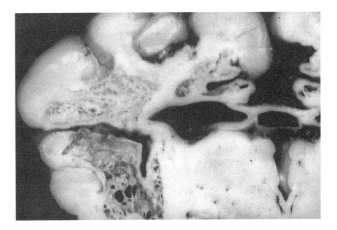

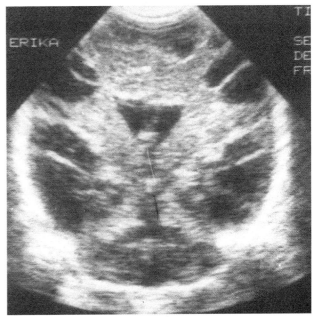

Fig. 1.4. 'Porencephaly' in 35-week fetus. *(Top)* Axial cut (back of fetal head on left of picture) showing destruction of posterior part of right hemisphere. *(Bottom)* Coronal cut showing dilated lateral ventricles and large cavity above right lateral ventricle, probably communicating with ventricular cavity. (Courtesy Dr M-C. Aubry, Maternité Port Royal, Paris.)

Fig. 1.5. Multicystic encephalomalacia. *(Top)* Brain of monozygotic twin whose stillborn co-twin was macerated. Note honeycomb appearance of subcortical white matter. *(Bottom)* Ultrasound image through anterior fontanelle (coronal cut). Note normal ventricular size and multiple cavities separated by thin septa.

PORENCEPHALY

The term porencephaly is often used loosely for any cavitating hemispheric lesion (Fig. 1.4). It is best, however, to restrict its use to circumscribed necrosis that occurs before the adult features of the hemisphere are manifest (Barth 1984, Friede 1989), as indicated by disturbances in the development of the adjoining cortex. The so-called schizencephaly is in fact an early form of porencephaly (Chapter 3). A later type is characterized by an abnormal disposition of the gyri adjacent to the cavity that converge toward the defect. The paucity of connective tissue scarring differentiates such a porencephaly from postnatal cavitation in which a similar topography of gyri occurs occasionally (Friede 1989). Most porencephalic lesions involve both the grey and white matter.

Multicystic encephalomalacia is also termed polyporencephaly or multicystic encephalopathy. Multiple cavities involve the greater part of both hemispheres. They may affect predominantly

either the white or the grey matter but may also involve the cortex and basal ganglia and usually are located mainly in the territories of the anterior and middle cerebral arteries (Fig. 1.5). Basal ganglia, cerebellum and brainstem may be spared (Takada *et al.* 1989, Larroche *et al.* 1990). The microscopic features are those of infarction with fat-laden macrophages and scattered glial scar tissue. The lesion is often associated with twin gestation but may also occur with perinatal asphyxia (Schmitt 1984, Frigieri *et al.* 1996) and less often with viral infections (Smith *et al.* 1977, Lyen *et al.* 1981) and metabolic disease (Rupar *et al.* 1996). Postnatal formation of such defects has been documented by sonograpy and CT scan (Pfister-Goedeke and Boltshauser 1982, Stannard and Jimenez 1983).

Hydranencephaly refers to massive necrosis of both hemispheres in the fetus, although postnatal cases may occur (Fig. 1.6). The hemispheres are replaced by fluid-filled cavities lined by a

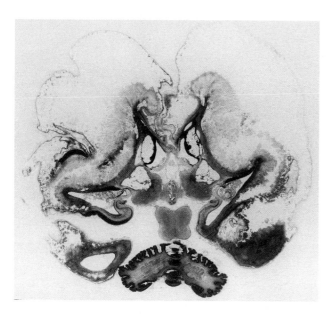

Fig. 1.6. Hydranencephaly: monozygotic twin with parabiotic syndrome (recipient twin). Dorsal part of both hemispheres is represented by thin membrane. Temporal lobes and central grey matter are better preserved, suggesting disturbances preferentially affecting the carotid circulation. (Courtesy Dr J-C. Larroche, by permission of Karger, Basel.)

thin membrane lying against the dura mater. The membrane may include small islands of relatively preserved cortex, and its inner surface may be covered by trabeculae or a continuous film of nervous tissue. The membrane is continuous with the molecular layer of preserved brain. The latter is usually in the territory of the posterior cerebral arteries, so that the occipital lobes and parts of the temporal lobes are preserved, as are, to some extent, the basal ganglia. Rare cases are associated with a progressive vasculopathy (Norman and McGillivray 1988). The head may be normal or enlarged, dilatation being due to aqueductal stenosis or obstruction of the foramina of Monro (Lyon and Robain 1967, Larroche 1986). In some cases a median–sagittal arch of relatively normal brain connects the occipital and frontal remnants of the brain, somewhat like the handle of a basket, a condition known as 'basket-brain' (Norman *et al.* 1958). Hydranencephaly is caused by the same factors as multicystic encephalopathy even though, in many cases, gestation appears to have been uneventful. Rare familial cases have been described (Fowler *et al.* 1972, Harper and Hockey 1983, Bordarier and Robain 1989).

Predominant grey matter involvement is less common with prenatal brain damage. However, it may occur and is probably not rare especially when there is conjunction of prenatal and perinatal aetiological factors. An example is bilateral symmetrical thalamic necrosis (Eicke *et al.* 1992) with or without calcification. A prenatal origin of this lesion is strongly supported by the absence of perinatal evidence of hypoxia, the high incidence of polyhydramnios which probably indicates prenatal swallowing difficulties, the early spasticity often present from the first days of life, and the frequent presence of early calcification (Govaert and de Vries 1997). Grey matter involvement may also predominate in the cortex or in the basal ganglia. Cohen and Roessmann

(1994) reviewed 10 published cases of prenatal damage to the basal ganglia, dividing them into those that had occurred before 24 gestational weeks and mainly consisted of pallidal necrosis, and those that had occurred between 24 and 36 weeks and were mainly thalamic and brainstem necrosis. Several patterns of prenatal cortical damage have been described, including the parasagittal pattern (Chapter 2), a central cortico-subcortical pattern involving mainly the central cortex and the basal ganglia (Barth *et al.* 1984) (Fig. 1.7), and a birolandic pattern selectively affecting the motor strips bilaterally (Maller *et al.* 1995). These patterns may also occur with perinatal damage and are described in Chapter 2. At a late stage they are responsible for so-called *ulegyria* or atrophic sclerotic scars involving one of several convolutions. The crown of the convolution is relatively preserved, while the depth of the gyri is severely affected, so that the appearance is of mushroom convolutions with a narrow base.

Some pathological features are highly suggestive of prenatal sclerotic lesions. These include the association of sclerotic lesions with malformations, especially microgyria (Bordarier and Robain 1992); in early lesions, the absence of a significant glial reaction when the insult was incurred before the 26th gestational week; and the presence of early calcification. However, prenatal infectious processes can produce a similar appearance. Some of these pathological features may be also clinical clues to a prenatal disorder, such as the presence of calcification in the first weeks of life.

CLINICAL MANIFESTATIONS AND DIAGNOSIS
During pregnancy there is often no obvious maternal illness or fetal distress. In severe cases, decrease in fetal movements may be noted clinically or by sonography. Stunting of fetal growth, identified by clinical and ultrasound examination, and hydramnios are inconstant and nonspecific. In cases of high-risk pregnancy or when abnormal events occur, the diagnosis can be made in some cases by sonographic examination or by other imaging procedures (Erasmus *et al.* 1982, Hughes and Miskin 1986, Larroche *et al.* 1990).

The diagnosis, in most cases, is postnatal, and it may be surprisingly late. The birth process itself may be difficult, thus leading to an erroneous diagnosis of perinatal hypoxic–ischaemic encephalopathy. The status of infants at birth is often completely normal. In some cases, the infant may appear to be in poor condition. Marked anaemia may be present in injuries resulting from fetomaternal or fetofetal haemorrhage and suggests the possibility of multicystic encephalomalacia in association with poor neurological condition with apathy and seizures, especially if a co-twin has died during late pregnancy (Aicardi *et al.* 1972). In rare cases, there may be microcephaly at birth and marked rigidity or spasticity with absence of normal reactivity, as in infants with bilateral thalamic calcification (Eicke *et al.* 1992). For infants with an abnormal neurological condition at birth, the diagnosis of the underlying abnormality can be suggested by EEG and made by ultrasonography or other form of imaging. An isoelectric EEG seems often to be associated with antepartum damage (Scher 1994). Barabas *et al.* (1993) found evidence for

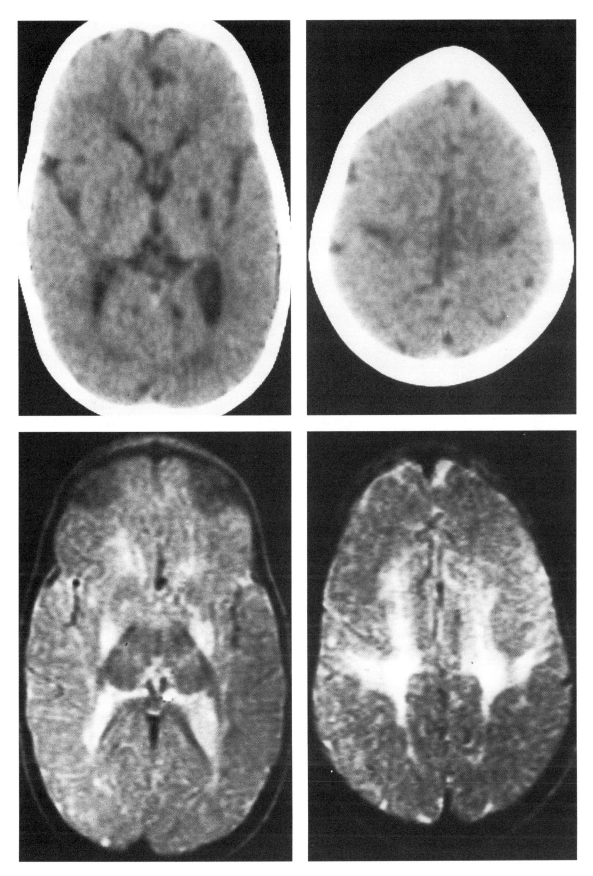

Fig. 1.7. Central cortico-subcortical pattern of brain damage associated with cavitation of both putamina in 16-month-old boy with history of prenatal hypoxia and cerebral palsy. *(Top)* CT scans showing cavitation of both putamina, more prominent on left side *(left)*, and linear areas of hypodensity in both central regions. In some patients such areas may be cystic *(right)* and are sometimes misdiagnosed as 'schizencephaly'. *(Bottom)* T$_2$-weighted spin-echo MRI demonstrates intense signal from areas that appeared hypodense on CT scan.

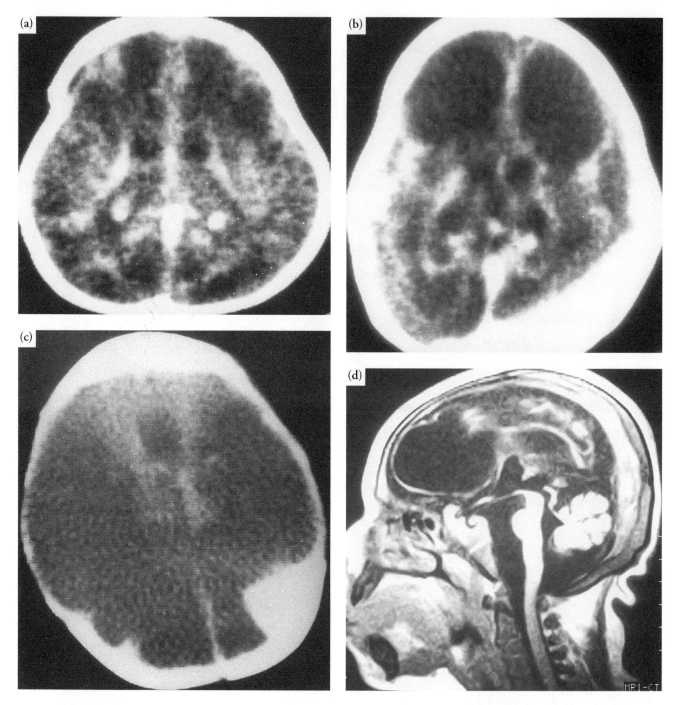

Fig. 1.8. Multicystic encephalomalacia. *(a–c)* CT scans in monozygotic twin. *(a)* Initial (non-enhanced) scan on second day of life showing multiple areas of hypodensity and blood in lateral ventricles and parenchyma. *(b)* Second scan at age 2 months showing multiple cavitation. *(c)* Third scan at 7 months demonstrating hydranencephaly. Supratentorial compartment contains only CSF. Posterior fossa structures are relatively better preserved. *(d)* MRI of another infant showing relative preservation of brainstem and cerebellum with extensive cavitation of cerebral hemisphere (courtesy Prof. Brian Neville, Great Ormond Street Hospital, London).

such damage in 17 of 20 infants (seven purely antepartum and ten with contribution of intrapartum problems). The EEG can help determine prenatal onset and timing of insult. Takeuchi and Watanabe (1989) and Watanabe (1992) showed that an acute insult produces a characteristic sequence of patterns, depression of the tracings being followed by recovery, whereas dysmaturity of the EEG (*i.e.* a pattern corresponding to a younger age) is more suggestive of a chronic insult. The CT and MRI features of porencephaly, multicystic encephalomalacia and focal ischaemic lesions are clear-cut (Fig. 1.8). However, small infarcts are poorly seen on ultrasound scans and often require MRI for diagnosis (Bouza *et al.* 1994). The presence of marked imaging abnormalities at birth or in the first few days of life helps rule out perinatally acquired damage and may be of considerable medicolegal value.

In infants with no obvious abnormality in the neonatal period, the diagnosis is often considerably delayed. Even hydranencephaly may be surprisingly silent and escape recognition for weeks or even months and be discovered only when there is enlargement of the head or abnormally fast head growth. Transillumination of the skull or neuroimaging will then reveal the damage (Naidich and Chakera 1984). A special problem of medicolegal consequences is raised by the occurrence of neurological abnormalities in infants born to mothers who have incurred various types of trauma during pregnancy. There seems to be a poor relation between the severity of maternal trauma and the occurrence of fetal brain damage (Larroche 1986, Pearlman *et al.* 1990). In rare cases of injury to the placenta (Eden *et al.* 1986) or of skull fracture in the fetus (Nakahara *et al.* 1989) the relationship is obvious.

The treatment of prenatally acquired brain lesions is mainly supportive. For hydranencephaly, shunting may be indicated to prevent excessive head growth. The possibility of preventing some prenatal insults with magnesium sulfate given during pregnancy is suggested by the observational study of Nelson and Grether (1995), but further study is necessary.

INHERITED METABOLIC AND NEURODEGENERATIVE DISORDERS WITH FETAL ONSET

Although metabolic disorders all have their origin prenatally, they usually have no obvious manifestations during pregnancy and early postnatal life. However, some peroxisomal disorders such as Zellweger syndrome, some mitochondrial disorders such as pyruvate dehydrogenase deficiency (Robinson *et al.* 1996), a few respiratory chain disorders (Samsom *et al.* 1994), and carbohydrate-deficient glycoprotein disease type I (Jensen *et al.* 1995) can impair prenatal brain development.

Recently, attention has been drawn to a heterogeneous group of diseases with fetal onset and continuing slow neonatal progression (Barth 1992, Albrecht *et al.* 1993). These disorders are described with other metabolic or degenerative disorders involving the same systems (Chapters 9, 10). A list of these diseases is given in Table 1.5. Despite their widely different causes, they share some clinical features, *e.g.* the presence of severe manifestations at birth and often of microcephaly and of systemic involvement. They may be a cause of early death because of the severity of multisystemic involvement. Their diagnosis is often difficult as other causes can produce similar features (Barth 1993). These include viral infections such as CMV disease, chromosomal aberrations, some types of cerebellar hypoplasia and some CNS malformations such as acrocallosal syndrome, otopalatodigital syndrome and Marden–Walker syndrome. Their prognosis is usually very poor.

EXOGENOUS AND ENDOGENOUS TOXIC DISORDERS

Although the placenta constitutes an effective barrier between

TABLE 1.5
Inherited neurodegenerative disorders with fetal onset

Disease	References
Peroxisomal diseases	Chapter 9
Zellweger syndrome	
Neonatal adrenoleukodystrophy	
Neonatal leukodystrophies	Barth (1992)
Wiedeman–Rautenstrauch type	Martin *et al.* (1984)
Pontocerebellar hypoplasias	Barth (1992)
Carbohydrate-deficient protein (CDG) syndromes; infantile types with olivopontocerebellar atrophy (OPCA)	Jensen *et al.* (1995), Pavone *et al.* (1996)
Type 1 (Barth–Brun syndrome) with microcephaly and extrapyramidal dyskinesia	Barth (1993)
Type 2 with anterior horn cell disease	Goutières *et al.* (1977)
PEHO syndrome (peripheral oedema, hypsarrhythmia, optic atrophy)	Salonen *et al.* (1991)
Neuroaxonal dystrophies	
Infantile type	Fitch *et al.* (1973), Aicardi and Castelein (1979)
Vasculopathies	
With hydranencephaly (Fowler syndrome)	Harding *et al.* (1995)
Calcific deposits	
Aicardi–Goutières syndrome (some cases)	Aicardi and Goutières (1984)
Lethal arthrogryposis with calcification	Illume *et al.* (1988)
Disordered axonal development with cataracts, myopathy and cardiomyopathy	Lyon *et al.* (1990)
Congenital neuropathy with cerebral maldevelopment/dysfunction	Neimann *et al.* (1973)
Dentato-olivary dysplasia with tonic seizures and suppression–burst EEG	Harding and Boyd (1991)

maternal and fetal circulations, various substances, therapeutic or otherwise, can reach the conceptus and produce malformations or other serious disturbances. Likewise, maternal metabolic dysregulation can adversely affect the offspring.

EXOGENOUS TOXIC SUBSTANCES
Table 1.6 lists some of the main substances that can be transmitted from mother to fetus and produce neurological damage.

THERAPEUTIC AGENTS
Since the thalidomide disaster, the potential adverse effects of drugs on the development of children of women treated during pregnancy have been widely recognized. The administration of drugs during pregnancy should be as parsimonious and cautious as possible, and no therapeutic agents that have not been extensively tested should ever be used.

Antiepileptic drugs
These can produce adverse effects on the fetus including malformations, intrauterine growth retardation and, possibly, behavioural and cognitive changes in postnatal life (for reviews, see Yerbi 1988, Delgado-Escueta *et al.* 1992, Vestermark 1993). For

TABLE 1.6
Main substances that can be transmitted from mother to fetus and produce neurological damage

Category	Pattern of damage	References
Therapeutic agents		
Antiepileptic drugs (phenytoin, barbiturates, carbamazepine, diones, sodium valproate)	Fetal growth retardation, small head, dysmorphism of face and fingers, facial clefts, congenital heart disease and other defects	See text
Benzodiazepines	Poorly defined	Laegreid *et al.* (1993)
Warfarin and other coumarin derivatives	Punctate chondrodystrophy, deafness	Pauli and Hahn (1993)
Vitamin A	Hydrocephalus, ear and heart anomalies (uncertain)	Elefant *et al.* (1987)
Retinoic acid, isotretinoin	CNS migration disorder	Lammer *et al.* (1985), Barth (1987)
Industrial pollutants		
Methylmercury	Abnormal neuronal migration, deranged cortical organization	Marsh *et al.* (1980), Peckham and Choi (1988)
Polychlorinated biophenyls (PCBs)	Microcephaly, large fontanelles, behavioural disturbances	Chen and Hsu (1994), Jacobson and Jacobson (1996)
Carbon monoxide	Hypoxic–ischaemic lesions	
Recreational substances		
Alcohol	Fetal growth retardation, facial dysmorphism, brain malformations with excess neuronal migration and other CNS defects	See text; Clarren *et al.* (1992), Majewski (1993)
Narcotics (heroin, codeine, methadone)	Virtually all such substances may produce fetal growth retardation, and narcotics may produce withdrawal symptoms in neonates. In addition, cocaine can induce abruptio placentae and fetal death and may be responsible for skull and brain malformations and vascular damage with infarcts or haemorrhage	See text
Other 'street drugs' (amphetamines, pyrobenzamine, phencyclidine)		
Cocaine		
Toluene and other inhalants	Microcephaly, minor craniofacial anomalies, limb anomalies	Hersh *et al.* (1985)
Tobacco	Growth retardation. Possible effects on cognitive development?	See text

unknown reasons possibly related to individual differences in drug metabolism (Yerbi 1988), adverse effects are observed only in some exposed fetuses, in an unpredictable manner. Although specific syndromes were formerly ascribed to one determined drug, such as the fetal hydantoin syndrome (Hanson and Buehler 1982) or the fetal dione syndrome (Feldman *et al.* 1977), it is now generally accepted that most anticonvulsant drugs, with the possible exception of sodium valproate, produce a similar pattern of malformations and a similar effect on fetal growth (Kelly 1984, Lyons Jones *et al.* 1989). This syndrome includes: growth retardation that may affect predominantly the increase in head circumference, this effect being possibly more marked with carbamazepine (Vestermark 1993); facial dysmorphism with hypertelorism and a flat nasal bridge; and digital anomalies, especially hypoplasia of the distal phalanges and nails (Gaily *et al.* 1988), these being perhaps more frequent with phenytoin treatment. More severe malformations may occur, among which facial or palatal clefts (Friis 1989), neural tube defects (Lindhout and Schmidt 1986) and congenital heart disease are most frequent. Although the effects on growth and head size appear to be reversible in most cases, lasting behavioural and/or cognitive changes have been reported (Holmes and Flannery 1988).

The frequency of the syndrome appears to vary with the individual drug, and combinations of drugs appear to be especially noxious (Vestermark 1993). Some investigators have reported a rate of abnormalities as high as 58 per cent among offspring of women who received a combination of carbamazepine, phenobarbitone and sodium valproate during pregnancy (Lindhout *et al.* 1984, 1992). However, the significance of many reported figures is open to debate because of the retrospective nature of most studies and the numerous possible biases.

The toxic effect of anticonvulsant drugs, especially phenytoin, might be related to the toxicity of drug epoxides. The concentration of these compounds is regulated enzymatically. A low epoxide activity in amniocytes of fetuses exposed to maternal phenytoin therapy seems to correlate with the occurrence of the fetal hydantoin syndrome, whereas a high activity may predict a normal infant (Buehler *et al.* 1990).

Valproic acid and sodium valproate seem to induce a specific malformation syndrome that includes abnormalities of the extremities and of the face distinct from those observed with other antiepileptic drugs, with epicanthal folds, a flat nasal bridge, a long upper lip, a thin vermilion border, a shallow philtrum and a downturned mouth. Affected children also have abnormal digits and long thin overlapping fingers and toes (Jager-Roman *et al.* 1986). Defects in the abdominal wall, stridor, tracheomalacia and urogenital anomalies have also been reported (Christianson *et al.* 1994). The incidence of spina bifida is probably increased in fetuses of mothers receiving sodium valproate (Lindhout and Schmidt 1986). According to Laegreid *et al.* (1993), the benzodiazepines might potentiate the teratogenic effects of valproate. They may also have a teratogenic effect of their own.

The possibility of such effects raises a major problem for the treatment of pregnant women (Chapter 16). Because teratogenesis is an early event, gestation in treated epileptic women should be carefully planned, although the balance of risks and benefits is hard to determine. The use of monotherapy or the simplification of therapeutic schemes has resulted in a possible decrease of malformations (Oguni *et al.* 1992). Nevertheless, no drug is completely safe, although the frequency of major malformations is low.

Other therapeutic agents
Many other pharmaceuticals have been indicted in the genesis of fetal defects (see Table 1.6). A review of drug effects in pregnancy is given by Koren and Nulman (1993). Coumarin derivatives can produce severe defects of the CNS and associated malformations (Pauli and Hann 1993) or a picture of punctate chondrodystrophy. The use of tocolytic drugs, especially indomethacin, may be associated with an increased incidence of enterocolitis and of cerebral lesions including intraventricular haemorrhage (Baerts *et al.* 1990, Norton *et al.* 1993).

In addition to chemical agents, ionizing radiation can induce microcephaly (Chapter 3).

'RECREATIONAL' DRUGS
Fetal alcohol syndrome
The frequency of the fetal alcohol syndrome (FAS), as originally described by Lemoine *et al.* (1968), depends on the population considered. Clarren and Smith (1978) suggested that the full-blown syndrome was present in 1–2 per cent of all newborn infants and that partial forms could occur is as many as 3–5 per cent of live births. It is difficult to determine a precise threshold for dangerous alcohol consumption. Majewski (1993) has observed the syndrome only in women with obvious chronic alcoholism. Daily doses in excess of 80 mL alcohol are clearly dangerous, but smaller doses may not be safe. In a prospective study (Day *et al.* 1990), the frequency of growth retardation and morphological abnormalities in infants was significantly related to use of alchohol throughout pregnancy or during the second and third trimesters. An occasional binge may be responsible for FAS (Clarren *et al.* 1992), although this is contested by others (Autti-Rämö and Granström 1991, Majewski 1993) and most investigators think that total abstinence is not necessary (Graham *et al.* 1988, Majewski 1993). Like all teratogenic agents, alcohol does not induce malformations regularly and uniformly (Choi *et al.* 1978). Alcohol has a direct toxicity for animal offspring, but indirect effects such as poor nutrition and associated habits, and especially smoking, probably play a role in humans (Gershoni-Baruch and Nelson 1988). Ethanol exposure may also induce impairment of the umbilical circulation and fetal hypoxia (Mukherjee and Hodgen 1982).

The *neuropathology* of FAS includes several types of brain malformation, especially excessive neuronal migration with leptomeningeal glioneuronal heterotopias (Wisniewski *et al.* 1983). Subtle developmental disorders such as dendritic spine abnormalities have been described (Ferrer and Galofré 1987), and

TABLE 1.7
Main features of the fetal alcohol syndrome

Growth and performance
Prenatal growth retardation (more in length than in weight)
Postnatal growth retardation
Developmental delay
Fine movement dysfunction

Craniofacial features
Microcephaly
Maxillary hypoplasia with relative prognathism
Epicanthal folds
No increase in interorbital distance
Apparent hypertelorism due to short palpebral fissures (blepharophimosis)
Thinning of vermilion border
Hypoplastic upper helix

Ocular features
Esotropy
Tortuous retinal vessels

Limbs
Joint anomalies (limitation of elbow extension, of interphalangeal joints)
Abnormal palmar creases

Visceral
Congenital heart disease
Excess neuronal migration
Other brain malformations

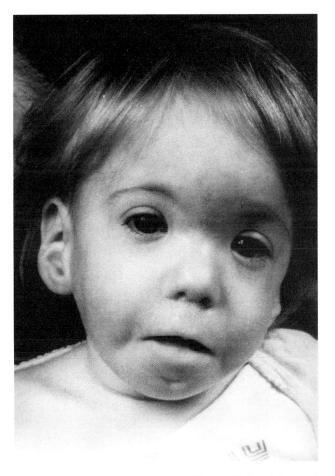

Fig. 1.9. Fetal alcohol syndrome. Typical facies with broad depressed nasal bridge, epicanthus, long philtrum, thin vermilion border and retrognathism.

21

gross malformations such as neural tube defects, abnormal gyration, agenesis of the corpus callosum and holoprosencephaly have been observed in a few cases (Ronen and Andrews 1991).

The *clinical manifestations* of the FAS (Table 1.7) include constant features, *viz.* retarded fetal growth and variable degrees of microcephaly (Majewski 1993). Affected infants usually have dysmorphic features including apparent hypertelorism (blepharophimosis), epicanthus and a thin upper lip (Fig. 1.9). Mild mental retardation is extremely frequent, being observed in up to 85 per cent of cases (Clarren and Smith 1978, Marcus 1987, Korkman *et al.* 1994). FAS may be responsible for up to 10 per cent of cases of mild mental retardation. Fundoscopic examination shows tortuous retinal vessels in many cases, and nerve hypoplasia was found in 19 of 25 infants by Strömland and Hellström (1996). The real frequency of mild forms is difficult to assess as diagnosis is somewhat subjective. Majewski described three stages of alcohol embryopathy: in stage 1, mental retardation was minimal and the face might be normal; in stages 2 and 3, the dysmorphic syndrome was clear-cut and the neurological features severe. Even in children with normal IQs, however, learning difficulties and behavioural disturbances, especially hyperactivity, seem to be an integral part of the syndrome (Shaywitz *et al.* 1980, Majewski 1993). Part of these may be related to hearing difficulties (Church and Gerkin 1988). Maturation of the EEG is delayed in alcohol-exposed infants (Ioffe and Chernick 1988).

Narcotic substances
Heroin, morphine and methadone do not appear to be teratogenic in humans. Chasnoff *et al.* (1982) found that 39 infants conceived when their mothers were using heroin and who subsequently were maintained on low-dose methadone, were lighter at birth and had significantly smaller heads than 27 children born to control mothers and 19 children born to women who were abusing various combinations of phenobarbitone, benzodiazepines, marijuana, pentazocine, pyribenzamine, codeine or phencycline, indicating the potential of narcotics for fetal impairment. Oro and Dixon (1987) also reported that narcotic drugs were associated with preterm birth and intrauterine growth retardation. The effects of narcotics are difficult to assess as abuse of these substances is often combined with underprivileged socioeconomic conditions and use of alcohol, heavy smoking and suboptimal nutrition.

Cocaine
Cocaine abuse is associated with the same effects as narcotics with respect to fetal growth (Volpe 1992). Withdrawal symptoms are similar to those observed in infants of narcotic-addicted mothers and should be treated along the same lines (American Academy of Pediatrics 1983). Cocaine abuse is, in addition, associated with abruptio placentae and stillbirth (Chasnoff *et al.* 1986, Hadeed and Siegel 1989). Cocaine is a potent vasoconstrictor, and cerebrovascular damage with porencephaly and small cavitations in the region of the basal ganglia have been described (for reviews, see Volpe 1992, 1995). Ischaemic damage could be the substrate of the neurological abnormalities repeatedly reported

in infants born to addicted mothers. Such abnormalities include microcephaly, dystonia (Beltran and Coker 1995), hypertonia, tremor, intellectual impairment and behavioural disturbances (Chiriboga *et al.* 1993, Gieron-Kothals *et al.* 1994, Mayes *et al.* 1995, Scafidi *et al.* 1996). The teratogenic potential of cocaine remains under discussion. Some investigators have reported eye and brain abnormalities (Dominguez *et al.* 1991). Bingol *et al.* (1987) have observed congenital heart disease, exencephaly and encephaloceles in four infants born to cocaine-addicted mothers and none in control infants or in those born to mothers abusing multiple substances, thus suggesting a possible teratogenic effect of cocaine. However, no agreement has been reached regarding the frequency and importance of fetal effects of cocaine (Dogra *et al.* 1994, Konkol 1994, King *et al.* 1995). This substance can provoke fetal vascular disruption leading to cavitary lesions of the nervous system or to limb reduction defects and intestinal atresia (Hoyme *et al.* 1990). It may also favour the occurrence of fetal intracranial haemorrhage by increasing cerebral blood-flow velocity (Van de Bor *et al.* 1990, Singer *et al.* 1994, Holzman *et al.* 1995). Gressens *et al.* (1992) have shown that cocaine induces disturbances of neuronal migration and corticogenesis in experimental animals and can also modify dopamine metabolism.

Tobacco-smoking
Smoking during pregnancy is well known to result in low birthweight infants, with the possible consequences that attach to intrauterine growth retardation. There is no report of specific malformations in such cases but intellectual impairment of infants has been reported (Olds *et al.* 1994).

Solvent abuse
Toluene used by inhalation ('glue sniffing') can produce an embryopathy (Pearson *et al.* 1994) and may produce micrencephaly, limb anomalies and minor facial dysmorphism.

INDUSTRIAL POLLUTANTS
Methylmercury discharged into the waters of Minamata Bay, Japan, was the source of an epidemic of brain malformations, and the same occurred following consumption of contaminated wheat in Iraq (Marsh *et al.* 1980, Peckham and Choi 1988). Severe migrational disorder and diffuse astrocytosis of the white matter was present in the brains of affected fetuses (Barth 1987). Affected infants displayed microcephaly, profound hypotonia, tremors or myoclonic jerks.

Polychlorinated biphenyls (PCBs) have been responsible for microcephaly and behavioural abnormalities in addition to intrauterine growth retardation, skin pigmentation and large fontanelles (Chen and Hsu 1994, Jacobson and Jacobson 1996).

ENDOGENOUS TOXICITY—CONSEQUENCES OF SOME MATERNAL METABOLIC DERANGEMENTS
The consequences of maternal metabolic errors on the fetus are of considerable importance. In addition to their frequency, they constitute the archetype of potentially familial, nongenetic disorders. Their prevention is possible if maternal disease is

diagnosed and appropriate counselling and monitoring of pregnancy are offered.

PHENYLKETONURIA AND HYPERPHENYLALANINAEMIA
Untreated phenylketonuria or imperfectly controlled hyperphenylalaninaemia have been shown to be responsible for neurological and other abnormalities in infants. These are described in Chapter 9.

DIABETES MELLITUS
Maternal diabetes mellitus is a significant cause of fetal and neonatal morbidity and mortality as the frequency of the disorder is 0.2–0.3 per cent of the population (Fraser 1994). All forms of diabetes can generate problems, but insulin-dependent (type 1) diabetes is especially dangerous. The main problems of infants of diabetic mothers include macrosomia and congenital malformations that particularly affect the brain (Barr et al. 1983) and the lower extremity of the vertebral column (Passarge and Lenz 1966). Other neurological complications such as intracranial venous thromboses are much less common (Ward 1977). Even though the mechanism of malformations in infants of diabetic mothers is incompletely understood, there is evidence that they are related to poor control of the diabetes. Elevated levels of maternal haemoglobin A1c in early pregnancy—which reflect insufficient control of glycaemia over a relatively long period—correlate with the occurrrence of major congenital anomalies in offspring (Miller et al. 1981, Freinkel et al. 1985), although the correlation is far from perfect. Despite the frequent presence of macrosomia that develops late in pregnancy, there is often fetal growth delay as shown by sonography early in gestation, which is associated with an increased risk of congenital malformations (Pedersen and Molsted-Pedersen 1981). Ultrasonography shows that the fetal behaviour is abnormal with a delayed pattern of eye and limb movements (Mulder 1993). It seems that prevention of congenital malformations can be achieved by careful control of the diabetes (Fuhrmann et al. 1983), provided it is obtained during the first seven or eight weeks of pregnancy when such defects are generated (Miller et al. 1981).

IMMUNOLOGICAL AND BLOOD DISEASES IN THE FETUS

The most common prenatal haematological disorder used to be *incompatibility in the rhesus blood system*. Erythroblastosis fetalis is now mostly of historical interest, as prevention of isoimmunization by administration of globulins following rhesus-incompatible pregnancies has become standard practice. This disease was the first to be treated by prenatal transfusions. However, *hydrops fetalis* remains common in countries where certain types of thalassaemia and haemoglobin E disease are frequent. Nonimmune hydrops may be due to infection with parvovirus B19 infection (Brown 1989). *Intrauterine thrombocytopenia*, whether idiopathic or due to isoimmunization against fetal platelets, may be responsible for prenatal brain damage (Naidu et al. 1983). While the disorder may be encountered in infants born to moth-

ers with apparently well-controlled disease, Burrows and Kelton (1993) found that those with severe disease and haemorrhage were born to mothers with significant thrombocytopenia. Haemorrhage may occur from the 20th week onwards (Jesurun et al. 1980, Herman et al. 1986), and diagnosis by sonography is possible (Bondurant et al. 1984). Up to 20 per cent of patients with congenital isoimmune thrombocytopenia will suffer prenatal haemorrhage. Such bleeding may be the origin of brain cavities in infants' brains (Manson et al. 1988, Govaert et al. 1995). Therefore, antenatal treatment especially with corticosteroids is important (Bussel et al. 1988). Full evaluation of the results of such therapy is not yet available but present results are encouraging.

Other intracranial haemorrhages of traumatic or unknown origin are occasionally observed prenatally and can be diagnosed by sonography (Kim and Elyaderani 1982, Donn et al. 1984). Bleeding may be in the subdural space (Gunn et al. 1985) or intraventricular (Zorzi et al. 1988), although this type of haemorrhage is much more frequently of postnatal origin.

INTRAUTERINE GROWTH RETARDATION AND PRETERM BIRTH

Although fetal growth retardation and preterm birth are not necessarily associated with neurological problems and are not a direct cause of brain damage, they play such an important indirect role in the aetiology of brain injury in the prenatal and perinatal periods that they deserve more than cursory mention.

INTRAUTERINE GROWTH RETARDATION
Intrauterine growth retardation (IUGR) is variably defined. Some investigators regard infants whose weight is below the 10th centile as being growth retarded, while others set the limit at the 3rd centile or at two standard deviations below the mean for age (Chiswick 1985). The group is very heterogeneous as many causes can be responsible (Harel et al. 1992). At least two major subgroups are defined (Kramer et al. 1990). *Proportionate*—incorrectly termed 'symmetrical'—growth retardation affects equally body length and weight as well as head circumference. It can be due to intrinsic defects of the fetus such as chromosomal abnormalities or dysmorphic syndromes, or to fetal deprivation from early in pregnancy in particular syndromes of dwarfism such as Russell–Silver syndrome. This type has also been observed in cases of placental mosaicism (Kalousek et al. 1991) and in infants born to mothers addicted to cocaine, although a degree of asymmetry is common in such cases (Volpe 1992). Asymmetrical, or rather *disproportionate* growth retardation affects growth in weight more than length and head growth, which may be completely normal. It is mainly observed in fetuses deprived during the later part of gestation as occurs with maternal toxaemia or preeclampsia. About 30 per cent of cases of asymmetrical growth retardation are idiopathic. In such cases, it is likely that uteroplacental vascular anomalies are an important factor (Fitzgerald and Stuart 1989). Harel et al. (1992) have emphasized the importance for the prognosis of the cephalic index (ratio of head

circumference to birth weight). A normal index often predicts a satisfactory neurological outcome. Infants with IUGR constitute up to 10 per cent of all livebirths and at least 30 per cent of low birthweight infants. As a group, their perinatal mortality is four to ten times higher than that of infants with normal growth.

Five to 15 per cent of fetuses with IUGR have malformations or dysmorphic syndromes. Approximately 2 per cent have chromosomal abnormalities, and less than 3 per cent have suffered intrauterine viral infections. Many of them have minor abnormalities (Lindhal and Michelsson 1986; Lindhal et al. 1988a,b).

In the disproportionate group, maternal haemorrhage, hypertension, renal disease, diabetes with microvascular changes, malnutrition, smoking and cardiac disease are important factors (Chiswick 1985, Tenovuo et al. 1988).

The neurodevelopmental progress of infants who suffered IUGR, especially those who belong to the asymmetrical group, is most often normal (Tenovuo et al. 1988). However, they are at increased risk of neonatal hypoxia (Levene et al. 1985, Soothill et al. 1987), hypoglycaemia and fetal hyperviscosity syndrome (Hakanson and Oh 1980), and attendant sequelae. Moreover, 10–35 per cent of them will have learning difficulties, and some will have deficient visual function (Stanley et al. 1989). Rapid head growth after birth is of favourable prognosis (Hack and Breslau 1986), while infants whose head growth is still insufficient at age 2 years have an unfavourable developmental outlook (Tenovuo et al. 1988). Veelken et al. (1992) studied a group of preterm infants with birthweights < 1501g, and compared 96 of them who were small for gestational age (SGA) with 275 with a birthweight appropriate for gestational age (AGA). The main aetiological factors in the SGA group included maternal toxaemia, alcohol consumption, placental insufficiency and signs of fetal stress. In the AGA group, the main gestational abnormalities were premature rupture of membranes and amnionitis. Cerebral palsy was found in only 7.5 per cent of the SGA infants but in 17.5 per cent of the AGA group, while minor abnormalities were more common in SGA (30 per cent) than in AGA infants (15.3 per cent). An important role in the mechanism of intrauterine growth retardation and associated brain damage is played by an imbalance between prostaglandins, especially prostacyclin which is a relaxant of smooth muscle fibres and thromboxane that has the reverse effect. Because of the likely vascular origin of IUGR, monitoring and early delivery are of importance as the duration of adverse conditions is probably critical.

PRETERM BIRTH
The essential role of preterm birth in the genesis of cerebral palsy, mental retardation and learning difficulties will be repeatedly emphasized in this book (Chapters 2, 7, 8, 23). An enormous amount of literature has been dedicated to the neurodevelopmental outcome of preterm infants (reviews in Dunn 1986, Piekkala et al. 1988, Amiel-Tison 1994, Stewart and Pezzani-Goldsmith 1994). Special attention has been paid in recent years to the very small preterm baby of < 1500g birthweight (Lefebvre et al. 1988, Lloyd et al. 1988, Portnoy et al. 1988). A high proportion of such children have learning difficulties, strabismus and other visual

problems or frank cerebral palsy, especially spastic or ataxic diplegia. In some studies (e.g. Vohr and Garcia-Col 1985) up to 54 per cent of low birthweight infants required special schooling. Adverse events during the neonatal period have a deleterious effect on later development, especially intracranial haemorrhage (Williams et al. 1987, Zubrick et al. 1988, Lewis and Bendersky 1989). On the other hand, a normal ultrasound scan and a normal neurological examination predict a satisfactory development (Stewart et al. 1988). Recent studies (e.g. Hagberg and Hagberg 1993) have shown that, despite the considerable improvement in the outcome of preterm birth, the increasing numbers of surviving preterm infants of very low birthweight represent a considerable burden and, indeed, have been responsible for an increase in frequency of cerebral palsy of the spastic type, often of particular severity. Hack et al. (1996) found that despite an increase in the survival rates of extremely low birthweight infants (500–750g), the morbidity remained unchanged, with 20 per cent subnormal cognitive function and 10 per cent cerebral palsy rates. Such data have led to discussion of the limits of viability (see Amiel-Tison 1994) and raised difficult ethical problems. The relationship between low birthweight and neurodevelopmental outcome in preterm infants is complex. Preterm birth and/or low birthweight are the ultimate consequence of preconceptional, prenatal and perinatal influences. They are more frequent in lower socioeconomic groups and with complicated pregnancies (Goldstein et al. 1995). Infection, particularly chorioamnionitis, is of especial significance in this regard (Hay et al. 1994). Conversely, they are associated with an increased rate of major or minor congenital anomalies, which suggests the possible role of genetic factors (Largo et al. 1989).

Because of the adverse impact of preterm birth on neurodevelopmental progress, its prevention is a high priority (Weisglas-Kuperus et al. 1993). Experience in industrialized countries has shown that regular medical examination of pregnant women and appropriate medico-social measures could significantly lessen the burden of preterm birth and consequent neurodevelopmental difficulties (Papiernik et al. 1985).

REFERENCES

Aalfs, C.M., van den Berg, H., Barth, P.G., Hennekam, R.C.M. (1995) 'The Hoyeraal–Hreidarsson syndrome: the fourth case of a separate entity with prenatal growth retardation, progressive pancytopenia and cerebellar hypoplasia.' European Journal of Pediatrics, 154, 304–308.

Abrams, E.J., Matheson, P.B., Thomas, P.A., et al. (1995) 'Neonatal predictors of infection status and early death among 332 infants at risk of HIV-1 infection monitored prospectively from birth.' Pediatrics, 96, 451–458.

Aicardi, J., Castelein, P. (1979) 'Infantile neuroaxonal dystrophy.' Brain, 102, 727–748.

—— Goutières, F. (1984) 'A progressive familial encephalopathy in infancy with calcifications of the basal ganglia and chronic cerebrospinal fluid lymphocytosis.' Annals of Neurology, 15, 49–54.

—— —— Hodebourg de Verbois, A. (1972) 'Multicystic encephalomalacia of infants and its relation to abnormal gestation and hydranencephaly.' Journal of the Neurological Sciences, 15, 357–373.

Albrecht, S., Schneider, M.C., Belmont, J., Armstrong, D.L. (1993) 'Fatal infantile encephalopathy with olivopontocerebellar hypoplasia and micrencephaly. Report of three siblings.' Acta Neuropathologica, 85, 394–399.

Al-Eissa, Y., Al-Mofada, S.M. (1992) 'Congenital brucellosis.' *Pediatric Infectious Disease Journal*, **11**, 667–671.

Alkalay, A.L., Pomerance, J.J., Rimoin, D.L. (1987) 'Fetal varicella syndrome.' *Journal of Pediatrics*, **111**, 320–323.

Altshuler, G. (1973) 'Toxoplasmosis as a cause of hydranencephaly.' *American Journal of Diseases of Children*, **125**, 251–252.

—— (1993) 'Some placental considerations related to neurodevelopmental and other disorders.' *Journal of Child Neurology*, **8**, 78–84.

Amato, M., Hüppi, P., Herschkowitz, N., Huber, P. (1991) 'Prenatal stroke suggested by intrauterine ultrasound and confirmed by magnetic resonance imaging.' *Neuropediatrics*, **22**, 100–102.

American Academy of Pediatrics, Committee on Drugs (1983) 'Neonatal drug withdrawal.' *Pediatrics*, **72**, 895–902.

—— Committee on Genetics (1994) 'Prenatal genetic diagnosis for pediatricians.' *Pediatrics*, **93**, 1010–1015.

Amiel-Tison, C. (1994) 'When is it best to be born? A pediatric perspective on behalf of the fetus.' *In:* Amiel-Tison, C., Stewart, A. (Eds.) *The Newborn Infant. One Brain for Life.* Paris: Editions INSERM, pp. 11–22.

Antonarakis, S.E. (1989) 'Diagnosis of genetic disorders at the DNA level.' *New England Journal of Medicine*, **320**, 153–163.

Aubry, J-P., Aubry, M-C. (1986) *Atlas d'Echo-anatomie Foetale Normale et Pathologique.* Paris: Masson.

Autti-Rämö, I., Granström, M-L. (1991) 'The psychomotor development during the first year of life of infants exposed to intrauterine alcohol of various duration. Fetal alcohol exposure and development.' *Neuropediatrics*, **22**, 59–64.

Baerts, W., Fetter, W.P.F., Hop, W.C.J., *et al.* (1990) 'Cerebral lesions in preterm infants after tocolytic indomethacin.' *Developmental Medicine and Child Neurology*, **32**, 910–918 + *erratum*, 1032.

Bale, J.F., Bray, P., Bell, W.E. (1985) 'Neuroradiographic abnormalities in congenital cytomegalovirus infection.' *Pediatric Neurology*, **1**, 42–47.

—— Sato, Y., Eisert, D. (1986) 'Progressive postnatal subependymal necrosis in an infant with congenital cytomegalovirus infection.' *Pediatric Neurology*, **2**, 367–370.

—— O'Neil, H.E., Hart, M.N., *et al.* (1989) 'Human cytomegalovirus nucleic acids in tissues from congenitally infected humans.' *Pediatric Neurology*, **5**, 216–220.

—— Blackman, J.A., Sato, Y. (1990) 'Outcome in children with symptomatic congenital cytomegalovirus infection.' *Journal of Child Neurology*, **4**, 131–136.

Barabas, R.E., Barmada, M.A., Scher, M.S. (1993) 'Timing of brain insults in severe neonatal encephalopathies with isoelectric EEG.' *Pediatric Neurology*, **9**, 39–44.

Barkovich, A.J., Lindan, C.E. (1994) 'Congenital cytomegalovirus infection of the brain: imaging analysis and embryologic considerations.' *American Journal of Neuroradiology*, **15**, 703–715.

—— Gressens, P., Evrard, P. (1992) 'Formation, maturation and disorders of brain neocortex.' *American Journal of Neuroradiology*, **13**, 423–446.

Barr, M., Hanson, J.W., Currey, K., *et al.* (1983) 'Holoprosencephaly in infants of diabetic mothers.' *Journal of Pediatrics*, **102**, 565–568.

Barth, P.G. (1984) 'Prenatal clastic encephalopathies.' *Clinical Neurology and Neurosurgery*, **86**, 65–75.

—— (1987) 'Disorders of neuronal migration.' *Canadian Journal of Neurological Sciences*, **14**, 1–16.

—— (1992) 'Inherited progressive disorders of the fetal brain: a field in need of recognition.' *In:* Fukuyama, Y., Suzuki, Y., Kamoshita, S., Casaer, P. (Eds.) *Fetal and Perinatal Neurology.* Basel: Karger, pp. 299–313.

—— (1993) 'Pontocerebellar hypoplasias. An overview of a group of inherited neurodegenerative disorders with fetal onset.' *Brain and Development*, **15**, 411–422.

—— van der Harten, J.J. (1985) 'Parabiotic twin syndrome with topical isocortical disruption and gastroschisis.' *Acta Neuropathologica*, **67**, 345–349.

—— Valk, J., Olislagers-De Slegte, R. (1984) 'Central cortico-subcortical pattern on CT in cerebral palsy: its relevance to asphyxia.' *Journal of Neuroradiology*, **11**, 65–71.

Beeram, M.R., Chopde, N., Dawood, Y., *et al.* (1996) 'Lumbar puncture in the evaluation of possible asymptomatic congenital syphilis in neonates.' *Journal of Pediatrics*, **128**, 125–129.

Bejar, R., Wozniak, P., Allard, M., *et al.* (1988) 'Antenatal origin of neurologic damage in newborn infants. I. Preterm infants.' *American Journal of Obstetrics and Gynecology*, **159**, 357–363.

Belman, A.L. (1992) 'Acquired immunodeficiency syndrome and the child's central nervous system.' *Pediatric Clinics of North America*, **39**, 691–714.

Beltinger, C., Saule, H. (1988) 'Sonography of subependymal cysts in congenital rubella syndrome.' *European Journal of Pediatrics*, **148**, 206–207.

Beltran, R.S., Coker, S.B. (1995) 'Transient dystonia of infancy, a result of intrauterine cocaine exposure?' *Pediatric Neurology*, **12**, 354–356.

Ben-Ami, T., Yousefzadeh, D., Backus, M., *et al.* (1990) 'Lenticulostriate vasculopathy in infants with infections of the central nervous system: sonographic and Doppler findings.' *Pediatric Radiology*, **20**, 575–579.

Best, J.M., Banatvala, J.E., Morgan-Capner, P., Miller, E. (1989) 'Fetal infection after maternal reinfection with rubella: criteria for defining reinfection.' *British Medical Journal*, 299, 773–775.

Biale, Y., Brawer-Ostrovsky, J., Insler, V. (1985) 'Fetal heart rate tracings in fetuses with congenital malformations.' *Journal of Reproductive Medicine*, **30**, 43–47.

Bianchi, D.W. (1995) 'Prenatal diagnosis by analysis of fetal cells in maternal blood.' *Journal of Pediatrics*, **127**, 847–856.

Bingol, N., Fuchs, M., Diaz, V., *et al.* (1987) 'Teratogenicity of cocaine in humans.' *Journal of Pediatrics*, **110**, 93–96.

Birnholz, J.C. (1989) 'Ultrasonic fetal neuro-ophthalmology.' *In:* Hill, A., Volpe, J.J. (Eds.) *Fetal Neurology.* New York: Raven Press, pp. 41–56.

Blanche, S., Mayaux, M-J., Rouzioux, C., *et al.* (1994) 'Relation of the course of HIV infection in children to the severity of the disease in their mothers at delivery.' *New England Journal of Medicine*, **330**, 308–312.

Bondurant, S., Boehm, F.H., Fleisher, A.C., Machin, J.E. (1984) 'Antepartum diagnosis of fetal intracranial hemorrhage by ultrasound.' *Obstetrics and Gynecology*, **63**, Suppl. 3, S25–S27.

Boppano, S.B., Pass, R.F., Britt, W.J., *et al.* (1992) 'Symptomatic congenital cytomegalovirus infection: neonatal morbidity and mortality.' *Pediatric Infectious Disease Journal*, **11**, 93–99.

Bordarier, C., Robain, O. (1989) 'Familial occurrence of prenatal encephaloclastic damage: anatomoclinical report of 2 cases.' *Neuropediatrics*, **20**, 103–106.

—— —— (1992) 'Microgyric and necrotic cortical lesions in twin fetuses: original cerebral damage consecutive to twinning?' *Brain and Development*, **14**, 174–178.

Bouza, H., Dubowitz, L.M.S., Rutherford, M., *et al.* (1994) 'Late magnetic resonance imaging and clinical findings in neonates with unilateral lesions on cranial ultrasounds.' *Developmental Medicine and Child Neurology*, **36**, 951–964.

Boyce, L.H., Khandji, A.G., DeKlerk, A.M., Nordli, D.R. (1994) 'Fetomaternal hemorrhage as an etiology of neonatal stroke.' *Pediatric Neurology*, **11**, 255–257.

Brar, H.S., Platt, L.D. (1989) 'Fetal biophysical score and fetal well-being.' *In:* Hill, A., Volpe, J.J. (Eds.) *Fetal Neurology.* New York: Raven Press, pp. 95–115.

Brown, K.E. (1989) 'What threat is human parvovirus B19 to the fetus? A review.' *British Journal of Obstetrics and Gynaecology*, **96**, 764–767.

Buehler, B.A., Delimont, D., Van Waes, M., Finnell, R.H. (1990) 'Prenatal prediction of risk of the fetal hydantoin syndrome.' *New England Journal of Medicine*, **322**, 1567–1572.

Burke, C.J., Tannenberg, A.E. (1995) 'Prenatal brain damage and placental infarction—an autopsy study.' *Developmental Medicine and Child Neurology*, **37**, 555–562.

Burn, J., Wickramasinghe, H.T., Harding, B., Baraitser, M. (1986) 'A syndrome with intracranial calcification and microcephaly in two sibs, resembling intrauterine infection.' *Clinical Genetics*, **30**, 112–116.

Burrows, R.F., Kelton, J.G. (1993) 'Fetal thrombocytopenia and its relation to maternal thrombocytopenia.' *New England Journal of Medicine*, **329**, 1463–1466.

Bussel, J.B., Berkowitz, R.L., McFarland, J.G., *et al.* (1988) 'Antenatal treatment of neonatal alloimmune thrombocytopenia.' *New England Journal of Medicine*, **319**, 1374–1378.

Callen, P.W. (1988) *Ultrasonography in Obstetrics and Gynecology, 2nd Edn.* London: Harcourt Brace Jovanovich.

Chamberlain, P.F., Manning, F.A., Morrison, I., *et al.* (1984) 'Ultrasound evaluation of amniotic fluid volume. 1: The relationship of marginal and decreased amniotic fluid volumes to perinatal outcome.' *American Journal of Obstetrics and Gynecology*, **150**, 245–249.

Chard, T., Macintosh, M. (1992) 'Antenatal diagnosis of congenital abnormalities.' *In:* Chard, T., Richards, M.P.M. (Eds.) *Obstetrics in the 1990s: Current Controversies. Clinics in Developmental Medicine No. 123/124.* London: Mac Keith Press, pp. 90–104.

Chasnoff, I.J., Hatcher, R.P., Burns, W.J. (1982) 'Polydrug and methadone-addicted newborns: a continuum of impairment?' *Pediatrics*, **70**, 210–213.
—— Bussey, M.E., Savitch, R., Stack, C.M. (1986) 'Perinatal cerebral infarction and maternal cocaine use.' *Journal of Pediatrics*, **108**, 456–459.
Chen, Y.-J., Hsu, C-C. (1994) 'Effects of prenatal exposure to PCBs on the neurological function of children: a neuropsychological and neuro-physiological study.' *Developmental Medicine and Child Neurology*, **36**, 312–320.
Chess, S. (1971) 'Autism in children with congenital rubella.' *Journal of Autism and Childhood Schizophrenia*, **1**, 33–47.
Chiriboga, C.A., Bateman, D.A., Brust, J.C.M., Hauser, W.A. (1993) 'Neurologic findings in neonates with intrauterine cocaine exposure.' *Pediatric Neurology*, **9**, 115–119.
Chiswick, M.L. (1985) 'Intrauterine growth retardation.' *British Medical Journal*, **291**, 845–848.
Choi, B.H., Lapham, L.W., Zaki, A.M., Saleem, T. (1978) 'Abnormal neuronal migration, deranged cerebral cortical organization, and diffuse white matter astrocytosis of human fetal brain: a major effect of methylmercury poisoning in utero.' *Journal of Neuropathology and Experimental Neurology*, **37**, 719–733.
Christianson, A.L., Chesler, N., Kromberg, J.G.R. (1994) 'Fetal valproate syndrome: clinical and neurodevelopmental features in two sibling pairs.' *Developmental Medicine and Child Neurology*, **36**, 361–369.
Church, M.W., Gerkin, K.P. (1988) 'Hearing disorders in children with fetal alcohol syndrome: findings from case reports.' *Pediatrics*, **82**, 147–154.
Clarren, S.K., Smith, D.W. (1978) 'The fetal alcohol syndrome.' *New England Journal of Medicine*, **298**, 1063–1067.
—— Astley, S.J., Gunderson, V.M., Spellman, D. (1992) 'Cognitive and behavioral deficits in nonhuman primates associated with very early embryonic binge exposures to ethanol.' *Journal of Pediatrics*, **121**, 789–796.
Cohen, M., Roessmann, U. (1994) '*In utero* brain damage: relationship of gestational age to pathological consequences.' *Developmental Medicine and Child Neurology*, **36**, 263–268.
Conboy, T.J., Pass, R.F., Stagno, S., et al. (1986) 'Intellectual development in school-aged children with asymptomatic congenital cytomegalovirus infection.' *Pediatrics*, **77**, 801–806.
Connor, E.M., Sperling, R.S., Gelber, R., et al. (1994) 'Reduction of maternal–infant transmission of human immunodeficiency virus type 1 with zidovudine treatment.' *New England Journal of Medicine*, **331**, 1173–1180.
Conry, J.A., Torok, T., Andrews, I. (1993) 'Perinatal encephalopathy secondary to in utero human parvovirus B19 (HPV) infection.' *Neurology*, **43**, Suppl. 2, A346. *(Abstract.)*
Cooper, L.Z., Krugman, S. (1967) 'Clinical manifestations of postnatal and congenital rubella.' *Archives of Ophthalmology*, **77**, 434–439.
Couture, A., Veyrac, C., Baud, C. (1994) *Echographie Cérébrale du Foetus au Nouveau-né. Imagerie et Hémodynamique.* Montpellier: Sauramps Médical.
Couvreur, J., Desmonts, G. (1988) 'Acquired and congenital toxoplasmosis.' *In:* Vinken, P.J., Bruyn, G.W., Klawans, H.L. (Eds.) *Handbook of Clinical Neurology. Revised Series Vol. 8. Microbial Disease.* Amsterdam: Elsevier, pp. 351–363.
—— —— Tournier, G., Collin, E. (1984) 'La production locale accrue d'immunoglobulines G dans le liquide céphalorachidien au cours de la toxoplasmose congénitale.' *Annales de Pédiatrie*, **31**, 829–835.
Cradock-Watson, J.E., Ridehalgh, M.K.S., Anderson, M.J., Pattison, J.R. (1985) 'Rubella reinfection and the fetus.' *Lancet*, **2**, 1039. *(Letter.)*
Daffos, F., Forestier, F., Capella Pavlovsky, M.C. (1984) 'Fetal blood sampling during the third trimester of pregnancy.' *British Journal of Obstetrics and Gynaecology*, **91**, 118–121.
—— —— —— et al. (1988) 'Prenatal management of 746 pregnancies at risk for congenital toxoplasmosis.' *New England Journal of Medicine*, **318**, 271–275.
D'Alton, M.E., DeCherney, A.H. (1993) 'Prenatal diagnosis.' *New England Journal of Medicine*, **328**, 114–120.
Day, N.L., Richardson, G., Robles, N., et al. (1990) 'Effect of prenatal alcohol exposure on growth and morphology of offspring at 8 months of age.' *Pediatrics*, **85**, 748–752.
Delgado-Escueta, A.V., Janz, D., Beck-Mannagetta, G. (1992) 'Pregnancy and teratogenesis in epilepsy.' *Neurology*, **42**, Suppl. 5, 1–160.
Desmond, M.M., Montgomery, J.R., Melnick, J.L., et al. (1969) 'Congenital rubella encephalitis: effects on growth and early development.' *American Journal of Diseases of Children*, **118**, 30–31.
Desmonts, G., Daffos, F., Forestier, F., et al. (1985) 'Prenatal diagnosis of congenital toxoplasmosis.' *Lancet*, **1**, 500–504.
—— Couvreur, J., Thuilliez, P. (1990) 'Cinq cas de transmission à l'enfant d'une infection toxoplasmique maternelle antérieure à la grossesse.' *Presse Médicale*, **19**, 1445–1449.
Dogra, V.S., Shyken, J.M.., Menon, P.A., et al. (1994) 'Neurosonographic abnormalities associated with maternal history of cocaine use in neonates of appropriate size for their gestional age.' *American Journal of Neuroradiology*, **15**, 697–702.
Dominguez, R., Aguirre Vila-Coro, A., Slopis, J.M., Bohan, T.P. (1991) 'Brain and ocular abnormalities in infants with in utero exposure to cocaine and other street drugs.' *American Journal of Diseases of Children*, **145**, 688–695.
Donn, S.M., Barr, M., McLeary, R.D. (1984) 'Massive intracerebral hemorrhage in utero: sonographic appearance and pathologic correlation.' *Obstetrics and Gynecology*, **63**, 28S–30S.
Dorfman, D.H., Glaser, J.H. (1990) 'Congenital syphilis presenting in infants after the newborn period.' *New England Journal of Medicine*, **323**, 1299–1302.
Dulième, A-M., Messiah, A., Blanche, S., et al. (1992) 'Natural history of human immunodeficiency virus type I infection in children: prognostic value of laboratory tests on the bimodal progression of the disease.' *Pediatric Infectious Disease Journal*, **11**, 630–635.
—— Amos, C.I., Felton, S., et al. (1995) 'Birth order, delivery route, and concordance in the transmission of human immunodeficiency virus type 1 from mothers to twins.' *Journal of Pediatrics*, **126**, 625–632.
Dunn, H.G. (Ed.) (1986) *Sequelae of Low Birthweight: the Vancouver Study. Clinics in Developmental Medicine No. 95/96.* London: Mac Keith Press.
Eden, R.D., Parker, R.T., Gall, S.A. (1986) 'Rupture of the pregnant uterus: a 53-year review.' *Obstetrics and Gynecology*, **68**, 671–674.
Eicke, M., Briner, J., Willi, U., et al. (1992) 'Symmetrical thalamic lesions in infants.' *Archives of Disease in Childhood*, **67**, 15–19.
Elefant, E., Bavous, F., Boyer, M. (1987) 'Médicaments et grossesse.' *In:* Tournaire, M. (Ed.) *Mises à Jour en Gynécologie et Obstétrique. Collège National des Gynécologues et Obstétriciens Français.* Paris: Vigot, pp. 287–344.
Ellis, W.G., Goetzman, B.W., Lindenberg, J.A. (1988) 'Neuropathologic documentation of prenatal brain damage.' *American Journal of Diseases of Children*, **142**, 858–866.
Enders, G., Miller, E., Cradock-Watson, J., et al. (1994) 'Consequences of varicella and herpes zoster in pregnancy: prospective study of 1739 cases.' *Lancet*, **343**, 1548–1551.
Erasmus, C., Blackwood, W., Wilson, J. (1982) 'Infantile multicystic encephalomalacia after maternal bee sting anaphylaxis during pregnancy.' *Archives of Disease in Childhood*, **57**, 785–787.
Erkkola, R., Grönroos, M., Pynnonen, R., Kilkku, P. (1984) 'Analysis of intrapartum fetal deaths: their decline with increasing electronic fetal monitoring.' *Acta Obstetricia et Gynecologica Scandinavica*, **63**, 459–462.
European Collaborative Study (1991) 'Children born to women with HIV-1 infection: natural history and risk of transmission.' *Lancet*, **337**, 253–260.
—— (1994a) 'Caesarian section and risk of vertical transmission of HIV-1 infection.' *Lancet*, **343**, 1464–1467.
—— (1994b) 'Natural hisory of vertically acquired human immunodeficiency virus infection.' *Pediatrics*, **94**, 815–819.
Evans, M.I., Schulman, J.D. (1989) 'Medical fetal therapy.' *In:* Evans, M.I., Fletcher, J.C., Dixler, A.O., Schulman, J.D. (Eds.) *Fetal Diagnosis and Therapy. Science, Ethics and the Law.* Philadelphia: Lippincott, pp. 403–412.
—— Drugan, A., Manning, F.A., Harrison, M.R. (1989) 'Fetal surgery in the 1990s.' *American Journal of Diseases of Children*, **143**, 1431–1436.
Evrard, P., De Saint Georges, P., Kadhim, H.J., Gadisseux, J.F. (1989) 'Pathology of prenatal encephalopathies.' *In:* French, J.H., Harel, S., Casaer, P. (Eds.) *Child Neurology and Developmental Disabilities.* Baltimore: P.H. Brookes, pp. 153–176.
Ewigman, B.G., Crane, J.P., Frigoletto, F.D., et al. (1993) 'Effects of prenatal ultrasound screening on perinatal outcome. RADIUS Study Group.' *New England Journal of Medicine*, **329**, 821–827.
Feldman, G.L., Weaver, D.D., Lovrien, E.W. (1977) 'The fetal trimethadione syndrome. Report of an additional family and further delineation of this syndrome.' *American Journal of Diseases of C'hildren*, **131**, 1389–1392.
Fernàndez, F., Pèrez-Higueras, A., Hernàndez, R., et al. (1986) 'Hydranencephaly after maternal butane-gas intoxication during pregnancy.' *Developmental Medicine and Child Neurology*, **28**, 361–363.
Ferrer, I., Galofré, E. (1987) 'Dendritic spine anomalies in fetal alcohol syndrome.' *Neuropediatrics*, **18**, 158–160.
Fitch, N., Carpenter, S., Lachance, R.C. (1973) 'Prenatal axonal dystrophy and

osteopetrosis.' *Archives of Pathology*, **95**, 298–301.

Fitzgerald, D.E., Stuart, B.T. (1989) 'Fetoplacental and uteroplacental blood flow in pregnancy.' *In:* Hill, A., Volpe, J.J. (Eds.) *Fetal Neurology.* New York: Raven Press, pp. 121–137.

Fowler, K.B., Stagno, S., Pass, R.F., *et al.* (1992) 'The outcome of congenital cytomegalovirus infection in relation to maternal antibody status.' *New England Journal of Medicine*, **326**, 663–667.

Fowler, M., Brown, C., Cabrera, K.F. (1971) 'Hydranencephaly in a baby after an aircraft accident to the mother: case report and autopsy.' *Pathology*, **3**, 21–30.

—— Dow, R., White, T.A., Greer, C.H. (1972) 'Congenital hydrocephalus–hydrencephaly in five siblings, with autopsy studies: a new disease.' *Developmental Medicine and Child Neurology*, **14**, 173–188.

Fraser, R. (1994) 'Diabetes in pregnancy.' *Archives of Disease in Childhood*, **71**, F224–F230.

Freeman, J.M. (1985) *Prenatal and Perinatal Factors Associated with Brain Disorders. NIH Publication No. 85-1149.* Washington, DC: NIH.

Freinkel, N., Dooley, S.L., Metzger, B.E. (1985) 'Care of the pregnant woman with insulin-dependent diabetes mellitus.' *New England Journal of Medicine*, **313**, 96–101.

Friede, R. (1989) *Developmental Neuropathology, 2nd Edn.* Berlin: Springer.

Frigieri, G., Guidi, B., Costa Zaccarelli, S., *et al.* (1996) 'Multicystic encephalo-malacia in term infants.' *Child's Nervous System*, **12**, 759–764.

Friis, M.L. (1989) 'Facial clefts and congenital heart defects in children of parents with epilepsy: genetic and environmental etiologic factors.' *Acta Neurologica Scandinavica*, **79**, 433–459.

Fuhrmann, K., Reiher, H., Semmler, K., *et al.* (1983) 'Prevention of congenital malformations in infants of insulin-dependent diabetic mothers.' *Diabetes Care*, **6**, 219–223.

Gaffney, G., Sellers, S., Flavell, V., *et al.* (1994) 'Case–control study of intra-partum care, cerebral palsy, and perinatal death.' *British Medical Journal*, **308**, 743–750.

Gaily, E., Granström, M.L., Hiilesmaa, V., Bardy, A. (1988) 'Minor anomalies in offspring of epileptic mothers.' *Journal of Pediatrics*, **112**, 520–529.

Garcia, A.G. (1968) 'Congenital toxoplasmosis in two successive sibs.' *Archives of Disease in Childhood*, **43**, 705–710.

Gershoni-Baruch, R., Nelson, M. (1988) 'The fetal alcohol syndrome: a review.' *Pediatric Reviews and Communications*, **3**, 45–59.

Gibbs, J.M., Weindling, A.M. (1994) 'Neonatal intracranial lesions following placental abruption.' *European Journal of Pediatrics*, **153**, 195–197.

Gibbs, R.S., Mead, P.B. (1992) 'Preventing neonatal herpes—current strategies.' *New England Journal of Medicine*, **326**, 946–947.

Gieron-Korthals, M.A., Helal, A., Martinez, C.R. (1994) 'Expanding spectrum of cocaine induced central nervous system malformations.' *Brain and Development*, **16**, 253–256.

Ginsberg, M.D., Myers, R.E. (1972) 'Clinical and neuropathological aspects of carbon monoxide intoxications in the primate: production of a leuko-encephalopathy.' *Transactions of the American Neurological Association*, **97**, 207–211.

Glaser, J.H., Dorfman, D. (1991) 'Congenital syphilis.' *New England Journal of Medicine*, **324**, 1065. *(Letter.)*

Goldstein, R.F., Thompson, R.J., Oehler, J.M., Brazy, J.E. (1995) 'Influence of acidosis, hypoxemia, and hypotension on neurodevelopmental outcome in very low birth weight infants.' *Pediatrics*, **95**, 238–243.

Gordon, N. (1993) 'Toxoplasmosis: a preventable cause of brain damage.' *Developmental Medicine and Child Neurology*, **35**, 567–573.

Goutières, F., Aicardi, J., Farkas, E. (1977) 'Anterior horn cell disease associated with ponto-cerebellar hypoplasia in infants.' *Journal of Neurology, Neurosurgery, and Psychiatry*, **40**, 370–378.

Govaert, P., de Vries, L.S. (1997) *An Atlas of Neonatal Brain Sonography. Clinics in Developmental Medicine No. 141/142.* London: Mac Keith Press.

—— Bridger, J., Wigglesworth, J. (1995) 'Nature of the brain lesion in fetal allo-immune thrombocytopenia.' *Developmental Medicine and Child Neurology*, **37**, 485–495.

Graham, J.M., Hanson, J.W., Darby, A.L., *et al.* (1988) 'Independent dys-morphology evaluations at birth and 4 years of age for children exposed to varying amounts of alcohol in utero.' *Pediatrics*, **81**, 772–778.

Gressens, P., Kosofsky, B.E., Evrard, P. (1992) 'Cocaine-induced disturbances of corticogenesis in the developing murine brain.' *Neuroscience Letters*, **140**, 113–116.

Griffiths, P.D., Stagno, S., Pass, R.F., *et al.* (1982) 'Congenital cytomegalovirus infection: diagnostic and prognostic significance of the detection of specific immunoglobulin M antibodies in cord serum.' *Pediatrics*, **69**, 544–549.

Grose, C., Meehan, T., Weiner, C.P. (1992) 'Prenatal diagnosis of congenital cytomegalovirus infection by virus isolation after amniocentesis.' *Pediatric Infectious Disease Journal*, **11**, 605–607.

Gunn, T.R., Mok, P.M., Becroft, D.M.O. (1985) 'Subdural hemorrhage in utero.' *Pediatrics,* **76**, 605–610.

Hack, M., Breslau, N. (1986) 'Very low birth weight infants: effects of brain growth during infancy on intelligence quotient at 3 years of age.' *Pediatrics*, **77**, 196–202.

—— Friedman, H., Fanaroff, A.A. (1996) 'Outcomes of extremely low birth weight infants.' *Pediatrics*, **98**, 931–937.

Haddad, J., Roth, S., Simeoni, J.P., *et al.* (1987) 'Varicelle et grossesse: aspects périnataux et prophylactiques.' *Archives Françaises de Pédiatrie*, **44**, 339–342.

Haddow, J.E., Palomaki, G.E., Knight, G.J., *et al.* (1992) 'Prenatal screening for Down's syndrome with use of maternal serum markers.' *New England Journal of Medicine*, **327**, 588–593.

Hadeed, A.J., Siegel, S.R. (1989) 'Maternal cocaine use during pregnancy: effect on the newborn infant.' *Pediatrics*, **84**, 205–210.

Hagberg, B., Hagberg, G. (1993) 'The origins of cerebral palsy.' *In:* David, T.J. (Ed.) *Recent Advances in Paediatrics, Vol.11.* London: Churchill Livingstone, pp. 67–83.

Hakanson, D.O., Oh, W. (1980) 'Hyperviscosity in the small-for-gestational age infant.' *Biology of the Neonate*, **37**, 109–112.

Hall, S.M. (1992) 'Congenital toxoplasmosis.' *British Medical Journal*, **305**, 291–297.

Hanshaw, J.B., Dudgeon, J.A., Marshall, M.D. (1985) *Viral Diseases of the Fetus and Newborn.* London: W.B. Saunders.

Hanson, J.W., Buehler, B.A. (1982) 'Fetal hydantoin syndrome: current status.' *Journal of Pediatrics*, **101**, 816–818.

Harding, B.N., Boyd, S.G. (1991) 'Intractable seizures from infancy can be associated with dentato-olivary dysplasia.' *Journal of the Neurological Sciences*, **104**, 157–165.

Harding, B.N., Ramani, P., Thurley, P. (1995) 'The familial syndrome of proliferative vasculopathy and hydranencephaly–hydrocephaly: immuno-cytochemical and ultrastructural evidence for endothelial proliferation.' *Neuropathology and Applied Neurobiology*, **21**, 61–67.

Harel, S., Goldin, E., Tomer, A., Yavin, E. (1992) 'Vascular-induced intrauterine growth retardation: animal and human models.' *In:* Fukuyama, Y., Suzuki, Y., Kamoshita, S., Casaer, P. (Eds.) *Fetal and Perinatal Neurology.* Basel: Karger, pp. 206–215.

Harper, C., Hockey, A. (1983) 'Proliferative vasculopathy and an hydranen-cephalic–hydrocephalic syndrome: a neuropathological study of two siblings.' *Developmental Medicine and Child Neurology*, **25**, 232–239.

Hay, P.E., Lamont, R.F., Taylor-Robinson, D., *et al.* (1994) 'Abnormal bacterial colonisation of the genital tract and subsequent preterm delivery and late miscarriage.' *British Medical Journal*, **308**, 295–298.

Hayward, J.C., Titelbaum, D.S., Clancy, R.R., Zimmerman, R.A. (1991) 'Lissencephaly–pachygyria associated with congenital cytomegalovirus infection.' *Journal of Child Neurology*, **6**, 109–114.

Herman, J.H., Jumbelic, M.I., Ancona, R.J., Kickler, T.S. (1986) 'In utero cerebral hemorrhage in alloimmune thrombocytopenia.' *American Journal of Pediatric Hematology and Oncology*, **8**, 312–317.

Hersh, J.H., Podruch, P.E., Rogers, G., Weisskopf, B. (1985) 'Toluene embryopathy.' *Journal of Pediatrics*, **106**, 922–927.

Higa, K., Dan, H., Manabe, H. (1987) 'Varicella-zoster virus infections during pregnancy: hypothesis concerning the mechanisms of congenital malformation.' *Obstetrics and Gynecology*, **69**, 214–222.

Hill, A., Volpe, J.J. (1989) *Fetal Neurology.* New York: Raven Press.

Hohlfeld, P., Daffos, F., Thulliez, P., *et al.* (1989) 'Fetal toxoplasmosis: outcome of pregnancy and infant follow-up after in utero treatment.' *Journal of Pediatrics*, **115**, 765–769.

—— Costa, J-M., *et al.* (1994) 'Prenatal diagnosis of congenital toxo-plasmosis with a polymerase-chain-reaction test on amniotic fluid.' *New England Journal of Medicine*, **331**, 695–699.

Holmes, G.L., Flannery, D.B. (1988) 'The effect of maternal seizures and anticonvulsants on fetal brain development.' *International Pediatrics*, **3**, 86–94.

Holzman, C., Paneth, N., Little, R., *et al.* (1995) 'Perinatal brain injury in premature infants born to mothers using alcohol in pregnancy.' *Pediatrics*, **95**, 66–73.

Hori, A., Fischer, G. (1982) 'Intrauterine purulent leptomeningitis.' *Acta Neuropathologica*, **58**, 78–80.

Hoyme, H.E., Jones, K.L., Dixon, S.D., *et al.* (1990) 'Prenatal cocaine exposure and fetal vascular disruption.' *Pediatrics*, **85**, 743 747.

Hreidarsson, S., Kristjansson, K., Johannesson, G., Johannesson, J.H. (1988) 'A syndrome of progressive pancytopenia with microcephaly, cerebellar hypoplasia and growth failure.' *Acta Paediatrica Scandinavica*, **77**, 773–775.

Hughes, H.E., Miskin, M. (1986) 'Congenital microcephaly due to vascular disruption: in utero documentation.' *Pediatrics*, **78**, 85–87.

Hughes, P., Weinberger, E., Shan, D.W.W. (1991) 'Linear areas of echogenicity in the thalami and basal ganglia of neonates: an expanded association.' *Radiology*, **179**, 103–105.

Hutto, C., Arvin, A., Jacobs, R., *et al.* (1987) 'Intrauterine herpes simplex virus infections.' *Journal of Pediatrics*, **110**, 97–101.

Iida, K., Takashima, S., Takeuchi, Y. (1992) 'Etiologies and distribution of neonatal leukomalacia.' *Pediatric Neurology*, **8**, 205–209.

Illume, N., Reske-Nielsen, E., Skovby, F., *et al.* (1988) 'Lethal autosomal recessive arthrogryposis multiplex congenita with whistling face and calcifications of the nervous system.' *Neuropediatrics*, **19**, 186–192.

Ioffe, S., Chernick, V. (1988) 'Development of the EEG between 30 and 40 weeks gestation in normal and alcohol-exposed infants.' *Developmental Medicine and Child Neurology*, **30**, 797–807.

Jacobson, J.L., Jacobson, S.W. (1996) 'Intellectual impairment in children exposed to polychlorinated biphenyls in utero.' *New England Journal of Medicine*, **335**, 783–789.

Jager-Roman, E., Deichl, A., Jakob, S., *et al.* (1986) 'Fetal growth, major malformations and minor anomalies in infants born to women receiving sodium valproate.' *Journal of Pediatrics*, **108**, 997–1004.

Jeannel, D., Costagliola, D., Niel, G., *et al.* (1990) 'What is known about the prevention of congenital toxoplasmosis.' *Lancet*, **336**, 359–361.

Jensen, P.R., Hansen, F.J., Skovby, F. (1995) 'Cerebellar hypoplasia in children with the carbohydrate-deficient glycoprotein syndrome.' *Neuroradiology*, **37**, 328–330.

Jesurun, C.A., Levin, G.S., Sullivan, W.R., Stevens, D. (1980) 'Intracranial hemorrhage in utero re thrombocytopenia.' *Journal of Pediatrics*, **97**, 695–696. *(Letter.)*

Johnson, K.P., Johnson, R.T. (1972) 'Granular ependymitis. Occurrence in myxovirus infected rodents and prevalence in man.' *American Journal of Pathology*, **67**, 511–525.

Jung, J.H., Graham, J.M., Schultz, N., Smith, D.W. (1984) 'Congenital hydranencephaly/porencephaly due to vascular disruption in monozygotic twins.' *Pediatrics*, **73**, 467–469.

Kalousek, D.K., Howard-Peebles, N., Olson, S.B., *et al.* (1991) 'Confirmation of CVS mosaicism in term placentae and high frequency of intrauterine growth retardation association with confined placental mosaicism.' *Prenatal Diagnosis*, **11**, 743–750.

Kelly, T.E. (1984) 'Teratogenicity of anticonvulsant drugs. I: Review of the literature.' *American Journal of Medical Genetics*, **19**, 413–434.

Kim, M.S., Elyaderani, M.K. (1982) 'Sonographic diagnosis of cerebroventricular hemorrhage in utero.' *Radiology*, **142**, 479–480.

King, T.A., Perlman, J.M., Laptook, A.R., *et al.* (1995) 'Neurologic manifestations of in utero cocaine exposure in near-term and term infants.' *Pediatrics*, **96**, 259–264.

Koeda, T., Inagaki, M., Kawahara, H., *et al.* (1993) 'Progressive encephalopathy associated with cytomegalovirus infection without immune deficiency.' *Journal of Child Neurology*, **8**, 373–377.

Konkol, R.J. (1994) 'Is there a cocaine baby syndrome?' *Journal of Child Neurology*, **9**, 225–226.

Koren, G., Nulman, I. (1993) 'Antenatal visualization of malformations associated with drugs and chemicals.' *Developmental Brain Dysfunction*, **6**, 305–316.

Korkman, M., Hilakivi-Clarke, L.A., Autti-Rämö, I., *et al.* (1994) 'Cognitive impairments at two years of age after prenatal alcohol exposure or perinatal asphyxia.' *Neuropediatrics*, **25**, 101–105.

Krägeloh-Mann, I., Petersen, D., Hagberg, G., *et al.* (1995) 'Bilateral spastic cerebral palsy. MRI, pathology and origin. Analysis from a representative series of 56 cases.' *Developmental Medicine and Child Neurology*, **37**, 379–397.

Kramer, M.S., Olivier, M., McLean, F.H., *et al.* (1990) 'Impact of intrauterine growth retardation and body proportionality on fetal and neonatal outcome.' *Pediatrics*, **85**, 707–713.

Kulhanjian, J.A., Soroush, V., Au, D.S., *et al.* (1992) 'Identification of women at unsuspected risk of primary infection with herpes simplex virus type 2 during pregnancy.' *New England Journal of Medicine*, **326**, 916–920.

Laegreid, L., Kyllerman, M., Hedner, T., *et al.* (1993) 'Benzodiazepine amplification of valproate teratogenic effects in children of mothers with absence epilepsy.' *Neuropediatrics*, **24**, 88–92.

Lahat, E., Aladjem, M., Schiffer, J., Starinsky, R. (1993) 'Hydrocephalus due to bilateral obstruction of the foramen of Monro: A "possible" late complication of mumps encephalitis.' *Clinical Neurology and Neurosurgery*, **95**, 151–154.

Lammer, E.J., Chen, D.T., Hoar, R.M., *et al.* (1985) 'Retinoic acid embryopathy.' *New England Journal of Medicine*, **313**, 837–840.

Landesman, S.H., Kalish, L.A., Burns, D.N., *et al.* (1996) 'Obstetrical factors and the transmission of human immunodeficiency virus type 1 from mother to child.' *New England Journal of Medicine*, **334**, 1617–1623.

Laneri, G.G., Claassen, D.L., Scher, M.S. (1994) 'Brain lesions of fetal onset in encephalopathic infants with nonimmune hydrops fetalis.' *Pediatric Neurology*, **11**, 18–22.

Largo, R.H., Pfister, D., Molinari, L., *et al.* (1989) 'Significance of prenatal, perinatal and postnatal factors in the development of AGA preterm infants at five to seven years.' *Developmental Medicine and Child Neurology*, **31**, 440–456.

Larroche, J-C. (1986) 'Fetal encephalopathies of circulatory origin.' *Biology of the Neonate*, **50**, 61–74.

—— Droullée, P., Delezoide, A.L., *et al.* (1990) 'Brain damage in monozygous twins.' *Biology of the Neonate*, **57**, 261–278.

Larsen, P.D., Chartrand, S.A., Tomashek, K.M., *et al.* (1993) 'Hydrocephalus complicating lymphocytic choriomeningitis virus infection.' *Pediatric Infectious Disease Journal*, **12**, 528–531.

Lefebvre, F., Bard, H., Veilleux, A., Martel, C. (1988) 'Outcome at school age of children with birthweights of 1000 grams or less.' *Developmental Medicine and Child Neurology*, **30**, 170–180.

Lemoine, P., Harousseau, H., Borteyru, J. (1968) 'Les enfants de parents alcooliques: anomalies observées.' *Ouest Médicale*, **25**, 476 482.

Levene, M.l., Kornberg, J., Williams, T.H.C. (1985) 'The incidence and severity of postasphyxial encephalopathy in full-term infants.' *Early Human Development*, **11**, 21–26.

Leveno, K.J., Cunningham, F.G., Nelson, S., *et al.* (1986) 'A prospective comparison of selective and universal electronic fetal monitoring in 34,995 pregnancies.' *New England Journal of Medicine*, **315**, 615–619.

Levi, S. (1976) 'Ultrasonic assessment of the high rate of human multiple pregnancy in the first trimester.' *Journal of Clinical Ultrasound*, **4**, 3–5.

Lewis, M., Bendersky, M. (1989) 'Cognitive and motor differences among low birth weight infants: impact of intraventricular hemorrhage, medical risk, and social class.' *Pediatrics*, **83**, 187–192.

Libman, M.D., Dascal, A., Kramer, M.S., Mendelson, J. (1991) 'Strategies for the prevention of neonatal infection with herpes simplex virus: a decision analysis.' *Reviews of Infectious Diseases*, **13**, 1093–1104.

Lindhout, D., Schmidt, D. (1986) 'In-utero exposure to valproate and neural tube defects.' *Lancet*, **1**, 1392–1393. *(Letter.)*

—— Meinardi, H., Meijer, J.N., Nau, H. (1992) 'Antiepileptic drugs and teratogenesis in two consecutive cohorts: changes in prescription policy paralleled by changes in pattern of malformations.' *Neurology*, **42**, Suppl. 5, 94–110.

Lloyd, B.W., Wheldall, K., Perks, D. (1988) 'Controlled study of intelligence and school performance of very low-birthweight children from a defined geographical area.' *Developmental Medicine and Child Neurology*, **30**, 36–42.

Lou, H.C., Hansen, D., Nordentoft, M., *et al.* (1994) 'Prenatal stressors of human life affect fetal brain development.' *Developmental Medicine and Child Neurology*, **36**, 826–832.

Low, J.A. (1989) 'Fetal acid-base status and outcome.' *In:* Hill, A., Volpe, J.J. (Eds.) *Fetal Neurology.* New York: Raven Press, pp. 195–217.

Lowichik, A., Siegel, J.D. (1995) 'Parasitic infections of the central nervous system in children. Part I: Congenital infections and meningoencephalitis.' *Journal of Child Neurology*, **10**, 4–17.

Luthy, D.A., Shy, K.K., Van Belle, G. (1987) 'A randomized trial of electronic fetal monitoring in preterm labor.' *Obstetrics and Gynecology*, **69**, 687–695.

Lyen, K.R., Lingam, S., Butterfill, A.M., *et al.* (1981) 'Multicystic encephalomalacia due to fetal viral encephalitis.' *European Journal of Pediatrics*, **137**, 11–16.

Lyon, G., Robain, O. (1967) 'Encéphalopathies circulatoires prénatales et paranatales.' *Acta Neuropathologica*, **9**, 79–98.

—— Arita, F., Le Galloudec, E., *et al.* (1990) 'A disorder of axonal development, necrotizing myopathy, cardiomyopathy, and cataracts: a new familial disease.' *Annals of Neurology*, **27**, 193–199.

Lyons Jones, K., Lacro, R.V., Johnson, K.A., Adams, J. (1989) 'Pattern of malformations in the children of women treated with carbamazepine during pregnancy.' *New England Journal of Medicine*, **320**, 1661–1666.

Macquart-Moulin, G., Julian, F., Chapel, S., Aymé, S. (1989) 'Sensibilité de l'échographie obstétricale dans le diagnostic anténatal des anomalies foetales majeures.' *Revue d'Epidémiologie et de Santé Publique*, **37**, 197–205.

Majewski, F. (1993) 'Alcohol embryopathy: experience in 200 patients.' *Developmental Brain Dysfunction*, **6**, 248–265.

Maller, A., Butler, I.J., Yeakley, J., Hankins, L. (1995) 'Rolandic cerebral palsy as a pattern of hypoxic–ischemic injury in full-term neonates.' *Paper presented at the 24th Meeting of the Child Neurology Society, Baltimore, October 26–28, 1995. (Abstract No. 201.)*

Manson, J., Speed, I., Abbott, K., Crompton, J. (1988) 'Congenital blindness, porencephaly and neonatal thrombocytopenia: a report of four cases.' *Journal of Child Neurology*, **3**, 120–124.

Marcus, J.C. (1982) 'Congenital neurosyphilis: a reappraisal.' *Neuropediatrics*, **13**, 195–199.

Marcus, J.C. (1987) 'Neurological findings in the fetal alcohol syndrome.' *Neuropediatrics*, **18**, 158 160.

Marques-Dias, M.J., Harmant-Van Rijckevorsel, G., Landrieu, P., Lyon, G. (1984) 'Prenatal cytomegalovirus disease and cerebral microgyria: evidence for perfusion failure, not disturbance of histogenesis, as the major cause of fetal cytomegalovirus encephalopathy.' *Neuropediatrics*, **15**, 18–24.

Marret, S., Gressens, P., Gadisseux, J-F., Evrard, P. (1995) 'Prevention by magnesium of excitotoxic neuronal death in the developing brain: an animal model for clinical intervention studies.' *Developmental Medicine and Child Neurology*, **37**, 473–484.

Marsh, D.O., Myers, G.J., Clarkson, T.W., *et al.* (1980) 'Fetal methylmercury poisoning: clinical and toxicological data on 29 cases.' *Annals of Neurology*, **7**, 348–353.

Martin, J.J., Ceuterick, C.M., Leroy, J.A., *et al.* (1984) 'The Wiedemann–Rautenstrauch or neonatal progeroid syndrome. Neuropathological study of a case.' *Neuropediatrics*, **15**, 43–48.

Mayes, L.C., Bornstein, M.H., Chawarska, K., Granger, R.H. (1995) 'Information processing and developmental assessments in 3-month-old infants exposed prenatally to cocaine.' *Pediatrics*, **95**, 539–545.

McCarthy, M. (1996) 'Timing of fetal membrane rupture predicts HIV risk.' *Lancet*, **347**, 1821.

Michie, C.A., Acolet, D., Charlton, R., *et al.* (1992) 'Varicella-zoster contracted in the second trimester of pregnancy.' *Pediatric Infectious Disease Journal*, **11**, 1050–1053.

Miller, E., Hare, J.W., Cloherty, J.P., *et al.* (1981) 'Elevated maternal hemoglobin A1c in early pregnancy and major congenital anomalies in infants of diabetic mothers.' *New England Journal of Medicine*, **304**, 1331–1334.

—— Cradock-Watson, J.E., Pollock, T.M. (1982) 'Consequences of confirmed maternal rubella at successive stages of pregnancy.' *Lancet*, **2**, 781–784.

Mito, T., Ando, Y., Takeshita, K., *et al.* (1989) 'Ultrasonographical and morphological examination of subependymal cystic lesions in maturely born infants.' *Neuropediatrics*, **20**, 211–214.

Mohide, P., Enkin, M. (1992) 'Are antenatal tests for fetal well-being worthwhile?' *In:* Chard, T., Richards, M.P.M. (Eds.) *Obstetrics in the 1990s: Current Controversies. Clinics in Developmental Medicine No. 123/124.* London: Mac Keith Press, pp. 132–142.

Mukherjee, A.B., Hodgen, G.D. (1982) 'Maternal ethanol exposure induces transient impairment of umbilical circulation and fetal hypoxia in monkeys.' *Science*, **218**, 700–702.

Mulder, E.J.H. (1993) 'Diabetes in pregnancy as a model for testing behavioural teratogenicity in man.' *Developmental Brain Dysfunction*, **6**, 210–228.

Müller, F., Moskophidis, M., Prange, M.W. (1984) 'Demonstration of locally synthesized immunoglobulin M antibodies to *Treponema pallidum* in the central nervous system of patients with untreated neurosyphilis.' *Journal of Neuroimmunology*, **7**, 43–54.

Murphy, D.J., Sellers, S., MacKenzie, I.Z., *et al.* (1995) 'Case–control study of antenatal and intrapartum risk factors for cerebral palsy in very preterm singleton babies.' *Lancet*, **346**, 1449–1454.

—— Squier, M.V., Hope, P.L., *et al.* (1996) 'Clinical associations and time of onset of cerebral white matter damage in very preterm babies.' *Archives of Disease in Childhood*, **75**, F27–F32.

Myers, R.E. (1972) 'Two patterns of brain damage and their conditions of occurrence.' *American Journal of Obstetrics and Gynecology*, **112**, 246–276.

Naeye, R.L., Peters, E.C. (1987) 'Antenatal hypoxia and low IQ values.' *American Journal of Diseases of Children*, **141**, 50–54.

Naidich, T.P., Chakera, T.M.H. (1984) 'Multicystic encephalomalacia: CT appearance and pathological correlation.' *Journal of Computer Assisted Tomography*, **8**, 631–636.

Naidu, S., Messmore, H., Caserta, V. (1983) 'CNS lesions in neonatal iso-immune thrombocytopenia.' *Archives of Neurology*, **40**, 552–554.

Nakahara, T., Sakoda, K., Uozumi, T., *et al.* (1989) 'Intrauterine depressed skull fracture. A report of two cases.' *Pediatric Neuroscience*, **15**, 121–124.

Neimann, W., Vidailhet, M., Martin, J.J., *et al.* (1973) 'Fragilité osseuse, amyotrophie, arriération et lésions dégénératives du système nerveux central.' *Archives Françaises de Pédiatrie*, **30**, 899–913.

Nelson, K.B., Ellenberg, J.H. (1981) 'Apgar scores as predictors of chronic neurologic disability.' *Pediatrics*, **68**, 36–44.

—— —— (1986) 'Antecedents of cerebral palsy. Multivariate analysis of risks.' *New England Journal of Medicine*, **315**, 81–86.

—— Grether, J.K. (1995) 'Can magnesium sulfate reduce the risk of cerebral palsy in very low birthweight infants?' *Pediatrics*, **95**, 263–269.

—— Dambrosia, J.M., Ting, T.Y., Grether, J.K. (1996) 'Uncertain value of electronic fetal monitoring in predicting cerebral palsy.' *New England Journal of Medicine*, **334**, 613–618.

Nigro, G., Clerico, A., Mondaini, C. (1993) 'Symptomatic congenital cytomegalovirus infection in two consecutive sisters.' *Archives of Disease in Childhood*, **69**, 527–528.

—— Scholz, H., Bartmann, U. (1994) 'Ganciclovir therapy for symptomatic congenital cytomegalovirus infection in infants: a two-regimen experience.' *Journal of Pediatrics*, **124**, 318–322.

Norman, M.G., McGillivray, B. (1988) 'Fetal neuropathology of proliferative vasculopathy and hydranencephaly–hydrocephaly with multiple limb pterygia.' *Pediatric Neuroscience*, **14**, 301–306.

Norman, R.M., Urich, H., Woods, G.E. (1958) 'The relationship between prenatal porencephaly and the encephalomalacias of early life.' *Journal of Mental Science*, **104**, 758–771.

Norton, M.E., Merrill, J., Cooper, B.A., *et al.* (1993) 'Neonatal complications after the administration of indomethacin for preterm labor.' *New England Journal of Medicine*, **329**, 1602–1607.

Oguni, M., Dansky, L., Andermann, E., *et al.* (1992) 'Improved pregnancy outcome in epileptic women in the last decade: relationship to maternal anticonvulsant therapy.' *Brain and Development*, **14**, 371–380.

Olds, D.L., Henderson, C.R., Tatelbaum, R. (1994) 'Intellectual impairment in children of women who smoke cigarettes during pregnancy.' *Pediatrics*, **93**, 221–227.

Ong, B.Y., Ellison, P.H., Browning, C. (1983) 'Intrauterine stroke in the neonate.' *Archives of Neurology*, **40**, 55–56.

Oro, A.S., Dixon, S.D. (1987) 'Perinatal cocaine and methamphetamine exposure: maternal and neonatal correlates.' *Journal of Pediatrics*, **111**, 571–578.

Papiernik, E., Bonyer, J., Dreyfus, J., *et al.* (1985) 'Prevention of preterm births: a perinatal study in Hagenau, France.' *Pediatrics*, **76**, 154–158.

Paryani, S.G., Arvin, A.M. (1986) 'Intrauterine infection with varicella-zoster virus after maternal varicella.' *New England Journal of Medicine*, **314**, 1542–1546.

Pass, R.F. (1992) 'Commentary: Is there a role for prenatal diagnosis of congenital cytomegalovirus infection?' *Pediatric Infectious Disease Journal*, **11**, 608–609.

Passarge, E., Lenz, W. (1966) 'Syndrome of caudal regression in infants of diabetic mothers: observations of further cases.' *Pediatrics*, **37**, 672–675.

Pastuszak, A.L., Levy, M., Schick, B., *et al.* (1994) 'Outcome after maternal varicella infection in the first 20 weeks of pregnancy.' *New England Journal of Medicine*, **330**, 901–905.

Pauli, R.M., Hann, J.M. (1993) 'Intrauterine effects of coumarin derivatives.' *Developmental Brain Dysfunction*, **6**, 229–247.

Pavone, L., Fiumara, A., Barone, R., *et al.* (1996) 'Olivopontocerebellar atrophy leading to recognition of carbohydrate-deficient glycoprotein syndrome type I.' *Journal of Neurology*, **243**, 700–705.

Pearl, K.N., Preece, P.M., Ades, A., Peckham, C.S. (1986) 'Neurodevelopmental assessment after congenital cytomegalovirus infection.' *Archives of Disease in Childhood*, **61**, 323–326.

Pearlman, M.D., Tintinalli, J.E., Lorenz, R.P. (1990) 'Blunt trauma during pregnancy.' *New England Journal of Medicine*, **323**, 1609–1613.

Pearson, M.A., Hoyme, H.E., Seaver, L.H., Rimsza, M.E. (1994) 'Toluene embryopathy: delineation of the phenotype and comparison with fetal alcohol syndrome.' *Pediatrics*, **93**, 211–215.

Peckham, C., Gibb, D. (1995) 'Mother-to-child transmission of the human immunodeficiency virus.' *New England Journal of Medicine*, **333**, 298–302.

—— Logan, G.S. (1988) 'Cytomegalovirus infection in pregnancy.' *In:* Cosmi, E.V., Di Renzo, G.C. (Eds.) *Proceedings of the XIth European Congress of Perinatal Medicine,* pp. 255–260.

Peckham, N.H., Choi, B.H. (1988) 'Abnormal neuronal distribution within the cerebral cortex after prenatal methylmercury intoxication.' *Acta Neuropathologica,* **76,** 222–226.

Pedersen, J.F., Mølsted-Pedersen, L. (1981) 'Early fetal growth delay detected by ultrasound marks increased risk of congenital malformation in diabetic pregnancy.' *British Medical Journal,* **283,** 269–271.

Perlman, J.M., Argyle, C. (1992) 'Lethal cytomegalovirus infection in preterm infants: clinical, radiological, and neuropathological findings.' *Annals of Neurology,* **31,** 64–68.

Pfister-Goedeke, L., Boltshauser, E. (1982) 'Postnatale Entwicklung einer multilokulären zystichen Enzophalopathie beim Neugeborenen. Ultraschall-Verlaufskontrolle multipler Hirninfarkte.' *Helvetica Paediatrica Acta,* **37,** 59–65.

Phelan, J.P., Smith, C.V. (1989) 'Antepartum fetal assessment: the contraction stress test.' *In:* Hill, A., Volpe, J.J. (Eds.) *Fetal Neurology.* New York: Raven Press, pp. 75–89.

Philipps, C.A., Maeck, J.vanS., Rogers, W.A., Savel, H. (1970) 'Intrauterine rubella infection following immunization with rubella vaccine.' *Journal of the American Medical Association,* **213,** 624–625.

Piekkala, P., Kero, P., Sillanpaa, M., Erkkola, R. (1988) 'The developmental profile and outcome of 325 unselected preterm infants up to two years of age.' *Neuropediatrics,* **19,** 33–40.

Portnoy, S., Callias, M., Wolke, D., Gamsu, H. (1988) 'Five-year follow-up study of extremely low-birthweight infants.' *Developmental Medicine and Child Neurology,* **30,** 590–598.

Prechtl, H.F.R. (1989) 'Fetal behavior.' *In:* Hill, A., Volpe, J.J. (Eds.) *Fetal Neurology.* New York: Raven Press, pp. 1–16.

Prober, C.G., Gershon, A.A., Grose, C., *et al.* (1990) 'Consensus: Varicella-zoster infections in pregnancy and the perinatal period.' *Pediatric Infectious Disease Journal,* **9,** 865–869.

Rademaker, K.J., de Vries, L.S., Barth, P.G. (1993) 'Subependymal pseudocysts: ultrasound diagnosis and findings at follow-up.' *Acta Paediatrica Scandinavica,* **82,** 394–399.

Randel, R.C., Kearns, D.B., Nespeca, M.P., *et al.* (1996) 'Vocal cord paralysis as a presentation of intrauterine infection with varicella-zoster virus.' *Pediatrics,* **97,** 127–128.

Rawstron, S.A., Jenkins, S., Blanchard, S., *et al.* (1993) 'Maternal and congenital syphilis in Brooklyn, NY. Epidemiology, transmission and diagnosis.' *American Journal of Diseases of Children,* **147,** 727–731.

Rayburn, W.F. (1989) 'Antepartum fetal monitoring: fetal movements.' *In:* Hill, A., Volpe, J.J. (Eds.) *Fetal Neurology.* New York: Raven Press, pp. 17–36.

Reardon, W., Hockey, A., Silberstein, P., *et al.* (1994) 'Autosomal recessive congenital intrauterine infection-like syndrome of microcephaly, intracranial calcifications and CNS disease.' *American Journal of Medical Genetics,* **52,** 58–65.

Remington, J.S., Desmonts, G. (1990) 'Toxoplasmosis.' *In:* Remington, J.S., Klein, D. (Eds.) *Infectious Disease of the Fetus and Newborn Infant, 3rd Edn.* Philadelphia: W.B. Saunders, pp. 89–195.

Riikonen, R., Donner, M. (1980) 'ACTH therapy in infantile spasms: side-effects.' *Archives of Disease in Childhood,* **55,** 664–672.

Robb, J.A., Benirschke, K., Barmeyer, R. (1986) 'Intrauterine latent herpes simplex virus infection. 1. Spontaneous abortion.' *Human Pathology,* **17,** 1196–1209.

Robinson, B.H., MacKay, N., Chun, K., Ling, M. (1996) 'Disorders of pyruvate carboxylase and the pyruvate dehydrogenase complex.' *Journal of Inherited Metabolic Diseases,* **19,** 452–462.

Robinson, R.O., Trounce, J.Q., Janota, I., Cox, T. (1993) 'Late fetal pontine destruction.' *Pediatric Neurology,* **9,** 213–215.

Roizen, N., Swisher, C.N., Stein, M.A., *et al.* (1995) 'Neurologic and developmental outcome in treated congenital toxoplasmosis.' *Pediatrics,* **95,** 11–20.

Ronen, G.M., Andrews, W.L. (1991) 'Holoprosencephaly as a possible embryonic alcohol effect.' *American Journal of Medical Genetics,* **40,** 151–154.

Rorke, L.B. (1973) 'Nervous system lesions in the congenital rubella syndrome.' *Archives of Otolaryngology,* **98,** 249–251.

Rupar, C.A., Gillett, J., Gordon, B.A., *et al.* (1996) 'Isolated sufite oxidase deficiency.' *Neuropediatrics,* **27,** 299–304.

Saari-Kemppainen, A., Karjalainen, O., Ylöstalo, P., Heinonen, O.P. (1990) 'Ultrasound screening and perinatal mortality: controlled trial of systematic one-stage screening in pregnancy. The Helsinki Ultrasound Trial.' *Lancet,* **336,** 387–391.

Salonen, R., Somer, M., Haltia, M., *et al.* (1991) 'Progressive encephalopathy with edema, hypsarrhythmia, and optic atrophy (PEHO syndrome).' *Clinical Genetics,* **39,** 287–293.

Samsom, J.F., Barth, P.G., de Vries, J.I.P., *et al.* (1994) 'Familial mitochondrial encephalopathy with fetal ultrasonographic ventriculomegaly and intracerebral calcifications.' *European Journal of Pediatrics,* **153,** 510–516.

Sánchez, P.J., Wendel, G.D., Grimprel, E., *et al.* (1993) 'Evaluation of molecular methodologies and rabbit infectivity testing for the diagnosis of congenital syphilis and neonatal central nervous system invasion by *Treponema pallidum.*' *Journal of Infectious Disease,* **167,** 148–157.

Scafidi, F.A., Field, T.M., Wheeden, A., *et al.* (1996) 'Cocaine-exposed preterm neonates show behavioral and hormonal differences.' *Pediatrics,* **97,** 851–855.

Scher, M.S. (1994) 'Neonatal encephalopathies as classified by EEG–sleep criteria: severity and timing based on clinical/pathologic correlations.' *Pediatric Neurology,* **11,** 189–200.

—— Belfar, H., Martin, J., Painter, M.J. (1991) 'Destructive brain lesions of presumed fetal onset: antepartum causes of cerebral palsy.' *Pediatrics,* **88,** 898–905.

Schifrin, B.S. (1989) 'The diagnosis and treatment of fetal distress.' *In:* Hill, A., Volpe, J.J. (Eds.) *Fetal Neurology.* New York: Raven Press, pp. 143–189.

Schlesinger, P.A., Duray, P.H., Burke, B.A., *et al.* (1985) 'Maternal–fetal transmission of the Lyme disease spirochete, *Borrelia burgdorferi.*' *Annals of Internal Medicine,* **103,** 67–69.

Schmitt, H.P. (1984) 'Multicystic encephalopathy. A polyetiologic condition in early infancy: morphologic, pathogenetic and clinical aspects.' *Brain and Development,* **6,** 1–9.

Sever, J.L., Ellenberg, J.H., Ley, A.C., *et al.* (1988) 'Toxoplasmosis: maternal and pediatric findings in 23,000 pregnancies.' *Pediatrics,* **82,** 181–192.

Shaul, W.L., Emery, H., Hall, J.G. (1975) 'Chondrodysplasia punctata and maternal warfarin use during pregnancy.' *American Journal of Diseases of Children,* **129,** 360–362.

Shaw, C.H., Alvord, E.C. (1974) 'Subependymal germinolysis.' *Archives of Neurology,* **31,** 374–381.

Shaywitz, S.E., Cohen, D.J., Shaywitz, B.A. (1980) 'Behavior and learning difficulties in children of normal intelligence born to alcoholic mothers.' *Journal of Pediatrics,* **96,** 978–982.

Singer, L.T., Yamashita, T.S., Hawkins, S., *et al.* (1994) 'Increased incidence of intraventricular hemorrhage and developmental delay in cocaine-exposed, very low birth weight infants.' *Journal of Pediatrics,* **124,** 765–771.

Sinha, S.K., D'Souza, S.W., Rivlin, E., Chiswick, M.L. (1990) 'Ischaemic brain lesions diagnosed at birth in preterm infants: clinical events and developmental outcome.' *Archives of Disease in Childhood,* **65,** 1017–1020.

Smith, C.V., Phelan, J.P. (1989) 'Antepartum fetal assessment: the nonstress test.' *In:* Hill, A., Volpe, J.J. (Eds.) *Fetal Neurology.* New York: Raven Press, pp. 61–74.

Smith, J.B., Groover, R.V., Klass, D.W., Hooser, O.W. (1977) 'Multicystic cerebral degeneration in neonatal herpes simplex virus encephalitis.' *American Journal of Diseases of Children,* **131,** 568–572.

Soothill, P.W., Nicolaides, K.H., Campbell, S. (1987) 'Prenatal asphyxia, hyperlacticacidaemia, hypoglycaemia and erythroblastosis in growth retarded foetuses.' *British Medical Journal,* **294,** 1051–1053.

Souza, I.E., Bale, J.F. (1995) 'The diagnosis of congenital infections: contemporary strategies.' *Journal of Child Neurology,* **10,** 271–282.

Squier, M., Keeling, J.W. (1991) 'The incidence of prenatal brain injury.' *Neuropathology and Applied Neurobiology,* **17,** 29–38.

Stagno, S. (1990) 'Cytomegalovirus.' *In:* Remington, J.S., Klein, O.J. (Eds.) *Infectious Disease of the Fetus and Newborn Infant, 3rd Edn.* Philadelphia: W.B. Saunders, pp. 241–281.

—— Whitley, R.J. (1985a) 'Herpesvirus infections of pregnancy. Part I: Cytomegalovirus and Epstein–Barr virus infections.' *New England Journal of Medicine,* **313,** 1270–1274.

—— —— (1985b) 'Herpesvirus infections of pregnancy. Part II: Herpes simplex virus and varicella-zoster virus infections.' *New England Journal of Medicine,* **313,** 1327–1330.

Stanley, O.H., Fleming, P.J., Morgan, M.H. (1989) 'Abnormal development of visual function following intrauterine growth retardation.' *Early Human Development,* **19,** 87–101.

Stannard, M.W., Jimenez, J.F. (1983) 'Sonographic recognition of multiple cystic encephalomalacia.' *American Journal of Radiology,* **141,** 1321–1324.

Steinlin, M.I., Nadal, D., Eich, G.F., *et al.* (1996) 'Late intrauterine cytomegalovirus infection: clinical and neuroimaging findings.' *Pediatric Neurology*, **15**, 249–253.

Stewart, A., Pezzani-Goldsmith, M. (1994) 'Long-term outcome of extremely low birth weight infants.' *In:* Amiel-Tison, C., Stewart, A. (Eds.) *The Newborn Infant: One Brain for Life.* Paris: Editions INSERM, pp. 151–166.

—— Hope, P.L., Hamilton, P., *et al.* (1988) 'Prediction in very preterm infants of satisfactory neurodevelopmental progress at 12 months.' *Developmental Medicine and Child Neurology*, **30**, 53–63.

Stoll, C., Dott, B., Roth, M.P., Alembik, Y. (1988) 'Aspects étiologiques et épidemiologiques des anomalies du tube neural.' *Archives Françaises de Pédiatrie*, **45**, 617–622.

Strömland, K., Hellström, A. (1996) 'Fetal alcohol syndrome—an ophthalmological and socioeducational prospective study.' *Pediatrics*, **97**, 845–850.

Szymonowicz, W., Preston, H., Yu, V.Y.H. (1986) 'The surviving monoamniotic twin.' *Archives of Disease in Childhood*, **61**, 454–458.

Takada, K., Shiota, M., Ando, M., *et al.* (1989) 'Porencephaly and hydranencephaly: a neuropathologic study of four autopsy cases.' *Brain and Development*, **11**, 51–56.

Takeuchi, T., Watanabe, K. (1989) 'The EEG evolution and neurological prognosis of neonates with perinatal hypoxia.' *Brain and Development*, **11**, 115–120 + *erratum*, 203.

Tardieu, M., Grospierre, B., Durandy, A., Griscelli, C. (1980) 'Circulating immune complexes containing rubella antigens in late-onset rubella syndrome.' *Journal of Pediatrics*, **97**, 370–373.

Tenovuo, A., Kero, P., Korvenranta, H., *et al.* (1988) 'Developmental outcome of 519 small-for-gestational age children at the age of two years.' *Neuropediatrics*, **19**, 41–45.

Tohyama, J., Kawahara, H., Inagaki, M., *et al.* (1992) 'Clinical and neuroradiologic findings of congenital hydrocephalus in infant born to mother with HTLV-1-associated myelopathy.' *Neurology*, **42**, 1406–1408.

Townsend, J.J., Baringer, J.R., Wolinsky, J.S., *et al.* (1975) 'Progressive rubella panencephalitis. Late onset after congenital rubella.' *New England Journal of Medicine*, **292**, 990–993.

Trudinger, B.J., Giles, W.B., Cook, C.M., *et al.* (1985) 'Fetal umbilical artery flow velocity waveforms and placental resistance: clinical significance.' *British Journal of Obstetrics and Gynaecology*, **92**, 23–30.

Truwit, C.L., Barkovich, A.J., Koch, T.K., Ferriero, D.M. (1992) 'Cerebral palsy: MR findings in 40 patients.' *American Journal of Neuroradiology*, **13**, 67–78.

Van de Bor, M., Walther, F.J., Sims, M.E. (1990) 'Increased cerebral blood flow velocity in infants of mothers who abuse cocaine.' *Pediatrics*, **85**, 733–736.

Veelken, N., Stollhof, K., Claussen, M. (1992) 'Development and perinatal risk factors of very low-birth-weight infants. Small versus appropriate for gestational age.' *Neuropediatrics*, **23**, 102–107.

Vestermark, V. (1993) 'Teratogenicity of carbamazepine: a review of the literature.' *Developmental Brain Dysfunction*, **6**, 266–278.

Visser, G.H.A. (1992) 'Abnormal antepartum fetal heart rate patterns and subsequent handicap.' *In:* Fukuyama, Y., Suzuki, Y., Kamoshita, S., Casaer, P. (Eds.) *Fetal and Perinatal Neurology.* Basel: Karger, pp. 216–222.

Vohr, B.R., Garcia-Coll, C.T. (1985) 'Neurodevelopmental and school performance of very low birthweight infants: a seven year longitudinal study.' *Pediatrics*, **76**, 345–350.

Volpe, J.J. (1992) 'Effect of cocaine use on the fetus.' *New England Journal of Medicine*, **327**, 399–407.

—— (1995) *Neurology of the Newborn, 3rd Edn.* Philadelphia: W.B. Saunders.

Ward, T.F. (1977) 'Multiple thromboses in an infant of a diabetic mother.' *Journal of Pediatrics*, **90**, 982–984.

Watanabe, K. (1992) 'The neonatal electroencephalogram and sleep cycle patterns.' *In:* Eyre, J.A. (Ed.) *The Neurophysiological Examination of the Newborn Infant. Clinics in Developmental Medicine No. 120.* London: Mac Keith Press, pp. 11–47.

Weber, K., Bratzke, H.J., Neubert, U., *et al.* (1988) '*Borrelia burgdorferi* in a newborn despite oral penicillin for Lyme borreliosis during pregnancy.' *Pediatric Infectious Disease Journal*, **7**, 286–289.

Weig, S.G., Marshall, P.C., Abroms, I.F., Gauthier, N.S. (1995) 'Patterns of cerebral injury and clinical presentation in the vascular disruptive syndrome of monozygotic twins.' *Pediatric Neurology*, **13**, 279–285.

Weil, M.L., Levin, M. (1995) 'Infections of the nervous system.' *In:* Menkes, J. (Ed.) *Textbook of Child Neurology, 5th Edn.*, pp. 379–509.

Weindling, M., Russell, G. (1992) 'Prenatal pathophysiology of brain damage. *In:* Fukuyama, Y., Suzuki, Y., Kamoshita, S., Casaer, P. (Eds.) *Fetal and Perinatal Neurology.* Basel: Karger, pp. 223–231.

Weisglas-Kuperus, N., Baerts, W., Smrkovsky, M., Sauer, P.J.J. (1993) 'Effects of biological and social factors on the cognitive development of very low birth weight children.' *Pediatrics*, **92**, 658–665.

Whittle, M.J. (1991) 'Routine fetal anomaly screening.' *In:* Drife, J.O., Donnai, D. (Eds.) *Antenatal Diagnosis of Fetal Abnormalities.* Berlin: Springer, pp. 35–43.

Williams, C.L., Benach, J.L., Curran, A.S., *et al.* (1988) 'Lyme disease during pregnancy: a cord blood serosurvey.' *Annals of the New York Academy of Sciences*, **539**, 504–506.

Williams, M.L., Lewandowski, L.J., Coplan, J., D'Eugenio, D.B. (1987) 'Neurodevelopmental outcome of preschool children born preterm with and without intracranial hemorrhage.' *Developmental Medicine and Child Neurology*, **29**, 243–249.

Williams, R.S., Caviness, V.S. (1984) 'Normal and abnormal development of the brain.' *In:* Tarter, R E., Goldstein, J. (Eds.) *Advances in Clinical Neuropsychology, Vol. 2.* New York: Plenum, pp. 1–62.

Williamson, W.D., Desmond, M.M., LaFevers, N., *et al.* (1982) 'Symptomatic congenital cytomegalovirus. Disorders of language, learning, and hearing.' *American Journal of Diseases of Children*, **136**, 902–905.

Winchester, B. (1990) 'Prenatal diagnosis of enzyme defects.' *Archives of Disease in Childhood*, **65**, 59–67.

Wisniewski, K., Dambska, M., Sher, J.H., Qazi, Q. (1983) 'A clinical neuropathological study of the fetal alcohol syndrome.' *Neuropediatrics*, **14**, 197–201.

Wladimiroff, J.W., Tonge, H.M., Stewart, P.A. (1986) 'Doppler ultrasound assessment of cerebral blood flow in the human fetus.' *British Journal of Obstetrics and Gynecology*, **93**, 471–475.

Wright, R., Johnson, D., Neumann, M., *et al.* (1997) 'Congenital lymphocytic choriomeningitis virus syndrome: a disease that mimics congenital toxoplasmosis or cytomegalovirus infection.' *Pediatrics electronic pages:* http://www.pediatrics.org/cgi/content/full/100/1/e9. (Abstract e9 in *Pediatrics*, **100**, 126–127.)

Yerbi, M.S. (1988) 'Teratogenicity of antiepileptic drugs.' *In:* Pedley, T.A., Meldrum, B.S. (Eds.) *Recent Advances in Epilepsy, Vol. 4.* Edinburgh: Churchill Livingstone, pp. 93–107.

Yoshioka, H., Kadamoto, Y., Mino, M. (1979) 'Multicystic encephalomalacia in liveborn twin with a stillborn macerated co-twin.' *Journal of Pediatrics*, **95**, 798–800.

Zorzi, C., Angonese, I., Nardelli, G.B., Cantarutti, F. (1988) 'Spontaneous intraventricular haemorrhage in utero.' *European Journal of Pediatrics*, **148**, 83–85.

Zubrick, S.R., Macartney, H., Stanley, F.J. (1988) 'Hidden handicap in school-age children who receive neonatal intensive care.' *Developmental Medicine and Child Neurology*, **30**, 145–152.

2
NEUROLOGICAL DISEASES IN THE PERINATAL PERIOD

This chapter deals with the period that extends from the onset of labour—covering abnormal intrapartum events—to the end of the neonatal period, conventionally limited to below 28 postnatal days. A majority of the neurological problems of that period arise during the first 10 days of life; a few late complications are possible and will be considered if their relationship to circumstances of birth or of the first few days is a direct one. Intracranial haemorrhages and hypoxic–ischaemic (or postasphyxial) encephalopathy dominate the neurology of the perinatal period, though it must be emphasized that they do not account for all the neurological problems of this period and that their predominance should not lead one to miss other important diagnoses such as metabolic or neuromuscular diseases.

Separation of perinatal from prenatal disorders is largely arbitrary. Indeed, prenatal factors such as intrauterine growth retardation, prenatal hypoxia of whatever origin, and preterm birth play a considerable role in the determination of many perinatal disorders, as the previous status of the brain and of the whole organism is a major factor of the response of the central nervous system (CNS) to the stress of birth and adaptation to extrauterine life. Likewise, prenatal factors profoundly influence the clinical presentation and prognosis of perinatal diseases.

The two major pathological conditions encountered in the perinatal period—haemorrhage and postasphyxial encephalopathy—are not totally separate entities. They often coexist and they share some common causes or precipitating factors. In particular, hypoxia and ischaemia can produce either or both conditions. However, other mechanisms such as mechanical trauma or coagulopathies can provoke haemorrhage without hypoxia, and the pathology and mechanisms are sufficiently different to warrant separate description.

INTRACRANIAL HAEMORRHAGE IN THE NEONATAL PERIOD

The epidemiology of intracranial haemorrhage has changed considerably over the past three decades. The incidence of traumatic haemorrhage, mainly subdural in location, has substantially decreased as a result of progress in obstetric practices. At the same time, the relative frequency of intraventricular haemorrhage has increased because it is mainly a disorder of preterm infants

and many more such babies survive than was the case previously. Furthermore, modern imaging techniques have made it possible to make an *in vivo* diagnosis of intraventricular and subarachnoid haemorrhage with a much greater precision than was previously possible. Indeed, many such haemorrhages would remain undetected without the use of such techniques.

There are two main groups of neonatal intracranial haemorrhage. Subdural haemorrhage is mainly of traumatic origin and occurs in term babies often of high birthweight (Welch and Strand 1986). Intraparenchymal haemorrhage is also occasionally traumatic in origin and occurs in the same category of infants (Pierre-Kahn *et al.* 1986). Intraventricular haemorrhage, on the other hand, is at least in part related to asphyxia and predominates in preterm babies (Volpe 1995). Other types of bleeding such as subarachnoid haemorrhage may have a dual mechanism and are often associated with intraventricular haemorrhage. Intraparenchymal haemorrhage may also occur spontaneously, especially thalamic haemorrhage. Subpial bleeding is often localized and is probably not associated with significant clinical abnormalities (Leviton *et al.* 1988).

INTRACRANIAL HAEMORRHAGE OTHER THAN INTRAVENTRICULAR HAEMORRHAGE
SUBDURAL HAEMORRHAGE
Subdural haemorrhage may result from tentorial tear with rupture of the straight sinus or the vein of Galen, or smaller afferent veins; from occipital osteodiastasis with damage to the occipital sinus or cerebellar veins; from tear of the falx with involvement of the inferior sagittal sinus; or from injury to the bridging veins between the convexity of the hemispheres and the superior sagittal sinus or between the tranverse or sigmoid sinus and the base of the brain (Govaert 1993, Volpe 1995). In the first two situations, bleeding is in the posterior fossa, whereas in the other cases it is supratentorial, located to the convexity in the case of injury to the bridging veins, to the hemispheral fissure in falx laceration, and at the base of the brain with rupture of the veins draining into the lateral sinus.

Rupture is caused by excessive head moulding in vertex presentation or to excessive traction on the aftercoming head in breech presentation (Pape and Wigglesworth 1979). Localized trauma with fracture by forceps application is rare (Pierre-Kahn *et al.* 1986). Tentorial haemorrhage can also occur as a consequence of vacuum extraction (Hanigan *et al.* 1990, Govaert 1993).

The *clinical features* are variable depending on the location and acuteness of the haemorrhagic process. In acute cases of *posterior fossa haemorrhage*, there is massive bleeding with compression of vital brainstem structures, manifested by stupor or coma, nuchal rigidity, opisthotonus, eye deviations, bradycardia and respiratory pauses. Seizures occur in 36 per cent of cases (Govaert 1993). A tense fontanelle, generalized hypotonia or hypertonia, skew eye deviation, facial palsy and unequal pupils may be observed. Of 90 cases reviewed by Govaert (1993), a fatal outcome occurred in 15 unoperated and three operated cases. Sequelae including hydrocephalus are not rare. In subacute cases, the onset of neurological symptoms is delayed for 12 hours or more. Irritability, stupor, a bulging fontanelle and respiratory irregularities may suggest the diagnosis (Menezes *et al.* 1983, Fenichel *et al.* 1984) Diagnosis by ultrasound scanning is possible; CT and especially MRI better define the size and exact location of the haematoma (Menezes *et al.* 1983, Govaert 1993). Surgical treatment is effective but adhesions may appear leading to the development of hydrocephalus, requiring insertion of a shunt.

Supratentorial haematoma of the convexity does not usually produce an immediately dramatic clinical picture. In typical cases, focal seizures or hemiparesis or both occur on the second or third day of life (Deonna and Oberson 1974). The occurrence of a IIIrd nerve palsy manifested by a dilated, nonreactive pupil on the side of the haematoma is characteristic. Minor subdural bleeding over the convexity may give only minimal clinical signs.

In cases of subdural haemorrhage, the CSF is usually bloody. Easy visualization of blood by neuroimaging techniques has made lumbar puncture unnecessary for the diagnosis of intracerebral haemorrhage. Rare cases of chronic infantile subdural haematoma are said to result from birth trauma (Govaert 1993).

Basal subdural haemorrhage due to lateral tentorial injury results in collection of blood underneath the temporal and/or occipital lobes. Govaert (1993) reviewed 21 cases confirmed by CT which presented in a similar way as convexity haematomas. Such cases are apt to be associated with arterial stroke due to compression of the middle cerebral artery (Govaert *et al.* 1992b). Similar cases have been seen involving the posterior cerebral artery (Deonna and Prod'hom 1980).

INTRACEREBELLAR HAEMORRHAGE

Intracerebellar haemorrhage has many features in common with posterior fossa subdural haematoma. Its mechanism is different, as it seems to be related to hypoxia and ischaemia rather than to mechanical trauma, although it may be caused by occipital osteodiastasis or traumatic cerebellar injury (Welch and Strand 1986, De Campo 1989). It is often associated with intraventricular haemorrhage. It is frequent in series of autopsied low birthweight preterm infants (Fig. 2.1), much less so in CT series (Volpe 1995) possibly because small haemorrhages may be difficult to diagnose by CT or ultrasound. It may originate as dissection from ventricular haemorrhage into the fourth ventricle

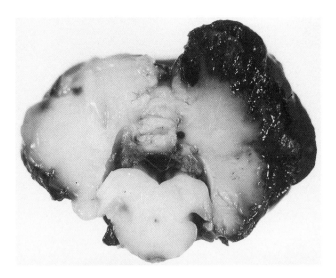

Fig. 2.1. Cerebellar haemorrage in infant born at 29 weeks gestational age, weighing 1500 g. Death at age 5 days. (Courtesy Dr J-C. Larroche, Maternité Port Royal, Paris.)

or from the subarachnoid space into the cerebellar parenchyma, or represent primary intracerebellar haematoma or haemorrhagic cerebellar infarction (Takashima and Becker 1989). Although a possible role of bands used for fixation of face masks in preterm infants has been suggested, this appears unlikely as the incidence was found to be similar when masks were not applied (Paneth *et al.* 1994). Onset usually occurs after the second day of life, and the neurological manifestations are generally overshadowed by symptoms and signs of hypoxia or respiratory distress. Apnoea, bradycardia and a falling haematocrit are frequent features. Ultrasonography or CT scan are diagnostic. Hydrocephalus is frequent, even following surgical evacuation of the collection, and may be associated with the development of a cerebellar cyst communicating with the fourth ventricle (Huang and Shen 1991). Clinically patent cerebellar deficit may be seen as a sequela (Williamson *et al.* 1985). Successful conservative management has been reported: with present day neuroimaging facilities it may become the most common form of treatment for those haematomas that do not provoke progressive hydrocephalus as judged by repeated sonographic examination (Fishman *et al.* 1981). Cerebellar haemorrhage has been seen as a complication of extracorporeal membrane oxygenation (Bulas *et al.* 1991) and in some infants with organic acidurias (Fischer *et al.* 1981, Dave *et al.* 1984).

INTRAPARENCHYMAL HAEMORRHAGE

Intraparenchymal haemorrhage is virtually always associated with subarachnoid haemorrhage. In most cases it involves a single lobe and may result from trauma or haemorrhagic infarction. In five cases studied by Pierre-Kahn *et al.* (1986) the haematoma communicated with the subdural space and the clot was surrounded by marked to massive cerebral oedema. Breech delivery and, in general, mechanically difficult delivery in term infants was a major causal factor, even though clotting defects or increased blood viscosity (Miller *et al.* 1981) may play an auxiliary role.

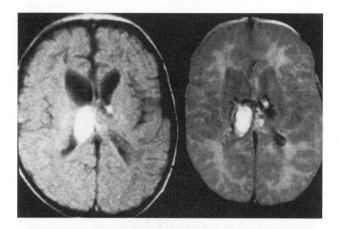

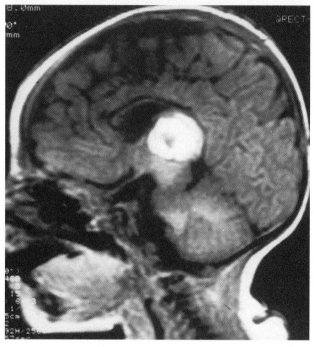

Fig. 2.2. Thalamic haemorrhage in 7-day-old infant. *(Top)* MRI, axial cut *(left:* T₁-weighted spin-echo sequence; *right:* T₂-weighted sequence). *(Bottom)* MRI, left paramedian sagittal cut.

bleeding can be thalamoventricular, in association with an asymmetrical ventricular haemorrhage (Roland *et al.* 1990, de Vries *et al.* 1992, Govaert *et al.* 1992a, Govaert 1993), or limited to the thalamus and neighbouring structures. The blood is visible by CT in the thalamus and occasionally also in the caudate nucleus on one side. In the few patients so far reported, the condition was manifested by seizures, occurring between 2 and 14 days of age in term infants, following a normal delivery. Eye signs could include vertical upward gaze palsy, deviation of the eyes toward the lesion, ipsilateral saccadic paresis and a flat visual evoked response, and they have been attributed to damage to the fronto-mesencephalic optic pathway (Trounce *et al.* 1985). Diagnosis is easily confirmed by ultrasonography, CT or MRI. No post-mortem examination has been reported, and the cause of the condition is obscure. The course was favourable in the few patients so far reported with only supportive treatment, although a less favourable outcome with severe sequelae was recently reported by Campistol *et al.* (1994). This relatively benign syndrome should be distinguished from acute *haemorrhagic necrosis of the thalamus and basal ganglia* (Kreusser *et al.* 1984, Voit *et al.* 1987), in which evidence of perinatal asphyxia is present, the haemorrhagic lesions are bilateral and symmetrical, and the prognosis is very poor.

Similar haemorrhages complicated by intraventricular irruption of blood may be a major cause of intraventricular haemorrhage in term infants (Roland *et al.* 1990) and may be associated with deep venous thrombosis.

Brainstem haemorrhage is rarely of traumatic origin. At least one case of spontaneous brainstem haemorrhage, with diaphragmatic paralysis and lower cranial nerve involvement, is on record (Blazer *et al.* 1989).

PRIMARY SUBARACHNOID HAEMORRHAGE
This heading refers to haemorrhage within the subarachnoid space that is not the result of extension from intraventricular, subdural or intraparenchymal haemorrhage and is not due to a structural vascular lesion. This is a common occurrence, as bloody or xanthochromic CSF containing several hundred red cells per mm³ is frequently found by lumbar puncture in newborn, especially term, infants. Significant subarachnoid haemorrhage, however, is much less frequent. Escobedo *et al.* (1975) found that only 29 per cent of infants <2000g at birth who had a bloody CSF at lumbar puncture had subarachnoid haemorrhage detectable by CT scan. Subarachnoid haemorrhage can be of either traumatic or asphyxic cause. These were found respectively in 16 and 17 of 48 cases reported by Govaert (1993), while 10 cases remained of undetermined origin.

Clinical manifestations are not uncommonly lacking. In other cases, seizures, usually focal in type, occur typically on the second day of life in otherwise well babies (Volpe 1995). These seizures, sometimes replaced by apnoeic attacks, have a favourable outcome. I have observed several newborn infants who developed a marked polymorphonuclear pleocytosis, with hypoglycorrhachia and clinical signs of meningeal irritation but a benign outcome, following subarachnoid bleeding. In such cases the

Hanigan *et al.* (1995) recently described four cases of lobar haemorrhage in term infants, two of them due to isoimmune thrombocytopenia. The symptomatology resembles that of subdural haematoma (Fenichel *et al.* 1984, Govaert 1993), with a symptom-free period of more than 24 hours, followed by focal signs and symptoms of high intracranial pressure. Variable focal signs depend on the lobe involved and may include convulsions, hemiparesis and ocular signs.

Surgical evacuation is indicated when symptoms of increased pressure are threatening. A residual cavity in the brain may cause no symptoms or may be associated with focal deficit (Chaplin *et al.* 1979, Pasternak *et al.* 1980). A similar syndrome may be due to haemorrhagic brain infarction.

Thalamic haemorrhage (Fig. 2.2) is a rare form of neonatal intraparenchymal haemorrhage (Fenichel *et al.* 1984, Primhak and Smith 1985, Trounce *et al.* 1985, Adams *et al.* 1988b). The diagnosis of purulent meningitis is often considered but the fluid is sterile and the course is of rapid resolution. Uncontrasted CT scan is now the cornerstone of diagnosis (Govaert *et al.* 1990), showing blood density images in the posterior interhemispheric fissure and in the region of the vein of Galen and on the tentorium. Ultrasound may also demonstrate the presence of blood in the basal cisterns (Paneth *et al.* 1994) but may be difficult to interpret.

The outcome is usually favourable, although some infants may develop posthaemorrhagic hydrocephalus (see Chapter 7). Except in that circumstance, no treatment beyond that of seizures is required.

Haemorrhagic disease of the newborn is a factor in at least some of the intracranial haemorrhages of term newborn infants. Prophylaxis by administration of vitamin K is effective (Matsuzaka *et al.* 1987) and should, therefore, be systematically performed.

Other coagulation disorders may be responsible for severe intracranial haemorrhage in the neonatal period. Haemophilia can produce subdural intraparenchymal or intraventricular haemorrhage (Kletzel *et al.* 1989). Thrombycotopenia has been reviewed in Chapter 1.

EPIDURAL HAEMATOMA AND RARE TYPES OF NEONATAL INTRACRANIAL HAEMORRHAGE.
Epidural haematoma is a rare condition in newborn infants (Gama and Fenichel 1985, Negishi *et al.* 1989) and is usually caused by mechanical trauma. Choux *et al.* (1975) reviewed 17 cases found in a series of 104 infants with epidural bleeding. Cephalhaematoma is commonly associated and communicates with the extradural blood collection through a skull fracture. Signs of progressive CNS dysfunction are usually delayed and may be absent altogether. Ultrasonography or CT shows the collection, which should be evacuated surgically. The collection tends to liquefy rapidly leading to a differential density within it (Aoki 1990). However, conservative treatment is possible in asymptomatic infants or in those with only mild difficulties (Pozzati and Tognetti 1986).

Other rare causes of haemorrhage in the newborn infant include venous thrombosis, vascular malformations, especially aneurysm of the vein of Galen (Chapter 15), and congenital tumours.

PERIVENTRICULAR–INTRAVENTRICULAR HAEMORRHAGE (PIVH)

PIVH is the most frequent type of intracranial haemorrhage in the neonate. It is overwhelmingly a disease of preterm infants although it does also occur, uncommonly, in term babies (Guekos-Thoeni *et al.* 1982, Lacey and Terplan 1982). The incidence is particularly high in very small preterm infants. Approximately 40 per cent of infants weighing < 1500 g studied in the 1970s had PIVH (Papile *et al.* 1978), but current incidence seems lower, of the order of about 15–20 per cent (Goddard-Finegold and Mizrahi 1987, Philip *et al.* 1989, Paneth *et al.* 1993). Perlman and Volpe (1986) found PIVH in 60 per cent of infants < 1000 g, as against 20 per cent in larger babies.

TABLE 2.1
Severity of periventricular–intraventricular haemorrhage

Severity	Staging of Papile et al. (1978)	Staging of Volpe (1995)
Grade I	Subependymal bleeding only	*Idem*, or < 10 per cent of ventricular area filled with blood
Grade II	< 50 per cent of ventricular area filled with blood. No ventricular dilatation	10–50 per cent of ventricular area filled with blood
Grade III	> 50 per cent of ventricular area filled with blood. Blood in the white matter of centrum semi-ovale	> 50 per cent of ventricular area filled with blood

The majority of cases of PIVH in preterm infants originate in the subependymal germinal matrix, the highly cellular area that gives rise to neurons and glia during gestation and involutes before term. In infants of less than 28 weeks gestational age, haemorrhage often is located to that part of the matrix overlying the body of the caudate nucleus, while in those over 28 weeks it more commonly overlies the head of the caudate. Haemorrhages are initially subependymal and are then clinically silent, although ventricular dilatation may occur (Fishman *et al.* 1984) with minor haemorrhage. Intraventricular haemorrhage results when the ependyma ruptures. Various staging systems have been devised (Papile *et al.* 1978, Volpe 1995) (Table 2.1). The presence of parenchymal blood (grade IV) probably does not correspond to extension of ventricular bleeding but to haemorrhagic infarction associated with PIVH (Guzzetta *et al.* 1986; Volpe 1989a,b). Such lesions are unilateral in two thirds of cases and are regularly located or predominate on the side of the larger PIVH. They probably represent infarction of venous origin (Gould *et al.* 1987) and may be due to impairment of venous circulation by compression resulting from the presence of a ventricular clot. They are different from haemorrhagic leukomalacia, which is usually bilateral and symmetrical and probably of ischaemic origin. Other commonly associated lesions (Skullerud and Westre 1986) include periventricular leukomalacia, which has been found in up to 75 per cent of infants who died with PIVH (Armstrong *et al.* 1987) and may be haemorrhagic or bland; and pontine neuronal necrosis that is encountered in up to 46 per cent of cases and is associated, in 20 per cent, with neuronal necrosis of the subiculum (*pontosubicular necrosis*). This constellation of lesions can be responsible for a large proportion of the neurological sequelae of PIVH.

Sequelae of PIVH include *hydrocephalus* that is due to posthaemorrhagic adhesive arachnoiditis. It occurs following irruption of blood through the aqueduct and the foramina of the fourth ventricle into the basal cisterns or as a result of granulous ependymitis at the level of the aqueduct. At the acute stage, the blood clot can obstruct the aqueduct or foramina.

When the haemorrhage remains limited to the subependymal area (grade I), periventricular cysts may develop but are probably of little clinical consequence. However, destruction of neuron and glial cell precursors may have deleterious consequences on subsequent brain development.

The pathogenesis of PIVH remains uncertain. Vascular rupture takes place in the capillaries of the richly vascularized germinal matrix (Pape and Wigglesworth 1979), which, in preterm infants, are tenuous and weak. A number of factors, especially obstetrical ones, may favour and precipitate the occurrence of haemorrhage (Shaver et al. 1992).

The capillary network at that age is involuting, and its vascular support may be deficient as the matrix is devoid of supporting mesenchymal elements. Moreover, an excessive amount of fibrinolytic activity has been found in the area and may facilitate bleeding.

Haemodynamic factors are probably essential. Critically ill preterm infants lack autoregulation of brain vessels, so that systemic changes in arterial pressure are passively transmitted to the cerebral vessels (Wimberley et al. 1982, Lou 1988). Cerebral blood flow varies directly with changes in arterial pressure (Van Bel et al. 1987, Miall-Allen et al. 1989, Bada et al. 1990), and an increase in systemic pressure can probably produce rupture of capillaries. This is especially likely to occur if a period of hypotension and ischaemia, with injury of the germinal matrix vessels, has preceded the peaks of hypertension. In experiments on newborn beagle puppies (Goddard-Finegold and Mizrahi 1987), hypotension followed by hypertension produced germinal matrix haemorrhage. Perlman et al. (1983) and Miall-Allen et al. (1989) have emphasized the importance of fluctuating cerebral blood flow, as estimated from the velocity of flux in the pericallosal branch of the anterior cerebral artery. A stable pattern with equal peaks and troughs in velocity of systolic and diastolic blood flow, in the first day of life, was not associated with PIVH, while an unstable pattern identified at-risk infants. This result, however, was not found in the study by Kuban et al. (1988). Blood flow velocity is highly sensitive to pulmonary mechanics. Pneumothorax, a frequent complication of artificial ventilation, is associated with both a dramatic increase in blood flow velocity —which returns to normal with resolution of the pneumothorax—and PIVH (Hill et al. 1982b, Kuban and Volpe 1993).

Increases in blood pressure which have been shown to occur in preterm infants during crying, feeding or suctioning (Lou and Friis-Hansen 1979) may conceivably precipitate bleeding, and the limit for the highest tolerable peak systolic blood pressure is lower for the low birthweight infant than for infants of normal birthweight.

Asphyxia, i.e. hypoxia with hypercapnia, is an important aetiological factor. It aggravates the circulatory disorders by increasing blood flow and disturbs autoregulation. It is also responsible for arterial hypertension and probably increases venous pressure (Perlman and Volpe 1987). Such an increase is facilitated by the anatomical disposition of the deep cerebral veins with reversal in the direction of flow between thalamostriate and internal cerebral veins.

Other possible factors in the aetiology of PIVH include coagulation abnormalities (Amato et al. 1988), agents such as benzylalcohol (Jardine and Rogers 1989), heparin used for flushing catheters (Lesko et al. 1986), and volume expansion particularly with bicarbonate administration (Pagano et al. 1990).

The multiplicity of causal factors (Leviton et al. 1988) and the important role of hypoxia account for the fact that PIVH is rarely an isolated lesion, as the same factors can also cause other anatomical damage (Takashima et al. 1989).

CLINICAL MANIFESTATIONS

PIVH occurs most commonly during the first 72 postnatal hours in preterm infants of less than 32 weeks gestational age, most of whom have suffered some degree of perinatal asphyxia or are mechanically ventilated or both (McDonald et al. 1984, Funato et al. 1992). Rare cases may occur prenatally (Govaert and de Vries 1997), and some investigators have proposed that PIVH could be the cause of some of the periventricular white matter lesions and ventricular dilatation found in children with hemiplegic cerebral palsy, even when born at term. Late onset, up to 8–10 days of age, is possible but rare.

Very small preterm infants (< 1000 g) tend to bleed earlier than larger ones. Perlman and Volpe (1986) found that the onset in such infants was at 10 ± 8 hours, as opposed to the second or third day in larger infants.

Two main clinical syndromes are observed. The classical acute presentation, with abrupt deterioration, periods of apnoea, abnormal ocular movements, opisthotonic attacks, bulging fontanelle, acidosis and a falling haematocrit, is easy to recognize. Many neonates present with a less dramatic syndrome, marked by decreased alertness, stupor or irritability, irregularities of respiratory rhythm and hypo- or hypertonia, with a fluctuating and protracted course that may extend over several days. Around 25 per cent of patients with PIVH remain asymptomatic (Papile et al. 1978). Some of these may insidiously develop hydrocephalus (Chapter 7).

The symptoms and signs of PIVH may be so subtle and nonspecific that diagnosis will rest mainly on ultrasound imaging, which is systematically indicated in all small preterm babies in intensive care units. Ultrasound diagnosis is accurate in 92 per cent of cases of ventricular bleeding and in 85 per cent of cases of subependymal haemorrhage (Szymonowicz et al. 1984). False positives are rare but may occur with vascular congestion.

CT scan is as effective as ultrasonography but more cumbersome and cannot be repeated, whereas ultrasound imaging (Fig. 2.3) is ideal for follow-up studies. The characteristic course of haemorrhage, from visible clots of variable size to progressive central then total resorption, has been described in detail (Levene et al. 1983, Pape et al. 1983, Trounce et al. 1986).

Other techniques are much less effective. Lumbar puncture is often inaccurate and is no longer indicated. Electroencephalography is more useful in assessing the severity of CNS dysfunction and determining prognosis rather than diagnosis (Watanabe et al. 1983, Connell et al. 1988). Positive rolandic sharp waves have a good correlation with PIVH (Clancy and Tharp 1984) but correlate even better with white matter lesions such as leukomalacia and are thus nonspecific (Marret et al. 1986).

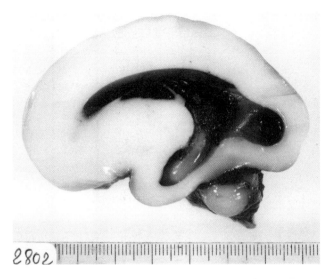

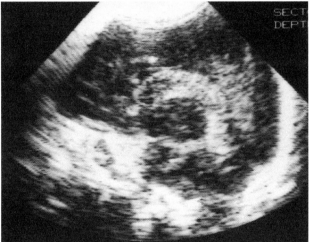

Fig. 2.3. Intraventricular haemorrhage in infant born at 27 weeks gestational age (birthweight 940 g; death at 36 hours after birth). *(Top)* Sagittal cut of brain demonstrates large clot occupying entire ventricular cavity. (Courtesy Dr J-C. Larroche, Maternité Port Royal, Paris.) *(Bottom)* Ultrasound scan shows hyperintense image representing blood clot in same location. (Courtesy Dr M. Monset-Couchard, Maternité Port Royal.)

COURSE AND SEQUELAE

Onset of PIVH is within five hours of birth in 40 per cent of infants (Paneth *et al.* 1993), and 90 per cent of cases can be detected by the fourth day of life (Volpe 1995). However, the haemorrhage may reach its maximal extent within only three to five days of diagnosis.

The course may be rapidly lethal especially when the haemorrhage is large or associated with large periventricular haemorrhagic infarction, when the mortality rate may be as high as 81 per cent (Volpe 1989b). Currently, the recovery rate is close to 70 per cent (Volpe 1995).

Hydrocephalus may appear immediately after the haemorrhage due to a large obstructing clot but more commonly develops progressively within one to three weeks of bleeding. Significant ventricular dilatation is not initially accompanied by an increase in head circumference, so ventricular dimensions

should be regularly followed by ultrasonography. The incidence of posthaemorrhagic hydrocephalus is less than 10 per cent after mild haemorrhage, 15–25 per cent after moderate haemorrhage, and 65–100 per cent after severe bleeding (Hill and Volpe 1981a). Of 87 infants with PIVH followed up by Hill and Volpe (1981b), 20 had rapidly progressive hydrocephalus with signs of increased intracranial pressure, 47 had no ventricular dilatation, and 20 had progressive hydrocephalus without evidence of increased intracranial pressure. In nine of these 20, hydrocephalus became arrested with or without resolution of ventriculomegaly. The remaining 11 had progressive dilatation following a stable period of two weeks to three months and ultimately required operation. Serial lumbar punctures may be useful as a temporary means of controlling hydrocephalus while waiting for the infant to reach a stable state but this does not avoid operation in progressive hydrocephalus (Ventriculomegaly Trial Group 1990, 1994). Some infants may require shunting because of secondary progression of hydrocephalus following a period of arrest (Perlman *et al.* 1990). Even with stable ventricular dilatation the prognosis is compromised. Shankaran *et al.* (1989) found neurodevelopmental sequelae in 19 of 33 infants with ventricular dilatation but in only three of 39 babies without ventriculomegaly.

Neurodevelopmental sequelae occur in 50–75 per cent of survivors of large haemorrhages (Papile *et al.* 1983). In contrast, the incidence of sequelae in infants with isolated germinal matrix bleeding is only 16 per cent (Catto-Smith *et al.* 1985). However, several studies (Weisglas-Kuperus *et al.* 1987, van de Bor *et al.* 1988, Fazzi *et al.* 1992, Vohr *et al.* 1992) have also shown that even infants with small PIVHs have a higher incidence of disability than those without. Krishnamoorthy *et al.* (1990) have confirmed in a large prospective study the association of PIVH with neurodevelopmental sequelae. They have stressed the importance of early ventriculomegaly as a predictor of motor sequelae. The extent to which neurodevelopmental sequelae are related to bleeding itself or to associated anomalies is uncertain. It has been shown that PIVH has significant metabolic consequences (Pranzatelli and Stumpf 1985) that may aggravate anatomical lesions. Periventricular leukomalacia probably plays an important role in the determination of *spastic diplegia* following intraventricular bleeding.

PREVENTION

The decreasing frequency of PIVH in most centres is difficult to attribute to any single factor. Because of the importance attributed to fluctuations of cerebral blood flow, increases in cerebral blood flow and venous pressure, and pressure-passive circulation, special attention has been given to events that affect systemic blood pressure during labour and delivery and during routine neonatal procedures such as suctioning in infants with respiratory distress.

Prevention strategies have focused on two types of measures. (1) Simple postnatal measures such as early intubation of infants with respiratory distress syndrome, avoidance of rapid volume infusions and minimal handling of infants are generally accepted (Volpe 1995). More complex measures aiming at controlling fluctuating blood flow velocity such as muscle paralysis with

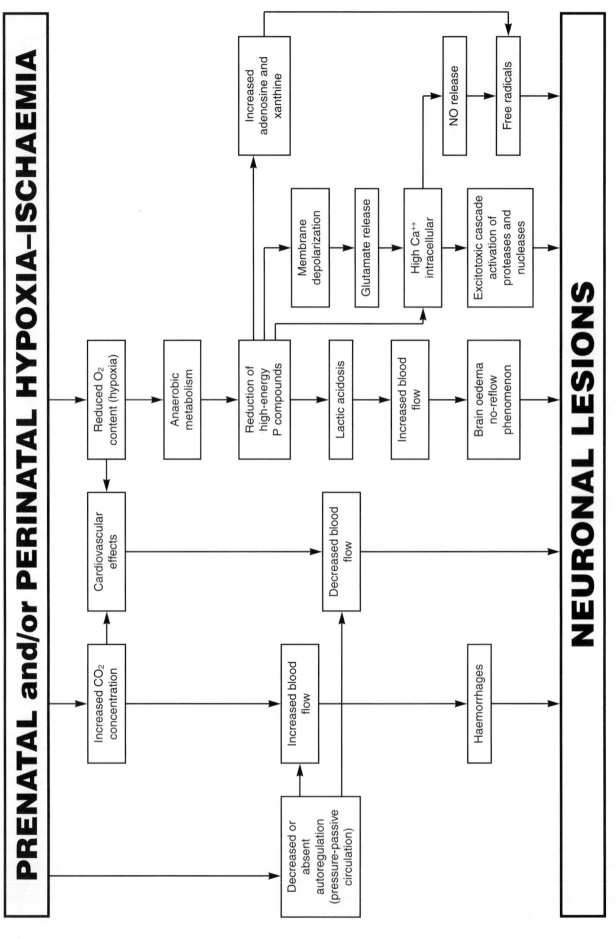

Fig. 2.4. Mechanisms of brain damage in hypoxic–ischaemic encephalopathy. Neuronal lesions are a consequence of various combinations of haemorrhage and necrosis. The latter is largely due to a cascade of events initiated by glutamate release that produces excessive calcium entry into the cells. Nitric oxide (NO) production seems also to be an important factor.

pancuronium in association with artificial ventilation have been shown to significantly reduce the incidence of PIVH (Perlman *et al.* 1985). Alterations in ventilatory methods with the use of systems automatically adjusting to the infants' efforts appear to be promising (Shaw *et al.* 1993). (2) Pharmacological interventions may be promising but the results of most techniques have yet to be confirmed. Vitamin E may have a protective effect, especially in very small infants, and may decrease the severity of PIVH (Fish *et al.* 1990). Phenobarbitone in doses sufficient to attain serum levels of 20-25 mg/L has been found effective by Donn *et al.* (1984) but not by others (Bedard *et al.* 1984, Kuban *et al.* 1986). Indomethacin has been found to reduce the incidence of PIVH, especially severe PIVH (Ment *et al.* 1994a,b). However, the effect is not entirely established (Volpe 1994), and the agent may lessen cerebral flow to a point that can conceivably produce hypoxia (Bandstra *et al.* 1988, Baerts *et al.* 1990). Ethamsylate may decrease the incidence of both mild and severe PIVH (Benson *et al.* 1986). The prophylactic administration of surfactant for prevention of the respiratory distress syndrome may reduce its incidence. However, the evidence is conflicting (Leviton *et al.* 1989), although neurological benefit has been observed (Amato *et al.* 1991) and the agent appears devoid of side-effects. Antenatal corticosteroids appear to reduce the risk of germinal matrix haemorrhage in small preterm infants (Leviton *et al.* 1993). A more complete assessment of such trials is necessary before the use of any form of drug prophylaxis can be recommended.

PIVH in Term Newborn Infants
PIVH in term babies is uncommon. There is some dispute about the site of origin (Pagano *et al.* 1990). Lacey and Terplan (1982) believe that bleeding originates in the choroid plexus of the lateral ventricle in most cases, whereas Guekos-Thoeni *et al.* (1982) think it is rare. In the experience of Roland *et al.* (1990), intraventricular haemorrhage in term neonates usually originates from a primary thalamic bleeding which may be of venous origin as indicated by the presence of predisposing factors for venous thrombosis (sepsis, cyanotic heart disease or coagulopathy).

The features and course of such secondary ventricular haemorrhage do not differ from those in primary cases but the incidence of subsequent cerebral palsy may be higher.

PIVH in term infants is often associated with cardiac or pulmonary disease. Symptoms and signs may be difficult to dissociate from those of accompanying hypoxia. Hydrocephalus and other complications are similar to those in preterm babies.

HYPOXIC–ISCHAEMIC ENCEPHALOPATHY (POSTASPHYXIAL ENCEPHALOPATHY)

Hypoxic–ischaemic encephalopathy (HIE) occurs in 1.5–6 per 1000 livebirths and is the single most important problem of neonatal neurology (Levene *et al.* 1985, Volpe 1995). This statement needs some qualification, as the incidence of HIE has probably decreased over the past two or three decades, and as the role of perinatal hypoxia in the causation of mental retardation and

cerebral palsy, which had been considerably overrated (Freeman and Nelson 1988, Bax and Nelson 1993), has been reassessed.

The definition of HIE is difficult and the role of birth asphyxia is difficult to define precisely, so the very term is being questioned; the noncommittal term of 'neonatal encephalopathy' has been proposed (Nelson and Leviton 1991, Leviton and Nelson 1992).The diagnosis of HIE should not be made without a serious historical and clinical basis, and alternative diagnoses should be carefully considered, especially because they may be important from the therapeutic and genetic points of view.

PATHOPHYSIOLOGY
The deficit in oxygen supply that produces HIE can result from two mechanisms: hypoxaemia, *i.e.* a reduced supply of oxygen in blood, and ischaemia, *i.e.* a reduced perfusion of the brain. In most cases, both are due to asphyxia, that is, hypoxia associated with hypercarbia (Altman *et al.* 1993) (Fig. 2.4). Acidosis, which is usually present with hypoxia, is largely related to increased production of lactate. Conversion of glucose to lactate is much less efficient than oxidation through the Krebs cycle and mitochondrial electron transport system. Oxidation of each molecule of glucose metabolized under anaerobic conditions generates only two molecules of adenosine diphosphate (ADP) as compared with 38 under aerobic conditions. Despite a considerable increase in the rate of glycolysis and an increase in cerebral blood flow due to acidosis and hypercapnia (Laptook *et al.* 1988), energy needs of the brain may not be satisfied. The increased rate of glycolysis results in a decline of brain glucose level. Prevention of this decline by prior administration of glucose increases adenosine triphosphate (ATP) production and improves survival (Vannucci and Yager 1992). However, abundant glucose also leads to increased lactate production which is deleterious in the adult brain though seemingly beneficial in the brain of the neonate (Hattori and Wasterlain 1990).

Ultimately, there is reduction of brain cell phosphocreatine and ATP as a consequence of the lack of oxygen, the final electron acceptor. This decrease has been demonstrated in human infants using phosphorus nuclear MRS (magnetic resonance spectroscopy) (Younkin *et al.* 1988, Laptook *et al.* 1989). The decrease in high energy phosphate compounds has been shown to occur even if cardiopulmonary function is stabilized (Hope *et al.* 1984). In experimental animals, ATP falls by more than 30 per cent in six minutes (Raichle 1983)

In fact, impairment of brain function precedes failure of energy metabolism (see Volpe 1995). When power failure appears imminent, the organism responds with a curtailment of neuronal activity through an undetermined mechanism, but this is not sufficient if hypoxia persists.

However, the neonatal brain is highly resistant to hypoxia. In experiments on monkey fetuses, reduction of oxygen saturation by 90 per cent, maintained for at least 25 minutes, is necessary to generate brain lesions. As a result, any episode of asphyxia severe enough to cause brain damage also produces disturbances in other organs, especially the heart, and ischaemia is constant under such circumstances.

Ischaemia has similar effects to asphyxia (Painter 1989). Glycolysis is increased but the uptake of glucose is prevented by impairment of the blood supply, hence the high-energy phosphates are depleted and lactate production rises.

The effects of hyperlactataemia are complex. It may be beneficial initially as it increases blood flow to the brain, but it becomes deleterious because it is, at least in part, responsible for brain oedema which, in turn, may compress the brain capillary bed and produce ischaemia (Myers 1972). At the same time, it impairs autoregulation of the cerebral blood flow resulting in a pressure-passive brain circulation (Lou 1988), thus rendering the brain more sensitive to changes in systemic blood pressure. The conjunction of brain oedema and systemic circulatory failure probably plays an essential role in the genesis of hypoxic brain damage. Hypoxia normally increases the proportion of cardiac output that is destined for the brain. With increasing hypoxia, there is diminished cardiac output with consequent inability to maintain blood pressure to sufficient levels. Mial-Allen *et al.* (1987) found a strong correlation between a mean systolic arterial pressure of less than 30 mmHg and the development of ischaemic brain lesions in the human newborn infant. However, heart rate and blood presure remain unchanged until arterial saturation is reduced by 65 per cent, then linearly decrease. This decline can be maintained for hours without the development of an encephalopathy if arterial oxygen concentration is not reduced by more than 85 per cent (Fenichel 1997).

The mechanism of brain oedema and hypoxic damage in hypoxic fetuses is unclear. Levene *et al.* (1989) found a good correlation between a high cerebral blood flow velocity—presumably reflecting cerebral hyperaemia that may, in turn, be responsible for increased intracranial pressure—and an unfavourable course. Lupton *et al.* (1988) have adduced evidence that oedema is a consequence, rather than a cause, of neuronal necrosis, thus accounting for the limited efficacy of anti-oedematous treatment of infants with HIE (Levene *et al.* 1987). The degree of intracranial hypertension was not found to be different in infants with HIE who survived and those who died (Goiten *et al.* 1983).

HIE is now known to consist of two successive stages, the second one, in which definitive brain damage occurs, being delayed for several hours. Prevention may therefore be possible. The mechanisms of cell damage and death with hypoxia or ischaemia are not simply the result of energy failure. This secondarily triggers a cascade of deleterious events when a critical level of energy deficit has been reached. Such events take place over several hours. Excessive membrane depolarization and the release of excitatory amino acid neurotransmitters, especially glutamate (Lipton and Rosenberg 1994), lead to calcium influx through NMDA and AMPA* membrane receptors (Morley *et al.* 1994) and to accumulation of cytosolic calcium. Calcium in turn activates various lipases, proteases and nucleases with resultant injury to essential cellular proteins. Free radicals are generated as

*NMDA = *N*-methyl-D-aspartate; AMPA = α-amino-3-hydroxy-5-methyl-4-isoxazole propionic acid.

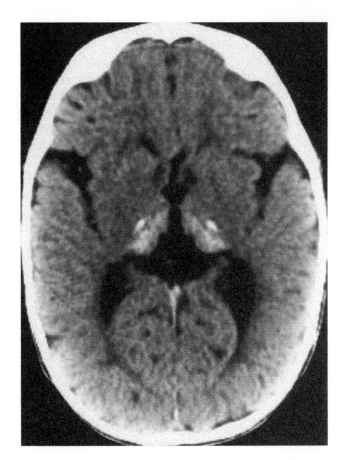

Fig. 2.5. Bilateral symmetrical calcification of the thalamus in a 3-month-old infant with history of pre- and perinatal hypoxia, quadriplegia and absence of neurodevelopmental progress.

a direct or indirect result of increased cytosolic calcium (McCord 1985), and nitric oxide (Dawson *et al.* 1992) plays a major role in their generation. This excitotoxic cascade ultimately results in membrane injury, cytoskeletal disruption and, finally, cell disintegration.

Many of these effects are theoretically preventable, and trials are being conducted with several agents including calcium channel blockers (Miller 1993, Palmer and Vannucci 1993); excitatory amino acid antagonists (Hattori *et al.* 1989), especially magnesium (Marret *et al.* 1995, Nelson and Grether 1995, Nelson 1996); inhibitors of nitric oxide synthesis (Dawson *et al.* 1992); free radical scavengers (Palmer and Vannucci 1993); and agents that inhibit free radical formation such as allopurinol (Palmer *et al.* 1990).

NEUROPATHOLOGY
Damage to the brain in experimental animals can follow two different patterns (Myers 1972). *Acute total asphyxia* rapidly leads to death because of circulatory collapse. Affected infant monkeys are stillborn or die in the perinatal period. Some may survive with evidence of brainstem and thalamic damage. Lesions similar to those in acutely asphyxiated monkeys or lambs occur in human fetuses and infants, often in association with other more diffuse damage. Such lesions are bilaterally symmetrical and are found

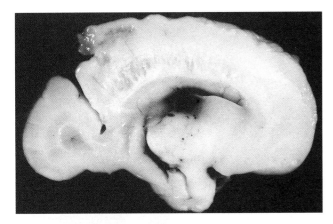

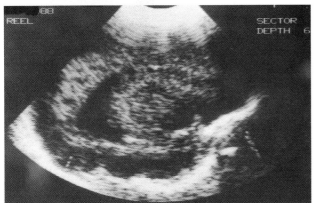

Fig. 2.6. Periventricular leukomalacia in infant born at 28 weeks gestational age (birthweight 945 g), who died age 2 weeks. *(Top)* Pathological specimen with multiple small cavities in periventricular location. (Courtesy Dr J-C. Larroche, Maternité Port Royal, Paris.) *(Bottom)* Ultrasound scan, sagittal cut: multiple cavities visible alongside ventricular cavity. (Courtesy Dr M. Monset-Couchard, Maternité Port Royal.)

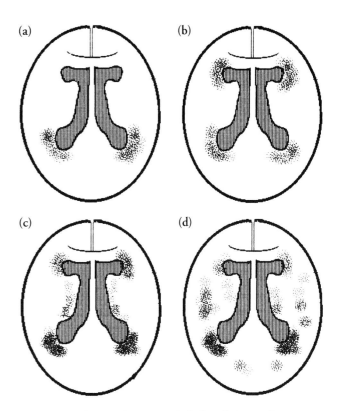

Fig. 2.7. Classification of periventricular leukomalacia according to extent of damage. *(a)* Grade 1: leukomalacia located alongside posterior horn of lateral ventricles. *(b)* Grade 2: located alongside both anterior and posterior horns of lateral ventricles. *(c)* Grade 3: extending entire length of lateral ventricles. *(d)* Grade 4: association with cavitary lesions of subcortical white matter.

particularly in the brainstem, the inferior colliculi, the superior olives, the lateral lemnisci and the nuclei of the lower cranial nerves (Leech and Brumback 1988, Natsume *et al.* 1995). Thalamic nuclei are also affected symmetrically, and the lesions may extend to involve the spinal cord (Schindler *et al.* 1975). Thalamic degeneration may be of prenatal or perinatal origin. Calcification is often seen at birth when degeneration is prenatal in origin, or develops within a few months in perinatal cases (Di Mario and Clancy 1989) (Fig. 2.5). This dorsal pattern of brainstem damage differs from the ventral pattern of pontine neuronal necrosis (Volpe 1995) which is often accompanied by neuronal necrosis in the subiculum of the hippocampus. The ventral pattern of *pontosubicular necrosis* (Friede 1989) is seen with chronic rather than acute asphyxia, and a possible role of hyperoxaemia in its causation has been suggested (Ahdab-Barmada *et al.* 1980).

Partial prolonged asphyxia is a more common cause of hypoxic-ischaemic damage. Brain lesions are then more diffuse, are associated with oedema, and affect mainly the cortex and basal ganglia.

The location of the most common lesions resulting from chronic ischaemia or hypoxia is highly dependent on gestational age (Hill 1991) and on multiple other factors such as the vascular response to injury, the local enzymatic equipment and its changes with maturation, which may explain in part the variable effects of disturbed energy metabolism in different areas of the CNS.

PERIVENTRICULAR LEUKOMALACIA
The most commonly occurring lesion of HIE in preterm infants is periventricular leukomalacia (Fig. 2.6). The term refers to bilateral, but not necessarily symmetrical, coagulation necrosis located adjacent to the external angle of the lateral ventricles. It may be limited to the region of the trigone and occipital horns, thus involving the optic radiations, or extend more anteriorly along the body and frontal ventricular horn (Fig. 2.7). Tissue destruction is followed by gliosis and may evolve into cavitated areas. Periventricular leukomalacia is haemorrhagic in about 25 per cent of cases (Hill *et al.* 1982a, Levene *et al.* 1983). The lesions, with or without cavitation, may extend into the white matter up to the arcuate fibres. They may rarely be extensive enough to produce a form of multicystic encephalomalacia (Dubowitz *et al.* 1985; Fawer *et al.* 1985, 1987; Cooke 1987; de Vries *et al.* 1987). Due to their location, they interrupt conduction in the fibres coming from the inner aspect and superior part of the hemisphere which are involved with the function of the lower limbs, and/or the optic radiations. This explains why they cause spastic diplegia and/or visual impairment. The latter is frequent with large cystic leukomalacias and can be predicted if

the infants do not fixate acuity cards at birth and at 3 months (Eken *et al.* 1996). Leukomalacia is often associated with PIVH (Trounce *et al.* 1986). It is not usually found in infants less than 6 days of age (Shuman and Selednik 1980) thus indicating the causal role of postnatal failure of cerebral perfusion (Calvert *et al.* 1987, Younkin *et al.* 1987). This is also supported by the occurrence of arterial hypotension in 21 per cent of affected infants (Perlman *et al.* 1996) and of leukomalacia in term infants with congenital cardiac disease (Glauser *et al.* 1990). Perfusion failure is thought to involve selectively the watershed areas between deep and superficial arterial supply (De Reuck *et al.* 1972), although this concept has been questioned (Kuban and Gilles 1985). Late-onset leukomalacia may occur in preterm infants with severe postnatal diseases such as necrotizing enterocolitis (de Vries *et al.* 1986, Perlman *et al.* 1996). Prolonged rupture of membranes and chorioamnionitis are also risk factors (Perlman *et al.* 1996). Although leukomalacia is regarded as being typical of preterm infants (Volpe 1995), recent studies suggest that similar lesions are not infrequently found in term infants with hemiplegia or diplegia (Niemann *et al.* 1994, Krägeloh-Mann *et al.* 1995). They are supposed to occur in the fetus at a similar gestational age to postnatal forms. Because of the vascular distribution of arterial supply and the high metabolic rate of the white matter at this period of development, hypoxic–ischaemic events of any cause would produce leukomalacia. Most cases would occur postnatally in ill preterm infants (especially with respiratory or cardiovascular distress), but prenatal cases would result from intrauterine ischaemic insult (Ellis *et al.* 1988, Gibbs and Weindling 1994). The proportion of prenatal cases is variably estimated, but proven prenatal cases have been described in infants dying within a few hours of birth and demonstrating clearcut lesions (Sinha *et al.* 1990, Iida *et al.* 1992).

The ultimate stage of periventricular leukomalacia is one of (centrolobar) sclerosis that may extend at a distance from the ventricle. In all cases the amount of white matter is decreased, especially in the posterior parts of the hemispheres, and ventricular dilatation is common. This seems to imply more extensive white matter damage than just periventricular necrosis (Leviton and Gilles 1996).

More diffuse lesions of the white matter may be observed in both preterm and term infants (Dambska *et al.* 1989) and have been termed *perinatal telencephalic leukoencephalopathy*. Hypertrophied glial cells, with or without PAS-positive granules disseminated in a background of rarefied tissue with perivascular exudates, represent the major change. Liquefaction of the white matter may occur locally. Infection may interact with asphyxia to produce such lesions (Leviton and Gilles 1984). The lesions resemble those in experimental cases of carbon monoxide poisoning during gestation. The histological pattern is observed mostly in infants dying of sepsis and may be caused by endotoxaemia.

SELECTIVE NEURONAL NECROSIS
In term infants, the cortex and the basal ganglia bear the brunt of hypoxic damage. However, postnatally acquired subcortical cavitated lesions with extensive cortical involvement resembling those in multicystic encephalomalacia have been reported in 15 preterm infants with cardiovascular compromise (Cross *et al.* 1992).

In the cortex, *selective neuronal necrosis* can be localized or diffuse, involving preferentially the left hemisphere (Volpe 1995). Initially, the lesion may be bland or haemorrhagic. The initial stage, at 24–36 hours, is marked by eosinophilia of the neuronal cytoplasm, loss of Nissl substance, and condensation and shrinking of nuclei. Later, cell necrosis is evident with reactive astrocytic gliosis. Neurons of the deep cortical layers and those located in the depth of sulci are preferentially affected (Friede 1989). At a late stage, the gyri become shrivelled and hard. These areas of *ulegyria* may be more or less extensive.

Diffuse lesions tend to involve the neocortex, the hippocampus, and Purkinje cells in the cerebellum. Circumscribed lesions are sometimes found in the territory of a major cortical vessel, mostly the middle cerebral artery.

Calcification of areas of necrosis is a common end stage of hypoxia. It was present in 39 of 99 brains with hypoxic lesions studied by Ansari *et al.* (1990) and involved mainly the white matter and brainstem. In four cases, the calcification was extensive enough to be radiologically detectable. Administration of parenteral calcium can favour the occurrence of brain calcification in severely stressed neonates (Changaris *et al.* 1984). Pasternak (1987) and Volpe and Pasternak (1977) have emphasized the predominance of neuronal necrosis and of resulting ulegyria in the parieto-occipital area, at the border between the territories of the anterior, middle and posterior cerebral arteries bilaterally. This *parasagittal pattern of neuronal necrosis* could be due to low perfusion pressure having its maximal effect in distal arterial territories. It involves also, to some extent, the white matter.

PARASAGITTAL PATTERN
The parasagittal pattern may be responsible for motor deficit in the proximal upper arms, as necrosis affects principally the corresponding area of the motor strip (Volpe 1995) (Fig. 2.8). The lesion can be clearly demonstrated by CT and especially by MRI in later life (Krägeloh-Mann *et al.* 1995). This pattern was not found by Lacey (1985). Volpe (1995) believes this is due to the fact that it is only rarely isolated in fatal cases.

LESIONS OF THE BASAL GANGLIA
Lesions of the basal ganglia were found at autopsy by Christensen and Melchior (1967) in 84 per cent of cases of cerebral palsy. They are often associated with cortical lesions that involve especially the rolandic area bilaterally (Pape and Wigglesworth 1979). Initially, hypoxic lesions appear on ultrasonography as hyperechogenic areas in the thalamus and basal ganglia which can be punctate, linear or mixed. These were shown to be located along the gangliothalamic vessels (Cabañas *et al.* 1994). At a later stage necrosis may manifest on CT as hypodense areas in the putamen and posterolateral part of the thalami (Rutherford *et al.* 1992) or as hypodensity of both putamina (Roig *et al.* 1993). Damage may predominate in the pallidum and subthalamic nucleus or extend

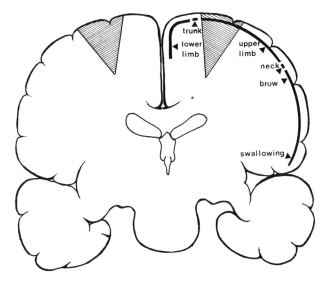

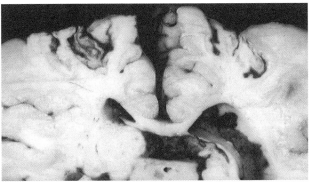

Fig. 2.8. Parasagittal pattern of ischaemic brain damage. *(Top)* Schematic representation of area of infarction at junction of anterior and middle artery territories (hatched triangles). Note infarcted areas correspond to motor area for upper part of arms. *(Bottom)* Pathological specimen showing presence of typical ulegyria in corresponding territory. (6-day-old infant with acute fetal distress and neonatal seizures.)

to the caudate and putamen. The first pattern is common in kernicterus and is known, in its late stage, as *status dysmyelinatus* (Friede 1989).The term *status marmoratus* applies to late post-asphyxial damage in which the basal ganglia have a marbled appearance due to an increase of myelinated fibres in the caudate, putamen and thalamus. This probably results from regeneration of myelinated fibres, formation of myelin around normally non-myelinated fibres, and redundant myelin formation or tissue shrinkage (Friede 1989). Friede and Schachenmayr (1977) found nerve fibres with essentially normal sheaths in the glial scars. Microscopically, small neurons in the putamen and caudate nuclei seem to be especially vulnerable. Cerebellar lesions are uncommon, whether in isolation or in association with damage to the basal ganglia, and laminar or focal cortical necrosis is associated in about 60 per cent of cases (Friede 1989).

FOCAL LESIONS
Focal lesions are due to arterial infarction and are located in a large majority of cases to the territory of the middle cerebral artery (Fujimoto *et al.* 1992). They are identical to cystic softening in

later life (Filipek *et al.* 1987). Most are probably of embolic origin (Coker *et al.* 1988), the clot originating in the ductus arteriosus or umbilical vessels. Some follow a difficult birth with at least some degree of asphyxia, but a majority supervene following uneventful delivery (Roodhooft *et al.* 1987, Coker *et al.* 1988). Occasionally, the softening is haemorrhagic (Chaplin *et al.* 1979). Focal lesions may communicate with the ventricle. They are often referred to as 'acquired' or 'clastic' porencephaly, although this term is better reserved for early acquired lesions (Chapters 1, 3).

CLINICAL AND NEUROIMAGING CORRELATES OF HYPOXIC–ISCHAEMIC PERINATAL LESIONS
Hypoxic–ischaemic lesions are usually the consequence of fetal distress before or during labour, and their prevention is a major reason for surgical or other types of obstetrical intervention (Schifrin1989). In many cases, it is difficult to determine the exact time when hypoxic lesions occurred, the more so as there is a correlation between abnormal pregnancy and perinatal difficulties (MacDonald *et al.* 1980, Barabas *et al.* 1993). In infants dying with a history of adverse perinatal factors such as meconium staining of the liquor or late fetal heart deceleration, autopsy often shows prenatal CNS lesions (Gaffney *et al.* 1994). Causes of intra-uterine hypoxia have been reviewed in Chapter 1. The present discussion is concerned only with intrapartum hypoxia, although clearly the status of the fetus before onset of the birth process is important in the causation and outcome of perinatal distress.

RELATIONSHIP OF STATUS DURING DELIVERY AND AT BIRTH TO HIE
Fetal distress during labour does not necessarily imply HIE, as many newborn infants with classical manifestations of distress do not develop neurological symptoms or sequelae. Nevertheless, assessment of the status of the fetus during the birth process, and of the neonate at birth, gives at least some idea about the risk of development of neurological damage and furnishes diagnostic arguments in favour of hypoxic–ischaemic encephalopathy (American Academy of Pediatrics 1992).

Fetal monitoring may be purely clinical but *electronic monitoring of fetal heart rate* has become routine practice in most developed countries (review in Schifrin 1989). Fetal heart rate monitoring permits precise assessment of heart rate, beat-to-beat variability and accelerations or decelerations in relation to uterine contractions. Abnormalities of each of these factors have been correlated to increased intrauterine death, to fetal acidosis and to low Agpar score at birth, and the management of delivery has been altered in consequence.

Whether electronic monitoring has decreased the incidence of neurological complications remains controversial (MacDonald *et al.* 1985, Luthy *et al.* 1987, Anthony and Levene 1990, Thacker *et al.* 1995). However, the technique has become standard practice at least for high-risk pregnancies. In a series of over 30,000 deliveries, Erkkolla *et al.* (1984) found an 80 per cent reduction in intrapartum fetal deaths, and a 40–50 per cent reduction in overall perinatal mortality, as utilization of monitoring increased from 9 per cent to almost 100 per cent of patients. In contrast, Shy *et al.* (1990) found no beneficial effect of monitoring on neurological development of small preterm infants. Indeed, the incidence of cerebral palsy was higher in monitored babies than in controls.

Nelson *et al.* (1996) found that the risk of cerebral palsy was significantly increased in children who had had multiple late decelerations or decreased beat-to-beat variability during labour, but that the vast majority of infants with such events do not have cerebral palsy. Thacker *et al.* (1995) reviewed 12 controlled trials and found only a minimal benefit from the procedure with no difference in the rate of cerebral palsy or neonatal deaths.

The use of near-infrared spectroscopy, a technique that allows measurement of the cerebral content of both oxygenated and de-oxygenated haemoglobin, can be implemented by attaching a probe to the fetal head after rupture of the membranes, but the technique is still in the experimental stage (Skov *et al.* 1993, Wyatt 1993, Peebles *et al.* 1994).

Fetal pH monitoring by scalp blood sampling (reviewed by Low 1989, Schifrin 1989) may be a critical adjunct to heart rate monitoring. Low pH correlates with an increased fetal risk of death or abnormality. The duration of fetal acidosis is very important. Recently, criticism has been raised about the value of acidosis, whether measured by scalp or cord blood sampling, as the relationship with neonatal neurological dysfunction has been found to be poor (Dijxhoorn *et al.* 1985, Ruth and Raivio 1988, Visser and Dijxhoorn 1988).

Meconium staining of the amniotic fluid has very little predictive value, even though heavy staining may be an indication for fetal scalp sampling (MacDonald *et al.* 1985).

Obtaining information from several techniques of monitoring is obviously important because indications for obstetrical intervention aimed at the prevention of brain damage rely heavily on them. Prediction of neurological damage, however, remains impossible on the sole basis of intrauterine assessment.

Clinical assessment of the infant at birth is another method—albeit a crude one—for judging the degree of hypoxia and of predicting neurological outcome. A low *Apgar score* indicates a need for resuscitation, but only a low Apgar score at 20 minutes is indicative of a significant risk of sequelae or death (Nelson and Ellenberg 1981). In fact, only a cluster of perinatal events, *including the presence of clinical signs of HIE,* will give reliable indications as to the likelihood of late sequelae (Ellenberg and Nelson 1988).

CLINICAL MANIFESTATIONS OF HIE

The symptoms and signs of HIE are different in term and preterm infants. However, typical postasphyxial encephalopathy similar to that seen in term babies can occur occasionally in the preterm infant, although in most, marked intraventricular haemorrhage and periventricular infarction are found (Hill and Volpe 1989, Volpe 1995).

In *term infants*, HIE varies in severity, and three main grades can be described (Sarnat and Sarnat 1976, Fenichel 1983, Hill 1991).

Mild HIE (grade 1) manifestations appear during the first 24 hours of life, then progressively diminish. Jitteriness, a 'hyperalert' state, irritability, and excessive responsiveness with low threshold for the Moro response, which may occur spontaneously, are the major symptoms. Examination shows a normal muscle tone with increased tendon reflexes and, frequently, ankle clonus. Consciousness is not impaired, except perhaps for a brief period of lethargy immediately after birth (Fenichel 1983).

Moderate HIE (grade 2) is characterized by lethargy and obtundation that lasts at least 24 hours. Efforts at arousing the infant result in jitteriness. Muscle tone is decreased at rest but hypertonus may appear on stimulation (Amiel-Tison *et al.* 1977). Spontaneous movements may be diminished. Weakness in the shoulders and proximal arm muscles may indicate predominant parasagittal involvement (Volpe 1995) but is difficult to evaluate. The clinical situation remains critical for 48–72 hours, following which it may either improve or develop into severe HIE.

Severe HIE (grade 3) is usually apparent immediately after birth. Infants are stuporous or comatose, and seizures develop within the first 12–24 hours of life. Some seizures are clearly epileptic in type. Others, presenting as opisthotonic attacks or 'subtle' convulsive manifestations, may represent either true seizures or 'release phenomena' due to cortical destruction or dysfunction (Chapter 16). There is profound hypotonia and unresponsiveness, and reflexes, including the Moro response, are abolished. Sucking and swallowing are depressed or absent and only oculovestibular reflexes persist. Periodic respiration and apnoea are common. Signs of increased intracranial pressure, with a bulging fontanelle and loss of pupillary and oculovestibular reflexes, appear after 24–72 hours and are of ominous significance (Lupton *et al.* 1988). If the infants do not die at this stage, signs subside progressively but neurological sequelae will result in over one-third of cases (Fenichel 1983, Hill and Volpe 1989).

Infants with preferential involvement of the brainstem and thalami may have bulbar manifestations such as sucking and swallowing difficulties out of proportion to impairment of other functions (Dambska *et al.* 1987, Roland *et al.* 1988, Di Mario and Clancy 1989).

Electroencephalography is of value in determining the prognosis of HIE (Scher and Beggarly 1989, Barabas *et al.* 1993, Wertheim *et al.* 1994). In mild HIE, the EEG is usually normal and regularly predicts a favourable outcome (Takeuchi and Watanabe 1989). In moderate or severe HIE, the background tracing is depressed. A flat EEG or a burst–suppression pattern ('*tracé paroxystique*') are of grave significance, especially if they persist for a week or more (Dreyfus-Brisac 1979, Lombroso 1985). Continuous EEG recording, when available, is of prognostic significance: discontinuity of the tracing and presence of paroxysmal EEG discharges may be associated with a poor outcome, whereas continuous tracing is regularly associated with a good outcome (Wertheim *et al.* 1994).

In *preterm infants*, HIE has no or only limited clinical manifestations. Most preterm infants who develop hypoxic brain lesions are sick babies with respiratory distress, necrotizing enterocolitis or sepsis as the primary clinical problem. Neuro-

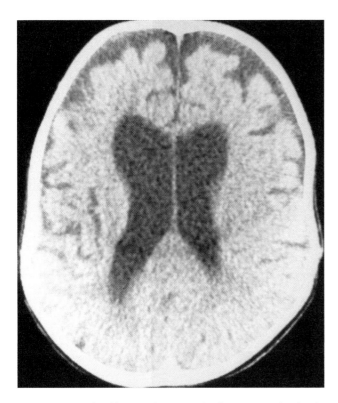

Fig. 2.9. Ventricular dilatation due to atrophy (here associated with subdural collection of fluid over both frontal lobes). Note predominant dilatation of anterior horns of lateral ventricles: such topography is suggestive of atrophy due to destructive processes, whereas dilatation due to mechanical factors (increased CSF pressure) predominates in posterior part of ventricles.

logical complications are discovered by systematic examination but especially by ultrasonography, regardless of clinical presentation. However, a clinical picture similar to that in term babies has been reported (Niijima and Levene 1989).

The EEG of the preterm infant is more difficult to interpret than that of term babies but it does give essential information with regard to the prognosis (Tharp *et al.* 1989). One important finding is that neurological sequelae are present in a majority of infants whose EEGs remained moderately abnormal for several weeks.

NEUROIMAGING CORRELATES OF PERINATAL
HYPOXIC–ISCHAEMIC LESIONS
Abnormal neuroimaging patterns in *term infants* may be diffuse or focal. Diffuse cortical lesions produce few ultrasonographic abnormalities. The presence of diffuse hyperdensities in a 'snowstorm' pattern is of uncertain value (Govaert and de Vries 1997). Likewise, white matter hypodensities on CT scans are normally observed during the first weeks of life (Fitzhardinge *et al.* 1982, Horie *et al.* 1988), and it is extremely difficult to determine at which point in time and intensity they can be considered abnormal. At a later stage, CT scans show the development of atrophy which usually predominates around the frontal horns (Barth 1984) and in the frontal cortex (Fig. 2.9). In the most severe cases, marked white matter hypodensities during the first days of life are followed by the development of multiple areas of

cavitation in the white matter. Calcification may develop (Kanarek and Gieron 1986) in the white matter, brainstem and cortex. Even the presence of extensive calcification does not necessarily imply an infectious process (Ansari *et al.* 1990).

Lesions of the basal ganglia can appear clearly on ultrasound scans, especially in cases of haemorrhagic necrosis of the central grey matter (Kreusser *et al.* 1984) but also in nonhaemorrhagic damage (Shen *et al.* 1986). Colamaria *et al.* (1988) found hyperdensities of the thalami in asphyxiated neonates and thought these might be the precursors of status marmoratus or thalamic calcification (Parisi *et al.* 1983). More diffuse hypervascularity may be a common feature of ischaemic brain damage at an early stage (Shewmon *et al.* 1981). Cavitation of the basal ganglia is a possible sequel to asphyxia (Rutherford *et al.* 1992, 1996). CT and especially MRI (Barkovich 1992) have revealed the frequency of basal ganglia abnormalities in HIE (Keeney *et al.* 1991; Pasternak *et al.* 1991; Rutherford *et al.* 1992, 1996; Natsume *et al.* 1995) (Fig. 2.10). Rutherford *et al.* have emphasized the frequency of hypersignal in the basal ganglia and thalami, most often in association with other lesions involving particularly the cortex. Serial imaging has shown the course of these lesions (Iwasaki *et al.* 1988, Byrne *et al.* 1990, Rutherford *et al.* 1996).

Focal ischaemic lesions are easily diagnosed by ultrasonography, CT (Bouza *et al.* 1994) or MRI scan (Mercuri *et al.* 1995).

The ultrasonographic appearance of *leukomalacia* in preterm infants has been extensively studied (Hill *et al.* 1982a, Adsett *et al.* 1985, Fawer *et al.* 1985, Rushton *et al.* 1985, Hope *et al.* 1988, Govaert and de Vries 1997). It appears initially as more or less well-defined areas of echodensity along the lateral ventricle usually between seven and 14 days after birth (Perlman *et al.* 1996). These may be located to the posterior horn and trigone, extend through the whole length of the ventricle, or be located anteriorly. Trounce *et al.* (1986) have described two patterns: 'prolonged flare' and cavitation. The 'flare' echodensities may disappear or be replaced by small cysts (Dubowitz *et al.* 1985, Cooke 1987, Monset-Couchard *et al.* 1988, Perlman *et al.* 1996). Dammann and Leviton (1997) propose that the term 'flare' applies only to those images that disappear without cavitation. Appleton *et al.* (1990) found neurological residua in four of 15 infants with only prolonged flare, suggesting that it may represent true leukomalacia. Cysts may remain limited to the juxtaventricular area or involve large areas of subcortical white matter. Even cystic lesions can rarely disappear without leaving radiologically visible residua though glial scar remains (Rodriguez *et al.* 1990). Large areas of leukomalacia are also visible on CT scan. At a late stage these appear as dilatation of the lateral ventricles, with irregular limits, as a result of the opening and 'absorption' of the cysts into the ventricular cavity (Van Bel *et al.* 1989). MRI appears to be a potent tool for the diagnosis of periventricular leukomalacia at all stages of its evolution (Wilson and Steiner 1986, Byrne *et al.* 1990) (Fig. 2.11). The reliability of sonography for the diagnosis of nonhaemorrhagic leukomalacia is not absolute. A high proportion of small lesions may escape recognition and the results are critically dependent on the timing of ultrasonographic examination (Nwaesei *et al.* 1988).

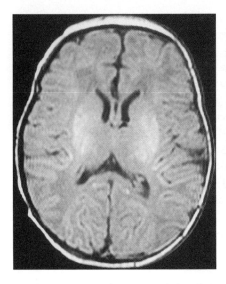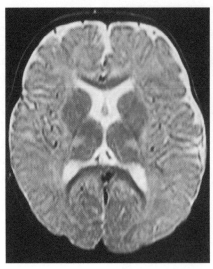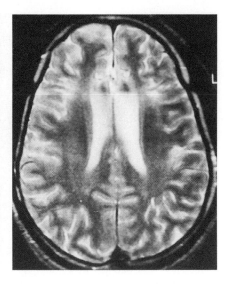

Fig. 2.10. Hypoxic–ischaemic encephalopathy in a term infant: MRI scans. *(Left)* Intense T_2 signal from the basal ganglia on axial cuts. *(Centre)* Extensive low T_1-weighted signal from basal ganglia and thalami. *(Right)* Multifocal cortico-subcortical damage in another infant.

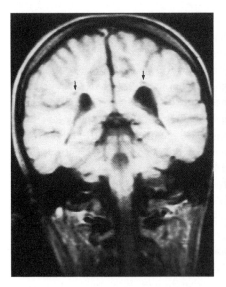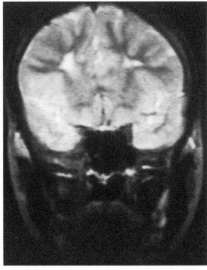

Fig. 2.11. Periventricular leukomalacia: MRI scans. *(Far left)* T_1-weighted sequence showing small areas of low signal alongside ventricular trigone *(arrowed)*. *(Left)* T_2-weighted image showing two areas of high signal immediately anterior to frontal horns.

The presence of cystic leukomalacia on ultrasound scan strongly correlates with the development of cerebral palsy, especially of spastic diplegia (Graziani *et al.* 1986, Graham *et al.* 1987, Costello *et al.* 1988, de Vries *et al.* 1993). Anteriorly located leukomalacia has a poorer prognosis than that found posteriorly (Fawer *et al.* 1987). In addition to cerebral palsy, the presence of cystic leukomalacia correlates with mental retardation and visual disturbances (Scher *et al.* 1989, Eken *et al.* 1996, Perlman *et al.* 1996). MRI provides superior morphological details but is difficult to use in the perinatal period (Dubowitz *et al.* 1985). Later on, it correlates well with previous ultrasound examination (de Vries *et al.* 1993). Sugita *et al.* (1990) found a good correlation between the extent of areas of high signal in T_2-weighted sequences and late neurological defects.

Focal ischaemic lesions (neonatal stroke) present in most cases with a characteristic syndrome of focal seizures with a fixed localization occurring in the first 48 hours of life (Coker *et al.*

1988), frequently in series lasting several hours without alteration of consciousness; these may be later followed by hemiplegia in about half the cases. In many cases, consciousness is preserved and there is no history of obstetric or prenatal difficulties. The EEG shows ictal focal discharges over the involved area. CT scan shows focal hypodense areas in a vascular distribution, sometimes with a mass effect (Fujimoto *et al.* 1992). Infarcts are often poorly demonstrated by ultrasound scanning.

The diagnosis of neonatal stroke can be considerably improved by the use of MRI, which is able to show small lesions not easily detected by ultrasound or even CT. The use of diffusion-weighted MRI (Cowan *et al.* 1994) can demonstrate early lesions that are not yet visualized by conventional techniques (L. Dubowitz, personal communication 1996). MRI with or without diffusion weighting also gives a precise idea of cortical lesions, which give a high T_2 signal in a diffuse or multifocal manner.

Other imaging techniques, *viz.* SPECT (single photon emission computed tomography) (Haddad *et al.* 1993, Shankaran 1993), PET (positron emission tomography) (Chugani 1993) and proton MRS (Peden *et al.* 1993), are currently used mainly as research tools.

Predominant involvement of the brainstem may be marked by oculomotor abnormalities, impairment of swallowing and tongue movements, and a remarkable facial appearance with facial weakness and a wide-open mouth (Roland *et al.* 1988). Involvement of the anterior horn of the spinal cord with loss of tendon reflexes and peripheral weakness may be associated (Clancy *et al.* 1989).

Symmetrical involvement of the parasagittal area (parasagittal pattern) according to Volpe (1995) presents with weakness in the proximal limbs, more prominent in the upper than in the lower extremities, as a result of the maximal involvement of the corresponding area of the motor strip. Other manifestations of HIE such as disturbances of awareness and diffuse hypotonia often make interpretation of weakness difficult.

Lesions of the basal ganglia are good indicators of late fetal or perinatal hypoxia. Hyperechogenicity in the thalami by colour Doppler flow imaging (Cabañas *et al.* 1994) is difficult to interpret.

DIAGNOSIS OF HIE

The diagnosis of HIE requires unequivocal evidence of fetal distress, depression at birth and clinical manifestations of encephalopathy. Like that of intracranial haemorrhage, it is made too often on insufficient evidence. It should be emphasized once more that prenatal or intrapartum difficulties are not a sufficient argument for making a diagnosis of HIE or intracranial haemorrhage and that clearcut neurological signs are an absolute requirement. Furthermore, neurological abnormalities in the neonatal period, even when they occur after fetal distress or a difficult birth, are not necessarily due to HIE. The differential diagnosis includes virtually all neonatal conditions. Some of them such as sepsis and metabolic diseases require urgent therapy and should always be thought of with high priority.

In particular, neonatal hypotonia is common to HIE and to many other conditions of cerebral or peripheral origin (see p. 55). In some cases it may be associated with evidence of CNS dysfunction or damage, as is frequent in myotonic dystrophy (Rutherford *et al.* 1989).

Depression of reactivity and tone may also be seen following absorption of drugs by mothers, especially benzodiazepines (Laegreid *et al.* 1987). Profound depression closely mimicking HIE and often associated with seizures is a major feature of accidental mepivacaine injection into the fetal scalp during paracervical or pudendal block (Hillman *et al.* 1979). In this case, the pupils are nonreactive to light and often dilated, and the doll's head oculocephalic reflex is absent.

Hypertonus and jitteriness that can be seen with mild HIE are also observed in many other neonatal conditions, as are convulsive seizures. Drug withdrawal is a common cause of jitteriness and irritability that may be asociated with true seizures. The symptoms of drug withdrawal can occur in infants of

mothers addicted to heroin, methadone, barbiturates or alcohol. Symptoms usually develop in the first 24–48 hours of life and subside in a few days. The determination of levels of aspartate aminotransferase and hydroxybutyrate dehydrogenase in serum is a sensitive test (Lackmann and Töllner 1995).

Imaging techniques have considerably improved the diagnosis of hypoxic–ischaemic lesions. These should be distinguished from developmental abnormalities whose frequency has been demonstrated by MRI (Chapter 3). Periventricular leukomalacia may be difficult to distinguish from subependymal pseudocysts due to hypoxic or posthaemorrhagic germinolysis. Rademaker *et al.* (1993) studied 24 such cases and precisely defined their characteristics. Although associated pathology is frequent in such cases, it is essential to recognize the benign nature of these lesions. In a prospective study, Shen and Huang (1985) found pseudocysts in 5 per cent of infants submitted to ultrasound scanning.

PROGNOSIS OF HIE

The prognosis of HIE in term infants depends mainly on the severity of the clinical picture during the first days of life. Intrapartum events and the status of the infant at birth, on the other hand, have a low prognostic value, although the presence of metabolic acidosis at birth in preterm infants ≤1500 g was recently shown to be a predictor of poor outcome (Goldstein *et al.* 1995). Indeed, neurodevelopmental sequelae due to hypoxia are not observed in the absence of clinical manifestations of HIE in the neonatal period (Freeman and Nelson 1988, Aylward *et al.* 1989). It seems unlikely that 'minor' disturbances such as learning difficulties or behavioural problems can be a sequel to hypoxia not clearly manifested in the neonatal period, and the concept of a continuum of casualties due to birth difficulties is no longer fashionable.

The prognosis for mild HIE is favourable and no sequelae are to be expected in such cases (Fenichel 1997). However, Rosenbloom (1994) reported that 10 of 17 infants with dyskinetic cerebral palsy attributed to birth hypoxia had only mild to moderate HIE at birth. The prognosis of severe HIE is poor (Mulligan *et al.* 1980, Finer *et al.* 1983), while that of moderate HIE is unpredictable. Fenichel (1983) indicates that the occurrence of prolonged or repeated convulsions in the first day of life implies a risk of sequelae of 50 per cent; that of a suppressed EEG at the end of one week, a risk of 64 per cent, and, at two weeks, of 100 per cent; and that of an Apgar score between 0 and 3 at 10 minutes, in addition to signs of moderate HIE, a risk of 50 per cent. The occurrence of resistant seizures is especially worrying (Mulligan *et al.* 1980, Watkins *et al.* 1988). A recent prospective follow-up study of 26 term infants with HIE (Gray *et al.* 1993) confirmed that all nine children with severe HIE had a poor outcome (death, or cerebral palsy and significant developmental delay), while nine of 13 with moderate HIE had a good outcome. Infants with diffusely increased echogenicity on ultrasound scans did poorly as did those with generalized hypodensity on CT scan. There was also a good correspondence between the results of Doppler ultrasound study of the middle cerebral artery and the outcome (Eken *et al.* 1995): an abnormal flow velocity and especially an abnormal resistance index were significantly related with a poor outcome. This is in conformity with the results of Levene *et al.* (1989). Microcephaly is a frequent sequela of HIE. A decrease in the ratio (actual head circumference)/(mean for age) of 3.1 per cent or greater between birth and 4 months of age is an accurate early predictor of poor outcome.

The prognosis for *term infants* with neonatal stroke is usually favourable (Trauner *et al.* 1993). Although a cystic cavity in the territory of the middle cerebral artery persists and may produce focal deficits, these are by no means constant and the overall neurodevelopment is often satisfactory.

The prognosis for *preterm infants* with diffuse subcortical hypoxic brain damage is serious (Szymonowicz *et al.* 1986, Fawer *et al.* 1987, Scher *et al.* 1989). The seriousness of cystic leukomalacia is well documented (Levene 1990, Ringelberg and van de Bor 1993). Van Bel *et al.* (1989) found that ventricular dilatation, probably attributable to cystic leukomalacia, could be observed in the absence of previous detectable periventricular echodensity, indicating the limitations of ultrasound examination. In the same infants, an increased cerebral blood flow velocity had been found during the first week of life. CT and MRI studies (Skranes *et al.* 1993) have confirmed the prognostic value of such examinations. Kuenzle *et al.* (1994) found a good correlation between the results of MRI examination with high field (2.35 T) in 43 neonates. All those with severe diffuse anomalies had severe sequelae; one third of those with moderate diffuse abnormalities, parasagittal or periventricular hyperintensity, and local necrosis or haemorrhage had mild sequelae, and all but one of the infants with normal MRI did well. Early decrease of head growth (Cordes *et al.* 1994) is strongly correlated to a poor outcome.

TREATMENT AND PREVENTION OF HYPOXIC–ISCHAEMIC BRAIN DAMAGE

No technique has proved effective in treating established HIE. On the other hand, utmost attention should be paid to disturbances in the functioning of other organs such as kidney and heart, and immediate correction of metabolic derangements is mandatory. Correction of acidosis should not be too rapid as rapid infusion of bicarbonate may precipitate the occurrence of intraventricular haemorrhage.

Control of the seizures may increase the chances of a favourable outcome (Volpe 1995) (Chapter 16). Attempts at reducing raised intracranial pressure (ICP) have been moderately successful. Levene and Evans (1985) found that repeated infusions of 20% mannitol were effective. They reported that a dose of 0.25 mg/kg given over 20 minutes and repeated every six hours for the first two days lowered ICP, without rebound effect. Lupton *et al.* (1988) considered that high ICP is due to cytotoxic oedema consequent upon neuronal necrosis and is therefore irreversible. Steroid therapy was widely used in the 1970s but its beneficial effect appears doubtful. Elevation of the head to 30° and 10 per cent fluid restriction may favourably influence ICP. The use of corticosteroids is not advised as their efficacy has not been properly assessed and their potential dangers are not negligible. Barbiturate therapy, meant to reduce the metabolic demand of

the brain and thus protect it against lack of oxygen, does not decrease the mortality rate or sequelae (Goldberg *et al.* 1986). Control of such factors as hypercapnia and hypoxaemia by assisted ventilation is of course essential (Shaw *et al.* 1993). Hypocapnia, however, is potentially detrimental (Greisen *et al.* 1987).

Prevention of hypoxic–ischaemic brain damage is a major issue that requires cooperation between obstetricians, paediatricians, child neurologists and neonatologists, as well as public health and social measures. For preterm infants, prevention of periventricular leukomalacia requires careful attention to risk factors (Calvert *et al.* 1987, Trounce *et al.* 1988), but the effectiveness of such measures has not been assessed. However, surfactant replacement therapy is associated with improvement of neurological function (Amato *et al.* 1991). Recent therapeutic trials (Vannucci 1990, Palmer and Vannucci 1993) have been briefly mentioned above (p. 40). Allopurinol may reduce brain damage (Palmer and Smith 1990). The use of glutamate antagonists is not recommended because of their possible effects on learning processes. The use of inhibitors of the production of prostaglandins and xanthine has no proven efficacy. Calcium channel blockers such as flunarizine and nimodipine are reported to have reduced the extent of hypoxic–ischaemic brain damage in adult animals (Alps and Hass 1987), but nicardipine administration may be associated with hypotension and reduction of cerebral blood flow (Levene *et al.* 1990). These and other agents are being intensively investigated (Levene 1993, Legido 1994). Administration of magnesium sulfate during pregnancy and labour may decrease the incidence of sequelae attributable to HIE (Nelson and Grether 1995).

LATE COMPLICATIONS OF NEONATAL RESPIRATORY DISTRESS

Acute respiratory distress of the neonate is sometimes followed, after prolonged periods of assisted ventilation, by a chronic lung disease known as *bronchopulmonary dysplasia*. This disorder often leads to congestive heart failure and death after several months. In such cases, Ellison and Farina (1980) first reported neurological involvement leading to clear progressive deterioration. Pathologically, the brainstem and cerebral hemisphere showed neuronal loss and gliosis. Systemic hypertension is frequent in infants with bronchopulmonary dysplasia. It is associated with high renin levels and may rarely induce neurological complications (Abman *et al.* 1984). Treatment of systemic hypertension in such infants with the angiotensin-I converting enzyme captopril has been associated with seizures, possibly due to haemorrhagic brain infarcts (Perlman and Volpe 1989a).

A peculiar movement disorder may develop at 3–4 months of age in some infants with bronchopulmonary dysplasia (Perlman and Volpe 1989b, Hadders-Algra *et al.* 1994). It features choreoathetotic movements, darting tongue motions and motor unrest (akathisia) and seems to disappear spontaneously by 18–30 months of age. Extracorporeal membrane oxygenation (ECMO), which is used in the treatment of the most severe forms of neonatal distress, may be associated with brain damage in 25–50 per cent of infants (Volpe 1995) with both haemorrhagic and ischaemic lesions. The neurological complications are described in Chapter 23.

KERNICTERUS

The term kernicterus was initially applied to the yellow staining of the basal nuclei found at autopsy of deeply jaundiced infants dying with severe erythroblastosis fetalis. Later, it was also used to designate the clinical picture of choreoathetosis and hearing loss that followed severe haemolytic disease. More recently the term has been applied to similarly stained brains of infants who died without blood group incompatibility and who had had only modest rises of blood bilirubin. Some authors have suggested that such modest rises could be associated with impairment of cognitive or other neurological functions, while others did not find such a relationship (Rubin *et al.* 1979). In agreement with Hansen and Bratlid (1986), I shall use the term kernicterus for the neuropathological findings of bilirubin staining of brainstem and basal nuclei and for the classical neurological picture, even though neuronal damage can be present without staining and, conversely, bilirubin staining may be an agonal phenomenon unrelated to bilirubin toxicity (Ahdab-Barmada and Moossy 1984, Watchko and Oski 1992). Some investigators have proposed a stricter definition requiring both staining and neuronal damage (see Volpe 1995), while simple staining of nuclei without neuronal lesions in preterm infants, often associated with only moderate hyperbilirubinaemia, is considered a different phenomenon. Similarly, I shall use the term bilirubin encephalopathy for all demonstrated or possible sequelae of bilirubin toxicity.

PATHOLOGY AND PATHOGENESIS

In addition to the macroscopic staining of the globus pallidus, dentate nuclei, cerebellar vermis, hippocampus and medullary nuclei, yellow pigment may be present in the meninges and choroid plexus. Microscopically, spongy degeneration and gliosis are present in the stained areas and in zones not macroscopically involved such as the cochlear nuclei and pathways. Pigment deposition is visible in neurons and glial cells. Neuronal necrosis generally involves the same structures as bilirubin staining, although some structures, *e.g.* Purkinje cells, may be severely affected without significant staining.

The mechanism of kernicterus is unclear. The relationship between albumin, free and bound bilirubin, and kernicterus or bilirubin encephalopathy is shown schematically in Figure 2.12. Bilirubin is undoubtedly toxic when it reaches neural tissue, perhaps by inhibiting phosphorylation and respiration in mitochondria (Hansen and Bratlid 1985, Perlman and Frank 1988, Stern and Cashore 1989). Normally, bilirubin is maintained within the vascular compartment where it is bound to albumin in an approximately equimolar concentration. The small unbound fraction may increase as a consequence of displacement from bilirubin-binding sites on albumin by exogenous agents such as certain drugs or endogenous substances like fatty acids. Bound bilirubin may not be harmless and it can cross the blood–brain barrier, especially when the latter is damaged by such factors as hypercarbia or hyperosmolarity (Bratlid *et al.* 1983), although unbound bilirubin is the major offender (Volpe 1995). In haemolytic disease, the high amount of free bilirubin accounts for the occurrence of kernicterus, at levels beyond 340 µmol/L (20 mg/dL), although much higher levels are not necessarily noxious. Determination of the binding capacity of albumin has not proved helpful in practice, the more so as many factors that increase the risk of bilirubin encephalopathy do not produce detectable increase in free levels (Ritter *et al.* 1982). Even though preterm infants with low albumin levels, acidosis, sepsis or PIVH (Amato *et al.* 1987, Epstein *et al.* 1988) are much more likely to develop kernicterus than those without such factors, it remains impossible to predict which infant will exhibit bilirubin toxicity (Watchko and Oski 1992).

Some evidence (Perlman and Frank 1988) suggests that bilirubin might enter the brain in a reversible manner and might be responsible for 'subclinical neurotoxicity' that may either be transient or evolve into definitive neuronal damage. This hypothesis is based mainly on alterations of auditory and visual evoked potentials with hyperbilirubinaemia (Nakamura *et al.* 1985). Evoked potentials may return to normal following exchange transfusion (Chin *et al.* 1985, Hung 1989, Deliac *et al.* 1990). If this hypothesis were confirmed, it would be possible to contemplate exchange transfusion on the basis of clinical and electrophysiological signs rather than solely on bilirubin levels (Perlman and Frank 1988), but the evidence is far from complete and the method difficult to use in practice. A similar attempt using MRI (Palmer and Smith 1990) remained inconclusive.

CLINICAL MANIFESTATIONS

The classical picture of the term infant with typical kernicterus is now rarely seen in developed countries. The first neurological signs develop between 48 hours and 4 days of age with feeding difficulties and a high pitched cry, followed by hypertonus, extensor spasms and, in rare cases, clonic seizures. Hyperthermia is frequent (Connolly and Volpe 1990). A similar, though less acute picture can occur in preterm infants between 4 and 7 days of age. Following the acute stage, hypotonia sets in. Later on, the classic tetrad of Perlstein (1960) including choreoathetosis, supranuclear ophthalmoplegia frequently affecting vertical more than horizontal eye movements, sensorineural hearing loss, and enamel hypoplasia may evolve progressively, although in many cases one or several features are absent and hearing loss may be isolated (De Vries *et al.* 1985). Deafness and choreoathetosis may appear later, even in the absence of neurological signs in the neonatal period. Abnormal MRI signal from the pallidum has been observed in one such case (Worley *et al.* 1996). Residual cognitive deficits are possible. Severe mental retardation is uncommon.

Several authors have entertained the possibility that bilirubin toxicity in preterm infants may remain inapparent in the neonatal period but be responsible for delayed development, hearing problems and motor or learning difficulties in childhood (Ritter *et al.* 1982, Nakamura *et al.* 1985). Van de Bor *et al.* (1989) found

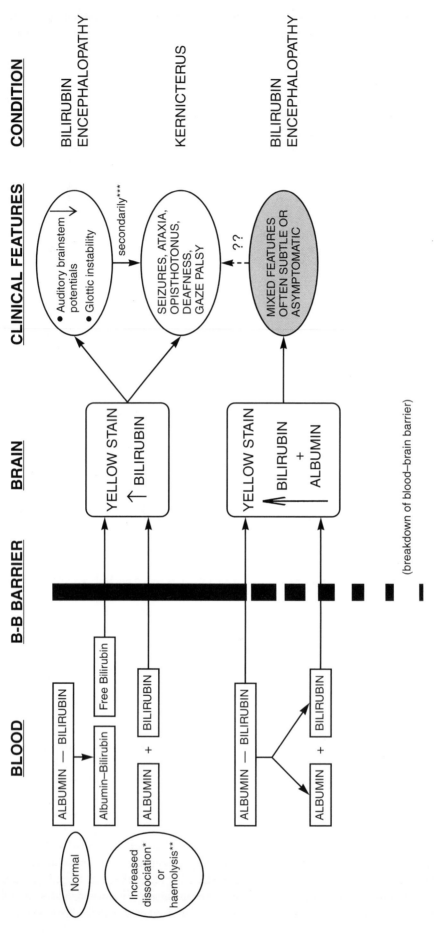

Fig. 2.12. Schematic representation of the relationship between albumin, free and bound bilirubin, and kernicterus or bilirubin encephalopathy. [Modified from Hansen and Bratild (1986).]

(*) May be due to drugs (*e.g.* sulfonamides), low albumin levels, and perhaps other factors such as acidosis; also observed in Crigler–Najjar syndrome (glucuronyl transferase deficiency). Except in the latter case is almost exclusively observed in preterm infants.

(**) Generally due to Rh haemolytic disease or ABO incompatibility.

(***) Intervention might be possible at this point to prevent neurological involvement.

a relationship between the occurrence of cerebral palsy (of undescribed type), as well as of minor developmental anomalies, and hyperbilirubinaemia in the first few days of life. In this large study, each increase in bilirubin level by 50 μmol/L (2.9 mg/dL) was associated with a small increase in the frequency of neurological sequelae. Later, the same group found such a relationship only in infants with intracranial haemorrhage (Van de Bor *et al.* 1992). Other recent large studies (Scheidt *et al.* 1991, Seidman *et al.* 1991, Graziani *et al.* 1992, O'Shea *et al.* 1992) did not confirm a relation between neonatal bilirubin concentrations and developmental problems or intelligence. A relationship with hearing loss seeems better established (de Vries *et al.* 1985).

The diagnosis of classical kernicterus is easy but the significance of a history of neonatal hyperbilirubinaemia, even moderate, in the neonatal period in a child with cerebral palsy, hearing loss or mental difficulties is impossible to interpret. Modern imaging has only rarely been used in kernicterus. In one study (Penn *et al.* 1994) it demonstrated high T_1-weighted signal from the hippocampus, thalamus and pallidum but not from the putamen, in agreement with pathological data.

THERAPY

The treatment of kernicterus in term infants with haemolysis rests on the prevention of excessive hyperbilirubinaemia. Exchange transfusion is indicated for infants with erythroblastosis at a level of 340 μmol/L (20 mg/dL). Prevention and prenatal treatment of blood group incompatibility (Whittle 1992) has resulted in almost complete disappearance of this problem. In a recent study (Watchko and Claassen 1994), only three of 81 infants had demonstrated kernicterus at relatively low bilirubin levels. Fifty per cent of the remaining 78 infants had bilirubin levels in excess of those recommended by the National Institute of Child Health and Human Development, so the indications for exchange remain uncertain. In preterm infants, exchange transfusion is of uncertain value and there is no agreement as to the levels at which it should be performed (Newman and Maisels 1992). Although relatively safe, the procedure carries certain risks (Keenan *et al.* 1985).

Phototherapy effectively limits the neonatal increase in bilirubin in preterm infants. The technique is safe (Brown *et al.* 1985, Lipsitz *et al.* 1985), and breakdown products do not seem to produce bilirubin encephalopathy (Scheidt *et al.* 1988) while lowering peak levels of bilirubin by an average of 70 μmol/L (4 mg/dL). The value of mesoporphyrin inhibitors of bilirubin production is being tested and encouraging results have been reported (Valaes *et al.* 1994, Kappas *et al.* 1995).

High levels of bilirubin may induce some behavioural changes in the absence of encephalopathy (Telzrow *et al.* 1980, Escher-Graub and Fricker 1986) but these are probably of limited significance.

METABOLIC INSULTS—NEONATAL ASPECTS

Metabolic disorders are considered in Chapter 9. Only the specific aspects of metabolic problems in the newborn infant are discussed here.

NEONATAL HYPOGLYCAEMIA

The conventional definition of significant hypoglycaemia in the neonate is a blood sugar level of less than 1.1 mmol/L (20 mg/dL). This is an arbitrary figure, however, as some infants may be symptomatic with levels of 1.6–2.2 mmol/L (30–40 mg/dL) while many others do not have symptoms even at levels well below 1.1 mmol/L (20 mg/dL). Other factors such as the rate of fall of glucose are thus important. Asymptomatic, transient hypoglycaemia can be detected in 11 per cent of all newborn babies during the first hours post partum before oral feeding is initiated (Fenichel 1988), especially in those with intrauterine growth retardation or birth asphyxia or in those born to diabetic or toxaemic mothers (Cornblath and Schwartz 1991). The incidence of symptomatic hypoglycaemia is certainly much lower.

MECHANISMS AND PATHOLOGY

The mechanisms of neonatal hypoglycaemia are diverse. Rare infants suffer from grave conditions like nesidioblastosis. In a majority, especially in small for gestational age neonates, an imbalance between a relatively large brain that consumes glucose as its primary fuel and a small liver depleted of glycogen reserves seems to compromise supply to the CNS. The absence of symptoms in many infants with hypoglycaemia may be related to the fact that the newborn brain can oxidize other fuels than glucose, such as ketone bodies, lactic acid and fatty acids. Brain dysfunction with seizures and coma is not associated with a significant fall in high-energy phosphate compounds, a situation that also obtains with hypoxia (Petroff *et al.* 1988).

The pathology of hypoglycaemia is reminiscent of that of hypoxia, with which it is often associated (Collins and Leonard 1984). Neuronal loss involves not only the brain but also anterior horn cells of the spinal cord, but it usually predominates in the posterior part of the cerebrum (Anderson *et al.* 1967).

CLINICAL FEATURES

Neurological manifestations of neonatal hypoglycaemia include apnoea, jitteriness, high-pitched cry, cyanosis, vomiting, seizures and coma, isolated or in any combination. The occurrence of symptoms seems to depend on the duration of hypoglycaemia more than on its degree (Koivisto *et al.* 1972). Several types can be observed. In the first few hours of life, an 'adaptive' hypoglycaemia frequently occurs in infants of diabetic mothers, those with erythroblastosis fetalis, and many preterm asphyxiated infants. Most cases with onset in the first 12 hours of life remain asymptomatic. Secondary hypoglycaemia usually occurs in the later part of the first day of life and is seen in infants born at or before term severely asphyxiated (Collins and Leonard 1984). The part played by hypoglycaemia in such cases is difficult to disentangle from that of the primary disorder. The classical type is seen primarily in small for gestational age infants. Symptoms are present in about 20 per cent of such cases. They appear in the latter part of the first day or in the second day. The outlook depends on severity and duration of hypoglycaemia and on therapy. Recurrent hypoglycaemia, on the other hand, is usually associated with hyperinsulinism, glycogenoses, fructose intolerance, or other disorders of carbohydrate metabolism or regulation. Congenital hypopituitarism, although infrequent, is an important cause because recognition is essential to avoid recurrences and mental retardation.

The *outcome* of neonatal hypoglycaemia is serious, with one study (Koivisto *et al.* 1972) showing mental or motor sequelae in about half of symptomatic patients, while only 6 per cent of asymptomatic children had neurodevelopmental abnormalities at follow-up. Pildes *et al.* (1974) found that the average IQ of patients with symptomatic hypoglycaemia was lower than that of controls. Focal epilepsy may be an isolated sequela (Boulloche *et al.* 1987). Recent studies suggest that lasting effects may follow relatively mild hypoglycaemia. Koh *et al.* (1988) reported delayed nerve conduction velocities in children with marginal hypoglycaemia which persisted after correction of the metabolic defect. Lucas *et al.* (1988) found that children who had prolonged biochemical hypoglycaemia had a 3–14 point disadvantage on the Bayley scale as compared with normoglycaemic children, although this was a retrospective study with consequent limitations.

TREATMENT
Treatment of neonatal hypoglycaemia consists of the intravenous administration of 0.5–1.0 g/kg of glucose as a 25% solution at a rate of 1 mL/min, followed by continuous infusion of 8–10 mg/kg/min. The bolus injection should be used only in case of emergency.

The underlying cause must be determined. Asymptomatic infants should probably have their glycaemia corrected by continuous infusion when blood glucose is below 2.2 mmol/L (40 mg/L) (Hawdon *et al.* 1994, Mehta 1994).

HYPOGLYCORRHACHIA WITHOUT HYPOGLYCAEMIA
Hypoglycorrhachia without hypoglycaemia (De Vivo *et al.* 1991) is a rare condition whose importance lies in the possibility of active treatment and in its diagnostic difficulties. The disorder is caused by deficiency of the carrier protein *GLUT1* that transports glucose from blood to CSF. It is transmitted as an autosomal recessive trait and usually manifests clinically from the end of the first month onwards. Truly neonatal cases are known (D.C. De Vivo, personal communication 1995). The major clinical features are seizures, but ataxia, paroxysmal disturbances of consciousness and even periodic weakness have been observed. A low CSF lactate level may be a clue. Treatment by ketogenic diet prevents neurological deficit and has been successsfully maintained for several years.

HYPERGLYCAEMIA
Marked hyperglycaemia occurs occasionally in neonates with CNS disturbances (Cornblath and Schwartz 1991) and has a grave prognostic significance. Idiopathic neonatal hyperglycaemia is exceptional (Lewis and Mortimer 1964).

DISTURBANCES OF ELECTROLYTE METABOLISM IN THE NEONATAL PERIOD

NEONATAL HYPOCALCAEMIA AND HYPOMAGNESAEMIA
Hypocalcaemia is defined as a blood calcium level below 1.75 mmol/L (7 mg/dL) and is often associated with hypomagnesaemia, a magnesium level below 0.6 mmol/L (1.5 mg/dL). Two distinct forms of neonatal hypocalcaemia form the bulk of the cases seen in the neonatal period.

Early hypocalcaemia occurs before 48 hours of age mainly in preterm infants, infants of diabetic mothers, and those who are small for gestational age or have suffered asphyxia. Between 21 and 60 per cent of such infants have calcium levels of less than 1.75 mmol/L (7 mg/dL) or ionized calcium levels of less than 0.75–0.85 mmol/L (3–3.5 mg/dL). This form has no symptoms of its own and any clinical manifestation observed is likely to be due to the primary condition of the infant. A possible explanation for the lack of correlation between symptoms and total calcium levels could be that clinical phenomena are due to low ionized calcium, possibly below 0.63 mmol/L (2.5 mg/dL) (Sorell and Rosen 1975). Exceptionally, cardiac complications, probably due to hypocalcaemia, have been reported in such cases. The mechanism of early hypocalcaemia is unknown. Parathyroid hormone levels are elevated and hypercalcitoninaemia may play a role. Therapeutic intravenous administration of calcium gluconate should be cautious. Changaris *et al.* (1984) observed a positive correlation between deposition of calcium into areas of pontosubicular necrosis and the administered dose of calcium gluconate in 17 infants with hypoxic encephalopathy.

Late hypocalcaemia presents at between 5 and 10 days of life, typically in infants fed cow milk formulae with a high phosphorus content. The excess phosphate load cannot be completely excreted by the immature kidney and the resulting hyperphosphataemia induces hypocalcaemia. Infants born in winter or early spring to mothers of low social class with subclinical vitamin D intake are at especial risk (Roberts *et al.* 1973). Late hypocalcaemia has become rare since modified formulae have been in common use.

The clinical features are those of classical '*neonatal tetany*'. Focal or multifocal clonic seizures (Chapter 16) appear in apparently normally alert and hungry infants. Jitteriness is almost universally present between seizures that occur repeatedly and may last intermittently for several days if untreated (Cockburn *et al.* 1973). About 15 per cent of infants have spread cranial sutures (Volpe 1995) and reflexes are abnormally brisk. Two-thirds of infants with late hypocalcaemia have high phosphorus blood levels and half of them have hypomagnesaemia.

The prognosis for late hypocalcaemia is good. Remarkably, the seizures, even when lasting for hours and days, do not leave residua (Lombroso 1996).

Treatment of the seizures can be accomplished by slow intravenous administration of 5% calcium gluconate (4 mL/kg) while monitoring the cardiac rate. Maintenance treatment is by oral administration of 75 mg/kg/d of elemental calcium. Magnesium has also been used successfully to correct both the hypomagnesaemia and the hypocalcaemia. It is given intramuscularly as a 50% solution of magnesium sulfate in a dose of 0.2 mL/kg every 8–12 hours (Cockburn *et al.* 1973). Prevention of late hypocalcaemia is easily realized by the avoidance of un-modified cow's milk formulae with consequent reduction of the phosphate load.

Late hypocalcaemia may also occur in infants born to mothers with hyperparathyroidism. Because maternal hyper-parathyroidism is often clinically silent, routine determination of calcium and phosphorus in maternal blood is in order if no obvious cause for the hypocalcaemia is present (Lynch and Rust 1994). Hypocalcaemia is also a manifestation of Di George syn-drome in which the seizures may precede the signs of immune deficiency which occur in association with cardiac and other malformations (Chapter 5). According to Lynch and Rust (1994), hypocalcaemia and hypomagnesaemia currently account for 5–13 per cent of neonatal seizures instead of a previous frequency of 20–34 per cent, and most cases are of the early onset variety. In their series of 15 infants, seven had congenital heart disease, six had idiopathic hypoparathyroidism, and seven were born to mothers with hyperparathyroidism.

Magnesium malabsorption is a rare familial disease. Serum magnesium level is below 0.08 mmol/L (0.2 mg/dL) as a result of specific intestinal malabsorption. Calcium levels are moderately low and the symptoms are much like those of hypocalcaemia. The patients respond favourably to high doses of magnesium (Stromme *et al.* 1969). Hypomagnesaemia may also occur with malnutrition and in the infantile tremor syndrome observed in India, some cases of which respond to magnesium supplementa-tion (Garewal *et al.* 1988).

HYPERCALCAEMIA AND HYPERMAGNESAEMIA
Hypercalcaemia in newborn infants may occur with fat necrosis, in some infants receiving intravenous infusion of calcium gluconate (Ramamurthy *et al.* 1975), and in rare patients with a defect of intestinal transport of tryptophan, the 'blue-diaper syn-drome'. It is also a feature of the Williams ('elfin face') syndrome although it often goes unrecognised during the neonatal period (Chapter 5).

Neonatal hyperparathyroidism is a rare, severe condition which features hypotonia, failure to thrive, respiratory distress associated with multiple rib fractures, and early death when untreated. The condition is familial in 50 per cent of cases (Harris and d'Ercole 1989). Hypercalcaemia may also be a feature of the more benign asymptomatic neonatal familial hypercalcaemia in which remis-sion occurs spontaneously (Orwoll *et al.* 1982).

Hypermagnesaemia may be observed following administration of large doses of magnesium sulfate to the mothers for treatment of toxaemia. Clinical features include weakness, depressed or absent tendon reflexes, hypotonia and stupor, and it may lead to respiratory failure (Tsang 1972). In severe cases, exchange trans-fusion may be lifesaving.

OTHER DISTURBANCES OF ELECTROLYTE METABOLISM
These are uncommon. *Hypernatraemia* may be observed with neonatal dehydration or in infants receiving breast milk with high

TABLE 2.2
Inherited metabolic diseases with neurological manifestations in the neonatal period*

Acute diseases
  Aminoacidopathies
    Leucinosis (maple syrup urine disease)
    Nonketotic hyperglycinaemia (glycine encephalopathy)
    Tyrosinaemia type I
    Sulfite oxidase deficiency
    Sulfite oxidase–xanthine oxidase deficiency (molybdenum cofactor defect)
  Disorders of metabolism of organic acids
    Propionate and methylmalonate metabolism
      Propionic acidaemia
      Methylmalonic acidaemia
    Disorders of branched-chain keto acid metabolism
      Isovaleric acidaemia
  Ammonia cycle defects (hyperammonaemia)
    Carbamylphosphate synthetase deficiency
    Ornithine transcarbamylase deficiency
    Arginosuccinic acid synthetase deficiency (citrullinaemia)
    Arginosuccinase deficiency (arginosuccinic aciduria)
    Arginase deficiency (hyperargininaemia)
    Congenital lysine intolerance
  Disorders of energy metabolism** (lactic acidosis)
    Disorders of pyruvate metabolism
      Pyruvate-dehydrogenase complex deficiencies
      Pyruvate carboxylase deficiency
    Disorders of respiratory chain (especially complex I and IV)
    Disorders of fatty acid oxidation
      Holocarboxylase deficiency
      Biotinidase deficiency
      Specific dehydrogenase defects
      ETF (electron transfer factor) dehydrogenase defects (glutaric aciduria type 2)
  Disorders of carbohydrate metabolism
    Glycogenosis types I and III
    Glycogen synthase deficiency
    Fructose diphosphatase deficiency
    Fructose intolerance
    Galactosaemia

Chronic diseases
  Zellweger syndrome and related diseases (Zellweger-like syndromes)
  Neonatal adrenoleukodystrophy
  Other disorders of peroxisomal function
  Pyridoxine dependency
  CDG (carbohydrate-deficient glycoprotein syndrome) (neonatal form)
  Sialidosis type 2 and galactosialidosis

*Electrolyte disorders and hypoglycaemia not included (see text).
**Some of these diseases are conventionally considered as organic acid disorders.

sodium concentration (Anand *et al.* 1980). Hyponatraemia with convulsions has been observed in a few neonates (Vanapruks and Prapaitrakul 1989). *Hyperkalaemia* may occur in asociation with severe neonatal distress of various origins. It may be respon-sible for disturbances of cardiac rhythm (Shortland *et al.* 1987).

OTHER METABOLIC DISTURBANCES IN THE NEONATAL PERIOD
This section deals with inherited metabolic disorders that manifest with acute neurological symptoms during the neonatal period (Table 2.2). These conditions are described fully in Chapter 9; this section is concerned only with the particular features they assume in newborn infants.

GENERAL MECHANISMS

The clinical manifestations of neonatal inherited metabolic diseases such as aminoacidaemias or organic acidaemias are the result of toxicity of metabolites that cannot be catabolized for want of a specific enzyme.

Most of these toxic products are diffusible substances that are cleared by the placenta during intrauterine life but accumulate after birth and produce symptoms when they have reached a critical level. This explains the delayed appearance of clinical manifestations following a free interval, which is an essential feature of neonatal metabolic diseases. Not infrequently, the first symptoms appear following the first milk feed.

In other conditions, an acute failure of energy production or utilization is at least partly responsible for the clinical manifestations, usually in association with accumulation of lactic acid in the body. In such cases also, the symptoms take some time to appear, as energy supply is provided by the maternal circulation in intrauterine life. However, prenatal abnormalities (malformations or clastic brain damage) may be found in some patients (Chapter 3), indicating that protection of the fetus may not be complete.

CLINICAL MANIFESTATIONS

Neurological deterioration manifesting after a symptom-free period of a few hours to a few days, often following the first feeds, occurs in newborn infants with disorders of intermediary metabolism that result in production of toxic metabolites. The first symptoms are often poor sucking followed by vomiting and marked disturbances of consciousness with lethargy, stupor and coma, and by abnormal muscular tone and movements. Profound hypotonia is most frequent but hypertonia with episodes of opisthotonus may occur, especially in leucinosis. Abnormal movements such as tremor, jitteriness, and boxing or pedalling movements may be a prominent feature. They are often loosely designated as seizures. However, true epileptic seizures with concomitant EEG paroxysmal activity are infrequent and seem to supervene more frequently in diseases of the ammonia cycle than in disorders of amino acid or organic acid metabolism (Aicardi 1992), with the notable exception of nonketotic hyperglycinaemia. Ophthalmoplegia may be seen in occasional patients (MacDonald and Sher 1977). Neurological deterioration is accompanied by systemic disturbances, including respiratory distress and tachypnoea, poor feeding, and vomiting. This *acute metabolic distress* is variably associated with ketoacidosis, hyperammonaemia or lactic acidosis, depending on its cause. Ketotic hyperglycinaemia, a combination of ketoacidosis and hyperglycinaemia, often associated with hyperammonaemia, neutropenia and thrombocytopenia, may occur secondary to the organic acidaemias and mimic sepsis. However, disturbances of energy metabolism may present in the same manner.

Nonketotic hyperglycinaemia has a distinctive clinical and EEG picture (Scher *et al.* 1986) with myoclonus and a suppression–burst EEG pattern (Chapters 9, 16). A transient form manifested by seizures and resolving spontaneously in less than six weeks has been described (Schiffmann *et al.* 1989).

Diseases interfering with the energy supply often present in a less suggestive manner and often without a free interval. Severe hypotonia is a common feature in association with progressive neurological deterioration, and cardiac failure, an enlarged liver or signs of hepatic disease are often present. Dysmorphic features are occasionally observed, indicating a prenatal onset of the disorders which can also result in visceral and brain malformations (Chapter 3).

DIAGNOSIS AND MANAGEMENT

The diagnosis of acute neonatal metabolic distress requires the exclusion of such common conditions as sepsis, meningitis and intracerebral haemorrhage. Acute cardiac distress which may be associated with neurological manifestations should also be excluded by appropriate investigations.

Metabolic investigation is best performed as a two-stage process (Saudubray *et al.* 1989, Poggi-Travert *et al.* 1995). The first stage is an emergency procedure that applies to all infants with acute neonatal distress with encephalopathic signs. Urine should be examined for reducing substances, presence of ketone bodies, pH, and presence of sulfite and keto acids by appropriate paper band tests. The presence of ketones is always abnormal in neonates. A positive DNPH (dinitrophenylhydrazine) test for keto acids is significant only in the absence of glycosuria and ketonuria. It is important to look for an abnormal smell of the urine as found in maple syrup urine disease and other organic acidurias. Blood tests include measurement of pH, lactate, ketone bodies, ammonia and organic and amino acids in addition to routine blood count and electrolytes. Lactate determination in CSF may be important for the diagnosis of disorders of energy metabolism. Results of the more rapidly available investigations should suggest the category of disorder and orientate management, even though an exact diagnosis may have to wait for several days. In all cases it is essential to store blood, urine and CSF for further, more specialized investigations.

Severe acidosis with an anion gap, mildly elevated ammonia and ketonuria favour a diagnosis of organic acidaemia.

Grossly elevated ammonia with slight acidosis suggests a urea cycle disorder, although high levels are also observed with organic acid disorders.

Hypoglycaemia and acidosis with a normal ammonia concentration and markedly elevated lactate suggest congenital lactic acidosis, even though hypoglycaemia also occurs with organic acidaemias, with disorders of fatty acid oxidation, and with disorders of carbohydrate metabolism such as fructose intolerance.

If neither hyperammonaemia nor acidosis is present, non-ketotic hyperglycinaemia is likely.

Increased lactate levels are present in multiple types of lactic acidosis, in mitochondrial diseases whether they involve pyruvate metabolism or respiratory chain enzymes, and in fructose diphosphatase deficiency, glycogenosis I and III, fructosaemia and galactosaemia.

The second stage includes more complex biochemical investigations such as mass spectroscopy of organic acids, identification of blood ketones, enzymatic assays and other specialized tests that should be performed in a referral laboratory.

The management of metabolic disorder is discussed in Chapter 9. Specific measures needed in the neonatal period include reduction of raised plasma levels of organic or amino acids, mostly by peritoneal dialysis, and in some cases general life support with assisted ventilation. Suppression of all protein feeding and vigorous measures to prevent tissue catabolism and to promote anabolism are essential. For example, an increase in body weight of 50 g corresponds to the incorporation of 1000 mg of leucine in newly formed tissue, thus clearing significant amounts from the blood and away from the brain.

CHRONIC METABOLIC DISORDERS IN THE NEONATAL PERIOD

These conditions are described in Chapter 9. It is important to realize that a few inherited metabolic diseases can manifest clinically at birth, in particular peroxisomal diseases (Stephenson 1988). Zellweger syndrome, neonatal adrenoleukodystrophy and related disorders are characterized from birth by extreme hypotonia, dysmorphism, skeletal anormalities and areflexia, that may simulate neuromuscular disorders.

CIRCULATORY DISORDERS IN THE NEONATAL PERIOD

Outside the cerebrovascular accidents described earlier in this chapter, or those related to neonatal intracranial infections, disorders of blood circulation are rare in the neonatal period. *Venous thromboses* are described in more detail in Chapter 15. Cases in newborn infants may present as neonatal sepsis (Wong *et al.* 1987). Thrombosis of the transverse sinus (Baram *et al.* 1988) or of the superior sagittal sinus (Konishi *et al.* 1987) can present with signs of raised intracranial pressure, seizures and intracranial haemorrhage. Although the outcome of most reported cases has been severe, more benign variants have been recognized with the help of modern imaging techniques. MRI is especially useful by showing absence of normal flow void within sinuses, the thrombus appearing hyperintense on both T_1- and T_2-weighted sequences (Baram *et al.* 1988, Rivkin *et al.* 1992).

Polycythaemia is present in around 1.5 per cent of newborn infants (Wiswell *et al.* 1986). About 85 per cent of affected infants have some clinical manifestations, including seizures and various and usually transient features such as jitteriness and focal deficits. Neurological sequelae have been reported (Delaney-Black *et al.* 1989) but are probably rare. Polycythaemia is the main cause of the hyperviscosity syndrome which is frequently present in infants who are small for gestional age (Wiswell *et al.* 1986).

NEONATAL HYPOTONIA AND HYPERTONIA

Neuromuscular diseases are described in Chapters 20–22. This section mentions only some peculiarities of neuromuscular disorders evident during the neonatal period.

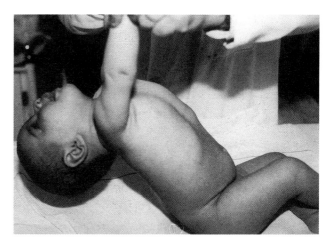

Fig. 2.13. 3-month-old infant with marked hypotonia not due to peripheral neuromuscular involvement.

HYPOTONIA

Hypotonia is one of the most frequent neurological signs in newborn babies. Its main causes are shown in Table 2.3. A majority of hypotonic neonates have *disorders of the CNS* (Fig. 2.13). In such cases, hypotonia is not accompanied by paralysis and there are usually other signs of CNS involvement such as lethargy, swallowing difficulties and abnormal primary reflexes. Such a picture obtains in HIE and in acute neonatal distress of metabolic or infectious origin. *Peripheral causes* of neonatal hypotonia generally produce some degree of paralysis and often respiratory and swallowing difficulties. In pure cases of peripheral hypotonia such as Werdnig–Hoffmann disease, the infants are alert and their behaviour is normal. However, in several situations such as neonatal myotonic dystrophy or the Prader–Willi syndrome, there is a mixture of central and peripheral involvement (Wharton and Bresnan 1989). *Neonatal myasthenia gravis* (Chapter 22), which occurs in the offspring of myasthenic mothers, should be thought of in all cases of neonatal hypotonia. Facial diplegia, ptosis and ophthalmoplegia are present in many but not all cases. Respiratory failure may result in death if no treatment is provided (Papazian 1992). Recovery occurs in three to four weeks. However, recovery may be delayed in some patients, necessitating prolongation of therapy for several months (Eymard *et al.* 1989). The diagnosis is easy when there is a clear-cut history or symptoms of maternal myasthenia. This is not always the case, and an edrophonium test is indicated whenever the possibility of congenital myasthenia is entertained. The test may be difficult to interpret, however, and demonstration of a decremental response to repetitive electrical stimulation may be more reliable in some cases (Hays and Michaud 1988).

The diagnosis of neonatal hypotonia also includes *hypotonia resulting from the administration of drugs to the mother*, especially diazepam (Laegreid *et al.* 1987). Inadvertent *injection of local anaesthetics* into the baby's scalp at the time of paracervical, pudendal or epidural block can produce a characteristic syndrome featuring hypotonia, respiratory depression and seizures on the

TABLE 2.3
Main causes of generalized hypotonia in the newborn infant

Site of major pathology	Disorder	Reference
Anterior horn cell	Werdnig–Hoffmann disease	Chapter 20
	Other anterior horn cell disease (in association with cerebellar atrophy)	Chapter 10
Peripheral nerves or roots	Congenital polyneuropathies (several types)	Chapter 21
Muscle	Congenital muscular dystrophy (several types including Fukuyama type and 'occidental' types with and without merosine deficiency)	Chapter 22
	Congenital myotonic dystrophy	
	Congenital myopathies	
	• Central core disease	
	• Centronuclear myopathy	
	• Nemaline myopathy	
	• Congenital fibre type disproportion	
	• Other structural myopathies	
	Glycogen storage disease types II and III	
	Mitochondrial myopathies (deficit in cytochrome c oxidase)	
	• Severe type	
	• Transient type	
Neuromuscular junction	Neonatal myasthenia (infants of myasthenic mothers)	Chapter 22
	Congenital myasthenia and myasthenic syndromes (several types)	
	Infantile botulism	Chapter 11
Central nervous system	Hypoxic–ischaemic encephalopathy	Chapters 2, 3, 9
	Brain malformations (including trisomy 21)	
	Haemorrhagic and other brain damage	
	Drug intoxication	Chapter 2
Mixed origin (mainly central nervous system)	Zellweger syndrome and related peroxisomal disorders	Chapters 4, 9
	Prader–Willi syndrome	Chapter 4
	Hypothyroidism	Chapter 23
Connective tissue abnormality	Marfan syndrome	Chapter 22
	Ehlers–Danlos syndrome	

first day of life. The prognosis is favourable if prompt supportive treatment is supplied (Volpe 1995).

HYPERTONIA

Hypertonia is rarely observed in the neonatal period outside acute neurological diseases such as HIE or kernicterus. *Hyperekplexia* or the 'stiff baby syndrome' (Tohier *et al.* 1991) is described in Chapter 17. Exceptionally, absence of the pyramidal tract results in markedly increased extensor tone (Roessmann *et al.* 1990). Some infants have an increased muscle tone with brisk tendon reflexes and a particularly intense Moro response in the absence of other obvious abnormality. Most develop normally but residual disability has been observed at follow-up in some of these infants (PeBenito *et al.* 1989). Such infants often have intense and long-lasting tremors and jitteriness (Parker *et al.* 1990, Kramer *et al.* 1994).

INFECTIOUS DISEASES IN THE NEONATAL PERIOD

Infections of the CNS and meninges are discussed in Chapter 11. Only a few general remarks about perinatally or postnatally acquired neonatal infections are provided here.

BACTERIAL INFECTIONS

These are suspected by clinicians more often than viral infections (see below) and are certainly of major importance though relatively uncommon. The majority are maternally transmitted, most often as ascending infection from the vagina, more rarely transplacentally. Their occurrence may be favoured by such factors as acute fetal distress, prolonged rupture of membranes, chorioamnionitis and preterm birth (Minkoff *et al.* 1984). The most common infecting organisms are group B streptococcus, *Escherichia coli* and *Listeria monocytogenes*, whose proliferation appears to be facilitated by the immature immunological defences of the newborn infant (Volpe 1995). Infection occurring later in the neonatal period may be due to nosocomial contamination by group B streptococcus (Davies and Rudd 1994), staphylococci, or hydrophilic gram-negative organisms that are occasionally found in the equipment of neonatal intensive care units, such as *Proteus* spp., *Serratia marcescens*, *Flavobacterium meningosepticum* and *Citrobacter* spp. (Klein *et al.* 1986).

VIRAL INFECTIONS

Viral infections are still diagnosed less frequently than the bacterial variety because they are less often considered. They only rarely involve the meninges and CNS in the newborn infant.

Coxsackie A and B viruses have been identified as being responsible for meningoencephalitis (Kaplan *et al.* 1983, Modlin 1986) and myocarditis. Echovirus infection may be more common but meningitis is rare (Morens 1978). A few cases of encephalitis are on record (Philip and Larson 1973; Chapter 11). Neonatal *herpes simplex encephalitis* is most often due to type 2 herpes virus, the organism usually being acquired during passage through the birth canal, although transplacental infection can also occur. When a maternal cervical lesion is present, delivery should be by caesarian section and prophylactic treatment with acyclovir is indicated. The disease is marked by lethargy and seizures with a severe course and sequelae. Skin vesicles may be present on the scalp and are of great diagnostic value. The disease is disseminated, affecting liver, kidney and retina (Chalhub *et al.* 1977). A remarkable periodic EEG pattern is often present (Mizrahi and Tharp 1982). The outcome is poor. Death or severe sequelae occur in most cases (Whitley *et al.* 1980).

SKULL FRACTURE, CEPHALHAEMATOMA AND OTHER CONSEQUENCES OF MECHANICAL SKULL TRAUMA

EXTRACRANIAL HAEMORRHAGE
Extracranial haemorrhage can be located between bone and periosteum (cephalhaematoma), or between periosteum and the aponeurosis covering the scalp (subgaleal haemorrhage), or above the aponeurosis (caput succedaneum). *Cephalhaematoma* occurs in 1–2 per cent of spontaneous births and is more frequent with mid-forceps and vacuum extraction deliveries (Govaert 1993, Volpe 1995). The haematoma is limited by the attachment of the periosteum to the periphery of bone, usually the parietal, rarely the occipital squama. The lesion is firm and tense. The elevated periosteum is palpable at the margin of bone, and may give the impression that there is a bony defect or a depressed fracture. In the rare occipital location, the haematoma can superficially resemble an encephalocele. Skull X-rays show an underlying linear fracture in up to 25 per cent of cases (Volpe 1995). The lesion spontaneously disappears in a few weeks or months. On late X-rays it may produce pseudolacunar images. Cephalhaematomas should not be tapped or evacuated as they disappear spontaneously and these manoeuvres imply a risk of infection.

Subgaleal haemorrhages are not limited to a single bone. The blood may spread beneath the entire scalp and even dissect into tissues of the neck, forehead and eyelids. It often occurs as a consequence of vacuum extraction (Govaert *et al.* 1992c). Coagulation defects, especially vitamin K deficiency, are a frequent complicating factor. When present, the lesion tends to increase in size during the first two to three days and may reach massive proportions with consequent acute anaemia and hyperbilirubinaemia (Govaert *et al.* 1992c, Govaert 1993). Subgaleal haemorrhage (also wrongly termed giant cephalhaematoma) may constitute a vital emergency requiring urgent transfusion. Vitamin K prophylaxis should prevent extensive lesions.

Caput succedaneum is of no pathological significance.

SKULL FRACTURES
Linear fractures of the skull are not rare in newborn babies. They are seldom associated with intracranial pathology and are therefore of limited significance and require no treatment. Depressed skull fracture (the so-called 'ping-pong lesion') usually involves the parietal bones. Palpation shows a localized depression but neurological complications rarely if ever occur. Surgical elevation is the classical treatment but spontaneous correction or elevation by other means such as breast pumps may be effective (Loeser *et al.* 1976). *Growing syndesmosal rupture* is caused by tear of the connective tissue bridges between individual skull bones and bone erosion by pulsatile arachnoid tissue (Govaert 1993). I have observed two babies with tears of the coronal suture associated with underlying cavitation of the brain of the type associated with growing skull fractures (Chapter 13). Occipital osteodiastasis with consequent contusion of the cerebellum is now rarely observed (Pape and Wigglesworth 1979).

NEONATAL DISORDERS OF THE SPINAL CORD

SPINAL CORD INJURY
Injury to the spinal cord is still observed in the newborn infant (Gould and Smith 1984). The frequency is difficult to evaluate. Towbin (1969) found cord lesions in over 10 per cent of all newborn necropsies. This figure is certainly much too high and may be due to inclusion of extreme congestion or haemorrhagic appearance of the epidural adipose tissue, which is a common finding (Friede 1989). Most lesions involve either the lower cervical and upper thoracic cord with breech delivery or the upper cervical region with cephalic presentation (MacKinnon *et al.* 1993). Vertebral lesions are uncommon. There may be laceration of the meninges and severe destruction of the cord, leaving it severely attenuated with gliosis, cavitation and destruction of tracts or cells that may affect the whole cord or part of it. Secondary necrosis due to circulatory disturbances has been observed (Adams *et al.* 1988a).

Cord injury occurs mostly in breech deliveries and mid-forceps extractions. Excessive longitudinal traction or rotation are the major mechanisms. Hyperextension of the fetal head is an important factor. When detected prenatally, caesarian section is indicated and usually avoids cord damage. Caterini *et al.* (1975) found that 15 of 73 babies with hyperextension of the head in breech presentation delivered vaginally died or had severe cord injury, whereas none of 35 such infants delivered by caesarian section had such problems. However, a few cases are on record of paraplegia following fetal neck hyperextension in infants born by caesarian section (Maekawa *et al.* 1976, Weinstein *et al.* 1983). In such cases, the lesion is prenatal and probably due to vascular insufficiency as a consequence of stretching of spinal vessels (Young *et al.* 1983).

The clinical manifestations are variable. Rapid death from respiratory failure may occur. The most common picture consists of *paraplegia* with massive hypotonia that may mimic a neuromuscular disorder and may be accompanied by paradoxical respiratory movements and respiratory insufficiency. The abdomen is soft and bulging, and the bladder is distended and empties with gentle suprapubic pressure. However, pyramidal tract signs are present (sometimes only secondarily) and a sensory level is detectable. The upper limbs may be affected, especially the lower roots of the brachial plexus. Hypotonia may persist or evolve into spasticity. The diagnosis is not always easy (Rehan and Seshia 1993), as extrinsic compression and congenital tumours, neuromuscular diseases and spinal cord necrosis secondary to intraarterial umbilical catheters (Muñoz *et al.* 1993) may present with similar symptoms. Somatosensory evoked potentials may help determine an equivocal sensory deficit (Bell and Dykstra 1985). Imaging of the cord confirms the diagnosis and allows a precise evaluation. Ultrasonography does not require transport of the infant and shows most lesions (Babyn *et al.* 1988, MacKinnon *et al.* 1993). MRI provides the best resolution (Lanska *et al.* 1990, Minami *et al.* 1994) and is clearly superior to CT myelography with metrizamide (Adams *et al.* 1988a).

The prognosis is poor with persistence of the deficits and occurrence of respiratory or urinary complications (De Léon *et al.* 1995). In occasional cases, more limited lesions may be responsible for suspended neurological signs with only mild spasticity of lower limbs. Such cases may evolve into true syringomyelia (Yamano *et al.* 1992). As no treatment is effective, emphasis must be placed on prevention. Patients with paraplegia should be meticulously taken care of and rehabilitated. Methylprednisolone treatment, as given with encouraging results to adults with spinal trauma (Bracken *et al.* 1992), has not been tried in neonates to the best of my knowledge.

A few cases are on record of probable *early prenatal damage to the spinal cord*, possibly of vascular origin. The extent of damage was variable from agenesis of the whole cord (Karpati *et al.* 1986) to segmental lesions usually in the cervical region (Darwish *et al.* 1981). Ramesh *et al.* (1989) have described segmental narrowing of the dorsal cord in association with vertebral abnormalities and congenital paraplegia which they attributed to an early insult to the developing spinal cord and vertebrae. Bode *et al.* (1994) reported congenital hypoplasia of the medulla oblongata.

SPINAL CORD INFARCTION
Spinal cord infarction following catheterization of the umbilical artery (very seldom the umbilical vein), with or without injection of drugs or fluids, is a rare but dramatic event (Muñoz *et al.* 1993), probably related to progressive thrombosis or spasm involving the main branch of the anterior spinal artery. A similar accident has been reported following inadvertent intraarterial injection of viscid material during intramuscular injection. Nontraumatic intramedullary haemorrhage has been recorded (Mutoh *et al.* 1989, De Léon *et al.* 1995).

INJURY TO NERVES, PLEXUSES AND ROOTS

Brachial plexus injury, the most common peripheral nerve injury in the neonatal period, is discussed in Chapter 21. Other injuries

to nerves, also described in Chapter 21, are rare in the neonatal period. A typical example is injury to the median nerve as a result of attempts at catheterization of the radial or humeral artery at the wrist or elbow for blood gas monitoring (Pape *et al.* 1978). Other examples are injury to the radial nerve as a result of subcutaneous fat necrosis of the upper arm (Lightwood 1951, Koenigsberger and Moessinger 1977) and laryngeal nerve palsy, probably related to abnormal intrauterine posture with rotation and lateral flexion of the head, causing the thyroid cartilage to compress the superior branch of the nerve against the thyroid bone, and the recurrent nerve against the cricoid cartilage (Chapple 1956). Palsy in the territory of the right laryngeal nerve has been reported following extracorporeal membrane oxygenation in neonates with severe respiratory distress (Schumacher *et al.* 1989).

Diaphragmatic paralysis is associated with brachial plexus injury in 80–90 per cent of cases. When isolated, its diagnosis as a cause of neonatal respiratory distress is made by chest X-rays showing elevation of one or both hemidiaphragms (Alvord *et al.* 1990). Artificial ventilation is often required, and plication of the diaphragm is later indicated.

REFERENCES

Abman, S.H., Warady, B.A., Lum, G.M., Koops, B.L. (1984) 'Systemic hypertension in infants with bronchopulmonary dysplasia.' *Journal of Pediatrics*, **104**, 928–931.

Adams, C., Babyn, P.S., Logan, W.J. (1988a) 'Spinal cord birth injury: value of computed tomographic myelography.' *Pediatric Neurology*, **4**, 105–109.

—— Hochhauser, L., Logan, W.J. (1988b) 'Primary thalamic and caudate hemorrhage in term neonates presenting with seizures.' *Pediatric Neurology*, **4**, 175–177.

Adsett, D.B., Fitz, C.R., Hill, A. (1985) 'Hypoxic–ischaemic cerebral injury in the term newborn: correlation of CT findings with neurological outcome.' *Developmental Medicine and Child Neurology*, **27**, 155–160.

Ahdab-Barmada, M., Moossy, J. (1984) 'The neuropathology of kernicterus in the premature neonate: diagnostic problems.' *Journal of Neuropathology and Experimental Neurology*, **43**, 45–56.

—— —— Painter, M. (1980) 'Pontosubicular necrosis and hyperoxemia.' *Pediatrics*, **66**, 840–847.

Aicardi J. (1992) 'Epilepsy and inborn errors of metabolism.' *In*: Roger, J., Bureau, M., Dravet, C., *et al.* (Eds.) *Epileptic Syndromes in Infancy, Childhood and Adolescence. 2nd Edn.* London: John Libbey, pp. 97–102.

Alps, B.J., Hass, W.K. (1987) 'The potential beneficial effect of nicardipine in a rat model of transient forebrain ischemia.' *Neurology*, **37**, 809–814.

Altman, D.I., Perlman, J.M., Volpe, J.J., Powers, W.J. (1993) 'Cerebral oxygen metabolism in newborns.' *Pediatrics*, **92**, 99–104.

Alvord, E.C., Austin, E.J., Larson, C.P. (1990) 'Neuropathologic observations in congenital phrenic nerve palsy.' *Journal of Child Neurology*, **5**, 205–209.

Amato, M., Fauchere, J.C., Von Muralt, G. (1987) 'Relationship between periventricular–intraventricular hemorrhage and neonatal hyperbilirubinemia in very low birth weight infants.' *American Journal of Perinatology*, **4**, 275–278.

—— Hermann, V. (1988) 'Coagulation abnormalities in low birth weight infants with periventricular hemorrhage.' *Neuropediatrics*, **19**, 154–157.

—— Hüppi, P., Markus, D., Herschkowitz, N. (1991) 'Neurological function of immature babies after surfactant replacement therapy.' *Neuropediatrics*, **22**, 43–44.

American Academy of Pediatrics, American College of Obstetricians and Gynecologists (1992) 'Relationship between perinatal factors and neurologic outcome.' *In:* Poland, R.L., Freeman, R.K. (Eds.) *Guidelines for Perinatal Care, 3rd Edn.* Elk Grove Village, IL: American Academy of Pediatrics, pp. 221–224.

Amiel-Tison, C., Korobkin, R., Esque-Vaucouloux, M.T. (1977) 'Neck extensor hypertonia: a clinical sign of insult to the central nervous system of the newborn.' *Early Human Development*, **1**,181–190.

Anand, S.K., Sandborg, C., Robinson, R.G., Lieberman, E. (1980) 'Neonatal hypernatremia associated with elevated sodium concentration in breast milk.' J*ournal of Pediatrics,* **96**, 66–68.

Anderson, J.M., Milner, R.D.G., Strich, S.J. (1967) 'Effects of neonatal hypoglycaemia on the nervous system: a pathological study.' *Journal of Neurology, Neurosurgery, and Psychiatry*, **30**, 295–310.

Ansari, M.Q., Chincanchan, C.A., Armstrong, D.L. (1990) 'Brain calcification in hypoxic–ischemic lesions: an autopsy review.' *Pediatric Neurology*, **6**, 94–101.

Anthony, M.Y., Levene, M.I. (1990) 'An assessment of the benefits of intrapartum fetal monitoring.' *Developmental Medicine and Child Neurology*, **32**, 547–553.

Aoki, N. (1990) 'Epidural haematoma in newborn infants: therapeutic consequences from the correlation between haematoma content and computed tomography features.' *Acta Neurochirurgica*, **106**, 65–67.

Appleton, R.E., Lee, R.E.J., Hey, E.N. (1990) 'Neurodevelopmental outcome of transient neonatal intracerebral echodensities.' *Archives of Disease in Childhood*, **65**, 27–29.

Armstrong, D.L., Sauls, C.D., Goddard-Finegold, J. (1987) 'Neuropathologic findings in short-term survivors of intraventricular hemorrhage.' *American Journal of Diseases of Children*, **141**, 617–621.

Aylward, G.P., Verhulst, S.J., Bell, S. (1989) 'Correlation of asphyxia and other risk factors with outcome: a contemporary view.' *Developmental Medicine and Child Neurology*, **31**, 329–340.

Babyn, P.S., Chuang, S.H., Daneman, A., Davidson, G.S. (1988) 'Sonographic evaluation of spinal cord birth trauma with pathologic correlation.' *American Journal of Roentgenology*, **151**, 763–766.

Bada, H.S., Korones, S.B, Perry, E.H., *et al.* (1990) 'Mean arterial blood pressure changes in premature infants and those at risk for ventricular hemorrhage.' *Journal of Pediatrics*, **117**, 607–614.

Baerts, W., Fetter, W.P.F., Hop, W.C.J., *et al.* (1990) 'Cerebral lesions in preterm infants after tocolytic indomethacin.' *Developmental Medicine and Child Neurology*, **32**, 910–918.

Bandstra, E.S., Montalvo, B.M., Goldberg, R.N., *et al.* (1988) 'Prophylactic indomethacin for prevention of intraventricular hemorrhage in premature infants.' *Pediatrics*, **82**, 533–542.

Barabas, R.E., Barmada, M.A., Scher, M.S. (1993) 'Timing of brain insults in severe neonatal encephalopathies with isoelectric EEG.' *Pediatric Neurology*, **9**, 39–44.

Baram, T.Z., Butler, I.J., Nelson, M.D., McArdle, C.B. (1988) 'Transverse sinus thrombosis in newborns: clinical and magnetic resonance imaging findings.' *Annals of Neurology*, **24**, 792–794.

Barkovich, A.J. (1992) 'MR and CT evaluation of profound neonatal and infantile asphyxia.' *American Journal of Neuroradiology*, **13**, 959–972.

Barth, P.G. (1984) 'Prenatal clastic encephalopathies.' *Clinical Neurology and Neurosurgery*, **86**, 65–75.

Bax, M., Nelson, K.B. (1993) 'Birth asphyxia: a statement.' *Developmental Medicine and Child Neurology*, **35**, 1022–1024.

Bedard, M.P., Shankaran, S., Slovis, T.L., *et al.* (1984) 'Effect of prophylactic phenobarbital on intraventricular hemorrhage in high-risk infants.' *Pediatrics*, **73**, 435–439.

Bell, H.J., Dykstra, D.D. (1985) 'Somatosensory evoked potentials as an adjunct to diagnosis of neonatal spinal cord injury.' *Journal of Pediatrics*, **106**, 298–301.

Benson, J.W.T., Hayward, C., Osborne, J.P. (1986) 'Multicentre trial of ethamsylate for prevention of periventricular haemorrhage in very low birthweight infants.' *Lancet*, **1**, 1297–1300.

Blazer, S., Hemli, J.A., Sujov, P.O., Braun, J. (1989) 'Neonatal bilateral diaphragmatic paralysis caused by brain stem haemorrhage.' *Archives of Disease in Childhood*, **64**, 50–52.

Bode, H., Bubl, R., Rutishauser, M., Nars, P.W. (1994) 'Congenital tetraplegia, respiratory insufficiency, and hypoplasia of medulla oblongata.' *Pediatric Neurology*, **10**, 161–163.

Boulloche, J., Mallet, E., De Menibus, C.H. (1987) 'Hypoglycémie néonatale par hyperinsulinisme et épilepsie ultérieure.' *Archives Françaises de Pédiatrie*, **44**, 85–89.

Bouza, H., Dubowitz, L.M.S., Rutherford, M., *et al.* (1994) 'Late magnetic resonance imaging and clinical findings in neonates with unilateral lesions on cranial ultrasound.' *Developmental Medicine and Child Neurology*, **36**, 951–964.

Bracken, M.B., Shepard, M.J., Collins, W.F., *et al.* (1992) 'Methylprednisolone or naloxone treatment after acute spinal cord injury: 1-year follow-up data.' *Journal of Neurosurgery*, **76**, 23–31.

Bratlid, D., Cashore, W.J., Oh, W. (1983) 'Effect of serum hyperosmolality on opening of blood–brain barrier for bilirubin in rat brain.' *Pediatrics*, **71**, 909–912.

Brown, A.K., Kim, M.H., Wu, P.Y.K., Bryla, D.A. (1985) 'Efficacy of photo-therapy in prevention and management of neonatal hyperbilirubinemia.' *Pediatrics*, **75** (Suppl.), 393–400.

Bulas, D.I., Taylor, G.A., Fitz, C.R., *et al.* (1991) 'Posterior fossa intracranial hemorrhage in infants treated with extracorporeal membrane oxygenation: sonographic findings.' *American Journal of Roentgenology*, **156**, 571–575.

Byrne, P., Welch, R., Johnson, M.A., *et al.* (1990) 'Serial magnetic resonance imaging in neonatal hypoxic–ischemic encephalopathy.' *Journal of Pediatrics*, **117**, 694–700.

Cabañas, F., Pellicer, A., Morales, C., *et al.* (1994) 'New pattern of hyperechogenicity in thalamus and basal ganglia studied by color Doppler flow imaging.' *Pediatric Neurology*, **10**, 109–116.

Calvert, S.A., Hopkins, E.M., Fong, K.W., Forsyth, S.C. (1987) 'Etiological factors associated with the development of periventricular leukomalacia.' *Acta Paediatrica Scandinavica*, **76**, 254–259.

Campistol, J., Pires, M., Poo, P., Iriondo, M. (1994) 'Hemorragia talámica e intraventricular en el recién nacido a término.' *Revista Neurologia*, **22**, 673–675.

Caterini, H., Langer, A., Sama, J.C., *et al.* (1975) 'Fetal risk in hyperextension of the fetal head in breech presentation.' *American Journal of Obstetrics and Gynecology*, **123**, 632–636.

Catto-Smith, A.G., Yu, V.Y.H., Bajuk, B., *et al.* (1985) 'Effect of neonatal periventricular haemorrhage on neurodevelopmental outcome.' *Archives of Disease in Childhood*, **60**, 8–11.

Chalhub, E.G., Baenziger, J., Feigen, R.D., *et al.* (1977) 'Congenital herpes simplex type II infection with extensive hepatic calcifications, bone lesions and cataracts: complete postmortem examination.' *Developmental Medicine and Child Neurology*, **19**, 527–534.

Changaris, D.G., Purohit, D.M., Balentine, J.D., *et al.* (1984) 'Brain calcification in severely stressed neonates receiving parenteral calcium.' *Journal of Pediatrics*, **104**, 941–946.

Chaplin, E.R., Goldstein, G.W., Norman, D. (1979) 'Neonatal seizures, intracerebral hematoma and subarachnoid hemorrhage in full-term infants.' *Pediatrics*, **63**, 812–815.

Chapple, C.C. (1956) 'A duosyndrome of the laryngeal nerve.' *American Journal of Diseases of Children*, **91**, 14–18.

Chin, K.C., Taylor, M.J., Perlman, M. (1985) 'Improvement in auditory and visual evoked potentials in jaundiced preterm infants after exchange transfusion.' *Archives of Disease in Childhood*, **60**, 714–717.

Choux, M., Grisoli, F., Peragut, J.C. (1975) 'Extradural hematomas in children.' *Child's Brain*, **1**, 337–347.

Christensen, E., Melchior, J. (1967) *Cerebral Palsy. A Clinical and Neuropathological Study. Clinics in Developmental Medicine No. 25.* London: Spastics International Medical Publications.

Chugani, H.T. (1993) 'Positron emission tomography scanning: applications in newborns.' *Clinics in Perinatology*, **20**, 395–409.

Clancy, R.R., Tharp, B.R. (1984) 'Positive rolandic sharp waves in the electroencephalograms of premature neonates with intraventricular hemorrhage.' *Electroencephalography and Clinical Neurophysiology*, **57**, 395–404.

—— Sladky, J.T., Rorke, L.B. (1989) 'Hypoxic–ischemic spinal cord injury following perinatal asphyxia.' *Annals of Neurology*, **25**, 185–189.

Cockburn, F., Brown, J.K., Belton, N.R., Forfar, J.O. (1973) 'Neonatal convulsions associated with primary disturbance of calcium, phosphorus and magnesium metabolism.' *Archives of Disease in Childhood*, **48**, 99–108.

Coker, S.B., Beltran, R.S., Myers, T.F., Hmura, L. (1988) 'Neonatal stroke: description of patients and investigation into pathogenesis.' *Pediatric Neurology*, **4**, 219–223.

Colamaria, V., Curatolo, P., Cusmai, R., Dalla Bernardina, B. (1988) 'Symmetrical bithalamic hyperdensities in asphyxiated full-term newborns: an early indicator of status marmoratus.' *Brain and Development*, **10**, 57–59.

Collins, J., Leonard, J.V. (1984) 'Hyperinsulinism in asphyxiated and small-for-dates infants with hypoglycaemia.' *Lancet*, **2**, 311–313.

Connell, J., De Vries, L., Oozeer, R., *et al.* (1988) 'Predictive value of early continuous electroencephalogram monitoring in ventilated preterm infants with intraventricular hemorrhage.' *Pediatrics*, **82**, 337–343.

Connolly, A.M., Volpe, J.J. (1990) 'Clinical features of bilirubin encephalopathy.' *Clinics in Perinatology*, **17**, 371–379.

Cooke, R.W.I. (1987) 'Early and late cranial ultrasonographic appearances and outcome in very low birthweight infants.' *Archives of Disease in Childhood*, **62**, 931–937.

Cordes, I., Roland, E.H., Lupton, B.A., Hill, A. (1994) 'Early prediction of the development of microcephaly after hypoxic–ischemic encephalopathy in the full-term newborn.' *Pediatrics*, **93**, 703–707.

Cornblath, M., Schwartz, R. (1991) *Disorders of Carbohydrate Metabolism in Infancy, 3rd Edn.* Oxford: Blackwell, pp. 225–246.

Costello, A.M.deL., Hamilton, P.A., Baudin, J., *et al.* (1988) 'Prediction of neurodevelopmental impairment at four years from brain ultrasound appearance of very preterm infants.' *Developmental Medicine and Child Neurology*, **30**, 711–722.

Cowan, F.M., Pennock, J.M., Hanrahan, J.D., *et al.* (1994) 'Early detection of cerebral infarction and hypoxic–ischemic encephalopathy in neonates using diffusion-weighted magnetic resonance imaging.' *Neuropediatrics*, **25**, 172–175.

Cross, J.H., Harrison, C.J., Preston, P.R., *et al.* (1992) 'Postnatal encephaloclastic porencephaly—a new lesion.' *Archives of Disease in Childhood*, **67**, 307–311.

Dambska, M., Laure-Kamionowska, M., Liebhart, M. (1987) 'Brainstem lesions in the course of chronic fetal asphyxia.' *Clinical Neuropathology*, **6**, 110–115.

—— —— Schmidt-Sidor, B. (1989) 'Early and late neuropathological changes in perinatal white matter damage.' *Journal of Child Neurology*, **4**, 291–298.

Dammann, O., Leviton, A. (1997) 'Duration of transient hyperechoic images of white matter in very-low-birthweight infants: a proposed classification.' *Developmental Medicine and Child Neurology*, **39**, 2–5.

Darwish, H., Sarnat, H., Archer, C., *et al.* (1981) 'Congenital cervical spinal atrophy.' *Muscle and Nerve*, **4**, 106–110.

Dave, P., Curless, R.G., Steinman, L. (1984) 'Cerebellar hemorrhage complicating methylmalonic and propionic acidemia.' *Archives of Neurology*, **41**, 1293–1296.

Davies, P.A., Rudd, P.T. (1994) *Neonatal Meningitis. Clinics in Developmental Medicine No. 132.* London: Mac Keith Press.

Dawson, T.M., Dawson, V.L., Snyder, S.H. (1992) 'A novel neuronal messenger molecule in brain: the free radical, nitric oxide.' *Annals of Neurology*, **32**, 297–311.

De Campo, M. (1989) 'Neonatal posterior fossa haemorrhage: a difficult ultrasound diagnosis.' *Australasian Radiology*, **33**, 150–153.

Delaney-Black, V., Camp, B.W., Lubchenco, L.O., *et al.* (1989) 'Neonatal hyperviscosity association with lower achievement and IQ scores at school age.' *Pediatrics*, **83**, 662–667.

de Léon, G.A., Radkowski, M.A., Crawford, S.E., *et al.* (1995) 'Persistent respiratory failure due to low cervical cord infarction in newborn babies.' *Journal of Child Neurology*, **10**, 200–204.

Deliac, P., Demarquez, J.L., Barberot, J.P., *et al.* (1990) 'Brainstem auditory evoked potentials in icteric fullterm newborns: alterations after exchange transfusion.' *Neuropediatrics*, **21**, 115–118.

Deonna, T., Oberson, R. (1974) 'Acute subdural hematoma of the newborn.' *Neuropädiatrie*, **5**, 181–190.

Deonna, T., Prod'hom, L-S. (1980) 'Temporal lobe epilepsy and hemianopsia in childhood of perinatal origin. An overlooked and potentially treatable disease? Report of two cases, one with a demonstrable etiology.' *Neuropädiatrie*, **11**, 85–90.

De Reuck, J., Chattha, A.S., Richardson, E.P. (1972) 'Pathogenesis and evolution of periventricular leukomalacia.' *Archives of Neurology*, **27**, 229–231.

De Vivo, D.C., Trifiletti, R.R., Jacobson, R.I., *et al.* (1991) 'Defective glucose transport across the blood–brain barrier as a cause of persistent hypoglycorrhachia, seizures, and developmental delay.' *New England Journal of Medicine*, **325**, 703–709.

De Vries, L.S., Lary, S., Dubowitz, L.M.S. (1985) 'Relationship of serum bilirubin levels to ototoxicity and deafness in high-risk low-birthweight infants.' *Pediatrics*, **76**, 351–354.

—— Regev, R., Dubowitz, L.M.S. (1986) 'Late onset cystic leucomalacia.' *Archives of Disease in Childhood*, **61**, 298–299.

—— Connell, J.A., Dubowitz, L.M.S., *et al.* (1987) 'Neurological, electrophysiological and MRI abnormalities in infants with extensive cystic leukomalacia.' *Neuropediatrics*, **18**, 61–66.

—— Smet, M., Goemans, N., *et al.* (1992) 'Unilateral thalamic haemorrhage in the pre-term and full-term newborn.' *Neuropediatrics*, **23**, 153–156.

—— Eken, P., Groenendaal, F., *et al.* (1993) 'Correlation between the degree of periventricular leukomalacia diagnosed using cranial ultrasound and MRI later in infancy in children with cerebral palsy.' *Neuropediatrics*, **24**, 263–268.

Dijxhoorn, M.J., Visser, G.H.A., Huisjes, H.J., *et al.* (1985) 'The relation between umbilical pH values and neonatal neurological morbidity in full-term appropriate for dates infants.' *Early Human Development*, **11**, 32–42.

DiMario, F.J., Clancy, R. (1989) 'Symmetrical thalamic degeneration with calcification of infancy.' *American Journal of Diseases of Children*, **143**, 1056–1060.

Donn, S.M., Barr, M., McLeary, R.D. (1984) 'Massive intracerebral hemorrhage in utero: sonographic appearance and pathologic correlation.' *Obstetrics and Gynecology*, **63**, 28S–30S.

Dreyfus-Brisac, C. (1979) 'Neonatal electroencephalography.' *In:* Scarpelli, E., Cosmi, E. (Eds.) *Reviews of Perinatal Medicine, Vol. 3.* New York: Raven Press, pp. 1397–1472.

Dubowitz, L.M.S., Bydder, G.M., Mushin, J. (1985) 'Development sequence of periventricular leucomalacia.' *Archives of Disease in Childhood*, **60**, 349–355.

Eken, P., Toet, M.C., Groenendaal, F., de Vries, L.S. (1995) 'Predictive value of early neuroimaging, pulsed Doppler and neurophysiology in fullterm infants with hypoxic–ischaemic encephalopathy.' *Archives of Disease in Childhood*, **73**, F75–F80.

—— de Vries, L.S., van Nieuwenhuizen, O., *et al.* (1996) 'Early predictors of cerebral visual impairment in infants with cystic leukomalacia.' *Neuropediatrics*, **27**, 16–25.

Ellenberg, J.H., Nelson, K.B. (1988) 'Cluster of perinatal events identifying infants at high risk for death or disability.' *Journal of Pediatrics*, **113**, 546–552.

Ellis, W.G., Goetzman, B.W., Lindenberg, J.A. (1988) 'Neuropathologic documentation of prenatal brain damage.' *American Journal of Diseases of Children*, **142**, 858–866.

Ellison, P.H., Farina, M.A. (1980) 'Progressive central nervous system deterioration: a complication of advanced chronic lung disease of prematurity.' *Annals of Neurology*, **8**, 43–46.

Epstein, M.F., Leviton, A., Kuban, K.C.K., *et al.* (1988) 'Bilirubin, intraventricular hemorrhage and phenobarbital in very low-birthweight babies.' *Pediatrics*, **82**, 350–354.

Erkkola, R., Grönroos, M., Pynnonen, R., Kilkku, P. (1984) 'Analysis of intrapartum fetal deaths: their decline with increasing electronic fetal monitoring.' *Acta Obstetricia et Gynecologica Scandinavica*, **63**, 459–462.

Escher-Graub, D., Fricker, H.S. (1986) 'Jaundice and behavioral organization in the full-term neonate.' *Helvetica Paediatrica Acta*, **41**, 425–435.

Escobedo, M., Barton, L.L., Volpe, J.J. (1975) 'Cerebrospinal fluid studies in an intensive care nursery.' *Journal of Perinatal Medicine*, **3**, 204–210.

Eymard, B., Morel, E., Dulac, O., *et al.* (1989) 'Myasthénie et grossesse: une étude clinique et immunologique de 42 cas.' *Revue Neurologique*, **145**, 696–701.

Fawer, C-L., Calame, A., Perentes, E., Anderegg, A. (1985) 'Periventricular leukomalacia: a correlation study between real-time ultrasound and autopsy findings.' *Neuroradiology*, **27**, 292–300.

—— Diebold, P., Calame, A. (1987) 'Periventricular leucomalacia and neurodevelopmental outcome in preterm infants.' *Archives of Disease in Childhood*, **62**, 30–36.

Fazzi, E., Lanzi, G., Gerardo, A., *et al.* (1992) 'Neurodevelopmental outcome in very-low-birth-weight infants with or without periventricular hemorrhage and/or leucomalacia.' *Acta Paediatrica*, **81**, 808–811.

Fenichel, G.M. (1983) 'Hypoxic–ischemic encephalopathy in the newborn.' *Archives of Neurology*, **40**, 261–266.

—— (1997) *Clinical Pediatric Neurology. A Signs and Symptoms Approach. 3rd Edn.* Philadelphia: W.B. Saunders.

—— Webster, D.L., Wong, K.T. (1984) 'Intracranial hemorrhage in the term newborn.' *Archives of Neurology*, **41**, 30–34.

Filipek, P.A., Krisnamoorthy, K.S., Davis, K.R., Kuehnle, K. (1987) 'Focal cerebral infarction in the newborn: a distinct entity.' *Pediatric Neurology*, **3**, 141–147.

Finer, N.N., Robertson, C.M., Peters, K.L., Coward, J.H. (1983) 'Factors affecting outcome in hypoxic–ischemic encephalopathy in term infants.' *American Journal of Diseases of Children*, **137**, 21–25.

Fish, W.H., Cohen, M., Franzek, D., *et al.* (1990) 'Effect of intramuscular vitamin E on mortality and intracranial hemorrhage in neonates of 1000 grams or less.' *Pediatrics*, **85**, 578–584.

60

Fischer, A.Q., Challa, V.R., Burton, B.K., McLean, W.T. (1981) 'Cerebellar hemorrhage complicating isovaleric acidemia: a case report.' *Neurology*, **31**, 746–748.

Fishman, M.A., Percy, A.K., Cheek, W.R., Speer, M.E. (1981) 'Successful conservative management of cerebellar hematomas in term neonates.' *Journal of Pediatrics*, **98**, 466–468.

—— Dutton, R.V., Okumura, S. (1984) 'Progressive ventriculomegaly following minor intracranial hemorrhage in premature infants.' *Developmental Medicine and Child Neurology*, **26**, 725–731.

Fitzhardinge, P.M., Flodmark, O., Fitz, C.R., Ashby, S. (1982) 'The prognostic value of computed tomography of the brain in asphyxiated premature infants.' *Journal of Pediatrics*, **100**, 476–481.

Freeman, J.M., Nelson, K.B. (1988) 'Intrapartum asphyxia and cerebral palsy.' *Pediatrics*, **82**, 240–249.

Friede, R. (1989) *Developmental Neuropathology, 2nd Edn.* Berlin: Springer.

—— Schachenmayr, W. (1977) 'Early stage of status marmoratus.' *Acta Neuropathologica*, **38**, 123–127.

Fujimoto, S., Yokochi, K., Togari, H., *et al.* (1992) 'Neonatal cerebral infarction: symptoms, CT findings and prognosis.' *Brain and Development*, **14**, 48–52.

Funato, M., Tamai, H., Noma, K., *et al.* (1992) 'Clinical events in association with timing of intraventricular hemorrhage in preterm infants.' *Journal of Pediatrics*, **121**, 614–619.

Gaffney, G., Sellers, S., Flavell, V., *et al.* (1994) 'Case–control study of intrapartum care, cerebral palsy, and perinatal death.' *British Medical Journal*, **308**, 743–750.

Gama, C.H., Fenichel, G.M. (1985) 'Epidural hematoma of the newborn due to birth trauma.' *Pediatric Neurology*, **1**, 52–53.

Garewal, G., Narang, A., Das, K.C. (1988) 'Infantile tremor syndrome: a vitamin B_{12} deficiency syndrome in infants.' *Journal of Tropical Pediatrics*, **34**, 174–178.

Gibbs, J.M., Weindling, A.M. (1994) 'Neonatal intracranial lesions following placental abruption.' *European Journal of Pediatrics*, **153**, 195–197.

Glauser, T.A., Rorke, L.B., Weinberg, P.M., Clancy, R.R. (1990) 'Acquired neuropathologic lesions associated with the hypoplastic left heart syndrome.' *Pediatrics*, **85**, 991–1000.

Goddard-Finegold, J., Mizrahi, E.M. (1987) 'Understanding and preventing perinatal, intracerebral, peri- and intraventricular hemorrhage.' *Journal of Child Neurology*, **2**, 170–185.

Goitein, K.J., Amit, Y., Mussaffi, H. (1983) 'Intracranial pressure in central nervous system infections and cerebral ischaemia in infancy.' *Archives of Disease in Childhood*, **58**, 184–186.

Goldberg, R., Moscoso, R., Bauer, C.R., *et al.* (1986) 'Use of barbiturate therapy in severe perinatal asphyxia: a randomized controlled trial.' *Journal of Pediatrics*, **109**, 851–856.

Goldstein, R.F., Thompson, R.J., Oehler, J.M., Brazy, J.E. (1995) 'Influence of acidosis, hypoxemia, and hypotension on neurodevelopmental outcome in very low birth weight infants.' *Pediatrics*, **95**, 238–243.

Gould, S.J., Smith, J.F. (1984) 'Spinal cord transection, cerebral ischemic and brainstem injury in a baby following a Kielland's forceps rotation.' *Neuropathology and Applied Neurobiology*, **10**, 151–158.

Gould, S.J., Howard, S., Hope, P.L., Reynolds, E.O.R. (1987) 'Periventricular intraparenchymal cerebral haemorrhage in preterm infants: the role of venous infarction.' *Journal of Pathology*, **151**, 197–202.

Govaert, P. (1993) *Cranial Haemorrhage in the Term Newborn Infant. Clinics in Developmental Medicine No. 129.* London: Mac Keith Press.

—— de Vries, L.S. (1997) *An Atlas of Neonatal Brain Sonography. Clinics in Developmental Medicine No. 141/142.* London: Mac Keith Press.

—— van de Velde, E., Vanhaesebrouck, P., *et al.* (1990) 'CT diagnosis of neonatal subarachnoid hemorrhage.' *Pediatric Radiology*, **20**, 139–142.

—— Achten, E., Van Haesebrouck, P., *et al.* (1992a) 'Deep cerebral venous thrombosis in thalamo-ventricular haemorrhage of the term newborn.' *Pediatric Radiology*, **22**, 123–127.

—— Vanhaesebrouck, P., de Praeter, C. (1992b) 'Traumatic neonatal intracranial bleeding and stroke.' *Archives of Disease in Childhood*, **67**, 840–845.

—— —— —— *et al.* (1992c) 'Vacuum extraction bone injury and neonatal subgaleal bleeding.' *European Journal of Pediatrics*, **151**, 532–535.

Graham, M., Levene, M.I., Trounce, J.Q., Rutter, N. (1987) 'Prediction of cerebral palsy in very low birth-weight infants: Prospective ultrasound study.' *Lancet*, **3**, 593–596.

Gray, P.H., Tudehope, D.I., Masel, J.P., *et al.* (1993) 'Perinatal hypoxic–ischaemic brain injury: prediction of outcome.' *Developmental Medicine and Child Neurology*, **35**, 965–973.

Graziani, L.J., Pasto, M., Stanley, C., *et al.* (1986) 'Neonatal neurosonographic correlates of cerebral palsy in preterm infants.' *Pediatrics*, **78**, 88–95.

—— Mitchell, D.G., Kornhauser, M., *et al.* (1992) 'Neurodevelopment of preterm infants: neonatal neurosonographic and serum bilirubin studies.' *Pediatrics*, **89**, 229–234.

Greisen, G., Munck, H., Lou, H. (1987) 'Severe hypocarbia in preterm infants and neurodevelopmental deficit.' *Acta Paediatrica Scandinavica*, **76**, 401–404.

Guekos-Thoeni, U., Boltshauser, E., Willi, U.V. (1982) 'Intraventricular haemorrhage in full-term neonates.' *Developmental Medicine and Child Neurology*, **24**, 704–705. *(Letter.)*

Guzzetta, F., Shackelford, G.D., Volpe, S., *et al.* (1986) 'Periventricular intraparenchymal echodensities in the premature newborn: critical determinant of neurologic outcome.' *Pediatrics*, **78**, 995–1006.

Haddad, J., Constantinesco, A., Facello, A., *et al.* (1993) 'Hexamethylpropylene amine oxime single-photon-emission computed tomography in perinatal asphyxia and ischemic hemorrhagic lesions.' *In:* Haddad, S., Saliba, E. (Eds.) *Perinatal Asphyxia.* Berlin: Springer, pp. 206–225.

Hadders-Algra, M., Bos, A.F., Martijn, A., Prechtl, H.F.R. (1994) 'Infantile chorea in an infant with severe bronchopulmonary dysplasia: an EMG study.' *Developmental Medicine and Child Neurology*, **36**, 177–182.

Hanigan, W.C., Morgan, A.M., Stahlberg, L.K., Hiller, J.L. (1990) 'Tentorial hemorrhage associated with vacuum extraction.' *Pediatrics*, **85**, 534–539.

Hanigan, W.C., Powell, F.C., Palagallo, G., Miller, T.C. (1995) 'Lobar hemorrhages in full-term neonates.' *Child's Nervous System*, **11**, 276–280.

Hansen, T.W.R., Bratlid, D. (1986) 'Bilirubin and brain toxicity.' *Acta Paediatrica Scandinavica*, **75**, 513–522.

Harris, S.S., d'Ercole, A.J. (1989) 'Neonatal hyperparathyroidism: the natural course in the absence of surgical intervention.' *Pediatrics*, **83**, 53–56.

Hattori, H., Morin, A.M., Schwartz, P.H., *et al.* (1989) 'Posthypoxic treatment with MK-801 reduces hypoxic–ischemic damage in the neonatal rat.' *Neurology*, **39**, 713–718.

Hattori, H., Wasterlain, C.G. (1990) 'Posthypoxic glucose supplement reduces hypoxic–ischemic brain damage in the neonatal rat.' *Annals of Neurology*, **28**, 122–128.

Hawdon, J.M., Ward Platt, M.P., Aynsley-Green, A. (1994) 'Prevention and management of neonatal hypoglycaemia.' *Archives of Disease in Childhood*, **70**, F60–F64.

Hayden, C.K., Shattuck, K.E., Richardson, C.J., *et al.* (1985) 'Subependymal germinal matrix hemorrhage in full-term neonates.' *Pediatrics*, **75**, 714–718.

Hays, R.M., Michaud, L.J. (1988) 'Neonatal myasthenia gravis: specific advantages of repetitive stimulation over edrophonium testing.' *Pediatric Neurology*, **4**, 245–247.

Hill, A. (1991) 'Current concepts of hypoxic–ischemic cerebral injury in the term newborn.' *Pediatric Neurology*, **7**, 317–325.

—— Volpe, J.J. (1981a) 'Seizures, hypoxic–ischemic brain injury and intraventricular hemorrhage in the newborn.' *Annals of Neurology*, **10**, 109–121.

—— —— (1981b) 'Normal pressure hydrocephalus in the newborn.' *Pediatrics*, **68**, 623–629.

—— —— (1989) 'Perinatal asphyxia: clinical aspects.' *Clinics in Perinatology*, **16**, 435–457.

—— Melson, G.L., Clark, H.B., Volpe, J.J. (1982a) 'Hemorrhagic periventricular leukomalacia: diagnosis by real-time ultrasound and correlation with autopsy findings.' *Pediatrics*, **69**, 282–284.

—— Perlman, J.M., Volpe, J.J. (1982b) 'Relationship of pneumothorax to occurrence of intraventricular hemorrhage in the premature newborn.' *Pediatrics*, **69**, 144–149.

Hillman, L.S., Hillman, R.E., Dodson, W.E. (1979) 'Diagnosis, treatment and follow-up of neonatal mepivacaine intoxication secondary to paracervical and pudendal blocks during labor.' *Journal of Pediatrics*, **95**, 472–477.

Hope, P., Costello, A.M.deL., Cady, E.B., *et al.* (1984) 'Cerebral energy metabolism studied with phosphorus NMR spectroscopy in normal and birth-asphyxiated infants.' *Lancet*, **2**, 366–370.

—— Gould, S.J., Howard, S., *et al.* (1988) 'Precision of ultrasound diagnosis of pathologically verified lesions in the brains of very preterm infants.' *Developmental Medicine and Child Neurology*, **30**, 457–471.

Horie, M., Yokochi, K., Inukai, K., *et al.* (1988) 'Computed tomographic findings in full-term infants with good prognosis.' *Brain and Development*, **10**, 100–105.

Huang, C.C., Shen, E.Y. (1991) 'Tentorial subdural hemorrhage in term newborns: ultrasonographic diagnosis and clinical correlates.' *Pediatric Neurology*, **7**, 171–177.

Hung, K.L. (1989) 'Auditory brainstem responses in patients with neonatal hyperbilirubinemia and bilirubin encephalopathy.' *Brain and Development*, **11**, 297–301.

Iida, K., Takashima, S., Takeuchi, Y. (1992) 'Etiologies and distribution of neonatal leukomalacia.' *Pediatric Neurology*, **8**, 205–209.

Iwasaki, Y., Kinoshita, M., Takamiya, K. (1988) 'Rapid development of basal ganglia calcification caused by anoxia.' *Journal of Neurology, Neurosurgery, and Psychiatry*, **51**, 449–450.

Jardine, D.S., Rogers, K. (1989) 'Relationship of benzyl alcohol to kernicterus, intraventricular hemorrhage and mortality in preterm infants.' *Pediatrics*, **83**, 153–160.

Kanarek, K.S., Gieron, M.A. (1986) 'Computed tomography demonstration of cerebral calcificatlon in postasphyxial encephalopathies.' *Journal of Child Neurology*, **1**, 56–60.

Kaplan, M.H., Klein, S.W., McPhee, J., Harper, R.G. (1983) 'Group B coxsackie virus infections in infants younger than three months of age: a serious childhood illness.' *Review of Infectious Diseases*, **5**, 1019–1032.

Kappas, A., Drummond, G.S., Henschke, C., Valaes, T. (1995) 'Direct comparison of Sn-mesoporphyrin, an inhibitor of bilirubin production, and phototherapy in controlling hyperbilirubinemia in term and near-term newborns.' *Pediatrics*, **95**, 468–474.

Karpati, F., Skolnik, M., Gati, J. (1986) 'Isolated absence of the spinal cord (amyelia) showing symptoms of respiratory distress syndrome.' *Orvosi Hetilap*, **127**, 833–834. *(Hungarian.)*

Keenan, W.J., Novak, K.K., Sutherland, J.M., *et al.* (1985) 'Mortality and morbidity associated with exchange transfusion.' *Pediatrics*, **75** (Suppl.), 417–421.

Keeney, S.E., Adcock, E.W., McArdle, C.B. (1991) 'Prospective observations of 100 high-risk neonates by high-field (1.5 Tesla) magnetic resonance imaging of the central nervous system. II. Lesions associated with hypoxic–ischemic encephalopathy.' *Pediatrics*, **87**, 431–438.

Klein, J.O., Feigin, R.D., McCracken, G.H. (1986) 'Report of the task force on diagnosis and management of meningitis.' *Pediatrics*, **78** (Suppl.), 959–982.

Kletzel, M., Miller, C.H., Becton, D.L., *et al.* (1989) 'Postdelivery head bleeding in hemophilic neonates.' *American Journal of Diseases of Children*, **143**, 1107–1110.

Koenigsberger, M.R., Moessinger, A.C. (1977) 'Iatrogenic carpal tunnel syndrome in the newborn infant.' *Journal of Pediatrics*, **91**, 443–445.

Koh, T.H.H.G., Aynsley-Green, A., Tarbit, M., Eyre, J.A. (1988) 'Neural dysfunction during hypoglycaemia.' *Archives of Disease in Childhood*, **63**, 1353–1358.

Koivisto, M., Blanco-Sequeiros, M., Krause, U. (1972) 'Neonatal symptomatic and asymptomatic hypoglycaemia: a follow-up study of 151 children.' *Developmental Medicine and Child Neurology*, **14**, 603–614.

Konishi, Y., Masanori, K., Masakatu, S. (1987) 'Superior sagittal sinus thrombosis in neonates.' *Pediatric Neurology*, **3**, 222–226.

Krägeloh-Mann, I., Petersen, D., Hagberg, G., *et al.* (1995) 'Bilateral spastic cerebral palsy. MRI pathology and origin. Analysis from a representative series of 56 cases.' *Developmental Medicine and Child Neurology*, **37**, 379–397.

Kramer, U., Nevo, Y., Harel, S. (1994) 'Jittery babies: a short-term follow-up.' *Brain and Development*, **16**, 112–114.

Kreusser, K.L., Schmidt, R.E., Shackelford, G.D., Volpe, J.J. (1984) 'Value of ultrasound for identification of acute hemorrhagic necrosis of thalamus and basal ganglia in an asphyxiated term infant.' *Annals of Neurology*, **16**, 361–363.

Krishnamoorthy, K.S., Kuban, K.C.K., Leviton, A., *et al.* (1990) 'Periventricular–intraventricular hemorrhage: sonographic localization, phenobarbital, and motor abnormalities in low birth weight infants.' *Pediatrics*, **85**, 1027–1033.

Kuban, K.C.K., Gilles, F.H. (1985) 'Human telencephalic angiogenesis.' *Annals of Neurology*, **17**, 539–548.

—— Volpe, J.J. (1993) 'Intraventricular hemorrhage: an update.' *Journal of Intensive Care Medicine*, **8**, 157–176.

—— Leviton, A., Krishnamoorthy, K.S., *et al.* (1986) 'Neonatal intracranial hemorrhage and phenobarbital.' *Pediatrics*, **77**, 443–450.

—— Skouteli, H., Chever, A., *et al.* (1988) 'Hemorrhage, phenobarbital and fluctuating cerebral blood flow velocity in the neonate.' *Pediatrics*, **82**, 548–553.

Kuenzle, C., Baenziger, O., Martin, E., *et al.* (1994) 'Prognostic value of early MR imaging in term infants with severe perinatal asphyxia.' *Neuropediatrics*, **25**, 191–200.

Lackmann, G.M., Töllner, U. (1995) 'The predictive value of elevation in specific serum enzymes for subsequent development of hypoxic–ischemic encephalopathy or intraventricular hemorrhage in full-term and premature asphyxiated newborns.' *Neuropediatrics*, **26**, 192–198.

Lacey, D.J. (1985) 'Inability to verify parasagittal cerebral injury as a neuropathologic entity in the asphyxiated term neonate.' *Pediatric Neurology*, **1**, 100–103.

—— Terplan, K. (1982) 'Intraventricular hemorrhage in full-term neonates.' *Developmental Medicine and Child Neurology*, **24**, 332–337.

Laegreid, L., Olegård, R., Wahlström, J., Conradi, N. (1987) 'Abnormalities in children exposed to benzodiazepines in utero.' *Lancet*, **1**, 108–109. *(Letter.)*

Lanska, M.J., Roessmann, U., Wiznitzer, M. (1990) 'Magnetic resonance imaging in cervical cord birth injury.' *Pediatrics*, **85**, 760–764.

Laptook, A.R., Peterson, J., Porter, A.M. (1988) 'Effects of lactic acid infusions and pH on cerebral blood flow and metabolism.' *Journal of Cerebral Blood Flow and Metabolism*, **8**, 193–200.

—— Corbett, R.J.T., Uauy, R., *et al.* (1989) 'Use of ^{31}P magnetic resonance spectroscopy to characterize evolving brain damage after perinatal asphyxia.' *Neurology*, **39**, 709–712.

Leech, R.W., Brumback, R.A. (1988) 'Massive brain stem necrosis in the human neonate: presentation of three cases with review of the literature.' *Journal of Child Neurology*, **3**, 258–262.

Legido, A. (1994) 'Perinatal hypoxic ischemic encephalopathy: recent advances in diagnosis and treatment.' *International Pediatrics*, **9**, 114–136.

Lesko, S.M., Mitchell, A.A., Epstein, M.F., *et al.* (1986) 'Heparin use as a risk factor for intraventricular hemorrhage in low-blrthweight infants ' *New England Journal ot Medicine*, **314**, 1156–1160.

Levene, M.I. (1990) 'Cerebral ultrasound and neurological impairment: telling the future.' *Archives of Disease in Childhood*, **65**, 469–471.

—— (1993) 'Management of the asphyxiated full term infant.' *Archives of Disease in Childhood*, **68**, 612–616.

—— Evans, D.H. (1985) 'Medical management of raised intracranial pressure after severe birth asphyxia.' *Archives of Disease in Childhood*, **60**, 12–16.

—— Wigglesworth, J.S., Dubowitz, V. (1983) 'Hemorrhagic periventricular leukomalacia in the neonate: a real-time ultrasound study.' *Pediatrics*, **71**, 794–797.

—— Kornberg, J., Williams, T.H.C. (1985) 'The incidence and severity of postasphyxial encephalopathy in full-term infants.' *Early Human Development*, **11**, 21–28.

—— Evans, D.H., Forde, A., Archer, L.N.J. (1987) 'Value of intracranial pressure monitoring of asphyxiated newborn infants.' *Developmental Medicine and Child Neurology*, **29**, 311–319.

—— Fenton, A.C., Evans, D.H., *et al.* (1989) 'Severe birth asphyxia and abnormal cerebral blood flow velocity.' *Developmental Medicine and Child Neurology*, **31**, 427–434.

—— Gibson, N.A., Fenton, A.C., *et al.* (1990) 'The use of a calcium-channel blocker, nicardipine, for severely asphyxiated newborn infants.' *Developmental Medicine and Child Neurology*, **32**, 567–574.

Leviton, A., Gilles, F.H. (1984) 'Acquired perinatal leukoencephalopathy.' *Annals of Neurology*, **16**, 1–8.

—— (1996) 'Ventriculomegaly, delayed myelination, white matter hypoplasia, and "periventricular" leukomalacia: how are they related?' *Pediatric Neurology*, **15**, 127–136.

—— Nelson, K.B. (1992) 'Problems with definitions and classification of newborn encephalopathy.' *Pediatric Neurology*, **8**, 85–90.

—— Pagano, M., Kuban, C.K. (1988) 'Etiologic heterogeneity of intracranial hemorrhages in preterm newborns.' *Pediatric Neurology*, **4**, 274–278.

—— Van Marter, L., Kuban, K.C.K. (1989) 'Respiratory distress syndrome and intracranial hemorrhage: cause or association? Inferences from surfactant clinical trials.' *Pediatrics*, **84**, 915–922.

—— Kuban, K.C., Pagano, M., *et al.* (1993) 'Antenatal corticosteroids appear to reduce the risk of germinal matrix hemorrhage in intubated low birthweight newborns.' *Pediatrics*, **91**, 1083–1088.

Lewis, S.R., Mortimer, P.E. (1964) 'Idiopathic neonatal hyperglycaemia.' *Archives of Disease in Childhood*, **39**, 618–624.

Lightwood, R. (1951) 'Radial nerve palsy associated with localized subcutaneous fat necrosis in the newborn.' *Archives of Disease in Childhood*, **32**, 436–437.

Lipsitz, P.J., Gartner, L.M., Bryla, D.A. (1985) 'Neonatal and infant mortality in relation to phototherapy.' *Pediatrics*, **75** (Suppl.), 422–426.

Lipton, S.A., Rosenberg, P.A. (1994) 'Excitatory aminoacids as a final common pathway for neurologic disorders.' *New England Journal of Medicine*, **330**, 613–622.

Loeser, J.D., Kilburn, H.L., Jolley, T. (1976) 'Management of depressed skull fracture in the newborn.' *Journal of Neurosurgery*, **44**, 62–64.

Lombroso, C.T. (1985) 'Neonatal polygraphy in full-term and premature infants: a review of normal and abnormal findings.' *Journal of Clinical Neurophysiology*, **2**, 105–155.

—— (1996) 'Neonatal seizures: a clinician's overview.' *Brain and Development*, **18**, 1–28.

Lou, H.C. (1988) 'The "lost autoregulation hypothesis" and brain lesions in the newborn—an update.' *Brain and Development*, **10**, 143–146.

—— Friis-Hansen, B. (1979) 'Elevations in arterial blood pressure during motor activity and epileptic seizures in the newborn.' *Acta Paediatrica Scandinavica*, **68**, 803–806.

Low, J.A. (1989) 'Fetal acid-base status and outcome.' *In:* Hill, A., Volpe, J.J. (Eds.) *Fetal Neurology.* New York: Raven Press, pp. 195–217.

Lucas, A., Morley, R., Cole, T.J. (1988) 'Adverse neurodevelopmental outcome of moderate neonatal hypoglycaemia.' *British Medical Journal*, **297**, 1304–1308.

Lupton, B.A., Hill, A., Roland, E.H., *et al.* (1988) 'Brain swelling in the asphyxiated term newborn: pathogenesis and outcome.' *Pediatrics*, **82**, 139–146.

Luthy, D.A., Shy, K.K., Van Belle, G. (1987) 'A randomized trial of electronic fetal monitoring in preterm labor.' *Obstetrics and Gynecology*, **69**, 687–695.

Lynch, B.J., Rust, R.S. (1994) 'Natural history and outcome of neonatal hypocalcemic and hypomagnesemic seizures.' *Pediatric Neurology*, **11**, 23–27.

MacDonald, D., Grant, A., Sheridan-Pereira, M., *et al.* (1985) 'The Dublin randomized controlled trial of intrapartum fetal heart rate monitoring.' *American Journal of Obstetrics and Gynecology*, **152**, 524–539.

MacDonald, H.M., Mulligan, J.C., Allen, A.C., Taylor, P.M. (1980) 'Neonatal asphyxia. I: Relationship of obstetric and neonatal complications to neonatal mortality in 38,405 consecutive deliveries.' *Journal of Pediatrics*, **96**, 898–903.

MacDonald, J.T., Sher, P.K. (1977) 'Ophthalmoplegia as a sign of metabolic disease in the newborn.' *Neurology*, **27**, 971–973.

MacKinnon, J.A., Perlman, M., Kirpalani, H., *et al.* (1993) 'Spinal cord injury at birth: diagnostic and prognostic data in twenty-two patients.' *Journal of Pediatrics*, **122**, 431–437.

Maekawa, K., Masaki, T., Kokubun, Y. (1976) 'Fetal spinal-cord injury secondary to hyperextension of the neck: no effect of caesarian section.' *Developmental Medicine and Child Neurology*, **18**, 229–232.

Marret, S., Parain, D., Samson-Dollfus, D., *et al.* (1986) 'Positive rolandic sharp waves and periventricular leukomalacia in the newborn.' *Neuropediatrics*, **17**, 199–202.

—— Gressens, P., Gadisseux, J-F., Evrard, P. (1995) 'Prevention by magnesium of excitotoxic neuronal death in the developing brain: an animal model for clinical intervention studies.' *Developmental Medicine and Child Neurology*, **37**, 473–484.

Matsuzaka, T., Yoshinaga, M., Tsuji, Y. (1987) 'Prophylaxis of intracranial hemorrhage due to vitamin K deficiency in infants.' *Brain and Development*, **9**, 305–308.

McCord, J.M. (1985) 'Oxygen-derived free radicals in postischemic tissue injury.' *New England Journal of Medicine*, **312**, 159–163.

McDonald, M.M., Koops, B.L., Johnson, M.L., *et al.* (1984) 'Timing and antecedents of intracranial hemorrhage in the newborn.' *Pediatrics*, **74**, 32–36.

Mehta, A. (1994) 'Prevention and management of neonatal hypoglycaemia.' *Archives of Disease in Childhood*, **70**, F54–F59.

Menezes, A.H., Smith, D.E., Bell, W.E. (1983) 'Posterior fossa hemorrhage in the term neonate.' *Neurosurgery*, **13**, 452–456.

Ment, L.R., Oh, W., Ehrenkranz, R.A., *et al.* (1994a) 'Low-dose indomethacin and prevention of intraventricular hemorrhage: a multicenter randomized trial.' *Pediatrics*, **93**, 543–550.

—— —— *et al.* (1994b) 'Low-dose indomethacin therapy and extension of intraventricular hemorrhage: a multicenter randomized trial.' *Journal of Pediatrics*, **124**, 951–955.

Mercuri, E., Cowan, F., Rutherford, M., *et al.* (1995) 'Ischaemic and haemorrhagic brain lesions in newborns with seizures and normal Apgar scores.' *Archives of Disease in Childhood*, **73**, F67–F74.

Miall-Allen, V.M., de Vries, L.S., Whitelaw, A.G.L. (1987) 'Mean arterial blood pressure and neonatal cerebral lesions.' *Archives of Disease in Childhood*, 62, 1068–1069.

—— —— Dubowitz, L.M.S., Whitelaw, A.G.L. (1989) 'Blood pressure fluctuation and intraventricular hemorrhage in the preterm infant of less than 31 weeks' gestation.' *Pediatrics*, **83**, 657–661.

Miller, G.M., Black, V.D., Lubchenco, L. (1981) 'Intracerebral hemorrhage in a term newborn with hyperviscosity.' *American Journal of Diseases of Children*, **135**, 377–378.

Miller, V.S. (1993) 'Pharmacologic management of neonatal cerebral ischemia and hemorrhage. Old and new directions.' *Journal of Child Neurology*, **8**, 7–18.

Minami, T., Ise, K., Kukita, J., *et al.* (1994) 'A case of neonatal spinal cord injury: magnetic resonance imaging and somatosensory evoked potentials.' *Brain and Development*, **16**, 57–60.

Minkoff, H., Grunebaum, A.N., Schwarz, R.H., *et al.* (1984) 'Risk factors for prematurity and premature rupture of membranes: a prospective study of the vaginal flora in pregnancy.' *American Journal of Obstetrics and Gynecology*, **150**, 965–972.

Mizrahi, E.M., Tharp, B.R. (1982) 'A characteristic EEG pattern in neonatal herpes simplex encephalitis.' *Neurology*, **32**, 1215–1220.

Modlin, J.F. (1986) 'Perinatal echovirus infection: insights from a literature review of 61 cases of serious infection and 16 outbreaks in nurseries.' *Review of Infectious Diseases*, **8**, 918–926.

Monset-Couchard, M., De Bethmann, O., Radvanyi-Bouvet, M.F., *et al.* (1988) 'Neurodevelopmental outcome in cystic periventricular leukomalacia (CPVL) (30 cases).' *Neuropediatrics*, **19**, 124–131.

Morens, D.M. (1978) 'Enteroviral disease in early infancy.' *Journal of Pediatrics*, **92**, 374–377.

Morley, F., Hogan, M.J., Hakim, A.M. (1994) 'Calcium-mediated mechanisms of ischemic injury and protection.' *Brain Pathology*, **4**, 37–47.

Mulligan, J.C., Painter, M.J., O'Donoghue, P.P., *et al.* (1980) 'Neonatal asphyxia. II: Neonatal mortality and long-term sequelae.' *Journal of Pediatrics*, **96**, 903–907.

Muñoz, M.E., Roche, C., Escribá, R., *et al.* (1993) 'Flaccid paraplegia as complication of umbilical artery catheterization.' *Pediatric Neurology*, **9**, 401–403.

Mutoh, K., Ito, M., Okuno, T., *et al.* (1989) 'Nontraumatic spinal intramedullary hemorrhage in an infant.' *Pediatric Neurology*, **5**, 53–56.

Myers, R.E. (1972) 'Two patterns of brain damage and their conditions of occurrence.' *American Journal of Obstetrics and Gynecology*, **112**, 246–276.

Nakamura, H., Takada, S., Shimabuku, R., *et al.* (1985) 'Auditory nerve and brainstem responses in newborn infants with hyperbilirubinemia.' *Pediatrics*, **75**, 703–708.

Natsume, J., Watanabe, K., Kuno, K., *et al.* (1995) 'Clinical, neurophysiologic, and neuropathological features of an infant with brain damage of total asphyxia type (Myers).' *Pediatric Neurology*, **13**, 61–64.

Negishi, H., Lee, Y., Itoh, K., *et al.* (1989) 'Nonsurgical management of epidural hematoma in neonates.' *Pediatric Neurology*, **5**, 253–256.

Nelson, K.B. (1996) 'Magnesium sulfate and risk of cerebral palsy in very low-birth-weight infants.' *Journal of the American Medical Association*, **276**, 1843–1844.

—— Ellenberg, J.H. (1981) 'Apgar scores as predictors of chronic neurologic disability.' *Pediatrics*, **68**, 36–44.

—— Grether, J.K. (1995) 'Can magnesium sulfate reduce the risk of cerebral palsy in very low birthweight infants?' *Pediatrics*, **95**, 263–269.

—— Leviton, A. (1991) 'How much of neonatal encephalopathy is due to birth asphyxia?' *American Journal of Diseases of Children*, **145**, 1325–1331.

—— Dambrosia, J.M., Ting, T.Y., Grether, J.K. (1996) 'Uncertain value of electronic fetal monitoring in predicting cerebral palsy.' *New England Journal of Medicine*, **334**, 613–618.

Newman, T.B., Maisels, M.J. (1992) 'Evaluation and treatment of jaundice in the term newborn: a kinder, gentler approach.' *Pediatrics*, **89**, 809–818.

Niemann, G., Wakat, J-P., Krägeloh-Mann, I., *et al.* (1994) 'Congenital hemiparesis and periventricular leukomalacia: pathogenetic aspects on magnetic resonance imaging.' *Developmental Medicine and Child Neurology*, **36**, 943–950.

Niijima, S., Levene, M.I. (1989) 'Post-asphyxial encephalopathy in a preterm infant.' *Developmental Medicine and Child Neurology*, **31**, 395–397.

Nwaesei, C.G., Allen, A.C., Vincer, M.J., *et al.* (1988) 'Effect of timing of cerebral ultrasonography on the prediction of later neurodevelopmental outcome in high-risk preterm infants.' *Journal of Pediatrics*, **112**, 970–975.

Orwoll, E., Silbert, J., McClung, M. (1982) 'Asymptomatic neonatal familial hypercalcemia.' *Pediatrics*, **69**, 109–111.

O'Shea, T.M., Dillard, R.G., Klinepeter, K.L., Goldstein, D.J. (1992) 'Serum bilirubin levels, intracranial hemorrhage, and the risk of developmental problems in very low birth weight neonates.' *Pediatrics*, **90**, 888–892.

Pagano, M., Leviton, A., Kuban, K. (1990) 'Early and late germinal matrix hemorrhage may have different antecedents.' *European Journal of Obstetrics and Gynecology and Reproductive Biology*, **37**, 47–54.

Painter, M.J. (1989) 'Fetal heart rate patterns, perinatal asphyxia and brain injury.' *Pediatric Neurology*, **5**, 137–144.

Palmer, C., Smith, M.B. (1990) 'Assessing the risk of kernicterus using nuclear magnetic resonance.' *Clinics in Perinatology*, **17**, 307–329.

—— Vannucci, R.C. (1993) 'Potential new therapies for perinatal cerebral hypoxia–ischemia.' *Clinics in Perinatology*, **20**, 411–432.

—— —— Towfighi, J. (1990) 'Reduction of perinatal hypoxic–ischemic brain damage with allopurinol.' *Pediatric Research*, **27**, 332–336.

Paneth, N., Pinto-Martin, J., Gardiner, J., *et al.* (1993) 'Incidence and timing of germinal matrix/intraventricular hemorrhage in low birth weight infants.' *American Journal of Epidemiology*, **137**, 1167–1176.

—— Rudelli, R., Kazam, E., Monte, W. (Eds.) (1994) *Brain Damage in the Preterm Infant. Clinics in Developmental Medicine No. 131.* London: Mac Keith Press.

Papazian, O. (1992) 'Transient neonatal myasthenia gravis.' *Journal of Child Neurology*, **7**, 135–141 + erratum, p. 325.

Pape, K.E., Wigglesworth, J.S. (1979) *Haemorrhage, Ischaemia and the Perinatal Brain. Clinics in Developmental Medicine No. 69/70.* London: Spastics International Medical Publications.

—— Armstrong, D.L., Fitzhardinge, P.M. (1978) 'Peripheral median nerve damage secondary to brachial arterial blood gas sampling.' *Journal of Pediatrics*, **93**, 852–856.

—— Bennett-Britton, M., Szymonowicz, W., *et al.* (1983) 'Diagnostic accuracy of neonatal brain imaging: a post-mortem correlation of computer tomography and ultrasound scans.' *Journal of Pediatrics*, **102**, 275–280.

Papile, L-A., Burstein, J., Burstein, R., Koffler, H. (1978) 'Incidence and evolution of subependymal and intraventricular hemorrhage: a study of infants with birthweights less than 1,500gm.' *Journal of Pediatrics*, **92**, 529–534.

—— Munsick-Bruno, G., Schaefer, A. (1983) 'Relationship of cerebral intraventricular hemorrhage and early childhood neurologic handicaps.' *Journal of Pediatrics*, **103**, 273–277.

Parisi, J.E., Collins, G.H., Kim, R.C., Crosley, C.J. (1983) 'Prenatal symmetrical thalamic degeneration with flexion spasticity at birth.' *Annals of Neurology*, **13**, 94–97.

Parker, S., Zuckerman, B., Bauchner, H., *et al.* (1990) 'Jitteriness in full-term neonates: prevalence and correlates.' *Pediatrics*, **85**, 17–23.

Pasternak, J.F. (1987) 'Parasagittal infarction in neonatal asphyxia.' *Annals of Neurology*, **21**, 202–204.

—— Mantovani, J.F., Volpe, J.J. (1980) 'Porencephaly from periventricular intracerebral hemorrhage in a premature infant.' *American Journal of Diseases of Children*, **134**, 673–675.

—— Predey, T.A., Mikhael, M.A. (1991) 'Neonatal asphyxia: vulnerability of basal ganglia, thalamus, and brainstem.' *Pediatric Neurology*, **7**, 147–149.

PeBenito, R., Santello, M.D., Faxas, T.A., *et al.* (1989) 'Residual developmental disabilities in children with transient hypertonicity in infancy.' *Pediatric Neurology*, **5**, 154–160.

Peden, C.J., Rutherford, M.A., Sargentoni, J., *et al.* (1993) 'Proton spectroscopy of the neonatal brain following hypoxic–ischaemic injury.' *Developmental Medicine and Child Neurology*, **35**, 502–510.

Peebles, D.M., Spencer, J.A.D., Edwards, A.D., *et al.* (1994) 'Relation between frequency of uterine contractions and human fetal cerebral oxygen saturation studied during labour by near infrared spectroscopy.' *British Journal of Obstetrics and Gynaecology*, **101**, 44–48.

Penn, A.A., Enzmann, D.R., Hahn, J.S., Stevenson, D.K. (1994) 'Kernicterus in a full term infant.' *Pediatrics*, **93**, 1003–1006.

Perlman, J.M., Frank, J.W. (1988) 'Bilirubin beyond the blood–brain barrier.' *Pediatrics*, **81**, 304–315.

—— Volpe, J.J. (1986) 'Intraventricular hemorrhage in extremely small premature infants.' *American Journal of Diseases of Children*, **140**, 1122–1124.

—— —— (1987) 'Are venous circulatory abnormalities important in the pathogenesis of hemorrhagic and/or ischemic cerebral injury?' *Pediatrics*, **80**, 705–711.

—— —— (1989a) 'Neurologic complications of captopril treatment of neonatal hypertension.' *Pediatrics*, **83**, 47–52.

—— —— (1989b) 'Movement disorder of premature infants with severe bronchopulmonary dysplasia: a new syndrome.' *Pediatrics*, **84**, 215–218.

—— McMenamin, J.B., Volpe, J.J. (1983) 'Fluctuating cerebral blood flow velocity in respiratory distress syndrome.' *New England Journal of Medicine*, **309**, 204–209.

—— Goodman, S., Kreusser, K.L., Volpe, J.J. (1985) 'Reduction in intraventricular hemorrhage by elimination of fluctuating cerebral blood flow velocity in preterm infants with respiratory distress syndrome.' *New England Journal of Medicine*, **312**, 1353–1357.

—— Lynch, B., Volpe, J.J. (1990) 'Late hydrocephalus after arrest and resolution of neonatal posthemorrhagic hydrocephalus.' *Developmental Medicine and Child Neurology*, **32**, 725–729.

—— Risser, R., Broyles, R.S. (1996) 'Bilateral cystic periventricular leukomalacia in the premature infant: associated risk factors.' *Pediatrics*, **97**, 822–827.

Perlstein, M.A. (1960) 'The late clinical syndrome of post-icteric encephalopathy.' *Pediatric Clinics of North America*, **7**, 665–687.

Petroff, O.A.C., Young, R.S.K., Cowan, B.E., Novotny, E.J. (1988) '¹H nuclear magnetic resonance spectroscopy study of neonatal hypoglycemia.' *Paediatric Neurology*, **4**, 31–34.

Philip, A.G.S., Larson, E.J. (1973) 'Overwhelming neonatal infection with ECHO 19 virus.' *Journal of Pediatrics*, **82**, 391–397.

—— Allan, W.C., Tito, A.M., Wheeler, L.R. (1989) 'Intraventricular hemorrhage in preterm infants: declining incidence in the 1980s.' *Pediatrics*, **84**, 797–801.

Pierre-Kahn, A., Renier, D., Sainte-Rose, C., Hirsch, J.F. (1986) 'Acute intracranial hematomas in term neonates.' *Child's Nervous System*, **2**, 191–194.

Pildes, R.S., Cornblath, M., Warren, I., *et al.* (1974) 'A prospective controlled study of neonatal hypoglycemia.' *Pediatrics*, **54**, 5–14.

Poggi-Travert, F., Billette de Villemeur, T., Hubert, P., *et al.* (1995) 'Diagnosis of metabolic disorders with acute neonatal onset.' *In:* Di Donato, S., Parini, R., Uziel, G. (Eds.) *Metabolic Encephalopathies—Therapy and Prognosis.* London: John Libbey, pp. 71–83.

Pozzati, E., Tognetti, E. (1986) 'Spontaneous healing of acute extradural hematomas. Study of 22 cases.' *Neurosurgery*, **18**, 696–700.

Pranzatelli, M.R., Stumpf, D.A. (1985) 'The metabolic consequences of experimental intraventricular hemorrhage.' *Neurology*, **35**, 1299–1303.

Primhak, R.A., Smith, M.F. (1985) 'Primary thalamic haemorrhage in first week of life.' *Lancet*, **1**, 635.

Rademaker, K.J., De Vries, L.S., Barth, P.G. (1993) 'Subependymal pseudocysts: ultrasound diagnosis and findings at follow-up.' *Acta Paediatrica*, **82**, 394–399.

Raichle, M.E. (1983) 'The pathophysiology of brain asphyxia.' *Annals of Neurology*, **13**, 2–10.

Ramamurthy, R.S., Harris, V., Pildes, R.S. (1975) 'Subcutaneous calcium deposition in the neonate associated with intravenous administration of calcium gluconate.' *Pediatrics*, **55**, 802–806.

Ramesh, V., Gardner-Medwin, D., Gibson, M., Colquhoun, I. (1989) 'Severe segmental narrowing of the spinal cord: an unusual finding in congenital spastic paraparesis.' *Developmental Medicine and Child Neurology*, **31**, 675–678.

Rehan, V.K., Seshia, M.M.K. (1993) 'Spinal cord birth injury—diagnostic difficulties.' *Archives of Disease in Childhood*, **69**, 92–94.

Ringelberg, J., van de Bor, M. (1993) 'Outcome of transient periventricular echodensities in preterm infants.' *Neuropediatrics*, **24**, 269–273.

Ritter, D.A., Kenny, J.D., Norton, H.J., Rudolph, A.J. (1982) 'A prospective study of free bilirubin and other risk factors in the development of kernicterus in premature infants.' *Pediatrics*, **69**, 260–266.

Rivkin, M.J., Anderson, M.L., Kaye, E.M. (1992) 'Neonatal idiopathic cerebral venous thrombosis: an unrecognized cause of transient seizures or lethargy.' *Annals of Neurology*, **32**, 51–56.

Roberts, R.A., Cohen, M.D., Forfar, J.O. (1973) 'Antenatal factors associated with neonatal hypocalcaemic convulsions.' *Lancet*, **2**, 809–811.

Rodriguez, J., Claus, D., Verellen, G., Lyon, G. (1990) 'Periventricular leukomalacia: ultrasonic and neuropathological correlations.' *Developmental Medicine and Child Neurology*, **32**, 347–352.

Roessmann, V., Horwitz, S.J., Kennell, J.H. (1990) 'Congenital absence of the corticospinal fibers: pathologic and clinical observations.' *Neurology*, **40**, 538–541.

Roig, M., Calopa, M., Rovira, A., *et al.* (1993) 'Bilateral striatal lesions in childhood.' *Pediatric Neurology*, **9**, 349–358.

Roland, E.H., Hill, A., Norman, M.G., *et al.* (1988) 'Selective brainstem injury in an asphyxiated newborn.' *Annals of Neurology*, **23**, 89–92.

—— Flodmark, O., Hill, A. (1990) 'Thalamic hemorrhage with intraventricular hemorrhage in the full-term newborn.' *Pediatrics*, **85**, 737–742.

Roodhooft, A.M., Parizel, P.M., Van Acker, K.J., et al. (1987) 'Idiopathic cerebral arterial infarction with paucity of symptoms in the full term neonate.' *Pediatrics*, **80**, 381–385.

Rosenbloom, L. (1994) 'Dyskinetic cerebral palsy and birth asphyxia.' *Developmental Medicine and Child Neurology*, **36**, 285–289.

Rubin, R.A., Balow, B., Fisch, R.O. (1979) 'Neonatal serum bilirubin levels related to cognitive development at ages 4 through 7 years.' *Journal of Pediatrics*, **94**, 601–604.

Rushton, D.I., Preston, P.R., Durbin, G.M. (1985) 'Structure and evolution of echo dense lesions in the neonatal brain.' *Archives of Disease in Childhood*, **60**, 798–808.

Ruth, J., Raivio, K.O. (1988) 'Perinatal brain damage: predictive value of metabolic acidosis and the Apgar score.' *British Medical Journal*, **297**, 24–27.

Rutherford, M.A., Heckmatt, J.Z., Dubowitz, V. (1989) 'Congenital myotonic dystrophy: respiratory function at birth determines survival.' *Archives of Disease in Childhood*, **64**, 191–195.

—— Pennock, J.M., Murdoch-Eaton, D.M., et al. (1992) 'Athetoid cerebral palsy with cysts in the putamen after hypoxic–ischaemic encephalopathy.' *Archives of Disease in Childhood*, **67**, 846–850.

—— Schwieso, J., et al. (1996) 'Hypoxic–ischaemic encephalopathy: early and late magnetic resonance imaging findings in relation to outcome.' *Archives of Disease in Childhood*, **75**, F145–F151.

Sarnat, H.B., Sarnat, M.S. (1976) 'Neonatal encephalopathy following fetal distress: a clinical and electroencephalographic study.' *Archives of Neurology*, **33**, 696–705.

Saudubray, J.M., Ogier, H., Bonnefont, J.P., et al. (1989) 'Clinical approach to inherited metabolic diseases in the neonatal period: a 20-year survey.' *Journal of Inherited Metabolic Diseases*, **12**, Suppl. 1, 25–41.

Scheidt, P.C., Bryla, D.A., Nelson, H.B., et al. (1988) 'NICHD phototherapy clinical trial: six year follow-up results.' *Pediatric Research*, **23**, 455A. (Abstract.)

—— Graubard, B.I., Nelson, K.B., et al. (1991) 'Intelligence at six years in relation to neonatal bilirubin level. Follow-up of the National Institute of Child Health and Human Development Clinical Trial on Phototherapy.' *Pediatrics*, **87**, 797–806.

Scher, M.S., Beggarly, M. (1989) 'Clinical significance of focal periodic patterns in the newborn.' *Journal of Child Neurology*, **4**, 175–185.

—— Bergman, I., Ahdab-Barmada, M., Fria, T. (1986) 'Neurophysiological and anatomical correlations in neonatal nonketotic hyperglycinemia.' *Neuropediatrics*, **17**, 137–143.

—— Dobson, V., Carpenter, N.A., Guthrie, R.D. (1989) 'Visual and neurological outcome of infants with periventricular leukomalacia.' *Developmental Medicine and Child Neurology*, **31**, 353–365.

Schiffmann, R., Kaye, E.M., Willis, J.K., et al. (1989) 'Transient neonatal hyperglycinemia.' *Annals of Neurology*, **25**, 201–203.

Schifrin, B.S. (1989) 'The diagnosis and treatment of fetal distress.' *In:* Hill, A., Volpe, J.J. (Eds.) *Fetal Neurology.* New York: Raven Press, pp. 143–189.

Schindler, H., Ballowitz, L., Schachinger, H. (1975) 'Anoxic encephalopathy with predominant involvement of basal ganglia, brain stem and spinal cord in the perinatal period.' *Acta Neuropathologica*, **32**, 287–298.

Schumacher, R.E., Weinfeld, I.J., Bartlett, R.H. (1989) 'Neonatal vocal cord paralysis following extracorporeal membrane oxygenation.' *Pediatrics*, **84**, 793–796.

Seidman, P.S., Paz, I., Stevenson, D.K., et al. (1991) 'Neonatal hyperbilirubinemia and physical and cognitive performance at 17 years of age.' *Pediatrics*, **88**, 828–833.

Shankaran, S., Koepke, T., Woldt, E., et al. (1989) 'Outcome after posthemorrhagic ventriculomegaly in comparison with mild hemorrhage without ventriculomegaly.' *Journal of Pediatrics*, **114**, 109–114.

—— Kottamasu, S.R., Kuhns, L. (1993) 'Brain sonography, computed tomography, and single-photon emission computed tomography in term neonates with perinatal asphyxia.' *Clinics in Perinatology*, **20**, 379–394.

Shaver, D.C., Bada, H.S., Korones, S.B., et al. (1992) 'Early and late intraventricular hemorrhage: the role of obstetric factors.' *Obstetrics and Gynecology*, **80**, 831–837.

Shaw, N.J., Cooke, R.W.I., Gill, A.B.L., et al. (1993) 'Randomised trial of routine versus selective paralysis during ventilation for neonatal respiratory distress syndrome.' *Archives of Disease in Childhood*, **69**, 479–482.

Shen, E-Y., Huang, F-Y. (1985) 'Subependymal cysts in normal neonates.' *Archives of Disease in Childhood*, **60**, 1072–1074.

—— Huang, C.C., Chyou, S.C., et al. (1986) 'Sonographic finding of the bright thalamus.' *Archives of Disease in Childhood*, **61**, 1096–1099.

Shewmon, D.A., Fine, M., Masdeu, J.C., Palacios, E. (1981) 'Post-ischemic hypervascularity of infancy: a stage in the evolution of ischemic brain damage with characteristic CT scan.' *Annals of Neurology*, **9**, 358–365.

Shortland, D., Trounce, J.Q., Levene, M.I. (1987) 'Hyperkalaemia, cardiac arrhythmias and cerebral lesions in high risk neonates.' *Archives of Disease in Childhood*, **62**, 1139–1143.

Shuman, R.M., Selednik, L.J. (1980) 'Periventricular leukomalacia: a one-year autopsy study.' *Archives of Neurology*, **37**, 231–235.

Shy, K.K., Luthy, D.A., Bennett, F.C., et al. (1990) 'Effects of electronic fetal-heart-rate monitoring, as compared with periodic auscultation, on the neurologic development of premature infants.' *New England Journal of Medicine*, **322**, 588–593.

Sinha, S.K., D'Souza, S.W., Rivlin, E., Chiswick, M.L. (1990) 'Ischaemic brain lesions diagnosed at birth in preterm infants: clinical events and developmental outcome.' *Archives of Disease in Childhood*, **65**, 1017–1020.

Skov, L., Pryds, O., Greisen, G., Lou, H. (1993) 'Estimation of cerebral venous saturation in newborn infants by near infrared spectroscopy.' *Pediatric Research*, **33**, 52–55.

Skranes, J.S., Vik, T., Nilsen, G., et al. (1993) 'Cerebral magnetic resonance imaging (MRI) and mental and motor function of very low birth weight infants at one year of corrected age.' *Neuropediatrics*, **24**, 256–262.

Skullerud, K., Westre, B. (1986) 'Frequency and prognostic significance of germinal matrix hemorrhage, periventricular leukomalacia and pontosubicular necrosis in preterm neonates.' *Acta Neuropathologica*, **70**, 257–261.

Sorell, M., Rosen, J.F. (1975) 'Ionized calcium: serum levels during symptomatic hypocalcemia.' *Journal of Pediatrics*, **87**, 67–70.

Stephenson, J.B.P. (1988) 'Inherited peroxisomal disorders involving the nervous system.' *Archives of Disease in Childhood*, **63**, 767–770.

Stern, L., Cashore, W.J. (1989) 'Cellular mechanisms of bilirubin encephalopathy in the newborn.' *In:* French, J.H., Harel, S., Casaer, P. (Eds.) *Child Neurology and Developmental Disabilities.* Baltimore: Paul Brookes, pp. 103–106.

Stromme, J.H., Nerbakken, R., Normann, T., et al. (1969) 'Familial hypomagnesemia.' *Acta Paediatrica Scandinavica*, **58**, 433–444.

Sugita, K., Takeuchi, A., Tanabe, Y. (1990) 'Neurologic sequelae and MRI in low birth weight patients.' *Pediatric Neurology*, **5**, 365–369.

Szymonowicz, G., Schaffler, K., Kussen, L.J., Yu, V.Y.H. (1984) 'Ultrasound and necropsy study of periventricular hemorrhage in preterm infants.' *Archives of Disease in Childhood*, **59**, 637–642.

—— Yu, V.Y.H., Bajuk, B., Astbury, J. (1986) 'Neurodevelopmental outcome of periventricular haemorrhage and leukomalacia in infants of 1250g or less at birth.' *Early Human Development*, **14**, 1–7.

Takashima, S., Becker, L.E. (1989) 'Relationship between abnormal respiratory control and perinatal brainstem and cerebellar infarctions.' *Pediatric Neurology*, **5**, 211–215.

—— Mito, T., Houdou, S., Ando, Y. (1989) 'Relationship between periventricular hemorrhage, leukomalacia and brainstem lesions in prematurely born infants.' *Brain and Development*, **11**, 121–124.

Takeuchi, T., Watanabe, K. (1989) 'The EEG evolution and neurological prognosis of perinatal hypoxia in neonates.' *Brain and Development*, **11**, 115–120.

Telzrow, R.W., Snyder, D.M., Tronick, E., et al. (1980) 'The behavior of jaundiced infants undergoing phototherapy.' *Developmental Medicine and Child Neurology*, **22**, 317–326.

Thacker, S.B., Stroup, D.F., Peterson, H.B. (1995) 'Efficacy and safety of intrapartum electronic fetal monitoring: an update.' *Obstetrics and Gynecology*, **86**, 613–620.

Tharp, B., Scher, M.S., Clancy, R.R. (1989) 'Serial EEGs in normal and abnormal infants with birthweights less than 1200 grams. A prospective study with long-term follow-up.' *Neuropediatrics*, **20**, 64–72.

Tohier, C., Roze, J.C., David, A., et al. (1991) 'Hyperexplexia or stiff baby syndrome.' *Archives of Disease in Childhood*, **66**, 460–461.

Towbin, A. (1969) 'Latent spinal cord and brain stem injury in newborn infants.' *Developmental Medicine and Child Neurology*, **11**, 54–68.

Trauner, D.A., Chase, C., Walker, P., Wulfeck, B. (1993) 'Neurologic profiles of infants and children after perinatal stroke.' *Pediatric Neurology*, **9**, 383–386.

Trounce, J.Q., Dodd, K.L., Fawer, C-L., et al. (1985) 'Primary thalamic haemorrhage in the newborn: a new clinical entity.' *Lancet*, **1**, 190–192.

—— Fagan, D., Levene, M.I. (1986) 'Intraventricular haemorrhage and periventricular leucomalacia: ultrasound and autopsy correlation.' *Archives of Disease in Childhood*, **61**, 1203–1207.

—— Shaw, D.E., Levene, M.I., Rutter, N. (1988) 'Clinical risk factors and periventricular leukomalacia.' *Archives of Disease in Childhood*, **63**, 17–22.

Tsang, R.C. (1972) 'Neonatal magnesium disturbances—a review.' *American Journal of Diseases of Children*, **124**, 282–293.

Valaes, T., Petmezaki, S., Henschke, C., *et al.* (1994) 'Control of jaundice in preterm newborns by an inhibitor of bilirubin production: studies with tin-mesoporphyrin.' *Pediatrics*, **93**, 1–11.

Vanapruks, V., Prapaitrakul, K. (1989) 'Water intoxication and hyponatraemic convulsions in neonates.' *Archives of Disease in Childhood*, **64**, 734–735.

Van Bel, F., van de Bor, M., Stijnen, T., *et al.* (1987) 'Aetiological rôle of cerebral blood-flow alterations in development and extension of peri-intraventricular haemorrhage.' *Developmental Medicine and Child Neurology*, **29**, 601–614.

—— den Ouden, L., van de Bor, M., *et al.* (1989) 'Cerebral blood-flow velocity during the first week of life of preterm infants and neurodevelopment at two years.' *Developmental Medicine and Child Neurology*, **31**, 320–328.

Van de Bor, M., Verloove-Vanhorick, S.P., Baerts, W., *et al.* (1988) 'Outcome of periventricular–intraventricular hemorrhage at 2 years of age in 484 very preterm infants admitted to 6 neonatal intensive care units in the Netherlands.' *Neuropediatrics*, **19**, 183–185.

—— Van Zeben-Van der Aa, T.M., Verloove-Vanhorick, S.P., *et al.* (1989) 'Hyperbilirubinemia in preterm infants and neurodevelopmental outcome at 2 years of age: results of a national collaborative survey.' *Pediatrics*, **83**, 915–920.

—— Ens-Dokkum, M., Schreuder, A.M., *et al.* (1992) 'Hyperbilirubinemia in low birth weight infants and outcome at 5 years of age.' *Pediatrics*, **89**, 359–364.

Vannucci, R.C. (1990) 'Current and potentially new management strategies for perinatal hypoxic–ischemic encephalopathy.' *Pediatrics*, **85**, 961–968.

—— Yager, J.Y. (1992) 'Glucose, lactic acid, and perinatal hypoxic–ischemic brain damage.' *Pediatric Neurology*, **8**, 3–12.

Ventriculomegaly Trial Group (1990) 'Randomised trial of early tapping in neonatal posthaemorrhagic ventricular dilatation.' *Archives of Disease in Childhood*, **65**, 3–10.

—— (1994) 'Randomised trial of early tapping in neonatal posthaemorrhagic ventricular dilatation: Results at 30 months.' *Archives of Disease in Childhood*, **70**, F129–F136.

Visser, G.H.A., Dijxhoorn, M.J. (1988) 'Intrapartum cardiotocogram, Apgar score and acidemia at birth: relationship to neonatal neurological morbidity.' *In:* Kubli, F., Patel, N., Schmidt, W. (Eds.) *Perinatal Events and Brain Damage in Surviving Children.* Berlin: Springer, pp. 168–174.

Vohr, B., Garcia-Coll, C., Flanagan, P., Oh, W. (1992) 'Effects of intraventricular hemorrhage and socioeconomic status on perceptual, cognitive, and neurologic status of low birth weight infants at 5 years of age.' *Journal of Pediatrics*, **121**, 280–285.

Voit, T., Lemburg, P., Neuen, E., *et al.* (1987) 'Damage of thalamus and basal ganglia in asphyxiated full-term neonates.' *Neuropediatrics*, **18**, 176–181.

Volpe, J.J. (1989a) 'Intraventricular hemorrhage in the premature infant: current concepts. Part I.' *Annals of Neurology*, **25**, 3–11.

—— (1989b) 'Intraventricular hemorrhage in the premature infant: current concepts. Part II.' *Annals of Neurology*, **25**, 109–116.

—— (1994) 'Brain injury caused by intraventricular hemorrhage: is indomethacin the silver bullet for prevention?' *Pediatrics*, **93**, 673–677.

—— (1995) *Neurology of the Newborn, 3rd Edn.* Philadelphia: W.B. Saunders.

—— Pasternak, J.F. (1977) 'Parasagittal cerebral injury in neonatal hypoxic–ischemic encephalopathy. Clinical and neuroradiologic features.' *Journal of Pediatrics*, **91**, 472–476.

Watanabe, K., Hakamada, S., Kuroyanagi, M., *et al.* (1983) 'Electroencephalographic study of intraventricular hemorrhage in the preterm newborn.' *Neuropediatrics*, **14**, 225–230.

Watchko, J.F., Oski, F.A. (1992) 'Kernicterus in preterm newborns: past, present, and future.' *Pediatrics*, **90**, 707–715.

—— Claassen, D. (1994) 'Kernicterus in premature infants: current prevalence and relationship to NICHD Phototherapy Study exchange criteria.' *Pediatrics*, **93**, 996–999.

Watkins, A., Szymonowicz, W., Jin, X., Yu, V.V.Y. (1988) 'Significance of seizures in very low-birthweight infants.' *Developmental Medicine and Child Neurology*, **30**, 162–169.

Weinstein, D., Margalioth, E.J., Navot, D., *et al.* (1983) 'Neonatal fetal death following cesarian section secondary to hyperextended head in breech presentation.' *Acta Obstetricia et Gynecologica Scandinavica*, **62**, 629–631.

Weisglas-Kuperus, N., Uleman-Vleeschdrager, M., Baerts, W. (1987) 'Ventricular haemorrhages and hypoxic–ischaemic lesions in preterm infants: neurodevelopmental outcome at 3½ years.' *Developmental Medicine and Child Neurology*, **29**, 623–629.

Welch, K., Strand, R. (1986) 'Traumatic parturitional intracranial haemorrhage.' *Developmental Medicine and Child Neurology*, **28**, 156–164.

Wertheim, D., Mercuri, E., Faundez, J,C., *et al.* (1994) 'Prognostic value of continuous electroencephalographic recording in full term infants with hypoxic ischaemic encephalopathy.' *Archives of Disease in Childhood*, **71**, F97–F102.

Wharton, R., Bresnan, M.J. (1989) 'Neonatal respiratory depression and delay in diagnosis in Prader–Willi syndrome.' *Developmental Medicine and Child Neurology*, **31**, 231–236.

Whitley, L.J., Nahmias, A.J., Visintine, A.M., *et al.* (1980) 'The natural history of herpes simplex virus infection of mother and newborn.' *Pediatrics*, **66**, 489–494.

Whittle, M.J. (1992) 'Rhesus haemolytic disease.' *Archives of Disease in Childhood*, **67**, 65–68.

Williamson, W.D., Percy, A.K., Fishman, M.A., *et al.* (1985) 'Cerebellar hemorrhage in the term neonate: developmental and neurologic outcome.' *Pediatric Neurology*, **1**, 356–360.

Wilson, D.A., Steiner, R.E. (1986) 'Periventricular leukomalacia: evaluation with MR imaging.' *Radiology*, **160**, 507–511.

Wimberley, P.D., Lou, H., Pedersen, H., *et al.* (1982) 'Hypertension peaks in the pathogenesis of intraventricular hemorrhage in the newborn. Abolition by phenobarbitone sedation.' *Acta Paediatrica Scandinavica*, **71**, 537–542.

Wiswell, T.E., Cornish, J.D., Northam, R.S. (1986) 'Neonatal polycythemia: frequency of clinical manifestations and other associated findings.' *Pediatrics*, **78**, 26 30.

Wong, V.K., Lemesurier, J., Franceschini, R., *et al.* (1987) 'Cerebral venous thrombosis as a cause of neonatal sepsis.' *Pediatric Neurology*, **3**, 235–237.

Worley, G., Erwin, C.W., Goldstein, R.F., *et al.* (1996) 'Delayed development of sensorineural hearing loss after neonatal hyperbilirubinemia: a case report with brain magnetic resonance imaging.' *Developmental Medicine and Child Neurology*, **38**, 271–277.

Wyatt, J.S. (1993) 'Near-infrared spectroscopy in asphyxial brain injury.' *Clinics in Perinatology*, **20**, 369–378.

Yamano, T., Fujiwara, S., Matsukawa, S., *et al.* (1992) 'Cervical cord birth injury and subsequent development of syringomyelia: a case report.' *Neuropediatrics*, **23**, 327–328.

Young, R.S.K., Towfighi, J., Marks, K.H. (1983) 'Focal necrosis of the spinal cord in utero.' *Archives of Neurology*, **40**, 654–655.

Younkin, D., Reivich, M., Jaggi, J.L. (1987) 'The effect of hematocrit and systolic blood pressure on cerebral blood flow in newborn infants.' *Journal of Cerebral Blood Flow and Metabolism*, **7**, 295–299.

Younkin, D., Medoff-Cooper, B., Guillet, R., *et al.* (1988) 'In vivo ^{31}P nuclear magnetic resonance measurement of chronic changes in cerebral metabolites following neonatal intraventricular hemorrhage.' *Pediatrics*, **82**, 331–336.

PART II

CNS MALFORMATIONS, CHROMOSOMAL ABNORMALITIES, NEUROCUTANEOUS SYNDROMES AND SKULL MALFORMATIONS

3

MALFORMATIONS OF THE CENTRAL NERVOUS SYSTEM

Malformations of the CNS have tended to be of interest only to neuropathologists and not to clinicians. The emergence of new concepts on teratogenesis drawn from experimental embryology, the study of animal models and other new techniques of investigation over the past two decades have excited the interest of other neurology specialists. With the advent of CT scanning, then of MRI, the diagnosis of many malformations has become feasible in the living patient and clinicians have become interested in their study. An early diagnosis has practical implications because it allows a precise prognosis to be made, and, in the case of genetically determined malformations, it is essential for genetic counselling. The development of techniques for prenatal diagnosis of fetal abnormalities (see Chapter 1) has coincided with a liberalization in attitudes toward abortion, allowing the possibility of preventing the birth of affected infants. This has raised considerable ethical and practical problems but the whole perspective of congenital brain defects has thus been transformed. Further advances in developmental neurobiology will enable us not only to answer fundamental questions about mammalian and, especially, human brain development but also hopefully to develop methods for the prevention, and perhaps the treatment, of at least some developmental brain defects (for reviews, see Caviness and Rakic 1978; Caviness et al. 1981; Rakic 1981; Evrard et al. 1984, 1989). A detailed account of the CNS malformations, their causes and pathology has recently been published (Harding and Copp 1997), to which the reader is referred for extensive review.

DEFINITIONS, FREQUENCY, AETIOLOGICAL FACTORS

The formation of the brain is such a fantastically complex process that it is not difficult to understand that it can be disturbed at any stage by a number of factors.

The term 'malformation', in this chapter, will designate any gross morphological abnormality of the CNS that dates to the embryonic or fetal period, regardless of its established or supposed mechanism (Evrard et al. 1984, Friede 1989). Some malformations are due to a deviation in the normal morphogenetic processes which may result from faulty genetic information or from interference with the harmonious development of correct genetic information. Another mechanism that can lead to malformation,

in the broad sense used in this text, is damage to normally formed structures followed by faulty repair. Malformations of this type generally occur late in pregnancy. However, purely destructive processes such as cystic softening or so-called 'clastic' porencephaly that do not modify the general structure of the nervous system do not belong in the group of malformations. Because repair mechanisms in the fetus are morphologically quite different from what they are later, in particular due to lack of glial proliferation, lesions incurred before the 20th week of pregnancy were often regarded in the past as resulting from 'arrest of development' or abnormal development. Such is the case of the so-called schizencephaly (see below) that was formerly thought to be due to arrest in development of the cerebral mantle but is now considered to result from an early destruction, perhaps of vascular origin. Secondary repair without evidence of cicatrization results in the formation of a cleft whose lips may be fused in a pial–ependymal 'seam' (Yakovlev and Wadsworth 1946). The cleft interferes with neuronal migration, if it is not yet completed, producing secondary abnormalities of migration (Menezes et al. 1988), thus illustrating the intricate relationship between external insults and errors of development, as well as the possible late consequences of temporally remote injuries.

Malformations are one of the commonest problems of child neurology. Statistical data suggest that 25 per cent of conceptuses are affected by a developmental CNS disturbance and such disturbances account for a high percentage of fetal deaths (Warkany et al. 1981, Kalter and Warkany 1983, Williams and Caviness 1984). In postnatal life, it has been estimated that 40 per cent of deaths in the first year of life are related in some way to CNS malformations (Evrard et al. 1989). In addition, recent studies indicate that many major neurological problems, such as cerebral palsy, are more frequently of prenatal than of postnatal origin (Nelson and Ellenberg 1986, Volpe 1995) and that a significant proportion of the prenatal cases are due to malformations. Likewise, prenatal abnormalities are often the origin of perinatal problems (Freeman and Nelson 1988).

The *aetiology* of CNS malformations remains obscure in most cases. It is generally held that the timing of an insult to the fetus is more important than the nature of the insult in determining the type of resulting malformations, and that the same noxious agent operating at different periods can produce distinct malformation patterns (Rodier 1980). However, some teratogenic agents tend preferentially to produce certain anomalies as shown by the effects of alcohol or of some antiepileptic drugs on the CNS. Thus sodium valproate tends to produce abnormal closure of the neural tube (Lindhout and Schmidt 1986), which is not the case with other anticonvulsant agents, although carbamazepine has also been incriminated (Rosa 1991).

Congenital malformations may be the result of *environmental causes* of infectious, toxic (Bingol *et al.* 1987), or physical (*e.g.* X-rays) nature; such account for about 5 per cent of malformations. Toluene encephalopathy (Hersh *et al.* 1985) and the fetal alcohol syndrome (Jones *et al.* 1973) are well-studied examples.

The exact role of *genetic factors* in the development of malformations is not entirely clear. According to Carter (1976), common malformations are seldom of monogenic (7.5 per cent) or chromosomal (6.0 per cent) origin, although new techniques will tend to increase the proportion of cases credited to minor chromosomal anomalies such as microdeletions. Polygenic inheritance, allowing for a multifactorial aetiology with interacting environmental and genetic factors, is the cause in 20 per cent of cases, whereas well-defined environmental teratogens have only a minor role (3.5 per cent), even though new teratogenic agents continue to be discovered, *e.g.* retinoic acid (Lammer *et al.* 1985).

About 60 per cent of all CNS malformations are of unknown cause (Cordero 1994).

The mechanisms of malformations are poorly understood despite recent important progress (Larroche 1977, Lyon and Beaugerie 1988, Evrard *et al.* 1989, Nelson and Holmes 1989, Walshe 1995). As already mentioned there are three major possibilities: (1) the programme of CNS development, in the form of DNA coding, is incorrect from the start because of inheritance, chromosomal anomaly, point mutations or larger DNA re-arrangements resulting in modified and improper instructions; (2) the basic design is normal but the instructions are incorrectly carried out because of traductional or post-traductional abnormalities, external interference with the processes of development, or haphazard accidents in the complex chain of events leading to a normal CNS; (3) the basic design is normal and it is normally carried out, only to be damaged secondarily with subsequent repair leading to major morphological changes in the CNS. Such changes may be difficult to distinguish morphologically from primary malformations.

From a didactic point of view, the likely date of occurrence of malformations allows one to separate them into two broad groups: (1) malformations that arise during the first five months of pregnancy—when major morphogenetic events, such as division of telencephalon into cerebral vesicles or neural tube closure, are taking place—and affect organogenesis and histogenesis, *i.e.* proliferation and migration of neurons leading to defective corticogenesis; (2) malformations that arise during the latter months of gestation, when all major cerebral components are in place and maturing. Most of these malformations are the secondary result of destructive processes such as ischaemia or infections (Larroche 1986). However, minor primary malformations can still arise because late migration, lamination and synaptogenesis can be interfered with (Sarnat 1987).

Peripheral malformations commonly accompany CNS abnormalities. For example, associated heart malformations are frequent and 7 per cent of children with congenital heart disease also have CNS malformations (Greenwood *et al.* 1975). Even outside well-defined malformation complexes, certain peripheral and visceral congenital anomalies tend to run together whereas other associations are rare (Natowicz *et al.* 1988, Khoury *et al.* 1989). Thus, neural tube defects are not associated with conotruncal abnormalities and are more frequent with spina bifida than with anencephaly or encephalocele. There exists also an association between CNS malformations and more general disturbances in development, abnormalities being 2.5 times more frequent in patients with intrauterine growth retardation than in the general population (Khoury *et al.* 1988).

NORMAL DEVELOPMENT OF THE CENTRAL NERVOUS SYSTEM

Only a brief outline of the embryological development of the CNS will be given. The reader is referred for more complete information to classical studies (Lemire *et al.* 1975, O'Rahilly and Müller 1987, Sarnat 1987, Barkovich *et al.* 1992, McConnell 1992). Table 3.1 presents a schematic overview of the main stages of CNS embryogenesis.

During the second week of embryogenesis, the three layers of ectoderm, mesoderm and entoderm are formed (Fig. 3.1). By two weeks the midline ectoderm, under the inductive influence of the underlying mesoderm, becomes the neural plate that further develops into the neural groove, then the neural tube. During the fourth week, the neural tube closes. The process of closure begins in the middle part of the tube and proceeds towards the extremities. Neural cell adhesion molecules play a central role in the process of closure (Waterman 1979). Closure of the neural tube is determined by dorsal induction from the mesoderm. Before closure of the tube, on day nine, the anlagen of the future rhombencephalon, mesencephalon, prosencephalon and otic placodes become apparent at its anterior part. Simultaneously, clusters of cells along the lateral margins of the neural tube separate to form the paired neural crests that will give rise to major structures of the peripheral nervous system, meninges, melanocytes and face.

The posterior part of the neural plate and notocord has a different fate: it forms a mass of cells which is going to canalize and to undergo the process of regressive differentation to form the lower spinal cord.

By 32–33 days, the prosencephalon has formed the telencephalic vesicles and the diencephalon has differentiated, so that four identifiable cellular masses are present by eight weeks, in the region of the basal ganglia. The process of vesicle formation probably results from ventral induction by the notocord, but intimate mechanisms of induction are poorly understood.

From about 30 days, the major inductive processes are completed and cellular differentiation begins. *Multiplication* of

TABLE 3.1
Major stages of CNS development

Stage	Peak time of occurrence	Major morphological events in cerebrum	Major morphological events in cerebellum	Main corresponding disorders*
Uterine implantation	1 wk			
Separation of 3 layers	2 wks	Neural plate		Enterogenous cysts and fistulae
Dorsal induction Neurulation	3–4 wks	Neural tube, neural crest and derivatives. Closure of anterior (d 24) and posterior (d 29) neuropores	Paired alar plates	Anencephaly, encephalocele, craniorachischisis, spina bifida, meningoceles
Caudal neural tube formation	4–7 wks	Canalization and regressive differentiation of cord	Rhombic lips (d 35), cerebellar plates	Diastematomyelia, Dandy–Walker syndrome, Cerebellar hypoplasia
Ventral induction	5–6 wks	Forebrain and face (cranial neural crest). Cleavage of prosencephalon into cerebral vesicles (d 33). Optic placodes (d 26), olfactory placodes. Diencephalon	Fusion of cerebellar plates	Holoprosencephaly, median cleft face syndrome
Neuronal and glial proliferation	8–16 wks	Cellular proliferation in ventricular and subventricular zone (interkinetic migration). Early differentiation of neuroblasts and glioblasts.	Migration of Purkinje cells (9–10 w). Migration of external granule layer (10–11 w)	Microcephaly, megalencephaly
Migration	12–20 wks	Radial migration and accessory pathways (e.g. corpus gangliothalamicum). Formation of corpus callosum	Dendritic tree of Purkinje cells (16–25 w)	Lissencephaly–pachygyria (types I and II), Zellweger syndrome, glial heterotopia, microgyria (some forms), agenesis of corpus callosum
Organization**	24 wks to postnatal	Late migration (to 5 months). Alignment, orientation and layering of cortical neurons. Synaptogenesis. Glial proliferation/differentiation well into postnatal life	Monolayer of Purkinje cells (16–28 w). Migration of granules to form internal granular layer (to postnatal life)	Minor cortical dysplasias, dendritic/synaptic abnormalities, microgyria (some forms)
Myelination	24 wks to 2 yrs postnatally			Dysmyelination, clastic insults

*Disorders do not necessarily correspond to abnormal development. They may also result from secondary destruction/disorganization.
**Programmed cellular death takes place throughout the second half of pregnancy and the first year of extrauterine life.

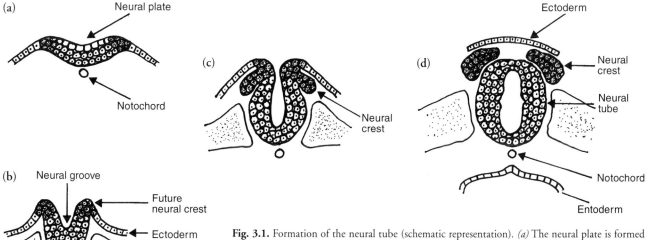

Fig. 3.1. Formation of the neural tube (schematic representation). (a) The neural plate is formed by thickening of the ectoderm under induction from the notochord. (b) The neural groove appears. The anlagen of the neural crest are visible. (c) The neural crest is well formed and its cells will migrate laterally to their targets. (d) Closure of the neural tube begins in the central region; the extremities (anterior and posterior neuropores) will close later. Closure allows the tube to be covered by ectoderm and mesenchymal tissue.

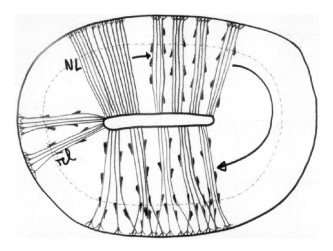

Fig. 3.2. Schematic representation of neuronal migration along radial glial guides. Transverse section of neural tube. (Courtesy Prof. P. Evrard, Cliniques Saint-Luc, Brussels.)
    NL: Embryonic stage—regularly aligned glial guides. *First arrow:* migration of neurons destined to deep cortical layers along glial guides now grouped in fascicles. *Curved arrow:* late stages of neuronal migration (layers II and III). Progressive defasciculation of glial guides.
    rl: Situation in the reeler mutant mouse in which no defasciculation takes place.

primitive cells that are going to form both neurons and glia occurs, mainly in the vicinity of the lumen of the neural tube. Mitoses take place in the deeper cellular layers (Caviness and Takahashi 1995). The resulting nuclei migrate toward the outside during telophase, then come back to the deep region to initiate another cycle, the so-called intrakinetic migration. Proliferation of cells exceeds the ultimate requirements so that it is intimately related to the poorly understood process of programmed cell death by apoptosis that affects some 30–50 per cent of the cells formed.

Corticogenesis has been particularly studied over the past two decades. In the embryonic period (45- to 50-day-old embryos), primitive corticopetal fibres arrive via the diencephalic sulcus and expand under the telencephalic pia; neurons appear within these fibres to form the primordial plexiform layer (PPL) (Marin-Padilla 1978, 1984) or preplate. The PPL precedes the migration of neurons that form the cortical plate and serves as scaffolding for subsequently migrating cells. These split the preplate into a superficial part that will constitute the molecular layer or layer I and a deep layer termed the subplate (or layer VII) that disappears before the end of intrauterine life. Subplate neurons act as a relay for corticopetal thalamic axons before cells of the cortical fourth layer are functional. They disappear by apoptosis before 1 year of age. Later migrating cells, that will form layers II to VI of the definitive cortex, migrate in an 'inside out' manner, that is to say the most recently generated late-migrating cells form the most superficial layer (layer II) of the cortical plate, whereas large pyramidal cells of layers V and VI migrate early.

Most neurons destined for the cerebral cortex migrate between the 10th and 18th gestational weeks, and the full complement of cortical neurons is essentially completed by 20 weeks.

However, cellular migration continues at a slower pace throughout pregnancy, and some cells, *e.g.* cerebellar and hippocampal granules, migrate postnatally (Sarnat 1987, 1991).

Neurons migrate radially along glial guides that extend from the ventricular (proliferative) zone to the pial surface of the neural tube and derived structures (Sidman and Rakic 1973; Rakic 1975, 1981; Williams and Caviness 1984) (Fig. 3.2). Glial guides are later converted into astrocytes, thus marking the end of migration. Several cells use the same glial fibre in their migration, which may be responsible for the columnar organization of the cortex universally found in mammals (Rockel *et al.* 1980), the column representing the functional units of the cortex. These functional units differ by their numbers rather than by their basic organization in different species. Not all neurons follow faithfully a particular glial guide. Twelve to 14 per cent leave their guide to migrate in a perpendicular direction (Caviness and Takahashi 1995, Walsh 1995) and a few may move to a neighbouring guide. In addition, precursor cells often move horizontally within the ventricular zone before radial migration begins, so there is a considerable mixing of neuron precursors which explains the dispersion of postmigratory neurons of a similar clonal origin over wide cortical areas (Walsh and Cepko 1993).

The second half of gestation is characterized by a rapid increase in the length and complexity of dendrites and axons, by the establishment of synapses, and by maturation and fine organization of the cortex. The result is a rapid increase in weight of the brain and the process of sulcation necessary to accomodate the massively increasing surface area of the cortex. Secondary and tertiary sulci appear between the seventh and ninth months of gestation, and most gyri are present by 28 weeks. The full laminar structure of the cortex is complete by birth.

Dendrites, axons and synapses develop at a tremendous rate, and many of the synapses then formed will eventually disappear. Development of dendrites, axonal arborizations and dendritic spines continues until the fourth year of life. Glial development is a complex process, various precursors having different fates. Some develop into radiating glial fibres used by migrating neurons. Many astrocytes are produced by the persisting periventricular proliferative zone after the end of neuronal migration (Gressens *et al.* 1992). Myelin begins to be deposited at about 30 weeks but most of the process of myelin formation is postnatal (Yakovlev and Lecours 1967, Brody *et al.* 1987).

DISTURBANCES OF NORMAL DEVELOPMENT

As expected from the complexity of the processes involved, there is an almost infinite variety of abnormalities of CNS development, only the most frequent of which will be considered.

DISORDERS OF NEURULATION AND CAUDAL NEURAL TUBE FORMATION (BLASTOPATHIES)
Disorders of neurulation and caudal neural tube formation include all forms of failure of the neural tube to fuse completely, with secondary abnormal development of the mesenchymal

structures enclosing the CNS, from anencephaly to sacral myelomeningocele and sacral agenesis (Peach 1965, Padget 1972, McLone and Naidich 1992). In the absence of tube closure, the posterior mesenchyme does not develop so that there is no bony structure covering the neuroectoderm.

The basic anomaly may be nondisjunction of the neural gutter from overlying epithelium, resulting in myelomeningocele or dermal sinus. Premature disjunction could be responsible for lipomyelocele or juxtamedullary or subpial lipoma. This in turn could result from a defect in the cell adhesion molecules. Other mechanisms include abnormal canalization or regression of the caudal end of the cord resulting in abnormalities of the filum (Tsukamoto *et al.* 1992) and abnormal splitting of the notochord responsible for spinal–enteric cysts and diastematomyelia.

The term *dysraphism* indicates, in its complete form, persistent continuity between posterior neuroectoderm and cutaneous ectoderm. Dysraphism comprises several varieties. *Cranial dysraphism* includes anencephaly and cephaloceles. *Spinal dysraphism* designates spina bifida cystica and occulta with several subtypes. The basic mechanism appears to be a lack of closure of the neural tube, perhaps related to a defect in the cell adhesion molecules, rather than secondary reopening or rupture of the neural tube.

The causes of dysraphism remain obscure. They seem to be sufficiently similar to allow all types to be considered together even though there may be some differences (for example the recurrence risks may not be equal for spina aperta, anencephaly or cephaloceles). Genetic factors are important. Usually, they fit in with a polygenic or multifactorial model (Carter 1976), but a small minority may follow a mendelian type of inheritance with recessive and even X-linked transmission (Holmes *et al.* 1976, Baraitser and Burn 1984). Environmental factors have been repeatedly stressed although the search for specific agents has been disappointing. Young maternal age and low socioeconomic level seem to play a role. The role of vitamin deficiency, especially folic acid, proposed by Smithells *et al.* (1981) is now accepted (Gordon 1995). A common polymorphism of the gene that codes for tetrahydrofolate reductase may significantly increase the risk of neural tube defect (van der Put *et al.* 1995). It has been confirmed that administration of multiple vitamin supplements containing folic acid sharply reduces the incidence of neural tube defects if given at least 28 days before conception and continued for the first two months of pregnancy (Smithells *et al.* 1983, Milunsky *et al.* 1989, MRC Study Research Group 1991, Czeizel and Dudás 1992). Maternal fever (Finnell *et al.* 1993), drugs (Lindhout and Schmidt 1986), other chemicals and X-irradiation (Giroud 1960) have also been incriminated. Valproic acid has been implicated (Robert and Guibaud 1982) although the evidence remains in dispute.

The empirical risks of recurrence for mothers who have given birth to a child with neural tube defects vary between 1.5 and 5 per cent (Nakano 1973, Milunsky 1980). The risk is about 6 per cent for women with two children with spina bifida. The risk may be higher for anencephaly, up to 10 per cent of siblings of anencephalics having neural tube defects of various types (Fedrick 1976). The transmission of anencephaly appears to be matrilineal, and the recurrence rate for maternal half-siblings is the same as for full siblings (James 1980).

The *incidence* of neural tube defects is widely variable in different parts of the world, being low in Japan and reaching 3 per cent in the British Isles (Luciano 1987). The incidence is 10 times higher in early abortuses (Bell 1979) and 24 times higher in stillborn infants (Wiswell *et al.* 1990). Secular changes in occurrence have long been known (Mortimer 1980, Windham and Edmonds 1982, Stone 1987). Anencephaly is three to seven times more frequent in girls than in boys (Nakano 1973), but the sex ratio is about equal in low spina bifida (Seller 1987). Currently, there is a sharp decrease in the frequency of neural tube defects in Western countries which may not be due entirely to prenatal diagnosis followed by termination.

The respective frequencies of the various types are variable. Stoll *et al.* (1988) in eastern France found an incidence of spina bifida of 0.62 per 1000. The incidence of anencephaly was 0.33 per 1000 and that of encephaloceles 0.14 per 1000. Wiswell *et al.* (1990) found a lower incidence for US populations. The total incidence for 763,364 births was 3.53 per cent in stillborn infants and 0.145 per cent in liveborn babies. The incidence of spina bifida was 68.9 per 100,000, that of anencephaly 36 per 100,000, and that of hydrocephalus, excluding haemorrhage and meningitis, 48.4 per 100,000.

Prenatal diagnosis of the open forms of neural tube defect is possible by ultrasonography and by determination of alpha-feto-protein (AFP) in the amniotic fluid obtained by amniocentesis (Wald and Cuckle 1984). AFP represents 90 per cent of total serum globulins in the fetus. With open tube defects, it leaks into the amniotic fluid and hence into maternal blood. Determination of AFP levels in amniotic fluid obtained by amniocentesis at 16–18 weeks gestational age permits detection of over 99 per cent of fetuses with neural tube defects. False positives are often, but not always, associated with other severe fetal abnormalities. Many false positives are avoided by simultaneous determination of acetyl-cholinesterase (Collaborative Acetylcholinesterase Study 1981).

AFP levels *in maternal serum* at 13–16 weeks gestation are used as a screening test for neural tube defects, and the routine determination of AFP is recommended, the more so as it is also used in the 'triple test' for the detection of Down syndrome. Normal adult levels are below 10 ng/mL and increase during pregnancy up to 500 ng/mL. Levels greater than 1000 ng/mL at 15–20 weeks gestational age are highly suggestive of neural tube defect. However, there is a high incidence of false positives, and even the finding of two abnormal levels of AFP without a 'benign' explanation (*i.e.* multiple pregnancy, wrong dates) is associated with a benign outcome of pregnancy in 40 per cent of instances and only 10 per cent of such fetuses have a neural tube defect (Burton and Dillard 1986). On the other hand, false negatives are also known to occur (Wald and Cuckle 1984), so the value is not absolute (Holtzman 1983). Nevertheless, screening by this method is now recommended by the American College of Gynecologists and Obstetricians.

Ultrasonography is used as a routine procedure for the detection of fetal malformations. It permits detection of over 98

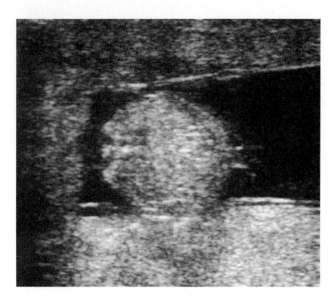

Fig. 3.3. Spina bifida aperta (antenatal diagnosis at 18 weeks of amenor-rhoea). Axial cut showing absence of neurulation of neural plate *(left side of photograph)*, which is denser than rest of fetal body and limited on both sides by a well-defined ridge. (Courtesy Dr M-C. Aubry, Maternité Port-Royal, Paris.)

per cent of cases of anencephaly from the age of about 12–14 weeks. For spina bifida (Fig. 3.3), similar figures are reached in the best hands at 16–20 weeks but qualified personnel and adequate material are not available everywhere (d'Alton and De Cherney 1993, Ewigman *et al.* 1993, Govaert and de Vries 1997). Careful search for a deformity of the frontal bone ('lemon sign') and of cerebellar compression due to the associated Chiari mal-formation ('banana sign') helps considerably to make a correct diagnosis (Nicolaides 1986), which is possible in most cases (Nadel *et al.* 1990, Van den Hof *et al.* 1990). False positive results occur uncommonly (Chard and Macintosh 1992). A recent study in a French department showed that the results of the *routine use* of ultrasonography are much less impressive (Stoll *et al.* 1988). The diagnosis of anencephaly was made in 88 per cent of cases but after 26 weeks in 60 per cent; that of spina bifida in only 53 per cent (11 per cent before 26 weeks); and that of encephaloceles in 64 per cent (50 per cent before 26 weeks). Antenatal diagnosis of encephaloceles and meningoceles is also relatively easy (Milunsky 1986). Currently, ultrasonography is probably the best tool for antenatal diagnosis of neural tube defects if performed by a well-trained operator. All at-risk women, *i.e.* those who have borne a previous fetus with tube defect, those who are taking sodium valproate, those with positive serum AFP screening and those in whom one ultrasound examination has been deemed suspect, should have ultrasonography in a reliable centre. If no certainty is gained, amniocentesis with AFP and acetylcholinesterase determination should be performed. In addi-tion, any examination of amniotic fluid taken for another indi-cation should include AFP determination. Some investigators think that amniocentesis can be avoided if a good ultrasonogram can be obtained (Nadel *et al.* 1990) but others are reluctant to abandon it completely (Drugan *et al.* 1988, Richards *et al.* 1988).

CRANIAL DYSRAPHISM
This heading includes anencephaly and encephaloceles or cephaloceles.

Anencephaly is a lethal condition that is progressively disap-pearing from most developed countries because its early antenatal diagnosis is easy. Anencephaly results from failure of the cephalic folds to fuse into a neural tube with resulting degeneration of the neural cells and absence of mesodermal tissue dorsal to the neural elements so that the bony skull does not develop. Partial forms with preservation of some telencephalic structures may be due to the fact that there are multiple sites of anterior neuropore closure (Golden and Chernoff 1995). Marin-Padilla (1980, 1991) pro-posed that the primary defect is in the segmental division of the anterior part of the embryo, with resultant hypoplasia of the sphenoid bone. This could produce secondary skull bone abnor-malities variably resulting in absence of formation of the skull vault or, in less severe cases, in a hypoplastic posterior fossa. In this view, CNS abnormalities are secondary: the defective skull results in failure of tube formation because of the wide gap between the lips of the neural gutter. Exposure then leads to secondary destruction of the brain.

The spinal cord, brainstem and cerebellum are present and part of the diencephalon may also be preserved. Failure of fusion of vertebrae (rachischisis) and herniation of cerebral tissue (exencephaly) are frequently associated. There may be evidence of secondary degeneration of some previously formed structures.

Automatisms of suction and Moro reflexes are usually present, and some infants exhibit seizures that may be similar to infantile spasms (André-Thomas and de Ajuriaguerra 1959). Anencephalic infants usually die in a few hours to weeks. The anterior hypophysis of anencephalic infants is ectopic or absent. The syndrome of panhypopituitarism with microphthalmia is probably related to anencephaly (Kaplowitz and Bodurtha 1993).

Atelencephaly differs from anencephaly by the presence of a normally formed skull (Garcia and Duncan 1977, Siebert *et al.* 1986). There is no organized neural structure above the dien-cephalic level, the telencephalon being reduced to a small mass of anarchically disposed neurons and glial cells. Surprisingly, such atelencephalic brains can occasionally produce typical epilep-tic EEG discharges, recordable from the scalp (Danner *et al.* 1985), a phenomenon also observed in cases of hydranencephaly. Accessory brains are a rare anomaly that may present with prenatal mass lesions (Harris *et al.* 1994a). Aprosencephaly is a more severe variant in which diencephalic structures are not preserved (Harris *et al.* 1994b).

Encephaloceles or cephaloceles and cranium bifidum
These abnormalities satisfy the criteria for dysraphism, *i.e.* a mesenchymal defect with herniation of dura, cerebral or cerebellar tissue, or ventricles is apparent (McLaurin 1987). Although anterior cephaloceles may be more closely related to disorders of ventral rather than dorsal induction (see below), they are considered here for convenience. Cephaloceles are frequently associated with other malformations such as agenesis of the corpus callosum or abnormal gyration (Martinez-Lage *et al.*

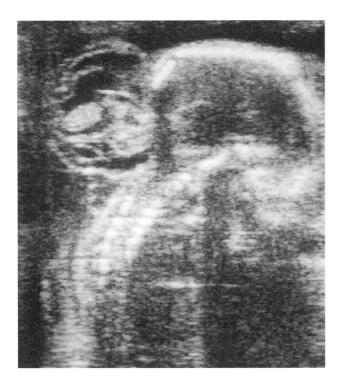

Fig. 3.4. Occipital encephalocele (antenatal diagnosis). Sagittal cut showing normal cranial vault anteriorly *(right side of photograph)* and large encephalocele protruding posteriorly with content of mixed echodensity *(left side)*. (Courtesy Dr M-C. Aubry, Maternité Port-Royal, Paris.)

1996). Cephaloceles are 3–16 times less common than spina bifida cystica. In Western countries, 85 per cent of encephaloceles are posteriorly located (Fig. 3.4), whereas in Asia anterior encephaloceles are more common. Isolated cranium bifidum, which is a simple skull defect without prolapse of meninges or brain, is rare and clinically insignificant (Naidich *et al.* 1992). Atretic encephaloceles are regarded as *formes frustes* of meningoencephaloceles. They commonly occur in the parietal and occipital regions (Yokota *et al.* 1988) and may present as a large posterior fontanelle. They may occur in the Walker–Warburg and Joubert syndromes. Most cephaloceles contain some brain tissue (encephaloceles). Cranial meningoceles contain only meninges and CSF without neural tissue.

Cranial meningoceles are less common than encephaloceles (Naidich *et al.* 1992). Small posterior meningocephaloceles are usually covered by a normal scalp. Larger ones may be covered by abnormal skin with angiomas or by a thin membrane. The presence of a hair collar may be a marker of cranial dysraphism (Drolet *et al.* 1995).

Meningoceles are genetically related to other neural tube defects. Forms that are part of mendelian syndromes are listed in Table 3.2.

Posterior encephaloceles may contain infratentorial or supratentorial brain structures or both (Simpson *et al.* 1984, Naidich *et al.* 1992). The bony defect may be of any size and is located above or below the tentorium. Cerebellar ectopia may be associated—the Chiari III malformation (see Table 3.3, p. 78). In the series of Lorber and Schofield (1979), comprising 147 occipital cephaloceles, only 25 per cent were pure meningoceles, hydrocephalus was present in half the cases and 16 per cent had other anomalies, especially agenesis of the corpus callosum. Parietal cephaloceles are much rarer and even more frequently associated with other malformations (McLaurin 1987). Posterior encephaloceles seem to result from dysraphism in most cases. However, postinductional occurrence is possible as in the case reported by Evrard and Caviness (1974).

Subtorcular occipital encephaloceles are usually associated with severe cerebellar developmental defects (Chapman *et al.* 1989).

The prognosis of posterior cephaloceles is poor (Brown and Sheridan-Pereira 1992). In one series (Lorber 1979), 90 per cent of infants died and 50 per cent of survivors were retarded. Fifty per cent of operated infants survived but two thirds of them remained disabled. Hydrocephalus is present in over half the cases (Lorber and Schofield 1979).

Anterior cephaloceles include several types: sphenoidal, protruding through the body of the sphenoid; and fronto-ethmoidal, subdivided into nasoethmoidal, nasofrontal, nasoorbital, interfrontal and posterior orbital types (David *et al.* 1984, Diebler and Dulac 1987). They are sometimes associated with supratentorial defects such as callosal agenesis (Barkovich *et al.* 1988). Their overall prognosis is considerably better than that of the posterior anomalies. There is no increased risk of recurrence in siblings.

They are usually revealed easily at birth by the presence of a visible deformity, especially in the nasofrontal and interfrontal types. Sphenoidal cephaloceles produce pharyngeal obstruction in association with hypertelorism and/or labial fissure and with optic nerve abnormalities (coloboma or optic atrophy). An endocrinological syndrome of deficit in somatotrophin, gonadotrophin or antidiuretic hormone secretion is noted in half the cases (Lieblich *et al.* 1978). Recurrent meningitis has been observed (Izquierdo and Gil-Carcedo 1988). Diagnosis is suggested by examination of the pharynx and is confirmed by skull X-rays and CT showing herniation of the third ventricle. Surgery is indicated. Basal cephaloceles (Morioka *et al.* 1995) may be associated with optic disc anomalies and hormonal disturbances.

Nasofrontal cephaloceles produce nasal obstruction and, rarely, CSF leakage. They may be detected only after 2 years of age. Their prognosis depends on the nature of the content. The so-called *nasal glioma* (Younus and Coode 1986) is a small nasal encephalocele that has become separated from the base of the brain.

Lipomas of the corpus callosum may have an anterosuperior extension that represents a mild form of cephalocele protruding in the region of the bregma (Kushnet and Goldman 1978). They should be distinguished from angiomas and dermoid cyst of the anterior fontanelle, melanotic progonoma and ectopic brain tissue (Naidich *et al.* 1992). Dermoid cysts of the anterior fontanelle can be adherent to the sagittal sinus, and great care should be exercised in their exeresis (Pannell *et al.* 1982).

Anterobasal temporal encephaloceles extending into the pterygopalatine fossa through a bony defect at the base of the greater wing of the sphenoid may be responsible for resistant epilepsy

TABLE 3.2
TABLE 3.2
Main syndromes with encephalocele

Syndrome	Main features*	Inheritance**	References
Meckel–Gruber syndrome	Polycystic kidneys, postaxial polydactyly, hydrocephalus, vermian agenesis, cleft lip and palate, clubfoot, genital anomalies, microphthalmia	AR (common: 1 per 30,000–50,000 births)	Hsia *et al.* (1971), Hori *et al.* (1980), Paetau *et al.* (1985)
Dandy–Walker syndrome	Vermal agenesis, hydrocephalus, heterotopia of lower olivary body, agenesis of corpus callosum	Sporadic	Hirsch *et al.* (1984), Pascual-Castroviejo *et al.* (1991)
Walker–Warburg syndrome	Hydrocephalus, vermian agenesis, severe neurological dysfunction from birth, type 2 lissencephaly (see text)	AR	Williams *et al.* (1984), Dobyns *et al.* (1989)
Joubert syndrome	Panting respiration and apnoeic episodes from birth, mental retardation, vermian agenesis, retinopathy or optic disc coloboma, cerebellar ataxia	AR	Aicardi *et al.* (1983), Edwards *et al.* (1988)
Tectocerebellar dysraphism with occipital encephalocele	Mental retardation	Sporadic	Friede 1978, Altman *et al.* (1992)
Goldenhar–Gorlin syndrome	Orofacial abnormalities, preauricular tags, epibulbar dermoids	Sporadic	Aleksic *et al.* (1983)
Chromosomal syndromes, in particular trisomy 13	See Chapter 5	Mainly sporadic	Holmes *et al.* (1976)
Occipital encephalocele, myopia and retinal dysplasia	Retinal detachment	Probably genetic, mode not established	Knobloch and Layer (1971)
Syndrome of cranial and limb defects secondary to aberrant tissue bands, amniotic bands syndrome	Congenital amputation of digits or limbs, facial clefts, circumferential scars around limbs	Nongenetic	Urich and Herrrick (1985), Moerman *et al.* (1992)
Median cleft face syndrome	Anterior encephalocele	AD (possibly)	De Myer (1967)
Roberts syndrome	Anterior encephalocele may be a part	AR	Freeman *et al.* (1974)

*All features are rarely present in each case. Encephalocele is not a constant feature.
**AR = autosomal recessive; AD = autosomal dominant.

(Leblanc *et al.* 1990) and for CSF otorrhoea and recurrent meningitis.

Cephaloceles are uncommonly *part of a defined syndrome* (Cohen and Lemire 1982), although they are frequently associated with other birth defects: cleft palate, microphthalmia, holoprosencephaly, agenesis of the corpus callosum and cerebellar defects. The most common of the many syndromes that include cephalocele as a necessary or prominent feature are listed in Table 3.2. The Meckel–Gruber syndrome is the most frequent of these (Hsia *et al.* 1971, Hori *et al.* 1980). It consists of polydactyly, polycystic kidneys, retinal dysplasia and hydrocephalus, in addition to the CNS features: prosencephalic dysgenesis, occipital encephalocele and rhombic roof dysgenesis (Ahdab-Barmada and Claassen 1990). The clinical expression of this autosomal recessive syndrome is variable, even within the same sibship, and cases may be wrongly diagnosed as Dandy–Walker syndrome or congenital hydrocephalus when the expression is incomplete (Seller 1981). Related syndromes have been reviewed by Naidich *et al.* (1992).

The treatment of cephaloceles is surgical. Surgery is sometimes indicated on an emergency basis when there is leakage of CSF. In other cases it is elective. The results depend on the volume of brain tissue contained in the cephalocele and on associated malformations (Brown and Sheridan-Pereira 1992).

SPINAL DYSRAPHISM
The term 'spinal dysraphism' applies to a heterogeneous group of spinal abnormalities with the common feature of imperfect formation of the midline mesenchymal, bony and neural structures.

In almost all cases spinal dysraphism manifests as *spina bifida* in which there is dysraphism of the osseous structures resulting in incomplete closure of the spinal canal. Some investigators have argued that secondary rupture, rather than absence of closure, is the cause in some cases (see Padget 1972).

Spina bifida cystica
Spina bifida cystica (Fig. 3.5) is the commonest type of spinal dysraphism and includes myeloschisis, myelomeningocele and meningocele. Except in the last of these, nervous structures are exposed without skin covering. In *spina bifida occulta* the neural elements are covered by skin and do not protrude above the level of the back.

Myelomeningocele and myeloschisis, which constitute 95 per cent of the cases of spinal dysraphism, are basically identical, the only difference being that myeloschisis is flat while myelomeningocele is bulging. There is no mesenchyme behind the spinal cord which has remained flat with a median groove corresponding to the open ependymal canal. The skin is in direct continuity with the meninges that attach to the lateral limits of

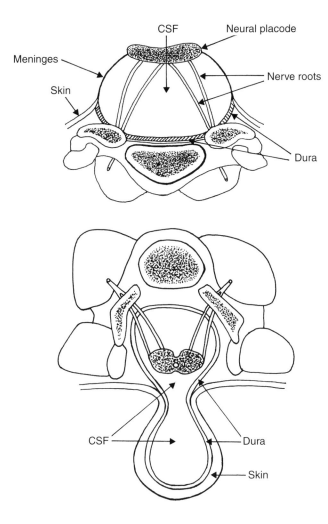

Fig. 3.5. *(Top)* Myelomeningocele. The neural placode has not undergone neurulation and is in direct continuity with the rest of the dorsal ectoderm. A thin membrane, representing the leptomeninx and easily torn open, connects the placode to the skin. Note the absence of the posterior arch of vertebra and of any form of mesenchymal derivate behind the neural tissue.

(Bottom) Meningocele. The spinal cord is completely formed. The meninges are covered with skin. In some cases, the neural roots may have an abnormal course and enter the meningocele before exiting from the spinal canal which remains uncovered with mesenchyma behind the neural tissue.

the plate (Naidich 1989). Variable abnormalities are associated. Diastematomyelia is present in 31–46 per cent of instances, the slit being cephalic to the cele in 31 per cent, at the level of the cele in 22 per cent and caudal to it in 25 per cent of cases (Emery and Lendon 1973). In rare patients, the cele is located to one hemicord or involves the two hemicords at different levels, producing very asymmetrical clinical findings. Hydrosyringomyelia is present in 33–75 per cent of cases and is often associated with severe scoliosis (Hall *et al.* 1975). Its incidence depends on the success of shunt therapy of accompanying hydrocephalus. Hydromyelia typically distends the entire length of the spinal canal from the obex down the central canal to the upper pole of the neural plate. CSF may remain within the central canal or disperse into the spinal cord, so the distinction between syringo-

myelia and hydromyelia is somewhat artificial (Schlesinger 1981, Breningstall *et al.* 1992).

In all cases, the cord is stuck in a low position. The meninges are extremely thin and rupture easily with a resulting high risk of infection. In cases left untreated, epithelialization takes place over the meningeal membrane and neural plate. The process may leave scarring with a fibrous band kinking and compressing the cord. In some cases, epidermoid or dermoid cysts result from skin cell inclusion in the scar, often associated with small lipomas detectable by MRI scan better than by CT. Segmental infarction of the cord may occur (Naidich 1989). Myeloceles are lumbar or thoracolumbar in more than half the cases, and lumbosacral in over 25 per cent. Cervical and thoracic locations together account for 11 per cent of cases (Matson 1969).

Cranial anomalies are often associated with myelomeningoceles, especially Chiari II malformation which is present in 70 per cent of cases (Table 3.3). Chiari I malformation (Fig. 3.6), on the other hand, is not associated with spina bifida and is rarely symptomatic during childhood (Dauser *et al.* 1989, Dure *et al.* 1989, Elster and Chen 1992). It may be associated with malformations of the base of the skull and upper cervical spine (Chapter 6), and with syringomyelia in about half the cases. The diagnosis can be made by ultrasonography (Govaert and de Vries 1997), but is determined more precisely by MRI, which shows the low position and elongation of the lower brainstem (Mikulis 1992). Symptoms may result from medullary compression and be precipitated by trauma. They variably include headache (Pascual *et al.* 1992), dysfunction of the lower cranial nerves, cerebellar signs, and pain in the neck and occipital region. Somnolence and episodes of apnoea are sometimes observed (Keefover *et al.* 1995, Yglesias *et al.* 1996).

Chiari II is the most common variant of the Cleland–Chiari malformation. It consists of partial dislocation of medulla and cerebellum, especially the vermis, into the cervical canal, overriding the upper spinal cord. The dorsal aspect of the medulla forms a kink at the bulbospinal junction (Naidich *et al.* 1980a). Cerebellar tissue may descend as far down as C3 level. The fourth ventricle is elongated and partially herniated into the cervical canal. There is often a defect in the posterior arch of the atlas, and a fibrous band is often present at the level of the foramen magnum and may compress the medulla. The posterior fossa is small, with scalloping and erosion of the posteromedial part of the petrous pyramids (Naidich *et al.* 1980c). The so-called lacunar skull (Luckenschädel) is present in up to 85 per cent of cases with Chiari II malformation (Peach 1965). It does not necessarily predict a low intelligence (Fishman *et al.* 1977). The brainstem is elongated and the colliculi are fused and beaked. The cerebellar hemispheres may develop anteriorly, surrounding the brainstem (Naidich *et al.* 1980a). There is a large massa intermedia and, not infrequently, heterotopias of hemispheral grey matter (Naidich *et al.* 1980b). A microgyric appearance of the cortex is often reported but microscopic examination indicates a normal cortical architecture, so the appearance is due to mechanical factors rather than a true malformation (Evrard *et al.* 1989). The falx cerebri and tentorium are hypoplastic (Naidich *et al.* 1980c). Extradural

TABLE 3.3
Chiari (Cleland–Chiari, Arnold–Chiari) malformations

Type	Main features	Associated abnormalities	Neurological features	References
Type I*	Downward displacement of lower cerebellum, especially tonsils, elongated 4th ventricle and lower brainstem, in the absence of intracranial space-occupying lesion	Platybasia, basilar impression, syringomyelia (20% of cases), hydrocephalus (40% of cases), no spina bifida or myelomeningocele	Mainly adolescents and adults. Features related to hydrocephalus or syringomyelia. Cervical compression with quadriplegia, apnoea, headaches possible even in young children (Itoh *et al.* 1988); rarely familial (Stovner *et al.* 1992)	Itoh *et al.* (1988), Tan *et al.* (1995)
Type II	Downward displacement of cerebellar vermis or tonsils along the dorsal aspect of cervical spinal cord. Kinking of posterior aspect of spinal cord at level of C2–C3 vertebrae	Myelomeningocele in over 95% of cases. Posterior fossa and midbrain abnormalities, aqueductal stenosis, meningeal anomalies (see text). Abnormal cortical gyration**	Manifest from newborn period by signs related to hydrocephalus and myelomeningocele. Dysfunction of lower cranial nerves, respiration and swallowing. Paralysis of upper limbs due to cervical compression	Naidich *et al.* (1980a,b,c), Friede (1989)
Type III	Downward displacement of cerebellum into a posterior encephalocele with elongation and herniation of 4th ventricle	Cervical spina bifida or posterior cranium bifidum or both	Manifest from newborn period. Analogous to type 2	Friede (1989)
Type IV	Cerebellar hypoplasia***			Friede (1989)

*Chronic tonsillar herniation (Friede 1989, Cama *et al.* 1995) secondary to hydrocephalus is difficult to separate completely from Chiari 1 deformity. Friede requires that cerebellar herniation is associated with one other component, *e.g.* elongated medulla. With or without brainstem elongation, quadriplegia or even sudden death following minor trauma may occur.
**Crowding of convolutions without architectonic abnormality.
***Although included in Chiari's original description, not a part of the Chiari deformity as understood now.

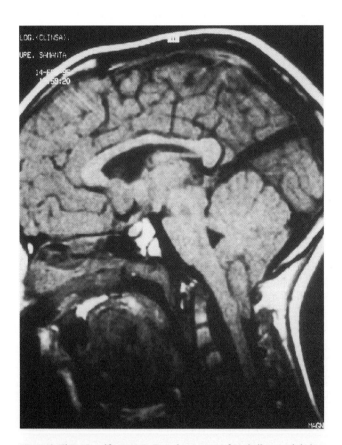

Fig. 3.6. Chiari I malformation. Dorsal extension of cerebellar tonsils below the level of the foramen magnum. The brainstem is elongated.

malformations of the duodenum, heart and oesophagus may accompany the neural deformity. The Chiari II malformation is associated with hydrocephalus in over 90 per cent of cases (Laurence 1964, Emery and MacKenzie 1973). Hydrocephalus is due to aqueductal stenosis in 30–73 per cent of cases (Stein *et al.* 1979). Its cause remains unclear in the remaining cases, although occlusion of the foramen of Magendie (Peach 1965, Naidich *et al.* 1980a) may be responsible. An imbalance between CSF production and resorption (Caviness 1976) is another possible mechanism. The choroid plexuses may be hypertrophic. Exceptionally, massive plexus hypertrophy can cause isolation of a lateral ventricle with consequent localized hydrocephalus (Chadduck and Glasier 1989). Ventricular dilatation is present from birth in 50–75 per cent of infants (Lorber 1974, Adams *et al.* 1985), suggesting that the apparent development of hydrocephalus following repair of myelomeningocele is probably not causally related to operation.

The mechanism of Chiari II malformation is unknown. Downward traction by the tethered spinal cord is no longer an accepted theory. An associated malformation is a more likely alternative. According to Marin-Padilla (1991), the primary defect is in the development of the mesenchyma of cephalic somites with hypoplasia of the basisphenoid resulting in a small posterior fossa, forcing the CNS out with secondary distortion.

The various abnormalities that accompany Chiari II deformity can be well demonstrated by CT scan and even better by MRI. A complete imaging study of the spinal lesion (Altman and

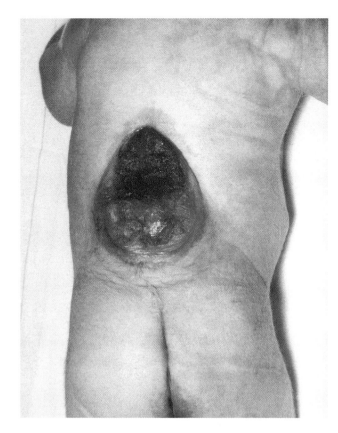

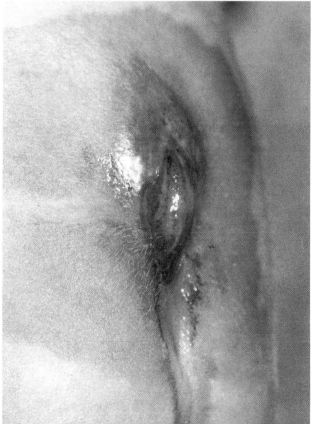

Fig. 3.7. Myelomeningoceles. *(Top)* Dorsolumbar lesion, associated with paraplegia and hydrocephalus. *(Bottom)* Lumbosacral lesion, clearly showing the non-neurulated cord. (Courtesy Dr F. Renault, Hôpital Trousseau, Paris.)

Altman 1987, Davis *et al.* 1988, Jaspan *et al.* 1988) is not necessary before primary repair, except when markedly asymmetrical signs are found. It is mandatory when reoperation on a previously treated patient is contemplated or when secondary deterioration occurs. MRI precisely indicates the relationship between the skin and the neural plate, root position, and intrinsic cord pathology such as diastematomyelia or hydromyelia (Lee *et al.* 1985).

• *Clinical features and complications.* At birth the appearance of the defect is that of a sac-like structure covered by a thin membrane which is often ruptured, with CSF leak. The surrounding skin is often angiomatous (Fig. 3.7). Older unrepaired lesions are partially epithelialized. The neurological manifestations of myelomeningocele include: (1) the direct consequences of the spinal malformation; (2) those of hydrocephalus and hindbrain anomalies; and (3) those of associated neural and extraneural abnormalities.

The consequences of the spinal lesion depend on the level of the myelocele, which in over 80 per cent of cases is located to the lumbosacral area. Children exhibit varying degrees of flaccid, areflexic paralysis and sensory deficits that may be asymmetrical, especially in high lesions. The pattern is usually a mixture of upper and lower motor neuron dysfunction. Motor deficit is often patchy. A sensory level is more constant and permits accurate determination of the upper limit of the lesion. After months and years, wasting, poor cutaneous circulation and trophic changes become prominent. Retractions lead to stiffness and deformities, and poor ossification is associated with fractures that may heal in awkward positions. The sphincter and detrusor functions are compromised in all cases. With lesions above L3 level, there is complete paraplegia. The lower limbs are completely flaccid but straight. Sensory deficits are present distal to the L3 or L4 dermatomes. Ambulation is impossible. In lower lumbar lesions, hip flexors, hip adductors and knee extensors are preserved. Hip dislocation is frequently present from birth, and flexion contracture of the hip results in flexion of the limbs at the hips with extension of the knee. With appropriate treatment, ambulation with aids is often possible. Lesions of the upper sacral roots are compatible with ambulation with minimal or no aids. However, there is variable involvement of the feet, so that most patients have at least some degree of deformity. With sacral lesions lower than S3, the function of the lower extremities is normal but there is saddle anaesthesia and sphincter dysfunction.

Sensory abnormalities may result in trophic changes of the skin, fractures with exuberant callus formation, or arthropathy.

Motor and sensory abnormalities are fixed following the early weeks of life. During the first 48 hours, a rapid deterioration of motor function is often noted (Stark and Drummond 1973), which is probably explained by mechanical trauma to the neural plate during the birth process and/or by exposure. Conversely, rapid improvement may occur following closure (Naidich 1989). Late postoperative deterioration is not part of the natural history of myelomeningoceles but is suggestive of complications. These include constriction of the reconstituted arachnoid tube, tethering of the spinal cord by scarring, hydrosyringomyelia, segmental cord infarction, and cord compression by a cyst or lipoma. In such cases, CT scan or MRI exploration may shed light on the cause of disturbances and lead to effective treatment.

Sphincter disturbances are of two major types, often coexisting. When the lesion is below S3 level, bladder and anal sphincters are paralysed and there is anaesthaesia of the rectum and lower urinary tract. Dribbling is present in one third of patients: the bladder is distended, with absent detrusor activity on cystometry (Stark 1971), and manual expression of urine is easy. In the larger group of higher lesions, detrusor contractions are weak and there is outlet obstruction at the external sphincter as a result of impaired coordination between its activity and that of the detrusor. Bladder sensation is variable. This results in high resting vesical pressure with bladder trabeculation and, eventually, dilatation of the upper urinary tract (Stark 1968). Bacteriuria is observed in 50 per cent of 2-year-old children; urinary tract infection leads to chronic pyelonephritis and is the most frequent cause of mortality and morbidity in these patients (Borzyskowski *et al.* 1982, McGuire 1985, Hunt and Whitaker 1987, Borzyskowski 1990).

Hydrocephalus is a major complication of meningomyelocele. Simple nonprogressive ventricular dilatation does not raise great difficulties. Progressive hydrocephalus is often present despite a normal head-growth curve. Normal pressure hydrocephalus may occur in some patients with myelomeningocele and these infants may benefit from shunting procedures. Hydrocephalus is present at birth in 85–95 per cent of cases as shown by ultrasonography. It is not observed with sacral defects.

Clinical manifestations of progressive hydrocephalus in myelocele patients usually have no special feature (Chapter 7). Peculiar manifestations, however, may result from involvement of lower cranial nerves, which appears to be due to a combination of brainstem abnormalities and hydrocephalus. Upper respiratory tract obstruction due to vocal cord paralysis, and central apnoea have long been recognized complications of the Chiari II malformation (Holinger *et al.* 1978) and represent a major cause of death in such patients (Papasozomenos and Roessmann 1981). Other respiratory difficulties can occur and are collectively known as central ventilatory dysfunction (CVD). CVD includes, in addition to obstruction of respiratory pathways, increased periodic breathing during sleep (Ward *et al.* 1986a) and central apnoea (Oren *et al.* 1986). Some children have a decreased or absent response to hypoxia and hypercapnia (Ward *et al.* 1986b, Petersen *et al.* 1995). The incidence of CVD in hydrocephalus patients varies from 5.7 per cent (Hays *et al.* 1989) to 30 per cent (McLone 1983). Onset of symptoms is within one month of birth in two-thirds of cases. In all cases of CVD, hydrocephalus is present. Symptoms may include stridor alone, or stridor associated with cyanotic spells and/or apnoeic episodes (Charney *et al.* 1987). The prognosis is poor: 19 of the 35 patients of Hays *et al.* died before 30 months of age. CVD may fluctuate and disappear. In several cases correction of shunt dysfunction has alleviated the symptoms of CVD suggesting that high intracranial pressure with brainstem compression may be a cause (Hays *et al.* 1989). In some cases, there appears to be a wider pattern of

dysfunction of lower cranial nerves, which includes dysphagia (Fernbach and McLone 1985), bradycardia, poor head control and weakness of the upper extremities that may be resolved by lowering intracranial pressure (Park *et al.* 1983, Bell *et al.* 1987).

Such cases of infantile brainstem syndrome require urgent investigation. Polygraphic sleep studies may be helpful in determining the frequency and types of apnoeic episodes. Deray *et al.* (1995) found abnormal polysomnographic study in 14 of 16 symptomatic patients, and severe abnormalities were associated with additional pathology such as myelomalacia and severe spinal stenosis. Most asymptomatic patients had normal studies and did well without surgery. However, Petersen *et al.* (1995) concluded that pneumogram and 10% CO_2 challenge did not reliably predict which infants will present symptoms. Barnet *et al.* (1993) and Taylor *et al.* (1996) emphasized the value of brainstem evoked potentials, whose abnormalities are well correlated to respiratory problems and neurological sequelae.

Treatment of CVD may require tonsillectomy or tracheostomy, alone or with surgical decompression of the posterior fossa (Pollack *et al.* 1992). Dysphagia alone does not require surgical treatment and is of favourable prognosis.

Another peculiar complication of hydrocephalus due to myelomeningocele is the late appearance of a marked and evolutive scoliosis with progressive paresis (Hall *et al.* 1975). Such neurological manifestations should be recognized early because revision of a malfunctioning shunt can improve dramatically the deficits (Hall *et al.* 1979, Hoffman *et al.* 1987).

Mental retardation is generally a consequence of hydrocephalus although *associated malformations* may play a role. The date of shunting, number of shunt revisions and, especially, the occurrence of CNS infections (McLone *et al.* 1982) have a major bearing on ultimate intelligence level. In the study of McLone *et al.*, the average IQ was 102 for patients who did not require a shunt, 95 for shunted, noninfected childen, and 72 for those with a history of ventriculitis. Seizures often occur in patients with hydrocephalus due to myelomeningocele (Talwar *et al.* 1995).

• *Management of spina bifida cystica.* The management of spina bifida cystica raises difficult problems, and no completely satisfactory solution is at hand (Liptak *et al.* 1988).

Prevention is certainly the best form of therapy. Primary prevention with vitamins and folic acid is efficacious and without danger. Multivitamin preparations containing folic acid are mandatory for pregnant women who have had an affected child, and are probably indicated for all pregnancies (MRC Study Research Group 1991). Prenatal diagnosis is currently the most effective means of preventing the birth of affected infants, but screening for spinal defect by ultrasound is not 100 per cent reliable, and screening of maternal serum for AFP, although recommended, is not cost-effective in areas where the incidence of spina bifida is relatively low. Preventive caesarian section is not universally recommended (Luthy *et al.* 1991) and vaginal delivery remains acceptable.

The *indications* for repair of myelomeningocele remain controversial. In the 1960s emergency repair was advocated for all cases. In the '70s, several investigators reported that cases with a very poor prognosis—*i.e.* high lumbar lesion with marked kyphosis, total flaccid paraplegia and bladder paralysis, major associated defects, and a head circumference at least 2 cm above the 90th centile—fared poorly despite modern techniques (Lorber 1972, 1974, 1975; Stark and Drummond 1973). Unoperated infants have a two-year survival rate of 0–4 per cent. Some clinicians are reluctant to 'select' patients for operation, unless perhaps in extreme cases such as small preterm, feeble infants. Indeed, long-term catastrophes can occur in unoperated infants (Charney *et al.* 1985), and a number of children with several adverse criteria have been able to live productive lives. In fact, operation aims essentially at preserving function rather than life and is indicated for most cases. Surgery may be performed in the neonatal period or be delayed for up to three months. The defect should then be dressed in a sterile way.

The *method* of surgical closure is also variable. New techniques (McLone 1980, Hobbins 1991) permit better mobility of the cord vis-a-vis the bony and cutaneous coverings. Closure of the defect makes the baby easier to handle, reduces the risk of ascending infection, and may improve motor and sensory function. Secondary tethering of the cord occurs in 10 per cent of patients who develop delayed symptoms, and will require further operation (Hunt 1990, McLone 1992).

Operation is but the first step in the management of spina bifida. The variety of problems that confront myelomeningocele patients is such that their successful management requires a team of specialists, including paediatric surgeon, paediatrician, urologist, physiotherapist and psychologist. Neurosurgical management following repair includes, in about 90 per cent of cases, shunting of progressive hydrocephalus and, occasionally, posterior fossa decompression in case of cervical spinal compression with respiratory difficulties and lower cranial nerve paralyses (see above).

Contracture deformities of the lower limbs demand physiotherapy, bracing, or orthopaedic operations such as muscle transplants or joint arthrodeses. The hips should be carefully monitored as dislocation is a common occurrence.

Urological problems are of paramount importance in the surveillance and treatment of spina bifida patients. The reader is referred to the guidelines formulated by the American Academy of Pediatrics (Action Committee on Myelodysplasia 1979) for their management as well as to the work of Eckstein and Molyneux (1982) and Borzyskowski (1990). Only a small proportion of patients will develop acceptable sphincter control. The rest will have to use different methods. Bladder expression, if the bladder capacity is sufficient and there is no vesico-ureteric reflux, may be effective in a small number of children (Borzyskowski 1990, Brett 1991, Kothari *et al.* 1995). Drug treatment with propantheline bromide or phenyloxybenzamine is of little value, and continuous catheter drainage (Minns *et al.* 1980) is variably evaluated. Transurethral resection may have a small place in treatment. Penile appliances, intermittent bladder catheterization (Eckstein and Molyneux 1982) and surgical urinary diversion are the main techniques for dealing with in-

continence. Infection and dilatation of the upper urinary tract are a major cause of morbidity and mortality in spina bifida patients. Therefore, early and regular monitoring of the urinary tract with urine cultures, intravenous pyelograms and cystograms are an essential part of management. Anal incontinence is less of a problem and can usually be managed successfully with enemas and training. Urodynamic assessment of children with neuropathic bladder (Rickwood 1990) is useful to determine the type of bladder dysfunction (Hunt and Whitaker 1987) and, consequently, the management. Conservative and surgical management has been reviewed in great detail by Borzyskowski (1990) and Stephenson and Mundy (1990).

The prognosis of myelomeningocele remains serious even though many individuals are able to live useful lives.

Meningoceles share the essential pathological features of myelomeningoceles but the mesenchymal defect is covered with skin and the spinal cord is normal. Herniation through the posterior bone and muscle defect is limited to the meninges. In some cases, roots may run in the wall of the meningocele or cross its cavity. At operation, the surgeon must carefully check any 'fibrous' tract, and the operating microscope and electrical stimulation are essential tools.

Meningoceles are never associated with hydrocephalus. The anatomical distribution is the same as that of myelomeningoceles. Meningoceles are sessile or pedunculated. In the latter case, the dura and arachnoid tend to fuse at the neck of the sac, and the development of adhesions may partially obliterate the communication that normally exists between the sac and the subarachnoid space (Friede 1989). In pedunculated lesions, the bony defect tends to be limited to one or two posterior arches.

Clinically, meningoceles are marked by protrusion of the skin over a fluctuating mass. Often the skin cover is abnormal and flat angiomas are present. Neurological examination is negative. Meningoceles do not require immediate repair and elective closure later in childhood is generally preferable.

Ventral meningoceles are much rarer. The main localization is sacral, and the lesions may be of large size and are associated with partial sacral aplasia. *Anterior sacral meningoceles* are dominantly inherited. They usually go unnoticed during childhood, although they may provoke rectal compression and chronic constipation (Say and Coldwell 1975, Anderson and Burke 1977).

Lateral meningoceles are herniations of an abnormally thin dura through the enlarged lateral foramina. They are seen with neurofibromatosis in association with scalloping of the vertebral bodies (Chapter 4).

Spina bifida occulta (occult spinal dysraphism)
The term 'spina bifida occulta' applies to cases of spinal dysraphism in which there is no herniation of the neural structures or envelopes through the mesenchymal defect (Fig. 3.8). This definition includes the split notochord syndrome, dorsal dermal sinuses, fibrolipomas of the filum terminale and diastematomyelia. Lipomas and lipomyelomeningoceles do not exactly fulfil the criteria for occult dysraphism as they produce definite protrusion of the skin and the cord lesion is very similar to that

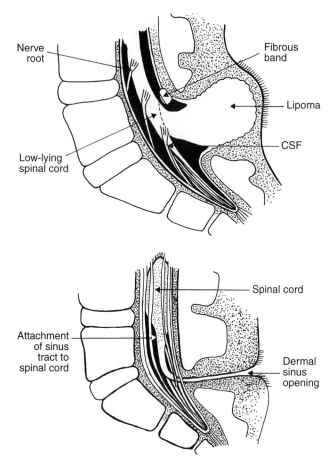

Fig. 3.8. Occult dysraphism. *(Top)* Lipomyelomeningocele. The lipoma is implanted on a low-lying spinal cord which is often incompletely neurulated. The intradural lipoma is in direct continuity with the subcutaneous lipoma. There is a variable degree of meningeal herniation through the bony defect. In most cases the lesion is asymmetrical. *(Bottom)* Congenital dermal sinus. The sinus tract ascends two or more vertebral bodies. It may end on the low-lying spinal cord, as shown here, or in a dermoid cyst.

Labels in figure (top): Nerve root, Fibrous band, Lipoma, CSF, Low-lying spinal cord. (bottom): Spinal cord, Attachment of sinus tract to spinal cord, Dermal sinus opening.

of classical myelomeningocele. However, they will be described in this section because their clinical symptomatology is not very different from that of other forms of occult dysraphism.

The clinical presentation of spina bifida occulta is variable (Anderson 1975). Lipomas, lipomeningoceles, diastematomyelia and the tethered cord syndrome share many common features, and their clinical manifestations will be described together. In all cases, detailed neuroradiological examination is necessary to assess the extent and nature of lesions. Plain X-rays, CT scan with and without metrizamide and MRI are all used. MRI is the best technique as it permits study in several planes (Bale *et al.* 1986, Altman and Altman 1987). Sonography of the spine and cord may also be useful although it is less precise (Scheible *et al.* 1983, Raghanendra and Epstein 1985). Hydrocephalus is not a feature of occult spinal dysraphism.

• *The split notochord syndrome.* This syndrome results from splitting of the notochord during embryogenesis with persistent communication between gut and the dorsal skin (Bentley and Smith 1960). Communication is usually only partial between gut

and vertebrae or the spinal cord. The total form (dorsal enteric fistula) is rare (Burrows and Sutcliffe 1968). *Intraspinal enteric cysts* are found mainly in the upper thoracic region. They are lined by digestive epithelium, can produce spinal compression and should be surgically treated (Kahn *et al.* 1971, Mohanty *et al.* 1979).

• *Dorsal dermal sinuses* are epithelium-lined dermal tubes that course from the skin surface toward the CNS. Many of them terminate on the dura. Others pierce the dura and terminate in an intradural dermoid cyst which is located two or more vertebrae above the cutaneous orifice (Martinez-Lage *et al.* 1995). Twenty to 30 per cent of intradural dermoids are associated with a dermal sinus. Dermal sinuses are mainly located at both extremities of the spinal canal. Of 127 sinuses reported by Wright (1971), 72 were in the lumbosacral region, 30 in the occipital area, and only 14 at the thoracic or cervical levels. Dermal sinuses are easily mistaken for pilonidal sinuses. If not clearly superficial, such tracts should be explored radiologically but never by a probe or by injection of contrast material. CT or MRI can visualize the tract as a line of increased density with an ascending orientation, and dermoid cysts are best shown by MRI (Scotti *et al.* 1980). The tract may pass between two spinous processes without producing any bony defect. Dermal sinuses are frequently revealed by a complication, mainly purulent meningitis that is often relapsing or recurrent. Intraspinal suppuration occasionally occurs (Bean *et al.* 1979). In any case of recurrent meningitis or meningitis due to unusual pathogens, careful examination of the spine and occipital region is mandatory. Shaving of the nuchal area may show a tiny, punctiform defect that may discharge fluid material. In some cases, chemical meningitis, with polymorphs in the CSF but no infecting organisms, results from fissuration of an intradural dermoid. I have seen chronic hydrocephalus as a result of basilar block, due to chemical meningitis, in two children. After antibiotic treatment of meningitis, resection of the tract should be performed after careful radiological assessment.

• *Spinal lipomas* are collections of fat and connective tissue partially encapsulated and, in most cases, are associated with failure of fusion of the posterior bony structures. Spinal lipomas may be of three types: intradural lipomas, lipomyelomeningocele, and fibrolipomas of the filum terminale.

Intradural lipomas (Chapman 1982, Tsuchiya *et al.* 1989) are rare tumours, representing less than 1 per cent of all spinal tumours, and may be cervical, thoracic or lumbar. They are of soft consistency and almost half of them have an extramedullary, extradural component. The spinal canal may be normal or expanded locally and there may be a narrow spina bifida. They can produce cord compression but there is no visible anomaly on the back.

Lipomyelomeningoceles consist of a lipoma or lipofibroma attached to the dorsal surface of the open, non-neurulated spinal cord, under an intact skin cover. The lipoma bulges in the lumbosacral region and merges peripherally with the normal subcutaneous fat. It is generally lateral to the midline and, in its most common location, deviates the buttock sulcus to one side.

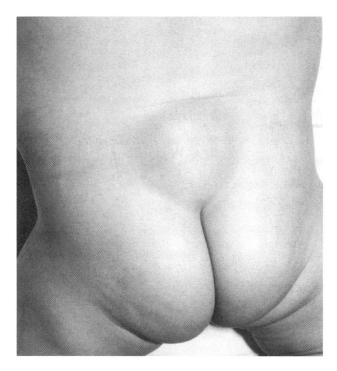

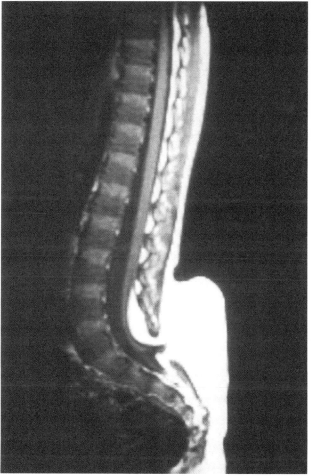

The lipoma may extend cephalad into the spinal canal, overriding the dorsal aspect of the neurulated cord, and is sometimes accompanied by a dermoid or epidermoid cyst. A meningocele is frequently associated with the lipoma (Fig. 3.9). The meningocele protrudes opposite an asymmetrical lipoma and produces a rotation of the neural plate. The spinal canal is open posteriorly so that the subcutaneous lipoma continues directly with the intraspinal part. There is usually a fibrous band or arch between the last lamina cephalad to the defect. The cord is often kinked on this band, which has to be divided to free the neural structures. In all cases, the caudal end of the cord is tethered in a low position below the L2 level (McLone *et al.* 1983b; Naidich *et al.* 1983a,b; Pierre-Kahn *et al.* 1983; Hirsch and Pierre-Kahn 1988). Bony abnormalities with errors of segmentation, osseous bars or partial sacral agenesis are present in over 40 per cent of cases. Cutaneous abnormalities in the form of tags, angiomas or blind sinuses are often present. CT and MRI are essential for determining, before surgical treatment, the exact anatomical details of the lesion.

Fibrolipomas of the filum terminale are due to abnormal canalization of the terminal cord and may be limited to the extradural portion of the filum or involve both the extra- and intradural portions in continuity. Intradural lipomas are distinct, lucent masses that taper where the filum pierces the dura. They may be associated with a small cyst. In a series of autopsies of children with otherwise normal spinal cords (Emery and Lendon 1973) fibrolipomas of the filum were found in 6 per cent of cases. Fibrolipomas are one possible cause of the *tight filum terminale syndrome*. In this syndrome neurological and orthopaedic abnormalities are associated with a thick, short filum terminale and a low position (below L2 level) of the conus medullaris (James and Lassman 1981). Traction on the spinal cord and repeated microtrauma may be responsible for the late appearance of neurological signs. The diagnosis of tight filum is difficult as the bony defect is of limited extent or absent altogether. CT and especially MRI (Bale *et al.* 1986) are most effective for diagnosis of a tight filum because it may be so closely applied to the posterior wall of the meningeal sac as to be invisible on myelography. Hendrick *et al.* (1977) found a lipoma in 23 per cent of their patients with tight filum, a cyst in 3 per cent, and scoliosis or kyphoscoliosis in 25 per cent. Cutaneous abnormalities in the form of angiomas of the saccrococcygeal area can be an important diagnostic clue, allowing the diagnosis to be suspected before any neurological damage is done (Albright *et al.* 1989).

• *Diastematomyelia.* This condition is marked by a sagittal cleft dividing the spinal cord into two 'half-cords' each surrounded by its own pia mater (Fig. 3.10). Diplomyelia or duplication of the spinal cord (Dryden 1980) is probably not a distinct entity. The cleft may extend through the full thickness of the cord or only partially through the dorsal half of the cord (partial syringomyelia) (Guthkelch 1974, Hilal *et al.* 1974). The cleft is usually located between T9 and S1 but cervical location has been reported (Simpson and Rose 1987). A bony spur is present in about half the cases (James and Lassman 1981). The spur may be partial,

Fig. 3.9. Lipomyelomeningocele. *(Top)* Skin-covered low-lying lipomatous mass. *(Bottom)* MRI scan: the intraspinal mass is in continuity with subcutaneous lipoma. Note low termination of spinal cord on upper pole of lipoma. (Courtesy Dr Kling Chong, Great Ormond Street Hospital, London.)

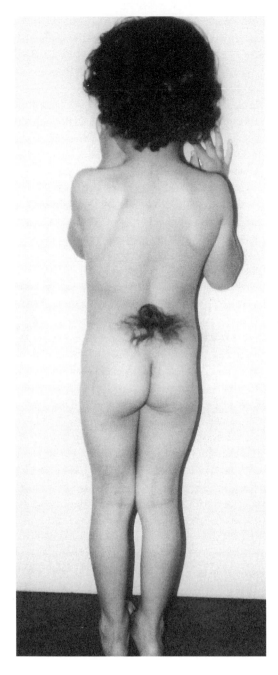

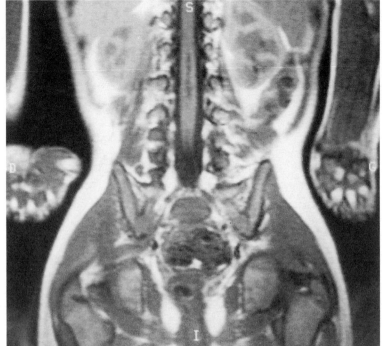

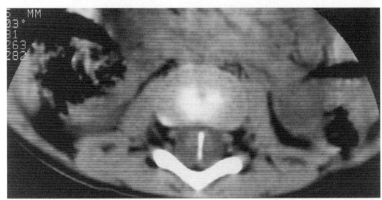

Fig. 3.10. Diastematomyelia in a 20-month-old boy. Note hair tuft on midline in the lumbar region. *(Top right)* MRI (T₁-weighted sequence, frontal cut). Cord is divided into two halves that reunite below midline septum. There is low attachment of the cord at L4–L5 level. *(Bottom right)* Axial cut demonstrates sagitally oriented bony septum. (Courtesy Dr D. Renier, Prof. J-F. Hirsh, Hôpital des Enfants Malades, Paris.)

purely cartilaginous or fibrous. It impales the cord or cauda equina so that the conus is fixed in a low position as a result of the differential growth between vertebral column and spinal cord. The two cords reunite below the cleft in 90 per cent of cases (Hilal *et al.* 1974).

There are two main forms of diastematomyelia (James and Lassman 1981). In about 40 per cent of cases, both the arachnoid and dura form separate tubes around each half-cord for a limited number of segments. There are thus two dural layers between the half-cords. It is in this form that there is a fibrous or bony spur that lies at the lowermost end of the cleft. If it does not, a second separate cleft should be sought at that location (Hilal *et al.* 1974).

In the remaining cases, the two half-cords lined by pia mater lie side-by-side in a single arachnoid tube surrounded by undivided dura. Such cases do not have a septum and usually remain asymptomatic (James and Lassman 1981). A tight filum is present in about half the patients and 5 per cent have multiple spurs.

The vertebral column is grossly abnormal in over 90 per cent of patients with diastematomyelia so that the plain X-ray picture is highly suggestive. The spinal canal is widened, errors of segmentation of the vertebral bodies are present in 85 per cent of cases, spina bifida is frequent, and scoliosis is marked in over half the cases. In the experience of Hilal *et al.* (1974), 4.9 per cent of 392 cases of scoliosis resulted from diastematomyelia.

Cutaneous abnormalities are present in 75 per cent of patients. Typically, a tuft of hair or a dimple overlies the defect, but a lipoma, angioma or dermal sinus may also occur.

Diastematomyelia, the tethered cord syndrome and lipo-myelomeningocele have many common neurological features. Two clinical neurological presentations are encountered. The first is a picture of congenital atrophy, weakness, and deformity of one lower limb, or of both limbs with a marked unilateral preponderance. Reflexes are depressed or abolished in the affected territory, and sphincter disturbances of the type seen in low spina bifida are present, especially with lipomyelomeningocele. The asymmetry is highly suggestive of spinal dysraphism, especially if associated with cutaneous anomalies, a palpable bony defect or kyposcoliosis. Such a picture demands plain X-ray and myelography, CT or MRI of the spinal canal.

The second presentation is a progressive neurological deficit that may appear at any age and can be superimposed on a previously fixed picture (Guthkelch 1974). In such patients, weakness and spasticity, an awkward gait and incontinence develop progressively. A mixture of peripheral and central signs and cutaneous abnormalities is characteristic. This syndrome may occur following trauma, or spontaneously following a growth spurt or a rapid increase in weight. The adipocytes in a lipoma tend to behave metabolically like those in the rest of the body (Giudicelli *et al.* 1986). Occasionally, a severe neurological syndrome develops suddenly with marked or massive paraplegia or quadriplegia. Following such an event, recuperation is far from good, even with early operation (Albright *et al.* 1989). This fact, together with improved microsurgical techniques, supports preventive operation at an early age.

• *The treatment of occult spinal dysraphism* is of variable difficulty. Its principal aim is to free the spinal cord from its low and posterior attachment without injury to the neural placode or roots. This aim is attained rather easily in diastematomyelia, for which liberation of the spur is usually sufficient (Logue and Edwards 1981). It is more difficult to divide a tight filum, as roots may be difficult to distinguish from fibrous tracts, and electric stimulation is invaluable. Lipomyelomeningoceles require careful preoperative radiological analysis; careful dissection of the lesion; location of neural tissue that must be respected, if necessary by leaving in place some fatty tissue; and division of posterior fibrous band and filum until the cord is freely movable (Naidich *et al.* 1983a, Pierre-Kahn *et al.* 1983, Hoffman *et al.* 1985, McLone *et al.* 1985). With present day techniques (James *et al.* 1984, Kanev *et al.* 1990), results are good and no deterioration takes place after operation. Prevention of neurological deficits by early operation in the frequent case where only cutaneous and osseous signs are present is therefore warranted even in young infants (Hirsch and Pierre-Kahn 1988, Harrison *et al.* 1990, Kanev *et al.* 1990). Urological complications are a major problem in many cases of spina bifida occulta (Fernandez *et al.* 1994). They should be systematically sought as early treatment is essential for prevention of upper urinary tract problems.

OTHER DEVELOPMENTAL ABNORMALITIES RELATED TO SPINAL DYSRAPHISM
Abnormalities that have more or less distant relation to spinal dysraphism include syringomyelia, sacral agenesis (Nievelstein *et al.* 1994), and congenital defects of the skull with or without defect of the scalp. These anomalies probably arise through different mechanisms and only superficially resemble dysraphic states.

Syringomyelia
Syringomyelia is defined as a tubular cavitation within the spinal cord. In theory, it differs from hydromyelia which is a dilatation of the cord central canal lined with ependyma, whereas the syringomyelic cavity is lined by glial cells. The distinction is, however, difficult in practice and it may be simpler to refer to all intraspinal cavities of nontumoural nature as hydrosyringomyelia (Gower *et al.* 1994), especially as the diagnosis is now frequently made by MRI scan demonstrating cavitation *in vivo* (Kokmen *et al.* 1985, Lee *et al.* 1985, Sherman *et al.* 1987, Van Hall *et al.* 1992, Gower *et al.* 1994). Hydrosyringomyelic cavities are of variable length. Tashiro *et al.* (1987) found a cervical cavity in 69 per cent of their cases, total length cavitation in 6 per cent, and cavitation limited to the lumbar cord in 3 per cent. The cavities may or may not be in communication with the fourth ventricle. Some may extend into the medulla and pons with resulting involvement of lower cranial nerves and nuclei (syringomyelo-bulbia). Cavitation may be of variable location and diameter within the cord, which is frequently distended by cyst fluid. Experience with CT has shown that most syringomyelic cavities are opacified by intrathecally injected contrast, even if only after a few hours, indicating communication with the subarachnoid space. Syringomyelia is often associated with Chiari I malformation and hydrocephalus which may play an important role in its mechanism. The thrust of the CSF wave has been thought to be responsible for the slow progressive downward extension of the cavity within the spinal cord (Gower *et al.* 1994). However, the exact mechanism that produces syringomyelia is uncertain (Morgan and Williams 1992). Syringomyelia can be a consequence of spinal trauma (McLean *et al.* 1973). It has also been reported in association with postmeningitic spinal arachnoiditis (Savoiardo 1976, Caplan *et al.* 1990).

Because most of the lesions involve the cervical cord, involvement of the upper limbs tends to be prominent. The central location of the cavity explains why temperature and pain sensation are electively disturbed, as the fibres that convey these sensations cross through the central white matter. Interference with fibres concerned with pain perception is responsible for the frequently observed trophic disturbances.

The condition is sporadic, although occasional familial forms have been reported (Busis and Hochberg 1985). The disease is rarely symptomatic in children, although symptoms have been observed as early as 2 years of age (Tashiro *et al.* 1987). Adolescent onset is common with up to 40 per cent of patients first seen in their second decade (Mariani *et al.* 1991).

The *clinical manifestations* (Morgan and Williams 1992) may include painless whitlows and occasionally Charcot's joints as a manifestation of the classical sensory disturbances in a suspended topography. Later paralysis and more complete sensory

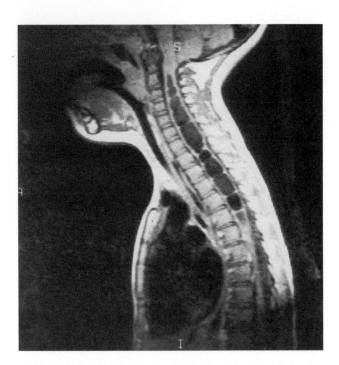

Fig. 3.11. Syringomyelia. Massive cavitation of the spinal cord in a 5½-year-old girl with only minimal symptoms and signs. (Courtesy Dr D. Renier, Prof. J-F. Hirsch, Hôpital des Enfants Malades, Paris.)

disturbances develop in the upper limbs, where abolition of deep tendon reflexes is an early sign. Pyramidal tract signs are frequently found in the lower limbs. With bulbar affectation, rotary nystagmus and other signs of hemibulbar syndrome may be present (Gower *et al.* 1994). Stridor and laryngospasm have been reported (Alcala and Dodson 1975). *Scoliosis* is a major and early manifestation. Tashiro *et al.* (1987) found scoliosis to be present before 10 years of age in 19 per cent of their cases.

Recent studies based on CT or MRI diagnosis indicate more variability of clinical features. Classical suspended dissociated hypoaesthesia appears to be uncommon, deep tendon reflexes may be preserved in the upper limbs, and nystagmus may be downbeating rather than rotatory (Tashiro *et al.* 1987, Pou-Serradel and Mares Segura 1988). Chiari I malformation was present in over half the cases in the latter series and basilar impression in 27 per cent of them. Symptoms tend to be uncharacteristic for a very long time and many cases are asymptomatic. Scoliosis is often the reason for imaging studies. Syringomyelia associated with myelomeningocele is usually asymptomatic (Breningstall *et al.* 1992). Acute presentation with sudden paraplegia is rare (Zager *et al.* 1990). *Syringobulbia* is often associated with spinal cord cavities but occasionally occurs alone. Onset is often many years before diagnosis. Symptoms and signs may include occipital headache, vertigo, auditory failure, nystagmus and lower nerve involvement (Morgan and Williams 1992).

The *diagnosis* of syringobulbomyelia is based on imaging techniques. Myelography has been supplanted by CT with metrizamide contrast and, lately, by MRI scanning (Kokmen *et al.* 1985, Sherman *et al.* 1987). This method allows full visualization of the cavity and separation of true syringomyelia from

intraspinal tumours (Goy *et al.* 1986). It also allows assessment of the efficacy of surgical treatment by measuring the size of the syrinx before and after operation (Grant *et al.* 1987a,b). MRI has shown clearly that even massive cavitation is often asymptomatic in children (Fig. 3.11), and spontaneous resolution has been reported (Sudo *et al.* 1990).

Treatment of syringomyelia is controversial. Regular monitoring of the patients is essential. In many cases, there is no or only very slow progression and operation is not indicated. In progressive disease, posterior fossa decompression is usually advised if Chiari I malformation is present (Mariani *et al.* 1991, Gower *et al.* 1994) and may be so effective that even treatment of asymptomatic patients is probably indicated. Recurrence is not infrequent (Mariani *et al.* 1991). For resistant cases, shunting of the cystic cavity may be considered (Barbaro *et al.* 1984, Suzuki *et al.* 1985). The exact value and complications of shunting treatment need further assessment.

Sacral agenesis

Agenesis of the sacrum and coccyx is part of the syndrome of caudal regression. Bony abnormalities are usually associated with major anomalies of the spinal cord (Tsukamoto *et al.* 1992, Nievelstein *et al.* 1994). Clinical manifestations include paraplegia with a flaccid neurogenic bladder, muscle hypoplasia and arthrogryposis. Recurrent urinary infections are a constant problem and the prognosis is poor. The aetiology is unclear but there is a strong association with maternal diabetes mellitus: about 1 per cent of the offspring of diabetic mothers have sacral agenesis (Passarge and Lenz 1966, Mills 1979) and 16 per cent of patients are born to diabetic mothers. An hereditary form of partial sacral agenesis has been reported (Say and Coldwell 1975).

Spinal intradural cysts and diverticula

Cysts of the arachnoid mater may develop dorsal to the spinal cord and may produce signs of compression (Wilkins and Odom 1976). The cysts often extend over several vertebral segments and communicate with the subarachnoid space by a small opening. Because of their posterior location they may go undetected by conventional myelography if the patient is not placed in the prone position. Such cysts are found in adolescents with kyphosis. They are better shown by MRI scanning. A syndrome of spinal arachnoid cyst, lymphoedema of the feet and a double row of eyelashes has been described (Schwartz *et al.* 1980). Richaud (1988) has reviewed in detail malformations of the spinal meninges in children.

Congenital defects of the skull and scalp

Aplasia of the scalp can occur alone or in combination with bone defects. Scalp defects are mainly located to the vertex. They are common in the trisomy 13 syndrome (Chapter 5).

Isolated skull defects may be located to the vertex in association with scalp aplasia (Little *et al.* 1990). A large posterior fontanelle is present in several conditions including the Walker–Warburg syndrome (see below) and represents a minor form of cephalocele. Symmetrical parietal foramina, sometimes referred to as the 'Catlin mark', may be large and palpable or are only visible on skull X-rays. They are transmitted as a dominant mendelian trait. Aplasia of the sphenoidal greater wing occurs in neurofibromatosis and can produce pulsatile exophthalmos.

Small scalp defects can be closed but large ones require grafting. Bony defects of small size may be left alone. Large defects require surgical closure.

DISORDERS OF VENTRAL INDUCTION
This term designates those malformations that seem to result from induction failure involving the three germ layers: cephalic mesoderm; adjacent neuroectoderm and associated neural crest derivatives; and entodermal anlagen for facial structures. Induction failure is probably time-specific as ventral induction is completed prior to the 33rd day of intrauterine life. The major defect is failure of the primary cerebral vesicle (telencephalon) to cleave and expand laterally. Midline facial defects that are frequently associated are a simultaneous consequence of the same defect involving the facial structures. The defect may have multiple causes. Genetic factors are known to be operative in a minority of cases (Roach *et al.* 1975). They include both mendelian inheritance with mainly dominant but sometimes recessive (Begleiter and Harris 1980) inheritance, and chromosomal abnormalities (Cohen and Lemire 1982, Leech and Shuman 1986a). The latter include trisomy or other anomalies of chromosome 13 and, less frequently, of chromosome 18, with deletion of its short arm or a ring chromosome; triploidy 69 XXX; mosaicism involving chromosome 13; and partial trisomy 7. Environmental influences are probably important, in particular maternal diabetes mellitus. About 1 per cent of diabetic mothers may bear children with holoprosencephaly, and the incidence of the condition among offspring of diabetic mothers is at least 200 times that in the general population (Barr *et al.* 1983) which is low, of the order of 1 per 18,000 (Myrianthopoulos and Chung 1974) to 6 per 10,000 livebirths (Matsunaga and Shiota 1987). The total frequency, including abortuses, is probably much higher (0.4 per cent of induced abortions in Japan). The empirical recurrence risk for a couple who have had an affected offspring is said to be 6 per cent (Roach *et al.* 1975). However, this figure is probably biased and results from the averaging of data from cases with different patterns of transmission.

Holoprosencephaly or Prosencephaly
These terms are used synonymously to designate the most common form of ventral induction defect. The term *arhinencephaly*, which is still often used as a synonym, is improper as abnormal development of the rhinencephalic structures and, in particular, absence of the olfactory bulbs and stems can exist in brains with complete separation of the hemispheres (Kobori *et al.* 1987), although they are virtually always lacking with incomplete forebrain division (Leech and Shuman 1986a). Holoprosencephaly means an undivided anterior brain (Fig 3.12*a*). The severity of the abnormality is variable (Probst 1979, Leech and Shuman 1986a, DeMyer 1987, Castillo *et al.* 1993, Oba and Barkovich 1995).

Alobar holoprosencephaly refers to a completely undivided, very small forebrain that assumes the shape of a horseshoe in the concavity of which lies a dorsal sac. This structure contains little neocortex, the concavity of the horseshoe being made of entorhinal cortex (Probst 1979, Friede 1989). The thalami are fused on the midline. The brainstem and cerebellum are well developed. Such brains are associated with extremely severe facial defects and ocular abnormalities. In *cyclopia*, a rapidly lethal condition, there is a single orbit with fused ocular globes. In cases of *ethmocephaly*, the nose is absent, replaced by a proboscis that is located above the level of the closely placed orbits. *Cebocephaly* patients present with an abnormal nose with single nostril. The most frequent type is *holoprosencephaly with median cleft lip* in which the premaxillary bone anlage is missing (Fig. 3.12*b*). There is marked osseous hypotelorism. Such patients may live for several months or years, in contrast with those affected by the previously mentioned types. Hydrocephalus may be associated.

In *semilobar holoprosencephaly*, there is no dorsal sac and the brain is divided into two hemispheres in its posterior part, while anteriorly abnormal transverse convolutions bridge the median fissure (Fig. 3.12*c,d*). The thalami are fused in the midline. In the most evolved forms, sometimes termed type A semilobar prosencephaly, the two hemispheres seem to be fully separated, even anteriorly. However, interhemispheric bridging is present in the anterior frontal region and there is no corpus callosum anteriorly, while the splenium may be present (Barkovich 1990). Anteriorly, the cerebral mantle invaginates deeply with both grey and white matter layers crossing the midline after having lined a more or less sinuous 'interhemispheric' fissure (Oba and Barkovich 1995). The sinuous fissure may be a cue for the diagnosis by CT of semilobar holoprosencephaly. MRI permits differentiation of the interhemispheric bridging from a true corpus callosum on sagittal cuts.

Lobar prosencephaly, in its fully developed forms, is characterized by almost complete separation of the hemispheres. Probst (1979) prefers not to classify it as holoprosencephaly, but it is included in the latter group by other investigators (Oba and Barkovich 1995). Barkovich and Quint (1993) reported on three patients with interhemispheric fusion limited to the middle part of the hemispheres. Barkovich (1990) used the term syntelencephaly to designate cases in which the hemispheric fissure was present in the anterior frontal region and in the occipital region without separation of the hemispheres in the posterior frontal and parietal regions.

Associated malformations (Jellinger *et al.* 1981) are common and include congenital heart disease; scalp defects; and polydactyly, in which case a chromosomal defect is likely. Holoprosencephaly may be a part of complex malformation syndromes, including Meckel–Gruber syndrome (Paetau *et al.* 1985) and Aicardi syndrome (Sato *et al.* 1987). Isolated forms are not, as a rule, part of a chromosomal syndrome.

The *diagnosis* of holoprosencephaly is easy when facial abnormalities are present (DeMyer *et al.* 1964, Burck *et al.* 1981). In addition to those described above, there may be bilateral cleft lip and palate with hypoplasia of the median tubercle (Couly and

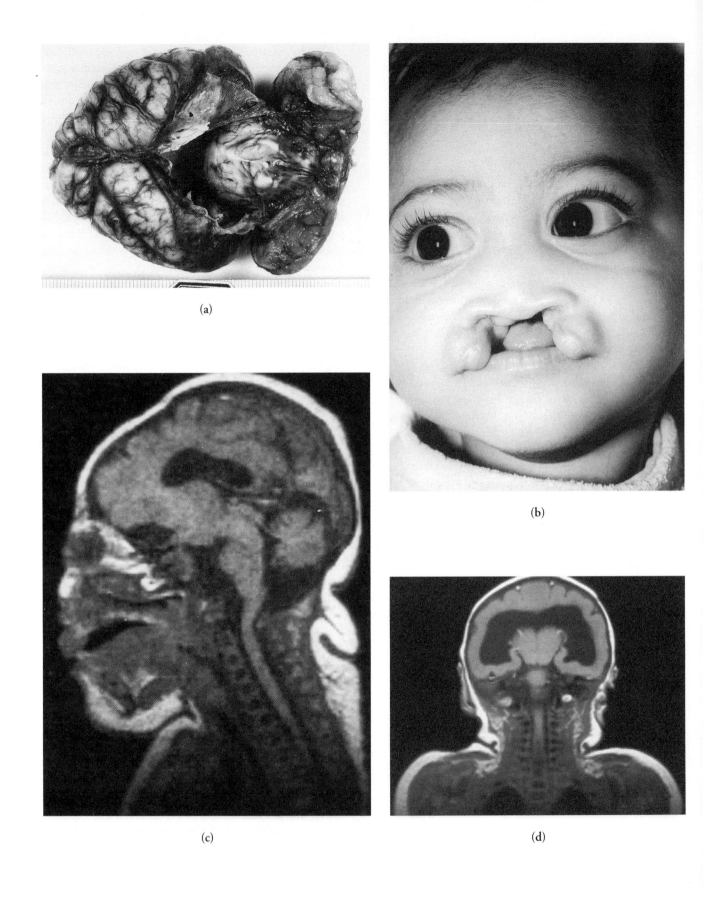

Fig. 3.12. Holoprosencephaly. *(a)* Holoprosencephalic brain of hypotrophic neonate (40 weeks gestational age, birthweight 1600 g) who died at 6 hours of life. (Courtesy Dr J-C. Larroche, Maternité Port Royal, Paris.) *(b)* Infant with holoprosencephaly with median cleft lip. Note absence of premaxillary bud. *(c,d)* Semilobar holoprosencephaly: MRI, T$_1$-weighted sequence. In *(c)* (sagittal cut), microcephaly, absence of corpus callosum and abnormal cortical gyri are evident. In *(d)* (frontal cut), there is a single telencephalic ventricle, fused thalami and broad gyri.

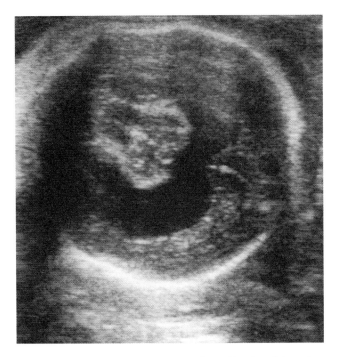

Fig. 3.13. Holoprosencephaly in a 29-week fetus: dilated single horseshoe ventricle (fetal forehead facing bottom of photograph). (Courtesy Dr M-C. Aubry, Maternité Port Royal, Paris.)

countered in the brains of retarded patients coming to autopsy. Other malformations, especially microgyrias or heterotopias, are associated (Kobori *et al.* 1987). It may be unilateral (Aleksic *et al.* 1975).

Telencephalic pseudo-monoventricle refers to a large cavum septum pellucidum in association with atresia of the frontal horns and various other abnormalities (Poll-Thé and Aicardi 1985). Cases on record displayed mental retardation and/or endocrinological disturbances.

Familial isolated agenesis of the olfactory stems, also known as Kallmann syndrome, is discussed with migration disorders (see below).

MEDIAN CLEFT FACE SYNDROMES
The median cleft face syndromes (DeMyer 1967) are a group of conditions whose visible common denominator is *hypertelorism*. Several cases are associated with other ventral induction abnormalities, the commonest of which is anterior cranium bifidum. Hypertelorism is a frequent feature in cases of corpus callosum agenesis, sometimes with cleft lip, bifid nose or similar anomalies (Aicardi *et al.* 1987). Anterior encephaloceles of various locations may be found, and these are frequently accompanied by extensive cortical and other malformations (Leech and Shuman 1986b). A similar picture can obtain with lipomas of the corpus callosum (Kushnet and Goldman 1978).

DISORDERS OF CORTICAL DEVELOPMENT
Abnormal development of the cortex (Table 3.4) is an extremely common cause of neurodevelopmental disorders. The high frequency of such abnormalities has become evident with the development of modern neuroimaging, especially MRI (Meencke 1994), and their role as a cause of epilepsy, cerebral palsy and mental retardation now appears greater than that of perinatally acquired damage. The terms commonly used for the description of these abnormalities are multiple and confusing. Pathological terms are often used to designate conditions diagnosed by imaging techniques. Such terms as 'cortical dysplasia' are used either in a general sense to refer to any type or abnormally developed cortex, or in the more restricted meaning of disorder of cortical organization. The term 'migration disorders' is often wrongly applied to abnormalities limited to final cortical organization. To avoid such confusion in this section I will use the term 'developmental cortical abnormalities' for all types of cortical developmental anomalies and the terms 'migration disorders' and 'organization disorders' for abnormalities of the corresponding stages of corticogenesis.

Table 3.4 lists the major disorders of corticogenesis and indicates their most likely mechanisms. The different stages of cortical formation are, in fact, interdependent and overlapping. The fate of precursor cells is determined before they migrate (McConnell and Kaznowski 1991), and this determination has a bearing on the subsequent processes of migration and organization. Thus, abnormal cells, *e.g.* in tuberous sclerosis or in some types of 'cortical dysplasia', often do not migrate to their normal position and/or fail to establish normal connectivity. Likewise,

Aicardi 1988) or trigonocephaly with orbital hypotelorism. However, the face may be normal in the semilobar forms. Microcephaly is a feature common to most forms unless aqueductal stenosis, with resulting hydrocephalus, is present (Nyberg *et al.* 1987). Diagnosis can also be made by ultrasonography when the fontanelle is open (Govaert and de Vries 1997). Infants with the most severe types rarely survive the neonatal period. Most surviving infants develop seizures that are often infantile spasms with hypsarrhythmia (Watanabe *et al.* 1976). Neurological manifestations are highly variable and some patients may survive into adulthood. A child presenting with spastic diplegia has been reported (Shanks and Wilson 1988). However, mental retardation, usually of a severe degree, is constant, particularly in cases that are symptomatic early. The occurrence of endocrinological abnormalities such as diabetes insipidus and growth hormone deficiency is possible (Begleiter and Harris 1980). Hydrocephalus is present in 40 per cent of patients with holoprosencephaly, especially when no facial abnormalities are associated.

Prenatal diagnosis of holoprosencephaly is relatively easy and can be made from the 16th week of pregnancy by ultrasonography (Chervenak *et al.* 1985) (Fig. 3.13). In the series of Nyberg *et al.* (1987) holoprosencephaly accounted for 19 per cent of all cases of hydrocephalus diagnosed prenatally. Twenty-nine per cent of the diagnosed cases had normal facial features, emphasizing the importance of not relying excessively on facial appearance. Orbital hypotelorism is the most reliable diagnostic feature for antenatal diagnosis.

CONDITIONS RELATED TO HOLOPROSENCEPHALY
Arhinencephaly without holoprosencephaly is occasionally en-

TABLE 3.4
Main disorders of cortical development*

Disorders of proliferation and differentiation
  Microcephaly
  Megalencephaly
  Hemimegalencephaly
  Tuberous sclerosis
  Taylor-type cortical dysplasia

Disorders of migration
  Periventricular heterotopias
    Nodular
    Laminar
  Subcortical heterotopias
    Nodular
    Laminar
  Lissencephaly (agyria)
  Pachygyria
  Polymicrogyria**
    Diffuse
    Bilateral
    Focal
  Excess migration (glioneuronal meningeal heterotopias)

Disorders of cortical organization
  Cortical dysplasias (several grades)
    Focal
    Unilateral
  Microdysgenesis

*Several mechanisms may be operative in a single case.
**May be a postmigrational anomaly.

disorders of cell proliferation are frequently associated with abnormal migration, e.g. in pachygyria or agyria. As a result, it may be difficult to determine which step of cortical development is mainly interfered with in individual cases and some classifications may be to some extent arbitrary. Thus, hemimegalencephaly or microcephaly are often associated with abnormal migration, and subcortical heterotopias frequently coexist with overlying cortical abnormalities. Several anomalies are often simultaneously present in the same brain, and microdysgenesis (Meencke and Veith 1992) may be present together with subcortical and cortical development abnormalities. I will describe successively the various anomalies that seem to result from the different mechanisms.

DISORDERS OF PROLIFERATION/DIFFERENTIATION
This section focuses on those cases in which disorders of proliferation and differentiation are the dominant abnormality, although they rarely occur in isolation. The phenomenon of programmed cell death, which normally affects between 30 and 50 per cent of formed neurons, may play an important role, while destructive processes may be responsible for loss of cerebral volume and may be difficult to distinguish from maldevelopment because of the peculiar features of the repair processes in fetal life.

Microcephaly/micrencephaly
Microcephaly is a difficult condition to define. Some authors refer to all children with head circumference more than two standard deviations below the mean (or below the 3rd centile) as having microcephaly (see Warkany 1981). Such a broad definition obviously includes normal individuals. Micrencephaly, on the other hand, theoretically refers to a small brain (Friede 1989) but in practice the two definitions are equivalent. All authors admit that children with moderately small heads (between 2 and 3 SD below the mean) are frequently normal (Sells 1977, Warkany 1981), but there is statistically an increased prevalence of mild microcephaly among children with learning disabilities (Smith 1981). Mental retardation may be more common when a small head is associated with growth retardation. However, even patients with head circumference between 3 and 4 SD below the mean may have a normal intelligence (Hecht and Kelly 1979).

Even when only cases of clearly pathological small heads (whether by measurement or because of associated features) are considered, the term microcephaly covers a wide range of heterogeneous cases due to multiple, although largely unknown, mechanisms. Insufficient cell proliferation is only one of these mechanisms, which conceivably can include excessive embryofetal cell death or later destruction from exogenous causes. A classical distinction is between *primary microcephaly*, e.g. microcephaly that is present by the seventh month of intrauterine life, including both genetic and nongenetic cases, and *secondary microcephaly* occurring after the seventh month of gestation. It is more useful, although sometimes difficult, to try to determine the causes and mechanisms in order to separate familial from sporadic forms. This section will focus on developmental microcephaly, *viz.* microcephalia vera and other genetic types of microcephaly. Sugimoto *et al.* (1993) found that 44 of 55 cases were of genetic origin, the rest being due to a variety of nongenetic developmental errors.

Microcephalia vera refers by definition to a genetic type of microcephaly. Whether it constitutes a single genetic entity is uncertain even though patients present in a similar manner. The degree of microcephaly is usually marked (at least 5–6 SD below the mean), with a narrow, receding forehead and a pointed vertex, giving a peculiar clinical and radiological appearance. Paradoxically, individuals with microcephalia vera do not exhibit gross neurological signs, but hyperkinetic behaviour and disturbances of fine motor coordination are frequently present (Accardo and Whitman 1988). Seizures may occcur in one-third of patients, most of whom are trainable and can acquire at least a simplified language. This is all the more remarkable as the brain weight may be as little as 500 g in the adult.

From a histological point of view, there is severe depletion of neurons in layers II and III (Evrard *et al.* 1989). In one case (Parain *et al.* 1985) early exhaustion of the germinative zone was evident in a 26-week old fetus.

The inheritance of mirocephalia vera is usually autosomal recessive (Kloepfer *et al.* 1964). In heterozygotes, the gene might be responsible for mild mental retardation, sometimes with a relatively small head (Qazi and Reed 1975). Dominant (Haslam and Smith 1979) and X-linked transmission (Renier *et al.* 1982) has also been recorded, although with slightly different clinical presentation, but is rare.

Indeed, the classical picture of microcephalia vera is fairly uncommon and the group of genetic microcephalies is highly heterogeneous. Tolmie *et al.* (1987) studied 29 isolated cases of microcephaly and nine families with several microcephalic members. Only one patient had the typical picture of microcephalia vera. The recurrence rate in affected families was 19 per cent, and several patients had marked pyramidal tract signs, quadriplegia, seizures or profound mental retardation.

A majority of patients have '*microcephaly plus*'. Tolmie *et al.* (1987) described a syndrome of genetic microcephaly with seizures and/or spasticity. In some of these cases the seizures were infantile spasms; severe microcephaly of more than 9 SD below the mean was present and was associated with profound mental retardation (Silengo *et al.* 1992). Other patients have retinal abnormalities and these forms have either autosomal dominant (Tenconi *et al.* 1981) or recessive transmission (Cantú *et al.* 1977, Norio *et al.* 1984, Mikati *et al.* 1985, Harbord *et al.* 1989). Others have short stature, dominantly inherited (Burton 1981), or an array of associated anomalies including congenital nephrotic syndrome (Shapiro *et al.* 1976, Nishikawa *et al.* 1997), a short jejuno-ileum (Nézelof *et al.* 1976), callosal agenesis or severe disturbances of migration (Neu *et al.* 1971).

Familial cases with intracranial calcification masquerading as intrauterine infection are of especial interest because the diagnosis of a familial condition is easily missed in such instances (Baraitser *et al.* 1983, Burn *et al.* 1986).

The neuropathology of such cases is variable. In some cases abnormalities of gyration are prominent (Barkovich *et al.* 1992), while the architecture of the brain in other cases is little deranged (Robain and Lyon 1972). MRI of the brain shows variable abnormalities of the cortical gyri in addition to the small size of the brain and poor development of the frontal lobes (Steinlin *et al.* 1991, Sugimoto *et al.* 1993).

At the opposite end of the spectrum are cases of clinically silent, dominantly transmitted microcephaly (Ramirez *et al.* 1983, Accardo and Whitman 1988), or cases without neurodevelopmental disturbances with chromosomal instability (Seemanova *et al.* 1985) or primary combined immunodeficiency (Berthet *et al.* 1994). An exhaustive list of syndromes with microcephaly is given by Friede (1989).

An extreme variant of microcephaly is that of *radial microbrain*. According to Evrard *et al.* (1989) the weight of brain in such cases can be as low as 16–50g. The radial brain columns are almost normal but their number is markedly decreased. Such cases are distinct from atelencephaly in which there is no cortical structure.

Microcephaly is also a feature of a vast number of chromosomal abnormalities, of dysmorphic syndromes with mental retardation, and of syndromes with dwarfism such as Seckel syndrome. The pathology of such cases is usually poorly known. Some of these syndromes are genetically determined.

Nongenetic microcephaly may result from a host of insults that can occur throughout gestation and even develop in postnatal life. X-irradiation (Miller and Mulvihill 1976), vascular disruption (Hughes and Miskin 1986), circulatory insufficiency (Larroche 1977), drugs and other chemicals (Jones *et al.* 1973, 1989) and hypoxic–ischaemic insult at birth can all induce microcephaly.

The *diagnosis* of microcephaly is easy in extreme cases but may be difficult in mild ones. The size of the head is normally highly variable on an individual and familial basis. Measurement of head size is imprecise, and the commonly used occipitofrontal circumference is only imperfectly correlated to brain volume, so that better indices have been sought using radiological measurements (Gooskens *et al.* 1989). However, head circumference remains the common simple method for evaluating brain size. In children, head circumference increases rapidly with the growth of the brain, so appropriate growth curves should be used for infants and children of average birthweight (Babson and Benda 1976) and for healthy and sick preterm infants (Sher and Brown 1975a,b; Gross *et al.* 1983). In normal infants, the weight of the brain trebles within the first year of life, and repeated measurements of head circumference are an essential part of examination.

The differential diagnosis with total craniosynostosis does not raise real problems, and the shape of skull, exophthalmia, normal development, signs of increased intracranial pressure and plain X-rays of the skull make the diagnosis obvious. The most important issue in diagnosis is to differentiate acquired (clastic) microcephaly from genetic types. Marked neurological involvement, severe mental retardation, and a history of abnormal prenatal or perinatal events in the face of moderate microcephaly support a clastic origin, while the reverse features favour a genetic microcephaly. However, clinical features leave considerable room for uncertainty. The demonstration of destructive changes on CT scan (Jaworski *et al.* 1986) is of great value. A normal CT, on the contrary, does not exclude an acquired origin.

Antenatal diagnosis is extremely difficult, especially in the absence of associated malformations, and errors by excess or by default have been frequent. Simple measurement of the biparietal diameter is not sufficient as it may be low in fetuses with sagittal craniosynostosis or marked intrauterine molding. Repeated examinations with full attention to skull shape are essential (Jaffe *et al.* 1987).

The *prognosis* of microcephaly is variable. Because certain children have relatively good intellectual potential, a sustained effort to educate them is worthwhile. Special schooling is unavoidable although an exceptional child will do well even with head circumference as low as 6 SD below the mean (personal case).

Macrocephaly and megalencephaly (Table 3.5)
The definition of macrocephaly raises problems comparable to those posed by microcephaly. The major diagnostic consideration is hydrocephalus or pericerebral collections because these may necessitate immediate treatment. A majority of the cases of macrocephaly are not due to abnormal brain development but will be considered here as the large head is a common and striking feature.

Macrocephaly, like microcephaly, is defined by reference to head circumference, the arbitrary limit of two standard deviations being often accepted. With this statistical criterion, the definition includes normal individuals as well as a collection of diverse and totally unrelated entities (see Table 3.5). Lorber and Priestley (1981) studied 510 children with head circumference above the 98th centile. Seventy-five per cent of these had hydrocephalus and

TABLE 3.5
Causes of macrocephaly other than internal hydrocephalus

Of extracerebral origin or due to the presence of alien tissue
    Pericerebral effusions, post-traumatic or of unknown origin (benign subdural effusions, external hydrocephalus)
        (Chapter 7)
    Congenital anomalies of intra- or extracerebral veins (aneurysm of the vein of Galen; other abnormalities of
        venous drainage) (Chapter 15)
    Achondroplasia and other skeletal dysplasias: osteopetrosis, Pyle disease, thanatophoric dwarfism (macrocephaly
        probably results in part from abnormal venous drainage and resulting hydrocephalus).
    Osteogenesis imperfecta (especially type III) (Tsipouras *et al.* 1986)
    Tumours, congenital or acquired (Chapter 14)
    Intracranial cysts, especially giant arachnoid cysts in infants (Chapter 14)
    Agenesis of corpus callosum*

Due to increased cerebral volume
    Megalencephaly of anatomical origin
        Tumours (diffuse astrocytomas or gliomatosis)
        Neurocutaneous syndromes (Chapter 4)
            Neurofibromatis type 1
            Tuberous sclerosis**
            Proteus syndrome
            Hemangiomatosis (Klippel–Trevaunay, Stürge–Weber, Shapiro–Shulman, Riley–Smith,
                Ruvalcaba–Myhre syndromes)
        Dysmorphic syndromes
            Cerebral gigantism (Sotos syndrome)
            Beckwith–Widemann syndrome
        Primary megalencephaly (usually nonfamilial, associated with abnormalities of brain architecture, including
            hemimegalencephaly***) (Chapter 3)
        Variant of normal (often familial and unassociated with brain abnormalities) (Chapter 3)
    Metabolic megalencephaly (Chapters 9, 10)
        Leukodystrophies (Canavan–van Bogaert and Alexander diseases)
        GM2 gangliosidosis (Tay–Sachs and Sandhoff diseases)
        Mucopolysaccharidoses
        Organic aciduria, especially glutaric aciduria type 1 and 2-oxyglutaric aciduria (Hoffmann *et al.* 1991, Barth
            et al. 1992, Martinez-Lage *et al.* 1994, Brismar and Ozaud 1995)

*Usually classified as hydrocephalus, often nonprogressive (see Chapter 3).
**Macrocephaly is unusual, in contrast to neurofibromatosis type 1.
***Hemimegalencephaly more commonly results in neurodevelopmental abnormalities than in macrocephaly.

increased intracranial pressure, 3 per cent had specific syndromes. and 20 per cent had primary megalencephaly with normal pressure. Only 13 per cent of the latter group were retarded, slow or neurologically abnormal. Males outnumbered girls by 4 to 1, and 50 per cent of the patients had a family history of macrocephaly.

The macrocephalies consist of two main groups: megalencephaly, and hydrocephalus and pericerebral collections. The latter group are considered in Chapter 7.

Megalencephaly implies an increased brain weight. Some authors (Friede 1989) separate patients with large heads but normal neurodevelopmental progress and function, from 'true' megalencephaly, *i.e.* with a brain significantly larger than the norm for age. Only the latter group belongs to the disorders of brain development. This distinction is to some extent artificial, as a large head—and even a heavy brain at autopsy—is not rare in normal individuals or in association with diseases such as neurofibromatosis, without any hint of brain dysfunction. For the purpose of this chapter, true megalencephaly will refer to excessive brain weight combined with various developmental anomalies with an increase in neural elements both neuronal and glial. This is usually associated with disturbances of migration and organization (Friede 1989) and, often, with giant abnormal cells reminiscent of those encountered in tuberous sclerosis and

indicative of a disturbance of cell differentiation. The gyral pattern of such brains is often abnormal. Some such brains may weigh twice as much as expected for age.

Even with a strict definition, megalencephaly includes several distinct pathological and clinical entities. It may be a part of specific syndromes such as Sotos syndrome (Chapter 5) or various neurocutaneous syndromes (Ross *et al.* 1989, Powell *et al.* 1993), or may be isolated (Stephan *et al.* 1975, Sakuta *et al.* 1989).

Clinical manifestations include mental retardation in virtually all cases, and diffuse neurological abnormalities and seizures in many patients.

The *mechanisms of megalencephaly* are poorly understood. Cell diploidy has been excluded (Robain *et al.* 1988, Friede 1989). Friede thinks that a dysregulation of cell proliferation of subneoplastic (or hamartomatous) nature, whether diffuse or more localized, is involved, and some cases are difficult to distinguish from gangliogliomas (Chapter 14). The significance of the elevated level of insulin-like growth factor (IGF) II in the brain of an infant with macrocephaly and grossly disturbed neocortical development remains in doubt (Schoenle *et al.* 1986).

The *differential diagnosis* of megalencephaly may be difficult. Hydrocephalus and intracranial collections should be excluded as they may require surgical treatment (Chapter 7).

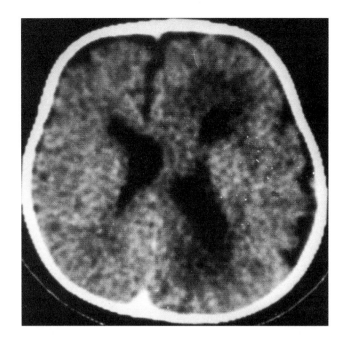

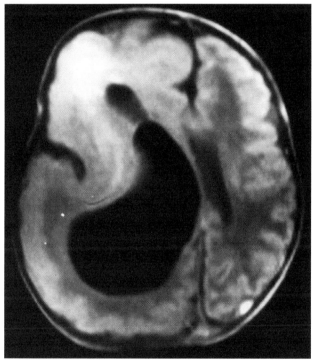

Fig. 3.14. Hemimegalencephaly. *(Top)* CT scan showing large left hemisphere with distorted ventricle and low density of frontal white matter (10-month-old patient with linear naevus). *(Bottom)* T$_1$-weighted MRI of another patient aged 5 months. Large right hemisphere, with abnormally thick cortex and few sulci. Greatly enlarged ventricle and abnormal signal from frontal white matter.

Patients with large heads and normal or near-normal neurodevelopmental function are also a heterogeneous group, although a majority appear to have genetically determined large heads. Lorber and Priestley (1981) found a high incidence of macrocephaly in the parents, especially the fathers, of such children. Day and Schutt (1979) and De Myer (1972) also suggested that

macrocephaly may be dominantly transmitted. Some of these macrocephalic children may have learning disorders, the incidence of which seems to be higher than among children of normal head size. The rate of head growth is particularly rapid in infants under 4 months of age (De Myer 1972, Lorber and Priestley 1981). At this stage the diagnosis of hydrocephalus is often suggested, and radiological examination is in order if the rate of increase does not slow down rapidly. In patients without any neurodevelopmental abnormality and a family history of large head, nothing more than careful follow-up is needed. However, the possibility of presymptomatic glutaric aciduria (Hoffmann *et al.* 1991) or another organic acid disorder frequently associated with macrocephaly should be excluded.

The shape of the skull is important to consider as patients with marked dolichocephaly (sagittal suture synostosis) usually have a head circumference 3 SD or more above the mean. In young infants with perinatal illnesses or in older infants who had nutritional problems, 'catch-up' growth may temporarily represent a diagnostic problem (Sher and Brown 1975a,b). CT scan should be obtained in cases with persistently divergent head curves or when signs of increased intracranial pressure are present.

No treatment of megalencephaly is available and in most cases none is necessary.

Hemimegalencephaly is a complex abnormality that includes both proliferation and migration disturbances (Fig. 3.14). It may involve only the cerebrum or both cererebrum and cerebellum. Involvement of the contralateral hemisphere may be present and should be carefully sought as it has a significant bearing on surgical decision (Chugani *et al.* 1996). The gyral pattern of the affected hemisphere is abnormal, resembling pachygyric or polymicrogyric cortex (Friede 1989). In cases that have been studied microscopically (Robain *et al.* 1988) the cortex was diffusely thickened with piling up of grey matter and absent laminar organization. Neurons are disoriented and widely spaced. Bosman *et al.* (1996) found a normal euploid DNA. Nodular heterotopias of grey matter are present in some cases. Giant neurons are frequently present (Bosman *et al.* 1996). Barkovich and Chuang (1990) found migration abnormalities in 11 of 12 cases. They proposed that polymicrogyria could be distinguished from lissencephaly and pachygyria by MRI, although the differences may be quite subtle. In one case, a hamartomatous process was present.

Clinical manifestations include variable degrees of mental retardation, and seizures, not infrequently infantile spasms, or the so-called Ohtahara syndrome (Chapter 16) in association with focal attacks. Hemiparesis may occur. In some cases, overgrowth of a hemiface or even of one side of the body is apparent, as in the linear naevus syndrome (Levin *et al.* 1984, Cavenagh *et al.* 1993, Dodge and Dobyns 1995), neurofibromatosis (Ross *et al.* 1989) or the Proteus syndrome (Cohen 1988). Suggestive EEG patterns include suppression–burst activity, alpha-like activity reminiscent of that seen in agyria–pachygyria, or repetitive triphasic complexes (King *et al.* 1985, Paladin *et al.* 1989, Vigevano *et al.* 1996). CT scan and especially MRI confirm the diagnosis by showing a thickened cortex with few sulci, absent or abnormal

TABLE 3.6
Main syndromes with agyria–pachygyria or pachygyria

Histological type	Syndrome	Genetics*	References
Type I (thick four-layered cortex)	Isolated lissencephaly sequence (no specific dysmorphism)	Sporadic?[1]	Dobyns et al. (1984)
	Miller–Dieker syndrome (specific dysmorphic syndrome)	Chromosomal anomaly (17p–) may be inherited	Dobyns et al. (1983)
	Norman–Roberts syndrome (microcephaly, dysmorphism)	AR	Norman et al. (1976), Dobyns et al. (1984)
	Lissencephaly, microcephaly and apnoea	AR?	Dobyns (1992)
Type II (Walker type, unlayered cortex)	Walker–Warburg syndrome (hydrocephalus, eye abnormalities)	AR	Dobyns et al. (1989), Dobyns (1993)
	Cerebro-oculo-muscular syndrome (COMS) (may be the same as Walker–Warburg syndrome)	AR Probably allelic to Walker–Warburg syndrome	Dambska et al. (1982), Towfighi et al. (1984), Dobyns (1993)
	Muscle, eye and brain syndrome[2] (severe myopia, probably related to other type II syndromes)	AR?	Santavuori et al. (1989)
Pachygyria	Milder form of type I with fast EEG rhythms	AR? or sporadic	Aicardi (1989)
	Other forms without EEG fast rhythms	AR?	Aicardi (1989)
	Fukuyama type muscular dystrophy	AR	Fukuyama et al. (1981)
	Palm syndrome (congenital nephrosis)	AR	Palm et al. (1986), Robain and Deonna (1983)
Other types	Cerebrocerebellar lissencephaly (microlissencephaly)	AR?	Dobyns et al. (1985), Kroon et al. (1996)
	Extreme neopallial hypoplasia	AR	Barth et al. (1982)
	Neu–Laxova syndrome	AR	Fitch et al. (1982)
Localized and atypical cases	Focal unilateral microgyria	Sporadic?	Andermann et al. (1987)
	Bilateral central macrogyria	Sporadic[3]	Kuzniecky et al. (1989)
	Diffuse laminar heterotopias	Sporadic or sex-linked dominant	Livingston and Aicardi (1990), Pinard et al. (1994)

*AR = autosomal recessive.
[1]Many cases are associated with abnormalities of the *LIS1* gene.
[2]No pathological confirmation of abnormal gyration is available.
[3]Rare familial cases.

operculation and often abnormal white matter on the affected side (Kalifa et al. 1987, Robain et al. 1988, Konkol et al. 1990). Positron emission tomography (PET) has been used to detect contralateral hemisphere involvement (Lee et al. 1994, Chugani et al. 1996). Vigevano and Di Rocco (1990) found that cases belonged to two distinct subgroups: infants with prenatal or perinatal onset of seizures and severe neonatal neurological anomalies have a poor outcome and often die early; infants with onset of seizures after the first six months of life tend to fare better and can become candidates for successful epilepsy surgery. A patient with normal intelligence and *epilepsia partialis continua* has been reported (Fusco et al. 1992).

The seizures of patients with hemimegalencephaly tend to be refractory to drug therapy (Pelayo et al. 1994). Hemispherectomy may control the seizures in up to 85 per cent of cases (Di Rocco 1996).

DISORDERS OF MIGRATION
The complex process of cell migration can be interfered with by acquired or genetic causes. Depending on the date and severity of the causal process, the spectrum of migration disorders will manifest as a major form (heterotopias, lissencephaly–pachygyria or polymicrogyria) or a minor disturbance (abnormal lamination of cortex, microdysgenesis) (Table 3.6). Both may be localized, multifocal or diffuse and variably associated (Barth 1987, Barkovich et al. 1996, Dobyns et al. 1996a). Localized areas of migration abnormalities are often associated with more diffuse brain changes (Sisodiya et al. 1995). An increasing number of familial migration disorders are recognized (see below) and may result from chromosomal deletions or gene mutations. These may affect the glial guides, the adhesion molecules between neurons and guides, or the growth cone function. Known or suspected acquired causes include intrauterine infections, especially cytomegalovirus disease and circulatory disorders (Dobyns et al. 1992). Any pathological process damaging the glial guides (e.g. haemorrhage, infarction, infection) can be a cause. Recent work has shown that some pathological abnormalities, formerly thought to be due to aberrations in development of the cortical plate, result in fact from destructive processes that occur after most of the process of corticogenesis has taken place (Caviness et al. 1981, Williams et al. 1984, Lyon and Beaugerie 1988, Evrard et al. 1989).

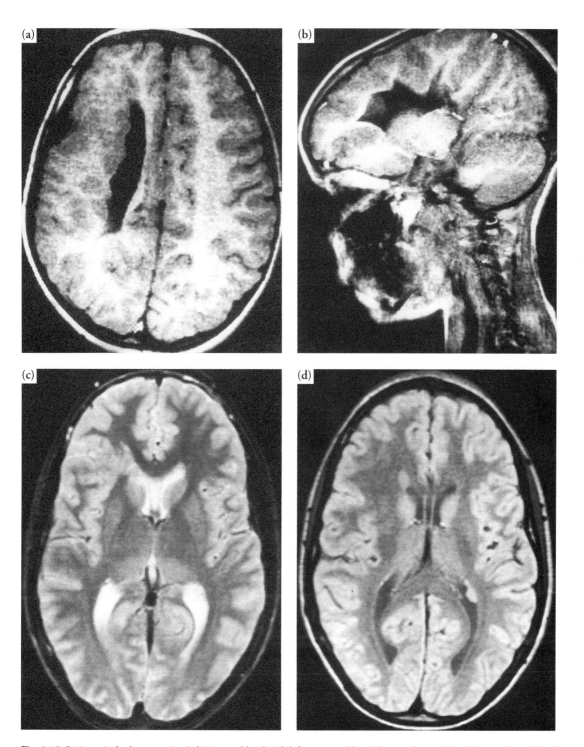

Fig. 3.15. Periventricular heterotopia. *(a,b)* 5-year-old girl with left congenital hemiplegia and normal intelligence. T$_1$-weighted MRI sequences show masses of heterotopic grey matter lining the right lateral ventricle and responsible for the festooned contour of its cavity. *(c,d)* Right frontal and left occipital heterotopia in 16-year-old boy with recent history of two seizures (normal neurological examination and development).

Periventricular heterotopias

Heterotopias are neuronal assemblies that have remained in a subependymal location corresponding to the primitive proliferative zone or have been arrested on their way to the cortical plates (Fig. 3.15). Their mechanism is poorly understood; they may result in part from failure of the normal mechanisms of pro-

grammed cell death (apoptosis). A rare, major form also features multiple abnormalities of migration affecting especially the basal ganglia and resulting in a partially undivided brain with no visible ventricles (Shaw and Alvord 1996).

Periventricular heterotopias are frequently part of complex malformation syndromes (Bergeron 1967) such as Aicardi

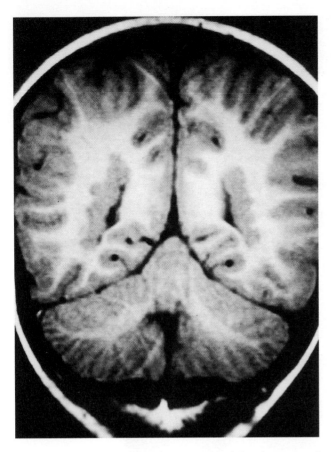

Fig. 3.16. Periventricular nodular heterotopia. Note bilateral, symmetrical nodules of grey matter lining the lateral ventricles.

sibship, in association with calcification of the choroid plexus (Lott *et al.* 1979).

Subcortical laminar heterotopias, also known as band heterotopias (Marchal *et al.* 1989, Barkovich *et al.* 1994, Franzoni *et al.* 1995) or 'double cortex' (Livingston and Aicardi 1990, Palmini *et al.* 1991a, Tohyama *et al.* 1992), are a generalized disorder of migration in which a superficial cortex, which may be grossly normal or show an aberrant gyration, is separated by a thin layer of white matter from a deep band of grey matter whose separation from the underlying white matter is straight as in agyria–pachygyria (Fig. 3.17). Patients with this anomaly often have seizures that may be focal or generalized, sometimes in the form of the Lennox–Gastaut syndrome, and EEG anomalies (Ricci *et al.* 1992, Hashimoto *et al.* 1993, Parmeggiani *et al.* 1994). The degree of mental involvement is quite variable and some patients develop normally (Livingston and Aicardi 1990, Ianetti *et al.* 1993). Barkovich *et al.* (1994) in a detailed study of 27 cases found a significant inverse correlation between the intellectual level and the thickness of the heterotopic band; an apparently normal cortex was associated with a better development. Genetic factors are an important cause of this syndrome that seems to be transmitted as an X-linked dominant trait. Only rare male cases are on record, and families in which females presented with double cortex and males with type I lissencephaly are on record (Pinard *et al.* 1994, Dobyns *et al.* 1996a). Unilateral and partial band heterotopias may be difficult to recognize and may require special cuts and reformatting on MRI for detection (Gallucci *et al.* 1991).

Agyria–pachygyria
The term agyria–pachygyria is preferable to that of lissencephaly, meaning a smooth brain, which applies only to extreme cases. In most cases, some gyri and sulci are present, and areas of polymicrogyria and of pachygyria can coexist in the same brain. There are several distinct forms of agyria–pachygyria with different pathological and clinical features (Dobyns *et al.* 1984, Dobyns 1987, Dobyns and Truwit 1995) (Table 3.6).

Dobyns *et al.* (1992) distinguish four grades of lissencephaly (I to IV) depending on the number of sulci visible on MRI scans. Only grade I actually deserves the name of lissencephaly, whereas grades II–IV are cases of pachygyria. Some cases of apparent pachygyria on MRI may in fact be examples of polymicrogyria (see below). For this reason, I will describe first those cases of lissencephaly whose histological structure can be safely surmised from the MRI scans, then cases of nonlissencephalic developmental cortical anomalies that may be either pachygyria (with a histological appearance similar to but less severe than lissencephaly) or polymicrogyria. Criteria for recognition of agyria–pachygyria on the basis of EEG and imaging features have been recently proposed (Sébire *et al.* 1995).

Type I lissencephaly is also known as classical lissencephaly or the Bielschowski type of lissencephaly. In this form, the brain is small with only the primary and sometimes a few secondary gyri. Cerebral vessels in the absence of sulci are tortuous so that angiography has been used as a diagnostic tool. On cutting, the

syndrome (Chevrie and Aicardi 1986; Aicardi 1994, 1996). They may also be isolated and give rise to epilepsy or neurological signs, or remain silent (Barkovich and Kjos 1992). Nodular heterotopias are preferentially localized in the posterior part of the brain and may be uni- or bilateral (Raymond *et al.* 1994, Dubeau *et al.* 1995). Bilateral, symmetrical bands of periventricular confluent nodules are often transmitted as a dominant trait but affect only females (Huttenlocher *et al.* 1994) (Fig. 3.16). This syndrome may resemble tuberous sclerosis (Di Mario *et al.* 1993). It is often responsible for epilepsy—frequently with generalized seizures—with onset in early adulthood (Kamuro and Tenokuchi 1993, Raymond *et al.* 1993, Dubeau *et al.* 1995) but also occasionally in the second decade. Some cases may remain asymptomatic for prolonged periods.

Subcortical heterotopias
Nodular heterotopias of grey matter are present in many patients with other migration abnormalities such as polymicrogyria or schizencephaly. Single or multifocal large heterotopic nodules may be a focus for partial seizures (Layton 1962). However, even giant heterotopias involving one hemisphere may remain asymptomatic (Jiménez *et al.* 1994). Detailed neuropsychological study of one such case demonstrated subtle deficits of hemispheric functions despite a normal intelligence (Calabrese *et al.* 1994). Familial subcortical heterotopias have also been reported, in one

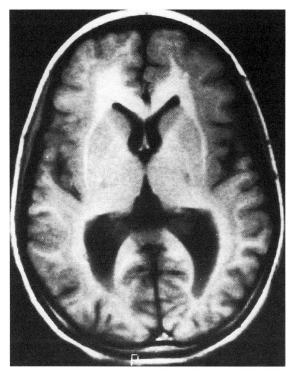

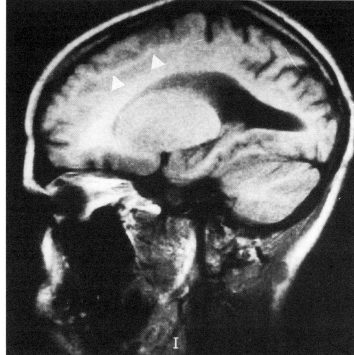

Fig. 3.17. Subcortical laminar heterotopia ('double cortex').
(Top) MRI, T_1-weighted sequence: *(left)* axial cut; *(right)* sagittal cut—a thin band of white matter lies between the true cortex and the thin laminar heterotopia of grey matter *(arrows)*.
(Opposite) Thick subcortical heterotopia in a mentally retarded child.

cortex is abnormally thick whereas the white matter appears as a narrow ribbon along the ventricles. Typically, the cortex consists of four layers: (1) a superficial, cell-sparse layer that corresponds to the molecular layer of the normal brain; (2) a narrow, cell-rich layer in which large pyramidal cells that should normally be located in the deeper layers are present; (3) a thin layer of white matter, below which (4) a thick band of small ectopic neurons extends almost to the ventricular wall (Stewart *et al.* 1975, Larroche 1977) (Fig. 3.18). Many of the neurons in both cellular layers are abnormally orientated, with an apical dendrite orientated down-wards or obliquely (Fabregues *et al.* 1984, Takashima *et al.* 1987). The deeper cellular layer is formed by ectopic neurons arrested in their migration from the germinal layer to the cortex at about 12 weeks gestation (Stewart *et al.* 1975) so that the cortex looks very much like that of a 13-week fetus. The neurons in this layer have an excessive columnar organization. In the medulla, ectopia of the olivary nuclei is characteristic. The dentate nuclei are abnormally convoluted and the pyramids are hypoplastic or absent (Friede 1989). Agenesis of the corpus callosum may be associated (Aicardi *et al.* 1987, Dobyns *et al.* 1992).

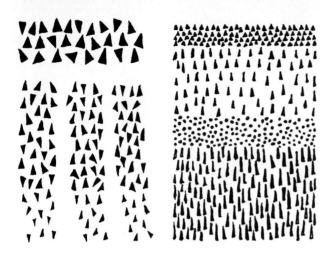

Fig. 3.18. *(Left)* Type I (classical) lissencephaly. Four-layer cortex. From surface *(top)* down: *(1)* molecular layer; *(2)* superficial cellular layer containing several types of cells, including large pyramids, normally more deeply located in layer 5; *(3)* thin, acellular or paucicellular layer; *(4)* broad band of heterotopic cells arrested in their migration—note columnar disposition. *(Right)* Normal disposition.

The causes of the migrational arrest responsible for type I lissencephaly are multiple (Dobyns *et al.* 1992). Most cases are sporadic. A significant proportion of cases result from a chromosomal abnormality, a deletion of the distal part of the short arm of chromosome 17 (17p13.3). Some such cases are part of a specific dysmorphic syndrome, the *Miller–Dieker syndrome,* which is characterized by a narrow forehead, long philtrum, absent notch of the upper lip, upturned nares, retrognathism, digital anomalies and hypervascularization of the retinae (Jones *et al.* 1980, Dobyns *et al.* 1983). In such cases, Dobyns and Truwit (1995) found a visible deletion of 17p13.3 in 14 of 25 patients, and submicroscopic deletion in 25 of 38 cases by cytogenetic techniques and in 35/38 using fluorescent *in situ* hybridization (FISH), and it appears likely that all cases of the Miller–Dieker syndrome are due to a deletion whether microscopic or submicroscopic.

Siblings with Miller–Dieker syndrome have been born to couples in which one parent carried a balanced translocation of the terminal fragment of chromosome 17p onto a chromosome in the 13–15 group, the translocation appearing in an unbalanced form in affected children (Greenberg *et al.* 1986, Goutières *et al.* 1987). In some pedigrees, male infants with type I lissencephaly have been born to mothers with subcortical heterotopias (Pinard *et al.* 1994, Dobyns *et al.* 1996a).

Most cases of type I lissencephaly are not part of the Miller–Dieker syndrome and are termed '*isolated lissencephaly sequence*' (Dobyns *et al.* 1983). Some of these cases have been shown to be associated with a submicroscopic deletion (37 per cent by cytogenetic techniques, 44 per cent by FISH—Dobyns and Truwit 1995) or with several mutations of a specific gene, the *LIS 1* gene (Dobyns *et al.* 1993) that codes for a hydrolase of a subunit of the platelet-activating factor (PAF) (Reiner *et al.*

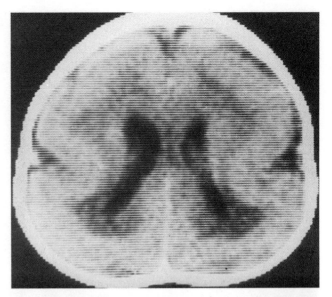

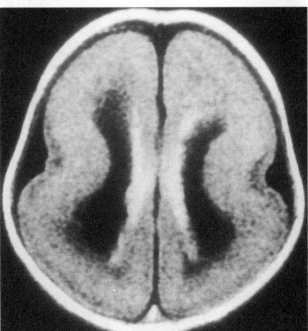

Fig. 3.19. Type I lissencephaly. *(Top)* CT scan: smooth cortex and interface between white and grey matter. Thick cortical ribbon and lack of operculation with open sylvian fissure. *(Bottom)* MRI scan showing smooth, thick cortical ribbon with dark line separating thin superficial layer from thick layer corresponding to heterotopic neurons arrested in their migration.

1993). It is not known how the excess of unhydrolyzed PAF induces the migration defect but interference with growth cone function is suspected. Not all cases of lissencephaly are due to *LIS 1* gene abnormalities. X-linked cases have been reported (Pavone *et al.* 1990, Berry-Kravis and Israel 1994, Dobyns *et al.* 1996a), and atypical cases with marked microcephaly and pulmonary insufficiency may be inherited in an autosomal recessive manner (Dobyns *et al.* 1992, Dobyns and Truwit 1995). An unknown proportion of cases may be due to intrauterine infections or ischaemic events.

The clinical presentation always features severe mental retardation and diplegia, often of the atonic type (Gastaut *et al.* 1987, De Rijk-Van Andel *et al.* 1990). Partial seizures and, especially, infantile spasms are the rule. Most patients have some degree of microcephaly, usually mild. In *nonchromosomal cases*, dysmorphism is minor although the forehead is narrow and retrognathism is frequent. The prognosis is poor with limited survival.

The *diagnosis* of type I lissencephaly has been made possible by modern imaging techniques. CT and MRI show the distinctive appearance of a thick cortical plate, with no or only a few sulci, separated from the hypodense white matter by a mildly undulating or almost rectilinear border (Barkovich *et al.* 1988, 1991). Layering of the cortex can be demonstrated with high-resolution CT or MRI (Fig. 3.19). Ultrasonography may demonstrate the smooth cortex in the fetus, the neonate or the young infant (Trounce *et al.* 1986, Cioni *et al.* 1996).

The EEG in most cases shows high-amplitude fast activity of alpha or beta frequency which may alternate, even on the same tracing, with high-amplitude delta or theta slow rhythms that may simulate slow spike–wave complexes or hypsarrhythmia (Hakamada *et al.* 1979; Dulac *et al.* 1983; Gastaut *et al.* 1987; De Rijk-Van Andel *et al.* 1988, 1992; Quirk *et al.* 1993; Mori *et al.* 1994; Dalla Bernardina *et al.* 1996; Pellicer *et al.* 1996) (Fig. 3.20).

The differential diagnosis is easy, as most conditions in which pachygyria is found, *e.g.* Zellweger syndrome or certain types of congenital nephrosis (Robain and Deonna 1983, Palm *et al.* 1986), have rather specific features. Certain fetal disorders can produce a pachygyric cortex, in particular cytomegalovirus infection. In such cases, periventricular calcification may be associated with abnormal gyration. Sudanophilic leukodystrophy with migrational disturbances may well be identical to type I lissencephaly or pachygyria (Norman *et al.* 1967).

Prenatal diagnosis is not possible by sonography before 30 weeks as tertiary sulci appear only at this date. DNA studies may show an abnormal or missing *LIS 1* gene. Chromosome studies and MRI of the parents (especially the mother) should be performed in search of laminar heterotopias in order to help determine the risk of recurrence.

Type II lissencephaly or Walker–Warburg syndrome (Pagon *et al.* 1983), also termed 'cobblestone' lissencephaly, is a completely different malformation from both the aetiological and morphological points of view (Williams *et al.* 1984; Dobyns *et al.* 1985, 1996a). The cortex has no sulci and its surface is granular, although areas of unlayered microgyria may be present (Bordarier *et al.* 1984). The meninges are thick and have a milky appearance due to massive mesenchymal proliferation, especially around the brainstem. The cerebellum is small and lacks a vermis. The pyramidal tracts are usually absent, and in 75 per cent of cases hydrocephalus is present. It is variably due to cisternal obstruction by abnormal meninges or to aqueductal stenosis (Bordarier *et al.* 1984). There is often fusion of the frontal poles and of the molecular surfaces of cerebellar lamellae. Microscopically, there is complete disruption of cortical architecture, the cortical plate consisting of a variable thickness of poorly oriented cells separated

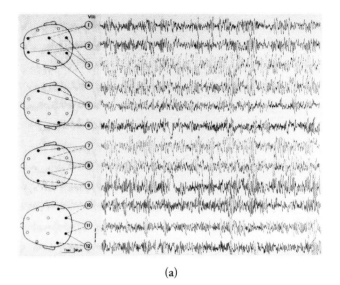

(a)

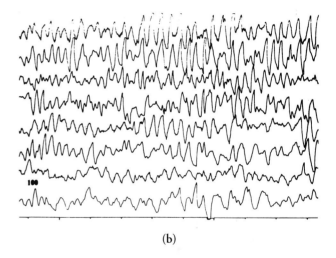

(b)

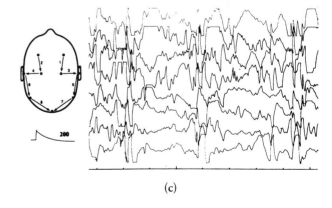

(c)

Fig. 3.20. *(a)* Lissencephaly–pachygyria in a 2-year-old girl: EEG showing typical fast rhythms at alpha and higher frequency.

(b) Miller–Dieker syndrome in a 14-week-old girl: runs of rhythmic activity of different frequencies but mostly in the theta range. (Courtesy Dr S. Boyd, Great Ormond Street Hospital, London.)

(c) Miller–Dieker syndrome in a 2-year-old boy: although some excess theta–alpha activity is present, the record is dominated by repetitive bursts of sharp waves reaching 500–600 µV. (Courtesy Dr S. Boyd, Great Ormond Street Hospital, London.)

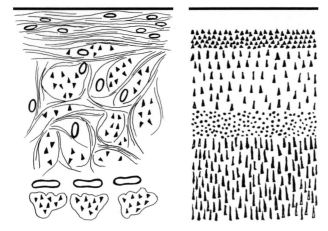

Fig. 3.21. Type II (Walker–Warburg) lissencephaly. *(Left)* Total disorganization of the cortex with neural cells separated by gliomesenchymal bundles originating in the thick fibrous meninges. These cells have apparently migrated beyond the molecular layer into the pial membrane. More deeply, a row of heterotopias are aligned under tangential vessels and are separated by a thin acellullar layer from the more superficial cells. *(Right)* Normal cortex.

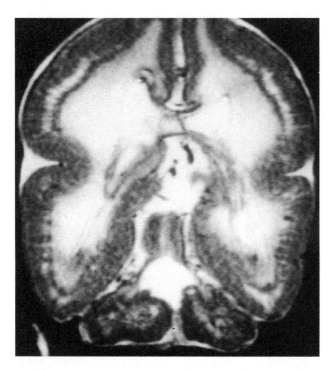

Fig. 3.22. Type II lissencephaly: T$_2$-weighted MR scan showing thick, smooth cortex. The thin white line probably corresponds to the acellular layer shown in Fig. 3.21. Note dilated ventricles and absence of cerebellar vermis.

by trabeculae of gliomesenchymal tissue in continuity with that of the meninges (Fig. 3.21). Multiple islands of heterotopic grey matter are aligned parallel to the cortical surface, separated from the overlying cortex by a thin layer of white matter in which thin blood vessels are tangentially aligned. These anomalies probably result from massive overmigration of neuroglial precursors through a disrupted pial–glial limiting membrane. This tissue

isolates glomerular or trabecular formations of neural cells (Takashima *et al.* 1987). The cerebellum is totally disorganized (Lyon and Beaugerie 1988) and the vermis is usually missing.

Type II lissencephaly is a genetic disorder transmitted as an autosomal recessive character (Dobyns *et al.* 1985, Dobyns 1987), although a protracted inflammatory (viral?) origin has been suggested (Williams *et al.* 1984) but seems unlikely.

The clinical features (Dobyns *et al.* 1989, Dobyns 1993, Yamaguchi *et al.* 1993) include severe neurological dysfunction from birth; eye abnormalities with retinal dysplasia in all cases, microphthalmia and anomalies of the anterior segment (Peters' anomaly, cataracts, persistence of primitive vitreous body) in most; and hydrocephalus or, less commonly, microcephaly. All infants with severe neurological abnormalities and hydrocephalus in association with eye anomalies are highly suspect of having type II lissencephaly, which is a relatively common cause of genetic hydrocephalus.

The diagnosis can be confirmed by CT or MRI, demonstrating agenesis of the cerebellar vermis and lissencephaly. The cortex is thinner than in type I lissencephaly, and fine trabeculae penetrating the cortex from the white matter are characteristic (Valanne *et al.* 1994), with the appearance of a double cortical layer due to the presence of the subcortical heterotopic islands that may be striking (Fig. 3.22). A posterior encephalocele or large posterior fontanelle is usually present. Walker–Warburg syndrome may be associated with adducted thumbs and aqueductal stenosis in some cases (Bordarier *et al.* 1984) and these should be distinguished from the X-linked Becker syndrome (Chapter 7) as the genetic implications are very different. Prenatal diagnosis is possible on the basis of hydrocephalus, encephalocele and eye abnormalities (microphthalmus and/or retinal detachment) (Farrel *et al.* 1987, Rhodes *et al.* 1992).

Muscle involvement is an integral part of type II lissencephaly syndrome (Dobyns *et al.* 1989, 1993), although a case with normal eyes and muscle is on record (Dobyns *et al.* 1996b). Widespread necrosis of fibres is present in all muscles, the appearance being reminiscent of that in severe muscular dystrophies. It appears likely at this juncture that the *cerebro-oculo-muscular syndrome* (COMS) (Dambska *et al.* 1982, Korithenberg *et al.* 1984, Towfighi *et al.* 1984, Dobyns 1993) is identical to the Walker–Warburg syndrome, while *Fukuyama-type muscular dystrophy* (Chapter 20; Takada *et al.* 1984) is a milder and genetically distinct but possibly allelic condition (Dobyns and Truwit 1995). Similar, though not identical, brain lesions with severe myopia and other ocular anomalies described by Santavuori *et al.* (1989) as *muscle, eye and brain disease* also seem possibly related to the Walker–Warburg syndrome. However, brain dysfunction is usually less, and eye abnormalities mainly consist of severe myopia. The condition seems to be genetically distinct from Fukuyama muscular dystrophy (Pihko *et al.* 1995).

The prognosis of type II lissencephaly is extremely poor. Most affected infants die in a few weeks or months, an occasional patient living to a few years. Patients with severe hydrocephalus should receive a shunt to avoid monstrous growth of the head but the ultimate prognosis remains dismal.

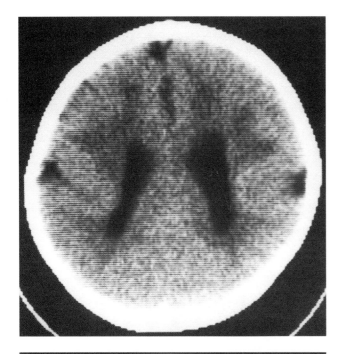

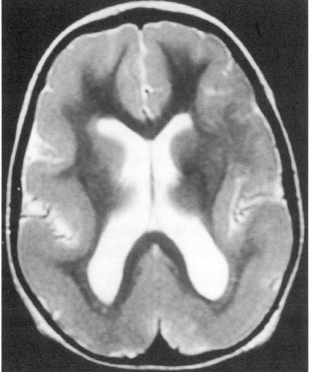

Fig. 3.23. Pachygyria. *(Top)* CT scan: abnormal appearance of both sylvian fissures; note also thickened cortical ribbon and straight border with white matter. *(Bottom)* MRI scan, T_1-weighted sequence: abnormally broad gyri with thick cortical ribbon in posterior half of brain.

Nonlissencephalic cortical dysgenesis

This includes pachygyria which is closely related to lissencephaly, of which it represents a minor grade and probably shares many aetiological factors, and polymicrogyria, a pathologically and aetiologically different condition. Although clearly distinct and having some differential imaging and EEG characteristics

(Sébire *et al.* 1995), both anomalies often share similar clinical and imaging features and may be difficult or impossible to separate.

Pachygyria (Fig. 3.23) histologically resembles type I lissencephaly, but the small neurons of layers II and IV are found (Stewart *et al.* 1975) and there is no deep cell sparse layer, indicating that migration has proceeded to a later stage. It may be diffuse or localized. Some other rare or poorly identified cortical abnormalities are shown in Table 3.6.

The terms *microgyria* and *polymicrogyria* refer to an abnormal appearance of cortical gyri that seem to be crowded, too narrow, and form an abnormal convolutional pattern. The macroscopical aspect, however, is variable. In some cases, broad convolutions are apparent that may be impossible to distinguish from areas of pachygyria by looking only at the surface of the brain, but the cortical ribbon is characteristically polymicrogyric with fusion of the molecular layers (Friede 1989). Polymicrogyria may affect the whole cortex. Much more frequently, it involves localized areas which may correspond to arterial territories, especially of the middle cerebral arteries (Lyon and Beaugerie 1988). Microgyria is consistently present in the immediate vicinity of schizencephalic defects. Areas of microgyria are lined on both sides of the cleft and extend down to the ventricle. Microgyria is often present on the contralateral side even in cases of unilateral cleft, particularly in the insular area. Microgyria may be associated with nodular heterotopia in the white matter (Friede 1989) or with other malformations such as agenesis of the corpus callosum or with evidence of fetal infections such as periventricular or parenchymal calcification.

Several histological types of polymicrogyria are observed. The most commonly encountered, clearly a developmental disorder, is *unlayered microgyria* (Harding and Copp 1997), in which a single cell layer undulates between the white matter and the molecular layer. This type often coexists with other developmental anomalies, *e.g.* agenesis of the corpus callosum. In *classical four-layer microgyria*, a first layer of small pyramidal cells underneath the molecular layer is separated by a cell-poor layer from the deep layer containing the large pyramids. The cell-poor layer corresponds to normal layers IV and V, with which it merges at the limits of the microgyric cortex (Richman *et al.* 1974, Williams and Caviness 1984, Lyon and Beaugerie 1988, Evrard *et al.* 1989). This appearance suggests a postmigrational disorder, occurring towards the fifth or sixth month of pregnancy, with secondary laminar necrosis that could be due to perfusion failure and resulting hypoxia (McBride and Kemper 1982, Goodlin 1984). The occurrence of classical polymicrogyria following abnormal events occurring after midgestation such as severe trauma, carbon monoxide intoxication or maternal asphyxia (Larroche 1986, Barth 1987), and its occurrence in only one member of a monozygous twin pair (Sugama and Kusaro 1994) support this interpretation. Evrard *et al.* (1989) found two peak periods for perfusion failure: between 20 and 24 weeks and during the last 10 weeks of gestation (Norman 1980). Perfusion failure may also be responsible for the microgyria that is seen with fetal infections (Marques-Dias *et al.* 1984), which can produce

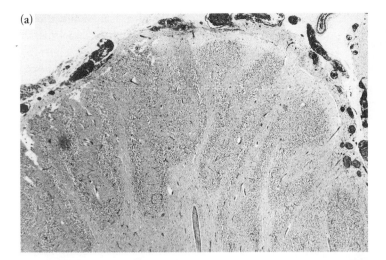

(a)

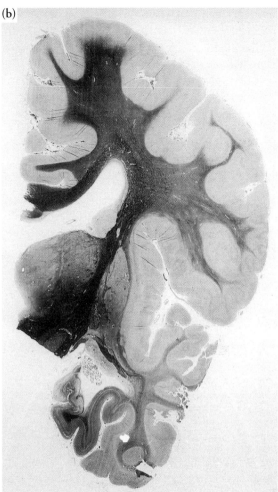

(b)

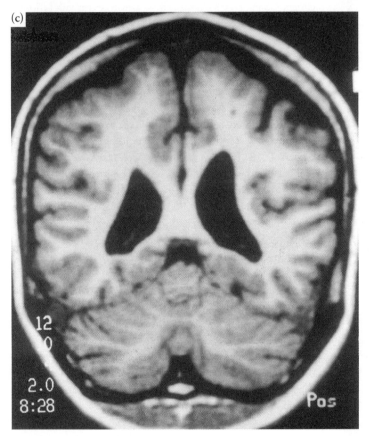

(c)

Fig. 3.24. Polymicrogyria. *(a)* Polymicrogyric cortex. Note undulating band of neurons without intervening sulci, indicating that the external appearance of the brain may be that of broad convolutions reminiscent of pachygyria. (Courtesy Dr J-C. Larroche, Maternité Port Royal, Paris.) *(b)* Low-power view of coronal section of one hemisphere at midthalamic level, showing the excessively folded and fused miniconvolutions of polymicrogyric cortex. (Courtesy Dr B. Harding, Institute of Neurology, London.) *(c)* MRI scan showing extensive areas of apparent polymicrogyria in upper part of both hemispheres predominating with striated appearance suggesting the existence of miniconvolutions. (Courtesy Dr Kling Chong, Great Ormond Street Hospital, London.)

vascular damage (Barkovich and Lindan 1994) or circulatory insufficiency, and for that located at the margin of porencephalic defects (Lyon and Robain 1967, Friede and Mikolasek 1978).

Another uncommon type of microgyria occurs probably slightly before the end of the migrational process. In this form, heterotopic neurons, arrested in their migration, are visible under the area of microgyric cortex (Lyon and Beaugerie 1988, Evrard *et al.* 1989). Arrest of migration may result from an insult to superficial layers, damaging the glial guides before later migrating cells have completed their migration. A similar lesion has been produced in fetal rats by freezing the superficial cortex (Dvorak and Feit 1977, Dvorak *et al.* 1978, Humphreys *et al.* 1991).

Microgyria found in the *Zellweger syndrome* (Chapter 9) is characterized by multiple areas of intracortical heterotopia consisting of a limited number of neurons that remain 'glued' in their migratory corridors at inappropriate pallial levels. As a result, large pyramidal cells are abnormally superficial, many radial columns are too broad, and adjacent columns are displaced downwards or upwards in relation to one another (Evrard *et al.* 1978, 1989; Della Giustina *et al.* 1981).

Polymicrogyria is also a feature of thanatophoric dwarfism (Hori *et al.* 1983, Shigematsu *et al.* 1985). It may also be associated with extraneurological abnormalities such as a short intestine (Nézelof *et al.* 1976). Rare familial cases are known, sometimes associated with cortical calcification (Baraitser *et al.* 1983).

Polymicrogyria may be diffuse, unilateral, multifocal or localized. Differentiation of diffuse forms of pachygyria and polymicrogyria is not clinically possible. Both present with epilepsy, mental retardation or neurological deficits of variable severity. In some cases, MRI can permit recognition of poly-microgyria when there is rippling of the brain surface and fine interdigitations can be made out at the interface of grey and white matter (Sébire *et al.* 1995, Raybaud *et al.* 1996) (Fig. 3.24). However, definite cases of polymicrogyria can present with a thick cortical band, *e.g.* in prenatal cytomegalovirus infection (Hayward *et al.* 1991). The presence of areas of high T_2 signal on MRI, underlying areas of abnormal cortex, may indicate gliosis and thus suggest a late event like microgyria, as gliosis does not occur before the 26th week of gestation (Barkovich and Kjos 1992, Dobyns *et al.* 1992). However, a similar signal may be present with Taylor-type cortical dysplasia (see below). EEG tracings of high-amplitude fast rhythms and alpha–theta pattern suggest true pachygyria (Aicardi 1991, 1994; Sébire *et al.* 1995; Dalla Bernardina 1996). Polymicrogyria should be distinguished from *ulegyria*, the sclerotic, atrophic convolutions occurring as a late result of hypoxic–ischaemic damage. These present in transverse sections as mushrooms because hypoxic damage is more prominent deep in sulci than on the crown of convolutions. They can occasionally be identified on MRI but clinical history is essential for diagnosis.

The *clinical manifestations* of microgyria are nonspecific and depend on the extent of the microgyric areas, their location and the presence of associated malformations. Small areas may not give rise to symptoms. Whether they may be causally related to dyslexia, as suggested by Galaburda *et al.* (1985), remains uncertain. Bilateral opercular polymicrogyria in association with agenesis of the septum pellucidum (Becker *et al.* 1989) represents a specific syndrome and can be diagnosed by CT or MRI. A few cases of familial diffuse dysplasia are on record (Kuzniecky 1994).

Localized cortical migration disorders are characterized by focal abnormal areas usually of polymicrogyria that may affect any part of the cortex and are often responsible for focal epilepsy (Guerrini *et al.* 1992a,b; Otsubo *et al.* 1993; Wyllie *et al.* 1994) (Fig. 3.25*a–c*). They are difficult to separate clinically or by imaging from localized disorders of organization, although differences are obvious pathologically. Bilateral focal migration abnormalities of variable extent are encountered. *Bifrontal dysgenesis* may occur as a familial syndrome (Dobyns and Truwit 1995). Two half-sisters born to the same mother showed a distinct MRI pattern of polymicrogyria (personal cases). Biooccipital cases with visual seizures have been reported (Sisodiya *et al.* 1995, Guerrini *et al.* 1997). A *bilateral perisylvian syndrome* has been repeatedly reported. Affected patients have a characteristic bilateral central rolandic and sylvian macrogyria with thickened cortex that may be more or less symmetrical (Fig. 3.25*d*). All patients have pseudobulbar palsy with dysarthria, dysphagia and limited ability to mimic facial expressions, and most have seizures (Kuzniecky *et al.* 1994a). Such cases were also described as devel-

opmental Foix–Chavany–Marie syndrome (Graff-Radford *et al.* 1986). Kuzniecky *et al.* (1994a,c) reported on 31 cases in which epilepsy subsequently developed in 85 per cent in the form of secondarily generalized or partial seizures or even infantile spasms (Kuzniecky *et al.* 1994b). Despite the thickened appearance of the abnormal cortex, biopsied cases demonstrated polymicrogyria (Becker *et al.* 1989, Shevell *et al.* 1992). Genetic factors are operative in at least some of these cases (Andermann and Andermann 1996). Arthrogryposis of central origin is present in some patients (Hageman *et al.* 1994, Kuzniecky *et al.* 1994a). Such cases may be related to the syndrome of septal agenesis with porencephalies in which a dysplastic cortex may be found in the absence of a cleft in the mantle (Menezes *et al.* 1988). *Posterior cortical dysgenesis* was described as a familial condition by Ferrie *et al.* (1995) in two siblings. In most such cases, the actual histological nature of the disturbance is not known, even though the MR images are suggestive of pachygyria. Cases of dysplasia involving a whole hemisphere are uncommon (Guerrini *et al.* 1992a,b, 1996a) and present in a similar fashion to other focal dysplasias. The affected hemisphere is usually small and the gyral pattern is abnormal throughout. Most patients have congenital hemiparesis but development is variably affected. Some children develop episodes of continuous spikes on EEG in slow sleep but this does not necessarily herald a poor mental outcome (Guerrini *et al.* 1996b). Some such cases histologically belong to the polymicrogyria group while others are more like disturbances of organization. They differ clearly from hemimegalencephaly by the reduced size of the involved hemispheres.

Unilateral opercular dysplasia is not rare (Ambrosetto 1992, Sébire *et al.* 1996). In fact, many cases of localized cortical dysplasia affect this area electively (Guerrini *et al.* 1992a). Some areas of localized cortical dysplasia may be associated with relatively benign forms of epilepsy (Guerrini *et al.* 1996b).

Some rare syndromes feature pachygyria-like cortex in association with extracerebral abnormalities: congenital nephrosis in male siblings (Robain and Deonna 1983, Palm *et al.* 1986); familial lymphoedema and vermian agenesis (Hourihane *et al.* 1993); congenital short bowel (Nézelof *et al.* 1976); and familial pachygyria with disseminated brain calcification and ataxia (Harbord *et al.* 1990).

Nodular cortical dysplasia, also called *status verrucosus*, consists of circumscribed cortical deformities presenting as hemispherical protrusions, 1–2 mm in diameter, on the cortical surface (Friede 1989). Each protrusion, or 'brain wart', comprises a core of radial myelinated fibres that projects into the superficial layers and splits as a fountain-head producing a bulge of the upper layers. These nodules, when limited in number, are probably asymptomatic. Similar deformities in large number are present in the brains of patients with *glutaric aciduria type 2* (Böhm *et al.* 1982, Goodman and Frerman 1984).

Glioneural heterotopia is common in malformed brains but may also occur in brains of normal individuals (Dambska *et al.* 1986, Choi and Matthias 1987, Hirano *et al.* 1992, Iida *et al.* 1994). These lesions consist of irregularly shaped nodules of variable size, sometimes of sheets of astrocytes and neurons

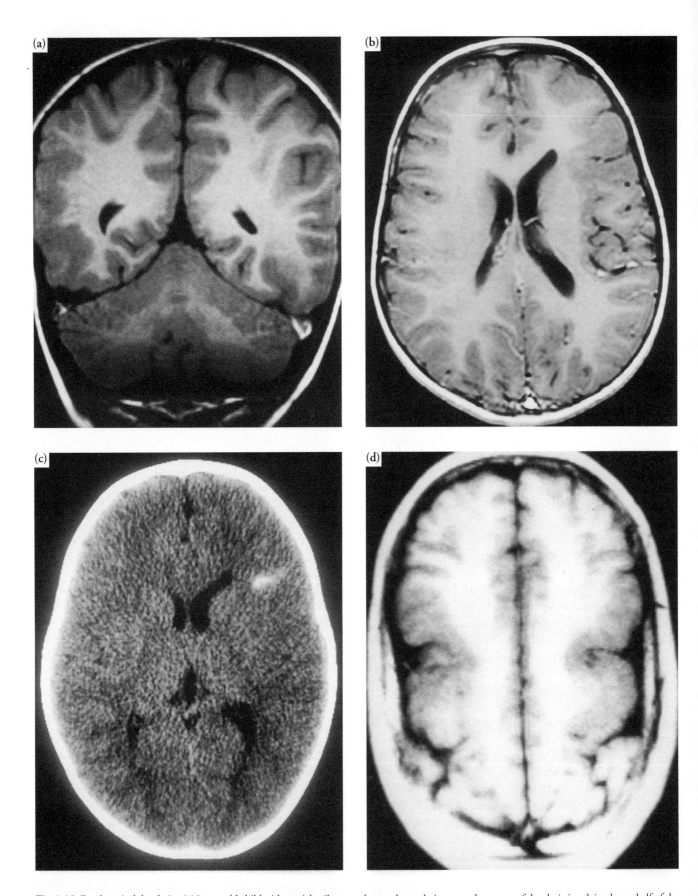

Fig. 3.25. Focal cortical dysplasia. *(a)* 8-year-old child with partial epilepsy and mental retardation: note large area of dysplasia involving lower half of the external aspect of right parietal lobe. *(b)* 6-year-old girl with partial epilepsy and moderate learning difficulties: T₁-weighted MRI scan shows dysplasia involving the left frontal lobe. *(c)* (Same child.) CT scan shows calcification of white matter underlying dysplastic area. *(d)* Bilateral perisylvian syndrome with bilateral central areas of polymicrogyria.

overlying the molecular layer. They seem to be due to excessive migration of neurons and glial cells into the subpial and subarachnoid space (Evrard *et al.* 1989). Together with other abnormalities, they are a common pathological feature of the fetal alcohol syndrome (Wisniewski *et al.* 1983). Massive extramolecular heterotopias (*i.e.* those comprising neurons that have migrated beyond the molecular layer of the cortex into the meninges) may be associated with mitochondrial diseases (Samson *et al.* 1994).

A peculiar migration abnormality is the cause of *Kallmann syndrome* of anosmia due to absence of olfactory bulb stalks and gyri, hypogonadism and often mild mental retardation (Christian 1982). This syndrome is genetically heterogeneous but usually transmitted as an X-linked recessive trait, and the gene (*KALIG-1*) has been localized to Xp22.3 (White *et al.* 1983). The migration defects involve the olfactory axons and gonadotrophin releasing hormone-secreting neurons that originate from the olfactory placode and normally migrate through the ethmoid to the olfactory bulbs that do not develop if not reached by axons. The migration of these cells in Kallmann syndrome is blocked in the nasal area because of lack of adhesion molecules that play a major role in olfactory axon development (Bick *et al.* 1992). Absence of the olfactory bulbs can be visualized by MRI (Truwit *et al.* 1993).

DISORDERS OF CORTICAL ORGANIZATION
Focal cortical 'dysplasia'
Less obvious developmental abnormalities can be the cause of severe neurological disturbances, especially epilepsy—usually focal but sometimes secondarily generalized (Janota and Polkey 1992; Guerrini *et al.* 1992a,b). The term 'cortical dysplasia', although confusing (see above), is often used for such abnormalities of cortical organization.

Several stages follow migration of neurons. They include laminar organization of postmigratory cells, differentiation of dendrites and axons, synaptogenesis with proliferation, then reduction in the number of synapses. Myelination is a late process that mainly takes place in postnatal life. Interference with these processes may be due to metabolic, genetic or unknown causes. The presence of abnormal cells (as in tuberous sclerosis or in Taylor-type cortical dysgenesis) impedes a normal cortical organization, even though the origin of the disturbance goes back to the initial stage of cell differentiation. Localized arrests of migration limited to a small number of radial columns with resulting small areas of heterotopia occur with Potter syndrome (Evrard *et al.* 1989). Synaptic dysgenesis may occur with hypothyroidism (Chapter 23), the fetal alcohol syndrome (Ferrer and Galofré 1987), malnutrition, Down syndrome, and trisomy 13 and 18 (Sumi 1970). It may play a role in mental deterioration of undetermined origin (Huttenlocher 1974).

Most of these dysplasias feature not only abnormal organization but also anomalies of migration. Insufficient programmed cell death may also play a role. They are described together because of their common macroscopical and clinical presentations.

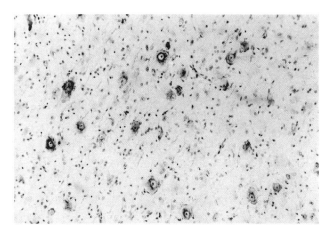

Fig. 3.26. Cortical biopsy of a child with focal dysplasia. Large neurons are irregularly located within cortex. Some neurons show characteristic peripheral condensation of chromatin. (Courtesy Dr B. Harding, Institute of Neurology, Queen Square, London.)

In areas of cortical dysplasia, the cortex is firm and the gyri are enlarged. Histologically, the picture varies from simple disorganization of laminae or columns with subcortical heterotopic neurons to more complex anomalies with giant neurons and 'balloon cells' as well as giant multinucleated astrocytes (Taylor *et al.* 1971) (Fig. 3.26). Such cases are closely related to focal pachygyria, and their relationship to tuberous sclerosis has been debated (Andermann *et al.* 1987). They are usually manifested by partial epileptic seizures. Kuzniecky *et al.* (1986) observed small focal areas of cortical dysplasia which were responsible for focal cortical myoclonus and focal motor seizures in four children. The lesions were demonstrated by MRI and could be treated surgically. Similar lesions were found in a case of status epilepticus (Desbiens *et al.* 1993). Variable degrees of mental retardation and focal neurological signs such as hemiparesis are often associated. The diagnosis rests heavily on MRI demonstration of the lesions (Palmini *et al.* 1991b). These are sometimes quite obvious, involving large cortical areas with or without infolding of the cortex (Guerrini *et al.* 1992b), or may be difficult to evidence requiring careful MRI study with thin slices, 3D acquisition and reformatting in various planes over the suspect area. The presence of intense epileptiform activity over abnormal cortical areas may be of diagnostic value (Palmini *et al.* 1996).

Resection of the abnormal areas may control the seizures (Palmini *et al.* 1991a,b; Wyllie *et al.* 1994). Palmini *et al.* (1993) suggested that the presence of abnormal balloon cells can be responsible for a high T_2 signal from the deep cortex and underlying white matter. Focal cortical dysplasia may be associated with developmental tumours (gangliogliomas and developmental neuroepithelial tumours) in the same area of brain.

Cortical microdysgenesis—minor cortical dysgenesis
Minor anomalies of cortical arrangement have long been known to pathologists. These include persistence of the subpial or Ranke–Brun subpial layer (Evrard *et al.* 1989); presence of aggregates of large neurons in the plexiform zone; fragmented

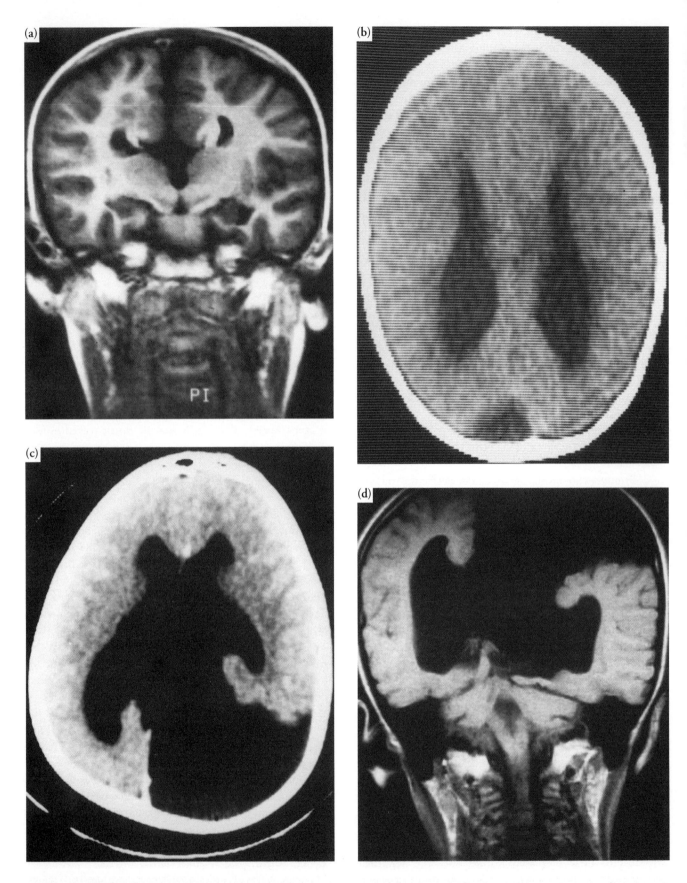

Fig. 3.27. Agenesis of the corpus callosum. *(a)* MRI (inversion–recovery sequence) clearly shows longitudinal corpora callosa (Probst bundles) alongside inner aspects of ventricular bodies. *(b)* Usual form. CT scan shows parallel lateral ventricles with dilatation of occipital horns (colpocephaly). *(c)* CT (axial cut) and *(d)* T$_1$-weighted MRI (coronal cut) showing agenesis associated with dorsal cyst of third ventricle in 14-year-old girl with large head (+6 SD) but normal intelligence and no evidence of hemispheric disconnection by appropriate neuropsychological tests.

appearance of superficial neuronal layers; excess number of 'ectopic' neurons subcortically and throughout the cortex; and excess number of cells in the molecular layer (Meencke and Janz 1984, Meencke 1987). Such anomalies are frequently found in the brain of epileptic or mentally retarded persons but they are also present in the cortex of normal individuals (Lyon and Gastaut 1985). Meencke and Janz (1984) have suggested that microdysgenesis could be the anatomical basis for cortical hyperexcitability in generalized epilepsy by modifying the normal cortical circuitry. Meencke and Veith (1992) found microdysgenesis in 32.7 per cent of 591 brains of persons with epilepsy as against 6 per cent of 7374 control brains, suggesting this anomaly plays a signficant role. Galaburda *et al.* (1985) and Kaufmann and Galaburda (1989) found an excess of foci of cortical dysgenesis with a left temporal predominance in four brains of dyslexic subjects as compared with ten control persons and thought they might play a role in the genesis of dyslexia. Cohen *et al.* (1989) attributed the dysphasia of their patient to bilateral minor dysgenesis involving the planum temporale and opercular area bilaterally. These provocative findings must await confirmation. Microdysgenesis is often associated with other epileptogenic lesions (Kuzniecky *et al.* 1991).

Other minor abnormalities of the cerebral hemispheres include abnormal synaptogenesis, and especially disturbances in the process of programmed cell death (apoptosis) that probably plays a major role in brain development but is currently poorly understood.

Other rare abnormalities include congenital Pick cell encephalopathy (De Léon *et al.* 1986), and localized dysgenesis (Tychsen and Hoyt 1985) resulting in hemianopsia or delayed operculation (Barth 1987). Delayed early myelination may occur in cases with abnormal gestation, *e.g.* maternal diabetes mellitus or placental insufficiency, as well as in infants with severe prolonged asphyxia or other damaging factors (Dambska and Laure-Kaminowska 1990).

ABNORMALITIES ASSOCIATED WITH DISORDERS OF CORTICAL DEVELOPMENT

Several deformities often coexist with migration disorders. However, they may also occur in isolation or in association with other malformations. They include agenesis of the corpus callosum, schizencephaly ('true' porencephaly), septo-optic dysplasia and colpocephaly.

Agenesis of the corpus callosum

This may be complete or partial. Atypical forms, difficult to separate from holoprosencephaly, may be encountered (Barkovich 1990). In the latter case, the posterior part is usually missing because the corpus callosum develops in an anteroposterior manner. Cases of anterior agenesis can however occur (Aicardi *et al.* 1987, Barkovich *et al.* 1988). Callosal agenesis is relatively common. It was present in 0.7 per cent of pneumoencephalographies and its recorded frequency must be higher with the introduction of CT scan and MRI. Jeret *et al.* (1985, 1986) found 33 cases in a series of 1447 CT scans. Myrianthopoulos and Chung (1974)

give an estimated figure of 1 in 20,000 individuals. Even now, the diagnosis is made preferentially in patients with neurological manifestations, so that the true frequency is not known. The absent callosal commissure is usually replaced by two longitudinal bundles, known as longitudinal corpora callosa or Probst bundles, that course on the inner aspect of the hemispheres (Fig. 3.27*a*). Sulci on the internal aspect have a radial disposition, and enlargement of the occipital horn that maintains their fetal morphology, the so-called *colpocephaly*, is common (Garg 1982, Noorani *et al.* 1988) (Fig. 3.27*b*). Other associated abnormalities frequently include the formation of cysts dorsal to the third ventricle, communicating or noncommunicating (Yokota *et al.* 1984a,b; Griebel *et al.* 1995) (Fig. 3.27*c,d*), and a miscellany of CNS malformations such as heterotopia, abnormalities of gyration, or cephaloceles (Jellinger *et al.* 1981; Atlas *et al.* 1986; Jeret *et al.* 1987; Serur *et al.* 1987, 1988; Barkovich and Norman 1988a). It is these associated anomalies that are responsible for the clinical manifestation. *Lipoma of the corpus callosum* (Fig. 3.28) is almost invariably associated with agenesis of the structure (Zee *et al.* 1981, Vade and Horowitz 1992). Peripheral malformations are common (Parrish *et al.* 1979). Eye abnormalities are especially frequent (Aicardi *et al.* 1987). Hypoplasia of the corpus callosum (Bodensteiner *et al.* 1994) (Fig. 3.29) may be a minor form of callosal dysgenesis but is more often the consequence of cortical neuronal loss.

The aetiology is multiple. In nonsyndromic forms, genetic transmission is rare, although a few autosomal recessive, X-linked recessive (Menkes et al, 1964, Kaplan 1983) and autosomal dominant cases are on record (Aicardi *et al.* 1987). Various chromosomal defects, including trisomy 18, trisomy 13 and trisomy 8, as well as a miscellany of less common chromosomal accidents have been found. Serur *et al.* (1988) reviewed 81 cases from the literature, of which 21 had trisomy 8, 14 had trisomy 13–15, and 18 involved abnormalities of chromosomes 17 or 18. Of 34 karyotypes they performed, two showed trisomy 8. Sumi (1970) reviewed the pathological findings of trisomy 18. Environmental factors include the fetal alcohol syndrome (Jones *et al.* 1973) and endogenous 'toxic' factors such as lactic acidosis (Chow *et al.* 1987), hyperglycinaemia (Dobyns 1989) and other metabolic defects (Bamforth *et al.* 1988). Up to 2 per cent of cases of callosal agenesis may be associated with a metabolic disease. Most cases are of unknown origin. Some investigators have suggested that vascular factors and other acquired factors can play a role in the determination of corpus callosum agenesis and are certainly important in the mechanism of hypoplasia and local thinning which are not infrequently found and may be mistaken for agenesis (Njiokiktjien *et al.* 1988).

The clinical manifestations of callosal agenesis can be described under two different headings: nonsyndromic and syndromic forms.

Nonsyndromic forms are the most common (Jeret *et al.* 1987, Serur *et al.* 1987). An unknown, though probably small, proportion of cases remain completely asymptomatic or are discovered only because of a large head. Most patients have mental retardation, seizures and/or a large head (Aicardi *et al.*

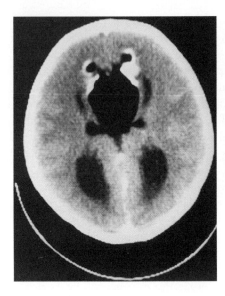
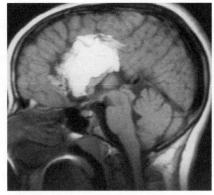
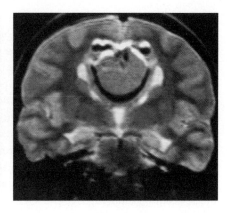

Fig. 3.28. Lipoma of the corpus callosum in an 8-year old girl with partial complex seizures but no neurodevelopmental abnormalities. *(Left)* CT scan showing large mass of fat density separating anterior horns of lateral ventricles, peripheral calcification and two small lateral expansions of the fatty mass. *(Centre)* MRI, sagittal cut showing replacement of corpus callosum by lipoma. *(Right)* MRI, T₂-weighted sequence showing complexity of mass and complete replacement of callosum by fatty tissue.

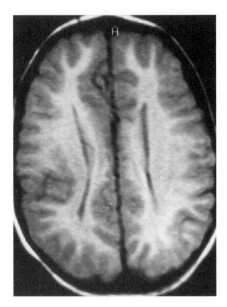
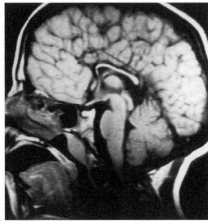
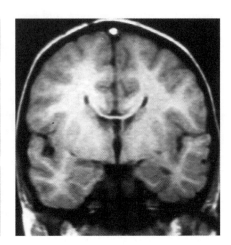

Fig. 3.29. Hypoplasia of the corpus callosum. *(Left)* MRI (axial cut) showing ventricular appearance consistent with callosal agenesis. *(Centre)* Sagittal cut showing complete callosum with genu and splenium, but short and thin. Note radial disposition of mesial gyri. *(Right)* Frontal cut showing wide separation of ventricular bodies by prolapsing limbic gyrus.

1987). Hypertelorism is a frequent finding. Eighty-two per cent of the patients of Jeret *et al.* (1987) had mental retardation or delayed development, 43 per cent had seizures, and 31 per cent had cerebral palsy. The seizures may be of any type, including infantile spasms, but more frequently are focal. Although a large head, sometimes as much as 5–7 SD above the mean, is common, indications for shunting should be extremely conservative as many of these cases of 'hydrocephalus' spontaneously stabilize without raising any problem. The macrocephaly may be due in part to the presence of giant cysts located dorsally to the third ventricle (Griebel *et al.* 1995). Specific disturbances of inter-hemispheric transfer are either totally lacking or only minimal (Jeeves and Temple 1987). Endocrinological abnormalities may be present in rare cases (Smith *et al.* 1986).

Syndromic forms are shown in Table 3.7.

Aicardi syndrome (Chevrie and Aicardi 1986, Donnenfeld *et al.* 1989, Aicardi 1996) accounts for 1–4 per cent of cases of infantile spasms and is probably due to an X-linked dominant mutation. It occurs almost exclusively in girls, although two cases in boys with an XXY chromosome complement have been reported, and only one familial case is known (Molina *et al.* 1989). Characteristic features of the syndrome include infantile spasms and specific choroidal lacunae, often in association with coloboma of the optic disc. Vertebrocostal abnormalities are present in half the cases. The outcome is poor, with persistence of seizures and severe retardation. However, the spectrum of severity is wider than previously thought (Menezes *et al.* 1994). In rare cases, the corpus callosum may be present (Aicardi 1994, 1996). The choroidal lacunae and associated MRI abnormalities (periventricular heterotopia, dysplastic cortex, ependymal cysts) permit the diagnosis (Fig. 3.30). Pathologically, there are multiple areas of heterotopia and polymicrogyria of the unlayered type in the brain (Billette de Villemeur *et al.* 1992), while the so-called lacunae represent thinning of the pigment epithelium and

TABLE 3.7
Syndromic forms of corpus callosum agenesis

Syndrome	Clinical features and genetics*	Associated malformations	References
Callosal agenesis constantly present[1]			
Aicardi syndrome	Infantile spasms and partial seizures, choroidoretinal lacunae and disc coloboma, severe retardation, vertebrocostal anomalies, 'split' brain EEG. Seen only in girls. *X-linked dominant*, lethal for males[2]	Periventricular heterotopia, cysts of choroid plexus, other intracranial cysts, microgyria, anomalies of posterior fossa	Chevrie and Aicardi (1986), Aicardi (1996)
Shapiro syndrome	Episodic hypothermia and diaphoresis. *Nonfamilial*	Hypothalamic lesion probably responsible for the syndrome that may occur with an intact callosum (Sheth *et al.* 1994)	Shapiro *et al.* (1969)
Reverse Shapiro syndrome	Hyperthermia, episodic		Hirayama *et al.* (1994)
Andermann syndrome	Neuropathy (mixed motor and sensory), peculiar facies. *Autosomal recessive*		Andermann (1981)
Acrocallosal syndrome	Mental retardation, dysmorphism. *Autosomal recessive*		Thyen *et al.* (1992)
Callosal agenesis inconstant feature			
Oro-facio-digital syndrome	Lingual hamartomas, abnormal buccal frenula, digital anomalies, sparse hair, mild retardation, limited to girls. *X-linked dominant*, lethal for males	Interhemispheric cysts	Baraitser (1986), Leão *et al.* (1995)
Dandy–Walker syndrome	Vermian agenesis, hydrocephalus. *Sporadic*[3]	Abnormal inferior olive	Hirsch *et al.* (1984)
Lissencephaly	*Usually sporadic*	Cortical malformation (see text)	Aicardi *et al.* (1987)
Apert syndrome	Acrocephalosyndactyly (see Chapter 5), callosal agenesis only occasional. *Autosomal dominant*		De Léon *et al.* (1987)
Trisomy 8	See Chapter 5. *Sporadic*		Serur *et al.* (1988)
Meckel–Gruber syndrome	Callosal agenesis only occasional (see also Aicardi *et al.* 1987). *Autosomal recessive*		Hsia *et al.* (1971)
Di George syndrome	Facial dysmorphism, hypocalcaemia with neonatal seizures due to aplasia of parathyroid glands. *Autosomal dominant (microdeletion)*		Conley *et al.* (1979)
Goldenhar syndrome	Epibulbar dermoids, ear malformations, preauricular fibrochondromas		Wilson (1983)
Microcephaly + cataracts	Dwarfism. *Autosomal recessive?*	Multiple CNS malformations	Scott-Emuakpor *et al.* (1977)

*Where known.
[1]However, may be absent in Shapiro syndrome and in rare cases of Aicardi syndrome.
[2]Only one familial case known.
[3]Rare familial cases.

choroid with loss of pigment granules. Ependymal cysts are frequently found around the third ventricle, and cysts or tumours of the choroid plexus may reach a large size (Aicardi 1996). They may permit prenatal diagnosis when found in association with callosal agenesis.

Other syndromic forms are rare or limited to certain ethnic groups like *Andermann syndrome* among French Canadians in the Lake St John region (Andermann 1981). Agenesis of the corpus callosum is often a part of oro-facio-digital syndrome type I (Aicardi 1994).

The syndrome of *periodic hypothermia and diaphoresis* (Shapiro *et al.* 1969) can be treated effectively with clonidine which was tried because of the discovery of an altered norepinephrine metabolism in this syndrome. However, half the cases are not accompanied by callosal agenesis (Sheth *et al.* 1994). Callosal agenesis with episodic hyperthermia ('reverse Shapiro syndrome') has been reported (Hirayama *et al.* 1994).

The *diagnosis* of callosal agenesis rests on neuroimaging. The diagnosis of complete agenesis is easy by ultrasonography, CT or MRI (Aicardi *et al.* 1987, Jeret *et al.* 1987, Serur *et al.* 1988). MRI is far superior for the diagnosis of partial agenesis (Atlas *et al.* 1986). *Antenatal diagnosis* is possible from about 20 weeks gestation (Klingensmith and Cioffi-Ragan 1986) (Fig. 3.31). A decision to terminate is difficult to take without reservation until more is known about the incidence of asymptomatic cases. Blum *et al.* (1990) recently reported that six of 12 infants in whom callosal agenesis had been diagnosed antenatally had a normal development at 2–8 years of age. Cases associated with other malformations or chromosomal anomalies all had a poor outcome. Fetal karyotyping and complete examination are therefore essential.

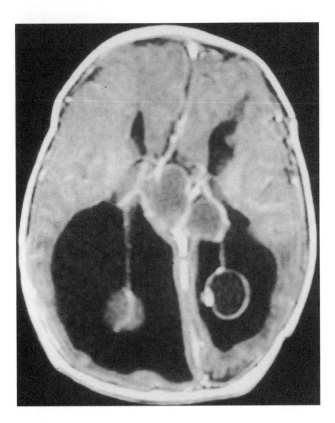

Fig. 3.30. Aicardi syndrome in a 3-month-old girl. Note hemisphere asymmetry, bilateral cysts of the choroid plexus, cysts around the third ventricle with a different fluid signal from the CSF, and periventricular heterotopia. The ependymal nature of choroid plexus cysts was verified histologically.

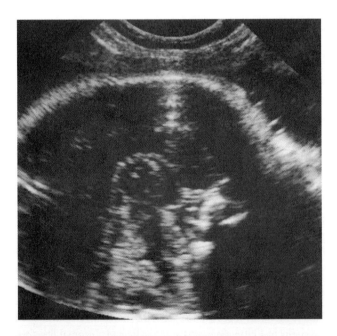

Fig. 3.31. Agenesis of the corpus callosum. Ultrasound antenatal scan, sagittal cut. Note normal fourth ventricle, absence of callosal echo, and dilated lateral ventricle. Back of fetal head is on left side of photograph. (Courtesy Dr M-C. Aubry, Maternité Port-Royal, Paris.)

Schizencephaly (porencephaly)

This anomaly is also knowns as *true porencephaly*. The term 'porencephaly', which is often used loosely to designate any cavity within brain parenchyma, refers here only to clefts or cavities of developmental origin that extend through the full depth of the mantle from the ventricle to the subarachnoid space (Friede 1989). Such clefts may be virtual, their two walls being apposed to form a pia–arachnoid seam (Yakovlev and Wadsworth 1946). Schizencephaly clearly dates to early pregnancy as the defects are surrounded and lined by an abnormal cortex with microgyria and neuronal heterotopia, indicating that the cleft existed before the end of migration and prevented neurons from reaching their normal location. This does not imply that they represent failure of the mantle to form, as implied by the term schizencephaly (Miller *et al.* 1984). True porencephaly is probably due to early destruction of the mantle, perhaps of circulatory origin, with faulty repair and interference with neuronal migration (Dekaban 1965, Aicardi and Goutières 1981, Menezes *et al.* 1988). Rare familiar cases are on record (Haverkamp *et al.* 1995). Some of the sporadic cases are associated with mutations in the homeobox gene *EMX 2* (Brunelli *et al.* 1996), and one familial case with the same mutation of this gene in two brothers is on record (Granata *et al.* 1997). Friede recognizes two types, with and without surrounding microgyria, which probably relates to the date of formation of the clefts. Late cases with evidence of scarring and calcification are on record (Menezes *et al.* 1988). The clefts are frequently bilateral but often asymmetrical. Even when unilateral, cortical dysplasia is often present in the opposite hemisphere. Large bilateral defects, so-called 'basket brain' (Dekaban 1965), constitute the most severe form of schizencephaly.

In most cases, the septum pellucidum is missing (Aicardi and Goutières 1981, Diebler and Dulac 1987, Menezes *et al.* 1988, Barkovich and Norman 1988a).

The *clinical features* of schizencephaly are extremely variable, and the severity of clinical features correlates with the importance of anatomical anomalies, with open-lip clefts giving rise to severe involvement (Barkovich and Kjos 1992). Some patients are profoundly retarded and quadriplegic. With the use of neuro-imaging it has been realized that many cases are much less severe, with mild retardation, congenital hemiplegia, a large head or even isolated partial seizures. The involvement of both sylvian and insular regions can be responsible for a biopercular syndrome with facial apraxia and speech difficulties (Becker *et al.* 1989). Epilepsy is present in about 80 per cent of patients (Granata *et al.* 1996).

The diagnosis is made by CT or MRI (Fig. 3.32), which not only show the clefts but also demonstrate the presence of hetero-topic grey matter alongside them, as well as gyral anomalies of the insular regions (Miller *et al.* 1984, Menezes *et al.* 1988, Aniskiewicz *et al.* 1990). Absence of the septum pellucidum may be the most obvious anomaly and should lead to careful search for narrow clefts or atypical gyration (Barkovich and Norman 1988a, Menezes *et al.* 1988).

Schizencephalies located to other brain areas—such as the ventral aspect of the brain (Stewart *et al.* 1978), the orbital fissure (Yakovlev and Wadsworth 1946), the posterior midline (Yokota

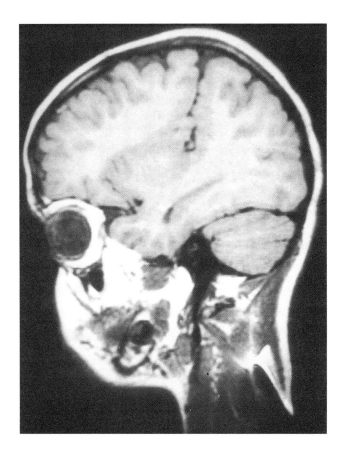

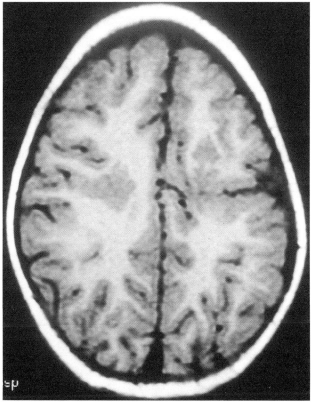

and Matsukado 1979) or the mesial occipital area (Granata *et al.* 1996)—are less common. Rare familial cases are on record (Haverkamp *et al.* 1995).

The diagnosis of schizencephaly is easy. However, large lesions may be difficult to distinguish from some cases of holoprosencephaly, while minor lesions with septal agenesis may be difficult to separate from septo-optic dysplasia, especially as a double-contoured papilla has been reported (Menezes *et al.* 1988). Holoprosencephaly is sometimes mistaken for bilateral schizencephaly (Miller *et al.* 1984, Noorani *et al.* 1988) because of the depth and vertical location of the sylvian fissures.

Septo-optic dysplasia
Septo-optic dysplasia is characterized by the association of optic nerve hypoplasia with absence of the septum pellucidum. The latter, however, is not constant (Williams *et al.* 1993). There are usually no associated clefts of the cerebral mantle or gyral abnormalities. In some cases, the floor of the third ventricle is abnormal. This structure is embryologically related to the development of the optic placodes, which explains the association (Friede 1989). This syndrome is not genetically determined. Environmental factors, in particular maternal diabetes mellitus (Donat 1991), play a role.

The clinical features include variable degrees of visual disturbances. Some patients may be mentally retarded (Morishima and Aranoff 1986, Williams *et al.* 1993). The optic discs have a characteristic appearance with a central part of less than half the normal diameter of the papilla, which represents the true disc, and a peripheral ring of about the size of a normal papilla. This double-contour is of great diagnostic value (Ouvrier and Billson 1986). Endocrine disturbances, especially growth hormone deficiency and diabetes insipidus, may occur (Hoyt *et al.* 1970) and should be searched for systematically because they may produce hypoglycaemia with its complications and sequelae.

A similar endocrinological syndrome may occur with other midline brain abnormalities, *e.g.* corpus callosum agenesis (Masera *et al.* 1994).

Other anomalies of the septum pellucidum include simple agenesis, cyst formation, and persistence of the septum beyond the first year of life. Most are asymptomatic but they may be a marker for other brain malformations (Barkovich and Norman 1988b, Bodensteiner *et al.* 1995). An occasional cyst may become symptomatic and compress the foramina of Monro with resulting hydrocephalus (Aoki 1986).

Colpocephaly
This is an abnormal shape of the lateral ventricles with symmetrical dilatation of the occipital horns and normal frontal horns. It is commonly associated with callosal agenesis and seldom occurs as a primary malformation of the occipital lobes. Hypoplasia of the optic nerves may be present in the latter cases (Coupland and Sarnat 1990). The diagnosis is easily made by neuroimaging, but periventricular leukomalacia may produce a superficially similar appearance (Bodensteiner and Gay 1990). Colpocephaly does not require shunting even when the dilatation is marked.

Fig. 3.32. Schizencephaly (true porencephaly). *(Top)* Sagittal cut shows right-sided cleft lined with heterotopic grey matter. *(Bottom)* Axial cut shows left-sided cleft and symmetrical area of heterotopic grey matter without visible cleft.

Absence of the corticospinal tracts may be a part of various malformation syndromes including congenital stenosis of the aqueduct. In rare cases it is the main malformation found (Roessmann *et al.* 1990).

MALFORMATIONS OF THE CEREBELLUM AND POSTERIOR FOSSA STRUCTURES

Abnormalities of cerebellar development are frequently associated with other disturbances in CNS organization but may also occur in isolation. They include major disturbances in cerebellar morphogenesis and less extensive disturbances affecting essentially cerebellar cortical organization (Friede 1989).

DISTURBANCES OF CEREBELLAR MORPHOGENESIS

Major morphological abnormalities of the cerebellum include the Dandy–Walker malformation and other types of dysgenesis of the cerebellar vermis, cerebellar aplasia or hypoplasia, and rare anomalies such as rhombencephalosynapsis and tectocerebellar dysraphia. The Chiari malformation has been described above (see pp. 77–78).

Dandy–Walker malformation and atresia of the cerebellar foramina

The main features of the classical Dandy–Walker malformation are: (1) complete or partial agenesis of the vermis; (2) large cystic formation in the posterior fossa corresponding to a diverticular expansion of an enormously dilated fourth ventricle; (3) hydrocephalus that is frequently lacking in neonates and young infants and occasionally until late adulthood. There is usually a marked enlargement of the posterior fossa and elevation of the torcular and lateral sinuses that course on the parietal bones instead of the occipital squama. The last two features are not found in other types of vermal agenesis and are, therefore, of diagnostic importance. Associated abnormalities, which are observed in up to 68 per cent of cases (Hart *et al.* 1972), include abnormal migration of the inferior olive (Hanaway and Netsky 1971), agenesis of the corpus callosum in 7–15 per cent of patients (Hart *et al.* 1972, Hirsch *et al.* 1984, Murray *et al.* 1985), and occipital encephaloceles in 17 per cent (Hirsch *et al.* 1984). Peripheral malformations are present in 25–30 per cent of cases (Hart *et al.* 1972) and include cleft lip and palate, cardiac malformations, urinary tract abnormalities and minor facial dysmorphism.

The classical form is now regarded as one end of a spectrum of abnormalities that also includes less severe types (Barkovich *et al.* 1989, Altman *et al.* 1992): Dandy-Walker variant in which part of the vermis is present and the posterior fossa is not enlarged; and megacisterna magna in which a large retrocerebellar pouch (Blake pouch) communicates with the fourth ventricle but a complete vermis is present. The latter entity is ill-defined and merges progressively with the common cases of prominent cisterna magna. However, some investigators think it is different from simple prominent cistern (see Barkovich 1990), and Bodensteiner *et al.* (1988) found that 62 per cent of patients with megacisterna magna had neurological abnormalities, suggesting it may be part of a malformation complex.

Atresia of the foramina of Magendie and Luschka was formerly thought to be the cause of the malformation. However, it is neither constant nor characteristic. The Dandy–Walker syndrome is currently attributed to a developmental arrest in the midbrain with persistence of the anterior membranous area of the fetal fourth ventricle. This structure normally disappears before the foramina open. The anomaly would seem to originate before the third fetal month (Friede 1989). Although occurrence in siblings has been reported in rare cases, the overwhelming majority of cases are sporadic, so that favourable genetic counselling may be given. Prenatal diagnosis is relatively easy (Newman *et al.* 1982) from the 18th to the 20th week. Differential diagnosis with a large cistern requires visualization of the vermis. Chromosomal anomalies have been encountered in a few cases (Murray *et al.* 1985, Bordarier and Aicardi 1990).

The clinical manifestations of the Dandy–Walker syndrome are mainly those of hydrocephalus. Therefore the diagnosis is made in 75 per cent of cases after 3 months of age and often only by the first birthday, as hydrocephalus usually becomes apparent by 1 year of age. The head may be elongated in the anteroposterior direction, with bulging of the occiput that may lead to fortuitous discovery of the anomaly. Remarkably, there are no cerebellar signs or disturbances of stance. Mental retardation is present in 30–50 per cent of patients and may be the reason for radiological examination.

Radiological diagnosis is generally straightforward (see Fig. 7.5, p. 195), with complete absence of the vermis, small cerebellar hemispheres, and enlargement of the posterior fossa by a huge collection that in half the cases extends upwards through the tentorial opening into the trigeminal cistern and/or downwards through the foramen magnum. Cases of Dandy–Walker variant (Sarnat and Alcala 1980) may be difficult to distinguish from a prominent magna or a retrocerebellar arachnoidal cyst. In such cases, sagittal MRI cuts are extremely useful. In variant forms, they show remnants of the vermis which are pushed upwards and anteriorly rotated. In megacisterna, the vermis is present with all its lobules, which may be atrophic and compressed against the brainstem.

The prognosis for patients with the Dandy–Walker syndrome is only moderately favourable even if the hydrocephalus is operated on early. The mortality rate in 144 cases reviewed by Hirsch *et al.* was 27 per cent, and only about half of the survivors had a normal IQ. Genetic prognosis, on the contrary, is good with a recurrence rate of 1–5 per cent.

Treatment involves shunting the hydrocephalus rather than opening the cystic fourth ventricle. Some surgeons advise inserting the shunt into the fourth ventricle but this is not a unanimous opinion. Additional shunting of the trapped fourth ventricle may be necessary (Raimondi *et al.* 1984) when the lateral ventricles have been shunted.

Complete atresia of the foramina of the fourth ventricle is uncommonly observed outside the Dandy–Walker complex (Amacher and Page 1971). It produces hydrocephalus that, in one of my patients, started and was much more marked in the fourth ventricle than in the rest of the ventricular system. Microscopic

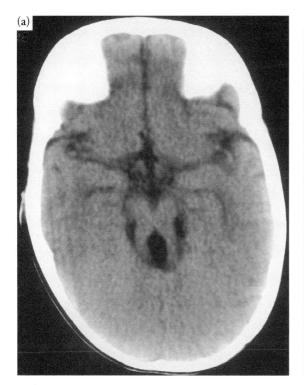

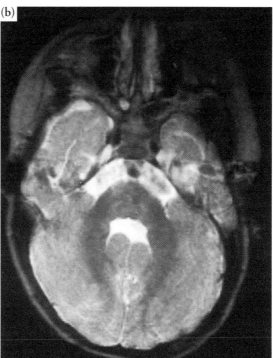

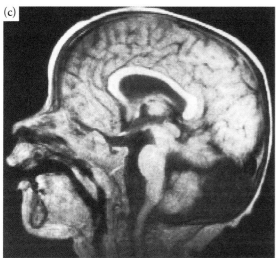

Fig. 3.33. Joubert syndrome. *(a)* CT scan showing increase of anteroposterior dimension of the upper fourth ventricle and characteristic 'molar tooth' appearance of brainstem. *(b)* T₂-weighted MRI scan showing the typical 'umbrella-shaped' lower fourth ventricle. The 'handle' of the umbrella appears as a white line resulting from opposition of the cerebellar hemispheres with absence of the vermis. *(c)* Sagittal end showing atrophic vermis with horizontal superior cerebellar peduncle.

examination of the membrane covering the fourth ventricle shows glial tisue, covered on its inner aspect by ependyma (Friede 1989). This glial membrane differentiates atresia of the foramina from fibrosis of the basal cisterns with consequent hydrocephalus. The origin of the membrane is unknown.

Joubert syndrome

Joubert syndrome consists of familial agenesis of the cerebellar vermis, episodic hyperpnoea, abnormal eye movements, ataxia and retardation (Joubert *et al.* 1969, Cantani *et al.* 1990). Facial asymmetry (Friede and Boltshauser 1978), retinal anomalies (King *et al.* 1984), choroidoretinal coloboma (Lindhout *et al.* 1980, Lindhout and Barth 1985) and various renal abnormalities may be associated. Respiratory disturbances include panting respiration interspersed with long pauses that are not associated

with changes in blood gases (Edwards *et al.* 1988). Respiratory abnormalities are prominent during the neonatal period when they allow an early diagnosis if metabolic diseases are excluded but may be absent in up to half the cases (Kendall *et al.* 1990) The radiological picture is variable, even within the same sibship (Aicardi *et al.* 1983). Some patients have a typical narrow cleft, extending sagittally from the fourth ventricle to the cisterna magna, while others have large fluid-filled collections that can mimic the variant Dandy–Walker malformation (Egger *et al.* 1982, Altman *et al.* 1992).

The vermis is dysplastic, the cerebellar peduncles small, and the superior cerebellar peduncles are almost at right angles to the brainstem. The floor of the fourth ventricle is convex towards the brainstem (Kendall *et al.* 1990) (Fig. 3.33). A flat or markedly depressed electoretinogram is present in many cases. Ultra-

TABLE 3.8
Main syndromes of agenesis of the cerebellar vermis

Syndrome	Features additional to vermian agenesis	Inheritance*	References
Dandy–Walker syndrome	High torcular, large posterior fossa, hydrocephalus	Sporadic[1]	Bordarier and Aicardi (1990)
Joubert syndrome	Abnormal respiratory rate from birth, mental retardation, eye anomalies (extinguished ERG, disc coloboma)	AR	Joubert *et al.* (1969)
Meckel–Gruber syndrome	Hydrocephalus, encephalocele, cystic kidneys	AR	Hori *et al.* (1980)
Dandy–Walker with facial angioma	Multiple vascular anomalies in CNS and peripheral vessels; aplasia of cerebellar hemispheres	Sporadic[2]	Pascual-Castroviejo (1985), Bordarier and Aicardi (1990)
Dekaban–Arima syndrome	Retinopathy, cystic kidneys	AR	Matsuzaka *et al.* (1986)
Walker–Warburg syndrome and cerebro-oculo-muscular disease (COMS)	Type II lissencephaly, hydrocephalus, retinal dysplasia and other eye abnormalities	AR	Towfighi *et al.* (1984)
COACH (cerebellar vermis, hypoplasia, oligophrenia, ataxia, coloboma and hepatic fibrosis)	Coloboma, ataxia, hepatic fibrosis	AR	Verloes and Lambotte (1989)
Mohr syndrome (oro-facio-digital syndrome type II, OFD II)	Hamartomata of tongue, abnormal frenula, postaxial polydactyly	AR	Baraitser (1986)
OFD III	Id. + abnormal eye movements	AR	Leão *et al.* (1995)
Jaeken syndrome	Autism, excretion of succinyl purine	AR	Jaeken and Van den Berghe (1984)
Coffin–Siris syndrome	Hypertrichosis, microcephaly, nail hypoplasia	AR?	Tunnessen *et al.* (1978)
Aase-Smith syndrome	Arthrogryposis	AD	Patton *et al.* (1985)
Aicardi syndrome	Callosal agenesis, choroidoretinal 'lacunae', infantile spasms, areas of periventricular heterotopia	XD[3]	Chevrie and Aicardi (1986, 1996)
Smith–Lemli–Opitz syndrome	Hypoplastic or absent vermis only occasional	AR	Tint *et al.* (1994)
Ruvalcaba–Myrhe–Smith syndrome	Large head, cutaneous pigmentation, papilloedema	AD	Ruvalcaba *et al.* (1971)
Goldenhar syndrome	Epibulbar dermoids, ear malformations, preauricular fibrochondromas	Sporadic	Aleksic *et al.* (1983)

*AR = autosomal recessive; AD = autosomal dominant; XD = X-linked dominant.
[1]If only cases of 'true' Dandy–Walker syndrome are considered (Bordarier and Aicardi 1990).
[2]May include several different types.
[3]Only one familial case known.

sonography may show renal cysts (King *et al.* 1984). Ataxia and mental retardation become manifest in late infancy and childhood, at a time when respiratory abnormalities decrease and become undetectable. Joubert syndrome is recessively inherited. Lindhout and Barth (1985) have proposed that there exists an X-linked variant (type II), associated with choroidoretinal coloboma, that might account for the excess of affected boys, but cases with coloboma have been observed in recessively inherited cases. Saraiva and Baraitser (1992) suggested that cases with retinal dystrophy tended to be associated with renal cysts and may represent a distinct subgroup.

The major features of Joubert syndrome, especially the respiratory abnormalities, are accounted for by developmental defects of the brainstem (Harmant-Van Rijckevorsel *et al.* 1983).

Other rare syndromes of vermal agenesis (Bordarier and Aicardi 1990) are shown in Table 3.8.

Aplasia and hypoplasia of the cerebellum
Major developmental defects of the cerebellum that affect predominantly the hemispheres (Robain *et al.* 1987) or about equally the hemispheres and vermis constitute a heterogeneous collection of rare anomalies with variable pathology and clinical manifestations (Sarnat and Alcala 1980, Robain *et al.* 1987, Altman *et al.* 1992). In fact, hypoplasia is difficult or impossible to distinguish from atrophy, even pathologically. Cases of probable atrophy and those of congenital pontocerebellar atrophies are discussed in Chapter 10. Proper classification of such defects is arduous. Friede (1989) argues that the classical separation into neocerebellar versus paleocerebellar hypoplasia is artificial and that it may be wiser, in many cases, to talk of aplasia of the anterior or posterior cerebellar lobes.

Total cerebellar aplasia is exceptional (Altman *et al.* 1992). Surprisingly, it is not always associated with clinical manifestations. Hypoplasia is less uncommon and may be predominantly unilateral. In some cases it is restricted to specific structures such as the flocculus (Vuia 1973). Abnormalities of deep cerebellar and brainstem nuclei and dysplasia of the inferior olivary body are frequent concomitants. In some cases hydrocephalus is present (Renier *et al.* 1983, Friede 1989) and other anomalies such as callosal agenesis or arhinencephaly may occur.

Unilateral aplasia (Boltshauser *et al.* 1996) is less rare and is often asymptomatic. It may be associated with ipsilateral facial

TABLE 3.9

Some syndromes featuring genetic nonprogressive cerebellar hypoplasia (excluding olivopontocerebellar atrophies)*

Syndrome	Features	Genetics†	References
Joubert syndrome	Ataxia, hyperpnoea, mental retardation, abnormal eye movements	AR	Aicardi *et al.* (1983)
Congenital cerebellar hypoplasia (CCH)	Congenital ataxia, mental retardation	AR	Wichman *et al.* (1985)
		XD	Fenichel and Phillips (1989)
		XR	Renier *et al.* (1983)
	Less severe, no or only mild mental retardation	AD	Rivier and Echenne (1992)
Sutherland–Gillespie syndrome	Congenital ataxia, iris hypoplasia, mental retardation	AR	Nevin and Lim (1990)
Congenital cerebellar hypoplasia with hypogonadism	Ataxia, hypogonadism, retinopathy in some cases	AR	De Michele *et al.* (1993)
PEHO syndrome	Peripheral oedema, ataxia, hypsarrhythmia, optic atrophy	AR	Salonen *et al.* (1991)
Congenital cerebellar ataxia with retinopathy	Ataxia, mental retardation, visual problems	AR	Dooley *et al.* (1992)
Malamud–Cohen syndrome	Cerebellar ataxia	XR	Young *et al.* (1987)
Norman syndrome**	Ataxia and mental retardation (severe or milder)	AR	Pascual-Castraviejo *et al.* (1994)
Congenital cerebellar ataxia with endosteal sclerosis	Ataxia and mental retardation	AR	Charrow *et al.* (1991)

†AR = autosomal recessive; AD = autosomal dominant; XR = X-linked recessive; XD = X-linked dominant.
*Only cerebellar hypoplasia with ataxia is shown here. Cases without cerebellar signs such as Dandy–Walker syndrome or Walker–Warburg syndrome omitted.
**Often regarded as a degeneration (see Chapter 10) although the course is static.

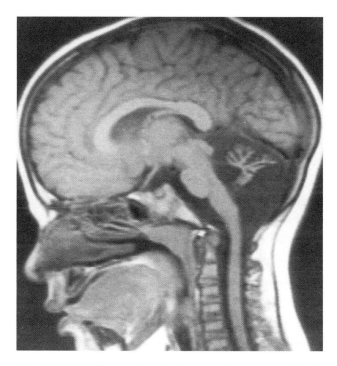

Fig. 3.34. Cerebellar atrophy of unknown origin in 8-year-old girl, affecting mostly the vermis. Part of the inferior vermis may be completely missing.

angioma and various abnormalities of cerebral and/or peripheral vessels (Chapter 15).

Clinical manifestations are extremely variable. They may be absent altogether or include ataxia, dysequilibrium and other cerebellar signs. Various degrees of mental retardation are common and may be the only feature. Many patients present as cases of ataxic cerebral palsy (Chapter 8). In most cases motor signs are prominent, but in some patients autistic features or microcephaly may be evident.

The diagnosis of cerebellar hypoplasia is mainly radiological (Fig. 3.34). Diffuse hypoplasia may be difficult to distinguish from Dandy–Walker variant by CT scanning, and megacistern is frequently mistaken for cerebellar hypoplasia. Differential signs include visualization of the falx cerebelli which is characteristic of a cisternal image, and the presence of a complete vermis on sagittal MRI.

Some of the cases of cerebellar hypoplasia are part of genetic syndromes but these are far from being well-defined. Some feature isolated congenital ataxia with various modes of transmission, while additional features are present in others (Al Shahwan *et al.* 1995) (Table 3.9). An association with chromosomal aberration has been reported (Arts *et al.* 1995).

Unusual cerebellar malformations
Tectocerebellar dysraphia (Friede and Boltshauser 1978) is a complex anomaly that includes an inverted cerebellum developed inside the fourth ventricle, hypoplasia of the vermis and occipital encephalocele.

Rhombencephalosynapsis (Schachenmayr and Friede 1982) designates congenital fusion of the cerebellar hemispheres with fusion of the dentate nuclei on the midline and aqueductal atresia. Mild cases may be compatible with prolonged survival with only mild symptoms.

Complex malformation of the cerebellum in association with encephalocele may result from ischaemic destruction of a previously normally formed cerebellum as a consequence of arterial compression by a diverticulum of the fourth ventricle (Evrard and Caviness 1974).

TABLE 3.10
CNS malformations that may be genetically determined*

Malformation	Mode of inheritance†	Recurrence risk
Neural tube defects (anencephaly spina bifida, encephaloceles)	Multifactorial	1–5% (up to 10% if two family members are affected
Holoprosencephaly	AD (AR or multifactorial in some cases)	6%[1]
Microcephaly	AR in most cases of isolated microcephaly. Syndromic forms may be AR or AD	Variable with type (see text)
Macrocephaly–megalencephaly	AD in simple macrocephaly	50%[2]
Agyria–pachygyria		
Type I	Rare familial (AR, XD or XR) cases	Low as a group
Miller–Dieker syndrome	17p deletion; may be inherited if parental translocation present	High risk if parental translocation
Type II (Walker–Warburg)	AR	25%[2]
Other cortical dysgenesis	Usually sporadic, familial cases of perisylvian syndrome. XD in subcortical band heterotopia	
Joubert syndrome	AR	25%[3]
Other vermian agenesis	AR, exceptionally AD (see Table 3.5)	25%
PEOH syndrome	AR	25%
CDG syndrome	AR	25%
Cerebellar hypoplasia	AR, AD, XD or XR	Variable with type
Agenesis of corpus callosum	AD, AR, X-linked cases, very rare in nonsyndromic forms	Very low as a group
Schizencephaly	?	Only rare cases

*Nongenetic types probably exist for all the malformations mentioned in the table.
†AR = autosomal recessive; AD = autosomal dominant; XR = X-linked recessive; XD = X-linked dominant.
[1]Represents a mixture of sporadic cases and of cases with various modes of transmission, hence of little practical value.
[2]Theoretical risk if all cases are inherited according to same mode.
[3]For unknown reasons there is a marked excess of affected males.

Dentato-olivary dysplasia responsible for neonatal tonic seizures reminiscent of Ohtahara syndrome has been found in a few patients (Harding and Boyd 1991, Robain and Dulac 1992). A genetic origin is likely (Harding and Copp 1997).

DISTURBANCES OF CEREBELLAR CORTICAL ORGANIZATION
Minor defects in microscopical organization of the cerebellar cortex are extremely common. Rorke *et al.* (1968) found them in 84 per cent of 147 cerebella. They have no clinical significance when not associated with other significant abnormalities. The so-called degeneration of the granular layer (Pascual-Castroviejo *et al.* 1994) is described in Chapter 10 even though its degenerative nature is far from certain.

Hypertrophy of the granular layer is probably a hamartomatous lesion intermediate between malformations and tumours. It is described in Chapter 14.

PRENATAL DIAGNOSIS, TREATMENT AND PREVENTION OF BRAIN MALFORMATIONS

The possibilities for active treatment of brain malformations are limited. Those malformations that induce hydrocephalus can be effectively managed by ventriculo-peritoneal shunt or other shunting operations. Even in such cases, however, neurodevelopmental dysfunction may persist after successful operation because diffuse abnormalities are present in addition to hydrocephalus. For most patients, only rehabilitation and physiotherapy are available. Special education is needed in many cases, and institutionalization may be necessary for the most severe cases.

Prevention of CNS malformations is one of the major challenges for child neurology in the coming years (Aicardi 1987). Primary prevention is not feasible at the present state of knowledge, one exception being the prevention of neural tube defects by administration of folic acid. Short of primary prevention, genetic counselling and prenatal diagnosis are the major preventive means available.

Genetic counselling requires that a precise diagnosis of fixed encephalopathies is made and that the rules of inheritance of the various types are known (Lie *et al.* 1994). Despite major advances in neuroimaging (Rosendahl and Kivinen 1989), such important malformation syndromes as polymicrogyria remain very difficult or impossible to diagnose, and the same obtains for 'minor' malformations. Ideally, a diagnosis of CNS malformation should

TABLE 3.11
CNS malformations associated with metabolic disorders

Metabolic error	Malformation	References
Fetal inborn errors of metabolism		
Nonketotic hyperglycinaemia	Agenesis of corpus callosum, abnormalities of gyration	Dobyns (1989)
Zellweger syndrome	Pachygyria and microgyria, agenesis of corpus callosum	Evrard et al. (1989)
Adrenoleukodystrophy (neonatal form)	Idem	Weinstein and Novotny (1987)
Trihydroxycholestanaemia	Cerebellar atrophy	Christensen et al. (1990)
Pyruvate dehydrogenase complex deficiency	Agenesis of corpus callosum, porencephaly	Weinstein and Novotny (1987), Matthews et al. (1993), Shevell et al. (1994)
Menkes disease	Agenesis of corpus callosum, abnormal gyration	Erdohazi et al. (1976)
Leigh syndrome	Abnormal gyration	Carleton et al. (1976)
Carbohydrate deficient glycoprotein (CDG) syndrome	Pontocerebellar hypoplasia	Jaeken and Carchon (1993)
Adenylsuccinase deficiency	Agenesis of cerebellar vermis	Jaeken and Van den Berghe (1984)
Glutaric aciduria type II (multiple acyl dehydrogenase deficiency)	Status verrucosus of cortex	Böhm et al. (1982)
Respiratory chain dysfunction	Cerebellar hypoplasia	Samson et al. (1994), Lincke et al. (1996)
Glutaric aciduria type I	Hypoplasia of temporal poles simulating arachnoid cysts, macrocephaly	Martinez-Lage et al. (1994)
Hurler disease	Agenesis of corpus callosum	Jellinger et al. (1981)
Multiple sulfatase deficiency	Agenesis of corpus callosum	(Two personal cases)
Smith–Lemli–Opitz syndrome (defective cholesterol biosynthesis)	Micrencephaly, hypoplasia of frontal lobe, abnormal gyration, cerebellar hypoplasia	Tint et al. (1994)
Metabolic disturbances of environmental (maternal) origin		
Phenylketonuria	Microcephaly	Lipson et al. (1984)
Fetal alcohol syndrome	Excess neuronal migration, agenesis of corpus callosum, abnormal gyration, holoprosencephaly	Wisniewski et al. (1983), Ronen and Andrews (1991)
Maternal diabetes mellitus	Holoprosencephaly, sacral agenesis, septo-optic dysplasia	Miller et al. (1981)

be not only precise but early if genetic counselling is to be effective (Evrard et al. 1985). The genetics of common CNS malformations do not follow simple mendelian rules (Carter 1976). Table 3.10 lists some of the main genetic malformations of the CNS and their mode of inheritance. Only a few malformation syndromes are firmly known to be nongenetic. This is the case for most nonsyndromic cases of agenesis of the corpus callosum, for Aicardi syndrome, Dandy–Walker syndrome and septo-optic dysplasia. Recognition of other syndromes of this type is obviously desirable. Unfortunately, it is more common for malformation syndromes to be either genetically or environmentally determined and, so far, we are not able to discriminate between the mechanisms. Chromosomal and MRI examination of parents, especially the mothers, can be helpful in some circumstances (see above).

Prenatal diagnosis of several brain malformations is feasible mainly by ultrasonography (Chard and McIntosh 1992, Platt et al. 1992, American Academy of Pediatrics 1994, Couture et al. 1994). Improvement in techniques makes earlier recognition possible, and techniques such as MRI may improve our ability to recognize developmental disturbances. Currently, the diagnosis is relatively late, except in gross abnormalities, with the consequence that only late termination is possible, which compares unfavourably with the earlier diagnosis of cases of metabolic diseases. Additionally, the reliability of ultrasonography depends heavily on the skill of examiners. Some abnormalities such as Dandy–Walker syndrome or agenesis of the corpus callosum may not be associated with neurodevelopmental dysfunction, thus raising difficult ethical issues.

Some developmental CNS anomalies may be associated with metabolic diseases (Table 3.11) (Erdohazi et al. 1976, Weinstein and Novotny 1987). Bamforth et al. (1988) found eight cases of callosal agenesis in 50 patients with inherited diseases of metabolism. Maternal diabetes mellitus is one major metabolic disorder capable of increasing considerably the incidence of certain CNS malformations. Moreover, the clear correlation that exists between high levels of glycosylated haemoglobin A1 in early pregnancy and the occurrence of severe defects in offspring

(Miller *et al.* 1981) supports the hypothesis that malformations in infants of diabetic mothers occur early during the first seven weeks of gestation. Such findings indicate that strict control of metabolic abnormalities such as maternal diabetes or phenylketonuria can prevent the occurrence of CNS malformations. The same probably applies to fetal alcoholism or cocaine use although prevention in such cases is clearly beyond the possibilities of medicine alone.

Careful monitoring of pregnancy is clearly important, and special attention should be given in cases involving higher risk factors such as maternal age over 35 years, multiple pregnancy, oligohydramnios or hydramnios, and to mothers with known disorders or who have previously given birth to a malformed infant. Fetuses that are small for gestational age are also at high risk. Khoury *et al.* (1988) found an incidence of malformation (of any type) of 8.0 per cent in small for gestational age babies compared to 3.3 per cent in infants appropriate for their gestational age. The discovery at ultrasonography of peripheral malformations, especially of cystic hygroma (Chervenak *et al.* 1983), is also an indication of high risk.

It is essential to inform future parents that even the best monitoring will miss a significant number of brain malformations whatever the technique used.

REFERENCES

Accardo, P., Whitman, B. (1988) 'Severe microcephaly with normal non-verbal intelligence.' *Pediatric Reviews and Communications*, **3**, 61–65.

Action Committee on Myelodysplasia, Section on Urology (1979) 'Current approaches to evaluation and management of children with myelomeningocele.' *Pediatrics*, **63**, 663–667.

Adams, M.M., Greenberg, F., Khoury, M.J., *et al.* (1985) 'Trends in clinical characteristics of infants with spina bifida—Atlanta 1972–1979.' *American Journal of Diseases of Children*, **139**, 514–517.

Ahdab-Barmada, M., Claassen, D. (1990) 'A distinctive triad of malformations of the central nervous system in the Meckel–Gruber syndrome.' *Journal of Neuropathology and Experimental Neurology*, **49**, 610–620.

Aicardi, J. (1987) 'The future of clinical child neurology.' *Journal of Child Neurology*, **2**, 152–159.

—— (1989) 'The lissencephaly syndromes.' *International Pediatrics*, **4**, 118–126.

—— (1991) 'The agyria–pachygyria complex: a spectrum of cortical malformations.' *Brain and Development*, **13**, 1–8.

—— (1994) 'The place of neuronal migration abnormalities in child neurology.' *Canadian Journal of Neurological Sciences*, **21**, 185–193.

—— (1996) 'Aicardi syndrome.' *In:* Guerrini, R., Andermann, F., Canapicchi, R., *et al.* (Eds.) *Dysplasias of Cerebral Cortex and Epilepsy.* Philadelphia: Lippincott–Raven, pp. 211–216.

—— Chevrie, J.J. (1994) 'Aicardi syndrome.' *In:* Lassonde, M., Jeeves, M.A. (Eds.) *The Natural Split-brain. Callosal Agenesis.* New York: Plenum, pp. 113–119.

—— Goutières, F. (1981) 'The syndrome of absence of the septum pellucidum with porencephalies and other developmental defects.' *Neuropediatrics*, **12**, 319–329.

—— Castello-Branco, M.E., Roy, C. (1983) 'Le syndrome de Joubert.' *Archives Françaises de Pédiatrie*, **40**, 625–629.

—— Chevrie, J.J., Baraton, J. (1987) 'Agenesis of the corpus callosum.' *In:* Vinken, P.J., Bruyn, G.W., Klawans, H.L. (Eds.) *Handbook of Clinical Neurology. Revised Series, Vol.6. Brain Malformation.* Amsterdam: North Holland, pp. 149–173.

Albright, A.L., Gartner, J.C., Wiener, E.S. (1989) 'Lumbar cutaneous hemangiomas as indicators of tethered spinal cord.' *Pediatrics*, **8**, 977–980.

Alcala, H., Dodson, W.E. (1975) 'Syringobulbia as a cause of laryngeal stridor in childhood.' *Neurology*, **25**, 875–878.

Aleksic, S., Budzilovich, G., Reuben, R., *et al.* (1975) 'Unilateral arhinencephaly in Goldenhar–Gorlin syndrome.' *Developmental Medicine and Child Neurology*, **17**, 498–504.

—— —— Greco, M.A., *et al.* (1983) 'Encephalocele (cerebellocele) in the Goldenhar–Gorlin syndrome.' *European Journal of Pediatrics*, **140**, 137–138.

Al Shahwan, S.A., Bruyn, G.W., Al Deeb, S.M. (1995) 'Non-progressive familial congenital cerebellar hypoplasia.' *Journal of the Neurological Sciences*, **128**, 71–77.

Altman, N.R., Altman, D.H. (1987) 'MR imaging of spinal dysraphism.' *American Journal of Neuroradiology*, **8**, 533–538.

—— Naidich, T.P., Braffman, B.H. (1992) 'Posterior fossa malformations.' *American Journal of Neuroradiology*, **13**, 691–724.

Amacher, A.L., Page, L.K. (1971) 'Hydrocephalus due to membranous obstruction of the fourth ventricle.' *Journal of Neurosurgery*, **35**, 672–676.

Ambrosetto, G. (1992) 'Unilateral opercular macrogyria and benign childhood epilepsy with centrotemporal (rolandic) spikes: report of a case.' *Epilepsia*, **33**, 499–503.

American Academy of Pediatrics, Committee on Genetics (1994) 'Prenatal genetic diagnosis for pediatricians.' *Pediatrics*, **93**, 1010–1015.

Andermann, E. (1981) 'Sensorimotor neuronopathy with agenesis of the corpus callosum.' *In:* Vinken, P.J., Bruyn, G.W. (Eds.) *Handbook of Clinical Neurology. Vol.42. Neurogenetic Directory, Part I.* Amsterdam: North Holland, pp. 100–103.

—— Andermann, F. (1996) 'Genetic aspects of neuronal migration disorders: X-linked inheritance in subcortical band and periventricular nodular heterotopia; familial occurrence of bilateral perisylvian polymicrogyria.' *In:* Guerrini, R., Andermann, F., Canapicchi, R., *et al.* (Eds.) *Dysplasias of Cerebral Cortex and Epilepsy.* New York: Lippincott–Raven, pp. 11–15.

—— Olivier, A., Melanson, D., Robitaille, Y. (1987) 'Epilepsy due to focal cortical dysplasia with macrogyria and the forme fruste of tuberous sclerosis: a study of 15 patients.' *In:* Wolf, P., Dam, M., Janz, D., Dreifuss, F.E. (Eds.) *Advances in Epileptology.* New York: Raven Press, pp. 35–38.

Anderson, F.M. (1975) 'Occult spinal dysraphism. A series of 73 cases.' *Pediatrics*, **55**, 826–835.

—— Burke, B.L. (1977) 'Anterior sacral meningocele.' *Journal of the American Medical Association*, **237**, 39–42.

André-Thomas, De Ajuriaguerra, J. (1959) 'Etude anatomo-clinique de l'anencéphalie.' *In:* Henger, G., Feld, M., Gruner, J. (Eds.) *Malformations Congénitales du Cerveau.* Paris: Masson, pp. 209–267.

Aniskiewicz, A.S., Frumkin, N.L., Brady, D.E., *et al.* (1990) 'Magnetic resonance imaging and neurobehavioral correlates in schizencephaly.' *Archives of Neurology*, **47**, 911–916.

Aoki, N. (1986) 'Cyst of the septum pellucidum presenting as hemiparesis.' *Child's Nervous System*, **2**, 326–328.

Arts, W.F.M., Hofstee, Y., Drejer, G.F., *et al.* (1995) 'Cerebellar and brainstem hypoplasia in a child with a partial monosomy for the short arm of chromosome 5 and partial trisomy for the short arm of chromosome 10.' *Neuropediatrics*, **26**, 41–44.

Atlas, S.W., Zimmerman, R.A., Bilaniuk, L.T., *et al.* (1986) 'Corpus callosum and limbic system: neuroanatomic MR evaluation of developmental anomalies.' *Radiology*, **160**, 355–362.

Babson, S.G., Benda, G.I. (1976) 'Growth graphs for the clinical assessment of infants of varying gestational age.' *Journal of Pediatrics*, **89**, 814–820.

Bale, J.F., Bell, W.E., Dunn, V., *et al.* (1986) 'Magnetic resonance imaging of the spine in children.' *Archives of Neurology*, **43**, 1253–1256.

Bamforth, F., Bamforth, S., Poskitt, K., *et al.* (1988) 'Abnormalities of corpus callosum in patients with inherited metabolic diseases.' *Lancet*, **2**, 451.

Baraitser, M. (1986) 'The oro-facio-digital (OFD) syndromes.' *Journal of Medical Genetics*, **23**, 116–119.

—— Burn, J. (1984) 'Neural tube defects as an X-linked condition.' *American Journal of Medical Genetics*, **17**, 383–385.

—— Brett, E.M., Piesowicz, A.T. (1983) 'Microcephaly and intracranial calcification in two brothers.' *Journal of Medical Genetics*, **20**, 210–212.

Barbaro, N.M., Wilson, C.B., Gutin, P.H. (1984) 'Surgical treatment of syringomyelia: favorable results with syringoperitoneal shunting.' *Journal of Neurosurgery*, **61**, 531–538.

Barkovich, A.J. (1990) 'Apparent atypical callosal dysgenesis: analysis of MR findings in six cases and their relationship to holoprosencephaly.' *American Journal of Neuroradiology*, **11**, 333–339.

—— Chuang, S.H. (1990) 'Unilateral megalencephaly: correlation of MR imaging and pathologic characteristics.' *American Journal of Neuroradiology*, **11**, 523–531.

—— Kjos, B.O. (1992) 'Schizencephaly: correlation of clinical findings with MR characteristics.' *American Journal of Neuroradiology*, **13**, 85–94.

—— Lindan, C.E. (1994) 'Congenital cytomegalovirus infection of the brain: imaging analysis and embryologic considerations.' *American Journal of Neuroradiology*, **15**, 703–715.

—— Norman, D. (1988a) 'Anomalies of the corpus callosum: correlation with further anomalies of the brain.' *American Journal of Neuroradiology*, **9**, 493–501.

—— —— (1988b) 'Absence of the septum pellucidum: a useful sign of the diagnosis of congenital brain malformations.' *American Journal of Neuroradiology*, **9**, 1107–1114.

—— Quint, D.J. (1993) 'Middle interhemispheric fusion: an unusual variant of holoprosencephaly.' *American Journal of Neuroradiology*, **14**, 431–440.

—— Chuang, S.H., Norman, D. (1988) 'MR of neuronal migration anomalies.' *American Journal of Roentgenology*, **150**, 179–187.

—— Jackson, D.E., Boyer, R.S. (1989) 'Band heterotopias: a newly recognized neuronal migration anomaly.' *Radiology*, **171**, 455–458.

—— Koch, T.K., Carrol, C.L. (1991) 'The spectrum of lissencephaly: report of ten patients analyzed by magnetic resonance imaging.' *Annals of Neurology*, **30**, 139–146.

—— Gressens, P., Evrard, P. (1992) 'Formation, maturation, and disorders of brain neocortex.' *American Journal of Neuroradiology*, **13**, 423–446.

—— Guerrini, R., Battaglia, G., et al. (1994) 'Band heterotopia: correlation of outcome with magnetic resonance imaging parameters.' *Annals of Neurology*, **36**, 609–617.

—— Kuzniecky, R.I., Dobyns, W.B., et al. (1996) 'A classification scheme for malformations of cortical development.' *Neuropediatrics*, **27**, 59–63.

Barnet, A.B., Weiss, I.P., Shaer, C. (1993) 'Evoked potentials in infant brainstem syndrome associated with Arnold–Chiari malformation.' *Developmental Medicine and Child Neurology*, **35**, 42–48.

Barr, M., Hanson, J.W., Currey, K., et al. (1983) 'Holoprosencephaly in infants of diabetic mothers.' *Journal of Pediatrics*, **102**, 565–568.

Barth, P.G. (1987) 'Disorders of neuronal migration.' *Canadian Journal of Neurological Sciences*, **14**, 1–16.

—— Van der Harten, J.J. (1985) 'Parabiotic twin syndrome with topical isocortical disruption and gastroschisis.' *Acta Neuropathologica*, **67**, 345–349.

—— Mullaart, R., Stam, F.C., Slooff, J.L. (1982) 'Familial lissencephaly with extreme neopallial hypoplasia.' *Brain and Development*, **4**, 145–151.

—— Hoffmann, G.F., Jaeken, J., et al. (1992) 'L-2-hydroxyglutaric acidemia: a novel inherited neurometabolic disease.' *Annals of Neurology*, **32**, 66–71.

Bean, J.R., Walsh, J.W., Blacker, H.M. (1979) 'Cervical dermal sinus and intramedullary spinal cord abcess: case report.' *Neurosurgery*, **5**, 60–62.

Becker, P.S., Dixon, A.M., Troncosi, J.C. (1989) 'Bilateral opercular polymicrogyria.' *Annals of Neurology*, **25**, 90–92.

Begleiter, M.L., Harris, D.J. (1980) 'Holoprosencephaly and endocrine dysgenesis in brothers.' *American Journal of Medical Genetics*, **7**, 315–318.

Bell, J.E. (1979) 'Central nervous system defects in early human abortuses.' *Developmental Medicine and Child Neurology*, **21**, 321–332.

Bell, W.O., Charney, E.B., Bruce, D.A., et al. (1987) 'Symptomatic Arnold–Chiari malformation: review of experience with 22 cases.' *Journal of Neurosurgery*, **66**, 812–816.

Bentley, J.F.R., Smith, J.R. (1960) 'Developmental posterior enteric remnants and spinal malformations. The split notochord syndrome.' *Archives of Disease in Childhood*, **35**, 76–86.

Bergeron, R.T. (1967) 'Pneumographic demonstration of subependymal heterotopic gray matter in children.' *American Journal of Roentgenology*, **101**, 168–177.

Berry-Kravis, E., Israel, J. (1994) 'X-linked pachygyria and agenesis of the corpus callosum: evidence for an X chromosome lissencephaly locus.' *Annals of Neurology*, **36**, 229–233.

Berthet, F., Caduff, R., Schaad, U.B., et al. (1994) 'A syndrome of primary combined immunodeficiency with microcephaly, cerebellar hypoplasia, growth failure and progressive pancytopenia.' *European Journal of Pediatrics*, **153**, 333–338.

Bick, D., Franco, B., Sherins, R.J., et al. (1992) 'Brief report: intragenic deletion of the *KALIG-1* gene in Kallmann's syndrome.' *New England Journal of Medicine*, **326**, 1752–1755.

Billette de Villemeur, T., Chiron, C., Robain, O. (1992) 'Unlayered polymicrogyria and agenesis of the corpus callosum: a relevant association?' *Acta Neuropathologica*, **83**, 265–270.

Bingol, N., Fuchs, M., Diaz, V., et al. (1987) 'Teratogenicity of cocaine in humans.' *Journal of Pediatrics*, **110**, 93–96.

Blum, A., André, M., Droullé, P., et al. (1990) 'Prenatal echographic diagnosis of corpus callosum agenesis. The Nancy experience 1982–1989.' *Genetic Counseling*, **1**, 115–126.

Bodensteiner, J.B. (1995) 'The saga of the septum pellucidum: a tale of unfunded clinical investigations.' *Journal of Child Neurology*, **10**, 227–231.

—— Gay, C.T. (1990) 'Colpocephaly: pitfalls in the diagnosis of a pathologic entity utilizing neuroimaging techniques.' *Journal of Child Neurology*, **5**, 166–168.

—— —— Marks, W.A., et al. (1988) 'Macro cisterna magna: a marker for maldevelopment of the brain.' *Pediatric Neurology*, **4**, 284–286.

—— Schaefer, G.B., Breeding, L., Cowan, L. (1994) 'Hypoplasia of the corpus callosum: a study of 445 consecutive MRI scans.' *Journal of Child Neurology*, **9**, 47–49.

Böhm, U., Uy, J., Kiessling, M., Lehnert, W. (1982) 'Multiple acyl-CoA-dehydrogenation deficiency (glutaric aciduria type II), congenital polycystic kidneys, and symmetric warty dysplasia of the cerebral cortex in two newborn brothers. II. Morphology and pathogenesis.' *European Journal of Pediatrics*, **139**, 60–65.

Boltshauser, E., Steinlin, M., Martin, E., Deonna, T. (1996) 'Unilateral cerebellar aplasia.' *Neuropediatrics*, **27**, 50–53.

Bordarier, C., Aicardi, J. (1990) 'Dandy–Walker syndrome and agenesis of the cerebellar vermis: diagnostic problems and genetic counselling.' *Developmental Medicine and Child Neurology*, **32**, 285–294.

—— —— Goutières, F. (1984) 'Congenital hydrocephalus and eye abnormalities with severe developmental brain defects: Warburg's syndrome.' *Annals of Neurology*, **16**, 60–65.

Borzyskowski, M. (1990) 'The conservative management of neuropathic vesicourethral dysfunction.' *In:* Borzyskowski, M., Mundy, A.R. (Eds.) *Neuropathic Bladder in Childhood. Clinics in Developmental Medicine No. 111.* London: Mac Keith Press, pp. 27–36.

—— Mundy, A.R., Neville, B.G.R., et al. (1982) 'Neuropathic vesicourethral dysfunction in children. A trial comparing clean intermittent catheterisation with manual expression combined with drug treatment.' *British Journal of Urology*, **54**, 641–644.

Bosman, C., Boldrini, R., Dimitri, L., et al. (1996) 'Hemimegalencephaly. Histological, immunohistochemical, ultrastructural and cytofluorimetric study of six patients.' *Child's Nervous System*, **12**, 765–775.

Breningstall, G.N., Marker, S.M., Tubman, D.E. (1992) 'Hydrosyringomyelia and diastematomyelia detected by MRI in myelomeningocele.' *Pediatric Neurology*, **8**, 267–271.

Brett, E.B. (Ed.) (1991) *Paediatric Neurology, 2nd Edn.* Edinburgh: Churchill Livingstone.

Brismar, J., Ozand, P.T. (1995) 'CT and MR of the brain in glutaric acidemia type 1: a review of 59 published cases and a report of 5 new patients.' *American Journal of Neuroradiology*, **16**, 675–683.

Brody, B.A., Kinney, H.C., Kloman, A.S., Gilles, F.H. (1987) 'Sequence of central nervous system myelination in human infancy. 1: Autopsy study of myelination.' *Journal of Neuropathology*, **46**, 283–301.

Brown, J.R. (1977) 'The Dandy–Walker syndrome.' *In:* Vinken, P.J., Bruyn, G.W. (Eds.) *Handbook of Clinical Neurology. Vol. 30. Congenital Malformations of the Brain and Skull, Part 1.* Amsterdam: North Holland, pp. 623–646.

Brown, M.S., Sheridan-Pereira, M. (1992) 'Outlook for the child with a cephalocele.' *Pediatrics*, **90**, 914–919.

Brunelli, S., Faiella, A., Capra, V., et al. (1996) 'Germline mutations in the homeobox gene *EMX2* in patients with severe schizencephaly.' *Nature Genetics*, **12**, 94–96.

Burck, U., Hayek, H.W., Zeidler, U. (1981) 'Holoprosencephaly in monozygotic twins—clinical and computer tomographic findings.' *American Journal of Medical Genetics*, **9**, 13–17.

Burn, J., Wickramasinghe, H.T., Harding, B., Baraitser, M. (1986) 'A syndrome with intracranial calcification and microcephaly in two sibs, resembling intrauterine infection.' *Clinical Genetics*, **30**, 112–116.

Burrows, F.G.O., Sutcliffe, J. (1968) 'The split notochord syndrome.' *British Journal of Radiology*, **41**, 844–847.

Burton, B.K. (1981) 'Dominant inheritance of microcephaly with short stature.' *Clinical Genetics*, **20**, 25–27.

—— Dillard, R.G. (1986) 'Outcome of infants born to mothers with unexplained elevations of maternal serum α-fetoprotein.' *Pediatrics*, **77**, 582–586.

Busis, N.A., Hochberg, F.H. (1985) 'Familial syringomyelia.' *Journal of Neurology, Neurosurgery, and Psychiatry*, **48**, 936–938.

119

Calabrese, P., Fink, G.R., Markowitsch, H.J., *et al.* (1994) 'Left hemispheric neuronal heterotopia: a PET, MRI, EEG, and neuropsychological investigation of a university student.' *Neurology*, **44**, 302–305.

Cama, A. Tortori-Donati, P., Piatelli, G.L., *et al.* (1995) 'Chiari complex in children—neuroradiological diagnosis, neurosurgical treatment and proposal of a new classification (312 cases).' *European Journal of Pediatric Surgery*, **5**, Suppl. 1, 35–38.

Cantani, A., Lucenti, P., Ronzani, G.A., Santoro, C. (1990) 'Joubert syndrome. Review of the fifty-three cases so far published.' *Annals of Genetics*, **33**, 96–98.

Cantú, J.M., Rojas, J.A., Garcia-Cruz, D., *et al.* (1977) 'Autosomal recessive microcephaly associated with chorioretinopathy.' *Human Genetics*, **36**, 243–247.

Caplan, L.R., Norohna, A.B., Amico, L.L. (1990) 'Syringomyelia and arachnoiditis.' *Journal of Neurology, Neurosurgery, and Psychiatry*, **53**, 106–113.

Carleton, G.C., Collins, G.H., Schimpff, R.D. (1976) 'Subacute necrotizing encephalopathy (Leigh's disease): two unusual cases.' *Southern Medical Journal*, **69**, 1301–1305.

Carter, C.O. (1976) 'Genetics of common single malformations.' *British Medical Bulletin*, **32**, 21–26.

Castillo, M., Bouldin, T.W., Scatliff, J.H., Suzuki, K. (1993) 'Radiologic–pathologic correlation: alobar holoprosencephaly.' *American Journal of Neuroradiology*, **14**, 1151–1156.

Cavenagh, E.C., Hart, B.L., Rose, D. (1993) 'Association of linear nevus syndrome and unilateral megalencephaly.' *American Journal of Neuroradiology*, **14**, 405–408.

Caviness, V.S. (1976) 'The Chiari malformations of the posterior fossa and their relation to hydrocephalus.' *Developmental Medicine and Child Neurology*, **18**, 103–116.

—— Rakic, P. (1978) 'Mechanism of cortical development: a view from mutations in mice.' *In:* Cowan, M.W., Hall, Z.W., Kandel, E.R. (Eds.) *Annual Reviews of Neuroscience*. Palo Alto: Annual Reviews, pp. 297–326.

—— Takahashi, T. (1995) 'Proliferative events in the cerebral ventricular zone.' *Brain and Development*, **17**, 159–163.

—— Pinto-Lord, M.C., Evrard, P. (1981) 'The development of laminated pattern in the mammalian neocortex.' *In:* Connelly, T.G. (Ed.) *Morphogenesis and Pattern Formation*. New York: Raven Press, pp. 102–126.

Chadduck, W.M., Glasier, C.M. (1989) 'Megachoroid as a cause of isolated ventricle syndrome.' *Pediatric Neurology*, **5**, 194–196.

Chapman, P.H. (1982) 'Congenital intraspinal lipomas: anatomic considerations and surgical treatment.' *Child's Brain*, **9**, 37–47.

—— Swearingen, B., Caviness, V.S. (1989) 'Subtorcular occipital encephaloceles. Anatomical considerations relevant to operative management.' *Journal of Neurosurgery*, **71**, 375–381.

Chard, T., Macintosh, M. (1992) 'Antenatal diagnosis of congenital abnormalities.' *In:* Chard, T., Richards, M.P.M. (Eds.) *Obstetrics in the 1990s: Current Controversies. Clinics in Developmental Medicine No. 123/124*. London: Mac Keith Press, pp. 90–104.

Charney, E.B., Weller, S.C., Sutton, L.N., *et al.* (1985) 'Management of the newborn with myelomeningocele. Time for a decision-making process.' *Pediatrics*, **75**, 58–64.

—— Rorke, L.B., Sutton, L.N., Schut, L. (1987) 'Management of Chiari II complications in infants with myelomeningocele.' *Journal of Pediatrics*, **111**, 364–371.

Charrow, J., Poznanski, A.K., Unger, F.M., Robinow, M. (1991) 'Autosomal recessive cerebellar hypoplasia and endosteal sclerosis: a newly recognized syndrome.' *American Journal of Medical Genetics*, **41**, 464–468.

Chervenak, F.A., Isaacson, G., Blakemore, K.J., *et al.* (1983) 'Fetal cystic hygroma. Cause and natural history.' *New England Journal of Medicine*, **309**, 822–825.

—— Isaacson, G., Hobbins, J.C., *et al.* (1985) 'Diagnosis and management of fetal holoprosencephaly.' *Obstetrics and Gynecology*, **66**, 322–326.

Chevrie, J.J., Aicardi, J. (1986) 'The Aicardi syndrome.' *In:* Pedley, T.A., Meldrum, B.S. (Eds.) *Recent Advances in Epilepsy, Vol.3*. Edinburgh: Churchill Livingstone, pp. 189–210.

Choi, B.H., Matthias, S.C. (1987) 'Cortical dysplasia associated with massive ectopia of neurons and glial cells within the subarachnoid space.' *Acta Neuropathologica*, **73**, 105–109.

Chow, C.W., Anderson, R.McD, Kenny, G.C.T. (1987) 'Neuropathology in cerebral lactic acidosis.' *Acta Neuropathologica*, **74**, 393–396.

Christensen, E., Van Eldere, J., Brandt, N.J., *et al.* (1990) 'A new peroxisomal disorder: di- and trihydroxycholestanaemia due to a presumed trihydroxy-cholestanoyl-CoA oxidase deficiency.' *Journal of Inherited Metabolic Diseases*, **13**, 363–366.

Christian, J.C. (1982) 'Kallmann syndrome (olfactogenital dysplasia).' *In:* Vinken, P.J., Bruyn, G.W. (Eds.) *Handbook of Clinical Neurology. Vol. 43. Neurogenetic Directory, Part II*. Amsterdam: North Holland, pp. 418–419.

Chugani, H.T. (1996) 'Functional imaging in cortical dysplasia: positron emission tomography.' *In:* Guerrini, R., Andermann, F., Canapicchi, R., *et al.* (Eds.) *Dysplasias of Cerebral Cortex and Epilepsy*. New York: Lippincott–Raven, pp. 169–174.

Cioni, G., Bartalena, L., Bagioni, E., *et al.* (1996) 'Prenatal and postnatal sonographic findings in cortical dysplasias.' *In:* Guerrini, R., Andermann, F., Canapicchi, R., *et al.* (Eds.) *Dysplasias of Cerebral Cortex and Epilepsy*. Philadelphia: Lippincott–Raven, pp. 105–113.

Cohen, M.M., (1988) 'Understanding Proteus syndrome, unmasking the Elephant Man, and stemming elephant fever.' *Neurofibromatosis*, **1**, 260–280.

—— Lemire, R.J. (1982) 'Syndromes with cephaloceles.' *Teratology*, **25**, 161–172.

—— Campbell, R., Yaghmai, F. (1989) 'Neuropathological abnormalities in develomental dysphasia.' *Annals of Neurology*, **25**, 567–570.

Collaborative Acetylcholinesterase Study (1981) 'Amniotic fluid acetylcholinesterase electrophoresis as a secondary test in the diagnosis of anencephaly and open spina bifida in early pregnancy.' *Lancet*, **2**, 321–324.

Conley, M.E., Beckwith, J.B., Mancer, J.F.K., Tenchkhoff, L. (1979) 'The spectrum of Di George syndrome.' *Journal of Pediatrics*, **94**, 883–890.

Cordero, J.F. (1994) 'Finding the causes of birth defects.' *New England Journal of Medicine*, **331**, 48–49.

Couly, G., Aicardi, J. (1988) 'Anomalies morphologiques associées de la face et de l'encéphale chez l'enfant.' *Archives Françaises de Pédiatrie*, **45**, 99–104.

Coupland, S.G., Sarnat, H.B. (1990) 'Visual and auditory evoked potential correlates of cerebral malformations.' *Brain and Development*, **12**, 466–472.

Couture, A., Veyrac, C., Baud, C. (1994) *Echographie Cérébrale du Foetus au Nouveau-né. Imagerie et Hémodynamique*. Montpelier: Sauramps Médical.

Czeizel, A.E., Dudás, I. (1992) 'Prevention of the first occurrence of neural-tube defects by periconceptional vitamin supplementation.' *New England Journal of Medicine*, **327**, 1832–1835.

Dalla Bernardina, B., Pérez-Jiménez, A., Fontana, E., *et al.* (1996) 'Electroencephalographic findings associated with cortical dysplasias. *In:* Guerrini, R., Andermann, F., Canapicchi, R., *et al.* (Eds.) *Dysplasias of Cerebral Cortex and Epilepsy*. Philadelphia: Lippincott–Raven, pp. 235–245.

D'Alton, M.E., DeCherney, A.H. (1993) 'Prenatal diagnosis.' *New England Journal of Medicine*, **328**, 114–120.

Dambska, M., Laure-Kaminowska, M. (1990) 'Myelination as a parameter of normal and retarded brain maturation.' *Brain and Development*, **12**, 214–220.

—— Wisniewski, K.E., Sher, J.H. (1986) 'Marginal glioneuronal heterotopias in nine cases with and without cortical abnormalities.' *Journal of Child Neurology*, **1**, 149–157.

Danner, R., Shewmon, A., Sherman, M.B. (1985) 'Seizures in an atelencephalic infant: is the cortex essential for neonatal seizures?' *Archives of Neurology*, **42**, 1014–1016.

Dauser, R.C., Di Pietro, M.A., Venes, J.L. (1989) 'Symptomatic Chiari I malformation in childhood. A report of 7 cases.' *Pediatric Neuroscience*, **14**, 184–190.

David, D.J., Sheffield, L., Simpson, D., White, J. (1984) 'Fronto-ethmoidal meningoencephaloceles: morphology and treatment.' *British Journal of Plastic Surgery*, **37**, 271–284.

Davis, P.C., Hoffman, J.C., Ball, T.I., *et al.* 1988) 'Spinal abnormalities in pediatric patients: MR imaging findings compared with clinical, myelographic and surgical findings.' *Radiology*, **166**, 679–685.

Day, R.E., Schutt, W.H. (1979) 'Normal children with large heads—benign familial megalencephaly.' *Archives of Disease in Childhood*, **54**, 512–517.

Dekaban, A. (1965) 'Large defects in cerebral hemisphere associated with cortical dysgenesis.' *Journal of Neuropathology and Experimental Neurology*, **24**, 512–530.

De Léon, G.A., Breningstall, G., Zaeri, N. (1986) 'Congenital Pick cell encephalopathy: a distinct disorder characterized by diffuse formation of Pick cells in the cerebral cortex.' *Acta Neuropathologica*, **70**, 235–242.

—— De Léon, G., Grover, W.D., *et al.* (1987) 'Agenesis of the corpus callosum and limbic malformation in Apert syndrome (type I acrocephalosyndactyly).' *Archives of Neurology*, **44**, 979–982.

Della Giustina, E., Goffinet, A.M., Landrieu, P., Lyon, G. (1981) 'A Golgi study of the brain malformation in Zellweger's cerebro-hepato-renal disease.' *Acta Neuropathologica*, **55**, 23–28.

De Michele, G., Filla, A., Striano, S., *et al.* (1993) 'Heterogeneous findings in four cases of cerebellar ataxia associated with hypogonadism (Holmes' type ataxia).' *Clinical Neurology and Neurosurgery*, **95**, 23–28.

De Myer, W. (1967) 'The median cleft face syndrome. Differential diagnosis of cranium bifidum, bifidum occultum, hypertelorism, and median cleft nose, lip, and palate.' *Neurology*, **17**, 961–971.

—— (1972) 'Megalencephaly in children. Clinical syndromes, genetic patterns, and differential diagnosis from other causes of megalencephaly.' *Neurology*, **22**, 634–643.

—— (1987) 'Holoprosencephaly (cyclopia–arhinencephaly).' *In:* Vinken, P.J., Bruyn, G.W. (Eds.) *Handbook of Clinical Neurology, Revised Series, Vol. 6. Brain Malformation.* Amsterdam: North Holland, pp. 225–244.

—— Zeman, W., Palmer, C.G. (1964) 'The face predicts the brain: diagnostic significance of median facial anomalies for holoprosencephaly (arhinencephaly).' *Pediatrics*, **34**, 256–263.

Deray, M., Duchowny, M., Papazian, O., *et al.* (1995) 'Sleep evaluation of respiratory abnormalities in children with Chiari II malformation.' *Acta Neuropediatrica*, **1**, 197–205.

De Rijk-Van Andel, J.F., Arts, W.F.M., De Weerd, A.W. (1988) 'EEG in type I lisssencephaly.' *Developmental Medicine and Child Neurology*, **30**, 126–127.

—— —— Barth, P.G., Loonen, M.C.B. (1990) 'Diagnostic features and clinical signs of 21 patients with lissencephaly type I.' *Developmental Medicine and Child Neurology*, **32**, 707–717.

—— —— de Weerd, A.W. (1992) 'EEG and evoked potentials in a series of 21 patients with lissencephaly type I.' *Neuropediatrics*, **23**, 4–9.

Desbiens, R., Berkovic, S.F., Dubeau, F., *et al.* (1993) 'Life-threatening focal status epilepticus due to occult cortical dysplasia.' *Archives of Neurology*, **50**, 695–700.

Diebler, C., Dulac, O. (1987) 'Cephaloceles.' *In: Pediatric Neurology and Neuroradiology.* Berlin: Springer, pp. 51–67.

Di Mario, F.J., Cobb, R.J., Ramsby, G.R., Leicher, C. (1993) 'Familial band heterotopias simulating tuberous sclerosis.' *Neurology*, **43**, 1424–1426.

Di Rocco, C. (1996) 'Surgical treatment of hemimegalencephaly.' *In:* Guerrini, R., Andermann, F., Canapicchi, R., *et al.* (Eds.) *Dysplasias of Cerebral Cortex and Epilepsy.* Philadelphia: Lippincott–Raven, pp. 295–304.

Dobyns, W.B. (1987) 'Developmental aspects of lissencephaly and the lissencephaly syndromes.' *Birth Defects Original Article Series*, **23**, 225–241.

—— (1989) 'Agenesis of the corpus callosum and gyral malformations are frequent manifestations of nonketotic hyperglycinemia.' *Neurology*, **39**, 817–820.

—— (1993) 'Classification of the cerebro-oculo-muscular syndrome(s). Commentary to Kimura's paper (pp. 182–191).' *Brain and Development*, **15**, 242–244.

—— Truwit, C.L. (1995) 'Lissencephaly and other malformations of cortical development: 1995 update.' *Neuropediatrics*, **26**, 132–147.

—— Stratton, R.F., Parke, J.T., *et al.* (1983) 'Miller–Dieker syndrome: lissencephaly and monosomy 17p.' *Journal of Pediatrics*, **102**, 552–558.

—— —— Greenberg, F. (1984) 'Syndromes with lissencephaly. I. Miller–Dieker and Norman–Roberts syndromes and isolated lisssencephaly.' *American Journal of Medical Genetics*, **18**, 509–526.

—— Kirkpatrick, J.B., Hittner, H.M., *et al.* (1985) 'Syndromes with lissencephaly. II. Walker–Warburg and cerebro-oculo-muscular syndromes and a new syndrome with type II lissencephaly.' *American Journal of Medical Genetics*, **22**, 157–195.

—— Pagon, R.A., Armstrong, D., *et al.* (1989) 'Diagnostic criteria for Walker–Warburg syndrome.' *American Journal of Medical Genetics*, **32**, 195–210.

—— Elias, E.R., Newlin, A.C., *et al.* (1992) 'Causal heterogeneity in isolated lissencephaly.' *Neurology*, **42**, 1375–1388.

—— Reiner, O., Carrozzo, R., Ledbetter, D.H. (1993) 'Lissencephaly. A human brain malformation associated with deletion of the *LIS1* gene located at chromosome 17p13.' *Journal of the American Medical Association*, **270**, 2838–2842.

—— Andermann, E., Andermann, F., *et al.* (1996a) 'X-linked malformations of neuronal migration.' *Neurology*, **46**, 831–839.

—— Patton, M.A., Stratton, R.F., *et al.* (1996b) 'Cobblestone lissencephaly with normal eyes and muscles.' *Neuropediatrics*, **27**, 70–75.

Dodge, N.N., Dobyns, W.B. (1995) 'Agenesis of the corpus callosum and Dandy–Walker malformation associated with hemimegalencephaly in the sebaceous nevus syndrome.' *American Journal of Medical Genetics*, **56**, 147–150.

Donat, J.F.G. (1981) 'Septo-optic dysplasia in an infant of a diabetic mother.' *Archives of Neurology*, **38**, 590–591.

Donnenfeld, A.E., Packer, R.J., Zackai, E.H., *et al.* (1989) 'Clinical, cytogenetic and pedigree findings in 18 cases of Aicardi syndrome.' *American Journal of Medical Genetics*, **32**, 461–467.

Dooley, J.M., LaRoche, G.R., Tremblay, F., Riding, M. (1992) 'Autosomal recessive cerebellar hypoplasia and tapeto-retinal degeneration: a new syndrome.' *Pediatric Neurology*, **8**, 232–234.

Drolet, B.A., Clowry, L., McTigue, M.K., Esterly, N.B. (1995) 'The hair collar sign: marker for cranial dysraphism.' *Pediatrics*, **96**, 309–315.

Drugan, A., Zador, I.E., Syner, F.N., *et al.* (1988) 'A normal ultrasound does not obviate the need for amniocentesis in patients with elevated serum alpha-fetoprotein.' *Obstetrics and Gynecology*, **72**, 627–630.

Dryden, R.J. (1980) 'Duplication of the spinal cord: a discussion of the possible embryogenesis of diplomyelia.' *Developmental Medicine and Child Neurology*, **22**, 234–243.

Dubeau, F., Tampieri, D., Lee, N., *et al.* (1995) 'Periventricular and subcortical nodular heterotopia. A study of 33 patients.' *Brain*, **118**, 1273–1287.

Dulac, O., Plouin, P., Perulli, L., *et al.* (1983) 'Aspects électroencéphalographiques de l'agyrie–pachygyrie classique.' *Revue d'Electroencéphalographie et de Neurophysiologie*, **13**, 232–239.

Dure, L.S., Percy, A.K., Cheek, W.R., Laurent, J.P. (1989) 'Chiari type 1 malformation in children.' *Journal of Pediatrics*, **115**, 573–576.

Dvorak, K., Feit, J. (1977) 'Migration of neuroblasts through partial necrosis of the cerebral cortex in newborn rats. Contribution to the problem of morphological development and developmental period of cerebral microgyria.' *Acta Neuropathologica*, **38**, 203–212.

—— Jurankova, Z. (1978) 'Experimentally induced focal microgyria and status verrucosus deformis in rats: pathogenesis and interrelation. Histological and autoradiographical study.' *Acta Neuropathologica*, **44**, 121–129.

Eckstein, H.B., Molyneux, M. (1982) 'Intermittent catheterization of the bladder for neuropathic incontinence.' *Zeitschrift für Kinderchirurgie*, **37**, 143–144.

Edwards, B.O., Fisher, A.Q., Flannery, D.B. (1988) 'Joubert syndrome: early diagnosis by recognition of the behavioral phenotype and confirmation by cranial sonography.' *Journal of Child Neurology*, **3**, 247–249.

Egger, J., Bellman, M.H., Ross, E.H., Baraitser, M. (1982) 'Joubert–Boltshauser syndrome with polydactyly in siblings.' *Journal of Neurology, Neurosurgery, and Psychiatry*, **48**, 737–739.

Elster, A.D., Chen, M.Y.M. (1992) 'Chiari I malformations: clinical and radiologic reappraisal.' *Radiology*, **183**, 347–353.

Emery, J.L., Lendon, R.G. (1973) 'The local cord lesion in neurospinal dysraphism (meningomyelocele).' *Journal of Pathology*, **110**, 83–96.

Emery, J.L., MacKenzie, N.G. (1973) 'Medullocervical dislocating deformity (Chiari II deformity) related to neurospinal dysraphism (meningomyelocele).' *Brain*, **96**, 155–162.

Erdohazi, M., Barnes, N.D., Robinson, M.J., Lake, B.D. (1976) 'Cerebral malformation associated with metabolic disorder: a report of two cases.' *Acta Neuropathologica*, **36**, 315–325.

Evrard, P., Caviness, V.S. (1974) 'Extensive developmental defect of the cerebellum associated with posterior fossa ventriculocele.' *Journal of Neuropathology and Experimental Neurology*, **33**, 385–390.

—— —— Prats-Viñas, J., Lyon, G. (1978) 'The mechanism of arrest of neuronal migration in the Zellweger malformation: an hypothesis based upon cytoarchitectonic analysis.' *Acta Neuropathologica*, **41**, 109–117.

—— Lyon, G., Gadisseux, J.F. (1984) 'Le développement prénatal du système nerveux et ses perturbations: mécanismes généraux.' *In: Progrès en Néonatologie, Vol. 4.* Basel: Karger, pp. 63–69.

—— Belpaire, M.C., Boog, G., *et al.* (1985) 'Diagnostic anténatal des affections du système nerveux central: résultats préliminaires d'une étude multicentrique européenne.' *Journal Français d'Echographie*, **2**, 123–126.

—— De Saint-Georges, P., Kadhim, H., Gadisseux, J.F. (1989) 'Pathology of prenatal encephalopathies.' *In:* French, J.H., Harel, S., Casaer, P. (Eds.) *Child Neurology and Developmental Disabilities.* Baltimore: P.H. Brookes, pp. 153–176.

Ewigman, B.G., Crane, J.P., Frigoletto, F.D., *et al.* (1993) 'Effect of prenatal ultrasound screening on perinatal outcome. RADIUS Study Group.' *New England Journal of Medicine*, **329**, 821–827.

Fabregues, I., Ferrer, I., Cusi, M.V., *et al.* (1984) 'Fine structure based on the Golgi method of the abnormal cortex and heterotopic nodules in pachygyria.' *Brain and Development*, **6**, 317–322.

Farrel, S.A., Toi, A., Leadman, M.L., *et al.* (1987) 'Prenatal diagnosis of retinal detachment in Walker–Warburg syndrome.' *American Journal of Medical Genetics,* **28**, 619–624.

Fedrick, J. (1976) 'Anencephalus in the Oxford Record Linkage Study Area.' *Developmental Medicine and Child Neurology,* **18**, 643–656.

Fenichel, G.M., Phillips, J.A. (1989) 'Familial aplasia of the cerebellar vermis— possible X-linked dominant inheritance.' *Archives of Neurology,* **46**, 582–583.

Fernandes, E.T., Reinberg, Y., Vernier, R., Gonzalez, R. (1994) 'Neurogenic bladder dysfunction in children: review of pathophysiology and current management.' *Journal of Pediatrics,* **124**, 1–7.

Fernbach, S.K., McLone, D.G. (1985) 'Derangement of swallowing in children with myelomeningocele.' *Pediatric Radiology,* **15**, 311–314.

Ferrer, I. (1984) 'A Golgi analysis of unlayered polymicrogyria.' *Acta Neuropathologica,* **65**, 69–76.

—— Galofré, E. (1987) 'Dendritic spine anomalies in fetal alcohol syndrome.' *Neuropediatrics,* **18**, 161–163.

Ferrie, C.D., Jackson, G.D., Giannakodimos, S., Panayiotopoulos, C.P. (1995) 'Posterior agyria–pachygyria with polymicrogyria. Evidence for an inherited neuronal migration disorder.' *Neurology,* **45**, 150–153.

Finnell, R.H., Taylor, L.E., Bennett, G.D. (1993) 'The impact of maternal hyperthermia on morphogenesis: clinical and experimental evidence for a fetal hyperthermia phenotype.' *Developmental Brain Dysfunction,* **6**, 199–209.

Fishman, M.A., Palkes, H.S., Schackelford, G.D., McAlister, W.H. (1977) 'Lacunar skull deformity and intelligence.' *Pediatrics,* **59**, 296–299.

Fitch, N., Resch, L., Rochon, L., (1982) 'The Neu–Laxova syndrome: comments on syndrome identification.' *American Journal of Medical Genetics,* **13**, 445–452.

Franzoni, E., Bernardi, B., Marchiani, V., *et al.* (1995) 'Band brain heterotopia. Case report and literature review.' *Neuropediatrics,* **26**, 37–40.

Freeman, J.M., Nelson, K.B. (1988) 'Intrapartum asphyxia and cerebral palsy.' *Pediatrics,* **82**, 240–249.

Freeman, M.V.R., Williams, D.W., Schimke, R.N., *et al.* (1974) 'The Roberts syndrome.' *Clinical Genetics,* **5**, 1–16.

Friede, R.L. (1978) 'Uncommon syndromes of cerebellar vermis aplasia. II: Tecto-cerebellar dysraphia with occipital encephalocele.' *Developmental Medicine and Child Neurology,* **20**, 764–772.

—— (1989) *Developmental Neuropathology, 2nd Edn.* Berlin: Springer.

—— Boltshauser, E. (1978) 'Uncommon syndromes of cerebellar vermis aplasia. I: Joubert syndrome.' *Developmental Medicine and Child Neurology,* **20**, 758–763.

—— Mikolasek, J. (1978) 'Postencephalitic porencephaly, hydranencephaly or polymicrogyria. A review.' *Acta Neuropathologica,* **43**, 161–168.

Fukuyama, Y., Osawa, M., Suzuki, H. (1981) 'Congenital progressive dystrophy of the Fukuyama type—clinical, genetic and pathological considerations.' *Brain and Development,* **3**, 1–29.

Fusco, L., Ferracuti, S., Fariello, G., *et al.* (1992) 'Hemimegalencephaly and normal intellectual development.' *Journal of Neurology, Neurosurgery, and Psychiatry,* **55**, 720–722.

Galaburda, A.M., Sherman, G.F., Rosen, G.D., *et al.* (1985) 'Developmental dyslexia: four consecutive patients with cortical anomalies.' *Annals of Neurology,* **18**, 222–233.

Gallucci, M., Bozzao, A., Curatolo, P., *et al.* (1991) 'MR imaging of incomplete band heterotopia.' *American Journal of Neuroradiology,* **12**, 701–702.

Garcia, C.A., Duncan, C. (1977) 'Atelencephalic microcephaly.' *Developmental Medicine and Child Neurology,* **19**, 227–232.

Garg, B.P. (1982) 'Colpocephaly: an error of morphogenesis.' *Archives of Neurology,* **39**, 243–246.

Gastaut, H., Pinsard, N., Raybaud, C., *et al.* (1987) 'Lissencephaly (agyria–pachygyria): clinical findings and serial EEG studies.' *Developmental Medicine and Child Neurology,* **29**, 167–180.

Giroud, A. (1960) 'Causes and morphogenesis of anencephaly.' *In:* Wolstenholme, G.E., O'Connor, C.M. (Eds.) *CIBA Foundation Symposium on Congenital Malformations.* Edinburgh: Churchill Livingstone, pp. 188–193.

Giudicelli, Y., Pierre-Kahn, A., Bourdeaux, A.M., *et al.* (1986) 'Are the metabolic characteristics of congenital intraspinal lipoma cells identical to, or different from normal adipocytes?' *Child's Nervous System,* **2**, 290–296.

Golden, J.A., Chernoff, G.F. (1995) 'Multiple sites of anterior neural tube closure in humans: evidence from anterior neural tube defects (anencephaly).' *Pediatrics,* **95**, 506–510.

Goodlin, R.C., Heidrick, W.P., Papenfuss, H.L., Kubitz, R.L. (1984) 'Fetal malformations associated with maternal hypoxia.' *American Journal of Obstetrics and Gynecology,* **149**, 228–229.

Goodman, S.I., Frerman, F.E. (1984) 'Glutaric acidaemia type II (multiple acyl-CoA dehydrogenation deficiency).' *Journal of Inherited Metabolic Diseases,* **7**, Suppl. 1, 33–37.

Gooskens, R.H.J.M., Willemse, J., Faber, J.A., Verdonck, A.F.M.M. (1989) 'Macrocephalies—a differential approach.' *Neuropediatrics,* **20**, 164–169.

Gordon, N. (1995) 'Folate metabolism and neural tube defects.' *Brain and Development,* **17**, 307–311.

Goutières, F., Aicardi, J., Rethoré, M.O., Lejeune, J. (1987) 'Syndrome de Miller–Dieker et translocation chromosomique (15;17).' *Archives Françaises de Pédiatrie,* **44**, 501–504.

Govaert, P., de Vries, L.S. (1997) *An Atlas of Neonatal Brain Sonography. Clinics in Developmental Medicine No. 141/142.* London: Mac Keith Press.

Gower, D.J., Pollay, M., Leech, R. (1994) 'Pediatric syringomyelia.' *Journal of Child Neurology,* **9**, 14–21.

Goy, A.M.C., Pinto, R.S., Raghavendra, B.N., *et al.* (1986) 'Intramedullary spinal cord tumors: MR imaging with emphasis on associated cysts.' *Radiology,* **161**, 381–386.

Graff-Radford, N.R., Bosch, E.P., Stears, J.C., Tranel, D. (1986) 'Developmental Foix–Chavany–Marie syndrome in identical twins.' *Annals of Neurology,* **20**, 632–635.

Granata, T., Battaglia, G., D'Incerti, L., *et al.* (1996) 'Schizencephaly: neuroradiologic and epileptologic findings.' *Epilepsia,* **37**, 1185–1193.

—— Farina, L., Faiella, A., *et al.* (1997) 'Familial schizencephaly associated with *EMX2* mutation.' *Neurology,* **48**, 1403–1406.

Grant, R., Hadley, D.M., Lang, D., *et al.* (1987a) 'MRI measurement of syrinx size before and after operation.' *Journal of Neurology, Neurosurgery, and Psychiatry,* **50**, 1685–1687.

—— Macpherson, P., *et al.* (1987b) 'Syringomyelia: cyst measurement by magnetic resonance imaging and comparision with symptoms, signs and disability.' *Journal of Neurology, Neurosurgery, and Psychiatry,* **50**, 1008–1014.

Greenberg, F., Stratton, R.F., Lockaart, L.H., *et al.* (1986) 'Familial Miller–Dieker syndrome associated with pericentric inversion of chromosome 17.' *American Journal of Medical Genetics,* **23**, 853–859.

Greenwood, R.D., Rosenthal, A., Parisi, L., *et al.* (1975) 'Extracardiac abnormalities in infants with congenital heart disease.' *Pediatrics,* **55**, 485–492.

Gressens, P., Richelme, C., Kadhim, H.J., *et al.* (1992) 'The germinative zone produces the most cortical astrocytes after neural migration in the developing mammalian brain.' *Biology of the Neonate,* **61**, 4–24.

Griebel, M.L., Williams, J.P., Russell, S.S., *et al.* (1995) 'Clinical and developmental findings in children with giant interhemispheric cysts and dysgenesis of the corpus callosum.' *Pediatric Neurology,* **13**, 119–124.

Gross, S.J., Oehler, J.M., Eckerman, C.O. (1983) 'Head growth and developmental outcome in very low-birth-weight infants.' *Pediatrics,* **71**, 70–75.

Guerrini, R., Dravet, C., Raybaud, C., *et al.* (1992a) 'Neurological findings and seizure outcome in children with bilateral opercular macrogyric-like changes detected by MRI.' *Developmental Medicine and Child Neurology,* **34**, 694–705.

—— *et al.* (1992b) 'Epilepsy and focal gyral anomalies detected by MRI: electroclinico-morphological correlations and follow-up.' *Developmental Medicine and Child Neurology,* **34**, 706–718.

—— Bureau, M., *et al.* (1996a) 'Diffuse and localized dysplasias of the cerebral cortex: clinical presentation, outcome, and proposal for a morphologic MRI classification based on a study of 90 patients.' *In:* Guerrini, R., Andermann, F., Canapicchi, R., *et al.* (Eds.) *Dysplasias of Cerebral Cortex and Epilepsy.* Philadelphia: Lippincott–Raven, pp. 255–269.

—— Parmeggiani, A., Bureau, M., *et al.* (1996b) 'Localized cortical dysplasia: good seizure outcome after sleep-related electrical status epilepticus.' *In:* Guerrini, R., Andermann, F., Canapicchi, R., *et al.* (Eds.) *Dysplasias of Cerebral Cortex and Epilepsy.* Philadelphia: Lippincott–Raven, pp. 329–335.

—— Dubeau, F., Dulac, O., *et al.* (1997) 'Bilateral parasagittal, parietooccipital polymicrogyria and epilepsy.' *Annals of Neurology,* **41**, 65–73.

Guthkelch, A.N. (1974) 'Diastematomyelia with median septum.' *Brain,* **97**, 729–742.

Hageman, G., Hoogenraad, T.U., Prevo, R.L. (1994) 'The association of cortical dysplasia and anterior horn arthrogryposis: a case report.' *Brain and Development,* **16**, 463–466.

Hakamada, S., Watanabe, K., Hari, K., Miyazaki, S. (1979) 'The evolution of electroencephalographic features in lissencephaly syndrome.' *Brain and Development,* **4**, 277–283.

Hall, P.V., Campbell, R.L., Kalsbeck, J.E. (1975) 'Meningomyelocele and progressive hydromyelia: progressive paresis in myelodysplasia.' *Journal of Neurosurgery*, **43**, 457–463.

—— Lindseth, R., Campbell, R., et al. (1979) 'Scoliosis and hydrocephalus in myelocele patients: the effects of ventricular shunting.' *Journal of Neurosurgery*, **50**, 174–178.

Hanaway, J., Netsky, M.G. (1971) 'Heterotopias of the inferior olive: relation to Dandy–Walker malformation and correlation with experimental data.' *Journal of Neuropathology and Experimental Neurology*, **3**, 380–381.

Harbord, M.G., Lambert, S.R., Kriss, A., et al. (1989) 'Autosomal recessive microcephaly, mental retardation with nonpigmentary retinopathy and a distinctive electroretinogram.' *Neuropediatrics*, **20**, 139–141.

—— Boyd, S., Hall-Crags, M.A., et al. (1990) 'Ataxia, developmental delay and an extensive neuronal migration abnormality in 2 siblings.' *Neuropediatrics*, **21**, 218–221.

Harding, B.N., Boyd, S.G. (1991) 'Intractable seizures from infancy can be associated with dentato-olivary dysplasia.' *Journal of the Neurological Sciences*, **104**, 157–165.

Harding, B.R., Copp, J.A. (1997) 'Malformations.' *In:* Graham, D.L., Lantos, P.L. (Eds.) *Greenfield's Neuropathology, 6th Edn.* London: Arnold, pp. 397–533.

Harmant-Van Rijkevorsel, G., Aubert-Tulkens, G., Moulin, D. (1983) 'Le syndrome de Joubert. Etude clinique et anatomo-pathologique.' *Revue Neurologique*, **139**, 715–724.

Harris, C.P., Townsend, J.J., Klatt, E.C. (1994a) 'Accessory brains (extracerebral heterotopias): unusual prenatal intracranial mass lesions.' *Journal of Child Neurology*, **9**, 386–389.

—— Norman, M.G., et al. (1994b) 'Atelencephalic holoprosencephaly.' *Journal of Child Neurology*, **9**, 412–416.

Harrison, M.J., Mitnick, R.J., Rosenblum, B.R., Rothman, A.S. (1990) 'Leptomyelolipoma: analysis of 20 cases.' *Journal of Neurosurgery*, **73**, 360–367.

Hart, M.N., Malamud, N., Ellis, W.G. (1972) 'The Dandy–Walker syndrome.' *Neurology*, **22**, 771–780.

Hashimoto, R., Seki, T., Takuma, Y., Suzuki, N. (1993) 'The 'double cortex' syndrome on MRI.' *Brain and Development*, **15**, 57–59.

Haslam, R., Smith, D.W. (1979) 'Autosomal dominant microcephaly.' *Journal of Pediatrics*, **95**, 701–705.

Haverkamp, F., Zerres, K., Ostertun, B., et al. (1995) 'Familial schizencephaly: further delineation of a rare disorder.' *Journal of Medical Genetics*, **32**, 242–244.

Hays, R.M., Jordan, R.A., McLaughlin, J.F., et al. (1989) 'Central ventilatory dysfunction in myelodysplasia: an independent determinant of survival.' *Developmental Medicine and Child Neurology*, **31**, 366–370.

Hayward, J.C., Titelbaum, D.S., Clancy, R.R., Zimmerman, R.A. (1991) 'Lissencephaly–pachygyria associated with congenital cytomegalovirus infection.' *Journal of Child Neurology*, **6**, 109–114.

Hecht, F., Kelly, J.V. (1979) 'Little heads: inheritance and early detection.' *Journal of Pediatrics*, **95**, 731–732.

Hendrick, E.B., Hoffman, H.J., Humphreys, R.P. (1977) 'Tethered cord syndrome.' *In:* McLaurin, R.L. (Ed.) *Myelomeningocele.* New York: Grune & Stratton, pp. 369–373.

Hersh, J.H., Podruch, P.E., Rogers, G., Weisskopf, B. (1985) 'Toluene embryopathy.' *Journal of Pediatrics*, **106**, 922–927.

Hilal, S.K., Marton, D., Pollack, E. (1974) 'Diastematomyelia in children: radiographic study of 34 cases.' *Radiology*, **112**, 609–621.

Hirano, S., Houdou, S., Hasegawa, M., et al. (1992) 'Clinicopathologic studies on leptomeningeal glioneuronal heterotopia in congenital anomalies.' *Pediatric Neurology*, **8**, 441–444.

Hirayama, K., Hoshino, Y., Kumashiro, M., Yamamoto, T. (1994) 'Reverse Shapiro's syndrome. A case of agenesis of the corpus callosum associated with periodic hyperthermia.' *Archives of Neurology*, **51**, 494–496.

Hirsch, J.F., Pierre-Kahn, A. (1988) 'Lumbosacral lipomas with spina bifida.' *Child's Nervous System*, **4**, 354–360.

—— —— Renier, D., et al. (1984) 'The Dandy–Walker malformation.' *Journal of Neurosurgery*, **61**, 515–522.

Hobbins, J.C. (1991) 'Diagnosis and management of neural-tube defects today.' *New England Journal of Medicine*, **324**, 690–691.

Hoffmann, G.F., Trefz, F.K., Barth, P.G., et al. (1991) 'Macrocephaly: an important indication for organic acid analysis.' *Journal of Inherited Metabolic Disease*, **14**, 329–332.

Hoffman, H.J., Taecholarn, C., Hendrick, E.B., Humphreys, R.P. (1985) 'Management of lipomyelomeningoceles. Experience at the Hospital for Sick Children, Toronto.' *Journal of Neurosurgery*, **62**, 1–8.

—— Neill, J., Crone, K.R., et al. (1987) 'Hydrosyringomyelia and its management in childhood.' *Neurosurgery*, **21**, 347–351.

Holinger, P.C., Holinger, L.D., Reichert, T.J., Holinger, P.H. (1978) 'Respiratory obstruction and apnea in infants with bilateral abductor vocal cord paralysis, meningomyelocele, hydrocephalus and Arnold–Chiari malformation.' *Journal of Pediatrics*, **92**, 368–373.

Holmes, L.B., Driscoll, S.G., Atkins, L. (1976) 'Etiologic heterogeneity of neural-tube defects.' *New England Journal of Medicine*, **294**, 365–369.

Holtzman, N.A. (1983) 'Prenatal screening for neural tube defects.' *Pediatrics*, **71**, 658–660.

Hori, A., Orthner, H., Kohlschütter, A., et al. (1980) 'CNS dysplasia in dysencephalia splanchnocystica (Gruber's syndrome). A case report.' *Acta Neuropathologica*, **51**, 93–97.

—— Friede, R.L., Fischer, G. (1983) 'Ventricular diverticula with localized dysgenesis of the temporal lobe in cloverleaf skull anomaly.' *Acta Neuropathologica*, **60**, 132–136.

Hourihane, J.O'B., Bennett, C.P., Chaudhuri, R., et al. (1993) 'A sibship with a neuronal migration defect, cerebellar hypoplasia and congenital lymphedema.' *Neuropediatrics*, **24**, 43–46.

Hoyt, W.F., Kaplan, S.L., Grumbach, M.M., Glaser, T.S. (1970) 'Septo-optic dysplasia in pituitary dwarfism.' *Lancet*, **1**, 893–894.

Hsia, Y.E., Bratu, M., Herbordt, A. (1971) 'Genetics of the Meckel syndrome (dysencephalia splanchnocystica).' *Pediatrics*, **48**, 237–247.

Hughes, H.E., Miskin, M. (1986) 'Congenital microcephaly due to vascular disruption: in utero documentation.' *Pediatrics*, **78**, 85–87.

Humphreys, P., Rosen, G.D., Press, D.M., et al. (1991) 'Freezing lesions of the developing rat brain: a model for cerebrocortical microgyria.' *Journal of Neuropathology and Experimental Neurology*, **50**, 145–160.

Hunt, G.M. (1990) 'Open spina bifida: outcome for a complete cohort treated unselectively and followed into adulthood.' *Developmental Medicine and Child Neurology*, **32**, 108–118.

—— Whitaker, R.H. (1987) 'The pattern of congenital renal anomalies associated with neural-tube defects.' *Developmental Medicine and Child Neurology*, **29**, 91–95.

Huttenlocher, P.R. (1974) 'Dendritic development in neocortex of children with mental defect and infantile spasms.' *Neurology*, **24**, 203–210.

—— Taravath, S., Mojtahedi, S. (1994) 'Periventricular heterotopia and epilepsy.' *Neurology*, **44**, 51–55.

Ianetti, P., Raucci, U., Basile, L.A., et al. (1993) 'Neuronal migrational disorders: diffuse cortical dysplasia or the "double cortex" syndrome.' *Acta Paediatrica*, **82**, 501–503.

Iida, K., Hirano, S., Takashima, S., Miyahara, S. (1994) 'Developmental study of leptomeningeal glioneuronal heterotopia.' *Pediatric Neurology*, **10**, 295–298.

Itoh, N., Mimaki, T., Tagawa, T., et al. (1988) 'Chiari I malformation with quadriplegia and respiratory disturbance in an infant.' *Brain and Development*, **10**, 189–190.

Izquierdo, J.M., Gil-Carcedo, L.M. (1988) 'Recurrent meningitis and transethmoidal intranasal meningoencephalocele.' *Developmental Medicine and Child Neurology*, **30**, 248–251.

Jaeken, J., Carchon, H. (1993) 'The carbohydrate-deficient glycoprotein syndromes: an overview.' *Journal of Inherited Metabolic Diseases*, **16**, 813–820.

—— Van den Berghe, G. (1984) 'An infantile autistic syndrome characterized by the presence of succinyl purines in body fluids.' *Lancet*, 2, 958–1061.

Jaffe, M., Tirosh, E., Oren, S. (1987) 'The dilemma in prenatal diagnosis of idiopathic microcephaly.' *Developmental Medicine and Child Neurology*, **29**, 187–189.

James, C.C.M., Lassman, L.P. (1981) *Spina Bifida Occulta. Orthopedic, Radiological and Neurosurgical Aspects.* New York: Grune & Stratton.

James, H.E., Williams, J., Brock, W., et al. (1984) 'Radical removal of lipomas of the conus and cauda equina with laser microneurosurgery.' *Neurosurgery*, **15**, 340–343.

James, W.H. (1980) 'The sex ratios of anencephalics born to anencephalic-prone women.' *Developmental Medicine and Child Neurology*, **22**, 618–622.

Janota, I., Polkey, C.E. (1992) 'Cortical dysplasia in epilepsy—a study of material from surgical resections for intractable epilepsy.' *In:* Pedley, T.R., Meldrum, B.S. (Eds.) *Recent Advances in Epilepsy.* Edinburgh: Churchill Livingstone, pp. 37–49.

Jaspan, T., Worthington, B.S., Holland, I.M. (1988) 'A comparative study of magnetic resonance imaging and computer tomography-assisted myelography in spinal dysraphism.' *British Journal of Radiology*, **61**, 445–453.

Jaworski, M., Hersh, J.H., Donat, J.A., *et al.* (1986) 'Computed tomography of the head in the evaluation of microcephaly.' *Pediatrics*, **78**, 1064–1069.

Jeeves, M.A., Temple, C.M. (1987) 'A further study of language function in callosal agenesis.' *Brain and Language*, **32**, 325–335.

Jellinger, K., Gross, N., Kaltenbäck, E., Grisold, W. (1981) 'Holoprosencephaly and agenesis of corpus callosum. Frequency of associated malformations.' *Acta Neuropathologica*, **55**, 1–10.

Jeret, J.S., Serur, D., Wisniewski, K., Fish, C. (1985–1986) 'Frequency of agenesis of the corpus callosum in the developmentally disabled population as determined by computerized tomography.' *Pediatric Neuroscience*, **12**, 101–103.

—— —— —— Lubin, R.A. (1987) 'Clinicopathological findings associated with agenesis of the corpus callosum.' *Brain and Development*, **9**, 255–264.

Jiménez, P., Colamaria, V., Avesani, E., *et al.* (1994) 'Studio elettroclinico e neuroradiologico di tre casi affetti da "Eterotopia Gigante" della sostanza grigia. Un nuevo disturbo della migrazione neuronale.' *In: XVI Congresso Nazionale Societa Italiana di Neuropsichiatria Infantile, Brescia, 21–24 Settembre 1994, Atti, Vol. III*, pp. 1061–1063.

Jones, K., Smith, D.W., Ulleland, C., Streissguth, A.P. (1973) 'Pattern of malformations in offspring of chronic alcoholic mothers.' *Lancet*, **1**, 1267–1271.

Jones, K.L., Gilbert, F., Kaveggia, E.G. (1980) 'The Miller–Dieker syndrome.' *Pediatrics*, **66**, 277–281.

—— Lacro, R.V., Johnson, K.A., Adams, J. (1989) 'Pattern of malformations in the children of women treated with carbamazepine during pregnancy.' *New England Journal of Medicine*, **320**, 1661–1666.

Joubert, M., Eisenring, J-J., Robb, J.P., Andermann, F. (1969) 'Familial agenesis of the cerebellar vermis. A syndrome of episodic hyperpnea, abnormal eye movements, ataxia, and retardation.' *Neurology*, **19**, 813–825.

Kahn, A.P., Hirsch, J.F., Da Lage, C., *et al.* (1971) 'Les kystes entériques intra-rachidiens (3 observations).' *Neurochirurgie*, **17**, 33–34.

Kalifa, G., Chiron, C., Sellier, N., *et al.* (1987) 'Hemimegalencephaly: MR imaging in five children.' *Radiology*, **165**, 29–34.

Kalter, H., Warkany, J. (1983) 'Congenital malformations: etiologic factors and their role in prevention.' *New England Journal of Medicine*, **308**, 424–431.

Kamuro, K., Tenokuchi, Y-I. (1993) 'Familial periventricular nodular heterotopia.' *Brain and Development*, **15**, 237–241.

Kanev, P.M., Lemire, R.J., Loeser, J.D., Berger, M.S. (1990) 'Management and long-term follow-up review of children with lipomyelomeningocele, 1952–1987.' *Journal of Neurosurgery*, **73**, 48–52.

Kaplan, P. (1983) 'X-linked recessive inheritance of agenesis of the corpus callosum.' *Journal of Medical Genetics*, **20**, 122–124.

Kaplowitz, P.B., Bodurtha, D. (1993) 'Congenital hypopituitarism and microphthalmia. Report of two cases.' *Acta Paediatrica*, **82**, 419–422.

Kaufmann, W.E., Galaburda, A.M. (1989) 'Cerebrocortical microdysgenesis in neurologically normal subjects: a histopathologic study.' *Neurology*, **39**, 238–244.

Keefover, R., Sam, M., Bodensteiner, J., Nicholson, A. (1995) 'Hypersomnolence and pure central sleep apnea associated with the Chiari I malformation.' *Journal of Child Neurology*, **10**, 65–67.

Kendall, B., Kingsley, D., Lambert, S.R., *et al.* (1990) 'Joubert syndrome: a clinico-radiological study.' *Neuroradiology*, **31**, 502–506.

Khoury, M.J., Erickson, J.D., Cordero, J.F., McCarthy, B.J. (1988) 'Congenital malformations and intrauterine growth retardation: a population study.' *Pediatrics*, **82**, 83–90.

—— Cordero, J.F., Mulinare, J., Opitz, J.M. (1989) 'Selected midline defect associations: a population study.' *Pediatrics*, **84**, 266–272.

King, M.D., Dudgeon, J., Stephenson, J.B.P. (1984) 'Joubert's syndrome with retinal dysplasia: neonatal tachypnoea as the clue to a genetic brain–eye malformation.' *Archives of Disease in Childhood*, **59**, 709–718.

—— Stephenson, J.B.P., Ziervogel, M., *et al.* (1985) 'Hemimegalencephaly— a case for hemispherectomy?' *Neuropediatrics*, **16**, 46–55.

Klingensmith, W.C., Cioffi-Ragan, D.T. (1986) 'Schizencephaly: diagnosis and progression in utero.' *Radiology*, **159**, 617–618.

Kloepfer, H.W., Platou, R.V., Hansche, W.J. (1964) 'Manifestations of a recessive gene for microcephaly in a population isolate.' *Journal de Génétique Humaine*, **13**, 52–59.

Knobloch, W.H., Layer, J.M. (1971) 'Retinal detachment and encephalocele.' *Journal of Pediatric Ophthalmology*, **8**, 181–184.

Kobori, J.A., Herrick, M.K., Urich, H. (1987) 'Arhinencephaly: the spectrum of associated malformations.' *Brain*, **110**, 237–260.

Kokmen, E., Marsh, W.R., Baker, H.L. (1985) 'Magnetic resonance imaging

in syringomyelia.' *Neurosurgery*, **17**, 267–270.

Konkol, R.J., Maister, B.H., Wells, R.G., Sty, J.R. (1990) 'Hemimegalencephaly: clinical, EEG, neuroimaging and IMP-SPECT correlation.' *Pediatric Neurology*, **6**, 414–418.

Korithenberg, R., Palm, D., Schlake, W., Klein, J. (1984) 'Congenital muscular dystrophy, brain malformation and ocular problems (muscle, eye and brain disease) in two German families.' *European Journal of Pediatrics*, **142**, 64–68.

Kothari, M.J., Kelly, M., Darbey, M., *et al.* (1995) 'Neurophysiologic assessment of urinary dysfunction in children with thoracic syringomyelia.' *Journal of Child Neurology*, **10**, 451–454.

Kroon, A.A., Smit, B.J., Barth, P.G., Hennekam, R.C.M. (1996) 'Lissencephaly with extreme cerebral and cerebellar hypoplasia. A magnetic resonance imaging study.' *Neuropediatrics*, **27**, 273–276.

Kushnet, M.W., Goldman, R.L. (1978) 'Lipoma of the corpus callosum associated with a frontal bone defect.' *American Journal of Roentgenology*, **131**, 517–518.

Kuzniecky, R. (1994) 'Familial diffuse cortical dysplasia.' *Archives of Neurology*, **51**, 307–310.

—— Berkovic, S., Andermann, F., *et al.* (1986) 'Focal cortical myoclonus and rolandic cortical dysplasia: clarification by magnetic resonance imaging.' *Annals of Neurology*, **23**, 317–325.

—— Andermann, F., Tampieri, D., *et al.* (1989) 'Bilateral central macrogyria: epilepsy, pseudobulbar palsy, and mental retardation—a recognizable neuronal migration disorder.' *Annals of Neurology*, **25**, 547–554.

—— Garcia, J.H., Faught, E., Morawetz, R.B. (1991) 'Cortical dysplasia in temporal lobe epilepsy: magnetic resonance imaging correlations.' *Annals of Neurology*, **29**, 293–298.

—— Andermann, F., and the CBPS Study Group (1994a) 'The congenital bilateral perisylvian syndrome: imaging findings in a muticenter study.' *American Journal of Neuroradiology*, **15**, 139–144.

—— —— Guerrini, R. (1994b) 'Infantile spasms: an early epileptic manifestation in some patients with the congenital bilateral perisylvian syndrome.' *Journal of Child Neurology*, **9**, 420–423.

—— —— —— and the CBPS Multicenter Collaborative Study (1994c) 'The epileptic spectrum in the congenital bilateral perisylvian syndrome.' *Neurology*, **44**, 379–385.

Kyllerman, M., Blomstrand, S., Månsson, J-E., *et al.* (1990) 'Central nervous system malformations and white matter changes in pseudo-neonatal adrenoleukodystrophy.' *Neuropediatrics*, **21**, 199–201.

Lammer, E.J., Chen, D.T., Hoar, R.M., *et al.* (1985) 'Retinoic acid embryopathy.' *New England Journal of Medicine*, **313**, 837–841.

Larroche, J.C. (1977) 'Cytoarchitectonic abnormalities (abnormalities of cell migration).' *In:* Vinken, P.J., Bruyn, G.W. (Eds.) *Handbook of Clinical Neurology. Vol. 30. Congenital Malformations of the Brain and Skull, Part I.* Amsterdam: North Holland, pp. 479–506.

—— (1986) 'Fetal encephalopathies of circulatory origin.' *Biology of the Neonate*, **50**, 61–74.

Laurence, K.M. (1964) 'Natural history of spina bifida cystica: detailed analysis of 407 cases.' *Archives of Disease in Childhood*, **39**, 41–57.

Layton, D.D. (1962) 'Heterotopic cerebral gray matter as an epileptogenic focus.' *Journal of Neuropathology and Experimental Neurology*, **21**, 244–249.

Leão, M.J., Ribeiro-Silva, M.L. (1995) 'Orofaciodigital syndrome type I in a patient with severe CNS defects.' *Pediatric Neurology*, **13**, 247–251.

Leblanc, E., Tampieri, D., Robitaille, Y., *et al.* (1990) 'Developmental anterobasal temporal encephaloceles and temporal lobe epilepsy: delineation of the syndrome and surgical considerations.' *In: Proceedings of the 2nd International Cleveland Clinic Epilepsy Symposium*, p. 46.

Lee, B.C.P., Zimmerman, R.D., Manning, J.J., Deck, M.D.F. (1985) 'MR imaging of syringomyelia and hydromyelia.' *American Journal of Neuroradiology*, **6**, 221–228.

Lee, N., Radtke, R.A., Gray, L., *et al.* (1994) 'Neuronal migration disorders: positron emission tomography correlations.' *Annals of Neurology*, **35**, 290–297.

Leech, R.W., Shuman, R.M. (1986a) 'Holoprosencephaly and related midline cerebral anomalies: a review.' *Journal of Child Neurology*, **1**, 3–18.

—— —— (1986b) 'Midline telencephalic dysgenesis: report of three cases.' *Journal of Child Neurology*, **1**, 224–232.

Lemire, R.J., Loeser, J.D., Leech, R.W., Alvord, E.C. (1975) *Normal and Abnormal Development of the Human Nervous System.* Hagerstown, MD: Harper & Row.

Levin, S., Robinson, R.O., Aicardi, J., Hoare, R.D. (1984) 'Computed tomographic appearance in the linear sebaceous nevus syndrome.' *Neuroradiology*, **26**, 469–472.

Lie, R.T., Wilcox, A.J., Skjaerven, R. (1994) 'A population-based study of the risk of recurrence of birth defects.' *New England Journal of Medicine*, **331**, 1–4.

Lieblich, J.M., Rosen, S.W., Guyda, H., *et al.* (1978) 'The syndrome of basal encephalocele and hypothalamic–pituitary dysfunction.' *Annals of Internal Medicine*, **89**, 910–916.

Lincke, C.R., van den Bogert, C., Nijtmans, L.G.J., *et al.* (1996) 'Cerebellar hypoplasia in respiratory chain dysfunction.' *Neuropediatrics*, **27**, 216–218.

Lindhout, D., Barth, P.G. (1985) 'Chorioretinal coloboma and Joubert syndrome.' *Journal of Pediatrics*, **107**, 158. *(Letter.)*

—— Schmidt, D. (1986) 'In-utero exposure to valproate and neural tube defects.' *Lancet*, **1**, 1392–1393.

—— Barth, P.G., Valk, J., Boen-Tan, T.N. (1980) 'Joubert syndrome associated with bilateral chorioretinal coloboma.' *European Journal of Pediatrics*, **134**, 173–176.

Lipson, A., Beuhler, B., Bartley, J., *et al.* (1984) 'Maternal hyperphenylalaninemia fetal effects.' *Journal of Pediatrics*, **104**, 216–220.

Liptak, G.S., Bloss, J.W., Briskin, H., *et al.* (1988) 'The management of children with spinal dysraphism.' *Journal of Child Neurology*, **3**, 3–20.

Little, B.B., Knoll, K.A., Klein, V.R., Heller, K.B. (1990) 'Hereditary cranium bifidum and symmetric parietal foramina are the same entity.' *American Journal of Medical Genetics*, **35**, 453–458.

Livingston, J.H., Aicardi, J. (1990) 'Unusual MRI appearance of diffuse subcortical heterotopia or 'double-cortex' in two children.' *Journal of Neurology, Neurosurgery, and Psychiatry*, **53**, 617–620.

Logue, V., Edwards, M.R. (1981) 'Syringomyelia and its surgical treatment. An analysis of 75 patients.' *Journal of Neurology, Neurosurgery, and Psychiatry*, **44**, 273–284.

Lorber, J. (1972) 'Spina bifida cystica: results of treatment of 270 consecutive cases with criteria for selection in the future.' *Archives of Disease in Childhood*, **47**, 854–873.

—— (1974) 'Selective treatment of myelomeningocele. To treat or not to treat.' *Pediatrics*, **53**, 307–310.

—— (1975) 'Ethical problems in the management of myelomeningocele and hydrocephalus.' *Journal of the Royal College of Physicians*, **10**, 47–60.

—— Priestley, B.L. (1981) 'Children with large heads: a practical approach to diagnosis in 557 children with special reference to 109 children with megalencephaly.' *Developmental Medicine and Child Neurology*, **23**, 494–504.

—— Schofield, J.K. (1979) 'The prognosis of occipital encephalocele.' *Zeitschrift für Kinderchirurgie*, **28**, 347–351.

Lott, I.T., Williams, R.S., Schnur, J.A., Hier, D.B. (1979) 'Familial amentia, unusual ventricular calcifications and increased cerebrospinal fluid protein.' *Neurology*, **29**, 1571–1577.

Luciano, R. (1987) 'Epidemiology and etiology of neural tube defects: an updating.' *Journal of Pediatric Neuroscience*, **3**, 57–71.

Luthy, D.A., Wardinsky, T., Shurtleff, D.B., *et al.* (1991) 'Cesarean section before the onset of labor and subsequent motor function in infants with meningomyelocele diagnosed antenatally.' *New England Journal of Medicine*, **324**, 662–666.

Lyon, G., Beaugerie, A. (1988) 'Congenital developmental malformations' *In:* Levene, M.I., Bennett, M.J., Punt, J. (Eds.) *Fetal and Neonatal Neurology and Neurosurgery*. Edinburgh: Churchill Livingstone, pp. 231–248.

—— Gastaut, H. (1985) 'Considerations on the significance attributed to unusual cerebral histological findings recently described in eight patients with primary generalized epilepsy.' *Epilepsia*, **26**, 365–367.

—— Robain, O. (1967) 'Encephalopathies circulatoires prénatales et paranatales.' *Acta Neuropathologica*, **9**, 79–98.

Marchal, G., Andermann, F., Tampieri, D., *et al.* (1989) 'Generalized cortical dysplasia manifested by diffusely thick cerebral cortex.' *Archives of Neurology*, **46**, 430–434.

Mariani, C., Cislaghi, M.G., Barbieri, S., *et al.* (1991) 'The natural history and results of surgery in 50 cases of syringomyelia.' *Journal of Neurology*, **238**, 433–438.

Marin-Padilla, M. (1978) 'Dual origin of the mammalian neocortex and evolution of the cortical plate.' *Anatomy and Embryology*, **152**, 109–126.

—— (1980) 'Morphogenesis of experimental encephalocele (cranioschisis occulta).' *Journal of the Neurological Sciences*, **46**, 83–89.

—— (1984) 'Neurons of layer I. A developmental analysis.' *In:* Peters, A., Jones, E.G. (Eds.) *Cerebral Cortex. Vol. 1. Cellular Components of the Cerebral Cortex*. New York: Plenum Press, pp. 447–478.

—— (1991) 'Cephalic axial skeletal–neural dysraphic disorders: embryology and pathology.' *Canadian Journal of Neurological Sciences*, **18**, 153–169.

Marques-Dias, M.J., Harmant-Van Rijckevorsel, G., Landrieu, P., Lyon, G. (1984) 'Prenatal cytomegalovirus disease and cerebral microgyria: evidence for perfusion failure, not disturbance of histogenesis, as the major cause of fetal cytomegalovirus encephalopathy.' *Neuropediatrics*, **15**, 18–24.

Martinez-Lage, J.F., Casas, C., Fernández, M.A., *et al.* (1994) 'Macrocephaly, dystonia, and bilateral temporal arachnoid cysts: glutaric aciduria type 1.' *Child's Nervous System*, **10**, 198–203.

—— Esteban, J.A., Poza, M., Casas, C. (1995) 'Congenital dermal sinus associated with an abscessed intramedullary epidermoid cyst in a child: case report and review of the literature.' *Child's Nervous System*, **11**, 301–305.

—— Poza, M., Sola, J., *et al.* (1996) 'The child with a cephalocele: etiology, neuroimaging, and outcome.' *Child's Nervous System*, **12**, 540–550.

Masera, N., Grant, D.B., Stanhope, R., Preece, M.A. (1994) 'Diabetes insipidus with impaired osmotic regulation in septo-optic dysplasia and agenesis of the corpus callosum.' *Archives of Disease in Childhood*, **70**, 51–53.

Matson, D.D. (1969) *Neurosurgery of Infancy and Childhood, 2nd Edn*. Springfield, IL: C.C. Thomas.

Matsunaga, E., Shiota, K. (1987) 'Holoprosencephaly in human embryos: epidemiologic studies of 150 cases.' *Brain Research*, **400**, 239–246.

Matsuzaka, T., Sakuragawa, N., Nakayama, H., *et al.* (1986) 'Cerebro-oculo-hepato-renal syndrome (Arima's syndrome): a distinct clinicopathological entity.' *Journal of Child Neurology*, **1**, 338–346.

Matthews, P.M., Brown, R.M., Otero, L., *et al.* (1993) 'Neurodevelopmental abnormalities and lactic acidosis in a girl with a 20-bp deletion in the X-linked pyruvate dehydrogenase E1α subunit gene.' *Neurology*, **43**, 2025–2030.

McBride, M.C., Kemper, T.L. (1982) 'Pathogenesis of four-layered microgyric cortex in man.' *Acta Neuropathologica*, **57**, 93–98.

McConnell, S. (1992) 'Perspectives on early brain development and the epilepsies.' *In:* Engel, J., Wasterlain, C., Cavalheiro, E.A., *et al.* (Eds.) *Molecular Neurobiology of Epilepsy. Epilepsy Research Supplement No. 9*. Amsterdam: Elsevier, pp. 183–191.

—— Kaznowski, C.E. (1991) 'Cell cycle dependence of laminar determination in developing neocortex.' *Science*, **254**, 282–285.

McGuire, E.J. (1985) 'Myelodysplasia: pathophysiology, applied neuroanatomy, and urologic manifestations.' *Journal of Pediatric Neuroscience*, **1**, 231–238.

McLaurin, R.L. (1987) 'Cranium bifidum and cranial cephaloceles.' *In:* Vinken, P.J., Bruyn, G.W. (Eds.) *Handbook of Clinical Neurology. Vol. 30. Congenital Malformations of the Brain and Skull, Part I*. Amsterdam: North Holland, pp. 209–217.

McLean, D.R., Miller, J.D.R., Allen, P.B.R., Ezzeddin, S.A. (1973) 'Posttraumatic syringomyelia.' *Journal of Neurosurgery*, **39**, 485–492.

McLone, D.G. (1980) 'Technique for closure of myelomeningocele.' *Child's Brain*, **6**, 65–73.

—— (1983) 'Results of treatment of children born with a myelomeningocele.' *Clinical Neurosurgery*, **30**, 407–412.

—— (1992) 'Continuing concepts in the management of spina bifida.' *Pediatric Neurosurgery*, **18**, 254–256.

—— Naidich, T.P. (1992) 'Developmental morphology of the subarachnoid space, brain vasculature, and contiguous structures, and the cause of the Chiari II malformation.' *American Journal of Neuroradiology*, **13**, 463–482.

—— Czyzewski, D., Raimondi, A.J., Sommers, R.C. (1982) 'Central nervous system infections as a limiting factor in the intelligence of children with meningomyelocele.' *Pediatrics*, **70**, 338–342.

—— Mutluer, S., Naidich, T.P. (1983) 'Lipomeningoceles of the conus medullaris.' *In:* Raimondi, J. (Ed.) *Concepts in Pediatric Neurosurgery, Vol. 3*. Basel: Karger, pp. 170–177.

—— Hayashida, S.F., Caldarelli, M. (1985) 'Surgical resection of lipomyelomeningoceles in 18 asymptomatic infants.' *Journal of Pediatric Neuroscience*, **1**, 239–244.

Meencke, H.J. (1987) 'Neuropathology of generalized primary epilepsy.' *In:* Wolf, P., Dam, D., Janz, D., Dreifuss, F.E. (Eds.) *Advances in Epileptology, Vol. 16*. New York: Raven Press, pp. 21–24.

—— (1994) 'Minimal developmental disturbances in epilepsy and MRI.' *In:* Shorvon, S.D., Fish, D.R., Andermann, F., *et al.* (Eds.) *Magnetic Resonance Scanning and Epilepsy*. New York: Plenum Press, pp. 127–136.

—— Janz, D. (1984) 'Neuropathological findings in primary generalized epilepsy. A study of eight cases.' *Epilepsia*, **25**, 8–21.

—— Veith, J. (1992) 'Migration disturbances in epilepsy.' *In:* Engel, J., Wasterlain, C., Cavalheiro, E.A., *et al.* (Eds.) *Molecular Neurobiology of Epilepsy. Epilepsy Research Supplement No. 9.* Amsterdam: Elsevier, pp. 31–40.

Menezes, A.V., MacGregor, D.L., Buncic, J.R. (1994) 'Aicardi syndrome: natural history and possible predictors of severity.' *Pediatric Neurology*, **11**, 313–318.

Menezes, L., Aicardi, J., Goutières, F. (1988) 'Absence of the septum pellucidum with porencephalia: a neuroradiologic syndrome with variable clinical expression.' *Archives of Neurology*, **45**, 542–545.

Menkes, J.H., Philippart, M., Clark, D.B. (1964) 'Hereditary partial agenesis of the corpus callosum.' *Archives of Neurology*, **11**, 198–208.

Mikati, M.A., Najjar, S.S., Sahli, I.F., *et al.* (1985) 'Microcephaly, hypergonadotrophic hypogonadism, short stature and minor anomalies: a new syndrome.' *American Journal of Medical Genetics*, **22**, 599–608.

Mikulis, D.J., Diaz, O., Egglin, T.K., Sanchez, R. (1992) 'Variance of the position of the cerebellar tonsils with age: preliminary report.' *Radiology*, **183**, 725–728.

Miller, E., Hare, J.W., Cloherty, J.P., *et al.* (1981) 'Elevated maternal hemoglobin A1c in early pregnancy and major congenital anomalies in infants of diabetic mothers.' *New England Journal of Medicine*, **304**, 1331–1334.

Miller, G.M., Stears, J.C., Guggenheim, M.A., Wilkening, G.N. (1984) 'Schizencephaly: a clinical and CT study.' *Neurology*, **34**, 997–1001.

Miller, R.W., Mulvihill, J.J. (1976) 'Small head size after atomic irradiation.' *Teratology*, **14**, 355–357.

Milunsky, A. (1980) 'Prenatal detection of neural tube defects. IV: Experience with 20,000 pregnancies.' *Journal of the American Medical Association*, **244**, 2731–2735.

—— (1986) 'The prenatal diagnosis of neural tube and other congenital defects.' *In:* Milunsky, A. (Ed.) *Genetic Disorders and the Fetus: Diagnosis, Prevention and Treatment. 2nd Edn.* New York: Plenum Press, pp. 453–519.

—— Jick, H., Jick, S.S., *et al.* (1989) 'Multivitaminic/folic acid supplementation in early pregnancy reduces the prevalence of neural tube defects.' *Journal of the American Medical Association*, **262**, 2847–2852.

Minns, R.A., Oag, J.C., Duffy, S.W., *et al.* (1980) 'In-dwelling urinary catheters in childhood spinal paralysis.' *Zeitschrift für Kinderchirurgie*, **31**, 387–397.

Moerman, P., Fryns, J-P., Vandenberghe, K., Lauweryns, J.M. (1992) 'Constrictive amniotic bands, amniotic adhesions, and limb–body wall complex: discrete disruption sequences with pathogenetic overlap.' *American Journal of Medical Genetics*, **42**, 470–479.

Mohanty, S., Rao, C.J., Shukla, P.K., *et al.* (1979) 'Intradural enterogenous cyst.' *Journal of Neurology, Neurosurgery, and Psychiatry*, **42**, 419–421.

Molina, J.A., Mateos, F., Merino, M., *et al.* (1989) 'Aicardi syndrome in two sisters.' *Journal of Pediatrics*, **115**, 282–283.

Morgan, D., Williams, B. (1992) 'Syringobulbia: a surgical appraisal.' *Journal of Neurology, Neurosurgery, and Psychiatry*, **55**, 1132–1141.

Mori, K., Hashimoto, T., Tayama, M., *et al.* (1994) 'Serial EEG and sleep polygraphic studies on lissencephaly (agyria–pachygyria).' *Brain and Development*, **16**, 365–373.

Morioka, M., Marubayashi, T., Masumitsu, T., *et al.* (1995) 'Basal encephaloceles with morning glory syndrome, and progressive hormonal and visual disturbances: case report and review of the literature.' *Brain and Development*, **17**, 196–201.

Morishima, A., Aranoff, G.S. (1986) 'Syndrome of septo-optic dysplasia: the clinical spectrum.' *Brain and Development*, **8**, 233–239.

Mortimer, E.A. (1980) 'The puzzling epidemiology of neural tube defects.' *Pediatrics*, **65**, 636–638.

MRC Study Research Group (1991) 'Prevention of neural tube defects: results of the Medical Research Council vitamin study.' *Lancet*, **338**, 131–137.

Murray, J.C., Johnson, J.A., Bird, T.D. (1985) 'Dandy–Walker malformation: etiologic heterogeneity and empiric recurrence risks.' *Clinical Genetics*, **28**, 272–283.

Myrianthopoulos, N.C., Chung, C.S. (1974) 'Congenital malformations in singletons: epidemiologic survey.' *Birth Defects Original Article Series*, **10** (4), 11–24.

Nadel, A.S., Green, J.K., Holmes, L.B., *et al.* (1990) 'Absence of need for amniocentesis in patients with elevated levels of maternal serum alpha-fetoprotein and normal ultrasonographic examinations.' *New England Journal of Medicine*, **323**, 557–561.

Naidich, T.P. (1989) 'Spinal dyraphism.' *International Pediatrics*, **4**, 89–97.

—— Pudlowski, R.M., Naidich, J.B. (1980a) 'Computed tomographic signs of the Chiari II malformation. Part II: Midbrain and cerebellum.' *Radiology*, **134**, 391–398.

—— —— —— (1980b) 'Computed tomographic signs of Chiari malformation. III: Ventricles and cisterns.' *Radiology*, **134**, 657–663.

—— —— —— *et al.* (1980c) 'Computed tomographic signs of the Chiari II malformation. I: Skull and dural partitions.' *Radiology*, **134**, 65–71.

—— McLone, D.G., Fulling, K.H. (1983a) 'The Chiari malformation. IV: The hindbrain deformity.' *Neuroradiology*, **25**, 179–197.

—— Mutluer, S. (1983b) 'A new understanding of dorsal dysraphism with lipoma (lipomyeloschisis): radiologic evaluation and surgical correction.' *American Journal of Neuroradiology*, **4**, 103–116.

—— Altman, N.R., Braffman, B.H., *et al.* (1992) 'Cephaloceles and related malformations.' *American Journal of Neuroradiology*, **13**, 655–690.

Nakano, K.K. (1973) 'Anencephaly: a review.' *Developmental Medicine and Child Neurology*, **15**, 383–400.

Natowicz, M., Chatten, J., Clancy, R., *et al.* (1988) 'Genetic disorders and major extracardiac anomalies associated with the hypoplastic left heart syndrome.' *Pediatrics*, **82**, 698–706.

Nelson, K., Ellenberg, J.H. (1986) 'Antecedents of cerebral palsy. Multivariate analysis of risk.' *New England Journal of Medicine*, **315**, 81–86.

—— Holmes, L.B. (1989) 'Malformations due to presumed spontaneous mutations in newborn infants.' *New England Journal of Medicine*, **320**, 19–23.

Neu, R.L., Kajii, T., Gardner, L.I., *et al.* (1971) 'A lethal syndrome of microcephaly with multiple congenital anomalies in three siblings.' *Pediatrics*, **47**, 610–612.

Nevin, N.C., Lim, J.H.K. (1990) 'Syndrome of partial aniridia, cerebellar ataxia, and mental retardation—Gillespie syndrome.' *American Journal of Medical Genetics*, **35**, 468–469.

Newman, G., Buschi, N., Sugg, N., *et al.* (1982) 'Dandy–Walker syndrome diagnosed in utero by ultrasonography.' *Neurology*, **32**, 180–184.

Nézelof, C., Jaubert, F., Lyon, G. (1976) 'Syndrome familial associant grêle court, malrotation interstinale, hypertrophie du pylore et malformations cérébrales. Etudes anatomo-clinique de trois observations' *Annales Anatomo-Pathologie*, **21**, 401–412.

Nicolaides, K.H., Campbell, S., Gabbe, S.G., Guidetti, R. (1986) 'Ultrasound screening for spina bifida: cranial and cerebellar signs.' *Lancet*, **2**, 72–74.

Nievelstein, R.A.J., Valk, J., Smit, L.M.E., Vermeij-Keers, C. (1994) 'MR of the caudal regression syndrome: embryologic implications.' *American Journal of Neuroradiology*, **15**, 1021–1029.

Njiokiktjien, C., Valk, J., Ramaekers, G. (1988) 'Malformation or damage of the corpus callosum? A clinical and MRI study.' *Brain and Development*, **10**, 92–99.

Nishikawa, M., Ichiyama, T., Hayashi, T., Furukawa, S. (1997) 'A case of early myoclonic encephalopathy with the congenital nephrotic syndrome.' *Brain and Development*, **19**, 144–147.

Noorani, P.A., Bodensteiner, J.B., Barnes, P.D. (1988) 'Colpocephaly: frequency and associated findings.' *Journal of Child Neurology*, **3**, 100–104.

Norio, R., Raitta, C., Lindahl, E. (1984) 'Further delineation of the Cohen syndrome; report on chorioretinal dystrophy, leukopenia and consanguinity.' *Clinical Genetics*, **25**, 1–14.

Norman, R.M. (1980) 'Bilateral encephaloclastic lesions in a 26-week gestation fetus: effect on neuroblast migration.' *Canadian Journal of Neurological Sciences*, **7**, 191–194.

—— Tingey, A.H., Valentine, J.C., Danby, T.A. (1967) 'Sudanophilic leucodystrophy in a pachygyric brain.' *Journal of Neurology, Neurosurgery, and Psychiatry*, **25**, 363–369.

—— Roberts, M., Sirois, J., Tremblay, L.J.M. (1976) 'Lissencephaly.' *Canadian Journal of Neurological Sciences*, **3**, 39–46.

Nyberg, D.A., Mack, L.A., Bronstein, A., *et al.* (1987) 'Holoprosencephaly: prenatal sonographic diagnosis.' *American Journal of Roentgenology*, **149**, 1051–1058.

Oba, H., Barkovich, A.J. (1995) 'Holoprosencephaly: an analysis of callosal formation and its relation to development of the interhemispheric fissure.' *American Journal of Neuroradiology*, **16**, 453–460.

Olson, D.M., Milstein, J.M. (1988) 'Hydromyelia associated with arrested hydrocephalus.' *Neurology*, **38**, 652–654.

Opitz, J.M., Penschaszadeh, V.B., Holt, M.C., Spano, L.M. (1987) 'Smith–Lemli–Opitz (RSH) syndrome bibliography.' *American Journal of Medical Genetics*, **28**, 745–750.

O'Rahilly, R., Müller, F. (1987) 'The developmental anatomy and histology of the human central nervous system.' *In:* Myrianthopoulos, N.C. (Ed.) *Handbook of Clinical Neurology. Vol. 6. No. 50. Malformations.* Amsterdam: North Holland, pp. 1–17.

Oren, J., Kelly, D.H., Todres, D., Shannon, D.C. (1986) 'Respiratory complications in patients with myelodysplasia and Arnold–Chiari malformation.' *American Journal of Diseases of Children*, **140**, 221–224.

Otsubo, H., Hwang, P.A., Jay, V., *et al.* (1993) 'Focal cortical dysplasia in children with localization-related epilepsy: EEG, MRI, and SPECT findings.' *Pediatric Neurology*, **9**, 101–107.

Ouvrier, R., Billson, F. (1986) 'Optic nerve hypoplasia: a review.' *Journal of Child Neurology*, **1**, 181–188.

Padget, D.H. (1972) 'Development of so-called dysraphism; with embryologic evidence of clinical Arnold–Chiari and Dandy–Walker malformations.' *Johns Hopkins Medical Journal*, **130**, 127–165.

Paetau, A., Salonen, R., Haltia, M. (1985) 'Brain pathology in the Meckel syndrome: a study of 59 cases.' *Clinical Neuropathology*, **4**, 56–62.

Pagon, R.A., Clarren, S.K., Millam, D.F., Hendrickson, A.E. (1983) 'Autosomal recessive eye and brain anomalies: Warburg syndrome.' *Journal of Pediatrics*, **102**, 542–546.

Paladin, F., Chiron, C., Dulac, O., *et al.* (1989) 'Electroencephalographic aspects of hemimegalencephaly.' *Developmental Medicine and Child Neurology*, **31**, 377–383.

Palm, I., Hagerstrand, I., Kristofferson, U., *et al.* (1986) 'Nephrosis and disturbances of neuronal migration in male siblings. A new hereditary disorder.' *Archives of Disease in Childhood*, **61**, 545–548.

Palmini, A., Andermann, F., Aicardi, J., *et al.* (1991a) 'Diffuse cortical dysplasia or the "double cortex" syndrome: the clinical and epileptic spectrum in 10 patients.' *Neurology*, **41**, 1656–1662.

—— —— Olivier, A., *et al.* (1991b) 'Neuronal migration disorders: a contribution of modern neuroimaging to the etiologic diagnosis of epilepsy.' *Canadian Journal of Neurological Sciences*, **18**, 580–587.

—— —— de Grissac, H., *et al.* (1993) 'Stages and patterns of centrifugal arrest of diffuse neuronal migration disorders.' *Developmental Medicine and Child Neurology*, **35**, 331–339.

—— Gambardella, A., Andermann, F., *et al.* (1996) 'The human dysplastic cortex is intrinsically epileptogenic.' *In:* Guerrini, R., Andermann, F., Canapicchi, R., *et al.* (Eds.) *Dysplasias of Cerebral Cortex and Epilepsy.* Philadelphia: Lippincott–Raven, pp. 43–52.

Pannell, B.W., Hendrick, E.B., Hoffman, H.J., Humphreys, R.P. (1982) 'Dermoid cysts of the anterior fontanelle.' *Neurosurgery*, **10**, 317–323.

Papasozomenos, S., Roessmann, U. (1981) 'Respiratory distress and Arnold–Chiari malformation.' *Neurology*, **31**, 97–100.

Parain, D., Gadisseux, J.F., Henocq, A., *et al.* (1985) 'Diagnostic prénatal et étude d'une microcéphalia vera à 26 semaines de gestation.' *In:* Szilwoski, H., Bormans, J. (Eds.) *Progrès en Neurologie Pédiatrique.* Bruxelles: Prodium, pp. 235–236.

Park, T.S., Hoffman, H.J., Hendrick, E.B., Humphreys, R.P. (1983) 'Experience with surgical decompression of the Arnold–Chiari malformation in young infants with myelomeningocele.' *Neurosurgery*, **13**, 147–152.

Parmeggiani, A., Santucci, M., Ambrosetto, P., *et al.* (1994) 'Interictal EEG findings in two cases with 'double cortex' syndrome.' *Brain and Development*, **16**, 320–324.

Parrish, M.L., Roessmann, U., Levinsohn, M.W. (1979) 'Agenesis of the corpus callosum: a study of the frequency of associated malformations.' *Annals of Neurology*, **6**, 349–354.

Pascual, J., Oterino, A., Berciano, J. (1992) 'Headache in type I Chiari malformation.' *Neurology*, **42**, 1519–1521.

Pascual-Castroviejo, I. (1985) 'The association of extracranial and intracranial vascular malformations in children.' *Canadian Journal of Neurological Sciences*, **12**, 139–148.

—— Velez, A., Pascual-Pascual, S-I., *et al.* (1991) 'Dandy–Walker malformation: analysis of 38 cases.' *Child's Nervous System*, **7**, 88–97.

—— Guttierez, M., Morales, C., *et al.* (1994) 'Primary degeneration of the granular layer of the cerebellum. A study of 14 patients and review of the literature.' *Neuropediatrics*, **25**, 183–190.

Passarge, E., Lenz, W. (1966) 'Syndrome of caudal regression in infants of diabetic mothers: observations of further cases.' *Pediatrics*, **37**, 672–675.

Patton, M.A., Sharma, A., Winter, R.M. (1985) 'The Aase–Smith syndrome.' *Clinical Genetics*, **28**, 521–525.

Pavone, L., Gullotta, F., Incorpora, G., *et al.* (1990) 'Isolated lissencephaly: report of four patients from two unrelated families.' *Journal of Child Neurology*, **5**, 52–59.

Peach, B. (1965) 'Arnold–Chiari malformation. Anatomic features of 20 cases.' *Archives of Neurology*, **12**, 527–535; 613–621.

Pelayo, R., Barasch, E., Kang, H., *et al.* (1994) 'Progressively intractable seizures, focal alopecia, and hemimegalencephaly.' *Neurology*, **44**, 969–971.

Pellicer, A., Cabañas, C., Pérez-Higueras, A., *et al.* (1996) 'Neural migration disorders studied by cerebral ultrasound and colour Doppler flow imaging.' *Archives of Disease in Childhood*, **73**, F55–F61.

Petersen, M.C., Wolraich, M., Sherbondy, A., Wagener, J. (1995) 'Abnormalities in control of ventilation in newborn infants with myelomeningocele.' *Journal of Pediatrics*, **126**, 1011–1015.

Pierre-Kahn, A., Renier, D., Sainte-Rose, C., Hirsch, J.F. (1983) 'Les lipomes lombo-sacrés avec spina-bifida. Corrélations anatomo-cliniques. Résultats thérapeutiques.' *Neurochirurgie*, **29**, 359–363.

Pihko, H., Lappi, M., Raitta, C., *et al.* (1995) 'Ocular findings in muscle–eye–brain (MEB) disease: a follow-up study.' *Brain and Development*, **17**, 57–61.

Pinard, J-M., Motte, J., Chiron, C., *et al.* (1994) 'Subcortical laminar heterotopia and lissencephaly in two families: a single X linked dominant gene.' *Journal of Neurology, Neurosurgery, and Psychiatry*, **57**, 914–920.

Platt, L.D., Feuchtbaum, L., Filly, R., *et al.* (1992) 'The California Maternal Serum α-Fetoprotein Screening Program—the role of ultrasonography in the detection of spina bifida.' *American Journal of Obstetrics and Gynecology*, **166**, 1328–1329.

Pollack, I.F., Pang, D., Albright, A.L., Krieger, D. (1992) 'Outcome following hindbrain decompression of symptomatic Chiari malformations in children previously treated with myelomeningocele closure and shunts.' *Journal of Neurosurgery*, **77**, 881–888.

Poll-Thé, B.T., Aicardi, J. (1985) 'Pseudomonoventricle due to a malformation of the septum pellucidum.' *Neuropediatrics*, **16**, 39–42.

Pou Serradell, A., Mares Segura, R. (1988) 'Corrélations clinico-morphologiques par I.R.M. dans la syringomyélie: étude de 22 cas.' *Revue Neurologique*, **144**, 181–193.

Powell, B.R., Budden, S.S., Buist, N.R.M. (1993) 'Dominantly inherited megalencephaly, muscle weakness, and myolipidosis: a carnitine-deficient myopathy within the spectrum of the Ruvalcaba–Myhre–Smith syndrome.' *Journal of Pediatrics*, **123**, 70–75.

Probst, F.P. (1979) *The Prosencephalies.* Berlin: Springer.

Qazi, Q.H., Reed, T.E. (1975) 'A possible major contribution to mental retardation in the general population by the gene for microcephaly.' *Clinical Genetics*, **7**, 85–90.

Quirk, J.A., Kendall, B., Kingsley, D.P.E., *et al.* (1993) 'EEG features of cortical dysplasia in children.' *Neuropediatrics*, **24**, 193–199.

Raghavendra, B.N., Epstein, F.J. (1985) 'Sonography of the spine and spinal cord.' *Radiologic Clinics of North America*, **23**, 91–105.

Raimondi, A.J., Sato, K., Takeyoshi, S. (1984) *The Dandy–Walker Syndrome.* Basel: Karger, pp. 1–75.

Rakic, P. (1975) 'Cell migration and neuronal ectopias in the brain.' *Birth Defects Original Articles Series*, **11**, 95–129.

—— (1981) 'Developmental events leading to laminar and areal organization of the neocortex.' *In:* Schmitt, F.O., Worden, F.G., Denis, S.G. (Eds.) *The Organization of Cerebral Cortex.* Cambridge, MA: MIT Press, pp. 7–28.

Ramirez, M.L., Rivas, F., Cantu, J.M. (1983) 'Silent microcephaly: a distinct autosomal dominant trait.' *Clinical Genetics*, **23**, 281–286.

Raybaud, C., Girard, N., Canto-Moreira, N., Poncet, M. (1996) 'High-definition magnetic resonance imaging identification of cortical dysplasias: micropolygyria versus lissencephaly.' *In:* Guerrini, R., Andermann, F., Canapicchi, R., *et al.* (Eds.) *Dysplasias of Cerebral Cortex and Epilepsy.* Philadelphia: Lippincott–Raven, pp. 131–143.

Raymond, A.A., Fish, D.R., Stevens, J.M., *et al.* (1994) 'Subependymal heterotopia: a distinct neuronal migration disorder associated with epilepsy.' *Journal of Neurology, Neurosurgery, and Psychiatry*, **57**, 1195–1202.

Reiner, O., Carrozzo, R., Shen, Y., *et al.* (1993) 'Isolation of a Miller–Dieker lissencephaly gene containing G protein β-subunit-like repeats.' *Nature*, **364**, 717–721.

Renier, W.O., Gabreels, F.J.M., Jasper, T.W.J., *et al.* (1982) 'X-linked syndrome with microcephaly, severe mental retardation, spasticity, epilepsy and deafness.' *Journal of Mental Deficiency Research*, **26**, 27–40.

—— —— Hustinx, T.W.J., *et al.* (1983) 'Cerebellar hypoplasia, communicating hydrocephalus and mental retardation in two brothers and a maternal uncle.' *Brain and Development*, **5**, 41–45.

Rhodes, R.E., Hatten, H.P., Ellington, K.S. (1992) 'Walker–Warburg syndrome.' *American Journal of Neuroradiology*, **13**, 123–126.

Ricci, S., Cusmai, R., Fariello, G., *et al.* (1992) 'Double cortex. A neuronal migration anomaly as a possible cause of Lennox–Gastaut syndrome.' *Archives of Neurology*, **49**, 61–64.

Richards, D.S., Seeds, J.W., Katz, V.L., *et al.* (1988) 'Elevated maternal serum alpha-fetoprotein with normal ultrasound: is amniocentesis always appropriate? A review of 26,069 screened patients.' *Obstetrics and Gynecology*, **71**, 203–207.

Richaud, J. (1988) 'Spinal meningeal malformations in children without meningoceles and meningomyeloceles.' *Child's Nervous System*, **4**, 79–87.

Richman, D.P., Stewart, R.M., Caviness, V.S. (1974) 'Cerebral microgyria in a 27-week fetus: an architectonic and topographic analysis.' *Journal of Neuropathology and Experimental Neurology*, **33**, 374–384.

Rickwood, A.M.K. (1990) 'Investigations.' *In:* Borzyskowski, M., Mundy, A.R. (Eds.) *Neuropathic Bladder in Childhood. Clinics in Developmental Medicine No. 111.* London: Mac Keith Press, pp. 10–26.

Rivier, F., Echenne, B. (1992) 'Dominantly inherited hypoplasia of the vermis.' *Neuropediatrics*, **23**, 206–208.

Roach, E., De Myer, W., Conneally, P.M., *et al.* (1975) 'Holoprosencephaly: birth data, genetic and demographic analyses of 30 families.' *Birth Defects*, **11**, 294–313.

Robain, O., Deonna, T. (1983) 'Pachygyria and congenital nephrosis: disorder of migration and neuronal orientation.' *Acta Neuropathologica*, **60**, 137–141.

—— Dulac, O. (1992) 'Early epileptic encephalopathy with suppression bursts and olivary–dentate dysplasia.' *Neuropediatrics*, **23**, 162–164.

—— Lyon, G. (1972) 'Les micrencéphalies familiales par malformation cérébrale.' *Acta Neuropathologica*, **20**, 96–109.

—— Dulac, O., Lejeune, J. (1987) 'Cerebellar hemispheric agenesis.' *Acta Neuropathologica*, **74**, 202–206.

—— Floquet, C. Heldt, N., Rozenberg, F. (1988) 'Hemimegalencephaly: a clinicopathological study of four cases.' *Neuropathology and Applied Biology*, **14**, 125–135.

Robert, E., Guibaud, P. (1982) 'Maternal valproic acid and congenital tube defects.' *Lancet*, **2**, 937. *(Letter.)*

Rockel, A.J., Hiorns, R.W., Powell, T.P.S. (1980) 'The basic uniformity in structure of the neocortex.' *Brain*, **103**, 221–244.

Rodier, P.M. (1980) 'Chronology of neuron development: animal studies and their clinical implication.' *Developmental Medicine and Child Neurology*, **22**, 525–545.

Roessmann, U., Horwitz, S.J., Kennell, J.H. (1990) 'Congenital absence of the corticospinal fibers: pathologic and clinical observations.' *Neurology*, **40**, 538–541.

Rorke, L.B., Fogelson, M.H., Riggs, H.E. (1968) 'Cerebellar heterotopia in infancy.' *Developmental Medicine and Child Neurology*, **10**, 644–650.

Ronen, G.M., Andrews, W.L. (1991) 'Holoprosencephaly as a possible embryonic alcohol effect.' *American Journal of Medical Genetics*, **40**, 151–154.

Rosa, F.W. (1991) 'Spina bifida in infants of women treated with carbamazepine during pregnancy.' *New England Journal of Medicine*, **324**, 674–677.

Rosendahl, H., Kivinen, S. (1989) 'Antenatal detection of congenital malformations by routine ultrasonography.' *Obstetrics and Gynecology*, **73**, 947–951.

Ross, G.W., Miller, J.Q., Persing, J.A., Urich, H. (1989) 'Hemimegalencephaly, hemifacial hypertrophy and intracranial lipoma: a variant of neurofibromatosis.' *Neurofibromatosis*, **2**, 69–77.

Ruvalcaba, R., Reichert, A., Smith, D. (1971) 'A new familial syndrome with osseous dysplasia and mental deficiency.' *Journal of Pediatrics*, **79**, 450–455.

Sakuta, R., Aikawa, H., Takashima, S., *et al.* (1989) 'Epidermal nevus syndrome with hemimegalencephaly: a clinical report of a case with acanthosis nigricans-like nevi on the face and neck, hemimegalencephaly and hemihypertrophy of the body.' *Brain and Development*, **11**, 191–194.

Salonen, R., Somer, M., Haltia, M., *et al.* (1991) 'Progressive encephalopathy with edema, hypsarrhythmia, and optic atrophy (PEHO syndrome).' *Clinical Genetics*, **39**, 287–293.

Samson, J.F., Barth, P.G., de Vries, J.I.P., *et al.* (1994) 'Familial mitochondrial encephalopathy with fetal ultrasonographic ventriculomegaly and intracerebral calcifications.' *European Journal of Pediatrics*, **153**, 510–516.

Santavuori, P., Somer, H., Sainio, K., *et al.* (1989) 'Muscle–eye–brain disease (MEB).' *Brain and Development*, **11**, 147–153.

Saraiva, J.M., Baraitser, M. (1992) 'Joubert syndrome: a review.' *American Journal of Medical Genetics*, **43**, 726–731.

Sarnat, H.B. (1987) 'Disturbances of late neuronal migrations in the perinatal period.' *American Journal of Diseases of Children*, **141**, 969–980.

—— (1991) 'Cerebral dysplasias as expressions of altered maturational processes.' *Canadian Journal of Neurological Sciences*, **18**, 196–204.

—— Alcala, H. (1980) 'Human cerebellar hypoplasia: a syndrome of diverse causes.' *Archives of Neurology*, **37**, 300–305.

Sato, N., Matsuishi, T., Utsunomya, H., *et al.* (1987) 'Aicardi syndrome with holoprosencephaly and cleft lip and palate.' *Pediatric Neurology*, **3**, 114–116.

Savoiardo, M. (1976) 'Syringomyelia associated with post-meningitic spinal arachnoiditis.' *Neurology*, **26**, 551–554.

Say, B., Coldwell, J.G. (1975) 'Hereditary defect of the sacrum.' *Human-genetik*, **27**, 231–234.

Schachenmayr, W., Friede, R.L. (1982) 'Rhombencephalosynapsis: a Viennese malformation?' *Developmental Medicine and Child Neurology*, **24**, 178–182.

Scheible, W., James, H.E., Leopold, G.R., Hilton, S. (1983) 'Occult spinal dysraphism in infants: screening with high-resolution real-time ultrasound.' *Radiology*, **145**, 743–746.

Schlesinger, E.B., Antunes, J.L., Michelsen, W.J., Louis, K.M. (1981) 'Hydromyelia: clinical presentation and comparison of modalities of treatment.' *Neurosurgery*, **9**, 356–365.

Schoenle, E.J., Haselbacher, G.K., Briner, J., *et al.* (1986) 'Elevated concentration of IGF II in brain tissue from an infant with macrencephaly.' *Journal of Pediatrics*, **108**, 737–740.

Schwartz, J.F., O'Brien, M.S., Hoffman, J.C. (1980) 'Hereditary spinal arachnoid cysts, distichiasis and lymphedema.' *Annals of Neurology*, **7**, 340–343.

Scott-Emuakpor, A.B., Heffelfinger, J., Higgins, J.V. (1977) 'A syndrome of microcephaly and cataracts in four siblings: a new genetic syndrome?' *American Journal of Diseases of Children*, **131**, 167–169.

Scotti, G., Harwood-Nash, D.C., Hoffman, H.J. (1980) 'Congenital thoracic dermal sinus: diagnosis by computer assisted metrizamide myelography.' *Journal of Computer Assisted Tomography*, **4**, 675–677.

Sébire, G., Goutières, F., Tardieu, M., *et al.* (1995) 'Extensive macrogyri or no visible gyri: distinct clinical, electroencephalographic, and genetic features according to different imaging patterns.' *Neurology*, **45**, 1105–1111.

—— Husson, B., Dusser, A., *et al.* (1996) 'Congenital unilateral perisylvian syndrome: radiological basis and clinical correlations.' *Journal of Neurology, Neurosurgery, and Psychiatry*, **61**, 52–56.

Seemanova, E., Passarge, E., Beneskova, D., *et al.* (1985) 'Familial microcephaly with normal intelligence, immunodeficiency and risk of lymphoreticular malignancies: a new autosomal recessive disorder.' *American Journal of Medical Genetics*, **20**, 639–648.

Seller, M.J. (1987) 'Neural tube defects and sex ratios.' *American Journal of Medical Genetics*, **26**, 699–707.

Sells, C.J. (1977) 'Microcephaly in a normal school population.' *Pediatrics*, **59**, 262–265.

Serur, D., Wisniewski, K.E., Lubin, R.A. (1987) 'Clinicopathological findings associated with agenesis of the corpus callosum.' *Brain and Development*, **9**, 255–264.

—— Jeret, J.S., Wisniewski, K. (1988) 'Agenesis of the corpus callosum: clinical, neuroradiological and cytogenetic studies.' *Neuropediatrics*, **19**, 87–91.

Shanks, D.E., Wilson, W.G. (1988) 'Lobar holoprosencephaly presenting as spastic diplegia.' *Developmental Medicine and Child Neurology*, **30**, 383–386.

Shapiro, L.P., Duncan, P.A., Farnsworth, P.B., Lefkowitz, M. (1976) 'Congenital microcephaly, hiatus hernia and nephrotic syndrome: an autosomal recessive syndrome.' *Birth Defects*, **12**, 275–278.

Shapiro, W.R., Williams, G.H., Plum, F. (1969) 'Spontaneous recurrent hypothermia accompanying agenesis of the corpus callosum.' *Brain*, **92**, 423–436.

Shaw, C.M., Alvord, E.C. (1996) 'Global cerebral dysplasia due to dysplasia and hyperplasia of periventricular germinal cells.' *Journal of Child Neurology*, **11**, 313–320.

Sher, P.K., Brown, S.B. (1975a) 'A longitudinal study of head growth in preterm infants.' I. Normal rates of head growth.' *Developmental Medicine and Child Neurology*, **17**, 705–710.

—— —— (1975b) 'A longitudinal study of head growth in pre-term infants. II. Differentiation between 'catch-up' growth and early infantile hydrocephalus.' *Developmental Medicine and Child Neurology*, **17**, 711–718.

Sherman, J.L., Barkovich, A.J., Citrin, C.M. (1987) 'The MR appearance of syringomyelia. New observations.' *American Journal of Neuroradiology*, **7**, 985–995.

Sheth, R.D., Barron, T.F., Hartlage, P.L. (1994) 'Episodic spontaneous hypothermia with hyperhydrosis: implications for pathogenesis.' *Pediatric Neurology*, **10**, 58–60.

Shevell, M.I., Carmant, L., Meagher-Villemure, K. (1992) 'Developmental bilateral perisylvian dysplasia.' *Pediatric Neurology*, **8**, 299–302.

—— Matthews, P.M., Scriver, C.R., *et al.* (1994) 'Cerebral dysgenesis and lactic acidemia: an MRI/MRS phenotype associated with pyruvate dehydrogenase deficiency.' *Pediatric Neurology*, **11**, 224–229.

Shigematsu, H., Takashima, S., Otani, K., Ieshima, A. (1985) 'Neuropathological and Golgi study on a case of thanatophoric dysplasia.' *Brain and Development*, 7, 628–632.

Sidman, R.L., Rakic, P. (1973) 'Neuronal migration with special reference to developing human brain: a review.' *Brain Research*, 62, 1–35.

Siebert, J.R., Warkany, J., Lemire, R.J. (1986) 'Atelencephalic microcephaly in a 21-week human fetus.' *Teratology*, 34, 9–19.

Silengo, M., Lerone, M., Martinelli, M., *et al.* (1992) 'Autosomal recessive microcephaly with early onset seizures and spasticity.' *Clinical Genetics*, 42, 152–155.

Simpson, D.A., David, D.J., White, J. (1984) 'Cephaloceles: treatment, outcome, and antenatal diagnosis.' *Neurosurgery*, 15, 14–21.

Simpson, R.K., Rose, J.E. (1987) 'Cervical diastematomyelia: report of a case and review of a rare congenital anomaly.' *Archives of Neurology*, 44, 331–335.

Sisodiya, S.M., Free, S.L., Stevens, J.M., *et al.* (1995) 'Widespread cerebral structural changes in patients with cortical dysgenesis and epilepsy.' *Brain*, 118, 1039–1050.

Smith, P.J., Hindmarsh, P., Kendall, B., Brook, C.G.D. (1986) 'Dysgenesis of the corpus callosum and hypopituitarism.' *Acta Paediatrica Scandinavica*, 75, 923–926.

Smith, R.D. (1981) 'Abnormal head circumference in learning-disabled children.' *Developmental Medicine and Child Neurology*, 23, 626–632.

Smithells, R.W., Sheppard, S., Schorah, C.J., *et al.* (1981) 'Apparent prevention of neural tube defects by periconceptional vitamin supplementation.' *Archives of Disease in Childhood*, 56, 911–918.

—— Nevin, N.C., Seller, M.J., *et al.* (1983) 'Further experience of vitamin supplementation for prevention of neural tube defect recurrences.' *Lancet*, 1, 1027–1031.

Stark, G. (1968) 'The pathophysiology of the bladder in myelomeningocele and its correlation with the neurological picture.' *Developmental Medicine and Child Neurology*, Suppl. 16, 76–86.

—— (1971) 'Prediction of urinary continence in myelomeningocele.' *Developmental Medicine and Child Neurology*, 13, 388–389.

—— Drummond, M. (1973) 'Result of selective early operation of myelomeningocele.' *Archives of Disease in Childhood*, 48, 676–683.

Stein, S., Schut, L., Borns, P. (1979) 'Hydrocephalus in myelomeningocele.' *Child's Brain*, 5, 413–419.

Steinlin, M., Zürrer, M., Martin, E., *et al.* (1991) 'Contribution of magnetic resonance imaging in the evaluation of microcephaly.' *Neuropediatrics*, 22, 184–189.

Stephan, M.J., Hall, B.D., Smith, D.W., Cohen, M.M. (1975) 'Macrocephaly in association with unusual cutaneous angiomatosis.' *Journal of Pediatrics*, 87, 353–359.

Stephenson, T.P., Mundy, A.R. (1990) 'Surgery of the neuropathic bladder.' *In:* Borzyskowski, M., Mundy, A.R. (Eds.) *Neuropathic Bladder in Childhood. Clinics in Developmental Medicine No. 111.* London: Mac Keith Press, pp. 37–58.

Stewart, R.M., Richman, D.P., Caviness, V.S. (1975) 'Lissencephaly and pachygyria; an architectonic and topographical analysis.' *Acta Neuropathologica*, 31, 1–12.

—— Williams, R.S., Kukl, P. (1978) 'Ventral porencephaly: a cerebral defect associated with multiple congenital anomalies.' *Acta Neuropathologica*, 42, 231–238.

Stoll, C., Dott, B., Roth, M.P., Alembik, Y. (1988) 'Aspects étiologiques et épidémiologiques des anomalies du tube neural.' *Archives Françaises de Pédiatrie*, 45, 617–622.

Stone, D.H. (1987) 'The declining prevalence of anencephalus and spina bifida: its nature, causes and implications.' *Developmental Medicine and Child Neurology*, 29, 541–546.

Stovner, L.J., Cappelen, J., Nilsen, G., Sjaastad, O. (1992) 'The Chiari type I malformation in two monozygotic twins and first-degree relatives.' *Annals of Neurology*, 31, 220–222.

Sudo, K., Doi, S., Maruo, Y., *et al.* (1990) 'Syringomyelia with spontaneous resolution.' *Journal of Neurology, Neurosurgery, and Psychiatry*, 53, 437–438.

Sugama, S., Kusaro, K. (1994) 'Monozygous twin with polymicrogyria and normal co-twin.' *Pediatric Neurology*, 11, 62–63.

Sugimoto, T., Yasuhara, A., Nishida, N., *et al.* (1993) 'MRI of the head in the evaluation of microcephaly.' *Neuropediatrics*, 24, 4–7.

Sumi, S.M. (1970) 'Brain malformations in the trisomy 18 syndrome.' *Brain*, 93, 821–830.

Suzuki, M., Davis, C., Symon, L., Gentili, F. (1985) 'Syringoperitoneal shunt for treatment of cord cavitation.' *Journal of Neurology, Neurosurgery, and Psychiatry*, 48, 620–627.

Takada, K., Nakamura, H., Tanaka, J. (1984) 'Cortical dysplasia in congenital muscular dystrophy with central nervous system involvement (Fukuyama type).' *Journal of Neuropathology and Experimental Neurology*, 43, 395–407.

Takashima, S., Becker, L.E., Chan, F., Takada, K. (1987) 'A Golgi study of the cerebral cortex in Fukuyama-type congenital muscular dystrophy, Walker-type "lissencephaly", and classical lissencephaly.' *Brain and Development*, 9, 621–626.

Talwar, D., Baldwin, M.A., Horbatt, C.I. (1995) 'Epilepsy in children with meningomyelocele.' *Pediatric Neurology*, 13, 29–32.

Tan, E-C., Takagi, T., Karasawa, K. (1995) 'Posterior fossa cystic lesions—magnetic resonance imaging manifestations.' *Brain and Development*, 17, 418–424.

Tashiro, K., Fukazawa, T., Morikawa, F., *et al.* (1987) 'Syringomyelic syndrome: clinical features in 31 cases confirmed by CT myelography or magnetic resonance imaging.' *Journal of Neurology*, 235, 26–30.

Taylor, D.C., Falconer, M.A., Bruton, C.J., Corsellis, J.A.N. (1971) 'Focal dysplasia of the cerebral cortex in epilepsy.' *Journal of Neurology, Neurosurgery, and Psychiatry*, 34, 369–387.

Taylor, M.J., Boor, R., Keenan, N.K., *et al.* (1996) 'Brainstem auditory and visual evoked potentials in infants with myelomeningocele.' *Brain and Development*, 18, 99–104.

Tenconi, R., Clementi, M., Moschini, B., *et al.* (1981) 'Chorioretinal dysplasia, microcephaly and mental retardation: an autosomal dominant syndrome.' *Clinical Genetics*, 20, 347–351.

Thyen, U., Aksu, F., Bartsch, O., Herb, E. (1992) 'Acrocallosal syndrome: association with cystic malformation of the brain and neurodevelopmental aspects.' *Neuropediatrics*, 23, 292–296.

Tint, G.S., Irons, M., Elias, E.R., *et al.* (1994) 'Defective cholesterol biosynthesis associated with the Smith–Lemli–Opitz syndrome.' *New England Journal of Medicine*, 330, 107–113.

Tolmie, J.L., McNay, M., Stephenson, J.B.P., *et al.* (1987) 'Microcephaly: genetic counselling and antenatal diagnosis after the birth of an affected child.' *American Journal of Medical Genetics*, 27, 583–594.

Towfighi, J., Sassani, J.W., Suzuki, K., Ladda, R.L. (1984) 'Cerebro-ocular dysplasia–muscular dystrophy (COD-MD) syndrome.' *Acta Neuropathologica*, 65, 110–123.

Tohyama, J., Kato, M., Koeda, T., *et al.* (1992) 'The 'double cortex' syndrome. Commentary to Hashimoto's paper (pp. 57–9).' *Brain and Development*, 15, 83–84.

Trounce, J.Q., Fagan, D.G., Young, I.D., Levene, M.I. (1986) 'Disorders of neuronal migration: sonographic features.' *Developmental Medicine and Child Neurology*, 28, 467–471.

Truwit, C.L., Barkovich, A.J., Grumbach, M.M., Martini, J.J. (1993) 'MR imaging of Kallmann syndrome, a genetic disorder of neuronal migration affecting the olfactory and genital system.' *American Journal of Neuroradiology*, 14, 827–838.

Tsipouras, P., Barabas, G., Matthews, W.S. (1986) 'Neurologic correlates of osteogenesis imperfecta.' *Archives of Neurology*, 43, 150–152.

Tsuchiya, K., Michikawa, M., Furuya, A., *et al.* (1989) 'Intradural spinal lipoma with enlarged intervertebral foramen.' *Journal of Neurology, Neurosurgery, and Psychiatry*, 52, 1308–1310.

Tsukamoto, H., Inagaki, M., Tomita, Y., Ohno, K. (1992) 'Congenital caudal spinal atrophy: a case report.' *Neuropediatrics*, 23, 260–262.

Tunnessen, W.N., McMillan, J.A., Levin, M.B. (1978) 'The Coffin–Siris syndrome.' *American Journal of Diseases of Children*, 132, 393–395.

Tychsen, L., Hoyt, W.F. (1985) 'Occipital lobe dysplasia: magnetic resonance findings in two cases of isolated congenital hemianopsia.' *Archives of Ophthalmology*, 103, 680–682.

Urich, H., Herrick, M.K. (1985) 'The amniotic band syndrome as a cause of anencephaly. Report of a case.' *Acta Neuropathologica*, 67, 190–194.

Vade, A., Horowitz, S. (1992) 'Agenesis of corpus callosum and intraventricular lipomas.' *Pediatric Neurology*, 8, 307–309.

Valanne, L., Pihko, H., Katevuo, K., *et al.* (1994) 'MRI of the brain in muscle–eye–brain (MEB) disease.' *Neuroradiology*, 36, 473–476.

Van den Hof, M.C., Nicolaides, K.H., Campbell, J., Campbell, S. (1990) 'Evaluation of the lemon and banana signs in one hundred thirty fetuses with open spina bifida.' *American Journal of Obstetrics and Gynecology*, 162, 322–327.

van der Put, N.M.J., Steegers-Theunissen, R.P.M., Frosst, P., *et al.* (1995)

'Mutated methylenetetrahydrofolate reductase as a risk factor for spina bifida.' *Lancet*, **346**, 1070–1071.

Van Hall, M.H.J.A., Beuls, E.A.M., Wilmink, J.T., *et al.* (1992) 'Magnetic resonance imaging of progresssive hydrosyringomyelia in two patients with meningomyelocele.' *Neuropediatrics*, **23**, 276–280.

Verloes, A., Lambotte, C. (1989) 'Further delineation of a syndrome of cerebellar vermis hypoplasia, oligophrenia, congenital ataxia, coloboma, and hepatic fibrosis.' *American Journal of Medical Genetics*, **32**, 227–232.

Vigevano, F., Di Rocco, C. (1990) 'Effectiveness of hemispherectomy in hemimegalencephaly with intractable seizures.' *Neuropediatrics*, **21**, 222–223.

—— Fusco, L., Granata, T., *et al.* (1996) 'Hemimegalencephaly: clinical and EEG characteristics.' *In:* Guerrini, R., Andermann, F., Canapicchi, R., *et al.* (Eds.) *Dysplasias of Cerebral Cortex and Epilepsy*. Philadelphia: Lippincott–Raven, pp. 285–294.

Volpe, J. (1995) *Neurology of the Newborn, 3rd Edn.* Philadelphia: W.B. Saunders.

Vuia, O. (1973) 'Malformation of the paraflocculus and atresia of the foramina of Magendie and Luschka in a child.' *Psychiatrie, Neurologie, Neurochirurgie*, **76**, 261–266.

Wald, N.J., Cuckle, M. (1984) 'Open neural tube defects.' *In:* Wald, N.J. (Ed.) *Antenatal and Neonatal Screening*. Oxford: Oxford University Press, pp. 25–73.

Walsh, C.A. (1995) 'Neuronal identity, neuronal migration, and epileptic disorders of the cerebral cortex.' *In:* Schwartzkroin, P.A., Moshé, S.L., Noebels, J.L., Swaun, J.W. (Eds.) *Brain Development and Epilepsy*. New York: Oxford University Press, pp. 122–143.

—— Cepko, C.L. (1993) 'Clonal dispersion in proliferative layers of developing cerebral cortex.' *Nature*, **362**, 632–635.

Ward, S.L.D., Jacobs, R.A., Gates, E.P., *et al.* (1986a) 'Abnormal ventilatory patterns during sleep in infants with myelomeningocele.' *Journal of Pediatrics*, **109**, 631–634.

—— Nickerson, B.G., Van der Hal, A., *et al.* (1986b) 'Absent hypoxic and hypercapneic arousal responses in children with mengingomyelocele and apnea.' *Pediatrics*, **78**, 44–50.

Warkany, J. (1981) 'Microcephaly.' *In:* Warkany, J., Lemire, R.J., Cohen, M.M. (Eds.) *Mental Retardation and Congenital Malformations of the Central Nervous System*. Chicago and London: Year Book Medical, pp. 13–40.

—— Lemire, R.J., Cohen, M.M. (1981) 'Spina bifida.' *In:* Warkany, J., Lemire, R.J., Cohen, M.M. (Eds.) *Mental Retardation and Congenital Malformations of the Central Nervous System*. Chicago and London: Year Book Medical, pp. 272–296.

Watanabe, K., Hara, K., Iwase, K. (1976) 'The evolution of neurophysiological features in holoprosencephaly.' *Neuropediatrics*, **7**, 19–41.

Waterman, R.E. (1979) 'Scanning electron microscope studies of central nervous system development.' *Birth Defects*, **15**, 55–79.

Weinstein, S.L., Novotny, E.J. (1987) 'Neonatal metabolic disorders masquerading as structural central nervous system anomalies.' *Annals of Neurology*, **22**, 406. *(Abstract.)*

White, B.J., Rogol, A.D., Brown, K.S., *et al.* (1983) 'The syndrome of anosmia with hypogonadotropic hypogonadism: a genetic study of 18 new families and a review.' *American Journal of Medical Genetics*, **15**, 417–435.

Wichman, A., Frank, L.M., Kelly, T.E. (1985) 'Autosomal recessive congenital cerebellar hypoplasia.' *Clinical Genetics*, **27**, 373–382.

Wilkins, R.H., Odom, G.L. (1976) 'Spinal intradural cyst.' *In:* Vinken, P.J., Bruyn, G.W. (Eds.) *Handbook of Clinical Neurology. Vol. 20. Tumours of the Spine and Spinal Cord, Part II*. Amsterdam: North Holland, pp. 53–102.

Williams, J., Brodsky, M.C., Griebel, M., *et al.* (1993) 'Septo-optic dysplasia: the clinical insignificance of an absent septum pellucidum.' *Developmental Medicine and Child Neurology*, **35**, 490–501.

Williams, R.S., Caviness, V.S. (1984) 'Normal and abnormal development of the brain.' *In:* Tarter, R.E., Goldstein, J. (Eds.) *Advances in Clinical Neuropsychology, Vol. 2*. New York: Plenum, pp. 1–62.

—— Swisher, C.N., Jennings, M., *et al.* (1984) 'Cerebro-ocular dysgenesis (Walker–Warburg syndrome): neuropathologic and etiologic analysis.' *Neurology*, **34**, 1531–1541.

Wilson, G.N. (1983) 'Cranial defects in the Goldenhar syndrome.' *American Journal of Medical Genetics*, **14**, 435–443.

Windham, G., Edmonds, L.D. (1982) 'Current trends in the incidence of neural tube defects.' *Pediatrics*, **70**, 333–337.

Wisniewski, K., Dambska, M., Sher, J., Qazi, Q. (1983) 'A clinical neuropathological study of the fetal alcohol syndrome.' *Neuropediatrics*, **14**, 197–201.

Wiswell, T.E., Tuttle, D.J., Northam, R.S., Simonds, G.R. (1990) 'Major congenital neurologic malformations. A 17-year survey.' *American Journal of Diseases of Children*, **144**, 61–67.

Wright, R.L. (1971) 'Congenital dermal sinuses.' *Progress in Neurological Surgery*, **4**, 175–191.

Wyllie, E., Baumgartner, C., Prayson, R., *et al.* (1994) 'The clinical spectrum of focal cortical dysplasia and epilepsy.' *Journal of Epilepsy*, **7**, 303–312.

Yakovlev, P.I., Lecours, A.R. (1967) 'The myelogenetic cycles of regional maturation of the brain.' *In:* Minkowski, A. (Ed.) *Regional Development of the Brain in Early Life*. Oxford: Blackwell, pp. 3–10.

—— Wadsworth, R.C. (1946) 'Schizencephalies: a study of congenital clefts in the cerebral mantle: I. Clefts with fused lips.' *Journal of Neuropathology and Experimental Neurology*, **5**, 116–130.

Yamaguchi, E., Hayashi, T., Kondoh, H., *et al.* (1993) 'A case of Walker–Warburg syndrome with uncommon findings. Double cortical layer, temporal cyst and increased serum IgM.' *Brain and Development*, **15**, 61–65.

Yglesias, A., Narbona, J., Vanaclocha, V., Artieda, J. (1996) 'Chiari type 1 malformation, glossopharyngeal neuralgia and central sleep apnoea in a child.' *Developmental Medicine and Child Neurology*, **38**, 1126–1130.

Yokota, A., Matsukado, Y. (1979) 'Congenital midline porencephaly. A new malformation associated with scalp anomaly.' *Child's Brain*, **5**, 380–397.

—— Oota, TR., Matsukado, Y. (1984a) 'Dorsal cyst malformations. Part I. Study and critical review of the definition of holoprosencephaly.' *Child's Brain*, **11**, 320–341.

—— —— Okudera, T. (1984b) 'Dorsal cyst malformations. Part II. Galenic dysgenesis and its embryological considerations.' *Child's Brain*, **11**, 403–417.

—— Kajiwara, H., Kohchi, M., *et al.* (1988) 'Parietal cephalocele: clinical importance of its atretic form and associated malformations.' *Journal of Neurosurgery*, **69**, 545–551.

Young, I.D., Moore, J.R., Tripp, J.H. (1987) 'Sex-linked recessive congenital ataxia.' *Journal of Neurology, Neurosurgery, and Psychiatry*, **50**, 1230–1232.

Younus, M., Coode, P.E. (1986) 'Nasal glioma and encephalocele: two separate entities. Report of two cases.' *Journal of Neurosurgery*, **64**, 516–519.

Zager, E.L., Ojemann, R.G., Poletti, C.E. (1990) 'Acute presentations of syringomyelia. Report of three cases.' *Journal of Neurosurgery*, **72**, 133–138.

Zee, C-S.L.I., McComb, J.G., Segall, H.D., *et al.* (1981) 'Lipomas of the corpus callosum associated with frontal dysraphism.' *Journal of Computer Assisted Tomography*, **5**, 201–205.

4
NEUROCUTANEOUS DISEASES AND SYNDROMES

Several diseases affect both the skin and the nervous system, which is probably a consequence of their common ectodermal origin. Most of these disorders are genetically determined and occur early in life, although late manifestations are frequent as many of the neurocutaneous syndromes are evolutive conditions.

The group of the neurocutaneous disorders is highly heterogeneous. The term 'phakomatosis' is sometimes used as a synonym. However, it has come to be applied mainly to those neurocutaneous diseases in which an excessive growth potential, with frequent development of hamartomas or tumours, is present. This applies to neurofibromatosis, tuberous sclerosis, von Hippel–Lindau disease and naevoid basal cell carcinoma syndrome. In this chapter, the term neurocutaneous syndrome is used for all diseases in which there is a nonfortuitous association of skin and nervous system abnormalities, even though the cutaneous manifestations may not be regularly present in all cases. Some of the neurocutaneous syndromes are considered in other chapters (*e.g.* those in which the nervous system involvement consists of vascular malformations). The grouping used is clearly arbitrary, but it is justified from a clinical point of view as the association of cutaneous and neurological manifestations raises specific problems. Neurocutaneous diseases are much more pleiotropic than suggested by their name as they may involve viscera as well as skull and CNS. Most neurocutaneous diseases are genetically determined, all three major mendelian types of inheritance being possible. Sporadic syndromes may be due to somatic mutations or to other, unknown mechanisms.

NEUROFIBROMATOSIS

Neurofibromatosis is not a single disorder. The term designates a spectrum of disorders that share many features but clearly differ from one another. There is no agreement as to how many entities belong to the neurofibromatoses.

Two distinct forms are generally recognized: type 1 (NF1), also termed von Recklinghausen's disease or peripheral type; and type 2 (NF2), also termed central neurofibromatosis. These two types are actually distinct diseases. The gene of NF1 is located in the pericentric region of the long arm of chromosome 17 (17q11.2), while that of NF2 is on the long arm of chromosome 22 (22q11.2). The clinical and pathological characteristics of these two diseases are also different (see below).

Other types of neurofibromatosis exist. Riccardi (1992) has proposed that seven distinct forms may be recognized. However, the individualization of some of these forms remains controversial.

The terms central and peripheral are better abandoned, because both NF1 and NF2 produce CNS lesions, albeit of different types.

Table 4.1 shows the criteria for the diagnosis of NF1/NF2.

The basic disturbance in neurofibromatosis appears to be an abnormality in development of the *neural crest* cells with resulting tendency to abnormal, excessive growth of affected tissues and the development of multiple tumours. Although increased levels of nerve growth factor have been reported in patients with NF2 (Fabricant and Todaro 1981) there is no consensus on this finding (Riccardi 1992), and normal levels of nerve growth factor are present in the classical von Recklinghausen type (Riopelle *et al.* 1984). The *NF1* gene codes for a protein, neurofibromin, which appears to be a GTPase-activating protein. GTPase converts the proto-oncogen *p21-ras* from active to inactive form, thus downregulating the production of oncogen and having a probable antioncogenic function (Gutmann and Collins 1992). Most NF1 cases with mental retardation are associated with large deletions of the gene. The *NF2* gene codes for merlin and acts as a tumour suppressor; several mutations are known (MacCollin 1995). Interestingly, a loss of chromosome 22, and hence of the *NF2* gene, is commonly found in schwannomas and meningiomas that occur outside NF2.

NEUROFIBROMATOSIS TYPE 1
NF1 accounts for at least 85 per cent of all cases of neurofibromatosis. The prevalence of the disease is about 1 in 3000 individuals. NF1 is inherited dominantly with a 98 per cent penetrance but with a high degree of phenotypic variability. According to Huson *et al.* (1988) and North (1993), approximately half the cases have only minor manifestations. Paternal transmission is more common than maternal inheritance. Occasional occurrence of a paternal germ line mosaicism may account for more than one affected offspring of clinically unaffected parents (Lazaro *et al.* 1994). About one third of cases are new

TABLE 4.1
Criteria for the diagnosis of the neurofibromatoses*

Neurofibromatosis type 1
1. Six or more café-au-lait spots > 5 mm in diameter in prepubertal patients and > 15 mm in postpubertal patients
2. Two or more neurofibromas (intracutaneous or subcutaneous) or one plexiform neurofibroma
3. Freckling in the axillary or inguinal region
4. Optic glioma
5. Two or more iris hamartomas (Lisch nodules)
6. Typical osseous lesion such as sphenoid dysplasia or tibial pseudarthrosis
7. One or more first degree relative with NF1

NF1 may be diagnosed if two or more of above criteria are present

Neurofibromatosis type 2
1. Bilateral VIIIth nerve neurofibromas
2. Unilateral VIIIth nerve mass in association with any two of the following: meningioma, neurofibroma, schwannoma, juvenile posterior subcapsular cataracts
3. Unilateral VIIIth nerve tumour or other spinal or brain tumour as above in first degree relative

NF2 may be diagnosed if one of the above criteria is present

*Modified from NIH Consensus Development Conference (1988).

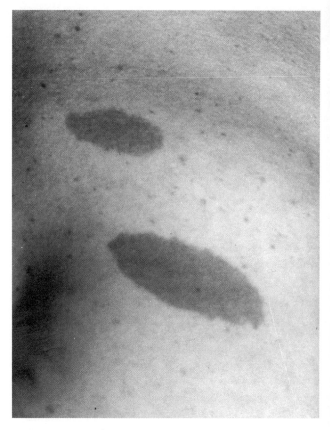

mutations, and the mutation rate is approximately one mutation per 10,000 gametes per generation.

CUTANEOUS MANIFESTATIONS

Skin features of NF1 consist of abnormalities of pigmentation and tumours (Fig. 4.1). *Café-au-lait spots* are the hallmark of NF1 and are found in virtually all cases. Their size varies with age; they are present from an early age but are not as readily visible in infancy as they are later. Ordinarily, at least six spots 0.5–1.0 cm are apparent by 1 year of age but an occasional patient may have less. Of 46 children with such spots prospectively followed by Korf (1992), 27 had developed other signs of NF1 (in the majority, within three years), six had segmental neurofibromatosis, three received other diagnoses, and eight remained without diagnosis. Axillary freckling was present in 84 per cent of 200 children followed by North (1993), and inguinal freckling was found in about half these patients. Diffuse pigmentation may overlie a plexiform neuroma. Xanthomas and angiomas are less common features. *Neurofibromas* may be intracutaneous and are then of a violaceous colour and a soft consistency, or subcutaneous and presenting as firm tumours along the trunk of peripheral nerves. They vary from a few millimeters to 3–4 cm at their greatest diameter. Neurofibromas are sometimes found in children under 10 years old, but they increase steadily in number with age, especially around puberty (Riccardi 1992). They can lead to peripheral neuropathy when they affect larger nerves. *Plexiform neurofibromas* combine cutaneous and subcutaneous elements to form tumours that may become huge and represent one of the most serious complications of NF1. They may be continuous with intracranial or intraspinal tumours. Plexiform tumours of the periorbital area, which occur in 5 per cent of patients, can produce proptosis and visual compromise. Large plexiform neurofibromas occur in 25–32 per cent of cases (Huson *et al.* 1988, North 1993) and tend to grow larger with age. The cosmetic

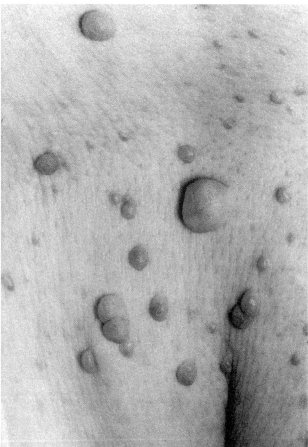

Fig. 4.1. Cutaneous manifestations of neurofibromatosis type I. *(Top)* Café-au-lait spots. *(Bottom)* Multiple neurofibromas.

burden may be considerable, and large cervical lesions may displace and compress vascular and respiratory structures and be life-threatening. Plexiform neurofibromas of the limbs may be associated with partial gigantism. Involvement of the face is possible and may be associated with exophthalmos and rarely with unilateral megalencephaly (Boltshauser *et al.* 1989, Ross *et al.* 1989). Such lesions may be associated with bony abnormalities of the orbit; they require rapid treatment if the eyelid completely covers the eye, to avoid secondary amblyopia. Most plexiform neurofibromas appear before 2 years of age and some may be present at birth.

Involvement of the iris by pigmented hamartomas known as *Lisch nodules* is specific for NF1. Lisch nodules are found in 22–30 per cent of NF1 patients by 6 years of age and in virtually all after age 12 years (Flueler *et al.* 1986, North 1993).

NEUROLOGICAL MANIFESTATIONS
Neurological manifestations of NF1 are protean and include macrocephaly which is present in 40–50 per cent of affected children, mental retardation, learning difficulties, and symptoms and signs due to intracranial and intraspinal tumours.

Macrocephaly (>98th centile) is present in only 16–45 per cent of children with NF1 (Huson *et al.* 1988, North 1993) and is not correlated with neurological or neuropyschological difficulties. It is due to megalencephaly and is not accompanied by symptoms of increased intracranial pressure. Headache occurs in over half the patients and may be migraine-like.

Mental retardation and learning difficulties are well known features of NF1 (Riccardi 1992). Mental retardation is uncommon: Riccardi put the frequency at 8 per cent but lower figures have been reported by other authors (North *et al.* 1994b, 1995; North 1997). However, the IQ of NF1 patients is on average lower than that of affected siblings (Eldridge *et al.* 1989). Specific learning difficulties are a common problem, being present in 32 per cent (Ferner and Hughes 1992, Hofman *et al.* 1994) to 65 per cent (North *et al.* 1994b), if impaired academic performance is taken as the criterion. Depressed performance in verbal tasks and a high incidence of language deficits are particularly obvious, but all areas of cognition can be affected. Attentional deficit disorder without hyperactivity is common and may respond to amphetamine therapy. A significant association of cognitive deficits with the presence of T_2-intense areas on MRI has been found by several investigators (North *et al.* 1994b, Denckla *et al.* 1996) but not by others (Moore 1995, Moore *et al.* 1996) and requires further study.

Epilepsy is more frequent in children with NF1 than in the general population but available figures vary between 3.5 per cent (North 1993) and 7.3 per cent (Huson *et al.* 1988). All types of seizures including infantile spasms (Motte *et al.* 1993, Fois *et al.* 1994) may occur.

Optic gliomas are present in 15–20 per cent of NF1 cases (Imes and Hoyt 1986, North 1993). Histologically, they may differ from other optic gliomas by the presence of an arachnoidal gliomatosis surrounding the optic nerve (Seiff *et al.* 1987) but otherwise they are typical pilocytic astrocytomas. They may be limited to the optic nerve or involve the chiasm and the retro-chiasmatic portion of the visual pathway. Between 10 and 60 per cent of optic gliomas are associated with NF1. The proportion tends to increase in the case of gliomas of the optic nerve, and especially of bilateral gliomas which are almost exclusively found in NF1 patients.

Clinical manifestations include proptosis and diminished visual acuity, but many gliomas are now discovered by systematic radiological evaluation of patients with known NF1 while they remain asymptomatic (Duffner and Cohen 1988, Packer *et al.* 1988a). Up to 39 per cent of cases present with precocious puberty (Habiby *et al.* 1995). The proportion of symptomatic cases is 20–30 per cent, and most symptomatic cases manifest early before age 6 and often by 2 years of age (Pascual-Castroviejo 1992, Listernick *et al.* 1994). Optic gliomas in NF1 fall into two groups: those that remain stable, and those that are active, increase in size and threaten vision. Only 52 per cent of patients whose optic gliomas were detected by MRI developed symptoms (Listernick *et al.* 1997). Emergence of symptoms after age 6 years is extremely rare. Progression beyond age 10 is rare. Intraorbital gliomas only rarely spread intracranially. The evolution of optic gliomas in NF1 may be more benign than in isolated cases (Listernick *et al.* 1994) but there is no universal agreement in this regard. Tumours anterior to the chiasm frequently remain stable, whereas more posteriorly located gliomas are more often invasive. The diagnosis of optic glioma may be suggested by finding an enlarged optic foramen, although this sign is not specific (Packer *et al.* 1988a) as elongation of the optic nerve and dural ectasia can simulate a tumour (Riccardi 1992, North 1997).

CT scan and MRI have transformed the conditions of the diagnosis of optic pathway tumours in NF1 patients (Fig. 4.2). On CT scan, the tumours appear as irregular enlargements that may extend into the chiasm with bulging in or filling of the chiasmatic cistern. MRI better demonstrates the tumours. There is an ongoing controversy about the indications for imaging in NF1. All agree that symptomatic cases should be scanned. For asymptomatic cases, the NIH Consensus Development Conference (1988) did *not* advise systematic study as no treatment is usually indicated. Riccardi (1992) is of the opposite opinion as some aggressive gliomas may progress silently for relatively long periods and may cause damage that could be prevented by early diagnosis. Monitoring of visual evoked potentials may permit early detection but there is a high level of false positives (North *et al.* 1994a). It often indicates extension into the optic tract and radiations (Bognanno *et al.* 1988, Di Mario *et al.* 1993). MRI often demonstrates high T_2 signal changes, especially in the optic tracts and radiations. The significance of this finding as well as that of noncontiguous areas of abnormal signal, especially in the basal ganglia and cerebellum, is not currently understood. In most cases it does not represent tumour extension, and such abnormal signals have been shown to remain stable or even disappear.

Similar areas of intense signal on T_2-weighted MRI scans are frequent in patients without optic pathway gliomas (Gray and Swaiman 1987, Bognanno *et al.* 1988, Duffner *et al.* 1989, Dunn and Roos 1989, North *et al.* 1994a). North (1997) found

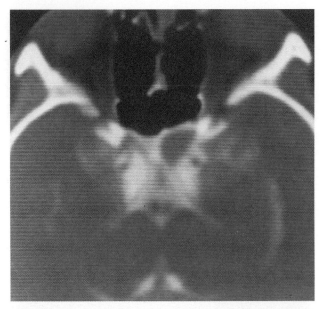

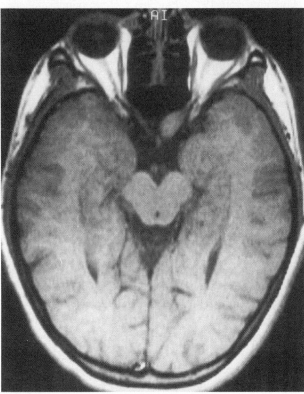

Fig. 4.2. NF1 in a 12-year-old girl. Unenhanced CT scan showed a possible anomaly of the preoptic cistern. *(Top)* CT scan after lumbar injection of metrizamide contrast shows a small mass at the origin of the left optic nerve. *(Bottom)* T₁-weighted MRI clearly delineates a small optic glioma.

with optic glioma had T_2-intense lesions, usually affecting diffusely the optic tracts, whereas lesions elsewhere were generally discrete and well-limited. T_2-intense areas tended to decrease and often disappeared before 12 years of age (Savick *et al.* 1992). The significance of these anomalies is not clear. Most of them do not seem to correspond to neoplastic changes. Their histological nature is unknown although the term 'hamartoma' is often applied to such lesions. They are more common in children and adolescents than in adults, and in patients with optic glioma than in those without. The 'hamartomas' of the optic tracts and the pallidum are larger than those located elsewhere and may give an abnormal signal, although a weak one, on T_1-weighted images (Inoue *et al.* 1997). The abnormally intense T_2 areas have been shown in a few cases to represent glial dyplasia or spongiotic changes rather than hamartomas (Di Paolo *et al.* 1995). The nature of the T_1-intensive lesions is unknown.

Treatment of optic glioma is still controversial (Packer *et al.* 1988b, Spitzer and Goodrich 1988, Dunn and Purvin 1990, Riccardi 1992). Most tumours that appear stable, especially if localized to the anterior optic pathways, should be watched carefully without surgical or other intervention. In a recent collaborative study, extension to the chiasm was seen in only four of 106 unilateral cases (North American Study Group for Optic Glioma 1989). For optic nerve gliomas that are growing and produce marked proptosis with complete unilateral loss of vision, surgical removal gives satisfactory results. For lesions that are not stable, X-ray therapy is effective (Packer *et al.* 1983). However, irradiation with doses of 5200 rads, as usually required, is associated in children with mental retardation and with endocrinological sequelae in one third of cases. For patients under 5 years of age, chemotherapy tends to be substituted for radiotherapy (Packer *et al.* 1988b). Combinations of actinomycin D and vincristine (Packer *et al.* 1988b) and carbiplatin (Charrow *et al.* 1993a) have been found effective and combined therapy with carbiplatin and vincristine is being evaluated (North 1997).

Other intracranial tumours are less common (Fig. 4.3). They are mostly astrocytomas that can involve the hemispheres, cerebellum, basal ganglia or brainstem. The latter are of interest because their prognosis is usually much better than that of brainstem tumours unassociated with NF1. Molloy *et al.* (1995) studied 17 patients. In only six of these was there evidence of progression by imaging and in only three was progression clinically detectable. The tumours involved the medulla in 14 cases. Fifteen of the patients were alive at follow-up after several years although no treatment other than a shunt when required was given. The authors concluded that these lesions are intermediate between 'hamartomas' and classical brainstem tumours and that aggressive treatment is best withheld unless there is evidence of progression on monitoring. Pollack *et al.* (1996) came to similar conclusions in a study of 21 cases.

Multiple brain tumours are not uncommon (Gray and Swaiman 1987, Hochstrasser *et al.* 1988) (Fig. 4.4). Intracranial calcification involving the central nuclei or the periventricular area is rare (Arts and Van Dongen 1986) and is not of tumoural origin.

high-intensity T_2 lesions in 32 of 50 systematically studied 8- to 16-year-old patients, 24 of whom had no tumour. The lesions were usually multiple, involved the optic tract in 20 patients, the basal ganglia in 24, the cerebellum in eight and the brainstem in six. The areas occasionally enhance with gadolinium. Hyperintense lesions in T_1-weighted sequences were present in 16 children, usually corresponding with T_2 abnormalities. All patients

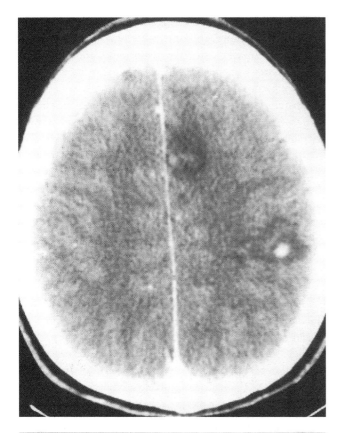

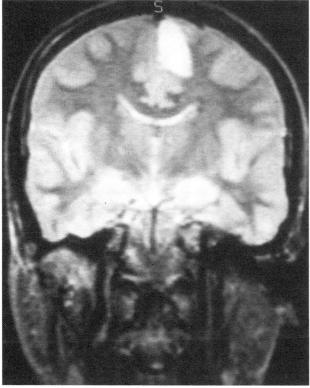

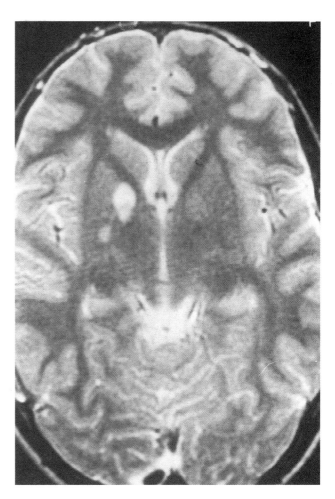

Fig. 4.4. NF1 in a 14-year-old girl. T₂-weighted MRI scan shows areas of increased signal ('hamartomas') in the right basal ganglia and in both thalami.

Fig. 4.3. 10-year-old girl with NF1 associated with right-sided partial motor seizures of recent onset. *(Top)* CT scan indicates two areas of decreased density in left hemisphere with central contrast enhancement in the posterior lesion. *(Bottom)* T₂-weighted MRI, coronal cut, shows intense signal from left frontomesial lesion. Two tumours (grade I–II astrocytomas) were subsequently removed at operation, with complete control of seizures for one year.

Intraspinal tumours, comprising mainly astrocytomas, are uncommon. Intraspinal neurofibromas occur mainly in the cervicothoracic region. These tumours not uncommonly are both intra- and extraspinal and may be in continuity with a subcutaneous plexiform neurofibroma. Intramedullary tumours such as ependymomas and astrocytomas are not a feature of NF1.

Major CNS malformations, especially disturbances of neuronal migration, are not common in NF1. However, hemimegalencephaly has been reported (Cusmai *et al.* 1990). Tumours of peripheral nerves may occur. One case of sudden death secondary to a neurofibroma of the Xth nerve is on record (Chow *et al.* 1993).

Hydrocephalus in a majority of cases is the result of aqueductal stenosis (Afifi *et al.* 1988, Riviello *et al.* 1988). It usually develops slowly and is recognized late. It is usually due to gliosis, diffuse or membranous, of the aqueduct. Small tumours of the peduncular region may be a cause, and MRI in the sagittal plane using both T₁- and T₂-weighted sequences should always be performed. An intense signal in T₂-weighted scans was present in seven of nine recent cases (Pou-Serradell and Ugarte-Elola 1989, Valentini *et al.* 1995). Other causes of ventriculomegaly in NF1 patients include Chiari I malformation (Afifi *et al.* 1988a), tumours of the posterior fossa and unknown causes.

Abnormalities of the skull are frequent in NF1. *Craniofacial dysplasia* can affect any portion of the cranial vault, most commonly the occipital regions along the lambdoid suture. Bones contributing to the orbit, especially the greater sphenoidal wing, are a site of election for dysplasia. The greater wing is missing in part, with resulting *pulsating exophthalmos* when the defect is large (Binet *et al.* 1969). The lesser wing and sella turcica are often involved in the dysplasia. *Dural ectasias* can produce bilateral enlargement of the auditory canal, which may suggest the diagnosis of NF2, but they are not associated with schwannoma of the VIIIth nerve (Inoue *et al.* 1997). *Calvarial defects* adjacent to the lambdoid suture (Joffe 1965) are clinically asymptomatic. *Scoliosis* is present in 20 per cent of cases and may be sufficiently severe to warrant surgical correction. It is occasionally associated with paraspinal neurofibromas and may also be associated with vertebral abnormalities. These are also frequent, and scalloping of the body of vertebrae is a common radiological finding in NF1, as is scoliosis. Lateral ectasia of the thinned dura through the intervertebral foramina (lateral meningoceles) is a rare complication of von Recklinghausen disease (Erkulvrawatr *et al.* 1979, Riccardi 1992). Tibial pseudoarthrosis is a common lesion (North 1997).

OTHER COMPLICATIONS OF NF1
These include growth retardation, which is present in about 25 per cent of patients (North 1993); eye disease, especially glaucoma and buphthalmos (Walsh and Hoyt 1969); osseous dysplasia; arachnoid cysts; and abnormalities of the EEG, seen in 15 per cent of patients (Riccardi 1992). Vascular manifestations include systemic hypertension with or without renal artery stenosis, which should always be looked for, and, rarely, cerebrovascular accidents (Tomsik *et al.* 1976, Pellock *et al.* 1980). Multiple stenoses of carotid arteries with the development of a moyamoya pattern has been reported (Rizzo and Lessell 1994). *Malignancies,* the most frequent of which are fibrosarcomas, are rare in childhood. *Leukaemia* especially of chronic myelogenous type can occur (Clark and Hutter 1982). It may be associated with the presence of cutaneous xanthomas. Visceral and endocrine tumours are relatively common in later life (Huson *et al.* 1988). Visceral autonomic localizations may be seen. In particular, intestinal ganglioneuromatosis with intestinal obstruction is recognized (Deschryver-Kecskemeti *et al.* 1983).

NEUROFIBROMATOSIS TYPE 2
NF2 is transmitted as a dominant autosomal trait. The gene has been mapped to chromosome 22 and several mutations have been found (Rouleau *et al.* 1993). *Bilateral acoustic neuromas (schwannomas)* are the essential feature, occurring in at least 90 per cent of cases (Evans *et al.* 1992a). These tumours develop mainly in late adolescence and early adulthood, and NF2 is rarely found in children. Loss of hearing is the first symptom. Cutaneous manifestations are uncommon and most patients have no café-au-lait spots, or only a small number of them. Lisch nodules are not found, but posterior subcapsular cataracts occur in 10 per cent or more of patients (Bouzas *et al.* 1993). *Other intracranial tumours* are frequent—especially meningiomas, often multiple—but optic nerve glioma has not been found in NF2 patients. The occurrence of astrocytoma also seems to be exceptional. Schwannomas of cranial nerves V to XII are common. They are frequently bilateral and multiple. Some authors indicate that atypical NF2 may occur sporadically and often present with multiple cranial or spinal schwannomas (Purcell and Dixon 1989, Pou-Serradell 1991). They have proposed separating a subgroup of NF2 under the term 'schwannomatosis', manifested by peripheral painful nerve schwannomas and often by multiple spinal root tumours (MacCollin *et al.* 1996). Such cases may be difficult to distinguish from paediatric cases of NF2 in which peripheral tumours may long precede the appearance of acoustic schwannomas (Mautner *et al.* 1993), and indeed have recently been shown to be a variant of NF2 (Evans *et al.* 1997).

Spinal cord tumours are of two types: schwannomas, which are of the same histological type as the acoustic neuroma, and ependymomas (Rubinstein 1986). The former may be multiple and lead to serious problems. Hamartomatous lesions resembling meningiomas, termed 'meningoangiomatosis' by Russell and Rubinstein (1977), may occur and be responsible for calcification, especially in the choroid plexus, at the periphery of one cerebellar hemisphere (Van Tassel *et al.* 1987), or as linear subependymal calcification (Arts and Van Dongen 1986) that may be associated with seizures (Clarke *et al.* 1990). Involvement of peripheral nerves can occur (Kilpatrick *et al.* 1992). Presymptomatic diagnosis is possible with chromosome 22 markers (Ruttledge *et al.* 1993).

NF2 is a separate disorder from NF1 (Wertelecki *et al.* 1988), and there is only one known patient with both NF1 and NF2 (inherited separately from each parent) (Sadeh *et al.* 1989, Evans *et al.* 1992b). The disease may be mistaken for NF1 in the rare patient with bilateral auditory canal enlargement without tumour (Kitamura *et al.* 1989). The presence of bilateral acoustic neuromas in NF1 has, however, been reported (Michels *et al.* 1989).

OTHER FORMS OF NEUROFIBROMATOSIS
SEGMENTAL NEUROFIBROMATOSIS (NF5)
NF5 is characterized by the unilateral occurrence of features that are typical of NF1 (café-au-lait spots and neurofibromas) in only one or in several dermal segments. The disorder is thought to result from a postzygotic event and any dermatome may be involved. Most cases are sporadic although familial transmission has been observed (Calzavara *et al.* 1988, Jung 1988). Roth *et al.* (1987) divide segmental neurofibromatosis into four subtypes, only one of which is genetically transmitted. The skin lesions are usually café-au-lait patches but neurofibromas may eventually develop. Other complications of neurofibromatosis do not occur so the prognosis is good.

OTHER POSSIBLE FORMS
Forms with only café-au-lait spots and other atypical forms are on record. Charrow *et al.* (1993b) found suggestive evidence of

non-linkage to the *NF1* locus, but Abeliovich *et al.* (1995) found close linkage to the *NF1* gene in a large pedigree. Intestinal neurofibromatosis may occur in isolation (Heimann *et al.* 1988) or form a part of syndromes related to neurofibromatosis (Hegstrom and Kircher 1985) and to the multiple endocrine neoplasia disorders (Fryns and Chrzanowska 1988, Griffiths *et al.* 1990). Type III or IIB multiple endocrine adenomatosis is characterized by a Marfan-like habitus, a lobulated tongue with multiple submucous neuromas, conjunctival nodules, thick lips, megacolon and multiple endocrine tumours.

A combination of NF1 with features of the Noonan phenotype (short stature, pectus carinatum, cardiac defect, ptosis and low intelligence) has been termed 'neurofibromatosis–Noonan syndrome' (Borochowitz *et al.* 1989), although whether it represents a distinct subtype is controversial. Watson syndrome (café-au-lait patches and pulmonic stenosis) which may include CNS involvement in the form of areas of increased T_2 signal (Leão and da Silva 1995), may also be closely related to NF1.

DIAGNOSIS AND MANAGEMENT OF THE NEUROFIBROMATOSES

The diagnosis of neurofibromatosis is essentially clinical and it is usually easy. Diagnostic criteria for NF1 and NF2 are shown in Table 4.1 (p. 132). Histological study of pigmented spots could show abnormalities in melanosomes (Martuza *et al.* 1985) but is not usually justified. Molecular genetic diagnosis is possible (see above).

Management of patients with neurofibromatosis should start with assessing the extent of the disease by a complete clinical, ophthalmological and radiological examination. A team approach, grouping specialists in the many different problems that often are associated with the condition, is essential as it has been shown that many patients are not appropriately diagnosed and treated for all their problems. Routine follow-up is mandatory. For those patients who have suspected brain tumours, yearly CT or MRI is required.

There is no drug treatment for NF. Surgical treatment is indicated for invasive tumours but the results are often disappointing. Surgery is also indicated for cosmetic deformities that in many cases amount to a major problem.

TUBEROUS SCLEROSIS

Tuberous sclerosis (TS) is a dominantly transmitted disorder with a variable expression and a high incidence of new mutations in the order of 58–68 per cent of recognized cases (Fleury *et al.* 1980, Hunt and Lindenbaum 1984). The prevalence of the disease is imperfectly known because of the frequency of paucisymptomatic forms. Population surveys indicate a prevalence of 1 in 6000 to 1 in 10,000 (Hunt and Lindenbaum 1984, Kuntz 1988, Webb and Osborne 1995). Occurrence of affected siblings with apparently unaffected parents is extremely rare (Michel *et al.* 1983). At least two mutant genes are responsible for tuberous sclerosis. In about half the families the gene maps to 9q34 (*TSC1*); in the remainder it is located on the short arm of

chromosome 16 (*TSC2*) and probably acts as a tumour-suppressor gene (Kandt *et al.* 1992). The gene on 16p has been identified and has homology to the GTPase-activating protein GAP3 (Nellist *et al.* 1993). Other previously suggested gene localizations have been refuted.

The mechanism of the disease is unkown. It involves an abnormality of differentiation of embryonic cells, with a tendency to hamartomatous proliferation, and a disturbance of the migrational process of CNS cells.

PATHOLOGY

The characteristic lesions found in the brain of patients with TS are cortical tubers, subependymal nodules, and giant cell tumours. *Tubers* are hard nodules of variable size which show disruption of normal lamination, increased astrocytic nuclei and a reduction of the number of neurons, which are replaced by bizarre giant cells (Huttenlocher and Heydemann 1984, Yamanouchi *et al.* 1997) that take both glial and neuronal markers. They may become calcified. Beneath the tubers, enlarged abnormal heterotopic neurons extend all the way to the ventricular walls. *Subependymal nodules* (Fig. 4.5*a*) are small excrescences on the ventricular walls that resemble solidified wax that has dripped down the side of a candle, hence the term 'candle guttering' which is traditionally used. They are composed of large round fusiform cells that are unanimously thought to be of astrocytic origin. *Subependymal giant cell astrocytomas* (Fig. 4.5*b*) are found in about 5 per cent of cases (Gomez 1988) and are consistently located to the region of the foramen of Monro. Unlike subependymal nodules, they grow, sometimes to a large size, but rarely, if ever, become malignant. The nature of the giant cells is still uncertain (Bonnin *et al.* 1984).

Visceral tumours arise from various viscera. *Rhabdomyomas* are found in the heart of 40–50 per cent of TS patients and are often multiple. *Renal lesions* include angiomyolipomas, which may be the only lesion of TS in some patients, and renal cysts (Robbins and Bernstein 1988). *Retinal phakomas* are benign astrocytic tumours that tend to calcify. Other hamartomatous lesions are seen less commonly (Gomez 1988).

CLINICAL MANIFESTATIONS

The clinical manifestations of TS vary considerably with the extent of involvement and age of onset. Table 4.2 groups the findings into those which are pathognomonic and those that are suggestive of diagnosis, according to the criteria proposed by Gomez (1988). The diagnosis is suspect if only one suggestive feature is present, presumptive if two are present, and highly probable if one of the two features is a relative with TS.

SEIZURES

In infants and children, seizures are the most common presenting complaint. They are generalized in about 85 per cent of cases. The most common seizures in infants are *infantile spasms* (Hunt 1983, Gomez 1988). Tonic or atonic seizures are also frequently seen. Complex partial seizures were observed in 17 of 25 patients with TS who had initially had infantile spasms and in 11 of 15 children

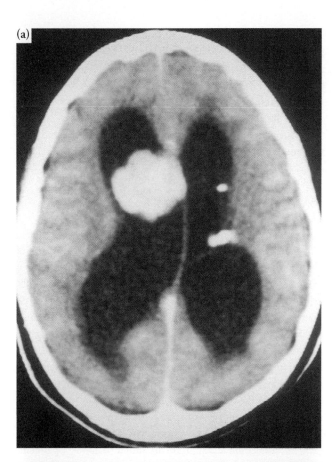

TABLE 4.2
Diagnostic criteria for tuberous sclerosis*

Pathognomonic features
Cortical tuber
Subependymal glial nodules
Retinal phakoma
Adenoma sebaceum
Periungual fibroma
Fibrous plaque of forehead or scalp
Multiple renal angiomyolipomas

Suggestive features
Immediate relative with TS
Hypomelanotic macules
Shagreen patches
Cardiac rhabdomyomas
Gingival fibroma
Multiple renal tumours
Renal cysts
Infantile spasms
Wedge-shaped areas of cortical/subcortical calcification
Multiple subcortical hypodense areas on CT (or high T_2 signal on MRI)
Peripapillary retinal hamartoma, indistinguishable from drüsen
Pulmonary lymphangiomyomatosis

*Modified from Gomez (1988).

who had had other types of seizure (Yamamoto *et al.* 1987). The unbiased frequency of seizures is about 60 per cent (Webb *et al.* 1991).

NEURODEVELOPMENTAL DIFFICULTIES

Mental subnormality is the rule in hospital-based series and was present in 82 per cent of children in one study (Monaghan *et al.* 1981). However, in the Mayo Clinic experience, only 47 per cent of patients and their affected relatives were mentally subnormal while 44 per cent had normal intelligence. Webb *et al.* (1991) give an even lower figure for mental retardation (40 per cent) in a population study. Mental retardation is found only in patients who have had seizures, especially if these had their onset before 2 years of age (Gomez 1988). The prognosis of infantile spasms in TS patients is thus serious. Riikonen and Simell (1990) found that infantile spasms due to tuberous sclerosis have an especially poor prognosis, while Yamamoto *et al.* (1987) reported that the mental outcome in such patients was significantly better than that of patients with symptomatic spasms due to other causes. In addition to mental subnormality, autism or other deviant behaviour such as hyperkinesia is not infrequently found in TS patients with infantile spasms (Hunt and Dennis 1987). Neurological deficits, on the other hand, are rare, with the exception of increased intracranial pressure that occurs in less than 3 per cent of cases and results from the development of intraventricular giant cell tumours and becomes symptomatic after the age of 5 years. These also may be responsible for a hemiplegia.

CUTANEOUS MANIFESTATIONS (Fig. 4.6)

The classical cutaneous lesions of TS are angiofibromas (adenoma sebaceum) that occupy symmetrical areas over the cheeks, naso-labial folds and chin. These red papular lesions are rare in infants and generally appear between 3 and 15 years of age (Rogers

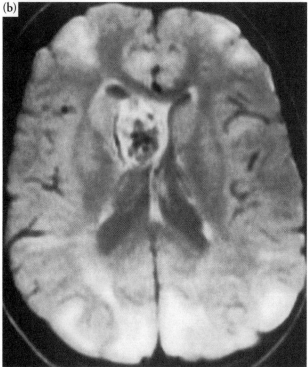

Fig. 4.5. Tuberous sclerosis. *(a)* CT scan showing calcified subependymal nodules projecting into the lateral ventricles and a calcified giant cell astrocytoma obstructing the foramina of Monro with resulting hydrocephalus. *(b)* MRI scan of an 11-year-old boy with clinically isolated cutaneous manifestations, normal intelligence and no seizures. Heterogeneous mass in the right foramen of Monro corresponds to a giant cell astrocytoma. Multiple areas of increased signal in cortex represent tubers.

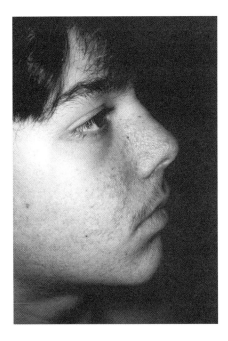
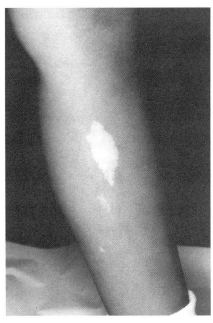
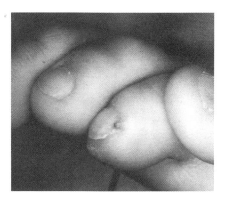

Fig. 4.6. Cutaneous manifestations of tuberous sclerosis. *(Left)* Facial angiofibromas (adenoma sebaceum). *(Centre)* Achromic naevus. *(Above)* Periungual fibroma. (Courtesy Dr D. Teillac, Prof. Y. de Prost, Hôpital des Enfants Malades, Paris.)

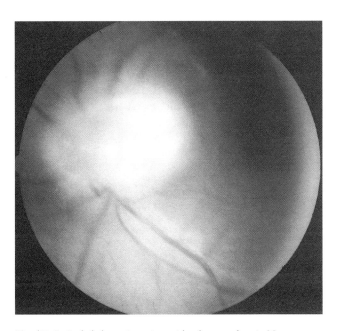

Fig. 4.7. Retinal phakoma in patient with tuberous sclerosis. Note tumour overlies retinal vessels.

1988). They are found only in half the cases of TS. Hypomelanotic macules (achromic patches or ash-leaf spots) are the earliest and most frequent cutaneous sign of TS (Hunt 1983) and occur in 90 per cent of cases (Fryer *et al.* 1990). They vary in number and size and are often present at birth, although they may become more visible and more numerous within a few months. They may be visible only under Wood's light in fair-skinned patients, especially infants. Isolated, small hypomelanotic spots are nonspecific. They are present in 0.8 per cent of normal newborn infants (Alper and Holmes 1983). The association of white spots with seizures, especially infantile spasms, is characteristic of

TS (Roth and Epstein 1971). A lock of *depigmented hair* may be an initial sign (McWilliam and Stephenson 1978). It results from the presence of a hypomelanotic spot on the scalp. Other cutaneous signs include *fibrous plaques*, usually on the forehead or scalp, that can occasionally be the sole manifestation of the disease; *shagreen patches* (20–40 per cent of cases) that consist of a slightly elevated plaque of epidermis with a granular surface and sometimes a yellowish-brown discolouration and appear after a few years of life, commonly in the lumbar region; *periungual fibromas* that are a pathognomonic lesion but one that seldom occurs before puberty and then only in about 50 per cent of patients; and molluscum pendulum in the cervical and lower facial region—not a specific lesion but quite unusual in childhood outside TS. Café-au-lait spots are not more frequent in TS than in the general population (Bell and McDonald 1985).

EYE ANOMALIES
Eye findings are represented by retinal astrocytomas (phakomas) (Fig. 4.7), which are found in half the cases and may be unique or multiple. They are round or oval in shape and become easy to diagnose when they calcify, assuming a typical mulberry appearance. Other ophthalmological findings in TS patients include depigmented retinal areas, hypopigmented iris spots (Gutman *et al.* 1982), hyaline or cystic nodules, cataracts and iris coloboma.

OTHER FINDINGS
In some patients, the presenting manifestations are visceral rather than CNS ones. Kidney tumours (angiolipomas) are present in 60 per cent of patients and may precede nervous system manifestations in infants, while hypertension may be the first feature in children (Robbins 1987). A search for other localizations of TS is always indicated in patients with renal disorders, as it is also in infants with abnormalities of cardiac rhythm or with heart

tumours detected by echography. These may occur prenatally or may only be revealed following administration of drugs such as carbamazepine (Weig and Pollack 1993). About half the cardiac rhabdomyomas are a manifestation of TS. Conversely, more than 50 per cent of TS patients have cardiac tumours. Many are asymptomatic but some may manifest as cardiac failure, although arrhythmia is more common. They may be the cause of embolic strokes although this is doubted by Gomez (1989).

Other visceral manifestations are rare or seen only in adults. Partial gigantism has been reported (Colamaria et al. 1988).

DIAGNOSIS

The diagnosis of TS is often clinically easy but, in infancy, the most characteristic manifestations have not yet appeared. By far the most powerful diagnostic tool is neuroimaging by CT or MRI. *CT scan* is abnormal in 89 per cent of patients. It shows subependymal calcified nodules, especially in the region of the foramen of Monro; cortical or subcortical areas of decreased attenuation which correspond to tubers and may be associated with widening of the adjacent gyrus; in some cases ventricular dilatation or cortical atrophy or both; focal areas of increased attenuation corresponding to calcified tubers; and occasionally cerebellar calcification (Kingsley et al. 1986). Gyriform calcification simulating that in Sturge–Weber syndrome may occur (Wilms et al. 1992). Contrast enhancement is useful if a giant cell astrocytoma is suspected as these take up contrast in 80 per cent of cases.

MRI scan does not show the calcified lesions well, but does show cortical and subcortical tubers much better than CT scan. They present as high signal areas in T_2-weighted sequences. These areas are generally much more numerous than hypodense areas evidenced by CT and are located in the cortex (Terwey and Doose 1987, Roach et al. 1991). They vary in number and localization, and there is some relationship between the number and localization of tubers and mental development and neuro-psychological findings (Shepherd et al. 1995, Curatolo 1996b, Goodman et al. 1997). Deep white matter cystic abnormalities have been rarely reported (Canapicchi et al. 1996). Radial bands or wedge-shaped areas extending from ventricle to cortex or to a cortical tuber (Braffman et al. 1992) are composed of clusters of heterotopic cells and are indicative of a disorder of migration associated with abnormal cell differentiation. According to Gomez (1988), a diagnosis of cerebral TS can probably be discarded if both CT and MRI are negative for cerebral abnormalities.

The *EEG* is of interest to better define the type of epilepsy associated with TS. Atypical hypsarrhythmia, often asymmetrical, is present in one third of cases. Focal signs are present in at least 40 per cent of tracings (Yamamoto et al. 1987). In later childhood, focal paroxysms or bilateral slow spike–wave complexes may be found.

MANAGEMENT

There is no specific treatment for the disease itself but several of its manifestations are amenable to therapy. Anticonvulsant drugs should be given for seizures, and infantile spasms may justify

ACTH or steroid treatment. Vigabatrin seems to be particularly effective in the treatment of infantile spasms due to TS (Chiron et al. 1990, Aicardi et al. 1996) and to a lesser extent for treatment of focal seizures (Curatolo 1994). Tumours should be removed surgically as far as possible, but in some cases palliative shunting may be necessary. Radiation therapy is not usually advised. Removal of a large tuber may be successful in controlling seizures in some patients. Disfiguring adenofibromas can be treated medically or surgically according to their nature.

Genetic counselling is an essential part of the management of TS patients and parents. Careful examination of both parents should be performed, especially clinical and ophthalmological assessment. If these are negative, Fryer et al. (1990) think that a CT scan is unlikely to help. Others systematically perform a CT scan and/or MRI, but the latter may be difficult to interpret (Braffman et al. 1992) and may not show calcification, although periventricular nodules can usually be made out easily. The nature of the disease should be explained in simple terms. In the usual case of an isolated patient without family history of the disease, a favourable genetic prognosis can be given with very few reservations, provided both parents have been carefully examined and have been found not to have any cutaneous, neurological or visceral feature of the disease. Such an assessment includes, in addition to clinical examination and search for possible cases in families, ophthalmological examination, renal ultrasonography and CT scan (Fleury et al. 1980). Prenatal diagnosis can be suspected on the basis of fetal ultrasound examination, showing cardiac rhabdomyomas or polycystic kidneys. Molecular genetic diagnosis is difficult because of genetic heterogeneity. Identification of a mutation of the *TS2* gene has been performed (Vrtel et al. 1996).

VON HIPPEL–LINDAU DISEASE

Although not a neurocutaneous disease, von Hippel–Lindau syndrome has many features in common with the phakomatoses, including a remarkable tendency to the development of non-vascular tumours. It is discussed in Chapter 15.

ATAXIA–TELANGIECTASIA

From a purely clinical point of view ataxia–telangiectasia (AT) can be regarded as a neurocutaneous syndrome although its pathological features and course are closer to those of the heredo-degenerative disorders, in particular the spinocerebellar degenerations. AT is defined as a heredofamilial disease of progressive cerebellar ataxia and choreoathetosis, progressive oculocutaneous telangiectasias, immunodeficiency with susceptibility to sino-pulmonary infections, impaired organ maturation, X-ray hypersensitivity, and a high incidence of malignancies (Waldmann et al. 1983). It has become clear that it is a multisystem genetic disorder with an autosomal recessive inheritance. The disease is probably heterogeneous, both clinically and genetically, as shown by the existence of four complementation groups. The responsible gene has been mapped to chromosome 11q22–23 in families with types A, C and D complementation groups (Shiloh 1995). Savitsky *et al.* (1995) isolated the gene that codes for a protein (ATM protein) with similarities to mammalian phosphatidylinositol-3′ kinases, and mutations in this gene have been found in all four complementation groups indicating that there is only one locus responsible for the condition.

MECHANISMS AND PATHOLOGY

One basic defect of the malady is the abnormal sensitivity of AT cells to X-rays and certain radiomimetic chemicals but not to ultraviolet irradiation (Paterson and Smith 1979). The AT cell resumes DNA synthesis with undue speed after insults to its enzymatic systems of damage repair (De Wit *et al.* 1981, Hanawalt and Painter 1985). It might then incorporate damage into its DNA that leads to chromosome and chromatid breaks (Kohn *et al.* 1982). Breakpoints are randomly distributed, but nonrandom chromosome rearrangements affect selectively chromosomes 7 and 14 at sites that are concerned with T-cell receptors and heavy-chain immunoglobulin coding and with the development of haematological malignancies (Aurias *et al.* 1980, Hecht and Hecht 1985, Aurias and Dutrillaux 1986). These sites include bands 7p14, 7p35, 14q2 and 14qter. Chromosomes 2 and 22 (at bands 2p11, 2p12 and 22q11) are also frequently involved (Gatti *et al.* 1985). In about 10 per cent of cases, a clone of cells with a 14–14 translocation with breakpoint at 14q32 develops which may be related to the emergence of malignancies.

Such disturbances could account for the frequency of infections and neoplasias. The mechanisms responsible for neurological disease, thymus aplasia, telangiectasias, growth retardation and impaired organ maturation have not been elucidated (Boder 1985). There is a general disturbance in tissue differentiation that accounts for the almost constant elevation of alpha-fetoprotein (AFP), a fetal serum protein of hepatic origin which indicates dedifferentiation of liver cells.

Recent work suggests that AT may be associated with dysregulation of the immunoglobulin gene superfamily which includes genes for T-cell receptors (Peterson and Funkhouser 1989). The normal switch from the production of IgM to IgG, IgA and IgE is defective, and the same may apply to the switch from immature T-cells that express the gamma/delta rather than the alpha/beta receptors (Carbonari *et al.* 1990). Conceivably, absence or mutation of a single protein coded for by chromosome 11 could explain the immunological and perhaps even the neurological features of the disease (Kastan 1995). The ATM protein apparently controls the cell cycle and plays a major role in the protection of the genome.

The major *pathological lesion* in the CNS is degeneration of Purkinje and granule cells in the cerebellum (De Léon *et al.* 1976, Paula-Barbosa *et al.* 1983). Usually, no vascular abnormalities are found except late degenerative gliovascular nodules in the white matter. Lesions of the basal ganglia are found only occasionally (Boder 1985). Degeneration of spinal tracts and anterior horn cells is often present in late cases. Nucleocytomegaly is a feature of several cell types throughout the body (De Léon *et al.* 1976).

CLINICAL FEATURES

NEUROLOGICAL FINDINGS

The main neurological manifestations of AT are ataxia and abnormal eye movements, which are present in virtually all cases, and choreoathetosis that occurs in 25 per cent of patients (Boder 1985). The ataxia has its onset in infancy, becoming apparent when the child begins to walk. From this early stage, the ataxia is associated with abnormal head movements, and affected children have a peculiar gait like 'little clowns' which is highly suggestive. The ataxia is relentlessly progressive but the pace is variable even in the same sibship. Intention tremor and myoclonus may be observed. Choreoathetosis may be so marked in some patients as to overshadow or mask the ataxia. A dystonic component is possible (Bodensteiner *et al.* 1980). Ocular motor signs are diagnostically important because they usually precede the appearance of telangiectasias. Saccades are slowly initiated and hypometric, so that fixation of a target is obtained by head rather than eye deviation, often in association with a head thrust or forced blinking as in Cogan's ocular motor apraxia (Baloh *et al.* 1978) but present in both horizontal and vertical gaze. Eye deviation, when obtained, is saccadic and often halts midway, and optokinetic nystagmus is absent. Dysarthria of cerebellar type, characteristic postures and a dull facies at rest with a slow-spreading smile contribute to the peculiar appearance of AT children. About 30 per cent of patients have mild mental retardation.

TELANGIECTASIAS

Telangiectasias are first noticed after 3 years of age, sometimes not until adolescence. They may be absent even later in some cases (Chung *et al.* 1994). Dilated conjunctival vessels, first noticed in the angles of both eyes, spread horizontally in the equatorial region of the conjunctivae toward the corneal limb. They may involve the ears, eyelids, and cubital and popliteal fossas. In late childhood and adolescence, progeric skin changes may appear as well as pigmentary changes and café-au-lait spots (Sedgwick and Boder 1972).

SENSITIVITY TO INFECTIONS

Repeated *sinopulmonary infections* are present in 48–81 per cent of patients (Chung *et al.* 1994). McFarlin *et al.* (1972) divided their patients into three groups with regard to the occurrence of infections. One third had frequent and severe infections with progressive lung disease, one third had infections but no progressive lung disease, and the remaining third had only a normal incidence of infections. There was a good correlation betwen the occurrence of infections and immunodeficiency as assessed by laboratory tests. Such a correlation was not found in other series (Roifman and Gelfand 1985).

Retardation of somatic growth is found in most patients, and many do not achieve normal puberty. In girls, this may be related to absence of ovary differentiation which is found in some cases.

COURSE AND PROGNOSIS

The neurological features of AT are relentlessly progressive. In addition to the classical early features, older patients tend to develop other signs of spinocerebellar degeneration such as posterior cord involvement with loss of deep tendon reflexes and spinal muscular atrophy (Boder 1985, Kwast and Ignatowicz 1990). Most patients are wheelchair dependent by 10–15 years of age, but mild forms are not rare.

Early death is frequently due to pulmonary disease but malignancies are now the most common cause. The incidence is 60–300 times higher than in normal persons (Swift *et al.* 1991), and 49 per cent of cases coming to autopsy had malignant tumours (Gatti and Good 1971). The most common tumours are lymphoreticular malignancies, especially non-Hodgkin lymphomas, lymphocytic leukaemia and Hodgkin lymphomas (Boder 1985), but other kinds of tumours also occur. Yoshitomi *et al.* (1980) found that lymphoreticular neoplasms and leukaemia predominate in patients under 15 years of age, while epithelial tumours predominate in older patients. Malignancies are also more common in obligate heterozygotes than in the general population (Swift *et al.* 1991). The frequency of cancers, especially breast carcinomas, is increased three to six times as compared with the general population, and this information has to be included in genetic counselling.

In older patients insulin-resistant diabetes develops in half the cases but is not responsible for ketosis (McFarlin *et al.* 1972).

DIAGNOSIS AND LABORATORY MARKERS
The clinical diagnosis of AT is easy when both cardinal features are present. Before the appearance of telangiectasias, the diagnosis of ataxic cerebral palsy is often made. However, ocular motor abnormalities and the 'little clown' gait are suggestive of AT.

Laboratory markers are important for both diagnosis and prognosis. The most constant markers are elevated levels of AFP (Waldmann and McIntire 1972) and carcinoembryonic antigen (Sugimoto *et al.* 1978), and chromosomal abnormalities, especially inversions and translocations involving chromosomes 7 and 14 (Aurias *et al.* 1980, Hecht and Hecht 1985), although neither of these abnormalities is always found (Richkind *et al.* 1982) and their demonstration requires specific techniques available in only a few centres.

The demonstration of humoral or cellular immunological defects may also permit an early diagnosis, although such defects are nonspecific and less frequently present (Roifman and Gelfand 1985). The dysgammaglobulinaemia of AT includes absence or low level of IgA including secretory IgA, normal or low level of IgG, and elevated or normal level of IgM. A deficit in Ig2 and Ig4 subclasses has been demonstrated in several patients, and IgE may also be absent or low (Oxelius *et al.* 1982). Defects of cellular immunity include a low lymphocyte count, a poor response to skin tests to common antigens, low T-lymphocyte proliferation in the presence of mitogens, and deficient antibody production to viral or bacterial antigens (McFarlin *et al.* 1972, Waldmann 1982). Excessive T-cell suppressor activity and intrinsic B-cell defects have been described in some patients, suggesting disturbances of immunoregulatory mechanisms.

Increased chromosomal breakage after exposure of cell cultures to ionizing radiation is of rapidly increasing diagnostic importance, although not yet a routine procedure. Such tests have been considered for the prenatal diagnosis of AT (Schwartz *et al.* 1985) but are being supplanted by DNA diagnosis.

Other investigations are of less importance. CT scan and MRI often show evidence of nonspecific cerebellar atrophy. Nerve conduction velocities may be slowed, and denervation of anterior horn cell type may be found in older patients (Dunn 1973).

ATYPICAL AND VARIANT FORMS OF ATAXIA–TELANGIECTASIA
Patients with atypical forms of AT are uncommon. Some cases are undoubtedly part of the spectrum of the disease, with a slow course and prolonged survival (Boder 1985). Others include markedly abnormal features such as mental retardation and spasticity (Meshram *et al.* 1986), peripheral neuropathy as a predominant sign (Terenty *et al.* 1978), absence of telangiectasia persisting into adulthood (Byrne *et al.* 1984), or even absence of neurological manifestations in the presence of elevated AFP, typical cytogenetic abnormalities and immunodeficiency (unpublished results). Some of these patients lack one or the other of the laboratory markers. They raise the question of the genetic heterogeneity of the disease, a question that will be solved by identifying the abnormal gene or genes. The syndrome of *ataxia–ocular motor apraxia* (Chapter 10) has a remarkably similar neurological presentation but does not show any feature of extraneurological involvement (Aicardi *et al.* 1988, Gascon *et al.* 1995). All biological markers for AT are absent, and in several cases cultured fibroblasts were normally resistant to irradiation (Gascon *et al.* 1995; and personal cases). The course is usually more benign, and it appears to represent a disease distinct from AT. The same probably applies to the *dysequilibrium–diplegia syndrome* (Hagberg *et al.* 1970, Graham-Pole *et al.* 1975) in which immunodeficiency is a major feature. This syndrome is associated with purine nucleotide phosphorylase deficiency (Soutar and Day 1991). Patients with this disorder have normal immunoglobulins and pyramidal tract signs, and in one case heterotopia and cortical dysplasia were present (Soutar and Day 1991). Other syndromes with neurological features, especially microcephaly, in association with chromosomal instability (Seemanova *et al.* 1985) may have some relationship to AT, especially the tendency to develop lymphoreticular malignancies.

MANAGEMENT
Although no specific treatment is available, several features of AT are accessible to active therapy. This applies especially to infections, and the life span of AT patients has been clearly prolonged by antibiotic treatment. Prevention of infections by regular injection of immunoglobulins is considered useful. Fetal thymus implants and stimulants of the immunological system have given inconclusive results.

Treatment of neurological manifestations is disappointing. Propanolol and sulpiride may improve fine motor coordination in a few cases. Rehabilitation and adequate educative support are always necessary.

The use of radiation therapy and chemotherapy in conventional doses is contraindicated in AT patients (Pritchard *et al.* 1982). Reduced doses of X-rays or chemicals, avoiding bleomycin, actinomycin D and cyclophosphamide, have given favourable results in a few cases (Abadir and Hakami 1983).

Regular surveillance of heterozygotes for cancer should be part of the family management.

LINEAR NAEVUS AND RELATED SYNDROMES

CLASSICAL LINEAR NAEVUS SYNDROME
In its complete form, this syndrome includes a cutaneous naevus with neurological and eye abnormalities. The skin lesion may be of several types. One typical appearance is that of the sebaceous naevus of Jadassohn. The lesion may be visible at birth or in infancy or become evident only after a few years (Clancy *et al.* 1985). It is a slightly raised, yellow-orange, smooth, linear plaque that abuts the midline of the forehead, nose or lips and often involves the scalp. It tends to become darker and verrucous as years pass. Early in life there is mainly acanthosis and little pigment, and sebaceous glands are often not prominent. Later, sebaceous glands proliferate and apocrine glands may be located aberrantly thoughout the thickness of skin.

A second type of naevus is the verrucous naevus which is formed of discrete papules, slightly darker than the surrounding skin, with a linear organization. Such naevi are more often located on the body and less on the face than the sebaceous naevus, and histologically there is only acanthosis and hyperkeratosis with abnormal dermis (Prensky 1987). It seems that either type of naevus may be associated with neurological abnormalities (Clancy *et al.* 1985), although most skin lesions are isolated. Associated cutaneous abnormalities such as ichthyosis, acanthosis nigricans, haemangiomas and café-au-lait spots are frequent, and linear naevus overlaps with other neurocutaneous syndromes with proliferative skin and subcutaneous tissue lesions (see below).

Neurological manifestations associated with both types of naevi (Feuerstein–Mims syndrome) consist of mental retardation, seizures, cranial nerve palsies, hydrocephalus and asymmetrical macrocephaly. Seizures are often partial, but infantile spasms have been observed in four of 11 patients in one series (Vigevano *et al.* 1984). From a pathological point of view, the most common brain abnormalities are disorders of proliferation and migration. Hemimegalencephaly (Pavone *et al.* 1991, Cavenagh *et al.* 1993) is particularly frequent and may be associated with hemihypertrophy of the ipsilateral face and body. Hamartomatous tumours were present in several patients (Levin *et al.* 1984, Clancy *et al.* 1985). Destructive lesions such as porencephaly have also been found (Baker *et al.* 1987, Prensky 1987) and may be of vascular origin as arterial aneurysms, arteriovenous malformations and abnormal venous return have been reported (Dobyns and Garg 1991). Similar lesions have been found in the spinal cord (Chatkupt *et al.* 1993). Other CNS abnormalities include arachnoid cysts, subtotal cerebellar agenesis (Wang *et al.* 1983),

and callosal agenesis with Dandy–Walker malformation (Dodge and Dobyns 1995).

The most common *eye abnormalities* are dermoids or epidermoids of the conjunctiva and colobomas of the iris, choroid, retina or optic nerve. Enlargement of the orbit and of the greater wing of the sphenoid on the side of the naevus may be present (Clancy *et al.* 1985). Familial cases are rare (Meschia *et al.* 1992).

The diagnosis may be difficult in early cases without visible naevus. The most common CT image is that of hypertrophy of one hemisphere, usually on the same side as the naevus with enlargement of the ipsilateral ventricle, and pachygyria with hypodense white matter (Vles *et al.* 1985). Such an image is consistent with pathological reports of hemimegalencephaly or other migration disorders.

The EEG usually shows paroxysmal activity over the involved hemisphere, sometimes with a hypsarrhythmic pattern. The prognosis is usually poor but mild cases exist with only seizures or mild learning difficulties. The syndrome is probably sporadic and the cause is unknown. The relatively frequent ocurrence of tumours suggests a close relationship with the phakomatoses. Treatment is symptomatic. Removal of the cutaneous lesion is possible in some patients.

RELATED SYNDROMES WITH PROLIFERATIVE SKIN AND SUBCUTANEOUS TISSUE LESIONS.
These syndromes and their main features are listed in Table 4.3.

ENCEPHALOCRANIOCUTANEOUS LIPOMATOSIS
This is a rare, apparently sporadic syndrome characterized by microcephaly, lipodermoids involving the conjunctiva, sclera or eyelids, and lipomatous swelling over the cranium or face. Convulsions and mental retardation may be present, and CT brain scan may show atrophy, cystic areas and intracranial calcification. In studies by Fishman (1987) and Bamforth *et al.* (1989) brain malformations in the form of porencephaly were present in all cases, eyelid excrescences in most, and iris abnormalities in two. The condition may be related to the Proteus syndrome (McCall *et al.* 1992).

PROTEUS SYNDROME
This term applies to a complex hamartomatous syndrome consisting of partial gigantism, asymmetry of the limbs, linear verrucous and intradermal naevi, shagreen patches and variable combinations of lymphangiomas, haemangiomas, macrocephaly and hyperostoses. Plantar skin hyperplasia (the so-called 'moccasin lesion') is a frequent and useful diagnostic feature. Epibulbar dermoids, colobomas, glaucoma and retinal detachment can occur. Hemimegalencephaly is frequent (Griffiths *et al.* 1994). The deformities resulting from the syndrome can reach extreme proportions, as in the case of Joseph Merick, the so-called 'Elephant Man' (Cohen 1988). The disease is still commonly misdiagnosed as neurofibromatosis. As the name implies, the Proteus syndrome has a very variable expresssion (Cohen 1988, Vaughn *et al.* 1993). Most proven cases to date have been sporadic. Somatic mosaicism may account for most features of

TABLE 4.3
Some rare neurocutaneous syndromes*

Syndrome	Main features	Genetics†	References
Syndromes with a hamartomatous tendency			
Encephalocraniocutaneous lipomatosis	Unilateral scalp lipomas, porencephaly, brain malformations	S	This chapter
Proteus syndrome	Hemihypertrophy, massive tissue overgrowth, plantar hypertrophy, multiple naevi and hamartomas	S	This chapter
Ruvalcaba–Myhre–Smith syndrome	Inconstant mental retardation, pigmented macules on penis, angiolipomas, intestinal polyposis, lipidic myopathy	AD?	DiLiberti *et al.* (1983)
Riley–Smith syndrome	Heredofamilial mesodermal hamartomas, macrocephaly + pseudopapilloedema	AD?	Dvir *et al.* (1988), Hoover *et al.* (1989)
Endocrine neoplasia type 2b	Submucous neuromas of lips, tongue and digestive tract; thickened, inverted eyelids; medullary thyroid cancer; phaeochromocytoma; marfanoid habitus; pes cavus; scoliosis; hypotonia; cutaneous neurofibromas		Fryns and Chrzanowska (1988), Griffiths *et al.* (1990)
Cowden syndrome	Multiple hamartomas and other tumours, Lhermitte–Duclos cerebellar ganglioglioma		Vinchon *et al.* (1994)
Cutis verticis gyrata–mental deficiency syndrome	Epilepsy, mental retardation		Striano *et al.* (1996)
Syndromes with abnormal pigmentation			
Naegeli type of incontinentia pigmenti	Skin pigmentation not preceded by inflammatory stage, reticular, widespread	AD?	Rosenfeld and Smith (1985)
Lentiginosis–deafness–cardiopathy syndrome	Lentigines, hypertrophic cardiomyopathy, conduction defects, mental retardation, deafness	AD	Schievink *et al.* (1995)
Leopard syndrome	*L*entigines, *e*lectrocardiographic abnormalities, *o*cular hypertelorism, *p*ulmonary artery stenosis, *a*bnormal genitalia, *r*etardation of growth, *d*eafness	AD	Gorlin *et al.* (1969)

Waardenburg syndrome	Frontal white forelock, heterochromia iridis
	  Type I: dystopia cantorum, 25 per cent deafness
	  Type II: no dystopia, 50 per cent deafness
		AD	De Saxe *et al.* (1984)

Chediak–Higashi syndrome	Partial albinism, recurrent infections, neurological deficits, neuropathy	AR	Van Hale (1987)
Carney complex	Spotty facial pigmentation, Cushing syndrome, peripheral nerve tumours	AD	Carney *et al.* (1985), Young *et al.* (1989)
Neuroectodermal melanolysosomal disease	Abnormal hair colour, severe developmental retardation, abnormally formed melanosomes	AR	Elejalde *et al.* (1979)
Familial spastic paraplegia with crural hypopigmentation	Paraplegia, slow nerve conduction velocities	AR	Abdallat *et al.* (1980), Stewart *et al.* (1981)
Neuroichthyosis syndromes			
Rud syndrome	Icthyosis, mental retardation, epilepsy, hypogonadism, retinitis pigmentosa, steroid sulfatase deficiency	AR	Münke *et al.* (1983), Marx-Miller *et al.* (1985), Larbrisseau and Carpenter (1982)
Ichthyosis with neutral lipid storage	Ataxia, sensorineural deafness	AR	Williams *et al.* (1985)
Sunohara syndrome	Anosmia, hypogonadism, neurological defects	XR	Sunohara *et al.* (1986)
Brittle hair, ichthyosis, dwarfism (BID)	Microcephaly, dwarfism, ichthyosis	AR	Jorizzo *et al.* (1980)
Keratitis, ichthyosis and deafness (KID)	Sensorineural deafness, ichthyosis, hypotrichosis	AR	Jurecka *et al.* (1985)
Miscellaneous			
Cerebello-trigeminal dermal dysplasia	Alopecia of parieto-occipital area, hypertelorism, anaesthesia in Vth nerve territory, cerebellar hypoplasia, fusion of vermis and pons	S?	Gomez (1979b), Lopez-Hernandez (1982)
Cutis verticis gyrata	Furrowed scalp and associated seizures and/or mental retardation		Rasmussen and Frias (1989), Striano *et al.* (1996)
Congenital alopecia, seizures and psychomotor retardation		AR	Wessel *et al.* (1987)

*Syndromes with mainly vascular intracranial abnormalities are not included (see Chapter 15).
†S = sporadic; AD = autosomal dominant; AR = autosomal recessive; XR = X-linked recessive.

the syndrome (Cohen 1993). Visceral tumours may occur (Gordon *et al.* 1995).

This syndrome is considered in Chapter 15 because of the prominence of vascular abnormalities. It is one common cause of hemihypertrophy that also occurs in some of the phakomatoses '*stricto sensu*'.

NEUROCUTANEOUS SYNDROMES CHARACTERIZED PRIMARILY BY ABNORMAL PIGMENTATION

INCONTINENTIA PIGMENTI (BLOCH–SCHULZBERGER TYPE)

Bloch–Schulzberger syndrome is a rare genetic disorder, observed almost exclusively in girls, probably transmitted as an X-linked dominant trait prenatally lethal in males. The gene is linked to Xq28 (Curtis *et al.* 1994).

SKIN FEATURES
These consist of three distinct but somewhat overlapping stages (Rosman 1992, Mangano and Barbagallo 1993). In the first stage, erythematous, papular, vesicular or bullous lesions are present at birth or during the first two weeks of life on the trunk and limbs. They are linear in distribution and last from days to months. In the second stage, between the second and the sixth weeks, the lesions are variably pustular, verrucous or keratotic. They may disappear without sequelae or are followed by the development of pigmentation, characteristic of the third stage of the disease. These pigmented lesions may be located outside the area of earlier lesions, and in 10 per cent of cases are not preceded by them. The pigmentation persists into adulthood but tends to fade with the passing of time. Histologically there is absent or decreased melanin in the basal epidermal cells with an accompanying excess in the dermis, thus suggesting a 'leakage' or 'incontinence' of the basal cells. In 50–80 per cent of cases, noncutaneous abnormalities are present.

CNS INVOLVEMENT
CNS involvement occurs in one third to one half of the cases, although unbiased frequency in familial cases may not exceed 10 per cent (Landy and Donnai 1993). Seizures may occur early and, generally, are focal or secondarily generalized. Infantile spasms have been reported (Simonsson 1972). Progression of the neurological disease may be by recurrent episodes suggestive of 'encephalomyelitis' (Siemes *et al.* 1978, Brunquell 1987), with obtundation, hemiparesis and areas of low absorption in the brain white matter on CT scan with subsequent atrophy (Avrahami *et al.* 1985). One patient had involvement of the anterior horn cells of the spinal cord (Larsen *et al.* 1987). Neuropathological study in one case showed a migrational disorder (O'Doherty and Norman 1968). Destructive encephalopathies of apparently perinatal onset were found by Hauw *et al.* (1977), Siemes *et al.* (1978) and Shuper *et al.* 1990). In all cases inflam-

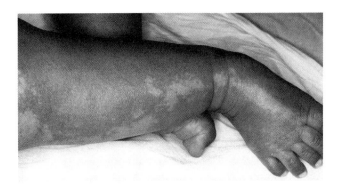

Fig. 4.8. Hypomelanosis of Ito. Note linear distribution of hypopigmented areas along axis of limb. (Courtesy Dr D. Teillac, Prof. Y. de Prost, Hôpital des Enfants Malades, Paris.)

matory lesions were visible. A syndrome of epidermolysis bullosa, encephalopathy and cyclic neutropenia (Grover *et al.* 1988) may be related.

EYE LESIONS
Various eye lesions are present in one third of cases, the most characteristic being a retrolental mass with detachment of a dysplastic retina (François 1984, Rosenfeld and Smith 1985). Dental abnormalities (peg-shaped teeth) occur in 70 per cent of patients. Treatment is symptomatic and includes ophthalmological interventions, antiepileptic agents, physiotherapy and orthopaedic measures as well as educational support. Genetic counselling is an important part of management.

Bloch–Schulzberger syndrome is probably different from the Naegeli type of incontinentia pigmenti rather than a subtype of the same disease (Rosman 1992). The latter occurs in boys and girls.

HYPOMELANOSIS OF ITO
Another condition that should be distinguished from Bloch–Schulzberger disease is hypomelanosis of Ito or *incontinentia pigmenti achromians*. This disorder is characterized by hypopigmented areas that have a peculiar streaked or whorled appearance and are often unilateral or with a strong unilateral predominance (Pascual-Castroviejo 1988, Griebel *et al.* 1989, Gordon 1994) (Fig. 4.8). The appearance is variable with the possibility of pigmented rather than achromic lesions and more commonly of an association of both. CNS involvement is extremely common. Glover *et al.* (1989) found psychomotor delay in 14 of their 19 patients, nine had seizures, and two had severe sensorineural deafness. Eye abnormalities include microphthalmia and related structural abnormalities and were present in three of Glover's patients. Macrocephaly, hemihypertrophy and scoliosis are commonly present. There is also a wide spectrum of EEG abnormalities from normal records to multifocal paroxystic features. Fast rhythm may be associated with areas of pachygyria (Esquivel *et al.* 1991, Ogino *et al.* 1994). Seizures may be of several types including infantile spasms. Ito disease is one of the causes of hemimegalencephaly (Pascual-Castroviejo *et al.* 1988).

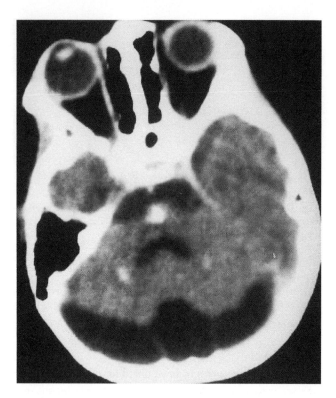

Fig. 4.9. Neurocutaneous melanosis in 3-year-old girl with giant hairy 'bathing suit' naevus and hydrocephalus. Note dilatation of cisterna magna and areas of increased density in pons and dentate nuclei. The latter may represent increased melanin content in these areas.

CT scan may show bilateral or unilateral hemispheric atrophy or areas of low attenuation in white matter (Rosemberg *et al.* 1984) or cerebellar atrophy (Pini and Faulkner 1995). MRI has shown the presence of neuronal heterotopia (Glover *et al.* 1989, Malherbe *et al.* 1993) and of white matter signal abnormalities (Bhushan *et al.* 1989), which is in agreement with the pathological findings of Ross *et al.* (1982) and Fujino *et al.* (1995).

Most confirmed cases of Ito's disease are sporadic (Moss and Burn 1988) although dominant transmission has been suggested. Girls are much more commonly affected than boys. Mosaicism for various chromosome aberrations appears to be a common cause of the disease (Miller and Parker 1985, Sybert *et al.* 1990). Moss *et al.* (1993) found such anomalies in two of four patients and suggested that chromosome analysis should ideally be performed on keratinocyte cultures whereas lymphocyte and fibroblast cultures are usually negative.

NEUROCUTANEOUS MELANOSIS

This rare nongenetic disorder is characterized by cutaneous pigmented naevi and variable involvement of the meninges and CNS (Fig. 4.9). The naevi may be multiple and of variable size. They must be of unusual size or number for the diagnosis to be considered, as small lesions are extremely common in normal persons. However, I have seen a child with biopsy-proven meningeal melanosis who had a single naevus of 5×5cm on one arm. A common presentation is the giant 'bathing suit' naevus that covers the lower part of the trunk, the pelvis and the upper part of the lower limbs. The naevi are heavily pigmented and hairy. More than half the patients with congenital hairy naevi develop CNS involvement, mainly in the form of progressive hydrocephalus, probably as a result of proliferation of meningeal melanocytes with consequent blockage of CSF reabsorption or circulation (Fox *et al.* 1964). There is often cystic dilatation of the cisterna magna (Humes *et al.* 1984, Barkovich *et al.* 1994). Seizures are common, and variable neurological deficits may result from parenchymal tumoural proliferation of melanocytes (Fox *et al.* 1964, Faillace *et al.* 1984, Rhodes *et al.* 1991), particularly at the base of the brain and brainstem.

The prognosis is poor, but hydrocephalus should be treated with a shunt. An occasional patient survives many years but malignant degeneration of CNS lesions is extremely common.

OTHER NEUROCUTANEOUS SYNDROMES WITH ABNORMAL PIGMENTATION

Albinism refers to a group of inherited disorders in which there is a reduction or absence of melanin formation. Many types of albinism are known (Witkop *et al.* 1983), and the main features of the condition are cutaneous and ocular rather than neurological. One remarkable finding is misrouting of the optic fibres, with an abnormally high proportion of crossed fibres and projection of only the most peripheral part of the temporal retina to the ipsilateral hemisphere, which may be demonstrated by study of the visual evoked potentials (Collewijn *et al.* 1985) and by special MRI techniques (Hedera *et al.* 1994). Albino children also have a special pattern of cognitive function with a much higher score on verbal than on performance items (Cole *et al.* 1987).

A syndrome associating partial albinism and immunodeficiency shares common features with Chediak–Higashi syndrome but also includes relapsing neurological symptoms and demyelination beginning in the posterior fossa and spreading to involve the whole white matter (Brismar and Harfi 1992). Defective immunodeficiency results in repeated infections.

Some other syndromes in this category are listed in Table 4.3.

NEUROICHTHYOSIS SYNDROMES

The term neuroichthyosis refers to the syndromes that associate ichthyosis or ichthyosiform dermatoses to central or peripheral nervous system involvement.

SJÖGREN–LARSSON SYNDROME

Sjögren–Larsson syndrome combines mental retardation and spastic diplegia with congenital ichthyosis. Spasticity becomes apparent between 4 and 30 months of age and mental retardation is severe (Jagell *et al.* 1981). Atypical retinitis pigmentosa with macular glistening dots is a frequent feature (Jagell and Heijbel 1982). Peripheral involvement may occur. The course is slowly progressive and no effective treatment is available. CT scan does not show any suggestive feature, but white matter changes can be demonstrated by MRI (Hussain *et al.* 1995). The disorder is transmitted as an autosomal recessive trait. It is associated with a defect of fatty alcohol metabolism, with deficiency of nicotinamide–adenine dinucleotide oxidoreductase in skin and leukocytes (Rizzo *et al.* 1989, De Laurenzi *et al.* 1996). Dietary treatment is not successful (Maaswinkel-Mooij *et al.* 1994). Prenatal diagnosis is possible (Rizzo *et al.* 1994). Somewhat similar syndromes, one without metabolic deficit (Scalais *et al.* 1992) and one with prominent myoclonus (Amano *et al.* 1995), have been observed.

NEUROTRICHOSIS
Morphological abnormalities of the hair are a feature of several metabolic neurological disorders, such as Menkes disease, biotin deficiency and arginosuccinic aciduria (Chapter 9).

TRICHOTHIODYSTROPHY
This disease is also known as Tay disease or Pollitt syndrome. Affected children have brittle and sparse hair, eyebrows and eyelashes. Microscopically, the hair shows trichorrhexis nodosa, and the sulfur content is reduced to about half the usual value, as is the cystine content (Price *et al.* 1980). Congenital ichthyosiform erythema is present in some patients (Tay 1971). Mental and physical retardation is associated with the cutaneous abnormalities (Rizzo *et al.* 1992, Tolmie *et al.* 1994). Microcephaly, ataxia and calcification of the basal ganglia have been reported (Crovato *et al.* 1984, Happle *et al.* 1984). The diagnosis of this syndrome has been discussed by Coulter *et al.* (1982). In two unrelated patients a peripheral neuropathy with marked slowing of nerve conduction velocities was present (unpublished data).

OTHER NEUROICHTHYOSIS SYNDROMES
Some other neuroichthyosis syndromes are listed in Table 4.3.

MISCELLANEOUS NEUROCUTANEOUS SYNDROMES

Among the rare neurocutaneous syndromes of this category, the most important is *naevoid basal cell carcinoma syndrome*. It is a complex disease with skin, bone and CNS manifestations, and a tendency to the development of neoplastic lesions, including medulloblastoma (Shanley *et al.* 1994).

Basal cell carcinomas are a feature of the syndrome before puberty in only 15 per cent of patients and are mainly located on the face, neck and upper trunk. Cysts of the jaw usually develop before 10 years of age. CNS abnormalities include, in addition to posterior fossa tumours, calcification of the falx cerebri and, less frequently, of the tentorium cerebelli and the petroclinoid ligament; agenesis of the corpus callosum (Naguib *et al.* 1982); bridging of the sella turcica; and occasionally mental retardation.

The disease, linked to chromosome 9q31, is transmitted as an autosomal recessive mendelian trait with complete penetrance and variable expressivity. The basal defect is unknown but there is an increased sensivity of the skin to X-irradiation. Basal cell carcinomas have developed in the scalp and paraspinal area exposed to the radiation portal after treatment of medulloblastoma in some patients.

Patients with this syndrome should be carefully watched for the possible development of an aggressive cancer. Small odontogenic cysts and skin tumours that show ulceration or haemorrhage should be removed.

Progressive hemifacial atrophy, also known as Parry–Romberg disease, may be associated with neurological manifestations (Chung *et al.* 1995). Seizures, often partial in type and localized on the side opposite the facial atrophy, are the most frequent symptoms. Unilateral or bilateral motor deficit, impaired sensory function, optic atrophy and involvement of cranial nerves may occur. Intracranial calcification is seen in some patients, and hemispheric atrophy has been demonstrated by CT scan (Klene *et al.* 1989, Terstegge *et al.* 1994). Vascular abnormalities are present in some cases (Strenge *et al.* 1996, Taylor *et al.* 1997). The neurological disease may be progressive and even dementia has been reported. Cortical dysplasia was shown by MRI in four recent cases (Dupont *et al.* 1997). The skin and facial atrophy is also progressive over several years but eventually stabilizes.

Lipoid proteinosis (*Urbach–Wiethe disease*), also known as cutaneomucous hyalinosis, is characterized by a peculiar infiltration of the skin and mucous membranes by a hyaline substance with resulting hoarseness and dysphonia. Neurological involvement may occur in the form of partial complex seizures. CT scan of the head (or even skull X-ray) may show calcification of the amygdalar region bilaterally (Özbek *et al.* 1994).

REFERENCES

Abadir, R., Hakami, N. (1983) 'Ataxia–telangiectasia with cancer: an indication for reduced radiotherapy and chemotherapy doses.' *British Journal of Radiology*, **56**, 343–345.

Abdallat, A., Davis, S.M., Farrage, J., McDonald, W.I. (1980) 'Disordered pigmentation, spastic paraparesis and peripheral neuropathy in three siblings: a new neurocutaneous syndrome.' *Journal of Neurology, Neurosurgery, and Psychiatry*, **43**, 962–966.

Abeliovich, D., Gelman-Kohan, Z., Silverstein S., *et al.* (1995) 'Familial café au lait spots: a variant of neurofibromatosis type 1.' *Journal of Medical Genetics*, **32**, 985–986.

Afifi, A.K., Dolan, K.D., Van Gilder, J., Fincham, R.W. (1988a) 'Ventriculomegaly in neurofibromatosis-1.' *Neurofibromatosis*, **1**, 299–305.

—— Jacoby, C.G., Bell, W.E., Menezes, A.H. (1988b) 'Aqueductal stenosis and neurofibromatosis: a rare association.' *Journal of Child Neurology*, **3**, 125–130.

Aicardi, J., Barbosa, C., Andermann, F., *et al.* (1988) 'Ataxia–ocular motor apraxia: a syndrome mimicking ataxia–telengiectasia.' *Annals of Neurology*, **24**, 497–502.

—— Sabril IS Investigator and Peer Review Groups, *et al.* (1996) 'Vigabatrin as initial therapy for infantile spasms: a European retrospective survey.' *Epilepsia*, **37**, 638–642.

Alper, J.C., Holmes, L.B. (1983) 'The incidence and significance of birthmarks in a cohort of 4,641 newborns.' *Pediatric Dermatology*, **1**, 56–58.

Amano, R., Ohtsuka, Y., Ohtahara, S. (1995) 'Monozygotic twin patients with congenital ichthyosis, microcephalus, spastic quadriplegia, myoclonus and EEG abnormalities.' *Pediatric Neurology*, **12**, 255–259.

Arts, W.F.M., Van Dongen, K.J. (1986) 'Intracranial calcified deposits in neurofibromatosis.' *Journal of Neurology, Neurosurgery, and Psychiatry*, **49**, 1317–1320.

Aurias, A., Dutrillaux, B. (1986) 'Probable involvement of immunoglobulin superfamily genes in most chromosomal rearrangements from ataxia–telengiectasia.' *Human Genetics*, **72**, 210–214.

—— —— Buriot, D., Lejeune, J. (1980) 'High frequencies of inversions and translocations of chromosomes 7 and 14 in ataxia–telengiectasia.' *Mutation Research*, **69**, 369–374.

Avrahami, E., Harel, S., Jurgenson, U., Cohn, D.F. (1985) 'Computed tomographic demonstration of brain changes in incontinentia pigmenti.' *American Journal of Diseases of Children*, **139**, 372–374.

Baker, R.S., Ross, P.A., Baumann, R.J. (1987) 'Neurologic complications of the epidermal nevus syndrome.' *Archives of Neurology*, **44**, 227–232.

Baloh, R., Yee, R.D., Boder, E. (1978) 'Eye movements in ataxia–telangiectasia.' *Neurology*, **28**, 1099–1104.

Bamforth, J.S.G., Riccardi, V.M., Thicon, D., *et al.* (1989) 'Encephalocranio-cutaneous lipomatosis: report of two cases and a review of the literature.' *Neurofibromatosis*, **2**, 166–173.

Barkovich, A.J., Frieden, I.J., Williams, M.L. (1994) 'MR of neurocutaneous melanosis.' *American Journal of Neuroradiology*, **15**, 859–867.

Bell, S.D., McDonald, D.M. (1985) 'The prevalence of café-au-lait patches in tuberous sclerosis.' *Clinical and Experimental Dermatology*, **10**, 562–565.

Bhushan, V., Gupta, R.R., Weinreb, J., Kairam, R. (1989) 'Unusual brain MRI findings in a patient with hypomelanosis of Ito.' *Pediatric Radiology*, **20**, 104–106.

Binet, E.F., Kieffer, S.A., Martin, S.H., Peterson, H.O. (1969) 'Orbital dysplasia in neurofibromatosis.' *Radiology*, **93**, 829–833.

Bodensteiner, J.B., Goldman, R.M., Goldblum, A.S. (1980) 'Progressive dystonia masking ataxia in ataxia–telangectasia.' *Archives of Neurology*, **37**, 464–465.

Boder, E. (1985) 'Ataxia–telangiectasia: an overview.' *In:* Gati, R.A., Swift, M. (Eds.) *Ataxia–Telangiectasia: Genetics, Neuropathology and Immunology of a Degenerative Disease of Childhood.* New York: Alan R. Liss, pp. 1–63.

Bognanno, J.R., Edwards, M.K., Lee, T.A., *et al.* (1988) 'Cranial MRI in neurofibromatosis.' *American Journal of Neuroradiology*, **9**, 461–468.

Boltshauser, E., Stocker, H., Sailer, H., Valavanis, A. (1989) 'Intracranial abnormalities associated with facial plexiform neurofibromas in neuro-fibromatosis type 1.' *Neurofibromatosis*, **2**, 274–277.

Bonnin, J.M., Rubinstein, L.J., Papasozomenos, S.C., Marangos, P.J. (1984) 'Subependymal giant-cell astrocytoma. Significance and possible cytogenetic implications of an immunohistochemical study.' *Acta Neuropathologica*, **62**, 185–193.

Borochowitz, Z., Berant, N., Dar, H., Berant, M. (1989) 'The neurofibro-matosis–Noonan syndrome: genetic heterogeneity versus clinical variability.' *Neurofibromatosis*, **2**, 309–314.

Bouzas, E., Parry, D.M., Eldridge, R., Kaiser-Kupfer, M.I. (1993) 'Visual impairment in patients with neurofibromatosis 2.' *Neurology*, **43**, 622–623.

Braffman, B.H., Bilaniuk, L.T., Naidich, T.P., *et al.* (1992) 'MR imaging of tuberous sclerosis: pathogenesis of this phakomatosis, use of gadopentetate dimeglumine, and literature review.' *Radiology*, **183**, 227–238.

Brismar, J., Harfi, H.A. (1992) 'Partial albinism with immunodeficiency: a rare syndrome with prominent posterior fossa white matter changes.' *American Journal of Neuroradiology*, **13**, 387–393.

Brunquell, P.J. (1987) 'Recurrent encephalomyelitis associated with incontin-entia pigmenti.' *Pediatric Neurology*, **3**, 174–177.

Byrne, E., Hallpike, J.F., Manson, J.L., *et al.* (1984) 'Ataxia-without-telan-giectasia. Progressive multisystem degeneration with IgE deficiency and chromosomal instability.' *Journal of the Neurological Sciences*, **66**, 307–317.

Calzavara, P.G., Carlino, A., Anzola, G.P., Pasolini, M.P. (1988) 'Segmental neurofibromatosis. Case report and review of the literature.' *Neurofibro-matosis*, **1**, 318–322.

Canapicchi, R., Abbuzzese, A., Guerrini, R., *et al.* (1996) 'Neuroimaging of tuberous sclerosis.' *In:* Guerrini, R., Andermann, F., Canapicchi, R., *et al.* (Eds.) *Dysplasias of Cerebral Cortex and Epilepsy.* New York: Lippincott–Raven, pp. 151–162.

Carbonari, M., Cherchi, M., Paganelli, R., *et al.* (1990) 'Relative increase of T cells expressing the gamma/delta rather than the alpha/beta receptors in ataxia–telangiectasia.' *New England Journal of Medicine*, **322**, 73–76.

Carney, J.A., Gordon, H., Carpenter, P.C., *et al.* (1985) 'The complex of myxomas, spotty pigmentation, and endocrine overactivity.' *Medicine*, **64**, 270–283.

Cavenagh, E.C., Hart, B.L., Rose, D. (1993) 'Association of linear sebaceous nevus syndrome and unilateral megalencephaly.' *American Journal of Neuroradiology*, **14**, 405–408.

Charrow, J., Listernick, R., Greenwald, M.J., *et al.* (1993a) 'Carboplatin-induced regression of an optic pathway tumor in a child with neurofibro-matosis.' *Medical Pediatric Oncology*, **21**, 680–684.

—— Ward, K. (1993b) 'Autosomal dominant multiple café-au-lait spots and neurofibromatosis 1: evidence of non-linkage.' *American Journal of Medical Genetics*, **45**, 606–608.

Chatkupt, S., Ruzicka, P.O., Lastra, C.R. (1993) 'Myelomeningocele, spinal

arteriovenous malformations and epidermal nevi syndrome: a possible rare association?' *Developmental Medicine and Child Neurology*, **35**, 737–741.

Chiron, C., Dulac, O., Luna, D., *et al.* (1990) 'Vigabatrin in infantile spasms.' *Lancet*, **335**, 363–364. *(Letter.)*

Chow, L.T.-C., Shum, B.S.-F., Chow, W-H. (1993) 'Intrathoracic vagus nerve neurofibroma and sudden death in a patient with neurofibromatosis.' *Thorax*, **48**, 298–299.

Chung, E.O., Bodensteiner, J.B., Noorani, P.A., Schochet, S.S. (1994) 'Cerebral white-matter changes suggesting leukodystrophy in ataxia telangiectasia.' *Journal of Child Neurology*, **9**, 31–35.

—— Sum, J., Morrell, M.J., Horoupian, D.S. (1995) 'Intracerebral involvement in scleroderma en coup de sabre: report of a case with neuropathologic findings.' *Annals of Neurology*, **37**, 679–681.

Clancy, R.R., Kurtz, M.B., Baker, D., *et al.* (1985) 'Neurologic manifestations of the organoid nevus syndrome.' *Archives of Neurology*, **42**, 236–240.

Clark, R.D., Hutter, J.J. (1982) 'Familial neurofibromatosis and juvenile chronic myelogenous leukemia.' *Human Genetics*, **60**, 230–232.

Clarke, A., Church, W., Gardner-Medwin, D., Sengupta, R. (1990) 'Intracranial calcification and seizures: a case of central neurofibromatosis.' *Developmental Medicine and Child Neurology*, **32**, 729–732.

Cohen, M. (1988) 'Understanding Proteus syndrome, unmasking the Elephant Man, and stemming elephant fever.' *Neurofibromatosis*, **1**, 260–280.

—— (1993) 'Proteus syndrome: clinical evidence for somatic mosaicism and selective review.' *American Journal of Medical Genetics*, **47**, 645–652.

Colamaria, V., Zambelli, L., Tinazzi, P., Dalla Bernardina, B. (1988) 'Tuberous sclerosis associated with partial gigantism in a child.' *Brain and Develop-ment*, **10**, 178–181.

Cole, G.F., Conn, P., Jones, R.B., *et al.* (1987) 'Cognitive functioning in albino children.' *Developmental Medicine and Child Neurology*, **29**, 659–665.

Collewijn, H., Apkarian, P., Spekreijse, H. (1985) 'The oculomotor behaviour of human albinos.' *Brain*, **108**, 1–28.

Coulter, D.L., Beals, T.F., Allen, R.J. (1982) 'Neurotrichosis: hair-shaft abnor-malities associated with neurological disease.' *Developmental Medicine and Child Neurology*, **24**, 634–644.

Crovato, F., Borrone, C., Rebora, A. (1984) 'The Tay syndrome (congenital ichthyosis with trichothiodystrophy).' *European Journal of Pediatrics*, **142**, 233–234. *(Letter.)*

Curatolo, P. (1994) 'Vigabatrin for refractory partial seizures in children with tuberous sclerosis.' *Neuropediatrics*, **25**, 55. *(Letter.)*

—— (1996a) 'Neurological manifestations of tuberous sclerosis complex.' *Child's Nervous System*, **12**, 515–521.

—— (1996b) 'Tuberous sclerosis: relationship between clinical and EEG findings and magnetic resonance imaging.' *In:* Guerrini, R., Andermann, F., Canapicchi, R., *et al.* (Eds.) *Dysplasias of Cerebral Cortex and Epilepsy.* New York: Lippincott–Raven, pp. 191–198.

Curtis, A.R., Lindsay, S., Boye, E., *et al.* (1994) 'A study of X chromosome activity in two incontinentia pigmenti families with probable linkage to Xq28.' *European Journal of Human Genetics*, **2**, 51–58.

Cusmai, R., Curatolo, P., Mangano, S., *et al.* (1990) 'Hemimegalencephaly and neurofibromatosis.' *Neuropediatrics*, **21**, 179–182.

De Laurenzi, V., Rogers, G.R., Hamrock, D.J., *et al.* (1996) 'Sjögren–Larsson syndrome is caused by mutations in the fatty aldehyde dehydrogenase gene.' *Nature Genetics*, **12**, 52–57.

De Léon, G.A., Grover, W.D., Huff, D.S. (1976) 'Neuropathologic changes in ataxia–telangiectasia.' *Neurology*, **26**, 947–951.

Denckla, M.B., Hofman, K., Mazzocco, M., *et al.* (1996) 'Relationship between T2-related hyperintensities (unidentified bright objects) and lower IQs in children with neurofibromatosis-1.' *American Journal of Medical Genetics*, **67**, 98–102.

De Saxe, M., Kromberg, J.G., Jenkins, T. (1984) 'Waardenburg syndrome in South Africa. Part 1. An evaluation of the clinical findings in 11 families.' *South African Medical Journal*, **66**, 256–261.

Deschryver-Kecskemeti, K., Clouse, R.L., Goldstein, M.N., *et al.* (1983) 'Intestinal ganglioneuromatosis: a manifestation of overproduction of nerve growth factor?' *New England Journal of Medicine*, **308**, 635–639.

De Wit, J., Jaspers, N.G., Bootsma, D. (1981) 'The rate of DNA synthesis in normal human and ataxia–telangiectasia cells after exposure to X-irradia-tion.' *Mutation Research*, **80**, 221–226.

DiLiberti, J.H., Weleber, R.G., Budden, S. (1983) 'Ruvalcaba–Myhre–Smith syndrome: a case with probable autosomal-dominant inheritance and additional manifestations.' *American Journal of Medical Genetics*, **15**, 491–495.

DiMario, F.J., Ramsby, G., Greenstein, R., *et al.* (1993) 'Neurofibromatosis type 1: magnetic resonance imaging findings.' *Journal of Child Neurology*, **8**, 32–39.

Di Paolo, D.P., Zimmerman, R.A., Rorke, L.B., *et al.* (1995) 'Neurofibromatosis type 1: pathologic substrate of high-signal-intensity foci in the brain.' *Radiology*, **195**, 721–724.

Dobyns, W.B., Garg, B.P. (1991) 'Vascular abnormalities in epidermal nevus syndrome.' *Neurology*, **41**, 276–278.

Dodge, N.N., Dobyns, W.B. (1995) 'Agenesis of the corpus callosum and Dandy–Walker malformation associated with hemimegalencephaly in the sebaceous nevus syndrome.' *American Journal of Medical Genetics*, **56**, 147–150.

Duffner, P.K., Cohen, M.E. (1988) 'Isolated optic nerve gliomas in children with and without neurofibromatosis.' *Neurofibromatosis*, **1**, 201–211.

—— —— Seidel, F.G., Shucard, D.W. (1989) 'The significance of MRI abnormalities in children with neurofibromatosis.' *Neurology*, **39**, 373–378.

Dunn, D.W., Purvin, V. (1990) 'Optic pathway gliomas in neurofibromatosis.' *Developmental Medicine and Child Neurology*, **32**, 820–824.

—— Roos, K.L. (1989) 'Magnetic resonance imaging evaluation of learning difficulties and incoordination in neurofibromatosis.' *Neurofibromatosis*, **2**, 1–5.

Dunn, H.G. (1973) 'Nerve conduction studies in children with Friedreich's ataxia and ataxia–telangiectasia.' *Developmental Medicine and Child Neurology*, **15**, 324–337.

Dupont, S., Catala, M., Hasboun, D., *et al.* (1997) 'Progressive facial hemiatrophy and epilepsy: a common underlying dysgenetic mechanism.' *Neurology*, **48**, 1013—1018.

Dvir, M., Beer, S., Aladjem, M. (1988) 'Heredofamilial syndrome of mesodermal hamartomas, macrocephaly and pseudopapilledema.' *Pediatrics*, **81**, 287–290.

Eldridge, R., Denckla, M.B., Bien, E., *et al.* (1989) 'Neurofibromatosis type 1 (Recklinghausen's disease). Neurologic and cognitive assessment with sibling controls.' *American Journal of Diseases of Children*, **143**, 833–837.

Elejalde, B.R., Holguin, J., Valencia, A., *et al.* (1979) 'Mutations affecting pigmentation in man. I: Neuroectodermal melanolysosomal disease.' *American Journal of Medical Genetics*, **3**, 65–80.

Erkulvrawatr, S., El Gammal, T., Hawkins, J., *et al.* (1979) 'Intrathoracic meningoceles and neurofibromatosis.' *Archives of Neurology*, **36**, 557–559.

Esquivel, E.E., Pitt, M.C., Boyd, S.G. (1991) 'EEG findings in hypomelanosis of Ito.' *Neuropediatrics*, **22**, 216–219.

Evans, D.G.R., Huson, S.M., Donnai, D., *et al.* (1992a) 'A clinical study of type 2 neurofibromatosis.' *Quarterly Journal of Medicine*, **84**, 603–618.

—— —— —— *et al.* (1992b) 'A genetic study of type 2 neurofibromatosis in the United Kingdom. Prevalence, mutation rate, fitness and confirmation of maternal transmission effect on severity.' *Journal of Medical Genetics*, **29**, 841–846.

—— Mason, S., Huson, S.M., *et al.* (1997) 'Spinal and cutaneous schwannomatosis is a variant of type 2 neurofibromatosis: a clinical and molecular study.' *Journal of Neurology, Neurosurgery, and Psychiatry*, **62**, 361–366.

Fabricant, R.N., Todaro, G.J. (1981) 'Increased serum levels of nerve growth factor in von Recklinghausen's disease.' *Archives of Neurology*, **38**, 401–405.

Faillace, W.J., Okawara, S.H., McDonald, J.V. (1984) 'Neurocutaneous melanosis with extensive intracerebral and spinal cord involvement. Report of two cases.' *Journal of Neurosurgery*, **61**, 782–785.

Ferner, R.E., Hughes, R.A.C. (1992) 'Intellectual impairment in NF1.' *In: Proceedings of the International Neurofibromatosis Convention, Vienna, 1992.*

Fishman, M.A. (1987) 'Encephalocraniocutaneous lipomatosis.' *Journal of Child Neurology*, **2**, 186–193.

Fleury, P., De Groot, W.P., Delleman, J.W., *et al.* (1980) 'Tuberous sclerosis: the incidence of sporadic cases versus familial cases.' *Brain and Development*, **2**, 107–117.

Flueler, U., Boltshauser, E., Kilchhofer, A. (1986) 'Iris hamartomata as diagnostic criterion in neurofibromatosis.' *Neuropediatrics*, **17**, 183–185.

Fois, A., Tiné, A., Pavone, L. (1994) 'Infantile spasms in patients with neurofibromatosis type 1.' *Child's Nervous System*, **10**, 176–179.

Fox, H., Emery, J.L., Goodbury, R.A. (1964) 'Neurocutaneous melanosis.' *Archives of Disease in Childhood*, **39**, 508–516.

François, J. (1984) 'Incontinentia pigmenti (Bloch–Schulzberger syndrome).' *British Journal of Ophthalmology*, **68**, 19–25.

Fryer, A.E., Chalmers, A.H., Osborne, J.P. (1990) 'The value of investigation for genetic counselling in tuberous sclerosis.' *Journal of Medical Genetics*, **27**, 217–223.

Fryns, J.P., Chrzanowska, K. (1988) 'Mucosal neuromata syndrome (MEN type IIb (III)).' *Journal of Medical Genetics*, **25**, 703–706.

Fujino, O., Hashimoto, K., Fujita, T., *et al.* (1995) 'Clinico-neuropathological study of incontinentia pigmenti achromians—an autopsy case.' *Brain and Development*, **17**, 425–427.

Gascon, G.G., Abdo, N., Sigut, D., *et al.* (1995) 'Ataxia–oculomotor apraxia syndrome.' *Journal of Child Neurology*, **10**, 118–122.

Gatti, R.A., Good, R.A. (1971) 'Occurrence of malignancy in immunodeficiency diseases.' *Cancer*, **28**, 89–98.

—— Aurias, A., Griscelli, C., Sparkes, R.S. (1985) 'Translocations involving chromosomes 2p and 22q in ataxia–telangiectasia.' *Disease Markers*, **3**, 169–175.

Glover, M.T., Brett, E.M., Atherton, D.J. (1989) 'Hypomelanosis of Ito: spectrum of the disease.' *Journal of Pediatrics*, **115**, 75–80.

Gomez, M.R. (1979a) 'Other visceral, vascular and osseous lesions.' *In:* Gomez, M.R. (Ed.) *Tuberous Sclerosis.* New York: Raven Press, pp. 171–192.

—— (1979b) 'Cerebello-trigeminal and focal dermal dysplasia: a newly recognized neurocutaneous syndrome.' *Brain and Development*, **1**, 253–256.

—— (Ed.) (1988) *Tuberous Sclerosis, 2nd Edn.* New York: Raven Press.

—— (1989) 'Strokes in tuberous sclerosis; are rhabdomyomas a cause?' *Brain and Development*, **11**, 14–19.

Goodman, M., Lamm, S.H., Engel, A., et al. (1997) 'Cortical tuber count: a biomarker indicating neurologic severity of tuberous sclerosis complex.' *Journal of Child Neurology*, **12**, 85–90.

Gordon, N. (1994) 'Hypomelanosis of Ito (incontinentia pigmenti achromians).' *Developmental Medicine and Child Neurology*, **36**, 271–274.

Gordon, P.L., Wilroy, R.S., Lasater, O.E., Cohen, M.M. (1995) 'Neoplasms in Proteus syndrome.' *American Journal of Medical Genetics*, **57**, 74–78.

Gorlin, R.J., Anderson, R.C., Blaw, M. (1969) 'Multiple lentigines syndrome. Complex comprising multiple lentigines, electrocardiographic conduction abnormalities, ocular hypertelorism, pulmonary stenosis, abnormalities of genitalia, retardation of growth, sensorineural deafness and autosomal dominant hereditary pattern.' *American Journal of Diseases of Children*, **117**, 652–662.

Graham-Pole, J., Ferguson, A., Gibson, A.A.M., Stephenson, J.B.P. (1975) 'Familial dysequilibrium–diplegia with T-lymphocyte deficiency.' *Archives of Disease in Childhood*, **50**, 927–933.

Gray, J., Swaiman, F. (1987) 'Brain tumors in children with neurofibromatosis: computed tomography and magnetic resonance imaging.' *Pediatric Neurology*, **3**, 335–341.

Griebel, V., Krägeloh-Mann, I., Michaelis, R. (1989) 'Hypomelanosis of Ito—report of four cases and survey of the literature.' *Neuropediatrics*, **20**, 234–237.

Griffiths, A.M., Mack, D.R., Byard, R.W., *et al.* (1990) 'Multiple endocrine neoplasia IIb: an unusual cause of chronic constipation.' *Journal of Pediatrics*, **116**, 285–288.

Griffiths, P.D., Welch, R.J., Gardner-Medwin, D., *et al.* (1994) 'The radiological features of hemimegalencephaly including three cases associated with Proteus syndrome.' *Neuropediatrics*, **25**, 140–144.

Grover, W.D., DeLéon, G., Riviello, J.J., *et al.* (1988) 'A new neurocutaneous syndrome: encephalopathy, epidermolysis bullosa, and cyclic neutropenia.' *Annals of Neurology*, **24**, 307. *(Abstract.)*

Gutman, I., Dunn, D., Behrens, M., *et al.* (1982) 'Hypopigmented iris spot. An early sign of tuberous sclerosis.' *Ophthalmology*, **89**, 1155–1159.

Gutmann, D.H., Collins, F.S. (1992) 'Recent progress toward understanding the molecular biology of von Recklinghausen neurofibromatosis.' *Annals of Neurology*, **31**, 555–551.

Habiby, R., Silverman, B., Listernick, R., Charrow, J. (1995) 'Precocious puberty in children with neurofibromatosis type 1.' *Journal of Pediatrics*, **126**, 364–367.

Hagberg, B., Hansson, O., Liden, S., Nilsson, K. (1970) 'Familial ataxic diplegia with deficient cellular immunity. A new clinical entity.' *Acta Paediatrica Scandinavica*, **59**, 545–550.

Hanawalt, P., Painter, R. (1985) 'On the nature of the "DNA-processing" defect in ataxia–telangiectasia.' *In:* Gatti, R.A., Swift, M. (Eds.) *Ataxia–Telangiectasia: Genetics, Neuropathology and Immunology of a Degenerative Disease of Childhood.* New York: Alan R. Liss, pp. 67–71.

Happle, R., Traupe, H., Gröbe, H., Bonsmann, G. (1984) 'The Tay syndrome (congenital ichthyosis with trichothiodystrophy).' *European Journal of Pediatrics*, **141**, 147–152.

Hauw, J-J., Perié, G., Bonnette, J., Escourolle, R. (1977) 'Les lésions cérébrales de l'incontinentia pigmenti. A propos d'un cas anatomique.' *Acta Neuropathologica*, **38**, 159–162.

Hecht, F., Hecht, B. (1985) 'Ataxia–telangiectasia breakpoints in chromosome rearrangements reflect genes important to T and B lymphocytes.' *In:* Gatti, R.H., Swift, M. (Eds.) *Ataxia–telangiectasia: Genetics, Neuropathology, and Immunology of a Degenerative Disease of Childhood.* New York: Alan R. Liss, pp. 189–195.

Hedera, P., Lais, S., Haacke, E.M., *et al.* (1994) 'Abnormal connectivity of the visual pathways in human albinos demonstrated by susceptibility-sensitized MRI.' *Neurology*, **44**, 1921–1926.

Hegstrom, J.L., Kircher, T. (1985) 'Alimentary tract ganglioneuromatosis–lipomatosis, adrenal myelolipomas, pancreatic telangiectasias and multinodular thyroid goiter. A possible neuroendocrine syndrome.' *American Journal of Clinical Pathology*, **83**, 744–747.

Heimann, R., Verhest, A., Vershraegen, J., *et al.* (1988) 'Hereditary intestinal neurofibromatosis. I. A distinctive genetic disease.' *Neurofibromatosis*, **1**, 26–32.

Hochstrasser, H., Boltshauser, E., Valavanis, A. (1988) 'Brain tumors in children with von Recklinghausen neurofibromatosis.' *Neurofibromatosis*, **1**, 233–239.

Hofman, K.J., Harris, E.L., Bryan, R.N., Denckla, M.B. (1994) 'Neurofibromatosis type 1: the cognitive phenotype.' *Journal of Pediatrics*, **124**, S1–S8.

Hoover, D.L., Robb, R.M., Petersen, R.A. (1989) 'Optic disc drusen and primary megalencephaly in children.' *Journal of Pediatric Ophthalmology and Strabismus*, **26**, 81–85.

Humes, R.A., Roskamp, J., Eisenbrey, A.B. (1984) 'Melanosis and hydrocephalus. Report of four cases.' *Journal of Neurosurgery*, **61**, 365–368.

Hunt, A. (1983) 'Tuberous sclerosis: a survey of 97 cases. I: Seizures, pertussis immunisation and handicap. II: Physical findings. III: Family aspects.' *Developmental Medicine and Child Neurology*, **25**, 346–349; 350–352; 353–357.

—— Dennis, J. (1987) 'Psychiatric disorder among children with tuberous sclerosis.' *Developmental Medicine and Child Neurology*, **29**, 190–198.

—— Lindenbaum, R.H. (1984) 'Tuberous sclerosis: a new estimate of prevalence within the Oxford region.' *Journal of Medical Genetics*, **21**, 272–277.

Huson, S.M., Harper, P.S., Compston, D.A.S. (1988) 'Von Recklinghausen neurofibromatosis: a clinical and population study in South-East Wales.' *Brain*, **111**, 1355–1381.

Hussain, M.Z., Aihara, M., Oba, H., *et al.* (1995) 'MRI of white matter changes in the Sjögren–Larsson syndrome.' *Neuroradiology*, **37**, 576–577.

Huttenlocher, P.R., Heydemann, R.T. (1984) 'Fine structure of cortical tubers in tuberous sclerosis.' *Annals of Neurology*, **16**, 595–602.

Imes, R.K., Hoyt, W.F. (1986) 'Childhood chiasmal gliomas: update on the fate of patients in the 1969 San Francisco study.' *British Journal of Ophthalmology*, **70**, 179–182.

Inoue, Y., Nemoto, Y., Tashiro, T., *et al.* (1997) 'Neurofibromatosis type 1 and 2: review of the central nervous system and related structures.' *Brain and Development*, **19**, 1–12.

Jagell, S., Heijbel, J. (1982) 'Sjögren–Larsson syndrome: physical and neurological features. A survey of 35 patients.' *Helvetica Paediatrica Acta*, **37**, 519–530.

—— Gutavson, K.H., Holmgren, G. (1981) 'Sjögren–Larsson syndrome in Sweden. A clinical, genetic and epidemiological study.' *Clinical Genetics*, **19**, 233–256.

Joffe, N. (1965) 'Calvarial bone defects involving the lambdoid suture in neurofibromatosis.' *British Journal of Radiology*, **38**, 23–27.

Jorizzo, J.L., Crounse, R.G., Wheeler, C.E. (1980) 'Lamellar ichthyosis: dwarfism, mental retardation and hair shaft abnormalities.' *Journal of the American Academy of Dermatology*, **2**, 309–317.

Jung, E.G. (1988) 'Segmental neurofibromatosis (NF-5).' *Neurofibromatosis*, **1**, 306–311.

Jurecka, W., Aberer, E., Mainitz, M., Jürgenson, O. (1985) 'Keratitis, ichthyosis, and deafness syndrome with glycogen storage.' *Archives of Dermatology*, **121**, 799–801.

Kandt, R.S., Haines, J.L., Smith, M., *et al.* (1992) 'Linkage of an important gene locus for tuberous sclerosis to a chromosome 16 marker for polycystic kidney disease.' *Nature Genetics*, **2**, 37–41.

Kastan, M. (1995) 'Ataxia–telangiectasia—broad implications for a rare disorder.' *New England Journal of Medicine*, **333**, 662–663.

Kilpatrick, T.J., Hjorth, R.J., Gonzales, M.F. (1992) 'A case of neurofibromatosis 2 presenting with a mononeuritis multiplex.' *Journal of Neurology, Neurosurgery, and Psychiatry*, **55**, 391–393.

Kingsley, D.P.E., Kendall, B.E., Fitz, C.R. (1986) 'Tuberous sclerosis. A clinicoradiological evaluation of 110 cases with particular reference to atypical presentation.' *Neuroradiology*, **28**, 38–46.

Kitamura, K., Senba, T., Kotmatzutaki, A. (1989) 'Bilateral internal auditory canal enlargement without acoustic nerve tumor in von Recklinghausen neurofibromatosis.' *Neurofibromatosis*, **2**, 47–52.

Klene, C., Massicot,, P., Ferrière-Fontan, I., *et al.* (1989) 'Sclérodermie "en coup de sabre" et hémi-atrophie faciale de Parry–Romberg. Problème nosologique. Complication neurologique.' *Annales de Pédiatrie*, **36**, 123–125.

Kohn, P.H., Whang-Peng, J., Levis, W.R. (1982) 'Chromosomal instability in ataxia–telangiectasia.' *Cancer*, **6**, 289–302.

Korf, B.R. (1992) 'Diagnostic outcome in children with multiple café au lait spots.' *Pediatrics*, **90**, 924–927.

Kuntz, N. (1988) 'Population studies.' *In:* Gomez, M.R. (Ed.) *Tuberous Sclerosis, 2nd Edn.* New York: Raven Press, pp. 213–215.

Kwast, O., Ignatowicz, R. (1990) 'Progressive peripheral neuron degeneration in ataxia–telangiectasia: an electrophysiologic study in children.' *Developmental Medicine and Child Neurology*, **32**, 800–807.

Landy, S.J., Donnai, D. (1993) 'Incontinentia pigmenti (Bloch–Schulzberger syndrome).' *Journal of Medical Genetics*, **30**, 53–59.

Larbrisseau, A., Carpenter, C. (1982) 'Rud syndrome: congenital ichthyosis, hypogonadism, mental retardation, retinitis pigmentosa and hypertrophic polyneuropathy.' *Neuropediatrics*, **13**, 95–98.

Larsen, R., Ashwal, S., Peckham, N. (1987) 'Incontinentia pigmenti: association with anterior horn cell degeneration.' *Neurology*, **37**, 446–450.

Lázaro, C., Ravella, A., Gaona, A., *et al.* (1994) 'Neurofibromatosis type 1 due to germ-line mosaicism in a clinically normal father.' *New England Journal of Medicine*, **331**, 1403–1407.

Leão, M., da Silva, M.L. (1995) 'Evidence of central nervous system involvement in Watson syndrome.' *Pediatric Neurology*, **12**, 252–254.

Levin, S., Robinson, R.O., Aicardi, J., Hoare, R.D. (1984) 'Computed tomography appearances in the linear sebaceous naevus syndrome.' *Neuroradiology*, **26**, 469–472.

Listernick, R., Charrow, J., Greenwald, M., Mets, M. (1994) 'Natural history of optic pathway tumors in children with neurofibromatosis type 1: a longitudinal study.' *Journal of Pediatrics*, **125**, 63–66.

—— Louis, D.N., Packer, R.J., Gutmann, D.H. (1997) 'Optic pathway gliomas in children with neurofibromatosis 1. Consensus statement from the NF1 Optic Pathway Glioma Task Force.' *Annals of Neurology*, **41**, 143–149.

Lopez-Hernandez, A. (1982) 'Craniosynostosis, ataxia, trigeminal anesthesia and partial alopecia with pons–vermis fusion anomaly (atresia of the fourth ventricle).' *Neuropediatrics*, **13**, 99–102.

Maaswinkel-Mooij, P.D., Brouwer, O.F., Rizzo, W.B. (1994) 'Unsuccessful dietary treatment of Sjögren–Larsson syndrome.' *Journal of Pediatrics*, **124**, 748–750.

MacCollin, M. (1995) 'Molecular analysis of the neurofibromatosis 2 tumor suppressor.' *Brain and Development*, **17**, 231–238.

—— Woodfin, W., Kronn, D., Short, M.P. (1996) 'Schwannomatosis: a clinical and pathologic study.' *Neurology*, **46**, 1072–1079.

Malherbe, V., Pariente, D., Tardieu, M., *et al.* (1993) 'Central nervous system lesions in hypomelanosis of Ito: an MRI and pathological study.' *Journal of Neurology*, **240**, 302–304.

Mangano, S., Barbagallo, A. (1993) 'Incontinentia pigmenti: clinical and neuroradiologic features.' *Brain and Development*, **15**, 362–366.

Martuza, R.L., Philippe, I., Fitzpatrick, T.B., *et al.* (1985) 'Melanin macroglobules as a cellular marker of neurofibromatosis: a quantitative study.' · *Journal of Investigative Dermatology*, **85**, 347–350.

Marxmiller, J., Trenkle, I., Ashwal, S. (1985) 'Rud syndrome revisited: ichthyosis, mental retardation, epilepsy and hypogonadism.' *Developmental Medicine and Child Neurology*, **27**, 335–343.

Mautner, V-F., Tatagiba, M., Guthoff, R., *et al.* (1993) 'Neurofibromatosis 2 in the pediatric age group.' *Neurosurgery*, **33**, 92–96.

McCall, S., Ramzy, M.I., Curé, J.K., Pai, G.S. (1992) 'Encephalocraniocutaneous lipomatosis and the Proteus syndrome: distinct entities with overlapping manifestations.' *American Journal of Medical Genetics*, **43**, 662–668.

McFarlin, D.E., Strober, W., Waldmann, T.A. (1972) 'Ataxia–telangiectasia.' *Medicine*, **51**, 281–314.

McWilliam, R.C., Stephenson, J.B.P. (1978) 'Depigmented hair, the earliest sign of tuberous sclerosis.' *Archives of Disease in Childhood*, **53**, 961–962.

Meschia, J.F., Junkins, E., Hofman, K.J. (1992) 'Familial systematized epidermal nevus syndrome.' *American Journal of Medical Genetics*, **44**, 664–667.

Meshram, C.M., Sawhney, I.M.S., Prabhakar, S., Chopra, J.S. (1986) 'Ataxia telangiectasia in identical twins: unusual features.' *Journal of Neurology*, **233**, 304–305.

Michel, J.M., Diggle, J.H., Brice, J., *et al.* (1983) 'Two half-siblings with tuberous sclerosis, polycystic kidneys and hypertension.' *Developmental Medicine and Child Neurology*, **25**, 239–244.

Michels, V.V., Whisnant, J.P., Garrity, J.A., Miller, G.M. (1989) 'Neurofibromatosis type 1 with bilateral acoustic neuromas.' *Neurofibromatosis*, **2**, 213–217.

Miller, C.A., Parker, W.D. (1985) 'Hypomelanosis of Ito: association with a chromosomal abnormality.' *Neurology*, **35**, 607–610.

Molloy, P.T., Bilaniuk, L.T., Vaughan, S.N., *et al.* (1995) 'Brainstem tumors in patients with neurofibromatosis type 1: a distinct clinical entity.' *Neurology*, **45**, 1897–1902.

Monaghan, H.P., Krafchik, B.R., MacGregor, D.L., Fitz, C.R. (1981) 'Tuberous sclerosis complex in children.' *American Journal of Diseases of Children*, **135**, 912–917.

Moore, B.D. (1995) 'NF1, cognition and MRI.' *Neurology*, **45**, 1029. *(Letter.)*
—— Slopis, J.M., Schomer, D., *et al.* (1996) 'Neuropsychological significance of areas of high signal intensity on brain MRIs of children with neurofibromatosis.' *Neurology*, **46**, 1660–1668.

Moss, C., Burn, J. (1988) 'Genetic counselling in hypomelanosis of Ito: case report and review.' *Clinical Genetics*, **34**, 109–115.
—— Larkins, S., Stacey, M., *et al.* (1993) 'Epidermal mosaicism and Blaschko's lines.' *Journal of Medical Genetics*, **30**, 752–755.

Motte, J., Billard, C., Fejerman, N., *et al.* (1993) 'Neurofibromatosis type one and West syndrome: a relatively benign association.' *Epilepsia*, **34**, 723–726.

Münke, M., Kruse, K., Goos, M., *et al.* (1983) 'Genetic heterogeneity of the ichthyosis, hypogonadism, mental retardation and epilepsy syndrome.' *European Journal of Pediatrics*, **141**, 8–13.

Naguib, M.G., Sung, J.H., Erickson, D.L., *et al.* (1982) 'Central nervous system involvement in the nevoid basal cell carcinoma syndrome: case report and review of the literature.' *Neurosurgery*, **11**, 52–56.

Nellist, M., Janssen, B., Ward, C.J., and the European Chromosome 16 Tuberous Sclerosis Consortium (1993) 'Identification and characterization of the tuberous sclerosis gene on chromosome 16.' *Cell*, **75**, 1305–1315.

NIH Consensus Development Conference (1988) 'Neurofibromatosis: conference statement.' *Archives of Neurology*, **45**, 575–578.

North, K. (1993) 'Neurofibromatosis type 1: review of the first 200 patients in an Australian clinic.' *Journal of Child Neurology*, **8**, 395–402.
—— (1997) *Neurofibromatosis Type 1.* London: Mac Keith Press for the International Child Neurology Association.
—— Cochineas, C., Tang, E., Fagan, E. (1994a) 'Optic gliomas in neurofibromatosis type 1: role of visual evoked potentials.' *Pediatric Neurology*, **10**, 117–123.
—— Joy, P., Yuille, D., *et al.* (1994b) 'Specific learning disability in children with neurofibromatosis type 1: significance of MRI abnormalities.' *Neurology*, **44**, 878–883.
—— —— —— *et al.* (1995) 'Cognitive function and academic performance in children with neurofibromatous type 1.' *Developmental Medicine and Child Neurology*, **37**, 427–436.

North American Study Group for Optic Glioma (1989) 'Tumor spread in unilateral optic glioma: study report No. 2.' *Neurofibromatosis*, **2**, 195–203.

O'Doherty, N.J., Norman, R.M. (1968) 'Incontinentia pigmenti (Bloch–Schulzberger syndrome) with cerebral malformation.' *Developmental Medicine and Child Neurology*, **10**, 168–174.

Ogino, T., Hata, H., Minakuchi, E., *et al.* (1994) 'Neurophysiologic dysfunction in hypomelanosis of Ito: EEG and evoked potential studies.' *Brain and Development*, **16**, 407–412.

Oxelius, A.V., Berkel, A.I., Hanson, L.A. (1982) 'IgG2 deficiency in ataxia–telangiectasia.' *New England Journal of Medicine*, **306**, 515–517.

Özbek, S.S., Akyar, S., Turgay, M. (1994) 'Computed tomography findings in lipoid proteinosis: report of two cases.' *British Journal of Radiology*, **67**, 207–209.

Packer, R.J., Savino, P.J., Bilaniuk, L.T., *et al.* (1983) 'Chiasmatic gliomas in childhood: reappraisal of natural history and effectiveness of cranial irradiation.' *Child's Brain*, **10**, 393–403.
—— Bilaniuk, L.T., Cohen, B.H., *et al.* (1988a) 'Intracranial visual pathway gliomas in childen with neurofibromatosis.' *Neurofibromatosis*, **1**, 212–222.
—— Sutton, L.N., Bilaniuk, L.T., *et al.* (1988b) 'Treatment of chiasmatic/hypothalamic gliomas of childhood with chemotherapy: an update.' *Annals of Neurology*, **23**, 79–85.

Pascual-Castroviejo, I. (1992) 'Complications of neurofibromatosis type 1 in a series of 197 children.' *In:* Fukuyama, Y., Suzuki, Y., Kamoshita, S., Casaer, P. (Eds.) *Fetal and Perinatal Neurology.* Basel: Karger, pp. 162–173.
—— López-Rodriguez, L., de la Cruz Medina, M., *et al.* (1988) 'Hypomelanosis of Ito. Neurological complications in 34 cases.' *Canadian Journal of Neurological Sciences*, **15**, 124–129.

Paterson, M.C., Smith, P.J. (1979) 'Ataxia–telangiectasia: an inherited human disorder involving hypersensitivity to ionizing radiation and related DNA-damaging chemicals.' *Annual Review of Genetics*, **13**, 291–318.

Paula-Barbosa, M.M., Ruela, C., Tavares, M.A., *et al.* (1983) 'Cerebellar cortex ultrastructure in ataxia–telangiectasia.' *Annals of Neurology*, **13**, 297–302.

Pavone, L., Curatolo, P., Rizzo, R., *et al.* (1991) 'Epidermal nevus syndrome: a neurologic variant with hemimegalencephaly, gyral malformation, mental retardation, seizures, and facial hemihypertrophy.' *Neurology*, **41**, 266–271.

Pellock, J.M., Kleinman, P.K., McDonald, B.M., Wixson, D. (1980) 'Childhood hypertensive stroke with neurofibromatosis.' *Neurology*, **30**, 656–659.

Peterson, R.D.A., Funkhouser, J.D. (1989) 'Speculations on ataxia–telangiectasia: defective regulation of the immunoglobulin gene superfamily.' *Immunology Today*, **10**, 313–315.

Pini, G., Faulkner, L.B. (1995) 'Cerebellar involvement in hypomelanosis of Ito.' *Neuropediatrics*, **26**, 208–210.

Pollack, I.F., Shultz, B., Mulvihill, J.J. (1996) 'The management of brain stem gliomas in patients with neurofibromatosis 1.' *Neurology*, **46**, 1652–1660.

Pou-Serradell, A. (1991) 'Lésions centrales dans les neurofibromatoses: corrélations cliniques, d'IRM et histopathologiques. Essai de classification.' *Revue Neurologique*, **147**, 17–27.
—— Ugarte-Elola, C. (1989) 'Hydrocephalus in neurofibromatosis: contribution of magnetic resonance imaging to its diagnosis, control and treatment.' *Neurofibromatosis*, **2**, 218–226.

Prensky, A.L. (1987) 'Linear sebaceous nevus.' *In:* Gomez, M.R. (Ed.) *Neurocutaneous Diseases: a Practical Approach.* London: Butterworths, pp. 335–344.

Price, V.H., Odom, R.B., Ward, W.H., Jones, F.T. (1980) 'Trichothiodystrophy: sulfur-deficient brittle hair as a marker for a neuroectodermal symptom complex.' *Archives of Dermatology*, **104**, 4–13.

Pritchard, J., Sandland, M.R., Breatnach, F.B., *et al.* (1982) 'The effects of radiation therapy for Hodgkin's disease in a child with ataxia–telangiectasia.' *Cancer*, **50**, 877–886.

Purcell, S.M., Dixon, S.L. (1989) 'Schwannomatosis. An unusual variant of neurofibromatosis or a distinct clinical entity?' *Archives of Dermatology*, **125**, 390–393.

Rasmussen, S.A., Frias, J.L. (1989) 'Cutis verticis gyrata: a proposed classification.' *Dysmorphology and Clinical Genetics*, **3**, 97–102.

Rhodes, R.E., Friedman, H.S., Hatten, H.P., *et al.* (1991) 'Contrast enhanced MR imaging of neurocutaneous melanosis.' *American Journal of Neuroradiology*, **12**, 380–382.

Riccardi, V.M. (1992) *Neurofibromatosis. Phenotype, Natural History and Pathogenesis. 2nd Edn.* Baltimore: Johns Hopkins University Press.

Richkind, K.E., Boder, E., Teplitz, R.L. (1982) 'Fetal proteins in ataxia–telangiectasia.' *Journal of the American Medical Association*, **248**, 1346–1347.

Riikonen, R., Simell, O. (1990) 'Tuberous sclerosis and infantile spasms.' *Developmental Medicine and Child Neurology*, **32**, 203–209.

Riopelle, R.J., Riccardi, V.M., Faulkner, S., Martin, M.C. (1984) 'Serum neuronal growth factor levels in von Recklinghausen's neurofibromatosis.' *Annals of Neurology*, **16**, 54–59.

Riviello, J.J., Marks, H.G., Lee, M.S., Mandell, G.A. (1988) 'Aqueductal stenosis in neurofibromatosis.' *Neurofibromatosis*, **1**, 312–317.

Rizzo, J.F., Lessell, S. (1994) 'Cerebrovascular abnormalities in neurofibromatosis type 1.' *Neurology*, **44**, 1000–1002.

Rizzo, R., Pavone, L., Micali, G. (1992) 'Trichothiodystrophy: report of a new case with severe nervous system impairment.' *Journal of Child Neurology*, **7**, 300–303.

Rizzo, W.B., Dammann, A.L., Craft, D.A., *et al.* (1989) 'Sjögren–Larsson syndrome: inherited defect in the fatty alcohol cycle.' *Journal of Pediatrics*, **115**, 228–234.
—— Craft, D.A., Kelson, T.L., *et al.* (1994) 'Prenatal diagnosis of Sjögren–Larsson syndrome using enzymatic methods.' *Prenatal Diagnosis*, **14**, 577–581.

Robbins, J. (1987) 'Xeroderma pigmentosum.' *In:* Gomez, M.R. (Ed.) *Neurocutaneous Diseases: a Practical Approach.* London: Butterworths, pp. 118–127.

Roach, E.S., Kerr, J., Mendelsohn, D., *et al.* (1991) 'Detection of tuberous sclerosis in parents by magnetic resonance imaging.' *Neurology*, **41**, 262–265.

Robbins, T.O., Bernstein, J. (1988) 'Renal involvement.' *In:* Gomez, M.R. (Ed.) *Tuberous Sclerosis, 2nd Edn.* New York: Raven Press, pp. 133–146.

Rogers, R.S. (1988) 'Dermatologic manifestations.' *In:* Gomez, M.R. (Ed.) *Tuberous Sclerosis, 2nd Edn.* New York: Raven Press, pp. 111–131.

Roifman, C.M., Gelfand, E.W. (1985) 'Heterogeneity of the immunological deficiency in ataxia–telangiectasia: absence of a clinical–pathological correlation.' *In:* Gatti, R.A., Swift, M. (Eds.) *Ataxia–telangiectasia: Genetics, Neuropathology, and Immunology of a Degenerative Disease of Childhood.* New York: Alan R. Liss, pp. 273–285.

Rosemberg, S., Arita, F.N., Campos, C., Alonso, F. (1984) 'Hypomelanosis of Ito. Case report with involvement of the central nervous system and review of the literature.' *Neuropediatrics*, **15**, 52–55.

Rosenfeld, S.I., Smith, M.E. (1985) 'Ocular findings in incontinentia pigmenti.' *Ophthalmology*, **92**, 543–546.

Rosman, N.P. (1992) 'Incontinentia pigmenti: presentations, pathology, pathogenesis and prognosis.' *In:* Fukuyama, Y., Suzuki, Y., Kamoshita, S., Casaer, P. (Eds.) *Fetal and Perinatal Neurology.* Basel: Karger, pp. 174–186.

Ross, D.L., Liwnicz, B.H., Chun, R.W.M., Gilbert, E. (1982) 'Hypomelanosis of Ito (incontinentia pigmenti achromians)—a clinicopathologic study: macrocephaly and gray matter heterotopias.' *Neurology*, **32**, 1013–1016.

Ross, G.W., Miller, J.Q., Persing, J.A., Urich, H. (1989) 'Hemimegalencephaly, hemifacial hypertrophy and intracranial lipoma: a variant of neurofibromatosis.' *Neurofibromatosis*, **2**, 69–77.

Roth, J.C., Epstein, C.J. (1971) 'Infantile spasms and hypopigmented macules. Early manifestations of tuberous sclerosis.' *Archives of Neurology*, **25**, 547–551.

Roth, R.R., Martines, R., James, W.D. (1987) 'Segmental neurofibromatosis.' *Archives of Dermatology*, **123**, 917–920.

Rouleau, G.A., Merel, P., Lutchman, M., *et al.* (1993) 'Alteration in a new gene encoding a putative membrane-organizing protein causes neuro-fibromatosis type 2.' *Nature*, 363, 515–521.

Rubinstein, L.J. (1986) 'The malformative central nervous system lesions in the central and the peripheral forms of neurofibromatosis.' *Annals of the New York Academy of Sciences*, **486**, 14–29.

Russell, D.S., Rubinstein, L.J. (1977) *Pathology of Tumors of the Nervous System, 4th Edn.* Baltimore: Williams & Wilkins.

Ruttledge, M.H., Narod, S.A., Dumanski, J.P., *et al.* (1993) 'Presymptomatic diagnosis for neurofibromatosis 2 with chromosome 22 markers.' *Neurology*, **43**, 1753–1760.

Sadeh, M., Martinovits, G., Goldhammer, Y. (1989) 'Occurrence of both neurofibromatoses 1 and 2 in the same individual with a rapidly progressive course.' *Neurology*, **39**, 282–283.

Savick, R.J., Barkovich, A.J., Edwards, M.S.B., *et al.* (1992) 'Evolution of white matter lesions in neurofibromatosis type 1: MR findings.' *American Journal of Roentgenology*, **159**, 171–175.

Savitsky, K., Bar-Shira, A., Gilad, S., *et al.* (1995) 'A single ataxia–telangiectasia gene with a product similar to P1-3 kinase.' *Science*, **268**, 1749–1753.

Scalais, E., Verloes, A., Sacre, J.P., *et al.* (1992) 'Sjögren–Larsson-like syndrome with bone dysplasia and normal fatty alcohol NAD+ oxidoreductase activity.' *Pediatric Neurology*, **8**, 459–465.

Schievink, W.I., Michels, V.V., Mokri, B., *et al.* (1995) 'A familial syndrome of arterial dissections with lentiginosis.' *New England Journal of Medicine*, **332**, 576–579.

Schwartz, S., Flannery, D.B., Cohen, M.M. (1985) 'Tests appropriate for the prenatal diagnosis of ataxia–telangiectasia.' *Prenatal Diagnosis*, **5**, 9–14.

Sedgwick, R.P., Boder, E. (1972) 'Ataxia–telangiectasia.' *In:* Vinken, P.J., Bruyn, G.W. (Eds.) *Handbook of Clinical Neurology. Vol.14. The Phakomatoses.* Amsterdam: North Holland, pp. 267–339.

Seemanova, E., Passarge, E., Beneskova, D., *et al.* (1985) 'Familial microcephaly with normal intelligence, immunodeficiency, and risk for lymphoreticular malignancies.' *American Journal of Medical Genetics*, **20**, 639–648.

Seiff, S.R., Brodsky, M.C., MacDonald, G., *et al.* (1987) 'Orbital optic glioma in neurofibromatosis. Magnetic resonance diagnosis of perineural arachnoidal gliomatosis.' *Archives of Ophthalmology*, **105**, 1689–1692.

Shanley, S., Ratcliffe, J., Hockey, A., *et al.* (1994) 'Nevoid basal cell carcinoma syndrome: review of 118 affected individuals.' *American Journal of Medical Genetics*, **50**, 282–290.

Shepherd, C.W., Houser, O.W., Gomez, M.R. (1995) 'MR findings in tuberous sclerosis complex and correlation with seizure development and mental impairment.' *American Journal of Neuroradiology*, **16**, 149–155.

Shiloh, Y. (1995) 'Ataxia–telangiectasia: closer to unraveling the mystery.' *European Journal of Human Genetics*, **3**, 116–138.

Shuper, A., Bryan, R.N., Singer, H.S. (1990) 'Destructive encephalopathy in incontinentia pigmenti: a primary disorder?' *Pediatric Neurology*, **6**, 137–140.

Siemes, H., Schneider, H., Dening, D., Hanefeld, F. (1978) 'Encephalitis in two members of a family with incontinentia pigmenti (Bloch–Schulzberger syndrome).' *European Journal of Pediatrics*, **129**, 103–115.

Simonsson, H. (1972) 'Incontinentia pigmenti: Bloch–Schulzberger syndrome associated with infantile spasms.' *Acta Paediatrica Scandinavica*, **61**, 612–614.

Soutar, R.L., Day, R.E. (1991) 'Dysequilibrium/ataxic diplegia with immunodeficiency.' *Archives of Disease in Childhood*, **66**, 982–983.

Spitzer, D.E., Goodrich, J.T. (1988) 'Optic gliomas and neurofibromatosis: neurosurgical management.' *Neurofibromatosis*, **1**, 223–232.

Stewart, R.M., Tunell, G., Ehle, A. (1981) 'Familial spastic paraplegia, peroneal neuropathy and crural hypopigmentation: a new neurocutaneous syndrome.' *Neurology*, **31**, 754–757.

Strenge, H., Cordes, P., Sticherling, M., Brossmann, J. (1996) 'Hemifacial atrophy: a neurocutaneous disorder with coup de sabre deformity, telangiectatic naevus, aneurysmatic malformation of the internal carotid artery and crossed hemiatrophy.' *Journal of Neurology*, **243**, 658–660.

Striano, S., Ruosi, P., Guzzetta, V., *et al.* (1996) 'Cutis verticis gyrata–mental deficiency syndrome: a patient with drug-resistant epilepsy and polyneurogyria.' *Epilepsia*, **37**, 284–286.

Sugimoto, T., Sawada, T., Tozawa, M., *et al.* (1978) 'Plasma levels of carcinoembryonic antigen in patients with ataxia–telangiectasia.' *Journal of Pediatrics*, **92**, 436–439.

Sunohara, N., Sakuragawa, N., Satoyoshi, E., *et al.* (1986) 'A new syndrome of anosmia, ichthyosis, hypogonadism and various neurological manifestations with deficiency of steroid sulfatase and arylsulfatase C.' *Annals of Neurology*, **19**, 174–181.

Swift, M., Morrell, D., Massey, R.B., Chase, C.L. (1991) 'Incidence of cancer in 161 families affected by ataxia–telangiectasia.' *New England Journal of Medicine*, **325**, 1831–1836.

Sybert, V.P., Pagon, R.A., Donlan, M., Bradley, C.M. (1990) 'Pigmentary abnormalities and mosaicism for chromosomal aberration: association with clinical features similar to hypomelanosis of Ito.' *Journal of Pediatrics*, **116**, 581–586.

Taylor, H.M., Robinson, R., Cox, T. (1997) 'Progressive facial hemiatrophy: MRI appearances.' *Developmental Medicine and Child Neurology*, **39**, 484–486.

Terenty, T.R., Robson, P., Walton, J.N. (1978) 'Presumed ataxia–telangiectasia in a man.' *British Medical Journal*, **2**, 802.

Terstegge, K., Kunath, B., Felber, S., *et al.* (1994) 'MR of brain involvement in progressive facial hemiatrophy (Romberg disease): reconsideration of a syndrome.' *American Journal of Neuroradiology*, **15**, 145–150.

Terwey, B., Doose, H. (1987) 'Tuberous sclerosis: magnetic imaging of the brain.' *Neuropediatrics*, **18**, 67–69.

Tolmie, J.L., de Berker, D., Dawber, R., *et al.* (1994) 'Syndromes associated with trichothiodystrophy.' *Clinical Dysmorphology*, **3**, 1–14.

Tomsik, T.A., Lukin, R.R., Chambers, A.A., Benton, C. (1976) 'Neurofibromatosis and intracranial arterial disease.' *Neuroradiology*, **11**, 229–234.

Valentini, L., Solero, C.L., Lasio, G., *et al.* (1995) 'Triventricular hydrocephalus: review of 71 cases evaluated at the Istituto Neurologico "C. Besta" Milan over the last 10 years.' *Child's Nervous System*, **11**, 170–172.

Van Hale, P. (1987) 'Chediak–Higashi syndrome.' *In:* Gomez, M.R. (Ed.) *Neurocutaneous Diseases: a Practical Approach.* London: Butterworths, pp. 209–213.

Van Tassel, P., Yeakley, J.W., Lee, K.F. (1987) 'Cerebellar calcification in central neurofibromatosis: CT in two cases.' *American Journal of Neuroradiology*, **8**, 913–915.

Vaughn, R.Y., Selinger, A.D., Howell, C.G., *et al.* (1993) 'Proteus syndrome: diagnosis and surgical management.' *Journal of Pediatric Surgery*, **28**, 5–10.

Vigevano, F., Aicardi, J., Lini, M., Pasquinelli, A. (1984) 'La sindrome del nevo sebaceo lineare: presentazione di una casistica multicentrica.' *Bollettino della Lega Italiana contra la Epilessia*, **45/46**, 59–63.

Vinchon, M., Blond, S., Lejeune, J.P., *et al.* (1994) 'Association of Lhermitte–Duclos and Cowden disease: report of a new case and review of the literature.' *Journal of Neurology, Neurosurgery, and Psychiatry*, **57**, 699–704.

Vles, J.S.H., Degraeuwe, P., De Cock, P., Casaer, P. (1985) 'Neuroradiological findings in Jadassohn nevus phakomatosis: a report of four cases.' *European Journal of Pediatrics*, **144**, 290–294.

Vrtel, R., Verhoef, S., Bouman, K., *et al.* (1996) 'Identification of a nonsense mutation at the 5′ end of the TSC2 gene in a family with a presumptive diagnosis of tuberous sclerosis complex.' *Journal of Medical Genetics*, **33**, 47–51.

Waldmann, T.A. (1982) 'Immunological abnormalities in ataxia–telangiectasia.' *In:* Harnden, D.G., Bridges, B.A. (Eds.) *Ataxia–Telangiectasia.* Chichester: John Wiley, pp. 37–51.

—— McIntire, K.R. (1972) 'Serum-alpha-fetoprotein levels in patients with ataxia–telangiectasia.' *Lancet*, **2**, 1112–1115.

—— Misiti, J., Nelson, D.L., Kraemer, K.H. (1983) 'Ataxia–telangiectasia: a multisystem hereditary disease with immunodeficiency, impaired organ maturation, X-ray hypersensitivity and a high incidence of neoplasia.' *Annals of Internal Medicine*, **99**, 367–379.

Walsh, F.B., Hoyt, W.F. (1969) 'Neurofibromatosis.' *In: Clinical Neuro-ophthalmology. Vol. 3. 3rd Edn.* Baltimore: Williams & Wilkins, pp. 1942–1957.

Wang, P.J., Maeda, Y., Izumi, T., *et al.* (1983) 'An association of subtotal cerebellar agenesis with organoid nevus—a possible new variety of neuro-cutaneous syndrome.' *Brain and Development*, **5**, 503–508.

Webb, D.W., Osborne, J.P. (1995) 'Tuberous sclerosis.' *Archives of Disease in Childhood*, **72**, 471–474.

—— Fryer, A.E., Osborne, J.P. (1991) 'On the incidence of fits and mental retardation in tuberous sclerosis.' *Journal of Medical Genetics*, **28**, 395–397.

Weig, S.G., Pollack, P. (1993) 'Carbamazepine-induced heart block in a child with tuberous sclerosis and cardiac rhabdomyoma: implications for evaluation and follow-up.' *Annals of Neurology*, **34**, 617–619.

Wertelecki, W., Rouleau, G.A., Superneau, D.W., *et al.* (1988) 'Neurofibro-matosis 2: clinical and DNA linkage studies of a large kindred.' *New England Journal of Medicine*, **319**, 278–283.

Wessel, H.B., Barmada, M.A., Hashida, Y. (1987) 'Congenital alopecia, seizures and psychomotor retardation in three siblings.' *Pediatric Neurology*, **3**, 101–107.

Williams, M.L., Koch, T.K., O'Donnell, J.J., *et al.* (1985) 'Ichthyosis and neutral lipid storage disease.' *American Journal of Medical Genetics*, **20**, 711–726.

Wilms, G., Van Wijck, E., Demaerel, P., *et al.* (1992) 'Gyriform calcifications in tuberous sclerosis simulating the appearance of Sturge–Weber disease.' *American Journal of Neuroradiology*, **13**, 295–297.

Witkop, C.J., Quevedo, W.C., Fitzpatrick, T.B. (1983) 'Albinism and other disorders of pigment metabolism.' *In:* Stanbury, J.B., Wyngaarden, J.B., Fredrickson, D.S. (Eds.) *The Metabolic Basis of Inherited Disease, 5th Edn.* New York: McGraw Hill, pp. 301–346.

Yamamoto, N., Watanabe, K., Negoro, T., *et al.* (1987) 'Long-term prognosis of tuberous sclerosis with epilepsy in children.' *Brain and Development*, **9**, 292–295.

Yamanouchi, H., Ho, M., Jay, V., Becker, L.E. (1997) 'Giant cells in cortical tubers in tuberous sclerosis showing synaptophysin-immunoreactive halos.' *Brain and Development*, **19**, 21–24.

Yoshitomi, F., Zaitsu, Y., Tanaka, K. (1980) 'Ataxia–telangiectasia with renal cell carcinoma and hepatoma.' *Virchow's Archive. A. Pathological Anatomy and Histology*, **389**, 119–125.

Young, W.F., Carney, J.A., Musa, B.U., *et al.* (1989) 'Familial Cushing's syndrome due to primary pigmented nodular adrenocortical disease. Re-investigation 50 years later.' *New England Journal of Medicine*, **321**, 1659–1664.

5
NEUROLOGICAL ASPECTS OF CHROMOSOMAL ANOMALIES AND DYSMORPHIC SYNDROMES

Neurological abnormalities, in particular impaired intellectual function, are extremely common in patients with chromosomal anomalies. These are responsible for approximately 6 per cent of CNS malformations (Carter 1976). The frequency of chromosomal abnormalities, usually with major brain malformations, is much higher in aborted fetuses and stillborn infants. In one study, chromosomal anomalies were found in 6.2 per cent of mentally retarded patients as opposed to 0.7 per cent of controls (Tharapel and Summit 1977). These figures are certainly underestimates as more subtle chromosome abnormalities such as small deletions or translocations may be detected only with modern sophisticated techniques. Chromosomal abnormalities and mental retardation are not always related. Abnormalities of sex chromosomes and minor anomalies of autosomal chromosomes are often compatible with a normal intelligence.

A vast number of syndromes associated with chromosomal abnormalities have been reported, and their description can be found in specialized texts (De Grouchy and Turleau 1984, Schinzel 1984, Jones 1988). An even greater number of dysmorphic syndromes with or without accompanying chromosomal anomalies are known, many of which also feature mental retardation and/or neurological signs. Only some chromosomal abnormalities or dysmorphic syndromes which are of special neurological importance are considered in this chapter.

ABNORMALITIES OF AUTOSOMAL CHROMOSOMES

DOWN SYNDROME (TRISOMY 21)
Trisomy 21 is the single most common cause of mental retardation. The condition occurs in about one in 650 births, although the frequency varies with maternal age, reaching one in 54 births in infants born to mothers aged 45 years or more. A high incidence is also observed in infants of very young mothers (Smith and Berg 1976).

AETIOLOGY
Down syndrome is caused by duplication of the genetic material localized on the long arm of chromosome 21 (Antonarakis 1993). Triplication of the 21q21–q22.3 region appears to be essential (Holtzman and Epstein 1992). Huret *et al.* (1987) found that a DNA fragment no larger than 3000 kb contains most of the genetic information involved in the pathogenesis of Down syndrome, and its presence in triplicate results in a similar phenotype.

The most common form, accounting for more than 90 per cent of cases, is associated with the presence of an extra chromosome 21. Eight per cent of cases are due to a translocation of chromosome 21 to another chromosome, usually 14 or 21. Rare cases are mosaics of normal and trisomic cells (Uchida and Freeman 1985). Most translocations resulting in Down syndrome arise *de novo* and are not associated with a familial occurrence. In less than a quarter of the cases with a translocation, the carrier of the translocation was a parent, usually the mother (Antonarakis *et al.* 1991, Antonarakis 1993). The recurrence rate for Down syndrome when a familial translocation is present varies between 5 and 15 per cent depending on the type of translocation and whether the father or the mother is the carrier, as compared with approximately 1 per cent in cases of nondisjunction. A higher risk exists for cases of 21q/21q translocation (Garver *et al.* 1982). Other mechanisms responsible for familial recurrence include parental mosaicism, found in 2.4 per cent of cases (Uchida and Freeman 1985), and a familial tendency to nondisjunction despite a normal karyotype.

PATHOLOGY AND PATHOGENESIS
Very little is known about how the presence of excess genetic material from chromosome 21 is responsible for the clinical picture of Down syndrome.

Brain pathology is rather minor. The brain is small, correlating with the small head circumference of the patients. The cerebellum is especially atrophic. The disproportionately small cerebellum is easily detectable on MRI scans, which also show a less marked volume reduction of the cerebrum (Becker *et al.* 1991, Golden and Hyman 1994). The first temporal gyrus is poorly developed and narrow. Microscopically, there is a reduction of granule cells in the cortex in some areas and curtailment

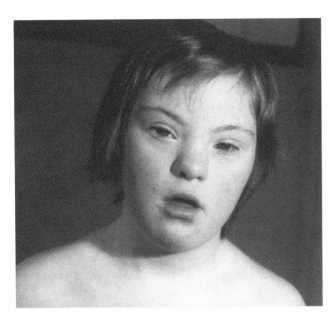

Fig. 5.1. Trisomy 21 (Down syndrome) in a 7-year-old-girl: classical features with upslanting palpebral fissures and epicanthus. (Courtesy Dr M-O. Réthoré, Hôpital des Enfants Malades, Paris.)

of a specific cell type, probably the aspinous stellate cells (Ross *et al.* 1984, Wisniewski *et al.* 1985). The number of spines on apical dendrites may be reduced (Marin Padilla 1976). Lamination of the superior temporal gyrus is delayed and disorganized, with increased cellular density in the upper layer (Golden and Hyman 1994). Histological abnormalities may be detectable as early as the 20th to 22nd week of intrauterine life (Wisniewski and Kida 1994).

A remarkable feature of trisomy 21 is the premature development of senile plaques and fibrillary tangles similar to those observed in Alzheimer disease. Such plaques are visible from age 30 years and correlate with the frequency of the development of dementia that occurs from 40 years of age in at least one-third of Down syndrome patients (St Clair and Blackwood 1985, Wisniewski *et al.* 1985). Interestingly, the gene for amyloid precursor protein is located just outside the duplicated area critical for Down syndrome and is expressed about four times normal in affected patients (Neve *et al.* 1988). This could conceivably lead to amyloid deposition, a hallmark of Alzheimer disease.

CLINICAL FEATURES
About 20 per cent of trisomy 21 fetuses are stillborn, and a trisomy 21 karyotype is found in 1 in 40 spontaneous abortions. Birthweight of Down syndrome infants is usually low, about 20 per cent of babies weighing < 2500 g. Physical growth in height, weight and head circumference remains subnormal, although with large interindividual variation.

The dysmorphic features of Down syndrome are very suggestive and the diagnosis is usually made at a glance even in newborn infants, although no individual dysmorphism is absolutely specific or constant (Fig. 5.1). Other malformations, especially atrioventricular canal and duodenal stenosis, are common.

The palpebral fissures are oblique and there is a complete median epicanthal fold. Brushfield spots, accumulations of fibrous tissue in the superficial layer of the iris, are present in 85 per cent of patients and differ from those observed in normal persons by their more central location. The external auditory meatus is narrow. The fifth finger is short and incurved, with a single flexion crease. A transverse palmar crease is seen in about half the patients and dermatoglyphics are characteristic (Smith and Berg 1976).

Down syndrome children are more sensitive than controls to infections and they have an increased risk of autoimmune diseases and leukaemia (Krivit and Good 1957).

From the neurological point of view, trisomy 21 patients manifest considerable hypotonia, and independent ambulation is delayed to about the age of 2 years. The degree of mental retardation is variable, the average IQ being about 50 though tending to decrease with age (Smith and Berg 1976). Mosaic patients may have higher IQ levels and verbal–perceptual skills (Fishler *et al.* 1976). Epilepsy is present in 5–6 per cent of patients (Stafstrom *et al.* 1991), a proportion lower than with most other causes of mental retardation in which 20–50 per cent of affected persons have seizures. Infantile spasms are clearly abnormally frequent (Pollack *et al.* 1978, Silva *et al.* 1996). Reflex seizures may be more common than in epilepsies of other causes (Guerrini *et al.* 1990b). Hearing loss is a common problem in children with Down syndrome but is mainly conductive in type (Balkany *et al.* 1979). Calcification of the basal ganglia is frequently present (Takashima and Becker 1985). Stroke may be more frequent in Down syndrome patients than in the general population and occurs even in childhood. The development of moyamoya disease (see Chapter 15) has been reported (Aylett *et al.* 1996).

Instability of the cervical column is frequent and may be a contraindication to some athletic activities (Chapter 6).

Antisocial behaviour is relatively uncommon; indeed, social adjustment tends to be ahead of that expected for the mental age (Chapter 28).

DIAGNOSIS AND MANAGEMENT
The diagnosis is usually made from birth on the basis of the dysmorphic syndrome. A karyotype is indicated in all cases to determine the type of trisomy present. If a translocation is present, the karyotype of parents should be obtained.

Antenatal diagnosis can be made by amniotic fluid cell culture or by biopsy of the trophoblast. It is indicated for pregnant women over 35–37 years of age and for young mothers who have had an affected child.

Prenatal screening for trisomy 21 is systematic in many countries for pregnant women aged 35 years or more at term and is also indicated for young women who have had an affected child. Screening for low-risk pregnancies is possible during the second trimester. The so-called 'triple test' shows low maternal serum alpha-fetoprotein, decreased unconjugated oestriol and elevated chorionic gonadotrophins in maternal serum in more than 60 per cent of cases of Down syndrome (Chard and Macintosh 1992). Ultrasound examination often shows short femora and cervical skin swelling. Amniocentesis is necessary to confirm the diagnosis by permitting demonstration of the trisomy. It is usually performed at 16 weeks gestational age. Early amniocentesis is possible but less effective. Chorionic villus biopsy, although it permits an earlier diagnosis, may be less reliable because of placental mosaicism (MRC 1991). Demonstration of abnormal numbers of gene copies in fetal cells by the polymerase chain reaction technique utilizing chromosome 21 markers is possible (Mansfield 1993) and may become a routine method of diagnosis.

There is no effective treatment for Down syndrome aside from the management of infections and hearing deficit and surgical treatment of correctable associated malformations. An adapted educational programme should be devised for each individual patient. Many children can be maintained within the family but the overall outlook for full autonomy is poor.

Complications of Down syndrome may require complex treatment. Neurological complications related to the unstable cervico-occipital junction of patients with trisomy 21 are discussed in Chapter 6.

OTHER TRISOMY SYNDROMES
Among the many trisomy syndromes currently known (De Grouchy and Turleau 1984), only trisomy 13, trisomy 18 and trisomy 8 will be considered.

TRISOMY 13 (PATAU SYNDROME)
The frequency of trisomy 13 is probably between 1 in 4000 and 1 in 10,000 births. Elevated maternal age increases the risk. Average birthweight is 2600 g (De Grouchy and Turleau 1984).

Affected children are profoundly retarded. The most characteristic features are hexadactyly, various types of facial clefts, most commonly bilateral cleft lip and palate, and microphthalmia. The feet are convex with protruding heels. Cryptorchidism and scrotal anomalies are the rule in boys, while bifid uterus and bifid vagina may be found in females.

Visceral malformations are common (Warkany et al. 1966). Heart disease is present in 80 per cent of patients and renal abnormalities in 30–50 per cent. Skin defects may occur, especially on the vertex. Eye abnormalities, in addition to microphthalmia, include cataracts, iris coloboma, retinal dysplasia and persistence of the primitive vitreous (Saraux et al. 1964).

The major neurological abnormality is *holoprosencephaly* (see Chapter 3) (Gulotta et al. 1981) which is usually accompanied by several other anomalies, especially in the cerebellum (Norman 1966). Arhinencephaly was found in 40 per cent of patients in the series of Gulotta et al. Severe neurological symptoms are present in most patients (Kunze 1980). Convulsions, often in the form of infantile spasms (Watanabe et al. 1976), are the rule. Most affected infants die before their first birthday.

The diagnosis is suggested by the striking external abnormalities. From a neurological point of view, trisomy 13 should be sought in cases of holoprosencephaly associated with visceral and limb abnormalities. Isolated holoprosencephaly is only rarely due to trisomy 13 (Kobori et al. 1987).

Partial trisomy 13 (De Grouchy and Turleau 1984) has a variable clinical expression depending on the triplicated segment.

TRISOMY 18 (EDWARDS SYNDROME)
The incidence of trisomy 18 is one in 8000 births, and there is a 4:1 female preponderance. Increased maternal age increases the frequency of the condition. Average duration of pregnancy is 42 weeks, and hydramnios, a small placenta and a single umbilical artery are frequently found. Mean birthweight is 2240 g (De Grouchy and Turleau 1984).

Affected children have a long narrow skull with prominent occiput. The bridge of the nose is protruding, the mandible is small and receding, and the ears are low set and imperfectly shaped. The index and fifth fingers cover the third and fourth fingers, and the fists are firmly closed. Cryptorchidism is constant in males.

Visceral malformations include congenital heart disease (patent ductus arteriosus or ventricular septal defect) in 95 per cent of cases. Meckel diverticulum, horseshoe kidneys, diaphragmatic hernia and hydronephrosis are also common.

Mental retardation is severe and is associated with hypotonia or hypertonia and weak sucking. Brain malformations (Norman 1966, Sumi 1970, Gulotta et al. 1981) include partial agenesis of the corpus callosum, abnormalities of the cerebellum, especially the inferior olivary bodies, and variable types of cortical dysplasia. In half the cases no abnormalities are detectable.

The diagnosis is confirmed by a karyotype that shows a homogeneous free trisomy (80 per cent of cases), a mosaic of trisomic and normal cells (10 per cent of cases) or (in the remaining 10 per cent) a translocation or complex abnormality (De Grouchy and Turleau 1984) such as a ring chromosome 18 (Amit et al. 1988).

TRISOMY 8
Trisomy 8 is less frequently recognized than trisomies 13 or 18 but its diagnosis may often be missed, as mental retardation is mild and dysmorphism is moderate. About one third of cases are not recognized before adulthood. The most suggestive facial feature is the thick and everted lower lip. Osteoarticular lesions such as brachydactyly, clinodactyly, club-feet and joint contractures are extremely common (Riccardi 1977).

From a neurological point of view, the most remarkable abnormality is agenesis of the corpus callosum which has been found in almost all cases in which it has been looked for (Aicardi et al. 1987). IQ is usually between 45 and 75.

The diagnosis should be systematically thought of in patients with callosal agenesis. Most cases are mosaics and all known cases have appeared *de novo*.

SYNDROMES CAUSED BY OTHER DEMONSTRATED OR SUSPECTED AUTOSOMAL ABNORMALITIES
Abnormalities of autosomal chromosomes other than trisomies are frequent and include a large number of syndromes with mental retardation, neurological symptoms and signs, and variable dysmorphism. Some of the associated syndromes are regularly associated with microscopically detectable chromosomal abnormalities that may be partial monosomy or trisomy, ring

chromosomes, or interstitial deletions or duplications. Not all interstitial deletions or duplications are microscopically visible, even using high-resolution banding of synchronized lymphocyte cultures. Molecular studies using DNA analysis with appropriate DNA probes (Ledbetter *et al.* 1989) or the FISH (fluorescent *in situ* hybridization) test have detected such abnormalities when none was cytogenetically apparent, *e.g.* in the Prader–Willi, Miller–Dieker and Angelman syndromes. Indeed, to be visible a deletion must involve about two million base pairs or 40–50 genes (Punnett and Zakai 1990). The smallest, submicroscopic deletions are often associated with the mildest forms of a particular syndrome, whereas large deletions are seen in the severe forms with other associated abnormalities. Such techniques have demonstrated that in many multisystem disorders, the phenotypic abnormalities are due to the involvement of closely spaced genes not related through their function, the 'contiguous gene syndromes'. Such is the case with X-chromosome microdeletions, *e.g.* the glycerate kinase deficiency syndrome, adrenal hypoplasia and muscular dystrophy (Darras and Francke 1988). Many of the currently identified dysmorphic syndromes are not always associated with detectable chromosomal abnormalities even using DNA analysis techniques. For most, however, evidence or strong suspicion of such abnormalities has been recognized in a variable proportion of cases so that it is artificial to establish a distinction between syndromes of detectable chromosomal origin and the others.

This section will therefore deal with some of the most common recognized syndromes and indicate for each of them the current knowledge about associated chromosomal or DNA abnormalities. Syndromes other than those considered may also be due to small deletions, duplications or other chromosomal abnormalities, and the transition between conventional genetic and chromosomal disorders is arbitrary as several dysmorphic syndromes can be transmitted according to mendelian laws, and as a large number of 'classical' genetic syndromes (*e.g.* Charcot–Marie–Tooth disease) are in fact the result of duplications or deletions of part of chromosomes.

Selected dysmorphic syndromes are described here. Less common syndromes regularly associated with cytogenetically detectable autosomal abnormalities are listed in Table 5.1, and other dysmorphic syndromes only occasionally associated with cytogenetic anomalies or with DNA abnormalities are listed in Table 5.2. This does not imply essential differences between the syndromes listed in the two tables.

PRADER–WILLI SYNDROME
Prader–Willi syndrome is relatively frequent. It is associated, in approximately half the patients, with an interstitial deletion of chromosome 15q11–13 (Ledbetter *et al.* 1982, Mattei *et al.* 1983, Caldwell and Taylor 1988). The deletion, in virtually all cases, is of paternal origin (Butler *et al.* 1986, Knoll *et al.* 1989). Approximately 40 per cent of cases without cytogenetic deletion have deletions detectable by DNA studies and 60 per cent have maternal disomy for all or part of chromosome 15 (Mascari *et al.* 1992). Prader–Willi syndrome and Angelman syndrome (see below) are classical examples of imprinting (*e.g.* the different

expression of a gene according to the sex of the transmitting parent). A gene for Prader–Willi syndrome was shown to be exclusively expressed when of paternal origin (Wevrick *et al.* 1994). Cases without chromosome 15 anomalies should be clinically reassessed and other conditions, such as the Smith–Magenis syndrome, considered (Greenberg *et al.* 1991). Patients with a deletion may be more typical than those without (Mattei *et al.* 1983), although atypical forms have been seen in patients with a demonstrated 15q deletion (Pauli *et al.* 1983, Schwartz *et al.* 1985, Miike *et al.* 1988). Butler *et al.* (1986) compared 21 children with deletion to 18 others with normal high resolution karyotype. The differences between the two groups were only minor. Just over half the deletion patients (11/21) walked by 24 months as compared to two-thirds of the nondeletion cases. Deletion patients were also blonder than nondeletion children and all were blue-eyed as compared to only 13/18 nondeletion patients (Lee *et al.* 1994).

The clinical features of the syndrome are highly suggestive, especially in the neonatal period, and in patients seen later, typical neonatal history is extremely useful for the diagnosis. Newborn infants with Prader–Willi syndrome are generally born at term but are small for gestational age. Thirty per cent are born by the breech. They demonstrate from birth a profound muscular hypotonia, so that a diagnosis of muscle disease is often entertained. Swallowing difficulties necessitate tube feeding for two to five weeks. The dysmorphic appearance is sufficient for a karyotype to be requested in virtually all cases (Stephenson 1980). Later on, the clinical picture changes. The most striking feature is the hyperphagia and obesity that develop in most children towards the end of the second year of life. At a late stage, there is marked obesity, persistent hypotonia and often proximal weakness and relatively mild mental retardation, with an average IQ of 65 (Butler *et al.* 1986), although up to 10 per cent of adult patients may have an IQ within the normal range (Greenswag *et al.* 1987). Hypogenitalism, often with cryptorchidism, and short stature and notable smallness of the face, nose, ears, hands and feet are also frequent features (Holm *et al.* 1993).

Adults with the Prader–Willi syndrome are short, overweight, cognitively impaired and emotionally labile. They have poor motor skills and hyperphagia (Greenswag 1987).

Atypical patients may have severe retardation (3 per cent) or be cognitively normal. Occasional patients may not be obese and, in rare cases, emaciation has been reported (Miike *et al.* 1988).

Diagnosis in the neonatal period should be considered in infants with low birthweight, marked hypotonia, swallowing difficulties requiring tube feeding, and dysmorphism. In older patients, obesity and an abnormal facies are suggestive. The differential diagnosis of Prader–Willi syndrome includes neuromuscular diseases and hypotonia due to cerebral disorders. Congenital muscular dystrophy, neonatal myotonic dystrophy and congenital myopathies are serious considerations. The dysmorphism, however, favours Prader–Willi syndrome, as does the prominent place of sucking and swallowing difficulties without significant respiratory impairment. Other causes of hypotonia of cerebral origin can raise a problem in older patients. Muscle

TABLE 5.1
Some uncommon chromosomal aberrations

Type of chromosome defect	Main features	References
Trisomy 9 mosaic syndrome	Severe mental retardation, sloping forehead with narrow bifrontal diameter, prominent nasal bridge, joint contractures, congenital heart defects in two-thirds of cases, absent optic tract (occasional)	Frohlich (1982), Golden and Schoene (1993)
4p– syndrome	Microcephaly, hypotonia, severe mental retardation, seizures, ocular hypertelorism with broad or beaked nose, low-set ears with preauricular dimple	Gottfried *et al.* (1981), Fagan *et al.* (1994)
Cri-du-chat (5p–) syndrome	Plaintive, acute cry; microcephaly; moon-like facies; severe mental retardation	de Grouchy and Turleau (1984)
Trisomy 9p	Growth deficiency, severe mental retardation, distal phalangeal hypoplasia, delayed closure of anterior fontanelle, ocular hypertelorism	Golden and Schoene (1993)
9p– syndrome	Trigonocephaly, mental retardation, hypoplastic supraorbital ridges, upslanting palpebral fissures	Alfi *et al.* (1976)
13q– syndrome	Microcephaly with high nasal bridge, mental retardation, thumb hypoplasia, eye defects that may include retinoblastoma, holoprosencephaly-type brain defects	Riccardi *et al.* (1979)
18q– syndrome	Hypotonia, mental retardation, microcephaly, midfacial hypoplasia, prominent antihelix, hypoplasia of labia minora in girls, long tapering fingers	Wertelecki and Gerald (1971)
18p– syndrome	Hypotonia, mental deficiency, ptosis, epicanthal folds, prominent auricles, holoprosencephaly–arhinencephaly in several cases	Schinzel *et al.* (1974)
Cat-eye syndrome (acrocentric extra chromosome ?22)	Mild mental deficiency, coloboma of iris (bilateral), anal atresia	Schinzel *et al.* (1981)
Aniridia–Wilms tumour association (11p13 deletion)	Aniridia, genitourinary anomalies, mental retardation, Wilms tumour. Demonstration of deletion may require FISH	Yunis and Ramsay (1980)
Smith–Magenis syndrome (17p11.2 deletion)	Mental retardation, sleep disturbances, hyperactivity, grossly destructive behaviour, brachycephaly, midface hypoplasia, hoarse voice, upper body squeeze stereotypy. Demonstration of deletion may require FISH	Smith *et al.* (1986), De Rijk-van Andel *et al.* (1991), Finucane *et al.* (1994)

biopsy (which should be avoided), serum creatine-kinase level and EMG are all normal. Treatment aims at preventing the development of obesity and at providing adequate specialized education. Fenfluramine therapy has been suggested for control of both weight gain and behaviour disturbances (Selikowitz *et al.* 1990; see also Chapter 16).

Cohen syndrome (Norio *et al.* 1984) may mimic Prader–Willi syndrome and is transmitted as an autosomal recessive trait. Ophthalmological signs (choroidoretinal dystrophy, optic atrophy when present) are of great diagnostic significance. Teeth abnormalities may be suggestive.

ANGELMAN SYNDROME

Angelman syndrome (formerly known as 'happy puppet syndrome') is caused in a majority of cases by a deletion of chromosome 15q11.2–12 which is similar, but not identical, to that found in children with Prader–Willi syndrome (Magenis *et al.* 1987, Knoll *et al.* 1989) and is maternally inherited (Knoll *et al.* 1989). The deletion includes a gene for the beta-3 subunit of GABA receptor (Saitho *et al.* 1994). Sixty to 75 per cent of patients have deletions or rearrangements in the long arm of chromosome 15 and the deletion is always on the maternal chromosome. A small proportion of cases have paternal disomy for chromosome 15 (Malcolm *et al.* 1991). At least 20 per cent of affected persons have normal chromosomes and no evidence of disomy. In some of these cases, recurrence in relatives may be observed (Clayton-Smith 1992). Such cases may be due to a dominant mutation at 15q11–13 resulting in an Angelman phenotype only when transmitted by females (Wystaff *et al.* 1993).

The clinical features consist of severe mental retardation with especially severe speech deficit, ataxia, and a remarkable jerky

TABLE 5.2
Selected dysmorphic syndromes with involvement of the central nervous system not usually associated with cytogenetic abnormalities

Syndrome (McKusick number)	Features	Genetic transmission* (gene location)	References
Cornelia de Lange (122470)	Short stature, mental retardation, special facies and limb anomalies (see text), hirsutism	AD?[1] (3q26/17q23)	Hawley et al. (1985)
Rubinstein–Taybi (268600)	Short stature, mental retardation, beaked nose, broad thumbs and toes, strabismus	S or AD[1] (16p13)	Rubinstein (1990), Stevens et al. (1990)
Dubowitz (223370)	Intrauterine growth retardation, prominent epicanthus, ptosis, short stature, mild microcephaly, shallow supraorbital ridge, short palpebral fissures with lateral telecanthus, severe eczema-like lesions on face and flexural areas, sparse hair, variable mental retardation, stubborness, hoarse cry	AR (?)	Ilyina and Lurie (1990), Hausen et al. (1995)
Seckel ('bird-headed dwarfism') (210600)	Intrauterine growth retardation, marked dwarfism, severe microcephaly, prominent nose, single transverse palmar crease, only 11 pairs of ribs, mental retardation	AR (?)	Majewski and Goecke (1982)
Williams (194050)	Prominent lips, hoarse voice, aortic stenosis (see text)	S (7q11)	Morris et al. (1988)
Smith–Lemli–Opitz (270400)	Short stature, ptosis of eyelids, anteverted nostrils, syndactyly of 2nd, 3rd toes, hypospadias and cryptorchidism in males, seizures, mental retardation. Disorder of cholesterol metabolism (see Chapter 9)	AR (7q32)	Curry et al. (1987), Tint et al. (1994)
Sotos (cerebral gigantism) (117550)	Variable mental deficiency, excessive head and body size with prenatal onset, large hands and feet, prognathism	AD?[1] (3p21?)	Cole and Hughes (1994)
Marshall–Smith (154780)	Accelerated growth, shallow orbits, broad middle phalanges, failure to thrive may suggest the diencephalic syndrome, unstable cranio-cervical junction	S	Roodhooft et al. (1988)
Beckwith–Wiedemann (130650)	Macrosomia, omphalocele, macroglossia usually mild–moderate mental retardation, neonatal hypoglycaemia, myoclonus, Wilms tumour or other neoplasms in some cases	AD?[1] (11p15)	Winter et al. (1986)
Coffin–Lowry (303600)	Severe mental deficiency, hypotonia, scoliosis, downslanting palpebral fissures, prominent brow and ears, bulbous nose, tapering fingers, cataplectic attacks	XR (Xp22)	Gilgenkrantz et al. (1988)
Freeman–Sheldon (whistling face syndrome) (195700)	Mask-like facies with small mouth giving a 'whistling' appearance, broad nasal bridge, telecanthus, aberrant positioning of hands and feet, rarely mental retardation	AD, AR? (severe form)	Kousseff et al. (1982)
Bardet–Biedl (209900)	Mental retardation, polydactyly, obesity hypogenitalism, retinitis pigmentosa, frequent renal abnormalties	AR (16q13–q22, 11q13, 3p11–p13 15q22)	Green et al. (1989), Lappert et al. (1994)
Laurence–Moon (245800)	Distinct from Bardet–Biedl syndrome, mental retardation, pigmentary retinopathy, hypogenitalism, spastic paraplegia	AR (?)	Farag and Teeby (1988)
Pallister–Hall (146510)	Imperforate anus, postaxial polydactyly, hypopituitarism, hypothalamic hamartoma, gelastic epilepsy	AR (3p/7q?)	Minns et al. (1994)
Pallister–Killian	Coarse features, hypertelorism, sparse hair	Tetrasomy 12p	Guerrini et al. (1990a), McLean et al. (1992)
Gingival fibromatosis–epilepsy–hypertrichosis (135400)	May simulate epilepsy treated with phenytoin	AD	Anavi et al. (1989)
	A related syndrome has been described		Pina–Nieto et al. (1986)

*AD = autosomal dominant, AR = autosomal recessive, S = sporadic, XR = X-linked recessive.
[1]Most cases are isolated. Only occasional familial cases reported.

movement disorder affecting the upper limbs and sometimes the trunk, that has been shown to be a special type of cortical myoclonus (Guerrini et al. 1996). Unmotivated bursts of laughter are characteristic but they may not be prominent, whereas a cheerful mood is constant (Williams and Frias 1982). Eighty-six per cent of affected children have seizures that are often repeated but of short duration and are more often atypical absences or tonic and atonic seizures than tonic–clonic ones (Dörries et al. 1988, Viani et al. 1995, Laan et al. 1997). Ambulation is acquired late, often after 5–6 years, and is very abnormal with the legs wide apart and with both ataxic and apraxic features (Sugimoto et al. 1992).

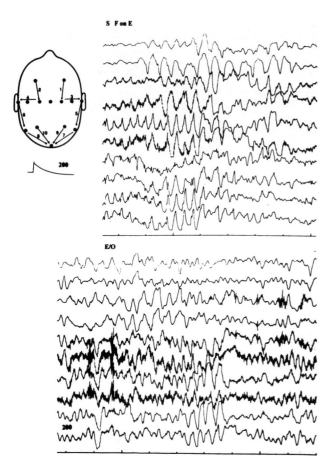

S F on E

E/O

200

Fig. 5.2. Typical EEG features in two children of different ages (*upper trace*, 7 years; *lower trace*, 2 years) with Angelman syndrome. Note the calibration. In both examples, there is excess rhythmic theta activity mixed with runs of slower components seen particularly over the anterior half of the two hemispheres. In *upper trace*, runs of 3–4/s activity mixed with ill-defined sharp waves are seen over the posterior third of the head when the eyes are held shut by an attendant. S = shut; F on E = 'finger on eyes'; E/O = eyes open. (Courtesy Dr S. Boyd, Great Ormond Street Hospital, London.)

The dysmorphic syndrome is moderate and may be unnoticeable in young patients. Prognathism usually develops only after a few years of age.

Most cases are isolated but familial cases are on record.

The diagnosis is often difficult in infants (van Lierde *et al.* 1990, Yamada and Volpe 1990). The combination of mental retardation with autistic features, a cheerful demeanour, ataxia and epileptic attacks, often of a 'minor' character, is highly suggestive. Because of the apraxic gait, manual stereotypies and sometimes hyperventilation, the diagnosis of Rett syndrome can be wrongly entertained in girls. However, the early onset of seizures before 1 year of age, the cheerful mood and the dysmorphism should rule out that possibility. The EEG is often very suggestive by showing runs of slow (3 Hz) waves, especially posteriorly, often notched and occasionally associated with actual spikes (Boyd *et al.* 1988) (Fig. 5.2). CT and MRI do not show any specific image, but mild dilatation of the ventricles and/or pericerebral spaces may be present (Dörries *et al.* 1988).

The prognosis is poor with severe mental retardation. Communicative language is not acquired.

WILLIAMS SYNDROME (WILLIAMS–BEUREN SYNDROME) (MCKUSICK 19405)

More than 200 cases of this syndrome have been reported. The clinical expression is variable. The full blown syndrome includes supravalvular aortic stenosis, multiple peripheral pulmonary arterial stenoses, elfin face, short stature, mental deficiency, characteristic dental malformations and infantile hypercalcaemia (Morris *et al.* 1988). Evidence of more diffuse vascular disease (renal and/or carotid and cerebral arteries) is present in some patients (Ardinger *et al.* 1994). As many as half the patients may have epilepsy, and most have difficulties with gross and fine motor coordination, oral motor skills and cerebellar function (Trauner *et al.* 1989). Joint contractures develop in many patients (Kaplan *et al.* 1989). An association with Chiari I malformation has been reported (Pober and Filiano 1995). Partial forms are common with predominance of heart, dysmorphic or metabolic (hypercalcaemia) features. An autosomal dominant inheritance for Williams syndrome has been suggested (Morris *et al.* 1993), but many cases appear to be sporadic. The mechanism of the hypercalcaemia does not seem to be related to the presence of a high plasma concentration of 1,25-dihydroxy vitamin D (Kruse *et al.* 1992).

Many patients with Williams syndrome have specific psychological profiles and speech or hearing difficulties (Meyerson and Frank 1987, Crisco *et al.* 1988, Udwin and Dennis 1995; see also Chapter 29).

The syndrome is associated with disruption of the elastin gene on chromosome 7q11, which accounts for the vascular abnormalities (Lowery *et al.* 1995, Nickerson *et al.* 1995). Most cases are sporadic although dominant transmission has been observed. Other features of the syndrome may be due to involvement of neighbouring genes. Diagnosis by FISH analysis is possible (Borg *et al.* 1995).

MILLER–DIEKER SYNDROME (17p– SYNDROME)

Miller–Dieker syndrome is a dysmorphic syndrome which features a distinctive facies with bitemporal hollowing, prominent forehead often with vertical furrows, upturned nares, a long philtrum with a thin vermilion border and a small jaw. Digital deformities, mainly camptodactyly and clinodactyly, are common (Dobyns *et al.* 1984). The most important pathological feature is the presence of type I lissencephaly (Chapter 3). There is deletion at the critical region of 17p13.3, detectable cytogenetically or by DNA analysis, and apparently of paternal origin.

Although most cases occur *de novo*, familial recurrence is possible in cases with parental translocation (Dobyns *et al.* 1984, Goutières *et al.* 1987) and as an X-linked trait (Chapter 3). The neurological features are those of type I lissencephaly.

DI GEORGE SYNDROME

Di George syndrome is due to a developmental defect of the third and fourth pharyngeal pouches and the fourth branchial arch.

The syndrome is genetically heterogeneous, with partial mono-somy of the proximal long arm of chromosome 22 detected microscopically in about one-third of cases, and a higher fre-quency of deletion (88 per cent) demonstrated by FISH studies (Driscoll *et al.* 1993). Uncommon cases have been associated with deletion of 17p and 10p (Levy-Mozziconacci *et al.* 1994). The thymus and parathyroids are absent and ectopic and the great vessels of the base of the heart are often malformed. Absence of the thymus may be associated with severe immunological defi-ciency, while that of the parathyroid glands may be responsible for severe hypocalcaemic convulsions in the neonatal period and later. Hypocalcaemia responds to parathyroid hormone. Cleft palate, micrognathia, low-set ears and hypertelorism are frequent (Conley *et al.* 1979).

An overlapping phenotype, known as the velo-cardio-facial or Schprintzen syndrome, features similar cardiovascular abnor-malities, facial dysmorphism, cleft palate and mental retardation, sometimes with late appearance of psychiatric disease, and is associated with the same 22q1 deletion. Cerebellar hypoplasia may be a feature (Devriendt *et al.* 1996). Both syndromes are dominantly transmitted, and their prenatal diagnosis is possible by DNA studies.

OTHER SELECTED DYSMORPHIC SYNDROMES WITH NEUROLOGICAL INVOLVEMENT

A huge number of dysmorphic syndromes have been identified, many of which include neurological abnormalities or brain malformations or both. These syndromes are reviewed in spe-cialized texts (Goodman and Gorlin 1979, Warkany *et al.* 1981, Smith 1982, Jones 1988). In addition, computerized data bases and retrieval systems can provide up-to-date information (*e.g.* POSSUM; Baraitser and Winter's London Neurogenetics Data-base)*. Only a few syndromes of special neurological interest will be briefly considered (Table 5.2). Other dysmorphic syndromes with well-defined brain malformations or neurological features have been described in other chapters of this book (see especially Chapter 3).

CORNELIA DE LANGE SYNDROME (BRACHMAN–DE LANGE SYNDROME, TYPUS DEGENERATIVUS AMSTELODAMENSIS) (McKUSICK 12247)

This syndrome is characterized by low birthweight, short stature, microcephaly, generalized hirsutism, a curious facies, with synophrys (eyebrows growing together), low hairline on neck and forehead, long eyelashes, depressed bridge of nose, a long philtrum and upturned nostrils. The hands have a flat, spade-like appearance and short tapering fingers. There is clinodactyly of the fifth finger. The thumbs are proximally implanted and the thenar eminence is inconspicuous. More marked abnormalities

*POSSUM—Murdoch Institute, Melbourne; London Neurogenetics Database (Baraitser and Winter)—Oxford University Press.

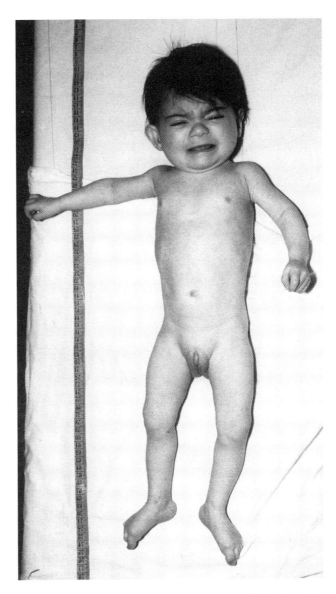

Fig. 5.3. Cornelia de Lange syndrome: depressed nasal bridge, low hair-line, synophris (eyebrows meeting on the midline), short arms and flexed fingers and toes. (Courtesy Dr M. Le Merrer, Hôpital des Enfants Malades, Paris.)

of limbs may be present, including radial hypoplasia or reduction of finger number, often unilaterally. Micrognathia is usually present (Hawley *et al.* 1985, Opitz 1985) (Fig. 5.3). Optic atrophy, coloboma of the optic nerve, proptosis and choanal atresia have been reported.

Various chromosomal anomalies have been found in patients with Cornelia de Lange syndrome (Jackson *et al.* 1993). Features suggestive of the de Lange syndrome are observed with partial trisomy of the distal portion of chromosome 3 (3q21–3ter). The syndrome of chromosome 3q duplication (dup(3q) syndrome) at least superficially simulates de Lange syndrome (Holder *et al.* 1994).

De Lange syndrome may be dominantly inherited, virtually all cases being new mutations. A recurrence risk of 2–5 per cent is quoted.

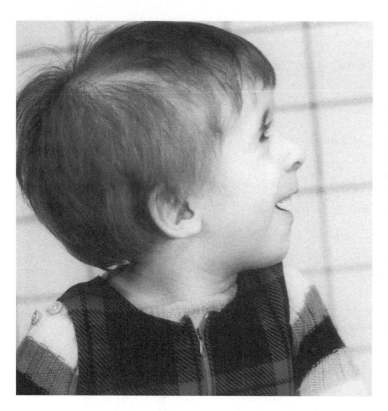

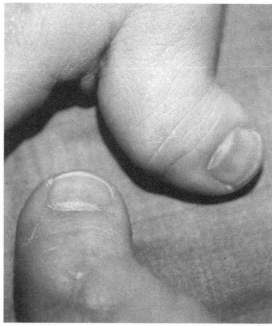

Fig. 5.4. Rubinstein–Taybi syndrome: *(left)* typical facies; *(above)* broad, abnormally oriented thumb. (Courtesy Dr M. Le Merrer, Hôpital des Enfants Malades, Paris.)

RUBINSTEIN–TAYBI SYNDROME
(McKUSICK 268600)

This syndrome is mainly characterized by the presence of broad thumbs and great toes, short stature, a peculiar facies, microcephaly and mental retardation. IQs range from 17 to 86 (Jones 1988). The palpebral fissures slant downwards, the maxilla is hypoplastic, and the nose is beaked with a nasal septum extending below the alae nasi. Epicanthal folds, strabismus and refractive errors are frequent (Fig. 5.4). There is an excess dermal ridge patterning in thenar and first interdigital areas of the palm. Pulmonary stenosis, large foramen magnum, vertebral anomalies and parietal foramina have been reported. There is a wide range of variability among affected individuals (Padfield *et al.* 1968). The incidence of this syndrome is probably underestimated (Sammito *et al.* 1988). Most cases are sporadic. Dominant transmission has been reported, and several sets of concordant monozygotic twins are on record. Submicroscopic deletions of 16p13 were found in 25 per cent of cases by Breuning *et al.* (1993).

SOTOS SYNDROME (CEREBRAL GIGANTISM)
(McKUSICK 11755)

Sotos syndrome commonly features mental retardation (83 per cent), the IQ of affected individuals varying from 18 to 119 with a mean of 72 (Jones 1988, Cole and Hughes 1994). The most striking feature is the excessively rapid somatic growth that begins before birth and is associated with advanced osseous maturation and with features reminiscent of acromegaly in adults (Sotos *et al.* 1977).

Neurological features may include seizures and strabismus. There is macrocephaly with mild dilatation of the lateral ventricles. Pigmentary abnormalities and intestinal polyps have been reported (Ruvalcaba *et al.* 1980) but may indicate a different syndrome.

Growth is especially fast during the first two or three years of life but then slows down so that the ultimate size may not always be outside the normal range (Cole and Hughes 1994). Even patients with a normal mental level usually have delay in expressive language and motor development (Bale *et al.* 1985).

Cases of Sotos syndrome are almost always sporadic, although there is evidence for dominant transmission in several cases (Bale *et al.* 1985). Under this hypothesis, most cases would represent new mutations. The mechanism of excessive growth is thought to be centrally determined but no precise data are available.

Other abnormalities such as deletion 10p13–14 or 17p13 have also been observed (Punnett and Zakai 1990).

Many other neurological syndromes associated with autosomal abnormalities are increasingly being recognized, *e.g.* epilepsy and anomalies of chromosomes 12, 14 and 20 (Holopainen *et al.* 1994; see also Chapter 16), and a complete list is beyond the scope of this book.

SMITH–LEMLI–OPITZ SYNDROME
(McKUSICK 27040)

The most striking features of this syndrome, in addition to mental retardation and marked hypotonia, are a peculiar facies with a high, square forehead, anteverted nostrils and micrognathia, and genital abnormalities in males including cryptorchidism and/or hypospadias and, in extreme instances, a complete failure of development of male genitalia despite a normal XY karyotype (Scarbrough *et al.* 1986). Other features include abnormal auricles, ptosis of the eyelids, inner epicanthal folds, transverse palmar crease, and various limb and visceral abnormalities (Opitz *et al.* 1994). Seizures are present in some patients, and feeding problems may be considerable. Mortality is high during the first year of life. Brain abnormalities may include micrencephaly, hypoplasia of the frontal lobes, abnormal gyration and cerebellar hypoplasia. The most severely affected cases are sometimes separated from the rest as type II Smith–Lemli–Opitz syndrome (Curry *et al.* 1987).

The syndrome is inherited as an autosomal recessive trait. The apparently increased frequency in males is probably related to the fact that diagnosis is easier in males because of the obvious genital abnormalities.

Plasma cholesterol concentrations are very low, while 7-dehydrocholesterol is raised, suggesting a defect in the enzyme that reduces the C-7,8 double bond in the latter compound (Tint *et al.* 1994). Survival correlates strongly with higher plasma cholesterol levels (Tint *et al.* 1995). Prenatal diagnosis by measurement of 7-dehydrocholesterol in amniotic fluid is possible (Dallaire *et al.* 1995). A high-cholesterol regime can normalize the level of cholesterol but is not clinically effective (Ullrich *et al.* 1996).

SEX CHROMOSOME ABNORMALITIES

Sex chromosome abnormalities are frequent, as determined by surveys of the newborn population. The incidence is about 2.5 per 1000 phenotypic boys and 1.4 per 1000 phenotypic girls (Grant and Hamerton 1976). The most common abnormalities are XXY (Klinefelter syndrome) and XYY complement in males and XXX and XO (Turner syndrome) in females.

The fragile X syndrome (sometimes referred to as Martin–Bell syndrome) is the second most common cause of mental retardation in the general population.

SEX CHROMOSOME ABNORMALITIES OTHER THAN THE FRAGILE X SYNDROME

These abnormalities are associated with a slightly increased risk of mental retardation. For example, Ratcliffe *et al.* (1994) found an XXY chromosome complement in 5.4 per 1000 phenotypic boys in institutions for the mentally retarded and that the mean IQ of such children was slightly lower than that of controls. The mean IQ of girls with three X chromosomes was 86.8; that of XXY boys 91.4 and that of XYY boys 101.7, all significantly lower than those of controls (respectively 109.1 and 115.8 for girls and boys). They also found that head circumference was smaller in the group with excess sex chromosomes, even at birth, implying an effect of extra gonosomes on brain growth pre- and postnatally. An XXX complement has been found in 4.3 per 1000 institutionalized phenotypic girls (Pennington *et al.* 1980). The mean IQ of XO (Turner) girls is normal, but many XO females do

exhibit right–left disorientation and defects in perceptual organization, and their verbal IQ tends to be higher than the performance IQ but with considerable interindividual variation (Temple and Carney 1993).

More severe mental retardation is probably more common in patients with more complex anomalies such as phenotypic males with three or more X chromosomes (Zalewski *et al.* 1966), or with duplication of both X and Y chromosomes (Schlegel *et al.* 1965). However, the main abnormalities encountered in such children are learning and perceptual disorders and behavioural difficulties (Bender *et al.* 1983, Ratcliffe *et al.* 1994). These are described in Chapter 28.

FRAGILE X SYNDROME

The fragile X syndrome is a genetic disorder initially characterized by a morphological abnormality of the X chromosome, the presence of a fragile site on the long arm at Xq27.3, which is apparent only when a medium deficient in folate is used for culture (Sutherland 1977). The disorder has now been shown to be due to the presence in the *FMR-1* gene of an expansion of a repeat trinucleotide (CGG) that normally contains six to 60 copies. In patients with the fragile X syndrome this repeat is expanded to more than 200 copies (full mutation), and 90 per cent of such persons have a cytogenetically detectable fragile site at Xq27.3. Transmission of the disease by asymptomatic males suggested the possibility of a premutation that is associated with expansion of the repeat to 50–200 copies. The premutation tends to remain stable during spermatogenesis but frequently expands to a full mutation during oogenesis, so that daughters of carrier males always carry only the premutation, while those of carrier females are often clinically affected. Males with a full mutation are mentally retarded, whereas only 30–50 per cent of females have mental deficiency, usually of a milder degree than males (Staley *et al.* 1993). Only 30–50 per cent have a demonstrable fragile site. The presence of a full mutation prevents the traduction of the gene into a protein (as a result of methylation) (Knight *et al.* 1993). The same absence of FMR-1 protein has now been reported in rare patients without trinucleotide expansion but with deletions or point mutations of the *FMR-1* gene (Hirst *et al.* 1995). Rare cases of males with normal mental functioning in the presence of a full mutation are on record (Smeets *et al.* 1995). The FMR-1 protein is expressed in many tissues and is most abundant in neurons. It appears to be normal in persons with the premutation (Devys *et al.* 1993). The functions of the FMR-1 protein are unknown. The fragile X syndrome is the most common heritable form of mental retardation (Mattei 1987). It is estimated that 1 in 1000 females are carriers and approximately 1 in 1300 to 1 in 3000 males are affected (Blomquist *et al.* 1983). The prevalence among children with moderate to severe learning difficulties without specific dysmorphic features ranges from 2 to 10 per cent (Slaney *et al.* 1995).

The common physical manifestations of the fragile X syndrome are listed in Table 5.3. The disorder is more easily recognizable in adolescents than in prepubertal children. The

TABLE 5.3
Clinical features of the fragile-X syndrome

Anthropometry	Normal weight and size
	Normal or large head (>75th centile)
	(>90th centile in 10 per cent)
Facial features	Long face
	High-arched palate
	Prominent jaw
	Epicanthal folds
	Mildly coarse facial features
	Strabismus
Genitalia	Macroorchidism (more common in, but not
	exclusive to, postpubertal boys)
Others	Hyperextensible fingers and other joints
	Hyperelastic skin
	Large floppy ears
Neurodevelopmental manifestations	Mental retardation (IQ<70)
	Autistic features
	Hyperactivity
	Poor coordination

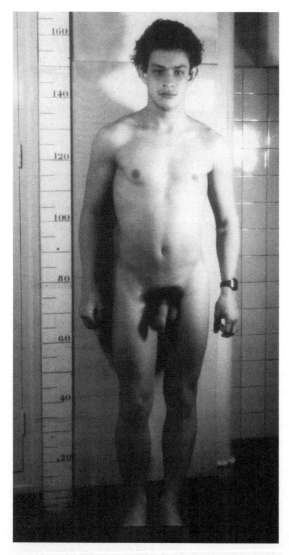

Fig. 5.5. Fragile X syndrome: elongated face, large ears, prognathism. General body development is good but the testicles are enlarged. (Courtesy Dr M-O. Réthoré, Hôpital des Enfants Malades, Paris.)

most important features are: the absence of retarded physical growth that is commonly found with many causes of mental retardation, and especially a normal or increased head circumference; a long face with prominent jaw; and macroorchidism (Ho *et al.* 1989) (Fig. 5.5). In prepubertal children, only a large head, large ears and high-arched palate are present. Joint hyperextensibility and floppy ears may be of diagnostic help. Despite the lack of prominence of macroorchidism in young patients, 15–40 per cent of them have some degree of testicular enlargement (Simko *et al.* 1989).

Mental retardation in fragile X syndrome is usually in the mild to moderate range but tends to become more severe in adolescence and adulthood (Borghgraef *et al.* 1987; Hagerman 1987, 1988; Wisniewski *et al.* 1989). Many patients have specific difficulties in speech, language, behaviour and social skills. 'Cluttered' speech is a suggestive feature (Hanson *et al.* 1986). Hyperactivity and attention deficit are common, and autism may be present in as many as 23 per cent of cases (Bregman *et al.* 1987, Thake *et al.* 1987, Vieregge and Froster-Iskenius 1989). However, the behavioural phenotype is different from that of other causes of autism and hyperactivity may be especially prominent (Baumgardner *et al.* 1995, Hagerman 1995).

Women carriers of the full mutation on one of their X chromosomes are usually phenotypically normal. Approximately 35 per cent appear to be retarded, generally in the mild range, and 15 per cent have borderline intelligence, learning disabilities or both (Kemper *et al.* 1986). The fragile X is thus an important cause of mild mental difficulties in women. In addition, about 10 per cent of cognitively normal carriers may have psychiatric conditions, especially affective or schizoid disorders (Reiss and Freund 1990).

The *diagnosis* of fragile X syndrome is difficult, especially in prepubertal boys and in female carriers who lack typical physical findings. Conversely, even macroorchidism or large ears are frequently unassociated with a fragile site on the X chromosome (Hagerman *et al.* 1988).

A family history of mental retardation is an important feature but is found in only two-thirds of cases (Simko *et al.* 1989).

Determination of the fragile site on the X chromosome on special culture medium is of value, but the proportion of chromosomes with the fragile site necessary for diagnosis is still debated, and no abnormality is found in some males and up to 50 per cent of females with a full mutation.

DNA studies are much more reliable and are clearly cost-effective (Rousseau *et al.* 1991, 1994; Oostra *et al.* 1993; Wang *et al.* 1993). A rapid antibody test for the detection of the FMR-1 protein in lymphocytes has been proposed as a screening procedure for the full mutation (Willemsen *et al.* 1995).

Prenatal diagnosis of X(fra)q27 is possible on cultured amniotic cells or chorionic villus cells and by DNA analysis. Highly difficult ethical problems arise, however, because only some carriers, especially among females, will be affected. Weaver and Sherman (1987) have computed the probability of retardation for offspring of affected carriers (Table 5.4) but precise counselling remains problematic.

TABLE 5.4
Probability of neurodevelopmental impairment in offspring of women carriers of the fragile Xq27 site and of normal transmitting males*

Offspring	Parent with fragile X			
	Normal woman	Mentally impaired woman	Normal transmitting male	Impaired male
Sons				
Mentally impaired	0.38	0.5	0	0
Asymptomatic carrier	0.12	0	0	0
Daughters				
Impaired carrier	0.16	0.28	0	>0.32[1]
Asymptomatic carrier	0.34	0.22	1.0	<0.68[1]

*Modified from Weaver and Sherman (1987).
[1]Estimates based on a known penetrance of 32 per cent of fragile X in females.

TABLE 5.5
Some common minor dysmorphic abnormalities

Third fontanelle or large posterior fontanelle
Abnormal scalp hair patterning (low hairline, absent or anteriorly displaced parietal hair whorl)
Epicanthal folds
Slanting of palpebral fissures
Ocular hypertelorism (dystopia canthorum)
Ptosis
Simplified earlobes, lack of lobulus
Posteriorly rotated ears, low-set ears
Preauricular pits or tags
Small nares, notched alae nasi
Borderline small mandible
Tongue frenulae
Branchial cleft fistula
Clinodactyly, camptodactyly
Simian crease (found in 4 per cent of normal infants unilaterally and in 1 per cent bilaterally)
Partial cutaneous syndactyly, broad nails, hypoplastic nails
Malproportion in length of particular segments of hands or digits
Minor degrees of hypospadias, hypoplasia of labia majora
Capillary haemangioma at nape of neck, central forehead and eyelids and lumbosacral area

The *treatment* for fragile X syndrome is based on socio-educational intervention, speech therapy and, if necessary, behaviour modification techniques. Methylphenidate may be useful in the treatment of hyperactivity. Folic acid therapy remains of unproven efficacy (see also Chapter 2).

OTHER SYNDROMES OF X-LINKED MENTAL RETARDATION

Fragile X syndrome accounts for only 50 per cent of the excess of mentally retarded boys. Many other more or less well-defined syndromes of X-linked mental retardation have been described (Opitz *et al.* 1986).

A second fragile X syndrome (FRAX-E) caused by an expanded GCC trinucleotide repeat in Xq28, 600 kb down from the *FMR-1* gene, has been found in several cases (Flynn *et al.*

1993). Mental retardation is usually mild and is absent altogether in many cases.

A third fragile X site (FRAX-F) that is also due to an expanded repeat and may be associated with mental retardation and seizures has been reported (Hirst *et al.* 1993).

Renpenning syndrome is characterized by moderate to severe mental retardation, mild microcephaly, short stature and normal chromosomes (Archidiacono *et al.* 1987).

Juberg–Marsidi syndrome features growth retardation, deafness and microgenitalism (Juberg and Marsidi 1980).

X-linked recessive mental retardation has also been reported in association with bodily overgrowth (Golabi and Rusen 1984), coarse features, short stature and macroorchidism (Atkin *et al.* 1985), and progressive complex neurological disorders (Davis *et al.* 1981, Schimke *et al.* 1984, Pfeiffer and Steffann 1985). Male relatives of patients with X-linked aqueductal stenosis may have moderate to severe mental retardation without hydrocephalus (Willems *et al.* 1987), sometimes in association with paraplegia, adducted thumbs and language disturbances (mental retardation–aphasia–shuffling gait–adducted thumbs syndrome or MASA). X-linked nerve deafness, optic nerve atrophy and dementia may constitute a specific X-linked recessive syndrome (Jensen 1981; see also Chapter 19).

MINOR MORPHOLOGICAL ANOMALIES AND VISCERAL MALFORMATIONS, AND THEIR RELATIONSHIP TO DYSMORPHIC SYNDROMES AND MAJOR CNS MALFORMATIONS

Minor anomalies are 'unusual morphologic features that are of no serious medical or cosmetic consequence to the patient' (Jones 1988). Some of the most common minor abnormalities are listed in Table 5.5. Such anomalies are extremely common. Marden *et al.* (1964) found a single abnormality in 14 per cent of all newborn babies, but this was not associated with an appreciable increase in the frequency of mental retardation or major malformations. However, when two minor anomalies were present,

11 per cent of the infants had major malformations and/or mental retardation, and the frequency rose to 90 per cent in those with three minor anomalies. Conversely, 42 per cent of patients with idiopathic mental retardation had three or more malformations of which 80 per cent were minor (Smith and Bostian 1964). A more recent study (Leppig *et al.* 1987) found a lower frequency of minor anomalies in retarded persons (19.6 per cent) but the same general trend, so that the discovery of multiple minor anomalies in an infant is of some prognostic significance. Likewise, the presence of minor dysmorphic defects in infants with seizures is associated with a relatively poor prognosis, probably as a result of associated brain malformations (Chevrie and Aicardi 1977).

Evaluation of the significance of minor anomalies should be careful. In particular, the presence of similar anomalies in blood relatives (*e.g.* camptodactyly or clinodactyly) often constitutes a satisfactory explanation for the presence of similar defects in patients.

A special place among the minor abnormalities should be given to the dermatoglyphics or dermal ridge patterns. These are formed between the 13th and 19th fetal weeks and reflect development at this period. Abnormal dermatoglyphic patterns are often associated with complex dysmorphic syndromes (*e.g.* distal axial palmar triradius in Down syndrome, an excess number of fingertips with an arch pattern in trisomy 18 or with a whorl pattern in the Smith–Lemli–Opitz syndrome) although no single pattern is specific.

Visceral malformations are frequently associated with CNS maldevelopment, either as part of malformation syndromes or associations, or in isolation, so their presence in patients with neurological disorders is an argument for a malformative origin. Even in nonsyndromal associations, some peripheral malformations tend to be electively associated with CNS abnormalities, *e.g.* choanal atresia (Rejjal *et al.* 1994) and certain cardiac malformations such as truncus arteriosus and hypoplastic left heart hypoplasia. Glauser *et al.* (1990) found that 29 per cent of children with left heart hypoplasia had brain maldevelopment such as holoprosencephaly or callosal agenesis and 27 per cent had microcephaly, while only 17 per cent had a recognized malformation syndrome. The recognition of such anomalies should therefore prompt a search for neurological abnormalities.

REFERENCES

Aicardi, J., Chevrie, J.J., Baraton, J. (1987) 'Agenesis of the corpus callosum.' *In:* Vinken, P.J., Bruyn, G.W., Klawans, H.L., Myrianthopoulos, N.C. (Eds.) *Handbook of Clinical Neurology. Vol.6. No. 50. Malformations.* Amsterdam: Elsevier, pp.149–173.

Alfi, O.S., Donnell, G.N., Allerdice, P.W., Derencsenyi, A. (1976) 'The 9p– syndrome.' *Annales de Génétique*, **19**, 11–16.

Amit, R., Gutman, A., Udassin, R., *et al.* (1988) 'Ring 18 chromosome with mental retardation, hemidysmorphism and mitochondrial encephalomyopathy.' *Pediatric Neurology*, **4**, 301–304.

Anavi, Y., Lerman, P., Mintz, S., Kiviti, S. (1989) 'Idiopathic familial gingival fibromatosis associated with mental retardation, epilepsy and hypertrichosis.' *Developmental Medicine and Child Neurology*, **31**, 538–542.

Antonarakis, S.E. (1993) 'Human chromosome 21: genome mapping and exploration, circa 1993.' *Trends in Genetics*, **9**, 142–148.

—— and the Down Syndrome Collaborative Group (1991) 'Parental origin of the extra chromosome in trisomy 21 as indicated by analysis of DNA polymorphisms.' *New England Journal of Medicine*, **324**, 872–876.

Archidiacono, N., Rocchi, M., Rinaldi, A., Filippi, G. (1987) 'X-linked mental retardation. II. Renpenning syndrome and other types (report of 14 families).' *Journal de Génétique Humaine*, **35**, 381–398.

Ardinger, R.H., Goertz, K.K., Mattioli, L.F. (1994) 'Cerebrovascular stenoses with cerebral infarction in a child with Williams syndrome.' *American Journal of Medical Genetics*, **51**, 200–202.

Atkin, J.F., Flaitz, K., Patil, S., Smith, W. (1985) 'A new X-linked mental retardation syndrome.' *American Journal of Medical Genetics*, **21**, 697–705.

Augusseau, S., Jouk, S., Jalbert, P., Prieur, M. (1986) 'DiGeorge syndrome and 22q11 rearrangements.' *Human Genetics*, **74**, 206. (*Letter.*)

Aylett, S.E., Britton, J.A., De Souza, C.M. (1996) 'Down syndrome and moyamoya disease: presentation with subarachnoid hemorrhage.' *Pediatric Neurology*, **14**, 259–261.

Bale, A.E., Drum, M.A., Parry, D.M., Mulvihill, J.J. (1985) 'Familial Sotos syndrome (cerebral gigantism): craniofacial and psychological characteristics.' *American Journal of Medical Genetics*, **20**, 613–624.

Balkany, T.J., Downs, M.P., Jafek, B.W., Krajicek, M.J. (1979) 'Hearing loss in Down's syndrome. A treatable handicap more common than generally recognized.' *Clinical Pediatrics*, **18**, 116–118.

Baumgardner, T.L., Reiss, A.L., Freund, L.S., Abrams, M.T. (1995) 'Specification of the neurobehavioral phenotype in males with fragile X syndrome.' *Pediatrics*, **95**, 744–752.

Becker, L., Mito, T., Takashima, S., Onodera, K. (1991) 'Growth and development of the brain in Down syndrome.' *Progress in Clinical and Biological Research*, **373**, 133–152.

Bender, B., Fry, E., Pennington, B., *et al.* (1983) 'Speech and language development in 41 children with sex chromososome anomalies.' *Pediatrics*, **71**, 262–267.

Blomquist, H.Q., Gustavson, K.H., Holingren, G., *et al.* (1983) 'Fra-X syndrome in mildly retarded children in Northern Swedish county.' *Clinical Genetics*, **24**, 393–398.

Borg, I., Delhany, J.D.A., Baraitser, M. (1995) 'Detection of hemizygosity at the elastin locus by FISH analysis as a diagnostic test in both classical and atypical cases of Williams syndrome.' *Journal of Medical Genetics*, **32**, 692–696.

Borghgraef, M., Fryns, J.P., Dielkens, A. (1987) 'Fragile X syndrome: a study of the psychological profile in 23 prepubertal patients.' *Clinical Genetics*, **32**, 179–186.

Boyd, S.G., Harden, A., Patton, M.A. (1988) 'The EEG in early diagnosis of Angelman (happy puppet) syndrome.' *European Journal of Pediatrics*, **147**, 508–513.

Bregman, J.D., Dykens, E., Watson, M., *et al.* (1987) 'Fragile X syndrome: variability of phenotypic expression.' *Journal of the American Academy of Child and Adolescent Psychiatry*, **26**, 463–471.

Breuning, M.H., Dauwerse, H.G., Fugazza, G., *et al.* (1993) 'Rubinstein–Taybi syndrome caused by submicroscopic deletions within 16p13.3.' *American Journal of Human Genetics*, **52**, 249–254.

Butler, M.G., Meaney, F.J., Palmer, C.G. (1986) 'Clinical and cytogenetic survey of 39 individuals with Prader–Labhart–Willi syndrome.' *American Journal of Medical Genetics*, **23**, 793–809.

Caldwell, M.L., Taylor, R.L. (1988) *Prader–Willi Syndrome. Selected Research and Management Issues.* Berlin: Springer.

Carter, C.O. (1976) 'Genetics of common single malformations.' *British Medical Bulletin*, **32**, 21–26.

Chard, T., Macintosh, M. (1992) 'Antenatal diagnosis of congenital abnormalities.' *In:* Chard, T., Richards, M.P.M. (Eds.) *Obstetrics in the 1990s: Current Controversies. Clinics in Developmental Medicine No. 123/124.* London: Mac Keith Press, pp. 90–104.

Chevrie, J.J., Aicardi, J. (1977) 'Convulsive disorders in the first year of life: etiologic factors.' *Epilepsia*, **18**, 489–498.

Clayton-Smith, J. (1992) 'Angelman's syndrome.' *Archives of Disease in Childhood*, **67**, 889–890.

Cole, T.R.P., Hughes, H.E. (1994) 'Sotos syndrome: a study of the diagnostic criteria and natural history.' *Journal of Medical Genetics*, **31**, 20–32.

Conley, M.E., Beckwih, J.B., Mancer, J.F.K., Tenckhoff, L. (1979) 'The spectrum of the DiGeorge syndrome.' *Journal of Pediatrics*, **94**, 883–890.

Crisco, J.J., Dobbs, J.M., Mulhern, R.K. (1988) 'Cognitive processing of children with Williams syndrome.' *Developmental Medicine and Child Neurology*, **30**, 650–656.

Curry, C.J.R., Carey, J.C., Holland, J.S., *et al.* (1987) 'Smith–Lemli–Opitz syndrome type II: multiple congenital anomalies with male pseudo-hermaphroditism and frequent early lethality.' *American Journal of Medical Genetics*, **26**, 45–57.

Dallaire, L., Mitchell, G., Giguère, R., *et al.* (1995) 'Prenatal diagnosis of Smith–Lemli–Opitz syndrome is possible by meaurement of 7-dehydro-cholesterol in amniotic fluid.' *Prenatal Diagnosis*, **15**, 855–858.

Darras, B.T., Francke, U. (1988) 'Myopathy in complex glycerol kinase deficiency patients is due to 3′ deletions of the dystrophin gene.' *American Journal of Human Genetics*, **4**, 126–130.

Davis, J.G., Silverberg, G., Williams, M.K., *et al.* (1981) 'A new X-linked recessive mental retardation syndrome with progressive spastic quadriparesis.' *American Journal of Human Genetics*, **33**, 75A. *(Abstract 1229.)*

De Grouchy, J., Turleau, C. (1984) *Clinical Atlas of Human Chromosomes, 2nd Edn.* New York: John Libbey.

De Rijk-van Andel, J.F., Cotsman-Berrevoets, C.E., van Hemel, J.O., Hamers, A.J.H. (1991) 'Clinical and chromosome studies of three patients with Smith–Magenis syndrome.' *Developmental Medicine and Child Neurology*, **35**, 343–347.

Devriendt, K., Van Thienen, M-N., Swillen, A., Fryns, J-P. (1996) 'Cerebellar hypoplasia in a patient with velo-cardio-facial syndrome.' *Developmental Medicine and Child Neurology*, **38**, 949–953.

Devys, D., Lutz, Y., Rouyer, N., *et al.* (1993) 'The FMR-1 protein is cytoplasmic, most abundant in neurons and appears normal in carriers of a fragile X premutation.' *Nature Genetics*, **4**, 335–340.

Dobyns, W.B., Stratton, R.F., Greenberg, F. (1984) 'Syndromes with lissencephaly. I: Miller–Dieker and Norman–Roberts syndromes and isolated lissencephaly.' *American Journal of Medical Genetics*, **18**, 509–526.

Dörries, A., Spohr, H.L., Kunze, J. (1988) 'Angelman (happy puppet) syndrome: seven new cases documented by cerebral computed tomography: review of the literature.' *European Journal of Pediatrics*, **148**, 270–273.

Driscoll, D.A., Salvin, J., Sellinger, B., *et al.* (1993) 'Prevalence of 22q11 microdeletions in DiGeorge and velocardiofacial syndromes: implications for genetic counselling and prenatal diagnosis.' *Journal of Medical Genetics*, **30**, 813–817.

Fagan, K., Colley, P., Partington, M. (1994) 'A practical application of fluorescent in situ hybridization in the Wolf–Hirschhorn syndrome.' *Pediatrics*, **93**, 826–827.

Farag, T.I., Teeby, A.S. (1988) 'Bardet–Biedl and Laurence–Moon syndromes in a mixed Arab population.' *Clinical Genetics*, **33**, 78–82.

Finucane, B.M., Konar, D., Haas-Givler, B., *et al.* (1994) 'The spasmodic upper body squeeze: a characteristic behaviour in Smith–Magenis syndrome.' *Developmental Medicine and Child Neurology*, **36**, 78–83.

Fishler, K., Koch, R., Donnell, G.N. (1976) 'Comparison of mental development in individuals with mosaic and trisomy 21 Down's syndrome.' *Pediatrics*, **58**, 744–748.

Flynn, G.A., Hirst, M.C., Knight, S.J.L., *et al.* (1993) 'Identification of the FRAXE fragile site in two families ascertained for X-linked mental retardation.' *Journal of Medical Genetics*, **30**, 97–100.

Frohlich, G.S. (1982) 'Delineation of trisomy 9.' *Journal of Medical Genetics*, **19**, 316–317.

Garver, K.L., Marchese, S.G., Steele, M.W., Ketterer, D.M. (1982) 'Recurrence risk in 21q/21q translocation Down syndrome.' *Journal of Pediatrics*, **100**, 243–245.

Gilgenkrantz, S., Mujica, P., Gruet, P, *et al.* (1988) 'Coffin–Lowry syndrome: a multicenter study.' *Clinical Genetics*, **34**, 230–245.

Glauser, T.A., Rorke, L.B., Weinberg, P.M., Clancy, R.R. (1990) 'Congenital brain anomalies associated with the hypoplastic left heart syndrome.' *Pediatrics*, **85**, 984–990.

Golabi, M., Rusen, L. (1984) 'A new X-linked mental retardation–overgrowth syndrome.' *American Journal of Medical Genetics*, **17**, 345–358.

Golden, J.A., Hyman, B.T. (1994) 'Development of the superior temporal neocortex is anomalous in trisomy 21.' *Journal of Neuropathology and Experimental Neurology*, **53**, 513–520.

—— Schoene, W.C. (1993) 'Central nervous system malformations in trisomy 9.' *Journal of Neuropathology and Experimental Neurology*, **52**, 71–77.

Goodman, R.M., Gorlin, R.J. (1979) *Atlas of the Face in Genetic Disorders, 2nd Edn.* St Louis: C.V. Mosby.

Gottfried, M., Lavine, M., Roessmann, U. (1981) 'Neuropathological findings in Wolf–Hirschhorn (4p–) syndrome.' *Acta Neuropathologica*, **55**, 163–165.

Goutières, F., Aicardi, J., Réthoré, M.O., Lejeune, J. (1987) 'Syndrome de Miller–Dieker familial et translocation chromosomique (15;17).' *Archives Françaises de Pédiatrie*, **44**, 501–504.

Grant, W.W., Hamerton, J. (1976) 'A cytogenetic survey of 14,069 newborn infants. II: Preliminary findings in children with sex chromosome abnormalities.' *Clinical Genetics*, **10**, 285–302.

Green, J.S., Parfrey, P.S., Harnett, J.D., *et al.* (1989) 'The cardinal manifestations of Bordet–Biedl syndrome, a form of Laurence–Moon–Biedl syndrome.' *New England Journal of Medicine*, **321**, 1002–1009.

Greenberg, F., Guzzetta, V., Montes de Oca-Luna, R., *et al.* (1991) 'Molecular analysis of the Smith–Magenis syndrome: a possible contiguous-gene syndrome associated with del (17) (p11.2).' *American Journal of Human Genetics*, **49**, 1207–1218.

Greenswag, L.R. (1987) 'Adults with Prader–Willi syndrome: a survey of 232 cases.' *Developmental Medicine and Child Neurology*, **29**, 145–152.

Guerrini, R., Bureau, M., Mattei, M-G., Battaglia, A., *et al.* (1990a) 'Trisomy 12p syndrome: a chromosomal disorder associated with generalized 3Hz spike and wave discharges.' *Epilepsia*, **31**, 557–566.

—— Genton, P., Bureau, M., *et al.* (1990b) 'Reflex seizures are frequent in patients with Down syndrome and epilepsy.' *Epilepsia*, **31**, 406–417.

—— DeLorey, T.M., Bonanni, P., *et al.* (1996) 'Cortical myoclonus in Angelman syndrome.' *Annals of Neurology*, **40**, 39–48.

Gullotta, F., Rehder, H., Gropp, A. (1981) 'Descriptive neuropathology of chromosomal disorders in man.' *Human Genetics*, **57**, 337–344.

Hagerman, R.J. (1987) 'Fragile X syndrome.' *Current Problems in Pediatrics*, **17**, 621–671.

—— (1995) 'Lessons from fragile X syndrome.' *In:* O'Brien, G., Yule, W. (Eds.) *Behavioural Phenotypes. Clinics in Developmental Medicine No. 138.* London: Mac Keith Press, pp. 59–74.

—— Berry, R., Jackson, A.W., *et al.* (1986) 'Institutional screening for the fragile X syndrome.' *American Journal of Diseases of Children*, **142**, 1216–1221.

Hansen, K.E., Kirkpatrick, S.J., Laxova, R. (1995) 'Dubowitz syndrome: long-term follow-up of an original patient.' *American Journal of Medical Genetics*, **55**, 161–164.

Hanson, D.M., Jackson, A.W., Hagerman, R.J. (1986) 'Speech disturbances (cluttering) in mildly impaired males with the Martin–Bell/fragile X syndrome.' *American Journal of Medical Genetics*, **23**, 195–206.

Hawley, P.D., Jackson, L.G., Kurnit, D.M. (1985) 'Sixty-four patients with Brachman–De Lange syndrome: a survey.' *American Journal of Medical Genetics*, **20**, 453–459.

Hirst, M.C., Barnicoat, A., Flynn, G., *et al.* (1993) 'The identification of a third fragile site, FRAXF, in Xq27–q28, distal to both FRAXA and FRAXE.' *Human Molecular Genetics*, **2**, 197–200.

—— Grewal, P., Flannery, A., *et al.* (1995) 'Two new cases of FMR1 deletion associated with mental impairment.' *American Journal of Human Genetics*, **56**, 67–74.

Ho, H-Z., Glahn, T.J., Ho, J-C. (1989) 'The fragile X syndrome.' *Developmental Medicine and Child Neurology*, **30**, 257–261.

Holder, S.E., Grimsley, L.M., Palmer, R.W., *et al.* (1994) 'Partial trisomy 3q causing mild Cornelia de Lange phenotype.' *Journal of Medical Genetics*, **31**, 150–152.

Holm, V.A., Cassidy, S.B., Butler, M.G., *et al.* (1993) 'Prader–Willi syndrome: consensus diagnostic criteria.' *Pediatrics*, **91**, 398–402.

Holopainen, I., Penttinen, M., Lakkala, T., Äärimaa, T. (1994) 'Ring chromosome 20 mosaicism in a girl with complex partial seizures.' *Developmental Medicine and Child Neurology*, **36**, 70–73.

Holtzman, D.M., Epstein, C.J. (1992) 'The molecular genetics of Down syndrome.' *Molecular Genetics Medicine*, **2**, 105–120.

Huret, J.L., Delabar, J.M., Marlhens, F. (1987) 'Down syndrome with duplication of a region of a chromosome 21 containing the CuZn superoxide dismutase gene without detectable karyotypic abnormality.' *Human Genetics*, **75**, 251–257.

Ilyina, H.G., Lurie, I.W. (1990) 'Dubowitz syndrome: possible evidence for a clinical subtype.' *American Journal of Medical Genetics*, **35**, 561–565.

Jackson, L., Kline, A.D., Barr, M.A., Koch, S. (1993) 'De Lange syndrome: a clinical review of 310 individuals.' *American Journal of Medical Genetics*, **47**, 940–946.

Jensen, P.K. (1981) 'Nerve deafness, optic nerve atrophy and dementia: a new X-linked recessive syndrome.' *American Journal of Medical Genetics*, **9**, 55–60.

Jones, K.L. (1988) *Smith's Recognizable Patterns of Human Malformation, 4th Edn.* Philadelphia: W.B. Saunders.

Juberg, R.C., Marsidi, I. (1980) 'A new form of X-linked mental retardation with growth retardation, deafness and microgenitalism.' *American Journal of Human Genetics*, **32**, 714–722.

Kaplan, P., Kirschner, M., Watters, G., Costa, T. (1989) 'Contractures in patients with Williams syndrome.' *Pediatrics*, **84**, 895–899.

Kemper, M.B., Hagerman, R.J., Ahmad, R.S., Mariner, R. (1986) 'Cognitive profiles and the spectrum of clinical manifestations in heterozygous fra (X) females.' *American Journal of Medical Genetics*, **23**, 139–156.

Knight, S.L.J., Flannery, A.V., Hirst, M.C., *et al.* (1993) "Trinucleotide repeat amplification and hypermethylation of a CpG island in FRAXE mental retardation.' *Cell*, **74**, 127–134.

Knoll, J.H.M., Nicholls, R.D., Magenis, R.E., *et al.* (1989) 'Angelman and Prader–Willi syndromes share a common chromosome 15 deletion but differ in parental origin of the deletion.' *American Journal of Medical Genetics*, **32**, 285–290.

Kobori, J.A., Herrick, M.K., Urich, H. (1987) 'Arhinencephaly. The spectrum of associated malformations.' *Brain*, **110**, 237–260.

Kousseff, B.G., McConnachie, P., Hadro, T.A. (1982) 'Autosomal recessive type of whistling face syndrome in twins.' *Pediatrics*, **69**, 328–331.

Krivit, W., Good, R.A. (1957) 'Simultaneous occurrence of mongolism and leukemia. Report of a nationwide survey.' *American Journal of Diseases of Children*, **94**, 289–293.

Kruse, K., Pankau, R., Gosch, A., Wohlfahrt, K. (1992) 'Calcium metabolism in Williams–Beuren syndrome.' *Journal of Pediatrics*, **121**, 902–907.

Kunze, J. (1980) 'Neurological disorders in patients with chromosomal anomalies.' *Neuropädiatrie*, **11**, 203–249.

Laan, A.E.M., Renier, W.O., Arts, W.F.M., *et al.* (1997) 'Evolution of epilepsy and EEG findings in Angelman syndrome.' *Epilepsia*, **38**, 195–199.

Ledbetter, D.H., Mascarello, J.T., Riccardi, V.M., *et al.* (1982) 'Chromosome 15 abnormalities and the Prader–Willi syndrome: a follow-up report of 40 cases.' *American Journal of Human Genetics*, **34**, 278–285.

—— Ledbetter, S.A., Van Tuinen, P., *et al.* (1989) 'Molecular dissection of a contiguous gene syndrome: frequent submicroscopic deletions: evolutionarily conserved sequences, and a hypomethylated "island" in the Miller–Dieker chromosome region.' *Proceedings of the National Academy of Sciences of the USA*, **86**, 5136–5140.

Lee, S-T., Nicholls, R.D., Bundey, S., *et al.* (1994) 'Mutations of the P gene in oculocutaneous albinism, ocular albinism, and Prader–Willi syndrome plus albinism.' *New England Journal of Medicine*, **330**, 529–534.

Leppert, M., Baird, L., Anderson, K.L., *et al.* (1994) 'Bardet–Biedl syndrome is linked to DNA markers on chromosome 11q and is genetically heterogeneous.' *Nature Genetics*, **7**, 108–112.

Leppig, K.A., Werler, M.M., Cann, C.I., *et al.* (1987) 'Predictive value of minor anomalies. I: Association with major malformations.' *Journal of Pediatrics*, **110**, 530–537.

Levy-Mozziconacci, A., Wernert, F., Scambler, P., *et al.* (1994) 'Clinical and molecular study of DiGeorge sequence.' *European Journal of Pediatrics*, **153**, 813–820.

Lowery, M.C., Morris, C.A., Ewart, A., *et al.* (1995) 'Strong correlation of elastin deletions, detection by FISH, with Williams syndrome: evaluation of 235 patients.' *American Journal of Human Genetics*, **57**, 49–53.

Magenis, R.E., Brown, M.G., Lacy, D.A., *et al.* (1987) 'Is Angelman syndrome an alternative result of del(15) (q11q13)?' *American Journal of Medical Genetics*, **28**, 829–838.

Majewski, F., Goecke, T. (1982) 'Studies of microcephalic primordial dwarfism. I: Approach to a delineation of the Seckel syndrome.' *American Journal of Medical Genetics*, **12**, 7–21.

Malcolm, S., Clayton-Smith, J., Nichols, M., *et al.* (1991) 'Uniparental paternal disomy in Angelman's syndrome.' *Lancet*, **1**, 694–697.

Mansfield, E.S., (1993) 'Diagnosis of Down syndrome and other aneuploidies using quantitative polymerase chain reaction and small tandem repeat polymorphisms.' *Human Molecular Genetics*, **2**, 43–50.

Marden, P.M., Smith, D.W., McDonald, M.J. (1964) 'Congenital anomalies in the newborn infant including minor variations.' *Journal of Pediatrics*, **64**, 358–371.

Marin Padilla, M. (1976) 'Pyramidal cell abnormalities in the motor cortex of a child with Down syndrome. A Golgi study.' *Journal of Comparative Neurology*, **167**, 63–81.

Mascari, M.J., Gottlieb, W., Rogan, P.K., *et al.* (1992) 'The frequency of uniparental disomy in Prader–Willi syndrome. Implications for molecular diagnosis.' *New England Journal of Medicine*, **326**, 1599–1607.

Mattei, J.F. (1987) 'Le retard mental lié à la fragilité du chromxome X.' *Archives Françaises de Pédiatrie*, **44**, 241–243.

—— Mattei, M.G., Giraud, F. (1983) 'Prader–Willi syndrome and chromosome 15. A clinical discussion of 20 cases.' *Human Genetics*, **64**, 356–362.

McKusick, V.A. (1988) *Mendelian Inheritance in Man, 8th Edn.* Baltimore: Johns Hopkins University Press.

McLean, S., Stanley, W., Stern, H., *et al.* (1992) 'Prenatal diagnosis of Pallister–Killian syndrome: resolution of cytogenetic ambiguity by use of fluorescent in situ hybridization.' *Prenatal Diagnosis*, **12**, 985–991.

Meyerson, M.D., Frank, R.A. (1987) 'Language, speech and hearing in Williams syndrome: intervention approaches and research needs.' *Developmental Medicine and Child Neurology*, **29**, 258–262.

Miike, T., Ogata, T., Ohtani, Y., *et al.* (1988) 'Atypical Prader–Willi syndrome with severe developmental delay and emaciation.' *Brain and Development*, **10**, 186–188.

Minns, R.A.M., Sterling, H.F., Wu, F.C.W. (1994) 'Hypothalamic hamartoma with skeletal malformations, gelastic epilepsy and precocious puberty.' *Developmental Medicine and Child Neurology*, **36**, 173–176.

Morris, C.A., Demsey, S.A., Leonard, C.O., *et al.* (1988) 'The natural history of Williams syndrome: physical characteristics.' *Journal of Pediatrics*, **113**, 318–326.

—— Thomas, I.T., Greenberg, F. (1993) 'Williams syndrome: autosomal dominant inheritance.' *American Journal of Medical Genetics*, **47**, 478–481.

MRC Working Party on the Evaluation of Chorion Villus Sampling (1991) 'Medical Research Council European trial of chorion villus sampling.' *Lancet*, **337**, 1481–1499.

Neve, R.L., Finch, E.A., Dawes, L.R. (1988) 'Expression of the Alzheimer amyloid precursor gene transcriptor in the human brain.' *Neuron*, **1**, 669–677.

Nickerson, E., Greenberg, F., Keating, M.T., *et al.* (1995) 'Deletions of the elastin gene at 7q11.23 occur in approximately 90% of patients with Williams syndrome.' *American Journal of Human Genetics*, **56**, 1156–1161.

Norio, R., Raitta, C., Lindahl, E. (1984) 'Further delineation of the Cohen syndrome; report on chorioretinal dystrophy, leukopenia and consanguinity.' *Clinical Genetics*, **25**, 1–14.

Norman, R.M. (1966) 'Neuropathological findings in trisomies 13–15 and 17–18 with special reference to the cerebellum.' *Developmental Medicine and Child Neurology*, **8**, 170–177.

Oostra, B.A., Jacky, P.B., Brown, W.T., Rousseau, F. (1993) 'Guidelines for the diagnosis of fragile X syndrome.' *Journal of Medical Genetics*, **30**, 410–413.

Opitz, J.M. (1985) 'The Brachmann–De Lange syndrome.' *American Journal of Medical Genetics*, **22**, 89–102.

—— Reynolds, J.F., Spano, L.M. (Eds) (1986) *X-linked Mental Retardation 2.* New York: Alan R. Liss.

—— Penchaszadeh, V.B., Holt, M.C., *et al.* (1994) 'Smith–Lemli–Opitz (RSH) syndrome bibliography: 1964–1993.' *American Journal of Medical Genetics*, **50**, 339–343.

Padfield, C.J., Partington, M.W., Simpson, N.E. (1968) 'The Rubinstein–Taybi syndrome.' *Archives of Disease in Childhood*, **43**, 94–101.

Pauli, R.M., Meisner, L.F., Szmanda, R.J. (1983) '"Expanded" Prader–Willi syndrome in a boy with an unusual 15q chromosome deletion.' *American Journal of Diseases of Children*, **137**, 1087–1089.

Pennington, B., Puck, M., Robinson, A. (1980) 'Language and cognitive development in 47 XXX females followed since birth.' *Behaviour Genetics*, **10**, 31–41.

Pfeiffer, R.A., Steffann, J. (1985) 'Familial congenital cataract, non-progressive neurological disorders and mental deficiency: a new X-linked syndrome?' *Ophthalmic Paediatrics and Genetics*, **5**, 201–203.

Pina-Nieto, J.M., Moreno, A.F.C., Silva, L.R., *et al.* (1986) 'Cherubism, gingival fibromatosis, epilepsy and mental deficiency (Ramon syndrome) with juvenile rheumatoid arthritis.' *American Journal of Medical Genetics*, **25**, 433–441.

Pober, B.R., Filiano, J.J. (1995) 'Association of Chiari 1 malformation and Williams syndrome.' *Pediatric Neurology*, **12**, 84–88.

Pollack, M.A., Golden, G.S., Schmidt, R., *et al.* (1978) 'Infantile spasms in Down syndrome: a report of 5 cases and review of the literature.' *Annals of Neurology*, **3**, 406–408.

Punnett, H.H., Zakai, E.H. (1990) 'Old syndromes and new cytogenetics.' *Developmental Medicine and Child Neurology*, **32**, 824–831.

Ratcliffe, S.G., Masera, N., Pan, H., McKie, M. (1994) 'Head circumference and IQ of children with sex chromosome abnormalities.' *Developmental Medicine and Child Neurology*, **36**, 533–544.

Reiss, A.L., Freund, L. (1990) 'Fragile X syndrome.' *Biological Psychiatry*, **7**, 223–240.

—— Aylward, E., Freund, L.S. (1991) 'Neuroanatomy of fragile X syndrome: the posterior fossa.' *Annals of Neurology*, **29**, 26–32.

Rejjal, A., Alaiyan, S., Coates, R., Abuzeid, M. (1994) 'The prevalence and spectrum of brain abnormalities in congenital choanal atresia.' *Neuropediatrics*, **25**, 85–88.

Riccardi, V.M. (1977) 'Trisomy 8: an international study of 70 patients.' *Birth Defects Original Articles Series*, **13** (3C), 171–184.

—— Hittner, H.M., Franceke, U., *et al.* (1979) 'Partial triplication and deletion of 13q: Study of a family presenting with bilateral retinoblastoma.' *Clinical Genetics*, **18**, 332–345.

Roodhooft, A.M., Van Acker, K.J., Van Thienen, M.N., *et al.* (1988) 'Marshall–Smith syndrome: new aspects.' *Neuropediatrics*, **19**, 179–182.

Ross, M.H., Galaburda, A.M., Kemper, T.L. (1984) 'Down's syndrome: is there a decreased population of neurons?' *Neurology*, **34**, 909–916.

Rousseau, F., Heitz, D., Biancalana, V., *et al.* (1991) 'Direct diagnosis by DNA analysis of the fragile X syndrome of mental retardation.' *New England Journal of Medicine*, **325**, 1673–1681.

—— —— Tarleton, J., *et al.* (1994) 'A multicenter study on genotype–phenotype correlations in the fragile X syndrome, using direct diagnosis with probe StB12.3: the first 2,253 cases.' *American Journal of Human Genetics*, **55**, 225–237.

Rubinstein, J.H. (1990) 'Broad thumb–hallux (Rubinstein–Taybi) syndrome 1957–1988.' *American Journal of Medical Genetics*, Suppl. 6, 3–16.

Ruvalcaba, R.H.A., Myhre, S., Smith, D.W. (1980) 'Sotos syndrome with intestinal polyposis and pigmentary changes of the genitalia.' *Clinical Genetics*, **18**, 413–416.

St-Clair, D., Blackwood, D. (1985) 'Premature senility in Down's syndrome.' *Lancet*, **2**, 34. *(Letter.)*

Saitoh, S., Harada, N., Jinno, Y., *et al.* (1994) 'Molecular and clinical study of 61 Angelman syndrome patients.' *American Journal of Medical Genetics*, **52**, 158–163.

Sammito, V., Romano, C., Ventimigilia, G., *et al.* (1988) 'High prevalence of the Rubinsten–Taybi syndrome in a group of mentally retarded, institutionalized subjects.' *Brain Dysfunction*, **1**, 176–186.

Saraux, H., Lafourcade, J., Lejeune, J., *et al.* (1964) 'La trisomie 13 et son expression ophtalmologique.' *Archives d'Ophtalmologie*, **24**, 581–602.

Scarbrough, P.R., Huddleston, K., Finley, S.C. (1986) 'An additional case of Smith–Lemli–Opitz syndrome in a 46,XY infant with female external genitalia.' *Journal of Medical Genetics*, **23**, 174–175.

Schimke, R.W., Horton, W.A., Collins, D.L., Therou, L. (1984) 'A new X-linked syndrome comprising progressive basal ganglion dysfunction, mental and growth retardation, external ophthamoplegia, postnatal microcephaly and deafness.' *American Journal of Medical Genetics*, **17**, 323–332.

Schinzel, A. (1984) *Catalogue of Unbalanced Chromosome Aberrations in Man.* New York: Walter de Gruyter.

—— Schmid, W., Luscher, U., *et al.* (1974) 'The 18p– syndrome.' *Archiv für Genetik*, **47**, 1–15.

—— —— Fraccaro, M., *et al.* (1981) 'The "cat eye syndrome": dicentric small marker chromosome probably derived from a No. 22 (tetrasomy 22pter→ q11) associated with a characteristic phenotype. Report of 11 patients and delineation of the clinical picture.' *Human Genetics*, **57**, 148–158.

Schlegel, R.J., Aspillaga, M.J., Neu, R., Gardner, L.I. (1965) 'Studies on a boy with XXYY chromosome constitution.' *Pediatrics*, **36**, 113–119.

Schwartz, S., Max, S.R., Panny, S.R., Cohen, M.M. (1985) 'Deletions of proximal 15q and non-classical Prader–Willi syndrome phenotypes.' *American Journal of Medical Genetics*, **20**, 255–263.

Selikowitz, M., Sunman, J., Pendergast, A., Wright, S. (1990) 'Fenfluramine in Prader–Willi syndrome: a double blind, placebo controlled trial.' *Archives of Disease in Childhood*, **65**, 112–114.

Silva, M.L., Cieuta, C., Guerrini, R., *et al.* (1996) 'Early clinical and EEG features of infantile spasms in Down syndrome.' *Epilepsia*, **37**, 977–982.

Simko, A., Hornstein, L., Soukup, S., Bagamery, N. (1989) 'Fragile X syndrome: recognition in young children.' *Pediatrics*, **83**, 547–552.

Slaney, S.F., Wilkie, A.O., Hirst, M.C., *et al.* (1995) 'DNA testing for fragile X syndrome in schools for learning difficulties.' *Archives of Disease in Childhood*, **72**, 33–37. (Comment, p. 544.)

Smeets, H.J.M., Smits, A.P.T., Verheij, C.E., *et al.* (1995) 'Normal phenotype in two brothers with a full *FMR1* mutation.' *Human Molecular Genetics*, **4**, 2103–2108.

Smith, A.C.M., McGavran, L., Robinson, J., *et al.* (1986) 'Interstitial deletion of (17) (p11.2p11.2) in nine patients.' *American Journal of Medical Genetics*, **24**, 393–414.

Smith, D.W. (1982) *Recognizable Patterns of Human Malformations.* Philadelphia: W.B. Saunders.

—— Bostian, K.E. (1964) 'Congenital anomalies associated with idiopathic mental retardation.' *Journal of Pediatrics*, **65**, 189–196.

Smith, G.F., Berg, J.M. (1976) *Down's Anomaly, 2nd Edn.* Edinburgh: Churchill Livingstone.

Sotos, J.F., Cutler, E.A., Dodge, P. (1977) 'Cerebral gigantism.' *American Journal of Diseases of Children*, **131**, 625–627.

Stafstrom, C.E., Patxot, O.F., Gilmore, H.E., Wisniewski, K.E. (1991) 'Seizures in children with Down syndrome: etiology, characteristics and outcome.' *Developmental Medicine and Child Neurology*, **33**, 191–200.

Staley, L.W., Hull, C.E., Mazzocco, M.M., *et al.* (1993) 'Molecular–clinical correlations in children and adults with fragile X syndrome.' *American Journal of Diseases of Children*, **147**, 723–726.

Stephenson, J.B.P. (1980) 'Prader–Willi syndrome: neonatal presentation and later development.' *Developmental Medicine and Child Neurology*, **22**, 792–795.

Stevens, C.A., Carey, J.C., Blackburn, B.L. (1990) 'Rubinstein–Taybi syndrome: a natural history study.' *American Journal of Medical Genetics*, Suppl. 6, 30–37.

Sugimoto, T., Yasuhara, A., Ohta, T., *et al.* (1992) 'Angelman syndrome in three siblings: characteristic epileptic seizures and EEG abnormalities.' *Epilepsia*, **33**, 1078–1082.

Sumi, S.M. (1970) 'Brain malformations in trisomy 18 syndrome.' *Brain*, **93**, 821–830.

Sutherland, G.R. (1977) 'Fragile sites on human chromosomes: demonstration of their dependence on the type of tissue culture medium.' *Science*, **197**, 265–266.

Takashima, S., Becker, L.E. (1985) 'Basal ganglia calcification in Down's syndrome.' *Journal of Neurology, Neurosurgery, and Psychiatry*, **48**, 61–64.

Temple, C.M., Carney, R.A. (1993) 'Intellectual functioning of children with Turner syndrome: a comparison of behavioural phenotypes.' *Developmental Medicine and Child Neurology*, **35**, 691–698.

Thake, A., Todd, J., Webb, T., Bundey, S. (1987) 'Children with fragile X chromosome at schools for the mildly mentally retarded.' *Developmental Medicine and Child Neurology*, **29**, 711–719.

Tharapel, A.T., Summit, R.L. (1977) 'A cytogenetic study of 200 unclassifiable mentally retarded children with congenital anomalies and 200 normal human subjects.' *Human Genetics*, **37**, 329–332.

Tint, G.S., Irons, H., Elias, E.R., *et al.* (1994) 'Defective cholesterol biosynthesis associated with the Smith–Lemli–Opitz syndrome.' *New England Journal of Medicine*, **330**, 107–113.

—— Salen, G., Batta, A.K., *et al.* (1995) 'Correlation of severity and outcome with plasma sterol levels in variants of the Smith–Lemli–Opitz syndrome.' *Journal of Pediatrics*, **127**, 82–87.

Trauner, D.A., Bellugi, U., Chase, C. (1989) 'Neurologic features of Williams and Down syndromes.' *Pediatric Neurology*, **5**, 166–168.

Uchida, I.A., Freeman, V.C.P. (1985) 'Trisomy 21 Down syndrome: parental mosaicism.' *Human Genetics*, **70**, 246–248.

Udwin, O., Dennis, J. (1995) 'Psychological and behavioural phenotypes in genetically determined syndromes: a review of research findings.' *In:* O'Brien, G., Yule, W. (Eds.) *Behavioural Phenotypes. Clinics in Developmental Medicine No. 138.* London: Mac Keith Press, pp. 90–208.

Ullrich, K., Koch, H-G., Meschede, D., *et al.* (1996) 'Smith–Lemli–Opitz syndrome: treatment with cholesterol and bile acids.' *Neuropediatrics*, **27**, 111–112. *(Letter.)*

Van Lierde, A., Atza, M.G., Giardino, D., Viani, F. (1990) 'Angelman's syndrome in the first year of life.' *Developmental Medicine and Child Neurology*, **32**, 1011–1016.

Viani, F., Romeo, A., Viri, M., *et al.* (1995) 'Seizures and EEG patterns in Angelman's syndrome.' *Journal of Child Neurology*, **10**, 467–471.

Vieregge, P., Froster-Iskenius, U. (1989) 'Clinico-neurological investigations in the fra(X) form of mental retardation.' *Journal of Neurology*, **236**, 85–92.

Wagstaff, J., Shugart, Y.Y., Lalande, M. (1993) 'Linkage analysis in familial Angelman syndsrome.' *American Journal of Human Genetics*, **53**, 105–112.

Wang, Q., Green, E., Barnicoat, A., *et al.* (1993) 'Cytogenetic versus DNA diagnosis in routine referrals for fragile X syndrome.' *Lancet*, **342**, 1025–1026.

Warkany, J., Passarge, E., Smith, L.B. (1966) 'Congenital malformations in autosomal trisomy syndromes.' *American Journal of Diseases of Children*, **112**, 502–517.

—— Lemire, R.J., Cohen, M.M. (1981) *Mental Retardation and Congenital Malformations of the Central Nervous System.* Chicago: Year Book.

Watanabe, K., Hara, K., Iwase, K. (1976) 'The evolution of neurophysiological features in holoprosencephaly.' *Neuropädiatrie*, **7**, 19–41.

Weaver, D.D., Sherman, S.L. (1987) 'A counseling guide to the Martin–Bell syndrome.' *American Journal of Medical Genetics*, **26**, 39–44. *(Letter.)*

Wertelecki, W., Gerald, P.S. (1971) 'Clinical and chromosomal studies of the 18q– syndrome.' *Journal of Pediatrics*, **78**, 44–52.

Wevrick, R., Kerns, J.A., Francke, U. (1994) 'Identification of a novel paternally expressed gene in the Prader–Willi syndrome region.' *Human Molecular Genetics*, **3**, 1877–1882.

Willems, P.J., Brouwer, O.F., Dijkstra, J., Wilrink, J. (1987) 'X-linked hydrocephalus.' *American Journal of Medical Genetics*, **27**, 921–928.

Willemsen, R., Mohkamsing, S., De Vries, B., *et al.* (1995) 'Rapid antibody test for fragile X syndrome.' *Lancet*, **345**, 1147–1148.

Williams, C.A., Frias, J.L. (1982) 'The Angelman ("happy puppet") syndrome.' *American Journal of Medical Genetics*, **11**, 453–460.

Winter, S.C., Curry, C.J.R., Smith, J.C., *et al.* (1986) 'Prenatal diagnosis of the Beckwith–Wiedemann syndrome.' *American Journal of Medical Genetics*, **24**, 137–141.

Wisniewski, K.E., Kida, E. (1994) 'Abnormal neurogenesis and synaptogenesis in Down syndrome brain.' *Developmental Brain Dysfunction*, **7**, 289–301.

—— Wisniewski, H.M., Wen, G.Y. (1985) 'Occurrence of neuropathological changes and dementia of Alzheimer's disease in Down's syndrome.' *Annals of Neurology*, **17**, 278–282.

—— French, J.H., Brown, W.T., *et al.* (1989) 'The fragile X syndrome and developmental disabilities.' *In:* French, J.H., Harel, P., Casaer, P. (Eds.) *Child Neurology and Developmental Disabilities.* Baltimore: P. Brookes, pp. 11–20.

Yamada, K.A., Volpe, J.J. (1990) 'Angelman's syndrome in infancy.' *Developmental Medicine and Child Neurology*, **32**, 1005–1011.

Yunis, J.J., Ramsay, N.K.C. (1980) 'Familial occurrence of the aniridia–Wilms tumor syndrome with deletion 11p13–14.1.' *Journal of Pediatrics*, **96**, 1027–1030.

Zalewski, W.A., Houston, C.S., Pozsonyi, J. (1966) 'The XXXXY chromosome anomaly: Report of three new cases and review of 30 cases from the literature.' *Canadian Medical Association Journal*, **94**, 1143–1154.

6
OSSEOUS MALFORMATIONS OF THE SKULL AND CERVICAL VERTEBRAE

This chapter reviews the abnormalities of the osseous skull and cervical vertebrae, as well as their consequences on the underlying central nervous system and associated CNS malformations.

CRANIOSYNOSTOSES AND CRANIOSTENOSES

Craniosynostosis is defined as the premature closure of one or more cranial sutures. The term craniostenosis refers to 'narrowing' of the skull as a result of fused sutures. This term is not exact since the cranial volume need not be lessened when fusion occurs early. With the exception of the metopic suture which closes antenatally, normal sutures in newborn infants are several millimeters wide. Fibrous union of suture lines occurs by age 6 months, and by 8 years ossification of the skull is complete. The causes of premature closure are unclear. Experimental immobilization of a suture can lead to its fusion (Nappen and Kokich 1983).

New membranous bone formation takes place along the sutures. Expansion of the bones of the cranial vault is in a direction perpendicular to the sutures. When sutures become obliterated before complete growth of the skull, growth is impeded in the corresponding direction and compensatory growth takes place at the remaining sutures with resulting deformity. The stimulus for growth is intracranial pressure (ICP) on the vault. Thus, obliteration of the sagittal suture will produce transverse narrowing of the vault with anteroposterior elongation of the skull, the so-called scaphocephaly, because of active growth at the coronal and lambdoid sutures; fusion of both halves of the coronal suture will produce a broad and shortened skull (brachycephaly); unilateral premature closure of the coronal suture will give rise to anteroposterior shortening of the affected half of the skull, while the opposite half will grow more or less normally, thus resulting in incurvation (scoliosis) of the base of the skull; closure of the metopic suture will produce a narrow forehead; and that of the lambdoid suture will result in flattening of the posterior part of the skull with growth directed anteriorly and superiorly as the sagittal and coronal sutures remain open (Fig. 6.1).

In the case of premature closure of several sutures (complex craniosynostosis), the ultimate skull deformity will depend on the topography of involved sutures and the timing of their fusion. Thus, more or less simultaneous obliteration of both the coronal and sagittal sutures tends to produce a pointed skull with marked vertical development as a result of the osteogenic activity of the lamboid and parietosquamous sutures (oxycephaly). However, if the coronal suture closes first, there will be brachycephaly with secondary upward expansion of the skull when the sagittal suture closes in turn (turricephaly).

Closure of the sutures is preceded by increased density along the line of the suture visible on plain X-rays. Despite obliteration of the sutures, the fontanelles often remain open—and bulging—with craniosynostosis for as long as normal (Duc and Largo 1986) and the cranial circumference is not necessarily diminished. In fact it is always increased in cases of scaphocephaly because the lengthening of the skull results in a smaller volume for the same circumference. Only in synostosis of all or at least of several sutures is microcephaly observed.

Anomalies of the skull base are frequent in patients with craniosynostosis. They include increased basilar angle in coronal fusion and diminished angle in sagittal fusion. Although a primary involvement of the base has been postulated (Moss 1975), results of surgery on the vault do not support that contention.

The *aetiology* of craniosynostosis is probably multifactorial. Acquired factors, such as intrauterine constraint, probably play a role (Graham *et al.* 1979, 1980; Graham and Smith 1980; Higginbottom *et al.* 1980) as suggested by the increased frequency of twinning in various types of craniosynostosis (Le Merrer *et al.* 1988). Genetic factors seem increasingly important, not only in syndromic forms of craniosynostosis but also in isolated types (Le Merrer *et al.* 1988), as shown in Table 6.1. Lajeunie *et al.* (1995) found 10–14 per cent of nonsyndromic forms to be familial and suggested that a dominant gene with a 60 per cent penetrance could be responsible. Hunter and Rudd (1977) found a positive family history in 12 of 104 families with an affected proband, with a recurrence risk of 2.7 per cent. For cases of sagittal synostosis, the same investigators (Hunter and Rudd 1976) found a positive family history in only five of 214 families and a recurrence risk of less than 2 per cent. Dominant inheritance has been found in cases of sagittal and of lambdoid synostosis (Fryburg *et al.* 1995) but this seems to be a rare occurrence. *Secondary craniosynostosis* can be due to abnormally low ICP as in cases of shunted hydrocephalus (see Chapter 7); to metabolic

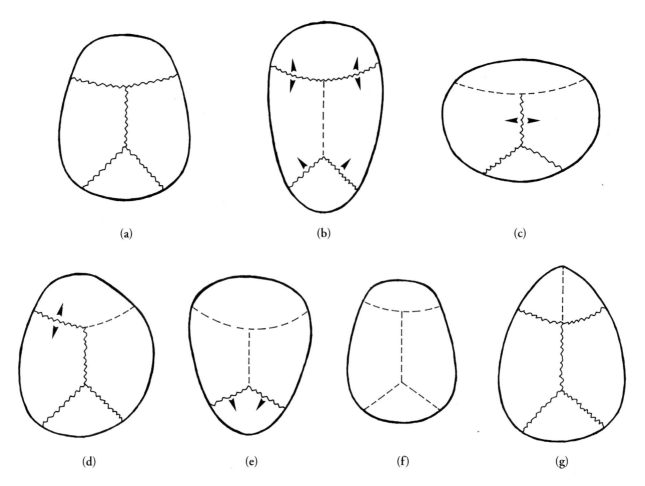

Fig. 6.1. Schematic representation of the main types of craniosynostosis. (*Solid, wavy lines* indicate normal sutures; *broken lines* indicate prematurely closed sutures; *arrows* show main direction of skull growth.) *(a)* Normal sutures and normal skull growth. *(b)* Premature closure of sagittal suture: scaphocephaly (elongated, narrow skull). *(c)* Premature closure of both arms of coronal suture: brachycephaly (short, broad skull). *(d)* Unilateral closure of coronal suture: plagiocephaly (skull flattened unilaterally). *(e)* Premature closure of both sagittal and coronal sutures. Skull shape may vary depending upon timing of closure of individual sutures. If roughly simultaneous, head is high and pointed (oxycephaly). If asynchronous, shape approximates that resulting from premature closure of individual suture that closes first. *(f)* Premature closure of all sutures: microcephalic synostosis (if sutures close simultaneously). *(g)* Premature closure of metopic suture: trigonocephaly (narrow, pointed forehead).

diseases interfering with control of bone growth such as hyperthyroidism (Penfold and Simpson 1975, Hirano *et al.* 1995), hypophosphatasia and vitamin D deficient rickets (Reilly *et al.* 1964), mucopolysaccharidoses and mucolipidosis III (Maroteaux 1982); to abnormal bone marrow proliferation as in haemolytic anaemia, thalassaemia or sickle cell disease; or to teratogenic agents such as aminopterin or hydantoin during pregnancy (Cohen 1979). *Increased ICP* is a frequent consequence of craniosynostosis (Hirsch *et al.* 1982). It may result from reduction of intracranial volume and/or from raised venous pressure (Thompson *et al.* 1995). It may be present even in synostosis of a single suture but is much more frequent with multiple fusion. Thompson *et al.* (1995) found high pressure (>15 mmHg) in 35 per cent, borderline pressure (10–15 mmgHg) in 37 per cent and normal pressure in 27 per cent of 136 cases. High pressure was significantly more common in syndromic (28/53) than in non-syndromic (20/83) cases. Occipital herniation occurs in rare cases. Following operation, ICP tends to decrease but not in all

cases. Moderate hydrocephalus developed in a few of the patients of Thompson *et al.*, perhaps as a result of increased venous pressure, and the rare cases of postoperative herniation remained asymptomatic. The consequences of long-standing high ICP on development remain imperfectly known. There is some correlation between the ultimate IQ level and the degree of intracranial hypertension (Hirsch *et al.* 1982, Thompson *et al.* 1995). It does not follow that mental defect is due to increased ICP, as both may occur in severe cases that feature several affected sutures and associated anomalies.

The incidence of craniosynostosis may be higher than the figure of 1 per 4500 to 1 per 30,000 births estimated by Myrianthopoulos (1977). Baraitser (1990) gives a figure of 1 per 2000, of which 20 per cent are syndromic forms.

ISOLATED CRANIOSYNOSTOSIS
The sagittal, coronal, metopic and lambdoid sutures can be affected (Table 6.1).

TABLE 6.1
TABLE 6.1
Nonsyndromic synostoses

Suture involved (skull shape)	Frequency among craniosynostoses %	Male/Female ratio*	Familial cases* %	Associated anomalies
Sagittal (scaphocephaly)	31.6**	0.823	2.0–9.2	13–31% of cases** (heart anomalies, other malformations, minor vertebral anomalies). Mental retardation unusual and mild
Coronal, unilateral and bilateral (brachycephaly, plagiocephaly)	25.2** (¹/₄ bilateral)	0.383	27* (may coexist within same family)	39–59% of cases** mostly optic atrophy (consequences of premature synostosis)
Coronal and sagittal (oxycephaly)	12*	0.611	26*	5–57% of cases**
Several sutures (complex)	5.5*	0.666	15.3*	28% of cases*
Cloverleaf skull	<1**	0.100	Very frequent	
Syndromic craniosynostoses	10–15**		Most (see text)	By definition present

*Data from Le Merrer *et al.* (1988).
**Combined data from Anderson and Geiger (1965), Shillito and Matson (1968), Hunter and Rudd (1976), Cohen (1979), Le Merrer *et al.* (1988).

SAGITTAL SUTURE

The sagittal suture is most commonly involved. Sagittal craniostenosis accounted for 30–50 per cent of cases in several large series (Anderson and Geiger 1965, Anderson and Gomes 1968, Shillito and Matson 1968, Hunter and Rudd 1976). Boys are much more often affected than girls. The appearance of the head is characteristic, with a long narrow skull (Fig. 6.2) and a normal face. An osseous ridge is palpable at the location of the sagittal suture. The head circumference is usually more than 2 or 3 SD above the mean for age. The deformity is recognizable at birth and is also visible on fetal X-rays (personal observations). The biparietal diameter of the fetal head is reduced in such cases, which should not be mistakenly diagnosed as microcephaly. Associated abnormalities are uncommon and are mainly minor ones. Surgical correction is relatively easy, and even without correction the physical appearance is less unusual than in other synostoses.

CORONAL SUTURE

Involvement of the coronal suture is next in frequency. Girls are more often affected than boys, and unilateral synostosis (plagiocephaly) is more common than bilateral closure (brachycephaly). Cases of both unilateral and bilateral synostosis can occur in the same sibship. In both forms, unusual physical appearance is marked and may be distressing. Unilateral closure normally has no or little effect on CNS function (Fig. 6.3), but bilateral stenosis is often associated with neurological complications. Optic atrophy, more often of primary than of postoedematous type, is frequent and should be systematically looked for. Optic atrophy can be due to intracranial hypertension, to traction on the nerve because of ascent of the chiasm related to increased vertical

diameter of the skull, or to direct compression in the optic canals. The latter, however, is unlikely, as operation on the vault suffices to prevent optic complications. Mental retardation is definitely more common than in sagittal craniosynostosis. It is related to increased ICP in some cases but the relative roles of associated brain abnormalities and intracranial hypertension are difficult to unravel. Results of surgical treatment are gratifying.

METOPIC SUTURE

Metopic craniosynostosis is of relatively little clinical significance. Although the frontal narrowing and associated midfrontal ridge are conspicuous in young children, the deformity appears uncommon in adults and no neurological consequences are known (Hunter *et al.* 1976). Most cases seem to be sporadic, and intrauterine cranial compression is a plausible hypothesis (Graham and Smith 1980). Associated malformations are usually minor and consist mainly of malpositions of fingers and toes. Metopic synostosis can also be part of a malformation syndrome that may include holoprosencephaly (Chapter 3) and its prognosis is then poor.

OTHER TYPES OF CRANIOSYNOSTOSIS

Oxycephalic craniosynostosis (Fig. 6.4) is especially frequent in North African populations and seems to be largely due to genetic factors (Le Merrer *et al.* 1988).

Cloverleaf skull is another type of complex synostosis that produces extreme deformity of the skull and restricts the normal expansion of the brain. It occurs in several different syndromes. The condition is never present at birth and synostosis of both the coronal and the sagittal sutures progresses during the first year of life. As in all cases of multiple craniosynostosis, increased ICP

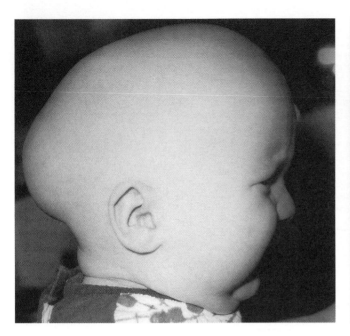
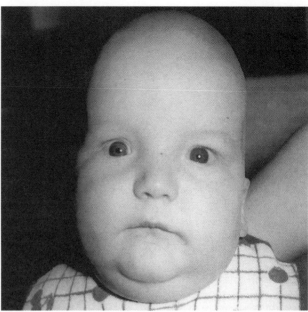

Fig. 6.2. Scaphocephaly due to premature closure of sagittal suture: note long, narrow skull. (Courtesy Dr D. Renier, Prof. J-F. Hirsch, Hôpital des Enfants Malades, Paris.)

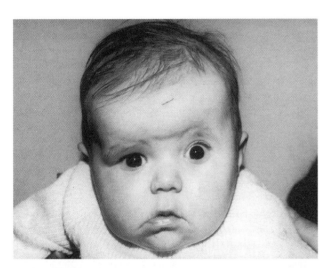
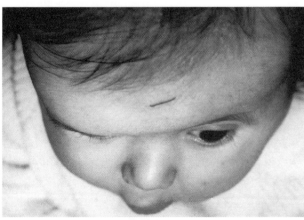

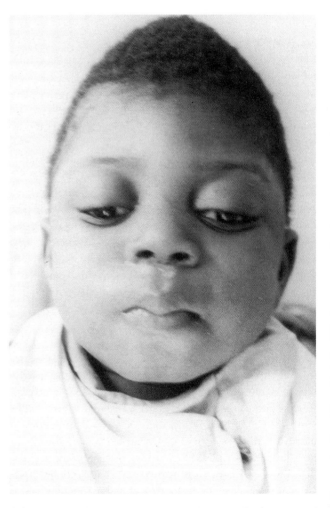

Fig. 6.3. Plagiocephalic craniosynostosis. There is closure of the left branch of the coronal suture, producing disappearance of the supraorbital ridge ipsilaterally and obliquity of the eyebrow. (Courtesy Dr D. Renier, Prof. J-F. Hirsch, Hôpital des Enfants Malades, Paris.)

Fig. 6.4. Oxycephaly resulting from premature closure of both the coronal and sagittal sutures. (Courtesy Dr D. Renier, Prof. J-F. Hirsch, Hôpital des Enfants Malades, Paris.)

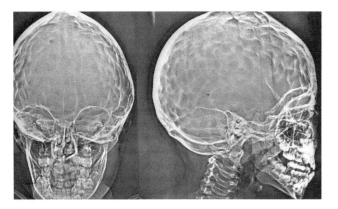

Fig. 6.5. Microcephalic synostosis (X-rays). All sutures are closed. Bones of the cranial vault are thin and digital markings are prominent. Venous sinuses are deeply grooved in bone. (7-year-old boy with intracranial hypertension and papilloedema. Two siblings were simultaneously affected. All had normal intelligence.)

is often a problem and papilloedema or primary optic atrophy often develop insidiously so that early intervention is mandatory.

Microcephalic craniosynostosis is rare and may be familial (personal cases). The shape of the skull is normal but ICP is often high and optic atrophy or papilloedema are frequently found.

Isolated lambdoid synostosis is rare. In the case of unilateral fusion, one form of plagiocephaly is produced.

DIAGNOSIS

The *radiological signs of craniosynostoses* include markedly increased digital markings that are especially prominent in cases with several sutures obliterated (Fig. 6.5). In sagittal synostosis, digital markings usually predominate in the frontal area bilaterally. Venous sinus grooves are deep and abnormally visible. The sella turcica may be greatly enlarged with erosion of the dorsum sellae. Such signs, which are present to some extent even in asymptomatic patients, indicate the presence of long-standing high ICP which can be confirmed by direct measurement. The sutures are not visible and hyperostosis is present along their normal course. At an early stage, however, the suture lines may remain visible in part or in totality. In such cases, the diagnosis is suggested by the narrow and straight appearance of the affected suture lines and the densification of their margins.

The diagnosis of craniosynostosis is usually easy as the skull deformities are fairly characteristic. Similarly misshapen skulls can exist in the absence of craniosynostosis, *e.g.* in secondary plagiocephaly due to positional stress in preterm or immobilized infants. In such cases no ridge is palpable over the involved sutures and the X-rays of the skull do not show digital markings or hyperdense or closed sutures. Plagiocephaly due to synostosis of one side of the coronal or lambdoid suture can be differentiated from that resulting from prolonged posturing by absence of the supraorbital ridge and obliquity of the eyebrow (Kane *et al.* 1996).

The diagnosis of hydrocephalus is sometimes wrongly suggested in patients with sagittal craniosynostosis because of the large head circumference.

Conversely, cases of primary microcephaly are not infrequently referred with a suggestion of craniosynostosis which is easily dismissed because of the usual presence of mental retardation and lack of radiological evidence of craniostenosis.

TREATMENT

The treatment of craniosynostosis has progressed considerably and the cosmetic results are quite satisfactory in cases of sagittal and unilateral coronal synostosis and in many cases of bilateral coronal and complex synostosis. The best results are obtained by early operation before the age of 6 months, but significant correction can be achieved later. Various complex procedures have been described (Anderson 1981, Marchac and Renier 1982, Marsh and Schwartz 1983) and all are major surgical operations. There is agreement that surgical treatment is indicated in the presence of ICP and/or incipient optic atrophy. For some types, such as sagittal synostosis or plagiocephaly, there is little if any risk of neurological complication and intervention aims only at correcting skull appearance. With current techniques, surgical risk is very small, and indications for surgery tend to be extended even to relatively benign cases such as sagittal synostosis as the cosmetic appearance is likely to generate significant embarassment and relational difficulties at school age or later. The aims of the procedure should be clearly explained to parents.

SYNDROMES WITH CRANIOSYNOSTOSIS

Approximately 20 per cent of the craniosynostoses occur in various syndromes, most of which are genetically determined. Comprehensive reviews of the syndromic craniosynostoses are available (Cohen 1979, 1986, 1988). Some of the most common syndromes are listed in Table 6.2. Such syndromes consist of multiple anomalies only one of which is the craniostenosis. Within the same syndrome, the type of craniosynostosis present is not always the same so the diagnosis should not rely mainly on determination of the sutures involved. Crouzon syndrome and Apert syndrome each account for roughly one third of cases of syndromic craniosynostosis. The last third consists of a miscellany of rare syndromes, some of them not yet definitely classified (Carter *et al.* 1982, Le Merrer *et al.* 1988, Lajeunie *et al.* 1995).

CROUZON SYNDROME

Crouzon syndrome follows an autosomal dominant mode of transmission. More than half of the 61 cases studied by Kreiborg (1981) represented new mutations, and the syndrome accounted for 3 per cent of the 370 craniosynostosis patients of Hunter and Rudd (1977). However, mild cases are frequent and the appearance of affected adults may be deceptively normal. Looking at early photographs of the parents may help recognize minimal involvement. The gene for Crouzon syndrome has been mapped to 10q25–q26 (Preston *et al.* 1994) and shown to code for fibroblast growth factor receptor 2 (FGFR2). Several mutations have been demonstrated (Reardon *et al.* 1994, Jabs *et al.* 1994, Oldridge *et al.* 1995).

Hypoplasia of the maxilla with shallow orbit and proptosis are essential components of the syndrome. Craniosynostosis is

TABLE 6.2
Main syndromes with craniosynostosis

Syndrome	Main features	Proportion of cases with craniosynostosis	Genetics (gene location)	Reference
Crouzon	Hypoplasia of maxilla, shallow orbits, proptosis	Almost all (coronal, then all sutures)	AD (10q25–q26, FGFR2)	Kreiborg (1981)
Apert type I acrocephalosyndactyly	Mental retardation, midface deficiency, proptosis, downslanting palpebral fissures, complete symmetrical syndactyly of hands and feet (digits II–IV)	Almost all (coronal first)	AD (10q25–q26, FGFR2) (most cases new mutations)	Cohen (1986)
Pfeiffer (type V acrocephalosyndactyly)	Strabismus, proptosis, hypertelorism, broad thumbs and great toes, mild variable cutaneous anomalies, syndactyly of fingers and toes	All cases (coronal)	AD (8p11–12; 10q25–26, FGFR1*)	Cohen (1988)
Saethre–Chotzen (type III acrocephalosyndactyly)	Facial asymmetry, low-set frontal hairline, ptosis, deviated nasal septum, variable brachydactyly and cutaneous syndactyly (esp. digits II–III). Normal thumbs and great toes. Parietal foramina	All cases (coronal, uni- or bilateral)	AD (7p21)	Friedman et al. (1977)
Carpenter	Preaxial polydactyly of the feet, obesity, short stature, congenital heart defect, soft tissue syndactyly, brachymesophalangy. Mental retardation frequent	All cases (complex)	AR	Robinson et al. (1985)
Baller–Gerold	Radial aplasia, radiohumeral synostosis, hypoplastic carpal bones	Common (coronal, lambdoid or metopic)	AR	Anyane-Yeboa et al. (1980)
Cranio-frontal-nasal dysplasia	Brachycephaly, ocular hypertelorism, clefting of nasal tip, skeletal abnormalities, hand and foot involvement, median cleft in some. Normal intelligence	Common (coronal)	AD or XD (10p11, ?Xpter-p22)	Slover and Sujansky (1979)
Chromosomal abnormalities and other rare or undescribed syndromes	Variable		S (sometimes dominant)	

*Mutation of FGFR1 gene on chromosome 8p11.2–p12 in some families. In others, mutation of exon B of FGFR2. (FGFR = fibroblast growth factor receptor.)

constant, begins in the first year of life, and most frequently affects first the coronal sutures. Eventually, all sutures become involved, but the shape of the skull is variable from cloverleaf skull (Rohatgi 1991) to scaphocephaly. Protuberance of the skull in the region of the closed anterior fontanelle is frequent. A high degree of variability is found among Crouzon patients. Conductive hearing loss is common and should be tested for. No consistent abnormalities of viscera or extremities are present but nasopharyngeal obstruction may lead to chronic respiratory insufficiency and cor pulmonale (Moore 1993). Seizures occurred in 12 per cent of patients in Kreiborg's series, but mental deficiency is rare (3 per cent). Hydrocephalus is also rare (Marchac and Renier 1982), but high ICP is found in 37 per cent of cases and chronic tonsillar herniation has been reported (Cinalli et al. 1995). Surgical treatment gives favourable results if undertaken early.

APERT SYNDROME
Apert syndrome virtually always results from a new dominant mutation. The disorder is allelic to Crouzon disease and due to different mutation of the FGFR2 gene (Wilkie et al. 1995). It is characterized by craniosynostosis, midfacial malformations and symmetrical syndactyly of the hands and feet, involving at least the second, third and fourth digits (Cohen 1986) (Fig. 6.6). The coronal suture is usually affected early, resulting in a brachycephalic high skull, but the synostosis pattern is variable. The anterior cranial fossa is short and the orbits are shallow. Cleft palate is common. Mental deficiency is very frequent and often severe. However, only half the patients in the series of Patton et al. (1988) were mentally retarded. Hydrocephalus is fairly common and abnormalities, especially partial agenesis of the corpus callosum, have been reported (Hogan and Bauman 1971, Aicardi et al. 1987, Cohen and Kreiborg 1990). Fusion of the fifth and sixth cervical vertebrae is present in 70 per cent of cases, and deafness and optic atrophy are frequent. Approximately 10 per cent of patients have visceral abnormalities. The prognosis is poor even with modern reconstructive techniques, and may be even more severe when associated malformations such as heart disease, scoliosis or microphthalmia are present.

OTHER SYNDROMIC CRANIOSYNOSTOSES (Table 6.2)
Saethre-Chotzen syndrome (Friedman et al. 1977) and Pfeiffer syndrome (Pfeiffer 1969, Vanek and Losan 1982) come next in

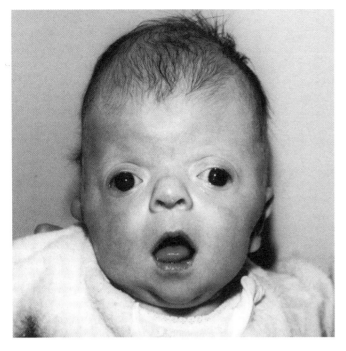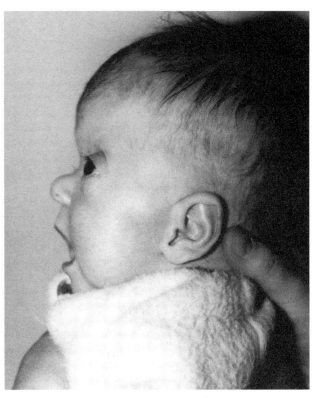

Fig. 6.6. Apert syndrome. There is hypoplasia of the maxillary bone, absence of supraorbital ridge and exophthalmos. (Courtesy Dr D. Renier, Prof. J-F. Hirsch, Hôpital des Enfants Malades, Paris.)

frequency. The mental prognosis is often favourable but there is marked variability both of neurological and of morphological features, at times with severe deformity.

In all studies there is a relatively high proportion of as yet unknown syndromes, even though currently at least 67 syndromes with craniosynostosis have been defined (Cohen 1986). Genetic counselling in such cases is obviously less precise, but seven of 11 undiagnosed syndromic craniosynostoses reported by Le Merrer *et al.* (1988) had a positive family history so that a high recurrence rate remains likely.

OTHER SKULL DYSPLASIAS

A large number of osseous dysplasias involve the skull and especially the base of the skull and can be responsible for neurological disturbances. Some of these conditions are listed in Table 6.3. In such cases, CNS involvement may be due to various mechanisms, the most common being compression of cranial nerves in the basal foramina, and intracranial hypertension as a result of encroachment of thickened bone on intracranial volume or of venous hypertension (Chapter 7). Other mechanisms include associated brain malformations and obscure processes such as intracerebral calcification. Aplasia of the greater wing of the sphenoid is associated with neurofibromatosis type 1 in approximately half the cases. It may be responsible for pulsatile exophthalmos (Chapter 4).

INVOLVEMENT OF CRANIAL NERVES
The IInd and VIIIth cranial nerves are those most frequently affected in patients with skull dysplasias. The facial nerve is also commonly involved. Cranial nerves V and IX to XII and the oculomotor nerves are less frequently interfered with.

Compression of the optic nerves generally results in primary optic atrophy that may develop very rapidly and can lead to complete blindness, as is often the case in *osteopetrosis* (Klintworth 1963, Lehman *et al.* 1977). Secondary optic atrophy following episodes of high ICP with papilloedema may also occur, perhaps as a result of venous obstruction. Episodes of high ICP with vomiting, fundal venous congestion and oedema sometimes respond dramatically to corticosteroid treatment, as I have observed in a patient with craniometaphyseal dysplasia.

Hearing loss is usually due to compression of the VIIIth nerve in its bony canal. However, involvement of the cochlea by thickening and densification of the petrous bone may also be a factor. Deafness is often progressive as are *palsies of other lower cranial nerves.*

Hyperostosis cranialis interna is a recently described hereditary syndrome with multiple cranial nerve involvement (Manni *et al.* 1990).

OTHER MECHANISMS
Other mechanisms of neural involvement are at play in some cases, even though compression by bony overgrowth is the most common. This applies especially to two diseases: osteopetrosis and deficit in carbonic anhydrase II.

In the severe form of *osteopetrosis* (Lehman *et al.* 1977), a progressive neurological disorder and choroidoretinal degeneration (Ruben *et al.* 1990) can evolve in addition to cranial nerve palsies. Gerritsen *et al.* (1994) reviewed 33 cases, half of which had optic nerve involvement. Three had associated retinal degeneration

TABLE 6.3
Some cranial osseous dysplasias with possible neurological consequences

Disease	Main features	References
Achondroplasia	Proximal dwarfism (short and thick long bones), normal intelligence, short base of skull with sunken nose root, short hands and feet	Hecht and Butler (1990)
Thanatophoric dwarfism	Resembles achondroplasia but early death by respiratory insufficiency	Langer *et al.* (1969)
Osteogenesis imperfecta	Bone fragility with multiple fractures, abnormal skull, blue sclerae (some types)	Tsipouras *et al.* (1986), Charnas and Marini (1993)
Craniometaphyseal dysplasia and Pyle's disease	Tall stature, hypertelorism, splayed metaphyses, sclerotic and thickened skull base	Carlson and Harris (1972), Heselson *et al.* (1979)
Osteopetrosis (mostly severe form)	Anaemia, enlarged liver and spleen, marble bones	Lehman *et al.* (1977), Gerritsen *et al.* (1994)
Carbonic anhydrase II deficiency	Marble bones, intracranial calcification	Sly *et al.* (1985)
Cranio-diaphyseal dysplasia and Camurati–Engelmann disease	Thickened long bones, thickened skull base, strabismus, exophthalmia	Yen *et al.* (1978), Maroteaux (1982)
Fibrous dysplasia	Intraosseous proliferation of fibrous tissue. May be monostotic or polyostotic. May include cutaneous naevi and endocrine signs (McCune–Albright syndrome), exophthalmos, nasal obstruction, deafness	Derome *et al.* (1983)
Generalized cortical hyperostosis (Van Buchem disease)	Sclerosis of diaphyses, skull, clavicles, ribs	Van Buchem (1971)
Cleidocranial dysostosis	Absent or rudimentary clavicles, large skull with many wormian bones	Siggers (1975)
Oro-facial-digital syndromes	Abnormalities of oral cavity (tongue hamartomas, abnormal frenula), disoriented fingers, enlarged skull	Toriello (1988), Leão and Ribeiro-Silva (1995)
Maroteaux–Lamy syndrome	Dwarfism, bone anomalies, normal intelligence	Young *et al.* (1980), Maroteaux (1982)

and two a progressive neurodegenerative disease. Five patients had histological evidence of ceroid–lipofuscinosis storage in neurons and may represent a separate subgroup of the disease (Ambler *et al.* 1983). Hydrocephalus is present in some cases but cannot explain the progressive deterioration which is seen in some patients with Albers–Schonberg disease and includes mental regression and pyramidal tract signs.

In *carbonic anhydrase II deficiency* extensive intracranial calcification is easily demonstrable by CT scan and even by plain X-rays in the central grey nuclei and throughout the white matter. Patients have, in addition, renal tubular acidosis. Some degree of mental retardation is commonly present. Isoenzyme II of carbonic anhydrase is lacking (Sly *et al.* 1985), but the exact mechanism of the disease remains to be elucidated.

In *thanatophoric dwarfism*, a lethal condition resembling severe achondroplasia, a specific malformation affecting especially the temporal lobes is regularly found at autopsy (Goutières *et al.* 1971).

Osteogenesis imperfecta, especially in its severe forms, may be associated with skull deformities, especially basilar invagination (see below) that may, in turn, be responsible for neurological disturbances (Tsipouras *et al.* 1986, Charnas and Marini 1993).

Macrocephaly is frequent and may be progressive since it is due to hydrocephalus and may require treatment.

Neurological involvement can be due to mechanical deformity of the skull produced by the development of a space-occupying lesion, as occurs in fibrous dysplasia of bone. The eyes are prominent and palsies may develop (Derome *et al.* 1983). In one type of *fibrous dysplasia*, pigmented areas are present on the skin, often in a unilateral distribution, and precocious puberty (of undetermined origin) is a part of the clinical picture (McCune–Albright syndrome).

The diagnosis of the skull dysplasias complicated by nerve involvement rests mainly on clinical and X-ray investigation of the skeleton. The reader is referred to Table 6.3 and to specialized books (*e.g.* Maroteaux 1982) for detailed information.

ABNORMALITIES OF THE CERVICO-OCCIPITAL JUNCTION AND VERTEBRAL COLUMN

Abnormalies of the cervico-occipital junction and cervical column account for some serious neurological problems in infants and children. The *Chiari malformations* and associated abnormalities

TABLE 6.4
Abnormalities of the cervico-occipital junction and cervical column which may be associated with neurological dysfunction

Bony abnormalities	Neural abnormalities	References
Basilar impression variably includes convexobasia, platybasia; partial and unilateral basilar impression; associated occipital vertebrae; occipitalization of atlas, hypoplasia of basiocciput; dehiscent posterior arch of atlas; dysplasia of occipital condyles	Chiari I malformation; dural bands and abnormal vessels at foramen magnum; kinking and compression by foramen magnum or odontoid process; syringomyelia; hydromyelia; hydrocephalus	Bull *et al.* (1955), Wackenheim (1967), Gardner *et al.* (1975), Stovner *et al.* (1992)
Narrowing of foramen magnum (without basilar impression) —achondroplasia —other osseous dysplasias	Compression of medulla or upper spinal cord; vascular compression (anterior spinal artery); hydrocephalus	Hecht *et al.* (1985)
Abnormalities of odontoid process (may be congenital or acquired) esp. trisomy 21 —hypoplasia or aplasia —atlanto-axial dislocation —absence of transverse ligament	Compression of upper spinal cord*	Stevens *et al.* (1994)
Cervical vertebral blocks —Klippel–Feil anomaly (Sprengel deformity may be associated)	Aberrant route of pyramidal tract? Mirror movements	Gunderson and Solitare (1968), Morrison *et al.* (1968), Schott and Wyke (1981)
—Goldenhar syndrome		Schrander-Stumpel *et al.* (1992)
—Others (*e.g.* Wildervanck syndrome with deafness)		Cohen *et al.* (1989), Keeney *et al.* (1992)

*Compression of upper spinal cord can occur with some metabolic diseases, *e.g.* Maroteaux–Lamy syndrome (Young *et al.* 1980) and chondrodystrophia punctata (Pascual-Castroviejo *et al.* 1994).

such as hydrosyringomyelia have already been considered (Chapter 3). They are often associated with abnormalities of the cervical column (Morgan and Williams 1992). Stevens *et al.* (1994) found that nine of 22 patients with a hypoplastic dens had a Chiari I malformation and six showed marked basilar invagination. This section is concerned with the neural complications of osseous and osteoarticular abnormalities, most of which are congenital and sometimes familial (Saltzman *et al.* 1991), but which may also be the consequence of trauma or inflammatory process (Greenberg 1968). Table 6.4 lists the main conditions in this group.

PATHOLOGICAL FEATURES
BASILAR IMPRESSION
Basilar impression is a deformity of the osseous structures at the base of the skull that produces an upward displacement of the edge of the foramen magnum. Most cases are congenital and may be familial (Bull *et al.* 1955, Coria *et al.* 1983a), but acquired cases occur, for instance in osteogenesis imperfecta. In extreme cases (convexobasia), the foramen may be likened to the crater of a volcano the slopes of which are constituted by the occipital and sphenoidal bones. The degree of impression is variable. In *platybasia*, the base of the skull is flat. Partial forms exist, and various abnormalities of the atlas and condylar processes are often associated (Bull *et al.* 1955, Wackenheim 1967). Ascension of the odontoid process, which may compress the anterior aspect

of the brainstem, and diverse abnormalities of the dens itself are often present. Underlying neural anomalies such as hydrosyringomyelia, fibrous bands compressing the lower brainstem, abnormal vessels and kinking of the medulla are almost always associated but their relationship to the bony deformities is unclear. There is evidence that decompression of the posterior fossa can improve considerably the anatomy of the spinal cord (Menezes *et al.* 1980).

NARROW FORAMEN MAGNUM
A narrow foramen magnum occurs with some of the skull dysplasias previously considered. It is a common accompaniment of *achondroplasia* in which the transverse diameter of the foramen is severely diminished in over three-quarters of cases (Reid *et al.* 1987, Nelson *et al.* 1988) as compared with normal values (Hecht *et al.* 1985). In achondroplastic children there may be an indentation of the posterior aspect of the spinal cord by the horizontalized occipital squama, although an hourglass appearance of the cervical cord due to atrophy is more common. The odontoid process may also be abnormal (Coria *et al.* 1983a).

ABNORMAL ODONTOID PROCESS
This can also exist in isolation. Hypoplasia occurs in 6 per cent of patients with Down syndrome (Braakhekke *et al.* 1985, Davidson 1988). The odontoid may not be fused with the body of the

axis (ossiculum terminale or os odontoideum). This anomaly was present in 24 of 62 patients with abnormalities of the odontoid process studied by Stevens *et al.* (1994), nine of whom were below 15 years of age. Chronic disunited fractures are more common in adults although they have been occasionally reported in infants (Hukuda *et al.* 1980), and hypoplasia of the dens is often part of a complex anomaly of the posterior fossa.

The more important abnormality in such cases is *atlantoaxial dislocation*, which may also occur as an isolated defect and may be spontaneous, traumatic or inflammatory (Greenberg 1968, Hukuda *et al.* 1980, Herring 1982) and is considerably facilitated by the ligamentous hyperlaxity that is present in persons with Down syndrome, especially girls (Davidson 1988).

Cervical vertebral blocks occur with several syndromes, the commonest being Klippel–Feil syndrome. Mirror movements can be present, although their mechanism is unclear (Gunderson and Solitaire 1968, Schott and Wyke 1981). Various associated defects, in particular deafness, spina bifida and hemivertebrae, can be present (Morrison *et al.* 1968).

CLINICAL FEATURES
Several clinical syndromes can obtain in patients with cervico-occipital abnormalities. Each clinical syndrome is not necessarily related to a specific type of osteoarticular anomaly even though definite preferential associations exist. For instance, basilar impression tends to be associated with a chronic, late-onset neurological picture, whereas atlantoaxial dislocation is mainly associated with acute complications.

CHRONIC, LATE-ONSET NEUROLOGICAL SYNDROME ASSOCIATED WITH BASILAR IMPRESSION
Children with basilar impression have usually no neurological symptoms or signs until adolescence even though the deformity is present from birth. However, many of these children have a low hairline, a head tilt or torticollis and limitation of head motion. Neurological symptoms may include vertiginous sensations, unsteady walking and occipital pain. Swallowing difficulties are usually a late symptom. Typical features include ataxia of lower limbs, bilateral pyramidal tract signs, loss of proprioception in the upper limbs, nystagmus and involvement of cranial nerves V to XII. Hydrocephalus can occur in association with Chiari I malformation. Syringomyelia is common but may be manifested early only by scoliosis despite impressive cavitation demonstrated by MRI (Chapter 3). Radiological landmarks of the region, especially for the odontoid process, have been reported (Bull *et al.* 1955; Stovner *et al.* 1992, 1993) and may be useful for diagnosis. Brainstem auditory evoked potentials are frequently abnormal. Sood *et al.* (1992) found them to be significantly more often abnormal in 22 patients with basilar impression than in seven with atlanto-axial dislocation. Barnet *et al.* (1993) found an abnormal N20 component of somatosensory evoked potentials from stimulation of the median nerve in 11 of 16 children with a Chiari malformation, often in association with clinical symptoms of brainstem involvement. CT scan with metrizamide and MRI now permit accurate assessment of both osseous and neural

abnormalities, thus allowing optimal planning of treatment. Surgical decompression of the posterior fossa is indicated when neurological symptoms and signs have occurred. The results are usually satisfactory.

NEUROLOGICAL FEATURES OF STENOSIS OF THE FORAMEN MAGNUM IN ACHONDROPLASIA (Fig. 6.7)
Achondroplasia can induce a neurological disorder through several mechanisms, the most usual being compression of the upper cervical cord and medulla by narrowing of the foramen magnum. The cord may also be compressed by stenosis of the cervical spinal canal and anteriorly by an abnormal odontoid process (Yamada *et al.* 1981). *Compression myelopathy* may produce overt quadriplegia or paraplegia (Morgan and Young 1980). Insidious neurological signs are more common than overt quadriplegia: ankle clonus, extensor plantar responses and hyper-reflexia are indications of spinal involvement, whereas hypotonia although frequent and marked is an unreliable sign as it is commonly observed in achondroplastic patients with ligament laxity (Reid *et al.* 1987). Syringomyelia has been only rarely encountered (Hecht and Butler 1990).

Respiratory insufficiency can give rise to chronic hypoxaemia, sometimes with bradycardia, to obstructive or central apnoea (Reid *et al.* 1987, Nelson *et al.* 1988, Pauli *et al.* 1995) or even to sudden death (Bland and Emery 1982). Apnoea may be the sole manifestation of myelopathy in some patients (Fremion *et al.* 1984). Complete assessment of achondroplastic children with apnoea or other respiratory difficulties should include blood gas measurements, electrocardiography, and, in selected cases, ultra-sonography and axial CT scan or MRI (sagittal and axial). A narrow foramen magnum or spinal canal and, especially, absence of both anterior and posterior perispinal subarachnoid spaces and an abnormal T_2 signal on MRI of the upper spinal cord seem to be the best indicators of imminent danger and should lead to consideration of the need for surgical treatment by decompression of the posterior fossa and cervical cord (Rimoin 1995). Surgery can prevent immediate and late complications including syringomyelia (Hecht *et al.* 1984).

Other neurological complications of achondroplasia include *macrocephaly* that is probably related mostly to increased venous pressure due to stenosis of the basal foramina, with resulting mild to moderate hydrocephalus (Chapter 7). Other mechanisms have been discussed (Hecht and Butler 1990).

Developmental delay, especially of muscle tone, is relatively frequent. Intellectual development may also be affected with 10–16 per cent of patients having an IQ < 80 (Hecht and Butler 1990). This may be related to respiratory insufficiency.

Vertebral canal stenosis in the lumbar region is a classical complication of achondroplasia and can produce root or spinal cord compression. Any deterioration in bladder or bowel function should lead to suspicion of spinal compression. Motor and sensory signs may also be found (Nelson *et al.* 1988). Lumbosacral lordosis may be at the origin of minor trauma to the cord and be associated with claudication of the cauda equina or conus medullaris (Hecht and Butler 1990).

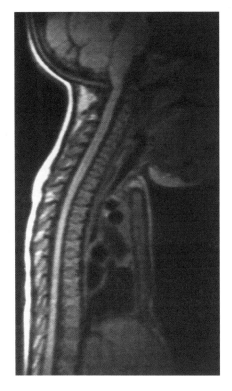
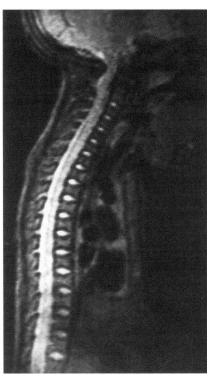

Fig. 6.7. Stenosis of the foramen magnum in 15-month-old boy with achondroplasia. Sagittal MRI cuts in *(left)* T₁-weighted and *(right)* T₂-weighted sequences show notch on posterior aspect of bulbospinal junction produced by edge of occipital squama. Such compression can be at the origin of quadriplegia. (Courtesy Dr D. Renier, Prof. J-F. Hirsch, Hôpital des Enfants Malades, Paris.)

Nerve root compression can affect the lower or upper limbs. *Occipital neuralgia* is not uncommon and can be treated by occipital neurectomy provided significant craniocervical junction compression has been excluded. The diagnosis of achondroplasia can now be easily confirmed by demonstration of mutation in the *FGFR3* gene (Stoilov *et al.* 1995), making the differential diagnosis with related conditions easy (Hall 1995).

ATLANTOAXIAL DISLOCATION

Atlantoaxial dislocation results from either incompetence of the transverse ligament or from abnormalities of the dens itself (Stevens *et al.* 1994). It can occur following cervical trauma, infection and inflammation of the pharynx, or rheumatoid arthritis. It is favoured by congenital abnormalities such as Morquio disease and by Down syndrome, owing to marked ligament laxity (Pueschel *et al.* 1987, 1988). Dislocation can produce quadriplegia with incontinence or paraplegia that may have a sudden onset but is often preceded by such manifestations as head tilt, abnormal staggering gait and the emergence of neurological signs. Hemiplegia is occasionally seen (Coria *et al.* 1983b). Diagnosis is confirmed by X-rays that show a distance of more than 5 mm between the anterior aspect of the odontoid and the atlas and by MRI or CT scans which also show the rotation and lateral displacement of the dens (Chaudry *et al.* 1987).

In *Down syndrome* the problem is to distinguish between simple asymptomatic atlantoaxial instability, which occurs in 19–31 per cent of patients (Pueschel *et al.* 1987, 1988), and dangerous subluxation and dislocation (Chaudry *et al.* 1987) that is found in 1–2 per cent of cases. Atlantoaxial dislocation is defined radiologically by an atlanto–dens interval ≥5 mm. CT scans may show additional abnormalities such as rotatory sub-luxation of C1–C2, an os odontoideum, atlanto-occipital fusion, or narrowing (<16 mm) of the cervical canal. Patients with atlantoaxial dislocation who are at risk of developing symptoms usually have a wide atlanto-dens interval (>7 mm) and may have mild pyramidal tract signs and gait disturbance. Their sensory evoked potentials from the wrist, especially the latency of N19 potential minus Erb latency, may be increased. Such children should not be allowed to practice somersaulting, trampolining or similar activities. For symptomatic cases, vertebral fusion is the preferred surgical method, whereas posterior decompression that produces further vertebral instability is contraindicated.

REFERENCES

Aicardi, J., Chevrie, J.J., Baraton, J. (1987) 'Agenesis of the corpus callosum.' *In:* Vinken, P.J., Bruyn, G.W. (Eds.) *Handbook of Clinical Neurology. Revised Series. Vol. 6. Brain Malformations.* Amsterdam: North Holland, pp. 149–173.

Ambler, M.W., Trice, J., Grauerholz, J., O'Shea, P.A. (1983) 'Infantile osteopetrosis and neuronal storage disease.' *Neurology*, **33**, 437–441.

Anderson, F.M. (1981) 'Treatment of coronal and metopic synostosis: 107 cases.' *Neurosurgery*, **8**, 143–149.

—— Geiger, L. (1965) 'Craniosynostosis: a survey of 204 cases.' *Journal of Neurosurgery*, **22**, 229–240.

Andersson, H., Gomes, S.P. (1968) 'Craniosynostosis. Review of the literature and indications for surgery.' *Acta Paediatrica Scandinavica*, **57**, 47–54.

Anyane-Yeboa, K., Gunning, L., Bloom, A.D. (1980) 'Baller–Gerold syndrome. Craniosynostosis–radial aplasia syndrome.' *Clinical Genetics*, **17**, 161–166.

Baraitser, M. (1990) *The Genetics of Neurological Disorders, 2nd Edn. Oxford Monographs on Medical Genetics, No. 18.* Oxford: Oxford University Press.

Barnet, A.B., Weiss, I.P., Shaer, C. (1993) 'Evoked potentials in infant brainstem syndrome associated with Arnold–Chiari malformation.' *Developmental Medicine and Child Neurology*, **35**, 42–48.

Bland, J.P., Emery, J.L. (1982) 'Unexpected death of children with achondroplasia after the perinatal period.' *Developmental Medicine and Child Neurology*, **24**, 489–492.

Braakhekke, J.P., Gabreëls, F.J.M., Renier, W.O., *et al.* (1985) 'Craniovertebral pathology in Down syndrome.' *Clinical Neurology and Neurosurgery*, **87**, 173–179.

Bull, J.S., Nixon, W.L., Pratt, R.T. (1955) 'Radiological criteria and familial occurrence of primary basilar impression.' *Brain*, **78**, 229–247.

Carlson, D.H., Harris, G.B.C. (1972) 'Craniometaphyseal dysplasia. A family with three documented cases.' *Radiology*, **103**, 147–151.

Carter, C.O., Till, K., Fraser, V., Coffey, R. (1982) 'A family study of cranio-synostosis, with probable recognition of a distinct syndrome.' *Journal of Medical Genetics*, **19**, 280–285.

Charnas, L.R., Marini, J.C. (1993) 'Communicating hydrocephalus, basilar invagination, and other neurologic features in osteogenesis imperfecta.' *Neurology*, **43**, 2603–2608.

Chaudry, V., Sturgeon, C., Gates, A.J., Myers, G. (1987) 'Symptomatic atlanto-axial dislocation in Down's syndrome.' *Annals of Neurology*, **21**, 606–609.

Cinalli, G., Renier, D., Sebag, G., *et al.* (1995) 'Chronic tonsillar herniation in Crouzon's and Apert's syndromes: the role of premature synostosis of the lambdoid suture.' *Journal of Neurosurgery*, **83**, 575–582.

Cohen, M.J., Kreiborg, S. (1990) 'The central nervous system in the Apert syndrome.' *American Journal of Medical Genetics*, **35**, 36–45.

Cohen, M.M. (1979) 'Craniostosis and syndromes with craniosynostosis. Incidence, genetics, penetrance, variability, and new syndrome updating.' *Birth Defects Original Article Series*, **15** (5B), 13–63.

—— (1986) 'Syndromes with craniosynostosis.' *In:* Cohen, M.M. (Ed.) *Craniosynostosis: Diagnosis, Evaluation and Management.* New York: Raven Press, pp. 413–590.

—— (1988) 'Craniosynostosis update, 1987.' *American Journal of Medical Genetics*, Suppl. 4, 99–148.

—— Rollnick, B.R., Kaye, C.I. (1989) 'Oculoauriculovertebral spectrum: an updated critique.' *Cleft Palate Journal*, **26**, 276–286.

Coria, F., Quintana, F., Rebollo, M., *et al.* (1983a) 'Occipital dysplasia and Chiari type I deformity in a family. Clinical and radiological study of three generations.' *Journal of the Neurological Sciences*, **62**, 147–158.

—— —— Villalba, M., *et al.* (1983b) 'Craniocervical abnormalities in Down's syndrome.' *Developmental Medicine and Child Neurology*, **25**, 252–255.

Davidson, R.G. (1988) 'Atlantoaxial instability in individuals with Down syndrome: a fresh look at the evidence.' *Pediatrics*, **81**, 857–865.

Derome, P.J., Visot, A., Akerman, M., *et al.* (1983) 'La dysplasie fibreuse cranienne.' *Neurochirurgie*, **29**, Suppl. 1, 1–117.

Duc, G., Largo, R.H. (1986) 'Anterior fontanel: size and closure in term and preterm infants.' *Pediatrics*, **78**, 904–908.

Fremion, A.S., Garg, B.P., Kalsbeck, J. (1984) 'Apnea as the sole manifestation of cord compression in achondroplasia.' *Journal of Pediatrics*, **104**, 398–401.

Friedman, J.M., Hanson, J.W., Graham, C.B., Smith, D.W. (1977) 'Saethre–Chotzen syndrome: a broad and variable pattern of skeletal malformations.' *Journal of Pediatrics*, **91**, 929–933.

Fryburg, J.S., Hwang, V., Lin, K.Y. (1995) 'Recurrent lambdoid synostosis within two families.' *American Journal of Medical Genetics*, **58**, 262–266.

Gardner, E., O'Rahilly, R., Prolo, D. (1975) 'The Dandy–Walker and Arnold–Chiari malformations.' *Archives of Neurology*, **32**, 393–396.

Gerritsen, E.J.A., Vossen, J.M., van Loo, I.H.G., *et al.* (1994) 'Autosomal recessive osteopetrosis: variability of findings at diagnosis and during the natural course.' *Pediatrics*, **93**, 247–253.

Goutières, F., Aicardi, J., Farkas-Bargeton, (1971) 'Une malformation cérébrale particulière associée au nanisme thanatophore.' *Revue Neurologique*, **125**, 435–440.

Graham, J.M., Smith, D.W. (1980) 'Metopic craniostenosis as a consequence of fetal head constraint: two interesting experiments of nature.' *Pediatrics*, **65**, 1000–1002.

—— De Saxe, M., Smith, D.W. (1979) 'Sagittal craniostenosis: fetal head constraint as one possible cause.' *Journal of Pediatrics*, **95**, 747–750.

—— Badura, R.J., Smith, D.W. (1980) 'Coronal craniostenosis: fetal head constraint as one possible cause.' *Pediatrics*, **65**, 995–999.

Greenberg, A.D. (1968) 'Atlanto-axial dislocations.' *Brain*, **91**, 655–684.

Gunderson, C.H., Solitare, G.B. (1968) 'Mirror movements in patients with Klippel–Feil syndrome.' *Archives of Neurology*, **18**, 675–678.

Hall, J.G. (1995) 'Information update on achondroplasia.' *Pediatrics*, **95**, 620. *(Letter.)*

Hecht, J.T., Butler, I.J. (1990) 'Neurologic morbidity associated with achondro-plasia.' *Journal of Child Neurology*, **5**, 84–97.

—— —— Scott, C.I. (1984) 'Long-term neurologic sequelae in achondroplasia.' *European Journal of Pediatrics*, **143**, 58–60.

—— Nelson, F.W., Butler, I.J., *et al.* (1985) 'Computerized tomography of the foramen magnum: achondroplastic values compared to normal standards.' *American Journal of Medical Genetics*, **20**, 355–360.

Herring, J.A. (1982) 'Cervical instability in Down's syndrome and juvenile rheumatoid arthritis.' *Journal of Pediatric Orthopedics*, **2**, 205–207.

Heselson, N.G., Raad, M.S., Hamersma, H., *et al.* (1979) 'The radiological manifestations of metaphyseal dysplasia (Pyle disease).' *British Journal of Radiology*, **52**, 431–440.

Higginbottom, M.C., Jones, K.L., James, H.E. (1980) 'Intrauterine constraint and craniosynostosis.' *Neurosurgery*, **6**, 39–44.

Hirano, A., Akita, S., Fujii, T. (1995) 'Craniofacial deformities associated with juvenile hyperthyroidism.' *Cleft Palate–Craniofacial Journal*, **32**, 328–333.

Hirsch, J.F., Renier, D., Sainte-Rose, C. (1982) 'Intracranial pressure in craniostenosis.' *Monographs in Paediatrics*, **15**, 114–118.

Hogan, G.R., Bauman, M.L. (1971) 'Hydrocephalus in Apert syndrome.' *Journal of Pediatrics*, **79**, 782–787.

Hukuda, S., Ota, H., Okabe, N., Tazima, K. (1980) 'Traumatic atlantoaxial dislocation causing os odontoideum in infants.' *Spine*, **5**, 207–210.

Hunter, A.G.W., Rudd, N.L. (1976) 'Craniosynostosis. I. Sagittal synostosis: its genetics and associated clinical findings in 214 patients who lacked involvement of the coronal suture(s).' *Teratology*, **14**, 185–193.

—— —— (1977) 'Craniosynostosis. II.Coronal synostosis: its familial characteristics and associated clinical findings in 109 patients lacking bilateral polysyndactyly or syndactyly.' *Teratology*, **15**, 301–310.

—— —— Hoffmann, H.J. (1976) 'Trigonocephaly and associated minor anomalies in mother and son.' *Journal of Medical Genetics*, **13**, 77–79.

Jabs, E.W., Li, X., Scott, A.F., *et al.* (1994) 'Jackson–Weiss and Crouzon syndromes are allelic with mutations in fibroblast growth factor receptor 2.' *Nature Genetics*, **8**, 275–279.

Kane, A.A., Mitchell, L.E., Craven, K.P., Marsh, J.L. (1996) 'Observations on a recent increase in plagiocephaly without synostosis.' *Pediatrics*, **97**, 877–885.

Keeney, G., Gebarski, S.S., Brunberg, J.A. (1992) 'CT of inner ear anomalies including aplasia, in a case of Wildervanck syndrome.' *American Journal of Neuroradiology*, **13**, 201–202.

Klintworth, G.K. (1963) 'The neurologic manifestations of osteopetrosis (Albers–Schönberg disease).' *Neurology*, **13**, 512–518.

Kreiborg, S. (1981) 'Crouzon syndrome. A clinical and roentgencephalometric study.' *Scandinavian Journal of Plastic and Reconstructive Surgery*, **18** (Suppl.), 1–198.

Lajeunie, E., Le Merrer, M., Bonaiti-Pellie, C., *et al.* (1995) 'Genetic study of nonsyndromic coronal craniosynostosis.' *American Journal of Medical Genetics*, **55**, 500–504.

Langer, L.O., Spranger, J.W., Greinacher, I., Herman, R.C. (1969) 'Thanatophoric dwarfism. A condition confused with achondroplasia in the neonate, with brief comments on achondrogenesis and homozygous achondroplasia.' *Radiology*, **92**, 285–295.

Leão, M.J., Ribeiro-Silva, M.L. (1995) 'Orofaciodigital syndrome type I in a patient with severe CNS defects.' *Pediatric Neurology*, **13**, 247–251.

Lehman, R.A.W., Reeves, J.D., Wilson, W.B., Wesenberg, R.I. (1977) 'Neurological complications of infantile osteopetrosis.' *Annals of Neurology*, **2**, 378–384.

Le Merrer, M., Ledinot, V., Renier, D., *et al.* (1988) 'Conseil génétique dans les craniosténoses: bilan d'une étude prospective réalisée avec le groupe d'études sur les malformations craniofaciales.' *Journal de Génétique Humaine*, **36**, 295–306.

Manni, J.J., Scaf, J.J., Huygen, P.L.M., *et al.* (1990) 'Hyperostosis cranialis interna. A new hereditary syndrome with cranial nerve entrapment.' *New England Journal of Medicine*, **322**, 450–454.

Marchac, D., Renier, D. (1982) *Craniofacial Surgery for Craniosynostosis.* Boston: Little Brown.

Maroteaux, P. (1982) *Maladies Osseuses de l'Enfant. 2ᵉᵐᵉ Edn.* Paris: Flammarion.

Marsh, J.L., Schwartz, H.G. (1983) 'The surgical correction of coronal and metopic craniosynostoses.' *Journal of Neurosurgery*, **59**, 245–251.

Menezes, A.H., VanGilder, J.C., Graf, C.J., McDonnell, D.E. (1980) 'Craniocervical abnormalities: a comprehensive surgical approach.' *Journal of Neurosurgery*, **53**, 444–455.

Moore, M.H. (1993) 'Upper airway obstruction in the syndromal craniosynostoses.' *British Journal of Plastic Surgery*, **46**, 355–362.

Morgan, D.F., Young, R.F. (1980) 'Spinal neurological complications of achondroplasia. Results of surgical treatment.' *Journal of Neurosurgery*, **52**, 463–472.

—— Williams, B. (1992) 'Syringobulbia: a surgical appraisal.' *Journal of Neurology, Neurosurgery, and Psychiatry*, **55**, 1132–1141.

Morrison, S.G., Perry, L.W., Scott, L.P. (1968) 'Congenital brevicollis (Klippel–Feil syndrome) and cardiovascular anomalies.' *American Journal of Diseases of Children*, **115**, 614–620.

Moss, M.L. (1975) 'Functional anatomy of cranial synostosis.' *Child's Brain*, **1**, 22–33.

Myrianthopoulos, N.C. (1977) 'Epidemiology of central nervous system malformations.' *In:* Vinken, P.J., Bruyn, G.W. (Eds.) *Handbook of Clinical Neurology. Vol. 30. Congenital Malformations of the Brain and Skull.* Amsterdam: North Holland, pp. 139–171.

Nappen, D.L., Kokich, V.G. (1983) 'Experimental craniosynostosis in growling rabbits.' *Journal of Neurosurgery*, **58**, 101–108.

Nelson, F.N., Hecht, J.T., Horton, W.A., *et al.* (1988) 'Neurological basis of respiratory complications in achondroplasia.' *Annals of Neurology*, **24**, 89–93.

Oldridge, M., Wilkie, A.O.M., Slaney, S.F., *et al.* (1995) 'Mutations in the third immunoglobulin domain of the fibroblast growth factor receptor 2 gene in Crouzon syndrome.' *Human Molecular Genetics*, **4**, 1077–1082.

Pascual-Castroviejo, I., Garcia-Peñas, J.J., Pascual-Pascual, S.I., Moneo, J.L.H. (1994) 'Cervical spinal cord compression in chondrodystroplasia punctata: report of two cases.' *Acta Neuropediatrica*, **1**, 118–123.

Patton, M.A., Goodship, J., Hayward, R., Lansdown, R. (1988) 'Intellectual development in Apert's syndrome: a long term follow up of 29 patients.' *Journal of Medical Genetics*, **25**, 164–167.

Pauli, R.M., Horton, V.K., Glinski, L.P., Reiser, C.A. (1995) 'Prospective assessment of risks for cervicomedullary-junction compression in infants with achondroplasia.' *American Journal of Human Genetics*, **56**, 732–744.

Penfold, J.L., Simpson, D.A. (1975) 'Premature craniosynostosis. A complication of thyroid replacement therapy.' *Journal of Pediatrics*, **86**, 360–363.

Pfeiffer, R.A. (1969) 'Associated deformities of the head and hands.' *Birth Defects*, **5**, 18–34.

Preston, R.A., Post, J.C., Keats, B.J.B., *et al.* (1994) 'A gene for Crouzon craniofacial dysostosis maps to the long arm of chromosome 10.' *Nature Genetics*, **7**, 149–153.

Pueschel, S.M. (1988) 'Atlantoaxial instability and Down syndrome.' *Pediatrics*, **81**, 879–880.

—— Findley, T.W., Furia, J., *et al.* (1987) 'Atlantoidal instability in persons with Down syndrome: roentgenographic, neurologic and somatosensory evoked potential studies.' *Journal of Pediatrics*, **110**, 515–521.

Reardon, W., Winter, R.M., Rutland, P., *et al.* (1994) 'Mutations in the fibroblast growth factor receptor 2 gene cause Crouzon syndrome.' *Nature Genetics*, **8**, 98–103.

Reid, C.S., Pyeritz, R.E., Kopits, S.E., *et al.* (1987) 'Cervicomedullary compression in young patients with achondroplasia: value of comprehensive neurologic and respiratory evaluation.' *Journal of Pediatrics*, **110**, 522–530.

Reilly, B.J., Leeming, J.M., Fraser, D. (1964) 'Craniosynostosis in the rachitic spectrum.' *Journal of Pediatrics*, **64**, 396–405.

Rimoin, D.L. (1995) 'Cervicomedullary junction compression in infants with achondroplasia: when to perform neurosurgical decompression.' *American Journal of Human Genetics*, **56**, 824–827.

Robinson, L.K., James, H.E., Mubarak, S.J., *et al.* (1985) 'Carpenter syndrome: natural history and clinical spectrum.' *American Journal of Medical Genetics*, **20**, 461–469.

Rohatgi, M. (1991) 'Cloverleaf skull—a severe form of Crouzon's syndrome: a new concept in aetiology.' *Acta Neurochirurgica*, **108**, 45–52.

Ruben, J.B., Morris, R.J., Judisch, G.F. (1990) 'Chorioretinal degeneration in infantile malignant osteopetrosis.' *American Journal of Ophthalmology*, **110**, 1–5.

Saltzman, C.L., Hensinger, R.N., Blane, C.E., Phillips, W.A. (1991) 'Familial cervical dysplasia.' *Journal of Bone and Joint Surgery*, **73**, 163–171.

Schott, G.D., Wyke, M.A. (1981) 'Congenital mirror movements.' *Journal of Neurology, Neurosurgery, and Psychiatry*, **44**, 586–599.

Schrander-Stumpel, T., de Die-Smulders, C.E., Hennekam, R.C., *et al.* (1992) 'Oculoauriculovertebral spectrum and cerebral anomalies.' *Journal of Medical Genetics*, **29**, 326–331.

Shillito, J., Matson, D.D. (1968) 'Craniosynostosis: a review of 519 surgical patients.' *Pediatrics*, **41**, 829–853.

Siggers, D.C. (1975) 'Cleidocranial dystostosis.' *Developmental Medicine and Child Neurology*, **17**, 522–524.

Slover, R., Sujansky, E. (1979) 'Frontonasal dysplasia with coronal craniosynostosis in three sibs.' *Birth Defects Original Article Series*, **15** (5B), 75–83.

Sly, W.S., Whyte, M.P., Sundaram, V., *et al.* (1985) 'Carbonic anhydrase II deficiency in 12 families with the autosomal recessive syndromes of osteopetrosis with renal tubular acidosis and cerebral calcification.' *New England Journal of Medicine*, **313**, 139–145.

Sood, S., Mahapatra, A.K., Bhatia, B. (1992) 'Somatosensory and brainstem auditory evoked potential in congenital craniovertebral anomaly: effect of surgical treatment.' *Journal of Neurology, Neurosurgery, and Psychiatry*, **55**, 609–612.

Stevens, J.M., Chong, W.K., Barber, C., *et al.* (1994) 'A new appraisal of abnormalities of the odontoid process associated with atlanto-axial subluxation and neurological disability.' *Brain*, **117**, 133–148.

Stoilov, I., Kilpatrick, M.W., Tsipouras, P. (1995) 'A common FGFR3 gene mutation is present in achondroplasia but not in hypochondroplasia.' *American Journal of Medical Genetics*, **55**, 127–133.

Stovner, L.J., Cappelen, J., Nilsen, G., Sjaastad, O. (1992) 'The Chiari type I malformation in two monozygotic twins and first-degree relatives.' *Annals of Neurology*, **31**, 220–222.

—— Bergan, U., Nilsen, G., Sjaastad, O. (1993) 'Posterior cranial fossa dimensions in the Chiari 1 malformation: relation to pathogenesis and clinical presentation.' *Neuroradiology*, **35**, 113–118.

Thompson, D.N.P., Harkness, W., Jones, B., Gonsalez, S., *et al.* (1995) 'Subdural intracranial pressure monitoring in craniosynostosis: its role in surgical management.' *Child's Nervous System*, **11**, 269–275.

Toriello, H.V. (1988) 'Heterogeneity and variability in the oro-facial-digital syndromes.' *American Journal of Medical Genetics*, Suppl. 4, 149–159.

Tsipouras, P., Barabas, G., Matthews, W.S. (1986) 'Neurologic correlates of osteogenesis imperfecta.' *Archives of Neurology*, **43**, 150–152.

Van Buchem, F.S.P. (1971) 'Hyperostosis corticalis generalisata. Eight new cases.' *Acta Medica Scandinavica*, **189**, 257–267.

Vanek, J., Losan, F. (1982) 'Pfeiffer's type of acrocephalosyndactyly in two families.' *Journal of Medical Genetics*, **19**, 289–292.

Wackenheim, A. (1967) 'Les dysplasies des condyles occipitaux.' *Annales de Radiologie*, **11**, 535–543.

Wilkie, A.O.M., Slaney, S.F., Oldridge, M. (1995) 'Apert syndrome results from localized mutations of FGFR2 and is allelic with Crouzon syndrome.' *Nature Genetics*, **9**, 165–172.

Yamada, H., Nakamura, S., Tajima, M., Kageyama, N. (1981) 'Neurological manifestations of pediatric achondroplasia.' *Journal of Neurosurgery*, **54**, 49–57.

Yen, J.K., Bourke, R.S., Popp, A.J., Wirth, C.R. (1978) 'Camurati–Engelmann disease (progressive hereditary craniodiaphyseal dysplasia). Case report.' *Journal of Neurosurgery*, **48**, 138–142.

Young, R., Kleinman, G., Ojemann, R.G., *et al.* (1980) 'Compressive myelopathy in Maroteaux–Lamy syndrome: clinical and pathological findings.' *Annals of Neurology*, **8**, 336–340.

PART III

NEUROLOGICAL CONSEQUENCES OF PRENATAL, PERINATAL AND EARLY POSTNATAL INTERFERENCE WITH BRAIN DEVELOPMENT: HYDROCEPHALUS, CEREBRAL PALSY

7
HYDROCEPHALUS AND NONTRAUMATIC PERICEREBRAL COLLECTIONS

HYDROCEPHALUS

Hydrocephalus is one of the possible consequences of some of the brain malformations or lesions described in the preceding chapters. It may also be acquired later in life as a result of tumours, infections or other causes. For convenience, all types of hydrocephalus of whatever cause in children of any age are studied in this chapter.

DEFINITION AND MECHANISMS

Hydrocephalus means an excess of fluid within the cranium. However, it is customary to reserve the term for the condition in which the volume of CSF is increased in all or part of the intracranial fluid spaces, and in which that increased volume is not the result of primary atrophy or dysgenesis of the brain. The abnormal accumulation of CSF results from an excessive pressure, at least in the initial stages of the disorder.

The greater part of the CSF is secreted actively by the choroid plexuses. Experiments in animals indicate that 35–70 per cent of CSF, depending on species, may come from extraplexic sources. In humans, it is estimated that 70–90 per cent of the fluid originates from the choroid plexuses (McComb 1983b), the remainder originating in brain parenchyma as a result of exchanges with cerebral extracellular spaces. The daily formation of CSF in children and adults is about 500 mL. The night and day rhythm of secretion is relatively stable and amounts to 0.35 mL/min in adults. The total volume of CSF in the head of an adult is about 120 mL, and the average ventricular volume is around 25 mL although individual variations occur. In the neonate, CSF volume is about 50 mL.

The hydrostatic pressure of the CSF (synonymous with intracranial pressure) originates from the CSF secretion pressure and from the resistances to its circulation and resorption. Secretion of CSF seems to result from a two-step process. The first step is the formation, by hydrostatic pressure, of a plasma ultrafiltrate through the choroidal capillary endothelium, which is devoid of tight junctions. The second step transforms the ultrafiltrate by an active metabolic process within the choroidal

epithelium. The rate of CSF formation is relatively independent of pressure. The rate of CSF resorption depends on CSF pressure and is relatively linear over the range of physiological pressures (Lorenzo et al. 1970, McComb 1983b).

CSF flows from the lateral ventricles through the third and fourth ventricles into the posterior fossa and then the basal cisterns (Bradley 1970). CSF flow then divides. Most of the CSF passes upward through the incisura and reaches the parasagittal arachnoid villi via the ambient cisterns, the sylvian fissures and the convexity cisterns. About 20 per cent of the fluid flows downward along the spinal subarachnoid space to the arachnoid villi along the nerve root sleeves. This flow is maintained by continuous entry of newly secreted CSF into the ventricles.

Most of the CSF is resorbed passively, through the arachnoid granulations along the superior sagittal sinus, into the sinus blood flow. The CSF pressure is normally greater than venous blood pressure. A pressure gradient of 20–50 mmH$_2$O is necessary for opening the valve mechanisms of the arachnoid villi (Welch and Friedman 1960). Thus, the mean CSF pressure normally depends on several factors: pressure secretion of the fluid, venous blood pressure, resistance of CSF pathways including cisterns and granulations, and distensibility of the walls of CSF spaces (that is, brain parenchyma, meninges and skull) or yield pressure which is important mainly in pathological situations (Naidich 1989). A significant amount of CSF may be resorbed via cervical lymph vessels (McComb et al. 1983) and this pathway may be of importance in hydrocephalus. Absorption of CSF by the brain in pathological circumstances (transependymal resorption) is suggested by CT scan or MR imaging (see below). However, the presence of subependymal fluid is no proof of its resorption as the fluid may simply move through the parenchyma to the pericerebral spaces (James et al. 1974).

This classical concept remains useful for the understanding of the causes and clinical features of hydrocephalus. However, recent work has shown that it has to be substantially modified to account for multiple aspects of the condition (see Sato et al. 1994). In particular, extrachoroidal sources of fluid, especially within the brain parenchyma which behaves in this respect as a sponge absorbing CSF (Hakim sponge), are of great importance; resorption is not exclusively through the granulations of Pacchioni but also into the brain extracellular space; and factors other than resistance to absorption are significant in determining CSF pressure.

Normal intracranial (or CSF) pressure at the level of the foramen of Monro is 100–150mm H_2O in children and adolescents at rest in the lying position. In the newborn, CSF pressure is lower, around 40–50 mmH_2O.

Except in the rare cases of CSF hypersecretion, hydrocephalus is virtually always due to an increase in the resistance of CSF circulation pathways. Such an increase may be located within the ventricular system, in the subarachnoid spaces or at the sites of resorption. CSF flow is a function of the difference between CSF and venous sinus pressures, divided by the resistance of pathways. As CSF production is stable over a relatively wide range or pressures, an increase in CSF pressure is inevitable to allow evacuation of newly formed CSF.

The magnitude of the effects of this increase in pressure will depend largely on the yield pressure or compliance of brain and skull. When the skull is distensible (low yield pressure), there is rapid ventricular enlargement, large final ventricular size, rapid decline in intraventricular pressure and relatively low final pressure after compensation. This is the situation in newborn babies and infants. In contrast, with low compliance (high yield pressure), ventricular enlargement is slow, final ventricular size is relatively small, intraventricular pressure remains high for long periods, and final pressure after compensation remains high. This situation obtains in older children and in adolescents and also in fetuses in which pressure from the uterine wall limits ventricular enlargement (Oi *et al.* 1990). In such cases, severe hydrocephalus with high pressure can develop *with deceptively little ventricular dilatation* (Jones 1987).

In addition to increase in mean intracranial pressure (ICP), *CSF pulse pressure* probably plays an important role in the determination of some aspects of hydrocephalus. CSF pulse pressure designates the systolic–diastolic variations in CSF pressure that result from those of arterial blood-pressure transmitted by arterial wall pulsations to the CSF. The amplitude of the CSF pulse pressure varies with the mean ICP and rises sharply with increasing mean CSF pressure (Naidich 1989). Pulse pressure also depends on ventricular compliance and on the rapidity with which outflow of venous blood and CSF can compensate for the instantaneous pressure rise. CSF pulse pressure has a significant role in determination of ventricular size. An experimental three-fold increase in the pulse amplitude causes hydrocephalus in animals. Conversely, removal of one plexus is associated with decrease of pulse pressure and of size of the corresponding ventricle (Di Rocco *et al.* 1979), and the same mechanism is probably responsible for the smaller size of shunted lateral ventricles. Pressure measurements have confirmed that in such cases, the pulse pressure is decreased in the ventricle where the tip of the catheter lies, probably as a result of damping of CSF pulsations by CSF outflow into the shunt.

Later effects of increased ICP and dilatation of the CSF spaces include the progressive development of cerebral atrophy that predominantly affects white matter and, in turn, facilitates further ventricular dilatation. There is splitting of the ependymal lining, spongy dissociation of nerve fibres and, eventually, development of astrocytosis (Weller and Shulman 1972). The grey matter, on the contrary, is long preserved. Reduction of cerebral blood flow, in particular in the anterior cerebral arteries, may play a role by inducing ischaemic injury to the cerebral hemispheres (Hill and Volpe 1982).

The eventual course of hydrocephalus will depend on the achievement of a new balance between CSF production, preservation of residual absorption capacity and development of alternative resorption pathways. If and when resorption and secretion of CSF equalize under a stable regime of pressure, stabilization of hydrocephalus occurs but at the expense of a variable degree of stable or slowly diminishing ventricular dilatation. Differentiating hydrocephalus that is stabilized or arrested from that which is slowly evolutive may be extremely difficult or even impossible, especially as several variables are at play at the same time. These include, for example, skull compliance, the CSF pressure which fluctuates with plateau waves occurring especially during REM sleep (Rosner and Becker 1983), and the development of new resorption pathways. It seems, however, that true arrest of hydrocephalus does occur in a small proportion of children (10–20 per cent) as shown by radionuclide clearing studies (Johnston *et al.* 1984).

The effects of hydrocephalus will also vary with the age of first development of the disorder. In addition to the differences resulting from the diverse yield pressures, one may observe modifications in the shape of the skull that may expand frontally with aqueductal stenosis, whereas a fourth ventricle cyst, as in Dandy–Walker malformation, may impede caudal migration of the tentorium that inserts on the parietal bones in an abnormally high situation. Similar mechanisms may be responsible for the skull changes that are present in hydrocephalus associated with spina bifida (Britton *et al.* 1988).

CLASSIFICATION OF HYDROCEPHALUS
Hydrocephalus comprises a highly heterogeneous group of conditions which have little in common aside from the dilatation of the CSF spaces. Several systems of classification can be used. One early approach separated 'communicating' hydrocephalus (*i.e.* those cases in which intraventricularly introduced dye was recovered in the lumbar cul-de-sac after a few minutes) from 'non-communicating' or 'blocked' hydrocephalus in which dye could not be detected by lumbar puncture. Such terms are now obsolete, and recent classifications are based on age of occurrence, aetiology and suspected mechanisms (Mori *et al.* 1995). The major mechanisms and causes are shown in Table 7.1. More detailed descriptions will be given in paragraphs dedicated to aetiological diagnosis in different age categories because age of occurrence has a major influence not only on prognosis and management but also on the likely causes of hydrocephalus (Table 7.2). In the series reported by Mori *et al.* (1995), 68 cases were of fetal onset, 316 were associated with myelomeningocele, 332 were congenital of

TABLE 7.1
Main mechanisms of hydrocephalus

Mechanism	Main causes
Oversecretion of CSF	Papilloma of choroid plexus, increased venous pressure (*e.g.* vein of Galen malformation)
Obstruction of CSF pathways	
Intraventricular block	
Foramen of Monro	Tumours (*e.g.* giant cell astrocytoma)
Third ventricle	Tumours (*e.g.* colloid cyst, craniopharyngioma)
Aqueduct of Sylvius	Tumours; malformations; inflammation (*e.g.* toxoplasmosis, meningitis, posthaemorrhagic granular ependymitis)
Fourth ventricle	Tumours and cysts; malformations (*e.g.* Chiari, Dandy–Walker*); haematoma; membranous obstruction of the foramen of Magendie
Extraventricular block**	
Basilar block	Inflammation (infectious or posthaemorrhagic); tumours (chiasmatic glioma, craniopharyngioma); malignant seeding of meninges; mucopolysaccharidosis
Convexity block	Mainly inflammation
Deficient resorption	
Venous hypertension	Compression of sinuses, abnormal basal foramina with compression; extracranial venous obstacles
Abnormalities of arachnnoid villi	Absence of villi; ?clogging of villi by high CSF protein
Unknown mechanism	Spinal cord tumours; Guillain–Barré syndrome

*The mechanism of hydrocephalus is not entirely clear. Aqueductal stenosis is often associated with Chiari malformation.
**For some causes, there may be both intraventricular and extraventricular block, or the precise mechanisms may be difficult to determine and be different in each case.

TABLE 7.2
Main causes of hydrocephalus in relation to age*

Fetal hydrocephalus	Aqueductal stenosis of genetic or acquired origin
	Dandy–Walker and related malformations
	Myelomeningocele, encephalocele
	Holoprosencephaly, corpus callosum agenesis
	Chromosomal abnormalities and multiple malformation syndromes
	Prenatal haemorrhage
	Prenatal infections (toxoplasmosis and others)
	Prenatal tumours
Infantile hydrocephalus	Late manifestation of prenatal causes, especially myelomeningocele, aqueductal stenosis, prenatal infections
	Perinatal intracranial haemorrhage, especially peri-intraventricular haemorrhage
	Purulent meningitis
	Tumours and cysts
	Aneurysm of vein of Galen and other vascular anomalies, *e.g.* venous anomalies or compression
	Mucopolysaccharidosis (Hurler)
Childhood hydrocephalus	Late manifestation of infantile (rarely antenatal) hydrocephalus
	Posterior fossa tumours (including periaqueductal tumours)
	Aqueductal stenosis or Dandy–Walker syndrome with delayed or very slow development of hydrocephalus

*In some cases, multiple mechanisms may be at play, *e.g.* aqueductal stenosis, basilar blockage due to infection or compression of posterior fossa in myelomingocele or encephalocele. The same causes may become symptomatic at widely different ages but there are clearcut statistical relationships between age and cause.

other causes, 152 were of posthaemorrhagic and 103 of post-meningitic origin.

EPIDEMIOLOGY

The incidence of hydrocephalus is imperfectly known. The figure of 3 per 1000 live births which is commonly quoted applies only to congenital (or early onset) hydrocephalus. Moreover, the practice of antenatal diagosis of malformations and systematic ultrasonographic examination during pregnancy has modified our knowledge of both the incidence and the distribution of causes of congenital hydrocephalus. For the period 1958–1981, Lorber (1984) found an incidence of 0.6 per 1000 live births. Recent studies in Sweden (Fernell *et al.* 1986, 1987a,b) found a mean prevalence of hydrocephalus manifesting during the first year of life of 0.53 per 1000 during the years 1967–1982, with a slightly increasing trend from 0.48 in 1967–1970 to 0.63 in 1979–1982 (cases of tumours and of neural tube defects were not included). Of the 202 infants studied, 30 per cent were born preterm. The increase did not continue after 1982 (Fernell *et al.* 1994). The increased prevalence was entirely ascribable to cases occurring in preterm infants, in whom it rose from 0.13 to 0.30 per 1000 during the study period. The origin of the hydrocephalus differed between term and preterm infants. Among term infants the origin was considered to be prenatal in 70 per cent, perinatal in 25 per cent and postnatal in 5 per cent, whereas among infants born preterm the corresponding proportions were 40 per cent, 60 per cent and less than 1 per cent respectively (Fernell *et al.* 1986, 1987a,c, 1994).

FETAL HYDROCEPHALUS

Antenatal diagnosis of hydrocephalus raises special diagnostic, prognostic and therapeutic problems.

DIAGNOSIS

The sonographic diagnosis of fetal hydrocephalus may be suspected sometimes as early as the 13th week (Hudgins *et al.* 1988), usually by the 16th week, and can be confirmed between the 20th and 22nd week. It is always difficult and should always be confirmed by an experienced observer.

The diagnosis is made by determining the ratio of the width of the lateral ventricles to that of the whole brain (Chervenak *et al.* 1984). The shape of the ventricles, an asymmetry of the choroid plexus, or abnormalities of the size and shape of the fourth ventricle may support diagnosis. Hydrocephalus can also be diagnosed by prenatal MRI but this is not a routine technique (Dinh *et al.* 1990). Differential diagnosis includes agenesis of the corpus callosum with dilatation of the posterior horns, cysts of the choroid plexus that are usually transient and insignificant, holoprosencephaly, and especially nonevolutive ventriculomegaly. Thus, the presence of ventriculomegaly cannot be equated with a diagnosis of hydrocephalus. Cases of isolated ventriculomegaly without other abnormalities (21 of 47 in the series of Hudgins *et al.* 1988) may resolve before birth and be compatible with normal development (Serlo *et al.* 1986). Conversely, a few cases are on record in which fetal ultrasonography did not reveal ventricular dilatation until the 24th week of gestation (Kelley *et al.* 1988, Ko *et al.* 1994, Brewer *et al.* 1996).

The presence of associated anomalies is of extreme diagnostic importance. A careful search for facial, limb, renal, cardiac, and other intracranial abnormalities should be part of the examination. Associated abnormalities are also of grave prognostic significance: in the series of Nyberg *et al.* (1987) they were present in 85 per cent of 61 fetuses with prenatal hydrocephalus and the mortality rate for these was 66 per cent. Similarly, associated malformations herald a poor prognosis in cases of apparently stable ventriculomegaly (Drugan *et al.* 1989).

When fetal hydrocephalus is suspected on sonographic examination, a complete investigation including karyotype, determination of alpha-fetoprotein and search for specific infectious agents by serology or by fetal blood sampling, as indicated, is in order.

AETIOLOGY

Malformations are the most common causes of antenatal hydrocephalus (Table 7.2). Most are also major causes of infantile hydrocephalus and are described below as they may become manifest only after birth. Several causes of antenatal hydrocephalus are responsible for neonatal or very early death. These include complex malformation syndromes such as the hydrolethalus syndrome (Salonen *et al.* 1981, Herva and Seppäinen 1984), which features microphthalmia, polydactyly, and heart and lung malformations, the Meckel–Gruber and Walker–Warburg syndromes (see Chapter 3), the 'VACTERL' association (Briard *et al.* 1984) and trisomies 13 and 18. Many of these are genetically

determined (see below). The main nongenetic causes are infectious diseases (*e.g.* toxoplasmosis), prenatal haemorrhage and congenital tumour (Catala *et al.* 1989, Fernell *et al.* 1994).

OUTCOME AND MANAGEMENT

The overall prognosis of antenatal hydrocephalus is poor. In many cases, spontaneous abortion or stillbirth results. The outcome of intrauterine shunting operations is at best uncertain, and most centres do not use the procedure. Termination of pregnancy is often performed for hydrocephalus of very early onset or with associated malformations and/or chromosome abnormalities (Serlo *et al.* 1986). In cases with a relatively thick mantle and slow progression, when parents decide to go on with pregnancy, delivery will usually be by caesarian section. Hydrocephalus present at birth, however, has, overall, a poor prognosis. Differences in evaluation depend, to a large extent, on the diagnostic criteria. Renier *et al.* (1988) included in their study only patients with head circumference at birth >2 SD above the mean. The survival rate of their 108 patients was 62 per cent at 10 years. Only 21 of the 75 survivors had an IQ ≥80, and 16 were of borderline intelligence. Kirkinen *et al.* (1996) found that seven of 25 infants diagnosed during pregnancy (excluding cases with associated malformations and/or lethal syndromes) were severely disabled and six had intermediate disability. They consider that termination should be considered if there are associated anomalies or chromosomal disorder, and if rapidly increasing ventricular dilatation is found on repeated echography.

HYDROCEPHALUS IN CHILDREN UNDER 2 YEARS OF AGE

DIAGNOSIS

The diagnosis of hydrocephalus is usually easy in this age group even though some cases escape recognition until late stages. An abnormally rapid development of the skull volume is the major and most striking manifestation. It is sometimes associated with irritability and unexplained vomiting. Not infrequently there is a delay in passing milestones, and this may be the first sign of alarm if the macrocephaly is moderate and has not drawn the attention of the family.

The skull volume is evaluated by measurement of (occipitofrontal) head circumference. Repeated measurements are especially important because the rapidity of growth gives some idea of the degree of severity of hydrocephalus. Comparison of the values obtained (preferably using a steel tape and ensuring that the maximum circumference has been obtained) should be displayed on an adequate head-growth chart (Raymond and Holmes 1994). A head circumference that crosses one or more grid lines over a period of a few weeks is evidence of definite abnormality in term infants, regardless of the absolute value, and any break in the normal slope of the curve is an absolute indication for further investigation. Interpretation of head growth may be difficult in preterm infants as ventricular size may increase without corresponding head enlargement. In such cases, comparison of ultrasound measurement with reference values (Saliba *et al.* 1990) is extremely useful.

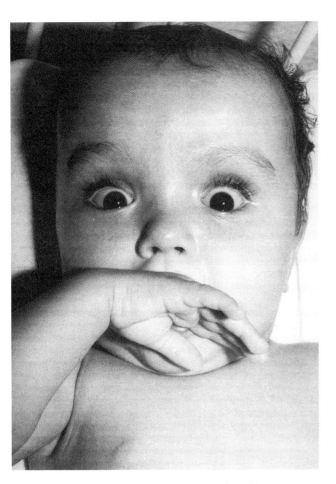

Fig. 7.1. 'Setting sun' phenomenon in boy with subdural haematoma, illustrating the fact that the phenomenon is not specific for hydrocephalus. Note retraction of upper eyelid and lowering of the globes, the iris being partly covered by the lower eyelid.

TABLE 7.3
Frequency of major clinical features of progressive hydrocephalus in 51 non-shunted patients*

Symptoms		
Asymptomatic	25	(49%)
Irritability or headache	17	(33%)
Vomiting	8	(16%)
Jitteriness		
Anorexia, drowsiness		(5–10%)
Signs		
Abnormally increased head circumference	39	(76%)
Tense anterior fontanelle	33	(65%)
Splayed sutures	20	(39%)
Scalp vein distension	17	(33%)
Sunsetting or loss of upward gaze	11	(22%)
Neck retraction or rigidity	7	(14%)
Decreased consciousness level		
Pupillary changes		
Decerebration		(5–10%)
Papilloedema		

*Data from Kirkpatrick et al. (1989).

or by removal of a bright light that had been placed in front of the eyes (Cernerud 1975). External strabismus is common and is probably related to involvement of the optic radiations rather than to VIth nerve paralysis. Optic atrophy is frequent in advanced cases, but papilloedema is rare unless the hydrocephalus is evolving rapidly such as occurs with papilloma of the choroid plexus (Pascual-Castroviejo *et al.* 1983). Seizures are a common manifestation of hydrocephalus. They may be due to the effects of hydrocephalus itself, with brain ischaemia resulting from increased ICP, to associated brain malformation, or to complications such as infections. They were observed in almost half the cases of Noetzel and Blake (1992).

The frequency of symptoms and signs of hydrocephalus in a series of 51 nonshunted patients (Kirkpatrick *et al.* 1989) is shown in Table 7.3. This series emphasizes the relative frequency of a complete absence of symptoms (49 per cent of cases, all infants) and that of a decreased level of consciousness. It also points to the rare occurrence of atypical features such as profuse sweating, neurogenic pulmonary oedema and stridor (Chapter 3). An interesting presentation is the *bobble-head doll syndrome* which is caused by dilatation of the third ventricle or by suprasellar cysts and consists of 2–3 Hz oscillatory movements of the head, usually in association with developmental delay (Tomasovic *et al.* 1975). A slow tremor in patients with hydrocephalus has been regarded as a possible equivalent of the bobble-head doll phenomenon (Russman *et al.* 1975).

SOME UNUSUAL PRESENTATIONS OF INFANTILE
HYDROCEPHALUS
The *late picture of chronic (nonshunted) hydrocephalus* has now become uncommon. It features a special neuropsychological profile with fluent speech but a low performance IQ resulting in what Hagberg and Sjögren (1966) have termed the 'cocktail party syndrome' because patients are extremely talkative even

Macrocephaly (*i.e.* a head circumference > 98th centile or > 2 SD above the mean for age) is usually symmetrical. It contrasts with the normal development of the face, lending an inverted triangular appearance to the head. The anterior fontanelle is usually large and tense or full in the sitting position. Splaying of the sutures of the cranial vault may be palpable. The scalp may appear abnormally thin and its veins dilated, strikingly so when the infant cries. This dilatation is the result of diversion of the intracranial venous drainage through emissary veins as a result of increased venous sinus pressure (Sainte-Rose *et al.* 1984).

Ocular manifestations are useful for the diagnosis. The 'setting sun' phenomenon is a downward conjugate deviation of gaze such that the iris is partially covered by the lower lid whilst the sclera is exposed above the upper rim of the iris. The latter is due in part to retraction of the upper eyelid. The mechanism of the setting sun phenomenon is not clear. It is a consequence of increased ICP probably compressing the mesencephalic tectum but it is not specific for hydrocephalus as it has been observed in children with subdural haematomas (Fig. 7.1). Moreover, retraction of the upper eyelids is occasionally present in otherwise normal infants at rest and can be regularly induced in neonates by sudden change from a vertical to a supine horizontal position

TABLE 7.4
Hydrocephalus of genetic origin

Type	Main features	Mode of transmission	References
Bickers–Adams syndrome	Aqueductal stenosis, flexion–adduction deformity of thumbs	XR	Adams *et al.* (1982)
Walker–Warburg syndrome (HARD+E syndrome)[1]	Lissencephaly, severe neurological dysfunction, eye abnormalities (retinal dysplasia, Peters anomaly, etc.), encephalocele	AR	Martinez-Lage *et al.* (1995)
Cerebro-oculo-muscular syndrome (COMS) and muscle–eye and brain disease	Closely related to Walker–Warburg syndrome	AR	Dobyns (1993)
Meckel syndrome	Polycystic kidneys, encephalocele, polydactyly	AR	Salonen (1984)
VACTERL association	Imperforate anus, congenital heart disease, tracheo-oesophageal fistula, vertebral and limb abnormalities	AR	Aleksic *et al.* (1984)
Hydrolethalus syndrome	Microphthalmia, polydactyly, external hydrocephalus, congenital heart disease, pulmonary hypoplasia	AR	Salonen *et al.* (1981)
Waaler–Aarskog syndrome	Costovertebral dysplasia, Sprengel deformity, communicating hydrocephalus	AD?, variable manifestations	Waaler and Aarskog (1980)
X-linked hydrocephalus without aqueductal stenosis[2]	Mental retardation, moderate hydrocephalus, clasped thumbs, spastic paraplegia	XR	Willems *et al.* (1987), Fryns *et al.* (1991)

*XR = X-linked recessive; AR = autosomal recessive; AD = autosomal dominant.
[1]HARD±E = *h*ydrocephalus, *a*gyria and *r*etinal *d*ysplasia ± *e*ncephalocele.
[2]Is probably a variant of Bickers–Adams syndrome due to mutation of *L1-CAM* gene at Xq28. Other variants include the so-called MASA syndrome and X-linked spastic paraplegia (SPG1) (see text).

though the semantic content of their language is rather limited. The syndrome also includes motor disturbances. Cerebellar ataxia was present in 65 per cent of the 63 patients of Hagberg and Sjögren, and bilateral spasticity was found in 17 per cent of these. The picture of ataxic diplegia is suggestive of hydrocephalus (Chapter 8). Hypothalamic and pituitary disturbances may also be a part of this syndrome (Tomono *et al.* 1983, Brauner *et al.* 1987). Short stature and obesity are frequent. *Precocious puberty* (before 10 years of age in girls and before 11 in boys) is frequent (15 per cent of patients in the series of Fernell *et al.* 1987c). It is not related to a specific cause of hydrocephalus, although it is common with suprasellar cysts (Pierre-Kahn *et al.* 1990). Late sequelae may also include specific learning disorders (Lonton 1979, Billard *et al.* 1987) and memory difficulties (Cull and Wyke 1984). This clinical syndrome may be seen in cases of arrested or of still slowly progressive hydrocephalus. It may also be seen as a sequela in late shunted cases.

Acute hydrocephalus is less common in infants than in older patients because of the low yield pressure of the skull and brain (Jones 1987). It is marked by intense symptoms, especially lethargy and stupor, and signs such as ocular motor palsies, extreme tension of the fontanelle, decerebration, or other signs of brainstem affectation. Papilloedema may be present in such cases. Rapid dilatation of the ventricular cavities may be the cause of secondary haemorrhage. Such patients require immediate surgical attention.

Very slowly evolving hydrocephalus, also termed 'occult' hydrocephalus (Di Rocco *et al.* 1989), is more frequent than acute forms. In such cases, the diagnosis may be made only by systematic serial measurements of head circumference or because of stagnation or regression of psychomotor development. In some cases, when hydrocephalus develops as a consequence of a previously known disease such as spina bifida, the occurrence of hydrocephalus is specifically looked for and, indeed, ventriculomegaly is usually detected by sonography or CT scan before symptoms or increase of head circumference are present (Chapters 2, 3). The problem then is to detect which of these cases of ventriculomegaly will result in progressive hydrocephalus. In cases of intraventricular haemorrhage or purulent meningitis, a significant proportion (up to 50 per cent of cases) will not. Such cases may be termed 'arrested' hydrocephalus but the distinction can be made only by follow-up examinations.

Localized forms of hydrocephalus can result from obstruction of one foramen of Monro by a tumour or, rarely, by postependymitis adhesions. Congenital atresia has also been reported (Wilberger *et al.* 1983). Even rarer is entrapment of the temporal horn resulting in focal obstructive hydrocephalus that can mimic an arachnoid cyst or an expansive porencephaly (Maurice-Williams and Choksey 1986). Reversible diencephalic dysfunction as a result of a trapped third ventricle has been reported (Darnell and Arbit 1993).

AETIOLOGY
The aetiological diagnosis of hydrocephalus is essential, especially as the prognosis depends largely on the causal mechanism.

In most cases a cause can be identified. However, it remained undetermined in 14 per cent of the series of 719 patients reported by Sainte-Rose *et al.* (1989). In the same series, *malformations*

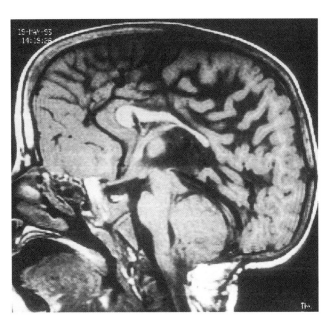

Fig. 7.2. Chiari II malformation. The brainstem is elongated and the medulla descends below the foramen magnum with kinking on the dorsal aspect of the cervical spinal cord. The 4th ventricle is very small. Note 'beaking' of the quadrigeminal plate, large interthalamic commissure and dysplastic corpus callosum.

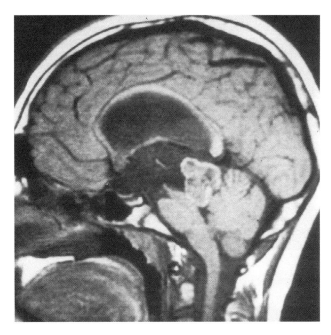

Fig. 7.3. Congenital stenosis of the sylvian aqueduct. T_1-weighted MRI, sagittal cut showing normal-sized 4th ventricle, dilated lateral ventricle and small tumour of quadrigeminal plate causing aqueduct obstruction. (Courtesy Dr Kling Chong, Great Ormond Street Hospital, London.)

accounted for 38.6 per cent of cases, tumours or other space-occupying processes for 20.4 per cent, haemorrhages for 15.6 per cent, meningitides for 7.4 per cent, and several miscellaneous other causes for 4.4 per cent of patients, with the cause being undetermined in the remaining 13.6 per cent. Genetic causes of hydrocephalus are relatively uncommon but are important for genetic counselling (Table 7.4).

Malformations
Chiari malformation, especially type II (Fig. 7.2; see also Chapter 3) formerly accounted for over 20 per cent of cases of hydroceph-alus—40 per cent in the series of Laurence (1959)—although the frequency of this cause is now declining. Hydrocephalus associated with Chiari II malformation and myelomeningocele may develop prenatally, and sonographic examination has shown that ventricular dilatation develops early before surgical closure (Chapter 3). The mechanisms of hydrocephalus suggested by Russell (1949) and Peach (1965) are still in dispute. Aqueductal stenosis is associated in one third of cases. Alternative mechanisms include atresia of the foramina of the fourth ventricle, or oblitera-tion of the subarachnoid space around the brainstem as a result of ascending infection. As indicated in Chapter 3, hydrocephalus associated with the Chiari II malformation is not infrequently accompanied by involvement of lower cranial nerves and res-piratory or swallowing difficulties that in some cases can be alleviated by treatment of the hydrocephalus alone. Chiari type I malformation is commonly associated with hydrocephalus in adults without meningomyelocele but with basilar osseous abnormalities (Levy *et al.* 1983). Such cases are rare in children (Vleck and Ito 1987).

Aqueductal stenosis is the cause of about 11 per cent of cases of hydrocephalus. The aqueduct may be reduced in size but histologically normal, but more often it is divided into several channels, most of them ending blindly, the so-called *forking* of the aqueduct (Russell 1949). Such cases are often associated with neighbouring anomalies such as 'beaking' of the collicular plate, suggesting that they may represent a mild form of dysraphism (McMillan and Williams 1977). In rare cases, obstruction of the aqueduct is due to a glial membrane. This anomaly seems to have a special relationship to neurofibromatosis type 1. The membrane is located at the intercollicular sulcus level, and the upper part of the aqueduct is widely dilated. Forking or stenosis of the aqueduct need not represent a primary abnormality. There is some evidence, in mice and humans, that it may be a secondary phenomenon, resulting from compression of the aqueduct by the cerebral hemispheres, dilated because of some other cause of hydrocephalus (Landrieu *et al.* 1979) or from inflammation due to viruses such as mumps virus. By the use of MRI it has become clear that many cases of the so-called 'idiopathic' aqueductal stenosis were in fact due to lesions encroaching on the aqueduct, especially slow growing tumours of the quadrigeminal plate or periaqueductal 'pencil' tumours (Fig. 7.3). In a series of 71 cases of triventricular hydrocephalus (Valentini *et al.* 1995), MRI revealed such lesions in 15 of the 25 cases studied. None of these lesions was progressive after one to five years of follow-up, but regular examination is clearly indicated.

Aqueductal stenosis may occur as a familial X-linked condition, the Bickers–Adams syndrome (Adams *et al.* 1982), affecting only boys. Patients are usually severely retarded. Most have a flexed and adducted thumb deformity which is neither

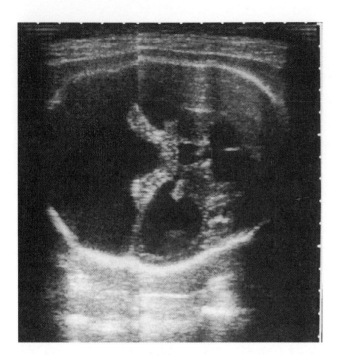

Fig. 7.4. Dandy–Walker malformation. Prenatal diagnosis by ultrasound scan at 33 weeks of amenorrhoea. Absence of cerebellar vermis and massive dilatation of posterior fossa (left side of picture) are clearly visible. (Courtesy Dr M-C. Aubry, Maternité Port Royal, Paris.)

constant nor specific. It may occur as an isolated defect and has been observed in the Walker–Warburg syndrome that has a probable autosomal recessive inheritance (Bordarier *et al.* 1984). Male relatives of patients with the Bickers–Adams syndrome may have severe mental retardation without hydrocephalus (Willems *et al.* 1987). Other types of hydrocephalus without aqueductal stenosis may have a similar X-linked transmission (Willems *et al.* 1987). X-linked hydrocephalus is usually associated with spastic paraplegia and failure of language development. It is due to multiple mutations at the *L1-CAM* gene locus at Xq28. The abnormal cell adhesion molecules that form thereby, apparently determine an anomaly of brainstem cell migration (Jouet *et al.* 1994, Jouet 1995). The same mutations can be expressed as X-linked spastic paraplegia without hydrocephalus (SPG1) or as the so-called MASA syndrome (*m*ental retardation, *a*phasia, *s*huffling gait, *a*dduction of the thumbs) which may coexist with X-linked hydrocephalus in the same lineages (Fryns *et al.* 1991, Jouet *et al.* 1994). X-linked hydrocephalus can be diagnosed prenatally in most cases. Difficulties may arise, however, because of late onset of ventricular dilatation (see above) and of features suggestive of a destructive process such as gross ventricular asymmetry (Brewer *et al.* 1996). A few cases of autosomal recessive congenital stenosis of the aqueduct have been reported (Barros-Nuñes and Rivas 1993), so a careful family history should be taken of all relatives when giving genetic counselling.

Dandy–Walker malformation is an uncommon cause of hydrocephalus, accounting for less than 2 per cent of cases (Hart *et al.* 1972, Hirsch *et al.* 1984). Prenatal diagnosis is possible because of absence of the cerebellar vermis (Fig. 7.4). In most cases, hydrocephalus is not present at birth but develops during the first year of life (Hirsch *et al.* 1984). The shape of the head, with a posterior bulge, may be suggestive, but the diagnosis rests on neuroimaging examination (Hanigan *et al.* 1985–86) (Fig. 7.5). The condition is not genetically determined but great care should be taken not to confuse the Dandy–Walker syndrome proper with other causes of agenesis or hypogenesis of the cerebellar vermis which often belong to genetic syndromes (Bordarier and Aicardi 1990; see Chapter 3).

Walker–Warburg syndrome comprises type II lissencephaly, congenital hydrocephalus, severe neurological dysfunction from the first days of life, retinal dysplasia, microphthalmia and abnormalities of the anterior chamber of the eye (Chapter 3). The association of eye anomalies and hydrocephalus may wrongly suggest a fetal infection but the condition is familial with a 25 per cent recurrence risk. The presence of Peters anomaly, retinal detachment or falciform fold of the retina should always raise the possibility of this syndrome which may also include an abnormal posterior fossa reminiscent of the Dandy–Walker syndrome (Bordarier *et al.* 1984).

Other malformations associated with hydrocephalus include encephaloceles (Diebler and Dulac 1987) which are approximately as common as the Dandy–Walker malformation, as well as a miscellany of malformation syndromes, some of which are of chromosomal origin (Chapter 5) and some are genetically determined (Waaler and Aarskog 1980, Aleksic *et al.* 1984, Herva and Seppainen 1984). *Agenesis of the corpus callosum* is often associated with marked ventricular dilatation and a large head (Chapter 3). Although virtually nothing is known about the hydrodynamics of such cases, experience indicates that many of these eventually stabilize so that shunting should be resorted to only in the face of evident progression in patients with callosal agenesis. Agenesis of the granulations of Pacchioni and arachnoid villi is exceptional.

Tumours

Tumours are not a common cause of hydrocephalus in infants, in contrast to their high frequency in older patients. Congenital tumours may be associated with hydrocephalus (Chapter 14), although macrocephaly in such cases may also be due to the bulk of the tumour itself. Craniopharyngiomas and optic nerve gliomas usually manifest later. Aqueductal tumours that may be difficult to distinguish from simple aqueductal stenosis (Raffel *et al.* 1988) have been described above. Meningeal leukaemia (Ricevuti *et al.* 1986) or gliomatosis (Civitello *et al.* 1988), as well as meningeal dissemination of primary brain tumours can produce hydrocephalus through basilar obstruction or blockage of arachnoid cisterns of the convexity. Some mucopolysaccharidoses, especially Hurler syndrome, commonly cause moderate hydrocephalus due to infiltration of the meninges and Virchow–Robin spaces by mucopolysaccharides.

Cysts of the meninges

In contrast to tumours, meningeal cysts are not uncommon.

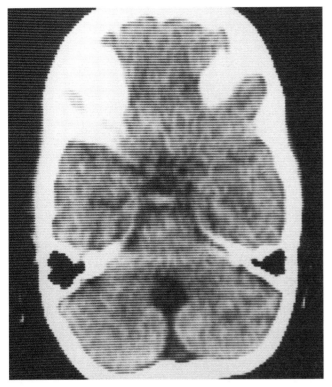

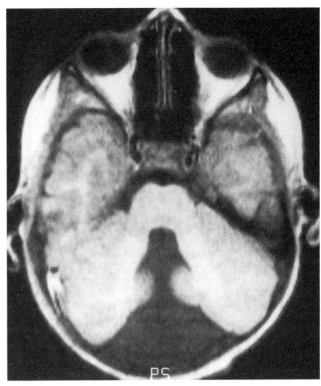

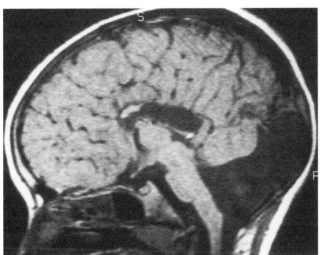

Fig. 7.5. Dandy–Walker malformation. *(Top left)* CT scan showing absence of lower vermis. *(Top right)* MRI in another patient showing absent vermis and posterior fossa cyst. *(Opposite)* Sagittal MRI cut of same patient. Note that this patient also had almost complete absence of the corpus callosum.

Posterior fossa cysts (Di Rocco *et al.* 1981, Barkovich *et al.* 1989), paramesencephalic arachnoid cysts (Grollmus *et al.* 1976) and suprasellar cysts (Hoffman *et al.* 1982, Pierre-Kahn *et al.* 1990) can all produce hydrocephalus. The latter type is often responsible, in addition, for a special endocrinological syndrome (Brauner *et al.* 1987).

Other space-occupying lesions
Other space-occupying lesions, *e.g.* retrocerebellar subdural haematoma (Gilles and Shillito 1970), can rarely cause hydrocephalus.

Haemorrhages
Haemorrhages can be the cause of acquired hydrocephalus by two distinct mechanisms. In the acute stage of an intraventricular or subarachnoid haemorrhage, the presence of a blood clot in the aqueduct or the cisterna magna, or the increased resistance resulting from the augmented viscosity of the CSF by admixture of blood, will induce ventricular dilatation. After the acute stage is over, the hydrocephalus may stabilize or regress. However, the development of meningeal adhesions or granular ependymitis can be responsible for the persistence or increase of chronic hydrocephalus, necessitating the placement of a permanent shunt.

The main causes of haemorrhage are preterm birth with peri-intraventricular haemorrhage (PIVH), trauma with subarachnoid or subdural bleeding, or bleeding from vascular malformations. PIVH is responsible for the rising incidence of hydrocephalus in preterm infants in recent years (Fernell *et al.*

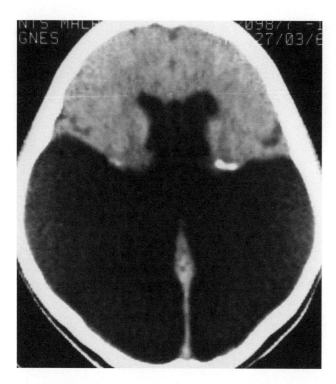

Fig. 7.6. Hydrocephalus due to toxoplasmic aqueductal stenosis. There is complete destruction of temporal, parietal and occipital cortex on both sides. Note also periventricular calcification.

1986, 1987b). Camfield *et al.* (1981) suggested that the incidence may be as high as 22 per cent in infants <1500g birthweight.

However, prospective studies have shown that progressive posthaemorrhagic hydrocephalus is less common than non-progressive or regressive ventricular dilatation following PIVH in preterm infants. Dykes *et al.* (1989) found that hydrocephalus developed in 53 of 409 infants with PIVH. In a majority of the cases progressive hydrocephalus remained asymptomatic. Hydrocephalus either regressed or was arrested in 35 of these 53 infants, only 18 having progressive hydrocephalus. Progressive hydrocephalus mainly follows grade III and IV haemorrhage. Hydrocephalus following grade II haemorrhage has a relatively favourable neurodevelopmental outcome (Krishnamoorthy *et al.* 1984). However, late hydrocephalus may develop after arrest and resolution of neonatal posthaemorrhagic hydrocephalus, so regular follow-up is essential (Perlman *et al.* 1990).

Infections
Bacterial infections are an important cause of hydrocephalus as a result of adhesive arachnoiditis or granulations that may develop following the bacteriological cure of acute meningitis or in the course of a subacute or chronic meningitis, especially tuberculous meningitis. In the latter case, ventricular dilatation is often the result of both brain atrophy and increased CSF pressure. CT or MRI show evidence of active arachnoiditis in the form of contrast enhancement of the meninges in the posterior fossa and basal cisterns (Chapter 11). Hydrocephalus may result from *chemical meningitis* due to fissuration of a dermoid cyst of the posterior

fossa or spinal canal. The resulting arachnoiditis may also be due in part to added infection. *Fungal infections* include crypto-coccosis and *Candida* meningitis, and occur especially in small preterm infants or immunosuppressed patients (Chapter 11).

Toxoplasmosis is a common cause of aqueductal stenosis (Fig. 7.6) that usually is recognized shortly after birth (Couvreur and Desmonts 1988; see also Chapter 1). In exceptional cases, a late flare-up of an old periaqueductal cystic lesion has produced aqueductal stenosis in adolescents (Ribierre *et al.* 1970).

Cysticercosis in its racemose type can result in obstruction of the aqueduct or the cavities of the third and fourth ventricles or basal cisterns, thus provoking acute hydrocephalus (Bittencourt *et al.* 1988).

Viral infections are only exceptionally a cause of aqueductal stenosis. A few cases following mumps infection have been reported (Ogata *et al.* 1992, Lahat *et al.* 1993). Cytomegalovirus infection is rarely responsible for prenatal aqueductal stenosis. Acute obstructive hydrocephalus has also been reported with Epstein–Barr virus infection (Yanofsky *et al.* 1981); with lymphocytic choriomeningitis (Green *et al.* 1949); in cases of cerebellar swelling associated with varicella (Chapter 11) or with Epstein–Barr virus infection (Roulet Perez *et al.* 1993); and with human T lymphotrophic virus 1 (HTLV-1) infection (Tohyama *et al.* 1992).

Rare causes of hydrocephalus
Among the rare causes of hydrocephalus in infants, special interest attaches to *venous causes*. Obstruction within the veins or sinuses or compression of these structures have long been held responsible for hydrocephalus due to deficient resorption of CSF although experimental ligation of veins is usually well tolerated in animals. Rosman and Shands (1978) have postulated that an increase in sinus blood pressure can be the cause either of the syndrome of benign intracranial hypertension (or pseudotumour cerebri) or of hydrocephalus, depending on the compliance of the skull. In infants with high compliance, hydrocephalus will result, whereas pseudotumour will obtain if the brain is rigidly encased in a virtually inextensible skull (Rosman and Shands 1978). Abnormal increases in sinus pressure may result from an anatomical obstacle or from functional factors (Young 1979). The former includes stenosis of the venous foramina at the base of the skull, such as occurs with achondroplasia (Pierre-Kahn *et al.* 1980, Yamada *et al.* 1981), certain types of craniostenosis (Scarfò *et al.* 1979, Sainte-Rose *et al.* 1984), tumours compressing or invading the sinuses (Kinal 1966), and thrombosis of jugular veins or superior vena cava (Haar and Miller 1975) as a result of catheterization (Newman *et al.* 1980) or surgical operations. Such cases can be improved by surgically widening the basal foramina (Lundar *et al.* 1990). Functional abnormalities resulting in high venous sinus pressure are mostly due to high-flow arteriovenous malformations (de Lange and de Vlieger 1970, Cronqvist *et al.* 1972, Lamas *et al.* 1977), especially *arteriovenous malformations of the vein of Galen* which may also act through direct compression of the aqueduct (Chapter 15). Rarely, a more distant arteriovenous shunt, such as produced by anastomosis of the right pulmonary

artery to the superior vena cava in the treatment of congenital heart disease, can produce a similar increase in intracranial venous pressure (Rosman and Shands 1978). Hydrocephalus produced by high venous pressure is generally of mild to moderate severity, although shunting has been necessary in a few cases (Hooper 1961, Haar and Miller 1975). Venous bypass between intracranial and extracranial circulations can also correct the hydrocephalus (Sainte-Rose *et al.* 1984) as does cure of an arteriovenous malformation.

Hypersecretion of CSF is mainly observed in choroid plexus papilloma or carcinoma (Pascual-Castroviejo *et al.* 1983). In this case, haemorrhage from the tumour and mechanical impairment of CSF circulation from the bulk of the intraventricular mass may also play a role in the development of hydrocephalus. The diagnosis of such lesions is easy with CT scan or MRI, and removal of the tumour may cure the hydrocephalus, although complementary shunting is often necessary.

Hydrocephalus of *unknown cause* may be due to unnoticed haemorrhage or infection or may be the late manifestation of a previously silent malformation.

HYDROCEPHALUS IN OLDER CHILDREN
DIAGNOSIS
The diagnosis of hydrocephalus in children and adolescents is that of intracranial hypertension. This is because the compliance of the skull is very limited so the increased pressure of CSF cannot be compensated for by the development of macrocrania.

The symptoms and signs will thus be those of high ICP with headache, lethargy, strabismus and papilloedema (Kirkpatrick *et al.* 1989; see Chapter 14).

Cases of slowly evolving hydrocephalus (*e.g.* aqueductal stenosis) may manifest with moderate macrocrania and progressive neurological signs such as disturbances of behaviour, neuropsychological regression, ataxia and pyramidal tract signs. Abnormal movements may result from decreased basal ganglia blood flow (Shahar *et al.* 1988). Ocular features are of diagnostic importance. The most characteristic is paresis of upward gaze (Parinaud syndrome), at times associated with *nystagmus retractorius*, deficient convergence and pupillary abnormalities. Ocular signs are a central part of *the sylvian aqueduct syndrome* (Chattha and De Long 1975) that also features memory disturbances and eventually decreased vigilance and coma. This syndrome is also observed with malfunctioning shunts and in patients with aqueductal stenosis, and, at onset, it may not include significant ventricular dilatation. Simultaneous pressure measurements in both the posterior fossa and the lateral ventricles have shown the presence of a marked pressure gradient (C. Sainte-Rose, personal communication 1991).

AETIOLOGY
The aetiological diagnosis of late hydrocephalus is dominated by *tumours* and other space-occupying lesions and by congenital stenoses of the aqueduct. Tumours of the posterior fossa are the commonest cause (Chapter 14). Aqueductal stenosis can decompensate very late, even in adulthood. Such patients have

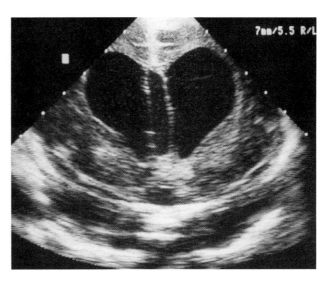

Fig. 7.7. Moderate hydrocephalus due to basilar block (transfontanelle ultrasonography): note presence of cyst in septum pellucidum.

often headaches and mild neurological signs such as pyramidal or cerebellar dysfunction. They frequently have optic atrophy attesting to the long-standing hypertension. Their heads are usually moderately enlarged, and skull X-rays show marked digital markings and ballooning of the sella turcica. Small periaqueductal tumours or slowly growing brainstem gliomas should be sought by careful neuroradiological examination, including MRI (Ho 1982, Sanford *et al.* 1982, Raffel *et al.* 1988, Valentini *et al.* 1995). *Neurofibromatosis type 1* may be associated with a diaphragm of the aqueduct or with periaqueductal gliosis or tumour (Balestrazzi *et al.* 1989, Valentini *et al.* 1995).

Hydrocephalus may occur in the absence of intracranial lesions in children with spinal cord tumours. Gelabert *et al.* (1990) reviewed 23 published cases and added one of their own. Onset was between 4 months and 16 years. Astrocytomas and ependymomas were most common, and the most frequent location of masses was thoracolumbar. High protein levels in CSF are regularly found and, together with compression of CSF outflow, have been thought to play a role in their mechanism. In five cases seen at our institution imaging showed evidence of basilar arachnoiditis similar to tuberculous meningitis, and seeding of the basilar meninges was demonstrated. This is a significant cause of apparently idiopathic hydrocephalus, and in such cases CT or MRI scanning of the cord is indicated.

NEUROIMAGING AND OTHER ANCILLARY EXAMINATIONS IN HYDROCEPHALUS
Modern progress in neuroimaging has radically modified the practice of neurology and neurosurgery and thus has transformed the evaluation and diagnostic methods for patients with hydrocephalus.

Ultrasonographic examination through the anterior fontanelle is safe and simple as long as the fontanelle is open. It is particularly well suited for repeated follow-up examinations. Approximate measurements of ventricular span can be obtained, and the sono-

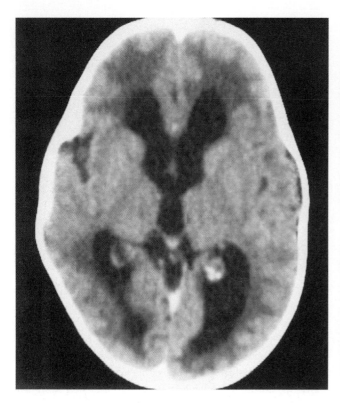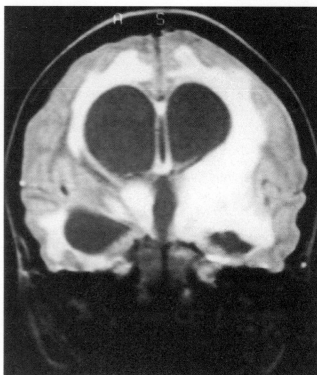

Fig. 7.8. Transependymal CSF resorption in active hydrocephalus. *(Left)* CT scan, axial cut, showing areas of decreased attenuation, most prominent around anterior and posterior ventricular horns. *(Right)* MRI, frontal cut, T_2-weighted image. Areas of transependymal absorption give an intense signal.

graphic characteristics of the ventricular walls and the presence of pericerebral effusions (if not located too high) can be verified (Fig. 7.7). Ultrasonography is better associated with another imaging technique (CT or MRI) to permit the continuation of follow-up after closure of the fontanelle and to try to determine the cause of ventricular dilatation.

CT scan allows for assessment of ventricular dilatation and for some rough quantification: measurement of the ventricular surface and of the ventricular surface index (ventricular surface/total surface on the same cut), and of Evan's index (distance between the two caudate nuclei/total width of brain). CT also explores the parenchyma, and the presence of periventricular hypodensities, especially around the anterior and, to a lesser extent, the posterior horns, indicates transependymal CSF absorption and is a good index of progression (Fig. 7.8). CT scan with contrast may help demonstrate the presence of tumours, arachnoiditis or other aetiological abnormalities.

MRI is more precise than CT and the possibility of obtaining multiplanar cuts allows for a detailed study of intracranial anatomy (Britton *et al.* 1988). Transependymal resorption is shown as areas of low T_1 and intense T_2 signal, and the status of myelination can be assessed. There are indications that MRI may permit measurement of CSF volume in the various compartments of the CNS (Condon *et al.* 1986) and also an evaluation of movements of fluid within the head.

Measurement of CSF pressure can be through the open fontanelle (Plandsoen *et al.* 1986, Bunegin *et al.* 1987), but intracranial determination is more reliable, if invasive, and may

be resorted to when other means of determining the progression of hydrocephalus have failed (Fig. 7.9). In some centres it has become a routine part of the management, although it can certainly be dispensed with in most cases. Normal pressure in the reclining patients is 50–120 mmH$_2$O at the level of the foramen of Monro. In the standing position it becomes negative (average = –50 mmH$_2$O). It fluctuates during the sleep–waking cycle with plateau waves of about 100 mmH$_2$O every 50–75 minutes during REM sleep (Miller 1991), and it appears that high plateau waves even with a normal resting pressure indicate that hydrocephalus is not arrested (Minns 1984, Allen 1986).

Techniques for the assessment of CSF dynamics, especially aqueductal CSF flow, have been developed (Nitz *et al.* 1992, Quencer 1992, Curless *et al.* 1992) but are not yet used as a routine investigation.

Assessment of blood flow velocity, which varies in inverse relationship to ICP (Goh and Minns 1993), is of interest as it is indicative of brain vascularization.

The *EEG* may be normal or slowed, and with high ICP may show runs of anterior delta waves, irrespective of the cause.

Auditory brainstem potentials are frequently abnormal, perhaps indicating a special sensitivity of this part of the brain to increased pressure.

DIFFERENTIAL DIAGNOSIS
The diagnosis of hydrocephalus has been considerably simplified by the availability of neuroimaging, especially sonography in young infants and CT/MRI at all ages.

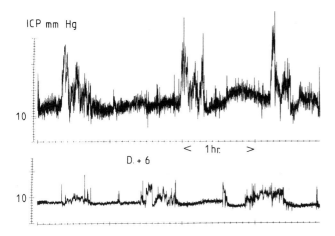

Fig. 7.9. Intracranial pressure curve in chronic hydrocephalus. Upper trace (preoperative) shows mild elevation of CSF pressure above 10 mmHg and very high peaks up to 40–50 mmHg, synchronous with phases of REM sleep. Lower trace (postoperative) shows normalization of basal pressure and low plateau waves. (Courtesy Prof. C. Sainte-Rose, Hôpital des Enfants Malades, Paris.)

In *older children* with symptoms and signs of increased ICP, the diagnostic evaluation is similar to that for tumour suspects (Chapter 14).

In *infants and younger children*, the problem is usually that of a large or enlarging head, often without symptoms. Causes of *macrocephaly*, aside from hydrocephalus and pericerebral collections, have been discussed in Chapter 3 (see Table 3.5, p. 92) and are easily diagnosed by neuroimaging. Agenesis of the corpus callosum is associated with ventricular enlargement, especially of the occipital and temporal horns. MRI shows incomplete development of the hippocampus (Baker and Barkovitch 1992).

Pericerebral collections are discussed later in this chapter. Such collections may be associated with some degree of ventricular dilatation thought to be secondary to the compression of the subarachnoid space. This secondary hydrocephalus usually disappears after treatment of the subdural effusion. The imaging appearance permits an easy differentiation.

The same applies to the *rapid head growth* that is often observed in *preterm or small for gestional age infants*, usually starting between 30 and 40 days of age (Sher and Brown 1975a,b). It is therefore important to use appropriate tables (Babson and Benda 1976, Raymond and Holmes 1994). When in doubt, sonograpy provides a rapid and precise answer. A similar phenomenon is sometimes observed in older infants up to 2–3 years of age when rapid 'catch-up' growth follows a prolonged period of caloric deprivation. Rapid growth can be associated with an increase in width of the pericerebral fluid spaces, and separation of the sutures may occur. Large congenital tumours can give rise to a large head mimicking hydrocephalus but imaging is totally different (Chapter 14).

In fact, real difficulties only arise in three sets of circumstances: one is represented by some cases of *brain atrophy*. Although, in principle, the head should be small in such cases, this does not universally apply and the head circumference can

be normal or even mildly increased. Whether this is related to a previous period of high CSF pressure cannot be determined in many cases. Pressure measurements in some such children have given normal figures.

The severity of neurodevelopmental defects is much greater in these cases than in true hydrocephalus. Moreover, brain imaging indicates that the distention of the ventricular system predominates in the frontal horns (Barth 1984), whereas in true hydrocephalus, dilatation is virtually always more marked in the temporal and occipital horns, at least early on. A combination of true hydrocephalus and atrophy may be seen in some patients. In such cases a marked dilatation of the anterior part of the lateral ventricles should lead one to suspect an associated destructive lesion process (Naidich 1989).

The second circumstance in which serious diagnostic difficulties arise is in infants who have had an intracranial haemorrhage or in infants or children following the acute state of bacterial meningitis. Repeated sonographic or CT scan examinations may be necessary before it can be decided whether one is dealing with acute temporary ventricular distension or progressive hydrocephalus. It should be noted that a considerable degree of ventricular dilatation can take place in preterm infants with obstructive hydrocephalus before any increase in head circumference is detectable.

A third difficulty is in distinguishing between arrested and slowly progressive hydrocephalus. Serial examinations, repeat neuroimaging studies and, in some cases, ICP monitoring can all be necessary to reach a decision. In infants, the ICP may be relatively normal even in the presence of progressive hydrocephalus because of the high compliance of the soft brain and unfused skull sutures. Continuous ICP recording in such cases often shows relatively normal basal pressure with abnormally high plateau waves (Di Rocco *et al.* 1975) especially during REM sleep (Pierre-Kahn *et al.* 1976). Therefore, many cases of hydrocephalus at this age are cases of 'normal pressure hydrocephalus', but the concept, as it applies to adults with disturbances of sphincter control and ambulation and progressive dementia, is not applicable to infants.

TREATMENT OF HYDROCEPHALUS
The treatment of hydrocephalus has been radically modified by the introduction of extracranial shunting procedures. Although these are by far the most common form of treatment they do not necessarily apply to the management of every case. The aims of treatment may include not only the diversion of CSF, but also the reduction of CSF production by medical or surgical means and the suppression of the cause of high CSF pressure.

INDICATIONS FOR TREATMENT
Medical treatment is rarely considered except in slowly progressive hydrocephalus and in the specific case of posthaemorrhagic hydrocephalus in preterm infants (see below).

As discussed previously, the decision to operate on a patient with hydrocephalus may not be easy because arrested hydrocephalus, even though it is rare, does exist and because complications of treatment are far from negligible. It seems reasonable to defer operation in infants over 3 years of age with apparently arrested hydrocephalus when intellectual performance is within normal limits and seems stable (McLone and Aronyk 1993). In younger children, the trend is to place a shunt because of the danger for normal development posed by persistent hydrocephalus.

The borderline between hydrocephalus and acute ventricular dilatation following haemorrhage or meningitis is difficult to draw, and various medical treatments such as drugs or repeated lumbar punctures have been used in such situations (Chapter 2).

The treatment of hydrocephalus in preterm infants following neonatal intraventricular haemorrhage poses a difficult problem. Shunts in such infants are technically difficult to place, and dysfunction and infection are frequent, especially when the CSF has a high protein content (Hislop *et al.* 1988). In addition, nonprogressive hydrocephalus is frequent and the course is unpredictable (Kreusser *et al.* 1984, Dykes *et al.* 1989).

For these reasons, alternative forms of treatment, especially repeated lumbar punctures (Ventriculomegaly Trial Group 1994) and external drainage (Kreusser *et al.* 1984), have been tried in infants with progressive hydrocephalus, as shown by weekly ultrasound examination and/or enlarging head (>2cm/week). The results of repeated lumbar punctures have been generally disappointing. Ninety per cent of children had poor mental development and the infection rate was 7 per cent in the Ventriculomegaly Trial Group study. External drainage usually does not remove the need for an internal shunt, and the risk of infection is not negligible. However, it may allow a delay in the placing of a shunt until the medical condition of the infant is less precarious (Kreusser *et al.* 1984).

The decision for surgical treatment may also be difficult in patients with long-standing hydrocephalus, spastic diplegia and neurodevelopmental problems. The degree of reversibility of such abnormalities is not really known. On the other hand, insidious deterioration certainly occurs in many cases, and surgical treatment is indicated whenever there is doubt about the progression of the disorder.

TREATMENT OF THE CAUSE
This applies to hydrocephalus secondary to space-occupying processes. Removal of a brain tumour will reestablish a normal CSF circulation. However, postoperative bleeding and aseptic meningitis may lead to the development of adhesions that will maintain active hydocephalus. Although some neurosurgeons advise shunting preliminary to tumour removal, a majority prefer to shunt only postoperatively when necessary. Excision or shunting of an arachnoid cyst is also a form of aetiological treatment but will be considered with shunting techniques.

MEDICAL TREATMENT
There is no satisfactory drug for hydrocephalus. *Acetazolamide* (up to 100 mg/kg/day) and *furosemide* (1 mg/kg/day) can reduce CSF production in humans by about 30 per cent (Bergman *et al.* 1980). *Isosorbide* also increases osmotic resorption of CSF. These drugs are mainly used as a temporizing measure, especially

in cases in which a decision about surgical intervention is uncertain and can be deferred for some time.

SURGICAL TREATMENT
Ventriculocisternostomy
In cases of isolated aqueductal stenosis a satisfactory circulation of CSF can be restored by establishing a patent communication between the anterior recess of the third ventricle and the chiasmatic cistern. The operation is possible in patients with a markedly dilated anterior recess that can be opened with a leukotome or ventriculoscope behind the posterior clinoid. Ventriculocisternostomy is effective in reducing intracranial hypertension but usually leaves a persistent dilatation of the ventricles (Hoffman *et al.* 1981, Hirsch 1982, Jaksche and Loew 1986). It avoids the problem of post-shunt pericerebral collections in patients with a large skull. Ventriculostomy should not be performed in patients with postmeningitic or posthaemorrhagic stenosis as these are likely to have some degree of basilar and/or convexity block.

Ventriculocisternostomy in a modified form (ventriculocystostomy) may be the treatment of choice for some types of intracranial cysts associated with hydrocephalus, especially suprasellar cysts (Pierre-Kahn *et al.* 1990a; see Chapter 14) and incisural cysts. In such cases, the operation may avoid a pressure dysequilibrium between the ventricular system and the cyst which can be responsible for postoperative dilatation of either cavity.

Shunting operations
These techniques aim at diverting the CSF that cannot reach its normal areas of resorption towards another site of drainage. This is achieved by inserting a unidirectional valve system with a specified level of opening pressure between a proximal catheter placed in the ventricular system (or other fluid-containing cavity) and a distal catheter that carries the outflow of the valve to the draining site.

Under special circumstances, for instance when there is infection of the CSF or the fluid is haemorrhagic and might obstruct the system, the distal catheter may be temporarily drained into a sterile pouch, external to the patient. *External drainage* is limited by the risk of infection and the consequent necessity to maintain the patient in strict aseptic conditions.

Internal shunts have become the standard treatment in the vast majority of cases of hydrocephalus. Numerous catheters and valve systems are available with different mechanisms and hydrodynamic characteristics. Residual ICP after shunting will depend on the opening pressure of the valve or the pressure within the drainage cavity and on the resistance of the shunt. Available valves are classified into low-pressure (opening pressure 20–50 mmH$_2$0), mid-pressure (50–80 mmH$_2$0) and high-pressure valves (80–120 mmH$_2$0). The flow once the valve is open will be determined by the ratio of the differential pressure between the two extremities of the system to its resistance. Most systems have a constant resistance so that the standing position inevitably produces overdrainage. Variable resistance systems have been proposed (review in Sainte-Rose *et al.* 1987) in order to avoid such problems.

Currently, drainage is generally into the peritoneal cavity (ventriculoperitoneal shunt), because this form of shunt is easier to insert and does not need lengthening with growth of the patient since a considerable length of catheter may be left within the peritoneum without serious problems (McComb 1983a). Ventriculoatrial shunts are now used only when the peritoneum does not absorb enough fluid or in cases of peritoneal or intraperitoneal infection.

In some patients, for instance those with the Dandy–Walker syndrome, the proximal shunt may be placed in the fourth ventricle rather than in the lateral ventricle.

Most systems include an inbuilt reservoir, placed subcutaneously over the skull, which theoretically allows shunt functioning to be assessed by pumping the reservoir. In fact, the correlation between response to pumping and functioning of the shunt is poor. According to Piatt (1992) only 18–20 per cent of blocked shunts cannot be pumped, and the ability to pump indicates shunt patency in only 65–81 per cent of cases. There is thus no simple manoeuvre for assessing shunt functioning. For this reason, some surgeons always use a separate fluid reservoir for pressure measurement and fluid collection (Leggate *et al.* 1988).

Lumboperitoneal and other shunts are now only rarely used. Some surgeons employ them for the treatment of pseudotumour cerebri. The catheter is introduced into the lumbar subarachnoid space and anchored to the lumbar fascia. The tube is then fed through a subcutaneous tunnel to exit through a small incision in the loin. Then, with or without interposition of a valve, the catheter is fed into another subcutaneous tunnel to the paraumbilical area where it is introduced into the peritoneal cavity as a ventriculoperitoneal catheter.

• *Incidents and accidents of internal CSF shunts.* In spite of considerable progress in the development and techniques of use of CSF shunts, numerous complications can and do occur (Hirsch and Hoppe-Hirsch 1988, Sainte-Rose *et al.* 1989, Di Rocco *et al.* 1994). They are more common in infancy and following operation for aqueductal stenosis (Di Rocco *et al.* 1994). Table 7.5 lists the main complications of shunts. *Infection* remains a serious complication of shunt procedures. Its incidence varies between 4 and 8 per cent in published series (Renier *et al.* 1984, Ammirati and Raimondi 1987, Hirsch and Hoppe-Hirsch 1988, Di Rocco *et al.* 1994) but is now declining. The rate is higher in infants under 6 months of age. The infecting organism is *Staphylococcus epidermidis* in half the cases, *S. aureus* in a quarter and gram-negative organisms in about a fifth (Bayston 1994). Rare pathogens may colonize shunts (Chapter 11). Infection is usually an early complication but can occur months or years after operation. Meningitis is the dominant infection (almost two-thirds of cases), while peritonitis occurs in about 20 per cent and wound infection in over 10 per cent. The clinical picture is often insidious, especially when *S. epidermidis* is the cause, and the diagnosis may be difficult, especially when eosinophilia is the prominent CSF anomaly (Vinchon *et al.* 1992). Death is possible, especially with gram-negative meningitis. Localized peritoneal infection can lead to ulceration of the bowel with exteriorization of the catheter through the anus. Septicaemia has become rare since ventriculoatrial shunt is now uncommon. The same applies to shunt nephritis (Wald and McLaurin 1978) and to cor pulmonale (Sleigh *et al.* 1993).

Prevention of infection by strict aseptic measures is essential (Hirsch and Hoppe-Hirsch 1988). Prophylactic antibiotics seem to reduce shunt infections and should be given on the day of operation and the following day (Haines and Taylor 1982, Hoffman *et al.* 1982a). Treatment of established infection includes aggressive antibiotic therapy for 10–20 days on average after removal of the shunt. The shunt is reinserted when CSF cultures are sterile and CSF glucose back to normal. Some authors advocate initial antibiotic treatment for five to six days before removal, and immediate replacement of the shunt. Antibiotics are then continued for two to three weeks (Hirsch and Hoppe-Hirsch 1988). In an occasional case antibiotic treatment with injections into the shunt may sterilize the CSF (Frame and McLaurin 1984, Bayston 1994). Removal of the shunt seems to give the lowest mortality (James *et al.* 1982). On the other hand, the incidental ocurrence of *Haemophilus influenzae* meningitis in a shunted child can often be successfully treated without removing the shunt (Rennels and Wald 1980). Peritonitis is usually cured by antibiotic therapy and removal of the infected catheter. Surgery is rarely necessary. Low-grade infection with formation of intraperitoneal cysts can be detected with the help of sonography (Briggs *et al.* 1984).

Shunt failure can result from primary misplacement of the shunt. In such cases, parenchymal haemorrhage, traumatic puncture of the internal capsule or puncture porencephaly can be responsible for hemiplegic sequelae (Boltshauser *et al.* 1980).

Most commonly, shunt failure occurs in correctly placed shunts. In the series of Sainte-Rose *et al.* (1989), 81 per cent of 1620 shunts had failed by 12 years after insertion. The risk of failure was highest, at 30 per cent, in the first postoperative year. Disappointingly, the risk was 7–14 per cent for each subsequent year and there was no indication of a trend toward improvement with time. *Blockage* of the shunt was the cause of failure in half the cases, most frequently at the ventricular end. *Migration, disconnection and fracture* were next in frequency, being observed in 14 per cent of cases. The mortality related to shunt failures was 1 per cent, and the incidence of subsequent epilepsy and of recurrent shunt failure was significantly increased. The symptoms and signs of obstruction may be overt or insidious. Parents should be advised to report immediately bouts of headaches or vomiting, lethargy, or the development of diplopia or other neurological signs.

In other patients, only vague symptoms and behavioural changes are present such as decreased spontaneity or poor school performance, perhaps in association with mild headaches. Still other children have intermittent shunt obstruction.

Sudden death can occur (Hyden *et al.* 1983), hence the need for rapid hospitalization. Nonfunctioning shunts need not be symptomatic. In the experience of Hayden *et al.* (1983), 23 per cent of 307 patients with nonfunctional shunts remained

TABLE 7.5
Main complications of ventricular shunts

Infection
Septicaemia (only with ventriculoatrial shunts)
Meningitis
Peritonitis
Shunt nephritis (only with ventriculoatrial shunts)
Wound infection

Primary misplacement
Intracranial
Intra-abdominal
Intravascular
Puncture porencephaly

Blockage and underdrainage
Proximal obstruction by choroid plexus, brain tissue, meninges, ependyma, pathological tissue or foreign material
Distal obstruction of abdominal or atrial catheter; development of intra-abdominal cyst; CSF ascites

Fractures of catheter or connectors

Migration of catheter
In hollow viscera (intestine, bladder, stomach)
In inguinal canal with hydrocele; coiling around intestine with intestinal obstruction
Isolated ventricles—especially trapped 4th ventricles with secondary stenosis of the sylvian aqueduct

Overdrainage
Intracranial hypotension
Shunt dependency
Post-shunt pericerebral collections
Slit ventricle syndrome
Post-shunt craniostenosis
Stenosis of the spinal canal

Epilepsy

---

asymptomatic for an average of 27 months. The diagnosis of blocked shunt is often difficult, and various techniques of assessment have been proposed, such as measurement of the Doppler pulsatility index (Pople *et al.* 1991) and MR flow study (Frank *et al.* 1990). Watkins *et al.* (1994) showed that a normal CT scan does not exclude blockage; percutaneous manometry in 26 cases gave no false positives or negatives but the results were equivocal in five children.

Migration of catheters following rupture of connectors may be particularly difficult to diagnose as CSF often continues to flow along the subcutaneous fibrous tunnel for prolonged periods.

Cortical visual impairment is a complication of shunt dysfunction. It is probably due to compression of the posterior cerebral arteries by the tentorium when there is a sudden increase of ventricular size with resultant downward displacement of the brain. CT scan shows bilateral occipital infarcts (Arroyo *et al.* 1985).

Isolated ventricles are due to blockage between the involved ventricle and the ventricular end of the shunt. They mainly involve the fourth ventricle (Coker and Anderson 1989), rarely the third ventricle (Darnell and Arbit 1993), and may be especially frequent when hydrocephalus in the Dandy–Walker syndrome is treated with lateral ventricle shunting (Hirsch and

Hoppe-Hirsch 1988). Blockage may also present as unilateral hydrocephalus following secondary obstruction of the foramen of Monro (Tamaki *et al.* 1985) or even affect only the temporal horn of one ventricle (Maurice-Williams and Choksey 1986). This complication is apt to occur after multiple shunt revisions (Coker and Anderson 1989). Overdrainage is also an important factor in the mechanism of trapped ventricles (Sainte-Rose *et al.* 1989). A trapped fourth ventricle can behave as any space-occupying posterior fossa lesion and requires placement of an additional shunt within the cavity. The diagnosis by neuroimaging is straightforward.

Overdrainage is a frequent complication of ventriculo-peritoneal shunts because of the 'siphon effect' that occurs in the upright position, due to the height of the hydrostatic column between the inlet and the outlet of the shunt. In standing patients, the draining capacity of the shunt exceeds the ventricular CSF secretion rate and overdrainage is constant. Overdrainage is more important with low-resistance valves (spring-ball type or silicone rubber diaphragm type) than with high-resistance valves (silicone rubber slit types).

Complications of overdrainage include subdural effusions, slit ventricle syndrome, orthostatic CSF hypotension, cranio-synostosis and shunt dependency (Gruber 1981, Kiekens *et al.* 1982, Serlo *et al.* 1985). Intracranial hypotension occurs especially after lumboperitoneal shunts (Rando and Fishman 1992) and can be responsible for headaches, vertigo and vomiting. MRI may show striking dural enhancement with gadolinium (Fishman and Dillon 1993, Pannulo *et al.* 1993, Mokri *et al.* 1995). The same phenomenon has also been reported following lumbar puncture (Krause *et al.* 1997). In rare cases, prolonged hypotension may result in spinal canal stenosis (Kobayashi and Hashi 1983). Overdrainage is also one of the causal factors of isolated ventricles (Matsumoto and Oi 1985, Tamaki *et al.* 1985) and may be associated with an increased incidence of epilepsy.

Post-shunt pericerebral collections occur in about 3 per cent of shunted patients but are symptomatic in only half the cases (Hoppe-Hirsch *et al.* 1987). A simple treatment is insertion of a valveless shunt into the subdural cavity draining it to the peritoneum in order to establish a temporary lower pressure in the subdural space than in the ventricle.

Slit ventricles are seen in about 20 per cent of cases but most remain asymptomatic. The slit ventricle syndrome is characterized by recurrent signs of increased ICP, due to intermittent obstruction of the shunt by the walls of the ventricle. It may also manifest as chronic headache (Epstein *et al.* 1978). CT scan shows only slightly larger ventricles in the presence of shunt obstruction than with a functioning shunt. This is because the slit ventricles are also usually stiff ventricles, in part because of the loss of CSF volumetric buffering reserve, necessary for instance in the case of vasodilatation, and in part because of periventricular gliosis as a result of previous infections and gliosis impairing reexpansion of previously collapsed ventricles (Hyde-Rowan *et al.* 1982). Prevention of the slit ventricle syndrome is difficult. Various techniques have been proposed such as antisiphon valves or constant flow valves (Sainte-Rose 1987).

Orthostatic CSF hypotension and shunt dependency are often associated with the presence of slit ventricles. They can be associated with headaches or behavioural changes but are more commonly asymptomatic. It sems that about 85 per cent of shunted patients will have to keep a shunt in place all their lives, and there is no simple means of determining in which patients the shunt can be removed despite the fact that various techniques have been proposed (Hayden *et al.* 1983). There is no reason to remove a shunt in asymptomatic patients, even if it is thought to be nonfunctional, as this can result in intracranial hypertension.

Post-shunt craniosynostoses (Kloss 1968) are in most cases limited to the premature fusion of the sagittal suture with resulting scaphocephaly. Only exceptionally do post-shunt synostoses represent more than a purely cosmetic problem, requiring surgical correction.

Epilepsy has been reported to be more common in shunted patients than in unoperated ones (Copeland *et al.* 1982). Ines and Markand (1977) found the frequency of seizures to be 18.2 per cent before operation and 65.4 per cent after. In a study of 171 patients, Di Rocco *et al.* (1985) found that 34 (19.9 per cent) had seizures, 25 of these having had fits before surgery. Saukkonen *et al.* (1990) reported that 48 per cent of their 168 shunt-treated patients had seizures, regardless of the aetiology of hydrocephalus. They were of the opinion that the mere presence of a shunt device in the brain parenchyma is of relatively little importance. Infections and parenchymal damage due to the cause of hydrocephalus were associated with an increased seizure rate as were multiple surgical procedures. High ICP may be a factor favouring the emergence of epilepsy (Faillace and Canady 1990).

COMPLICATIONS UNRELATED TO SHUNT PROCEDURES

These are rarely observed now as virtually all cases of definitely progressive hydrocephalus are shunted. However, some complications can develop insidiously before treatment, including *hemiplegia*. There is an established relationship between hydrocephalus and the hemiplegic type of cerebral palsy. In 28 cases of cerebral palsy secondary to hydrocephalus investigated by O'Reilly and Walentynowicz (1981), 11 were of the hemiplegic type. In rare cases a *puncture porencephaly* can develop along the track of a ventricular needle or of a nonfunctioning catheter. In other children, hemiplegia may result from ependymal rupture with CSF dissection into the centrum semi-ovale (Russell 1949) or from the development of a *diverticulum of the lateral ventricle*, located in most cases at the level of the trigone on the internal aspect of the hemisphere, that may enter the posterior fossa (Adams 1975, Naidich *et al.* 1982). Such diverticula may rupture into cisternal spaces and realize a spontaneous ventriculo-cisternostomy with stabilization of the hydrocephalus. Occasional complications of unoperated hydrocephalus include *intra-ventricular haemorrhage* in the case of rapidly evolutive hydrocephalus, and *hydrosyringomyelia* as a consequence of stabilized hydrocephalus (Olson and Milstein 1988). The latter may be associated with marked scoliosis that may improve with treatment of the hydrocephalus.

OUTCOME

Before the introduction of shunt treatment, less than half of liveborn term infants with hydrocephalus survived (Foltz and Shurtleff 1963), whereas currently the mortality rate is between 10 and 15 per cent (Fernell *et al.* 1986, 1994). At the same time, the characteristic sequelae of chronic untreated hydrocephalus have all but disappeared (Ingram and Naughton 1962). In a recent series (Fernell *et al.* 1988), the frequency of ataxic cerebral palsy had fallen to 8 per cent and that of other forms of cerebral palsy to 18 per cent. Mild mental retardation occurred in 21 per cent and severe retardation in 16 per cent. Epilepsy was present in 25 per cent of survivors and visual difficulties with optic atrophy in 11 per cent. The incidence of the 'cocktail party syndrome' (Hagberg 1962, Tew 1979) was only 3 per cent as compared with a frequency of 27 per cent in the preshunting era. It seems likely that cerebral palsy other than the ataxic form, mental retardation, epilepsy and precocious puberty, none of which has decreased significantly since shunting was introduced, are attributable mainly to the brain pathology associated with hydrocephalus. In contrast, ataxia, squint and the cocktail party syndrome seem more directly related to unchecked long-standing intracranial hypertension and ventricular distension. Similar results are found in most series (Riva *et al.* 1994).

Results of shunting operations are still far from fully satisfactory. Kokkonen *et al.* (1994) had seven deaths among 42 children, and five of the survivors were institutionalized for severe mental impairment. Only one-third of these patients had vocational training while a quarter stayed at home without meaningful activity. In the recent series of Mori *et al.* (1995), 22 per cent of 1450 patients had mental retardation. Poor results were correlated with age and cause of hydrocephalus (see below), with the presence of epilepsy, of shunt complications and delay in their treatment, and with the degree of ventricular dilatation before shunt.

Even in children with shunted hydrocephalus who develop relatively normally, there is an overrepresentation of clumsiness and poor motor coordination. In most cases, the results on performance scales of IQ tests are lower than those on the verbal items (Billard *et al.* 1987, Fernell *et al.* 1988).

It is still unclear whether treatment should aim at achieving a normal ventricular size. Overall, children with moderate or severe ventricular dilatation do less well than those with normal sized ventricles (Fernell *et al.* 1988). However, a number of factors can be responsible for ventricular dilatation such as operational delay and associated atrophy, and there may be little correlation between ventricular size and intellectual function (Lonton 1979). Some patients who have a very large head and a thin cerebral mantle may be quite normal. Multivariate analysis of prognostic factors indicates that ventricular dilatation in itself explains only 20 per cent of the ultimate variance of the results. Children with large ventricular size after shunting seem to do less well on nonverbal and visuospatial function tests, but the rest of their functions seem normal when aetiology and age at operation are taken into account (Billard *et al.* 1987).

The cause of hydrocephalus and the age of presentation are major prognostic factors (Hirsch 1994).

Fetal hydrocephalus has a particularly poor outcome (Mori *et al.* 1995). Preterm infants with ventricular haemorrhage currently represent a large group with a rather poor prognosis. Hislop *et al.* (1988) found that of 19 infants shunted for posthaemorrhagic ventricular dilatation, 14 developed shunt complications and several had severe sequelae such as hypsar-rhythmia and infantile spasms. Seventy-three per cent of the very preterm infants studied by Fernell *et al.* (1994) developed cerebral palsy, 55 per cent had mental retardation, 52 per cent epilepsy and 22 per cent severe visual impairment. The prognosis is largely determined by the presence of other lesions associated with intraventricular haemorrhage such as periventricular leuko-malacia (Ventriculomegaly Trial Group 1994). These are much more difficult to detect by ultrasonography than are haemorrhages (Hope *et al.* 1988), so that the outcome may be difficult to predict.

Patients with postmeningitic or toxoplasmic hydrocephalus also do rather poorly because of the usual occurrence in such cases of diffuse brain damage. It is difficult in many cases to assess the role of high pressure itself irrespective of the cause.

A significant part of the sequelae are no doubt due to repeated episodes of shunt dysfunction, and improvement of the material and methods of shunting is a high priority. Prevention of hydro-cephalus can be achieved by measures such as earlier and better treatment of bacterial meningitis and prevention of haemorrhage. Prevention of preterm birth is a major target, as it is among small preterm infants that the majority and the most severe cases of hydrocephalus occur.

NONTRAUMATIC PERICEREBRAL COLLECTIONS

Nontraumatic pericerebral collections of fluid represent one of the most common causes of large head in infants and children. Since the widespread use of modern neuroimaging, they have been recognized both in symptomatic and asymptomatic patients and can be divided into two broad groups: symptomatic cases that are associated with brain damage or genetic syndromes, and cryptogenetic cases that have been variously designated as benign subdural collections (Robertson *et al.* 1979, Briner and Boden-steiner 1980, Rothenberger and Brandl 1980), benign external hydrocephalus (Kendall and Holland 1981, Alvarez *et al.* 1986, Maytal *et al.* 1987), and benign extracerebral or extraaxial collections (Carolan *et al.* 1985/86, Hamza *et al.* 1987). Reported frequencies for these groups vary. Symptomatic cases accounted for 13 of 94 patients (14 per cent) in the series of Hamza *et al.* (1987) and for 36 of 63 patients (57 per cent) in that of Alvarez *et al.* (1986).

The exact location of fluid is controversial. Those authors who think these effusions are within the subarachnoid space (Ment *et al.* 1981) speculate that there is impairment of CSF re-sorption into the venous system as a result of increased venous pressure or increased resistance of the arachnoid villi (Barlow 1984). Other investigators are of the opinion that the fluid is collected in the subdural space and that its persistence may be explained by a subarachnoid–subdural fistula with a one-way

valve effect (Baraton *et al.* 1989) or by other, undefined mechanisms. Baraton *et al.* have shown that contrast injected into the lumbar space in 26 cases never contaminated the pericerebral collections but remained limited to the anterior part of the subarachnoid space underneath the pericerebral collection which is therefore subdural. It is likely that both subdural and subarachnoid collections occur.

The fluid is usually clear and the protein level normal or only slightly elevated. Ventricular dilatation of variable, but usually mild, degree may be associated.

PERICEREBRAL COLLECTIONS OF KNOWN CAUSE
These are usually associated with ICP and some degree of internal hydrocephalus.

ABNORMAL VENOUS RETURN
This is an obvious cause of increased venous pressure within the cranium. Abnormal constriction and/or aberrant venous pathways rarely exist in isolation, but they may be associated with certain types of craniosynostosis (Sainte-Rose *et al.* 1984, Tanaka *et al.* 1985). Thrombosis of the superior vena cava, of jugular veins or of intracranial sinuses may also be a cause. Vena cava thrombosis is most often caused by indwelling central catheters used for drug infusion or parenteral feeding (Couch *et al.* 1985). Hydroceph-alus from such causes is virtually always mixed internal and external. The 'external part' may however actually be within the subdural space. Increase in pressure from large arteriovenous malformations, especially aneurysms of the vein of Galen, also pro-duce external as well as internal hydrocephalus (Lamas *et al.* 1977).

ACHONDROPLASIA
This disease is regularly associated with external hydrocephalus as well as ventricular dilatation (Pierre-Kahn *et al.* 1980, Yamada *et al.* 1981). Increase in venous pressure is due to narrowing of the basal venous foramina. Such narrowing may also prevent dampening of CSF pulse pressure waves by immediate outflow of blood from the cranium (Naidich 1989). Treatment of external hydrocephalus of venous origin is based on reduction of venous pressure by cure of its cause or by bypass operation (Sainte-Rose *et al.* 1984).

CRYPTOGENIC PERICEREBRAL COLLECTIONS
Cryptogenic pericerebral effusions are manifested clinically by a large head. All affected children have head circumference above the 95th centile by 1 year of age. Eventually, velocity of head growth decreases and the head growth curve becomes parallel to the normal growth pattern (Pettit *et al.* 1980) or tends toward normal. This phenomenon may be particularly striking in preterm infants. In 12 such patients followed by Al-Saedi *et al.* (1996), the head circumference stabilized between 15 and 18 months at the 95th centile.

There are usually no abnormal neurological signs, but motor and sometimes language development may be delayed (Alvarez *et al.* 1986).

The radiological signs include moderate enlargement of the pericerebral spaces especially in the frontal or frontoparietal regions bilaterally and symmetrically, with interhemispheric sulcus dilatation extending posteriorly to the middle third of the brain (Briner and Bodensteiner 1980, Rothenberger and Brandl 1980, Maytal *et al.* 1987).

Although the causes of cryptogenic effusion are, by definition, unknown, a relationship to simple megalencephaly (Lorber and Priestley 1981, Gooskens *et al.* 1988) has been suggested. Alvarez *et al.* (1986) found a family history of large head in 32 of their 36 cases and suggested the existence of a continuum between collections and the familial megalencephaly studied by Day and Schutt (1979). The occurrence of 'external hydrocephalus' in twins has been reported (Cundall *et al.* 1989).

The diagnosis of cryptogenic pericerebral effusion should exclude all known causes, particularly chronic traumatic subdural haematoma (Chapter 13), venous hypertension, and various genetic syndromes such as the Sotos, Beckwith–Wiedemann, Goldenhar and Weaver syndromes (Alvarez *et al.* 1986). The large clear pericerebral space present in preterm infants is physiological.

The course of pericerebral collections is usually benign. A few patients are left with mild or, rarely, moderate mental retardation (Nickel and Gallenstein 1987, Hamza *et al.* 1987). Although surgical treatment has sometimes been performed (Andersson *et al.* 1984), spontaneous resorption is the rule and no treatment is justified.

REFERENCES

Adams, C., Johnston, W.P., Nevin, N.C. (1982) 'A family study of congenital hydrocephalus.' *Developmental Medicine and Child Neurology*, 24, 493–498.

Adams, R.D. (1975) 'Diverticulation of the cerebral ventricles. A cause of progressive focal encephalopathy.' *Developmental Medicine and Child Neurology*, Suppl. 35, 17, 135–137.

Aleksic, S., Budzilovich, G., Greco, A., *et al.* (1984) 'Neural defects in Say–Gerald (Vater) syndrome.' *Child's Brain*, 11, 255–260.

Allen, R. (1986) 'Intracranial pressure: a review of clinical problems, measurement techniques and monitoring methods.' *Journal of Medical Engineering and Technology*, 10, 299–320.

Al-Saedi, S.A., Lemke, R.P., Debooy, V.D., Casiro, O. (1996) 'Subarachnoid fluid collections: a cause of macrocrania in preterm infants.' *Journal of Pediatrics*, 128, 234–236.

Alvarez, L.A., Maytal, J., Shinnar, S. (1986) 'Idiopathic external hydrocephalus: natural history and relationship to benign familial macrocephaly.' *Pediatrics*, 77, 901–907.

Ammirati, M., Raimondi, A.J. (1987) 'Cerebrospinal fluid shunt infections in children. A study on the relationship between the etiology of hydrocephalus, age at the time of shunt placement, and infection rate.' *Child's Nervous System*, 3, 106–109.

Andersson, H., Elfverson, J., Svendsen, P. (1984) 'External hydrocephalus in infants.' *Child's Brain*, 11, 398–402.

Arroyo, H.A., Jan, J.E., McCormick, A.Q., Farrell, K. (1985) 'Permanent visual loss after shunt malfunction.' *Neurology*, 35, 25–29.

Babson, S.G., Benda, G.I. (1976) 'Growth graphs for the clinical assessment of infants of varying gestational age.' *Journal of Pediatrics*, 89, 814–820.

Baker, L.L., Barkovich, A.J. (1992) 'The large temporal horn: MR analysis in developmental brain anomalies versus hydrocephalus.' *American Journal of Neuroradiology*, 13, 115–122.

Balestrazzi, P., De Gressi, S., Donadio, A., Lenzini, S. (1989) 'Periaqueductal gliosis causing hydrocephalus in a patient with neurofibromatosis type 1.' *Neurofibromatosis*, 2, 322–325.

Baraton, J., Brunelle, F., Pierre-Kahn, A., *et al.* (1989) 'Tomodensitométrie couplée à la cisternographie dans les épanchements péri-cérébraux chroniques du jeune enfant.' *Neurochirurgie*, 35, 395–400.

Barkovich, A.J., Kjos, B.B., Norman, D. (1989) 'Revised classification of posterior fossa cysts and cystlike malformations based on the results of multiplanar MR imaging.' *American Journal of Neuroradiology*, 10, 977–988.

Barlow, C.F. (1984) 'CSF dynamics in hydrocephalus. With special attention to external hydrocephalus.' *Brain and Development*, 6, 119–127.

Barros-Nuñes, P., Rivas, F. (1993) 'Autosomal recessive congenital stenosis of aqueduct of Sylvius.' *Genetic Counseling*, 4, 19–23.

Barth, P.G. (1984) 'Prenatal clastic encephalopathies.' *Clinical Neurology and Neurosurgery*, 86, 65–75.

Bayston, R. (1994) 'Hydrocephalus shunt infections.' *Journal of Antimicrobial Chemotherapy*, 34, Suppl. A, 75–84.

Bergman, E.W., Freeman, J., Epstein, M.H. (1980) 'Treatment of infantile hydrocephalus with acetazolamide and furosemide: three-to-four-year follow-up.' *Annals of Neurology*, 8, 227A. *(Abstract.)*

Billard, C., Santini, J.J., Nargeot, M.C., *et al.* (1987) 'Quel avenir pour les enfants hydrocéphales? Pronostic neurologique, visuel et intellectuel d'une série de 77 hydrocéphalies non tumorales.' *Archives Françaises de Pédiatrie*, 44, 849–854.

Bittencourt, P.R.M., Gracia, C.M., Lorenzana, P. (1988) 'Epilepsy and parasitosis of the central nervous system.' *In:* Pedley, T.A., Meldrum, B.S. (Eds.) *Recent Advances in Epilepsy, Vol.4.* Edinburgh: Churchill Livingstone, pp. 123–159.

Boltshauser, E., Hirsig, J., Isler, W., Rickham, P.P. (1980) 'Hemiparesis—an uncommon symptom of hydrocephalus or shunt dysfunction.' *Zeitschrift für Kinderchirurgie und Grenzgebiete*, 30, 191–197.

Bordarier, C., Aicardi, J. (1990) 'Dandy–Walker syndrome and agenesis of the cerebellar vermis: diagnostic problems and genetic counselling.' *Developmental Medicine and Child Neurology*, 32, 285–294.

—— —— Goutières, F. (1984) 'Congenital hydrocephalus and eye abnormalities with severe developmental brain defects: Warburg's syndrome.' *Annals of Neurology*, 16, 60–65.

Bradley, K.C. (1970) 'Cerebrospinal fluid pressure.' *Journal of Neurology, Neurosurgery, and Psychiatry*, 33, 387–397.

Brauner, R., Pierre-Kahn, A., Nemedy-Sandor, E., *et al.* (1987) 'Pubertés précoces par kyste arachnoïdien suprasellaire. Analyse de 6 observations.' *Archives Françaises de Pédiatrie*, 44, 489–493.

Brewer, C.M., Fredericks, B.J., Pont, J.M.W., *et al.* (1996) 'X-linked hydrocephalus masquerading as spina bifida and destructive porencephaly in successive generations of one family.' *Developmental Medicine and Child Neurology*, 38, 632–636.

Briard, M.L., Le Merrer, M., Plauchu, H., *et al.* (1984) 'Association VACTERL et hydrocéphalie: une nouvelle entité familiale.' *Annales de Génétique*, 27, 220–223.

Briggs, J.R., Hendry, G.M.A., Minns, R.A. (1984) 'Abdominal ultrasound in the diagnosis of cerebrospinal fluid pseudocysts complicating ventriculoperitoneal shunts.' *Archives of Disease in Childhood*, 59, 661–664.

Briner, S., Bodensteiner, J. (1980) 'Benign subdural collections of infancy.' *Pediatrics*, 67, 802–804.

Britton, J., Marsh, H., Kendall, B., Kingsley, D. (1988) 'MRI and hydrocephalus in childhood.' *Neuroradiology*, 30, 310–314.

Bunegin, L., Albin, M.S., Rauschhuber, R., Marlin, A.E. (1987) 'Intracranial pressure measurement from the anterior fontanelle utilizing a pneumoelectronic switch.' *Neurosurgery*, 20, 726–731.

Camfield, P.R., Camfield, C.S., Allen, A.C., *et al.* (1981) 'Progressive hydrocephalus in infants with birth weight less than 1500 g.' *Archives of Neurology*, 38, 653–655.

Carolan, P.L., McLaurin, R.L., Towbin, R.B., *et al.* (1985–1986) 'Benign extra-axial collections of infancy.' *Pediatric Neurosciences*, 12, 140–144.

Catala, M., Jeannin, C., Zerah, M., *et al.* (1989) 'Hydrocéphalie congénitale après hémorragie intraventriculaire in utero.' *Revue Neurologique*, 145, 228–230.

Cernerud, L. (1975) 'The setting-sun eye phenomenon in infancy.' *Developmental Medicine and Child Neurology*, 17, 447–455.

Chattha, A.S., Delong, G.R. (1975) 'Sylvian aqueduct syndrome is a sign of acute obstructive hydrocephalus in children.' *Journal of Neurology, Neurosurgery, and Psychiatry*, 38, 288–296.

Chervenak, F., Berkowitz, R.L., Tortora, M., *et al.* (1984) 'Diagnosis of ventriculomegaly before fetal viability.' *Obstetrics and Gynecology*, 64, 652–656.

Civitello, L.A., Packer, R.J., Rorke, L.B., *et al.* (1988) 'Leptomeningeal dissemination of low-grade gliomas in childhood.' *Neurology,* **38,** 562–566.

Coker, S.B., Anderson, C.L. (1989) 'Occluded fourth ventricle after multiple shunt revisions for hydrocephalus.' *Pediatrics,* **83,** 981–985.

Condon, B.R., Patterson, J., Wyper, D., *et al.* (1986) 'A quantitative index of ventricular CSF volumes, using MR imaging.' *Journal of Computer Assisted Tomography,* **10,** 784–792.

Copeland, G.P., Foy, P.M., Shaw, M.D.M. (1982) 'The incidence of epilepsy after ventricular shunting operations.' *Surgical Neurology,* **17,** 279–281.

Couch, R., Camfield, P.R., Tibbles, J.A.R. (1985) 'The changing picture of pseudotumor cerebri in children.' *Canadian Journal of Neurological Sciences,* **12,** 48–50.

Couvreur J., Desmonts, G. (1988) 'Acquired and congenital toxoplasmosis.' *In:* Vinken, P.J., Bruyn, G.W., Klavans, H.L. (Eds.) *Handbook of Clinical Neurology. Revised Series, Vol.8. Microbial Disease.* Amsterdam: Elsevier, pp. 351–363.

Cronqvist, S., Granholm, L., Lundström, N.R. (1972) 'Hydrocephalus and congestive heart failure caused by intracranial arteriovenous malformations in infants.' *Journal of Neurosurgery,* **36,** 249–254.

Cull, C., Wyke, M.A. (1984) 'Memory function of children with spina bifida and shunted hydrocephalus.' *Developmental Medicine and Child Neurology,* **26,** 177–183.

Cundall, D.B., Lamb, J.T., Roussounis, S.H. (1989) 'Identical twins with idiopathic external hydrocephalus.' *Developmental Medicine and Child Neurology,* **31,** 678–681.

Curless, R.G., Quencer, R.M., Katz, D.A., Campanioni, M. (1992) 'Magnetic resonance demonstration of intracranial CSF flow in children.' *Neurology,* **42,** 377–381.

Darnell, R.B., Arbit, E. (1993) 'Reversible diencephalic dysfunction: episodic hyperhidrosis due to a trapped third ventricle.' *Neurology,* **43,** 579–582.

Day, R.E., Schutt, W.H. (1979) 'Normal children with large heads—benign familial megalencephaly.' *Archives of Disease in Childhood,* **54,** 512–517.

De Lange, S.A., De Vlieger, M. (1970) 'Hydrocephalus associated with raised venous pressure.' *Developmental Medicine and Child Neurology,* **12,** Suppl. 22, 28–32.

Diebler, C., Dulac, O. (1987) *Pediatric Neurology and Neuroradiology.* Berlin: Springer.

Dinh, D.H., Wright, R.M., Hanigan, W.C. (1990) 'The use of magnetic resonance imaging for the diagnosis of fetal intracranial anomalies.' *Child's Nervous System,* **6,** 212–215.

Di Rocco, C., McLone, D.G., Shimosi, T., Raimondi, A.J. (1975) 'Continuous intraventricular cerebrospinal fluid pressure recording in hydrocephalic children during wakefulness and sleep.' *Journal of Neurosurgery,* **42,** 683–689.

—— Di Trapani, G. Pettorossi, V.E., Caldarelli, M. (1979) 'On the pathology of experimental hydrocephalus induced by artificial increase in endoventricular CSF pulse pressure.' *Child's Brain,* **5,** 81–95.

—— Caldarelli, M., Di Trapani, G. (1981) 'Infratentorial arachnoid cysts in children.' *Child's Brain,* **8,** 119–133.

—— Iannelli, A., Pallini, R., Rinaldi, A. (1985) 'Epilepsy and its correlation with cerebral ventricular shunting procedures in infantile hydrocephalus.' *Journal of Pediatric Neurosciences,* **1,** 255–263.

—— Cardarelli, M., Ceddia, A. (1989) '"Occult" hydrocephalus in children.' *Child's Nervous System,* **5,** 71–75.

—— Marchese, E., Velardi, F. (1994) 'A survey of the first complication of newly implanted CSF shunt devices for the treatment of nontumoral hydrocephalus. Cooperative survey of the 1991–1992 Education Committee of the ISPN.' *Child's Nervous System,* **10,** 321–327.

Dobyns, W.B. (1993) 'Classification of the cerebro-oculo-muscular syndromes.' *Brain and Development,* **15,** 242–244.

Drugan, A., Krause, B., Canady, A., *et al.* (1989) 'The natural history of prenatally diagnosed ventriculomegaly.' *Journal of the American Medical Association,* **261,** 1785–1788.

Dykes, F.D., Dunbar, B., Lazzara, A., Ahmann, P.A. (1989) 'Posthemorrhagic hydrocephalus in high-risk preterm infants: natural history, management and long-term outcome.' *Journal of Pediatrics,* **114,** 611–618.

Epstein, F., Marlin, A.E., Wald, A. (1978) 'Chronic headache in the shunt dependent adolescent with nearly normal ventricular volume: diagnosis and treatment.' *Neurology,* **3,** 351–355.

Faillace, W.J., Canady, A.I. (1990) 'Cerebrospinal fluid shunt malfunction signaled by new or recurrent seizures.' *Child's Nervous System,* **6,** 37–40.

Fernell, E., Hagberg, B., Hagberg, G., Von Wendt, L. (1986) 'Epidemiology of infantile hydrocephalus in Sweden. I. Birth prevalence and general data.' *Acta Paediatrica Scandinavica,* **75,** 975–981.

—— —— —— —— (1987a) 'Epidemiology of infantile hydrocephalus in Sweden. II. Origin in infants born at term.' *Acta Paediatrica Scandinavica,* **76,** 411–417.

—— —— —— —— (1987b) 'Epidemiology of infantile hydrocephalus in Sweden. III. Origin in preterm infants.' *Acta Paediatrica Scandinavica,* **76,** 418–423.

—— Uvebrant, P., Von Wendt, L. (1987c) 'Overt hydrocephalus at birth—origin and outcome.' *Child's Nervous System,* **3,** 350–353.

—— Hagberg, B., Hagberg, G., *et al.* (1988) 'Epidemiology of infantile hydrocephalus in Sweden: a clinical follow-up study of children born at term.' *Neuropediatrics,* **19,** 135–142.

—— Hagberg, G., Hagberg, B. (1994) 'Infantile hydrocephalus epidemiology: an indicator of enhanced survival.' *Archives of Disease in Childhood,* **70,** F123–F128.

Fishman, R.A., Dillon, W.P. (1993) 'Dural enhancement and cerebral displacement secondary to intracranial hypotension.' *Neurology,* **43,** 609–611.

Foltz, E.L., Shurtleff, D.B. (1963) 'Five-year comparative study of hydrocephalus in children with and without operation (113 cases).' *Journal of Neurosurgery,* **20,** 1064–1079.

Frame, P.T., McLaurin, R.L. (1984) 'Treatment of CSF shunt infections with intrashunt plus oral antibiotic therapy.' *Journal of Neurosurgery,* **60,** 354–360.

Frank, E., Buonocore, M., Hein, L. (1990) 'The use of magnetic resonance imaging to assess slow fluid flow in a model cerebrospinal fluid shunt system.' *British Journal of Neurosurgery,* **4,** 53–57.

Fryns, J-P., Spaepen, A., Cassiman, J.J., Van den Berghe, H. (1991) 'X linked complicated spastic paraplegia, MASA syndrome, and X linked hydrocephalus owing to congenital stenosis of the aqueduct of Sylvius: variable expression of the same mutation at Xq28.' *Journal of Medical Genetics,* **28,** 429–431. (*Letter.*)

Gelabert, M., Bollar, A., Paseiro, M.J., Allut, A.G. (1990) 'Hydrocephalus and intraspinal tumor in childhood.' *Child's Nervous System,* **6,** 110–112.

Gilles, F.H., Shillito, J. (1970) 'Infantile hydrocephalus: retrocerebellar subdural hematoma.' *Journal of Pediatrics,* **76,** 529–537.

Goh, D., Minns, R.A. (1993) 'Cerebral blood flow velocity monitoring in pyogenic meningitis.' *Archives of Disease in Childhood,* **68,** 111–119.

Gooskens, R.H.J.M., Willemse, J., Bijlsma, J.B., Hanlo, P.W. (1988) 'Megalencephaly: definition and classification.' *Brain and Development,* **10,** 1–7.

Green, W.R., Sweet, L.K., Prichard, R.W. (1949) 'Acute lymphocytic choriomeningitis. A study of 21 cases.' *Journal of Pediatrics,* **35,** 688–701.

Grollmus, J.M., Wilson, C.B., Newton, T.H. (1976) 'Paramesencephalic arachnoid cysts.' *Neurology,* **26,** 128–134.

Gruber, R. (1981) 'The relationship of ventricular shunt complications to the chronic overdrainage syndrome. A follow-up study.' *Zeitschrift für Kinderchirurgie,* **34,** 346–352.

Haar, F.L., Miller, C.A. (1975) 'Hydrocephalus resulting from superior vena cava thrombosis in an infant. Case report.' *Journal of Neurosurgery,* **42,** 597–601.

Hagberg, B. (1962) 'The sequelae of spontaneously arrested infantile hydrocephalus.' *Developmental Medicine and Child Neurology,* **4,** 583–587.

—— Sjögren, I. (1966) 'The chronic brain syndrome of infantile hydrocephalus.' *American Journal of Diseases of Children,* **112,** 189–196.

Haines, S.J., Taylor, F. (1982) 'Prophylactic methicillin for shunt operations: effects on incidence of shunt malfunction and infection.' *Child's Brain,* **9,** 10–22.

Hamza, M., Bodensteiner, J.B., Noorani, P.A., Barnes, P.D. (1987) 'Benign extracerebral fluid collections: a cause of macrocrania in infancy.' *Pediatric Neurology,* **3,** 218–221.

Hanigan, W.C., Wright, R., Wright, S. (1985–1986) 'Magnetic resonance imaging of the Dandy–Walker malformation.' *Pediatric Neurosciences,* **12,** 151–156.

Hart, M.N., Malamud, N., Ellis, W.G. (1972) 'The Dandy–Walker syndrome. A clinicopathological study based on 28 cases.' *Neurology,* **22,** 771–780.

Hayden, P.W., Shurtleff, D.B., Stuntz, T.J. (1983) 'A longitudinal study of shunt function in 360 patients with hydrocephalus.' *Developmental Medicine and Child Neurology,* **25,** 334–337.

Herva, R., Seppäinen, U. (1984) 'Roentgenologic findings of the hydrolethalus syndrome.' *Pediatric Radiology,* **14,** 41–43.

Hill, A., Volpe, J.J. (1982) 'Decrease in pulsatile flow in the anterior cerebral arteries in infantile hydrocephalus.' *Pediatrics*, **69**, 4–7.

Hirsch, J.F. (1982) 'Percutaneous ventriculocisternostomies in noncommunicating hydrocephalus.' *In: Shunts and Problems with Shunts. Monographs in Neural Sciences, Vol. 8.* Basel: Karger, pp. 21–25.

—— (1994) 'Consensus: long-term outcome in hydrocephalus.' *Child's Nervous System*, **10**, 64–69.

—— Hoppe-Hirsch, E. (1988) 'Shunts and shunt problems in childhood.' *In:* Symon, L. (Ed.) *Advances and Technical Standards in Neurosurgery, Vol.16.* Wien: Springer, pp. 177–196.

—— Pierre-Kahn, A., Renier, D. *et al.* (1984) 'The Dandy–Walker malformation.' *Journal of Neurosurgery*, **61**, 515–522.

Hislop, J.E., Dubowitz, L.M.S., Kaiser, A.M., *et al.* (1988) 'Outcome of infants shunted for post-haemorrhagic ventricular dilatation.' *Developmental Medicine and Child Neurology*, **30**, 451–456.

Ho, K.L. (1982) 'Tumors of the cerebral aqueduct.' *Cancer*, **49**, 154–162.

Hoffman, H.J., Harwood-Nash, D., Gilday, D.L (1981) 'Percutaneous third ventriculostomy in the management of noncommunicating hydrocephalus.' *Concepts in Pediatric Neurosurgery*, **1**, 87–106.

—— Bruce, E., Humphreys, R.P. (1982a) 'Management of hydrocephalus.' *In: Shunts and Problems with Shunts. Monographs in Neural Sciences, Vol. 8.* Basel: Karger, pp. 21–25.

—— Hendrick, E.B., Humphreys, R.P., Armstrong, E.A. (1982b) 'Investigation and management of suprasellar arachnoid cysts.' *Journal of Neurosurgery*, **57**, 597–602.

Hoppe-Hirsch, E., Sainte-Rose, C., Renier, D., Hirsch, J.F. (1987) 'Pericerebral collections after shunting.' *Child's Nervous System*, **3**, 97–102.

Hooper, R. (1961) 'Hydrocephalus and obstruction of the superior vena cava in infancy. Clinical study of the relationship between cerebrospinal fluid pressure and venous pressure.' *Pediatrics*, **28**, 792–799.

Hope, P.L., Gould, S.J., Howard, S., *et al.* (1988) 'Precision of ultrasound diagnosis of pathologically verified lesions in the brains of very preterm infants.' *Developmental Medicine and Child Neurology*, **30**, 457–471.

Hudgins, R.J., Edwards, M.S.B., Goldstein, R., *et al.* (1988) 'Natural history of fetal ventriculomegaly.' *Pediatrics*, **82**, 692–697.

Hyde-Rowan, M.D., Recate, H.L., Nulsen, F.E. (1982) 'Reexpansion of previously collapsed ventricles: the slit ventricle syndrome.' *Journal of Neurosurgery*, **56**, 536–539.

Ines, D.F., Markand, O.N. (1977) 'Epileptic seizures and abnormal electroencephalographic findings in hydrocephalus and their relation to the shunting procedures.' *Electroencephalography and Clinical Neurophysiology*, **42**, 761–768.

Ingram, T.T.S., Naughton, J.A. (1962) 'Paediatric and psychological aspects of cerebral palsy associated with hydrocephalus.' *Developmental Medicine and Child Neurology*, **4**, 287–292.

Jaksche, H., Loew, F. (1986) 'Burr hole third ventriculo-cisternostomy. An unpopular but effective procedure for treatment of certain forms of occlusive hydrocephalus.' *Acta Neurochirurgica*, **79**, 48–51.

James, A.E., Strecker, E-P., Sperber, E., *et al.* (1974) 'An alternative pathway of cerebrospinal fluid absorption in communicating hydrocephalus. Transependymal movement.' *Radiology*, **111**, 143–146.

James, H.E., Walsh, J.W., Wilson, H.D., Connor, J.D. (1982) 'Management of cerebrospinal fluid infections. A clinical experience.' *In: Shunts and Problems with Shunts. Monographs in Neural Sciences, Vol.8.* Basel: Karger, pp. 75–77.

Johnston, I.H., Howman-Giles, R., Whittle, I.R. (1984) 'The arrest of treated hydrocephalus in children. A radionuclide study.' *Journal of Neurosurgery*, **61**, 752–756.

Jones, H.C. (1987) 'The pathophysiology of congenital hydrocephalus.' *Journal of Pediatric Neurosciences*, **3**, 9–20.

Jouet, M. (1995) 'The pathogenesis of X-linked hydrocephalus.' *European Journal of Pediatric Surgery*, **5**, Suppl. 1, 5–7.

—— Rosenthal, A., Armstrong, G., *et al.* (1994) 'X-linked spastic paraplegia (SPG1), MASA syndrome and X-linked hydrocephalus result from mutations in the *L1* gene.' *Nature Genetics*, 7, 402–407.

Kelley, R.I., Mennuti, M.T., Hickey, W.F., Zackai, E.H. (1988) 'X-linked recessive aqueductal stenosis without macrocephaly.' *Clinical Genetics*, **33**, 390–394.

Kendall, B., Holland, I. (1981) 'Benign communicting hydrocephalus in children.' *Neuroradiology*, **21**, 93–96.

Kiekens, R., Mortier, W., Pothmann, R., *et al.* (1982) 'The slit-ventricle syndrome after shunting in hydrocephalic children.' *Neuropediatrics*, **13**, 190–194.

Kinal, M.E. (1966) 'Infratentorial tumors and the dural venous sinuses.' *Journal of Neurosurgery*, **25**, 395–401.

Kirkinen, P., Serlo, W., Jouppila, P., *et al.* (1996) 'Long-term outcome of fetal hydrocephaly.' *Journal of Child Neurology*, **11**, 189–192.

Kirkpatrick, M., Engleman, H., Minns, R.A. (1989) 'Symptoms and signs of progressive hydrocephalus.' *Archives of Disease in Childhood*, **64**, 124–128.

Kloss, J.L. (1968) 'Craniosynostosis secondary to ventriculo-atrial shunt.' *American Journal of Diseases of Children*, **116**, 315–317.

Ko, T-M., Hwa, H-L., Tseng, L-H., *et al.* (1994) 'Prenatal diagnosis of X-linked hydrocephalus in a Chinese family with four successive affected pregnancies.' *Prenatal Diagnosis*, **14**, 57–60.

Kobayashi, A., Hashi, K. (1983) 'Secondary spinal canal stenosis associated with long-term ventriculoperitoneal shunting.' *Journal of Neurosurgery*, **59**, 854–860.

Kokkonen, J., Serlo, W., Saukkonen, A-L., Juolasmaa, A. (1994) 'Long-term prognosis for children with shunted hydrocephalus.' *Child's Nervous System*, **10**, 384–387.

Krausse, I., Kornreich, L., Waldman, D., Garty, B.Z. (1997) 'MRI meningeal enhancement with intracranial hypotension caused by lumbar puncture.' *Pediatric Neurology*, **16**, 163–165.

Kreusser, K.L., Tarby, T.J., Taylor, D., *et al.* (1984) 'Rapidly progressive post-hemorrhagic hydrocephalus: treatment with external ventricular drainage.' *American Journal of Diseases of Children*, **138**, 633–637.

Krishnamoorthy, K.S., Kuehnle, K.J., Todres, I.D., DeLong, G.R. (1984) 'Neurodevelopmental outcome of survivors with posthemorrhagic hydrocephalus following grade II neonatal intraventricular hemorrhage.' *Annals of Neurology*, **15**, 201–204.

Lahat, E., Aladjem, M., Schiffer, J., Starinsky, R. (1993) 'Hydrocephalus due to bilateral obstruction of the foramen of Monro: a 'possible' late complication of mumps encephalitis.' *Clinical Neurology and Neurosurgery*, **95**, 151–154.

Lamas, E., Lobato, R.D., Esparza, J. (1977) 'Dural posterior fossa AVM producing raised sagittal sinus pressure.' *Journal of Neurosurgery*, **46**, 804–810.

Landrieu, P., Ninane, J., Ferrière, G., Lyon, G. (1979) 'Aqueductal stenosis in X-linked hydrocephalus: a secondary phenomenon?' *Developmental Medicine and Child Neurology*, **21**, 637–642.

Laurence, K.M. (1959) 'The pathology of hydrocephalus.' *Annals of the Royal College of Surgeons of England*, **24**, 388–401.

Leggate, J.R.S., Baxter, P., Minns, R.A., *et al.* (1988) 'Role of a separate subcutaneous cerebrospinal fluid reservoir in the management of hydrocephalus.' *British Journal of Neurosurgery*, **2**, 327–337.

Levy, W.J., Mason, L., Hahn, J.F. (1983) 'Chiari malformation presenting in adults: a surgical experience in 127 cases.' *Neurosurgery*, **12**, 377–389.

Lonton, A.P. (1979) 'The relationship between intellectual skills and the computerized tomograms of children with spina bifida and hydrocephalus.' *Zeitschrift für Kinderchirurgie*, **28**, 368–374.

Lorber, J. (1984) 'The family history of uncomplicated hydrocephalus: an epidemiological study based on 270 probands.' *British Medical Journal*, **289**, 281–284.

—— Priestley, B.L. (1981) 'Children with large heads: a practical approach to diagnosis in 557 children with special reference to 109 children with megalencephaly.' *Developmental Medicine and Child Neurology*, **23**, 494–504.

Lorenzo, A.V., Page, L.K., Watters, G.V. (1970) 'Relationship between cerebrospinal fluid formation: absorption and pressure in human hydrocephalus.' *Brain*, **93**, 679–692.

Lundar, T., Bakke, S.J., Nornes, H. (1990) 'Hydrocephalus in an achondroplastic child treated by venous decompression at the jugular foramen.' *Journal of Neurosurgery*, **73**, 138–140.

Martinez-Lage, J.F., Garcia Santos, J.M., Poza, M., *et al.* (1995) 'Neurosurgical management of Walker–Warburg syndrome.' *Child's Nervous System*, **11**, 145–153.

Matsumoto, S., Oi, S. (1985) 'Slit-like ventricle and isolation of CSF pathway as complications of the shunt procedure in childhood hydrocephalus. Part 4. The slit ventricle syndrome.' *Annual Review of Hydrocephalus*, **3**, 108–109.

Maurice-Williams, R.S., Choksey, M. (1986) 'Entrapment of the temporal horn: a form of focal obstructive hydrocephalus.' *Journal of Neurology, Neurosurgery, and Psychiatry*, **49**, 238–242.

Maytal, J., Alvarez, L.A., Elkin, C.M., Shinnar, S. (1987) 'External hydrocephalus: radiologic spectrum and differentiation from cerebral atrophy.' *American Journal of Roentgenology*, **48**, 1223–1230.

McComb, J.G. (1983a) 'Colonic complications of ventriculoperitoneal shunts.' *Neurosurgery*, **13**, 169. (*Comment on paper by* Abu-Dalu *et al.*, pp. 167–169.)

—— (1983b) 'Recent research into the nature of cerebrospinal fluid formation and absorption.' *Journal of Neurosurgery*, **59**, 369–383.

—— Hyman, S., Weiss, M.H. (1983) 'Lymphatic drainage of cerebrospinal fluid in the cat.' *In:* Schneider, D. (Ed.) *Workshop in Hydrocephalus.* New York: Raven Press, pp. 169–183.

McLone, D.G., Aronyk, K.E. (1993) 'An approach to the management of arrested or compensated hydrocephalus.' *Pediatric Neurosurgery*, **19**, 101–103.

McMillan, J.J., Williams, B. (1977) 'Aqueduct stenosis: case review and discussion.' *Journal of Neurology, Neurosurgery, and Psychiatry*, **40**, 521–532.

Ment, L.R., Duncan, C.C., Geehr, R. (1981) 'Benign enlargement of the subarachnoid spaces in the infant.' *Journal of Neurosurgery*, **54**, 504–508.

Miller, J.D. (1991) 'Basic intracranial dynamics.' *In:* Minns, R.A. (Ed.) *Problems of Intracranial Pressure in Childhood. Clinics in Developmental Medicine No. 113/114.* London: Mac Keith Press, pp. 1–12.

Minns, R.A. (1984) 'Intracranial pressure monitoring.' *Archives of Disease in Childhood*, **59**, 486–488.

Mokri, B., Parisi, J.E., Scheithauer, B.W., *et al.* (1995) 'Meningeal biopsy in intracranial hypotension: meningeal enhancement on MRI.' *Neurology*, **45**, 1801–1807.

Mori, K., Shimada, J., Kurisaka, M., *et al.* (1995) 'Special Task Committee Report. Classification of hydrocephalus and outcome of treatment.' *Brain and Development*, **17**, 338–348.

Naidich, T.P. (1989) 'Hydrocephalus.' *International Pediatrics*, **4**, 137–140.

—— McLone, D.G., Hahn, Y.S., Hanaway, J. (1982) 'Atrial diverticula in severe hydrocephalus.' *American Journal of Neuroradiology*, **3**, 257–266.

Newman, L.J., Heitlinger, L., Hiesiger, E., *et al.* (1980) 'Communicating hydrocephalus following total parenteral nutrition.' *Journal of Pediatric Surgery*, **15**, 215–217.

Nickel, R.E., Gallenstein, J.S. (1987) 'Developmental prognosis for infants with benign enlargement of the subarachnoid spaces.' *Developmental Medicine and Child Neurology*, **29**, 181–186.

Nitz, W.R., Bradley, W.G., Watanabe, A.S., *et al.* (1992) 'Flow dynamics of cerebrospinal fluid: assessment with phase contrast velocity MR imaging performed with retrospective cardiac gating.' *Radiology*, **183**, 395–405.

Noetzel, M.J., Blake, J.N. (1992) 'Seizures in children with congenital hydrocephalus: long-term outcome.' *Neurology*, **42**, 1277–1281.

Nyberg, D.A., Mack, L.A., Hirsch, J., *et al.* (1987) 'Fetal hydrocephalus: sonographic detection and clinical significance of associated anomalies.' *Radiology*, **163**, 187–191.

Ogata, H., Oka, K., Mitsudome, A. (1992) 'Hydrocephalus due to acute aqueductal stenosis following mumps infection: report of a case and review of the literature.' *Brain and Development*, **14**, 417–419.

Oi, S., Matsumoto, S., Katayama, K., Mochizuki, M. (1990) 'Pathophysiology and postnatal outcome of fetal hydrocephalus.' *Child's Nervous System*, **6**, 338–345.

Olson, D.M., Milstein, J.M. (1988) 'Hydromyelia associated with arrested hydrocephalus.' *Neurology*, **38**, 652–654.

O'Reilly, D.E., Walentynowicz, J.E. (1981) 'Etiological factors in cerebral palsy: an historical review.' *Developmental Medicine and Child Neurology*, **23**, 633–642.

Pannullo, S.C., Reich, J.B., Krol, G., *et al.* (1993) 'MRI changes in intracranial hypotension.' *Neurology*, **43**, 919–926.

Pascual-Castroviejo, I., Villareso, F., Perez-Higueras, A., *et al.* (1983) 'Childhood choroid plexus neoplasms: a study of 14 cases less than 2 years old.' *European Journal of Pediatrics*, **140**, 51–56.

Peach, B. (1965) 'Arnold–Chiari malformation. Morphogenesis.' *Archives of Neurology*, **12**, 527–535.

Perlman, J.M., Lynch, B., Volpe, J.J. (1990) 'Late hydrocephalus after arrest and resolution of neonatal post-hemorrhagic hydrocephalus.' *Developmental Medicine and Child Neurology*, **32**, 725–729.

Pettit, R.E., Kilroy, A.W., Allen, J.H. (1980) 'Macrocephaly with head growth parallel to normal growth pattern.' *Archives of Neurology*, **37**, 518–521.

Piatt, J.H. (1992) 'Physical examination of patients with cerebrospinal fluid shunts: is there useful information in pumping the shunt?' *Pediatrics*, **89**, 470–473.

Pierre-Kahn, A., Gabersek, V., Hirsch, J.F. (1976) 'Intracranial pressure and rapid eye movement sleep in hydrocephalus.' *Child's Brain*, **2**, 155–166.

—— Hirsch, J.F., Renier, D., *et al.* (1980) 'Hydrocephalus and achondroplasia. A study of 25 observations.' *Child's Brain*, **7**, 205–219.

—— Capelle, L., Brauner, C., *et al.* (1990) 'Presentation and management of suprasellar arachnoid cysts. Review of 20 cases.' *Journal of Neurosurgery*, **73**, 355–359.

Plandsoen, W.C.G., De Jong, D.A., Van Eijndhoven, J.H.M., Stroink, H. (1986) 'Non-invasive ICP monitoring in the anterior fontanelle in newborn children, using the Rotterdam teletransducer.' *Clinical Neurology and Neurosurgery*, **88**, 321–322.

Pople, I.K., Quinn, M.W., Bayston, R., Hayward, R.D. (1991) 'The Doppler pulsatility index as a screening test for blocked ventriculo-peritonal shunts.' *European Journal of Pediatric Surgery*, **1**, Suppl. 1, 27–29.

Quencer, R.M. (1992) 'Intracranial CSF flow in pediatric hydrocehpalus: evaluation with cine–MR imaging.' *American Journal of Neuroradiology*, **13**, 601–608.

Raffel, C., Hudgins, R., Edwards, M.S.B. (1988) 'Symptomatic hydrocephalus: initial findings in brainstem gliomas not detected on computed tomographic scans.' *Pediatrics*, **82**, 733–737.

Rando, T.A., Fishman, R.A. (1992) 'Spontaneous intracranial hypotension: report of two cases and review of the literature.' *Neurology*, **42**, 481–487.

Raymond, G.V., Holmes, L.B. (1994) 'Head circumference standards in neonates.' *Journal of Child Neurology*, **9**, 63–66.

Renier, D., Lacombe, J., Pierre-Kahn, A., *et al.* (1984) 'Factors causing acute shunt infection. Computer analysis of 1174 operations.' *Journal of Neurosurgery*, **61**, 1072–1078.

—— Sainte-Rose, C., Pierre-Kahn, A., Hirsch, J.F. (1988) 'Prenatal hydrocephalus: outcome and prognosis.' *Child's Nervous System*, **4**, 213–222.

Rennels, M.B., Wald, E.R. (1980) 'Treatment of *Haemophilus influenzae* type b meningitis in children with cerebrospinal fluid shunts.' *Journal of Pediatrics*, **97**, 424–426.

Ribierre, M., Couvreur, J., Canetti, J. (1970) 'Les hydrocéphalies par sténose de l'aqueduc de Sylvius dans la toxoplasmose congénitale.' *Archives Françaises de Pédiatrie*, **27**, 501–510.

Ricevuti, G., Savoldi, F., Piccolo, G., *et al.* (1986) 'Meningeal leukemia diagnosed by cytocentrifuge study of cerebrospinal fluid. A study of 631 cerebrospinal fluid samples from 87 patients.' *Archives of Neurology*, **43**, 466–470.

Riva, D., Milani, N., Giorgi, C., *et al.* (1994) 'Intelligence outcome in children with shunted hydrocephalus of different etiology.' *Child's Nervous System*, **10**, 70–73.

Robertson, W.C., Chun, R.W.M., Orrison, W.W., Sackett, J.F. (1979) 'Benign subdural collections of infancy.' *Journal of Pediatrics*, **94**, 382–385.

Rosman, N.P., Shands, K.N. (1978) 'Hydrocephalus caused by increased intracranial venous pressure: a clinicopathological study.' *Annals of Neurology*, **3**, 445–450.

Rosner, M.J., Becker, D.P. 1983) 'The etiology of plateau waves: a theoretical model and experimental observations.' *In:* Ishii, S, Nagai, H., Brock, M. (Eds.) *Intracranial Pressure.* Berlin: Springer, pp. 301–305.

Rothenberger, A., Brandl, H. (1980) 'Subdural effusions in children under two years—clinical and computer-tomographical data.' *Neuropädiatrie*, **11**, 139–150.

Roulet Perez, E., Maeder, P., Cotting, J., *et al.* (1993) 'Acute fatal parainfectious cerebellar swelling in two children. A rare or an overlooked situation?' *Neuropediatrics*, **24**, 346–351.

Russell, D.S. (1949) *Observations on the Pathology of Hydrocephalus. Medical Research Council Special Report Series, 265.* London: HMSO.

Russman, B.S., Tucker, S.H., Schut, L. (1975) 'Slow tremor and macrocephaly: expanded version of the bobble-head doll syndrome.' *Journal of Pediatrics*, **87**, 63–66.

Sainte-Rose, C., Lacombe, J., Pierre-Kahn, A., *et al.* (1984) 'Intracranial venous sinus hypertension: cause or consequence of hydrocephalus in infants?' *Journal of Neurosurgery*, **60**, 727–736.

—— Hooven, M.D., Hirsch, J.F. (1987) 'A new approach in the treatment of hydrocephalus.' *Journal of Neurosurgery*, **66**, 213–226.

—— Hoffman, H.J., Hirsch, J.F. (1989) 'Shunt failure.' *Concepts in Pediatric Neurosurgery*, **9**, 7–20.

Saliba, E., Bertrand, P., Gold, F., *et al.* (1990) 'Area of lateral ventricles measured on cranial ultrasonography in preterm infants: reference range.' *Archives of Disease in Childhood*, **65**, 1029–1032.

Salonen, R. (1984) 'The Meckel syndrome: clinicopathological findings in 67 patients.' *American Journal of Medical Genetics*, **18**, 671–689.

—— Herva, R., Norio, R. (1981) 'The hydrolethalus syndrome: delineation of a "new" lethal malformation syndrome based on 28 patients.' *Clinical Genetics*, **19**, 321–330.

Sanford, R.A., Bebin, J., Smith, R.W. (1982) 'Pencil gliomas of the aqueduct of Sylvius. Report of two cases.' *Journal of Neurosurgery*, 57, 690–696.

Sato, O., Takei, F., Yamada, S. (1994) 'Hydrocephalus: is impaired cerebrospinal fluid circulation only one problem involved?' *Child's Nervous System*, 10, 151–155.

Saukkonen, A-L., Serlo, W., Von Wendt, L. (1990) 'Epilepsy in hydrocephalic children.' *Acta Paediatrica Scandinavica*, 79, 212–218.

Scarfò, G.B., Tomaccini, D., Gambacorta, D., Capaccioli, L. (1979) 'Contribution to the study of craniostenosis: disturbance of the cerebrospinal fluid flow in oxycephaly.' *Helvetica Paediatrica Acta*, 34, 235–243.

Serlo, W., Heikkinen, E., Saukkonen, A-L., Von Wendt, L. (1985) 'Classification and management of the slit ventricle syndrome.' *Child's Nervous System*, 1, 194–199.

—— Kirkinen, P., Jouppila, P., Herva, R. (1986) 'Prognostic signs in fetal hydrocephalus.' *Child's Nervous System*, 2, 93–97.

Shahar, E., Lambert, R., Hwang, P.A., Hoffman, H.J. (1988) 'Obstructive hydrocephalus-induced Parkinsonism. I: Decreased basal ganglia regional blood flow.' *Pediatric Neurology*, 4, 117–119.

Sher, P.K., Brown, S.B. (1975a) 'A longitudinal study of head growth in pre-term infants. I: Normal rates of head growth.' *Developmental Medicine and Child Neurology*, 17, 705–710.

—— —— (1975b) 'A longitudinal study of head growth in pre-term infants. II: Differentiation between 'catch-up' head-growth and early infantile hydrocephalus.' *Developmental Medicine and Child Neurology*, 17, 711–718.

Sleigh, G., Dawson, A., Penny, W.J. (1993) 'Cor pulmonale as a complication of ventriculo-atrial shunts reviewed.' *Developmental Medicine and Child Neurology*, 35, 74–78.

Tamaki, N., Nagashima, T., Matsumoto, S. (1985) 'Pathophysiology of hydrocephalus. Part 1. Slit-like ventricle, normal volume hydrocephalus, isolated fourth ventricle, and isolated unilateral hydrocephalus.' *Annual Review of Hydrocephalus*, 3, 104–105.

Tanaka, Y., Nakamura, S., Yamada, H., Kageyama, N. (1985) 'Pathogenesis of hydrocephalus in craniosynostosis.' *Annual Review of Hydrocephalus*, 3, 139–140.

Tew, B. (1979) 'The "cocktail party" syndrome in children with hydrocephalus and spina bifida.' *British Journal of Disorders of Communication*, 14, 89–101.

Tohyama, J., Kawahara, H., Inagaki, M., *et al.* (1992) 'Clinical and neuroradiologic findings of congenital hydrocephalus in infant born to mother with HTLV-1-associated myelopathy.' *Neurology*, 42, 1406–1408.

Tomasovic, J.A., Nellhaus, G., Moe, P.G. (1975) 'The bobble-head doll syndrome: an early sign of hydrocephalus. Two new cases and a review of the literature.' *Developmental Medicine and Child Neurology*, 17, 777–783.

Tomono, Y., Maki, Y., Ito, M., Nakada, Y. (1983) 'Precocious puberty due to postmeningitic hydrocephalus.' *Brain and Development*, 5, 414–417.

Valentini, L., Solero, C.L., Lasio, G., *et al.* (1995) 'Triventricular hydrocephalus: review of 71 cases evaluated at the Istituto Neurologico "C. Besta" Milan over the last 10 years.' *Child's Nervous System*, 11, 170–172.

Ventriculomegaly Trial Group (1994) 'Randomised trial of early tapping in neonatal post haemorrhagic ventricular dilatation: results at 30 months.' *Archives of Disease in Childhood*, 70, F129–F136.

Vinchon, M., Vallée, L., Prin, L., *et al.* (1992) 'Cerebro-spinal fluid eosinophilia in shunt infections.' *Neuropediatrics*, 23, 235–240.

Vleck, B.W., Ito, B. (1987) 'Acute paraparesis secondary to Arnold–Chiari type 1 malformation and neck hyperflexion.' *Annals of Neurology*, 21, 100–101.

Waaler, P.E., Aarskog, D. (1980) 'Syndrome of hydrocephalus, costovertebral dysplasia and Sprengel anomaly with autosomal dominant inheritance.' *Neuropediatrics*, 11, 291–297.

Wald, S.L., McLaurin, R.L. (1978) 'Shunt-associated glomerulonephritis.' *Neurosurgery*, 3, 146–149.

Watkins, L., Hayward, R., Andar, U., Harkness, W. (1994) 'The diagnosis of blocked cerebrospinal fluid shunts: a prospective study of referral to a paediatric neurosurgical unit.' *Child's Nervous System*, 10, 87–90.

Welch, K., Friedman, V. (1960) 'The cerebrospinal fluid valves.' *Brain*, 83, 454–469.

Weller, R.O., Shulman, K. (1972) 'Infantile hydrocephalus: clinical, histological, and ultrastructural study of brain damage.' *Journal of Neurosurgery*, 36, 255–265.

Wilberger, J.E., Vertosick, F.T., Vries, J.K. (1983) 'Unilateral hydrocephalus secondary to congenital atresia of the foramen of Monro. Case report.' *Journal of Neurosurgery*, 59, 899–901.

Willems, P.J., Brouwer, O.F., Dijkstra, J., Wilrink, J. (1987) 'X-linked hydrocephalus.' *American Journal of Medical Genetics*, 27, 921–928.

Yamada, H., Nakamura, S., Tajima, M., Kageyama, N. (1981) 'Neurological manifestations of pediatric achondroplasia.' *Journal of Neurosurgery*, 54, 49–57.

Yanofsky, C.S., Hanson, P.A., Lepow, M. (1981) 'Parainfectious acute obstructive hydrocephalus.' *Annals of Neurology*, 10, 62–63.

Young, B. (1979) 'Hydrocephalus and elevated intracranial venous pressure. Case report.' *Child's Brain*, 5, 73–80.

8
CEREBRAL PALSY

Jean Aicardi and Martin Bax

DEFINITION

Cerebral palsy (CP) is a persistent disorder of movement and posture caused by nonprogressive defects or lesions of the immature brain. The absence of progression of brain pathology may not be absolute. The natural course of lesions incurred during the late prenatal or perinatal period is of extended duration, and cicatrization, progressive atrophy, retractile gliosis or cavitation can take place in the postnatal period. Such changes can be visualized by imaging techniques (Lütschg *et al.* 1983). The lesions responsible for CP differ with the clinical syndrome and especially with the degree of maturity of the infant at the time of insult. Those incurred before 20 weeks gestation result in brain malformations (see Chapter 3). Insults incurred at 26–30 weeks postconceptional age cause mainly damage to the white matter in the periventricular areas, ultimately resulting in periventricular leukomalacia, whether they occur prenatally, or postnatally in the preterm infant. Cortical and basal ganglia damage occurs towards the end of the first trimester of pregnancy in term babies (Barkovich and Truwit 1990, Rorke and Zimmerman 1992). Such differences in vulnerability are related to the metabolic demands of specific brain areas which vary with maturation of the brain, and to the characteristics of fetal circulation, as hypoperfusion is probably a frequent mechanism. However, it is not always possible to differentiate *a posteriori* lesions of different timing. Bouza *et al.* (1994b) found discrepancies between the types of lesion found by ultrasound scanning in the neonatal period and those found by magnetic resonance imaging in later childhood. Moreover, additional damage may appear as a consequence of an episode of status epilepticus initiated by a previous epileptogenic brain lesion (Aicardi and Chevrie 1983).

From a clinical viewpoint, the symptoms and signs of CP are not unchanging. During infancy and childhood, modifications in muscle tone and function are readily apparent, and, indeed, a diagnosis of the type of CP and even of its existence may have to wait until 3–4 years of age (Nelson and Ellenberg 1982, Piper *et al.* 1988). Such changes may result from the fact that deficits from damaged brain areas that normally should become functional at predetermined ages become manifest only at those ages. For example, involvement of the upper limb in congenital hemiplegia becomes evident at 4–5 months of age, at a time when prehension normally develops. Other changes, however, are not well understood, for example the development of late dystonia after several years of stable spastic CP (Burke *et al.* 1980, Mutch *et al.* 1992, Bhatt *et al.* 1993).

The concept of CP is to some extent an artificial one because the causes, mechanisms and consequences of the pathological lesions are multiple and the very nature of the various conditions that constitute CP is highly heterogeneous. Some definitions do not include an upper age limit for the onset of signs/symptoms (Brett 1997), while others set limits at 3–4 years. Clearly, any such strict limitation is arbitrary. However, the diagnostic problems and therapeutic requirements are common to all cases of what is termed cerebral palsy, and this applies essentially to lesions occurring in the young, immature brain, before 3–4 years of age.

The limits of the concept of CP are not clear-cut. Some slowly progressive conditions, *e.g.* Rett syndrome, may for long periods be difficult to separate, and this also applies to cases with minimal motor symptoms and signs with associated mental retardation or learning difficulties. Indeed, lesions of a similar cause (*e.g.* malformations of the brain) may produce isolated mental retardation or CP depending on the extent and location of the lesions.

INCIDENCE

Data on the incidence of CP vary with the series studied and the periods over which they were collected. Known figures apply only to industrialized countries. There is no doubt that the incidence in the Third World is much higher and that potentially preventable causes, especially perinatal ones, are much more common in developing countries. The overall incidence remains fairly stable in Western countries at between 1.5 and 2.5 per 1000 (Hensleigh *et al.* 1986) and does not reflect the large reduction in neonatal mortality that has taken place over the past 20 years. In Sweden, the incidence of CP was 2.24 per 1000 in the years 1954–1959 and went down to 1.3 per 1000 in the period 1950–1970. Since then, the incidence increased in the periods 1971–1978 and, especially, 1979–1982, to 2.17 per 1000, of which 1.23 per 1000 were term infants and 0.94 per 1000 were preterm infants. The increase started in 1970 and was mainly due to a rising number of cases of spastic and ataxic diplegia (Hagberg *et al.* 1975a, 1984, 1989a, 1993). Similar trends have been reported from Western Australia (Blair and Stanley 1982, Stanley

1987), Denmark (Glenting 1976) and the USA (Hensleigh *et al.* 1986). The diminished incidence in the 1960s apparently resulted from better neonatal care. The recent increase in frequency is probably due to the survival of very preterm babies of less than 1000g birthweight (Hagberg *et al.* 1989b). However, a decreasing prevalence of spastic CP was found by Krägeloh-Mann *et al.* (1994) despite an increasing survival rate in the years 1983–1986.

AETIOLOGY AND RISK FACTORS

CP is a condition with multiple aetiologies. Many of these have been reviewed in Chapters 1 and 2. The causes are variable with the type of CP, and these will be dealt with later in this chapter, together with the pathological lesions that are largely dependent on the form. However, some common risk factors for CP in general deserve comment.

The aetiology of CP is often impossible to determine in the individual patient; indeed, CP usually has a multifactorial origin and selection of one factor may be arbitrary. Some factors often are operative only in infants predisposed by other conditions, such as preterm birth or fetal malnutrition (Hagberg and Hagberg 1993, Kuban and Leviton 1994). In many cases, no significant aetiological factors are found. In one large study (Krägeloh-Mann *et al.* 1995a), no definite aetiological factor was found in 217 of 487 infants (44 per cent). The causes of different forms of CP are differently distributed as indicated below.

Recently, the attribution of CP to birth trauma and asphyxia has been questioned (Freeman and Nelson 1988, Shields and Shifrin 1988, Aylward *et al.* 1989, Kuban and Leviton 1994). Convincing evidence for the role of brain malformations (Truwit *et al.* 1992, Sugimoto *et al.* 1995) and for the prenatal origin of many destructive lesions by imaging and pathological studies (Scher *et al.* 1991) has been brought forward. There is good evidence that only a minority of cases result from the action of perinatal factors (Nelson and Ellenberg 1986, Blair and Stanley 1988, Nelson 1988, Painter 1989), and postnatal factors play only a minor role.

Prenatal factors include genetic (Gustavson *et al.* 1969, Bundey 1992, Petterson *et al.* 1993) and chromosomal disorders, congenital infections, cerebral maldevelopment, periventricular leukomalacia, and noncerebral maldevelopments in association with mental retardation (Krägeloh-Mann *et al.* 1995b). Such factors are most commonly found in term babies and rarely in very preterm infants. It seems likely that prenatal factors are predominant in cases of CP of undetermined cause without an abnormal perinatal history.

Perinatal factors refer to those that were operative between the onset of labour and the end of the first week of life and include demonstrated brain oedema and neonatal shock, confirmed intracerebral haemorrhage, confirmed sepsis or CNS infection, and clear evidence of hypoxic–ischaemic encephalopathy with both abnormal neonatal neurological signs and poor neonatal cardiorespiratory condition. Perinatal factors seem to be particularly important in preterm infants with spastic CP (Krägeloh-Mann *et al.* 1995a).

Postnatal factors are responsible for less than 10 per cent of cases (Blair and Stanley 1982, Arens and Molteno 1989). The most common type of CP in these cases is hemiplegia (Lademan 1976) with both postconvulsive and vascular aetiologies.

The timing of insult is dependent on the type of CP and on the time of delivery. Prenatal factors are most common in term infants and in cases of ataxic or hemiplegic CP. Perinatal factors are frequent in dyskinetic CP in term infants and in diplegic CP in preterm babies.

PREDISPOSING FACTORS
Preterm birth and intrauterine growth retardation are of major importance in the aetiology of CP although they are not in themselves the determining cause.

Preterm birth is mainly associated with bilateral spastic CP (Dunn 1986, Stanley and English 1986, Hagberg and Hagberg 1993). According to Stanley and Alberman (1984), there is no excess of preterm birth among infants of other groups. Within the spastic group, a recent study found about 20–25 per cent of infants to be of very low birthweight (<1500g) and 38–39 per cent of low birthweight (1500–2499g). Among diplegic cases the proportion of very low birthweight and low birthweight infants reached 60–76 per cent of cases (Krägeloh-Mann *et al.* 1993). These figures are in general agreement with previous literature (Dunn 1986, Stanley and English 1986, Hagberg *et al.* 1989b).

Intrauterine growth retardation (Stanley and English 1986, Largo *et al.* 1989) is a significant risk factor. Hagberg *et al.* (1976) found that 13 per cent of 376 term infants with CP were small for gestational age whereas the expected figure was only 2.3 per cent. Prenatal and perinatal factors are frequently intermixed. However, the exact mechanisms responsible for CP in infants who are small for gestational age remain largely undetermined. Largo *et al.* (1989) found that the presence of minor morphological abnormalities was correlated with adverse events during gestation and the birth process. In general, CP is often associated with a series of suboptimal conditions between conception and the perinatal period rather than with a single insult (Hagberg *et al.* 1976, Ellenberg and Nelson 1988).

PREDICTIVE FACTORS
Some factors increase the risk of CP. These include maternal factors such as maternal diabetes mellitus, threatened abortion, pre-eclampsia and twin pregnancy (Chapter 1). However, it is difficult to predict which infants will be affected, even though patients with severe perinatal events such as intraventricular haemorrhage (Van de Bor *et al.* 1988), ventricular dilatation (Shankaran *et al.* 1989), chronic lung disease (Perlman and Volpe 1989), polycythaemia (Amit and Camfield 1980) and clinically manifest hypoxic–ischaemic encephalopathy (Fenichel 1983, Levene *et al.* 1986) are at especially high risk. As indicated in Chapter 2, late fetal heart-rate deceleration during labour, intrapartum and neonatal pH, and Apgar scores are not reliable predictors of developmental disturbances. A study from Ireland (Grant *et al.* 1989) did not show any decrease in CP with systematic electronic monitoring of delivery.

Nelson and Ellenberg (1987) found that 68 per cent of childen with CP had a normal Apgar score and a normal neurological examination during the neonatal period. Only 13 per cent of their term children with CP had an Apgar score of 5 or less. All had in addition abnormal neurological signs in the neonatal period. Thus, most of the children with CP have no history of perinatal abnormality.

Results of neurological examination at 36 weeks in preterm babies (Allen and Capute 1989) and at 4 months in all infants (Ellenberg and Nelson 1981) bear a reasonable, although imperfect, relationship to the occurrence of CP, as do some specific neurological patterns (Harris 1987) such as neck extensor hypertonia (Amiel-Tison et al. 1977). Clusters of neonatal abnormalities are more reliable than isolated signs (Ellenberg and Nelson 1988, Morgan and Aldag 1996).

Ultrasound examination has proved reliable to detect extensive periventricular leukomalacia (Chapter 2). Cystic or haemorrhagic lesions predict a high probability of neuromotor sequelae (Graziani et al. 1986; Guzzetta et al. 1986; Cooke 1987; Graham et al. 1987; Bozynski et al. 1988; Scher et al. 1989; Bouza et al. 1994b,c). A recent study of 206 infants born before 33 weeks showed that only 4 per cent of those with a normal ultrasound scan had major sequelae at 8 years as against 27 per cent of those with ventricular dilatation and 69 per cent of those with atrophy (Roth et al. 1993). CT scan seems to be of less predictive value (Adsett et al. 1985) in the newborn period (Lütshg et al. 1983, Houdou et al. 1988). CT scans, however, are abnormal in 60–80 per cent of cases of CP (Kotlarek et al. 1981, Taudorf et al. 1984). In infants with motor delay but no definitive neurological signs, MR imaging may help predict the development of CP by showing abnormalities of myelination (Candy et al. 1993). Van Bogaert et al. (1992) also reported predictively abnormal MRI sequences in patients with normal CT scans who later developed CP. Taudorf and Vorstrup (1989) have shown that cerebral blood flow abnormalities can be detected by dynamic techniques (SPECT) in patients with CP, despite a normal CT scan. MR imaging is capable of demonstrating abnormalities that are undetectable by CT scan (van Bogaert et al. 1992), especially cortical malformations and white matter changes.

The value of EEG as a predictor of normal or abnormal development has been extensively studied (Takeuchi and Watanabe 1989, Tharp et al. 1989, Watanabe 1992; see Chapter 2). Evoked potentials are also of some value (Willis et al. 1989). The study of regional cerebral glucose metabolism using PET scanning may have some predictive value (Kerrigan et al. 1991) but is limited to a few centres.

In neonates with a normal neurological examination, normal EEG and normal ultrasonography, the probability of normal development is extremely high. However, the presence of abnormalities suggestive of CP is much less reliable. Some childen apparently 'outgrow' CP (Nelson and Ellenberg 1982, Taudorf et al. 1984, Piper et al. 1988, Niemann et al. 1996), that is to say they develop early motor signs that mimic those found in CP patients to the point of receiving an early diagnosis, only to develop normal motor patterns later on. About 25 per cent of

such infants have later learning difficulties and hyperactivity (PeBenito et al. 1989). Such an outcome is also observed in some of the children who had risk factors for CP without ever developing neurological hard signs. Transient dystonia (Willemse 1986, Crouchman 1987, Angelini et al. 1988) with a favourable outcome may also mimic CP during the first year of life.

CLASSIFICATION OF CEREBRAL PALSY

Attempts at classification of CP have been multiple (see Ingram 1964, 1966) and no system is fully satisfactory. A pathological classification is clearly impractical as very few cases come to autopsy and as different lesions frequently produce a similar clinical picture. Clinical classifications (Minear 1956) are more important as there is at least some correlation between the type of neurological involvement, the outcome, and therapy, even though many factors other than the gross distribution of motor disturbances may be more important for determining prognosis and treatment. For that reason, associated impairments such as epilepsy, visual disturbances, hearing difficulties and neurodevelopmental deficits have to be taken into account in the individual assessment of the patient and the multidisciplinary therapeutic approach. The changing nature of the symptoms and signs during the first years of life also makes clinical classification difficult: in many cases the pattern of movements and posture will change completely, e.g. from hypotonia and dystonia to spasticity or ataxia. An aetiological classification is not useful because similar aetiological factors can produce different pathological lesions and clinical features. Thus, preterm birth may be associated with diplegia, ataxia or hemiplegia, depending upon the brain lesion present.

The five major types of CP are: hemiplegia, spastic diplegia and ataxic diplegia, tetraplegia, dystonic/dyskinetic CP, and ataxic CP. Some investigators recognize in addition a spastic–dystonic group and a three-limb spastic type observed especially in very preterm infants (Hagberg and Hagberg 1993, Krägeloh-Mann et al. 1993). Other forms, less common and difficult to classify, will be briefly discussed. Distinction between the various forms may be difficult, especially the differentiation of quadriplegia from diplegia as some upper limb involvement is present in the latter and only a quantitative difference may separate these types.

VARIOUS CLINICAL FORMS
OF CEREBRAL PALSY

The reported incidences of the various forms of CP vary with the published series. Hagberg et al. (1989a) found the incidence of hemiplegia to be 0.79 per 1000, that of tetraplegia 0.16 per 1000, that of spastic diplegia 0.90 per 1000, that of dyskinetic forms 0.21 per 1000, and that of ataxic forms 0.11 per 1000, for a total incidence of 2.17 per 1000. The corresponding figures from the same authors for the period 1967–1970 (Hagberg et al. 1975a,b), were respectively 0.55, 0.07, 0.41, 0.16 and 0.15 for a total incidence of 1.34 per 1000 live births. In their recent series (Hagberg et al. 1993b), hemiplegia accounted for 59 per cent of cases, tetraplegia for 13 per cent, diplegia for 79 per cent, and dyskinesia and ataxia for 13 per cent each. Thus, bilateral spastic CP is the most common form. The three-limb dominated type (spastic triplegia) represented 11 per cent of such cases in a recent study (Krägeloh-Mann *et al.* 1995a) and poses especially difficult problems. In an earlier series, Crothers and Paine (1959) found that 64.6 per cent of patients had spastic CP, 40.5 per cent had hemiplegia, 22 per cent had an extrapyramidal disorder and 13.1 per cent had mixed forms.

HEMIPLEGIA OR HEMIPARESIS
Hemiplegia is a unilateral motor disability mostly spastic in type.

CONGENITAL HEMIPLEGIA
Congenital hemiplegia, defined as a hemiplegia whose causal lesion is present before the end of the neonatal period (28 days), accounts for 70–90 per cent of cases of hemiplegic CP. Its incidence remained stationary in Sweden over the years 1959–1978 but decreased in Denmark from 0.58 to 0.41 per 1000 live births between 1950 and 1969 (Glenting 1976) and in Western Australia from 0.63 to 0.25 per 1000 live births between the periods 1966–1970 and 1971–1975 (Dale and Stanley 1980).

Aetiology
The aetiology is thought to be prenatal in about 75 per cent of cases (Goutières *et al.* 1972, Michaelis *et al.* 1980, Powell *et al.* 1988a, Kyllerman 1989), but the proportion of cases in which the lesion was caused by demonstrated perinatal brain damage is a matter of controversy (Kotlarek *et al.* 1981). Familial cases are rare. A few cases of dominant porencephaly with hemiplegia are on record (Haar and Dyken 1977, Berg *et al.* 1983, Zonana *et al.* 1986), and a syndrome of congenital hemiplegia and cataract has been reported as a sporadic (Schachat *et al.* 1957) or familial (Blumel *et al.* 1960) occurrence. This association may be a separate entity (Uvebrandt 1988). Around 25 per cent of patients are born preterm (Goutières *et al.* 1972, Uvebrandt 1988).

Obvious prenatal factors (*e.g.* brain malformations) were present in 7.6 per cent of Uvebrandt's patients, but the proportion is higher in some series (Diebler and Dulac 1987, Wiklund *et al.* 1990). Obvious perinatal factors, mainly intracerebral haemorrhage, were found in 4.5 per cent of term and 8.1 per cent of preterm infants, and postnatal factors in 10.7 per cent of cases in Uvebrandt's series. Aetiology remained unspecified in one third to one quarter of cases even though abnormal prenatal events were much more frequent in patients than in control infants (Uvebrandt 1988). Boys are more commonly affected than girls, and the right side is involved in 53–58 per cent of cases.

Pathology
The neuropathology of congenital hemiplegia is mostly inferred from imaging findings, and only a limited number of pathological studies are available (Christensen and Melchior 1967, Lyon and Robain 1967).

Cystic softenings in the territory of the middle cerebral artery are one common cause (Fig. 8.1). They may be of prenatal (Ong

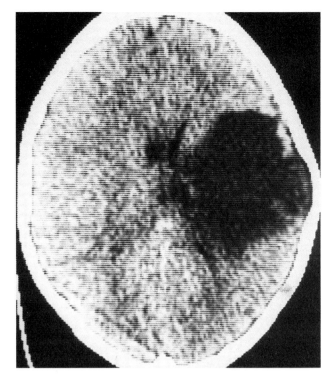

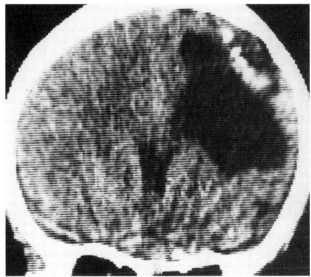

Fig. 8.1. Cystic softening in territory of left middle cerebral artery in 6-year-old girl with right congenital hemiplegia: CT scan (*top*—axial cut; *bottom*—frontal cut). Note expansion of cranial vault, thinning of bone at level of cavity, and areas of calcification at upper and external border.

et al. 1983, Asindi *et al.* 1988) or perinatal origin (Claeys *et al.* 1983, Baumann *et al.* 1987, Amato *et al.* 1991). Recent MRI studies in newborn infants have shown the frequency of strokes with focal infarction of variable extent (Bouza *et al.* 1994a, Koelfen *et al.* 1995). Some of these strokes are associated with difficult birth and evidence of hypoxia but a majority have no recognized cause (Coker *et al.* 1988). In both cases, the cause of vascular obstruction remains unknown, although embolism from the placental vessels or ductus arteriosus has been suggested (Asindi *et al.* 1988).

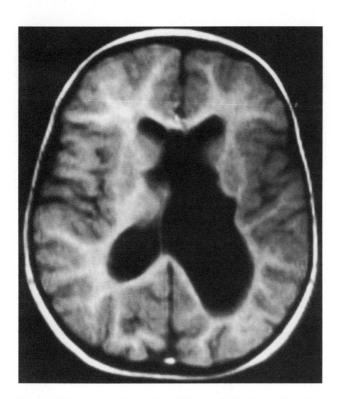

Fig. 8.2. Right congenital hemiplegia. Subcortical brain damage. Note that left hemisphere is smaller than right, in addition to marked ventricular dilatation.

Subcortical lesions, as shown by focal enlargement of one lateral ventricle, are common (Kotlarek *et al.* 1981, Claeys *et al.* 1983, Taudorf *et al.* 1984, Wiklund *et al.* 1990) (Fig. 8.2). Such periventricular lesions have emerged as the largest subgroup of children with congenital hemiplegia (Wiklund *et al.* 1990). At least some of these lesions are probably the result of periventricular leukomalacia or other ischaemic events in the prenatal period (Chapter 2). They are regarded as being caused by ischaemia occurring between 28 and 35 weeks gestation (Volpe 1995). Diffuse enlargement of a lateral ventricle with irregularities of the walls is commonly seen (Claeys *et al.* 1983). Brain maldevelopment is found almost exclusively in term children. Schizencephaly, hemimegalencephaly and polymicrogyria are most common (Krägeloh-Mann *et al.* 1995b).

Less common lesions include haemorrhagic brain damage, whether haemorrhagic leukomalacia, periventricular haemorrhagic infarction (Guzzetta *et al.* 1986), or disruption of the central white matter by blood from a ventricular haemorrhage. Prenatal parenchymal haemorrrhages are an uncommon lesion that can result from prenatal haemorrhagic diseases such as maternal thrombocytopenic purpura (Donn *et al.* 1984, Herman *et al.* 1986). Perinatal haemorrhagic infarcts or haematomas (Chaplin *et al.* 1979) are also a possible cause of congenital hemiplegia. Extensive unilateral cystic leukomalacia may be found. Diencephalic lesions were found in 18 of 33 patients reported by Steinlin *et al.* (1993). They involved the basal ganglia, thalami and internal capsule and were the predominant lesion in 10 patients.

The CT changes found in children with congenital hemiplegia have been variously classified. Maldevelopment accounted for 17 per cent of the cases of Wiklund *et al.* (1990) and for 15 per cent of those of Steinlin *et al.* (1993). Wiklund *et al.* found that among 111 children from a population-based study, 42 per cent had periventricular atrophy and 12 per cent had cortical/subcortical atrophy, while 29 per cent had a normal scan. The proportion of normal CTs was much lower (7.5–13 per cent) in most other series (Kotkarek *et al.* 1981, Claeys *et al.* 1983, Uvebrandt 1988).

MRI studies evidence in many cases lesions undetectable by CT (van Bogaert *et al.* 1992). They showed polymicrogyria in eight of 40 cases of Truwit *et al.* (1992). MRI also shows that deep lesions are often bilateral and asymmetrical (Barkovich and Truwit 1990; Truwit *et al.* 1992; Steinlin *et al.* 1993; Bouza *et al.* 1994b,c; Barkovich *et al.* 1995; Krägeloh-Mann *et al.* 1995b).

Ultrasonography in the neonatal period also enables detection of infarcts and of periventricular lesions (Bouza *et al.* 1994c, Govaert and de Vries 1997). The predictive value of ultrasonography is good, but some change in the appearance of the lesions can be observed after several years so that it may not always be possible to retrospectively diagnose their time of occurrence and exact type.

The various types of brain lesion, as indicated by neuroimaging studies, have some prognostic value. Generally, lesions involving the cortex, such as cystic softening, are associated with a higher frequency of epilepsy and mental deficit than mainly subcortical lesions (Kotlareck *et al.* 1981, Taudorf *et al.* 1984, Molteni *et al.* 1987). However, individual prediction on the basis of CT images is unreliable.

Clinical features
Unilateral paresis and spasticity are the characteristic features of hemiplegia. Weakness usually predominates in the distal part of limbs. Hemiplegia is rarely diagnosed at birth. Indeed, *hemisyndromes* of unilateral motor deficit observed during the neonatal period generally disappear without hemiparetic sequelae. Hemiplegia was recognized in the neonatal period in 10 of 93 cases in the series of Crothers and Paine (1959) and in 9 per cent of the 185 cases in the series of Goutières *et al.* (1972). A free interval is present in more than 90 per cent of cases and lasts until the age of 4–9 months. That this period is really symptom-free has been demonstrated by repeatedly normal neurological examination in the face of known extensive hemispheric lesions in several patients (Bouza *et al.* 1994a). The first manifestations become apparent by 4–5 months in a majority of cases, when attempts at reaching are always on the same side. An early 'hand preference' should lead one to suspect congenital hemiplegia. Fisting and an abnormal posture of the arm with flexion at the elbow are usually present. However, diagnosis is often very late. It was established by 10 months of age in only 53 per cent of the cases of Uvebrandt and by 18 months in only 67 per cent of the cases of Goutières *et al.* In severe cases, there is delay in passing milestones but approximately half the affected children walk at the average age.

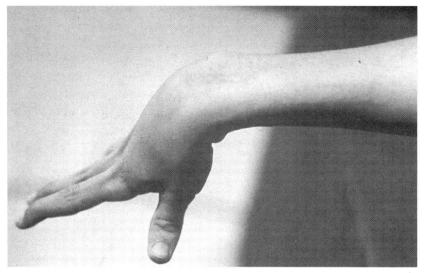

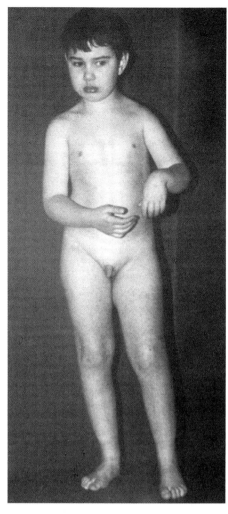

Fig. 8.3. Congenital hemiplegia. *(Right)* 7-year-old boy with left hemiplegia predominating markedly in upper limb. *(Above)* Typical attitude of hand in patient with right hemiplegia. (Courtesy Dr J-P. Padovani, Hôpital des Enfants Malades, Paris.)

Involvement of the lower limb often becomes apparent only with ambulation.

Prehension of hemiplegic children is characteristic: there is excessive abduction of the arm, flexion at the wrist and hyperextension of the fingers, which are spread apart (Fig. 8.3). No pincer grasp develops in many patients (Brown *et al.* 1987). The upper limb is usually much more involved than the leg (Crothers and Paine 1959; Ingram 1964, 1966; Brown *et al.* 1987). However, Uvebrandt (1988) found that the lower limb was predominantly affected in about half his patients, and Bouza *et al.* (1994a) also found some evidence for predominant lower limb involvement in preterm infants. This may be due to the increased survival of very preterm infants in whom the predominant lesion is hydrocephalus or periventricular leukomalacia which preferentially involve the periventricular pyramidal fibres that control the lower limb. The face is not affected or there is only a mild deficit predominating on the lower VIIth nerve, in contrast to the marked facial palsy usually seen with acquired hemiplegia (Goutières *et al.* 1972, Brown *et al.* 1987). Growth of the affected side of the body is usually less than that of the opposite side. This dwarfism predominantly involves the hand and upper limb. It may also be observed in acquired hemiplegia incurred before the end of the growth period. Associated move-

ments are prominent and tend to persist indefinitely. Physical signs include 'pyramidal' type spasticity, increased tendon reflexes, and Babinski and Rossolimo signs (Lin *et al.* 1994). Weakness is usually mild, overshadowed by spasticity and associated movements. Frank choreoathetosis is not rare (Dooling and Adams 1975), and in some cases the term *hemidystonia* is more appropriate than that of hemiplegia (Nardocci *et al.* 1996).

Contractures tend to develop if appropriate measures are not taken. *Cortical sensory abnormalities* were present in 68 per cent of the patients examined by Tizard *et al.* (1954), and 25 per cent of them had a *visual field defect* sparing the macula. Brown *et al.* (1987) indicated that sensory abnormalities are difficult to test and may be less common than previously suggested. Mercuri *et al.* (1996) found that visual field defects, decreased visual acuity or deficient stereopsis were present in 11 of 14 children studied.

The severity of hemiplegia can be graded functionally (Claeys *et al.* 1983). In mild cases, there is a pincer grasp and individual finger movements are possible. In moderate hemiplegia the hand can be used globally, while in severe cases it is not used at all. In such cases there is usually relatively severe involvement of the lower limb. Strabismus is frequent, and optic atrophy is occasionally observed (Brett 1997). *Congenital cataract* has been reported in assocation with congenital hemiplegia.

Epilepsy is a major complication of congenital hemiplegia. It was present in 27 per cent (Diebler and Dulac 1987), 34 per cent (Uvebrandt 1988) and 44 per cent of cases (Goutières *et al.* 1972), the frequency depending mainly on the type of referral to any particular centre. Epilepsy may be focal or secondarily generalized. It is not necessarily intractable. and approximately 80 per cent of cases are successfully treated medically (Uvebrandt 1988). Rare cases of benign rolandic epilepsy have been reported in patients with congenital hemiplegia (Santanelli *et al.* 1989). Startle epilepsy (Chauvel *et al.* 1992) is a frequent type and should always lead to a careful search for mild pyramidal signs or body hemiatrophy as it is commonly seen in patients with minimal hemiparesis.

Mental retardation is present in 18–50 per cent of patients. The prevalence of mental retardation is strongly correlated to the presence of epilepsy (Aicardi 1990). Epilepsy is five times more common in patients with mental retardation than in those without (Uvebrandt 1988), and 71.4 per cent of children with epilepsy in the series of Goutières *et al.* (1972) had mental retardation as against 28.6 per cent of nonepileptic children with hemiplegia. Vargha-Khadem *et al.* (1992) have shown that epileptogenic lesions of similar extent and location have a significantly more deleterious effect on intelligence and language than those unassociated with seizures. The prevalence of mental retardation is also correlated with the severity of hemiplegia. Thus, there is a strong tendency for cases of hemiplegia to separate into two subgroups: severe cases with multiple disabilities and a poor outlook for social and professional integration, and mild cases that interfere relatively little with everyday life. Speech and language defects are also related to the severity of mental retardation. Although there is no gross difference in language with the hemisphere affected, impairment of both verbal and nonverbal IQ is greater in children with left hemisphere lesions, while visuospatial functions are equally affected with lesions of either side (Vargha-Khadem *et al.* 1985, Carlsson *et al.* 1994). Such effects may be due to the lesion itself or from the 'crowding effect' resulting from transfer of functions to preserved brain areas. They were not found by Goodman and Yude (1996) who confirmed the selective involvement of visuospatial skills.

The role of plasticity in the reorganization of the brain following an early insult is imperfectly explored. Nass (1985) has shown that transcranial magnetic stimulation can induce ipsilateral hand responses in addition to the normal contralateral ones. This may be one mechanism of the mirror movements seen in some children with congenital hemiplegia. Animal and human studies (Benecke *et al.* 1991, Farmer *et al.* 1991, Carr *et al.* 1993, Chugani *et al.* 1996) suggest that considerable functional and even anatomical changes are possible in neonates and infants.

Differential diagnosis
The differential diagnosis of congenital hemiplegia is not difficult. In the first months of life, the main differential diagnoses include temporary neonatal hemisyndromes and obstetrical brachial palsy. The latter can be differentiated by the absence of deep tendon reflexes and of any involvement of the lower limb

just by careful clinical examination. Later, pure hemidystonia or athetosis can raise difficult problems. Indeed, a mixture of dystonic and spastic signs is more common than either alone. Congenital monoplegia is rare when careful examination is performed. In our experience the lower limb is the one affected in such cases. Mild hemiparesis is often missed for years and diagnosed only because of the discovery of mild neurological signs or hypoplasia of one side of the body often in relation to the investigation of epileptic seizures.

Treatment
The treatment of CP, including congenital hemiplegia, is dealt with below. Special attention should be paid to therapy of epilepsy, which represents a major problem (Aicardi 1990). In rare cases, progressive motor deficit is seen in patients with porencephalies, and in such cases shunting of the porencephalic cavity has been reported to bring about significant improvement (Tardieu *et al.* 1981). The mechanism of expanding porencephalies is unclear. Some probably communicate with a ventricular cavity that becomes distended as a result of hydrocephalus but some are not associated with hydrocephalus.

ACQUIRED HEMIPLEGIA
Acquired hemiplegia can result from multiple causes. Cases of acute onset can result from inflammatory disorders, demyelinating diseases, migraine, trauma and, especially, vascular disease and unilateral or predominantly unilateral status epilepticus, the so-called hemiconvulsion–hemiplegia or HH syndrome (Gastaut *et al.* 1960) or acute postconvulsive hemiplegia (Aicardi *et al.* 1969, Isler 1971, Okuno 1994). Cases of progressive onset mainly suggest neoplastic disease, especially gliomas of the brainstem, basal ganglia or thalamus, and degenerative disorders (Chapters 12, 14).

Although *acute acquired hemiplegia* can occur at any age, the vast majority of cases start during the first three years of life. The onset is often acute and dominated by the features of the causative illness such as convulsions and coma. The hemiplegia is generally maximal from onset and flaccid with marked facial involvement. Spasticity develops later in most cases. Aphasia is present in left-sided cases, in contrast with congenital hemiplegia (Rapin 1995). The degree and rate of recovery are quite variable, some patients being left with severe, persistent weakness, while others make an almost complete recovery. The cause of hemiplegia largely determines the prognosis. Postepileptic hemiplegia has a bleak outcome with 75 per cent of patients developing residual epilepsy and more than 80 per cent having some degree of mental impairment (Aicardi *et al.* 1969, Aicardi and Chevrie 1983). Vascular hemiplegia has a more favourable prognosis. The CT scan findings are also dependent on the cause. Postepileptic hemiplegia cases exhibit a characteristic sequence of predominantly unilateral hemispheric oedema, followed by global atrophy of the affected hemisphere which is a virtually specific finding (Gastaut *et al.* 1960, Aicardi 1994, Kataoka *et al.* 1988).

Acquired hemiplegia may be difficult to distinguish from

congenital hemiplegia when it occurs in infants, especially as seizures may reveal previously unrecognized deficit. Flaccidity and facial involvement are strong arguments in favour of an acquired hemiplegia.

Acquired hemiplegia resulting from vascular disease, especially arterial thrombosis or embolism, is dealt with in Chapter 15.

BILATERAL SPASTIC CEREBRAL PALSY

This term is used for forms of CP in which both sides of the body are involved. The most common form of bilateral spastic CP is spastic diplegia, defined as a type in which the lower limbs are much more affected than the arms. Involvement of the upper limbs is constant, however, even though it may be very mild and detectable only by careful examination. The incidence of diplegia has varied over the years. It is nowadays the most frequent form of CP (41 per cent of cases in the series of Hagberg and Hagberg 1989). Two subtypes, pure diplegia and ataxic diplegia, are recognized. Tetraplegia, also termed quadriplegia, bilateral hemiplegia or four-limb dominated CP, is characterized by bilateral spasticity predominating in the upper limbs or equally affecting all four limbs. It is less commoon than diplegia (86 cases *vs* 300 in the series of Krägeloh-Mann *et al*. 1995a).

Several investigators (Hagberg and Hagberg 1993, Krägeloh-Mann *et al*. 1995a) recognize two additional forms: a three-limb dominated type (triplegia) amounting to 55 cases in the series of Krägeloh-Mann *et al*. and a dyskinetic–spastic type seen in 46 patients in the same study. This form, also termed tetraplegia dystonica in the Scandinavian literature, is intermediate between spastic and dyskinetic–dystonic CP.

SPASTIC DIPLEGIA
Aetiology
The aetiology of spastic diplegia is dominated by the high frequency of preterm birth among affected children and by a relatively high frequency of perinatal factors. Of 78 children reported by Ingram (1964), 34 were preterm, and diplegia accounts for up to 81 per cent of cases of CP in preterm infants. Approximately 5–10 per cent of preterm babies with a birthweight <1500g will develop diplegia (Bennett *et al*. 1981), but the proportion is much lower among heavier preterm babies. However, the latter account for a large majority of cases of spastic diplegia because of their overwhelmingly higher frequency. Infants with spastic diplegia who were not born preterm are globally more severely disabled than those who were (Hagberg *et al*. 1975b). In a recent series (Krägeloh-Mann *et al*. 1995a), 33 per cent of infants with diplegia were born before 32 weeks gestational age and 35 per cent between 32 and 36 weeks. Only 32 per cent were term infants.

Over one half of affected children have a history of abnormal labour or delivery but its significance remains debated (Cooke 1987, Powell *et al*. 1988b). Veelken *et al*. (1983) found that only 31 per cent of their patients with diplegia had had birth asphyxia, and this was never an isolated event. Krägeloh-Mann *et al*. (1995a) found that aetiology differed with maturity of the infants. Perinatal factors (see definition, p. 211) were predominant in very

preterm babies (61 per cent), whereas prenatal factors were present in only 1 per cent of them. The same factors were found respectively in 32 and 34 per cent of moderately preterm infants and in 13 and 25 per cent of term infants. In a high proportion of their patients, no definite aetiological factor could be found. The predominance of perinatal factors in preterm children is probably explained by cardiorespiratory instability, exposing them to periods of hypoperfusion (Krägeloh-Mann *et al*. 1995b) that selectively affect the parieto-occipital white matter. Even minor events—not clinically detectable—might be responsible, thus explaining the frequency of a negative history.

Diplegia in term infants is more frequently related to prenatal factors. It seems likely that the same circulatory disturbances that occur in preterm infants in the perinatal period take place *in utero* at a similar gestational age. The prenatal origin of some cases of periventricular leukomalacia has been well demonstrated (Sinha *et al*. 1990, Iida *et al*. 1993).

Predisposing prenatal factors have also been suspected. Drillien (1964) found that mothers of diplegic children had more reproductive failures than mothers of normal children and that siblings of diplegic children had a higher than expected incidence of seizures or mental retardation. Cases observed in recent years have been increasingly often in very small preterm infants who are more severely disabled than earlier patients (Hagberg *et al*. 1989b).

Pathology
The pathology of diplegia is related to periventricular lesions which are the predominant type of brain damage in preterm babies. Intraventricular haemorrhage, especially when followed by ventricular dilatation (Papile *et al*. 1983, Van de Bor *et al*. 1988), is a possible cause of diplegia. Indeed, the occurrence of a large head in association with diplegic CP—especially ataxic diplegia—should always raise the suspicion of hydrocephalus. *Periventricular leukomalacia* is the most common lesion responsible for spastic diplegia. This is easily understandable as the involved areas are located along the external angle of the lateral ventricles thus damaging the fibres from the internal aspect of the hemisphere which include the motor fibres to the lower limbs (Fig. 8.4). The location of leukomalacia along the posterior part of the lateral ventricles, interrupting the optic radiations, is responsible for visual difficulties and strabismus (Van Nieuwenhuizen and Willemse 1984, Scher *et al*. 1989, Schenk-Rootlieb *et al*. 1994).

Other pathological lesions may be found in some cases of diplegia. Pasternak (1987) has indicated the possible role of parasagittal cerebral injury (Chapter 2). However, such lesions located at the border zone between vascular territories in the upper part of the motor strip are more commonly associated with involvement of the upper limbs in tetraplegic patients.

Diffuse ulegyria (Christensen and Melchior 1967), the central corticosubcortical pattern of atrophy described by Barth *et al*. (1984), and extensive cystic encephalomalacia are also associated with four-limb dominated bilateral CP (Hagberg *et al*. 1989a,b).

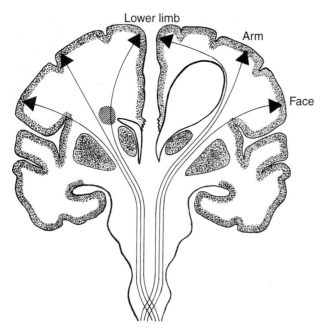

Lower limb   Arm

Face

Fig. 8.4. Schematic representation of relationship of corticospinal fibres to periventricular leukomalacia *(left side of schema)* and to dilated lateral ventricle in hydrocephalus *(right side of schema)*. In both cases, fibres from the mesial cortex (leg area) are preferentially involved, the leukomalacic area interrupting leg fibres *(left side)* or stretching leg fibres around the dilated ventricle *(right side)*. This explains predominant location of neurological signs (diplegia).

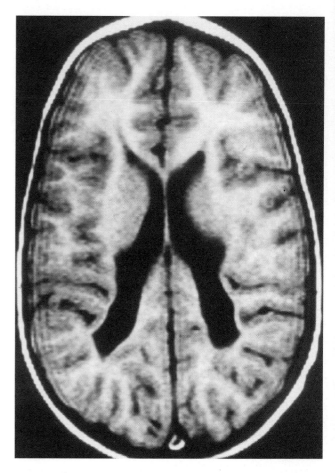

Fig. 8.5. T$_1$-weighted MRI scan of a child with spastic diplegia. The posterior horns of the lateral ventricles are irregularly dilated and there is considerable loss of white matter around them. This image is characteristic of the late stage of periventricular leukomalacia and is observed mainly in preterm infants.

CT scan studies of patients with spastic diplegia usually show a reduction in the bulk of the white matter symmetrically in both parieto-occipital areas with consequent dilatation of the posterior horn. The dilated ventricles have irregular contours. In severe cases, the lesions extend more anteriorly with global increase in ventricular size. Periventricular hypodensities of the centrum semi ovale are sometimes seen (Kanda *et al.* 1982, Taudorf *et al.* 1984). Yokochi *et al.* (1989) found a good correlation between the extent of CT lesions and the severity of clinical impairment. In mild cases CT scan may be normal. MRI, however, demonstrates even small lesions as areas of low T$_1$ and high T$_2$ signal of the lateral angles at the ventricles with variable reduction in the volume of the white matter. Recent work has shown that up to a quarter of cases demonstrated by MRI in infants born preterm had no clinical abnormality (Olsén *et al.* 1997). MRI also permits precise assessment of the extent of leukomalacia (Fig. 8.5) and occasionally demonstrates unilateral involvement (Flodmark *et al.* 1989, Konishi *et al.* 1991, Krägeloh-Mann *et al.* 1992, van Bogaert *et al.* 1992). Sequential studies, from neonatal ultrasonography to later MRI, support the concept of a peri/neonatal timing of lesions in preterm children (Dubowitz *et al.* 1985, Skranes *et al.* 1992, de Vries *et al.* 1993). Cavitated leukomalacia usually results in severe diplegia. However, diplegia can occur without any detectable lesion in the newborn period, and noncavitated echogenic areas may disappear without sequelae (Graziani *et al.* 1986, Scher *et al.* 1989).

Clinical features
The most striking feature of spastic diplegia is the increased muscle tone in the lower extremities. Some patients demonstrate hypotonia, lethargy and feeding difficulties during the neonatal period. In a majority of infants, however, there is a latent period up to 6–12 weeks of age after which hypotonia may be sufficiently marked to arouse suspicion (Ingram 1964, 1966). A 'dystonic' stage follows which is characterized by involuntary mass movements and diffuse increase in tone whenever the child's position is altered. When the infant is held vertically, the legs extend and assume a scissored position as a result of adductor spasm (Fig. 8.6). However, many cases are not diagnosed until 8–9 months of age because of the subtlety of early abnormalities of tone. In the next, spastic, stage, flexion of the hips and knees becomes predominant. In the standing posture, the legs are often internally rotated. When independent walking is achieved, it tends to be on tiptoes with maintained semiflexion of the lower limb joints. Some diplegic children walk on everted feet. In the most severe cases, independent walking is not possible because of lack of balance, truncal hypotonia or contractures.

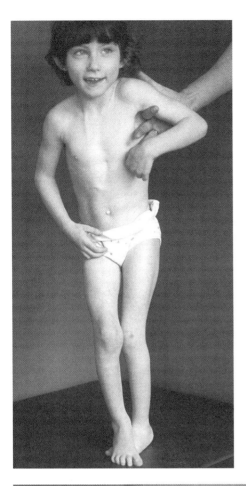

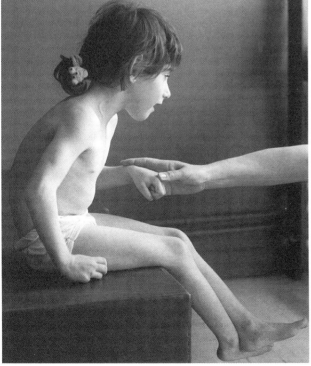

Fig. 8.6. Spastic diplegia. Child born preterm with both intraventricular haemorrhage and periventricular leukomalacia. *(Top)* Standing: note equinus feet, scissoring of legs and relative underdevelopment of lower half of body. *(Bottom)* Sitting: note truncal hypotonia and incomplete flexion of knees. (Courtesy Dr F. Renault, Hôpital Trousseau, Paris.)

The upper limbs are variably affected. The elbows tend to be flexed when walking, but manipulative skills are much less impaired than locomotion. Impaired coordination of rapid movement is, however, common. Deep tendon reflexes are hyperactive in all extremities and pyramidal signs are easily elicited.

The condition is not infrequently asymmetrical, and some cases with monoplegia of a lower limb probably represent the consequence of unilateral leukomalacia. Some children have associated dystonia and involuntary movements that may be incapacitating. Rarely, incapacitating secondary progressive dystonia appears after several years of stable course (Bhatt *et al.* 1993).

Epilepsy is relatively uncommon; it was observed in 16 per cent of the patients of Veelken *et al.* (1983) and in 27 per cent of those of Ingram (1964). It is often fairly easy to control. Strabismus is especially common in patients with diplegia. Visuo-perceptual problems are also common in children with diplegia (Schenk-Rootlieb *et al.* 1994). Posterior brain lesions are much more common in the presence of visual difficulties than in their absence, and there is a positive correlation between the extent of peritrigonal white matter atrophy and the severity of visual problems (Koeda and Takeshita 1992, Fedrizzi *et al.* 1996).

The intellectual function of diplegic patients is relatively preserved in most cases. Sixty-nine per cent of the patients of Hagberg *et al.* (1975b) had normal or borderline intelligence. Impairment of upper limb function tends to be associated with lower intelligence levels (Ingram 1964) and, in general, with severe motor dysfunction. Performance IQ is more affected than verbal function and correlates with the extent of white matter lesions (Fedrizzi *et al.* 1996).

According to Hagberg *et al.* (1989a), however, the previously expressed opinion that the average preterm child with CP is mildly diplegic with a rather discrete motor disability, normally gifted or only slightly retarded, no longer holds. A shift towards more cases with mental retardation, epilepsy and marked motor disability has now taken place as a result of increased survival of very immature infants.

Spastic diplegia occasionally raises difficult *diagnostic problems*. A transient dystonic stage has long been recognized in preterm infants (Drillien 1964), especially those of less than 32 weeks gestation and of less than 2000 g birthweight. They frequently show extensor posturing, increased adductor tone, poor head control and persistence or excess of primitive reflexes. D'Eugenio *et al.* (1993) followed 135 preterm infants of ≤32 weeks gestational age and found this transient dystonia to be associated with low DQ levels on the Bayley scale at 15 and 24 months but normal cognitive and motor function at 4 years.

Differential diagnosis
Familial spastic paraplegia (Chapter 10) of early onset may be impossible to separate from spastic diplegia, although the absence of preterm birth and of perinatal problems, together with the lack of any involvement of the upper limbs, should arouse suspicion. Undiagnosed familial paraplegia is probably a major cause of the relatively high rate of familial recurrence in patients with bilateral

spasticity (Bundey 1992). Some rare metabolic disorders can mimic spastic diplegia, especially the chronic form of hyperargininaemia (Scheuerle *et al.* 1993), and should be thought of in familial and atypical cases. Atypical forms of dopa-responsive dystonia can present with some spasticity, brisk tendon reflexes and upgoing toes (striatal toe). In the absence of appropriate birth history, and especially when a dystonic component is marked, a trial of L-dopa is indicated (Chapter 10).

ATAXIC DIPLEGIA
Ataxic diplegia, also termed spastic–ataxic diplegia, accounts for 5–7 per cent of cases of CP (Sanner 1979). Ataxic diplegia is mostly of congenital origin but acquired cases occur. Its fluctuations in incidence approximately parellel those of spastic diplegia (Hagberg *et al.* 1975a, 1989a). Of 31 cases described by Hagberg *et al.*, 14 weighed less than 2500g at birth. Prenatal causes appear to be at play in a majority of cases, although nine of Hagberg's patients had a history of perinatal asphyxia. Ataxic diplegia is the characteristic postnatally acquired CP syndrome of infantile hydrocephalus (Hagberg and Sjögren 1966), although congenital hydrocephalus can also provoke spastic diplegia. Clinically, the infants are initially markedly hypotonic. The hypotonia progressively gives way to spasticity and increased tendon reflexes. After the first birthday, tremor and titubation in the sitting position become apparent. Standing and walking independently may not be possible, and the use of the arms is made difficult by ataxia. Staccato speech is common, and the mental level is normal in 70 per cent of cases (Hagberg *et al.* 1975a).

TRIPLEGIA (THREE-LIMB-DOMINATED BILATERAL SPASTIC CEREBRAL PALSY)
This form of bilateral spastic CP has recently attracted attention, probably because it has become more common as a result of increased survival of very preterm infants (Hagberg *et al.* 1989b). In the series of Krägeloh-Mann *et al.* (1993), 47 per cent of children with triplegia had a perinatal aetiology and this applied especially to the very preterm children. Intraventricular haemorrhage is electively associated with triplegia and this is probably explained by the frequent occurrence of asymmetrical haemorrhagic infarction in association with severe intraventricular bleeding.

The clinical picture is severe with marked motor disability in 80 per cent of infants, mental retardation in 63 per cent and epilepsy in 48 per cent (Krägeloh-Mann *et al.* 1993). Variable and sometimes bizarre combinations of deficits are observed, and the outcome is generally poor.

TETRAPLEGIA
Tetraplegia is the most severe type of CP. The borderline between tetraplegia and dystonic CP may be difficult to draw, and the term spastic–dyskinetic CP reflects the possible interaction of dystonic and spastic features. The condition is characterized by bilateral spasticity predominating in the upper limbs with involvement of the bulbar muscles, almost always in association with severe mental subnormality and microcephaly. This form accounts for approximately 5 per cent of all cases of CP (Brett 1997) but it represents a significant problem, as affected children are totally dependent and pose the most difficult problems of care, feeding and prevention of deformities.

In a recent Swedish series of 96 cases (Edebol-Tysk 1989, Edebol-Tysk *et al.* 1989), only 5 per cent were born before term but 21 per cent were small for gestational age and another 25 per cent were at the lower limit of birthweight for age. The cause was deemed to be prenatal in 30 per cent, pre- and perinatal in 16 per cent, postnatal in 18 per cent and untraceable in 12 per cent. There is a high incidence of brain malformations in this group, and destructive processes of pre- or perinatal origin such as multicystic encephalomalacia (Chutorian *et al.* 1979, Lyen *et al.* 1981) or hydranencephaly (Jung *et al.* 1984, Larroche 1986) are common. A syndrome of autosomal recessive quadriplegia and macrocephaly is on record (McKusick 1988). CNS infections were the cause of 17 of the 96 cases of Edebol-Tysk, including six cases of early herpes simplex virus encephalitis. The predominance of term children is confirmed in other series, but some investigators (Stanley *et al.* 1993, Krägeloh-Mann *et al.* 1995a) have found a higher frequency of perinatal causes.

Extensive bilateral parasagittal insult which can be severe enough to amount to multicystic encephalomalacia is also found (Krägeloh-Mann *et al.* 1995a,b).

In addition to cortical and subcortical lesions, in most cases there is associated damage to the brainstem (Wilson *et al.* 1982) and the basal nuclei, sometimes with the development of thalamic calcification (Parisi *et al.* 1983). Eicke *et al.* (1992) studied six cases of this syndrome and found evidence for a prenatal origin.

From a clinical point of view, very gross retardation is the dominant feature. Bilateral spasticity, cranial nerve palsies, bulbar paralysis, absence of speech or gross dysarthria make these infants totally helpless, and feeding, prevention of aspiration and nutrition are major problems (Morton *et al.* 1993). The outlook is very poor and most affected infants do not develop beyond a neonatal stage. The dyskinetic–spastic type has a similar distribution of aetiological factors but clinically features a greater dystonic or athetoid component.

DYSKINETIC CEREBRAL PALSY (EXTRAPYRAMIDAL OR ATHETOID CP)
CLASSIFICATION
Dyskinetic forms of CP constitute a rather well-defined group from the aetiological and clinical points of view (Kyllerman 1977, 1981; Foley 1992). However, there is considerable confusion with respect to the terms used. Those of athetosis, chorea, dystonia and dyskinesia have been employed for similar cases, and multiple denominations have been used for abnormal movements. Up to 17 different types have been described (Minear 1956). Even though the use of many different terms reflects the existence of several different types of abnormal motion, it does not correspond to any practical necessity because abnormal movements of various types may have the same cause and because several types are frequently present in the same patient. Kyllerman's classification (1981,1983) defines dyskinetic CP as one that

is dominated by abnormal movements or postures secondary to defective coordination of movements or regulation of muscle tone, or both. The essential disability in dystonic–dyskinetic CP is an inability to organize and properly execute intended movements, and also to coordinate automatic movements and to maintain a posture. This results in major disability, all the more so as persistence of primitive motor patterns, such as the asymmetrical tonic neck reflex, is usually present and some degree of spasticity is often associated.

Kyllerman distinguished two subtypes of dyskinetic CP on a clinical basis, the hyperkinetic and the dystonic forms. These types also depend on different aetiological factors and correspond to distinct outcomes. In the *hyperkinetic subgroup*, the motor pattern is dominated by massive, apparently purposeless, involuntary movements. These may be of several types. *Athetosis* affects mainly the distal part of the limbs. The movements are slow and often writhing, with hyperextension of fingers. *Choreic movements* are quicker and more jerky and involve mainly the proximal muscles. They may be difficult to distinguish from myoclonus. *Dystonic postures* normally designate sustained tonic contractions often of a writhing and slow nature, involving a whole limb or the axial musculature. The term dystonic movements is sometimes used to describe the slow changes of such postures which result in forceful movements. *Tremor and other forms of hyperkinesia* (tensions, myoclonus, ataxia) are sometimes associated. All these abnormal movements share the common feature of being induced by attempted movements or efforts at maintaining a posture. In fact one basic feature of the dyskinetic patients is their inability to restrict movements to the intended pattern and location with resultant overflow of movements to antagonist and agonist muscles, well beyond the territory that should have been involved. Rare cases of intention myoclonus are on record (Sugama and Kusano 1995).

In the *dystonic subgroup*, the motor disorder is characterized by sudden, abnormal shifts of general muscle tone, especially increases of muscle tone in trunk extensors induced by emotional stimuli and changes in posture of neck muscles on intended acts or movements. In such cases, there is always strong, primitive reflex activity that interferes with any voluntary motor effort. These patients also have a tendency repeatedly to assume and retain distorted, twisted postures in the same stereotyped pattern (Kyllerman 1981). Dystonic patients often exhibit abnormal movements but not to the same extent as hyperkinetic ones. Such patients often have some spasticity as well.

Mixed dystonic–hyperkinetic cases were uncommon in Kyllerman's experience, representing only 7–8 per cent of all cases.

Of 116 cases of dyskinetic CP studied by Kyllerman (1981, 1983), 35 (30 per cent) belonged to the hyperkinetic group and 81 (70 per cent) were classified as dystonic cases. Eight of the 35 hyperkinetic patients also had signs of dystonia that manifested by a stiff and twisted character of positionally released motor patterns and by sudden increase of muscle tone in trunk extensors. Forty-three (53 per cent) of the dystonic patients also had some hyperkinesia.

Dystonic patients, especially when they show spastic signs, may be difficult to distinguish from those with spastic tetraplegia. They may correspond to the generalized and the mixed forms of CP of other classifications.

AETIOLOGY

The incidence of dyskinetic CP is about 10 per cent of all CP cases. A slight decrease in incidence has been observed recently among term infants, but a similar increase in incidence has been apparent in preterm infants (Hagberg *et al.* 1975b, Kyllerman 1983). The incidence of perinatal factors is higher than in other types of CP, with 67 per cent of factors referrable to the perinatal period, 21 per cent to the prenatal period, and a small proportion of postnatally acquired or untraceable cases. Among hyperkinetic cases there is a very high proportion of preterm, appropriate for gestational age, infants, many with hyperbilirubinaemia, often in combination with hypoxia (Hagberg *et al.* 1975b). Hyperkinetic cases are seen both in term infants of normal birthweight who suffer severe asphyxia at birth and in small for gestational age infants with hypoxia (Foley 1992). In term infants, dyskinetic CP often follows severe hypoxia at birth especially in the late stage of delivery. Rosenbloom (1994) emphasized that recovery from initial severe depression may be relatively good, and reported that eight of 10 children with dyskinetic CP had mild (n = 3) or moderate (n = 5) hypoxic–ischaemic encephalopathy with rapid and substantial recovery which could have predicted later normal development. The basic risk factors of hypoxia and hyperbilirubinaemia are more often combined than found in isolation, and a reduced optimality score (Prechtl 1980) is equally distributed in all dyskinetic cases of CP (Kyllerman 1983). Despite the frequency of hyperbilirubinaemia, kernicterus is now rarely demonstrated and the classic tetrad is virtually never encountered.

The role of hyperbilirubinaemia in preterm infants remains obscure and clinicopathological studies have indicated that no reliable predictive factors for kernicterus are currently known (Turkel *et al.* 1980). Van de Bor *et al.* (1989) found a higher incidence of CP in infants who had had hyperbilirubinaemia in the neonatal period as compared with a control group. Individual prediction, however, is not possible.

In some children with dyskinetic CP, no aetiological factor is apparent. In a few of these, CT scan shows calcification of the basal ganglia (Billard *et al.* 1989). A genetic origin may be suspected in such cases in which late increase in symptoms and signs is sometimes observed (Fletcher and Marsden 1996).

PATHOLOGY

The pathology of dyskinetic CP is characterized by a remarkably selective involvement, with atrophy and sclerosis, of the central grey nuclei. This is referred to as status dysmyelinatus when it affects mainly the pallidum and is the classic lesion following kernicterus (Christensen and Melchior 1967, Ahdab-Barmada and Moossy 1984, Volpe 1995). In preterm babies, however, this lesion may be less clearly individualized and combine with ponto-subicular necrosis and other brain damage (Ahdab-Barmada *et*

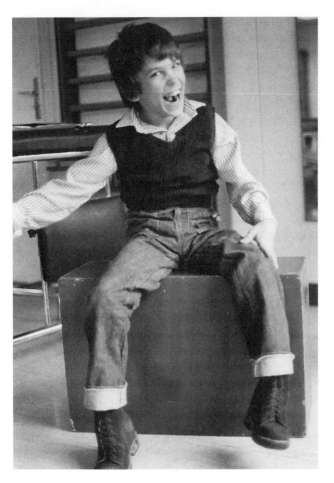

Fig. 8.7. Dyskinetic cerebral palsy. (Courtesy Dr F. Renault, Hôpital Trousseau, Paris.)

al. 1980). Status marmoratus refers to a marbled appearance of the basal ganglia, especially the striatum and thalamus, which results from diffuse gliosis associated with abnormal deposition of myelin (Friede 1989, Volpe 1995). Status marmoratus is the classical lesion of posthypoxic choreoathetosis, although involvement of the pallidum may also occur (Kyllerman 1983). Associated lesions of ulegyria of the central convolutions are common. Neuroimaging by CT is often difficult to interpret. MR imaging can show cystic lesions in the putamen and/or thalamus (Yokochi *et al.* 1991; Rutherford *et al.* 1992, 1994) which may also be associated with signs of cortical involvement and/or the presence of oedema. Isolated lesions of the basal ganglia correlate well with extrapyramidal CP; the presence of cortical lesions may indicate more diffuse damage with a more severe outcome (Rutherford *et al.* 1994). In the neonatal period, enhancement of the thalamus has been reported as an early indicator of later status marmoratus (Colamaria *et al.* 1988).

CLINICAL FEATURES
The pattern of abnormal muscle tone and movement in dyskinetic CP is never present during the first months of life but progressively appears between 5 and 10 months of age, and the full picture may not be completed before age 2 years. However,

affected infants are usually hypotonic from birth and there is no clear-cut free interval before the development of dystonia. The first abnormalities are reminiscent of those of the dystonic stage of spastic diplegia and mainly involve the trunk and lower limbs. Dystonic movements of excessive opening of the mouth are often the first suggestion of an evolving dystonic CP. Later, the involuntary movements of the limbs become evident, but the rate and extent of evolution varies with the patients. Muscle tone at rest is normal or diminished. Control of truncal tone is often deficient, which is one of the main difficulties for acquiring a standing position and ambulation. Severe hypotonia is positively correlated to the severity of the dystonia, and the persistence of primary reflexes is also a predictor of severity. Tendon reflexes are normal or increased in the lower limbs. The plantar responses are often unassessable because of the athetoid movements. Speech is almost always impaired as a result of involvement of the buccopharyngo-laryngeal muscles (O'Dwyer and Neilson 1988) and, at times, of associated hearing loss. Swallowing difficulties are common and may pose nutritional problems. Drooling may be a major problem (Harris and Purdy 1987). The general appearance of the children is striking with grimacing face and bizarre contractions at each attempted movement that easily lead one to regard them as mentally abnormal (Fig. 8.7). Most patients are very thin. Fixed contractures are unusual but dislocation of the hips is not rare. Only a minority of patients are able to walk independently. Life-threatening episodes of ballismus can be induced by intercurrent fevers in rare patients. They may require emergency treatment with haloperidol, pimozide or phenytoin (Harbord and Kobayashi 1991).

Intelligence was normal or within the dull–normal range (IQ 70–80) in 86 per cent of Kyllerman's hyperkinetic patients and in 64 per cent of his dystonic children. Even with a normal intelligence, however, these patients have difficulties related to the abnormality of fine movements, especially for writing, but most can learn to type using a modified keyboard. Epilepsy is relatively uncommon (about 25 per cent of cases) and is usually easy to control. Visual problems are common, strabismus being found in one-third of cases.

The classic tetrad of Perlstein (1960), which is characteristic of the late stage of kernicterus, includes athetosis, perceptive high-tone deafness, supranuclear palsy of upward gaze, and enamel hypoplasia of incisor teeth. It is now very rare in industrialized countries. It can be dissociated with only deafness or one or two other features. Supranuclear palsy may affect both vertical and horizontal movements, mimicking ocular motor apraxia.

DIFFERENTIAL DIAGNOSIS
The differential diagnosis of dyskinetic CP includes degenerative conditions such as the Pelizaeus–Merzbacher and Lesch–Nyhan syndromes that may present at about the same age with very similar features (Chapter 9); glutaric aciduria type I that usually has a sudden onset following an infectious episode but can also evolve in a slow, progressive way; and other organic acid disorders (Gascon *et al.* 1994). Rarer metabolic conditions, *e.g.* molybdenum cofactor deficiency, may be a cause. Complicated forms

of spastic paraplegia with dystonia may raise difficult problems (Fletcher and Marsden 1996). Minimal cases of dyskinetic CP may be difficult to distinguish from the choreiform syndrome described by Prechtl and Stemmer (1962) in patients with learning and behavioural problems. Diplegic CP at its early stage can resemble closely the onset of the dyskinetic type. Dystonia musculorum deformans is usually excluded because, in such cases, there are no abnormal personal antecedents and the CT scan is normal.

However, cases of delayed-onset dystonia due to perinatal or early childhood brain injury (Burke *et al.* 1980, Saint-Hilaire *et al.* 1991) can pose a difficult problem when only minimal neurological signs were present before dystonia appeared, which may be as late as 21 years of age. Moreover, the dystonia in such cases may remain progressive for several years. The finding of CT, MRI or EEG abnormalities excludes primary dystonia, but as these are not present in all cases a chance association between idiopathic dystonia and early static encephalopathy cannot be totally ruled out (Saint-Hilaire *et al.* 1991). Dopa-responsive dystonia usually differs in its age of onset, initial normal development, normal imaging and fluctuating course. Because atypical cases occur (Nygaard *et al.* 1994), a trial of L-dopa at the least suspicion is indicated. Perlman and Volpe (1989) and Hadders-Algra *et al.* (1994) have reported a syndrome of abnormal movements, mainly choreic and akathisic in type, with orolingual dyskinesia which they observed in 10 preterm infants with severe pulmonary dysplasia. The onset was at 3–4 months of age and the dyskinesia subsided in the second or third year in most cases, but the long-term outcome is not known.

Transient dystonia may occur in apparently normal infants during the first year of life (Willemse 1986, Deonna *et al.* 1991). It usually affects one or more limbs, does not involve the trunk or neck, presents after 4 months of age and interferes relatively little with the child's activities. The limb posturing may be intermittent or permanent and disappears in weeks or months. A form involving the trunk has been tentatively attributed to maternal cocaine use (Beltran and Coker 1995). A paroxysmal form has been described (Angelini *et al.* 1988).

ATAXIC CEREBRAL PALSY (NONPROGRESSIVE CEREBELLAR ATAXIA)

Ataxic CP accounts for about 7–15 per cent of all cases of CP (Sanner 1979, Hagberg *et al.* 1984). Nonprogressive ataxia is an obviously heterogeneous condition. Its pathogenetic mechanisms are poorly known and its nosological interpretation is controversial. The term is used here to designate only those cases in which cerebellar symptoms and signs are clearly in the forefront, not ataxic diplegia that has been reviewed above. Most cases of nonprogressive cerebellar ataxia are congenital even though the clinical manifestations often do not become suggestive before 1 or 2 years of age, at the time when children normally begin to walk.

AETIOLOGY
Prenatal factors play a dominant role in the aetiology of non-

progressive cerebellar ataxia (Hagberg *et al.* 1975b, Sanner 1979, Clement *et al.* 1984). Obvious prenatal factors were present in 25 per cent of the cases of Hagberg *et al.* (1975b) and, in 41 per cent of patients, no cause was obvious but a prenatal origin was probable. Genetic factors were found in many series (Hagberg *et al.* 1972, Sanner 1973, Sanner and Hagberg 1974, Clement *et al.* 1984, Kvistad *et al.* 1985, Wichman *et al.* 1985, Tomiwa *et al.* 1987), in some cases in association with specific syndromes, such as Gillespie syndrome (Chapter 10) or the syndrome of congenital ataxia with fixed mydriasis that appears to be transmitted as an autosomal dominant character, or in association with 'nonsyndromic' forms. Hagberg *et al.* (1972) described in detail the *dysequilibrium syndrome* (see below) which appears to be recessively inherited but to be limited to certain areas of Sweden (Sanner 1973).

Familial congenital nonprogressive ataxia has been reported from many parts of the world, and autosomal recessive (Mathews *et al.* 1989, Pascual-Castroviejo *et al.* 1994), autosomal dominant (Furman *et al.* 1985, Tomiwa *et al.* 1987) and X-linked dominant (Fenichel and Phillips 1989) or recessive (Young *et al.* 1987) cases are on record. The correspondence between pathology (atrophic or dysplastic) and mode of inheritance is poorly documented (Guzzetta *et al.* 1993). Sporadic cases are common. The clinical and pathological differentiation between the various forms described is difficult, and such disorders as Norman disease and the dysequilibrium syndrome share many common characteristics although they occur in different populations (Chapters 3, 10), so the exact nosological situation of the dysequilibrium syndrome is not clear. Likewise, simple or predominantly hemispheral cerebellar atrophy can be genetically determined (Clement *et al.* 1984), sometimes with an X-linked inheritance (Young *et al.* 1987).

PATHOLOGY
The pathology of ataxic CP is imperfectly known (Chapter 3). Both dysplastic and destructive (or atrophic) lesions can be responsible but are not practically possible to differentiate on the basis of imaging. The true nature of lesions may be impossible to determine without pathological examination. Aplasia of the vermis (Bordarier and Aicardi 1990) may be the cause of congenital ataxia, but even total absence of the vermis may not give rise to clinical symptoms, as is the case in the Dandy–Walker malformation (Chapter 3). In contrast, most patients with Joubert syndrome, in which large remnants of vermis are often present, usually display ataxia and dysequilibrium. The same poor correlation between pathological and clinical findings is found with hemispheral dysgenesis. Absence of one cerebral hemisphere is rarely associated with clinical manifestations, and even bilateral extreme hypoplasia or absence of hemispheres has remained asymptomatic in rare cases (Friede 1989). Miller and Cala (1989) found that CT examination of 29 patients with ataxic CP gave normal results in 38 per cent of cases and showed an abnormal posterior fossa in 28 per cent, whereas the cerebral hemispheres, especially the parietal regions, were abnormal in 55 per cent of patients.

TABLE 8.1
Main causes of chronic ataxia

Cause	Remarks	References
Brain tumours		
Mostly posterior fossa tumours including brainstem; sometimes supratentorial tumours	Progressive ataxia; high intracranial pressure common but not constant	Chapter 14
Other tumours		
Neuroblastoma with opsomyoclonic syndrome	May disappear even with persisting tumour	Chapter 12
Metabolic diseases		
Sphingolipidoses		Chapter 9
Metachromatic leukodystrophy		
Krabbe leukodystrophy		
GM2 gangliosidosis (juvenile)		
Niemann–Pick C disease and variants	Ophthalmoplegia and splenomegaly may be present	
Gaucher disease (juvenile)		
Ceroid-lipofuscinosis, especially late infantile form	Myoclonic epilepsy a dominant feature	Chapter 10
Abnormalities of DNA repair		Chapters 4, 9
Ataxia–telangiectasia	Ataxia and extrapyramidal features are dominant features (telangiectasia may be absent)	
Cockayne syndrome		Chapter 9
Scleroderma pigmentosum	Ataxia uncommon	Chapter 9
Energy metabolism		Chapter 9
Leigh syndrome	} Ataxia often recurrent	
Pyruvate dehydrogenase deficiency		
Respiratory chain diseases (especially MERFF)	Myoclonic epilepsy a dominant feature	
Other mitochondrial disorders		
Fatty acid metabolism		Chapter 9
Adrenoleukodystrophy and adrenomyeloneuropathy	Occasional cases may present as 'spinocerebellar degeneration'	Kurihara *et al.* (1993)
Refsum disease and other peroxisomal disorders	Treatable condition	
Other metabolic defects		Chapter 9
Abetalipoproteinaemia	Vitamin E defiency or malabsorption produces a simlilar syndrome	Chapter 10
Hypobetalipoproteinaemia		
Lafora disease	Progressive deterioration; prominent myoclonus	
Cholestanol disease (cerebrotendinous xanthomatosis)	Cataracts, tendon xanthomas	
Mevalonic aciduria	Profound delay, cataracts, marked cerebellar atrophy	Hoffmann *et al.* (1993)
Carbohydrate-deficient glycoprotein (CDG) syndrome	Mental retardation, microcephaly, retinopathy, systemic involvement, dysmorphism	Jaeken and Carchon (1993)
L-2-hydroxyglutaric aciduria		Barbot *et al.* (1997)

continues ↗

Atrophic lesions include postasphyxic cerebellar damage of prenatal or postnatal origin (Friede 1989) and also possible 'degenerative' conditions such as congenital atrophy of the granular layer (Pascual-Castroviejo *et al.* 1994) which is a genetic condition in many cases. The possibility of an acquired origin of the disease has been suggested as a similar disorder occurs in kittens born to dams infected with the virus of feline pancytopenia. Atrophy of the cerebellar hemisphere may coexist with posterior encephaloceles (Evrard and Caviness 1974).

CLINICAL FEATURES
The overall clinical features vary from case to case. In some children, typical ataxia affecting both lower and upper limbs, with dysmetria and intention tremor, is apparent by 2–3 years of age. These cases, termed 'simple' ataxic CP by Hagberg *et al.* (1972, 1975b), generally do not have pyramidal tract signs. Many such children are able to walk by 3–4 years of age although they may fall frequently. Many have some degree of intellectual impairment but severe retardation is rare (Clement *et al.* 1984) and most patients can adjust to their disability, even though writing is a problem and relatively few are able to attend regular schools. In some children, microcephaly, seizures and marked mental retardation are associated (Pascual-Castroviejo *et al.* 1994). In other cases, the major disturbance is in control of postural tone and especially with balance in the standing position. When stood upright these children tend to fall without being able to use any of

TABLE 8.1
(continued)

Cause	Remarks	References
Heredodegenerative diseases		Chapter 10
Progressive myoclonic epilepsies	Myoclonic component in forefront, cerebellar syndrome often mild	
Leukodystrophies		
Pelizaeus–Merzbacher disease	} Progressive ataxia is often a feature	
Other 'orthochromatic' leukodystrophies		
Other leukoencephalopathies (childhood ataxia with diffuse CNS hypomyelination)		Schiffman *et al.* (1994)
Multisystem disorders		
Intranuclear neuronal inclusion disease	} Multiple neurological symptoms and signs	
Machado–Joseph disease		Rosenberg *et al.* (1992)
Spinocerebellar degenerations		
Friedreich ataxia	Well defined clinical features	
Early onset ataxia with retained deep tendon reflexes	In all atypical cases, careful search for a metabolic cause (*e.g.* adrenoleukodystrophy, Leigh syndrome, ataxia–telangiectasia) is mandatory (see Chapter 10)	
Olivopontocerebellar atrophy		
Behr syndrome		
Dominant and X-linked cerebellar ataxias		
Ataxia–ocular motor apraxia		Aicardi *et al.* (1988)
Leber optic atrophy		Chapter 19
Diplegia–dysequilibrium syndrome		Chapter 11
Cerebellar parenchymal degenerations especially of the granular layer	Mental retardation more prominent than ataxia	Chapters 3, 10
Nonprogressive congenital cerebellar ataxias (ataxic cerebral palsy)		Present chapter, and Chapters 3, 10
Cerebellar aplasia and hypoplasia	May be paucisymptomatic	
Vermian aplasia/hypoplasia		
Joubert and related syndromes	Dandy–Walker syndrome does not induce ataxia	
Gillespie syndrome	Ataxia and aniridia	
Chiari I malformation	} May induce ataxia through hydrocephalus	Chapters 3, 6
Basilar impression		
Destructive lesions and encephaloceles		Present chapter
Congenital hypothyroidism	Systemic features and dysmorphism	Chapter 24
Nonprogressive acquired cerebellar ataxias		
After acute hypoxia		Chapter 13
Near-drowning		
Cardiac arrest	In some cases, syndrome of posthypoxic action and intention myoclonus	
Near-miss sudden death		
Hypoglycaemia		
Heat stroke		

the mechanisms that normally maintain equilibrium and prevent the consequences of the loss of stance. In some patients, there is no dysmetria or ataxia in the upper limbs. Such cases correspond to the dysequilibrium syndrome as described by Hagberg *et al.* (1972). In most patients, however, the static cerebellar syndrome is associated with at least some dysfunction of the cerebellar hemispheres, and the separation between both types of cerebellar ataxia may be difficult. Children with predominantly static cerebellar syndrome tend to walk very late, after 6 years of age, or not at all, and many of them are severely retarded or display autistic features (Sanner and Hagberg 1974, Clement *et al.* 1984). Although Hagberg *et al.* (1972) found vermal atrophy to be a regular feature of the dysequilibrium syndrome, recent studies have

shown that CT scans may be normal in all forms of ataxic CP and that correlations between the clinical and radiological features are rather inconsistent (Wüllner *et al.* 1993). Only 25 per cent of the Miller and Cala (1989) cases of predominant disturbance of equilibrium had an abnormal vermis.

DIFFERENTIAL DIAGNOSIS (Table 8.1)
Ataxic CP should not be confused with physiological incoordination of young infants or of children with global retardation of milestones. Simple clumsiness may be responsible for diagnostic errors (Gubbay 1985). The most difficult differential diagnosis is with the progressive ataxias and this problem may take a long time to clarify as some of the progressive cerebellar ataxias have

a very slow course. Indeed, such disorders as the Marinesco–Sjögren syndrome are sometimes classified as forms of CP. However, the appearance of cataracts and, later, of a special type of myopathy militates against such classification. Degeneration of the granular layer, although it has sometimes been regarded as a degenerative disease, is not associated with any progression of the clinical symptoms and signs and is indistinguishable from several other forms of CP due to atrophy or hypoplasia of the cerebellum. Pelizaeus–Merzbacher disease is a special diagnostic consideration as the clinical features may closely mimic non-progressive ataxic CP and as its X-linked transmission makes diagnosis extremely important for genetic counselling. MRI is of great help by showing absent or extremely limited myelination in T_1-weighted sequences and an intense signal from the white matter on T_2-weighted sequences (Silverstein *et al.* 1990).

MIXED FORMS OF CEREBRAL PALSY

The proportion of cases of CP assigned to mixed types varies considerably depending on the defining criteria used. If one considers that the presence of dystonic or athetotic movements of the hand in congenital hemiplegia is enough to talk of mixed forms, then their frequency is extremely high, but other associations such as ataxia and dystonia or spasticity are common. Dyskinetic–dystonic forms are frequently associated with bilateral spastic CP, especially in postasphyxic cases. Regardless of attribution to a particular type, functional analysis of each individual patient is the basis for therapy and is therefore more important than classification (Mulligan *et al.* 1980).

UNUSUAL MANIFESTATIONS OF CEREBRAL PALSY

Many investigators include in the descriptions of cerebral palsies a *hypotonic or atonic type* that is characterized by general muscular hypotonia which persists beyond 2–3 years of age and does not result from a primary disorder of muscle or peripheral nerve. A majority of these infants later develop spastic, dyskinetic and, especially, ataxic CP, but in some cases generalized hypotonia persists well into childhood. These may simply constitute the most severe forms of CP, where the maturational changes in the brain do not occur that would normally lead to dystonic or spastic patterns developing (Brett 1997). Clancy *et al.* (1989) think that hypoxic–ischaemic involvement of the spinal cord, and especially of the anterior horn cells, is common in perinatal hypoxia and may be responsible for at least some of the motor symptoms in many cases of CP. Sladky and Rorke (1986) also underline the frequency of spinal damage in perinatal hypoxia. However, in most cases of 'atonic' diplegia the electromyogram does not indicate denervation and the deep tendon reflexes are increased rather than depressed. Major malformations of the brain such as agyria–pachygyria are an important cause of hypotonic CP. Some infants with severe perinatal or prenatal hypoxia may develop selective symptoms and signs of involvement of the brainstem nuclei such as absence of eye movements and pupillary responses to light, absent gag reflex, ptosis and facial diplegia (Roland *et al.* 1988). A similar clinical picture may be seen in association

with bilateral symmetrical calcification of the thalami (Ambler and O'Neill 1975, Parisi *et al.* 1983) which in rare cases may be familial (Abuelo *et al.* 1981). In experiments on animals, acute hypoxia produces selective necrosis of brainstem and thalamic nuclei (Myers 1972), and lesions in the same areas have been reported in humans under similar conditions (Friede 1989).

A pseudobulbar type of CP, known as Worster-Drought type, occurs with bilateral lesions limited to the opercular regions (Worster-Drought 1974). The clinical picture is one of severe disturbances of speech, lingual movements, and intentional facial motility with preservation of automatic and affective movements. Drooling is a serious problem and swallowing difficulties may be present. Most cases seem to be due to bilateral opercular disturbances of migration (Chapter 3) but some result from acquired damage to the same areas due to perinatal hypoxia (Koeda *et al.* 1995) or to the sequelae of herpes encephalitis. Partial forms are not uncommon.

DIAGNOSIS AND DIFFERENTIAL DIAGNOSIS

The correct diagnosis of CP is highly dependent on knowledge of normal development and its variants. It is relatively easy to exclude the diagnosis of CP early if the developmental pattern of a suspected infant is normal. On the other hand, a positive diagnosis of CP of whichever type will have to await, in most cases, the appearance of definitive signs and these can be very late. In one study from Finland (Kruus *et al.* 1989), the incidence of CP in two prospective series of infants was initially estimated to be as high as 3.9 per 1000 and 5.9 per 1000, respectively, only to finally settle at about 2.0 per 1000 after the infants were over 4 years of age. Such figures indicate how much the diagnosis can err if infants are not followed up and how one should be careful in evaluating the 'effect' of early intervention. Modern imaging techniques can contribute to an early diagnosis. In one series (Truwit *et al.* 1992) 37 of 40 CP patients had an abnormal MRI, and in another (Candy *et al.* 1993) 17 of 22 infants with apparently isolated motor delay had MRI anomalies suggesive of CP.

The diagnosis of CP can be delayed in children with variants of normal development. Robson and Mac Keith (1971) showed that the diagnosis of spastic diplegia was significantly delayed in 'shufflers' with hypotonia of the lower limbs and axial muscles.

It is often stated that a history of abnormal factors in pregnancy, birth or the neonatal period is an important argument in favour of the diagnosis of CP. However, the relationship between such factors and the occurrence of later CP is not a close one and they should be accepted as supporting the diagnosis only in cases of major anomalies such as preterm birth and, especially, clinically manifest hypoxic–ischemic encephalopathy.

The diagnosis of CP is essentially clinical. Neuroimaging can have a confirmatory value in some cases. Electromyography, that may shed some light on the mechanisms (Harrison 1988, Kanda *et al.* 1988), has no place in practical diagnosis except for the exclusion of other conditions that share with CP some weakness or hypotonia.

The differential diagnosis of specific types of CP has already been discussed. Only problems common to most types of CP are reviewed here.

An essential diagnostic consideration is the differentiation of progressive neurological disorders, especially treatable ones, from CP. Spinal cord tumour in the cervical region and slow growing brain tumours should always be excluded (Haslam1975).

Many metabolic or heredodegenerative diseases run a slow course and their clinical manifestations can mimic all types of CP (Aicardi *et al.* 1988). The leukodystrophies for example may be initally impossible to distinguish from spastic diplegia, and ataxia–telangiectasia has features indistinguishable from those of many nonprogressive ataxias. Some cases of dopa-sensitive dystonia may simulate diplegia or athetoid CP, and a trial of L-dopa is indicated when history and examination make this a realistic possibility. Leigh disease (Fryer *et al.* 1994), organic acidaemias (Gascon *et al.* 1994), mitochondrial diseases (Tsao *et al.* 1994) and carbohydrate-deficient glycoprotein syndrome (Stibler *et al.* 1993) can also mimic any type of CP, and differentiation of fixed from progressive metabolic disorders is becoming increasingly difficult, so that indications for investigations may need to be reviewed.

The diagnosis of progressive neurological diseases can be helped by laboratory tests (Chapters 9, 10). However, these should be used only in cases selected on a clinical basis. In some cases, laboratory tests may be misleading. One patient with paraplegia due to a congenital spinal tumour (J.A., personal case) had for several years a diagnosis of metachromatic leukodystrophy, on the basis of a pseudodeficiency in arylsulfatase A (Chapter 9).

Patients with mental retardation without motor abnormalities are often given a diagnosis of CP because, in both situations, normal milestones are attained late. Yet it is essential not to consider children with CP as being mentally retarded on this basis.

Hypotonia is a feature common to most early cases of CP but also to different diseases that are not infrequently misdiagnosed as CP. The Prader–Willi syndrome is especially likely to be confused with CP because of the mental retardation, difficulties with swallowing, respiratory depression and frequent low birthweight (Wharton and Bresman 1989). The same applies to congenital myotonic dystrophy (Chapter 22), which indeed often coexists with actual hypoxic encephalopathy due to early asphyxia resulting from respiratory muscle involvement (Rutherford *et al.* 1989).

Hypertonia which is also a common early feature of several forms of CP may also occur in infants with other problems or in otherwise normal infants (PeBenito *et al.* 1989). Neck extensor hypertonia in particular is often a precursor of CP (Amiel-Tison *et al.* 1977, Ellenberg and Nelson 1981). Touwen and Hadders-Algra (1983) found this to apply only when other abnormalities were associated with hyperextension of the neck and trunk. The marked hypertonia observed in hyperekplexia (Chapter 17) may simulate diplegia or tetraplegia but there is progressive improvement and touch stimuli frequently produce a consider-able hypertonic response with apnoea. Georgieff and coworkers have emphasized increased muscle trunk tone as a marker of development in low-birthweight infants, not followed by CP (Georgieff and Bernbaum 1986, Georgieff *et al.* 1986).

MANAGEMENT

Given the protean manifestations of CP, its management presents a challenge to health services. Most would agree that children with such chronic and complex neurological disabilities need to be seen at a multidisciplinary centre. Bax and Whitmore (1991) have suggested that the minimum disciplines required to be involved would be paediatrics, physiotherapy, occupational therapy, speech therapy, psychology, community nursing, social work and education. As the child grows, the way this team functions would vary: in the preschool years the child might attend a preschool centre or nursery class at a child development centre, usually situated in association with a hospital, whereas during school years, s/he may be placed at a special school or be integrated in a normal school. The problem of providing a service for these young people as they reach adolescence and leave school is a difficult one, and few countries have adequate services.

A second issue is that while motor disorder is a prerequisite for the diagnosis of CP, other manifestations of static encephalopathies occur very commonly in the child with CP, including epilepsy, visual problems, learning disorders, mental retardation and incontinence. Both visual acuity problems and strabismus are more common among people with CP than in the general population, and they require identification and treatment. 'Learning disorders' may range from profound mental retardation to difficulties with specific tasks, such as reading or mathematics, in children of otherwise normal intelligence.

Because the child with CP presents to the health services at or soon after birth, a lot of emphasis in the medical, health and therapeutic literature has been on the early management of the child. Indeed, one subject of debate is how far the early treatment can influence the outcome (Palmer *et al.* 1988). Early support and help for the parents and family is very important, but equally one has to recognize that while there is some increase in mortality, in general people with CP will live the full life span. Therefore, when considering the management of CP one has to think about providing a service to meet health needs from infancy through to adulthood.

CP is defined as a nonprogressive disorder, but it has also been described as a not unchanging disorder. Unfortunately, there are few studies on the natural history of CP. Reports on populations are mostly cross-sectional. In one classic text, Crothers and Paine (1959) recounted their experience at the clinic which they had run together. While this did look, in rather general terms, at the outcomes and produce some life expectancy tables, the accounts were somewhat anecdotal (this applies to a number of other studies). Some cross-sectional studies have looked at cerebral-palsied people at older ages. Thomas *et al.* (1989) reported one such study and in general found a poor outcome in adult life. It is difficult to know whether these findings, which have been replicated (*e.g.* Stevenson *et al.* 1997), represent changes (and this very often implies deterioration), are a consequence of the original static encephalopathy, or represent an inadequate level of care. It is clear that the level of care for young people with CP tends to drop when they leave school, but equally, a recent report revealed that in one hospital-based population some people who had been diagnosed as having athetoid CP in fact had a degenerating condition (Fletcher and Marsden 1996). Anecdotally, anyone who sees young adults with CP is aware of such deterioration, for example it is common to find people who had been able to feed themselves losing that ability in early adult life, and certainly the movement disorder has secondary consequences, such as osteoarthritis, which may be more prevalent in this population than in others. In planning services, therefore, problems of providing continuity of care are very significant.

Of course, a diagnosis of CP has implications not only for the health services but also for education. At least half of the children with CP in most studies have moderate or severe learning disorders, while even those whose cognitive levels are in the normal range may have specific problems in school such as a reading difficulty. In the past, in developed countries, children with CP have often been educated in special schools, either specifically for such children or more generally for those with motor disabilities. In recent years, there has been great emphasis on integrating or, to use the American term, 'mainstreaming' children with CP, and the pros and cons of the situation have been much discussed (*e.g.* Butler 1996). Perhaps more important than whether the child is in a normal or special school, is that the teachers and other personnel around the child know enough about the condition(s) that the child is suffering from and can plan and programme her/his education accordingly. Doing this effectively in a mainstream school is probably more expensive than in a special school, but of course that is not a reason for not trying to put the child among her/his ordinary peers.

The child with CP will also need a good preschool facility, and in assessing educational status and making plans as discussed above, a period of observation in a nursery may be extremely helpful. A properly planned preschool program may help the child integrate into a mainstream school when s/he reaches 5 or 6 years of age. One would hope that, as discussed below, within any nursery provision for such a child, there would be good speech, physio- and occupational therapy available at the site.

MEETING THE NEEDS OF THE DISABLED CHILD
The child needs: (i) diagnosis; (ii) assessment; (iii) treatment; (iv) management; (v) care and counselling; (vi) periodic diagnostic review and assessment.

The diagnostic issues have been discussed earlier in this chapter. In so far as the diagnosis, to some extent, is one of exclusion, this will often mean that there is a period of anxiety for the parents when they are not sure what diagnosis is going to be given them. In some instances, for example with a child who suffers an intraventricular haemorrhage during the perinatal period, the situation may become clearer at an earlier age. In any

case, parents will wish to have as much information about the cause of their child's disability as early as possible. The view on disclosure, *i.e.* telling the parents about the nature of their child's condition, has been much discussed, and a useful summary has been produced by the UK charity Scope (Leonard 1994).

ASSESSMENT
It goes without saying that any child with CP needs regular assessment of their health status. Upper respiratory tract infections are just as common in children with CP as in the normal population, but because of poor swallowing they may be more unpleasant for the child with CP. Some milestones may be passed later in the child with CP, for example control of bowel or bladder may be achieved late or never achieved at all. One should also bear in mind that a proportion of children with CP have neuropathic bladders (Reid and Borzyskowski 1993), and this problem will need appropriate investigation and management (Borzyskowski and Mundy 1990, Borzyskowski 1996).

The diagnostic labels, such as 'spastic diplegia' or 'hemiplegia', give a broad indication of the nature of the child's problems, but to plan a management programme one needs to know what the child is actually able to do. Assessment of the child involves comparing function and all aspects of development with the expected norms for age (Bax *et al.* 1990). The child with CP will commonly have delayed development as well as abnormal development. S/he may be late to roll, crawl, sit and walk, and the delay of these motor milestones may well be the first thing that worries the parents and brings the child to the physician. When the child is not mentally retarded, there may be a very uneven developmental profile, with delayed motor development but evidence of near-normal speech and language. If there is mental retardation there may be global delay in all aspects of development. Obviously, the more functions that are involved, the worse the likely prognosis, but prediction in the first year or so of life is difficult. As the child becomes older, however, it begins to be possible to predict what the eventual performance will be like. By 2 years, for instance, one can predict future ambulatory ability with around 90 per cent accuracy (Sala and Grant 1995) (Table 8.2).

Assessment therefore involves looking at all aspects of the child's development: gross and fine motor function, vision, hearing, speech and language, perceptual and intellectual function and, most importantly, social and emotional development.

Difficulties in assessing the child with CP may arise if the motor disorder interferes with the assessment of other aspects of function. For example, a simple form-board test requires a 2-year-old child to place various shapes into same-shaped spaces: the child with CP may have the ability to match the shapes correctly but, lacking the motor skills to make the required movements, be unable either to make those movements or to indicate that s/he wants to. The most prominent difficulty that arises involves the assessment of communication, where motor interference with the organs of communication makes it extremely difficult for a child to use speech or to use nonverbal forms of communication such as pointing or making other gestures. Given such complex-

TABLE 8.2
Prediction of future ambulation at age 2 years*

1. Physical signs
The child is unlikely to walk if there is:
Persistence of: Extensor thrust ①
              Asymmetrical tonic neck reflex ③
              Moro reflex ④
              Neck-righting response ⑤
Failure to develop a parachute reaction ②

2. Type of cerebral palsy

Hemiplegia	All walk
Spastic diplegia	~90% walk
Spastic quadriplegia	? Probably around 50% walk
Athetosis	? ~70% walk
Ataxia	All walk

3. Developmental assessment at around 2 years
The child is likely to walk if the following milestones are achieved by this age:
Arm propping (parachutes)
Sitting from prone
Reciprocal crawling
Maintaining sitting

*Adapted from Sala and Grant (1995).
At around 2 years of age, three factors enable one to predict future walking ability: *first*, physical signs (figures in circles represent significance of signs); *second*, type of cerebral palsy; and *third*, developmental status.

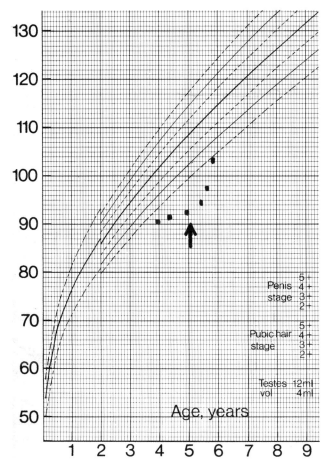

Fig. 8.8. Height chart from a child, showing return to 3rd centile within nine months of commencement of vigorous dietary supplementation *(arrowed).* His weight followed rather more slowly.

ities, it is often helpful to have the child in a nursery situation with skilled teachers and therapists around so that a continuous assessment can be made of the child's function.

Aside from function, it is also important to look at other aspects of the child's physical development. The child with CP often has disturbances of growth: in the hemiplegic child this will be unilateral, but in the spastic diplegic child there may be normal growth in the arms and in the upper extremities, but diminished growth in the legs. Most of this delay will probably occur within the first two years of life. A difficulty here is that children with CP commonly have feeding difficulties, and every care has to be taken to maintain adequate nutrition, bearing in mind that their basal metabolic rates may be different to those of children without disabilities. Malnutrition, of course, can itself lead to growth failure, and it is often difficult to be certain what causes suppressant growth. Figure 8.8 shows a height chart from a child whose failure to grow was thought to be an intrinsic part of his condition until more vigorous dietary supplementation showed that this was not the case.

Other aspects of development may also be affected, for example cryptorchidism is more common among children with CP than in the general population. Children with CP will suffer all the normal problems of childhood, such as frequent respiratory infections, but in a child whose physical difficulties make breathing and coughing difficult and sometimes ineffective, these may be of serious consequence. A particular problem in CP is drooling which can occur in as many as 50 per cent of cases. It is a very unpleasant problem and difficult to treat. Various drugs have been tried, of which scopolamine patches are probably the most useful (Lewis *et al.* 1994); benzehexol (Blasco *et al.* 1992) and glycopyrrolate (Blasco and Stansbury 1996) are also worth a try. Redirection of the salivary ducts and removal of a salivary gland is another possibility with a good rate of success in experienced hands (Burton 1991).

The assessment of epilepsy in children with CP presents particular problems. The EEG in CP is often disorganized, and unusual movements are common so that the decision as to whether or not the child is having a convulsive episode is difficult. Equally, epilepsy in brain-damaged children tends to be persistent, and its treatment is 'often an integral part of the comprehensive care of the children with cerebral palsy' (Aicardi 1990). The use of video recording by the parents is often helpful in coming to some decision about the nature of the phenomenon they are describing. It is sometimes necessary to admit the child to hospital for observation to determine the nature of the seizures. Details of the treatment are discussed elsewhere in this text (Chapter 16).

Various techniques have been developed to aid in assessing the child with CP. One significant advance in recent years has been the development of the gait laboratory, in which the use of video tape, EMG and force-plates allows one to study objectively the origins of the child's abnormal gait. Standardized measures of normal gait have been developed, and these have been applied to decision-making in the treatment of abnormal gait in CP (Sutherland 1984, Sutherland *et al.* 1988, Gage 1991). A more simple but apparently as effective a technique of studying gait, by measurement of instantaneous foot velocities, has been described by Law and Minns (1987).

One problem with the motor assessment of the child with CP has been the difficulty in knowing which standard measures to employ. When the well-known scales of infant development such as the Griffiths or Bayley scales are used, the child with CP is placed very low on the scale and it is difficult to measure any improvement over time. The Gross Motor Function Measure (Russell *et al.* 1993) is an advance here, and other infant measures are also reported (*e.g.* Harris *et al.* 1984).

TREATMENT
'Treatment' often implies 'cure', so it is important to emphasize to the parents that while one can modify the manifestations of CP, as yet there is no curative treatment for it and the child will have a persistent abnormality. Of course there are some aspects of the child's condition that can be effectively treated—in at least 50 per cent of cases epilepsy can be stopped (Aicardi 1990), spectacles may deal with visual problems, and a squint may be corrected—but in general all one can offer is a management programme that ameliorates the condition and allows the child to develop the best possible function.

Prevention of contracture may also be seen as an effective treatment. It is important to have some understanding of the origins of the contracture. The spasticity in the muscle means that the limb is held in abnormal posture. Muscle growth depends to some extent on stretch, so if abnormal postures are maintained for long periods, muscle growth will be abnormal and eventually the muscle will become short and contractures will develop. Also, the abnormal muscle movements tend to interfere with joint function and this is particularly true around the ankle, so that the child may develop varus or valgus deformities around the foot. A tendency to internal rotation and adduction at the hips means that abnormalities may develop around the hip joint; the joint is likely to be dysplastic and eventually may dislocate completely, and should therefore be viewed radiographically regularly during the early years of life. Clinical assessment of the hip has been very fully discussed by both Scrutton (1984) and Bleck (1987). Good management hopefully will prevent the dislocation developing.

In general, deformities can be prevented by maintaining the joints and muscles in neutral positions. Thus, in the child with spastic diplegia or hemiplegia, the gastrocnemius and soleus are spastic, the ankle is kept in extension and the child toe-walks. Varus or valgus deformity should be preventable by early splinting with a lightweight ankle–foot orthosis to maintain the foot in a neutral position. Deformities in the upper limbs can be prevented in a similar way.

MANAGEMENT OF THE MOTOR DISORDER
Numerous ways have been tried to moderate the abnormalities found in the different varieties of CP. The protean nature of the condition attracts enthusiasts who believe there must be some way of reversing the inevitable consequences of the damage in the motor areas of the brain. Sometimes in association with a medical centre, but more often not, many unorthodox treatments have been tried. In the following sections discussion will be limited to physiotherapy, surgical (largely orthopaedic) management, and drug treatment. In general, most of the treatments relate to the spastic forms of the disorder; athetoid problems are mentioned separately. While the cause of the disorder is central, it is clear the effects are peripheral, and it is important to have an understanding of the neurophysiology of movement and the qualities of muscles. This subject has been well reviewed by Walsh (1993).

PHYSIOTHERAPY
It seems commonsensical to suggest that disordered movements might be improved by some sort of manipulation of or exercises with the affected muscles. Notions of such treatment were derived in the 1940s and '50s from the experience of treating children who had suffered from anterior poliomyelitis. During the 1960s a number of therapists with experience of treating CP emerged in different parts of the world, often with different and sometimes conflicting ideas about how the condition could be managed. The issues have been well reviewed by Scrutton (1984). Broadly, the therapist aims to prevent the development of deformity, suppress unwanted or abnormal movements and promote optimal function.

Early treatment methods often involved a child being brought on a regular basis to a treatment centre where, for a period of time (rarely more than an hour a day) exercises would be carried out. However, it was soon realized that an hour's exercise a day is unlikely to change the abnormal motor pattern, and that in order to achieve any success it was necessary for suggested patterns of movement to be carried out throughout the day by carers (usually the parents but also teachers).

The first task of the therapist is to prevent the development of contractures. Most therapists would then aim to prevent unwanted movements and promote normal active ones. The spastic child, though stiff, is often weak because it is difficult to exercise spontaneously. The pragmatic therapist tries to draw on personal experience of different therapeutic techniques (discussed briefly below) to develop a specific programme to meet the needs of each individual child.

Every activity one carries out has a motor component. Whereas in a normal child such activity would occur spontaneously, in the child with CP every activity has to be reviewed to see that it is carried out as normally as possible. Thus, many children with CP have feeding difficulties, and the whole process of eating may be interrupted by abnormal posturing which interferes with the movements of deglutition. The child must be seated in an adequate and controlled position so that s/he can use the hands and move lips, teeth and palate to eat in a normal fashion. For many activities, *e.g.* writing or using some sort of tool, seating and standing postures have to be reviewed before the activity itself can be studied and planned. Thus the task of the physiotherapist and occupational therapist is to review with the parents all the activities of the day and to try to ensure that movements are made as effectively and easily as possible.

We give here one example of such a programme, developed to deal with an abnormal pattern of behaviour emerging in a child described by Scrutton (1984):

Problem: Consistent preferred head turning (PHT) and asymmetric tonic neck response (ATNR) in an infant with quadriplegic cerebral palsy—probably rigid/dystonic.

Consideration: We cannot treat the ATNR as such—it will diminish or remain depending on factors within the child. We can usually prevent the PHT and ATNR from being perfected through practice—leading to unnecessarily retained asymmetry long after the response has disappeared—and so reduce the effect this has on gross movement and posture.

Aim: To encourage head turning to the opposite side and movements and postures against the asymmetric response.

Action:

(1) Parents to approach, play, and feed the child from the opposite side.

(2) Use a foam cut-out to hold his head to the neutral or opposite side when supine or in a 'baby relax'.

(3) Use a prone wedge: some infants lose all preferred head turning in a supported prone position, others spontaneously turn to the opposite side.

(4) Corner seat: placed high in the room (on a table) to encourage looking down and positioned so that the preferred side is to a blank wall. Preferred head turning is often less in sitting than supine.

(5) Supported sitting propping on an extended 'occipital' arm.

(6) Creeping: facilitating jaw-side leg flexion and abduction followed by symmetrical creeping facilitated through shoulder girdle or head/neck.

(7) Jaw-side upper limb exploring face, sucking fingers, *etc.*

(8) Any symmetrical activity.

Scrutton's book includes chapters by several practitioners who have developed 'systems of therapy'. The best known (and probably the best thought out) are the techniques developed by the Bobaths (Bobath 1980, Bobath and Bobath 1984). Their approach is often referred to as a neurodevelopmental one. It aims by an understanding of the abnormal patterns of motor development observed in children with CP to inhibit these patterns, and through understanding of the normal patterns of development to promote normal movement. In recent years their programmes have emphasized the integration of the treatment into daily living. Other well-known systems of therapy include those of Vojta (1984) and the Peto School (Hári and Ákos 1971). The latter is an educational approach to motor disability and believes that constant training will lead to improvement. A problem with all these approaches is the failure to recognize the extent to which normal motor development follows morphological development within the CNS.

A danger with some of these systems of therapy (such as those advocated by Glen Doman and Cari Delacato—see Cummins 1988) is that they place great strains on the child and parents, disrupting the normal patterns of family life to no proven benefit. A working party of the European Academy of Childhood Disability (McConachie *et al.* 1997) recently stressed the importance of moving away from a system of therapy devised to be applied to a child, to a child-centred approach—that is, devising a programme to help the child which relates to the child's needs rather than any theoretical position of the health carers. The authors wrote: 'management of a child's programme should be goal orientated, and specifically adapted to that child's wishes and circumstances'. There was some discussion of the question, 'Should life adapt to therapy, or therapy adapt to life?', with general agreement on the latter position. One corollary is that the traditional division between different methods of therapy is inappropriate, and that professionals should select from different approaches, the techniques needed for meeting the goals set for a particular child.

ORTHOPAEDIC MANAGEMENT

It has already been mentioned that many contractures and the abnormal growth of muscles and hence of joints can be prevented by early splinting to maintain joints in neutral positions. This management will often be the coresponsibility of the orthopaedist and the physiotherapist. The orthopaedic surgeon can help the child in a number of ways. Where fixed deformities have developed, corrective surgery may be carried out, and there are surgical procedures that can also help with movement.

In general, the orthopaedic surgeon may carry out bony operation and/or lengthen and transfer muscles. For a full discussion of orthopaedic management in CP, readers are referred to the comprehensive volume by Bleck (1987). The bony operation of choice may be arthrodesis because stability at a joint may be more important than the range of movement. The very common instability of the ankle joint with either valgus or varus deformity can be corrected by such surgery. Where contracture has occurred, lengthening of the muscle may restore the situation. This—and in particular, lengthening of the Achilles tendon—is probably the most common surgery performed on patients with CP. Where contractures have occurred in the hips and knees, the surgeon may carry out soft tissue surgery around the hip, knee and ankle in a single operation. Function may be improved by transferring a tendon so that the muscle is acting differently on a joint. Thus, with an overflexed wrist, the surgeon may transplant a wrist flexor onto the dorsum of the hand to increase extension. Interestingly, the transferred muscle will adopt a new role.

NEW APPROACHES

One problem that arises with the management of CP is that new approaches constantly emerge that are greeted with a wave of enthusiasm and show preliminary results which appear encouraging. An example of this was in the 1970s when cerebellar implants were in vogue and a large number were placed in children with CP, but in time it was demonstrated that no improvement occurred. There are some recent developments to which one should draw attention. The first is the use of dorsal rhizotomy. The technique, which has been known for a long time and was taken up by Peacock in the '80s, involves cutting selective dorsal roots (Peacock and Staudt 1990). A number of recent studies of reasonably controlled trials demonstrate some benefits. However, one problem with most of these reports is that the patient selection and identification is not well described; nor have many of the studies looked at alternative possibilities in terms of management. An exception to this is a recent study by McLaughlin *et al.* (1997, 1998) which compared patients treated by dorsal rhizotomy or by physiotherapy and found little difference in outcome between the two patient groups.

DRUG THERAPY

In general, the use of drugs in CP has proved disappointing, and many doctors limit their use to the control of severe spasms seen in the worst cases. Many drugs have been tried, and diazepam has proved particularly effective, although finding the optimum dosage in each case is often difficult.

Currently the most widely used drug is probably baclofen. It may be given intrathecally by continuous perfusion or in boluses (Armstrong *et al.* 1997). Drugs which seem to be effective when tested on animals often prove disappointing in treating humans.

A more recent development has been the use of botulinum toxin, which in a similar fashion to the alcohol–phenol injections reported by Tardieu and his colleagues in the '70s (Tardieu and Hariga 1972, Tardieu *et al.* 1973), decreases spasticity by blocking the release of acetylcholine at the neuromuscular junction. This is theoretically tempting because the effects are temporary. At the time of writing, the number of reports which are of adequate controlled trials of the use of botulinum toxin are rather few (for a review, see Forssberg and Tedroff 1997). However, papers by Cosgrove and his colleagues (Cosgrove *et al.* 1994, Corry *et al.* 1997), with reasonable trials in both upper and lower limbs, lend quite powerful support to its use as an adjunct to other forms of management of the motor disorder.

In patients with athetoid CP, contractures and fixed deformities are not usually a problem, and the main difficulties relate to their involuntary movements. Sometimes these can be very powerful and extremely difficult to interrupt, making all purposeful movement impossible. Again, various drugs have been tried but with no great success. Many patients report that a small amount of alcohol significantly reduces the unwanted movements.

Motor control has to be achieved by patient therapeutic work. The use of visual feedback, where the individual can observe the unwanted movements and attempt to control them, is one technique that has achieved some success.

COMMUNICATION

Many individuals with CP have communication problems, and this may present a more serious challenge than their movement difficulties. The early emphasis will be to try and develop speech, but as with walking, where it is important to realize that this may not be achieved, so too by the age of 4 or 5 years a decision should be taken as to whether the child's level of comprehensibility in speech will mean that s/he is never going to be an oral communicator. From early on, alternative methods of communication can be considered. These may vary from low-tech aids such as picture boards or Bliss symbol charts, to high-tech aids with computers providing the person with an output through a voice synthesizer.

Another possibility is use of a sign language, but the problem here is that the child may have difficulty in signing because of her/his motor difficulties (Decoste and Glennen 1997).

FEEDING PROBLEMS

It is curious that the older textbooks on CP (*e.g.* Crothers and Paine 1959, lngram 1964) make no mention of the problem for the child with CP of feeding, whereas in fact, in a very significant proportion of people with CP feeding difficulties occur and persist through into adult life. The child may never develop beyond the suck–swallow pattern of infancy and may never be able to chew. Difficulties arise, therefore, in both the oral and swallowing parts of feeding. Also, issues concerning the stomach arise, with a high incidence of reflux. For many of the most severely disabled children there has recently been a move to gastrostomy where the long-term results are in some doubt (Strauss *et al.* 1997). However, the use of a peg gastrostomy (Eltumi and Sullivan 1997) means that such treatment can be considered, for a short time, to help with the nutrition of the child, while efforts to help their feeding skills can go on without the pressure and anxiety of having to provide nutrition through the oral route alone. Most experts regard prolonged use of nasogastric tubes as a factor leading to difficulties.

The situation is complicated by the fact that poor growth may be partially a feature of the condition, as is clearly demonstrated in hemiplegia. Many CP clinics and child development centres now have specialist feeding clinics with dietitians, speech therapists and physicians as part of the team trying to maintain adequate nutrition and a satisfactory feeding pattern. It is important to remember also that, apart from their nutritional role, meal times are significant social occasions in most societies.

LEARNING DISORDERS

The child with CP may have global mental retardation or specific learning problems, *e.g.* difficulty with reading (sometimes called dyslexia), or with mathematics, or some other specific problem. These difficulties will emerge as the child reaches school age. It is often hard to predict which children will have such problems. Thus, although the child with speech and language delay is more likely to have difficulties in reading, many late language developers do learn to read. There may be particular patterns of problems with particular types of CP, for instance the hemiplegic child may be particularly prone to specific learning problems, but data on this are currently not firmly established.

The proportion of children with CP and global retardation varies according to the different aetiological reports and the inclusion or exclusion of severely disabled children who barely reach beyond the 3-month level of function. It seems likely that developments in perinatal care over the last decade have led to an increasing number of children with spastic quadriplegia who are severely mentally retarded. In addition to the continuing management of their movement disorders, such children will obviously require all the services needed by other mentally retarded children, including some special educational provision.

Whatever the nature of the learning disorder, efforts must be made to try to assess the child's level of functioning as early as possible. Sometimes remarkable intellectual function remains intact despite very severe motor and communication difficulties (see for example Christy Brown's account of himself in *My Left Foot*). However, such instances are the exception rather than the rule, and one is usually faced with trying to help the parents understand that their child is not just physically disabled but also has severe mental disability. Determining intellectual function at a single assessment may be difficult, but serial measurements over time will demonstrate the learning capacity or lack of it, and this too may help the parents appreciate their child's severe disability.

BEHAVIOURAL PROBLEMS
Rutter *et al.* (1970) firmly established the fact that the child with CNS damage is much more likely than a normal child to have a behaviour problem. Early studies showed that behaviour problems were five or six times as common in children with CP as in the normal population. In general, the pattern of behaviour problems tends to be the same as that found in normal children, and the main effect of the brain damage seems to be to make the child more vulnerable to disordered behaviour rather than to initiate particular types of problems. Thus, a family psychopathology may play a part in generating such problems, and it may be possible to plan potential remediation within the family. However, the family with a disabled child may find it hard to accept that they have a role in the child's behaviour difficulties, and psychiatric referral to a centre which uses a family therapy approach to problems may initially prove unhelpful.

There are various crisis points for the family where their stress may be extreme. These include: (i) the prediagnostic and diagnostic periods; (ii) going to school—the realization that the child is not going to attend or function in an ordinary way in a normal school; (iii) the attainment of puberty; and (iv) the young adult's need to achieve independence. The family and the child will need more support and counselling on these occasions.

Of course, there are certain behaviours that relate specifically to the child's disability. For instance, neuropathic bladder (Borzyskowski and Mundy 1990) may occur as a result of some dysfunction of the control mechanisms associated with the more common developmental difficulty of achieving bladder competence.

Hyperactive or hyperkinetic behaviour is associated with brain damage (Taylor 1986). Equally, hyperactive behaviour can be iatrogenically induced, and barbiturates should be avoided in the treatment of epilepsy in brain-injured children.

While much behavioural symptomatology is similar to that seen in normal children, that is not to say that the disability itself is not a factor in causing the behaviour. This applies equally to the child and to the family. Thus, while divorce is no more common among the parents of disabled children than in the general population, when it occurs in such a family the parents frequently cite problems with the child as a factor in the divorce. Similarly, children (particularly adolescents) will report their disability as a cause of their depression.

ADOLESCENT AND ADULT LIFE
As has been indicated, the outcome for the child with CP, as revealed by studies which have looked at young disabled adults, is often not very satisfactory. In addition to the continuation of all the problems that have been described, reaching adulthood imposes new problems for the individual with CP. The tasks of the adolescent include the achievement of independence, self-image or identity, expression of sexuality, and vocation. We deliberately use the word vocation rather than work because for many people with CP, employment may be difficult to find, and one may have to face the situation that the young person is not going to have a job but nevertheless needs to have a purposeful life plan. All aspects of independence obviously pose problems. Society has only recently accepted the sexuality of disabled people, and far too little work has been done on the implications of the physical disability itself for ordinary sexual activity. Communication systems developed in the early teenage years may be less appropriate as the young person gets older, and it has been shown that many young adults have inadequate communication systems (Thomas *et al.* 1989).

CONCLUSION
The World Health Organization has attempted to clarify some of the words used to discuss the problems of people with developmental disorders (WHO 1980), and their definitions can equally be applied to children with CP. Thus, the term *impairment* is used to describe the actual pathology or lesion the individual has (*e.g.* brain damage), *disability* describes the functional effect of that impairment, and *handicap* describes the practical consequences of the impairment or disability. A handicap is thus a social phenomenon, and very much 'in the eye of the beholder'. For example, a man in a wheelchair may not regard himself as being disabled; however, he may be unable to operate a lift (elevator) because he cannot reach the buttons, and so we would say that he is thereby handicapped.

A young child is unaware of the implications of her/his disability, while parents and professionals make the judgement that s/he is handicapped. As s/he gets older, s/he realizes the social consequences of the disability. The physician caring for children with CP has to try to help them accept their disability, while encouraging them to see that society does not 'handicap' them.

REFERENCES

Abuelo, D.N., Barsel-Bowers, G., Tutschka, G., *et al.* (1981) 'Symmetrical infantile thalamic degeneration in two sibs.' *Journal of Medical Genetics*, **18**, 448–450.

Adsett, A.B., Fitz, C.R., Hill, A. (1985) 'Hypoxic–ischaemic cerebral injury in the term newborn: correlation of CT findings with neurological outcome.' *Developmental Medicine and Child Neurology*, **27**, 155–160.

Ahdab-Barmada, M., Moossy, J. (1984) 'The neuropathology of kernicterus in the premature neonate: diagnostic problems.' *Journal of Neuropathology and Experimental Neurology*, **43**, 45–56.

—— —— Painter, M. (1980) 'Pontosubicular necrosis and hyperoxemia.' *Pediatrics*, **66**, 840–847.

Aicardi, J. (1990) 'Epilepsy in brain-injured children. A review.' *Developmental Medicine and Child Neurology*, **32**, 191–202.

—— (1994) *Epilepsy in Children. 2nd Edn.* New York: Raven Press.

—— Chevrie, J.J. (1983) 'Consequences of status epilepticus in infants and children.' *In:* Delgado-Escueta, A.V., Wasterlain, C.G., Treiman, D.M., Porter, R.J. (Eds.) *Status Epilepticus. Advances in Neurology, Vol. 34.* New York: Raven Press, pp. 115–125.

—— Amsili, J., Chevrie, J.J. (1969) 'Acute hemiplegia in infancy and childhood.' *Developmental Medicine and Child Neurology,* **11,** 162–173.

—— Barbosa, C., Andermann, E., *et al.* (1988) 'Ataxia–ocular motor apraxia: a syndrome mimicking ataxia–telangiectasia.' *Annals of Neurology,* **24,** 497–502.

Allen, M.C., Capute, A.J. (1989) 'Neonatal neurodevelopmental examination as a predictor of neuromotor outcome in premature infants.' *Pediatrics,* **83,** 498–506.

Amato, M., Hüppi, P., Herschkowitz, N., Huber, P. (1991) 'Prenatal stroke suggested by intrauterine ultrasound and confirmed by magnetic resonance imaging.' *Neuropediatrics,* **22,** 100–102.

Ambler, M., O'Neill, W. (1975) 'Symmetrical infantile thalamic degeneration with focal cytoplasmic calcification.' *Acta Neuropathologica,* **33,** 1–8.

Amiel-Tison, C., Korobkin, R., Esque-Vaucouloux, M.T. (1977) 'Neck extensor hypertonia: a clinical sign of insult to the central nervous system of the newborn.' *Early Human Development,* **1,** 181–190.

Amit, M., Camfield, P. (1980) 'Neonatal polycythemia causing multiple cerebral infarcts.' *Archives of Neurology,* **37,** 109–110.

Angelini, L., Rumi, V., Lamperti, E., Nardocci, N. (1988) 'Transient paroxysmal dystonia in infancy.' *Neuropediatrics,* **19,** 171–174.

Arens, L.J., Molteno, C.D. (1989) 'A comparative study of postnatally acquired cerebral palsy in Cape Town.' *Developmental Medicine and Child Neurology,* **31,** 246–254.

Armstrong, R.W., Steinbok, P., Cochrane, D.D., *et al.* (1997) 'Intrathecally baclofen for treatment of children with spasticity of cerebral origin.' *Journal of Neurosurgery,* **87,** 409–414.

Asindi, A.A., Stephenson, J.B.P., Young, D.G. (1988) 'Spastic hemiparesis and presumed prenatal embolisation.' *Archives of Disease in Childhood,* **63,** 68–69.

Aylward, G.P., Verhulst, S.J., Bell, S.(1989) 'Correlation of asphyxia and other risk factors with outcome: a contemporary view.' *Developmental Medicine and Child Neurology,* **31,** 329–340.

Barbot, C., Fineza, I., Diogo, L., *et al.* (1997) 'L-2-hydroxyglutaric aciduria: clinical, biochemical and magnetic resonance imaging in six Portuguese pediatric patients.' *Brain and Development,* **19,** 268–273.

Barkovich, A.J., Truwit, C.L. (1990) 'Brain damage from perinatal asphyxia: correlation of MR findings with gestational age.' *American Journal of Neuroradiology,* **11,** 1087–1096.

—— Westmark, K., Partridge, C., *et al.* (1995) 'Perinatal asphyxia: MR findings in the first 10 days.' *American Journal of Neuroradiology,* **16,** 427–438.

Barth, P.G., Valk, J., Olislagers-De Slegte, R. (1984) 'Central cortico–subcortical pattern on CT in cerebral palsy. Its relevance to asphyxia.' *Journal of Neuroradiology,* **11,** 65–71.

Baumann, R.J., Carr, W.A., Shuman, R.M. (1987) 'Patterns of cerebral arterial injury in children with neurological disabilities.' *Journal of Child Neurology,* **2,** 298–306.

Bax, M.C.O., Whitmore, K. (1991) 'District Handicap Teams in England: 1983–1988.' *Archives of Disease in Childhood,* **66,** 656–664.

—— Hart, H., Jenkins, S.M. (1990) *Child Development and Child Health. The Preschool Years.* Oxford: Blackwell Scientific.

Beltran, R.S., Coker, S.B. (1995) 'Transient dystonia of infancy, a result of intrauterine cocaine exposure?' *Pediatric Neurology,* **12,** 354–356.

Benecke, R., Meyer, B-U., Freund, H-J. (1991) 'Reorganisation of descending motor pathways in patients after hemispherectomy and severe hemispheric lesions demonstrated by magnetic brain stimulation.' *Experimental Brain Research,* **83,** 419–426.

Bennett, F.C., Chandler, L.S., Robinson, N.M., Sells, C.J. (1981) 'Spastic diplegia in premature infants. Etiologic and diagnostic considerations.' *American Journal of Diseases of Children,* **135,** 732–737.

Berg, R.A., Aleck, K.A., Kaplan, A.M. (1983) 'Familial porencephaly.' *Archives of Neurology,* **40,** 567–569.

Bhatt, M.H., Obeso, J.A., Marsden, C.D. (1993) 'Time course of postanoxic akinetic–rigid and dystonic syndromes.' *Neurology,* **43,** 314–317.

Billard, C., Dulac, O., Boulloche, J., *et al.* (1989) 'Encephalopathy with calcification of the basal ganglia in children. A reappraisal of Fahr's syndrome with respect to 14 new cases.' *Neuropediatrics,* **20,** 12–19.

Blair, E., Stanley, J.J. (1982) 'An epidemiological study of cerebral palsy in Western Australia. III: Postnatal aetiology.' *Developmental Medicine and Child Neurology,* **24,** 575–585.

—— —— (1988) 'Intrapartum asphyxia: a rare cause of cerebral palsy.' *Journal of Pediatrics,* **112,** 515–519.

Blasco, P.A., Stansbury, J.C.K. (1996) 'Glycopyrrolate treatment of chronic drooling.' *Archives of Paediatrics and Adolescent Medicine,* **150,** 932–935.

—— Allaire, J.H., and the participants of the Consortium on Drooling (1992) 'Drooling in the developmentally disabled: management practices and recommendations.' *Developmental Medicine and Child Neurology,* **34,** 849–862.

Bleck, E.E. (1987) *Orthopaedic Management in Cerebral Palsy. Clinics in Developmental Medicine No. 99/100.* London: Mac Keith Press.

Blumel, J., Evans, E.B., Eggers, G.W.N. (1960) 'A combination of congenital cataract and cerebral palsy in a brother and a sister.' *Archives of Ophthalmology,* **63,** 246–253.

Bobath, K. (1980) *A Neurophysiological Basis for the Treatment of Cerebral Palsy. Clinics in Developmental Medicine No. 75.* London: Spastics International Medical Publications.

—— Bobath, B. (1984) 'The neuro-developmental treatment.' *In:* Scrutton, D. (Ed.) *Management of the Motor Disorders of Children with Cerebral Palsy. Clinics in Developmental Medicine No. 90.* London: Spastics International Medical Publications, pp. 6–18.

Bordarier, C., Aicardi, J. (1990) 'Dandy–Walker syndrome and agenesis of the cerebellar vermis: diagnostic problems and genetic counselling. A review.' *Developmental Medicine and Child Neurology,* **32,** 285–294.

Borzyskowski, M. (1996) 'An update on the investigation of the child with a neuropathic bladder.' *Developmental Medicine and Child Neurology,* **38,** 744–748.

—— Mundy, A.R. (Eds.) (1990) *Neuropathic Bladder in Childhood. Clinics in Developmental Medicine No. 111.* London: Mac Keith Press.

Bouza, H., Dubowitz, L.M.S., Cowan, F., Pennock, J.M. (1994a) 'Late magnetic resonance imaging and clinical findings in neonates with unilateral lesions on cranial ultrasound.' *Developmental Medicine and Child Neurology,* **36,** 951–964.

—— —— Rutherford, M., Pennock, J.M. (1994b) 'Prediction of outcome in children with congenital hemiplegia: a magnetic resonance imaging study.' *Neuropediatrics,* **25,** 60–66.

—— Rutherford, M., Acolet, D., *et al.* (1994c) 'Evolution of early hemiplegic signs in full-term infants with unilateral brain lesions in the neonatal period: a prospective study.' *Neuropediatrics,* **25,** 201–207.

Bozynski, M.E.A., Nelson, M.N., Genaze, D. *et al.* (1988) 'Cranial ultrasonography and the prediction of cerebral palsy in infants weighing <1200 grams at birth.' *Developmental Medicine and Child Neurology,* **30,** 342–348.

Brett, E.M. (Ed.) (1997) *Pediatric Neurology, 3rd Edn.* Edinburgh: Churchill Livingstone.

Brown, C. (1954) *My Left Foot.* London: Secker & Warburg.

Brown, J.K., Van Rensburg, F., Walsh, G., *et al.* (1987) 'A neurological study of hand function of hemiplegic children.' *Developmental Medicine and Child Neurology,* **29,** 287–304.

Bundey, S. (1992) *Genetics in Neurology, 2nd Edn.* Edinburgh: Churchill Livingstone.

Burke, R.E., Fahn, S., Gold, A.P. (1980) 'Delayed onset dystonia in patients with 'static' encephalopathy.' *Journal of Neurology, Neurosurgery, and Psychiatry,* **43,** 789–797.

Burton, M.J. (1991) 'The surgical management of drooling.' *Developmental Medicine and Child Neurology,* **33,** 1110–1116.

Butler, C. (1996) 'Mainstreaming experience in the United States: is it the appropriate educational placement for every disabled child?' *Developmental Medicine and Child Neurology,* **38,** 861–866.

Candy, E.J., Hoon, A.H., Capute, A.J., Bryan, R.N. (1993) 'MRI in motor delay: important adjunct to classification of cerebral palsy.' *Pediatric Neurology,* **9,** 421–429.

Carlsson, G., Uvebrandt, P., Hugdahi, K., *et al.* (1994) 'Verbal and non-verbal function of children with right- versus left-hemiplegic cerebral palsy of pre- or perinatal origin.' *Developmental Medicine and Child Neurology,* **36,** 503–512.

Carr, L.J., Harrison, L.M., Evans, A.L., Stephens, J.A. (1993) 'Patterns of central motor reorganization in hemiplegic cerebral palsy.' *Brain,* **116,** 1223–1247.

Chaplin, E.R., Goldstein, G.W., Norman, D. (1979) 'Neonatal seizures, intracerebral hematoma, and subarachnoid hemorrhage in full-term infants.' *Pediatrics,* **63,** 812–815.

Chauvel, P., Trottier, S., Wignal, J.P., Bancaud, J. (1992) 'Somatomotor seizures of frontal lobe origin.' *In:* Chauvel, P., Delgado–Escueta, A.V., Halgren, E.,

234

Bancaud, J. (Eds.) *Frontal Lobe Seizures and Epilepsies.* New York: Raven Press, pp. 185–232.

Christensen, E., Melchior, J. (1967) *Cerebral Palsy—a Clinical and Neuropathological Study. Clinics in Developmental Medicine No. 25.* London: Spastics International Medical Publications.

Chugani, H.T., Miller, R.A., Chugani, D.C. (1996) 'Functional brain reorganization in children.' *Brain and Development*, **18**, 347–356.

Chutorian, A.M., Michener, R.C., Defendini, R., *et al.* (1979) 'Neonatal polycystic encephalomalacia: four new cases and review of the literature.' *Journal of Neurology, Neurosurgery, and Psychiatry*, **42**, 154–160.

Claeys, V., Deonna, T., Chrzanowski, R. (1983) 'Congenital hemiparesis: the spectrum of lesions. A clinical and computerized tomographic study of 37 cases.' *Helvetica Paediatrica Acta*, **38**, 439–455.

Clancy, R.R., Sladky, J.T., Rorke, L.B. (1989) 'Hypoxic–ischemic spinal cord injury following perinatal asphyxia.' *Annals of Neurology*, **25**, 185–189.

Clement, M.C., Briard, M.L., Ponsot, G., Arthuis, M. (1984) 'Ataxies cérébelleuses congénitales non progressives.' *Archives Françaises de Pédiatrie*, **41**, 685–700.

Coker, S.B., Beltran, R.S., Myers, T.F., Hmura, L. (1988) 'Neonatal stroke: description of patients and investigation into pathogenesis.' *Pediatric Neurology*, **4**, 219–223.

Colamaria, V., Curatolo, P., Cusmai, R., Dalla Bernardina, B. (1988) 'Symmetrical bithalamic hyperdensities in asphyxiated full-term newborns: an early indicator of status marmoratus.' *Brain and Development*, **10**, 57–59.

Cooke, R.W.I. (1987) 'Early and late cranial ultrasonographic appearances and outcome in very low birthweight infants.' *Archives of Disease in Childhood*, **62**, 931–937.

Corry, I.S., Cosgrove, A.P., Walsh, E.G., *et al.* (1997) 'Botulinum toxin A in the hemiplegic upper limb: a double-blind trial.' *Developmental Medicine and Child Neurology*, **39**, 185–193.

Cosgrove, A.P., Corry, I.S., Graham, H.K. (1994) 'Botulinum toxin in the management of the lower limb in cerebral palsy.' *Developmental Medicine and Child Neurology*, **36**, 386–396.

Crothers, B., Paine, R.S. (1959) *The Natural History of Cerebral Palsy.* (Reprinted 1988 as *Classics in Developmental Medicine No. 2.* London: Mac Keith Press.)

Crouchman, M. (1987) 'Environmentally induced transient motor signs in infancy.' *Developmental Medicine and Child Neurology*, **29**, 685–687.

Cummins, R.A. (1988) *The Neurologically-Impaired Child: Doman–Delacato Techniques Reappraised.* London: Croom Helm.

Dale, A., Stanley, F.J. (1980) 'An epidemiological study of cerebral palsy in Western Australia 1956–1975. II: Spastic cerebral palsy and perinatal factors.' *Developmental Medicine and Child Neurology*, **22**, 13–25.

Decoste, D.C., Glennen, S.L. (Eds.) (1997) *The Handbook of Augmentative and Alternative Communication.* San Diego: Singular Publishing.

Deonna, T-W., Ziegler, A-L., Nielsen, J. (1991) 'Transient idiopathic dystonia in infancy.' *Neuropediatrics*, **22**, 220–224.

D'Eugenio, D.B., Slagle, T.A., Mettelman, B.B., Gross, S.J. (1993) 'Developmental outcome of preterm infants with transient neuromotor abnormalities.' *American Journal of Diseases of Children*, **147**, 570–574.

de Vries, L.S., Eken, P., Groenendaal, F., *et al.* (1993) 'Correlation between the degree of periventricular leukomalacia diagnosed using cranial ultrasound and MRI later in infancy in children with cerebral palsy.' *Neuropediatrics*, **24**, 263–268.

Diebler, C., Dulac, O. (1987) *Pediatric Neurology and Neuroradiology.* Berlin: Springer.

Donn, S.M., Barr, M., McLeary, R.D. (1984) 'Massive intracerebral hemorrhage in utero: sonographic appearance and pathologic correlation.' *Obstetrics and Gynecology*, **63** (Suppl.), 28S–30S.

Dooling, E.C., Adams, R.D. (1975) 'The pathological anatomy of posthemiplegic athetosis.' *Brain*, **98**, 29–48.

Drillien, C.M. (1964) *The Growth and Development of the Prematurely Born Infant.* Edinburgh: Churchill Livingstone.

Dubowitz, L.M.S., Bydder, G.M., Mushin, J. (1985) 'Developmental sequence of periventricular leukomalacia. Correlation of ultrasound, clinical, and nuclear magnetic resonance functions.' *Archives of Disease in Childhood*, **60**, 349–355.

Dunn, H.G. (1986) *Sequelae of Low Birthweight: the Vancouver Study. Clinics in Developmental Medicine No. 95/96.* London: Mac Keith Press.

Edebol-Tysk, K. (1989) 'Epidemiology of spastic tetraplegic cerebral palsy in Sweden. I. Impairments and disabilities.' *Neuropediatrics*, **20**, 41–45.

—— Hagberg, B., Hagberg, G. (1989) 'Epidemiology of spastic tetraplegic cerebral palsy in Sweden. II. Prevalance, birth data and origin.' *Neuropediatrics*, **20**, 46–52.

Eicke, M., Briner, J., Willi, U., *et al.* (1992) 'Symmetrical thalamic lesions in infants.' *Archives of Disease in Childhood*, **67**, 15–19.

Ellenberg, J.H., Nelson, K.B. (1981) 'Early recognition of infants at high risk for cerebral palsy: examination at age four months.' *Developmental Medicine and Child Neurology*, **23**, 705–716.

—— —— (1988) 'Cluster of perinatal events identifying infants at high risk for death or disability.' *Journal of Pediatrics*, **113**, 546–552.

Eltumi, M., Sullivan, P.B. (1997) 'Nutritional management of the disabled child: the role of percutaneous endoscopic gastrostomy.' *Developmental Medicine and Child Neurology*, **39**, 66–68.

Evrard, P., Caviness, V.S. (1974) 'Extensive developmental defect of the cerebellum associated with posterior fossa ventriculocele.' *Journal of Neuropathology and Experimental Neurology*, **33**, 385–390.

Farmer, S.F., Harrison, L.M., Ingram, D.A., Stephens, J.A. (1991) 'Plasticity of central motor pathways in children with hemiplegic cerebral palsy.' *Neurology*, **41**, 1505–1510.

Fedrizzi, E., Inverno, M., Bruzzone, M.G., *et al.* (1996) 'MRI features of cerebral lesions and cognitive functions in preterm spastic diplegic children.' *Pediatric Neurology*, **15**, 207–212.

Fenichel, G.M. (1983) 'Hypoxic–ischemic encephalopathy in the newborn.' *Archives of Neurology*, **40**, 261–266.

—— Phillips, J.A. (1989) 'Familial aplasia of the cerebellar vermis. Possible X-linked dominant inheritance.' *Archives of Neurology*, **46**, 582–583.

Fletcher, N.A., Marsden, C.D. (1996) 'Dyskinetic cerebral palsy: a clinical and genetic study.' *Developmental Medicine and Child Neurology*, **38**, 873–880.

Flodmark, O., Lupton, B., Li, D., *et al.* (1989) 'MR imaging of periventricular leukomalacia in childhood.' *American Journal of Roentgenology*, **152**, 583–590.

Foley, J. (1992) 'Dyskinetic and dystonic cerebral palsy and birth.' *Acta Paediatrica*, **81**, 57–60.

Forssberg, H., Tedroff, K.B. (1997) 'Botulinum toxin treatment in cerebral palsy: intervention with poor evaluation?' *Developmental Medicine and Child Neurology*, **39**, 635–640.

Freeman, J.M., Nelson, K.B. (1988) 'Intrapartum asphyxia and cerebral palsy.' *Pediatrics*, **82**, 240–249.

Friede, R.L. (1989) *Developmental Neuropathology, 2nd Edn.* Berlin: Springer.

Fryer, A., Appleton, R., Sweeney, M.G., *et al.* (1994) 'Mitochondrial DNA 8993 (NARP) mutation presenting with a heterogeneous phenotype including 'cerebral palsy'.' *Archives of Disease in Childhood*, **71**, 419–422.

Furman, J.M., Baloh, R.W., Chugani, H., *et al.* (1985) 'Infantile cerebellar atrophy.' *Annals of Neurology*, **17**, 399–402.

Gage, J.R. (1991) *Gait Analysis in Cerebral Palsy. Clinics in Developmental Medicine No. 121.* London: Mac Keith Press.

Gascon, G.G., Ozand, P.T., Brismar, J. (1994) 'Movement disorders in childhood organic acidurias—clinical, neuroimaging and biochemical correlations.' *Brain and Development*, **16** (Suppl.), 94–103.

Gastaut, H., Poirier, F., Payan, H., *et al.* (1960) 'H.H.E. syndrome. Hemiconvulsions, hemiplegia, epilepsy.' *Epilepsia*, **1**, 418–447.

Georgieff, M.K., Bernbaum, J.C. (1986) 'Abnormal shoulder girdle muscle tone in premature infants during their first 18 months of life.' *Pediatrics*, **77**, 664–669.

—— Hoffman-Williamson, M., Daft, A. (1986) 'Abnormal truncal muscle tone as a useful early marker for developmental delay in low birth weight infants.' *Pediatrics*, **77**, 659–663.

Glenting, P. (1976) 'Variations in the population of congenital (pre- and perinatal) cases of cerebral palsy in Danish countries east of the Little Belt during the years 1950–1969.' *Ugeskrift for Laeger*, **138**, 2984–2991. *(Danish.)*

Goodman, R., Yude, C. (1996) 'IQ and its predictors in childhood hemiplegia.' *Developmental Medicine and Child Neurology*, **38**, 881–890.

Goutières, F., Challamel, M.J., Aicardi, J., Gilly, R. (1972) 'Les hémiplégies congénitales: sémiologie, étiologie et pronostic.' *Archives Françaises de Pédiatrie*, **29**, 839–851.

Govaert, P., de Vries, L.S. (1997) *An Atlas of Neonatal Brain Sonography. Clinics in Developmental Medicine No. 141/142.* London: Mac Keith Press.

Graham, M., Levene, M.I., Trounce, J.Q., Rutter, N. (1987) 'Prediction of cerebral palsy in very low birth-weight infants: prospective ultrasound study.' *Lancet*, **2**, 593–596.

Grant, A., O'Brien, N., Joy, M-T., *et al.* (1989) 'Cerebral palsy among children born during the Dublin randomised trial of intrapartum monitoring.' *Lancet*, **2**, 1233–1236.

Graziani, L.J., Pasto, M., Stanley, C., *et al.* (1986) 'Neonatal neurosonographic correlates of cerebral palsy in preterm infants.' *Pediatrics,* **78**, 88–95.

Gubbay, S.S. (1985) 'Clumsiness.' *In:* Vinken, P.J., Bruyn, G.W., Klawans, H.L. (Eds.) *Handbook of Clinical Neurology. Revised Series, Vol. 2. Neurobehavioral Disorders.* Amsterdam: Elsvier, pp. 159–167.

Gustavson, K.H., Hagberg, B., Sanner, G. (1969) 'Identical syndromes of cerebral palsy in the same family.' *Acta Paediatrica Scandinavica,* **58**, 330–340.

Guzzetta, F., Shackelford, G.D., Volpe, S., *et al.* (1986) 'Periventricular intra-parenchymal echodensities in the premature newborn: critical determinant of neurologic outcome.' *Pediatrics,* **78**, 995–1006.

—— Mercuri, E., Bonanno, S., *et al.* (1993) 'Autosomal recessive congenital cerebellar atrophy. A clinical and neuropsychological study.' *Brain and Development,* **15**, 439–445.

Haar, F., Dyken, P. (1977) 'Hereditary nonprogressive athetotic hemiplegia: a new syndrome.' *Neurology,* **27**, 849–854.

Hadders-Algra, M., Bos, A.F., Martin, A., Prechtl, H.F.R. (1994) 'Infantile chorea in an infant with severe bronchopulmonary dysplasia: an EMG study.' *Developmental Medicine and Child Neurology,* **36**, 177–182.

Hagberg, B., Hagberg, G. (1989) 'The changing panorama of infantile hydro-cephalus and cerebral palsy over forty years—a Swedish survey.' *Brain and Development,* **11**, 368–373.

—— —— (1993) 'The origins of cerebral palsy.' *In:* David, T.J. (Ed.) *Recent Advances in Paediatrics, Vol. 11.* London: Churchill Livingstone, pp. 67–83.

—— Sjorgen, I. (1966) 'The chronic brain syndrome of infantile hydro-cephalus. A follow-up study of 63 spontaneously arrested cases.' *American Journal of Diseases of Children,* **112**, 189–196.

—— Hagberg, G., Olow, I. (1975a) 'The changing panorama of cerebral palsy in Sweden 1954–1970. I. Analysis of general changes.' *Acta Paeditrica Scandinavica,* **64**, 187–192.

—— —— —— (1975b) 'The changing panorama of cerebral palsy in Sweden 1954–1970. II. Analysis of the various syndromes.' *Acta Paediatrica Scandinavica,* **64**, 193–200.

—— —— —— (1976) 'The changing panorama of cerebral palsy in Sweden. III. The importance of foetal deprivation of supply.' *Acta Paediatrica Scandinavica,* **65**, 403–408.

—— —— —— (1984) 'The changing panorama of cerebral palsy in Sweden. IV. Epidemiological trends 1959–1978.' *Acta Paediatrica Scandinavica,* **73**, 433–440.

—— —— Von Wendt, L. (1989a) 'The changing panorama of cerebral palsy in Sweden. V. The birth year period 1979–1982.' *Acta Paediatrica Scandinavica,* **78**, 283–290.

—— —— Zetterström, R. (1989b) 'Decreasing perinatal mortality: increase in cerebral palsy morbidity.' *Acta Paediatrica Scandinavica,* **78**, 664–670.

—— —— Olow, I. (1993) 'The changing panorama of cerebral palsy in Sweden. VI. Prevalence and origin during the birth year period 1983–86.' *Acta Paediatrica Scandinavica,* **82**, 387–393.

Hagberg, G., Sanner, G., Steen, M. (1972) 'The dysequilibrium syndrome in cerebral palsy. Clinical aspects and treatment.' *Acta Paediatrica Scandinavica,* Suppl. 226.

Harbord, M.G., Kobayashi, J.S. (1991) 'Fever producing ballismus in patients with choreoathetosis.' *Journal of Child Neurology,* **6**, 49–52.

Hári, M., Ákos, K. (1971; translated 1988) *Conductive Education.* London: Routledge.

Harris, S.R. (1987) 'Early neuromotor predictors of cerebral palsy in low-birthweight infants.' *Developmental Medicine and Child Neurology,* **29**, 508–519.

—— Purdy, A.H. (1987) 'Drooling and its management in cerebral palsy.' *Developmental Medicine and Child Neurology,* **29**, 805–814.

—— Swanson, M.W., Andrews, M.A., *et al.* (1984) 'Predictive validity of the Movement Assessment of Infants.' *Journal of Developmental and Behavioural Pediatrics,* **5**, 336–342.

Harrison, A. (1988) 'Spastic cerebral palsy: possible spinal interneuronal contributions.' *Developmental Medicine and Child Neurology,* **30**, 769–780.

Haslam, R.H.A. (1975) "Progressive cerebral palsy' or spinal cord tumour? Two cases of mistaken identity.' *Developmental Medicine and Child Neurology,* **17**, 232–237.

Hensleigh, P.A., Fainstat, T., Spencer, R. (1986) 'Perinatal events and cerebral palsy.' *American Journal of Obstetrics and Gynecology,* **154**, 978–981.

Herman, J.H., Jumbelic, M.I., Ancona, R.J., Kickler, T.S. (1986) 'In utero cerebral hemorrhage in alloimmune thrombocytopenia.' *American Journal of Pediatric Hematology and Oncology,* **8**, 312–317.

Hoffmann, G.F., Charpentier, C., Mayatepek, E., *et al.* (1993) 'Clinical and biochemical phenotype in 11 patients with mevalonic aciduria.' *Pediatrics,* **91**, 915–921.

Houdou, S., Takashima, S., Takeshita, K., Ohta, S. (1988) 'Infantile subcor-tical leukohypodensity demonstrated by computed tomography.' *Pediatric Neurology,* **4**, 165–167.

Iida, K., Takashima, S., Takeuchi, Y., *et al.* (1993) 'Neuropathologic study of newborns with prenatal-onset leukomalacia.' *Pediatric Neurology,* **9**, 45–48.

Ingram, T.T.S. (1964) *Paediatric Aspects of Cerebral Palsy.* Edinburgh: E. & S. Livingstone.

—— (1966) 'The neurology of cerebral palsy.' *Archives of Disease in Childhood,* **41**, 337–357.

Isler, W. (1971) *Acute Hemiplegias and Hemisyndromes in Childhood. Clinics in Developmental Medicine No. 41/42.* London: Spastics International Medical Publications.

Jaeken, J., Carchon, H. (1993) 'The carbohydrate-deficient glycoprotein syn-dromes: an overview.' *Journal of Inherited Metabolic Diseases,* **16**, 813–820.

Jung, J., Graham, J.M., Schultz, N., Smith, D.W. (1984) 'Congenital hydra-nencephaly/porencephaly due to vascular disruption in monozygotic twins.' *Pediatrics,* **73**, 467–469.

Kanda, T., Ashida, H.M., Fukase, H. (1988) 'Electromyography in spastic diplegia.' *Brain and Development,* **10**, 120–124.

—— Suzuki, J., Yamion, Y., Fusuki, H. (1982) 'CT findings of spastic diplegia with special reference to grade of motor disturbance.' *Brain and Develop-ment,* **4**, 239. *(Abstract.)*

Kataoka, K., Okuno, T., Mikawa, H., Hojo, H. (1988) 'Cranial computed tomographic and electroencephalographic abnormalities in children with post-hemiconvulsive hemiplegia.' *European Neurology,* **28**, 279–284.

Kerrigan, J.F., Chugani, H.T., Phelps, M.E. (1991) 'Regional cerebral glucose metabolism in clinical subtypes of cerebral palsy.' *Pediatric Neurology,* **7**, 415–425.

Koeda, T., Takeshita, K. (1992) 'Visuo-perceptual impairment and cerebral lesions in spastic diplegia with preterm birth.' *Brain and Development,* **14**, 239–244.

—— —— Kisa, T. (1995) 'Bilateral opercular syndrome: an unusual complica-tion of perinatal difficulties.' *Brain and Development,* **17**, 193–195.

Koelfen, W., Freund, M., Varnholt, V. (1995) 'Neonatal stroke involving the middle cerebral artery in term infants: clinical presentation, EEG and imaging studies, and outcome.' *Developmental Medicine and Child Neurology,* **37**, 204–212.

Konishi, Y., Kuriyama, M., Hayakawa, K., *et al.* (1991) 'Magnetic resonance imaging in preterm infants.' *Pediatric Neurology,* **7**, 191–195.

Kotlarek, F., Rodewig, R., Brüll, D., Zeumer, H. (1981) 'Computed tomo-graphic findings in congenital hemiparesis in childhood and their relation to etiology and prognosis.' *Neuropediatrics,* **12**, 101–109.

Krägeloh-Mann, I., Hagberg, B., Petersen, D., *et al.* (1992) 'Bilateral spastic cerebral palsy—pathogenetic aspects from MRI.' *Neuropediatrics,* **23**, 46–48.

Krägeloh-Mann, I., Hagberg, G., Meisner, C., *et al.* (1993) 'Bilateral spastic cerebral palsy—a comparative study between South-west Germany and West Sweden. I. Clinical patterns and disabilities.' *Developmental Medicine and Child Neurology,* **35**, 1037–1047.

—— —— —— *et al.* (1994) 'Bilateral spastic cerebral palsy—a comparative study between South-west Germany and West Sweden. II. Epidemiology.' *Developmental Medicine and Child Neurology,* **36**, 473–483.

—— —— —— *et al.* (1995a) 'Bilateral spastic cerebral palsy—a collaborative study between South-west Germany and West Sweden. III. Etiology.' *Developmental Medicine and Child Neurology,* **37**, 191–203.

—— Peterson, D., Hagberg, G., *et al.* (1995b) 'Bilateral spastic cerebral palsy—MRI pathology and origin. Analysis from a representative series of 56 cases.' *Developmental Medicine and Child Neurology,* **37**, 379–397.

Kruus, S., Louhimo, T., Granström, M.L. (1989) 'Prevalence of cerebral palsy in Finland.' *Communication to the Congress of the European Federation of Child Neurology Societies, Prague, June 25–28, 1989.*

Kuban, K.C.K., Leviton, A. (1994) 'Cerebral palsy.' *New England Journal of Medicine,* **330**, 188–195.

Kurihara, M., Kumagi, K., Yagishita, S., *et al.* (1993) 'Adrenomyeloneuropathy presenting as cerebellar ataxia in a young child: a probable variant of adrenoleukodystrophy.' *Brain and Development,* **15**, 377–380.

Kvistad, P.H., Dahl, A., Skre, H. (1985) 'Autosomal recessive nonprogressive ataxia with an early childhood debut.' *Acta Neurologica Scandinavica,* **71**, 295–302.

236

Kyllerman, M. (1977) 'Dyskinetic cerebral palsy. An analysis of 115 Swedish cases.' *Neuropädiatrie*, **8** (Suppl), S28–S32.
—— (1981) 'Dyskinetic cerebral palsy.' MD thesis, Department of Pediatrics, University of Göteborg.
—— (1983) 'Reduced optimality in pre- and perinatal conditions in dyskinetic cerebral palsy—distribution and comparison to controls.' *Neuropediatrics*, **14**, 29–36.
—— (1989) 'The epidemiology of chronic neurologic diseases of children in Sweden.' *In:* French, J.H., Harel, S., Casaer, P. (Eds.) *Child Neurology and Developmental Disabilities.* Baltimore: Paul Brookes, pp. 137–143.
Lademan, A. (1976) 'Postneonatally acquired cerebral palsy. A study of the aetiology, clinical findings and prognosis in 170 cases.' *Acta Neurologica Scandinavica*, **57**, Suppl. 65, 3–148.
Largo, R.H., Pfister, D., Molinari, L., *et al.* (1989) 'Significance of prenatal, perinatal and postnatal factors in the development of AGA preterm infants at five to seven years.' *Developmental Medicine and Child Neurology*, **31**, 440–486.
Larroche, J.C. (1986) 'Fetal encephalopathies of circulatory origin.' *Biology of the Neonate*, **50**, 61–74.
Law, H.T., Minns, R.A. (1987) 'Assessment of abnormalities of gait in children from measurements of instantaneous foot velocities during the swing phase.' *Child: Care, Health and Development*, **13**, 311–327.
Leonard, A. (1994) *Right From the Start.* London: Scope.
Levene, M.I., Sands, C., Grindulis, H., Moore, J.R. (1986) 'Comparison of two methods of predicting outcome in perinatal asphyxia.' *Lancet*, **1**, 67–69.
Lewis, D.W., Fontana, C., Mehallick, L.K., Everett, Y. (1994) 'Transdermal scopolamine for reduction of drooling in developmentally delayed children.' *Developmental Medicine and Child Neurology*, **36**, 484–486.
Lin, J-P., Brown, J.K., Brotherstone, R. (1994) 'Assessment of spasticity in hemiplegic cerebral palsy. II: Distal lower-limb reflex excitability and function.' *Developmental Medicine and Child Neurology*, **36**, 290–303.
Lütschg, J., Hänggeli, C., Huber, P., (1983) 'The evolution of cerebral hemispheric lesions due to pre- or perinatal asphyxia (clinical and neuroradiological correlation).' *Helvetica Paediatrica Acta*, **38**, 245–254.
Lyen, K.R., Lingam, S., Butterfill, A.M., *et al.* (1981) 'Multicystic encephalomalacia due to fetal viral encephalitis.' *European Journal of Pediatrics*, **137**, 11–16.
Lyon, G. Robain, O. (1967) 'Encéphalopathies circulatoires prénatales et paranatales.' *Acta Neuropathologica*, **9**, 79–98.
Mathews, K.D., Afifi, A.K., Hanson, J.W. (1989) 'Autosomal recessive cerebellar hypoplasia.' *Journal of Child Neurology*, **4**, 189–194.
McConachie, H., Smyth, D., Bax, M. (1997) 'Services for children with disabilities in European countries.' *Developmental Medicine and Child Neurology*, **39**, Suppl. 76, 1–72.
McKusick, V.A. (1988) *Mendelian Inheritance in Man, 7th Edn.* Baltimore: Johns Hopkins University Press.
McLaughlin, J.F., Bjornson, K.F., Astley, S., *et al.* (1997) 'Efficacy of selective dorsal rhizotomy in spastic diplegia: changes in spasticity and mobility after 24 months.' *Developmental Medicine and Child Neurology*, **39**, Suppl. 75, 15. *(Abstract.)*
—— —— —— *et al.* (1998) 'Selective dorsal rhizotomy: efficacy and safety in a investigator masked randomized clinical trial.' *Developmental Medicine and Child Neurology. (In press.)*
Mercuri, E., Spanò, M., Bruccini, G., *et al.* (1996) 'Visual outcome in children with congenital hemiplegia: correlation with MRI findings.' *Neuropediatrics*, **27**, 184–188.
Michaelis, R., Rooschütz, B., Dopfer, R. (1980) 'Prenatal origin of congenital spastic hemiparesis.' *Early Human Development*, **4**, 243–255.
Miller, G., Cala, L.A. (1989) 'Ataxic cerebral palsy—clinico-radiologic correlations.' *Neuropediatrics*, **20**, 84–89.
Minear, W.L. (1956) 'A classification of cerebral palsy.' *Pediatrics*, **18**, 841–852.
Molteni, B., Oleari, G., Fedrizzi, E., Bracchi, M. (1987) 'Relation between CT patterns, clinical findings and etiological factors in children born at term, affected by congenital hemiparesis.' *Neuropediatrics*, **18**, 75–80.
Morgan, A.M., Aldag, J.C. (1996) 'Early identification of cerebral palsy using a profile of abnormal motor patterns.' *Pediatrics*, **98**, 692–697.
Morton, R.E., Bonas, R., Fourie, B., Minford, J. (1993) 'Videofluoroscopy in the assessment of feeding disorders of children with neurological problems.' *Developmental Medicine and Child Neurology*, **35**, 388–395.
Mulligan, J.C., Painter, M.J., O'Donoghue, P.A., *et al.* (1980) 'Neonatal asphyxia. II. Neonatal mortality and long-term sequelae.' *Journal of Pediatrics*, **96**, 903–907.

Mutch, L., Alberman, E., Hagberg, B., *et al.* (1992) 'Cerebral palsy epidemiology: where are we now and where are we going?' *Developmental Medicine and Child Neurology*, **34**, 547–555.
Myers, R.E. (1972) 'Two patterns of brain damage and their conditions of occurrence.' *American Journal of Obstetrics and Gynecology*, **112**, 246–276.
Nardocci, N., Zorzi, G., Grisoli, M., *et al.* (1996) 'Acquired hemidystonia in childhood: a clinical and neuroradiological study of thirteen patients.' *Pediatric Neurology*, **15**, 108–113.
Nass, R. (1985) 'Mirror movement asymmetries in congenital hemiparesis: the inhibition hypothesis revisited.' *Neurology*, **35**, 1059–1062.
Nelson, K.B. (1988) 'What proportion of cerebral palsy is related to birth asphyxia?' *Journal of Pediatrics*, **112**, 572–574.
—— Ellenberg, J. (1982) 'Children who "outgrew" cerebral palsy.' *Pediatrics*, **69**, 529–536.
—— —— (1986) 'Antecedents of cerebral palsy. Multivariate analysis of risk.' *New England Journal of Medicine*, **315**, 81–86.
—— —— (1987) 'The asymptomatic newborn at risk of cerebral palsy.' *American Journal of Diseases of Children*, **141**, 1333–1335.
Niemann, G., Grodd, W., Schöning, M. (1996) 'Late remission of congenital hemiparesis: the value of MRI.' *Neuropediatrics*, **27**, 197–201.
Nygaard, T.G., Waran, S.P., Levine, R.A., *et al.* (1994) 'Dopa-responsive dystonia simulating cerebral palsy.' *Pediatric Neurology*, **11**, 236–240.
O'Dwyer, N.J., Neilson, P.D. (1988) 'Voluntary muscle control in normal and athetoid dysarthric speakers.' *Brain*, **111**, 877–899.
Okuno, T. (1994) 'Acute hemiplegia syndrome in childhood.' *Brain and Development*, **16**, 16–22.
Olsén, P., Pääkkö, E., Vainionpää, L., *et al.* (1997) 'Magnetic resonance imaging of periventricular leukomalacia and its clinical correlation in children.' *Annals of Neurology*, **41**, 754–761.
Ong, B.Y., Ellison, P.H., Browning, C. (1983) 'Intrauterine stroke in the neonate.' *Archives of Neurology*, **40**, 55–56.
Painter, M.J. (1989) 'Fetal heart rate patterns, perinatal asphyxia, and brain injury.' *Pediatric Neurology*, **5**, 137–144.
Palmer, F.B., Shapiro, B.K., Wachtel, R.C., *et al.* (1988) 'The effect of physical therapy on cerebral palsy.' *New England Journal of Medicine*, **318**, 803–808.
Papile, L-A., Munsick-Bruno, G., Schaefer, A. (1983) 'Relationship of cerebral intraventricular hemorrhage and early childhood neurologic handicaps.' *Journal of Pediatrics*, **103**, 273–277.
Parisi, J.E., Collins, G.H., Kim, R.C., Crosley, C.J. (1983) 'Prenatal symmetrical thalamic degeneration with flexion spasticity at birth.' *Annals of Neurology*, **13**, 94–97.
Pascual-Castroviejo, I., Guttierez, M., Morales, C., *et al.* (1994) 'Primary degeneration of the granular layer of the cerebellum. A study of 14 patients and review of the literature.' *Neuropediatrics*, **25**, 183–190.
Pasternak, J.F. (1987) 'Parasagittal infarction in neonatal asphyxia.' *Annals of Neurology*, **21**, 202–204.
Peacock, W.J., Staudt, L.A., (1990) 'Spasticity in cerebral palsy and the selective posterior rhizotomy procedure.' *Journal of Child Neurology*, **5**, 179–185.
PeBenito, R., Santello, M.D., Faxas, T.A., *et al.* (1989) 'Residual developmental disabilities in children with transient hypertonicity in infancy.' *Pediatric Neurology*, **5**, 154–160.
Perlman, J.M., Volpe, J.J. (1989) 'Movement disorder of premature infants with severe bronchopulmonary dysplasia: a new syndrome.' *Pediatrics*, **84**, 215–218.
Perlstein, M.A. (1960) 'The late clinical syndrome of post-icteric encephalopathy.' *Pediatric Clinics of North America*, **7**, 665–687.
Petterson, B., Stanley, F.J., Garner, B.J. (1993) 'Spastic quadriplegia in Western Australia. II: Pedigrees and family patterns of birthweight and gestational age.' *Developmental Medicine and Child Neurology*, **35**, 202–215.
Piper, M.C., Mazer, B., Silver, K.M., Ramsay, M. (1988) 'Resolution of neurological symptoms in high-risk infants during the first two years of life.' *Developmental Medicine and Child Neurology*, **30**, 26–35.
Powell, T.G., Pharoah, P.O.D., Cooke, R.W.I., Rosenbloom, L. (1988a) 'Cerebral palsy in low birthweight infants. I. Spastic hemiplegia: associations with intrapartum stress.' *Developmental Medicine and Child Neurology*, **36**, 11–18.
—— —— —— —— (1988b) 'Cerebral palsy in low-birthweight infants. II. Spastic diplegia: associations with fetal immaturity.' *Developmental Medicine and Child Neurology*, **30**, 19–25.
Prechtl, H.F.R. (1980) 'The optimality concept.' *Early Human Development*, **4**, 201–205.
—— Stemmer, C.J. (1962) 'The choreiform syndrome in children.' *Developmental Medicine and Child Neurology*, **4**, 119–127.

Rapin, I. (1995) 'Acquired aphasia in children.' *Journal of Child Neurology*, **10**, 267–270.

Reid, C.J.D., Borzyskowski, M. (1993) 'Lower urinary tract dysfunction in cerebral palsy.' *Archives of Disease in Childhood*, **68**, 739–742.

Robson, P., Mac Keith, R.C. (1971) 'Shufflers with spastic cerebral palsy: a confusing clinical picture.' *Developmental Medicine and Child Neurology*, **13**, 651–659.

Roland, E.H., Hill, A., Norman, M.G., et al. (1988) 'Selective brainstem injury in an asphyxiated newborn.' *Annals of Neurology*, **23**, 89–92.

Rorke, L.B., Zimmerman, R.A. (1992) 'Prematurity, postmaturity, and destructive lesions in utero.' *American Journal of Neuroradiology*, **13**, 517–536.

Rosenberg, R.N. (1992) 'Machado–Joseph disease: an autosomal dominant motor system degeneration.' *Movement Disorders*, **7**, 193–203.

Rosenbloom, L. (1994) 'Dyskinetic cerebral palsy and birth asphyxia.' *Developmental Medicine and Child Neurology*, **36**, 285–289.

Roth, S.C., Baudin, J., McCormick, D.C., et al. (1993) 'Relation between ultrasound appearance of the brain of very preterm infants and neurodevelopmental impairment at eight years.' *Developmental Medicine and Child Neurology*, **35**, 755–768.

Russell, D., Rosenbaum, P., Gowland, C., et al. (1993) *Gross Motor Function Measure Manual, 2nd Edn.* Hamilton, Ontario: Children's Developmental Rehabilitation Programme, Chedoke–McMaster Hospitals, McMaster University.

Rutherford, M.A., Heckmatt, J.Z., Dubowitz, V. (1989) 'Congenital myotonic dystrophy: respiratory function at birth determines survival.' *Archives of Disease in Childhood*, **64**, 191–195.

—— Pennock, J.M., Murdoch-Eaton, D.M., et al. (1992) 'Athetoid cerebral palsy with cysts in the putamen after hypoxic–ischaemic encephalopathy.' *Archives of Disease in Childhood*, **67**, 846–850.

—— —— Dubowitz, L.M.S. (1994) 'Cranial ultrasound and magnetic resonance imaging in hypoxic–ischaemic encephalopathy: a comparison with outcome.' *Developmental Medicine and Child Neurology*, **36**, 813–825.

Rutter, M., Graham, P., Yule, W. (1970) *A Neuropsychiatric Study in Childhood. Clinics in Developmental Medicine No. 35/36.* London: Spastics International Medical Publications.

Saint-Hilaire, M.H., Burke, R.E., Bressman, S.B., et al. (1991) 'Delayed-onset dystonia due to perinatal or early childhood asphyxia.' *Neurology*, **41**, 216–222.

Sala, D.A., Grant, A.D. (1995) 'Prognosis for ambulation in cerebral palsy.' *Developmental Medicine and Child Neurology*, **37**, 1020–1026.

Sanner, G. (1973) 'The dysequilibrium syndrome. A genetic study.' *Neuropädiatrie*, **4**, 403–413.

—— (1979) 'Pathogenetic and preventive aspects of non-progressive ataxic syndromes.' *Developmental Medicine and Child Neurology*, **21**, 663–671.

—— Hagberg, B. (1974) '188 cases of non-progressive ataxic syndromes in childhood. Aspects of etiology and classification.' *Neuropädiatrie*, **5**, 224–235.

Santanelli, P., Bureau, M., Magaudda, A., et al. (1989) 'Benign partial epilepsy with centrotemporal (or rolandic) spikes and brain lesion.' *Epilepsia*, **30**, 182–188.

Schachat, W.S., Wallace, H.M., Palmer, M., Slater, B. (1957) 'Ophthalmological findings in children with cerebral palsy.' *Pediatrics*, **19**, 623–628.

Schenk-Rootlieb, A.J.F., van Nieuwenhuizen, O., van Waes, P.F.G.M., van der Graaf, Y. (1994) 'Cerebral visual impairment in cerebral palsy: relation to structural abnormalities of the cerebrum.' *Neuropediatrics*, **25**, 68–72.

Scher, M.S., Dobson, V., Carpenter, N.A., Guthrie, R.D. (1989) 'Visual and neurological outcome of infants with periventricular leukomalacia.' *Developmental Medicine and Child Neurology*, **31**, 353–365.

—— Belfar, H., Martin, J., Painter, M.J. (1991) 'Destructive brain lesions of presumed fetal onset: antepartum causes of cerebral palsy.' *Pediatrics*, **88**, 898–906.

Scheuerle, A.E., McVie, R., Beaudet, A.L., Shapira, S.K. (1993) 'Arginase deficiency presenting as cerebral palsy.' *Pediatrics*, **91**, 995–996.

Schiffmann, R., Moller, J.R., Trapp, B.D., et al. (1994) 'Childhood ataxia with diffuse central nervous system hypomyelination.' *Annals of Neurology*, **35**, 331–340.

Scrutton, D. (Ed.) (1984) *Management of the Motor Disorders of Children with Cerebral Palsy. Clinics in Developmental Medicine No. 90.* London: Spastics International Medical Publications.

Shankaran, S., Koepke, T., Woldt, E., et al. (1989) 'Outcome after post-hemorrhagic ventriculomegaly in comparison with mild hemorrhage without ventriculomegaly.' *Journal of Pediatrics*, **114**, 109–114.

Shields, J.R., Schifrin, B.S. (1988) 'Perinatal antecedents of cerebral palsy.' *Obstetrics and Gynecology*, **71**, 899–905.

Silverstein, A.M., Hirsh, D.K., Trobe, J.D., Gebarski, S.S. (1990) 'MR imaging of the brain in five members of a family with Pelizaeus–Merzbacher disease.' *American Journal of Neuroradiology*, **11**, 495–499.

Sinha, S.K., D'Souza, S.W., Rivlin, E., Chiswick, M.L. (1990) 'Ischaemic brain lesions diagnosed at birth in preterm infants: clinical events and developmental outcome.' *Archives of Disease in Childhood*, **65**, 1017–1020.

Skranes, J.S., Nilsen, G., Smevik, O., et al. (1992) 'Cerebral magnetic resonance imaging (MRI) of very low birth weight infants at one year of corrected age.' *Pediatric Radiology*, **22**, 406–409.

Sladky, J.T., Rorke, L.B. (1986) 'Perinatal hypoxic/ischemic spinal cord injury.' *Pediatric Pathology*, **6**, 87–101.

Stanley, F.J. (1987) 'The changing face of cerebral palsy.' *Developmental Medicine and Child Neurology*, **29**, 263–265.

—— Alberman, E. (1984) 'Birthweight, gestational age and the cerebral palsies.' *In:* Stanley, F., Alberman, E. (Eds.) *The Epidemiology of the Cerebral Palsies. Clinics in Developmental Medicine No. 87.* London: Spastics International Medical Publications, pp. 57–68.

—— English, D.R. (1986) 'Prevalence and risks factors for cerebral palsy in a total population cohort of low-birthweight infants.' *Developmental Medicine and Child Neurology*, **28**, 559–568.

—— Blair, E., Hockey, A., et al. (1993) 'Spastic quadriplegia in Western Australia: a genetic epidemiological study. I: Case population and perinatal risk factors.' *Developmental Medicine and Child Neurology*, **35**, 191–201.

Steinlin, M., Good, M., Martin, E., et al. (1993) 'Congenital hemiplegia: morphology of cerebral lesions and pathogenetic aspects from MRI.' *Neuropediatrics*, **24**, 224–229.

Stevenson, C.J., Pharoah, P.O.D., Stevenson, R. (1997) 'Cerebral palsy—the transition from youth to adulthood.' *Developmental Medicine and Child Neurology*, **39**, 336–342.

Stibler, H., Westerberg, B., Hanefeld, F., Hagberg, B. (1993) 'Carbohydrate-deficient glycoprotein (CDG) syndrome—a new variant, type III.' *Neuropediatrics*, **24**, 51–52.

Strauss, D., Kastner, T., Ashwal, S., White, J. (1997) 'Tubefeeding and mortality in children with severe disabilities and mental retardation.' *Pediatrics*, **99**, 358–362.

Sugama, S., Kusano, K. (1995) 'A case of dyskinetic cerebral palsy resembling post-anoxic action myoclonus.' *Brain and Development*, **17**, 210–212.

Sutherland, D.H. (1984) *Gait Disorders in Childhood and Adolescence.* Baltimore: Williams & Wilkins.

—— Olshen, R.A., Biden, E.N., Wyatt, M.P. (1988) *The Development of Mature Walking. Clinics in Developmental Medicine No. 104/105.* London: Mac Keith Press.

Sugimoto, T., Woo, M., Nishida, N., et al. (1995) 'When do brain abnormalities in cerebral palsy occur? An MRI study.' *Developmental Medicine and Child Neurology*, **37**, 285–292.

Takeuchi, T., Watanabe, K (1989) 'The EEG evolution and neurological prognosis of perinatal hypoxia in neonates.' *Brain and Development*, **11**, 115–120.

Tardieu, G., Hariga, J. (1972) 'Selective partial denervation by alcohol injections and their results in spasticity.' *Reconstructive Surgery and Traumatology*, **13**, 18–36.

—— Got, C., Lespargot, A. (1975) 'Indications d'un nouveau type d'infiltration au point moteur (alcool à 96°). Applications cliniques d'une étude expérimentale.' *Annales de Medecine Physique*, **18**, 539–557.

Tardieu, M., Evrard, P., Lyon, G. (1981) 'Progressive expanding congenital porencephalies: a treatable cause of progressive encephalopathy.' *Pediatrics*, **68**, 198–202.

Taudorf, K, Vorstrup, S. (1989) 'Cerebral blood flow abnormalities in cerebral palsied children with a normal CT scan.' *Neuropediatrics*, **20**, 33–40.

—— Melchior, J.C., Pederson, H. (1984) 'CT findings in spastic cerebral palsy. Clinical, aetiological and prognostic aspects.' *Neuropediatrics*, **15**, 120–124.

Taylor, E.A. (1986) *The Overactive Child. Clinics in Developmental Medicine No. 97.* London: Mac Keith Press.

Tharp, B.R., Scher, M.S., Clancy, R.R. (1989) 'Serial EEGs in normal and abnormal infants with birthweights less than 1200 grams. A prospective study with long-term follow-up.' *Neuropediatrics*, **20**, 64–72.

Thomas, A.P., Bax, M.C.O., Smyth, D.P.L. (1989) *The Health and Social Needs of Young Adults with Physical Disabilities. Clinics in Developmental Medicine No. 106.* London: Mac Keith Press.

Tizard, J.P.M., Paine, R.S., Crothers, B. (1954) 'Disturbances of sensation in children with hemiplegia.' *Journal of the American Medical Association*, **155**, 628–632.

Tomiwa, K., Baraitser, M., Wilson, J. (1987) 'Dominantly inherited congenital cerebellar ataxia with atrophy of the vermis.' *Pediatric Neurology*, **3**, 360–362.

Touwen, B.C.L., Hadders-Algra, M. (1983) 'Hyperextension of neck and trunk and shoulder retraction in infancy. A prognostic study.' *Neuropediatrics*, **14**, 202–205.

Truwit, C.L., Barkovich, A.J., Koch, T.K., Ferriero, D.M. (1992) 'Cerebral palsy: MR findings in 40 patients.' *American Journal of Neuroradiology*, **13**, 67–78.

Tsao, C.Y., Wright, F.S., Boesel, C.P., Luquette, M. (1994) 'Partial NADH dehydrogenase defect presenting as spastic cerebral palsy.' *Brain and Development*, **16**, 393–395.

Turkel, S.B., Guttenberg, M.E., Moynes, D.R., Hodgman, J.E. (1980) 'Lack of identifiable risk factors for kernicterus.' *Pediatrics*, **66**, 502–506.

Uvebrandt, P. (1988) 'Hemiplegic cerebral palsy. Aetiology and outcome.' *Acta Paediatrica Scandinavica*, Suppl. 345, 5–100.

van Bogaert, P., Baleriaux, D., Christophe, C., Szliwowski, H.B. (1992) 'MRI of patients with cerebral palsy and normal CT scan.' *Neuroradiology*, **34**, 52–56.

Van de Bor, M., Verloove-Vanhorick, S.P., Baerts, W., *et al.* (1988) 'Outcome of periventricular–intraventricular hemorrhage at 2 years of age in 484 very preterm infants admitted to 6 neonatal intensive care units in the Netherlands.' *Neuropediatrics*, **19**, 183–185.

—— van Zeben-van der Aa, T.M., Verloove-Vanhorick, S.P., *et al.* (1989) 'Hyperbilirubinemia in preterm infants and neurodevelopmental outcome at 2 years of age: results of a national collaborative survey.' *Pediatrics*, **83**, 915–920.

Van Nieuwenhuizen, O., Willemse, J. (1984) 'CT-scanning in children with cerebral visual disturbance and its possible relation to hypoxia and ischaemia.' *Behavioural Brain Research*, **14**, 143–145.

Vargha-Khadem, F., O'Gorman, A.M., Watters, G.V. (1985) 'Aphasia and handedness in relation to hemispheric side, age at injury and severity of cerebral lesion during childhood.' *Brain*, **108**, 677–696.

—— Isaacs, E., van der Werf, S., *et al.* (1992) 'Development of intelligence and memory in children with hemiplegic cerebral palsy. The deleterious consequences of early seizures.' *Brain*, **115**, 315–329.

Veelken, N., Hagberg, B., Hagberg, G., Olow I. (1983) 'Diplegic cerebral palsy in Swedish term and preterm children—differences in reduced optimality, relations to neurology and pathogenetic factors.' *Neuropediatrics*, **14**, 20–28.

Vojta, V. (1984) 'The basic element of treatment according to Vojta.' *In:* Scrutton, D. (Ed.) *Management of the Motor Disorders of Children with Cerebral Palsy. Clinics in Developmental Medicine No. 90.* London: Spastics International Medical Publications, pp. 75–85.

Volpe, J.J. (1995) *Neurology of the Newborn, 3rd Edn.* Philadelphia: W.B. Saunders.

Walsh, E.G. (1993) *Muscles, Masses and Motion. The Physiology of Normality, Hypotonicity, Spasticity and Rigidity. Clinics in Developmental Medicine No. 125.* London: Mac Keith Press.

Watanabe, K. (1992) 'The neonatal electroencephalogram and sleep cycle patterns.' *In:* Eyre, J.A. (Ed.) *The Neurophysiological Examination of the Newborn Infant. Clinics in Developmental Medicine No. 120.* London: Mac Keith Press, pp. 11–47.

Wharton, R.H., Bresman, M.J. (1989) 'Neonatal respiratory depression and delay in diagnosis in Prader–Willi syndrome.' *Developmental Medicine and Child Neurology*, **31**, 231–236.

WHO (1980) '*International Classification of Impairments, Disabilities and Handicaps.* Geneva: World Health Organization.

Wichman, A., Frank, L.M., Kelly, T.E. (1985) 'Autosomal recessive congenital cerebellar hypoplasia.' *Clinical Genetics*, **27**, 373–382.

Wiklund, L.M., Uvebrandt, P., Flodmark, O. (1990) 'Morphology of cerebral lesions in children with congenital hemiplegia: a study with computed tomography.' *Neuroradiology*, **32**, 179–186.

Willemse, J. (1986) 'Benign idiopathic dystonia with onset in the first year of life.' *Developmental Medicine and Child Neurology*, **28**, 355–363.

Willis, J., Duncan, M.C., Bell, R., *et al.* (1989) 'Somatosensory evoked potentials predict neuromotor outcome after periventricular hemorrhage.' *Developmental Medicine and Child Neurology*, **31**, 435–439.

Wilson, E.R., Mirra, S., Schwartz, J.F. (1982) 'Congenital diencephalic and brain stem damage: neuropathologic study of three cases.' *Acta Neuropathologica*, **57**, 70–74.

Worster-Drought, C. (1974) 'Suprabulbar paresis.Congenital suprabulbar paresis and its differential diagnosis with special reference to acquired suprabulbar paresis.' *Developmental Medicine and Child Neurology*, **16**, Suppl. 30, 1–33.

Wüllner, U., Klockgether, T., Petersen, D., *et al.* (1993) 'Magnetic resonance imaging in hereditary and idiopathic ataxia.' *Neurology*, **43**, 318–325.

Yokochi, K., Horie, M., Inukai, K., *et al.* (1989) 'Computed tomographic findings in children with spastic diplegia: correlation with the severity of their motor abnormality.' *Brain and Development*, **11**, 236–240.

—— Aiba, K., Kodama, M., Fujimoto, S. (1991) 'Magnetic resonance imaging in athetotic cerebral palsied children.' *Acta Paediatrica Scandinavica*, **80**, 818–823.

Young, I.D., Moore, J.R., Tripp, J.H. (1987) 'Sex-linked recessive congenital ataxia.' *Journal of Neurology, Neurosurgery, and Psychiatry*, **50**, 1230–1232.

Zonana, J., Adornato, B.T., Glass, S.T., Webb, M.J. (1986) 'Familial porencephaly and congenital hemiplegia.' *Journal of Pediatrics*, **109**, 671–674.

PART IV

METABOLIC AND HEREDODEGENERATIVE DISORDERS OF THE CENTRAL NERVOUS SYSTEM

Diseases due to inborn errors of metabolism account for a large proportion of CNS disorders. Well over 250 such genetic diseases are currently known and the list is rapidly growing as a result of progress in biochemistry and molecular biology.

Metabolic and heredodegenerative CNS disorders can be divided into three groups. The first includes those diseases for which a definite enzymatic defect has been demonstrated, thus allowing for a firm and usually prenatal diagnosis as well as some understanding of the mechanisms. The second group consists of those diseases in which accumulation of storage material within neural cells clearly indicates the presence of a catabolic defect and is also of practical use for the diagnosis. The third group comprises a heterogeneous collection of progressive neurological diseases that have a clinical presentation similar to that of the first two groups but for which no biochemical or molecular error has been identified or suggested by the presence of storage products. It is highly likely that these disorders also result from an abnormal metabolism. Indeed, Canavan disease and rare cases of neuro-axonal dystrophy (van Diggelen *et al.* 1988, Schindler *et al.* 1989) have recently been shown to be associated with biochemical anomalies, and the same is likely to occur for many diseases in the group. Recent advances in molecular genetics have allowed mapping of the responsible genes for many of these diseases, and cloning has been performed for a substantial proportion of them; the proteins coded for by these genes are of many types, including cytoskeletal and signalling proteins, regulatory and growth factors, and membrane receptors. Despite cloning of the abnormal gene and determination of the protein structure, the mechanisms of most disorders remain unknown, although these discoveries permit a precise classification and sometimes diagnosis—including in a few cases prenatal diagnosis—of these disorders, through direct testing for abnormal DNA or protein or through linkage studies.

For all metabolic and degenerative diseases, an early diagnosis is of more than academic interest, as in some cases a specific therapy is available, for many a prenatal diagnosis is feasible, and, for all, prognosis and genetic counselling critically depend on a correct recognition. In some cases, it has become possible to detect not only actual diseases but also individual susceptibility to certain diseases by determining the genotype of individuals (*e.g.* susceptibility to vascular thrombosis in heterozygotes for homocystinuria, increased liability to some cancers in heterozygotes for the gene of ataxia–telangiectasia), thus opening a completely new domain whose limits and consequences are currently difficult to predict.

This part is divided into two chapters. Chapter 9 deals with defined inborn errors of metabolism. The main subgroups of neurological importance are disorders of amino acid and organic acid metabolism, lysosomal diseases, the peroxisomal disorders, and errors in energy metabolism especially the mitochondrial diseases, but many other defects can also involve the CNS.

Chapter 10 is concerned with storage disorders without known biochemical error and diseases of the third group. A biochemical error has now been recognized in an increasing proportion of these, and the distinction between the various groups is becoming increasingly blurred and is bound ultimately to disappear. Some of the diseases considered may have completely different mechanisms but are included for convenience even though in a few cases their progressive nature may not be established.

Virtually all metabolic and degenerative CNS diseases are genetically determined, and they are generally transmitted as autosomal recessive traits, less commonly as autosomal dominant or X-linked ones. In recent years, other modalities of genetic transmission have been uncovered, such as trinucleotide repeats with anticipation, imprinting or uniparental disomy, and this knowledge makes genetic counselling more precise. For diseases with specific biochemical defects a variety of tests are available, and many can be diagnosed before birth by study of cultured amniotic cells or chorionic villus biopsy. This is also feasible for an increasing number of conditions in which specific DNA abnormalities can be demonstrated. Systematic screening techniques are available for some disorders.

For other disorders, a morphological diagnosis may be feasible using in most cases peripheral rather than brain biopsy. Skin and conjunctival biopsy (Arsenio-Nunes *et al.* 1981, Ceuterick and Martin 1992, Prasad *et al.* 1996), rectal biopsy (Brett and Lake 1975, Goutières *et al.* 1990) and, less commonly, other biopsies (*e.g.* gingival) are sufficient for most diagnoses. Brain biopsy (Boltshauser and Wilson 1976) is seldom indicated except when an inflammatory disease is a serious consideration because in this case, practical conclusions may result. This is rarely, if ever, the case with degenerative diseases, as a suspected genetic disease cannot be excluded by a negative biopsy (because of possible sampling error), whereas a positive biopsy does not add much to the genetic counselling because recessive autosomal inheritance is very likely if the progressive character of the disease is established. The current development of stereotactic brain biopsy (Thomas and Kitchen 1993) may widen the indications because of its ease and relative innocuity.

The diagnosis of heredodegenerative diseases without known molecular or metabolic errors raises special problems as it rests exclusively on clinical grounds, if clinical medicine is defined as 'an intellectual process whereby data from all sources, whether strictly clinical (in the restricted sense) or from the laboratory and other technical tools, is integrated and shaped into a meaningful profile' (Aicardi 1987). In many instances, there is no technical tool capable of providing the clinician with a yes-or-no answer. Even determination of genotypic abnormalities may not be totally reliable because of genetic heterogeneity. A typical example is tuberous sclerosis that is caused by mutations of at least two different genes (Chapter 4) without any associated specific clinical feature. For diagnostic and prognostic purposes, diseases cannot be defined without reference to their phenotype.

The most important clinical feature of a large majority of the metabolic and heredodegenerative CNS diseases is their progressive character. A progressive encephalopathy in a child is, for all practical purposes, a genetic disease, even though no precise diagnostic tag can be affixed, *provided a subacute or chronic inflammatory disorder can be ruled out* (the commonest of these now being AIDS).

The progressive character is not always easily affirmed. Two essential arguments are drawn from history: (1) the notion of a free interval during which development had been normal; (2) the loss of already acquired skills. These features may be obvious in late-onset disease with abrupt deterioration. They may be difficult to discern in diseases of very early (or neonatal) onset, in those in which deterioration sets in insidiously, and in those in which the initial development had never been normal. The associated occurrence of epileptic attacks, heavy drug treatment or other intervening pathological events may further compound the problem.

TABLE IV.1
Investigations in children with clinically progressive encephalopathies

Neuroimaging
Ultrasound may be useful in infants mainly to exclude structural lesions
CT scan without and with enhancement
MRI scan, especially for white matter disorders using both T_1- and T_2-weighted sequences
Angiography (MRA) in rare cases
Functional imaging (MR spectroscopy) in rare cases (Tzika *et al.* 1993)

Neurophysiological investigations
EEG including sleep tracing and slow photic stimulation routinely. Cassette recordings and/or polygraphic recordings in selected cases
Electroretinogram (ERG)
Evoked potentials (visual, auditory, sensory) in selected patients
Electromyography (EMG) and nerve conduction velocity studies (sensory and motor) especially for diagnosis of peripheral myelin involvement

CSF examination including pressure measurement, cell count and cytological examination, protein assay including electrophoresis for determination of protein profile, looking for a 'degenerative' or 'inflammatory' profile

Haematology, microbiology, immunology
Search for abnormal red cells (acanthocytes)
Search for inclusions or vacuoles in white blood cells
Marrow examination in selected cases
Immunological studies in some cases
Microbial studies especially for HIV, *Borrelia*, measles, syphilis

Biochemical studies*
pH determination, search for ketone bodies
Amino acid and organic acid chromatography**
Lysosomal enzymes
Lactate in blood and CSF following muscular exercise and/or glucose load in selected cases, pyruvate, special mitochondrial investigations
Screening for peroxisomal disease (very-long-chain fatty acids)
Liver function studies

Tissue examination
Skin and/or conjunctival biopsy
Rectal biopsy (shows neurons)
Nerve biopsy
Brain biopsy
Muscle biopsy for morphological and chemical examination when mitochondrial disease is suspected
Culture fibroblasts for possible further examinations

Genetic studies
Karyotype in rare cases (search for breakage as in ataxia–telangiectasia or xeroderma pigmentosum)
Molecular genetics (DNA studies)

*More complex studies including loading tests may be indicated in specific cases. (Always keep urine and blood samples for further more sophisticated studies.)
**Routine testing may not be useful, and more precise studies in selected cases are probably more rewarding.

The appearance of new neurological signs should not necessarily be interpreted as indicating progression as it is commonly observed in the first two or three years of life in children with various types of cerebral palsy.

Some forms of actual deterioration do not indicate a relentlessly destructive process in the brain. Loss of acquired skills does occur with epilepsy, especially with West and Lennox–Gastaut syndromes, but the deterioration stops after a few months or years and resumption of progress can be observed. Similarly, the regression associated with some cases of autism is different from the degenerative diseases as there is apparently no progressive brain pathology.

In all cases, deterioration of known, nonmetabolic cause should be ruled out, as effective treatment is often available. Such include inflammatory diseases, some cases of brain tumours, obstructive hydrocephalus, vascular disorders such as moyamoya disease or sickle cell disease with repeated strokes, and arteriovenous malformations responsible for deterioration as a result of blood 'steal' through the malformation with consequent neighbouring ischaemia.

A genetic cause of CNS disease is not excluded by the apparent lack of clinical progression. It is now well established that genetic degenerative conditions can be very difficult to separate from fixed encephalopathies caused by malformations or prenatally acquired insults. Barth (1992) has drawn attention to the progressive disorders of the fetal brain present at birth, often in the form of an apparently static encephalopathy. An increasing number of such slowly progressive congenital conditions are known, such as peroxisomal diseases (Brown *et al.* 1993), lactic acidosis and other organic acid diseases (Brown *et al.* 1988, De Meirleir *et al.* 1993) and mitochondrial disorders (Barkovich *et al.* 1993). Some of these conditions are responsible for true CNS (and peripheral) malformations, thus blurring the limits between domains classically considered separate. This may result in the temptation to investigate extensively a vast number of cases with a view to recognizing genetic diseases. The cost of such a policy, not only in economic but also in human terms (*e.g.* pain, hospitalization, anxiety generated) is an obvious limiting factor, but the 'reasonable' indications and limitations are impossible to define precisely, and physicians have to rely heavily on common sense and clinical acumen.

Investigations that may be indicated in children suspected of progressive disorders of the CNS are shown in Table IV.1. The choice of tests used is heavily dependent on the clinical features, and the number of tests performed should be kept to a minimum (Stephenson and King 1989). The specificity and reliability of the tests is variable (see later chapters). For instance, an extinguished ERG is of considerable value for the diagnosis of ceroid–lipofuscinosis or of peroxisomal diseases, while the ERG may be normal in some patients with these disorders. Even enzymatic tests are fallible with both false positive (arylsulfatase pseudodeficiency) and false negative tests. Close clinical supervision and control of interpretation of laboratory examination is essential in all cases.

REFERENCES

Aicardi, J. (1987) 'The future of clinical child neurology.' *Journal of Child Neurology*, **2**, 152–159.

Arsenio-Nunes, M.L., Goutières, F., Aicardi, J. (1981) 'An ultramicroscopic study of skin and conjunctival biopsies in chronic neurological disorders of childhood.' *Annals of Neurology*, **9**, 163–173.

Barkovich, A.J., Good, W.V., Koch, T.K., Berg, B.O. (1993) 'Mitochondrial disorders: analysis of their clinical and imaging characteristics.' *American Journal of Neuroradiology*, **14**, 1119–1137.

Barth, P.G. (1992) 'Inherited progressive disorders of the fetal brain: a field in need of recognition.' *In:* Fukuyama, Y., Suzuki, Y., Kamoshita, S., Casaer, P. (Eds.) *Fetal and Perinatal Neurology.* Basel: Karger, pp. 299–313.

Boltshauser, E., Wilson, J. (1976) 'Value of brain biopsy in neurodegenerative disease in childhood.' *Archives of Disease in Childhood*, **51**, 264–268.

Brett, E.M., Lake, B.D. (1975) 'Reassessment of rectal approach to neuropathology in childhood. Review of 307 biopsies over 11 years.' *Archives of Disease in Childhood*, **50**, 753–762.

Brown, F.R., Voigt, R., Singh, A.K., Singh, I. (1993) 'Peroxisomal disorders: neurodevelopmental and biochemical aspects.' *American Journal of Diseases of Children*, **147**, 617–626.

Brown, G.K. Haan, E.A., Kirby, D.M., *et al.* (1988) '"Cerebral" lactic acidosis: defects in pyruvate metabolism with profound brain damage and minimal systemic acidosis.' *European Journal of Pediatrics*, **147**, 10–14.

Ceuterick, C., Martin, J-J. (1992) 'Electron microscopic features of skin in neurometabolic disorders.' *Journal of the Neurological Sciences*, **112**, 15–29.

De Meirleir, L., Lissens, W., Denis, R., *et al.* (1993) 'Pyruvate dehydrogenase deficiency: clinical and biochemical diagnosis.' *Pediatric Neurology*, **9**, 216–220.

Goutières, F., Mikol, J., Aicardi, J. (1990) 'Neuronal intranuclear inclusion disease in a child: diagnosis by rectal biopsy.' *Annals of Neurology*, **27**, 103–106.

Prasad, A., Kaye, E.M., Alroy, J. (1996) 'Electron microscopic examination of skin biopsy as a cost-effective tool in the diagnosis of lysosomal storage disease.' *Journal of Child Neurology*, **11**, 301–308.

Schindler, D., Bishop, D.F., Wolfe, D.E., *et al.* (1989) 'Neuroaxonal dystrophy due to lysosomal alpha-*N*-acetylgalactosaminidase deficiency.' *New England Journal of Medicine*, **320**, 1735–1740.

Stephenson, J.B.P., King, M.D. (1989) *Handbook of Neurological Investigations in Children.* London: Wright.

Thomas, D.G.T., Kitchen, N.D. (1993) 'Stereotactic techniques for brain biopsies.' *Archives of Disease in Childhood*, **69**, 621–622.

Tzika, A.A., Ball, W.S., Vigneron, D.B., *et al.* (1993) 'Clinical proton MR spectroscopy of neurodegenerative disease in childhood.' *American Journal of Neuroradiology*, **14**, 1267–1281.

van Diggelen, O.P., Schindler, D., Willemsen, R., *et al.* (1988) 'α-*N*-acetylgalactosaminidase deficiency, a new lysosomal storage disorder.' *Journal of Inherited Metabolic Disease*, **11**, 349–357.

9
METABOLIC DISEASES

Hélène Ogier and Jean Aicardi

Metabolic diseases of the nervous system comprise a vast group of heterogeneous conditions which have in common only the presence of a known metabolic deficit at their origin but which differ enormously in pathology, clinical presentation and diagnostic problems.

Several broad subgroups of metabolic diseases will be considered successively.

(1) *Disorders involving subcellular organelles.* These include diseases of lysosomes, the Golgi and pre-Golgi apparatus and peroxisomes. The classical example is that of lysosomal disorders that are due to lack of lysosomal enzymes and result in *storage disorders*. In such cases, an enzymatic block produces accumulation of storage substances that may interfere with the function and/or survival of neural cells. The metabolic block may also act by inducing deficiency of metabolites normally produced beyond the block or by interfering with other metabolic pathways as a result of deviation from normal to accessory or normally unused pathways. However, some disorders of subcellular organelles (*e.g.* peroxisomal diseases) do not produce accumulation of storage substances but interfere in various ways with essential metabolic processes.

(2) *Disorders of intermediary metabolism.* These diseases are extremely diverse but here the metabolic blocks do not generate storage. Interference with numerous metabolic pathways leads to disturbances of energy production, amino acid and organic acid catabolism with endogenous intoxication, and interference with neurotransmitter synthesis.

(3) *Disorders of metallic, especially copper, metabolism.*

(4) *Miscellaneous metabolic diseases.* Progressive metabolic CNS disorders are individually rare. However, their prevalence in Sweden was found to be 0.58 per 1000, a frequency similar to that of neural tube defects or congenital hemiplegia (Uvebrant *et al.* 1992).

A number of metabolic diseases involve only occasionally or secondarily the nervous system and will be only alluded to.

Several disorders of carbohydrate metabolism can affect the CNS indirectly by inducing hypoglycaemia, *e.g.* various types of glycogenosis, especially type I, and fructose intolerance. Fructose 1-6-diphosphate deficiency can be associated with severe ventricular dilatation and hypoplasia of the vermis and cerebellar hemispheres, and alpha-ketoglutarate dehydrogenase deficiency and pyruvate dehydrogenase deficiency are often responsible also

for basal ganglia abnormalities (Brismar and Ozand 1994a,b). Isolated hypoglycorrhachia caused by deficit of specific glucose carrier is described in Chapter 2. The effects on the brain can be prevented by a ketogenic diet.

Galactosaemia resulting from deficit of galactose-uridyltransferase or rarely of epimerase is associated with CNS toxicity and growth failure, in addition to cataracts (Segal 1993). The gene is located to chromosome 9q13 and several mutations are known which in 90 per cent of cases result in complete absence of enzymatic activity. Even in cases correctly treated by low galactose diet, significant visual–perceptual deficits and EEG abnormalities are found in one-third to one-half of the patients. This may be due to the continuing endogenous formation of toxic galactose-1-phosphate from glucose-1-phosphate through the action of epimerase. A few patients have more definite neurological signs, including cerebellar or extrapyramidal features (Böhles *et al.* 1986, Friedman *et al.* 1989) that can be progressive (Koch *et al.* 1992, Bohu *et al.* 1995). Waggoner and Buist (1993) found that 18 per cent of 175 patients had cerebellar signs. Cognitive deficits are frequent and may be progessive. Verbal dyspraxia with disturbances of speech rhythm without receptive deficit was found in 13 of 24 patients of Nelson *et al.* (1991) and in 50 per cent of the 175 cases reviewed by Waggoner and Buist (1993) and was usually of a severe degree. Pseudotumour cerebri (Huttenlocher *et al.* 1970) and skeletal muscle involvement (Bresolin *et al.* 1993) have been reported. In contrast, galactokinase deficiency (Gitzelmann *et al.* 1974) is associated with cataracts but does not generate neurodevelopmental deficits.

Cystinosis primarily affects the kidney with progressive renal insufficiency. However, with successful management of renal disease neurological manifestations may become apparent. Cognitive defects, progressive dementia and spasticity (Trauner *et al.* 1988) may be associated with cerebral atrophy and multifocal calcification of the internal capsules and periventricular white matter (Fink *et al.* 1989a). A vacuolar myopathy may develop in the late stages of the disease (Charnas *et al.* 1994).

Lowe syndrome is marked by congenital cataracts, hypotonia, absent deep tendon reflexes, mental retardation, generalized aminoaciduria and renal tubular acidosis with hypophosphataemia (Charnas *et al.* 1991). Although 12 of 47 patients studied by Kenworthy *et al.* (1993) had an IQ >70, tantrums and irritability were frequent. MRI may show periventricular lesions

(Ono *et al.* 1996). The oculocerebrorenal syndrome is a sex-linked genetic disease affecting only males. Female carriers can be detected by the presence of multiple fine lens opacities. The gene codes for a 105kD protein which may be related to the Golgi complex (Olivos-Glander *et al.* 1995). Although clearly a metabolic disorder, Lowe syndrome is currently difficult to classify.

DISORDERS OF SUBCELLULAR ORGANELLES: 1. LYSOSOMAL DISEASES

Lysosome function is to hydrolyse a large number of complex molecules. When this function fails, *storage disorders* within the lysosomes result. Most lysosomal diseases are due to a genetic defect of one of the lysosomal enzymes involved in the degradation of a specific substance. However, some diseases, including mucolipidoses II and III, result from post-traductional abnormalities affecting normally synthesized proenzymes. Others (*e.g.* Salla disease and cystinosis) are due to defective transport of substrates across lysosomal membrane.

All lysosomal diseases (currently about 30 are known) are inherited as recessive—mostly autosomal recessive—traits. New diseases (*e.g.* infantile ceroid–lipofuscinosis) are still being added to the list.

The clinical presentation is variable with the defective enzyme. Even for the same enzyme deficit, the phenotypic manifestations are variable, reflecting the possible existence of multiple different abnormalities of the same gene and/or occurrence of joint effects of other genes, alternative messenger RNA splicing, or post-traductional modifications. These, in turn, result in absence or in different abnormalities of proteins, with variable activity and therefore different clinical features.

SPHINGOLIPIDOSES
The sphingolipidoses are lysosomal diseases with absent or imperfect degradation of the sphingolipids which are essential components of CNS membranes. The major steps of sphingolipid catabolism and the corresponding enzymes and enzymatic blocks are represented in Figure 9.1.

GANGLIOSIDOSES
These are important diseases that result from enzymatic blocks which involve the removal of *N*-acetylgalactose from the complex ganglioside molecules. Gangliosides are found mainly in nuclear areas of grey matter and not, in any great amount, in myelin. Their normal functions are incompletely understood. Although many gangliosides have been isolated from the brain, four major components, GM1 to GM4, account for over 90 per cent of the total ganglioside fraction.

GM2 gangliosidoses
GM2 gangliosidoses are the commonest diseases of this group. Several varieties are known depending on the nature of the enzyme defect. Three isozymes of hexosaminidase have been recognized. Hexosaminidase A is composed of one alpha and 2 beta subunits (A1, B2), hexosaminidase B solely of B units (B2 B2) and hexosaminidase S only of A units (A2). In classical Tay–Sachs disease or B variant, hexosaminidase A (HexA) and S are inoperative as a result of a mutation at the A locus on chromosome 15 (15q22–q25.1). Hexosaminidase B is normal but unable to hydrolyse gangliosides *in vivo*. Different mutations at the alpha locus are known (Budde-Steffen *et al.* 1988, Nakano *et al.* 1990). Thus GM2 gangliosidosis in French Canadians (Palomaki *et al.* 1995) may be due to a different DNA defect (deletion of intron 1 and promoter region) to that in Ashkenazi Jews, which in 73 per cent of cases comprises a four-base insertion in exon 11. However, some French Canadians have the same mutation as Ashkenazi Jews and within a single population different mutations can be observed (Boustany *et al.* 1991). B1 mutation results in an altered substrate specificity of HexA (Gordon *et al.* 1988). In this variant, the mutated enzyme displays an essentially normal activity when tested with conventional methylumbelliferyl substrates but is unable to hydrolyse GM2 or sulfated methyl-umbelliferyl synthetic substrate (Specola *et al.* 1990). The O variant (Sandhoff disease) is characterized by deficiency of both beta-hexosaminidase isoenzymes A and B due to a mutation at the beta locus on chromosome 5 (5q13). Variant AB is caused by the deficiency of an activator protein (saponin) required for the interaction of HexA with its natural substrate (Kotagal *et al.* 1986). There is, thus, a considerable clinical and biochemical heterogeneity of GM2 gangliosidoses.

The pathological changes in the CNS are common to all forms of gangliosidosis with some variations related to the length of the course and undefined factors. The main finding is the presence in neurons of lipid-soluble material within the cytoplasm with later disappearance of many neurons and the development of extensive gliosis. Purkinje cells and neurons in brainstem nuclei, and neurons in visceral plexus are also affected (Ushiyama *et al.* 1985). Visceral involvement, especially of the kidney, is marked in Sandhoff disease in which a large accumulation of globoside is characteristic.

Electron microscopy shows multiple membranous cytoplasmic bodies (Terry bodies) composed essentially of lipids with 10 per cent protein. The processes of involved neurons are massively expanded, and this excess of probably excitable membranes may be responsible for abnormal neuronal function (Purpura and Suzuki 1976).

Tay–Sachs disease is by far the most frequent form of gangliosidosis, affecting 1 in 2000 persons among Ashkenazi Jewish populations of eastern European background. The gene frequency is estimated to be 1 in 27 among Jews and 1 in 380 in non-Jews.

The onset is between 3 and 9 months, with loss of acquired milestones and of muscle tone following an essentially normal initial development. Acoustic startles may precede all other symptoms and persist for several months. Neurological symptoms rapidly progress. Initial hypotonia is replaced by spastic tetraparesis, and epileptic seizures may appear late in the course. After the first year of life, the infants are helpless, blind and unre-

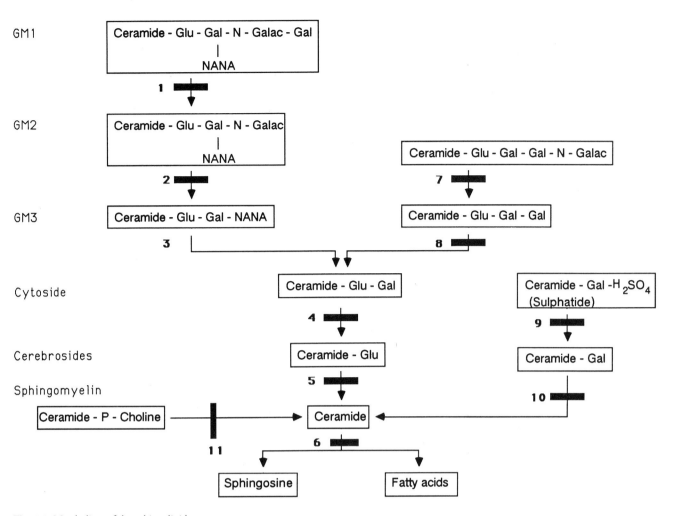

Fig. 9.1. Metabolism of the sphingolipids.

Key: Gal = galactose. Glu = glucose. N-Galac = *N*-acetylgalactosamine. NANA = neuraminic acid (*N*-acetylneuraminic acid).

1 = β-galactosidase. 2 = β-hexosaminidase A (Tay–Sachs disease) and other GM2 gangliosidoses. 3 = GM3 sialidase. 4 = lactosylceramidase (lactosylceramidosis). 5 = β-glucosidase (glucocerebrosidase) (Gaucher disease). 6 = ceramidase (Farber disease). 7 = β-hexosaminidase B (Sandhoff disease and other O variants of GM2 gangliosidosis). 8 = ceramide-trihexosidase/α-galactosidase (Fabry disease). 9 = cerebroside sulfatase/arylsulfatase* (metachromatic leukodystrophy). 10 = β-galactosidase/β-galactocerebrosidase (Krabbe disease). 11 = sphingomyelinase (Niemann–Pick disease A and B).

*Activity measured on artificial substrates, not always parallel to cerebroside sulfatase activity.

sponsive and often develop a progressive macrocephaly. MRI in the early stages of the disease shows increased T_2 signal from the basal ganglia. The caudate nuclei often protrude into the lateral ventricles. Later, T_2 signal is increased throughout the white matter (Yoshikawa *et al.* 1992).

Death usually occurs before 3 years of age. From early in the course, a cherry-red spot is present in both macular areas, surrounded by a zone of milky whitish retina (Kivlin *et al.* 1985). This whitish zone is due to lipid storage in the retinal ganglion cells that are especially dense in the posterior pole, whereas the red spot represents the normal macula which is devoid of ganglion cells and appears abnormally red by contrast with the surrounding retina. Although characteristic of Tay–Sachs disease, the cherry-red spot may also be seen in other types of gangliosidosis, in sialidosis, in Niemann–Pick disease, in infantile Gaucher disease and in rare cases of metachromatic leukodystrophy and of Krabbe's disease (Naidu *et al.* 1988b).

Sandhoff disease (type O gangliosidosis) is clinically indistinguishable from classical Tay–Sachs but represents only 7 per cent of cases of GM2 gangliosidosis.

The diagnosis of Tay–Sachs disease is easily confirmed by absence of hexosaminidase A or both Hex A and Hex B assay in serum or leukocytes. Patients with a B1 mutation have intermediate levels of Hex A activity when tested with a nonsulfated umbilliferyl substrate. For them the use of sulfated 4-Mu-gal-*N*-Ac-6-sulfate (4-MUG) substrate is necessary for diagnosis (Maia *et al.* 1990, Specola *et al.* 1990). Prenatal diagnosis by Hex A assay is possible in the second trimester of gestation.

Carrier detection using blood is possible and has been automated for mass screening surveys (Kaback *et al.* 1993). Fibroblast testing is required if the woman is pregnant, or if either partner is diabetic, has had a myocardial infarct or has hepatitis. Also, pseudodeficiency of Hex A occurs in compound heterozygotes who carry one common disease-causing mutation on one allele and one of two benign mutations on the second allele. Such individuals are clinically normal although they cannot hydrolyse synthetic 4-MUG substrates. These benign mutations have significant implications for heterozygote screeening programmes and for prenatal diagnosis. Their frequency was found to be respectively 3 per cent and 38 per cent in Ashkenazi Jewish and non-Jewish enzyme-defined carriers (Cao *et al.* 1993).

Juvenile GM2 gangliosidosis is rare. Onset is between 2 and 6 years by gait instability and often speech disturbances, followed by ataxia and pyramidal tract signs. Intellectual deterioration is present at end stage (Maia *et al.* 1990). Many patients have seizures, and a few have ataxia (Streifler *et al.* 1993) or dystonia and choreoathetotic movements (Specola *et al.* 1990, Nardocci *et al.* 1992). There is no racial predilection.

Chronic GM2 gangliosidosis is often termed 'adult form' although the onset is before 10 years in 35 per cent of cases. Onset is with a special dysarthria followed by gait difficulties, pyramidal tract signs, ataxia and lower motor neuron involvement. Psychiatric disturbances occur later in half the cases. Dystonia is present in some patients (Oates *et al.* 1986), and supranuclear ophthalmoplegia has been reported (Harding *et al.* 1987, Specola *et al.* 1990).

Atypical forms may present as anterior horn cell disease of juvenile onset (Navon *et al.* 1995), as isolated dystonia, or as atypical spinocerebellar degeneration (Willner *et al.* 1981).

A clinical picture of Tay–Sachs disease may be seen in patients with normal amounts of Hex A and B (AB variant) (Gravel *et al.* 1995) and is difficult to diagnose as it requires direct study of marked natural gangliosides catabolism. The B1 variants usually present as infantile disease but may also be found in patients with juvenile and chronic forms (Specola *et al.* 1990), although in the latter type an AB variant may be more common.

No treatment for the GM2 gangliosidoses is known. The process of ganglioside accumulation and consequent brain degeneration is already well-established by midtrimester of fetal life, so the prospects for enzyme replacement therapy are not favourable.

GM1 gangliosidosis

This disorder is due to deficiency of acid beta-galactosidase whose gene is located on 3pter–3p21 (see Fig. 9.1). In addition to lipid storage closely similar to that in GM2 gangliosidoses, the stored material also includes vacuolar inclusions with accumulation of numerous mannose-containing oligosaccharides, resulting from defective terminal beta-galactose residue removal during glycoprotein catabolism. Several beta-galactosidase isoenzymes are recognized. The three isoenzymes (A1, A2, A3) are defective in all forms of GM1 gangliosidosis, and the various phenotypes are probably explained by different mutations (at least eight are known) resulting in proteins with different residual substrate specificities (Suzuki *et al.* 1991).

GM1 gangliosidosis type 1 (pseudo-Hurler disease, Landing disease) is a rare autosomal recessive disease, clinically present at birth. Affected infants are markedly hypotonic, suck poorly, fail to thrive and do not make any psychomotor progress. They have frontal bossing, coarse facial features, macroglossia and hirsutism.

Half of them have a retinal cherry-red spot, and hepatosplenomegaly is usually evident. The skeletal deformities are similar to those of Hurler syndrome. The course is severe. Blindness, quadriplegia and epileptic seizures appear and death usually supervenes before 2 years of age.

GM1 gangliosidosis type 2 has a later onset between 6 months and 3 years of age. No marked skeletal abnormalities are present, although the first or second lumbar vertebrae are abnormally shaped, so that the presentation is one of progressive neurological deterioration with spasticity, cerebellar and extrapyramidal signs. Optic atrophy and a cherry-red spot may be present, and acoustic startles occur in half the cases although usually late in the course. The gene is the same as for infantile type 1 but there is heterozygosity for two separate mutations, one of which is that commonly found in homozygous form in type 1 (Boustany *et al.* 1993).

GM1 gangliosidosis type 3 has its onset in late childhood, adolescence or even in adulthood. Its presentation is variable. A picture of spinocerebellar degeneration is possible. Variants include a dystonic form (Guazzi *et al.* 1988, Tanaka *et al.* 1995) and atypical cases, *e.g.* with myopathy and cardiomyopathy (Charrow and Hvizd 1986). Intellectual deterioration may be late or absent in such forms. Low T_1 signal from the pallidum and putamen has been reported (Tanaka *et al.* 1995).

The *diagnosis* of GM1 gangliosidosis can be helped by the absence of urinary excretion of mucopolysaccharides, by the presence of bony abnormalities, especially of the lumbar vertebrae, and by the presence of foamy cells in the bone marrow. It is confirmed by the absence or marked reduction of beta-galactosidase activity in leukocytes or fibroblasts. In the late (type 3) forms, beta-galactosidase deficiency is partial (5–20 per cent normal). Prenatal diagnosis can be made on cultured amniotic cells or trophoblasts.

Beta-galactosidase is also deficient in Morquio type B disease (p. 252) which is a skeletal disorder without neurological involvement, and in galactosialidosis which is described with the sialidoses (p. 253).

GM3 gangliosidosis is an exceptional condition characterized by poor physical development, abnormal facies, rapid neurological deterioration and early death. The nosological situation of this disease remains unsettled (Tanaka *et al.* 1975).

Deficiency in lysosomal alpha-*N*-acetylgalactosaminidase (Chapter 10) may pathologically resemble neuroaxonal dystrophy (van Diggelen *et al.* 1988, Wang *et al.* 1988).

GAUCHER DISEASE

Gaucher disease is a relatively frequent recessive disease due to deficiency of beta-glucocerebrosidase (see Fig. 9.1). The gene coding for beta-glucocerebrosidase is located on chromosome 1q21–q31. The different types may correspond to allelic mutations at this locus. More than 35 mutations are currently known (Horowitz and Zimram 1994). It has been proposed that patients with a homozygous leucine → proline 444 mutation have neurological manifestations while heterozygotes do not. However, some patients with homozygous 444 mutation have no neurological signs while some patients with other mutations (*e.g.* 601) do. Patients with a 370 mutation may have ophthalmoplegia without neurological signs but with aggressive systemic disease (Horowitz *et al.* 1993). Phenotypic variations may be due to compound heterozygosity, which is frequent, or to post-transcriptional abnormalities (Tsuji *et al.* 1987). Homoallelism is common in types 3 and 2 but not in type 1. Three main phenotypes are encountered: chronic adult form, neuropathic infantile form and juvenile type.

Type 1 Gaucher disease is the most common type but is only occasionally observed in children. It is mainly marked by hepatosplenomegaly, bone abnormalities, and sometimes hypersplenism and pulmonary manifestations. There is no involvement of the CNS except perhaps in rare late cases. Glucocerebrosides accumulate throughout the reticuloendothelial system. The major marker is the Gaucher cell that has a lacy, striated cytoplasm and is found in the bone marrow, spleen, liver and lymph nodes. Electron microscopy shows inclusion bodies containing tubular elements (Kaye *et al.* 1986). Increased acid phosphatase is a constant finding of some diagnostic value.

Type 2 Gaucher disease (acute infantile Gaucher disease or neuronopathic type) is also due to glucosyl ceramide beta-glucosidase deficiency. There is some suggestion of heterogeneity as the glycolipid content of the liver is variable and the composition of the glycolipids may also be variable.

The clinical onset is at 3–5 months of age with muscle hypotonia and loss of interest in surroundings. Spasticity gradually sets in. Neck retraction and bulbar signs are often prominent and result in marked feeding difficulties. Splenomegaly is usually pronounced but, in one personal patient, it was hardly detectable clinically. Cherry-red spots are sometimes present. Convulsions may occur during the second semester. Death usually occurs before 2 years of age.

The pathological changes in the CNS include foci of cell loss and neuronophagia (Kaye *et al.* 1986). A few perivascular Gaucher cells may be present but there is usually no marked degree of cytoplasmic storage in this form (Willemsen *et al.* 1987, Grafe *et al.* 1988). An even more severe neonatal form, associated with congenital ichthyosis, has been reported (Ince *et al.* 1995).

Type 3 Gaucher disease (juvenile Gaucher disease) becomes apparent during the first decade of life, the major features at this period being slowly progressive hepatosplenomegaly, rapidly associated with intellectual deficiency (Winkelman *et al.* 1983). Cerebellar ataxia and extrapyramidal signs frequently develop. The most suggestive features include supranuclear horizontal ophthalmoplegia that may be the initial feature (Gross-Tsur *et al.* 1989) and in some myoclonic epilepsy (Nishimura *et al.* 1980). Moderate bony changes such as widening of humeral and femoral diaphyses may be present. A phenotypic variant of type 3, known as the Norrbottnian type, is frequently encountered in northern Sweden (Dreborg *et al.* 1980). The onset is early, around 1 year of age, with progressive hepatosplenomegaly and hypersplenism. Mental deterioration, ataxia and spastic tetraplegia evolve slowly after age 3 years. Splenectomy often precipitates

appearance or aggravation of neurological signs. This type is regularly associated with a homozygous 444 mutation. Some investigators separate type IIIa with progressive neurological disease and mild systemic manifestations and type IIIb with severe systemic disease (Mistry 1995). A type IIIc with onset of oculomotor apraxia, splenomegaly, cardiac valve anomalies and corneal opacities has recently been described (Mistry 1995).

In fact, the neurological features are quite variable. Some patients have early features such as ophthalmoplegia starting in the first few years and may keep a normal intellect to adulthood with only extrapyramidal signs without epilepsy or deterioration, and many intermediate forms exist (Lyon *et al.* 1996).

Pathologically, intraneuronal storage disease is obvious and glucosylceramide is detected chemically (Wenger *et al.* 1983). Treatment of subacute forms with bone marrow transplantation has been tried. Enzyme infusion therapy (Bembi *et al.* 1994, Erikson *et al.* 1995) is extremely costly but is effective on systemic manifestations. It does not improve neurological signs but may stabilize them. It is ineffective in acute type II cases. Splenectomy is contraindicated in type III cases.

Lactosyl ceramidosis is an exceptional disease caused by deficient ceramide lactosyl beta-galactosidase. There is mental and motor regression from 1 or 2 years of age with associated hepatosplenomegaly and a rapidly lethal course (Watts and Gibbs 1986).

NIEMANN–PICK DISEASE
Niemann–Pick disease is a heterogeneous group of diseases linked by an accumulation of sphingomyelin in the reticuloendothelial system. Of the three main types A, B and C, types A and B are due to a deficiency of sphingomyelinase and constitute type I, while other forms without sphingomyelinase deficit form group II in the new classification proposed by Schuchman and Desnick (1995). Type C will be studied with disorders of cholesterol metabolism.

Niemann–Pick disease type A (acute neuronopathic type, type I) is transmitted as an autosomal recessive character and occurs especially in Ashkenazi Jews. The gene maps to 11p15, and three mutations account for 92 per cent of cases (Schuchman 1995). The pathological hallmark of the condition is the presence in the reticuloendothelial system of large vacuolated cells. Foam cells and ballooned ganglion cells are found in the CNS. Biochemically, there is a marked storage of sphingomyelin, a major component of normal myelin, in association with cholesterol in the spleen, liver and kidney. Storage is also present in the brain although usually at moderate level.

The clinical onset of the disease is during the first year of life, with hepatosplenomegaly and poor physical and mental development. Jaundice, diarrhoea and pulmonary infiltrates are common.

Neurological features are prominent in approximately one-third of infants and appear eventually in most. Myoclonic seizures, spasticity and blindness are the major manifestations. One-quarter of the patients have retinal cherry-red spots. A peripheral neuropathy occurs in 10 per cent of cases with slowing of conduction velocities (Gumbinas *et al.* 1975). Death occurs before age 5 years.

The diagnosis is suggested by the presence of vacuolated cells in the bone marrow. Sphingomyelinase deficiency in leukocytes or fibroblasts is definitive confirmation of the diagnosis.

Niemann–Pick disease type B is characterized by visceral involvement without neurological features and occurs mainly in older children and adults. An occasional patient may develop neurological signs.

FABRY DISEASE

This rare, sex-linked disorder is due to a deficiency (absence, low activity or fast catabolism) of the A isoenzyme of alpha-galactosidase (ceramide trihexosidase) caused by several mutations of the gene mapping at Xq22 (Eng *et al.* 1994). However, detectable mutations are found in only a minority of patients (Ploos van Amstel *et al.* 1994). As a result, large amounts of trihexoside accumulate in various organs, especially the kidneys. Foam cells with vacuolated cytoplasm are found in smooth and striated muscle, in marrow and renal glomeruli. In the CNS, storage is confined to walls of the blood vessels and, to a lesser extent, to the autonomic nervous system (Kaye *et al.* 1988). MRI scans may show periventricular high signal and discrete lesions suggestive of demyelination (Menzies *et al.* 1988).

Clinical manifestations of the disease usually begin in childhood. Skin abnormalities may be the presenting feature, in the form of punctate angiectatic lesions (angiokeratoma corporis diffusum) that are commonly found on the genitalia or umbilicus or about the hips, but may rarely involve the face. Episodes of pain in the limbs and sometimes in the abdomen are often the first symptoms. Pain is deep, of a burning character and occurs in episodes lasting from hours to weeks. These are often associated with unexplained fever. Cornea verticillata is seen by slit lamp examination and is often present in heterozygotes (Watts and Gibbs 1986). Peripheral neuropathy involving small fibres has been reported. Approximately 30 per cent of patients have cardiac defects including mitral valve prolapse and cardiomyopathy, and transient ischaemic attacks commonly occur.

The disease runs a progressive course and CNS and visceral vascular accidents often occur with focal neurological signs, hypertension or myocardial infarcts. Renal involvement is the usual cause of death. Women carriers usually display late and milder symptoms.

The diagnosis is confirmed early by determination of alpha-galactosidase in plasma, leukocytes or fibroblasts. Antenatal diagnosis and carrier detection are possible.

Treatment includes prevention of painful episodes which can usually be achieved with carbamazepine or phenytoin (Filling-Katz *et al.* 1989), and therapy for renal insufficiency. Renal transplants have little effect on the CNS lesions, although sensory symptoms and renal function may be improved.

CERAMIDOSIS (LIPOGRANULOMATOSIS, FARBER DISEASE)

This rare disease is due to deficient activity of lysosomal ceramidase and is transmitted as an autosomal recessive character. The onset is during the first weeks of life, with irritability, a hoarse cry and the appearance of nodular erythematous swellings around the wrists and other joints. Severe motor and mental retardation is frequent and convulsions are common. Cardiac valvular lesions may be present. Death occurs before 2–3 years of age although a mild form may allow survival for several years.

The basic lesion is a granuloma that forms around mesenchymal cells containing large amounts of ceramide. Neurons and glial cells are swollen by storage material (Moser and Chen 1983).

SULFATIDOSIS (METACHROMATIC LEUKODYSTROPHY)

Metachromatic leukodystrophy is an autosomal recessive disease due to deficiency of cerebroside sulfatase, although, for practical reasons, artificial substrates are used which test the arylsulfatase A activity. Diffuse demyelination and accumulation of metachromatic material (metachromasia), caused by the presence of sulfatides, produces an unusual staining with the use of certain dyes when they combine with storage material. Sulfatides are stored in the CNS and in many peripheral tissues including skin and gall bladder. There are two major phenotypes: an infantile form with a population prevalence of approximately 1 in 40,000 and a juvenile form with a 1 in 150,000 population prevalence. In addition, rare cases are due to a different mutation involving an activator protein (saponin B) that is coded for by a gene at 10q21–q22. The gene for cerebroside sulfatase maps to 22q13–22qter. A mutation on exon 2 (459.1G) is responsible for most cases of the late infantile form, whereas a mutation on exon 8 (P426L) is commonly found in later onset form (Barth *et al.* 1994a), but the phenotype/genotype correspondence is imperfect. Complex arylsulfatase A alleles can cause various types of metachromatic leukodystrophy (Kappler *et al.* 1994). Compound heterozygosity seems to be responsible for juvenile forms (Polten *et al.* 1991, Gieselmann *et al.* 1994).

In the *late infantile form*, onset of symptoms is usually between 10 and 25 months with a mean of 17 months (MacFaul *et al.* 1982). Irritability and floppiness are often the first manifestations. In children who had started to walk, a gait disorder that may be related predominantly to either poor balance or stiffness precedes loss of ambulation. Spasticity of the lower limbs is consistently observed and progresses gradually. This contrasts with the usual reduction or abolition of deep tendon reflexes. Mental regression is relatively late, and seizures are uncommon and late. Strabismus frequently appears and optic atrophy may develop. Death occurs one to four years after onset. In almost all cases there is an increased protein level in the CSF and a marked slowing of motor and sensory nerve conduction velocities. In some infants, involvement of the peripheral nervous system may remain isolated for several weeks, thus masquerading for polyradiculoneuritis or heredodegenerative neuropathy. Convulsions are exceptional and the EEG shows some slowing without paroxysmal features.

The *juvenile form* begins between 4 and 10 years of age and is often marked by mental regression and behaviour disturbances. In other cases, motor disturbances are the first symptom although nerve conduction velocity may be normal in some children. Convulsion and movement disorders can occur. Adult forms may present as psychiatric disease (Fisher *et al.* 1987).

The EEG is slow without paroxysmal features. The ERG is normal.

In all forms, CT or MRI scans show changes in the periventricular white matter which may initially be slight. Confirmation of the diagnosis is easily obtained by measurement of arylsulfatase A activity which is usually totally absent in infantile forms and between 0 and 10 per cent in juvenile cases (Polten *et al.* 1991). In the rare activator protein deficiency, study of sulfatide catabolism *in vitro* by radioactive assay is necessary for the diagnosis. Sulfatides can be found in urine, and metachromasia has been found on peripheral nerve biopsy although this is no longer advised.

Problems in diagnosis may arise because pseudodeficiency occurs in 7–15 per cent of the general population and results in absence or very low levels of arylsulfatase activity (Barth *et al.* 1994b). Pseudodeficiency is caused by two different mutations in the cerebroside-sulfatase gene and can be detected directly by polymerase chain reaction without requiring a radioactive assay. Because of its frequency, it may often be present in relatives of persons with metachromatic leukodystrophy or in coincidence with unrelated neurological diseases (Clarke *et al.* 1989). Cerebroside-sulfatase activity in such cases may be present, but lack of arylsulfatase activity has also been found in association with impaired cerebroside sulfate hydrolysis in fibroblasts (Hreidarsson *et al.* 1983). Such cases do not represent the preclinical stage of adult leukodystrophy, and the reason why no symptoms are present remains obscure. *Pseudodeficiency* may raise a difficult problem in antenatal diagnosis (Francis *et al.* 1993). A majority of the cases of arylsulfatase A pseudodeficiency are due to homozygosity for the arylsulfatase A pseudodeficiency allele, but some may result from compound heterozygosity between a pseudodeficiency and one of the metachromatic leukodystrophy alleles (Polten *et al.* 1991). No clinical manifestation is apparent when arylsulfatase A activity is 10 per cent of normal or higher. Prenatal diagnosis thus requires a full study of the enzymatic features or both parents. It can be made early on chorionic villus sampling (Poenaru *et al.* 1988). Determination of the molecular mutation will eventually solve this problem.

Although no satisfactory treatment is known, attempts at bone marrow transplant have met with some success (Krivit *et al.* 1990).

Mucosulfatidosis (Multiple Sulfatase Deficiency, Austin Disease)

Mucosulfatidosis is a rare disease characterized by absence of arylsulfatase A, B and C and of mucopolysaccharide sulfatase activity. As a result, patients accumulate sulfatides, mucopolysaccharides and cholesterol sulfate in CNS and viscera and there is increased excretion of heparan sulfate in urine.

Clinical manifestations include coarse features, hepatosplenomegaly and skeletal changes in association with progressive neurodevelopmental deterioration and peripheral neuropathy. Ichthyosis is a frequent suggestive feature. Early severe retinal degeneration (Harbord *et al.* 1991) and cervical cord compression may occur. The course is similar to that of metachromatic leuko-

dystrophy. This is an autosomal recessive disease that may result from a mutation of a regulatory gene, although precise data are not available. The condition may be present at birth (Burch *et al.* 1986), and a case with associated agenesis of the corpus callosum has been seen at our institution.

Globoid Cell Leukodystrophy (Krabbe Disease)

This disease results from deficiency of beta-galactocerebrosidase and is transmitted as an autosomal recessive trait. The gene maps to 14q24–q32 (Cannizzaro *et al.* 1994), and a number of molecular defects have been identified (Tatsumi *et al.* 1995). Several forms are known (Hagberg 1984): the infantile form is most common, but rare juvenile, late infantile and adult forms have been observed.

Pathologically, there is marked atrophy of the brain with extensive demyelination of the white matter. Large, multinucleated cells (globoid cells) are seen around blood vessels and store a protein-bound cerebroside. On electron microscopy, there are crystalline needle-like inclusions which correspond to the globoid cell material. Such inclusions are also present in Schwann cells of peripheral nerves that display considerable segmental demyelination.

Clinical features vary with the age of onset. The classical infantile form (Hagberg *et al.* 1970) begins virtually always before 6 months of age and often before 3 months or even during the first weeks or days of life. Restlessness, irritability and progressive stiffness are the initial symptoms and may develop rather acutely. Increased muscle tone and pyramidal tract signs are found on examination, and opisthotonic spasms are often precipitated by external stimuli. Loss of acquired skills may be difficult to assess because of the young age at onset. Deep tendon relfexes are often absent or weak due to peripheral neuropathy. Convulsions are not exceptional and may present as infantile spasms with an atypical hypsarrhythmic EEG pattern (Williams *et al.* 1979). The course is rapid and death usually occurs at 1–2 years of age.

Clinical variants are occasionally observed (Hagberg 1984). One presentation is with massive hypotonia, the infant lying in the frog position. A retinal cherry-red spot is occasionally present (Naidu *et al.* 1988b).

In all cases, a high CSF protein is found and nerve conduction velocities are considerably lowered. CT scan generally does not show hypodensity of the white matter, but rather generalized brain atrophy. Discrete symmetrical areas of increased density are often seen in the deep grey matter of hemispheres and brainstem, in periventricular and capsular white matter and in the cerebellum. Relatively limited areas of decreased white matter density are sometimes seen in late-onset cases. MRI shows a low signal in the same areas on T_1-weighted sequences and large zones of high signal in the centrum semi-ovale on T_2-weighted sequences (Darras *et al.* 1986, Farley *et al.* 1992, Tada *et al.* 1992) (Fig. 9.2). Evoked potentials are considerably delayed and abnormal. A final diagnosis is easily obtained by enzymatic assay.

Juvenile globoid cell leukodystrophy has a more variable clinical picture (Hagberg 1984, Loonen *et al.* 1985, Phelps *et al.* 1991). Some children present with primarily motor symptoms in the

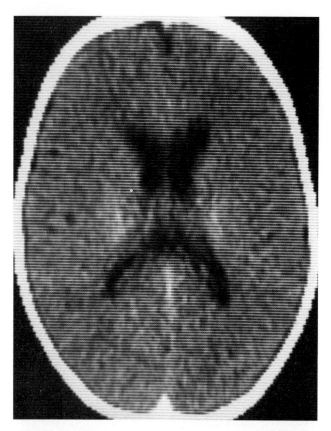

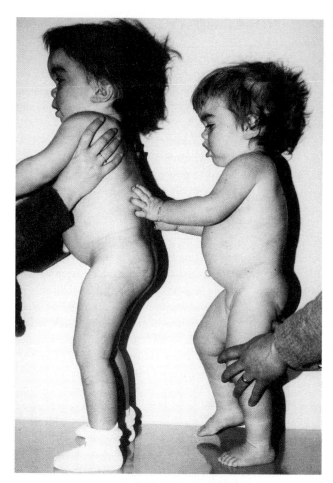

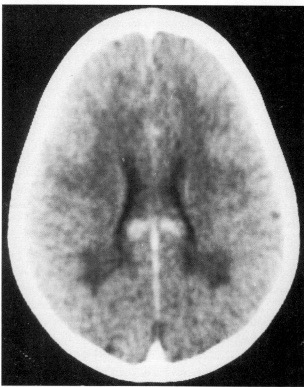

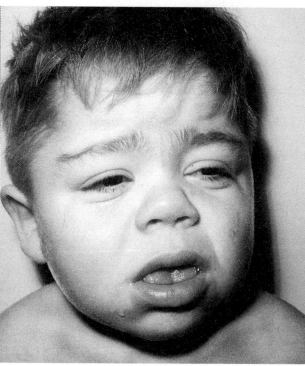

Fig. 9.2. Krabbe leukodystrophy. *(Top)* 13-month-old girl with progressive deterioration and rigidity from age 9 months. CT scan showing little or no hypodensity of the white matter, but high density in the central grey matter and internal capsule. *(Bottom)* Juvenile Krabbe disease: enhanced CT scan. Note moderate demyelination around the posterior ventricular horns with contrast enhancement involving the splenium of the corpus callosum, a finding usually suggestive of adrenoleukodystrophy.

Fig. 9.3. Type I mucopolysaccharidosis (Hurler disease). *(Top)* Two sisters aged 7 and 3 years, demonstrating enlarged head with scaphocephaly, typical profile, umbilical hernia and short hands with broad, partially flexed fingers. *(Bottom)* 12-year-old boy with typical facies. (Courtesy Dr P. Maroteaux, Hôpital des Enfants Malades, Paris.)

TABLE 9.1
Main characteristics of the mucopolysaccharidoses

Type	Eponym	Osseous visceral abnormalities	Neurological features	Urinary excretion of MPS*	Mode of inheritance**	Enzyme deficiency (gene location)
IH	Hurler	Marked. Severe dwarfism	Severe	DS + HS	AR	α-L-iduronidase (4p16)
IS or V	Scheie	Mild***	Mild	DS + HS	AR	*Idem*
II	Hunter	Marked. Severe dwarfism	Mild or moderate	HS	XR	Iduronosulfate-sulfatase (Xq28)
III	Sanfilippo	Mild. May be lacking at onset	Severe with progressive mental deterioration and seizures	HS	AR	A: Heparan-*N*-sulfamidase B: α-*N*-glucosamine-*N*-acetylglucosaminidase C: α-glucosamine-*N*-acetyl transferase D: *N*-acetyl-α-glucosaminido-6-sulfatase (12q14)
IV	Morquio (B milder)	Marked osseous anomalies	Absent (except as complication of bony lesions)	KS	AR	A: *N*-acetylgalactosamine-6-sulfatase (3p21–p14) B: β-galactosidase (16q24)
VI	Maroteaux–Lamy	Severe dwarfism and bony abnormalities	Absent (except as complication of meningeal involvement)	DS	AR	*N*-acetylgalactosamine-4-sulfatase (5p11–5q13)
VII	Sly	Mild to severe	Absent to severe	DS + HS	AR	β-glucuronidase (7q21–q22)

*DS = dermatan sulfate; HS = heparan sulfate; KS = keratan sulfate.
**AR = autosomal recessive; XR = X-linked recessive.
***Limited to carpal tunnel syndrome.

form of diplegia. In others the onset is with mental deterioration, loss of vision, dystonia or cerebellar manifestations. Visual failure is a major symptom. Peripheral neuropathy may or may not be present, and CSF protein is often normal. Marked variability in clinical presentation may be present in the same family (Phelps *et al.* 1991). A partial remission has been observed in one patient (Goebel *et al.* 1990).

A *late infantile or early childhood form* is recognized by some investigators (Loonen *et al.* 1985). The onset is between 1 and 3 years, with motor symptoms, failing vision and progressive mental deterioration. A neuropathy is present. Atypical manifestations such as hemiplegia may mark the onset of the disease (Ashwal *et al.* 1988). Rare cases can present with features suggestive of spinocerebellar degeneration (Thomas *et al.* 1984).

MUCOPOLYSACCHARIDOSES (MPS) (Table 9.1)

The mucopolysaccharidoses are inborn errors of metabolism due to deficiency of a lysosomal glucosidase or sulfatase which leads to the accumulation of mucopolysaccharides or glycosaminoglycans in the lysosomes. Table 9.1 indicates the main characteristics of the diseases of this group. These disorders will be dealt with only briefly as the neurological manifestations are often overshadowed by the dysmorphic features. Details can be found in specialized books (McKusick 1972, Maroteaux 1974).

HURLER AND SCHEIE DISEASES (MPS IH AND IS)

In *Hurler disease*, visceral alterations are widespread and mucopolysaccharide-containing cells are present in the reticuloendothelial system and connective tissue. The CNS is severely affected with infiltration of the meninges, leading to hydrocephalus.

Neurons are distended by inclusions that on electron microscopy appear as 'zebra bodies'. The stored material in the brain is mainly composed of GM2 and GM3 gangliosides, whereas, in peripheral tissues, the stored material is mainly formed of dermatan and heparan sulfates, which are also excreted in the urine in large quantities.

Hurler disease is an autosomal recessive disorder that occurs in 1 in 100,000 births. Affected infants appear normal at birth but develop slowly with bony changes becoming apparent between 6 months and 2 years of age. Hepatosplenomegaly, nasal discharge and umbilical hernia are evident. Characteristic skeletal deformities set in progressively, together with coarsening of facial features, kyphoscoliosis, articular contractures and mental deterioration. Corneal opacities are seen, and marked dwarfism is consistently present (Fig. 9.3). The head is large, often dolichocephalic. CT and MRI scans show ventricular dilatation and hypodensity of hemispheral white matter (Afifi *et al.* 1990, Lee *et al.* 1993). Cystic arachnoiditis is often found in the hypothalamic region (McKusick and Neufeld 1983) and is responsible for hydrocephalus. Death supervenes before 20 years of age.

The diagnosis can be confirmed by L-iduronidase assay. The presence of azurophilic granules in granulocytes, Reilly granules, vacuolated lymphocytes (Gasser I cells), and basophilic cells in the bone marrow (Gasser II cells) is a strong argument for the diagnosis. Prenatal diagnosis is possible (Fensom and Benson 1994). The gene is located at 4p16.3. Multiple mutations are known, two of them being responsible for 80 per cent of cases (Scott *et al.* 1992).

Enzyme replacement therapy by bone marrow transplantation has met with partial success (Hopwood *et al.* 1993). Corneal clouding may disappear, but effects on growth and neurological development remain to be assessed.

In *Scheie disease*, formerly known as MPS type V, a clinical picture analogous to that in Hurler disease obtains and dysmorphism may be marked, but neurological involvement is limited to a high incidence of the carpal tunnel syndrome and mentation is unaffected. Genetic compounds of Hurler and Scheie mutations are known as Hurler–Scheie disease. Some patients develop hydrocephalus (Winters *et al.* 1976).

HUNTER DISEASE (MPS II)
This disorder is transmitted as an X-linked trait and is about five times less frequent than MPS I. Depending on the presence or absence of mental retardation, a mild and a severe form are recognized. Neurological abnormalities in the mild type may include sensorineural deafness, retinitis pigmentosa and moderate hydrocephalus. Nerve entrapment syndromes are common (Karpati *et al.* 1974) as a result of thickening of connective tissue. Enzyme assay permits antenatal and postnatal diagnosis. The gene is located to Xq28 and a deletion is found in 30 per cent of cases (Adinolfi 1993).

SANFILIPPO DISEASE (MPS III)
The clinical presentation of Sanfilippo disease is that of a progressive neurological and mental retardation beginning between 2 and 6 years of age. Corneal opacities are absent, and abnormally coarse features and thick hair, although present early, are superseded by the neurological disturbances. Convulsions are not uncommon.

The course is inexorably progressive and most patients die before the age of 20 years.

The diagnosis is often difficult initially because of the predominantly neurological manifestations. Urine screening for excretion of mucopolysaccharides is routinely indicated in patients with unexplained regression. Enzyme assay permits differentiation of four types which are phenotypically indistinguishable. Antenatal diagnosis is feasible (Fensom and Benson 1994).

MORQUIO DISEASE (MPS IV).
Morquio disease consists of bony abnormalities and corneal opacities without mental deficiency. In the severe or A type, hypoplasia of the odontoid process is regularly present and bulbospinal compression may occur. Meningeal and neuronal involvement has been reported (Koto *et al.* 1978). In the mild or B form, neurological features are absent. Atlantoaxial instability is frequent and may be responsible for spinal compression.

MAROTEAUX–LAMY DISEASE (MPS VI)
This disorder has a variable severity with diverse degrees of dwarfism and visceral involvement. Mental dysfunction is mild or absent. The main neurological complication is spinal compression, usually at cervical level, that may produce quadriplegia. This complication results from thickening of the meninges due to deposition of MPS and is difficult to treat surgically (Young *et al.* 1980).

SLY DISEASE (MPS VII)
Sly disease is a very rare disease that may mimic Hurler disease with severe neurodevelopmental involvement or have only a limited expression without neurological features (Bernsen *et al.* 1987).

OTHER FORMS OF MPS
Atypical and unclassified types rarely occur. Maroteaux (1973) described a new type in which prominent athetosis is associated with the excretion of keratan sulfate.

DISORDERS OF SUBCELLULAR ORGANELLES: 2. MUCOLIPIDOSES, SIALIDOSES AND DISORDERS OF GLYCOPROTEIN METABOLISM

MUCOLIPIDOSES
The mucolipidoses are rare diseases that have features of both the mucopolysaccharidoses and the lipidoses. Four types are described (Table 9.2), although types 2 and 3 may be regarded as two degrees (severe and mild) of the same disease. They are transmitted as autosomal recessive characters.

SIALIDOSIS I (CHERRY-RED SPOT MYOCLONUS SYNDROME)
Sialidosis I has a juvenile or adult onset and produces a rather pure intention and action myoclonus with a slow progression and no or only very slow mental deterioration (Rapin *et al.* 1978, Young *et al.* 1987).

MUCOLIPIDOSIS IV
Mucolipidosis IV is a rare disease that affects mainly but not exclusively Ashkenazi Jews. Failing vision and mental delay develop simultaneously following a normal neonatal period. Corneal opacities may be absent despite poor vision in the first months of life (Amir *et al.* 1987). Dystonia has been observed in some patients (Goutières *et al.* 1979). A mild variant with mainly ophthalmological features has been reported (Casteels *et al.* 1992).

DISORDERS OF GLYCOPROTEIN METABOLISM
These disorders (Fig. 9.4) overlap with the mucolipidoses. Sialidoses I and II belong to both groups. Three main conditions are described.

MANNOSIDOSIS
Mannosidosis is due to deficiency of alpha-mannosidase A and B, resulting in neuronal storage of mannose-rich oligosaccharides. A severe type (type I) has an infantile onset and is characterized by a Hurler-like appearance, mental retardation, hearing loss and hepatosplenomegaly. Type II form has a juvenile onset and a milder course, but there is considerable overlap between the two types (Bennet *et al.* 1995). Cognitive deficit may be mild and nonprogressive (Noll *et al.* 1989).

TABLE 9.2
The mucolipidoses (ML) and sialidoses

Type	Age of onset	Clinical features	Enzyme deficiency (gene location)	References
Sialidosis I (cherry-red spot –myoclonus syndrome)	Late childhood to adulthood	Action and intention myoclonus, retinal cherry-red spot, normal intelligence, no dysmorphism	Sialidase (α-neuraminidase) (6p21)	Rapin *et al.* (1978)
Sialidosis II	Neonatal period to second decade	Myoclonus, dysmorphic features, coarsening of facies, sometimes visceromegaly, possibly angiokeratoma and renal failure	α-neuraminidase (6p21)	Winter *et al.* (1980)
Sialidosis III (Goldberg syndrome, ML1)	Childhood or adolescence	Short stature, mild developmental delay; deterioration at adolescence	Sialidase (α-neuraminidase)	Spranger and Cantz (1978), Young *et al.* (1987)
ML II (I-cell disease)	First year	Marked dysmorphism, gingival hyperplasia, severe neurodevelopmental deterioration	N-acetylglucosaminyl-phosphotransferase, resulting in post-traductional abnormalities leading to defective internalization of terminal mannose in oligosaccharide chain	Leroy *et al.* (1972)
ML III (pseudo-Hurler polydystrophy)	After age 2 years	Moderate facial dysmorphism, dysostosis, mild mental deficiency		Zammarchi *et al.* (1994b)
ML IV	Before 6–12 months	Visual disturbances, corneal opacity, retinal degeneration, motor delay and lack of mental progress. Self-mutilation	Ganglioside sialidase	Amir *et al.* (1987)
		Possible mild variant with only visual disturbances		Casteels *et al.* (1992)

FUCOSIDOSIS

Fucosidosis is caused by deficiency of the enzyme fucosidase. The severe form, type I, is characterized by progressive intellectual deterioration, spasticity, coarse facial features and bony changes. Dystonia may be a prominent feature (Gordon *et al.* 1995). Type II has a similar presentation but is milder and the clinical picture includes angiokeratoma of the skin, especially affecting the genitalia and gingivae (Willems *et al.* 1991). However, as more cases have become known, the gap between types I and II has been gradually filled by a continuum of intermediate cases (Willems *et al.* 1991). Cases of both types have coexisted within the same pedigree and the reasons for phenotypic discrepancies are not understood.

GALACTOSIALIDOSIS

Galactosialidosis results from a combined deficiency of neuraminidase and beta-galactosidase. The onset of the *juvenile form* is between 5 and 10 years of age with cerebellar and extrapyramidal signs. Myoclonic seizures and action myoclonus usually develop after several years, and mental deterioration is late. There are no bony changes except for frequent wedging of the first lumbar vertebra. Coarse features progressively develop. An infantile form has been reported that closely resembles type I gangliosidosis (Galjaard *et al.* 1984). This disease is due to absence of a 'protective protein' that prevents proteolysis of the active enzyme. Galactosialidosis is genetically heterogeneous (Suzuki *et al.* 1988).

DISORDERS RELATED TO THE MUCOLIPIDOSES AND MPS

Salla disease is a disorder of the transport of sialic acid across lysosomal membranes. As a result, lysosomes store a large quantity of free sialic acid (Renlund *et al.* 1986). Clinical manifestations include psychomotor retardation of early onset during the first year of life, later followed by slowly progressive cerebellar and extrapyramidal dysfunction with severe cognitive deterioration (Renlund 1984). The disease is frequent in Finland but cases occur outside this country (Mancini *et al.* 1992, Robinson *et al.* 1997). Diagnosis can be helped by finding vacuolated leukocytes in blood and vacuolated cells in skin or conjunctival biopsy samples, and is confirmed by demonstration of high levels of sialic acid in urine. Prenatal diagnosis is possible by determination of sialic acid in amniotic fluid.

Other disorders of sialic acid metabolism include *infantile sialuria* without evidence of lysosomal storage (Wilcken *et al.* 1987); *French-type sialuria* (Montreuil *et al.* 1968) and variants (Ylitalo *et al.* 1986); and *infantile sialic acid storage disease* (Cameron *et al.* 1990), in which there is marked storage in lysosomes with fetal hydrops, severe retardation and bone defects. The clinical presentation of these patients varies from progressive deterioration with death in early childhood to a mild disease with normal life span. In rare cases, no lysosomal sialic acid storage could be demonstrated (Roesel *et al.* 1987). In severe forms, renal disease may be associated (Pueschel *et al.* 1988).

Aspartylglucosaminuria, consequent to a deficit of aspartyl-glucosaminidase, is also frequent in Finland. It is marked by

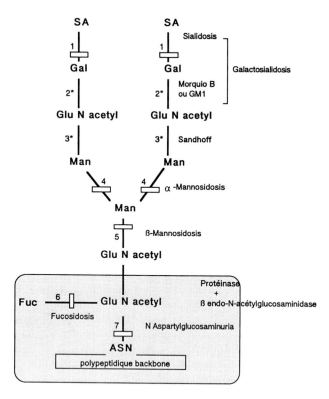

Fig. 9.4. Oligosaccharidoses: catabolism of glycoproteins. The two parts of the chain are degraded after the action of proteinases and β-endo-*N*-acetylglucosaminidase.

Key: 1 = sialidase = α-neuraminidase. 2* = β-galactosidase (see Fig. 9.1: sphingolipid catabolism = GM1 gangliosidosis). 1+2 = galactosialidosis. 3* = hexosaminidase A or B (see Fig. 9.1: sphingolipid catabolism = Sandhoff disease). 4 = α-mannosidase. 5 = β-mannosidase. 6 = α-fucosidase. 7 = *N*-aspartylglucosaminidase.

mental deterioration that begins in childhood or adolescence, lenticular opacities, bony changes reminiscent of the mucopolysaccharidoses, and mitral insufficiency (Arvio *et al.* 1993). Increased excretion of a variety of glycoasparagines can be detected by chromatography.

Storage of glutamyl-ribose-5-phosphate has been reported in one patient with progressive neurological deterioration, facial dysmorphism and renal failure, possibly inherited as an X-linked recessive trait (Williams *et al.* 1984).

CARBOHYDRATE-DEFICIENT GLYCOPROTEIN SYNDROME
Carbohydrate-deficient glycoprotein syndrome (CDG) comprises a group of inherited multisystemic disorders characterized by a deficiency of carbohydrate moieties in a number of sialoproteins. This is most readily detected in transferrin, which can be used as the biochemical marker. So far, four different types are described that differ in their carbohydrate-deficient transferrin patterns (Jaeken *et al.* 1991). Type I is the most frequent with more than two hundred known cases and has a fairly well delineated symptomatology. The previous reports of olivopontocerebellar atrophy of neonatal onset and disialotransferrin developmental deficiency (DDD) syndrome undoubtedly belong to this group (Horslen *et al.* 1991).

Biochemical background and pathogenesis
Glycosylation of proteins is an essential step in the posttranslational maturation of nascent polypeptides. It takes place in the endoplasmic reticulum and Golgi apparatus, and is part of cotranslational translocation of proteins through the cellular endomembrane system. In the processing of *N*-linked glycoproteins a preformed oligosaccharide (containing glucose, mannose and *N*-acetylglucosamine) is transferred from a membrane-bound dolicholpyrophosphate lipid carrier to asparagine residues of the polypeptide backbone.

The sugar residues which constitute the oligosaccharides are derived from nucleotide sugars such as guanosine diphosphatase (GDP) mannose. CDG type I is due in 80 per cent of cases to a deficiency in phosphomannomutase which prevents formation of mannose-1-phosphate and of GDP-mannose needed for the synthesis of dolichol-pyrophosphate-oligosaccharides in the endoplasmic reticulum (Van Schaftingen and Jaeken 1995) (Figs. 9.4, 9.5).

The Golgi apparatus receives proteins from the endoplasmic reticulum and processes the *N*-linked oligosaccharides to more complex forms by enzymatic stepwise removal and addition of sugar moities. *N*-acetylglucosaminyltransferase II is deficient in the rare CDG type II and prevents addition of the outer *N*-acetylglucosamine residue in the complex oligosaccharide (Jaeken *et al.* 1994). The basis of other types has not yet been determined.

The proteins concerned in this glycosylation process include transport proteins, glycoprotein hormones, complement factors, immunoglobulins, enzymes and enzyme inhibitors. Some are membrane proteins such as receptors in specialized cells. Thus defective glycolysation results in varying multisystem involvement.

Genetic background
Inheritance of CDG types I and II is autosomal recessive. CDG type I is panethnic. The true incidence is not known; in Sweden, it has been estimated to be around 1 in 40,000–60,000. Linkage analysis has enabled mapping of the CDG type I gene to chromosome 16p13.3–p13.12 and that of CDG type II to chromosome 14q21.

Prenatal diagnosis is possible in types I and II by assaying amniocytes for phosphomannomutase (CDG type I) or *N*-acetylglucosaminyltransferase II (CDG type II) (Martinsson *et al.* 1994, Van Schaftingen and Jaeken 1995).

Neuropathology
Nearly all cases exhibit olivopontocerebellar atrophy (OPCA) and myelin-like lysosomal storage (Eyskens *et al.* 1994). In two twins who died at ages 4 months and 6 years the atrophy was more marked in the longer surviving brother, suggesting a progressive degenerative process. Localized cerebral infarction suggests vascular occlusion. Microscopy reveals a complete loss of Purkinje cells, a subtotal loss of granular cells throughout the cerebellar cortex, and gliosis of pontine nuclei (Stromme *et al.* 1991). Sural nerve biopsies have shown abnormal myelin sheaths (Nordborg *et al.* 1991), and lysosomal storage has been found in anterior

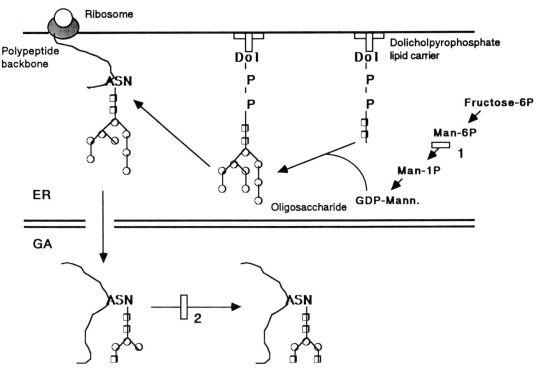

Fig. 9.5. Schematic representation of glycosylation process indicating the sites of the defects in CDG types I and II.
Key: □ = *N*-acetylglucosamine; O = mannose; ER = endoplasmic reticulum; GA = Golgi apparatus; ASN = asparagine.
1 = phosphomannomutase (CDG type I); 2 = *N*-acetylglucosaminyltransferase II (CDG type II).

horn cells (Eyskens *et al.* 1994) and also in hepatocytes, indicating a change in myelin turnover.

Clinical features
• *CDG type 1.* The manifestations of CDG type I are progressive and have been divided into four stages representing the evolution with age (Jaeken *et al.* 1991, Hagberg *et al.* 1993, Stibler *et al.* 1994).

The infantile stage is dominated by an alarming multisytemic involvement that progresses from the neonatal period through late infancy. It is characterized by poor feeding, failure to thrive and floppiness. Early psychomotor retardation is present in all patients, with severe gross motor delay, pronounced axial hypotonia, muscular weakness and later signs of dysequilibrium or of true cerebellar ataxia. A normal head circumference at birth can progress to acquired microcephaly. Tendon reflexes are initially weak, and areflexia appears within the first two to three years of life. Visual inattention, roving eye movements and internal strabismus are frequent. Congenital cataracts have been noted in a few patients (Eyskens *et al.* 1994). The majority of patients have some facial dysmorphism, inverted nipples, and peculiar body morphology with limb joint restrictions, thorax deformity and unusual lipodystrophy with fat pads above the buttocks (Fig. 9.6), over parts of the perineal region and/or on the fingers. Lipoatrophic streaks or patches on the lower limbs are frequently present. Mild hepatomegaly is associated with hepatic fibrosis or giant cell hepatitis. Enlarged kidneys and proteinuria have been noted. In many cases, alarming episodes of multiple organ system failure may occur: these include severe infections, hepatic failure, cardiac effusion with tamponade, and stupor occasionally associated with seizures and intracerebral haemorrhage. These acute episodes of deterioration are responsible for the high infantile mortality (15–20 per cent).

The childhood stage is dominated by a nonprogressive mental deficiency of variable degree. Most patients have DQ/IQ around 50. Cerebellar ataxia and peripheral neuropathy, responsible for muscular atrophy, prevent independent ambulation in most cases. Recurrent episodes of dyskinetic or choreoathetotic movements may occur. Strabismus and retinitis pigmentosa regularly develop. Stroke-like episodes, related to partial cerebrovascular thrombosis, occur in half the patients after the age of 4–5 years with coma, seizures and transient blindness. About one-half of patients develop epilepsy.

During adolescence and adulthood the condition is static. Most patients achieve some social functioning but remain dependent.

Mildly elevated CSF protein levels can be present in the early stages. EEG patterns are nonspecific. ERGs are abnormal with progressive decrease of rod responses (Andréasson *et al.* 1991). Visual, auditory brainstem and somatosensory evoked potential studies may be abnormal. Nerve conduction velocities are reduced in both motor and sensory nerves, with gradual slowing until adolescence.

Neuroimaging of the brain shows rapidly progressive cerebellar and brainstem hypoplasia in most patients during the first year of life. Supratentorial structures are usually normal, although

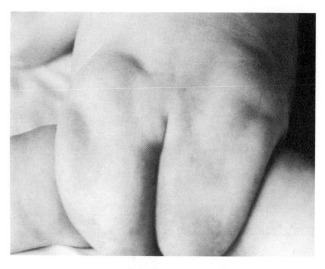

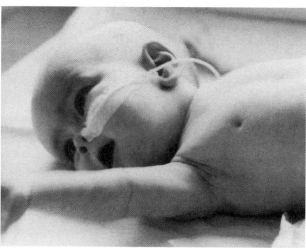

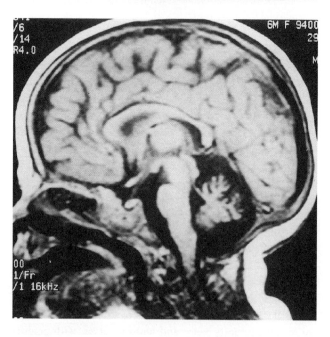

Fig. 9.6. Carbohydrate-deficient glycoprotein syndrome type 1. *(Top)* Abnormal fat pads on the buttocks *(Centre)* Inverted nipples; note also feeding difficulties (tube feeding). *(Bottom)* MRI, sagittal cut, showing marked cerebellar atrophy and relatively thin brainstem. (Courtesy Prof. Billette de Villemeur, Hôpital Trousseau, Paris.)

one third of patients have central and/or cortical atrophy. There is no indication of hypo- or dysmyelination on MRI or MRS studies (Akaboshi *et al.* 1995, Holzbach *et al.* 1995).

The *diagnosis* is usually made by demonstrating markedly reduced amounts of tetrasialotransferrin and increased amounts of di-, mono- and asialotransferrin. All the serum glycoproteins may be altered. Anomalies of various clotting factors and inhibitors could explain the stroke-like episodes (Van Geet and Jaeken 1993). Due to nonspecific leakage to serum, several lysosomal enzymes (*e.g.* arylsulfatase A, beta-hexosaminidase) and non-lysosomal enzymes (*e.g.* transaminases) are elevated. Many transport proteins (*e.g.* apoprotein B), glycoprotein hormones (*e.g.* IGF1) and complement factors are involved as well.

• *CDG type II.* The two patients described with CDG type II (Ramaekers *et al.* 1991)had very severe developmental delay but no peripheal neuropathy and a normal cerebellum on MRI. Dysmorphic features were more pronounced and both had stereotypic handwashing movements as seen in Rett syndrome.

Biochemically, the carbohydrate deficiency of transferrin is more marked, and transferrin isoform pattern shows near-absence of tetra-, penta- and asialotransferrin and more marked increase of disialotransferrin (Ramaekers *et al.* 1991, Jaeken *et al.* 1994).

• *CDG type III.* Two unrelated patients presenting with neonatal floppiness and dystrophic appearance have been described. Later in infancy they displayed areas of patchy skin depigmentation similar to the lesions of incontinentia pigmenti, severe visual, motor and mental impairments, and epilepsy with infantile spasms and hypsarrhythmia. MRI/CT scan studies showed marked generalized dysmyelination and atrophy (Holzbach *et al.* 1995). Flaccid tetraparesis, areflexia, optic atrophy, café-au-lait spots and scoliosis later evolved. The carbohydrate deficiency of transferrin was not as prominent as in CDG type I or II and the isoform pattern was different (Stibler *et al.* 1993).

• *CDG type IV.* A putative fourth type has been described in two unrelated patients presenting with a neonatal onset of severe seizures (Eyskens *et al.* 1994, Stibler *et al.* 1995).

It is clear that this group of disorders is far from being completely investigated and that phenotypic variability among already described types as well as additional forms will probably be delineated when all enzymes and their corresponding genes implicated in the complex processing of glycosylation are known.

DISORDERS OF SUBCELLULAR ORGANELLES: 3. PEROXISOMAL DISORDERS

The peroxisomal disorders are a group of diseases caused by inherited defects of peroxisomal biogenesis which result in generalized peroxisomal enzyme defects, or by dysfunction of either a single or multiple peroxisomal enzymes. These disorders may present with a wide range of phenotypes. The prototypes are

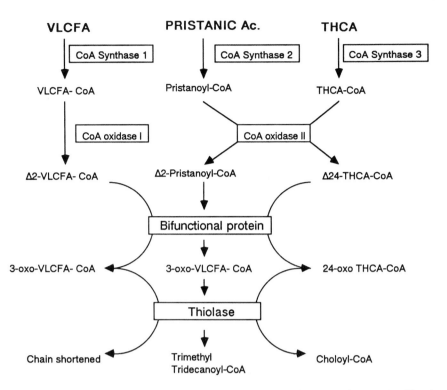

Fig. 9.7. Peroxisomal β-oxidation system of very-long-chain fatty acids (VLCFAs), pristanic acid and trihydroxycholestanoic acid (THCA).

Zellweger syndrome, rhizomelic chondrodysplasia punctata, X-linked adrenoleukodystrophy and Refsum disease, which combine all characteristic symptoms. Besides these 'classical' syndromes, many patients present with variant forms which lack one or more clinical characteristic signs and may be more difficult to diagnose without an adequate biochemical screening (for extensive reviews see Brown *et al.* 1993, Fournier *et al.* 1994, Lazarow and Moser 1995, Poggi-Travert *et al.* 1995, Wanders *et al.* 1995a).

PEROXISOMES AND THEIR METABOLIC FUNCTIONS

DEFINITION AND IDENTIFICATION OF PEROXISOMES

Peroxisomes are ubiquitous organelles containing integral membrane proteins, membrane-associated proteins and more than 50 matrix enzymes that participate in multiple metabolic processes. They are biochemically defined by the presence of a catalase and several oxidases used to stain these organelles for light and electron microscopy (Roels *et al.* 1988). The specificity of histochemical identification can be improved by the use of immunocytochemical procedures with antibodies raised against peroxisomal enzymes or specific peroxisomal membrane proteins (Kamei *et al.* 1993, Espeel *et al.* 1995). Peroxisomes are more numerous in cells that specialize in the metabolism of complex lipids (very-long-chain fatty acids and plasmalogens) and in the developing nervous system than they are in mature cells, suggesting that they serve important physiological functions in the CNS.

BIOCHEMICAL PEROXISOMAL PATHWAYS

Peroxisomal disorders are characterized by a build-up of metabolites normally degraded by peroxisomal enzymes or by decreased amounts of metabolites normally synthesized by peroxisomes, depending on the specific enzyme defects involved. Only those which are of direct diagnostic relevance are described.

Peroxisomal beta-oxidation
Peroxisomal beta-oxidation is a major metabolic route along which several inborn errors can occur. The main substrates oxidized in peroxisomes are saturated very-long-chain fatty acids (VLCFAs), di- and trihydroxycholestanoic acids (DHCA, THCA) which are intermediate substrates in bile acid synthesis from cholesterol, pristanic acid and the long-chain dicarboxylic acids. The peroxisomal beta-oxidation system of VLCFAs, THCA and pristanic acid includes three main steps. The first step, leading to the formation of CoA-substrates, is mediated by three distinct acyl-CoA synthetases. The second step is catalysed by two specific peroxisomal oxidases. The subsequent oxidation of VLCFAs, THCA and pristanic acid proceeds via the same beta-oxidation enzymes: bifunctional protein and peroxisomal thiolase (Fig. 9.7). Absence of peroxisomes is responsible for generalized beta-oxidation impairment (Zellweger syndrome, neonatal leukodystrophy, infantile Refsum disease), while isolated defects may involve each step of this peroxisomal beta-oxidation system with specific biochemical abnormalities.

Plasmalogen biosynthesis
Plasmalogens are a special class of ether phospholipids. Their role is unknown, but they are especially abundant in the CNS. The first two steps in plasmalogen synthesis are catalysed by

TABLE 9.3
Classification of human peroxisomal disorders

Disorders	Peroxisomes in liver	Peroxisomal enzyme defects
Group I: Peroxisomal biogenesis defects		
Zellweger syndrome	Absent	
Neonatal adrenoleukodystrophy	Scarce/Absent	Generalized defects
Infantile Refsum disease	Scarce/Absent	
Rhizomelic chondrodysplasia punctata	Present and abnormal	Plasmalogens synthesis, phytanic oxidase, unprocessed thiolase
Zellweger-like syndrome	Present and normal	VLCFA oxidation, bile acid synthesis, plasmalogen synthesis
Group II: Single peroxisomal enzyme deficiencies involving β-oxidation defects		
X-linked adrenoleukodysrophy	Present and normal	ALD protein
Pseudo-neonatal adrenoleukodystrophy	Present and abnormal	Acyl-CoA oxidase
Pseudo-Zellweger	Present and abnormal	Thiolase
Bifunctional enzyme deficiency	Present and normal	Bifunctional protein
Group III: Single peroxisomal enzyme deficiencies without β-oxidation involvement		
Refsum disease	Unknown	Phytanic acid oxidase
Pseudo-rhizomelic chondrodysplasia	Unknown	Plasmalogen synthesis
Di-(tri-)hydroxycholestanoic acidaemia	Unknown	Bile acid synthesis
Mevalonic aciduria	Unknown	Cholesterol synthesis

peroxisomal enzymes: dihydroxyacetonephosphate acyltransferase and alkyldihydroxyacetone phosphate synthase. Their deficient activity is responsible for low plasmalogen synthesis in patients affected with either peroxisomal biogenesis defects or isolated deficiency of one of these enzymes.

Phytanic oxidation

Phytanic acid is a branched-chain fatty acid derived from dietary sources. Its degradation is via an alpha-oxidative pathway to yield pristanic acid. Further oxidation occurs via peroxisomal beta-oxidation. Due to defective phytanic and pristanic oxidation, both derivatives accumulate with several peroxisomal disorders. Subcellular localization of the phytanic alpha-oxidation system is controversial. However, at least one of the enzymes involved is localized in peroxisomes (Wanders *et al.* 1995b).

Pipecolic catabolism

L-pipecolate oxidase is a peroxisomal enzyme which catalyses the hydrogenation of L-pipecolate. Its deficiency explains high levels of pipecolic acid in plasma, CSF and urine of patients with Zellweger syndrome.

Peroxisomes contain various enzymes involved in early steps of *cholesterol biosynthesis*, and some disorders such as mevalonic aciduria may also belong to the peroxisomal disorders (see pp. 298–299).

MOLECULAR AND GENETIC BACKGROUND

The peroxisomal disorders can be subdivided into two main groups (Table 9.3). The first group is characterized by loss of multiple peroxisomal enzyme activities often associated with morphological abnormalities of the organelle. These enzymes, synthesized on free polyribosomes, are directed toward the organelle by targeting sequences which are recognized by receptors and/or peroxisomal membrane proteins allowing their import

into the peroxisome. Most generalized peroxisomal disorders may be due to defects in these targeting and import mechanisms. Within this group, complementation studies in cell lines from patients have demonstrated at least 11 complementation groups; these have no clear relationship with clinical phenotypes except for the eleventh one which correlates with the rhizomelic chondrodysplasia punctata phenotype. Complementation analyses have already led to the identification of five peroxisomal membrane proteins or targeting signals with their corresponding genes, mutations and chromosomal localizations (Braverman *et al.* 1995; Moser, A.B. *et al.* 1995; Yahraus *et al.* 1996). All generalized peroxisomal disorders are inherited as autosomal recessive traits with an aggregate incidence of approximately 1 in 50,000 live births.

In the second group, the structure of the organelle is intact and the defects involve only one peroxisomal enzyme activity. Each disorder represents a complementation group. The gene of X-linked adrenoleukodystrophy (X-ALD) has been cloned and mapped to the terminal segment of the long arm of the X chromosome (Xq28), and multiple mutations are known (Krasemann *et al.* 1996), 80 per cent of which result in a total absence of the protein normally coded for. This protein is a member of the ATP-binding transporter family (Shani *et al.* 1996), and the disorder results from deficient transport of lignoceroyl-CoA-ligase to the peroxisome rather than from deficiency of this catabolic enzyme. The human peroxisomal thiolase gene, responsible for pseudo-Zellweger disease, has been mapped to chromosome 3p23–p22. Except for X-ALD, all these single peroxisomal enzyme deficiencies are inherited in an autosomal recessive manner.

All peroxisomal disorders can be prenatally detected on chorionic villi or amniocytes using tests similar to those described for postnatal diagnosis. VLCFA assays in plasma and/or fibroblasts can identify almost 80 per cent of the female carriers, while molecular biology would allow more acurate identification.

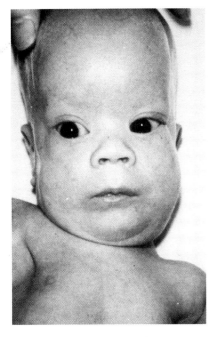
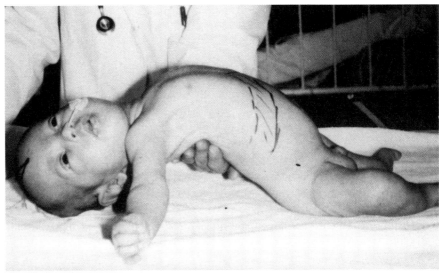

Fig. 9.8. Zellweger syndrome. *(Left)* Note high forehead, epicanthus, slanting palpebral fissures. *(Above)* Marked hypotonia, hepatomegaly and swallowing difficulties (nasal feeding tube). (Courtesy Dr B-T. Poll-Thé, Academisch Ziekenhuis, Utrecht.)

CLINICAL CONSEQUENCES OF PEROXISOMAL DYSFUNCTION

GROUP I: DISORDERS WITH MULTIPLE PEROXISOMAL ENZYME DEFECTS

This group mostly derives from errors in peroxisomal biogenesis. Five disorders belong to this group and share several morphological and biochemical abnormalities (Table 9.3).

The cerebrohepatorenal syndrome of Zellweger

Zellweger syndrome, the most severe disorder in this group, presents in the newborn baby with typical facial dysmorphism including high forehead, widely patent fontanelles and sutures, shallow orbital ridges, low and broad nasal bridge, epicanthus, external ear deformity, micrognathia and redundant neck skin folds (Fig. 9.8). Neurological manifestations are dominated by severe hypotonia with depressed or absent tendon reflexes and poor sucking and swallowing. Generalized seizures frequently start during the first days of life. Absence of psychomotor development, failure to thrive and retinal degeneration with extinguished ERG are always present. Optic atrophy, cataracts or glaucoma may occur. Hepatomegaly and liver dysfunction are constant findings, and polycystic kidneys are frequent. Skeletal deformities may result in equinovarus of the feet and flexion contractures. Stippled calcification most frequently involves the patella but may affect other areas of the skeleton and resembles that of chondrodysplasia punctata. Disturbed adrenocortical function is frequently observed following an ACTH stimulation test, even in the absence of clinical signs of adrenal insufficiency. The EEG is always abnormal with multifocal paroxystic activity, and evoked potentials are grossly disturbed. Nerve conduction velocities and EMG are normal. CT scans and cerebral MRI show gyral abnormalities, especially extensive pachygyria, low density of the white matter and, in some cases, vermian hypoplasia. Post-

mortem studies of the brain show a striking and characteristic disorder of neuronal migration. A sudanophilic leukodystrophy of variable severity may be associated. Variable organ involvement is the rule, including hepatic cirrhosis/fibrosis, renal cysts, and striated adrenal cells similar to those found in X-ALD. Absence of demonstrable peroxisomes or presence of peroxisomal membrane 'ghosts' in liver and other tissues with generalized biochemical peroxisomal impairment characterize this disorder. Zellweger-like syndrome has been described in two patients who, clinically and biochemically, were indistinguishable from patients with Zellweger syndrome but had structurally intact peroxisomes.

Neonatal adrenoleukodystrophy (NALD)

NALD is a less severe form. Craniofacial dysmorphism is absent or mild, and patients may show some developmental progress before progressive deterioration and death, which occurs within the first decade of life. The main clinical features include developmental delay or deterioration, hypotonia, seizures, sensorineural deafness, and poor vision usually due to retinal degeneration, sometimes associated with cataracts or optic atrophy. Failure to thrive is frequent, as are subclinical adrenal insufficiency and liver dysfunction. CT scan may show contrast enhancement around hypodense areas of the white matter as described in X-ALD. The main neuropathological findings are demyelination (cerebral hemispheres, cerebellum and brainstem), neuronal migration disturbances less consistent and less marked than in Zellweger syndrome (polymicrogyria and neuronal heterotopias), perivascular lymphocytic infiltrates, and PAS-positive macrophages. Ultrastructurally, these macrophages contain bilamellar inclusions similar to those found in adrenal cortex, liver, lymph nodes, thymus and spleen. Hepatic peroxisomes are morphologically undetectable or rare and much smaller than in control livers. NALD patients also have biochemical evidence of multiple peroxisomal dysfunction resembling that found in Zellweger syndrome.

Infantile Refsum disease

First described as a phytanic acid storage disorder, infantile Refsum disease has subsequently proved to be the mildest form of peroxisomal disease with absence of identifiable liver peroxisomes. The clinical course is characterized by a normal neonatal period followed by a few months of nonspecific features, with digestive signs resembling a malabsorption syndrome, hepatomegaly with impaired liver function, low plasma levels of cholesterol and apolipoproteins, and mild facial dysrmorphism. Developmental delay with hypotonia and ataxic gait, choroidoretinopathy and sensorineural hearing loss become evident by the age of 1–3 years. Patients may survive until the second decade of life with severe cognitive dysfunction. Milder forms of the disorder, with normal intellectual progress, seem possible (MacCollin *et al.* 1990). CT scans show moderate atrophy without signs of cortical malformation or hypodense lesions. Post-mortem study in one case has revealed micronodular liver cirrhosis, adrenal hypoplasia, and absence of macroscopic brain malformation but a severe cerebellar granular layer hypoplasia with ectopic Purkinje cells in the molecular layer (Moser 1989). Hepatic peroxisomes are morphologically absent, and patients display multiple peroxisomal dysfunction.

Rhizomelic chondrodysplasia punctata (RCDP)

RCDP is a bone dysplasia, characterized by rhizomelic dwarfism, facial dysmorphism, congenital cataract, joint contractures, severe epiphyseal and extraepiphyseal calcification, mental retardation, hepatomegaly and ichthyosis. Peroxisomal structures appear to be intact in fibroblasts, whereas in liver the organelles may be absent in some hepatocytes and enlarged in others. A remarkable clinical heterogeneity occurs, and variant forms lacking the classical clinical set along with typical biochemical abnormalities have been described. Complementation analyses and molecular studies have demonstrated that both classical and variant forms belong to the eleventh complementation group due to defective PTS2 receptor (Braverman *et al.* 1995; Moser, A.B. *et al.* 1995; Motley *et al.* 1996).

Hyperpipecolic acidaemia

Hyperpipecolataemia is characterized by hypotonia, retinopathy, hepatomegaly and severe developmental delay, and belongs to the generalized peroxisomal disorders.

These disorders are associated with either generalized or multiple loss of peroxisomal functions. Increased levels of VLCFAs, notably C26:0 (hexacosanoic acid), in plasma is the most useful diagnostic test in Zellweger syndrome, NALD, and infantile Refsum disease. These results are confirmed by studies in cultured fibroblasts, in which oxidation of VLCFAs is severely impaired. Elevated levels of bile acid intermediates (DHCA and THCA) in plasma and urine are due to defective beta-oxidation of bile acids. Elevated blood levels of phytanic and pristanic acids are due

to their impaired alpha- and beta-oxidations respectively. However, plasma phytanic acid accumulation is much less marked than in adult Refsum disease. Decreased plasmalogen content in red blood cells and in cultured fibroblasts, and defective dihydroxyacetone phosphate acyltransferase activity in fibroblasts, leukocytes or thrombocytes are major features in these disorders. High pipecolate levels in plasma and CSF are present in nearly all patients. In contrast, the biochemical abnormalities of RCDP include impaired plasmalogen biosynthesis and accumulation of phytanic acid, but normal plasma levels of VLCFAs despite the fact that the peroxisomal thiolase is present only in precursor form.

GROUP II: DISORDERS INVOLVING A SINGLE PEROXISOMAL ENZYME DEFECT

X-linked adrenoleukodystrophy

X-ALD (Moser, H.W. *et al.* 1995) is a relatively common disease that features combined involvement of the CNS and adrenals. Adrenal involvement is clinically manifest only in a minority of cases.

Over half the patients have the childhood form of the disorder, approximately 25 per cent have a late-onset presentation with adrenomyeloneuropathy, and 10 per cent have isolated Addison disease. In some studies, adrenomyeloneuropathy is the most common phenotype (Van Geel *et al.* 1997). One of the remarkable features of X-ALD is the intensity of the CNS inflammatory reaction. The cause is unclear but is probably related to the presence of abnormal lipids. This reaction may play an important role in the pathogenesis of the disease. It is absent in patients with adrenomyeloneuropathy.

Onset of X-ALD is commonly between 4 and 8 years, although adolescent onset is not rare, with progressive disturbances of gait and subtle cognitive decline. An apparently acute onset with focal seizures, often of long duration, may be observed (Zammarchi *et al.* 1994a). Spasticity, pseudobulbar symptoms and dementia eventually develop. Extrapyramidal features or ataxia may be present. Cortical disturbances of vision and hearing are highly suggestive but are seldom observed. The rate of deterioration is extremely variable and transient improvement of symptoms may occur, but a helpless state eventually sets in and death results after a few months to several years.

Features suggestive of adrenocortical insufficiency were present in only 12 per cent of the 303 cases of Moser *et al.* (1984). The least uncommon is cutaneous pigmentation that is rarely the first manifestation of the disease. It may be limited to mild pigmentation of scars.

The CSF protein content is often elevated. CT scan usually shows a symmetrical decrease in white matter density, most often located posteriorly. Enhancement occurs at the periphery of the hypodense areas and in the splenium of the corpus callosum after injection of contrast material, but may disappear in the late stages of the disease (Fig. 9.9). MRI can detect small areas of high signal in T_2-weighted images, especially in the internal capsules, even in presymptomatic patients (Aubourg *et al.* 1989, 1990). VLCFAs are regularly elevated, and a C26:C22 ratio of

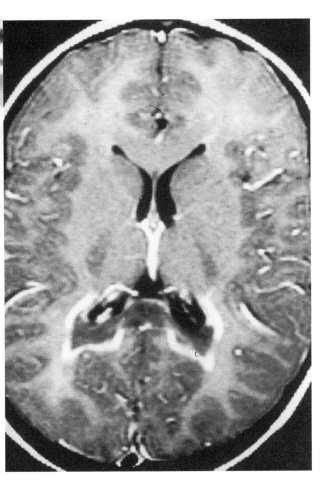

Fig. 9.9. X-linked adrenoleukodystrophy. T₁-weighted gadolinium enhanced MRI scan showing contrast uptake in demyelinated areas around the posterior horns and in the splenium of the corpus callosum.

1.6 ± 0.84 in plasma and of 0.42 ± 0.15 in fibroblasts is characteristic (Moser *et al.* 1984). Heterozygotes also have increased C20:C23 ratios, with little overlap with nonaffected persons. The exceptional finding (Kennedy *et al.* 1994) of nondiagnostic levels of VLCFAs suggests that the limit between heterozygotes and patients may overlap, requiring caution in interpretation of negative results. Antenatal diagnosis is possible in amniocytes and chorionic cells, based on VLCFA levels.

Variant forms of X-ALD with isolated features of adrenal insufficiency represent perhaps 40 per cent of cases of Addison disease. Rare variants may present in adolescents or young adults as spinocerebellar degeneration (Kobayashi *et al.* 1986, Miyai *et al.* 1990), and marked variability between siblings has been reported. Progressive cerebellar ataxia may be an isolated manifestation of X-ALD (Kurihara *et al.* 1993). An X-linked neonatal form, with a much more prolonged course than the recessive neonatal disease, has been reported in two patients (Nigro *et al.* 1993). Three cases apparently arrested for periods of 5–12 years in the absence of therapy have been recently reported (Korenke *et al.* 1996). Rare cases of X-ALD in women are on record (Simpson *et al.* 1987), and one girl with early manifestations has been reported (Naidu *et al.* 1988a).

Adrenomyeloneuropathy (AMN)

AMN is the second most common manifestation of the *ALD* gene, observed in 21 per cent of affected kindreds (Moser *et al.* 1984), and may be even more frequent in some populations (Van Geel *et al.* 1994). Both X-ALD and AMN can occur in the same pedigree. AMN is rare in childhood, the mean age of onset being 28 years. Male patients have paraparesis in all cases, sensory involvement and abnormal nerve conduction velocities in most cases, and subclinical or manifest adrenal dysfunction in some. Mixed forms with features of both X-ALD and AMN may occur (Willems *et al.* 1990). Most AMN patients have no neurological or cognitive anomalies. However, MRI of the brain is abnormal with disseminated white matter involvement in up to 45 per cent of cases which may resemble that seen in multiple sclerosis. Such patients may have some degree of cognitive impairment, and those with very extensive white matter lesions may exhibit cognitive difficulties or even dementia (Edwin *et al.* 1996). Thirty to 50 per cent of female carriers may have paraparesis and sensory disturbances in adulthood.

Other isolated peroxisomal beta-oxidation defects

Several cases resembling NALD or Zellweger syndrome have been described with isolated deficiency of one of the specific enzymes involved in the peroxisomal beta-oxidation system (see Fig. 9.7). Whatever the site of the defect patients all have high plasma levels of VLCFAs, other peroxisomal functions are normal, and usually peroxisomes are found in liver. Immunoblot and enzymatic studies have enabled recognition of isolated acyl-CoA oxidase defect (pseudo-NALD), isolated thiolase deficiency (pseudo-Zellweger), and isolated bifunctional protein deficiency. In the latter two conditions, THCA and DHCA accumulation coexist with high levels of VLCFAs. Within this group an apparently restricted biochemical defect leads to multiorgan involvement analogous to that observed in the disorders of peroxisome biogenesis, suggesting that defects in the peroxisomal beta-oxidation system can cause profound developmental disturbances (Powers 1995).

Isolated peroxisomal enzymes defects other than beta-oxidation

Classical Refsum disease (Chapter 21) is characterized by accumulation of phytanic acid in tissue and body fluids due to phytanic oxidation defect. Liver peroxisomes are present and other peroxisomal functions are intact (Steinberg 1995).

Pseudorhizomelic chondrodysplasia punctata with biochemical abnormalities limited to a deficiency of either dihydroxyacetone phosphate acyltransferase or alkyl-dihydroxyacetone phosphate synthase has been described in three patients with a clinical phenotype similar to that of the 'classical' RCDP syndrome. This identification emphasizes the functional importance of plasmalogens.

Dihydroxycholestanaemia and trihydroxycholestanaemia have been described in four patients with neurological involvement. Enzymatic defect has not yet been identified unequivocally.

Hyperoxaluria type 1 and acatalasaemia are other isolated peroxisomal enzyme deficiencies due to deficiency in alanineglyoxylate aminotransferase and catalase respectively. Neither disorder shows any involvement of the CNS.

TREATMENT

For classical Refsum disease, dietary restriction of phytanic acid, with or without with plasmapheresis, can prevent further progression of the disease (Steinberg 1995). Therapeutic options for patients with disorders of peroxisomal biogenesis are limited by severe abnormalities already present *in utero*. Thus, dietary manipulations that normalize phytanic acid and VLCFA levels combined with oral administration of plasmalogens may not be justified. In several patients oral docosahexaenoic supplementation may have improved both the neurological status and the blood levels of VLCFAs and plasmalogens (Martinez 1996).

In X-ALD, dietary treatment with a mixture of glycerol esters of oleic and erucic acids (Lorenzo's oil) is effective in normalizing VLCFA levels (Korenke *et al.* 1995). However, the clinical efficacy of the diet is uncertain and it has not prevented aggravation of the condition, although some suggestion to the contrary has been offered. The possibility of preventing deterioration in boys treated at the presymptomatic stage remains to be explored (Moser 1993). Erucic acid does not enter the brain which probably explains these limited results (Aubourg *et al.* 1993). Bone marrow transplantation has occasionally given spectacular results (Aubourg *et al.* 1990), and improvement has been observed in seven of 52 boys treated. Mortality is high if no compatible donor is available. It may be indicated in the absence of clinical symptoms when early MRI abnormalities appear in the internal capsules or corpus callosum (Aubourg *et al.* 1992; Moser, H.W. *et al.* 1995). A different approach, currently being tried, is with anti-inflammatory agents (beta-interferon, thalidomide and cyclosporine) in an effort to suppress the intense inflammatory response that may be responsible for at least some of the clinical manifestations of the disease.

DISORDERS OF AMINO ACID AND ORGANIC ACID CATABOLISM

PHENYLKETONURIA AND HYPERPHENYLALANINAEMIA

Hyperphenylalaninaemia (HPA) is defined as elevated fasting levels of phenylalanine in blood as compared with values obtained from healthy subjects of identical age. HPA represents a group of disorders, of which phenylalanine-hydroxylase (PAH) deficiency is the most common. A small number are due to defects in the biopterin cofactor system.

THE METABOLIC DERANGEMENT

Hydroxylation of phenylalanine to tyrosine requires three enzymes, PAH, pterin-carbinolamine dehydratase (PCD) and dihydropterine reductase (DHPR), and two cofactors, tetradihydrobiopterin (THB) and reduced NAD (Fig. 9.10). Based on plasma phenylalanine levels and residual PAH activity in liver, three different inherited phenotypes of HPA due to PAH defiency are described: classical phenylketonuria (PKU), atypical PKU,

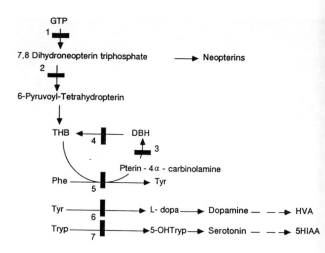

Fig. 9.10. Synthesis and recycling of pterins.
Key: GTP = guanosine triphosphate; TBH = 5,6,7,8-tetrahydrobiopterin; DBH = q-dihydrobiopterin.
1 = GTP cyclohydrolase; 2 = PTPS (6-pyruvoyl-tetrahydropterin synthase); 3 = pterin-4-α-carbinolamine dehydratase (PCD); 4 = dehydropteridine reductase (DHPR); 5 = phenylalanine hydroxylase (PAH); 6 = tyrosine hydroxylase; 7 = tryptophane hydroxylase.

TABLE 9.4
The different hyperphenylalaninaemia (HPA) phenotypes due to phenylalanine hydroxylase (PAH) deficiency

	Residual PAH activity	Blood phenylalanine
HPA type I (classical PKU)	<1%	>1200 µmol/L
HPA type II ('atypical PKU')	1–5%	600–1200 µmol/L
HPA type III (mild HPA, non-PKU HPA)	>5%	<600µmol/L

PKU = phenylketonuria.

and non-PKU HPA (Table 9.4) (Smith and Brenton 1995). Defects in THB synthesis and recycling are responsible for both HPA and neurotransmitter disorders (see pp. 275–276).

Accumulation of phenylalanine in the body increases alternative metabolic pathways, whose metabolites are excreted: transamination to phenylpyruvate, phenyllactate, phenylacetate and phenylacetylglutamine, and decarboxylation to phenylethylamine. Orthohydroxylation is not affected, and increased amounts of orthohydroxyphenyl metabolites (orthohydroxyphenylacetate) are synthesized.

GENETICS

HPA is one of the most prevalent disorders of amino acid metabolism in the White population, occurring in approximately 1 in 10,000 live births. This autosomal recessively inherited disorder is caused by more than 200 mutations at the PAH locus. High phenotypic complexity results from the multiplicity of these mutations and from the fact that most patients are genetic compounds at the PAH locus. Different groups of mutations predominate in a given ethnic population, allowing prenatal diagnosis, carrier detection and the prediction of the PKU phenotype linked with a particular haplotype (Güttler and Gulberg 1996).

PATHOGENESIS

The clinical manifestations of HPA are thought to result from phenylalanine accumulation and its secondary effects on brain chemistry. The fact that PKU is most often accompanied by mental retardation whilst non-PKU HPA is not, suggests that there is a threshold level of phenylalanine in extracellular fluids above which persistent postnatal (or fetal) HPA causes irreversible brain damage. If the threshold value is exceeded only later in life, after diet discontinuation in the early-treated PKU patients, reversible chemical changes appear which may affect neuropsychological function (Waisbren *et al.* 1994).

Patients with PKU exhibit a reduction of amine neurotransmitter synthesis when plasma phenylalanine levels are high. Secondary effects of HPA upon serotonin and catecholamine precursors tyrosine and tryptophan must be important. Excess phenylalanine interferes with tyrosine and tryptophan metabolism at different sites. Defective neurotransmitter synthesis may be due both to a competitive inhibition of transport of large amino acids (tyrosine, tryptophan and branched-chain amino acids) into the brain across the blood–brain barrier and from the CSF back into blood—resulting in low tyrosine and tryptophan concentrations in the brain of PKU patients despite high levels in the CSF—and to a possible direct or competitive inhibition of hydroxylation of tyrosine by high levels of phenylalanine. The prefrontal dysfunction (executive function deficit) described in PKU patients supports the hypothesis that dopaminergic synthesis is impaired by high phenylalanine levels (Welsh 1996).

Abnormal myelination, reduction of brain weight and decreased myelin content are found in the brains of untreated older PKU patients (Bauman and Kemper 1982). These detrimental effects have been confirmed using the HPH-5 mouse model. Current and previous observations have led to the hypothesis that myelin reduction is due to inhibition of an oligodendroglial cell-specific ATP-sulfurylase which results in low content of sulfatides in myelin that in turn is exposed to proteolytic degradation. Consequently, neuronal loss and decreased interneuronal connections occur, a fact that has been demonstrated by quantitative evaluation of neurotransmitter receptor density. If the results obtained in animals can be extrapolated to humans, special involvement of the hippocampus and the occipital area of the cortex could explain some of the neurophysiological disturbances observed in non- or poorly treated PKU patients (Hommes 1994).

Abnormal brain protein synthesis due to polysome disaggregation and slowed polypeptide chain elongation may result in low brain weight. (Polysome disaggregation also occurs in heart and brain of fetal rats exposed to maternal HPA, a finding that bears on the fetopathy associated with human maternal HPA.)

Decreased DNA content and synthesis in neurons exposed to high levels of phenylalanine can also account for decreased proliferation of neurons, neuronal loss and impaired brain growth.

CLINICAL FINDINGS
Untreated PKU

The clinical features of untreated PKU include mental retardation, neurological abnormalities and extraneural symptoms (although the timing varies from patient to patient). Retarded intellectual development, the most important and constant clinical feature, is often associated with microcephaly. EEG abnormalities are frequent (78–95 per cent of cases), but only 25 per cent of patients have seizures, most often either of grand mal type or infantile spasms. Psychotic behaviour with hyperactivity, destructiveness, self-injury, impulsiveness, and uncontrolled behaviour with episodes of excitement is not infrequent. A majority of patients have blond hair, blue eyes and lightly pigmented or eczematous skin. A peculiar musty odour has been repeatedly mentioned. The general physical development is usually good.

This clinical phenotype is largely a matter of historical interest because the disease is now prevented by early diagnosis and treatment. However, patients with HPA continue to be missed in the neonatal period because testing is not done or because false negative results are obtained.

Early-treated PKU

Children with PKU detected by routine neonatal screening and started on a phenylalanine-controlled diet soon after birth generally have an intelligence within the normal range (Azen *et al.* 1996). However, retrospective studies indicate that even with the best treatment, children tend to have an IQ below those of their first-degree relatives and an educational performance inferior to their siblings and age-matched controls (Weglage *et al.* 1993). The higher incidence of abnormal behaviour, notably hyperactivity, noted by some authors (Smith *et al.* 1990) has been interpreted as due to the stress associated with chronic disease (Burgard *et al.* 1994). However, subclinical neuropsychological and neurophysiological (evoked potential and nerve velocity) disturbances are frequent, especially in those patients who do not adhere strictly to the diet (Ludolph *et al.* 1996, Weglage *et al.* 1996a). The frequency of an abnormal EEG increases with age despite early and strict dietary control (Pietz *et al.* 1993), and MRI studies indicate that dysmyelination is almost universal in older patients affected with both classical PKU and HPA type II. MRI changes involve the occipital–parietal regions and extend into the frontal and temporal lobes in the most severe cases. They have no clear relationship with the clinical or neuropsychological status, nor with the phenylalanine control in early childhood, but are correlated with the blood phenylalanine level at the time of imaging and are partially reversible by reducing blood phenylalanine concentrations (Clearly *et al.* 1994, Ullrich *et al.* 1994).

TREATMENT

In patients with classical and atypical HPA, a phenylalanine-restricted diet must be initiated shortly after birth to prevent irreversible brain damage. For many years, discontinuation of the diet after 4–8 years of age was considered safe, but because of the described intellectual, neurological and neuropsychological degradation after diet relaxation, treatment for life is becoming a universal policy (Smith and Brenton 1995). In patients with persistent non-PKU HPA (serum phenylalanine levels below 600 μmol/L), intellectual, neurological and neuropsychological outcome is not impaired and dietary treatment is not necessary (Weglage et al. 1996b).

With treatment initiated later in childhood or in adulthood, some improvement in behaviour can occur, but follow-up of these patients suggests that they are more susceptible to develop behavioural changes after withdrawal of the diet than are early-treated patients. Gene therapy based on somatic gene transfer is not yet possible in humans (Eisensmith and Woo 1996).

Discontinuation of the diet
Despite adequate biochemical control during childhood, deficits are often more marked in adolescents and adults who have discontinued their diet than in those who maintain blood phenylalanine levels below 1000 μmol/L. Brisk tendon reflexes, intention tremor, delayed visual evoked responses, psychological problems, IQ loss, minor impairment in cognitive abilities and even neurological deterioration have been reported in several such individuals. The extent to which these are related to subtle neurological damage occurring in childhood or result from the effect of higher phenylalanine levels on neurotransmitter metabolism is unclear, but these symptoms improve when the patients return to a controlled diet and are largely prevented by continuous treatment (Welsh et al. 1990, Stemerdink et al. 1995, Weglage et al. 1996a). Consequently, an increasing number of centres advise patients with classical PKU to remain on a diet which keeps plasma phenylalanine levels below 600 μmol/L.

MATERNAL PKU
Maternal PKU syndrome occurs in children of untreated phenylketonuric women, despite the fact that usually the children do not themselves have PKU.

PHENOTYPE
The syndrome is characterized by low birthweight, microcephaly, dysmorphism, congenital defects and developmental retardation. There is evidence that an increased risk is directly correlated to maternal phenylalanine level during pregnancy without obvious threshold in effect. When maternal plasma phenylalanine concentrations are above 1200 μmol/L (classical PKU), 92 per cent of children have mental retardation, 73 per cent microcephaly, 40 per cent intrauterine growth delay, and 12 per cent congenital heart malformations. Children born to atypical PKU women (blood phenylalanine levels between 600 and 1200 μmol/L) also have increased incidence of microcephaly, mental subnormality and other congenital anomalies, such as cardiac defects (Lenke and Levy 1980). When maternal phenylalanine is below 900 μmol/L congenital abnormalities are uncommon but the risks for microcephaly and mental retardation remain high. Microcephaly is the most constant clinical finding, therefore its presence must always suggest maternal HPA even when the mother is of normal intelligence. MRI studies have revealed abnormal development of the corpus callosum without the white matter changes noted in PKU children (Levy et al. 1996). Offspring of women with mild HPA (160–600 μmol/L) have normal early IQs. However, head size, birthweight and intelligence scores may be inversely correlated to the maternal phenylalanine concentrations, a finding suggesting the absence of a threshold for adverse effects of phenylalanine on the fetal brain (Levy et al. 1994).

PATHOGENESIS
Fetal damage and postnatal PKU probably have a similar pathogenesis, phenylalanine being the initiator of harm. In all species, fetal amino acid concentrations are higher than maternal levels (average ratio = 1.48). Thus a 'safe' maternal phenylalanine level could lead to an 'unsafe' level in the fetus.

Phenylalanine probably competes with other neutral amino acids for placental and brain transport, which may contribute to decreased fetal growth and abnormal CNS maturation. Tyrosine and tryptophan deficiencies may have a central role in this process: the pattern of congenital abnormalities seen in maternal PKU is characteristic of damage to neural crest derivatives (heart, aortic arch and face), and it seems possible that failure of normal crest migration and development is associated with insufficient neurotransmitter fetal biosynthesis from tyrosine and tryptophan (Kudo and Boyd 1996).

PREVENTION
There is now good evidence that, provided maternal blood phenylalanine levels can be controlled both before conception and during the course of pregnancy, the outcome for the fetus is good. From current collaborative studies, the level at which the maternal blood phenylalanine must be kept is certainly below 600 μmol/L or even lower (<360 or <250 μmol/L). Therefore, prevention requires compliance to a strict low-phenylalanine diet along with adequate caloric and micronutrient provision. Tyrosine supplementation must be carefully controlled, since by inhibiting the transport of other neutral amino acids, high levels of tyrosine may also be responsible for fetal damage (Smith and Brenton 1995, Hanley et al. 1996).

TYROSINAEMIA TYPE I
Hereditary tyrosinaemia type I is characterized by progressive hepatorenal dysfunction and accumulation of tyrosine and its metabolites. In both acute and chronic forms, most untreated patients die from liver failure or hepatoma. However, in infants and children recurrent acute peripheral neuropathy may be responsible for death independently from liver failure. This neuropathy, mainly described among patients from Quebec, may arise whatever the ethnic origin of patients (Kvittingen 1991, Kvittingen et al. 1995).

BIOCHEMICAL AND GENETIC ASPECTS
Tyrosinaemia is an autosomal recessive disorder caused by a deficiency of fumarylacetoacetase, the final enzyme in the catabolic pathway of tyrosine (Fig. 9.11). Maleylacetoacetate

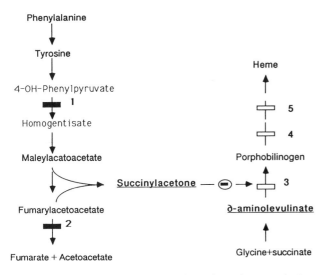

```
Phenylalanine
      │
      ▼
   Tyrosine                           Heme
      │                                 ▲
      ▼                                 │
4-OH-Phenylpyruate              ╪══ 5
      ┃ 1                              │
      ▼                          ╪══ 4
 Homogentisate                         ▲
      │                                │
      ▼
Maleylacatoacetate              Porphobilinogen
      │                                 ▲
      ▼        Succinylacetone ─ ⊖ → ╪══ 3
Fumarylacetoacetate             δ-aminolevulinate
      ┃ 2                              ▲
      ▼                                │
Fumarate + Acetoacetate        Glycine+succinate
```

Fig. 9.11. Tyrosine metabolism and its relationship to haem synthesis.
Key: 1 = para-OH-phenylpyruvate dioxygenase (the site of NTBC inhibition); 2 = fumarylacetoacetase; 3 = δ-aminolaevulinate dehydratase; 4 = acute intermittent porphyria; 5 = other porphyrias.

and fumarylacetoacetate accumulate and are metabolized to succinylacetone, which is found in the blood and urine of affected individuals. Succinylacetone inhibits delta-aminolaevulinate dehydratase (ALDH) activity and is responsible for abnormally high urinary excretion of delta-aminolaevulinic acid (δ-ALA). Accumulation of succinylacetone and δ-ALA in plasma and urine permits the diagnosis, which is confirmed by the measurement of fumarylacetoacetase activity in lymphocytes or fibroblasts. Antenatal diagnosis relies on succinylacetone determination in amniotic fluid and/or fumarylacetoacetase in chorionic villus samples. Several mutations of the gene have been described (Phaneuf *et al.* 1992, St-Louis *et al.* 1994).

PATHOGENESIS
The pathogenesis is not fully understood. For unexplained reasons, not all patients experience neurological crises. Comparison with other pathological conditions in which δ-ALA is increased, such as acute intermittent porphyria, hereditary ALDH deficiency (Kappas *et al.* 1995) and lead poisoning, suggests that the recurrent onset of neuropathy is linked to δ-ALA accumulation and/or hepatic haem deficiency (*Lancet* 1990). Liver transplantation and treatment with NTBC, which both correct the δ-ALA accumulation, prevent neurological crises (Mitchell *et al.* 1990, Lindstedt *et al.* 1992, Gibbs *et al.* 1993).

CLINICAL FEATURES
Symptoms may start within a few weeks (acute forms) or months (subacute forms) after birth, or in the following years (chronic forms). Patients present with signs of hepatic and tubular dysfunction (Debré–de Toni–Fanconi syndrome). In acute and subacute forms, liver dysfunction may be prominent and tubulopathy only biologically expressed. If untreated, death from liver failure occurs within a few months. In chronic forms, liver disease

is milder, and renal involvement is expressed as a tubulopathy with hypophosphataemic rickets. Hepatoma and end-stage renal failure are late complications.

Neurological crises, described as porphyria-like symptoms, may arise in patients affected with either the acute or subacute forms, even well controlled by dietary therapy. Most episodes are preceded by intercurrent infections. Features include rapid progression of diffuse pain, mainly localized in legs and abdomen, associated with vomiting, irritability, hypertonia, painful attacks of opisthotonic posturing and brisk tendon reflexes. A rapidly ascending paralysis associated with areflexia may follow and results in respiratory insufficiency and death in the absence of assisted ventilation. Throughout this course patients are conscious. Oral self-mutilation, such as tongue-biting, and grinding and avulsion of the teeth, is observed especially during the initial phase.

Seizures secondary to metabolic disturbances (hyponatraemia, hypoxia) and sustained hypertension may occur. Duration of recovery varies greatly from one crisis to another. A full recovery is most often noted, but multiple recurrences lead to chronic and disabling peripheral neuropathy with amyotrophy. EEG and CSF are normal. Sequential motor and sensory nerve conduction studies have shown progressive alteration in motor action potentials and nerve conduction velocities with histopathological axonal degeneration and demyelination (Mitchell *et al.* 1990, Gibbs *et al.* 1993).

TREATMENT
NTBC is a powerful inhibitor of the para-hydroxyphenylpyruvate dioxygenase activity, the second step of tyrosine catabolism (see Fig. 9.11). Its administration to tyrosinaemic patients prevents toxic metabolite accumulation with further increase in tyrosinaemia. The latter is avoided by a phenylalanine/tyrosine-restricted diet. Such a regimen has been applied to more than 100 patients with clear beneficial effects. It normalizes liver and renal function and prevents neurological crises. More data, however, are required to confirm that long-term use of NTBC is not harmful and that it is effective to prevent hepatocarcinoma (Lindstedt *et al.* 1992). The promising results of NTBC treatment reduce the need for liver transplantation which is still required in patients who have already developed hepatocarcinoma at the time of diagnosis.

BRANCHED-CHAIN AMINO ACIDS (BCAAs)
Maple syrup urine disease (MSUD), methylmalonic aciduria, propionic aciduria, isovaleric aciduria and other organic acidurias secondary to BCAA catabolism defects collectively comprise the most commonly encountered inborn errors of amino acid metabolism. They have many symptoms in common and usually present with one of three clinical types: severe neonatal form, intermittent late-onset form and chronic progressive form. Recurrent coma, the main feature of these disorders, appears to be due to direct toxicity of the accumulated metabolites, while chronic accumulation may interfere with CNS development or cerebral metabolism leading to developmental delay (Surtees *et al.* 1992; Hilliges *et al.* 1993; Lehnert *et al.* 1994; Peineman and Danner 1994; van der Meer *et al.* 1994, 1996).

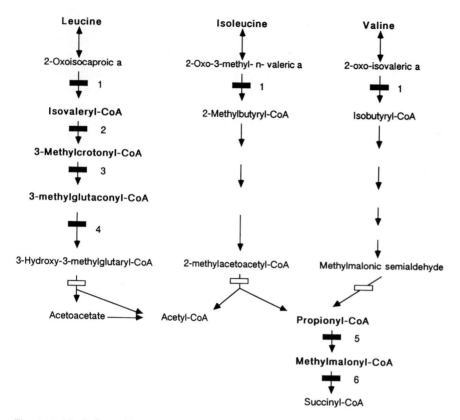

Fig. 9.12. Metabolism of branched-chain amino acids, indicating origin of some known inherited metabolic disorders.

Key: 1 = BCAA decarboxylase (maple syrup urine disease); 2 = isovaleryl-CoA dehydrogenase (isovaleric aciduria); 3 = 3-methylcrotonyl-CoA carboxylase (3-methylcrotonylglycinuria); 4 = 3-methylglutaconyl-CoA hydratase (3-methylglutaconic aciduria type I); 5 = propionyl-CoA carboxylase (propionic aciduria); 6 = methylmalonyl-CoA mutase (methylmalonic aciduria).

BIOCHEMICAL BACKGROUND

These diseases result from defects of enzymes involved in the catabolism of leucine, valine and isoleucine (Fig. 9.12). The three neutral BCAAs are initially metabolized through a common pathway: a transamination is followed by a thiamine-dependent decarboxylation, which is deficient in MSUD (step 1). The decarboxylation defect is responsible for accumulation of BCAAs and their corresponding keto acids. Subsequently the catabolic pathways of the BCAAs diverge. Leucine is further metabolized to acetoacetate and acetyl-CoA. Specific enzyme deficiencies may occur at every step. Isovaleryl-CoA dehydrogenase deficiency is responsible for isovaleric aciduria (step 2), isovalerate being a highly toxic substrate. Deficiency of 3-methylcrotonyl-CoA carboxylase, a biotin-dependent enzyme, (step 3) produces 3-methylcrotonyl-glycinuria, as a result of either apoenzyme decarboxylase mutation or of abnormal biotin metabolism (see p. 285). The catabolism of valine and isoleucine produces propionyl-CoA and methylmalonyl-CoA. Methionine and threonine, fatty acids with odd-number carbons and the side-chain of cholesterol, are other precursors of propionyl-CoA. Propionyl-CoA forms methyl-malonyl-CoA through a biotin-dependent decarboxylase (step 5) whose deficiency is due to apoenzyme decarboxylase mutation (propionic aciduria) or to abnormal biotin metabolism. Methyl-malonyl-CoA is converted to succinyl-CoA by the B_{12}-dependent

methylmalonyl-CoA mutase (step 6). Deficient activity of the mutase enzyme leads to methylmalonic aciduria. Abnormal B_{12} metabolism is responsible for variant forms of methylmalonic aciduria. Many of the intramitochondrial CoA metabolites accumulated are substrates for carnitine esterification, a process which allows the transformation of neurotoxic metabolites into nontoxic by-products and leads to secondary carnitine deficiency (Burns *et al.* 1996)

GENETIC BACKGROUND

Each disorder of this group is inherited in an autosomal recessive manner. Antenatal diagnosis can be performed through the measurement of specific enzyme activity in fresh chorionic villus samples or cultivated amniotic cells and through the direct determination of abnormal intermediates in amniotic fluid (Jakobs *et al.* 1991). Many different mutations cause the metabolic phenotype of these disorders and their variants (Crane *et al.* 1992, Tahara *et al.* 1993, Peinemann and Danner 1994).

NEUROPATHOLOGY

A limited number of available autopsy studies indicate cerebral atrophy and a variety of histological changes including swelling, demyelination and spongy degeneration. A few cases of cerebellar haemorrhage are known (Dave *et al.* 1984, Brismar *et al.* 1990a).

Specific involvement of the globus pallidus in methylmalonic aciduria and generalized involvement of all basal ganglia in propionic aciduria have been reported in some autopsied cases (Korf *et al.* 1986).

PATHOGENESIS

The pathogenesis of cerebral involvement in branched-chain acid disorders is poorly understood. Direct toxicity of accumulated intermediates may explain some reversible changes. In MSUD, branched-chain keto acids are potential inhibitors for pyruvate and alpha-ketoglutarate dehydrogenases, two enzymes important for brain mitochondrial energy production. Similar effects of propionic and methylmalonic acids on brain energy production are possible. In addition, these metabolites could reduce gamma-aminobutyric acid (GABA) synthesis (Heidenreich *et al.* 1988, Roodhooft *et al.* 1990).

Irreversible changes may be the result of interaction with myelin synthesis. This would occur in the postnatal period, since antenatal placental epuration of toxic substrates is effective. Propionyl-CoA and methylmalonyl-CoA are utilized in the synthesis of odd-numbered and methyl-branched long-chain fatty acids (Wendel *et al.* 1993). By incorporating these abnormal fatty acids into lipids, chronic accumulation of propionyl-CoA and methylmalonyl-CoA may be responsible for abnormal lipid membrane synthesis in the CNS. This process may be relevant for the genesis of basal ganglia necrosis. The roles of hypoxia, hypovolaemia and ketoacidosis have also been discussed; however, from clinical data it appears that the occurrence of this lesion is not systematically linked with any of those disturbances (Heidenreich *et al.* 1988).

CLINICAL FEATURES

Severe neonatal forms

A typical clinical presentation is with relentless deterioration without apparent cause in newborn infants following an initial symptom-free period. The first symptoms are poor sucking and difficulty feeding, followed by unexplained and progressive coma. During the comatose state axial hypotonia contrasts with limb hypertonia. Abnormal movements are frequent, including bouts of hypertonus with opisthotonus, gross tremors, myoclonic jerks and repetitive flexion–extension movements of the limbs. Convulsions may inconsistently occur later in the course. Affected babies may have cerebral oedema with bulging fontanelle, arousing suspicion of CNS infection. EEGs often show a burst–suppression pattern. A unique pattern (comb-like rhythm) has been observed in neonatal MSUD (Tharp 1992). Biochemical abnormalities include metabolic acidosis and ketonuria. Secondary hyperammonaemia and hyperlactacidaemia may accompany organic acidurias. The overall short-term prognosis is improving. Later, despite the treatment, acute life-threatening intercurrent episodes often occur, with clinical manifestations resembling those of late intermittent forms.

Intermittent late-onset forms

In approximatively one-third of patients, BCAA disorders present in childhood, or even in adolescence or adulthood. Recurrent attacks are frequent, though in between these the patient may seem entirely normal. In most cases, the onset is precipitated by conditions which enhance protein catabolism (infection, trauma, etc.) or by excessive protein intake, but may occur without overt cause. Recurrent attacks of coma, or lethargy with ataxia are the main presentations. Most often, coma is not accompanied by other abnormal neurological signs. Ketoacidosis and various glycaemic abnormalities indicate a metabolic origin. A few patients, however, may present with acute hemiplegia and hemianopia, or signs and symptoms of cerebral oedema mimicking a cerebrovascular accident or CNS tumour.

Abnormal EEGs with slow delta-waves, loss of normal alpharhythm, mild nonspecific irregularities or grossly aberrant patterns are often encountered. Focal activity, when present, is usually localized in the temporal regions.

Patients may die during these episodes. Severe cerebral oedema with brainstem compression has been reported in several MSUD patients (Riviello *et al.* 1991, Levin *et al.* 1993). This complication, which is worsened by intemperate rehydration, may, however, be a major cause of death in all BCAA patients presenting with acute decompensation. Some recover without sequelae. Many children who survive severe, prolonged or recurrent metabolic disturbances are left with brain damage. Seizures are a common sequela. In infancy and early childhood they tend to be generalized, often myoclonic in type. During later childhood, tonic–clonic or atypical absence seizures are common. Neuroimaging usually shows cerebral atrophy and some delay in myelination. In untreated or poorly treated MSUD, cerebral oedema may persist, confined to the posterior limb of the internal capsule, cerebral peduncles, posterior fossa and dorsal brainstem (Brismar *et al.* 1990a). An increasing number of patients with methylmalonic and propionic aciduria present with an acute or progressive extrapyramidal syndrome due to bilateral necrosis of the basal ganglia (Fig. 9.13). These lesions mainly affect the globus pallidus in methylmalonic patients, and both the lentiform nuclei and the caudate heads in propionic acidaemia (Surtees *et al.* 1992; Stöckler *et al.* 1992; Brismar and Ozand 1994a,b; Hamilton *et al.* 1995).

Chronic progressive forms

Hypotonia, muscular weakness, nonspecific developmental delay and seizures are rarely the only revealing signs, and most often they coexist with digestive and nutritional symptoms such as persistent anorexia, chronic vomiting and failure to thrive. These rather nonspecific presentations are often misdiagnosed for months or years until an acute neurological attack or an unexplained episode of dehydration leads to the diagnosis. Movement disorders such as chorea associated with mental deterioration may reveal progressive forms of organic acidurias (Gascon *et al.* 1994).

BIOCHEMICAL DIAGNOSIS

The diagnosis is based on the recognition of abnormal intermediate substrates and their by-products which result from the

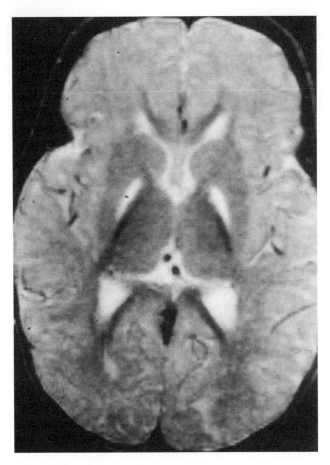

Fig. 9.13. Methylmalonic acidaemia. T_2-weighted MRI showing symmetrical areas of high signal from the globus pallidus of an 8-month-old child. Delayed myelination is also evident.

metabolic block. In MSUD patients, amino acid chromatography is characterized by high plasma and urine levels of leucine, valine and isoleucine and the presence of alloisoleucine. In contrast, all other enzymatic blocks result in plasma accumulation and urinary excretion of organic acids and are diagnosed using gas–liquid chromatography and mass spectrometry, while amino acid chromatography does not permit the diagnosis. The final diagnosis is made by measuring specific enzymatic activities in cultured fibroblasts or leukocytes.

TREATMENT

Treatment is aimed at reducing toxic metabolites (Ogier de Baulny *et al.* 1995b, Ogier de Baulny and Saudubray 1995). In the neonatal period, most acutely ill babies require exogenous detoxification procedures. Long-term dietary treatment involves restriction in protein intake and an otherwise well-balanced diet. Because some vitamins are cofactors of specific enzymatic steps, megadoses of these vitamins must be systematically tested in each case. This therapeutic trial allows the recognition of vitamin-responsive patients who are less severely affected and may do well with a less strict diet. L-carnitine supplementation is systematically used in the treatment of organic acidurias. In isovaleric aciduria, L-glycine and L-carnitine supplementation to increase

isovaleryl-glycine and isovaleryl-carnitine urinary excretions are effective means of treatment (Fries *et al.* 1996).

Despite early diagnosis and treatment, at any age, these children are at risk for life-threatening metabolic imbalances and neurological sequelae. In addition, other complications may involve kidney, pancreas and heart. All these long-term complications raise the question of more aggressive therapy such as liver transplantation (Schlenzig *et al.* 1995).

GLUTARIC ACIDURIA TYPE I (GA-I)

GA-I is an inborn error of lysine and tryptophan catabolism characterized clinically by an extrapyramidal syndrome with dystonia and choreoathetosis, pathologically by striatal degeneration, and biochemically by deficiency of glutaryl-CoA dehydrogenase (GDH) (Amir *et al.* 1989, Haworth *et al.* 1991, Hoffmann *et al.* 1991).

BIOCHEMICAL AND GENETIC BACKGROUNDS

GA-I is an autosomal recessive disorder caused by a defect in GDH, a riboflavin-requiring enzyme that catalyses the dehydrogenation of glutaryl-CoA to glutaconyl-CoA and further to crotonyl-CoA (Fig. 9.14). Both substrates accumulate, leading to abnormal urinary excretion of glutaric and 3-hydroxyglutaric acids. Patients can be identified by measuring GDH activity in fibroblasts, leukocytes or liver biopsies, although correlation between residual activity and clinical phenotype is poor. Prenatal diagnosis is available by determination of glutaric acid concentration in amniotic fluid, and GDH activity in cultured amniotic cells or chorionic villus samples.

PATHOPHYSIOLOGY

Neurotransmitter dysmetabolism was thought to be the main pathophysiological process. The structural similarity of glutamic and glutaric acids may promote abnormal glutaminergic synaptic activity with decreased synthesis of GABA secondary to glutamate decarboxylase inhibition (Fig. 9.14). However, this hypothesis is not supported by the finding of normal or only slightly elevated CSF-GABA levels contrasting with the low GABA levels found in previous biochemical analysis of brain in two children (Hoffmann *et al.* 1991).

CLINICAL PRESENTATION

Intially, affected children develop normally for several months, although they may have mild hypotonia, irritability and jitteriness. Macrocephaly, present at birth or acquired in the first few months of life, is an important early sign. Chronic subdural effusions and haematomas can be the presenting features in infancy (Hoffmann *et al.* 1995a) and may wrongly suggest child abuse (Hoffmann *et al.* 1996). In typical cases, an acute neurological deterioration resembling encephalitis occurs during the first two years of life, with lethargy, hypotonia, loss of head control, seizures, opisthotonus, grimacing, tongue thrusting, rigidity and dystonia. Recovery is slow and incomplete, with marked residual dystonic and/or choreoathetotic movements, while mental retardation appears relatively mild. Progressive developmental delay

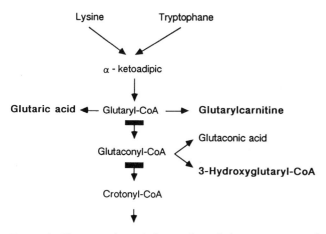

Fig. 9.14. Glutaric acid metabolism and metabolic consequences of glutaryl-CoA dehydrogenase deficiency *(solid bars).*

Lysine → α-ketoadipic ← Tryptophane

Glutaric acid ← Glutaryl-CoA → Glutarylcarnitine

Glutaconyl-CoA → Glutaconic acid / 3-Hydroxyglutaryl-CoA

Crotonyl-CoA

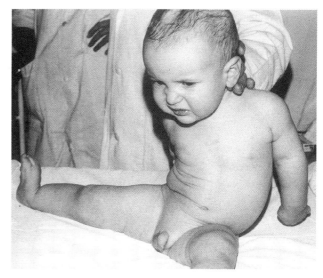

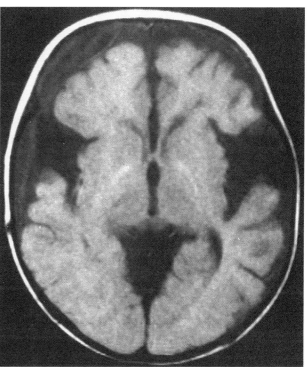

Fig. 9.15. *(Top)* Glutaric aciduria type I in a boy with marked dystonia of axial muscles and limbs. Note severe scoliosis. *(Bottom)* MRI scan of another child showing high signal from basal ganglia and marked temporal lobe atrophy with 'pseudocystic' widening of both sylvian fissures. (Courtesy Dr Barthez-Carpentier, Tours.)

with choreoathetosis is a less common presentation. After the onset of neurological symptoms the clinical presentation of both acute and chronic forms is similar. The course may be punctuated by acute episodes of coma, seizures, ketosis, hypoglycaemia or Reye-like syndrome during intercurrent infections or trauma. The risk for encephalopathic crises, however, declines after the age of 3 years. Asymptomatic homozygotes have been identified because of a positive family history or minor neurological symptoms. Hoffmann *et al.* (1996) reported 21 such cases in which preventive therapy was associated with normal development.

The EEG is most often normal, except during acute episodes when nonspecific patterns may be registered. CSF and neurophysiological investigations are normal. Serial CT and MRI studies performed in patients followed since birth show a progressive CNS involvement. Frontotemporal atrophy is a consistent finding even in asymptomatic patients. In symptomatic patients a more marked frontotemporal atrophy that may mimic bilateral arachnoid cysts (Martinez-Lage *et al.* 1994) is associated with diffuse cortical atrophy and areas of hypodensity in white matter, caudate and putamen (Brismar and Ozand 1994a, 1995) (Fig. 9.15).

These findings are in agreement with neuropathological reports which show that minimal striatal changes noted in young affected patients are much more marked in older children, with neuronal loss and extensive fibrous gliosis. Degeneration of the globus pallidus and marked spongiosis of subcortical white matter have also been reported (Soffer *et al.* 1992).

BIOCHEMICAL DIAGNOSIS
The diagnosis is made by urinary organic acid analysis demonstrating abnormal excretion of glutaric and 3-hydroxyglutaric acids. This finding, however, may be present only during crises or even absent altogether. In such cases determination of urinary organic acid in CSF, and in urine after alkaline hydrolysis, and measurement of plasma and urinary acylcarnitine appear to support the diagnosis (Campistol *et al.* 1992). Definitive diagnosis may require determination of GDH activity in fibroblasts.

TREATMENT
Lowering of glutaric acid levels may be achieved through: (1) a controlled lysine and tryptophan diet; (2) enhancement of GDH residual activity by riboflavin supplementation; (3) enhancement of glutaric acid urinary excretion by L-carnitine supplementation. This regimen gives unsatisfactory results in symptomatic children, but could halt progression of the disease in patients diagnosed during the presymptomatic phase. Baclofen and valproic acid, which increase GABA concentration in brain, have been used

with questionable effects (Hoffmann *et al.* 1991, 1995a). Early treatment of intercurrent illnesses, and fluid and glucose administration are important.

CANAVAN DISEASE (*N*-ACETYLASPARTIC ACIDURIA)

Canavan disease, also known as spongy degeneration of the brain, is an infantile neurodegenerative disorder which primarily affects the white matter, caused by aspartoacylase deficiency. Urine or plasma analysis for *N*-acetylaspartic acid (NAA) can now be considered as the biochemical marker of a disorder which was previously diagnosed by brain biopsy (Divry *et al.* 1988, Matalon *et al.* 1988).

BIOCHEMICAL BACKGROUND AND PATHOGENESIS

Canavan disease is caused by deficiency of the activity of the aspartoacylase enzyme which normally hydrolyses NAA to aspartate and acetate. Enzyme activity is present in various tissues (brain, leukocytes, liver, kidneys, adrenals, lungs and fibroblasts). Deficiency leads to NAA accumulation in brain and in all biological fluids.

In the brain, NAA is the second most abundant free amino acid after glutamic acid. However its function is still unknown. NAA and its synthesizing enzyme are found in high concentration in the cortical grey matter, while degradation of NAA by aspartoacylase mainly occurs in white matter. It has been suggested that NAA could be essential in the conversion of lignoceric acid to cerebronic and glutamic acids that serve the synthesis of myelin and could also be implicated in neurotransmission (Matalon *et al.* 1993, 1995b).

GENETIC BACKGROUND

Canavan disease is an autosomal recessive disorder. It is prevalent among Ashkenazi Jews (carrier frequency = 1:37.7), but also affects other ethnic groups. The true incidence is not known. However, since the use of NAA and/or aspartoacylase measurements for diagnosis, more than 125 patients have been identified (Matalon *et al.* 1995b).

The gene maps to chromosome 17p13–ter. Several mutations have already been reported with *E285A* point mutation being the most prevalent among the Ashkenazi Jewish population and *A305E* point mutation the most common among the European non-Jewish patients. Homozygosity for both *A305E* and *E285A* mutations has been identified in patients with both the severe and the mild forms of the disease, indicating that clinical course is not related to molecular heterogeneity (Shaag *et al.* 1995).

Prenatal diagnosis based on aspartoacylase assay in cultured amniocytes or chorionic villus samples is unreliable. Assay for NAA in amniotic fluid using the stable isotope dilution method is more efficient (Bennett *et al.* 1993). Mutation analysis can be more accurate for those families with known genotype (Shaag *et al.* 1995; Matalon *et al.* 1993, 1995a).

NEUROPATHOLOGY

Spongy degeneration of the subcortical white matter, with

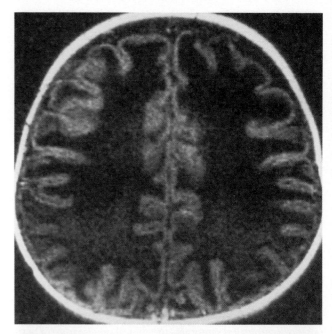

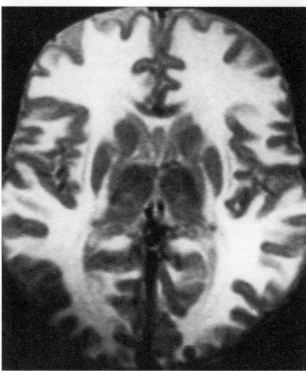

Fig. 9.16. Canavan–van Bogaert disease. *(Top)* T_1-weighted MRI sequence. Note absence of myelin signal and involvement of deep cortical layers. *(Bottom)* T_2-weighted sequence showing intense signal from white matter and deep cortical layers.

vacuoles within the myelin sheaths, is associated with astrocytic swelling and elongated mitochondria on electron microscopic examination. A fine network of fluid-containing cystic spaces also involves the deeper layers of the grey matter.

CLINICAL FEATURES

In the infantile form, affected babies are usually symptom-free

TABLE 9.5
Some rare organic acidurias associated with neurological signs

Inborn errors	Enzyme deficiency	Possible neurological signs	Other features	References
3-Hydroxybutyric aciduria	Combined semialdehyde dehydrogenase?	Brain dysgenesis, seizures	Congenital malformations, recurrent bouts of ketoacidosis	Boulat et al. (1995)
D-2-hydroxyglutaric aciduria	D-2-hydroxyglutaric dehydrogenase?	Macrocephaly, severe developmental delay, hypotonia, pyramidal signs, cortical atrophy ± leukodystrophy, myoclonic seizures	Cardiomyopathy, dysmorphism	Nyhan et al. (1995)
Malonic aciduria	Malonyl-CoA decarboxylase	Developmental delay, hypotonia	Cardiomyopathy	MacPhee et al. (1993)
3-Methyl-glutaconic aciduria				
Type I	3-Methylglutaconic hydratase	Speech delay	Bouts of acidosis ± hypoglycaemia	Duran et al. (1982)
Type II	Unknown	—	Growth retardation, cardiomyopathy, neutropenia	Gibson et al. (1993)
Type III	Unknown	Developmental delay, seizures, movement disorder. Basal ganglia involvement	Acidosis, liver failure, tubulopathy, cardiomyopathy, ophthalmological involvement	Gibson et al. (1993)
'Optic atrophy plus' syndrome	Unknown	Bilateral optic atrophy; extrapyramidal dysfunction; progressive spasticity, ataxia and cognitive deficit	—	Al Aqeel et al. (1994), Elpeleg et al. (1994)
D-glyceric aciduria	D-glycerate kinase	Nonketotic hyperglycinaemia-like signs or encephalopathy, microcephaly, seizures	—	van Schaftingen (1989), Largillière et al. (1991)
Sjögren–Larsson disease	Fatty alcohol oxidoreductase	Spastic di- or tetraplegia, mental retardation, leukodystrophy	Retinopathy, congenital ichthyosis	Rizzo et al. (1994)
Pyroglutamic aciduria	Glutathione synthetase	Progressive neurological damage: ataxia, seizures, mental retardation	Neonatal haemolysis, acidosis	Jain et al. (1994)

at birth and in early life. By the age of 3–6 months, developmental delay with hypotonia, head lag and acquired macrocephaly insidiously appear. Later on, patients develop hypertonia with spasticity, seizures and cerebral blindness, often with optic atrophy. Most patients die within the first decade. Rare congenital and occasional late-onset cases are on record. It seems, however, that their genotype is the same as that of infantile forms (Matalon 1995b, Shaag et al. 1995).

Typically, CT or MR imaging of the brain reveal diffuse, symmetrical subcortical white matter degeneration with relative sparing of the internal capsule, the centrum semi-ovale, the cerebellum and the brainstem (Fig. 9.16). Demyelination progresses with age. In a few patients, early neuroimaging failed to demonstrate leukodystrophy (Toft et al. 1993), and on T_2-weighted images high-signal lesions have been found to affect the lentiform and caudate nuclei (Toft et al. 1993). MR spectroscopy reveals accumulation of NAA in the brain with elevated ratios of NAA/phosphocreatine + creatine and/or of NAA/choline. These results probably indicate early myelin dysmetabolism (Toft et al. 1993).

BIOCHEMICAL DIAGNOSIS
The diagnosis is established by gas chromatography/mass spectroscopy for measurement of NAA in urine, plasma and CSF. It is further confirmed by enzymatic determination of aspartoacylase in cultured fibroblasts.

L-2-HYDROXYGLUTARIC ACIDURIA
L-2-hydroxyglutaric aciduria, a recently described disorder, is associated with a progressive neurodegenerative process with subcortical leukodystrophy, cerebellar atrophy and basal ganglia involvement. The metabolic fate of L-2-hydroxyglutaric acid and the pathogenesis of the disorder are unknown. However, the homogeneous clinical and neuroimaging features clearly delineate a neurometabolic disease with autosomal inheritance (Barth et al. 1992, 1993).

During infancy and early childhood, mental and motor development appear normal or slightly delayed. Thereafter, the presenting symptoms vary with walking or speech delay, seizures or learning disabilities. Progressive cerebellar ataxia and mental retardation become the most prominent features by the end of the first decade. Mild extrapyramidal and pyramidal symptoms may coexist, and generalized epileptic seizures may occur. Raised CSF protein has been reported. Neuroimaging reveals progressive subcortical white matter changes with loss of myelin in the arcuate fibres and preservation of central myelin. Basal ganglia may be involved with atrophy of the caudate nuclei and signal changes in the putamen. The cerebellum is affected with folial

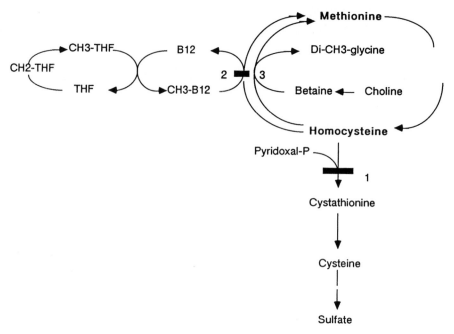

Fig. 9.17. Biochemical pathways in homocystinuria.
Key: THF = tetrahydrofolate; 1 = cystathionine β-synthase; 2 = methionine synthetase; 3 = betaine-homocysteine methyltransferase.

atrophy mainly of the vermis and signal changes in the dentate nuclei. In one patient, proton magnetic resonance of the brain has revealed signs suggesting a neurodegenerative process (Hanefeld *et al.* 1994).

Neuropathology shows loss of myelin with reactive astrocytes and enlarged perivascular spaces in white matter (Wilcken *et al.* 1993) and even polycystic white matter degeneration (Kaabachi *et al.* 1993). Olivopontocerebellar atrophy with neuronal loss in the cerebellum, dentate, pontine and inferior olivary was found in one patient (Chen *et al.* 1996)

The biochemical pattern is characterized by accumulation of L-2-hydroxyglutaric acid and lysine in body fluids with usually higher concentrations in the CSF than in the plasma (Hoffmann *et al.* 1995b). This disorder should be distinguished from D-2-hydroxyglutaric aciduria, another rare neurometabolic disorder responsible for early-onset encephalopathy associated with myoclonic epilepsy, cortical blindness and static periventricular leukodystrophy (Nyhan *et al.* 1995, Sugita *et al.* 1995). Rare disorders of metabolism of other organic acids are shown in Table 9.5.

HOMOCYSTINURIA

Cystathionine beta-synthase deficiency is the most common cause of homocystinuria. Clinically, the disease involves the eyes, skeleton, brain and vascular system. Mental retardation is a major feature, but a substantial proportion of patients have normal intelligence. Neurological signs include seizures, spasticity and psychiatric disorders. Homocystinuria and high plasma levels of methionine biochemically characterize the disease. (For reviews, see Mudd *et al.* 1985, 1995; Andria and Sebastio 1995).

BIOCHEMICAL BACKGROUND
BIOCHEMICAL BACKGROUND
In humans, methionine is catabolized to homocysteine through the transmethylation pathway (Fig. 9.17). Homocysteine is further degraded via the transulfuration route, yielding the end-products sulfite and sulfate. Cystathionine beta-synthase catalyses the first step of this degradative pathway and requires vitamin B$_6$ as a cofactor. Deficient activity of cystathionine beta-synthase is responsible for accumulation of homocysteine and methionine and decreased synthesis of cysteine.

About 50 per cent of the homocysteine formed is remethylated to methionine. Enzymatic defects which affect remethylation are responsible for homocystinuria and hypomethionaemia (see p. 288)

GENETIC BACKGROUND
Based on neonatal screening, the incidence of this autosomal recessive disease is about 1 in 335,000 live births. This may be an underestimate as hypermethioninaemia may be absent during the neonatal screening period. Enzymatic studies and biological B$_6$-responsiveness suggest much heterogeneity among the mutations that underlie cystathionine beta-synthase defects. Three biochemically determined groups of patients are defined following B$_6$ administration: one group is unresponsive, the second is clearly reponsive and the last has intermediate responsiveness. The human cystathionine beta-synthase gene maps to chromosome 21, and several disease-causing mutations have been described with complete lack of correlation between genotype and phenotype.

Cystathionine beta-synthase deficiency is expressed in cultured fibroblasts, lymphoblasts, amniotic fluid cells and chorionic villus samples, allowing postnatal and prenatal diagnosis (Fowler *et al.* 1982). Heterozygotes for the trait may metabolize homocysteine at a lower rate than controls. The risk for thromboembolic disease in affected persons and the incidence of heterozygosity in patients with thromboembolic events are not agreed upon (Kang *et al.* 1992).

PATHOPHYSIOLOGY
While some data are available concerning homocystinuria, thrombosis and atherosclerosis, the relationship between the biochemical abnormalities and the development of mental retardation, ectopia lentis or skeletal abnormalities remains obscure (Selhub and Miller 1992; for a review, see Mudd *et al.* 1995).

CLINICAL FEATURES
Homocystinuria is a progressive multisystem disorder. The risk of developing manifestations of the disease increases with age. B_6-responsive patients are more mildly affected than B_6-unresponsive ones. Four organ systems show major involvement: the eye, the skeleton, the CNS and the vascular system. Ectopia lentis is the most consistent finding. It is rarely present before the age of 2 years. Fifty per cent of B_6-unresponsive and responsive untreated patients have ectopia lentis by 6 and 10 years respectively. However, a normal ophthalmological examination at any age is no reason for rejecting the diagnosis. Optic atrophy, retinal degeneration or detachment, cataracts and corneal opacities appear to be secondary to lens dislocation. The most consistent skeletal findings are osteoporosis and scoliosis. Dolichostenomelia is responsible for the marfanoid aspect. Other frequently associated deformities include pectus carinatum, pes cavus, genu valgum, biconcave vertebrae and epimetaphyseal widening.

Mental retardation is often the first recognized feature. Walking may be delayed and some patients have a 'Charlie Chaplin-like' gait. The IQ varies widely. B_6-responsive patients have higher IQs (median 78) than B_6-unresponsive ones (median 56). Twenty-one per cent of untreated patients have experienced grand mal seizures, but EEGs are most often abnormal even without seizures (Del Giudice *et al.* 1983). Hemiparesis or focal neurological signs suggest cerebrovascular occlusion. Dystonia has been observed in a few patients as well as other extrapyramidal signs such as resting tremor (Arbour *et al.* 1988). Psychiatric abnormalities are frequent, and prevail among patients with lower IQs, who often present with disturbed behaviour and obsessive–compulsive disorder (Abbott *et al.* 1987).

Homocystinuric patients have potentially life-threatening thromboembolic events. Vascular occlusions occur in any vessel at any age and may be the first manifestation. Cerebrovascular accidents may be responsible for optic atrophy, hemiparesis, seizures or focal neurological signs. Occlusions also occur in kidney, pulmonary artery, iliac vein, vena cava or coronary vessels. The risk of thromboembolic complications seems higher following intercurrent infections and surgery, and is responsible for a high mortality rate. Other features include fair hair, thin skin with malar flush and livedo reticularis, inguinal hernia, myopathic

EMG, fatty liver, hyperinsulinism and increased level of growth hormone.

BIOLOGICAL FINDINGS
Various abnormalities of clotting factors and platelets, and mildly low levels of folates and B_{12} may be found. Usually, the cyanide–nitroprusside test (Brand reaction) in urine is positive. Definitive diagnosis is based on plasma and urine amino acid chromatography which shows homocysteine, excess methionine and reduced cysteine. In some B_6-responsive cases homocystinaemia may be mild and determination of total homocysteine is more reliable for evaluation of homocysteine accumulation.

TREATMENT
The management of homocystinuria should be directed towards lowering the body accumulation of homocystine and increasing the cystine content. This is easily achieved in B_6-responsive patients by oral administration of 100–500 mg/d of pyridoxine, folate and B_{12} depletions being appropriately corrected. B_6-unresponsive patients require a low-methionine diet with cysteine and betaine supplementation. Prevention of thromboembolic episodes is best achieved through strict metabolic control, administration of antiaggregant molecules (dipyramidol and/or aspirin), and with hydration.

Early treatment of patients detected in the neonatal period is effective in preventing mental retardation and seizures, and in delaying lens dislocation. Late treatment may improve development and behaviour.

SULFITE OXIDASE DEFICIENCY
Sulfite oxidase deficiency, isolated or in association with xanthine oxidase deficiency (SO-XO deficiency or molybdenum cofactor deficiency) is a rare metabolic disorder. The chemical diagnosis is based on detection of sulfituria. Both disorders appear to be inherited in an autosomal recessive manner.

METABOLIC PATHWAYS AND BIOCHEMICAL HALLMARKS
The terminal step in the methionine transulfuration pathway is conversion of sulfite to sulfate catalysed by sulfite oxidase (Fig. 9.18). Sulfite oxidase is a complex enzyme which requires a pterin-containing molybdenum cofactor. Thus sulfite oxidase deficiency can arise as a result of a defect in sulfite oxydase apoenzyme or in molybdenum cofactor synthesis. Both conditions are characterized by low sulfaturia and sulfituria associated with a peculiar amino acid profile. Sulfituria can be detected using 'sulfitest strips'. This method may, however, gives false negative and false positive results (van der Klei-van Moorsel *et al.* 1991, Hansen *et al.* 1993). Plasma and urine amino acid chromatography shows accumulation of thiosulfate, *S*-sulfocysteine and taurine. Xanthine oxidase being another molybdenoenzyme, in combined SO-XO deficiency the previous pattern is associated with hypouricaemia and xanthinuria.

Sulfite oxidase activity and the level of molybdenum cofactor can be measured on cultured fibroblasts and other tissues for further confirmation of the diagnosis. Prenatal diagnosis can

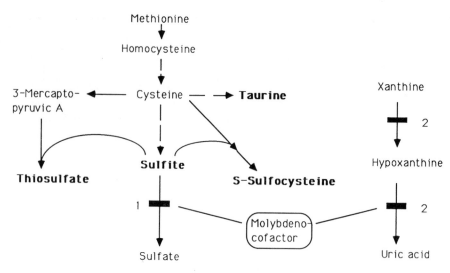

Fig. 9.18. Disturbed metabolism due to molybdenum cofactor deficiency.
Key: 1 = sulfite oxidase; 2 = xanthine oxidase.

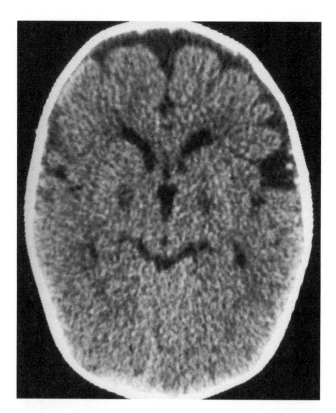

Fig. 9.19. CT scan of a 2-month-old infant with sulfite oxidase deficiency and convulsions since birth. There is symmetrical cavitation of both pallida and frontal cortical atrophy.

be performed by measuring sulfite oxidase activity in amniotic cells or chorionic villus samples and by *S*-sulfocysteine analysis in amniotic fluid (Gray *et al.* 1990).

PATHOGENESIS
The pathogenesis of the disease is only speculative. Accumulated sulfite may have direct CNS toxicity. Lack of sulfate is another possible pathogenic factor as inorganic sulfate is required for the synthesis of sulfate esters and of mucopolysaccharides (van der Klei-van Moorsel *et al.* 1991). *S*-sulfocysteine may have neuroexcitatory properties and may be responsible for seizures (Kurlemann *et al.* 1996).

CLINICAL ASPECTS
Most patients present soon after birth with intractable seizures (Slot *et al.* 1993). The EEG may show a suppression–burst pattern (Aukett *et al.* 1988, van Gennip *et al.* 1994b). Further course is characterized by severe developmental delay, spastic tetraplegia, axial hypotonia and microcephaly. Seizures most often remain unchanged but spasms and choreoathetoid movements may appear. Peculiar facial dysmorphism is often mentioned, with a large, coarse face, broad nasal bridge, enophthalmia, long philtrum, large ears and sagging skin. Ectopia lentis is mentioned in about 50 per cent of the cases. It may be present soon after birth or occur as late as 4 years. Xanthine urolithiasis is an inconstant feature. Most patients die within the first two years of life (Arnold *et al.* 1993, Hansen *et al.* 1993, Slot *et al.* 1993, van Gennip *et al.* 1994b).

CT and MRI studies show multicystic leukoencephalopathy (Rupar *et al.* 1996) but a normal neonatal pattern of myelination in the brainstem, an abnormal shape of the frontal horns, and a severe volume loss or cavitation of basal ganglia and corpus callosum (Schuierer *et al.* 1995) (Fig. 9.19). Pathologically there is severe cerebral atrophy, ulegyria and multicystic subcortical lesions in the white matter. Microscopically both grey and white matter are involved. Severe neuronal loss, astrocytic gliosis, microcavitations and spongiosis affect the whole cortex. In the cerebellum granular and Purkinje cells are rare. Demyelination and marked axonal loss are found. The similarities between isolated sulfite oxidase deficiency and molybdenum cofactor deficiency suggest that encephalopathy is linked to the sulfite oxidase defect (Roth *et al.* 1985, Arnold *et al.* 1993).

A less severe form with prolonged survival has been described in two patients with combined sulfite and xanthine oxidase deficiency and in one patient with isolated sulfite oxidase deficiency (Barbot *et al.* 1995, Mize *et al.* 1995). Their development was normal for a few months, followed by unexplained episodes simulating encephalitis with hemiplegic sequelae in two. Exuberant choreoathetoid movements and atonic seizures were observed. Dislocated lenses were found in the two patients affected with combined deficiency, which in one was associated with a Marfan-like habitus. MRI has revealed increased signal in the globus pallidus.

TREATMENT
Several therapeutic attempts aimed at lowering sulfite accumulation or preventing sulfate and molybdenum depletion have been unsuccessful (Boles *et al.* 1993). Dextrometorphan, by counteracting the neuroexcitatory effect of *S*-sulfocysteine, has been tried with some success in a patient (Kurlemann *et al.* 1996).

DISORDERS OF NEUROTRANSMITTER METABOLISM

TETRAHYDROBIOPTERIN (THB) DEFICIENCY
Evidence that THB deficiency is responsible for atypical HPA (also called malignant HPA) arose following the description of children with neonatal HPA who, despite early dietary control, experienced severe and progressive neurological deterioration. Since then, hundreds of patients have been observed, most of them recognized after the use of neonatal screening for PKU (Dhondt 1991, Blau *et al.* 1996).

In mammals, THB is the cofactor of the aromatic amino acid hydroxylases—phenylalanine, tyrosine and tryptophan hydroxylases—and for all known isoforms of nitric oxide synthase. Consequently, a defect in the metabolism of THB results in high blood levels of phenylalanine and failure to hydroxylize tyrosine and tryptophan, the subtrates for serotonin and catecholamine synthesis. The severe neurological outcome of these patients thus appears to be linked to neurotransmitter deficiencies. In addition, nitric oxide formation is impaired and the CNS is subjected to increased oxidative stress (Brand *et al.* 1995).

METABOLIC PATHWAY AND ENZYMATIC DEFICIENCIES
The metabolic pathway comprises a synthetic and a regenerating route (see Fig. 9.10). Two enzyme defects affect the synthetic pathway of THB, guanosine triphosphate cyclohydrolase (GTP-ch) deficiency and pyruvoyl-tetrahydropterin synthase (PTPS) deficiency. Two other enzyme defects affect regeneration of TBH in the liver, dihydropteridine reductase (DHPR) and pterin-4α-carbinolamine dehydratase (PCD) deficiencies (Kaufman 1993).

HPA is often the first biochemical manifestation of these disorders. The failure of the tyrosine and tryptophan hydroxylating systems is not evident in the newborn period, and the erroneous diagnosis of PKU may prevent application of specific treatment.

TABLE 9.6
Pterin patterns in tetrahydrobiopterin deficiencies

	DHPR	GTP-ch	PTPS	PCD*
Neopterin (N)	Normal	Low	High	Normal
Biopterin (B)	High to normal**	Low	Low	Low
N/B ratio	Low to normal**	Normal	High	High
% (B/B+N)	High to normal	Normal	Low	Low

DHPR = dihydropteridine reductase; GTP-ch = guanosine triphosphate cyclohydrolase; PTPS = pyruvoyl-tetrahydropteridin synthetase; PCD = pteridine carbinolamine dehydratase.
*Presence of 7-biopterin characterizes this form.
**Contrary to what would theoretically be expected, normal values are often found.

Therefore, THB deficiency should be looked for in any neonate screening positive for HPA. DHPR deficiency, despite different molecular defects, is the most clinically homogeneous group. In contrast, PTPS deficiency shows heterogeneity in the intensity of the block, and partial, peripheral and transient forms have been described (Shintaku *et al.* 1988). Partial forms are characterized by the normalization within months of an initially typical biochemical pattern associated with normal development. Peripheral forms are defined by an abnormal biochemical pattern in urine contrasting with the absence of any abnormality in the CSF. However, this diagnosis must be cautious as some infants with peripheral forms have developed neurological signs by the age of 6 months. Most of the transient forms could be partial PAH deficiency associated with delayed maturation of THB synthesis.

Each enzyme deficiency is responsible for a specific abnormal pattern of pterins and catecholamine metabolites (HVA, 5-HIAA) in urine, plasma and CSF (Table 9.6). However, in DHPR deficiency, the neopterin/biopterin (N/B) ratio may be normal, and PKU patients with high blood levels of phenylalanine may have a low N/B ratio which is corrected as the phenylalanine level normalizes. Neurotransmitter metabolites HVA and 5-HIAA are usually < 10 per cent of normal value in the CSF of patients with severe cofactor deficiency. This biochemical pattern leads to suspicion of the diagnosis which must be later confirmed by specific enzymatic studies.

GENETIC BACKGROUND
All biopterin metabolism defects are inherited as autosomal recessive traits. Based on neonatal screening, they account for 1–3 per cent of patients with HPA. The true incidence is probably higher, since THB deficiency may occur with normal phenylalanine levels (Tanaka *et al.* 1987). Almost two-thirds of all THB-deficient patients are affected with PTPS, one third have DHPR, and only a few patients have either GTP-ch or PCD defects. Antenatal diagnosis of THB deficiency uses quantification of pterins in amniotic fluid and specific enzyme activity in fetal and extrafetal tissue. The genes coding for these human enzymes have been cloned, allowing molecular characterization of mutations (Blau *et al.* 1993, 1994).

CLINICAL MANIFESTATIONS

Severe deficiency of THB results in a progressive encephalopathy (Hyland 1993, Smith and Brenton 1995). Birth is uneventful except for a higher incidence of low birthweight and microcephaly in typical biopterin synthetase deficiency (Dhondt 1991). In the neonatal period, minor neurological signs such as hypotonia, decreased spontaneous movements and poor sucking may be present. Developmental delay is usually noted by the age of 4 months. Poor head control, truncal hypotonia, lead-pipe rigidity of the limbs and spastic paresis are prominent. Dystonic posturing, abnormal movements, oculogyric crises and choreoathetosis are frequent. Drowsiness, irritability, swallowing difficulties, excessive drooling and unexplained hyperthermia may be features. Acquired microcephaly and seizures, often myoclonic in type, are common. Sudden or rapid unexplained death may occur. The EEG often shows abnormal slow or disorganized background, epileptic discharges or hypsarrhythmia. CT scan or cerebral MRI may reveal cortical or subcortical atrophy and white matter disease (Brismar *et al.* 1990b). DHPR deficiency is noteworthy for the incidence of brain calcification involving the white matter and/or the basal ganglia resembling CNS changes of methotrexate toxicity.

BIOCHEMICAL DIAGNOSIS

Neonatal blood phenylalanine levels are usually high. However, around one-fifth of all neonates are near the positive cut-off value of the HPA screening test, so all neonates with HPA must be screened for THB deficiency whatever the phenylalanine level. Several methods have been proposed for prompt biochemical diagnosis of these cases. Pterin and neurotransmitter metabolite profiles and THB loading test are sufficient for diagnosis of GTP-ch, PTPS and PCD. In contrast, DHPR deficiency is more difficult to assess, and all HPA patients should be systematically screened by enzyme assay in erythrocytes using dry blood spot on Guthrie card (Dhondt 1991, Ponzone *et al.* 1993).

TREATMENT

Treatment of THB-deficient patients has two main goals: control of HPA and restoration of monoamine neurotransmission for which supplementation with biopterin could appear the logical therapy. However, THB is an unstable molecule readily oxidized to dihydrobiopterin (DHB), and entry of THB into the brain is inadequate to correct the hydroxylating system in the CNS.

In biopterin synthesis (GTP-ch, PTPS) and PCD defects, HPA can usually be corrected by the use of TBH supplementation (1–5 mg/kg/d) because integrity of the regenerating system allows the reduction of the oxidized form. In contrast, the regenerating system is missing in DHPR deficiency, and biopterin supplementation could be insufficient to correct the HPA, so a phenylalanine-controlled diet is usually necessary.

Neurotransmitter replacement therapy is achieved by giving neurotransmitter precursors—L-dopa (5–10 mg/kg/d) in combination with an inhibitor of peripheral aromatic amino acid decarboxylase (carbidopa) in a ratio of 10:1—and the serotonin precursor 5-hydroxytryptophan (5-HT, 5–10 mg/kg/d). The dosage should be adjusted based on CSF neurotransmitter metabolite evaluation and on serum prolactin levels which indirectly reflect central dopamine effectiveness (Spada *et al.* 1996). Addition of deprenyl (selegiline) may decrease L-dopa and 5-HT requirements and may result in greater clinical improvement (Schuler *et al.* 1995).

Treatment with folinic acid in cases of DHPR deficiency should also be considered. Folate deficiency has been documented in DHPR-deficient patients, and folinic acid administration has led to significant improvement in clinical signs and neurotransmitter metabolite levels in the CSF (Smith and Brenton 1995).

Long-term effectiveness of treatment is still unknown. In patients who present neurological abnormality, neurological signs can be reversed (muscular tone, seizures and alertness), but some developmental delay remains. Early-treated patients may have a near-normal developmental course.

NONKETOTIC HYPERGLYCINAEMIA (NKH)

NKH is an inborn error of amino acid catabolism in which large amounts of glycine accumulate in body fluids. The classical phenotype is a life-threatening illness that develops in the neonatal period, during which most patients die. Survivors are severely retarded and usually have seizures.

BIOCHEMICAL BASIS

Glycine is implicated in numerous biochemical reactions, among which glycine–serine interconversion appears to be the most important for maintaining glycine homeostasis. This reaction involves two reversible enzymatic steps, one subserved by serine hydromethyltransferase, the other by the glycine cleavage system, this last step serving the catabolism:

$$Serine + THF \rightleftharpoons Glycine + CH_2THF;$$
$$Glycine + THF + H_2O \rightleftharpoons CH_2THF + CO_2 + NH_3.*$$

The glycine cleavage system localized in liver and brain includes four protein components named P, H, T and L. Deficiency in this system has been demonstrated to be due to deficiency in either P, T or H protein. A majority of NKH patients have a specific defect in P-protein (Hayasaka *et al.* 1987, Tada and Kure 1993).

Primary deficiency leads to glycine accumulation in plasma, urine, CSF and brain tissue. Inhibition of the glycine cleavage system by several metabolites (*e.g.* organic acids, valproate) is responsible for secondary hyperglycinaemia and hyperglycinuria without abnormal CSF concentration.

GENETIC BACKGROUND

NKH is inherited in an autosomal recessive manner. Antenatal diagnosis is efficiently performed using direct enzymatic assay from fresh chorionic villus samples and is also possible by DNA analysis. Measurement of glycine/serine ratio in amniotic fluid is unreliable (Tada and Kure 1993, Nanao *et al.* 1994, Toone *et al.* 1994).

---

*THF = tetrahydrofolate; CH$_2$THF = methylenetetrahydrofolate.

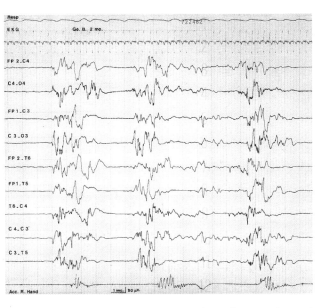

Fig. 9.20. Glycine encephalopathy (nonketotic hyperglycinaemia): typical suppression–burst EEG tracing in 2-month-old boy. Note myoclonic jerks of right hand synchronous with EEG bursts *(lower trace)*. (By permission of John Libbey Eurotext, London.)

NEUROPATHOLOGY

The most striking feature is lack of myelination, frequently associated with abnormal brain morphology. Ten of 16 brains studied by Dobyns (1989) showed an abnormal gyral pattern, hypoplasia, agenesis of the corpus callosum, colpocephaly or cerebellar hypoplasia. A severe spongy leukodystrophy is present. Similar brain malformations have been reported in several other inborn errors of metabolism (Chapter 3).

PATHOGENESIS

Although the mechanism underlying the neurological dysfunction is not fully understood, glycine itself has an important role in the pathogenesis (Tada and Kure 1993). Glycine is an inhibitory neurotransmitter whose receptors are mainly located in the spinal cord and brainstem. These glycine receptors are specifically antagonized by strychnine and competitively inhibited by benzodiazepines. However, inhibitory neurotransmission and the location of glycine receptors in brainstem and spinal cord poorly explain seizures which are a major factor in NKH patients. Another, strychnine-insensitive, site with high affinity for glycine exists in the brain. This site is associated with the *N*-methyl-D-aspartate (NMDA) receptor, one of the main glutamate receptors that plays a major role in excitatory transmission in the cortex and diencephalon. NMDA-mediated neurotoxicity is markedly potentiated by glycine, and excessive activation of NMDA receptors may directly result in neurotoxicity (D'Souza *et al.* 1993).

Brain dysmyelination could also result from the defective glycine–serine interconversion with decreased production of one-carbon units, a metabolism which has higher activity in the period of myelination (Hayasaka *et al.* 1987).

CLINICAL FEATURES

Classical early-onset phenotype

This is the most frequently occurring type of NKH. In the severe form, also known as early or neonatal myoclonic encephalopathy (Chapter 16), symptoms may appear from 7 hours postpartum to the eighth day of life. Lethargy and muscular weakness appear first. Shallow breathing follows and rapidly yields to apnoeic spells. Affected infants are flaccid and unresponsive to stimuli but often present erratic myoclonias and subtle partial seizures. Rapid screening of urine and blood excludes most other metabolic disorders with neonatal onset: there is no ketoacidosis, and no hyperlactataemia or hyperammonaemia. The 'burst–suppression' pattern on the EEG (Fig. 9.20), though nonspecific, is an important diagnostic feature.

A majority of patients die in this early period. For some infants, episodes of apnoea and respiratory depression are transient difficulties, and they may survive. However, no effective treatment is known, and early survivors invariably develop a severe epileptic encephalopathy and die within the first years of life. They display spastic cerebral palsy, associated in most cases with infantile spasms or less often with partial convulsions. The periodic EEG pattern most often disappears after a few months and changes to atypical hypsarrhythmia or multifocal epileptic discharges (Mises *et al.* 1982).

CT and MRI scans show progressive cerebral atrophy and delayed myelination of the supratentorial white matter (Press *et al.* 1989). An abnormally thin corpus callosum may be found (Dobyns 1989).

Atypical cases

There are two major types: an infantile type generally symptomatic during the first year of life, and a late-onset form observed in childhood or adolescence. The infantile type of NKH has been reported in about 30 patients and can be easily misdiagnosed as static encephalopathy (Christodoulou *et al.* 1993, Steiner *et al.* 1996). After an uneventful neonatal period, these children have developmental delay that can progress to moderate or profound intellectual disability. Most have some upper motor neuron signs, poor fine motor coordination, expressive speech deficit, hyperactivity and aggressive behaviour, and some have episodic tonic–clonic seizures. Following intercurrent febrile illness or trauma, they may present with acute deterioration, seizures that are often difficult to control, or unusual symptoms such as myoclonic jerks, abnormal twitching movements, agitated delirium, chorea, ataxia and vertical gaze palsy. In one case, developmental regression was reminiscent of the lysosomal storage diseases (Trauner *et al.* 1981). The EEG shows a slow pattern with prominent high voltage of up to 200 mV (2–3 Hz waves) (Cole and Meek 1985, Palmer and Oberholzer 1985).

The late-onset form is very rare and presents as a spinocerebellar degeneration with optic atrophy (Bank and Morrow 1972, Steiman *et al.* 1979).

Transient neonatal forms have been described that clinically and biologically resemble the classical type. The biochemical abnormalities are reported to resolve within one to six weeks but clinical outcome is uncertain and enzymatic assay has never been reported in these cases (Eyskens *et al.* 1992).

DIAGNOSIS

The diagnosis is confirmed by demonstration of elevated plasma and CSF glycine levels, with a high glycine CSF/plasma ratio which is the most specific abnormality. Definitive diagnosis relies on enzymatic studies on liver or transformed lymphoblasts. Most of the neonatal-onset forms have no residual activity; in late-onset forms residual activity varies from zero to 25 per cent (Kure *et al.* 1992).

TREATMENT

There is no known effective therapy. Treatment with high-dosage sodium benzoate, a substance that promotes more efficient urinary excretion of glycine, decreases the frequency of seizures, but is insufficient to prevent developmental delay (Van Hove *et al.* 1995). New therapeutic approaches have used various molecules that would antagonize the excitatory effect of glycine on NMDA receptors. Dextromethorphan, ketamine and tryptophan have been used occasionally with some developmental improvement. Attempts to block glycinergic inhibition by strychnine have proved ineffective (Matsuo *et al.* 1995, Tegtmeyer-Metzdorf *et al.* 1995).

INBORN ERRORS OF GABA METABOLISM

Gamma-aminobutyric acid (4-aminobutyric acid), a major inhibitory neurotransmitter amino acid, is synthesized from glutamic acid in a reaction catalysed by a pyridoxine-dependent glutamate decarboxylase. The catabolic steps comprise a pyridoxine-dependent transamination which yields succinate semialdehyde and an oxidation to succinate which finally enters the Krebs cycle. A secondary route, catalysed by a dehydrogenase, converts succinate semialdehyde to gamma-hydroxybutyrate which is futher oxidized (Fig. 9.21). The inherited disorders of GABA metabolism include: pyridoxine-dependent seizures, GABA transaminase deficiency, succinic semialdehyde dehydrogenase deficiency, and homocarnosinosis (Table 9.7) (Jakobs *et al.* 1993).

4-HYDROXYBUTYRIC ACIDURIA

This rare condition, inherited in an autosomal recessive manner, is characterized by the accumulation of gamma-hydroxybutyric acid (GHB) and succinate semialdehyde (SSA) in body fluids secondary to succinic semialdehyde dehydrogenase (SSA-DH) deficiency. Deficient SSA-DH activity has been demonstrated in isolated lymphocytes and cultured lymphoblasts or fibroblasts (Jakobs *et al.* 1993). Prenatal diagnosis can use evaluation of GHB accumulated in amniotic fluid and measurement of SSA-DH activity in cultured amniocytes (Gibson *et al.* 1994).

Pathophysiology

The disorder results in accumulation of GHB, a neuropharmacologically active compound used as an intravenous anaesthetic drug which acts as a direct or indirect GABA-receptor agonist. In animals, dose-dependent effects of GHB resemble some clinical

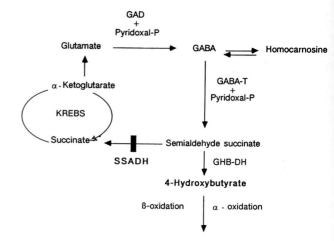

Fig. 9.21. Metabolism of γ-aminobutyric acid (GABA).
Key: GAD = glutamic acid decarboxylase; GABA-T = GABA-transaminase; SSADH = succinic semialdehyde dehydrogenase; GHB-DH = γ-hydroxybutyric acid dehydrogenase.

manifestations recorded in patients (Jakobs *et al.* 1993). High plasma levels of GHB in CSF probably reflect an abnormally high concentration in the brain, which may have neurotoxicity and may impair the neurophysiological role of GABA in development and function.

Clinical features

About 40 cases are known with a variable clinical phenotype (Jakobs *et al.* 1993). The most frequent features are mild psychomotor delay associated with muscular hypotonia, areflexia, significant ataxia of the trunk and limbs, and delayed speech. Ocular dyspraxia, mild intention tremor and episodic seizures are present in some cases. Lethargy and choreoathetosis have been mentioned. Less severe cases with mild motor retardation and abnormal speech development have also been reported. Imaging is usually normal or reveals mild atrophy. In three cases, MRI studies have revealed bilateral abnormal signal in the globus pallidus and necrosis of the dentate nuclei (DeVivo *et al.* 1988, Uziel *et al.* 1993, Brismar and Ozand 1994a).

Biochemical diagnosis

The diagnosis is confirmed by high levels of GHB in plasma, CSF and urine, in association with abnormal urinary excretion of several GHB by-products. Persistent hyperglycinuria has been reported in three affected sibs. CSF free-GABA is high or in the normal control range (Jakobs *et al.* 1993).

Treatment

Administration of gamma-vinyl-GABA, a GABA transaminase inhibitor, decreases GHB accumulation in CSF and results in some mild clinical improvement (Gibson *et al.* 1995).

PYRIDOXINE DEPENDENCY

Pyridoxine dependency is a rare disease characterized by the occurrence of intractable seizures that are controlled only by the

TABLE 9.7
TABLE 9.7
Some inborn errors of neurotransmitter metabolism

Inborn error	Deficiency	Main neurological features	Diagnostic tests	References
I—Disorders of monoamines				
'Malignant' hyperphenylalaninaemia	Disorders of tetrahydrobiopterin synthesis	Convulsions, mental retardation, peripheral hypertonia, central hypotonia, dysautonomia	Abnormal urinary and CSF pteridine profiles. Increased phenylalanine. Decreased CSF HVA and 5-HIAA. DHPR* assay (dry blood spots)	Smith and Brenton (1995)
Hereditary dopa-responsive dystonia (Segawa disease, dominant)	GTP-cyclohydrolase	Dystonia with diurnal fluctuations	Decreased CSF HVA, 5-HIAA, biopterin and neopterin	Ichinose et al. (1994)
Hereditary dopa-responsive dystonia (Segawa disease, recessive)	Tyrosine hydroxylase	Dystonia with diurnal fluctuations	Responsiveness to small dose of L-dopa. Decreased CSF HVA, normal CSF 5-HIAA	Knappskog et al. (1995), Lüdecke et al. (1995)
Aromatic L-amino acid decarboxylase defects	L-amino acid decarboxylase	Central hypotonia, oculogyric crises, seizures, dystonia	Decreased CSF HVA and 5-HIAA	Hyland et al. (1992)
Dopamine β-hydroxylase defect	Dopamine β-hydroxylase	Bilateral ptosis, hypotonia, hypotension	Increased CSF L-dopa and HVA	Man in't Veld et al. (1987)
Monoamine oxidase defect (X-linked)	Monoamine oxidase A	Behavioural disturbances, mental retardation	Low urinary excretion of HVA and 5-HIAA	Abeling et al. (1994)
II—Nonketotic hyperglycinaemia	Glycine cleavage system	Hypotonia, myoclonus. EEG: 'burst–suppression'/hypsarrhythmia. Microcephaly, mental retardation	Increased CSF/plasma glycine ratio. Enzyme assay (liver)	Hayasaka et al. (1987)
III—GABA disorders				
4-Hydroxybutyric aciduria	Succinic semialdehyde dehydrogenase	Ataxia, hypotonia, speech retardation, mental retardation	Increased 4-hydroxybutyrate and succinic semialdehyde (urine), increased CSF GABA. Enzyme assay (lymphocytes)	Jakobs et al. (1993)
Pyridoxine dependency	Glutamic acid dehydrogenase?	Seizures (onset neonatal to 1.5y)	Responsiveness to pyridoxine (50–200 mg i.v.) during EEG monitoring	Baxter et al. (1996)
GABA transaminase	GABA transaminase	Severe mental retardation, hypotonia, excessive growth	High CSF and plasma GABA levels. Increased plasma growth hormone level. Enzyme assay (lymphocytes)	Jaeken et al. (1984b)
Homocarnosinosis		Spastic paraplegia, mental retardation, retinal pigmentation	High CSF homocarnosine	Sjaastad et al. (1976)
Hereditary hyperekplexia (Startle disease)	Glycine receptor α1 subunit mutation with high affinity for GABA	Exaggerated startle reflex, hypertonia, apnoea	Low free GABA levels in CSF	Berthier et al. (1995)

*DHPR = dihydropteridine reductase.

administration of pyridoxine. It is transmitted as an autosomal recessive character.

The disease is thought to result from an abnormality of the glutamate-decarboxylase (GAD) apoenzyme (Kaufman et al. 1987) preventing correct binding with its coenzyme, pyridoxal-5-phosphate, the activated form of pyridoxine (vitamin B₆). GAD is the rate-limiting enzyme in the synthesis of GABA, a major inhibitory neurotransmitter whose deficiency is responsible for the syndrome.

The typical clinical presentation of pyridoxine dependency is usually with neonatal seizures that occur repetitively and lead to death or to brain damage (Gordon 1997). Intrauterine convulsions from the fifth month onwards have been reported

(Haenggeli et al. 1991). Frequently associated features include irritability, screaming, jitteriness, feeding difficulties, distended abdomen, hypotonia, dystonia and hepatomegaly (Baxter et al. 1996). Death occurs on average at 3.5 months (Haenggeli et al. 1991). Atypical, late-onset forms can begin at up to 18 months of age (Bankier et al. 1983, Goutières and Aicardi 1985). Any type of seizures, including infantile spasms (Bankier et al. 1983) and myoclonic attacks (Krishnamoorthy 1983) can be observed.

The diagnosis rests entirely on the intravenous administration of pyridoxine at doses of 40–300mg which immediately stop the seizures. Caution should be exerted during administration as hypotonia and apnoea with flattening of the EEG have been reported (Kroll 1985, Mikati et al. 1991).

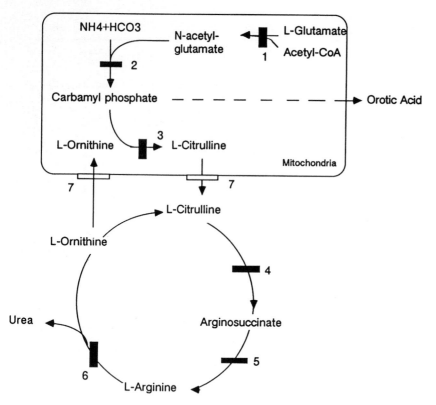

Fig. 9.22. The urea cycle, indicating site of each inherited enzyme defect.
   Key: 1 = *N*-acetylglutamate synthetase (NAGS); 2 = carbamyl phosphate synthetase (CPS); 3 = ornithine trancarbamylase (OTC); 4 = argininosuccinate synthetase (ASS); 5 = argininosuccinate lyase (ASL); 6 = arginase; 7 = intramitochondrial transport defect (HHH syndrome).

Therapy should be maintained indefinitely. Prenatal oral administration of pyridoxine to women who have had an affected child may be indicated in the second half of pregnancy. Relapses following discontinuation of pyridoxine usually supervene in less than 10 days. In some cases, especially late-onset ones, relapses can occur only after several weeks or even months, and a partial response to antiepileptic agents may be seen. Although neuro-imaging generally gives normal results, abnormalities of the white matter, polymicrogyria and hydrocephalus have been reported (Jardim *et al.* 1994, Baxter *et al.* 1996). Baumeister *et al.* (1994) have suggested that the dose of pyridoxine that controls seizures does not lower levels of glutamate in CSF to normal values, and persistently high glutamate levels might be responsible for sequelae. They suggest the use of larger doses, which is supported by the clinical experience of Baxter *et al.* (1996) who noted psychological improvement by increasing pyridoxine dosage over the dose that controlled the seizures. Determination of CSF glutamate level is probably indicated to permit adjustment of pyridoxine dose.

OTHER GABA-RELATED DISORDERS
GABA transaminase deficiency, homocarnosinosis and *hyperekplexia* are other GABA-related disorders which have been described in a few patients but have not been fully investigated (Table 9.7).

UREA CYCLE DISORDERS

Patients with urea cycle disorders (UCDs) can present from birth to adulthood with symptoms depending on the degree of the enzyme defect. Hyperammonaemia, the common biological hallmark, clearly has a toxic effect on the CNS. At any age, hyperammonaemia may be responsible for acute toxicity, which can be fatal or result in severe CNS sequelae. In less severe forms, mild and chronic hyperammonaemia may lead to cerebral impairment (Batshaw 1994, Brusilow and Horwich 1995, Leonard 1995, Brusilow and Maestri 1996).

BIOCHEMICAL BACKGROUND AND METABOLIC CONSEQUENCES
The urea cycle subserves the incorporation of nitrogen not used for protein synthesis, into urea, the waste nitrogen substrate in mammals. The complete cycle—illustrated in Figure 9.22—is localized in the liver, which alone contains the first three required enzymes. The following steps are expressed both in liver and in other tissues. The urea cycle is also part of the biochemical route for *de novo* arginine synthesis. Hereditary disorders have been described at each enzymatic step. In addition, a defect of ornithine transport across the mitochondrial membrane causes the HHH syndrome (*h*yperammonaemia, *h*yperornithinaemia, *h*omocitrullinuria). In lysinuric protein intolerance, disturbed

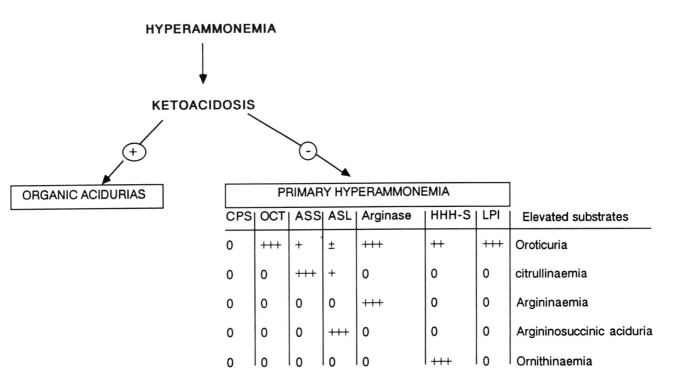

Fig. 9.23. Flow diagram illustrating the diagnosis of hyperammonaemia.
Key: 0 = absent; ± = not always present; + = present (low concentration); ++ = present (moderate concentration); +++ = present (high concentration). LPI = lysinuric protein intolerance; HHH-S = HHH syndrome. (See Fig. 9.22 for other abbreviations).

transport of dibasic amino acids (lysine, arginine, ornithine) across the cell membrane results in urea cycle disruption.

In UCDs, the major biochemical finding is hyperammonaemia. Figure 9.23 outlines the diagnostic approach, which is based on determination of the acid-base status, plasma and urinary amino acids, and oroticuria. In the case of carbamylphosphate accumulation (ornithine carbamyltransferase (OCT) deficiency, lysinuric protein intolerance, HHH syndrome) or overproduction (hyperargininaemia), orotic acid is produced through activated cytosolic pyrimidine synthesis. Definitive diagnosis requires enzymatic assays in appropriate tissues.

GENETIC BACKGROUND

The *OCT* gene is located on the X chromosome. Female heterozygotes have a mosaic of normal and affected liver cells and may present various clinical manifestations from the asymptomatic state to severe chronic symptomatology and unexpected acute metabolic crises occurring at any age. For genetic counselling, screening for carriers is essential. Heterozygotes can be detected by protein load or allopurinol test and by molecular genetic techniques. All the other UCDs are inherited in an autosomal recessive mode.

For fetuses at risk, antenatal diagnosis is available by several methods specific for each disease, including amino acid measurement in amniotic fluid, and enzymatic assays in amniocytes, fetal liver biopsy and fetal red blood cells. Only OCT deficiency can be diagnosed using molecular biology (Kamoun *et al.* 1995).

NEUROPATHOLOGY

Most autopsy studies have been on newborn infants with advanced disease. Cerebral oedema and uncal herniation, with histopathological changes such as cortical neuronal loss, spongiosis or cavitation, may result from episodes of hypotension or cardiac arrest. Alzheimer II cells are a more specific feature, probably correlated with the stage of the disease and/or level of hyperammonaemia. Rare reports of hypomyelination, cerebellar heterotopias and cortico-subcortical cystic necrosis due to infarction may reflect antenatal CNS damage (Harding *et al.* 1984, Filloux *et al.* 1986).

PATHOPHYSIOLOGY

Ammonia appears to be the major cause of the acute encephalopathy. Isolated hyperammonaemia experimentally induced in primates reproduces all the clinical, biological, neurophysiological and neuropathological changes that occur in hyperammonaemic patients. Neurological symptoms appear to be secondary to swelling of astrocytes, responsible for cerebral oedema and alteration of cerebral blood flow, which in turn could explain most of the reported biochemical abnormalities. Astrocyte swelling is thought to be due to the intracellular osmotic effect of glutamine, whose concentration increases during experimental hyperammonaemia. Some manifestations of chronic hyperammonaemia such as anorexia, vomiting and sleep disturbances might be due to increased brain uptake of tryptophan and thus increased brain serotonin turnover. The latter may also be produced by benzoate, which is used for alternative waste nitrogen excretion in patients. This toxic effect could theoretically be reversed by selective serotonin 2-receptor antagonists or with controlled tryptophan intake.

Neurotoxic effects of the other accumulated metabolites such as citrulline and argininosuccinate are still in debate. Arginase deficiency is a disorder characterized by progressive paresis and accumulation of arginine and guanidine compounds which are potential neurotoxins (Marescau *et al.* 1990).

CLINICAL MANIFESTATIONS
NEONATAL-ONSET FORMS
The majority of patients present with symptoms in the neonatal period. Every UCD may be expressed in the newborn infant, but severe neonatal-onset forms are commonly due to OCT or carbamylphosphate synthetase deficiencies, or to citrullinaemia or argininosuccinic aciduria. The most important diagnostic features in neonates are vomiting, hypotonia, lethargy progressing to coma, and seizures developing within hours or days after a symptom-free period of 24 hours or more. Severe hyperammonaemia (>700 µmol/L) and respiratory alkalosis are the characteristic biological signs leading to specific biochemical investigations: amino acid chromatography and urinary orotate levels (see Fig. 9.23). Severe CNS depression and cardiorespiratory failure result in death. Neuroimaging reveals cerebral oedema. Affected infants have a poor neurological outcome even if rapidly treated, but medical care should be continued while a precise diagnosis is made—with exclusion of the rare transient hyperammonaemia of the newborn infant (Hudak *et al.* 1985)—to facilitate genetic counselling.

LATE-ONSET FORMS
An increasing number of patients are diagnosed later in childhood or even in adulthood. Whatever the defect, most of the clinical symptomatology is secondary to hyperammonaemia, but some additional signs may indicate specific disorders.

Symptomatology common to all forms of hyperammonaemia
Acute hyperammonaemia may be responsible for variously associated signs such as episodes of lethargy and ataxia, coma with infrequent seizures, recurrent vomiting or altered mental state manifested by irritability, combativeness, agitation, incoherent speech and confusion. Such episodes are often associated with high protein intake or intercurrent infections, although not infrequently there is no overt cause. Mild crises abate with cessation of protein intake. Severe or persistent hyperammonaemia can be responsible for severe cerebral oedema, which can progress to diffuse or localized cortical or subcortical atrophy and diffuse grey and white matter hypodensity. One patient affected with a late-onset form of OTC deficiency presented with an unusual neurological course due to central pontine myelinolysis (Mattson *et al.* 1995), and we are aware of a second similar case (G. Mitchell, personal communication 1997). These features can to some extent be reversible, and their severity is usually correlated with the duration of hyperammonaemic coma. Acute manifestations often

lead to the misdiagnosis of encephalitis, cerebral tumour or vascular accident. Hepatomegaly and hepatic failure are frequent, and Reye-like syndrome or drug toxicity are often discussed. Chronic hyperammonaemia may result in protein avoidance, anorexia, vomiting and failure to thrive, mimicking various food intolerances. Hyperactivity, nocturnal episodes of restlessness, destructive behaviour and progressive mental retardation are often misdiagnosed as psychiatric problems.

In both acute and chronic forms, the diagnosis is based on plasma ammonia levels. Marked hyperammonaemia accompanies acute episodes. In milder forms, ammonaemia levels may be normal after an overnight fast, so that determinations should be made following protein intake.

Specific clinical signs
Argininosuccinic aciduria and some cases of *citrullinaemia* may present with brittle hair, trichorrhexis nodosa and prominent hepatomegaly. In *arginase deficiency* the major features include early progressive spastic diplegia predominating in the lower limbs, associated with loss of mental skills. Seizures, ataxia and athetosis can be additional signs. This progressive neurological impairment is often accompanied by minor signs of chronic hyperammonaemia, while acute episodes of metabolic decompensation are rarely noted (Antonozzi and Leuzzi 1987, Brockstedt *et al.* 1990). *HHH syndrome* may present in the neonatal period or late in childhood with mild symptoms of hyperammonaemia associated with muscle hypotonia. Progressive spastic paresis commonly develops during adolescence (Shih 1995). Mental development varies widely from normal intelligence to severe retardation. *Lysinuric protein intolerance* presents in infants with anorexia, recurrent vomiting, lethargy, growth failure, muscular hypotonia, hepatosplenomegaly, pancytopenia and osteoporosis. Drowsiness or coma often result from forced feeding with high-protein foods.

TREATMENT
Neonatal-onset forms and some acute cases of decompensation require rapid exogenous detoxification procedures (Ogier de Baulny and Saudubray 1995). Long-term therapy aims at limiting the endogenous and exogenous nitrogen load, supplying deficient metabolites (*e.g.* citrulline, arginine, ornithine, aspartate), and increasing the disposal of nitrogen by means other than urea formation.

Nitrogen load is reduced by restricting protein intake and reversing catabolic situations. Disposal of ammonia by means of benzoate and phenylacetate, which conjugate respectively with endogenous glycine and glutamine, helps eliminate waste nitrogen as hippurate and phenylacetylglutamine. Because arginine becomes an indispensable amino acid for patients affected with UCD, supplemental arginine is needed for all but hyperargininaemia patients. Arginine supplementation represents the basic treatment of argininosuccinic aciduria. In hyperargininaemia, arginine intake needs to be kept low to control the production of toxic guanidine compounds (Lambert *et al.* 1991). The rare patients with *N*-acetylglutamate synthetase deficiency and some patients with partial carbamylphosphate synthetase deficiency may be effectively treated with *N*-carbamylglutamate supplementation.

Therapy has to be tailored to the specific UCD, and each individual patient must be evaluated for metabolic profile before an optimal therapy can be instituted. Despite careful management, liver transplantation may represent the only available therapeutic approach for children with severe recurrent acute decompensation.

DISORDERS OF VITAMIN METABOLISM

The main vitamin disorders with neurological presentations are outlined in Table 9.8 (overleaf).

BIOTIN METABOLISM: MULTICARBOXYLASE DEFICIENCY

Defects in biotin metabolism responsible for multicarboxylase deficiency (MCD) result in severe neurological impairment with hyperlactataemia. Because they are treatable with megadoses of biotin, early diagnosis is of importance. Skin rashes, alopecia and breathing problems are hallmark manifestations. However, they are inconstant and the diagnosis should be considered in any case of hyperlactataemia (Baumgartner and Suormala 1995, Wolf 1995).

BIOCHEMICAL AND GENETIC BACKGROUND
Biotin acts as a cofactor in four carboxylases in humans: acetyl-CoA carboxylase, propionyl-CoA carboxylase, beta-methyl-crotonyl-CoA carboxylase and pyruvate carboxylase (Fig. 9.24). Isolated defects are known for the last three enzymes (see p. 228). Two defects in the intracellular utilization of biotin are responsible for MCD: *holocarboxylase synthetase (HCS) deficiency* is a disorder of biotinylation of apocarboxylases; and *biotinidase deficiency* is a disorder of biotin recycling. MCD leads to a characteristic organic aciduria comprising lactate, methylcrotonyl-glycine and propionyl-CoA derivatives. Enzyme defects are demonstrable in leukocytes or cultured fibroblasts, and biotinidase activity can be determined in serum. Prenatal diagnosis of these two autosomal recessive disorders is feasible. cDNA for both biotinidase and HCS have been characterized, and disease-causing mutations recognized. The genes for biotinidase and HCS map to chromosomes 3p25 and 21q22.1 respectively (Aoki *et al.* 1995, Pomponio *et al.* 1995).

PATHOPHYSIOLOGY
The pathogenesis of neurological involvement is not clear. Brain energy deficit due to pyruvate carboxylase dysfunction and diverse toxic effects of organic acid accumulation are two potential mechanisms common to both biotinidase and HCS deficiencies. In biotinidase deficiency, impairment of the biotin recycling pathway may be responsible for early biotin deprivation in the CNS, which may explain why neurological impairment is more severe in biotinidase deficiency than in HCS deficiency (Baumgartner *et al.* 1989, Duran *et al.* 1993).

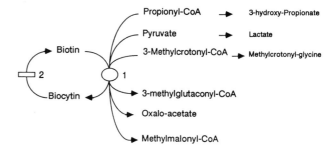

Fig. 9.24. Enzymatic blocks involved in multiple carboxylase defect. Apocarboxylases are propionyl-CoA carboxylase, pyruvate carboxylase and β-methylcrotonyl-CoA carboxylase.
Key: 1 = holocarboxylase synthetase; 2 = biotinidase.

CLINICAL FEATURES
MCD is characterized by neurological symptoms, skin rashes and ketoacidosis, occurring either in the neonatal period or later in infancy or childhood. Although there is an overlap in the age of onset, most neonatal forms are due to HCS deficiency, and the late-onset forms to biotinidase deficiency. The neonatal forms share clinical and biological features with neonatal-onset forms of other organic acidurias (see p. 228). The late-onset forms may present with either acute or insidious manifestations. In acute-onset forms, progressive lethargy with hypotonia and ataxia occurs following intercurrent infections. Refractory seizures are the most common manifestation and can remain isolated for long periods (Wolf 1995). Erythematous rashes, alopecia, conjunctivitis or blepharitis may be present at any time in the course, which is progressive even though transient recovery may occur. Chronic forms present with either a steady progression or a series of acute accidents separated by periods of apparent normality. The most common neurological features are unsteady gait, episodes of ataxia, hypotonia and developmental regression. Tonic–clonic or myoclonic seizures or abnormal movements may develop at any time. Respiratory problems with recurrent infections, unexplained episodes of tachypnoea or recurrent stridor may suggest Leigh syndrome.

Biochemical diagnosis is easy when lactic acidosis is associated with specific organic aciduria. Mild intellectual impairment, persistent ataxia, optic atrophy, abnormal visual evoked potentials, retinal impairment and sensorineural hearing loss may persist despite treatment, especially in biotinidase deficiency patients. CT and MRI studies may be normal or show some cerebral oedema and cortical atrophy. Basal ganglia calcification has been noted, and basal ganglia hypodensities compatible with Leigh syndrome may occur after several months of neurological deterioration. Autopsy may show pathological features of Leigh syndrome and many other signs usually encountered in other organic acidurias (Hanavar *et al.* 1992, Wolf 1995).

TREATMENT
Megadoses of oral biotin reverse all the clinical and biological signs within a few days. Biotin requirement is usually around 5–10 mg/d. However, some patients with severe HCS deficiency

TABLE 9.8

Inborn errors	Enzyme deficiency	Possible neurological signs	Other features	Diagnostic tests
Multiple carboxylase	Holocarboxylase deficiency (neonatal-onset form). Biotinidase deficiency (late-onset form)	Episodes of coma or progressive encephalopathy (Leigh), ataxia, basal calcification, sensorineural deafness, optic atrophy	Skin rashes, alopecia, conjunctivitis	Ketoacidosis + lactic acidosis; organic aciduria; response to biotin; serum biotinidase; holocarboxylase assay in leukocytes/fibroblasts
Vitamin B$_{12}$				
Absorption defects	Intrinsic factor deficiency. R-binding protein deficiency	Developmental retardation, subacute combined degeneration	Megaloblastic anaemia, gastrointestinal disorders, failure to thrive	Low serum cobalamin; methylmalonic aciduria and homocystinuria; Shilling test; intrinsic factor/transcobalamin II assays
Immerslund–Gräsbeck syndrome	Unknown			
Transport defect	Transcobalamin II deficiency			
Intracellular metabolism				
CblA, CblB	Adenosylcobalamin synthesis defect	cf. Methylmalonic aciduria		Methylmalonic aciduria
CblC, CblD, CblF	Adenosyl + methylcobalamin synthesis defect	Developmental delay, seizures, microcephaly, retinopathy, dementia (in older patients)	Anaemia (macrocytic), multivisceral disorders (early onset)	Methylmalonic aciduria and homocystinuria; hypomethioninaemia
CblE, CblG	Methylcobalamin synthetase defect	Idem + subacute combined degeneration of the cord	Anaemia (macrocytic)	Homocystinuria, hypomethioninaemia
Folates				
Malabsorption	Specific protein-carrier defect	Mental retardation, seizures, ataxia, athetosis, peripheral neuropathy, cerebral calcification	Anaemia (macrocytic), failure to thrive	Homocystinuria; low folate levels (serum erythrocytes, CSF)
Homocystinuria 'variant'	Methylenetetrahydrofolate	Mental retardation, seizures, microcephaly, psychosis	Thrombosis	Homocystinuria + hypomethioninaemia
Pyridoxine dependency	Unknown (glutamic acid dehydrogenase?)	Seizures (onset neonatal to 1 year)		Therapeutic response to pyridoxine (50–200 mg i.v. during EEG monitoring)
Vitamin E (Muller et al. 1983)	Selective malabsorption? (Harding et al. 1985) Secondary malabsorption (Muller et al. 1985)	Peripheral neuropathy, myopathy, ataxia	Retinopathy	Low serum levels of vitamin E
Hartnup disease (Jonas and Butler 1989)	Intestinal and renal neutral amino acid transport	Ataxia, psychosis, lethargy; usually asymptomatic	Eczema	Aminoaciduria; response to nicotinamide therapy (50 mg/d)

may require restriction of protein intake and higher doses of biotin (Baumgartner and Suormala 1995).

VITAMIN B$_{12}$ METABOLISM DISORDERS

The description of inherited disorders at each step of the vitamin B$_{12}$ (cobalamin) metabolic pathway has allowed new insights into the pathogenesis of both cobalamin and folate deficiencies (Hall 1990). Clinical features are broadly similar for all inborn errors of cobalamin metabolism, with the exception of isolated adenosylcobalamin deficiency whose expression is identical to methylmalonic aciduria (see p. 228) (Stabler et al. 1990, Fenton and Rosenberg 1995, Linnell and Bhatt 1995).

BIOCHEMICAL BACKGROUND

The term cobalamin designates a group of compounds which function as coenzymes in two cellular reactions in humans: the generation of methionine from homocysteine with methyl-

cobalamin as coenzyme; and the conversion of methylmalonyl-CoA to succinyl-CoA using adenosylcobalamin as coenzyme. Dietary cobalamin, mostly obtained from animal proteins, is absorbed bound to intrinsic factor, then enters the blood flow bound to transcobalamin-II to be taken up by cells via a specific surface recognition site. Once within the cell, cobalamin undergoes a series of modifications resulting in methylcobalamin and adenosylcobalamin. Deficiencies of cobalamin can be classified into four groups: children born to mothers deficient in cobalamin; deficiency in the cobalamin absorption system; defective transport of the vitamin; and disorders of intracellular utilization. The fourth group correspond to a series of complementation groups designated CblA to CblG, each related to specific enzymatic blocks in intracellular metabolism. Depending on the site of the enzymatic defect, affected patients display methylmalonic aciduria or homocystinuria or a combination of both, as summarized in Figure 9.25. Plasma levels of cobalamin are always in

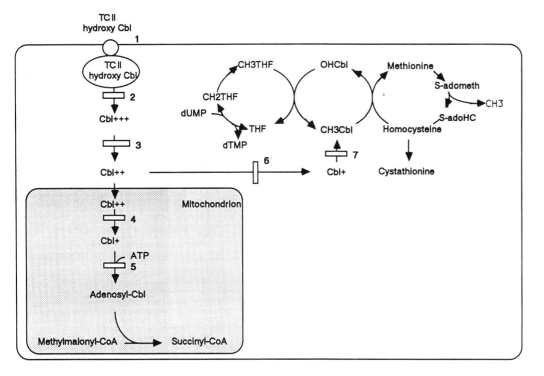

Fig. 9.25. Intracellular metabolism of cobalamin (Cbl).

Key: TC = transcobalamin; ATP = adenine triphosphate; THF = tetrahydrofolate; d-UMP = d-uridine monophosphate; d-TMP = d-thymidine monophosphate; S-adometh = *S*-adenosylmethionine; S-adoHC = *S*-adenosylhomocysteine.

TC II deficiency (1), ClbF (2) and CblC or CblD (3) impair both adenosyl- and methyl-Cbl cofactor synthesis, resulting in combined methylmalonic aciduria and homocystinuria associated with hypomethioninaemia. CblA (4) and ClbB (5) impair only adenosyl-Cbl synthesis, resulting in isolated methylmalonic aciduria. CblE (6) and CblG (7) impair only methyl-Cbl synthesis, resulting in homocystinuria and hypomethioninaemia. (CblA, B, C, D, E, F and G are the different complementation groups of methylmalonic acidurias: see text.)

the normal range in intracellular defective cobalamin metabolism as well as in transcobalamin II defect. Conversely, they are low in congenital B$_{12}$ deficiency and in absorption defects.

GENETIC BACKGROUND
All defects of intracellular cobalamin metabolism are inherited in an autosomal recessive manner. Prenatal diagnosis can be performed by assaying amniotic fluid for amino acids and organic acids. Futher confirmation can be obtained by measuring appropriate enzymes in chorionic villus samples (Parvy *et al.* 1995).

PATHOPHYSIOLOGY
Many neurological, haematological and biochemical features are common to acquired cobalamin and folate deficiencies, to congenital defects in absorption or transport of cobalamin and folate, and to intracellular defects in cobalamin and folate metabolism. All defects result in deficiency in methionine synthetase which plays a central role in the pathogenesis of both cobalamin and folate metabolism disturbances (Hall 1990, Weir and Scott 1995). Methionine synthetase deficiency has several putative secondary effects including the storage of folates as methyltetrahydrofolate (CH$_3$THF) (folate trap theory), thus preventing their use in folate coenzyme synthesis which appears essential for DNA

synthesis and haematopoiesis. Methionine synthetase deficiency also results in defective synthesis of methionine and of adenosyl-methionine, which is the main methyl donor for methylation of many substrates such as neurotransmitters, myelin basic protein and phospholipids of plasma membranes. This defective methylation is thought to be the cause of *subacute combined degeneration of the cord* described in both acquired and congenital defects. Other factors may disturb the structure and function of the CNS in acquired and congenitally impaired cobalamin metabolism, *e.g.* toxicity of accumulated homocysteine which may be responsible for vascular injury and thromboembolism (see p. 275), and for the accumulation of methylmalonyl-CoA and propionyl-CoA due to defective mutase activity (see p. 228).

CLINICAL FEATURES
Congenital vitamin B$_{12}$ deficiency
Vitamin B$_{12}$ deficiency in breast-fed infants of mothers who have subclinical pernicious anaemia or who are on a vegan diet without adequate B$_{12}$ supplementation may result in neurological regression, abnormal movements and coma associated with megaloblastic anaemia. Vitamin B$_{12}$ administration rapidly improves the neurological status, but further developmental progress may remain delayed (Graham *et al.* 1992; see Chapter 23).

Cobalamin absorption and transport deficiencies

Defects in cobalamin absorption and transport are responsible for a cobalamin deficiency syndrome characterized by a progressive disease with onset from 1 month to a few years of age. Usually the first symptoms are gastrointestinal, with failure to thrive, muscular weakness, drowsiness and megaloblastic anaemia. A few months later, peripheral neuropathy, myelopathy and encephalopathy develop, with marked developmental delay. Defects in absorption are due either to intrinsic factor deficiency or to selective malabsorption (Immerslund–Grasbeck syndrome). Defective transport is essentially due to transcobalamin II deficiency which may, despite treatment, lead to severe neurological impairment (Monagle and Tauro 1995).

Defects in intracellular metabolism

Intracellular cobalamin deficiencies impairing the synthesis of methylcobalamin alone (CblE/G/F) or of both methyl- and adenosylcobalamin (CblC/D) present with three main types. The most frequent is a severe early-onset form described in newborn babies and young infants below 3 months of age. These show progressive lethargy, hypotonia, abnormal movements, and/or seizures associated with pancytopenia and megaloblastic anaemia. Some patients also have multisystemic involvement including renal failure with haemolytic uraemic syndrome, cardiomyopathy and interstitial pneumonia. Retinal involvement with granular dyspigmentation of the macula and further peripheral pigmentary retinitis is an early sign in many CblC patients. Communicating hydrocephalus can be a further complication (Chenel *et al.* 1993). A small number of patients present, in childhood, with progressive neurological deterioration, microcephaly, episodic seizures and megaloblastic anaemia which usually leads on to the diagnosis. If untreated, acute neurological deterioration may occur with signs and symptoms resembling subacute degeneration of the cord. Rare affected adolescents and adults have presented similar subacute degeneration of the cord preceded by an acute deterioration of intellectual function and, sometimes, behavioural disturbances (Gold *et al.* 1996). In older patients, megaloblastic anaemia may be subtle, and borderline macrocytosis should be viewed with particular attention. CT and MRI studies reveal cerebral atrophy and/or demyelination.

TREATMENT

Responsiveness to cobalamin supplementation must be systematically tested. Depending on the defect implicated, use of parenteral versus oral routes, pharmacological versus minute doses and hydroxycobalamin versus natural cobalamin substrates (methyl-, adenosylcobalamin) should be discussed (Linnell and Bhatt 1995). In both transport and intracellular defects, methionine replenishment with oral betaine could be essential. As predicted by the metabolic pathway of betaine, addition of folic acid could be helpful in long-term betaine therapy (Allen *et al.* 1993). Because endogenous carnitine synthesis depends on methionine, carnitine supplementation could be useful in these conditions of methionine synthesis impairment. Dietary protein restriction and adjuvants such as pyridoxine and folinic acid have no logical support.

DEFECTS IN FOLATE METABOLISM

Folate metabolism is complex and still incompletely known. Two inherited disorders are well recognized. One involves the intestinal transport of the vitamin and probably represents the sole situation in which pure folate deficiency occurs. The second disease, CH_2THF reductase deficiency involves intracellular folate–coenzyme interconversion. Both disorders are inherited as autosomal recessive traits. A third defect, glutamate formiminotransferase deficiency, may result in severe CNS involvement. The existence of other suspected disorders, such as inherited dihydrofolate reductase deficiency, has not been proved (Rosenblatt 1995, Zittoun 1995).

BIOCHEMICAL AND GENETIC BACKGROUND

Folates are derived from a parent compound, folic acid. Dietary folates are transported inside the intestinal cells by a specific carrier system, then transfered into the circulation, mainly in the form of CH_3THF. Circulating CH_3THF enters the tissues through a high-affinity carrier linked to intracellular methionine synthetase activity, which generates tetrahydrofolate (THF). Within the cell, a series of reactions (Fig. 9.26) lead to the formation of the various folate coenzymes that constitute the donors or acceptors of single carbon units required for several metabolic processes. Hereditary defect in the specific folate receptor impairs both intestinal absorption and CNS uptake, resulting in low levels of folates in serum and CSF and secondary deficiencies in folate-dependent reactions. Purine and pyrimidine synthesis defect result in megaloblastic anaemia; deficiency in glutamate formiminotransferase explains forminimoglutamic acid (FIGLU) excretion; and defective methionine synthesis is responsible for combined homocystinuria and hypomethioninaemia. Glutamate formiminotransferase and formimino-THF-cyclodeaminase activities are performed by a single protein, whose defect results in histidine catabolism deficiency with urinary excretion of FIGLU without involvement of crucial folate-coenzymes which may be supplied by dietary sources. CH_2THF reductase deficiency leads to defective synthesis of CH_3THF, the methyl donor for methionine synthesis from homocysteine, resulting in combined homocystinuria and hypomethioninaemia. Megaloblastic anaemia is usually absent because normal amounts of CH_2THF, the coenzyme of thymidylate synthase, permits a normal biosynthesis of DNA. The gene of CH_2THF reductase has been isolated, and various mutations responsible for the severe form of CH_2THF reductase deficiency have been described (Goyette *et al.* 1995). Antenatal diagnosis can be made by measuring CH_2THF reductase activity in chorionic villus samples (Marquet *et al.* 1994). A common polymorphism, which confers thermolability to the reductase, is associated with significantly increased risk for neural tube defect (van der Put *et al.* 1995, Whitehead *et al.* 1995) and cardiovascular disease (Kluijtmans 1996).

The two main identified disorders involve the interrelation between folate and cobalamin metabolisms, and most of the

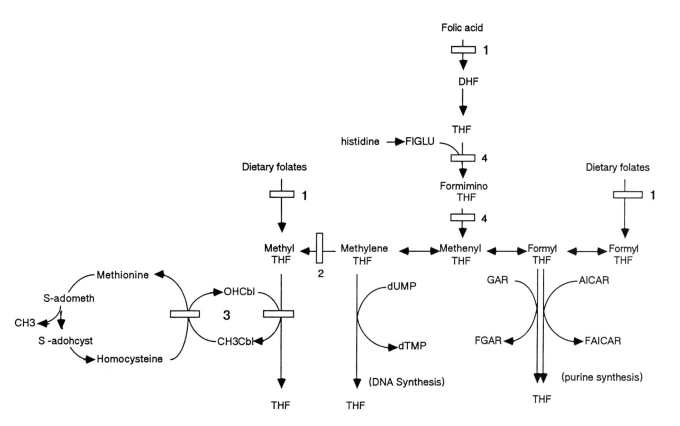

Fig. 9.26. Major metabolic interconversions of folates.

Vertical reactions depict the main route of formation of tetrahydrofolate (THF) and attachment of a single carbon unit to THF. Horizontal reactions represent the interconversion of the various THF derivatives: below these are the biosynthetic reactions that regenerate THF, which can then be recycled.

Key: DHF = dihydrofolate; FIGLU = formiminoglutamate; GAR = glycinamide ribonucleotide; FGAR = formylglycinamide ribonucleotide; AICAR = aminoimidazole-carboxamide ribonucleotide; FAICAR = formiminoimidazole-carboxamide ribonucleotide. (See Fig. 9.25 for other abbreviations.)

1 = congenital malabsorption defect; 2 = CH₂THF reductase; 3 = methionine synthetase; 4 = glutamate formiminotransferase and formimino-THF cyclodeaminase.

pathogenic theories described in relation to cobalamin deficiency also apply (Hall 1990, Weir and Scott 1995).

CLINICAL FEATURES
Methylenetetrahydrofolate reductase deficiency
Patients present with many neurological signs and symptoms similar to those described in intracellular cobalamin defects involving methionine synthase. However, they do not have megaloblastic anaemia. In the neonatal-onset form, multiorgan involvement and retinopathy have not been described. Onset in childhood, with progressive neurological deterioration, is the most frequent. A period of a few months normal development is followed by several months to several years of developmental slowing or arrest with poor head growth. Episodic seizures of various types are the rule. Hypotonia, ataxic gait and extrapyramidal movements are encountered in a few patients. In the absence of effective treatment, a third period of rapidly progressive deterioration follows with unexplained bouts of apathy, lethargy or coma often accompanied by central respiratory failure leading to death. Preceding or following these attacks, the neurological signs worsen with further mental deterioration, gait disturbances, muscular weakness, spastic paresis and sometimes extrapyramidal

symptoms with parkinsonian rigidity and tremors. In a few young patients the second period is not observed, and they deteriorate abruptly following an acute event such as generalized tonic–clonic seizures. In adolescence and adulthood, many signs are similar to the late stage described above, except that most patients have normal development before the onset, the first sign being rapid mental deterioration and in a very few patients signs of schizophrenia (Pasquier *et al.* 1994, Walk *et al.* 1994). Less commonly, cerebrovascular complications may reveal the disorder (Visy *et al.* 1991). Biological investigations reveal mild homocystinuria and hypomethioninaemia in association with low to normal folate levels. Low CSF neurotransmitter levels have been reported (Haworth *et al.* 1993). CT and MRI reveal nonspecific cortical and subcortical atrophy and periventricular demyelination (Walk *et al.* 1994). Results of neurophysiological investigations are all in accordance with a diffuse process of demyelination (Clayton *et al.* 1986, Haworth *et al.* 1993, Walk *et al.* 1994). The pathological changes in autopsied young infants include dilated cerebral ventricles, internal hydrocephalus, microgyria, demyelination and gliosis (Beckman *et al.* 1987). In some cases, vascular changes resemble those described in 'classic' homocystinuria (Kanwar *et al.* 1976, Wendel *et al.* 1983). In children, the presence of classical findings of subacute combined degeneration of the cord supports the hypothesis of methionine and adenosylmethionine deficiencies in the genesis of neurological changes (Surtees *et al.* 1991).

Hereditary folate malabsorption
Congenital folate malabsorption presents in infants below 1 month of age with severe megaloblastic anaemia, diarrhoea, failure to thrive, and progressive neurological deterioration with convulsions. The diagnosis is based on low levels of folate in serum, red blood cells and CSF, with undetectable amounts of CH3THF. Oral or intramuscular folic acid, folinic acid or methylfolate supplementation usually leads to haematological and general improvement, with normalization of serum folate content but inconstant correction in CSF. Some patients have remained mentally retarded with variously combined neurological signs such as recurrent seizures, ataxia, athetosis and peripheral neuropathy. Calcification affecting the parietal cortex and basal ganglia has been reported (Wevers *et al.* 1994, Zittoun 1995).

Glutamate formiminotransferase deficiency
The clinical expression of this disorder is variable (Zittoun 1995). In type I, mental retardation, hypotonia, abnormal EEG, and cortical atrophy are reported in half the cases, in association with folate-responsive megaloblastic anaemia. These features appear between the ages of 2 weeks and 18 months. In type II, mental retardation and neurological abnormalities are absent or mild, with only speech defect present. There is no evidence of folate deficiency, and the biochemical hallmark is spontaneously high excretion of FIGLU.

TREATMENT
Supplementation with different forms of folate must be systematically tested with either oral or intramuscular administration. Addition of methionine or betaine may benefit patients whose CSF abnormalities are not normalized by folate supplementation. Their administration may be the only available means to correct methionine levels in CNS and to prevent further neurological deterioration (Surtees *et al.* 1991, Walk *et al.* 1994).

LACTIC ACIDOSIS

RESPIRATORY CHAIN DISORDERS
Respiratory chain disorders constitute an increasingly recognized group of diseases with extremely variable clinical, biochemical and neuropathological presentations (DiMauro and Moraes 1993, Shoffner and Wallace 1994, Grossman 1995, Jackson *et al.* 1995, Brown and Squier 1996, Tein 1996).

Ragged red fibres are a histological hallmark and are usually associated with mitochondrial ultrastructural alterations. However, they are not specific for primary respiratory chain defect and may be present in other diseases. They are inconstantly found in true primary respiratory chain disorders, and they do not characterize a specific defect within the respiratory chain.

There is a striking clinical and biological heterogeneity among this group of disorders. Clinical presentations include infantile lactic acidosis with failure to thrive, progressive external ophthalmoplegia (PEO), proximal myopathy and multisystem neurological syndromes mainly affecting the CNS, with seizures, ataxia, dementia, movement disorders and stroke-like episodes. Short stature, retinopathy, deafness, peripheral neuropathy, cardiac conduction defects, cardiomyopathy, renal and endocrine dysfunction, and diabetes associated with deafness also occur. *In vitro* studies of mitochondrial metabolism using polarography, enzymatic assays, immunoblotting, *in situ* hybridization and DNA analysis have identified a variety of defects without clear correlation with symptoms and signs and the different biochemical lesions. Some authors (*e.g.* Petty *et al.* 1986) consider that mitochondrial disorders may present variably without constituting well-defined syndromes. Others (*e.g.* Pavlakis *et al.* 1984) propose that many can be classified into specific syndromes such as the Kearns–Sayre syndrome, the syndrome of mitochondrial myopathy, encephalopathy, lactic acidosis and stroke-like episodes (MELAS), and that of myoclonic epilepsy with ragged red fibres (MERRF), although many cases remain difficult to classify.

FUNCTIONAL ORGANIZATION OF THE RESPIRATORY CHAIN
The respiratory chain is the terminal step for energy production after metabolic substrates have undergone glycolysis and fatty acid oxidation and then entered the Krebs cycle which produces reduced metabolites (NADH2, FADH2) (Fig. 9.27, p. 292). Respiratory chain enzymes, located to the inner mitochondrial membrane, transfer electrons through an oxidoreductive pathway. This oxygen-consuming process creates an electrochemical gradient across the inner mitochondrial membrane, which in turn supplies the energy required for mitochondrial transport of ions, proteins and substrates, and drives conversion of ADP and phosphate to ATP. The respiratory chain comprises five enzyme complexes, including ubiquinone (CoQ) and cytochrome *c* (cyt-c) (Table 9.9). Each complex is formed by a functional association of different protein subunits and cytochromes whose mutations are responsible for defects of the various complexes.

GENETIC BACKGROUND
Mitochondria are exclusively maternally transmitted and possess their own double-stranded circular DNA molecules (mt-DNA), which replicate with every cell cycle. Sequencing of the human mitochondrial genome has shown that mt-DNA codes for 13 proteins which are components of the mitochondrial respiratory chain, as well as for two ribosomal RNAs and 22 transfer RNAs. Primary point mutations occurring within the mt-genome may be responsible for maternally transmitted disorders, while single deletion or duplication in mt-DNA often appear as sporadic cases. The main phenotypic expressions of mitochondrial deletions or duplications are Kearns–Sayre syndrome, PEO, Pearson syndrome and the syndrome of diabetes mellitus with deafness. Missense point mutations involving genes encoding for protein

TABLE 9.9
Composition and genetic control of the mitochondrial respiratory chain

Respiratory chain complex	Polypeptide subunits and prosthetic groups*	Number of mt-DNA encoded subunits
NADH coenzyme Q reductase (complex I)	42 8 iron-sulfur proteins FMN	7 (ND 1, 2, 3, 4, 4L, 5, 6)
Succinate coenzyme Q (complex II)	4–5 Few iron-sulfur proteins FAD	0
Ubiquinol cytochrome c (cyt-c) reductase (complex III)	11 (cyt-b, cyt-c1) 2 iron-sulfur proteins	1 (cyt-b)
Cyt-c reductase (complex IV)	13 (cyt-a, cyt-a3)	3 (CoI, II, III)
ATP synthase (complex V)	12–14 (adenine)	2 (ATP 6, 8)

*FMN = flavine mononucleotide; FAD = flavine adenine nucleotide.

subunits are responsible for Leber hereditary optic neuropathy which most often involves complex I, and for the NARP syndrome (*n*europathic muscle weakness, *a*taxia, *r*etinitis *p*igmentosa) of which the most severe phenotype is maternally inherited Leigh syndrome. A second group of point mutations affect the tRNA genes and are mainly, but not exlusively, associated with progressive encephalomyopathies such as MERRF and MELAS. Some principles may in part explain the heterogeneity and the progressive course of these disorders. Mixed populations of mutant and wild type mt-DNA (heteroplasmy) segregate during cellular replication into pure populations (homoplasmy). When the mutation is a large deletion, the deleted molecules become enriched over time. Involvement of t-RNA, due to either mitochondrial deletion or t-RNA gene mutations, is responsible for defective mt-DNA translation. Cells will express an mt-DNA mutant phenotype only when the cellular energy level falls below the minimum required for normal function. Table 9.10 (p 291) lists the known mutations, insertions and deletions of mt-DNA and the associated phenotypes.

The nuclear genome encodes for the approximately 50 remaining polypeptides of the respiratory chain, and it is to be expected that many mitochondrial diseases will be due to mutations of nuclear genes. In addition, n-DNA controls polypeptide transport and mt-genome replication, transcription and translation, whose defects could be responsible for multiple mt-DNA deletions and depletions which are either recessively or dominantly transmitted. At least two such defects are associated with clinical disturbances (myopathy or more diffuse diseases): mitochondrial DNA depletion and multiple mitochondrial DNA deletions (DiMauro and Moraes 1993, Grossman 1995, Tein 1996). Except for one nuclear gene encoding for one protein subunit of complex II, none of the nuclear genes have yet been defined (Bourgeron *et al.* 1995). They are undoubtedly involved in many cases as evidenced by *in situ* hybridization studies on skeletal muscle which reveal specific decrease in nuclear encoded subunits (Possekel *et al.* 1995, Lombès *et al.* 1996). These recessively inherited mutations have highly variable phenotypic

expressions with multisystem disorders and various isolated organ involvements due, in part, to the existence of tissue-specific isoforms of nuclear encoded subunits.

BIOLOGICAL FEATURES
Metabolic screening by body fluid analyses and *in vivo* functional tests may be useful in determining mitochondrial dysfunction (Touati *et al.* 1997). Measurements of lactate and pyruvate in plasma, urine and CSF, and of lactate/pyruvate and beta-hydroxybutyrate/acetoacetate ratios (redox ratios) point to disturbances of energy metabolism. Apart from the usual lactaturia, rare patients have abnormal urinary excretion of Krebs-cycle intermediates such as fumarate, malate, alpha-ketoglutarate and succinate or 3-methylglutaconic acid. Carnitine deficiency in serum and muscle may reflect inefficient fatty acid oxidation. MR spectroscopy, by measuring the phosphocreatine/P_i* ratio, indicates ATP-synthesis defect during muscle exercise.

Biochemical investigations may localize more precisely the metabolic block. For this purpose, skeletal muscle biopsy specimens are most often used. However, specific studies can be performed on fibroblasts, blood cells, liver, kidney or brain. Polarographic studies, using a fresh muscle specimen, localize the defect to one or more of the cytochrome complexes. Cytochrome spectra, cytochrome content, and assay of the enzymatic activities allow further elucidation of the defect.

CLINICAL FEATURES
Whatever the defect involved, clinical findings can be grouped under two major headings: myopathic forms and multisystem disorders including encephalopathy. Among the latter group, some cases present as defined neurological disorders such as Kearns–Sayre syndrome, MELAS, MERFF, NARP, Leigh and Alpers diseases. However, not all patients with respiratory chain disease may be so easily categorized and many overlaps between categories have been documented. Moreover, similar clinical

*P_i = inorganic phosphorus.

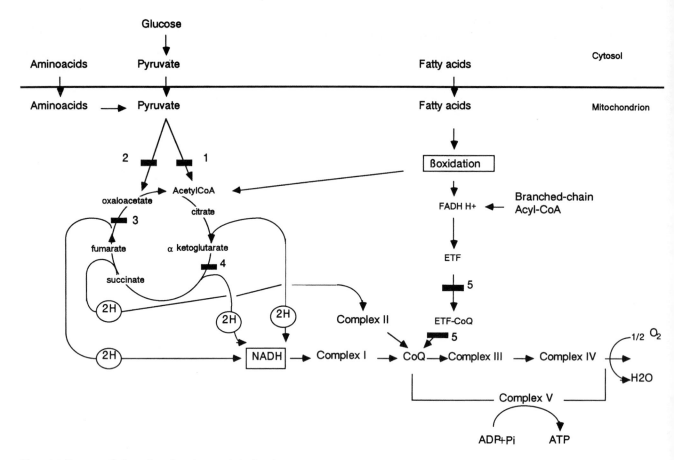

Fig. 9.27. Pyruvate, Krebs cycle and respiratory chain disorders.
Key: 1 = pyruvate dehydrogenase; 2 = pyruvate carboxylase; 3 = fumarase; 4 = α-ketoglutarate dehydrogenase; 5 = electron transfer factor (ETF) and ETF-CoQ dehydrogenase.

presentations can result from mitochondrial disorders not due to respiratory chain abnormalities.

Myopathic forms
Myopathic forms are characterized by progressive weakness of the limbs with variable exertional intolerance, muscle pain, breathlessness, tiredness and nausea. Symptoms may appear within the first two years of life, with hypotonia and delayed motor skills, or later in childhood, adolescence or adulthood. The myopathy may remain isolated or become associated with various additional signs such as PEO and retinopathy. Patients can die from early cardiorespiratory failure or remain stable for years. Lactataemia at rest can be normal or mildly increased. Short aerobic exercises can provoke severe lactic acidosis. Except in very young children, morphological and histochemical abnormalities in biopsied muscle are often characteristic. These isolated myopathic forms are associated with mt-DNA point mutations or with defects in various complexes, complex I and complex III deficiencies being the most frequent. In association with PEO, they may be due to a large deletion of mt-DNA similar to those described in Kearns–Sayre syndrome.

Among this group, *neonatal cytochrome-c-oxidase (complex IV) deficiency* may present with peculiar phenotypes: fatal and benign myopathies both present with severe progressive and generalized

weakness, respiratory distress and lactic acidosis. Patients with the fatal form die of respiratory failure before 1 year of age. Coexistence of a tubulopathy (De Toni–Debré–Fanconi type), cardiomyopathy or liver disease leads to different clinical subtypes. Patients with the benign form improve spontaneously despite initial severe weakness and are usually normal by age 2–3 years.

Multisystem disorders
These involve mainly the CNS and present in the neonatal period or later in childhood, adolescence or even in adulthood.

• *Fatal infantile form.* This features neonatal lactic acidosis with hypotonia, seizures and respiratory distress, and results in death within a few months. As in complex IV deficiency, renal, cardiac and hepatic involvement may be seen. Severe hyperlactataemia is present, while morphological studies of muscle can be normal or reveal a nonspecific lipid–glycogen storage. CT and MRI scans may show cortical and subcortical atrophy and dysmyelination. This syndrome is frequently, but not exclusively, associated with complex I and complex IV deficiencies.

• *Progressive encephalopathy.* Severe encephalopathy may start later in childhood after a period of apparently normal development. Such 'undefined' types can feature various proportions of

TABLE 9.10
Phenotypes commonly associated with some mitochondrial mutations

Phenotypes

Mitochondrial DNA insertion–deletion mutations
KSS
CPEO + other organ involvement
CPEO, isolated
Pearson syndrome
Maternally inherited DM + deafness

	Mutation	Gene
Missense base substitutions		
LHON	nt11778	ND4
	nt3460	ND1
	nt4160	ND1
	nt1448	ND6
	nt7444	COX1
	nt15257	Cyt-b
	(several others)	
LHON + dystonia	nt14459	ND6
NARP/Leigh disease	nt8993	ATP-6 (A6)
MELAS	nt11084	ND4
Base substitutions (impairing mitochondrial protein synthesis)		
MERRF (± cardiomyopathy)	nt8344	tRNA^{Lys}
MERRF/MERRF–MELAS	nt8656	
MELAS/KSS/CPEO/	nt3243	tRNA$^{Leu(UUR)}$
Encephalopathy ± RRF/Myopathy/		
DM + deafness		
MELAS	nt3271	
Cardiomyopathy	nt3303	
Myopathy + cardiomyopathy/	nt3260	
Myopathy + RRF/DM + cataracts +		
Wolff–Parkinson–White syndrome		
Myopathy	nt3302	
	nt3250	
Myopathy (childhood)	nt15990	tRNA^{Prol}
Multisystemic disorder +	nt4269	tRNA^{Ileu}
cardiomyopathy	nt4317	

Key: KSS = Kearns–Sayre syndrome; CPEO = chronic progressive external ophthalmoplegia; DM = diabetes mellitus; LHON = Leber hereditary optic neuropathy; NARP = neuropathy, ataxia and retinitis pigmentosa; MELAS = mitochondrial encephalomyopathy, lactic acidosis and stroke-like episodes; MERRF = myoclonic epilepsy and ragged red fibres; nt = nucleotide; ND = NADH dehydrogenase; ATP = ATP synthase; COX = cytochrome *c* oxidase; Cyt-b = cytochrome b; tRNA = transfer RNA; Lys = lysine; Leu = leucine; Prol = proline; Ileu = isoleucine.

the following manifestations: developmental delay, hypotonia, weakness, ataxia, pyramidal signs, seizures, myoclonia, retinopathy, ptosis, PEO, sensorineural deafness, mild dysmorphism and growth retardation. Plasma lactate levels are mildly elevated or normal. In such cases, high CSF lactate and lactaturia are of great diagnostic value. Some patients present with bouts of drowsiness following intercurrent infections during which high plasma lactate levels and redox ratios may be found. Ragged red fibres are frequently associated with lipid–glycogen storage. CT and MRI scans may be normal or reveal cerebral and/or cerebellar atrophy and bilateral hyperdensity in the basal ganglia or white matter. Altered EMG, nerve conduction velocities and visual or brainstem evoked potentials can be found. Cases have been described with defects in all complexes of the respiratory chain.

• *Subacute necrotizing encephalopathy: Leigh syndrome.* No clear boundaries seem to exist between Leigh syndrome and some of the 'undefined' encephalomyopathies. However, the term refers to a relatively consistent constellation of pathological findings which may be associated with widely variable clinical manifestations and can be determined by several distinct primary or secondary disturbances of energy metabolism. Pyruvate carboxylase and pyruvate dehydrogenase deficiencies were the first defects described, but the syndome appears to be frequently associated with respiratory chain disorders. Rahman *et al.* (1996) studied 67 patients from 56 pedigrees and found enzymatic defects in 29 (13 complex I, 9 complex IV, 7 pyruvate dehydrogenase complex). Eleven patients had mt-DNA mutations at nt 8993. Complex IV deficiency is most frequently reported and seems to be expressed in fibroblasts, opening a way to prenatal diagnosis. Other deficiencies such as of complexes V, III, II and I and biotinidase deficiency (Baumgartner *et al.* 1989) have also been reported with features of Leigh syndrome.

The vast majority of cases are transmitted as an autosomal recessive trait. The form associated with complex V deficiency is due to a point mutation at the nucleotide 8993 of mt-DNA and is maternally inherited: Leigh syndrome represents the most severe clinical phenotype linked to this mt-DNA mutation, while milder forms are expressed as the NARP syndrome.

The *neuropathological changes* involve most consistently the brainstem in a bilateral, roughly symmetrical distribution. The lesions are sharply delineated and cut across grey and white matter with a preponderance in the former. The pathological complex of Leigh syndrome consists of a marked spongiosis involving mainly the neuropil while neurons are relatively preserved. White matter lesions include loss of myelin and, eventually, of axons. An intense capillary proliferation with endothelial swelling is an essential feature (Fig. 9.28). The lesions are typically ischaemic in type but do not correspond to any vascular territory (Cavanagh and Harding 1996).

Lesions of this type characteristically affect the tegmentum of midbrain and pons, the periaqueductal grey matter, the substantia nigra and posterior colliculi, the floor of the fourth ventricle, and the dentate nuclei. Lesions of the basal ganglia, especially the putamen and caudate nucleus, are common. Cortical lesions are only uncommonly severe. Extensive leuko-encephalopathy is found in rare cases (Bourgeois *et al.* 1992, Zafeiriou *et al.* 1995). The mamillary bodies are exceptionally involved, which is important for distinguishing the condition from Wernicke disease in which similar lesions are present but regularly involve these structures. Abnormal mitochondria have been observed in rare cases. Ragged red fibres are not found (Nagai *et al.* 1992).

The *clinical manifestations* are extremely variable, and the diagnosis is very difficult as no biochemical markers are available in a majority of cases. Some common features such as deterioration with slow recovery following infections, exercise intolerance, poor somatic growth and abrupt changes in respiratory or cardiac rate may suggest the diagnosis of mitochondrial disorder.

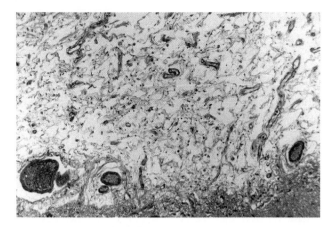

Fig. 9.28. Leigh syndrome. Typical histological appearance of tissues: note sharply demarcated area of marked spongiosis with intense capillary proliferation.

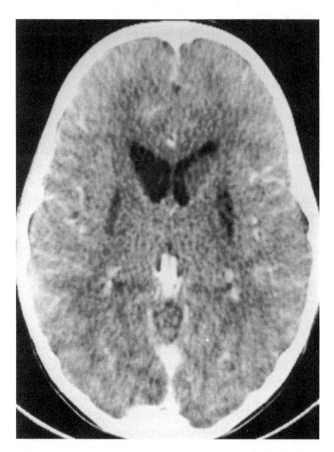

Fig. 9.29. Leigh necrotizing encephalomyelopathy. Cavitation of both lenticular nuclei. Head of left caudate nucleus is hypodense. There is marked atrophy of head of right caudate nucleus with widening of corresponding frontal horn.

In the *infantile form*, the onset is during the first two years, often in the first semester of life. Hypotonia and psychomotor regression may be preceded or accompanied by poor feeding and vomiting. Neurological signs may include ataxia, pyramidal tract signs that may be initially unilateral, dystonia or rigidity and optic atrophy. Movement disorders, including choreoathetosis,

dystonia and sometimes myoclonus, are frequent and may even be paroxysmal (De Vivo and van Coster 1991, Macaya *et al.* 1993). Signs of affectation of the brainstem, especially ocular motor palsies with strabismus, ptosis or more extensive ophthalmoplegia, and respiratory difficulties with hypoventilation and recurrent apnoea, are especially suggestive. Episodes of stupor may supervene. They are not always related to apnoea or hypoventilation. Seizures occur in some patients and may present as infantile spasms (Santorelli *et al.* 1993). The course is often rapidly progressive but remissions and exacerbations are common. These are often precipitated by infections or fasting. Acute fulminating cases with rapid respiratory deficiency or lethal apnoea are on record. Protracted forms with prolonged periods of stabilization are not infrequent and may be difficult to distinguish from static encephalopathies. Cases with very slow progression presenting as cerebral palsy are on record (Fryer *et al.* 1994, Coker and Thomas 1995). In some cases, swallowing dificulties and or digestive disturbances may suggest gastrointestinal disease. Involvement of the peripheral nervous system is not rare (Jacobs *et al.* 1990). In a few cases, it may be the predominant manifestation, and cases simulating Guillain–Barré syndrome are on record (Coker 1993). Hypertrophic cardiomyopathy has been reported (Grunnet *et al.* 1991).

Later forms are less commonly encountered but may occur throughout childhood and adolescence and well into adulthood (Kalimo *et al.* 1979). A *juvenile form* has been tentatively isolated, with predominant extrapyramidal manifestations such as dystonia or abnormal movements. Cases in which hypokinesia and rigidity were predominant have been reported (Van Erven *et al.* 1989). In some cases, mild psychomotor retardation with slight neurological abnormalities may remain unchanged for years until rapid deterioration occurs, sometimes only in adulthood (Whetsell and Plaitakis 1978).

Rare neonatal forms have been reported (Coker and Thomas 1995). Sex-linked forms (Old and De Vivo 1989) may be rapidly lethal but mild forms probably exist.

Some features may be correlated to specific biochemical and genetic abnormalities. Forms associated with the nt 8993 mutation may be especially severe: seizures including infantile spasms may be more common, and a pigmentary retinopathy is present in 40 per cent of cases (Santorelli *et al.* 1993). Pyruvate dehydrogenase complex deficiency is associated with clinical onset in early infancy, and profound hypotonia and seizures in 50 per cent of cases. Cytochrome *c* oxidase deficiency is associated with clinical onset in late infancy, profound hypotonia in all patients, and ataxia, nystagmus, ophthalmoplegia, optic atrophy and peripheral neuropathy in about half the cases (Van Coster *et al.* 1991). However, Rahman *et al.* (1996) did not find a strong correlation between the basic defect and clinical features.

The *differential diagnosis* of Leigh syndrome includes a vast number of progressive or acute neurological conditions from the leukodystrophies (Bourgeois *et al.* 1992) through extrapyramidal diseases and ataxia to hereditary neuropathies (Jacobs *et al.* 1990). The demonstration of an enzyme deficit can be made in 25–30 per cent of cases. Increased levels of blood lactate and pyruvate are only inconstantly present. Increased CSF lactate is more frequent but not constant. CT scan shows hypodense areas in the putamina and/or caudate nuclei in a majority of cases (Schwartz *et al.* 1981). Such lesions are also well demonstrated by MRI (Medina *et al.* 1990, Heckmann *et al.* 1993) (Fig. 9.29) and may be detectable in infants by ultrasonography (Yamagata *et al.* 1990). *In vivo* MR spectroscopy may show increased lactate concentration in affected brain areas and may represent a diagnostic aid in the near future (Detre *et al.* 1991). High lactate levels in the basal nuclei can be found even in cases in which CSF lactate levels are normal (Krägeloh-Mann *et al.* 1992, 1993). The presence of raised CSF protein levels, sometimes with an oligoclonal profile, is not rare, and conduction velocities are slowed in 15–20 per cent of cases (Jacobs *et al.* 1990). Abnormal brainstem auditory evoked potentials are frequently demonstrated even in the absence of clinical signs or symptoms of brainstem involvement. Muscle biopsy is usually unrevealing except for biochemical study.

• *Kearns–Sayre syndrome and progressive external ophthalmoplegia.* This multisystemic disorder is characterized by an invariant triad: onset in childhood or adolescence; PEO and pigmentary retinal degeneration; plus at least one of the following: heart block, elevated CSF protein content and cerebellar dysfunction. Still other clinical abnormalities are present in many cases, and two constant pathological features have been described: ragged red fibres and spongy degeneration of the brain. The signs and symptoms may progress in various sequences.

Children with Kearns–Sayre syndrome usually appear normal at birth. Early development may be normal or mildly delayed. In early childhood, some patients may display episodes of drowsiness, fever and headaches with aseptic meningitis. Severe sideroblastic anaemia isolated or associated with exocrine pancreatic failure is rare but transient features resembling those described in Pearson syndrome, which is due to a similar mitochondrial deletion, may occur (Bernes *et al.* 1996). Ptosis and PEO are usually the first neurological manifestation of the disease, often associated with evidence of asymptomatic retinal degeneration. Later, mild visual loss with pigmentary retinopathy and sometimes with optic atrophy may occur. The most common neurological feature is a cerebellar syndrome which may become severe. Mental retardation or regression may be present. Usually seizures do not occur, unless there is concomitant hypoparathyroidism. Pyramidal signs restricted to an extensor plantar response, myopathy or peripheral neuropathy are not prominent. Heart block is a late sign which may be responsible for syncopal episodes or sudden death despite pacemaker insertion. Rarely, congestive heart failure and supraventricular tachycardia are encountered. Associated endocrine disorders include short stature with growth hormone defect in some cases, latent diabetes and hypoparathyroidism. Renal dysfunction often includes a proximal tubular defect, distal tubulopathy, glomerulopathy, and renal failure. Elevated CSF levels of lactic acid, although mild and variable, are frequently observed in plasma, urine and CSF. Elevated protein levels, sometimes with mild pleocytosis, are often an early sign

in Kearns–Sayre syndrome. A rise of lactacidaemia on graded exercise and abnormal results in muscle MR spectroscopy can give indirect evidence of mitochondrial dysfunction.

Neuroimaging shows a progressive leukoencephalopathy with cortical and/or cerebellar atrophy and calcification in the basal ganglia or deep white matter. An extinguished ERG and abnormal visual evoked potentials may precede ophthalmoloscopic evidence of retinopathy. EMG and nerve conduction velocity studies in some cases may indicate peripheral neuropathy or myopathic changes.

Histochemical and electron microscopic studies of skeletal muscle demonstrate ragged red fibres and altered mitochondria. Altered type I fibres lack histochemical cytochrome *c* oxidase activity and coexist with normal fibres. Muscle mt-DNA analysis has shown that 80 per cent of patients with Kearns–Sayre syndrome have deleted mt-DNA. However, Kearns–Sayre syndrome without deletion has been demonstrated and not all patients with deleted mt-DNA have Kearns–Sayre syndrome.

• *Myoclonic epilepsy with ragged red fibres.* MERRF is a maternally inherited encephalomyopathy, characterized by myoclonus, ataxia and mitochondrial myopathy. Tonic–clonic seizures, hearing loss and dementia are frequently associated.

In most cases, symptoms begin between the ages of 5 and 13 years with a cerebellar syndrome with ataxia, tremor and myoclonic jerks, particularly induced by action or intended movement. Many patients have generalized or massive myoclonic seizures, and some become demented. Hearing loss, optic atrophy and proprioceptive sensory loss may occur. PEO, retinal degeneration or stroke-like episodes are not present. The severity of symptoms along a maternal lineage varies greatly from severe to mild manifestations, sometimes with only abnormal visual evoked response and EEG. CSF and serum lactate levels may be slightly increased. Endocrine disorder may occur.

The EEG records abnormal background activity, variously associated with spike–wave patterns and a photoparoxysmal response. Visual, auditory and somatosensory evoked response studies may show abnormal latencies, while EMG shows myopathic changes. CT and MRI may indicate cerebral and cerebellar atrophy. At post-mortem examination, degeneration of the cerebral hemispheres, cerebellum, posterior spinal column and spinocerebellar tracts has been found.

Ragged red fibres and ultrastructurally abnormal mitochondria in biopsed muscle are constant and may be the only sign in asymptomatic individuals within a family.

• *Mitochondrial myopathy, encephalopathy, lactic acidosis and stroke-like episodes.* Aside from these leading features, the MELAS syndrome is also characterized by the absence of PEO, retinal degeneration, heart block and raised CSF protein levels. However, such signs may not be found, and stroke-like episodes may represent the hallmark of this syndrome.

Symptoms can begin between the ages of 3 and 35 years. All patients have stroke-like episodes reminiscent of those in ischaemic accidents. Hemiparesis, isolated or associated with hemianopsia, and cortical blindness are prominent features. These episodes occur either spontaneously or following a bout of vomiting, headache, abdominal pain, drowsiness, or focal or generalized seizures. *Epilepsia partialis continua* or myoclonic seizures are relatively common. Intellectual regression and behavioural problems are prominent. The myopathy is often clinically asymptomatic or expressed as muscular weakness and mild amyotrophy. Additional features include short stature, diabetes mellitus, sensorineural hearing loss, mild retinal degeneration and cardiac involvement. Lactate levels in plasma and CSF are usually high, and creatine kinase is inconsistently increased. The CSF protein content is normal.

The EEG is usually abnormal, with occasional spike and wave or focal spike discharges. Neuroimaging shows focal lucencies or increased T_2 signal, generally not in a vascular distribution, affecting various sites of the white matter, cortex or brainstem, and areas of calcification or high T_2 signal in the basal ganglia. Cerebral and cerebellar atrophy may be associated. Autopsies have shown spongy degeneration, focal encephalomalacia and basal ganglia calcification. Ragged red fibres, lipid droplets and abnormal mitochondria are present in muscles.

• *Alpers disease.* This autosomal recessive degenerative disease primarily affects the cerebral grey matter. Biochemically, it has been associated with deficiencies of pyruvate carboxylase, pyruvate dehydrogenase and respiratory chain compounds, *e.g.* coenzyme Q and complexes I and IV (Fischer *et al.* 1986, DiMauro *et al.* 1990). The clinical manifestations are considered in Chapter 10. Seizures and EEG abnormalities are much more prominent than in Leigh syndrome, which is a reflection of the extensive involvement of cortical grey matter. Variable visceral involvement may be associated.

TREATMENT
Most attempts to improve respiratory chain function use naturally occuring vitamins, coenzymes and metabolic intermediates. Metabolic therapies reported to produce a positive effect include coenzyme Q10, phylloquinone or menadione in conjunction with ascorbate, succinate, and thiamine or riboflavin. Pharmaceutical therapies include idebenone, corticosteroids and dichloroacetate. These approaches, however, produce only mild degrees of symptomatic improvement (Shoffner and Wallace 1994).

PYRUVATE DEHYDROGENASE DEFICIENCY
Pyruvate dehydrogenase (PDH) deficiency is an important cause of encephalopathy associated with lactic acidosis (Brown 1992; Robinson 1993, 1995; Robinson *et al.* 1996). PDH deficiency has been reported in infants and children with congenital fatal infantile lactic acidosis, progressive neurological deterioration and Leigh syndrome, Alpers disease, carbohydrate-sensitive ataxia and other hereditary ataxic syndromes, myopathy and neuropathy.

NORMAL PDH ACTIVITY AND IMPLICATIONS OF PDH DEFICIENCY
PDH controls the entry of pyruvate, the glycolytic end-product,

into mitochondria for oxidative metabolism and thus plays an important regulatory role in cellular energy metabolism in glycolytic-dependent organs such as the CNS. In the brain, PDH is required for the formation of acetylcholine from acetyl-CoA. Thus PDH defects are expected to involve the nervous system.

PDH is a mitochondrial multienzyme complex comprising three catalytic enzymes (E1, E2, E3), two regulatory enzymes (PDH kinase and phosphatase), and three coenzymes (thiamine, lipoic acid, FADH$_2$). Another component, the X-protein, probably has a structural function.

Most patients with PDH deficiency have a defect in the E1 component, with a lesser number of defects occuring in the E2, E3, and X components (Robinson *et al.* 1990, 1996; Brown 1992). E1 is a tetrameric ($\alpha_2\beta_2$) enzyme whose alpha-polypeptide gene is located on the X chromosome. All E1 defects reported to date are due to various *E1α* gene mutations (Lissens *et al.* 1996). Despite this X-linkage, there are equal numbers of affected males and females with similar clinical expression. This fact results from the high incidence of neomutations, the pattern of X-inactivation in females, and the nature of the mutation which in general differs in males and females. Males have a high representation of missense mutations, while females are much more likely to have DNA rearrangements. A missense mutation conferring true thiamine responsiveness has been reported.

E3 is shared by two other dehydrogenases involved in Krebs cycle and branched-chain amino acid catabolism. Lactic acidosis, alpha-ketoglutaric aciduria and high plasma levels of branched-chain amino acids permit the biological diagnosis of E3 deficiency.

CLINICAL FEATURES
Patients with PDH deficiency may present with symptoms at any time from birth. In the *neonatal form*, severe lactic acidosis, hypotonia and apnoeic spells are the most frequent features. Most patients die within the first few months of life after a clinical course marked by failure to thrive, developmental delay, hypotonia, respiratory difficulties and seizures. E1 and X-component defects have been documented in the neonatal period (Sperl *et al.* 1990, Geoffroy *et al.* 1996).

In a second group of patients, symptoms occur after an apparently uneventful period of a few months. Seizures or episodes of weakness, respiratory failure or ataxia are the first manifestations. Later, these episodes may recur, and variable degrees of progressive neurological impairment are seen. Optic atrophy, ptosis, ophthalmoplegia and retinal degeneration have been mentioned. West syndrome may occur in a few girls (Matsuda *et al.* 1995). Many patients die within a few years but some survive with severe disability. E1 defects are the most frequent abnormality within this group. However, the rare reported cases of E3 and PDH phosphatase deficiencies can be associated with these clinical forms (Elpeleg *et al.* 1995). Facial dysmorphism resembling that seen in the fetal alcohol syndrome has been described in both groups of patients with E1 deficiency (Robinson *et al.* 1987, Old and DeVivo 1989).

A third group comprises mentally normal patients with chronic or episodic ataxia, myopathy or neuropathy (Bonne *et al.* 1993, Robinson *et al.* 1996).

In some neonatal-onset forms, MRI studies have shown severe abnormalities including agenesis or dysgenesis of the corpus callosum, generalized atrophy with striking ventriculomegaly and hypomyelination (Otero *et al.* 1995). Neuropathological findings confirm this brain dysgenesis. Dysplasia and ectopia of the inferior olivary nuclei, dysplasia of dentate nuclei, absence or hypoplasia of the medullary pyramids, periventricular neuronal heterotopia and deficient myelination are other findings. Most children with the progressive form present with radiological and neuropathological signs of Leigh syndrome. Olivopontocerebellar atrophy associated with signs of Leigh syndrome has been described in one patient with intermittent ataxia (Brismar and Ozand 1994a, Shevell *et al.* 1994, van der Knaap *et al.* 1996).

BIOLOGICAL AND BIOCHEMICAL FEATURES
Accumulation of lactate in blood and CSF and increased excretion in urine are the common biological features. These can be severe during the neonatal period or during episodes of deterioration, while patients in the third group have only a mild hyperlactataemia which may rise after glucose loading and exertional tests. Redox ratios are usually normal.

Due to the multiple defective component of the PDH complex that can be involved and the possibility of a high residual activity, especially in females, the final diagnosis relies on full biochemical investigations including Western blot and molecular approaches (Lissens *et al.* 1996), besides enzymatic studies in fibroblasts or muscle.

TREATMENT
Because they are PDH cofactors, thiamine and lipoate treatment may be effective in a few patients (Byrd *et al.* 1989, Old and DeVivo 1989, Pastoris *et al.* 1996). Ketogenic diets and dichloroacetate may decrease lactate accumulation without clear improvement of the progressive neurological impairment (Yoshida *et al.* 1990, Tóth *et al.* 1993).

PYRUVATE CARBOXYLASE DEFICIENCY
This is a rare autosomal recessive disorder marked by hyperlactataemia and severe CNS involvement (Robinson 1995, Robinson *et al.* 1996).

BIOCHEMICAL BACKGROUND
Pyruvate carboxylase is a biotin-containing protein whose function in the brain is to maintain intermediates of the Krebs cycle. If the neurotransmitter pool is replenished from *de novo* synthesis in presynaptic terminals, pyruvate carboxylase defects, through Krebs cycle disruption, could be responsible for aspartate, glutamate and GABA deficiency (Perry *et al.* 1985). Pyruvate carboxylase activity is expressed in fibroblasts and amniocytes allowing prenatal diagnosis (Robinson *et al.* 1985).

Pyruvate carboxylase deficiency exists in at least two clinical and biochemical phenotypes. In general, the enzymatic defect in the more severe form is associated with the absence of apoprotein on Western blot and missplicing mutation at the DNA level. In the milder form, a detectable apoprotein is present but carries a point DNA mutation.

CLINICAL FEATURES
The neonatal-onset form presents as an overwhelming lactic acidosis with hepatic failure and death before 3 months of age. A late-onset form presents in the first semester after the neonatal period with mild hyperlactacidaemia and psychomotor retardation and has longer survival. Both groups have less than 5 per cent residual activity in their fibroblasts. The biochemical pattern in neonatal forms is notable for the presence of a secondary hyperammonaemia with citrullinaemia and a very high lactate/pyruvate ratio contrasting with low beta-hydroxybutyrate/acetoacetate ratio.

Based on rare MRI reports, the most specific change is a diffuse white matter abnormality associated with periventricular cysts which are almost invariably haemorrhagic. The CNS pathology shows poor myelination involving cerebral and cerebellar white matter and sometimes the base of the pons, loss of neurons in the cerebral cortex, ventricular enlargement, thinning of the corpus callosum and proliferation of astrocytes (van der Knaap *et al.* 1996).

TREATMENT
Therapeutic trials have attempted to replenish the Krebs cycle using glutarate, aspartate and citrate supplementation, but all have failed to prevent neurological degradation.

DEFECTS OF THE KREBS CYCLE
These include fumarase and alpha-ketoglutarate dehydrogenase deficiencies. Fumarase deficiency has been reported in eight children with severe neurological impairment. The defect involves both cytosol and mitochondrial isoforms and appears to be autosomal recessive (Elpeleg *et al.* 1992, Remes *et al.* 1992). Alpha-ketoglutarate deficiency has been described in one family (Bonnefont *et al.* 1992). The clinical presentation resembles that of early-onset PDH deficiency or the mitochondrial encephalomyopathies. Normal or mild hyperlactataemia is associated with abnormal fumaric aciduria in patients with fumarase deficiency, and alpha-glutaric aciduria in alpha-ketoglutarate dehydrogenase deficiency. All patients in the studies mentioned had cortical atrophy, and three patients with fumarase deficiency had evidence of *in utero* involvement with hydrocephalus and dysmorphism (Remes *et al.* 1992). Agenesis of the corpus callosum, and small cysts in an occipital horn have been described in one case (Walker *et al.* 1989). Autopsy in another case revealed hypomyelination and heterotopia located in cerebellum, occipital and parietal areas (Gellera *et al.* 1990).

MITOCHONDRIAL FATTY ACID BETA-OXIDATION DEFECTS

Inborn errors in mitochondrial fatty acid oxidation represent a

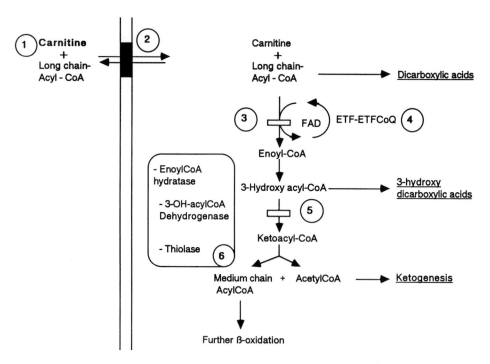

Fig. 9.30. Simplified schema of long-chain fatty acid beta-oxidation indicating sites of major inborn defects.
   Key: 1 = primary carnitine deficiency; 2 = carnitine acylcarnitine shuttle (carnitine palmityl transferase I and II, carnitine translocase); 3 = long- and very-long-chain acyl-CoA dehydrogenase (LCAD/VLCAD); 4 = electron transfer system (MAD, glutaric aciduria type II); 5 = long-chain 3-hydroxy-acyl-CoA dehydrogenase (LCHAD); 6 = trifunctional protein.

group of disorders which affect energy metabolism during fasting and metabolic stress. As a consequence, common features include metabolic decompensation associated with fasting, recurrent hypoglycaemia, Reye-like syndrome and unexplained sudden infant death. Chronic involvement of fatty-acid-dependent tissues may result in myopathy and cardiomopathy. About 15 different defects are known (Hale and Bennett 1992, Vockley 1994, Pollitt 1995, Roe and Coates 1995, Stanley 1995, Tein 1996).

BIOCHEMICAL BACKGROUND
The general pathways of mitochondrial fatty acid oxidation and the sites of the different known enzymatic defects are shown in Figure 9.30. Long-chain fatty acids are converted to their CoA-esters in the cytosol and transported into the mitochondria by a specific carnitine-acyl-carnitine shuttle which comprises carnitine palmitoyltransferase I and II (CPT-I, CPT-II), and carnitine acyl-carnitine translocase. Medium- and short-chain acyl-CoA readily diffuse into the mitochondria. Primary carnitine deficiency, CPT-I, CPT-II and translocase deficiencies impair mitochondrial transport of long-chain fatty acids and consequently beta-oxidation and ketogenesis. Further beta-oxidation involves four sequential steps with chain-length-specific enzymes. The first step requires four distinct acyl-CoA dehydrogenases, the very-long-, long-, medium- and short-chain acyl-CoA dehydrogenases (VLCAD, LCAD, MCAD, SCAD), which transform fatty acyl-CoA to enoyl-CoA. All four acyl-CoA dehydrogenases release electrons which pass to the respiratory chain via the electron-transfer flavoprotein system. The latter specific electron transfer sytem is shared with other flavoprotein dehydrogenases: glutaryl CoA-, isovaleryl CoA-, and sarcosine dehydrogenases. The three remaining steps of long-chain beta-oxidation can be performed by either a single trifunctional protein or unifunctional enzymes which are active on short- and medium-chain substrates. Each four-step beta-oxidation cycle releases acetyl-CoA which enters the Krebs cycle in tissues such as heart and muscle. In liver, during the fasting state, acetyl-CoA is converted to ketones (ketogenesis) which are exported to peripheral organs, such as the brain, for final oxidation (ketolysis). Known defects in intramitochondrial beta-oxidation are secondary to VLCAD, LCAD, MCAD, SCAD, long-chain 3-hydroxy-acylCoA dehydrogenase (LCHAD), short-chain 3-hydroxy-acyl-CoA dehydrogenase (SCHAD), and trifunctional protein deficiencies. Multiple acyl-CoA dehydrogenase (MAD) deficiency, also called *glutaric aciduria type II*, is caused by a defect in the electron transfer system. Several alternative pathways become important when mitochondrial beta-oxidation is impaired. Beta-oxidation in microsomes results in the production of characteristic dicarboxylic acids, and conjugation of acyl-CoA to glycine and carnitine is an important mechanism of detoxification.

   The biochemical diagnosis is based on the identification of abnormal dicarboxylic acids and their by-products (glycine, carnitine) in urine. Glutaric and branched-chain organic acid-urias are associated in MAD deficiency. It should be emphasized that these specific patterns are best detected during an acute crisis, while in the basic state the most reliable tests are the determination of total and esterified carnitine and the identification of an abnormal acyl-carnitine profile in plasma. Measurement of fatty acid oxidation rate in fresh lymphocytes or cultured fibroblasts is a useful tool to narrow the search for the specific defect involved. Direct enzymatic assay may then be performed for definitive diagnosis. Most defects are expressed in cultured fibroblasts; however, certain of these defects, such as muscle CPT-I and SCHAD deficiencies, may be tissue-specific.

GENETIC BACKGROUND

Overall, these disorders are frequent, but MCAD deficiency is the most common. More than 200 cases have been reported, and the estimated heterozygote frequency may be 1–2 per cent in White populations. All are inherited as autosomal recessive traits. Antenatal diagnosis is available from culture of amniocytes or a chorionic villus sample using techniques similar to those applied for postnatal diagnosis (Ogier de Beaulny *et al.* 1995a,b; Nada *et al.* 1996). Complementary DNAs have been cloned for most of these enzymes, and various disease-causing mutations are described. The most recently recognized concern the infantile form of CPT-II deficiency (Bonnefont *et al.* 1996, Yamamoto *et al.* 1996), VLCAD deficiency (Strauss *et al.* 1995, Souri *et al.* 1996), and defects in both the alpha and beta subunits of the trifunctional protein (Ushikubo *et al.* 1996) and the electron-transfer flavoprotein system (Colombo *et al.* 1994, Beard *et al.* 1995). Prevalent mutations have been described in the *MCAD* gene, the gene of the adult (muscular) form of CPT-II and the alpha subunit gene of trifunctional protein.

CLINICAL FINDINGS

NEONATAL-ONSET FORMS

Neonatal presentation may occur with almost all fatty acid oxidation defects with the exception of primary carnitine deficiency. In the first few days of life, babies may manifest unexpected cardiorespiratory collapse or rapidly progressive lethargy with profound hypotonia. In most but not all cases, this abrupt deterioration is associated with hypoketotic hypoglycaemia. Lactic acidosis, mild to severe hyperammonaemia and various degree of liver involvement are the rule. Cardiomyopathy with arrhythmia and mild to severe muscular involvement with increased creatine kinase occurs in many long-chain oxidation defects. Unexplained neonatal death occurs in some patients, and in such cases this may also have occurred in earlier siblings. Abnormal organogenesis with dysmorphic features, cystic dysplasia of the brain and kidneys, and polymicrogyria are encountered in some MAD and CPT-II-deficient patients (North *et al.* 1995). One patient with CPT-II deficiency presented with severe neonatal myopathy without other organ involvement (Land *et al.* 1995). In SCAD deficiency, primary neurological signs such as hypertonia, hyperactivity, nystagmus and developmental delay suggest severe impairment of cerebral maturation (Bhala *et al.* 1995). The prognosis is variable. MAD and LCAD deficiencies appear the most life-threatening. Many patients who have survived the neonatal period die a few months later during intercurrent decompensation

or after an unremitting course with severe encephalopathy, failure to thrive and muscular weakness. Some rare patients, however, are doing well after several years (Largillière *et al.* 1991).

INFANTILE-ONSET FORMS

These are the most common. Most often they occur within the first two years of life, but they may arise at any time up till adulthood. They share many signs and symptoms with the neonatal forms. They are characterized by potentially life-threatening episodes of hypoketotic hypoglycaemia, coma and multiorgan failure following an intercurrent catabolic state. Despite correction of blood glucose levels, some patients may display persistent lethargy, seizures, dystonic movements or opisthotonos due to concomitant cerebral oedema which suggests that elevated levels of fatty acid intermediates are neurotoxic agents. Liver involvement with hepatic failure, lactic acidosis and hyperammonaemia has frequently been misdiagnosed as Reye syndrome. Various degrees of myolysis and/or cardiomyopathy are frequently associated. In some cases, rapid unexpected death may suggest sudden infant death syndrome. Between episodes many patients, especially children with MCAD deficiency, may appear asymptomatic. Others may display chronic involvement of muscle and heart or suffer neurological sequelae.

Chronic muscle weakness with lipid storage myopathy has been described in all these defects with the exception of CPT-I deficiency, and may be the presenting sign in some. Among these, the mild 'adult' form of CPT-II deficiency is a unique entity characterized by attacks of rhabdomyolosis without other organ involvement. These attacks occur in the second or third decade of life and are triggered by prolonged exercise, fasting or cold exposure. This may also be seen with trifunctional protein deficiency (Schaefer *et al.* 1996).

Cardiomyopathy is associated with several long-chain fatty acid disorders, but is the main sign of primary carnitine deficiency which is otherwise characterized by a severe lipidic myopathy.

In the course of their disease, some patients with trifunctional protein or LCAD deficiency develop progressive axonal neuropathy and pigmentary retinopathy. Neurological sequelae have been observed with MCAD, a disorder which is otherwise considered as the least severe form of fatty oxidation defect. Patients may suffer developmental delay (21 per cent), behavioural disturbances (15 per cent), chronic seizure disorder (17 per cent), and motor defects reported as cerebral palsy (10 per cent). Few neuroimaging studies have been reported; brain atrophy, periventricular demyelination and basal ganglia lesions may be the major radiological signs (Brismar and Ozand 1994a).

TREATMENT

The main therapy is prevention of fasting and catabolic states. In acute situations, intravenous glucose infusion (8–10 mg/kg/min) should be started without delay. There is no clear evidence that restricting fat is useful in MCAD deficiency. In contrast, in patients with defects in LCAD metabolism low-fat diet supplemented with medium triglycerides may be beneficial. In patients

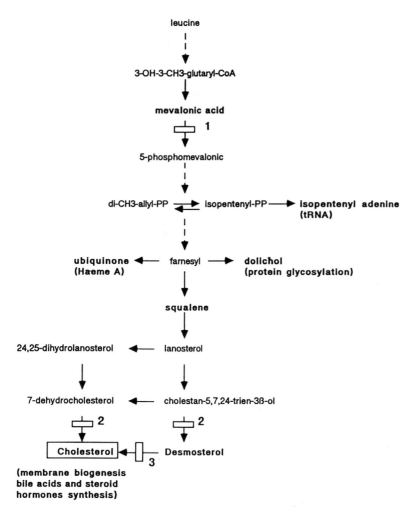

Fig. 9.31. Schematic representation of cholesterol biosynthesis and main metabolic relationships with other pathways (see text).

Key: 1 = mevalonate kinase (mevalonic aciduria); 2 = 7-dehydrocholesterol dehydrogenase (Smith–Lemli–Opitz syndrome); 3 = C24–C25 double-bound reductase (possible defect in desmosterolosis).

with primary carnitine deficiency, carnitine supplementation (100–200 mg/kg/d) improves cardiac and muscle function within a few months. The role of carnitine supplementation in other beta-oxidation defects remains controversial. Some patients with mild variants of MAD and SCAD deficiencies may respond to riboflavin supplementation (100 mg/kg/d) (Stanley 1995).

DEFECTS OF INTRACELLULAR CHOLESTEROL METABOLISM

MEVALONIC ACIDURIA
Mevalonic aciduria is a rare inborn error of the biosynthesis of isoprenoid groups. It is a multisystemic disorder with great variability in severity. CNS involvement with progressive cerebellar atrophy is an important sign (Hoffmann *et al.* 1993).

BIOCHEMICAL BACKGROUND AND PATHOGENESIS
Mevalonic aciduria results from deficiency of mevalonate kinase, a peroxisomal enzyme in the biosynthetic pathway of both sterol

and nonsterol isoprenes (Fig. 9.31). This pathway is crucial for cell proliferation and cellular function. The respective pathogenic roles of end-product defects and toxicity of mevalonate accumulation are unclear. Either appears sufficient to explain multiorgan involvement and the teratogenic aspects of the disorder suggested by the high rate of miscarriages and stillbirths of malformed fetuses in affected families.

GENETIC BACKGROUND
The gene of this autosomal recessive disorder has been cloned, and a disease-causing mutation has been identified (Goebel-Schreiner *et al.* 1995). Mevalonate kinase activity is expressed in fibroblasts, lymphoblasts, amniotic cells and chorionic villi. Prenatal diagnosis has already been performed by assaying chorionic villus samples for enzymatic activity and amniotic fluid for mevalonic acid.

NEUROPATHOLOGY
Neuropathological examination in one patient has revealed

agenesis of the cerebellar vermis, necrosis of granule cells and neuronal necrosis in the cerebral cortex (Hoffman *et al.* 1993).

CLINICAL FEATURES

The disorder may manifest from infancy to childhood with marked phenotypic heterogeneity: four children died before their fourth year, while one 12-year-old patient is mildly impaired. Psychomotor retardation of varying degree is a constant finding. Most patients over 2 years develop progressive ataxia, dysarthria and cerebellar atrophy. Muscular hypotonia with weakness is present in all patients. Failure to thrive, anaemia, hepatospleno-megaly and lymphadenopathy are common. Mild dysmorphism was present in eight of 11 cases reported by Hoffman *et al.* (1993); and cataracts, uveitis and retinitis pigmentosa may occur. Neuroimaging shows progressive cerebellar atrophy.

All patients suffer frequent bouts of fever, vomiting and diarrhoea, accompanied by increased blood sedimentation, arthralgia, subcutaneous oedema, morbilliform rash, anaemia, and worsening of muscular hypotonia with high levels of serum creatine kinase, hepatosplenomegaly and lymphadenopathy. Some patients may have seizures or die during such crises.

BIOCHEMICAL DIAGNOSIS

The diagnosis relies on organic acid analysis to identify meval-onic acid accumulation in body fluids and on mevalonate kinase assay in fibroblasts or lymphocytes

TREATMENT

No effective therapy is available. Supplementation with pre-sumably deficient end-products such as cholesterol, bile acids and ubiquinone has not produced any clinical or biochemical improvement. Blocking mevalonate hyperproduction by low doses of HMG-CoA reductase inhibitor (lovastatin) has resulted in severe crises in two patients. The best therapeutic approach seems to be intermittent corticosteroid therapy (prednisone, 2 mg/kg/d) especially during intercurrent crises.

SMITH–LEMLI–OPITZ SYNDROME

Smith–Lemli–Opitz syndrome (SLOS) is a syndrome of multiple congenital anomalies and mental retardation (Opitz 1994). Recently, a defect of cholesterol biosynthesis associated with this disease has been found (Tint *et al.* 1994). The combination of elevated plasma 7-dehydrocholesterol (7-DHC) levels and reduced cholesterol concentration can now be considered as the biochemical marker of a disorder which was previously diagnosed from its clinical defects.

BIOCHEMICAL BACKGROUND AND PATHOGENESIS

In the last part of the biosynthetic pathway of cholesterol, lanosterol is demethylated, isomerized, and the side-chain reduced (see Fig. 9.31). Depending on the order of the reduction step the synthesis proceeds along two branches which both require a 3-beta-hydroxysteroid Δ^7-reductase capable of saturating the 7 double bond. In plasma and in various tissues the coexistence of a low concentration of cholesterol and a marked accumulation

TABLE 9.11
Clinical manifestations in Smith–Lemli–Opitz syndrome

Microcephaly, mental retardation
Poor growth
Dysmorphic features:
  Epicanthal folds, ptosis, blepharoptosis, low-set retroverted ears, micrognathia, cleft palate, anteverted nares.
Urogenital malformations:
  Genital hypoplasia, cryptorchidism, hypospadias, micropenis, ambiguous genitalia, urinary tract anomalies, hydronephrosis, renal cystic dysplasia
Limb abnormalities:
  Syndactyly, postaxial polydactyly, digital whorls
Digestive tract:
  Poor feeding, frequent vomiting, Hirschsprung disease, pancreatic anomalies
Hepatic dysfunction:
  Hepatomegaly, fibrosis
Congenital heart disease
Adrenal enlargement
Epiphyseal dysplasia
Cataracts
High infant mortality rate

of 7-DHC and other sterols such as 8-DHC suggests a block at the level of 3-beta-hydroxysteroid Δ^7-reductase which has been confirmed in the liver (Tint *et al.* 1995a,b). Secondary to the cho-lesterol defect, the bile acid pattern is abnormal (Natowicz and Evans 1994), and the overflow of isoprenoids leads to 3-methyl-glutaconic overproduction (Kelley and Kratz 1995).

The teratogenic aspect of SLOS could be due in part to a block sufficient to deprive the embryo or fetus of cholesterol and prevent normal development, whereas the incorporation of 7-DHC into all membranes may interfere with proper membrane function. This does not imply that cholesterol supplementation would benefit newborn infants with SLOS, especially as CNS cholesterol provision is probably different in early fetal life (maternal origin) and in postnatal life (endogenous synthesis). Recent description of tissue accumulation of desmosterol (desmosterolosis) in a severely malformed baby emphasizes the importance of this endogenous cholesterol pathway during fetal life (Clayton *et al.* 1996).

GENETIC BACKGROUND

SLOS is an autosomal recessive disorder with a high birth preval-ence among North American Whites. The gene is located on chromosome 7 (7q32) but has not yet been cloned. Prenatal diagnosis is available by assaying amniotic fluid and/or chorionic villus samples for 7-DHC or by measuring cholesterol synthesis from radiolabelled precursors (McGaughran *et al.* 1995, Wanders *et al.* 1996). These techniques can also apply for post-mortem diagnosis in a grossly malformed fetus.

NEUROPATHOLOGY

Gross examination of the brain shows varying abnormalities such as hypoplasia of the corpus callosum, frontal lobes, cerebellum, brainstem and spinal cord. There is widespread demyelination in the central and peripheral nervous system.

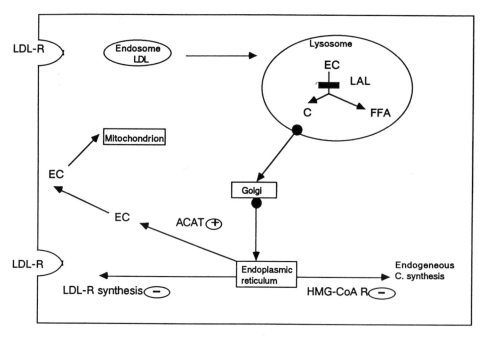

Fig. 9.32. Intracellular metabolism of exogenous cholesterol. Esterified cholesterol (EC) enters the cell at the low-density lipoprotein receptors (LDL-R). The endosome joins the lysosome where EC is submitted to hydrolysis through lysosomal acid lipase (LAL). Defect in LAL results in Wolman and cholesterol ester storage diseases. Free cholesterol (C) is directed through the Golgi and endoplasmic apparatus and is responsible for three retro-controlled reactions: HMG-CoA reductase (HMG-CoA-R) inhibition, LDL-R synthesis inhibition, and activation of acetylcholesterol acyl transferase (ACAT). Niemann–Pick type C disease could be due to defective transport of cholesterol through the lysosome or through the Golgi apparatus.

Neuronal loss and heterotopias affect the cerebral and cerebellar cortex, the dentate nuclei, and the anterior and posterior horns (Cherstvoy *et al.* 1984).

CLINICAL FEATURES (Table 9.11)
SLOS features microcephaly, mental retardation, growth retardation, distinctive facial dysmorphism, postaxial polydactyly, and syndactyly of the second and third toes. A wide spectrum of other abnormalities has been observed and the phenotype ranges from relatively mild to severe lethal forms. None of the clinical findings indicated in Table 9.11 is either specific or obligatory. The suggestion that two types could exist—type I comprising the milder manifestations and type II embracing the severe forms—is no longer relevant as both types have qualitatively similar biochemical profiles. CNS imaging may show hypoplasia of the frontal lobes, corpus callosum, cerebellum and brainstem, associated with poor myelination. Periventricular grey matter heterotopias and polymicrogyria or pachygyria have been reported (Marion *et al.* 1987).

BIOCHEMICAL DIAGNOSIS
The diagnosis relies on plasma sterol measurements by gas chromatography or mass spectrometry. Plasma concentration of cholesterol is reduced, while 7-DHC and its isomer 8-DHC are markedly elevated. Determination of plasma cholesterol using cholesterol oxidase is unreliable for SLOS diagnosis because it measures cholesterol, 7-DHC and 8-DHC all together. The

diagnosis can be further confirmed by measuring these compounds and *de novo* cholesterol synthesis in various tissues and fibroblasts (Tint *et al.* 1995b)

TREATMENT
Cholesterol and bile acid supplementation should theoretically result in suppression of *de novo* cholesterol biosynthesis and decreased accumulation of 7-DHC. Some authors have described some improvement with this regime, while others have reported that, despite normalization of plasma cholesterol levels, plasma 7-DHC remained high and clinical status was not improved (Ullrich *et al.* 1996).

NIEMANN–PICK DISEASE TYPE C
BIOCHEMICAL AND GENETIC BACKGROUND
In contrast with Nieman–Pick disease types A and B, type C disease is characterized by normal sphingomyelinase activity in most tissues although decreased activity can be demonstrated in fibroblasts in three-quarters of cases. Sphingomyelin storage remains mild or moderate, while a striking increase in nonesterified cholesterol is characteristic. Defective intracellular cholesterol esterification is regularly found (Vanier *et al.* 1988), and the disorder is currently classified as a cholesterol metabolism defect (Fig. 9.32). Fibroblasts are deeply coloured by Filipin dye, indicating an excess of free cholesterol. Prenatal diagnosis is possible by study of cholesterol esterification (Vanier *et al.* 1992). Niemann–Pick C disease has been mapped to 18p11 (Carstea *et*

al. 1993) but genetic heterogeneity is possible. However, the primary metabolic defect remains unknown so that the diagnosis is less reliable than the demonstration of sphingomyelinase deficiency which allows a firm prenatal diagnosis in types A and B.

CLINICAL FEATURES
A cholestatic icterus with hepatomegaly may be present in half the cases during the neonatal period, disappearing before the age of 3 months. During the first three months 6–20 per cent of patients develop a severe cholestatic disease with hepatosplenomegaly and ascites, leading to death before the appearance of neurological symptoms and signs (Fink *et al.* 1989b, Kelly *et al.* 1993).

In the remaining patients, neurodevelopmental failure becomes prominent. In severe cases, deterioration is rapid, marked mainly by hypotonia and delay in developmental motor milestones, followed by loss of acquired skills, spasticity and, sometimes, atonic episodes of a cataplectic nature but without epilepsy. Many of these patients die before 3–5 years of age without developing ophthalmoplegia.

In less severe forms, with onset after 3 years of age, poor school progress and unsteady gait are usually the first manifestations. The average age of onset in the cases of Kelly (1993) was 4.5 years, and some patients may have no neurological signs up to late adolescence or early adulthood. Cerebellar ataxia is increasingly prominent, and many patients display dystonic features. Movement disorder and grimacing may be the most striking manifestations. The so-called *juvenile dystonic lipidosis* (Martin *et al.* 1984) appears to be a form of Niemann–Pick type C. Supranuclear palsy of vertical gaze, especially downward, is a cardinal sign, and the cases of neurovisceral storage disease with vertical supranuclear ophthalmoplegia are also linked with type C disease (Neville *et al.* 1973). Cataplectic attacks are common (Kandt *et al.* 1982). Eventually, spasticity sets in and mental deterioration progresses but at a variable pace. A few patients are still alive in their twenties.

The diagnosis can be confirmed by demonstrating limited degradation of sphingomyelin in fibroblasts or defective intracellular esterification of cholesterol (Vanier *et al.* 1988). Skin biopsy (Ceuterick and Martin 1992) may be of some help but the inclusions are nonspecific.

Other reported types of Niemann–Pick disease include type D, which is found in Nova Scotia and is very similar to type C, as well as a number of cases described in adults (types E and F) or in children and which are now grouped with type C (Filling-Katz *et al.* 1992).

WOLMAN DISEASE AND CHOLESTEROL ESTER STORAGE DISEASE
Wolman disease and cholesterol ester storage disease (CESD) are two phenotypic expressions of lysosomal acid lipase (LAL) deficiency which results in massive accumulation of cholesteryl esters and triglycerides in most tissues. Wolman disease represents the early-onset form which is uniformly fatal, while CESD is a more benign type with late onset (Assmann and Seedorf 1995).

BIOCHEMICAL BACKGROUND AND PATHOGENESIS
LAL hydrolyses cholesteryl esters and triglycerides after they have been removed from the plasma into cells via low-density lipoprotein (LDL) receptors. After hydrolysis, free cholesterol is mainly directed to the endoplasmic reticulum where three types of regulatory reactions are induced: (i) inhibition of endogenous synthesis of cholesterol; (ii) repression of the gene that governs LDL-receptor synthesis; and (iii) activation of acyl-CoA-cholesterol transferase (ACAT), which esterifies cholesterol in cytoplasm. With LAL deficiency, there is a lysosomal accumulation of cholesteryl ester-rich lipids, a process that is worsened by the absence of feedback (see Fig. 9.31). The tissue distribution of abnormal lipid storage is related to the quantitative importance of this LAL-dependent degradation which mainly occurs in liver, macrophages and adrenals. These intracellular defects are responsible for secondary alterations of plasma lipoprotein homeostasis with increased levels of LDL-cholesterol, triglycerides and apobetalipoproteins.

GENETIC BACKGROUND
Both disorders are autosomal recessive. Structural mutations of the *LAL* gene, which has been localized to chromosome 10 (10q23.2–23.3), have already been identified without clear genotype/phenotype relations (Muntoni *et al.* 1995). Prenatal diagnosis is available by assaying LAL activity in amniotic cells or chorionic villus samples.

NEUROPATHOLOGY
In Wolman disease, a mild lipid storage can involve neurons and foamy histiocytes in the leptomeninges, the endothelium of capillaries and the choroid plexus. Despite early atheroma, no cerebral strokes have been reported in CESD.

CLINICAL FEATURES
Wolman disease presents in the first weeks of life with severe diarrhoea that rapidly causes wasting associated with massive hepatosplenomegaly, anaemia and acanthocytosis. Affected infants have an early normal development but progressively display developmental delay with loss of interest and hypotonia. Adrenal calcification is a constant feature which can be associated with subclinical adrenal failure. Vacuolization of peripheral lymphocytes and foam cells in bone marrow aspiration have been noted. Despite supportive nutritional measures death occurs within months.

CESD is most often diagnosed following fortuitous discovery of hepatosplenomegaly in childhood or even in adulthood. The clinical course is dominated by liver disease and hypercholesterolaemia. There is no adrenal calcification and the CNS is not involved.

BIOCHEMICAL DIAGNOSIS
Diagnosis is based on the demonstration of LAL deficiency in cultured fibroblasts, lymphocytes or other tissues. Hyperlipoproteinaemia is common in CESD but absent in Wolman disease.

TREATMENT

No specific treatment is available for Wolman disease. Combined cholestyramine and HMG-CoA reductase inhibitor treatment which alters the dyslipoproteinaemia in CESD has never been tried in Wolman disease. Liver transplantation has been successfully performed in CESD patients with severe liver fibrosis (Leone *et al.* 1995).

DISORDERS OF COPPER METABOLISM

WILSON DISEASE (HEPATOLENTICULAR DEGENERATION)

PATHOLOGY AND PATHOPHYSIOLOGY

Wilson disease is an autosomal recessive disorder of the CNS, affecting especially the basal ganglia, associated with cirrhosis of the liver. The disease is related to a derangement of the metabolism of copper, specifically with high levels of liver copper and copper accumulation within the brain substance, in particular within the central grey matter.

Normally 20–50 per cent of ingested copper is absorbed from the intestine and transported as an albumin complex to the liver (Walshe 1986). In the liver, the copper is incorporated into newly synthesized ceruloplasmin for transport to the rest of the body, excreted into the biliary system, or incorporated into copper storage proteins such as metallothionein. More than 95 per cent of serum copper is normally in the form of ceruloplasmin. Normal concentratation of ceruloplasmin in the plasma of children older than 2 years is 200–430 μmol/L (30–65 mg/dL). Low levels are frequent in younger children and are of no diagnostic value. Plasma level is elevated during pregnancy, with high oestrogen concentration, liver cirrhosis, malignant disease and hyperthyroidism. Ninety-five per cent of patients with Wilson disease have markedly diminished ceruloplasmin levels. However, this is not a constant finding and ceruloplasmin levels as low as those in Wilson disease (*e.g.* in nephrosis patients) may not be associated with symptoms. The same applies to familial ceruloplasmin deficiency in which there are no clinical manifestations or these are limited to blepharospasm and retinal degeneration (Miyajima *et al.* 1987).

Radioisotope studies after intravenous administration of ^{64}Cu to patients with Wilson disease show an initial rise of serum copper which is more marked than in controls but is not followed by the appearance of the tracer in the globulin fraction where ceruloplasmin is normally found. In addition, plasma levels of nonceruloplasmin copper are increased and the biliary excretion of copper is reduced considerably, accounting for decreased faecal excretion. The basic molecular defect is absence or reduced function of a protein which has copper-transporting ATPase activity and a marked amino acid homology with the copper transport protein that is mutated in Menkes kinky hair disease (Tanzi *et al.* 1993). This impedes transport of copper from hepatocytes to bile and results in accumulation of copper. The gene coding for this protein maps to 13q14.3 and a large number of mutations are known (Thomas *et al.* 1995). Most patients appear to be compound heterozygotes for different mutations, and the genotype

seems to affect clinical findings, particularly the age of onset (Houwen *et al.* 1995). Although direct identification of the mutation is sometimes possible, the large number of mutations makes it difficult.

Accumulation of copper initially damages hepatocyte mitochondria and peroxisomes. Eventually, excess copper leaks from liver into blood and is taken up by tissues, especially brain, with secondary damage.

Pathologically, the liver shows focal necrosis with secondary postnecrotic cirrhosis. Copper is initially diffusely spread within the cytoplasm and secondarily becomes sequestered within lysosomes. In the brain, the basal ganglia show spongy degeneration, loss of neurons and large numbers of large protoplasmic astrocytes (Alzheimer type II glia). The frontal lobe cortex is similarly involved. Lesser changes are found in other parts of the CNS.

Copper is present in the cornea and is deposited in clumps close to the endothelial surface of Descemet's membrane, which is responsible for the Kayser–Fleischer ring.

CLINICAL FEATURES

Wilson disease is transmitted as an autosomal recessive trait with a frequency of 1 in 100,000 in homozygous form. In about one-third of cases, the disorder presents at 3–5 years of age with hepatic manifestations. Another 30 per cent present after 8 years of age with neurological symptoms, and the rest may show a mixture of hepatic and cerebral changes. In about 10 per cent of children, Wilson disease first presents as an acute or intermittent haemolytic anaemia (Werlin *et al.* 1978).

Neurological manifestations usually begin from 10 years of age onwards. Rare patients may have neurological symptoms as early as 3 years. The clinical features are extremely variable and, according to Walshe (1986), 'no two patients are ever quite the same and there is no such thing as a typical case of Wilson's disease'. Four major clinical types are recognized: the dystonic form, the 'pseudosclerotic' type, a parkinsonian–rigid form (Oder *et al.* 1991, 1993), and a choreic form.

Most cases of the neurological form with onset before adulthood are of the 'dystonic' type with faciolinguopharyngeal involvement causing facial masking, dysarthria and dysphagia, associated with or preceded by mental deterioration or psychiatric problems (Medalia *et al.* 1988). Speech is often severely impaired. Choreic and myoclonic movements are frequently observed, and painful spasms are common. Pyramidal signs are infrequent. The course may be acute, but in most cases it is slowly progressive. During late stages, muscular rigidity is generalized, bizarre dyskinesias often appear and the patients are severely incapacitated. Psychiatric manifestations are often prominent and may constitute the sole or most prominent feature for months or even years (Jackson *et al.* 1994, Akil and Brewer 1995).

The pseudosclerotic form of Wilson disease is rare in adolescents but intermediate types are not uncommon. In such cases, dysarthria, intention tremor and asterixis are prominent.

Hypokinesia and rigidity, sometimes with tremor at rest are features of the rigid–akinetic type. In many cases, several different syndromes coexist or occur in succession. In a few cases, tongue

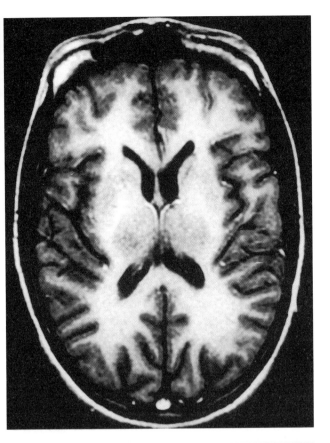

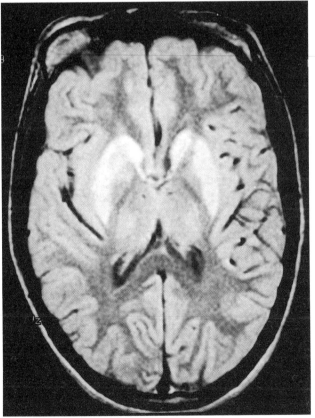

Fig. 9.33. Wilson disease. *(Top)* T₁-weighted MRI showing bilaterally low signal from the basal ganglia and thalami. Global atrophy of brain is also evident. *(Bottom)* T₂-weighted MRI scan of another patient showing intense signal from both putamina.

dyskinesia (Liao *et al.* 1991) or tongue tremor with dysarthria (Topaloglu *et al.* 1990) were the sole manifestations.

Almost all patients with neurological features have a Kayser–Fleischer ring that may be seen with the naked eye or require slit-lamp examination. It may be complete or incomplete and may be present even in the presence of normal liver function. Rare cases of neurological disease in the absence of a corneal ring are known to occur (Demirkiran *et al.* 1996).

DIAGNOSIS

The diagnosis of Wilson disease rests on a high index of suspicion. Wilson disease must be thought of first in any child or adolescent with dystonia and extrapyramidal syndrome, and in those with deterioration and behavioural disorders, because this is a treatable disease (Walshe and Yealland 1992).

The Kayser–Fleischer ring is an essential clue as it is almost never absent in cases with neurological symptoms. Neuroimaging shows, in about half the cases, symmetrical areas of hypodensity in the thalamus and basal ganglia which are visible both with CT scan (Williams and Walshe 1981) and with MRI (Selwa *et al.* 1993, Roh *et al.* 1994) as low T_1 and high T_2 signal (Fig. 9.33). Such abnormalities may decrease or disappear with chelating treatment. Urinary copper is high (in excess of 0.8 μmol/d), as is non-ceruloplasmin-bound copper.

Serum ceruloplasmin level is generally <13–17 μmol/L (100 mg/L), and serum copper is <9 μmol/L (50 mg/dL; normal values: 14–30 μmol/L, 90–160 mg/dL). Low ceruloplasmin levels found on routine family screening unaccompanied by any abnormality of liver function usually indicate a heterozygous condition. In dubious cases, liver biopsy and determination of liver copper is mandatory. Levels in excess of 250 μg/g dry weight indicate Wilson disease.

Prenatal diagnosis and detection of presymptomatic cases is sometimes possible, especially when a deletion is present (Tümer *et al.* 1994). However, the large number of mutations makes it difficult in many cases (Thomas *et al.* 1995). Exclusion of the diagnosis is feasible in many cases by haplotype determination of the patient and parents and known affected family members.

TREATMENT

Therapy of Wilson disease aims at removing excess copper from tissues in symptomatic patients and to prevent accumulation in presymptomatic cases.

D-penicillamine (0.5–0.75 g/d for children under 10 years, 1 g/d in older patients) is given orally in divided doses. Treatment is best monitored by measuring urinary copper excretion which often increases dramatically upon starting treatment then returns to normal over a few months. When effective, the Kayser–Fleischer rings begin to fade in a few weeks and should disappear completely in about a year. A significant decrease of CT/MRI abnormalities should also be obtained as both indicate effective 'de-copperization'. Pyridoxine, 25 mg/kg/d, is added because of the antivitamin effect of penicillamine. Treatment should be started progressively as worsening of symptoms can occur in up to 40 per cent of patients at onset of therapy (Brewer *et al.* 1987):

the dose should be slowly increased while carefully watching clinical condition and copper excretion. Side-effects include fever, rashes, nephrotic syndrome, pyridoxine deficiency, thrombocytopenia and, rarely, myasthenic symptoms. Steroids may help overcome some of these problems.

Alternative therapies include triethylene tetramine (triene), although this seems less effective than penicillamine (Walshe 1996), and oral zinc sulfate, 300–600 mg/d (Brewer *et al.* 1983, Hoogenraad *et al.* 1987), which may be effective when penicillamine is poorly tolerated or as initial treatment in very sick patients. Both these agents can cause initial deterioration (Walshe and Munro 1995). With zinc therapy, gastrointestinal intolerance may occur and the effect is modest. BAL rescue (i.m. dimercaprol) has been used in some resistant cases. A low-copper diet is recommended. Tetrahydromolybdate is theoretically an excellent therapeutic agent and very good results have been reported followed by maintenance zinc therapy (Brewer *et al.* 1996). In the present state of knowledge, such therapies are probably best reserved for asymptomatic or mildly symptomatic cases, whereas penicillamine remains indicated for more severe cases.

Most children who have isolated hepatic disease usually do well. Approximately 40–50 per cent of those with neurological manifestations become asymptomatic, but those with mixed forms have a more severe outlook than purely hepatic forms (Starosta-Rubinstein *et al.* 1987). Patients with advanced liver disease can benefit from liver transplantation.

VARIANTS AND RELATED DISORDERS
A few cases with features reminiscent of Wilson disease but with a different disturbance in copper metabolism have been reported.

Sibs with neurological signs, splenomegaly, absent Kayser–Fleischer ring, associated palsy of vertical gaze and an accumulation of copper in the mucosa of the lower intestine, clearly had a different condition to Wilson disease (Godwin-Austen *et al.* 1978). A few patients with prepubertal onset of neurological symptoms and some atypical features had marginally low ceruloplasmin, no Kayser–Fleischer rings and only mild accumulation of copper in their liver without hepatotoxic effect (Willvonseder *et al.* 1973, Pall *et al.* 1987, Ono *et al.* 1988). One similar patient had massive hepatic accumulation of copper without cirrhosis (Heckmann and Saffer 1988). The mechanism of such cases is not understood. Some patients may respond to penicillamine. Hereditary ceruloplasmin deficiency may cause clinical and neuroimaging anomalies reminiscent of Wilson disease (Morita *et al.* 1995).

MENKES DISEASE (KINKY HAIR DISEASE, STEELY HAIR DISEASE, TRICHOPOLIODYSTROPHY)
Menkes disease is an uncommon X-linked disease (incidence 1 in 50,000 births) characterized pathologically by multiple focal involvement of the grey matter and chemically by low serum copper and ceruloplasmin. The gene is located at Xq13.3 and codes for a copper-transporting ATPase. Deficiency of this protein results in lack of transport of copper to cellular organelles. There is secondary deficit of several enzymes including cytochrome *c*

oxidase and lysine oxidase, accounting for bone and connective tissue abnormalities.

PATHOLOGY AND PATHOPHYSIOLOGY
Copper levels are low in the liver and brain but are elevated in intestinal mucosa and kidneys. Orally administered copper is poorly absorbed but intravenous copper produces a brisk rise of serum copper. The copper content of fibroblasts is markedly elevated. This suggests maldistribution of copper that becomes unavailable for the synthesis of copper-containing enzymes. Excessive uptake of copper by fibroblasts is the basis for prenatal diagnosis of this disease (Horn 1981) which can also be done by measurement of copper in chorionic villus samples (Tønnesen *et al.* 1985). DNA analysis may permit first-trimester diagnosis (Tümer *et al.* 1994).

Defective activity of metalloenzymes produces diffuse disturbances that particularly affect arteries in the brain and elsewhere, and extensive focal degeneration of the grey matter with neuronal loss and gliosis. There is profound involvement of the cerebellar cortex (Robain *et al.* 1988) with loss of Purkinje cells. Remaining cells show abnormal dendritic arborization and axonal swellings.

CLINICAL MANIFESTATIONS
Clinical manifestations become evident from the neonatal period or after 2–3 months. Hypothermia and poor weight gain are prominent. Seizures soon occur, and a profound deterioration with hypotonia becomes apparent. The cherubic appearance of affected infants is striking. The hair is sparse, brittle and colourless (Menkes 1988). Microscopic examination easily confirms the diagnosis by showing pili torti (Fig. 9.34) and occasionally trichorrhexis nodosa. In the first few weeks of life, however, the primary hair may be normal. Hydroureters and hydronephrosis are common. Generalized osteoporosis, metaphyseal spurring, diaphyseal periosteal reaction, scalloping of the posterior aspect of the vertebral bodies and multiple wormian bones are often present. Angiography shows elongated and tortuous arteries but is not routinely indicated. However, tortuosity of intracranial arteries is well demonstrated by MR angiography. Neuroimaging techniques show diffuse brain atrophy, defective myelination and often subdural haematoma. In some cases, more focal abnormalities with areas of cortical atrophy and associated hypodensity are seen (Takahashi *et al.* 1993) (Fig. 9.35).

The course is rapidly downhill and the mean age at death is 19 months. The diagnosis is easy, although bony lesions can suggest scurvy or the battered baby syndrome, the more so as subdural effusions are not unusual.

Copper level is low but this may occur normally in the neonatal period so that one may have to wait a few weeks to confirm the diagnosis, although increased uptake by culture of fibroblasts is already present. Heterozygotes may be suspected by the presence of pili torti (Taylor and Green 1981) and by DNA studies.

Variants of kinky hair disease may present with ataxia and mild mental retardation (Haas *et al.* 1981, Procopis *et al.* 1981,

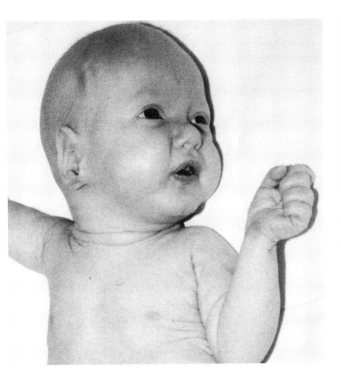

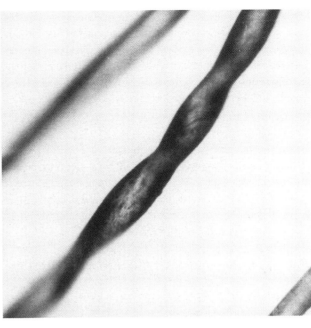

Fig. 9.34. Menkes kinky hair disease. Note chubby appearance of face. Head has a paucity of short, steely, twisted hair.

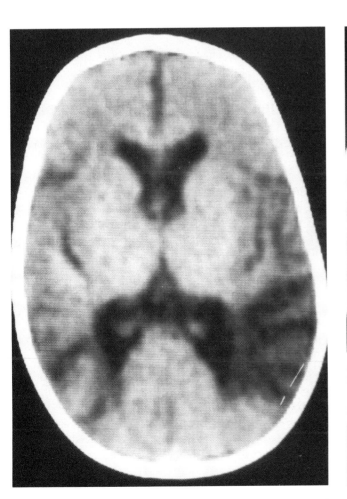

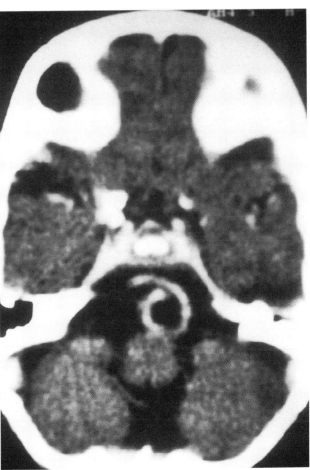

Fig. 9.35. Menkes kinky hair disease. *(Left)* CT scan showing extensive destructive lesions of vascular origin in both parietal regions. *(Right)* Enhanced CT scan showing dilatation, tortuosity and irregular calibre of basilar artery.

Danks 1988) and run a less malignant course. Other atypical cases have presented with hypotonia and hair anomalies but without seizures or hypothermia (Inagaki *et al.* 1988). The condition reported by Dinno *et al.* (1981) which is unassociated with copper abnormalities and affects both sexes is probably a different disorder.

TREATMENT
Treatment with parenterally administered copper restores blood levels but does not correct the neurological disease. Administration of copper-histidine may favourably influence the neurological disease in some cases, particularly if commenced early at 35 weeks gestational age (Tümer *et al.* 1996), but negative results have also been reported (Kaler *et al.* 1995).

MISCELLANEOUS METABOLIC DISORDERS

DISORDERS OF PURINE METABOLISM
LESCH–NYHAN SYNDROME
Lesch–Nyhan syndrome is an X-linked disorder due to deficiency of the enzyme hypoxanthine-guanine phosphoribosyltransferase (HGPRT). As a consequence of this defect, hypoxanthine cannot be reutilized and hypoxanthine formed is catabolized to xanthine and uric acid or excreted. Depletion of hypoxanthine, which acts as a feedback regulator of uric acid synthesis, leads to markedly increased production of uric acid, resulting In hyperuricaemia and its consequences.

The mechanism of neurological disturbances is still obscure and is unrelated to uric acid. The concentration of dopamine and the activity of enzymes involved in its synthesis are lessened, and this and other alterations in neurotransmitter balance within the basal ganglia are probably important (Jankovic *et al.* 1988).

There is a striking degree of heterogeneity of HGPRT defects, and many variants have been recognized variably due to small deletions or point mutations in the gene located at Xq26–q27 (Wilson *et al.* 1983), some of them with distinctive clinical concomitants.

Pathologically, no definite lesions have been recognized (Watts *et al.* 1982).

Clinical manifestations
The clinical manifestations become apparent during the first year of life in the form of psychomotor retardation and generalized muscular hypotonia (Christie *et al.* 1982, Watts *et al.* 1982). Torsion dystonia, chorea or athetosis are subsequently superimposed on hypotonia but become progressively less obvious as spasticity progressively develops. Seizures occur in about half the children. Self-mutilation with biting of fingers, lips and tongue appears usually between 2 and 4 years of age but sometimes later (Hatanaka *et al.* 1990). Affected children are variably retarded, usually mildly or moderately, but most suffer from attention deficit and difficulties of comprehension of complex or lengthy speech and in multistep reasoning (Matthews *et al.* 1995). They are severely disturbed by their compulsion to self-mutilate and appear happier when maintained in restraints.

In late childhood or adolescence haematuria, renal calculi and ultimately renal failure develop. Gouty arthritis and urate tophi can also be observed.

The diagnosis is suggested by a high level of serum uric acid. However, urinary uric acid content is a better indicator, as serum uric acid may occasionally be normal. Antenatal diagnosis is possible by enzymatic analysis of blood, skin fibroblasts or amniotic cells, which is easily carried out, and by mutation identification which can also be used to detect female carriers (Alford *et al.* 1995).

Treatment
Treatment with allopurinol is effective in relieving symptoms due to high uric acid but has no action on neurological manifestations. Attempts at gene therapy using a retrovirus to deliver the missing enzyme to bone marrow cells are being pursued.

PARTIAL DEFICITS IN HGPRT AND VARIANTS OF LESCH–NYHAN SYNDROME
Deficits in HGPRT less complete than those in the classical Lesch–Nyhan syndrome (less than 1.3 per cent of normal) can produce various clinical pictures. Patients with a level of more than 8.5 per cent of normal have no neurological symptoms but may have uric acid-related problems. At intermediate range, a neurological picture similar to Lesch–Nyhan syndrome but without mental retardation and self-mutilation may be observed (Bakay *et al.* 1979). Other variants with mild mental retardation, spasticity and skeletal malformations (Page *et al.* 1987), choreoathetosis (Gottileb *et al.* 1982), developmental retardation and deafness have been described. A neurodevelopmentally similar syndrome with some features reminiscent of the Lesch–Nyhan syndrome with hyperuricaemia due to deficiency of phosphoribosyl pyrophosphate synthetase has been reported (Simmonds *et al.* 1982). Rare cases of typical Lesch–Nyhan syndrome in girls are on record (Ogasawara *et al.* 1989).

SYNDROME OF INFANTILE AUTISM WITH PRESENCE OF SUCCINYLPURINES IN BODY FLUIDS
Jaeken and Van den Berghe (1984) have reported on an autistic syndrome with severe mental retardation in association with the presence of large amounts of succinyladenosine and succinylaminoimidazole carboxamide riboside in body fluids. CSF protein was low in affected children and there was hypoplasia of the cerebellar vermis (Chapter 3). A fast, inexpensive diagnostic test has been developed (Maddocks and Reed 1989).

PURINE NUCLEOSIDE PHOSPHORYLASE DEFICIENCY
This rare disease is characterized by severe immunodeficiency. A neurological syndrome consisting of an association of diplegia and dysequilibrium syndrome seems to be an integral part of the disease (Simmonds *et al.* 1987; see also Chapter 11).

DISORDERS OF PYRIMIDINE DEGRADATION
Cases of probable defects of pyrimidine dehydrogenase (van Gennip *et al.* 1994a) and of dihydropyrimidinase (Putman *et al.*

1997) can present with convulsions, mental retardation or choreo-athetosis, sometimes associated with dysmorphism. This group of conditions may represent a novel category of neurodevelopmental disorders and should be thought of in the investigation of obscure neurological conditions.

GUANIDOACETATE METHYLTRANSFERASE DEFICIENCY

This rare disease is marked by arrested development, extrapyramidal features and sometimes seizures (Ganesan *et al.* 1997). MRI may show high signal from the globus pallidus. The diagnosis is suggested by a low plasma creatinine level (5–10 µmol/L) which is, however, often overlooked as the lower limit for the normal range for creatinine is undefined. Treatment is by oral supplementation with 500–2000 mg of creatinine.

PORPHYRIAS

This group of disorders is uncommon in childhood. The main clinical features of acute intermittent porphyria and of hereditary coproporphyria are described in Chapter 21.

DISORDERS OF DNA REPAIR

Defects in DNA repair mechanisms play an important role in several neurological diseases (Mazzarello *et al.* 1992). These include ataxia–telangiectasia (Chapter 4) and xeroderma pigmentosum. Xeroderma pigmentosum is an autosomal recessive disease characterized by acute sensitivity of the skin to sun, leading to the development of cutaneous malignancies. At least nine genetic forms of the disease exist, eight of them with defective DNA nucleotide excision repair (Robbins 1987). Some patients develop a progressive neurodegeneration starting in infancy or before adolescence with intellectual impairment or dementia, microcephaly, abnormal movements or cerebellar signs. Deafness and peripheral neuropathy may occur (Robbins *et al.* 1991).

CEREBROTENDINOUS XANTHOMATOSIS

Cerebrotendinous xanthomatosis is a rare inherited disorder of bile acid metabolism leading to accumulation of cholestanol and cholesterol in most tissues including the CNS. It is responsible for xanthomas, early cararact, severe neurological deterioration and premature atherosclerosis. In spite of its rarity, diagnosis is important because early treatment can halt and in some cases reverse the neurological impairment (Meiner *et al.* 1994).

BIOCHEMICAL AND GENETIC BACKGROUND

Cerebrotendinous xanthomatosis is an autosomal recessive disorder due to defective 27-hydroxylase enzyme activity. The defect impairs the mitochondrial part of bile acid synthesis from cholesterol and results in accumulation of cholestanol and cholesterol. In serum, cholesterol levels are normal but increased cholestanol levels result in an abnormal cholestanol/cholesterol ratio. The defect is responsible for a low synthesis of chenodeoxycholic acid, the end-product of bile acid synthesis. This, in turn, results in upregulation of the cholesterol 7-alpha-hydroxyl-ase, the rate-limiting enzyme in bile acid synthesis, and further accumulation of bile acid intermediates. The enzymatic activity is expressed in cultured fibroblasts and liver.

A cDNA encoding human 27-hydroxylase has been characterized allowing its location to chromosome 2 and the identification of various disease-causing mutations. Molecular biology would enable genetic counselling by permitting early detection of presymptomatic cases and carriers (Leitersdorf *et al.* 1993, Garuti *et al.* 1996, Okuyama *et al.* 1996).

NEUROPATHOLOGY

The cerebellar white matter, the optic pathways and the long tracts of the brainstem, spinal cord and spinal roots are most involved. Lesions are due to axonal degeneration with loss of myelinated fibres and accumulation of lipids. Cystic spaces and crystalline clefts surrounded by foamy cells, gliosis, axonal spheroids and multinucleated foreign giant cells are found in many parts of the CNS but especially in the cerebellum (Soffer *et al.* 1995). The sterol fraction from affected parts of the CNS and peripheral nerves is essentially made up of cholestanol.

CLINICAL FEATURES

The major clinical signs include xanthomas in the tendons and tuberous xanthomas, juvenile cataracts, progressive neurological dysfunction and dementia, and premature coronary heart disease or atherosclerosis. Some patients have respiratory insufficiency and endocrinological disturbances. The development of the symptoms is highly variable with neurological involvement occurring in the second or third decade of life although in many patients early signs may precede the onset of neurological signs by several years (Wevers *et al.* 1992). The early clinical course is characterized by intractable diarrhoea and mild to moderate developmental delay in some affected children. Juvenile bilateral cataracts, sometimes associated with optic neuropathy, xanthomas and progressive neurological impairment, are seen in the second stage of the disease (Cruysberg *et al.* 1995, Verrips *et al.* 1995). Neurological signs include peripheral neuropathy, pyramidal and cerebellar signs with spasticity and ataxia, and convulsions in some cases (Kuriyama *et al.* 1991). Some patients may present with prominent psychiatric disorders (Berginer *et al.* 1988). Xanthomas may be absent in early stages of the disorder or even never develop (Arpa *et al.* 1995, Slebner *et al.* 1996), and a few patients have had normal intelligence in spite of neurological impairment such as ataxia, paresis or peripheral neuropathy (Blorkhem *et al.* 1987). In the late and final stage, neurological deterioration is severe, speech becomes difficult, and swallowing difficulties and sphincter incontinence develop. MRI studies of the brain and spinal cord have revealed cerebral, cerebellar and spinal cord atrophy (Bencze *et al.* 1990) and demyelination in the cerebrum, cerebellum and brainstem (Bencze *et al.* 1990, Arpa *et al.* 1995, Okada *et al.* 1995). Nodular, bilateral symmetrical lesions in the cerebellar white matter, strongly suggestive of calcification, have been noted in one case (Arpa *et al.* 1995). Results of neurophysiological studies are consistent with axonal and peripheral neuropathy (Arpa *et al.* 1995).

DIAGNOSIS

Biochemical diagnosis is made by the determination of excessive urinary excretion of bile alcohols and by the cholestanol/cholesterol ratio in serum (Björkhem *et al.* 1987, Arpa *et al.* 1995). The definitive diagnosis relies on measurement of 7-alpha-hydroxylase in cultured fibroblasts.

TREATMENT

By supplying the end-product of bile acid synthesis, supplementation with chenodeoxycholic acid decreases cholestanol accumulation and results in clear clinical, radiological and neurophysiological improvement (Berginer *et al.* 1984, Björkhem *et al.* 1987, Verrips *et al.* 1995). Addition of simvastatin, an inhibitor of 3-hydroxy-3-methyl-glutaryl-CoA reductase, may further improve the therapeutic effects (Watts *et al.* 1996).

REFERENCES

Abbott, M.H., Folstein, S.E., Abbey, H., Pyeritz, R.E. (1987) 'Psychiatric manifestations of homocystinuria due to cystathionine β-synthase deficiency: prevalence, natural history, and relationship to neurologic impairment and vit B6-responsiveness.' *American Journal of Medical Genetics*, **26**, 959–969.

Abeling, N.G.G.M., van Gennip, A.H., Overmars, H., *et al.* (1994) 'Biogenic amine metabolite patterns in the urine of monoamine oxidase A-deficient patients. A possible tool for diagnosis.' *Journal of Inherited Metabolic Disease*, **17**, 339–341.

Adinolfi, M. (1993) 'Hunter syndrome: cloning of the gene, mutations and carrier detection.' *Developmental Medicine and Child Neurology*, **35**, 79–85.

Afifi, A.K., Sato, Y., Waziri, M.H., Bell, W.E. (1990) 'Computed tomography and magnetic resonance imaging of the brain in Hurler's disease.' *Journal of Child Neurology*, **5**, 235–241.

Akaboshi, S., Ohno, K., Takeshita, K. (1995) 'Neuroradiological findings in the carbohydrate-deficient glycoprotein syndrome.' *Neuroradiology*, **37**, 491–495.

Akil, M., Brewer, G.J. (1995) 'Psychiatric and behavioral abnormalities in Wilson's disease.' *In:* Weiner, W.J., Lang, A.E. (Eds.) *Behavioral Neurology of Movement Disorders. Advances in Neurology, Vol. 65.* New York: Raven Press, pp. 171–178.

Al Aqeel, A., Rashed, M., Ozand, P.T., *et al.* (1994) '3-Methylglutaconic aciduria: ten new cases with a possible new phenotype.' *Brain and Development*, **16** (Suppl.), 23–32.

Alford, R.L., Redman, J.B., O'Brien, W.E., Caskey, C.T. (1995) 'Lesch–Nyhan syndrome: carrier and prenatal diagnosis.' *Prenatal Diagnosis*, **15**, 329–338.

Allen, R.H., Stabler, S., Lindenbaum, J. (1993) 'Serum betaine, N,N-dimethylglycine and N-methylglycine levels in patients with cobalamin and folate deficiency and related inborn errors of metabolism.' *Metabolism*, **42**, 1448–1460.

Amir, N., Zlotogora, J., Bach, G. (1987) 'Mucolipidosis type IV: clinical spectrum and natural history.' *Pediatrics*, **79**, 953–959.

—— Elpeleg, O.N., Shalev, R.S., Christensen, E. (1989) 'Glutaric aciduria type I: enzymatic and neuroradiologic investigations of two kindreds.' *Journal of Pediatrics*, **114**, 983–989.

Andréasson, S., Blennow, G., Ehinger, B., Strömland, K. (1991) 'Full-field electroretinograms in patients with the carbohydrate-deficient glycoprotein syndrome.' *American Journal of Ophthalmology*, **112**, 83–86.

Andria, G., Sebastio, G. (1995) 'Homocystinuria due to β-cystathionine synthase deficiency and related disorders.' *In:* Fernandes, J., Saudubray, J.M., van den Berghe, G. (Eds.) *Inborn Metabolic Diseases. Diagnosis and Treatment. 2nd Edn.* Berlin: Springer-Verlag, pp. 177–182.

Antonozzi, I., Leuzzi, V. (1987) 'Case report. Hyperargininaemia.' *Journal of Inherited Metabolic Disease*, **10**, 200.

Aoki, Y., Suzuki, Y., Sakamoto, O., *et al.* (1995) 'Molecular analysis of holocarboxylase synthetase deficiency: a missense mutation and a single base deletion are predominant in Japanese patients.' *Biochimica et Biophysica Acta*, **1272**, 168–174.

Arbour, L., Rosenblatt, B., Clow, C., Wilson, G.N. (1988) 'Postoperative dystonia in a female patient with homocystinuria.' *Journal of Pediatrics*, **113**, 863–864.

Arnold, G.L., Greene, C.L., Stout, J.P., Goodman, S.I. (1993) 'Molybdenum cofactor deficiency.' *Journal of Pediatrics*, **123**, 595–598.

Arpa, J., Sánchez, C., Vega, A., *et al.* (1995) 'Cerebrotendinous xanthomatosis diagnosed after traumatic subdural haematoma.' *Revue Neurologique*, **23**, 675–678.

Arvio, M., Autio, S., Louhiala, P. (1993) 'Early clinical symptoms and incidence of aspartylglucosaminuria in Finland.' *Acta Paediatrica*, **82**, 587–589.

Ashwal, S., Rorke, L.B., Epstein, M.A., *et al.* (1988) 'Rapid deterioration in a three-year-old with left hemiparesis.' *Pediatric Neuroscience*, **14**, 124–133.

Assmann, G., Seedorf, U. (1995) 'Acid lipase deficiency: Wolman disease and cholesterol ester storage disease.' *In:* Scriver, C.R., Beaudet, A.L., Sly, W.S., Valle, D. (Eds.) *The Metabolic and Molecular Bases of Inherited Disease, 7th Edn.* New York: McGraw Hill, pp. 2563–2587.

Aubourg, P., Sellier, N., Chaussain, J.L., Kalifa, G. (1989) 'MRI detects cerebral involvement in neurologically asymptomatic patients with adrenoleucodystrophy.' *Neurology*, **39**, 1619–1621.

—— Blanche, S., Jambaqué, I., *et al.* (1990) 'Reversal of early neurologic and neuroradiologic manifestations of X-linked adrenoleukodystrophy by bone marrow transplantation.' *New England Journal of Medicine*, **322**, 1860–1866.

—— Adamsbaum, C., Lavallard-Rousseau, M.C., *et al.* (1992) 'Brain MRI and electrophysiologic abnormalities in preclinical and clinical adrenomyeloneuropathy.' *Neurology*, **42**, 85–91.

—— Adamsbaum, C., Lavallard-Rousseau, M-C., *et al.* (1993) 'A two-year trial of oleic and erucic acids ("Lorenzo's oil") as treatment for adrenomyeloneuropathy.' *New England Journal of Medicine*, **329**, 745–752.

Aukett, A., Bennett, M.J., Hosking, G.P. (1988) 'Molybdenum cofactor deficiency: an easily missed inborn error of metabolism.' *Developmental Medicine and Child Neurology*, **30**, 531–535.

Azen, C., Koch, R., Friedman, E., *et al.* (1996) 'Summary of findings from the United States Collaborative Study of children treated for phenylketonuria.' *European Journal of Pediatrics*, **155**, Suppl. 1, S29–S32.

Bakay, B., Nissinen, E., Sweetman, L., *et al.* (1979) 'Utilization of purines by an HPRT variant in an intelligent, nonmutilative patient with features of the Lesch–Nyhan syndrome.' *Pediatric Research*, **13**, 1365–1370.

Bank, W., Morrow, G. (1972) 'A familial spinal cord disorder with hyperglycinemia.' *Archives of Neurology*, **27**, 136–144.

Bankier, A., Turner, M., Hopkins, I.J. (1983) 'Pyridoxine dependent seizures: a wider clinical spectrum.' *Archives of Disease in Childhood*, **58**, 415–418.

Barbot, C., Martins, E., Vilarinho, L., *et al.* (1995) 'A mild form of infantile isolated sulphite oxidase deficiency.' *Neuropediatrics*, **26**, 322–324.

Barth, M.L., Fensom, A., Harris, A. (1994a) 'The arylsulphatase A gene and molecular genetics of metachromatic leucodystrophy.' *Journal of Medical Genetics*, **31**, 663–666.

—— Ward, C., Harris, A., *et al.* (1994b) 'Frequency of arylsulfatase A pseudodeficiency associated mutations in a healthy population.' *Journal of Medical Genetics*, **31**, 667–671.

Barth, P.G. Hoffmann, G.F., Jaeken, J., *et al.* (1992) 'L-2-hydroxyglutaric acidemia: a novel inherited neurometabolic disease.' *Annals of Neurology*, **32**, 66–71.

—— —— *et al.* (1993) 'L-2-hydroxyglutaric acidaemia: clinical and biochemical findings in 12 patients and preliminary report on L-2-hydroxyacid dehydrogenase.' *Journal of Inherited Metabolic Disease*, **16**, 753–761.

Batshaw, M.L. (1994) 'Inborn errors of urea synthesis.' *Annals of Neurology*, **35**, 133–141.

Bauman, M.L., Kemper, T.L. (1982) 'Morphologic and histoanatomic observations of the brain in untreated human phenylketonuria.' *Acta Neuropathologica*, **58**, 55–63.

Baumeister, F.A.M., Gsell, W., Shin, Y.S., Egger, J. (1994) 'Glutamate in pyridoxine-dependent epilepsy: neurotoxic glutamate concentration in the cerebrospinal fluid and its normalization by pyridoxine.' *Pediatrics*, **94**, 318–321.

Baumgartner, E.R., Suormala, T.M. (1995) 'Biotin-responsive multipole carboxylase deficiency.' *In:* Fernandes, J., Saudubray, J.M., van den Berghe, G. (Eds.) *Inborn Metabolic Diseases. Diagnosis and Treatment. 2nd Edn.* Berlin: Springer Verlag, pp. 239–245.

—— —— Wick, H., *et al.* (1989) 'Biotinidase deficiency: a cause of subacute necrotizing encephalomyelopathy (Leigh syndrome). Report of a case with lethal outcome.' *Pediatric Research*, **26**, 260–266.

Baxter, P., Griffiths, P., Kelly, T., Gardner-Medwin, D. (1996) 'Pyridoxine-dependent seizures: demographic, clinical, MRI and psychometric features, and effect of dose on intelligence quotient.' *Developmental Medicine and Child Neurology*, **38**, 998–1006.

Beard, S.E., Goodman, S.I., Bemelen, K., Frerman, F.E. (1995) 'Characterization of a mutation that abolishes quinone reduction by electron transfer flavoprotein–ubiquinone oxidoreductase.' *Human Molecular Genetics*, **4**, 157–161.

Beckman, D.R., Hoganson, G., Berlow, S., Gilbert, E.F. (1987) 'Pathological findings in 5,10-methylenetetrahydrofolate reductase deficiency.' *Birth Defects*, **23**, 47–50.

Bembi, B., Zanatta, M., Carrozzi, M., *et al.* (1994) 'Enzyme replacement treatment in type 1 and type 3 Gaucher's disease.' *Lancet*, **344**, 1679–1682.

Bencze, K.S., Vande Polder, D.R., Prockop, L.D. (1990) 'Magnetic resonance imaging of the brain and spinal cord in cerebrotendinous xanthomatosis.' *Journal of Neurology, Neurosurgery, and Psychiatry*, **53**, 166–167.

Bennet, J.K., Dembure, P.P., Elsas, L.J. (1995) 'Clinical and biochemical analysis of two families with type I and type II mannosidosis.' *American Journal of Medical Genetics*, **55**, 21–26.

Bennett, M.J., Gibson, K.M., Sherwood, W.G., *et al.* (1993) 'Reliable prenatal diagnosis of Canavan disease (aspartoacylase deficiency): comparison of enzymatic and metabolite analysis.' *Journal of Inherited Metabolic Disease*, **16**, 831–836.

Berginer, V.M., Salen, G., Shefer, S. (1984) 'Long-term treatment of cerebrotendinous xanthomatosis with chenodeoxycholic acid.' *New England Journal of Medicine*, **311**, 1649–1652.

—— Foster, N.L., Sadowsky, M., *et al.* (1988) 'Psychiatric disorders in patients with cerebrotendinous xanthomatosis.' *American Journal of Psychiatry*, **145**, 354–357.

Bernes, S.M., Bacino, C., Prezant, T.R., *et al.* (1996) 'Identical mitochondrial DNA deletion in mother with progressive external ophthalmoplegia and son with Pearson marrow–pancreas syndrome.' *Journal of Pediatrics*, **123**, 598–602.

Bernsen, P.L.J.A., Wevers, R.A., Gabreëls, F.J.M., *et al.* (1987) 'Phenotypic expression in mucopolysaccharidosis VII.' *Journal of Neurology, Neurosurgery, and Psychiatry*, **50**, 699–703.

Berthier, M., Oriot, D., Bonneau, D., Jaeken, J. (1995) 'Does a mutation of the glycine receptor modify GABA metabolism in startle disease?' *Acta Paediatrica*, **84**, 5. (Letter.)

Bhala, A., Willi, S.M., Rinaldo, P., *et al.* (1995) 'Clinical and biochemical characterization of short-chain acyl-coenzyme A dehydrogenase deficiency.' *Journal of Pediatrics*, **126**, 910–915.

Björkhem, I., Skrede, S., Buchmann, M.S., *et al.* (1987) 'Accumulation of 7-α-hydroxy-4-cholesten-3-one and cholesta-4,6-dien-3-one in patients with cerebrotendinous xanthomatosis: effect of treatment with chenoxycholic acid.' *Hepatology*, **7**, 266–271.

Blau, N., Thöny, B., Heizmann, C.W., Dhondt, J.L.. (1993) 'Tetrahydrobiopterin deficiency: from phenotype to genotype.' *Pteridines*, **4**, 1–10.

—— Kierat, L., Matasovic, A., *et al.* (1994) 'Antenatal diagnosis of tetrahydrobiopterin deficiency by quantification of pterins in amniotic fluid and enzyme activity in fetal and extrafetal tissue.' *Clinica Chimica Acta*, **226**, 159–169.

—— Barnes, I., Dhondt, J.L. (1996) 'International database of tetrahydrobiopterin deficiencies.' *Journal of Inherited Metabolic Disease*, **19**, 8–14.

Böhles, H., Wenzel, D., Shin, Y.S. (1986) 'Progressive cerebellar and extrapyramidal motor disturbances in galactosemic twins.' *European Journal of Pediatrics*, **145**, 413–417.

Bohu, P.A., Hannequin, D., Hemet, C., *et al.* (1995) 'Complications neurologiques tardives de la galactosémie: étude de trois cas.' *Revue Neurologique*, **151**, 136–138.

Boles, R.G., Ment, L.R., Meyn, M.S., *et al.* (1993) 'Short-term response to dietary therapy in molybdenum cofactor deficiency.' *Annals of Neurology*, **34**, 742–744.

Bonne, G., Benelli, C., De Meirler, L., *et al.* (1993) 'E1 pyruvate dehydrogenase deficiency in a child with motor neuropathy.' *Pediatric Research*, **33**, 284–288.

Bonnefont, J-P., Chretien, D., Rustin, P., *et al.* (1992) 'Alpha-ketoglutarate dehydrogenase deficiency presenting as congenital lactic acidosis.' *Journal of Pediatrics*, **121**, 255–258.

—— Taroni, F., Cavadini, P., *et al.* (1996) 'Molecular analysis of carnitine palmitoyltransferase II deficiency with hepatocardiomuscular expression.' *American Journal of Human Genetics*, **58**, 971–978.

Boulat, O., Benador, N., Girardin, E., Bachmann, C. (1995) '3-Hydroxy-isobutyric aciduria with a mild clinical course.' *Journal of Inherited Metabolic Disease*, **18**, 204–206.

Bourgeois, M., Goutieres, F., Chretien, D., *et al.* (1992) 'Deficiency in complex II of the respiratory chain, presenting as a leukodystrophy in two sisters with Leigh syndrome.' *Brain and Development*, **14**, 404–408.

Bourgeron, T., Rustin, P., Chretien, D., *et al.* (1995) 'Mutation of a nuclear succinate dehydrogenase gene results in mitochondrial respiratory chain deficiency.' *Nature Genetics*, **11**, 144–149.

Boustany, R-M.N., Tanaka, A., Nishimoto, J., Suzuki, K. (1991) 'Genetic cause of a juvenile form of Tay–Sachs disease in a Lebanese child.' *Annals of Neurology*, **29**, 104–107.

—— Qian, W-H., Suzuki, K. (1993) 'Mutations in acid β-galactosidase cause GM₁-gangliosidosis in American patients.' *American Journal of Human Genetics*, **53**, 881–888.

Brand, M.P., Heales, S.J.R., Land, J.M., Clark, J.B. (1995) 'Tetrahydrobiopterin deficiency and brain nitric oxide synthase in *hph1* mouse.' *Journal of Inherited Metabolic Disease*, **18**, 33–39.

Braverman, N., Dodt, G., Gould, S.J., Valle, D. (1995) 'Disorders of peroxisome biogenesis.' *Human Molecular Genetics*, **4**, 1791–1798.

Bresolin, N., Comi, G.P., Fortunato, F., *et al.* (1993) 'Clinical and biochemical evidence of skeletal muscle involvement in galactose-1-phosphate uridyl transferase deficiency.' *Journal of Neurology*, **240**, 272–277.

Brewer, G.J., Hill, G.M., Prasad, A.S. (1983) 'Oral zinc therapy for Wilson's disease.' *Annals of Internal Medicine*, **99**, 314–320.

Brewer, G.J., Terry, C.A., Aisen, A.M., Hill, G.M. (1987) 'Worsening of neurologic syndrome in patients with Wilson's disease with initial penicillamine therapy.' *Archives of Neurology*, **44**, 490–493.

—— Johnson, V., Dick, R.D., *et al.* (1996) 'Treatment of Wilson disease with ammonium tetrathiomolybdate. II: Initial therapy in 33 neurologically affected patients and follow-up with zinc therapy.' *Archives of Neurology*, **53**, 1017–1025.

Brismar, J., Ozand, P.T. (1994a) 'CT and MR of the brain in the diagnosis of organic acidemias: experiences from 107 patients.' *Brain and Development*, **16** (Suppl.), 104–124.

—— —— (1994b) 'CT and MR of the brain in disorders of the propionate and methylmalonate metabolism.' *American Journal of Neuroradiology*, **15**, 1459–1473.

—— —— (1995) 'CT and MR of the brain in glutaric acidemia type I: a review of 59 published cases and a report of 5 new patients.' *American Journal of Neuroradiology*, **16**, 675–683.

—— Aqeel, A., Brismar, G., *et al.* (1990a) 'Maple syrup urine disease: findings on CT and MR scans of the brain in 10 infants.' *American Journal of Neuroradiology*, **11**, 1219–1228.

—— Gascon, G., Ozand, P. (1990b) 'Malignant hyperphenylalaninemia.' *American Journal of Neuroradiology*, **11**, 135–138.

Brockstedt, M., Smit, L.M.E., de Grauw, A.J.C., *et al.* (1990) 'A new case of hyperargininaemia: neurological and biochemical findings prior to and during dietary treatment.' *European Journal of Pediatrics*, **149**, 341–343.

Brown, F.R., Voigt, R., Singh, A.K., Singh, I. (1993) 'Peroxisomal disorders: neurodevelopmental and biochemical aspects.' *American Journal of Diseases of Children*, **147**, 617–626.

Brown, G.K. (1992) 'Pyruvate dehydrogenase E1α deficiency.' *Journal of Inherited Metabolic Disease*, **15**, 625–633.

—— Squier, M.V. (1996) 'Neuropathology and pathogenesis of mitochondrial diseases.' *Journal of Inherited Metabolic Disease*, **19**, 553–572.

Brusilow, S.W., Horwich, A.L. (1995) 'Urea cycle enzyme.' *In:* Scriver, C.R., Beaudet, A.L., Sly, W.S., Valle, D. (Eds.) *The Metabolic and Molecular Bases of Inherited Disease, 7th Edn.* New York: McGraw Hill, pp. 1187–1232.

—— Maestri, N.E. (1996) 'Urea cycle disorders: diagnosis, pathophysiology, and therapy.' *Advances in Pediatrics*, **43**, 127–170.

Budde-Steffen, C., Steffen, M., Siegel, D.A., Suzuki, K. (1988) 'Presence of β-hexosaminidase A α-chain mRNA in two different variants of G_{M2}-gangliosidosis.' *Neuropediatrics*, **19**, 59–61.

Burch, M., Fensom, A.H., Jackson, M., *et al.* (1986) 'Multiple sulphatase deficiency presenting at birth.' *Clinical Genetics*, **30**, 409–415.

Burgard, P., Armbruster, M., Schmidt, E., Rupp, A. (1994) 'Psychopathology of patients treated early for phenylketonuria: results of the German collaborative study of phenylketonuria.' *Acta Paediatrica*, Suppl. 407, 108–110.

Burns, S.P., Iles, R.A., Saudubray, J-M., Chalmers, R.A. (1996) 'Propionyl-carnitine excretion is not affected by metronidazole administration to patients with disorders of propionate metabolism.' *European Journal of Pediatrics*, **155**, 31–35.

Byrd, D.J., Krohn, H.P., Winkler, L., *et al.* (1989) 'Neonatal pyruvate dehydrogenase deficiency with lipoate responsive lactic acidaemia and hyperammonaemia.' *European Journal of Pediatrics*, **148**, 543–547.

Cameron, P.D., Dubowitz, V., Besley, G.T.N., Fensom, A.H. (1990) 'Sialic acid storage disease.' *Archives of Disease in Childhood*, **65**, 314–315.

Campistol, J., Ribes, A., Alvarez, L., *et al.* (1992) 'Glutaric aciduria type I: unusual biochemical presentation.' *Journal of Pediatrics*, **121**, 83–86.

Cannizzaro, L.A., Chen, Y.Q., Rafi, M.A., Wenger, D.A. (1994) 'Regional mapping of the human galactocerebrosidase gene (GALC) to 14q31 by in situ hybridization.' *Cytogenetics and Cell Genetics*, **66**, 244–245.

Cao, Z., Natowicz, M.R., Kaback, M.M., *et al.* (1993) 'A second mutation associated with apparent β-hexosaminidase A pseudodeficiency: identification and frequency estimation.' *American Journal of Human Genetics*, **53**, 1198–1205.

Carstea, E.D., Polymeropoulos, M.H., Parker, C.C., *et al.* (1993) 'Linkage of Niemann–Pick disease type C to human chromosome 18.' *Proceedings of the National Academy of Sciences of the USA*, **90**, 2002–2004.

Casteels, I., Taylor, D.S., Lake, B.D., *et al.* (1992) 'Mucolipidosis type IV. Presentation of a mild variant.' *Ophthalmic Paediatrics and Genetics*, **13**, 205–210.

Cavanagh, J.B., Harding, B.N. (1994) 'Pathogenic factors underlying the lesions in Leigh's disease. Tissue responses to cellular energy deprivation and their clinico-pathological consequences.' *Brain*, **117**, 1357–1376.

Ceuterick, C., Martin, J-J. (1992) 'Electron microscopic features of skin in neurometabolic disorders.' *Journal of the Neurological Sciences*, **112**, 15–29.

Charnas, L.R., Bernardini, I., Rader, D., *et al.* (1991) 'Clinical and laboratory findings in the oculocerebrorenal syndrome of Lowe, with special reference to growth and renal function.' *New England Journal of Medicine*, **324**, 1318–1325.

—— Luciano, C.A., Dalakas, M., *et al.* (1994) 'Distal vacuolar myopathy in nephropathic cystinosis.' *Annals of Neurology*, **35**, 181–188.

Charrow, J., Hvizd, M.G. (1986) 'Cardiomyopathy and skeletal myopathy in an unusual variant of G_{M1} gangliosidosis.' *Journal of Pediatrics*, **108**, 729–732.

Chen, E., Nyhan, W.L., Jakobs, C., *et al.* (1996) 'L-2-hydroxyglutaric aciduria: neuropathological correlations and first report of severe neurodegenerative disease and neonatal death.' *Journal of Inherited Metabolic Disease*, **19**, 335–343.

Chenel, C., Wood, C., Gourrier, E., *et al.* (1993) 'Syndrome hémolytique et urémique néonatal, acidurie méthylmalonique et homocystinurie par déficit intracellulaire de la vitamine B12. Intérêt du diagnostic étiologique.' *Archives Françaises de Pédiatrie*, **50**, 749–754.

Cherstvoy, E.D., Lazjuk, G.I., Ostrovskaya, T.I., *et al.* (1984) 'The Smith–Lemli–Opitz syndrome: a detailed pathological study as a clue to a etiological heterogeneity.' *Virchows Achiv A. Pathological Anatomy and Histopathology*, **404**, 413–425.

Christie, R., Bay, C., Kaufman, I.A., *et al.* (1982) 'Lesch–Nyhan disease: clinical experience with nineteen patients.' *Developmental Medicine and Child Neurology*, **24**, 293–306.

Christodoulou, J., Kure, S., Hayasaka, K., Clarke, J.T.R. (1993) 'Atypical non-ketotic hyperglycinemia confirmed by assay of the glycine cleavage system in lymphoblasts.' *Journal of Pediatrics*, **123**, 100–102.

Clarke, J.T., Skomorowski, M.A., Chang, P.L. (1989) 'Marked clinical difference between two sibs affected with juvenile metachromatic leukodystrophy.' *American Journal of Medical Genetics*, **33**, 10–13.

Clayton, P.T., Smith, I.S., Harding, B., *et al.* (1986) 'Subacute combined degeneration of the cord, dementia and parkinsonism due to an inborn error of folate metabolism.' *Journal of Neurology, Neurosurgery, and Psychiatry*, **49**, 920–927.

—— Mills, K., Keeling, J., Fitz Patrick, D. (1996) 'Desmosterolosis: a new inborn error of cholesterol biosynthesis.' *Lancet*, **348**, 404. *(Letter.)*

Clearly, M.A., Walter, J.H., Wraith, J.E., *et al.* (1994) 'Magnetic resonance imaging of the brain in phenylketonuria.' *Lancet*, **344**, 87–90.

Coker, S.B. (1993) 'Leigh disease presenting as Guillain–Barré syndrome.' *Pediatric Neurology*, **9**, 61–63.

—— Thomas, C. (1995) 'Connatal Leigh disease.' *Clinical Pediatrics*, **34**, 349–352.

Cole, D.E.C., Meek, D.C. (1985) 'Juvenile non-ketotic hyperglycinaemia in three siblings.' *Journal of Inherited Metabolic Disease*, **8**, Suppl. 2, 123–124.

Colombo, I., Finocchiaro, G., Garavaglia, B., *et al.* (1994) 'Mutations and polymorphisms of the gene encoding the b-subunit of the electron transfer flavoprotein in three patients with glutaric acidemia type II.' *Human Molecular Genetics*, **3**, 429–435.

Crane, A.M., Martin, L.S., Valle, D., Ledley, F.D. (1992) 'Phenotype of disease in three patients with identical mutations in methylmalonyl CoA mutase.' *Human Genetics*, **89**, 259–264.

Cruysberg, J.R.M., Wevers, R.A., van Engelen, B.G.M., *et al.* (1995) 'Ocular and systemic manifestations of cerebrotendinous xanthomatosis.' *American Journal of Ophthalmology*, **120**, 597–604.

Danks, D.M. (1988) 'The mild form of Menkes disease: progress report on the original case.' *American Journal of Medical Genetics*, **30**, 859–864.

Darras, B.T., Kwan, E.S., Gilmore, H.E., *et al.* (1986) 'Globoid cell leukodystrophy: cranial computed tomography and evoked potentials.' *Journal of Child Neurology*, **1**, 126–130.

Dave, P., Curless, R.G., Steinman, C. (1984) 'Cerebellar hemorrhages complicating methylmalonic and propionic acidemia.' *Archives of Neurology*, **41**, 1293–1296.

Del Giudice, E., Striano, S., Andria, G. (1983) 'Electroencephalographic abnormalities in homocystinuria due to cystathionine synthase deficiency.' *Clinical Neurology and Neurosurgery*, **85**, 165–168.

Demirkiran, M., Jankovic, J., Lewis, R.A., Cox, D.W. (1996) 'Neurologic presentation of Wilson disease without Kayser–Fleischer rings.' *Neurology*, **46**, 1040–1043.

Detre, J.A., Wang, Z., Bogdan, A.R., *et al.* (1991) 'Regional variation in brain lactate in Leigh syndrome by localized ^{1}H magnetic resonance spectroscopy.' *Annals of Neurology*, **29**, 218–221.

De Vivo, D.C., van Coster, R.N. (1991) 'Leigh syndrome: clinical and biochemical correlates.' *In:* Fukuyama, Y., Kamoshita, K.S., Ohtsuka, C., Suzuki, Y., (Eds.) *Modern Perspectives in Child Neurology.* Tokyo: Japanese Society of Child Neurology, pp. 27–37.

—— Gibson, K.M., Resor, L.D., *et al.* (1988) '4-Hydroxybutyric acidemia: clinical features, pathogenetic mechanisms and treatment strategies.' *Annals of Neurology*, **24**, 304. *(Abstract.)*

Dhondt, J-L. (1991) 'Strategy for the screening of tetrahydrobiopterin deficiency among hyperphenylalaninaemic patients: 15-years experience.' *Journal of Inherited Metabolic Disease*, **14**, 117–127.

DiMauro, S., Moraes, C.T. (1993) 'Mitochondrial encephalomyopathies.' *Archives of Neurology*, **50**, 1197–1208.

—— Lombes, A., Nakase, H., *et al.* (1990) 'Cytochrome c oxidase deficiency.' *Pediatric Research*, **28**, 536–541.

Dinno, N.D., Yacoub, U., Holmes, W., Weisskopf, B. (1981) 'Pseudo-Menkes syndrome.' *Journal of Pediatrics*, **99**, 325. *(Letter.)*

Divry, P., Vianey-Liaud, C., Gay, C., *et al.* (1988) 'N-acetylaspartic aciduria: report of three new cases in children with a neurological syndrome associating macrocephaly and leukodystrophy.' *Journal of Inherited Metabolic Disease*, **11**, 307–308.

Dobyns, W.B. (1989) 'Agenesis of the corpus callosum and gyral malformations are frequent manifestations of non-ketotic hyperglycinemia.' *Neurology*, **39**, 817–820.

Dreborg, S., Erickson, A., Hagberg, B. (1980) 'Gaucher disease–Norbottnian type: I. General clinical description.' *European Journal of Pediatrics*, **133**, 107–118.

D'Souza, S.W., McConnell, S.E., Slater, P., Barson, A.J. (1993) 'Glycine site of the excitatory amino acid N-methyl-D-aspartate receptor in neonatal and adult brain.' *Archives of Disease in Childhood*, **69**, 212–215.

Duran, M., Beemer, F.A., Tibosch, A.S. *et al.* (1982) 'Inherited 3-methylglutaconic aciduria in two brothers—Another defect of leucine metabolism.' *Journal of Pediatrics*, **101**, 551–554.

—— Baumgartner, E.R., Suormala, T.M., *et al.* (1993) 'Cerebrospinal fluid organic acids in biotinidase deficiency.' *Journal of Inherited Metabolic Disease*, **16**, 513–516.

Edwin, D., Speedie, L.J., Kohler, W., *et al.* (1996) 'Cognitive and brain magnetic resonance imaging findings in adrenomyeloneuropathy.' *Annals of Neurology*, **40**, 675–678.

Eisensmith, R.C., Woo, S.L.C. (1996) 'Gene therapy for phenylketonuria.' *European Journal of Pediatrics*, **155**, Suppl. 1, S16–S19.

Elpeleg, O.N., Amir, N., Christensen, E. (1992) 'Variability of clinical presentation in fumarate hydratase deficiency.' *Journal of Pediatrics*, **121**, 752–754.

—— Costeff, H., Joseph, A., *et al.* (1994) '3-Methylglutaconic aciduria in the Iraqi–Jewish 'optic atrophy plus' (Costeff) syndrome.' *Developmental Medicine and Child Neurology*, **36**, 167–172.

312

—— Ruitenbeek, W., Jakobs, C., *et al.* (1995) 'Congenital lacticacidemia caused by lipoamide dehydrogenase deficiency with favorable outcome.' *Journal of Pediatrics*, **126**, 72–74.

Eng, C.M., Desnick, R.J. (1994) 'Molecular basis of Fabry disease: mutations and polymorphisms in the human alpha-galactosidase A gene.' *Human Mutations*, **3**, 103–111.

Erikson, A., Åström, M., Månsson, J.E. (1995) 'Enzyme infusion therapy of the Norrbottnian (type 3) Gaucher disease.' *Neuropediatrics*, **26**, 203–207.

Espeel, M., Roels, F., Giros, M., *et al.* (1995) 'Immunolocalization of a 43kDa peroxisomal membrane protein in the liver of patients with generalized peroxisomal disorders.' *European Journal of Cell Biology*, **67**, 319–327.

Eyskens, F.J.M., Van Doorn, J.W.D., Mariën, P. (1992) 'Neurologic sequelae in transient nonketotic hyperglycinemia of the neonate.' *Journal of Pediatrics*, **121**, 620–621.

—— Ceuterick, C., Martin, J-J., *et al.* (1994) 'Carbohydrate-deficient glycoprotein syndrome with previously unreported features.' *Acta Paediatrica*, **83**, 892–896.

Farley, T.J., Ketonen, L.M., Bodensteiner, J.B., Wang, D.D. (1992) 'Serial MRI and CT findings in infantile Krabbe disease.' *Pediatric Neurology*, **8**, 455–458.

Fensom, A.H., Benson, P.F. (1994) 'Recent advances in the prenatal diagnosis of the mucopolysaccharidoses.' *Prenatal Diagnosis*, **14**, 1–12.

Fenton, W.A., Rosenberg, L.E. (1995) 'Inherited disorders of cobalamin transport and metabolism.' *In:* Scriver, C.R., Beaudet, A.L., Sly, W.S., Valle, D. (Eds.) *The Metabolic and Molecular Bases of Inherited Disease, 7th Edn.* New York: McGraw Hill, pp. 3129–3149.

Filling-Katz, M.R., Merrick, H.F., Fink, J.K., *et al.* (1989) 'Carbamazepine in Fabry's disease: effective analgesia with dose-dependent exacerbation of autonomic dysfunction.' *Neurology*, **39**, 598–600.

—— Miller, S.P.F., Merrick, H.F., *et al.* (1992) 'Clinical, pathologic, and biochemical features of a cholesterol lipidosis accompanied by hyperlipidemia and xanthomas.' *Neurology*, **42**, 1768–1774.

Filloux, F., Townsend, J.J., Leonard, C. (1986) 'Ornithine transcarbamylase deficiency: neuropathologic changes acquired in utero.' *Journal of Pediatrics*, **108**, 942–945.

Fink, J.K., Brouwers, P., Barton, N., *et al.* (1989a) 'Neurologic complications in long-standing nephropathic cystinosis.' *Archives of Neurology*, **46**, 543–548.

—— Filling-Katz, M.R., Sokol, J., *et al.* (1989b) 'Clinical spectrum of Niemann–Pick disease type C.' *Neurology*, **39**, 1040–1049.

Fischer, J.C., Ruitenbeek, W., Gabreëls, F.J.M., *et al.* (1986) 'A mitochondrial encephalomyopathy: the first case with an established defect at the level of coenzyme Q.' *European Journal of Pediatrics*, **144**, 441–444.

Fisher, N.R., Cope, S.J., Lishman, W.A. (1987) 'Metachromatic leukodystrophy: conduct disorder progressing to dementia.' *Journal of Neurology, Neurosurgery, and Psychiatry*, **50**, 488–489.

Fournier, B., Smeitink, J.A.M., Dorland, L., *et al.* (1994) 'Peroxisomal disorders: a review.' *Journal of Inherited Metabolic Disease*, **17**, 470–486.

Fowler, B., Børresen, A.L., Boman, N. (1982) 'Prenatal diagnosis of homocystinuria.' *Lancet*, **2**, 875. *(Letter.)*

Francis, G.S., Bonni, A., Shen, N., *et al.* (1993) 'Metachromatic leukodystrophy: multiple nonfunctional and pseudodeficiency alleles in a pedigree: problems with diagnosis and counseling.' *Annals of Neurology*, **34**, 212–218.

Friedman, J.H., Levy, H.L., Boustany, R.M. (1989) 'Late onset of distinct neurologic syndromes in galactosemic siblings.' *Neurology*, **39**, 741–742.

Fries, M.H., Rinaldo, P., Schmidt-Sommerfeld, E., *et al.* (1996) 'Isovaleric acidemia: response to a leucine load after three weeks of supplementation with glycine, L-carnitine, and combined glycine–carnitine therapy.' *Journal of Pediatrics*, **129**, 449–452.

Fryer, A., Appleton, R., Sweeney, M.G., *et al.* (1994) 'Mitochondrial DNA 8993 (NARP) mutation presenting with a heterogeneous phenotype including 'cerebral palsy'.' *Archives of Disease in Childhood*, **71**, 419–422.

Galjaard, H., d'Azzo, A., Hoogeveen, A., Verheiven, F.W. (1984) 'Combined beta-galactosidase-sialidase deficiency in man: genetic defect of a protective protein.' *In:* Barranger, J.A., Brady, R.B. (Eds.) *The Molecular Basis of Lysosomal Storage Disorders.* London: Academic Press, pp. 113–132.

Ganesan, V., Johnson, A., Connelly, A., *et al.* (1997) 'Guanidoacetate methyltransferase deficiency: new clinical features.' *Pediatric Neurology*, **17**, 155–157.

Garuti, R., Lelli, N., Barozzini, M., *et al.* (1996) 'Partial deletion of the gene encoding sterol 27-hydroxylase in a subject with cerebrotendinous xanthomatosis.' *Journal of Lipid Research*, **37**, 662–672.

Gascon, G.G., Ozand, P.T., Brismar, J. (1994) 'Movement disorders in childhood organic acidurias. Clinical, neuroimaging, and biochemical correlations.' *Brain and Development*, **16** (Suppl.), 94–103.

Gellera, C., Uziel, G., Rimoldi, M., *et al.* (1990) 'Fumarase deficiency is an autosomal recessive encephalopathy affecting both the mitochondrial and the cytosolic enzymes.' *Neurology*, **40**, 495–499.

Geoffroy, V., Fouque, F., Benelli, C., *et al.* (1996) 'Defect in the X-lipoyl-containing component of the pyruvate dehydrogenase complex in a patient with a neonatal lactic acidemia.' *Pediatrics*, **97**, 267–272.

Gibbs, T.C., Payan, J., Brett, E.M., *et al.* (1993) 'Peripheral neuropathy as the presenting feature of tyrosinaemia type I and effectively treated with an inhibitor of 4-hydroxyphenylpyruvate dioxygenase.' *Journal of Neurology, Neurosurgery, and Psychiatry*, **56**, 1129–1132.

Gibson, K.M., Elpeleg, O.N., Jakobs, C., *et al.* (1993) 'The multiple syndromes of 3-methylglutaconic aciduria.' *Pediatric Neurology*, **9**, 120–123.

—— Baumann, C., Ogier, H., *et al.* (1994) 'Pre- and postnatal diagnosis of succinic semialdehyde dehydrogenase deficiency using enzyme and metabolite assays.' *Journal of Inherited Metabolic Disease*, **17**, 732–737.

—— Jakobs, C., Ogier, H., *et al.* (1995) 'Vigabatrin therapy in six patients with succinic semialdehyde dehydrogenase deficiency.' *Journal of Inherited Metabolic Disease*, **18**, 143–146.

Gieselmann, V., Zlotogora, J., Harris, A., *et al.* (1994) 'Molecular genetics of metachromatic leukodystrophy.' *Human Mutations*, **4**, 233–242.

Gitzelmann, R., Wells, H.J., Segal, S. (1974) 'Galactose metabolism in a patient with hereditary galactokinase deficiency.' *European Journal of Clinical Investigation*, **4**, 79–85.

Godwin-Austen, R.B., Robinson, A., Evans, K., Lascelles, P.T. (1978) 'An unusual neurological disorder of copper metabolism clinically resembling Wilson's disease but biochemically a distinct entity.' *Journal of the Neurological Sciences*, **39**, 85–98.

Goebel, H.H., Harzer, K., Ernst, J.P., *et al.* (1990) 'Late-onset globoid cell leukodystrophy: unusual ultrastructural pathology and subtotal beta-galactocerebrosidase deficiency.' *Journal of Child Neurology*, **5**, 299–307.

Goebel-Schreiner, B., Schreiner, R., Hoffmann, G.F., Gibson, K.M. (1995) 'Segregation of the N301T mutation in the family of the index patient with mevalonate kinase deficiency.' *Journal of Inherited Metabolic Disease*, **18**, 197–200.

Gold, R., Bogdahn, U., Kappos, L., *et al.* (1996) 'Hereditary defect of cobalamin metabolism (homocystinuria and methylmalonic aciduria) of juvenile onset.' *Journal of Neurology, Neurosurgery, and Psychiatry*, **60**, 107–108. *(Letter.)*

Gordon, B.A., Gordon, K.E., Hinton, G.G., *et al.* (1988) 'Tay–Sachs disease: B1 variant.' *Pediatric Neurology*, **4**, 54–57.

—— Seo, H.C., *et al.* (1995) 'Fucosidosis with dystonia.' *Neuropediatrics*, **26**, 325–327.

Gordon, N. (1997) 'Pyridoxine dependency: an update.' *Developmental Medicine and Child Neurology*, **39**, 63–65.

Gottlieb, R.P., Koppel, M.M., Nyhan, W.L., *et al.* (1982) 'Hyperuricaemia and choreoathetosis in a child without mental retardation or self-mutilation—a new HPRT variant.' *Journal of Inherited Metabolic Disease*, **5**, 183–186.

Goutières, F., Aicardi, J. (1985) 'Atypical presentations of pyridoxine-dependent seizures: a treatable cause of intractable epilepsy in infants.' *Annals of Neurology*, **17**, 117–120.

—— Arsenio-Nunes, M.L., Aicardi, J. (1979) 'Mucolipidosis type IV.' *Neuropediatrics*, **10**, 321–331.

Goyette, P., Frosst, P., Rosenblatt, D.S., Rozen, R. (1995) 'Seven novel mutations in the methylenetetrahydrofolate reductase gene and genotype/phenotype correlations in severe methylenetetrahydrofolate reductase deficiency.' *American Journal of Human Genetics*, **56**, 1052–1059.

Grafe, M., Thomas, C., Schneider, J., *et al.* (1988) 'Infantile Gaucher's disease: A case with neuronal storage.' *Annals of Neurology*, **23**, 300–303.

Graham, S.M., Arvela, O.M., Wise, G.A. (1992) 'Long-term neurologic consequences of nutritional vitamin B_{12} deficiency in infants.' *Journal of Pediatrics*, **121**, 710–714.

Gravel, R.A., Clarke, J.T.R., Kaback, M.M., *et al.* (1995) 'The GM2 gangliosidoses.' *In:* Scriver, C.R., Beaudet, A.L., Sly, W.S., Valle, D. (Eds.) *The Metabolic and Molecular Bases of Inherited Disease, 7th Edn.* New York: McGraw Hill, pp. 2839–2879.

Gray, R.G.F., Green, A., Basu, S.N., *et al.* (1990) 'Antenatal diagnosis of molybdenum cofactor deficiency.' *American Journal of Obstetrics and Gynecology*, **163**, 1203–1204.

Grossman, L. (1995) 'Mitochondrial mutations and human disease.' *Environmental and Molecular Mutagenesis*, **25**, Suppl. 26, 30–37.

Gross-Tsur, V., Har-Even, Y., Gutman, I., Amir, N. (1989) 'Oculomotor apraxia: the preseting sign of Gaucher disease.' *Pediatric Neurology*, **5**, 128–129.

Grunnet, M.L., Zalneraitis, E.L., Russman, B.S., Barwick, M.C. (1991) 'Juvenile Leigh's encephalomyelopathy with peripheral neuropathy, myopathy, and cardiomyelopathy.' *Journal of Child Neurology*, **6**, 159–163.

Guazzi, G.C., D'Amore, I., Van Hoof, F., *et al.* (1988) 'Type 3 (chronic) GM1 gangliosidosis presenting as infanto-choreo-athetotic dementia, without epilepsy, in three sisters.' *Neurology*, **38**, 1124–1127.

Gumbinas, M., Larsen, M., Liu, H.M. (1975) 'Peripheral neuropathy in classic Niemann–Pick disease, ultrastructure of nerves and skeletal muscles.' *Neurology*, **25**, 107–109.

Güttler, F., Guldberg, P. (1996) 'The influence of mutations on enzyme activity and phenylalanine tolerance in phenylalanine hydroxylase deficiency.' *European Journal of Pediatrics*, **155**, Suppl. 1, S6–S10.

Haas, R.H., Robinson, A., Evans, K., *et al.* (1981) 'An X-linked disease of the nervous system with disordered copper metabolism and features differing from Menkes' disease.' *Neurology*, **31**, 852–859.

Haenggeli, C-A., Girardin, E., Paunier, L. (1991) 'Pyridoxine-dependent seizures, clinical and therapeutic aspects.' *European Journal of Pediatrics*, **150**, 452–455.

Hagberg, B. (1984) 'Krabbe's disease: clinical presentation of neurological variants.' *Neuropediatrics*, **15** (Suppl.), 11–15.

—— Kollberg, H., Sourander, P., Akerson, H.O. (1970) 'Infantile globoid cell leucodystrophy (Krabbe's disease): a clinical, morphological and genetical study of 32 Swedish cases.' *Neuropädiatrie*, **1**, 74–88.

—— Blennow, G., Kristiansson, B., Stibler, H. (1993) 'Carbohydrate-deficient glycoprotein syndromes: peculiar group of new disorders.' *Pediatric Neurology*, **9**, 255–262.

Hale, D.E., Bennett, M.J. (1992) 'Fatty acid oxidation disorders: a new class of metabolic diseases.' *Journal of Pediatrics*, **121**, 1–11.

Hall, C.A. (1990) 'Function of vitamin B$_{12}$ in the central nervous system as revealed by congenital defects.' *American Journal of Hematology*, **34**, 121–127.

Hamilton, R.L., Haas, R.H., Nyhan, W.L., *et al.* (1995) 'Neuropathology of propionic acidemia: a report of two patients with basal ganglia lesions.' *Journal of Child Neurology*, **10**, 25–30.

Hanavar, M., Janota, I., Neville, B.G.R., Chalmers, R.A. (1992) 'Neuropathology of biotinidase deficiency.' *Acta Neuropathologica*, **84**, 461–464.

Hanefeld, F., Kruse, B., Bruhn, H., Frahm, J. (1994) '*In vivo* proton magnetic resonance spectroscopy of the brain in a patient with L-2-hydroxyglutaric acidemia.' *Pediatric Research*, **35**, 614–616.

Hanley, W.B., Koch, R., Levy, H.L., *et al.* (1996) 'The North American Maternal Phenylketonuria Collaborative Study, develomental assessment of the offspring: preliminary report.' *European Journal of Pediatrics*, **155**, Suppl. 1, S169–S172.

Hansen, L.K., Wulff, K., Dorche, C., Christensen, E. (1993) 'Molybdenum cofactor deficiency in two siblings: diagnostic difficulties.' *European Journal of Pediatrics*, **152**, 662–664.

Harbord, M., Buncic, J.R., Chuang, S.A., *et al.* (1991) 'Multiple sulfatase deficiency with early severe retinal degeneration.' *Journal of Child Neurology*, **6**, 229–235.

Harding, A.E., Matthews, S., Jones, S., *et al.* (1985) 'Spinocerebellar degeneration associated with a selective defect of vitamin E absorption.' *New England Journal of Medicine*, **313**, 32–35.

—— Young, E.P., Schon, F. (1987) 'Adult onset supranuclear ophthalmoplegia, cerebellar ataxia, and neurogenic proximal muscle weakness in a brother and sister: another hexosaminidase A deficiency syndrome.' *Journal of Neurology, Neurosurgery, and Psychiatry*, **50**, 687–690.

Harding, B.N., Leonard, J.V., Erdohazi, M. (1984) 'Ornithine carbamoyl transferase deficiency: a neuropathological study.' *European Journal of Pediatrics*, **141**, 215–220.

Hatanaka, T., Higashino, H., Woo, M., *et al.* (1990) 'Lesch–Nyhan syndrome with delayed onset of self-mutilation: hyperactivity of interneurons at the brainstem and blink reflex.' *Acta Neurologica Scandinavica*, **81**, 184–187.

Haworth, J.C., Booth, F.A., Chudley, A.E., *et al.* (1991) 'Phenotypic variability in glutaric aciduria type I: report of fourteen cases in five Canadian Indian kindreds.' *Journal of Pediatrics*, **118**, 52–58.

—— Dilling, L.A., Surtees, R.A.H., *et al.* (1993) 'Symptomatic and asymptomatic methylenetetrahydrofolate reductase deficiency in two adult brothers.' *American Journal of Medical Genetics*, **45**, 572–576.

Hayasaka, K., Tada, K., Fueki, N., *et al.* (1987) 'Nonketotic hyperglycinemia: analyses of glycine cleavage system in typical and atypical cases.' *Journal of Pediatrics*, **110**, 873–877.

Heckmann, J., Saffer, D. (1988) 'Abnormal copper metabolism: another "non-Wilson's" case.' *Neurology*, **38**, 1493–1495.

—— Eastman, R., Handler, L., *et al.* (1993) 'Leigh disease (subacute necrotizing encephalomyelopathy): MR documentation of the evolution of an acute attack.' *American Journal of Neuroradiology*, **14**, 1157–1159.

Heidenreich, R., Natowicz, M., Hainline, B.E., *et al.* (1988) 'Acute extrapyramidal syndrome in methylmalonic acidemia: "metabolic stroke" involving the globus pallidus.' *Journal of Pediatrics*, **113**, 1022–1027.

Hilliges, C., Awiszus, D., Wendel, U. (1993) 'Intellectual performance of children with maple syrup urine disease.' *European Journal of Pediatrics*, **152**, 144–147.

Hoffmann, G.F., Trefz, F.K., Barth, P.G., *et al.* (1991) 'Glutaryl coenzyme A dehydrogenase deficiency: a distinct encephalopathy.' *Pediatrics*, **88**, 1194–1203.

—— Charpentier, C., Mayatepek, E., *et al.* (1993) 'Clinical and biochemical phenotype in 11 patients with mevalonic aciduria.' *Pediatrics*, **91**, 915–921.

—— Böhles, H.J., Burlina, A., *et al.* (1995a) 'Early signs and course of disease of glutaryl-CoA dehydrogenase deficiency.' *Journal of Inherited Metabolic Disease*, **18**, 173–176.

—— Jakobs, C., Holmes, B., *et al.* (1995b) 'Organic acids in cerebrospinal fluid and plasma of patients with L-2-hydroxyglutaric aciduria.' *Journal of Inherited Metabolic Disease*, **18**, 189–193.

—— Athanassopoulos, S., Burlina, A.B., *et al.* (1996) 'Clinical course, early diagnosis, treatment, and prevention of disease in glutaryl-CoA dehydrogenase deficiency.' *Neuropediatrics*, **27**, 115–123.

Holzbach, U., Hanefeld, F., Helms, G., *et al.* (1995) 'Localized proton magnetic resonance spectroscopy of cerebral abnormalities in children with carbohydrate-deficient glycoprotein syndrome.' *Acta Paediatrica*, **84**, 781–786.

Hommes, F.A. (1994) 'Loss of neurotransmitter receptors by hyperphenylalaninemia in the HPH-5 mouse brain.' *Acta Paediatrica*, Suppl. 407, 120–121.

Hoogenraad, T.U., Van Hattum, J., Van den Hamer, C.J.A. (1987) 'Management of Wilson's disease with zinc sulphate. Experience in a series of 27 patients.' *Journal of the Neurological Sciences*, **77**, 137–146.

Hopwood, J.J., Vellodi, A., Scott, H.S., *et al.* (1993) 'Long-term clinical progress in bone marrow transplanted mucopolysaccharidosis type I patients with a defined genotype.' *Journal of Inherited Metabolic Disease*, **16**, 1024–1033.

Horn, N. (1981) 'Menkes X-linked disease: prenatal diagosis of hemizygous males and heterozygous females.' *Prenatal Diagnosis*, **1**, 107–120.

Horowitz, M., Zimram, A. (1994) 'Mutations causing Gaucher disease.' *Human Mutations*, **3**, 1–11.

—— Tzuri, G., Eyal, N., *et al.* (1993) 'Prevalence of nine mutations among Jewish and non-Jewish Gaucher disease patients.' *American Journal of Human Genetics*, **53**, 921–930.

Horslen, S.P., Clayton, P.T., Harding, B.N., *et al.* (1991) 'Olivopontocerebellar atrophy of neonatal onset and disialotransferrin developmental deficiency syndrome.' *Archives of Disease in Childhood*, **66**, 1027–1032.

Houwen, R.H.J., Juyn, J., Hoogenraad, T.U., *et al.* (1995) 'H714Q mutation in Wilson disease is associated with late, neurological presentation.' *Journal of Medical Genetics*, **32**, 480–482.

Hreidarsson, S.J., Thomas, G.H., Kihara, H., *et al.* (1983) 'Impaired cerebroside sulfate hydrolysis in fibroblasts of sibs with "pseudo" arylsulfatase A deficiency without metachromatic leukodystrophy.' *Pediatric Research*, **17**, 701–704.

Hudak, M.L., Jones, M.D., Brusilow, S.W. (1985) 'Differentiation of transient hyperammonemia of the newborn and urea cycle enzyme defects by clinical presentation.' *Journal of Pediatrics*, **107**, 712–719.

Huttenlocher, P.R., Hillman, R.E., Hsia, Y.E. (1970) 'Pseudotumor cerebri in galactosemia.' *Journal of Pediatrics*, **76**, 902–905.

Hyland, K. (1993) 'Abnormalities of biogenic amine metabolism.' *Journal of Inherited Metabolic Disease*, **16**, 676–690.

—— Surtees, R.A.H., Rodeck, C., Clayton, P.T. (1992) 'Aromatic L-amino acid decarboxylase deficiency: clinical features, diagnosis, and treatment of a new inborn error of neurotransmitter amine synthesis.' *Neurology*, **42**, 1980–1988.

Ichinose, H., Ohye, T., Takahashi, E-i., *et al.* (1994) 'Hereditary progressive dystonia with marked diurnal fluctuation caused by mutations in the GTP cyclohydrolase I gene.' *Nature Genetics*, **8**, 236–242.

Inagaki, M., Hashimoto, K., Yoshino, K., *et al.* (1988) 'Atypical form of Menkes kinky hair disease with mitochondrial NADH-CoQ reductase deficiency.' *Neuropediatrics*, **19**, 52–55.

Ince, Z., Çoban, A., Peker, Ö., *et al.* (1995) 'Gaucher disease associated with congenital ichthyosis in the neonate.' *European Journal of Pediatrics*, **154**, 418. *(Letter.)*

Jackson, G.H., Meyer, A., Lippmann, S. (1994) 'Wilson's disease. Psychiatric manifestations may be the clinical presentation.' *Postgraduate Medicine*, **95**, 135–138.

Jackson, M.J., Schaefer, J.A., Johnson, M.A., *et al.* (1995) 'Presentation and clinical investigation of mitochondrial respiratory chain disease. A study of 51 patients.' *Brain*, **118**, 339–357.

Jacobs, J.M., Harding, B.N., Lake, B.D., *et al.* (1990) 'Peripheral neuropathy in Leigh's disease.' *Brain*, **113**, 447–462.

Jaeken, J., Van den Berghe, G. (1984) 'An infantile autistic syndrome characterised by the presence of succinylpurines in body fluids.' *Lancet*, **2**, 1058–1061.

—— Casaer, P., DeCock, P., *et al.* (1984) 'Gamma-aminobutyric acid-transaminase deficiency: a newly recognized inborn error of neurotransmitter metabolism.' *Neuropediatrics*, **15**, 165–169.

—— Stibler, H., Hagberg, B. (1991) 'The carbohydrate-deficient glycoprotein syndrome. A new inherited multisystemic disease with severe nervous system involvement.' *Acta Paediatrica Scandinavica*, Suppl. 375, 5–71.

—— Schachter, H., Carchon, H., *et al.* (1994) 'Carbohydrate deficient glycoprotein syndrome type II: a deficiency in Golgi localised *N*-acetylglucosaminyltransferase II.' *Archives of Disease in Childhood*, **71**, 123–127.

Jain, A., Buist, N.R.M., Kennaway, N.G., *et al.* (1994) 'Effect of ascorbate or *N*-acetylcysteine treatment in a patient with hereditary glutathione synthetase deficiency.' *Journal of Pediatrics*, **124**, 229–233.

Jakobs, C., Ten Brink, H.J., Stellaard, I. (1991) 'Prenatal diagnosis of inherited metabolic disorders by quantitation of characteristic metabolites in amniotic fluid: facts and future.' *Prenatal Diagnosis*, **10**, 265–271.

—— Jaeken, J., Gibson, K.M. (1993) 'Inherited disorders of GABA metabolism.' *Journal of Inherited Metabolic Disease*, **16**, 704–715.

Jankovic, J., Caskey, T.C., Stout, T., Butler, I.J. (1988) 'Lesch–Nyhan syndrome: a study of motor behavior and cerebrospinal fluid neurotransmitters.' *Annals of Neurology*, **23**, 466–469.

Jardim, L.B., Pires, R.F., Martins, C.E.S., *et al.* (1994) 'Pyridoxine-dependent seizures associated with white matter abnormalities.' *Neuropediatrics*, **25**, 259–261.

Jonas, A.J., Butler, I.J. (1989) 'Circumvention of defective aminoacid transport in Hartnup disease using tryptophan ethyl-ester.' *Journal of Clinical Investigation*, **84**, 200–204.

Kaabachi, N., Larnaout, A., Rabier, D., *et al.* (1993) 'Familial encephalopathy and L-2-hydroxyglutaric aciduria.' *Journal of Inherited Metabolic Disease*, **16**, 893.

Kaback, M., Lim-Steele, J., Dabholkar, D., *et al.* (1993) 'Tay–Sachs disease—carrier screeening, prenatal diagnosis, and the molecular era. An international perspective, 1970–1993.' *Journal of the American Medical Association*, **270**, 2307–2315.

Kaler, S.G., Buist, N.R.M., Holmes, C.S., *et al.* (1995) 'Early copper therapy in classic Menkes disease patients with a novel splicing mutation.' *Annals of Neurology*, **38**, 921–928.

Kalimo, H., Lundberg, P.O., Olsson, Y. (1979) 'Familial subacute necrotizing encephalomyelopathy of the adult form (adult Leigh syndrome).' *Annals of Neurology*, **6**, 200–206.

Kamei, A., Houdou, S., Takashima, S., *et al.* (1993) 'Peroxisomal disorders in children: immunohistochemistry and neuropathology.' *Journal of Pediatrics*, **122**, 573–579.

Kamoun, P., Fensom, A.H., Shin, Y.S., *et al.* (1995) 'Prenatal diagnosis of the urea cycle diseases: a survey of the European cases.' *American Journal of Medical Genetics*, **55**, 247–250.

Kandt, R.S., Emerson, R.G., Singer, H.S., *et al.* (1982) 'Cataplexy in variant forms of Niemann–Pick disease.' *Annals of Neurology*, **12**, 284–288.

Kang, S.S., Wong, P.W.K., Malinow, M.R. (1992) 'Hyperhomocyst(e)inemia as a risk factor for occlusive vascular disease.' *Annual Review of Nutrition*, **12**, 279–288.

Kanwar, Y.S., Manaligod, J.R., Wong, P.W.K. (1976) 'Morphologic studies in a patient with homocystinuria due to 5,10-methylenetetrahydrofolate reductase deficiency.' *Pediatric Research*, **10**, 598–609.

Kappas, A., Sassa, S., Galbraith, R.A., Nordmann, Y. (1995) 'The porphyrias.' *In:* Scriver, C.R., Beaudet, A.L., Sly, W.S., Valle, D. (Eds.) *The Metabolic and Molecular Bases of Inherited Disease, 7th Edn.* New York: McGraw Hill, pp. 2103–2159.

Kappler, J., Sommerlade, H.J., von Figura, K., Gieselmann, V. (1994) 'Complex arylsulfatase A alleles causing metachromatic leukodystrophy.' *Human Mutations*, **4**, 119–127.

Karpati, G., Carpenter, S., Eisen, A.A., *et al.* (1974) 'Multiple peripheral nerve entrapments. An unusual phenotypical variant of the Hunter syndrome (mucopolysaccharidosis II) in a family.' *Archives of Neurology*, **31**, 418–422.

Kaufman, D.L., Lederman, J.N., Wong, A.M., *et al.* (1987) 'A new method to detect point mutations in the gene for glutamic acid decarboxylase in patients with pyridoxine-dependent seizures.' *Annals of Neurology*, **22**, 446–447. *(Abstract.)*

Kaufman, S. (1993) 'New tetrahydrobiopterin-dependent systems.' *Annual Review of Nutrition*, **13**, 261–286.

Kaye, E.M., Ullman, M.D., Wilson, E.R., Barranger, J.A. (1986) 'Type 2 and type 3 Gaucher disease: a morphological and biochemical study.' *Annals of Neurology*, **20**, 223–230.

—— Kolodny, E.H., Logigian, E.L., Ullman, M.D. (1988) 'Nervous system involvement in Fabry's disease: clinicopathological and biochemical correlation.' *Annals of Neurology*, **23**, 505–509.

Kelley, R.I., Kratz, L. (1995) '3-Methylglutaconic acidemia in Smith–Lemli–Opitz syndrome.' *Pediatric Research*, **37**, 671–674.

Kelly, D.A., Portmann, B., Mowat, A.P., *et al.* (1993) 'Niemann–Pick disease type C: diagnosis and outcome in children, with particular reference to liver disease.' *Journal of Pediatrics*, **123**, 242–247.

Kennedy, C.R., Allen, J.T., Fensom, A.H., *et al.* (1994) 'X-linked adrenoleukodystrophy with non-diagnostic plasma very long chain fatty acids.' *Journal of Neurology, Neurosurgery, and Psychiatry*, **57**, 759–761.

Kenworthy, L., Park, T., Charnas, L.R. (1993) 'Cognitive and behavioral profile of the oculocerebrorenal syndrome of Lowe.' *American Journal of Medical Genetics*, **46**, 297–303.

Kivlin, J.D., Sanborn, G.E., Myers, G.G. (1985) 'The cherry-red spot in Tay–Sachs and other storage diseases.' *Annals of Neurology*, **17**, 356–360.

Kluijtmans, L.A., van den Heuvel, L.P.W.J., Boers, G.H.J., *et al.* (1996) 'Molecular genetic analysis in mild hyperhomocysteinemia: a common mutation in the methylenetetrahydrofolate reductase gene is a genetic risk factor for cardiovascular disease.' *American Journal of Human Genetics*, **58**, 35–41.

Knappskog, P.M., Flatmark, T., Mallet, J., *et al.* (1995) 'Recessively inherited L-DOPA-responsive dystonia caused by a point mutation (Q381K) in the tyrosine hydroxylase gene.' *Human Molecular Genetics*, **4**, 1209–1212.

Kobayashi, T., Noda, S., Umezaki, H., *et al.* (1986) 'Familial spinocerebellar degeneration as an expression of adrenoleukodystrophy.' *Journal of Neurology, Neurosurgery, and Psychiatry*, **49**, 1438–1440.

Koch, T.K., Schmidt, K.A., Wagstaff, J.E., *et al.* (1992) 'Neurologic complications in galactosemia.' *Pediatric Neurology*, **8**, 217–220.

Korenke, G.C., Hunneman, D.H., Kohler, J., *et al.* (1995) 'Glyceroltrioleate/glyceroltrierucate therapy in 16 patients with X-chromosomal adrenoleukodystrophy/adrenomyeloneuropathy: effect on clinical, biochemical and neurophysiological parameters.' *European Journal of Pediatrics*, **154**, 64–70.

—— Pouwels, P.J.W., Frahm, J., *et al.* (1996) 'Arrested cerebral adrenoleukodystrophy: a clinical and proton magnetic resonance spectroscopy study in three patients.' *Pediatric Neurology*, **15**, 103–107.

Korf, B., Wallman, J.K., Levy, H.L. (1986) 'Bilateral lucency of the globus pallidus complicating methylmalonic acidemia.' *Annals of Neurology*, **20**, 364–366.

Kotagal, S., Wenger, D.A., Alcala, H., *et al.* (1986) 'AB variant GM2 gangliosidosis: cerebrospinal fluid and neurologic characteristics.' *Neurology*, **36**, 438–440.

Koto, A., Horwitz, A.L., Suzuki, K., *et al.* (1978) 'The Morquio syndrome: neuropathology and biochemistry.' *Annals of Neurology*, **4**, 26–36.

Krägeloh-Mann, I., Grodd, W., Niemann, G., *et al.* (1992) 'Assessment and therapy monitoring of Leigh disease by MRI and proton spectroscopy.' *Pediatric Neurology*, **8**, 60–64.

—————— Schöning, M., *et al.* (1993) 'Proton spectroscopy in five patients with Leigh's disease and mitochondrial enzyme deficiency.' *Developmental Medicine and Child Neurology*, **35**, 769–776.

Krasemann, E.W., Meier, V., Korenke, G.C. *et al.* (1996) 'Identification of mutations in the ALD-gene of 20 families with adrenoleukodystrophy/adrenomyeloneuropathy.' *Human Genetics*, **97**, 194–197.

Krishnamoorthy, K.S. (1983) 'Pyridoxine-dependency seizure: report of a rare presentation.' *Annals of Neurology*, **13**, 103–104.

Krivit, W., Shapiro, E., Kennedy, W., *et al.* (1990) 'Treatment of late infantile metachromatic leukodystrophy by bone marrow transplantation.' *New England Journal of Medicine*, **322**, 28–32.

Kroll, J.S. (1985) 'Pyridoxine for neonatal seizures: an unexpected danger.' *Developmental Medicine and Child Neurology*, **27**, 377–379.

Kudo, Y., Boyd, C.A.R. (1996) 'Plasma tyrosine transport and maternal phenylketonuria.' *Acta Paediatrica*, **85**, 109-110.

Kure, S., Narisawa, K., Tada, K. (1992) 'Enzymatic diagnosis of nonketotic hyperglycinemia with lymphoblasts.' *Journal of Pediatrics*, **120**, 95–98.

Kurihara, M., Kumagai, K., Yagishita, S., *et al.* (1993) 'Adrenoleukomyeloneuropathy presenting as cerebellar ataxia in a young child: a probable variant of adrenoleukodystrophy.' *Brain and Development*, **15**, 377–380.

Kuriyama, M., Fujiyama, J., Yoshidome, H., *et al.* (1991) 'Cerebrotendinous xanthomatosis: clinical and biochemical evaluation of eight patients and review of the literature.' *Journal of the Neurological Sciences*, **102**, 225–232.

Kurlemann, G., Debus, O., Schuierer, G. (1996) 'Dextrometorphan in molybdenum cofactor deficiency.' *European Journal of Pediatrics*, **155**, 422–423.

Kvittingen, E.A. (1991) 'Tyrosinemia type I—an update.' *Journal of Inherited Metabolic Disease*, **14**, 554–562.

—— Clayton, P.T., Leonard, J.V. (1995) 'Tyrosine.' *In:* Fernandes, J., Saudubray, J.M., van den Berghe, G. (Eds.) *Inborn Metabolic Diseases: Diagnosis and Treatment. 2nd Edn.* Berlin: Springer Verlag, pp. 161–166.

Lambert, M.A., Marescau, B., Desjardins, M., *et al.* (1991) 'Hyperargininemia: intellectual and motor improvement related to changes in biochemical data.' *Journal of Pediatrics*, **118**, 420–424.

Lancet (1990) 'Hereditary tyrosinaemia.' *Lancet*, **335**, 1500–1501. *(Editorial.)*

Land, J.M., Mistry, S., Squier, M., *et al.* (1995) 'Neonatal carnitine palmitoyltransferase-2 deficiency: a case presenting with myopathy.' *Neuromuscular Disorders*, **5**, 129–137.

Largillière, C., Van Schaftingen, E., Fontaine, M., Farriaux, J.P. (1991) 'D-glyceric acidaemia: clinical report and biochemical studies in a patient.' *Journal of Inherited Metabolic Disease*, **14**, 263–264.

Lazarow, P.B., Moser, H.W. (1995) 'Disorders of peroxisomes biogenesis.' *In:* Scriver, C.R., Beaudet, A.L., Sly, W.S., Valle, D. (Eds.) *The Metabolic and Molecular Bases of Inherited Disease, 7th Edn.* New York: McGraw Hill, pp. 2287–2324.

Lee, C., Dineen, T.E., Brack, M., *et al.* (1993) 'The mucopolysaccharidoses: characterization by cranial MR imaging.' *American Journal of Neuroradiology*, **14**, 1285–1292.

Lehnert, W., Sperl, W., Suormala, T., Baumgartner, E.R. (1994) 'Propionic acidaemia: clinical, biochemical and therapeutic aspects. Experience in 30 patients.' *European Journal of Pediatrics*, **153**, Suppl. 1, S68–S80.

Leitersdorf, E., Reshef, A., Meiner, V., *et al.* (1993) 'Frameshift and splice-junction mutations in the sterol 27-hydroxylase gene cause cerebrotendinous xanthomatosis in Jews of Moroccan origin.' *Journal of Clinical Investigations*, **91**, 2488–2496.

Lenke, R.R., Levy, H.L. (1980) 'Maternal phenylketonuria and hyperphenylalaninemia: an international survey of the outcome of untreated and treated pregnancies.' *New England Journal of Medicine*, **303**, 1202–1208.

Leonard, J.V. (1995) 'Urea cycle disorders.' *In:* Fernandes, J., Saudubray, J.M., van den Berghe, G. (Eds.) *Inborn Metabolic Diseases: Diagnosis and Treatment. 2nd Edn.* Berlin: Springer Verlag, pp. 167–176.

Leone, L., Ippoliti, P.F., Antonicelli, R., *et al.* (1995) 'Treatment and liver transplantation for cholesterol ester storage disease.' *Journal of Pediatrics*, **127**, 509–510.

Leroy, L.G., Mae, W.H., McBrinn, M.C., *et al.* (1972) 'I-cell disease: biochemical studies.' *Pediatric Research*, **6**, 752–757.

Levin, M.L., Scheimann, A., Lewis, R.A., Beaudet, A.L. (1993) 'Cerebral edema in maple syrup urine disease.' *Journal of Pediatrics*, **122**, 167. *(Letter.)*

Levy, H.L., Waisbren, S.E., Lobbregt, D., *et al.* (1994) 'Maternal mild hyperphenylalaninaemia: an international survey of offspring outcome.' *Lancet*, **344**, 1589–1594.

—— Lobbregt, D., Barnes, P.D., Young Poussaint, T. (1996) 'Maternal phenylketonuria: magnetic resonance imaging of the brain in offspring.' *Journal of Pediatrics*, **128**, 770–775.

Liao, K-K., Wang, S-J., Kwan, S-Y., *et al.* (1991) 'Tongue dyskinesia as an early manifestation of Wilson disease.' *Brain and Development*, **13**, 451–453.

Linnell, J.C., Bhatt, H.R. (1995) 'Inherited errors of cobalamin and their management.' *Baillière's Clinical Haematology*, **8**, 567–601.

Lindstedt, S., Holme, E., Lock, E.A., *et al.* (1992) 'Treatment of hereditary tyrosinaemia type I by inhibition of 4-hydroxyphenylpyruvate dioxygenase.' *Lancet*, **340**, 813–817.

Lissens, W., DeMeirler, L., Seneca, S., *et al.* (1996) 'Mutation analysis of the pyruvate dehydrogenase E1 alpha gene in eight patients with a pyruvate dehydrogenase complex deficiency.' *Human Mutations*, **7**, 46–51.

Lombès, A., Romero, N.B., Touati, G., *et al.* (1996) 'Clinical and molecular heterogeneity of cytochrome c oxidase deficiency in the newborn.' *Journal of Inherited Metabolic Disease*, **19**, 286–295.

Loonen, M.C.B., van Diggelen, O.P., Janse, O.P., *et al.* (1985) 'Late-onset globoid cell leucodystrophy (Krabbe's disease). Clinical and genetic delineation of two forms and their relation to the early-infantile form.' *Neuropediatrics*, **16**, 137–142.

Lüdecke, B., Dworniczak, B., Bartholomé, K. (1995) 'A point mutation in the tyrosine hydroxylase gene associated with Segawa's syndrome.' *Human Genetics*, **95**, 123–125.

Ludolph, A.C., Vetter, U., Ullrich, K. (1996) 'Studies of multimodal evoked potentials in treated phenylketonuria: the pattern of vulnerability.' *European Journal of Pediatrics*, **155**, Suppl. 1, S64–S68.

Lyon, G., Adams, R.D., Kolodny, E.H. (1996) *Neurology of Hereditary Metabolic Diseases of Children, 2nd Edn.* New York: McGraw Hill.

Macaya, A., Munell, F., Burke, R.E., De Vivo, D.C. (1993) 'Disorders of movement in Leigh syndrome.' *Neuropediatrics*, **24**, 60–67.

MacCollin, M., De Vivo, D.C., Moser, A.B., Beard, M. (1990) 'Ataxia and peripheral neuropathy: a benign variant of peroxisome dysgenesis.' *Annals of Neurology*, **28**, 833–836.

MacFaul, R., Cavanagh, N., Lake, B.D., *et al.* (1982) 'Metachromatic leucodystrophy: review of 38 cases.' *Archives of Disease in Childhood*, **57**, 168–175.

MacPhee, G.B., Logan, R.W., Mitchell, J.S., *et al.* (1993) 'Malonyl coenzyme A decarboxylase deficiency.' *Archives of Disease in Childhood*, **69**, 433–436.

Maddocks, J., Reed, T. (1989) 'Urine test for adenylosuccinase deficiency in autistic children.' *Lancet*, **1**, 158–159. *(Letter.)*

Maia, M., Alves, D., Ribeiro, G., *et al.* (1990) 'Juvenile GM2 gangliosidosis variant B1: clinical and biochemical study in seven patients.' *Neuropediatrics*, **21**, 18–23.

Mancini, G.M.S., Hu, P., Verheijen, F.W., *et al.* (1992) 'Salla disease variant in a Dutch patient. Potential value of polymorphonuclear leucocytes for heterozygote detection.' *European Journal of Pediatrics*, **151**, 590–595.

Man in't Veld, A.J., Boomsma, F., Moleman, P., Schalekamp, M.A.D.H. (1987) 'Congenital dopamine-beta-hydroxylase deficiency. A novel orthostatic syndrome.' *Lancet*, **1**, 183–188.

Marescau, B., De Deyn, P.P., Lowenthal, A., *et al.* (1990) 'Guanidino compound, analysis as a complementary diagnostic parameter for hyperargininemia: follow-up of guanidino compound levels during therapy.' *Pediatric Research*, **27**, 297–303.

Marion, R.W., Alvarez, L.A., Marans, Z.S., *et al.* (1987) 'Computed tomography of the brain in the Smith–Lemli–Opitz syndrome.' *Journal of Child Neurology*, **2**, 198–200.

Maroteaux, P. (1973) 'Un nouveau type de mucopolysaccharidose avec athétose et élimination urinaire de kératan sulfate.' *Nouvelle Presse Médicale*, **2**, 975–979.

—— (1974) *Les Maladies Osseuses de l'Enfant.* Paris: Flammarion.

Marquet, J., Chadefaux, B., Bonnefont, J.P., *et al.* (1994) 'Methylenetetrahydrofolate reductase deficiency: prenatal diagnosis and family studies.' *Prenatal Diagnosis*, **14**, 29–33.

Martin, J.J., Lowenthal, A., Ceuterick, C., Vanier, M.T. (1984) 'Juvenile dystonic lipidosis (variant of Niemann–Pick disease type C).' *Journal of the Neurological Sciences*, **66**, 33–45.

Martinsson, T., Bjursell, C., Stibler, H., *et al.* (1994) 'Linkage of a locus for carbohydrate-deficient glycoprotein syndrome type I (CDG1) to chromosome 16p, and linkage disequilibrium to microsatellite marker D16S406.' *Human Molecular Genetics*, **3**, 2037–2042.

Martinez, M. (1996) 'Docosahexaenoic acid therapy in docosahexaenoic acid-deficient patients with disorders of peroxisomal biogenesis.' *Lipids*, **31** (Suppl.), S145–S152.

Martinez-Lage, J.F., Casas, C., Fernández, M.A., *et al.* (1994) 'Macrocephaly, dystonia, and bilateral temporal arachnoid cysts: glutaric aciduria type I.' *Child's Nervous System*, **10**, 198–203.

Matalon, R., Michals, K., Sebesta, D., *et al.* (1988) 'Aspartoacylase deficiency and N-acetylaspartic aciduria in patients with Canavan disease.' *American Journal of Medical Genetics*, **29**, 463–471.

—— Kaul, R., Michals, K. (1993) 'Canavan disease: biochemical and molecular studies.' *Journal of Inherited Metabolic Disease*, **16**, 744–752.

———— Gao, G.P., *et al.* (1995a) 'Prenatal diagnosis for Canavan disease: the use of DNA markers.' *Journal of Inherited Metabolic Disease*, **18**, 215–217.

—— Michals, K., Kaul, R. (1995b) 'Canavan disease: from spongy degeneration to molecular analysis.' *Journal of Pediatrics*, **127**, 511–517.

Matsuda, J., Ito, M., Naito, E., *et al.* (1995) 'DNA diagnosis of pyruvate dehydrogenase deficiency in female patients with congenital lactic acidaemia.' *Journal of Inherited Metabolic Disease*, **18**, 534–546.

Matthews, W.S., Solan, A., Barabas, G. (1995) 'Cognitive functioning in Lesch–Nyhan syndrome.' *Developmental Medicine and Child Neurology*, **37**, 715–722.

Mattson, L.R., Lindor, N.R., Goldman, D.H., *et al.* (1995) 'Central pontine myelinolysis as a complication of partial ornithine carbamoyl transferase deficiency.' *American Journal of Medical Genetics*, **60**, 210–213.

Matsuo, S., Inoue, F., Takeuchi, Y., *et al.* (1995) 'Efficacy of tryptophan for the treatment of nonketotic hyperglycinemia: a new therapeutic approach for modulating the *N*-methyl-D-aspartate receptor.' *Pediatrics*, **95**, 142–146.

Mazzarello, P., Poloni, M., Spadari, S., Focher, F. (1992) 'DNA repair mechanisms in neurological disease: facts and hypotheses.' *Journal of the Neurological Sciences*, **112**, 4–14.

McGaughran, J.M., Clayton, P.T., Mills, K.A., *et al.* (1995) 'Prenatal diagnosis of Smith–Lemli–Opitz syndrome.' *American Journal Of Medical Genetics*, **56**, 269–271.

McKusick, V.A. (1972) *Heritable Disorders of Connective Tissue, 4th Edn.* St Louis: C.V. Mosby.

—— Neufeld, E.F. (1983) 'The mucopolysaccharide storage diseases.' *In:* Stanbury, J.B., Wyngaarden, J.B., Frederickson, J.L. *et al.* (Eds.) *The Metabolic Nature of Inherited Diseases, 5th Edn.* New York: McGraw Hill, pp. 751–787.

Medalia, A., Isaacs-Glaberman, K., Scheinberg, H. (1988) 'Neuropsychological impairment in Wilson's disease.' *Archives of Neurology*, **45**, 502–504.

Medina, L., Chi, T.L., De Vivo, D.C., Hilal, S.K. (1990) 'MR findings in patients with subacute necrotizing encephalomyelopathy (Leigh syndrome): correlation with biochemical defect.' *American Journal of Neuroradiology*, **11**, 379–384.

Meiner, V., Meiner, Z., Reshef, A., *et al.* (1994) 'Cerebrotendinous xanthomatosis: molecular diagnosis enables presymptomatic detection of a treatable disease.' *Neurology*, **44**, 288–290.

Menkes, J.H. (1988) 'Kinky hair disease: twenty five years later.' *Brain and Development*, **10**, 77–79.

Menzies, D.G., Campbell, I.W., Kearn, D.M. (1988) 'Magnetic resonance imaging in Fabry's disease.' *Journal of Neurology, Neurosurgery, and Psychiatry*, **51**, 1240–1241.

Mikati, M.A., Trevathan, E., Krishnamoorthy, K.S., Lombroso, C.T. (1991) 'Pyridoxine-dependent epilepsy: EEG investigations and long-term follow-up.' *Electroencephalography and Clinical Neurophysiology*, **78**, 215–221.

Mises, J., Moussali Salefranque, F., Laroque, M.L., *et al.* (1982) 'EEG findings as an aid to the diagnosis of neonatal nonketotic hyperglycinaemia.' *Journal of Inherited Metabolic Disease*, **5**, Suppl. 2, 117–120.

Mistry, P.K. (1995) 'Genotype/phenotype correlations in Gaucher's disease.' *Lancet*, **346**, 982–983.

Mitchell, G., Larochelle, J., Lambert, M., *et al.* (1990) 'Neurologic crises in hereditary tyrosinemia.' *New England Journal of Medicine*, **322**, 432–437.

Miyai, I., Fujimura, H., Umekage, T., *et al.* (1990) 'Magnetic resonance imaging in adrenoleukodystrophy presenting as spinocerebellar degeneration.' *Journal of Neurology, Neurosurgery, and Psychiatry*, **53**, 623–624. *(Letter.)*

Miyajima, H., Nishimura, Y., Mizoguchi, K., *et al.* (1987) 'Familial apoceruloplasmin deficiency associated with blepharospasm and retinal degeneration.' *Neurology*, **37**, 761–767.

Mize, C., Johnson, J.L., Rajagopalan, K.V. (1995) 'Defective molybdopterin biosynthesis: clinical heterogeneity associated with molybdenum cofactor deficiency.' *Journal of Inherited Metabolic Disease*, **18**, 283–290.

Monagle, P.T., Tauro, G.P. (1995) 'Long term follow up of patients with transcobalamin II deficiency.' *Archives of Disease in Childhood*, **72**, 237–238.

Montreuil, J., Biserte, G., Strecker, G., *et al.* (1968) 'Description d'un nouveau type de meliturie: la sialurie.' *Clinica Chimica Acta*, **21**, 61–69.

Morita, H., Ikeda, S-i., Yamamoto, K., *et al.* (1995) 'Hereditary ceruloplasmin deficiency with hemosiderosis: a clinicopathological study of a Japanese family.' *Annals of Neurology*, **37**, 646–656.

Moser, A.B., Rasmussen, M., Naidu, S., *et al.* (1995) 'Phenotype of patients with peroxisomal disorders subdivided into sixteen complementation groups.' *Journal of Pediatrics*, **127**, 13–22.

Moser, H.W. (1989) 'Peroxisomal diseases.' *Advances in Pediatrics*, **36**, 1–38.

—— (1993) 'Lorenzo oil therapy for adrenoleukodystrophy: a prematurely amplified hope.' *Annals of Neurology*, **34**, 121–122.

—— Chen, W.W. (1983) 'Ceramidase deficiency. Farber's lipogranulomatosis.' *In:* Stanbury, J.B., Wyngaarden, J.B., Fredrikson, J.L., *et al.* (Eds.) *The Metabolic Basis of Inherited Disease, 5th Edn.* New York: McGraw Hill, pp. 820–830.

—— Moser, A.E., Singh, I., O'Neill, B.P. (1984) 'Adrenoleukodystrophy: survey of 303 cases: biochemistry, diagnosis, and therapy.' *Annals of Neurology*, **16**, 628–641.

—— Smith, K.D., Moser, A.B. (1995) 'X-linked adrenoleukodystrophy.' *In:* Scriver, C.R., Beaudet, A.L., Sly, W.S., Valle, D. (Eds.) *The Metabolic and Molecular Bases of Inherited Disease, 7th Edn.* New York: McGraw Hill, pp. 2325–2349.

Motley, A.M., Tabak, H.F., Smeitink, J.A., *et al.* (1996) 'Non-rhizomelic and rhizomelic chondrodysplasia punctata within a single complementation group.' *Biochimica et Biophysica Acta*, **1315**, 153–158.

Mudd, S.H., Skovby, F., Levy, H.L., *et al.* (1985) 'The natural history of homocystinuria due to cystathionine beta-synthase deficiency.' *American Journal of Human Genetics*, **37**, 1–31.

—— Levy, H.L., Skovby, F. (1995) 'The disorders of transulfuration.' *In:* Scriver, C.R., Beaudet, A.L., Sly, W.S., Valle, D. (Eds.) *The Metabolic and Molecular Bases of Inherited Disease, 7th Edn.* New York: McGraw Hill, pp. 1279–1327.

Muller, D.P.R., Lloyd, J.K., Wolff, O.H. (1983) 'Vitamin E and neurological function.' *Lancet*, **1**, 225–228.

———— (1985) 'The role of vitamin E in the treatment of the neurological features of abetalipoproteinemia and other disorders of fat absorption.' *Journal of Inherited Metabolic Disease*, **8**, Suppl. 1, 88–92.

Muntoni, S., Wiebusch, H., Funke, H., *et al.* (1995) 'Homozygosity for a splice junction mutation in exon 8 of the gene encoding lysosomal acid lipase in a Spanish kindred with cholesterol ester storage disease (CESD).' *Human Genetics*, **95**, 491–494.

Nada, M.A., Vianey-Saban, C., Roe, C.R., *et al.* (1996) 'Prenatal diagnosis of mitochondrial fatty acid oxidation defects.' *Prenatal Diagnosis*, **16**, 117–124.

Nagai, T., Goto, Y.I., Matsuoka, T., *et al.* (1992) 'Leigh encephalopathy: histologic and biochemical analyses of muscle biopsies.' *Pediatric Neurology*, **8**, 328–332.

Naidu, S., Hoefler, G., Watkins, P.A., *et al.* (1988a) 'Neonatal seizures and retardation in a girl with biochemical features of X-linked adrenoleukodystrophy.' *Neurology*, **38**, 1100–1107.

—— Hofmann, K.J., Moser, H.W., *et al.* (1988b) 'Galactosylceramide-β-galactosidase deficiency in association with cherry red spot.' *Neuropediatrics*, **19**, 46–48.

Nakano, T., Nanba, E., Tanaka, A., *et al.* (1990) 'A new point mutation within exon 5 of beta-hexosaminidase alpha gene in a Japanese infant with Tay–Sachs disease.' *Annals of Neurology*, **27**, 465–473.

Nanao, K., Okamura-Ikeda, K., Motokawa, Y., *et al.* (1994) 'Identification of the mutations in the T-protein gene causing typical and atypical nonketotic hyperglycinemia.' *Human Genetics*, **93**, 655–658.

Nardocci, N., Bertagnolio, B., Rumi, V., Angelini, L. (1992) 'Progressive dystonia symptomatic of juvenile GM2 gangliosidosis.' *Movement Disorders*, **7**, 64–67.

Natowicz, M.R., Evans, J.E. (1994) 'Abnormal bile acids in the Smith–Lemli–Opitz syndrome.' *American Journal of Medical Genetics*, **50**, 364–367.

Navon, R., Khosravi, R., Korczyn, T., *et al.* (1995) 'A new mutation in the HEXA gene associated with a spinal muscular atrophy phenotype.' *Neurology*, **45**, 539–543.

Nelson, C.D., Waggoner, D.D., Donnell, G.N., *et al.* (1991) 'Verbal dyspraxia in treated galactosemia.' *Pediatrics*, **88**, 346–350.

Neville, B.G.R., Lake, B.D., Stephens, R., Sanders, M.D. (1973) 'A neuro-visceral storage disease with vertical nuclear ophthalmoplegia and its relationship to Niemann–Pick disease. A report of nine patients.' *Brain*, **96**, 97–120.

Nigro, M.A., Wishnow, R., Moser, A.B. (1993) 'An X-linked recessive form of neonatal adrenoleukodystrophy.' *Annals of Neurology*, **34**, 465. *(Abstract.)*

Nishimura, R., Omos-Lau, N., Ajmone-Marsan, C., Baranger, J.A. (1980) 'Electroencephalographic findings in Gaucher disease.' *Neurology*, **30**, 152–159.

Noll, R.B., Netzloff, M.L., Kulkarni, R. (1989) 'Long-term follow-up of biochemical and cognitive functioning in patients with mannosidosis.' *Archives of Neurology*, **46**, 507–509.

Nordborg, C., Hagberg, B., Kristiansson, B. (1991) 'Sural nerve pathology in the carbohydrate-deficient glycoprotein syndrome.' *Acta Paediatrica Scandinavica*, Suppl. 375, 39–49.

North, K.N., Hoppel, C.L., De Girolami, U., *et al.* (1995) 'Lethal neonatal deficiency of carnitine palmitoyltransferase II associated with dysgenesis of the brain and kidneys.' *Journal of Pediatrics*, **127**, 414–420.

Nyhan, W.L., Shelton, G.D., Jakobs, C., *et al.* (1995) 'D-2-hydroxyglutaric aciduria.' *Journal of Child Neurology*, **10**, 137–142.

Oates, C.E., Bosch, E.P., Hart, M.N. (1986) 'Movement disorders associated with chronic GM2 gangliosidosis: case report and review of the literature.' *European Neurology*, **25**, 154–159.

Oder, W., Grimm, G., Kollegger, H., *et al.* (1991) 'Neurological and neuro-psychiatric spectrum of Wilson's disease: a prospective study of 45 cases.' *Journal of Neurology*, **238**, 281–287.

—— Prayer, L., Grimm, G., *et al.* (1993) 'Wilson's disease: evidence of subgroups derived from clinical findings and brain lesions.' *Neurology*, **43**, 120–124.

Ogasawara, N., Stout, J.T., Goto, H., *et al.* (1989) 'Molecular analysis of a female Lesch–Nyhan patient.' *Journal of Clinical Investigation*, **24**, 1024–1027.

Ogier de Baulny, H., Saudubray, J.M. (1995) 'Emergency treatments.' *In:* Fernandes, J., Saudubray, J.M., van den Berghe, G. (Eds.) *Inborn Metabolic Diseases: Diagnosis and Treatment. 2nd Edn.* Berlin: Springer Verlag, pp. 47–55.

—— Slama, A., Touati, G., *et al.* (1995a) 'Neonatal hyperammonemia caused by a defect of carnitine-acylcarnitine translocase.' *Journal of Pediatrics*, **127**, 723–728.

—— Wendel, U., Saudubray, J.M. (1995b) 'Branched chain organic acidurias.' *In:* Fernandes, J., Saudubray, J.M., van den Berghe, G. (Eds.) *Inborn Metabolic Diseases: Diagnosis and Treatment. 2nd Edn.* Berlin: Springer Verlag, pp. 207–221.

Okada, J., Oonishi, H., Tamada, H., *et al.* (1995) 'Gallium uptake in cerebro-tendinous xanthomatosis.' *European Journal of Nuclear Medicine*, **22**, 1069–1072.

Okuyama, E., Tomita, S., Takeuchi, H., Ichikawa, Y. (1996) 'A novel muta-tion in the cytochrome P450$_{27}$ (*CYP27*) gene caused cerebrotendinous xanthomatosis in a Japanese family.' *Journal of Lipid Research*, **37**, 631–639.

Old, S.E., De Vivo, D.C. (1989) 'Pyruvate dehydrogenase complex deficiency: biochemical and immunoblot analysis of cultured skin fibroblasts.' *Annals of Neurology*, **26**, 746–751.

Olivos-Glander, I.M., Jänne, P.A., Nussbaum, R.L. (1995) 'The oculocerebro-renal syndrome gene product is a 105-kD protein localized to the Golgi complex.' *American Journal of Human Genetics*, **57**, 817–823.

Ono, J., Harada, K., Mano, T., *et al.* (1996) 'MR findings and neurologic manifestations in Lowe oculocerebrorenal syndrome.' *Pediatric Neurology*, **14**, 162–164.

Ono, S., Kurisaki, H. (1988) 'An unusual neurological disorder with abnormal copper metabolism.' *Journal of Neurology*, **235**, 397–399.

Opitz, J.M. (1994) 'RSH/SLO ("Smith–Lemli–Opitz") syndrome: historical, genetic, and developmental considerations.' *American Journal of Human Genetics*, **50**, 344–346.

Otero, L.J., Brown, G.K., Silver, K., *et al.* (1995) 'Association of cerebral dysgenesis and lactic acidemia with X-linked PDH E1α subunit mutations in females.' *Pediatric Neurology*, **13**, 327–332.

Page, T., Nyhan, W.L., Morena de Vega, V. (1987) 'Syndrome of mild mental retardation, spastic gait and skeletal malformations in a family with partial deficiency of hypoxanthine-guanine phosphoribosyl transferase.' *Pediatrics*, **79**, 713–717.

Pall, H.S., Williams, A.C., Blake, D.R., *et al.* (1987) 'Movement disorder associated with abnormal copper metabolism and decreased blood anti-oxidants.' *Journal of Neurology, Neurosurgery, and Psychiatry*, **50**, 1234–1235.

Palmer, T., Oberholzer, V.G. (1985) 'Aminoacid loading tests in a patient with nonketotic hyperglycinaemia.' *Journal of Inherited Metabolic Disease*, **8**, Suppl. 2, 125–126.

Palomaki, G.E., Williams, J., Haddow, J.E., Natowicz, M.R. (1995) 'Tay–Sachs disease in persons of French-Canadian heritage in northern New England.' *American Journal of Medical Genetics*, **56**, 409–412.

Parvy, P., Bardet, J., Chadefaux-Vekemans, B., *et al.* (1995) 'Free amino acids in amniotic fluid and the prenatal diagnosis of homocystinuria with methyl-malonic aciduria.' *Clinical Chemistry*, **41**, 1663–1664.

Pasquier, F., Lebert, F., Petit, H., *et al.* (1994) 'Methylenetetrahydrofolate reductase deficiency revealed by a neuropathy in a psychotic adult.' *Journal of Neurology, Neurosurgery, and Psychiatry*, **57**, 765–766. *(Letter.)*

Pastoris, O., Savasta, S., Foppa, P., *et al.* (1996) 'Pyruvate dehydrogenase deficiency in a child responsive to thiamine treatment.' *Acta Paediatrica*, **85**, 625–628.

Pavlakis, S.G., DiMauro, S., DeVivo, D.C., Rowland, L.P. (1984) 'Mito-chondrial myopathy, encephalopathy, lactic acidosis and stroke-like episodes: a distinctive clinical syndrome.' *Annals of Neurology*, **16**, 481–488.

Peinemann, F., Danner, D.J. (1994) 'Maple syrup urine disease 1954 to 1993.' *Journal of Inherited Metabolic Disease*, **17**, 3–15.

Perry, T.L., Haworth, J.C., Robinson, B.H. (1985) 'Brain amino acid abnor-malities in pyruvate carboxylase deficiency.' *Journal of Inherited Metabolic Disease*, **8**, 63–66.

Petty, R.K.H., Harding, A.E., Morgan-Hughes, J.A. (1986) 'The clinical features of mitochondrial myopathy.' *Brain*, **109**, 915–938.

Phaneuf, D., Lambert, M., Laframboise, R., *et al.* (1992) 'Type I hereditary tyrosinemia. Evidence for molecular heterogeneity and identification of a causal mutation in a French Canadian patient.' *Journal of Clinical Investiga-tions*, **90**, 1185–1192.

Phelps, M., Aicardi, J., Vanier, M. (1991) 'Late-onset Krabbe leukodystrophy. A report of four cases.' *Journal of Neurology, Neurosurgery, and Psychiatry*, **54**, 293–296.

Pietz, J., Schmidt, E., Matthis, P., *et al.* (1993) 'EEGs in phenylketonuria. I: Follow-up to adulthood; II: Short term diet-related changes in EEGs and cognitive function.' *Developmental Medicine and Child Neurology*, **35**, 54–64.

Ploos van Amstel, J.K., Jansen, R.P.M., de Jong, J.G.M., *et al.* (1994) 'Six novel mutations in the alpha-galactosidase A gene in families with Fabry disease.' *Human Molecular Genetics*, **3**, 503–505.

Poenaru, L., Castelnau, L., Besançon, A.M., *et al.* (1988) 'First trimester prenatal diagnosis of metachromatic leukodystrophy on chorionic villi with immunoprecipitation electrophoresis.' *Journal of Inherited Metabolic Disease*, **11**, 123–130.

Poggi-Travert, F., Fournier, B., Poll-Thé, B.T., Saudubray, J.M. (1995) 'Clinical approach to inherited peroxisomal disorders.' *Journal of Inherited Metabolic Disease*, **18**, Suppl. 1, 1–18.

Pollitt, R.J. (1995) 'Disorders of mitochondrial long-chain fatty acid oxidation.' *Journal of Inherited Metabolic Disease*, **18**, 473–490.

Polten, A., Fluharty, A.L., Fluharty, C.B., *et al.* (1991) 'Molecular basis of different forms of metachromatic leukodystrophy.' *New England Journal of Medicine*, **324**, 18–22.

Ponzone, A., Guardamagna, O., Spada, M., *et al.* (1993) 'Differential diagnosis of hyperphenylalaninaemia by a combined phenylalanine–tetrahydro-biopterin loading test.' *European Journal of Pediatrics*, **152**, 655–661.

Pomponio, R.J., Reynolds, T.R., Cole, H., *et al.* (1995) 'Mutational hotspot in the human biotinidase gene causes profound biotinidase deficiency.' *Nature Genetics*, **11**, 96–98.

Possekel, S., Lombès, A., Ogier de Baulny, H., *et al.* (1995) 'Immunohisto-chemical analysis of muscle cytochrome *c* oxidase deficiency in children.' *Histochemistry*, **103**, 59–68.

Powers, J.M. (1995) 'The pathology of peroxisomal disorders with pathogenic considerations.' *Journal of Neuropathology and Experimental Neurology*, **54**, 710–719.

Press, G.A., Barshop, B.A., Haas, R.H., *et al.* (1989) 'Abnormalities of the brain in non-ketotic hyperglycinemia: MR manifestations.' *American Journal of Neuroradiology*, **10**, 315–321.

Prick, M.J.J., Gabreëls, F.J.M., Renier, W.O., *et al.* (1981) 'Progressive infantile poliodystrophy: association with disturbed pyruvate oxidation in muscle and liver.' *Archives of Neurology*, **38**, 767–772.

Procopis, P., Camakaris, S., Danks, D. (1981) 'Mild forms of Menkes steely hair syndrome.' *Journal of Pediatrics*, **98**, 97–99.

Pueschel, S.M., O'Shea, P.A., Alroy, J., *et al.* (1988) 'Infantile sialic acid storage disease associated with renal disease.' *Pediatric Neurology*, **4**, 207–212.

Purpura, D.P., Suzuki, K. (1976) 'Distortion of neuronal geometry and forma-tion of aberrant synapses in neuronal storage disease.' *Brain Research*, **116**, 1–21.

Putman, C.W.M.M., Rotteveel, J.J., Wevers, R.A., *et al.* (1997) 'Dihydro-pyrimidinase deficiency, a progressive neurological disorder.' *Neuropediatrics*, **28**, 106–110.

Rahman, S., Blok, R.B., Dahl, H-H.M., *et al.* (1996) 'Leigh syndrome: clinical features and biochemical and DNA abnormalities.' *Annals of Neurology*, **39**, 343–351.

Ramaekers, V.T., Stibler, H., Kint, J., Jaeken, J. (1991) 'A new variant of the carbohydrate deficient glycoproteins syndrome.' *Journal of Inherited Metabolic Disease*, **14**, 385–388.

Rapin, I., Goldfisher, S., Katzman, R., *et al.* (1978) 'The cherry-red spot myoclonus syndrome.' *Annals of Neurology*, **3**, 234–242.

Remes, A.M., Rantala, E., Hiltunen, K., *et al.* (1992) 'Fumarase deficiency: two siblings with enlarged cerebral ventricles and polyhydramnios in utero.' *Pediatrics*, **89**, 730–734.

Renlund, M. (1984) 'Clinical and laboratory diagnosis of Salla disease in infancy and childhood.' *Journal of Pediatrics*, **104**, 232–236.

—— Kovanen, P.T., Raivio, K.O., *et al.* (1986) 'Studies on the defect underlying the lysosomal storage of sialic acid in Salla disease.' *Journal of Clinical Investigation*, **77**, 568–574.

Riviello, J.J., Rezvani, I., DiGeorge, A.M., Foley, C.M. (1991) 'Cerebral edema causing death in children with maple syrup urine disease.' *Journal of Pediatrics*, **119**, 42–45.

Rizzo, W.B., Dammann, A.L., Craft, D.A., *et al.* (1989) 'Sjögren–Larsson syndrome: inherited defect in the fatty alcohol cycle.' *Journal of Pediatrics*, **115**, 228–234.

Robain, O., Aubourg, P., Routon, M.C., *et al.* (1988) 'Menkes disease: a Golgi and electron microscopic study of the cerebellar cortex.' *Clinical Neuropathology*, **7**, 47–52.

Robbins, J.H. (1987) 'Xeroderma pigmentosum.' *In:* Gomez, R. (Ed.) *Neurocutaneous Diseases: a Practical Approach.* London: Butterworths, pp. 118–127.

—— Brumback, R.A, Mendiones, M., *et al.* (1991) 'Neurological disease in xeroderma pigmentosum. Documentation of a late onset type of the juvenile onset form.' *Brain*, **114**, 1335–1361.

Robinson, B.H. (1993) 'Lacticacidemia.' *Biochimica et Biophysica Acta*, **1182**, 231–244.

—— (1995) 'Lactic acidemia (disorders of pyruvate carboxylase, pyruvate dehydrogenase).' *In:* Scriver, C.R., Beaudet, A.L., Sly, W.S., Valle, D. (Eds.) *The Metabolic and Molecular Bases of Inherited Disease, 7th Edn.* New York: McGraw Hill, pp. 1479–1499.

—— Toone, J.R., Petrova-Benedict, R., *et al.* (1985) 'Prenatal diagnosis of pyruvate carboxylase deficiency.' *Prenatal Diagnosis*, **5**, 67–71.

—— MacMillan, H., Petrova-Benedict, R., Sherwood, W.G. (1987) 'Variable clinical presentation in patients with defective E$_1$ component of pyruvate dehydrogenase complex.' *Journal of Pediatrics*, **111**, 525–533.

—— MacKay, N., Petrova-Benedict, R., *et al.* (1990) 'Defects in the E$_2$ lipoyl transacetylase and the X-lipoyl containing component of the pyruvate dehydrogenase complex in patients with lactic acidemia.' *Journal of Clinical Investigation*, **85**, 1821–1824.

—— —— Chun, K., Ling, M. (1996) 'Disorders of pyruvate carboxylase and the pyruvate dehydrogenase complex.' *Journal of Inherited Metabolic Disease*, **19**, 452–462.

Robinson, R.O., Fensom, A.H., Lake, B.D. (1997) 'Salla disease—rare or under-diagnosed?' *Developmental Medicine and Child Neurology*, **39**, 153–157.

Roe, C.R., Coates, P.M. (1995) 'Mitochondrial fatty acid oxidation disorders.' *In:* Scriver, C.R., Beaudet, A.L., Sly, W.S., Valle, D. (Eds.) *The Metabolic and Molecular Bases of Inherited Disease, 7th Edn.* New York: McGraw Hill, pp. 1501–1533.

Roels, F., Pauwels, M., Poll-Thé, B.T., *et al.* (1988) 'Hepatic peroxisomes in adrenoleukodystrophy and related syndromes. Cytochemical and morphometric data.' *Virchows Archiv für Pathologische Anatomie*, **413**, 275–285.

Roesel, R.A., Byrne, K.M., Hommes, F., *et al.* (1987) 'Infantile free sialuria without lysosomal storage.' *Pediatric Neurology*, **3**, 40–43.

Roh, J.K., Lee, T.G., Wie, B.A., *et al.* (1994) 'Initial and follow-up brain MRI findings and correlation with the clinical course in Wilson's disease.' *Neurology*, **44**, 1064–1068.

Roodhooft, A.M., Baumgartner, E.R., Martin, J.J., *et al.* (1990) 'Symmetrical necrosis of the basal ganglia in methylmalonic acidemia.' *European Journal of Pediatrics*, **149**, 582–584.

Rosenblatt, D.S. (1995) 'Inherited disorders of folate transport and metabolism.' *In:* Scriver, C.R., Beaudet, A.L., Sly, W.S., Valle, D. (Eds.) *The Metabolic and Molecular Bases of Inherited Disease, 7th Edn.* New York: McGraw Hill, pp. 3111–3128.

Roth, A., Nogues, C., Monnet, J.P., *et al.* (1985) 'Anatomo-pathological findings in a case of combined deficiency of sulphite oxidase and xanthine oxidase with a defect of molybdenum cofactor.' *Virchows Archiv. A. Pathological Anatomy and Histopathology*, **405**, 379–386.

Rupar, C.A., Gillett, J., Gordon, B.A., *et al.* (1996) 'Isolated sulfite oxidase deficiency.' *Neuropediatrics*, **27**, 299–304.

Santorelli, F.M., Shanske, S., Macaya, A., *et al.* (1993) 'The mutation at nt 8993 of mitochondrial DNA is a common cause of Leigh's syndrome.' *Annals of Neurology*, **34**, 827–834.

—— Tanji, K., Sano, M., *et al.* (1997) 'Maternally inherited encephalopathy associated with a single-base insertion in the mitochondrial tRNA^{Trp} gene.' *Annals of Neurology*, **42**, 256–260.

Schaefer, J., Jackson, S., Dick, D.J., Turnbull, R. (1996) 'Trifunctional enzyme deficiency: adult presentation of a usually fatal β-oxidation defect.' *Annals of Neurology*, **40**, 597–602.

Schlenzig, J.S., Poggi-Travert, F., Laurent, J., *et al.* (1995) 'Liver transplantation in two cases of propionic acidaemia.' *Journal of Inherited Metabolic Disease*, **18**, 448–461.

Schuchman, E.H. (1995) 'Two new mutations in the acid sphingomyelinase gene causing type A Niemann–Pick disease: N389T and R441X.' *Human Mutations*, **6**, 352–357.

—— Desnick, R.J. (1995) 'Niemann–Pick diseases types A and B: acid sphingomyelinase deficiency.' *In:* Scriver, C.R., Beaudet, A.L., Sly, W.S., Valle, D. (Eds.) *The Metabolic and Molecular Bases of Inherited Disease, 7th Edn.* New York: McGraw Hill, pp. 2601–2624.

Schuierer, G., Kurlemann, G., Bick, U., Stephani, U. (1995) 'Molybdenum-cofactor deficiency: CT and MR findings.' *Neuropediatrics*, **26**, 51–54.

Schuler, A., Blau, N., Ponzone, A. (1995) 'Monoamine oxidase inhibitors in tetrahydrobiopterin deficiency.' *European Journal of Pediatrics*, **154**, 997. *(Letter.)*

Schwartz, W.J., Hutchinson, H.T., Berg, B.O. (1981) 'Computerized tomography in subacute necrotizing encephalomyelopathy (Leigh disease).' *Annals of Neurology*, **10**, 268–270.

Scott, H.S., Guo, X-H., Hopwood, J.J., Morris, C.P. (1992) 'Structure and sequence of the human α-L-iduronidase gene.' *Genomics*, **13**, 1311–1313.

Segal, S. (1993) 'The challenge of galactosemia.' *International Pediatrics*, **8**, 125–132.

Selhub, J., Miller, J.W. (1992) 'The pathogenesis of homocysteinemia: interruption of the coordinate regulation by S-adenosylmethionine of the remethylation and transsulfuration of homocysteine.' *American Journal of Clinical Nutrition*, **55**, 131–138.

Selwa, L.M., Vanderzant, C.W., Brunberg, J.A., *et al.* (1993) 'Correlation of evoked potential and MRI findings in Wilson's disease.' *Neurology*, **43**, 2059–2064.

Shaag, A., Anikster, Y., Christensen, E., *et al.* (1995) 'The molecular basis of Canavan (aspartoacylase deficiency) disease in European non-Jewish patients.' *American Journal of Human Genetics*, **57**, 572–580.

Shani, N., Sapag, A., Valle, D. (1996) 'Characterization and analysis of conserved motifs in a peroxisomal ATP-binding cassette transporter.' *Journal of Biological Chemistry*, **271**, 8725–8730.

Shevell, M.I., Matthews, P.M., Scriver, C.R., *et al.* (1994) 'Cerebral dysgenesis and lactic acidemia: an MRI/MRS phenotype associated with pyruvate dehydrogenase deficiency.' *Pediatric Neurology*, **11**, 224–229.

Shih, V.E. (1995) 'Ornithine.' *In:* Fernandes, J., Saudubray, J.M., van den Berghe, G. (Eds.) *Inborn Metabolic Errors. Diagnosis and Treatment. 2nd Edn.* Berlin: Springer Verlag, pp. 183–190.

Shintaku, H., Niederwieser, A., Leimbacher, W., Curtius, H-C. (1988) 'Tetrahydrobiopterin deficiency: assay for 6-pyruvoyl-tetrahydropterin synthase activity in erythrocytes, and detection of patients and heterozygous carriers.' *European Journal of Pediatrics*, **147**, 15–19.

Shoffner, J.M., Wallace, D.C. (1994) 'Oxidative phosphorylation diseases and mitochondrial DNA mutations: diagnosis and treatment.' *Annual Review of Nutrition*, **14**, 535–568.

Siebner, H.R., Berndt, S., Conrad, B. (1996) 'Cerebrotendinous xanthomatosis without tendon xanthomas mimicking Marinesco–Sjögren syndrome: a case report.' *Journal of Neurology, Neurosurgery, and Psychiatry*, **60**, 582–585.

Simmonds, H.A., Webster, D.R., Wilson, J., Lingham, S. (1982) 'An X-linked syndrome characterized by hyperuricemia, deafness and neurodevelopmental abnormalities.' *Lancet*, **2**, 68–70.

—— Fairbanks, L.D., Morris, G.S., *et al.* (1987) 'Central nervous system dysfunction and erythrocyte guanosine triphosphate depletion in purine nucleoside phosphorylase deficiency.' *Archives of Disease in Childhood*, **62**, 385–391.

Simpson, R.H.W., Rodda, J., Reinecke, C.J. (1987) 'Adrenoleukodystrophy in a mother and son.' *Journal of Neurology, Neurosurgery, and Psychiatry*, **50**, 1165–1172.

Sjaastad, O., Berstad, J., Gjesdahl, P., Gjessing, L. (1976) 'Homocarnosinosis 2. A familial metabolic disorder associated with spastic paraplegia, progressive mental deficiency, and retinal pigmentation.' *Acta Neurologica Scandinavica*, **53**, 275–290.

Slot, H.M.J., Overweg-Plandsoen, W.C.G., Bakker, H.D., *et al.* (1993) 'Molybdenum-cofactor deficiency: an easily missed cause of neonatal convulsions.' *Neuropediatrics*, **24**, 139–142.

Smith, I., Brenton, D.P. (1995) 'Hyperphenylalaninaemias.' *In:* Fernandes, J., Saudubray, J.M., van den Berghe, G. (Eds.) *Inborn Metabolic Diseases. Diagnosis and Treatment. 2nd Edn.* Berlin: Springer Verlag, pp. 147–160.

—— Beasley, M.G., Ades, A.E. (1990) 'Intelligence and quality of dietary treatment in phenylketonuria.' *Archives of Disease in Childhood*, **65**, 472–478.

Soffer, D., Amir, N., Elpeleg, O.N., *et al.* (1992) 'Striatal degeneration and spongy myelinopathy in glutaric acidemia.' *Journal of Neurological Sciences*, **107**, 199–204.

—— Benharroch, D., Berginer, V. (1995) 'The neuropathology of cerebrotendinous xanthomatosis revisited: a case report and review of the literature.' *Acta Neuropathologica*, **90**, 213–220.

Souri, M., Aoyama, T., Orii, K., *et al.* (1996) 'Mutation analysis of very-long-chain acyl-coenzyme A dehydrogenase (VLCAD) deficiency: identification and characterization of mutant VLCAD cDNAs from four patients.' *American Journal of Human Genetics*, **58**, 97–106.

Spada, M., Ferraris, S., Ferrero, G.B., *et al.* (1996) 'Monitoring treatment in tetrahydrobiopterin deficiency by serum prolactin.' *Journal of Inherited Metabolic Disease*, **19**, 231–233.

Specola, N., Vanier, M.T., Goutières, F., *et al.* (1990) 'The juvenile and chronic forms of GM2 gangliosidosis: clinical and enzymatic heterogeneity.' *Neurology*, **40**, 145–150.

Sperl, W., Ruitenbeek, W., Kerkhof, C.M.C., *et al.* (1990) 'Deficiency of the α and β subunits of pyruvate dehydrogenase in a patient with lactic acidosis and unexpected sudden death.' *European Journal of Pediatrics*, **149**, 487–492.

Spranger, J., Cantz, M. (1978) 'Mucolipidosis I, the cherry-red spot–myoclonus syndrome and neuraminidase deficiency.' *Birth Defects: Original Articles Series*, **14** (6B), 105–112.

Stabler, S.P., Allen, R.H., Savage, D.G., Lindenbaum, J. (1990) 'Clinical spectrum and diagnosis of cobalamin deficiency.' *Blood*, **76**, 871–881.

Stanley, C.A. (1995) 'Disorders of fatty acid oxidation.' *In:* Fernandes, J., Saudubray, J.M., van den Berghe, G. (Eds.) *Inborn Metabolic Diseases: Diagnosis and Treatment. 2nd Edn.* Berlin: Springer Verlag, pp. 133–143.

Starosta-Rubinstein, S., Young, A.B., Kluin, K., *et al.* (1987) 'Clinical assessment of 31 patients with Wilson's disease.' *Archives of Neurology*, **44**, 365–370.

Steiman, G.S., Yudkoff, M., Bearman, P.H. (1979) 'Late onset non-ketotic hyperglycinemia and spinocerebellar degeneration.' *Journal of Pediatrics*, **94**, 907–911.

Steinberg D. (1995) 'Refsum disease.' *In:* Scriver, C.R., Beaudet, A.L., Sly, W.S., Valle, D. (Eds.) *The Metabolic and Molecular Bases of Inherited Disease, 7th Edn.* New York: McGraw Hill, pp. 2351–2369.

Steiner, R.D., Sweetser, D.A., Rohrbaugh, J.R., *et al.* (1996) 'Nonketotic hyperglycinemia: atypical clinical and biochemical manifestations.' *Journal of Pediatrics*, **128**, 243–246.

Stemerdink, B.A., van der Meere, J.J., van der Molen, M.W., *et al.* (1995) 'Information processing in patients with early and continuously-treated phenylketonuria.' *European Journal of Pediatrics*, **154**, 739–746.

Stibler, H., Westerberg, B., Hanefeld, F., Hagberg, B. (1993) 'Carbohydrate-deficient glycoprotein (CDG) syndrome—a new variant, type III.' *Neuropediatrics*, **24**, 51–52.

—— Blennow, G., Kristiansson, B., *et al.* (1994) 'Carbohydrate-deficient glycoprotein syndrome: clinical expression in adults with a new metabolic disease.' *Journal of Neurology, Neurosurgery, and Psychiatry*, **57**, 552–556.

—— Stephani, U., Kutsch, U. (1995) 'Carbohydrate-deficient glycoprotein syndrome—a fourth subtype.' *Neuropediatrics*, **26**, 235–237.

St-Louis, M., Leclerc, B., Laine, J., *et al.* (1994) 'Identification of a stop mutation in five Finnish patients suffering from hereditary tyrosinemia type I.' *Human Molecular Genetics*, **3**, 69–72.

Stöckler, S., Slavc, I., Ebner, F., Baumgartner, R. (1992) 'Asymptomatic lesions of the basal ganglia in a patient with methylmalonic aciduria.' *European Journal of Pediatrics*, **151**, 920. *(Letter.)*

Strauss, A.W., Powell, C.K., Hale, D.E., *et al.* (1995) 'Molecular basis of human mitochondrial very-long-chain acyl-CoA dehydrogenase deficiency causing cardiomyopathy and sudden death in childhood.' *Proceedings of the National Academy of Sciences of the USA*, **92**, 10496–10500.

Streifler, J.Y., Gornish, M., Hadar, H., Gadoth, N. (1993) 'Brain imaging in late-onset GM2 gangliosidosis.' *Neurology*, **43**, 2055–2058.

Stromme, P., Maehlen, J., Strom, E.H., Torvik, A. (1991) 'Postmortem findings in two patients with carbohydrate-deficient glycoprotein syndrome.' *Acta Paediatrica Scandinavica*, Suppl. 375, 55–62.

Sugita, K., Kakinuma, H., Okajima, Y., *et al.* (1995) 'Clinical and MRI findings in a case of D-2-hydroxyglutaric aciduria.' *Brain and Development*, **17**, 139–141.

Surtees, R., Leonard, J., Austin, S. (1991) 'Association of demyelination with deficiency of cerebrospinal-fluid S-adenosylmethionine in inborn errors of methyl-transfer pathway.' *Lancet*, **338**, 1550–1554.

—— Matthews, E.E., Leonard, J.V. (1992) 'Neurologic outcome of propionic acidemia.' *Pediatric Neurology*, **8**, 333–337.

Suzuki, Y., Shimozawa, N., Orii, T., *et al.* (1988) 'Molecular analysis of peroxisomal β-oxidation enzymes in infants with Zellweger-like syndrome: further heterogenicity of the peroxisomal disorder.' *Clinica Chimica Acta*, **172**, 65–76.

—— Sakuraba, H., Oshima, A., *et al.* (1991) 'Clinical and molecular heterogeneity in hereditary beta-galactosidase deficiency.' *Developmental Neuroscience*, **13**, 299–303.

Tada, K., Kure, S. (1993) 'Non-ketotic hyperglycinaemia: molecular lesion, diagnosis and pathophysiology.' *Journal of Inherited Metabolic Disease*, **16**, 691–703.

—— Taniike, M., Ono, J., *et al.* (1992) 'Serial magnetic resonance imaging studies in a case of late onset globoid cell leukodystrophy.' *Neuropediatrics*, **23**, 306–309.

Tahara, T., Kraus, J.P., Ohura, T., *et al.* (1993) 'Three independant mutations in the same exon of the *PCCB* gene: differences between Caucasian and Japanese propionic acidaemia.' *Journal of Inherited Metabolic Disease*, **16**, 353–360.

Takahashi, S., Ishii, K., Matsumoto, K., *et al.* (1993) 'Cranial MRI and MR angiography in Menkes' syndrome.' *Neuroradiology*, **35**, 556–558.

Tanaka, J., Garcia, J.H., Max, S.R., *et al.* (1975) 'Cerebral sponginess and GM3 gangliosidosis: ultrastructure and probable pathogenesis.' *Journal of Neuropathology and Experimental Neurology*, **34**, 249–262.

Tanaka, K., Yoneda, H., Nakajima, T., *et al.* (1987) 'Dihydrobiopterin synthesis defect: an adult with diurnal fluctuation of symptoms.' *Neurology*, **37**, 519–522.

Tanaka, R., Momoi, T., Yoshida, A., *et al.* (1995) 'Type 3 GM1-gangliosidosis: clinical and neuroradiological findings in an 11-year-old girl.' *Journal of Neurology*, **242**, 299–303.

Tanzi, R.E., Petrukhin, K., Chernov, I., *et al.* (1993) 'The Wilson disease gene is a copper transport ATPase with homology to the Menkes disease gene.' *Nature Genetics*, **5**, 344–350.

Tatsumi, N., Inui, K., Sakai, N., *et al.* (1995) 'Molecular defects in Krabbe disease.' *Human Molecular Genetics*, **4**, 1865–1868.

Taylor, C.J., Green, S.H. (1981) 'Menkes' syndrome (trichopoliodystrophy): use of scanning electron-microscope in diagnosis and carrier identification.' *Developmental Medicine and Child Neurology*, **23**, 361–368.

Tegtmeyer-Metzdorf, H., Roth, B., Günther, M., *et al.* (1995) 'Ketamine and strychnine treatment of an infant with nonketotic hyperglycinaemia.' *European Journal of Pediatrics*, **154**, 649–653.

Tein, I. (1996) 'Metabolic myopathies.' *Seminars in Pediatric Neurology*, **3**, 59–98.

Tharp, B.R. (1992) 'Unique EEG pattern (comb-like rhythm) in neonatal maple syrup urine disease.' *Pediatric Neurology*, **8**, 65–68.

Thomas, G.R., Forbes, J.R., Roberts, E.A., *et al.* (1995) 'The Wilson disease gene: spectrum of mutations and their consequences.' *Nature Genetics*, **9**, 210–217.

Thomas, P.K., Halpern, J-P., King, R.H.M., Patrick, D. (1984) 'Galactosylceramide lipidosis: novel presentation as a slowly progressive spinocerebellar degeneration.' *Annals of Neurology*, **16**, 618–620.

Tint, G.S., Irons, M., Elias, E.R., *et al.* (1994) 'Defective cholesterol biosynthesis associated with the Smith–Lemli–Opitz syndrome.' *New England Journal of Medicine*, **330**, 107–113.

—— Salen, G., Batta, A.K., *et al.* (1995a) 'Correlation of severity and outcome with plasma sterol levels in variants of the Smith–Lemli–Opitz syndrome.' *Journal of Pediatrics*, **127**, 82–87.

—— Seller, M., Hughes-Benzie, R., *et al.* (1995b) 'Markedly increased tissue concentrations of 7-dehydrocholesterol combined with low levels of cholesterol are characteristic of the Smith–Lemli–Opitz syndrome.' *Journal of Lipid Research*, **36**, 89–95.

Toft, P.B., Geib-Holtorff, R., Rolland, M.O., *et al.* (1993) 'Magnetic resonance imaging in juvenile Canavan disease.' *European Journal of Pediatrics*, **152**, 750–753.

Tønnesen, T., Horn, N., Sondergaard, F., *et al.* (1985) 'Measurement of copper in chorionic villi for first-trimester diagnosis of Menkes' disease.' *Lancet*, **1**, 1038–1039.

Toone, J.R., Applegarth, D.A., Levy, H.L. (1994) 'Prenatal diagnosis of non-ketotic hyperglycinaemia: experience in 50 at-risk pregnancies.' *Journal of Inherited Metabolic Disease*, **17**, 342–344.

Topaloglu, H., Gücüyener, K., Orkun, C., Renda, Y. (1990) 'Tremor of tongue and dysarthria as the sole manifestation of Wilson's disease.' *Clinical Neurology and Neurosurgery*, **92**, 295–296.

Tóth, P.P., El-Shanti, H., Eivins, S., *et al.* (1993) 'Transient improvement of congenital lactic acidosis in a male infant with pyruvate decarboxylase deficiency treated with dichloroacetate.' *Journal of Pediatrics*, **123**, 427–430.

Touati, G., Rigal, O., Lombès, A., *et al.* (1997) 'In vivo functional investigations of lactic acid in patients with respiratory chain disorders.' *Archives of Disease in Childhood*, **76**, 16–21.

Trauner, D.A., Page, T., Greco, C., *et al.* (1981) 'Progressive neurodegenerative disorder in a patient with nonketotic hyperglycinemia.' *Journal of Pediatrics*, **98**, 272–275.

—— Chase, C., Scheller, J., *et al.* (1988) 'Neurologic and cognitive defects in a child with cystinosis.' *Journal of Pediatrics*, **112**, 912–914.

Tsuji, S., Choudari, P.V., Martin, B.M., *et al.* (1987) 'A mutation in the human glucocerebrosidase gene in neuronopathic Gaucher's disease.' *New England Journal of Medicine*, **316**, 570–575.

Tümer, Z., Tønnesen, T., Böhmann, J., *et al.* (1994) 'First trimester prenatal diagnosis of Menkes disease by DNA analysis.' *Journal of Medical Genetics*, **31**, 615–617.

—— Horn, N., Tønnesen, T., *et al.* (1996) 'Early copper-histidine treatment for Menkes disease.' *Nature Genetics*, **12**, 11–13.

Ullrich, K., Möller, H., Weglage, J., *et al.* (1994) 'White matter abnormalities in phenylketonuria: results of magnetic resonance measurements.' *Acta Paediatrica*, Suppl. 407, 78–82.

—— Koch, H-G., Meschede, D., Flotmann, U, Seedorf, U. (1996) 'Smith–Lemli–Opitz syndrome: treatment with cholesterol and bile acids.' *Neuropediatrics*, **27**, 111–112. *(Letter.)*

Ushikubo, S., Aoyama, T., Kamijo, T., *et al.* (1996) 'Molecular characterization of mitochondrial trifunctional protein deficiency: formation of the enzyme complex is important for stabilization of both α- and β-subunits.' *American Journal of Human Genetics*, **58**, 979–988.

Ushiyama, M., Ikeda, S-i., Nakayama, J., *et al.* (1985) 'Type III (chronic) G_{M1}-gangliosidosis. Histochemical and ultrastructural studies of rectal biopsy.' *Journal of the Neurological Sciences*, **71**, 209–223.

Uvebrant, P., Lanneskog, K., Hagberg, B. (1992) 'The epidemiology of progressive encephalopathies in childhood. I. Live birth prevalence in West Sweden.' *Neuropediatrics*, **23**, 209–211.

Uziel, G., Bardelli, P., Pantaleoni, C., *et al.* (1993) '4-hydroxybutyric aciduria: clinical findings and vigabatrin therapy.' *Journal of Inherited Metabolic Disease*, **16**, 520–522.

Van Coster, R., Lombès, A., De Vivo, D.C., *et al.* (1991) 'Cytochrome c oxidase-associated Leigh syndrome: phenotypic features and pathogenetic speculations.' *Journal of the Neurological Sciences*, **104**, 97–111.

van der Klei-van Moorsel, J.M., Smit, L.M.E., Brockstedt, M., *et al.* (1991) 'Infantile isolated sulphite oxidase deficiency: report of a case with negative sulphite test and normal sulphate excretion.' *European Journal of Pediatrics*, **150**, 196–197.

van der Knaap, M.S., Jakobs, C., Valk, J. (1996) 'Magnetic resonance imaging in lactic acidosis.' *Journal of Inherited Metabolic Disease*, **19**, 535–547.

van der Meer, S.B., Poggi, F., Spada, M., *et al.* (1994) 'Clinical outcome of long-term management of patients with vitamin B_{12}-unresponsive methylmalonic acidemia.' *Journal of Pediatrics*, **125**, 903–908.

—— —— —— *et al.* (1996) 'Clinical outcome and long-term management of 17 patients with propionic acidaemia.' *European Journal of Pediatrics*, **155**, 205–210.

van der Put, N.M.J., Steegers-Theunissen, R.P.M., Frosst, P., *et al.* (1995) 'Mutated methylene tetrahydrofolate reductase as a risk factor for spina bifida.' *Lancet*, **346**, 1070–1071

van Diggelen, O.P., Schindler, D., Willemsen, R., *et al.* (1988) 'α-N-acetylgalactosaminidase deficiency, a new lysosomal storage disorder.' *Journal of Inherited Metabolic Disease*, **11**, 349–357.

Van Erven, P.M.M., Renier, W.O., Gabreëls, F.J.M., *et al.* (1989) 'Hypokinesia and rigidity as clinical manifestations of mitochondrial encephalomyopathy: report of three cases.' *Developmental Medicine and Child Neurology*, **31**, 81–91.

Van Geel, B.M., Assies, J., Weverling, G.J., Barth, P.G. (1994) 'Predominance of the adrenomyeloneuropathy phenotype of X-linked adrenoleukodys-trophy in the Netherlands: a survey of 30 kindreds.' *Neurology*, **44**, 2343–2346.

—— —— Wanders, R.J.A., Barth, P.G. (1997) 'X linked adrenoleukodystrophy: clinical presentation, diagnosis, and therapy.' *Journal of Neurology, Neurosurgery, and Psychiatry*, **63**, 4–14.

Van Geet, C., Jaeken, J. (1993) 'A unique pattern of coagulation abnormalities in carbohydrate-deficient glycoprotein syndrome.' *Pediatric Research*, **33**, 540–541.

van Gennip, A.H., Abeling, N.G.G.M., Stroomer, A.E.M., *et al.* (1994a) 'Clinical and biochemical findings in six patients with pyrimidine degradation defects.' *Journal of Inherited Metabolic Disease*, **17**, 130–132.

—— —— —— *et al.* (1994b) 'The detection of molybdenum cofactor deficiency: clinical symptomatology and urinary metabolite profile.' *Journal of inherited Metabolic Disease*, **17**, 142–145.

Van Hove, J.L.K., Kishnani, P., Muenzer, J., *et al.* (1995) 'Benzoate therapy and carnitine deficiency in non-ketotic hyperglycinemia.' *American Journal of Medical Genetics*, **59**, 444–453.

Vanier, M.T., Wenger, D.A., Comly, M.E., *et al.* (1988) 'Niemann–Pick disease group C: clinical variability and diagnosis based on defective cholesterol esterification: a collaborative study on 70 patients.' *Clinical Genetics*, **33**, 331–348.

—— Rodriguez-Lafrasse, C., Rousson, R., *et al.* (1992) 'Prenatal diagnosis of Niemann–Pick type C disease: current strategy from an experience of 37 pregnancies at risk.' *American Journal of Human Genetics*, **51**, 111–122.

Van Schaftingen, E. (1989) 'D-glycerate kinase deficiency as a cause of D-glyceric aciduria.' *FEBS Letters*, **243**, 127–131.

—— Jaeken, J. (1995) 'Phosphomannomutase deficiency is a cause of carbohydrate-deficient glycoprotein syndrome type I.' *FEBS Letters*, **377**, 318–320.

Verrips, A., Renier, W.O., van Heyst, A.F.J., *et al.* (1995) 'Cerebrotendinous xanthomatosis in children.' *Developmental Medicine and Child Neurology*, **37**, Suppl. 72, 130–131.

Visy, J.M., LeCoz, P., Chadefaux, B., *et al.* (1991) 'Homocystinuria due to 5,10-methylenetetrahydrofolate reductase deficiency revealed by stroke in adult siblings.' *Neurology*, **41**, 1313–1315.

Vockley, J. (1994) 'The changing face of disorders of fatty acid oxidation.' *Mayo Clinic Proceedings*, **69**, 249–257.

Waggoner, D.D., Buist, N.R.M. (1993) 'Long-term complications in treated galactosemia—175 U.S. cases.' *International Pediatrics*, **8**, 97–100.

Waisbren, S.E., Brown, M.J., deSonneville, L.M.J., Levy, H.L. (1994) 'Review of neuropsychological functioning in treated phenylketonuria: an information processing approach.' *Acta Paediatrica*, Suppl. 407, 98–103.

Walk, D., Kang, S-S., Horwitz, A. (1994) 'Intermittent encephalopathy, reversible nerve conduction slowing, and MRI evidence of cerebral white matter disease in methylenetetrahydrofolate reductase deficiency.' *Neurology*, **44**, 344–347.

Walker, V., Mills, G.A., Hall, M.A., *et al.* (1989) 'Case report. A fourth case of fumarase deficiency.' *Journal of Inherited Metabolic Disease*, **12**, 331–332.

Walshe, J.M. (1986) 'Wilson's disease.' In: Vinken, P.J., Bruyn, G.W., Klawans, H.L. (Eds.) *Handbook of Clinical Neurology. Vol. 49. Extrapyramidal Disorders.* Amsterdam: Elsevier, pp. 248–257.

—— (1996) 'Treatment of Wilson's disease: the historical background.' *Quarterly Journal of Medicine*, **89**, 553–555.

—— Munro, N.A.R. (1995) 'Zinc-induced deterioration in Wilson's disease aborted by treatment with penicillamine, dimercaprol, and a novel zero copper diet.' *Archives of Neurology*, **52**, 10–11. *(Letter.)*

—— Yealland, M. (1992) 'Wilson's disease: the problem of delayed diagnosis.' *Journal of Neurology, Neurosurgery, and Psychiatry*, **55**, 692–696.

Wanders, R.J.A., Schutgens, R.B.H., Barth, P.G. (1995a) 'Peroxisomal disorders: a review.' *Journal of Neuropathology and Experimental Neurology*, **54**, 726–739.

—— van Roermund, C.W., Schor, D.S., *et al.* (1995b) '2-Hydroxyphytanic acid oxidase activity in rat and human liver and its deficiency in the Zellweger syndrome.' *Biochimica et Biophysica Acta*, **1227**, 177–182.

—— Romeijn, W., Hennekan, R.C.M., *et al.* (1996) 'Smith–Lemli–Opitz syndrome: impaired de novo cholesterol synthesis due to deficient Δ^7-reductase activity in cultured skin fibroblasts and its application to pre- and postnatal detection.' *Journal of Inherited Metabolic Disease*, **19**, Suppl. 1, 4. *(Abstract.)*

Wang, A.M., Schindler, D., Bishop, D.F., *et al.* (1988) 'Schindler disease: biochemical and molecular characterization of a new neuroaxonal dystrophy due to α-N-acetylgalactosaminidase deficiency.' *American Journal of Human Genetics*, **43** (Suppl.), A99. *(Abstract.)*

Watts, G.F., Mitchell, W.D., Bending, J.J., *et al.* (1996) 'Cerebrotendinous xanthomatosis: a family study of sterol 27-hydroxylase mutations and pharmacotherapy.' *Quarterly Journal of Medicine*, **89**, 55–63.

Watts, R.W.E., Gibbs, D.A. (1986) 'Sphingolipidoses.' *In:* Watts, R.W.E, Gibbs, D.A. (Eds.) *Lysosomal Diseases: Biochemical and Clinical Aspects.* London: Taylor & Francis, pp. 43–117.

—— Spellacy, E., Gibbs, D.A., *et al.* (1982) 'Clinical, post-mortem, biochemical and therapeutic observations on the Lesch–Nyhan syndrome with particular reference to the neurological manifestations.' *Quarterly Journal of Medicine*, **51**, 43–78.

Weglage, J., Fünders, B., Wilken, B., *et al.* (1993) 'School performance and intellectual outcome in adolescents with phenylketonuria.' *Acta Paediatrica*, **81**, 582–586.

—— Pietsch, M., Fünders, B., *et al.* (1996a) 'Deficits in selective and sustained attention processes in early treated children with phenylketonuria—result of impaired frontal lobe functions?' *European Journal of Pediatrics*, **155**, 200–204.

—— Ullrich, K., Pietsch, M., *et al.* (1996b) 'Untreated non-phenylketonuric-hyperphenylalaninaemia: intellectual and neurological outcome.' *European Journal of Pediatrics*, **155**, Suppl. 1, S26–S28.

Weir, D.G., Scott, J.M. (1995) 'The biochemical basis of the neuropathy in cobalamin deficiency.' *Baillière's Clinical Haematology*, **8**, 479–497.

Welsh, M.C. (1996) 'A prefrontal dysfunction model of early-treated phenylketonuria.' *European Journal of Pediatrics*, **155**, Suppl. 1, S87–S89.

—— Pennington, B.F., Ozonoff, S., *et al.* (1990) 'Neuropsychology of early-treated phenylketonuria: specific executive function deficits.' *Child Development*, **61**, 1697–1713.

Wendel, U., Claussen, U., Dieckmann, E. (1983) 'Prenatal diagnosis of methylene tetrahydrofolate reductase deficiency.' *Journal of Pediatrics*, **102**, 938–940.

—— Zass, R., Leupold, D. (1993) 'Contribution of odd-numbered fatty acid oxidation to propionate production in neonates with methylmalonic and propionic acidaemias.' *European Journal of Pediatrics*, **152**, 1021–1023.

Wenger, D.A., Roth, S., Kudoh, T., *et al.* (1983) 'Biochemical studies in a patient with subacute neuropathic Gaucher disease without visceral glucosylceramide storage.' *Pediatric Research*, **17**, 344–348.

Werlin, S.L., Grand, R.J., Perman, J.A., Watkins, J.B. (1978) 'Diagnostic dilemmas of Wilson's disease: diagnosis and treatment.' *Pediatrics*, **62**, 47–51.

Wevers, R.A., Cruysberg, J.R.M., van Heijst, A.F.J., *et al.* (1992) 'Paediatric cerebrotendinous xanthomatosis.' *Journal of Inherited Metabolic Disease*, **15**, 374–376.

—— Hansen, S.I., van Hellenberg Hubar, J.L.M., *et al.* (1994) 'Folate deficiency in cerebrospinal fluid associated with a defect in folate binding protein in the central nervous system.' *Journal of Neurology, Neurosurgery, and Psychiatry*, **57**, 223–226.

Whetsell, W.O., Plaitakis, A. (1978) 'Leigh's disease in an adult with evidence of "inhibitor factors" in family members.' *Annals of Neurology*, **3**, 519–524.

Whitehead, A.S., Gallagher, P., Mills, J.L., *et al.* (1995) 'A genetic defect in 5, 10 methylenetetrahydrofolate reductase in neural tube defects.' *Quarterly Journal of Medicine*, **88**, 763–766.

Wilcken, B., Don, N., Greenaway, R., *et al.* (1987) 'Sialuria: a second case.' *Journal of Inherited Metabolic Disease*, **10**, 97–102.

—— Pitt, J., Heath, D., *et al.* (1993) 'L-2-hydroxyglutaric aciduria: three Australian cases.' *Journal of Inherited Metabolic Disease*, **16**, 501–504.

Willems, P.J., Vits, L., Wanders, R.J.A., *et al.* (1990) 'Linkage of DNA marker at Xq28 to adrenoleukodystrophy and adrenomyeloneuropathy present within the same family.' *Archives of Neurology*, **47**, 665–669.

—— Gatti, R., Dabry, J.K., *et al.* (1991) 'Fucosidosis revisited: a review of 77 patients.' *American Journal of Medical Genetics*, **38**, 111–131.

Willemsen, R., Van Dongen, J.M., Ginns, E.I., *et al.* (1987) 'Ultrastructural localization of glucocerebrosidase in cultured Gaucher's disease fibroblasts by immunocytochemistry.' *Journal of Neurology*, **234**, 44–51.

Williams, F.J.B., Walshe, J.M. (1981) 'Wilson's disease. An analysis of the cranial computerised tomographic appearances found in 60 patients and the changes in response to treatment with chelating agents.' *Brain*, **104**, 735–752.

Williams, J.C., Butler, I.J., Rosenberg, H.S., *et al.* (1984) 'Progressive neurologic deterioration and renal failure due to storage of glutamyl ribose-5-phosphate.' *New England Journal of Medicine*, **311**, 152–155.

Williams, R.S., Ferrante, R.J., Caviness, V.S. (1979) 'The isolated human cortex. A Golgi analysis of Krabbe's disease.' *Archives of Neurology*, **36**, 134–139.

Willner, J.P., Grabowski, G.A., Gordon, R.E., *et al.* (1981) 'Chronic GM2 gangliosidosis masquerading as atypical Friedreich ataxia: clinical, morphologic, and biochemical studies of nine cases.' *Neurology*, **31**, 787–798.

Willvonseder, R., Goldstein, N.P., McCall, J.T., *et al.* (1973) 'A hereditary disorder with dementia, spastic dysarthria, vertical eye movement paresis, gait disturbance, splenomegaly, and abnormal copper metabolism.' *Neurology*, **23**, 1039–1049.

Wilson, J.M., Young, A.B., Kelley, W.N. (1983) 'Hypoxanthine-guanine phosphoribosyltransferase deficiency. The molecular basis of the clinical syndromes.' *New England Journal of Medicine*, **309**, 900–910.

Winkelman, M.D., Banker, B.Q., Victor, M., Moser, H.W. (1983) 'Non-infantile neuropathic Gaucher's disease.' *Neurology*, **33**, 994–1008.

Winter, R.W., Swallow, D.M., Baraitser, M., Purkiss, P. (1980) 'Sialidosis type 2 (acid neuraminidase deficiency): clinical and biochemical features of a further case.' *Clinical Genetics*, **18**, 203–210.

Winters, P.R., Harrod, M.J., Molenich-Heetred, S.A., *et al.* (1976) 'Alpha-L-iduronidase deficiency and possible Hurler–Scheie genetic compound.' *Neurology*, **26**, 1003–1007.

Wolf, B. (1995) 'Disorders of biotin metabolism.' *In:* Scriver, C.R., Beaudet, A.L., Sly, W.S., Valle, D. (Eds.) *The Metabolic and Molecular Bases of Inherited Disease, 7th Edn.* New York: McGraw Hill, pp. 3151–3177.

Yahraus, T., Braverman, N., Dodt, G., *et al.* (1996) 'The peroxisome biogenesis disorder group 4 gene, *PXAAA1*, encodes a cytoplasmic ATPase required for stability of the PTS1 receptor.' *The EMBO Journal*, **15**, 2914–2923.

Yamagata, T., Yano, S., Okabe, I., *et al.* (1990) 'Ultrasonography and magnetic resonance imaging in Leigh disease.' *Pediatric Neurology*, **6**, 326–329.

Yamamoto, S., Abe, H., Kohgo, T., *et al.* (1996) 'Two novel gene mutations (Glu174→Lys, Phe383→Tyr) causing the "hepatic" form of carnitine palmitoyltransferase II deficiency.' *Human Genetics*, **98**, 116–118.

Ylitalo, V., Hagberg, B., Rapola, J., *et al.* (1986) 'Sella disease variants. Sialoyl-aciduric encephalopathy with increased sialidase activity in two non-Finnish children.' *Neuropediatrics*, **17**, 44–47.

Yoshida, I., Sweetman, L., Kulovich, S., *et al.* (1990) 'Effect of lipoic acid in a patient with defective activity of pyruvate dehydrogenase and branched-chain ketoacid dehydrogenase.' *Pediatric Research*, **27**, 75–79.

Yoshikawa, H., Yamada, K., Sakuragawa, N. (1992) 'MRI in the early stage of Tay–Sachs disease.' *Neuroradiology*, **34**, 394–395.

Young, I.D., Young, E.P., Mossman, J., *et al.* (1987) 'Neuraminidase deficiency: case report and review of the phenotype.' *Journal of Medical Genetics*, **24**, 283–290.

Young, R., Kleinman, G., Ojemann, R.G., *et al.* (1980) 'Compressive myelopathy in Maroteaux–Lamy syndrome: clinical and pathological findings.' *Annals of Neurology*, **8**, 336–340.

Zafeiriou, D.I., Koletzko, B., Mueller-Felber, W., *et al.* (1995) 'Deficiency in complex IV (cytochrome *c* oxidase) of the respiratory chain, presenting as a leukodystrophy in two siblings with Leigh syndrome.' *Brain and Development*, **17**, 117–121.

Zammarchi, E., Donati, M.A., Tucci, F., *et al.* (1994a) 'Acute onset of X-linked adrenoleukodystrophy mimicking encephalitis.' *Brain and Development*, **16**, 238–240.

—— Savelli, A., Donati, A., Pasquini, E. (1994b) 'Self-mutilation in a patient with mucolipidosis III.' *Pediatric Neurology*, **11**, 68–70.

Zittoun, J. (1995) 'Congenital errors of folate metabolism.' *Baillière's Clinical Haematology*, **8**, 603–616.

10
HEREDODEGENERATIVE DISORDERS

A significant proportion of genetically transmitted neurological diseases has not yet been linked with demonstrated metabolic errors, especially known enzymatic deficits. Many are characterized by early degeneration of one or more specific CNS areas or systems, perhaps related to defective maintenance of vital elements of certain neurons. Some demonstrate morphological evidence of storage at the microscopic or ultramicroscopic level. There is little doubt, however, that they are caused by as yet unknown genetic abnormalities of structural or enzyme proteins, many of which will be recognized in the near future. These disorders share most of the clinical features of recognized metabolic diseases; in particular, they are progressive illnesses in the sense indicated in the introduction to Part IV, with a free interval and a loss of previously acquired skills, even though the progressive nature of some may be difficult to determine. Heredodegenerative disorders can have their onset at any age, and age of onset is an important diagnostic clue (Lyon *et al.* 1996). Barth (1991, 1993) has drawn attention to the prenatal origin of a group of degenerative diseases that manifest clinically at birth (see Table 1.5, p. 19). Recognition of the progressive character of such conditions may be difficult in the absence of a free interval, especially as many are very slowly progressive.

Because no specific biological disturbance for such conditions is known, their diagnosis rests essentially on clinical grounds, especially careful history taking, family investigation and neurological examination, and on certain laboratory tests—radiological, neurophysiological, ophthalmological or biochemical—as is the case, for example, with Huntington disease, the leukodystrophies or several spinocerebellar degenerations.

Brain biopsy has been used for the diagnosis of progressive CNS disorders (Boltshauser and Wilson 1976). It has been largely replaced, over the past two decades, by peripheral biopsies of muscle, appendix, gingiva, etc. Conjunctival and skin biopsy on the one hand (Martin and Ceuterick 1978, Arsenio-Nunes *et al.* 1981) and rectal biopsy on the other (Brett and Lake 1975) have met with considerable success in the diagnosis of some heredodegenerative disorders. The latter has the advantage of allowing direct study of neuronal cells and may be the only way of confirming the diagnosis of disorders such as intraneuronal inclusion disease (Goutières *et al.* 1990) and some of the ceroid–lipofuscinoses (Barthez-Carpentier *et al.* 1991). Skin or conjunctival biopsy may be more efficient for the diagnosis of neuroaxonal dystrophy and related conditions.

Study of this group of disorders is benefitting from the progress of DNA techniques and the use of DNA probes. These permit identification of mutations within or close to the relevant gene, making reliable diagnosis possible either directly or through linkage studies. When the gene has been cloned and localized by the techniques of positional cloning ('reverse genetics'), appropriate methods can be applied to help determine the abnormal gene product and, hopefully, understand the mechanisms of the disease and eventually prepare possible therapies. DNA studies may permit prenatal diagnosis. However, with linkage methods, study of nonaffected as well as affected family members is required, and the degree of reliability depends on the proximity to the causal gene of the marker gene under study, as recombination by meiotic crossover is more likely for relatively distant markers (Antonarakis 1989, American Academy of Pediatrics 1994). With direct study of the gene sequence, mutations or deletions can be detected, enabling precise determination of the genotype and consequently exact determination of the subtype and genetic origin of the disorder.

Diagnosis by molecular genetic techniques has medical and ethical implications that have to be carefully considered. There is no doubt though that they have opened exciting new perspectives in the field of heredodegenerative disease.

The group of heredodegenerative CNS disorders is defined mainly by negative findings. It is thus highly heterogeneous, including for the sake of convenience many disorders with no real link between them. In this chapter, the various conditions studied will be grouped mainly according to gross pathological criteria, *e.g.* on the system or part of the CNS that bears the brunt of the disease, although topographic delimitation is far from being always precise. Pathological location of the process is relatively well correlated with the clinical features (Lyon *et al.* 1996).

For convenience, a few diseases which are not progressive but have similar clinical presentations and are also of genetic origin will be included in this discussion.

LEUKODYSTROPHIES

The leukodystrophies are a group of degenerative diseases that affect principally the myelin of the brain—and sometimes also of the peripheral nerves—thus producing widespread involvement of the white matter. In many cases some involvement of grey nuclei coexists but is clearly overshadowed by that of white matter (Lyon *et al.* 1996). The leukodystrophies may be classified according to the enzymatic defect when known (*e.g.* metachro-

TABLE 10.1
Causes of bilateral images of abnormal density or signal in the white matter of the cerebral hemispheres

Cause	References
Leukodystrophies	
With known metabolic defect	Chapter 9
Metachromatic leukodystrophy	
Globoid cell (Krabbe) leukodystrophy[1]	
Adrenoleukodystrophy (classical and neonatal)	
Zellweger syndrome, neonatal adrenoleukodystrophy[2]	
Spongy degeneration of CNS (Canavan–van Bogaert disease[3])	
Without defined metabolic defect	
Sudanophilic leukodystrophies	
Pelizaeus–Merzbacher disease[4]	
Cockayne disease[5]	See text
Alexander disease	
Leukodystrophy with calcification of central grey matter (Aicardi–Goutières syndrome)	Aicardi and Goutières (1984)
Leukodystrophy with megalencephaly, mild course and cystic formation	van der Knaap *et al.* (1995)
Leukodystrophy with vanishing white matter	van der Knaap *et al.* (1997)
Mitochondrial encephalomyopathies[6]	
Pyruvate dehydrogenase deficiency	Chapter 9
Cytochrome oxidase deficiency	Zafeiriou *et al.* (1995)
Leigh disease (forms with extensive white matter involvement)	Bourgeois *et al.* (1992)
Amino acid and organic acid disease	
Glutaric aciduria types 1, 2	Brismar and Ozand (1994), Uziel *et al.* (1995)
2-hydroxyglutaric aciduria	Sugito *et al.* (1995)
4-hydroxybutyric and other organic acidurias	Brismar and Ozand (1994)
Phenylketonuria	Chapter 9
Others	Brismar and Ozand (1994)
Congenital muscular dystrophies	Chapter 22
Fukuyama type	
Merosine-negative congenital dystrophy	
Periventricular leukomalacia (extensive forms) and posthypoxic leukoencephalopathy, *e.g.* with CO intoxication	Chapter 2
Toxic leukoencephalopathy (methotrexate and X-ray therapy, metronidazole and other immunosuppressive agents)	Small *et al.* (1996); Chapter 13
Viral infections, *e.g.* acute disseminated encephalomyelitis, subacute panencephalitis in rare cases, congenital infections	Chapter 11
Hydrocephalus (transependymal resorption of CSF)	Chapter 7
Vascular diseases (CADASIL)[8]	Hutchinson *et al.* (1995)

[1] Intense signal on T_2-weighted MRI sequences in thalami, cerebellum and sometimes centrum ovale, no abnormal density of white matter on CT.
[2] Gyration abnormalities associated.
[3] Acylaspartase deficiency.
[4] Intense signal on T_2-weighted sequences, low signal on T_1-weighted sequences, no abnormal density on CT.
[5] Calcification of central grey matter and marked ventricular dilatation often associated.
[6] Central calcification often associated.
[7] Calcification at grey–white junction in most cases.
[8] CADASIL = *c*erebral *a*utosomal *d*ominant *ar*teriopathy with *s*ubcortical *i*nfarcts and *l*eukoencephalopathy.

matic leukodystrophy or arylsulfatase deficiency, Krabbe leukodystrophy or galactocerebroside-beta-galactosidase deficiency) or according to pathology, taking into account staining characteristics of myelin breakdown products, presence of multinucleated cells and topography of myelin involvement. Leukodystrophies with known enzymatic defects have been described in Chapter 9.

In general, the leukodystrophies are characterized clinically by the predominance of motor disturbances, especially pyramidal and cerebellar symptoms and signs, with slow mental deterioration and low incidence of seizures, myoclonus and paroxysmal EEG abnormalities.

SUDANOPHILIC LEUKODYSTROPHIES
In this group, myelin breakdown products are stained normally by Sudan black. The diagnosis of these disorders ultimately rests on pathological examination. However, the clinical features and

pattern of inheritance in some cases strongly suggest the diagnosis during life, thus allowing for effective genetic counselling. CT and MRI have considerably facilitated the tentative diagnosis of leukodystrophy but also raise diagnostic problems as the correspondence between imaging and pathology is not strict (Table 10.1). For example, hypodensities of the white matter can be seen with sequelae of extensive periventricular leukomalacia, in hydrocephalus, in some cases of congenital muscular dystrophy (Chapter 22), and in metabolic disorders, *e.g.* in cases of Leigh syndrome with extensive white matter involvement.

PELIZAEUS–MERZBACHER DISEASE (PMD)
This rare, X-linked condition is due to deletions or mutations of the gene of the proteolipid protein (PLP), a major component of CNS myelin, localized to the long arm of the X chromosome (Xq21.2–q22). This gene also encodes, by alternative splicing, another myelin protein (DM20) that is also abnormal in most cases of PMD (Carango *et al.* 1995). Forty different mutations have been described (Pratt *et al.* 1995, Nezu *et al.* 1996). Deletions were found in some families. Duplication of the gene is frequent, accounting for about 50 per cent of familial forms, but is less common in sporadic cases (Boespflug-Tanguy *et al.* 1994, 1996). PMD is allelic to one form of X-linked hereditary spastic paraplegia termed SPG-2 (Saugier-Veber *et al.* 1994).

Pathologically, there is paucity or absence of myelin in the hemispheres with preservation of islands of normal myelination especially around small vessels. The axons are relatively preserved, and oligodendrocytes are abnormal, containing laminar inclusions (Watanabe *et al.* 1973). In the severe congenital (often termed 'connatal') form, there is virtually no myelin and the amount of fat in the white matter is reduced, suggesting absence of myelination rather than myelin destruction. This so-called 'tigroid' pattern of myelin is no longer regarded as being specific for PMD. Present criteria also include X-linked inheritance and suggestive clinical features (Boulloche and Aicardi 1986).

Two main forms of the disease are recognized: a classical type and the connatal variant of Seitelberger. Differentiation of these two forms does not depend on the age of onset, which is in all cases in the first few months of life, but on the rate of progression and severity of the clinical picture (Scheffer *et al.* 1991). Both forms may coexist in the same family (Boespflug-Tanguy *et al.* 1996).

The first clinical manifestations usually consist of rotatory nystagmus or roving eye movements appearing within three months of birth. Laryngeal stridor may also be present (Renier *et al.* 1981, Boulloche and Aicardi 1986, Scheffer *et al.* 1991). Hypotonia is present early but the disorder runs at a variable pace. Some children may even start walking and develop some meaningful language before slow regression sets in, with dystonic, pyramidal and cerebellar signs and optic atrophy. Some adult patients may still walk and talk, albeit at a simplified level (Silverstein *et al.* 1989). More often, the course is more severe, with only limited development before deterioration, leading to a stage of helplessness and decortication (Boulloche and Aicardi 1986).

Nystagmus disappears before age 2 years in 20 per cent of patients (Huygen *et al.* 1992). CSF and other laboratory exam-

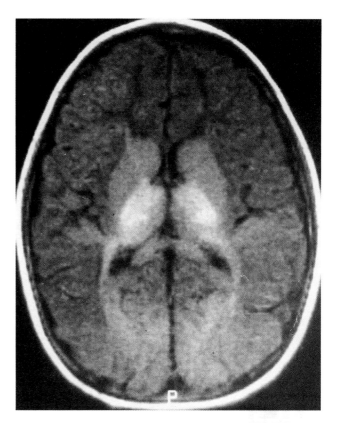

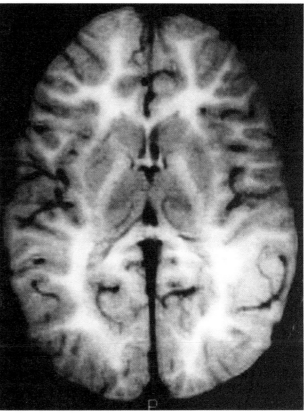

Fig. 10.1. Pelizaeus-Merzbacher disease. *(Top)* T₁-weighted MRI sequence shows almost total absence of myelin signal except in thalami and, faintly, in thalamo-occipital fibres. *(Bottom)* T₂-weighted sequence shows intense signal from white matter, confirming absence of normal myelin. (5-year-old boy with nystagmus from age 4 months and very slowly progressive ataxic diplegia, initially diagnosed as cerebral palsy.)

inations are to no avail, with the exception of evoked potentials which are abnormal early in the course (Apkarian *et al.* 1993, Nezu 1995, Wang *et al.* 1995).

In the congenital form (Cassidy *et al.* 1987, Haenggeli *et al.* 1989) the course is more severe, with severe feeding problems and extrapyramidal symptoms, the infants having no or very little development and dying within a few years. Convulsions are possible.

The diagnosis rests on the pattern of inheritance (with the knowledge that the disease may vary between members of the same sibship so that affected maternal uncles may be only mildly affected and remain undiagnosed), the eye and vestibular involvement (Huygen *et al.* 1992, Nezu 1995) and the slowly progressive course. CT scans show only mild to moderate brain atrophy without abnormal attenuation of the white matter. The diagnosis of spinocerebellar atrophy or of cerebellar cerebral palsy is often considered. T_2-weighted MRI gives an intense signal from the white matter (Penner *et al.* 1987, Shimonura *et al.* 1988, Van der Knaap and Valk 1989), while T_1-weighted images show no myelin signal (Fig. 10.1). Prenatal diagnosis is possible by DNA or linkage studies.

Only symptomatic treatment is available.

Atypical forms presenting as spinal muscular atrophy are on record (Kaye *et al.* 1994). Cases reported as PMD in girls (Cassidy *et al.* 1987, Haenggeli *et al.* 1989, Nezu *et al.* 1996) although with a similar clinical presentation probably belong to other disorders.

OTHER SUDANOPHILIC DYSTROPHIES

Currently, many conditions presenting as leukodystrophy from clinical and neuroimaging points of view remain unclassified (Fig. 10.2). These conditions have to be separated from other diseases involving the white matter but not genetically determined (see Table 10.1). Helpful markers for defining distinct white matter disorders include head circumference growth patterns, MRI and MRS patterns (Van der Knaap 1992) and clinical presentation. Pathologically, there is extensive orthochromatic de-myelination with normal, orthochromatic, breakdown products, and without preservation of myelinated 'islands'.

Van der Knaap *et al.* (1995) have described an apparently familial disease with extensive MRI abnormalities limited to the white matter but a discrepantly mild clinical course with late appearance of mild spastic and cerebellar signs and macrocephaly. Analysis of MRI scans and an MRS pattern that showed a very low brain content of the normal chemical constituents of the white matter suggested increased water content. Indeed, cavitation in the frontal and/or temporal poles was a suggestive feature of these cases (Fig. 10.3). Five similar patients have been reported by Goutières *et al.* (1996). Singhal *et al.* (1996) described 30 similar patients from India with a prolonged course. Convulsions were frequent in these patients.

Hanefeld *et al.* (1993) reported on three siblings with similar imaging findings but with normal head size, no cyst formation and a more rapid course. Schiffman *et al.* (1992) described children with progressive ataxia and diplegia, hypomyelination and an MRS pattern of low *N*-acetylaspartate, low choline and

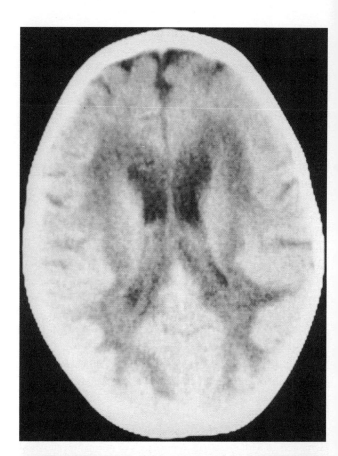

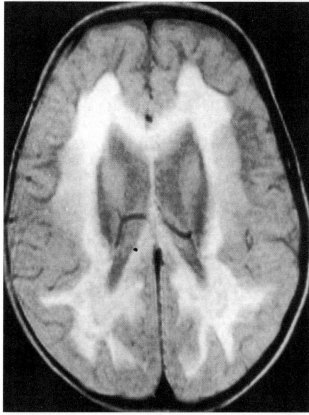

Fig. 10.2. 'Sudanophilic' leukodystrophy without more specific diagnosis. 4-year-old girl with progressive bilateral spasticity and neurodevelopmental deterioration. *(Top)* CT scan. *(Bottom)* MRI, T_2-weighted axial cut showing diffuse intense signal from the whole of the white matter.

326

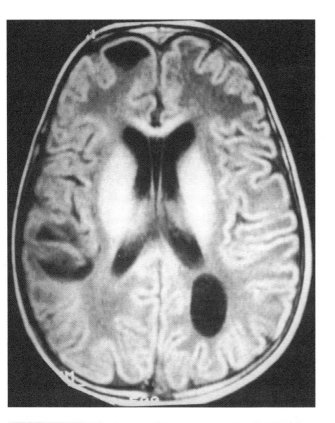

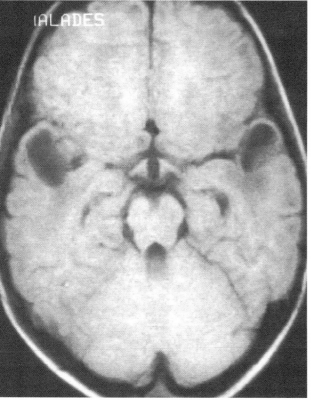

Fig. 10.3. Leukodystrophy with megalencephaly and cavitation of white matter. *(Top)* T₁-weighted MRI shows extensive demyelination with preservation of some central myelin in the corpus callosum and internal capsule. Cavitation is evident in the right frontal pole and both parietal regions. *(Bottom)* Bilateral temporal cyst formation in another child. Both patients have macrocephaly and slowly progressive spasticity. (Courtesy Dr F. Goutières, Hôpital des Enfants Malades, Paris.)

low creatinine in white matter. Many further cases have been reported (van der Knaap *et al.* 1997) with onset in infancy or early childhood, a progressive downhill course punctuated by episodes of acute deterioration following infection or minor head trauma, and a neurological picture of ataxia and spasticity. Myelin signal from the white matter was progressively replaced by CSF-like signal. Extensive cavitation of the white matter was found in one autopsy case. The disease is also known as 'vanishing white matter' or childhood ataxia with central nervous system hypomyelination (CACH).

A form of leukodystrophy with pigmented glial cells and macrophages (van Bogaert–Nyssen disease) has been reviewed by Belec *et al.* (1988). The disease has been only exceptionally observed in children (Seiser *et al.* 1990). Leukodystrophy with palmoplantar keratosis has been described in adults (Lossos *et al.* 1995). Skin abnormalities were also present in the cases of '*dermatoleukodystrophy*' described by Matsuyama *et al.* (1978) in which spheroids were prominent in the white matter. Rare cases known as *noncalcifying meningeal angiomatosis of Divry and van Bogaert* (Hooft *et al.* 1965) appear to be the consequence of cortical microangiomatosis rather than true leukodystrophies. Such cases may be associated with cutaneous livedo reticularis. Cases of associated *pachygyria and leukodystrophy* are on record (Norman *et al.* 1962). It is not clear whether these represent primary leukodystrophy, as the white matter in pachygyria may look abnormal. Recently, Labrune *et al.* (1996) reported three sporadic cases of diffuse white matter disease, extensive calcification and cyst formation with resulting hydrocephalus, and suggested that a diffuse vasculopathy was responsible.

Most cases of *sudanophilic leukodystrophy* seem to be inherited as an autosomal recessive character and it is probably wise to include in this group those cases reported as Pelizaeus–Merzbacher disease with recessive inheritance, as the preservation of islands of myelin is nonspecific and is also found in several other leukodystrophies.

The rate of progression of the various types of sudanophilic leukodystrophy is quite variable. Some are slowly progressive (Sugama and Kusano 1995). A rare type of prenatal leukodystrophy, probably autosomal recessive, known as Wiedeman–Rautenstrauch syndrome features progeroid features in association with demyelination of early onset (Martin *et al.* 1984).

COCKAYNE SYNDROME AND RELATED DISORDERS
Cockayne syndrome is a rare but clinically characteristic entity that features a leukodystrophy with preservation of islands of myelin, retinal degeneration, dwarfism, deafness, unusual facies, skin hypersensitivity to sunlight (Leech *et al.* 1985, Nance and Berry 1992) and a peripheral neuropathy (Grunnet *et al.* 1983). There is often calcification of the basal nuclei and marked ventricular dilatation. The condition is transmitted as an autosomal recessive trait. The basic defect is unknown but fibroblasts grown from patients with Cockayne syndrome show an inhibition of DNA and RNA synthesis after ultraviolet irradiation (Leech *et al.* 1985). On the basis of this abnormal sensitivity, three complementation groups have been delineated, suggesting genetic

heterogeneity (Lehmann 1982). This defect is also the proposed basis for prenatal diagnosis of the disease (Cleaver *et al.* 1994).

The clinical features are distinctive (Nance and Berry 1992). In type 1, after a normal first year, there is slowing of growth and neurodevelopmental retardation with the slowly progressive appearance of cerebellar and pyramidal tract signs and microcephaly. After a few years, patients have short stature, cachexia with sunken eyes, sensitivity of the skin to sunshine, a progeric appearance and large ears. The diagnosis rests on the demonstration of pigmentary retinopathy and of abnormalities of white matter and basal ganglia by CT scan or MRI (Dabbagh and Swaiman 1988). The CSF is normal. Nerve conduction velocities are decreased in most cases (Grunnet *et al.* 1983). The course is frequently complicated by the development of hypertension and renal failure (Nance and Berry 1992). No treatment is available. Fryns *et al.* (1991) reported in one case an interstitial deletion of chromosome 10.

There is an early type (type 2) in which infants fail to thrive and have the same RNA synthesis abnormality (Torillo 1990). Occasional cases are on record which share some of the dysmorphic features of Cockayne syndrome, such as small size, prominent ears and beaked nose, sometimes with basal ganglia calcification (Billard *et al.* 1989).

LEUKODYSTROPHY WITH CALCIFICATION OF THE BASAL GANGLIA AND LYMPHOCYTOSIS OF CEREBROSPINAL FLUID (AICARDI–GOUTIÈRES SYNDROME)

This is probably an autosomal recessive condition, and its pathology is poorly known. In similar cases, an inflammatory meningeal reaction was found in addition to patchy leukodystrophy with preserved islands of myelin. The clinical features include a very early onset in the first weeks or months of life so that deterioration, if any, is far from obvious. The general condition of the patient is poor, there is marked hypotonia interrupted by opisthotonic episodes, failure to develop and death in a state of decerebration within a few years although some children survive for several years (Aicardi and Goutières 1984, Cardenas-Mera *et al.* 1995, Tolmie *et al.* 1995). The two major diagnostic features are: (1) the presence of calcification of the basal nuclei and sometimes also of dentate nuclei associated with hypodensities of the white matter and brain atrophy (Fig. 10.4); and (2) a persistent mild CSF lymphocytosis (10–80 cells/mm³). Moderately elevated levels of interferon alpha are present in CSF (Lebon *et al.* 1988). Similar cases have been reported from highly inbred Indian communities of Northern Quebec (Black *et al.* 1988a,b). The disease should be distinguished from cases of calcification of the basal ganglia without evidence of white matter disease sometimes with brain atrophy and without pleocytosis, as the cells eventually disappear. Such cases are not rare (Billard *et al.* 1989) and probably represent a sequela to several nonprogressive, nongenetic disorders, although they may also occur with metabolic diseases (see Table 10.1). Infection with human immunodeficiency virus (HIV) can produce an identical picture, and HIV infection should be systematically looked for in such cases (Belman *et al.* 1986).

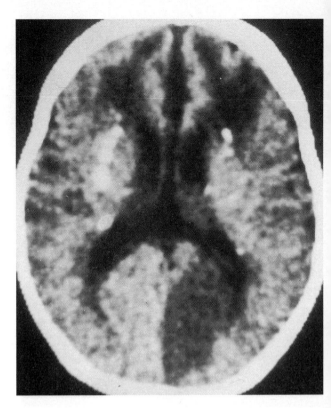

Fig. 10.4. Leukodystrophy with calcification of central grey nuclei and chronic CSF lymphocytosis (Aicardi-Goutières syndrome). Note extensive parenchymal atrophy and marked hypodensities in frontal and occipital white matter. (By permission of Adis Health Science Press, Sydney.)

The cases of disseminated calcification involving the basal ganglia, cerebellum and white matter reported by Razavi-Encha *et al.* (1988), Boltshauser *et al.* (1991) and Sabatino *et al.* (1994) may belong to the same disorder.

LEUKODYSTROPHY WITH ROSENTHAL FIBRES (ALEXANDER DISEASE)

This disease is defined by diffuse demyelination and sometimes cavitation of the white matter with little or no sparing of the arcuate fibres. Rosenthal fibres are astrocytic processes containing fibrillary aggregates. These are nonspecific findings (Goebel *et al.* 1981) but their large number, subpial and perivascular distribution and association with abnormal oligodendrocytes are characteristic (Borrett and Becker 1985). This pathological picture may be accompanied by variable clinical manifestations. Pridmore *et al.* (1993) studied 10 patients and reviewed 30 cases from the literature. Seventeen of the 40 had hydrocephalus and seven had ataxia. Spastic paraparesis, seizures and papilloedema, choreoathetosis, marked feeding difficulties and bulbar symptoms were encountered. Two of nine patients in whom head circumference was measured had no macrocephaly. Although onset is most commonly in infancy with the slow emergence of mental deficiency, pyramidal tract signs and a large head, cases with juvenile or even late onset up to adulthood and with virtually no progression have been recorded (Russo *et al.* 1976). The possibility of a localized form has been discussed (Goebel *et al.* 1981), and atypical clinical manifestations such as hiccup (Wilson *et al.* 1981) may be the presenting feature. No biochemical anomaly has been found, so that the pathological findings may well represent a pathological syndrome rather than a specific disease. Virtually all cases with pathological confirmation were sporadic. The diagnosis is suggested by the presence of a large head and CT scan features of white matter hypodensity often with an anterior location or predominance (Holland and Kendall 1980). MRI shows abnormally intense signal from the white matter on T$_2$-weighted sequences (Hess *et al.* 1990). The EEG can show spikes or sharp waves of frontocentral location. The electroretinogram is normal (Pridmore *et al.* 1993). The diagnosis can be pathologically proved only by cerebral biopsy but it is difficult to give favourable genetic advice on the sole basis of pathology. It appears likely that most leukodystrophies with macrocephaly belong to other entities (Naidu *et al.* 1993, van der Knaap *et al.* 1995, Singhal *et al.* 1996).

The relationship between the cases of megalencephalic leukodystrophy mentioned above and those of pathologically verified Alexander disease is still unclear (Torreman *et al.* 1993). Harbord *et al.* (1990) reported a familial case in which biopsy showed neither Rosenthal fibres nor spongiosis. These patients had frequent spikes and polyspikes and brief bursts of polyspikes on their EEGs.

DISORDERS INVOLVING PREDOMINANTLY THE GREY MATTER

These include the poliodystrophies and the neuronal ceroid–lipofuscinoses, although, in the latter, involvement of the CNS is more diffuse.

POLIODYSTROPHIES

Poliodystrophies form a heterogeneous collection of disorders also known collectively as Alpers disease. They are characterized pathologically by predominant involvement of the grey matter, which is reduced in volume and of abnormally firm consistency. At a late stage, the brain is usually grossly atrophic. Neurons are greatly reduced or lacking altogether in a focal or laminar topograpy. There is marked glial proliferation, sometimes associated with a spongy appearance of the neuropil, hence the term glioneuronal spongy degeneration used by some authors (*e.g.* Janota 1974). At an early stage, the focal distribution of lesions is remarkable and they may be minimal. Such grey matter degeneration is difficult to differentiate from other conditions such as hypoxic sequelae, hypoglycaemia or postepileptic encephalopathy (Lyon *et al.* 1996), and undoubtedly such cases have been included among reports of poliodystrophy. Therefore, the diagnosis should be based not only on pathological findings but also on the notion of a progressive illness. Most authentic cases of poliodystrophy have an established or probable genetic origin with an autosomal recessive inheritance.

The best defined group among the poliodystrophies is the *progressive neuronal degeneration of childhood (PNDC) with hepatic involvement* (Harding 1990, Harding *et al.* 1995). The onset of this disorder is usually wihin the first two years of life and in most cases before 6 years. Seizures and developmental regression appear insidiously, often in a child whose initial development had been somewhat slow. Generalized or focal myoclonus is a frequent feature, and epilepsia partialis continua is suggestive of the diagnosis. Bilateral spasticity, opisthotonus and decerebration eventually set in, often after several episodes of partial status epilepticus (Franco *et al.* 1994). Blindness is common and may be due either to occipital cortical involvement, which is often prominent, or to optic atrophy. The EEG is always severely abnormal with multifocal paroxysmal activity. Boyd *et al.* (1986) emphasized the occurrence of large slow waves mixed with small-amplitude polyspikes often asymmetrically located over the occipital regions. Visual evoked potentials are grossly abnormal with a normal ERG. CSF protein may be increased. Neuroimaging indicates progressive brain atrophy without signal change. PNDC runs a fatal course. Signs of hepatic disease that may end in terminal liver failure often become obvious late in the course (Kendall *et al.* 1987, Harding 1990).

Similar cases without hepatic failure occur (Bourgeois *et al.* 1992). The age of onset is variable, and late cases with atypical features may suggest spinocerebellar degeneration (Harding 1990).

Although PNDC is probably heterogeneous, its features are suggestive of a mitochondrial disorder. Cases with abnormal energy metabolism, affecting the Krebs cycle (Prick *et al.* 1981, 1982) or the respiratory chain (Prick *et al.* 1983, Gabreëls *et al.* 1984) have long been known, and morphological mitochondrial abnormalities have been reported (Shapira *et al.* 1975).

Such cases may be easily mistaken for valproate hepatotoxicity and may account for some of the reported cases in which an early age of onset and the presence of seizures and severe neurological signs are often prominent (Bicknese *et al.* 1992; personal cases).

Other cases of poliodystrophy may have different causes. It has been suggested that some cases with spongy degeneration resembled the spongiform encephalopathies caused by prions. However, an unconventional agent has been recovered only once from the brain of an affected child (Manuelidis and Rorke 1989).

THE CEROID–LIPOFUSCINOSES (NEURONAL CEROID–LIPOFUSCINOSES, BATTEN DISEASE)

The ceroid–lipofuscinoses are characterized by the storage of certain lipopigments that present morphological and tinctorial similarities with ceroid and lipofuscin, autofluorescent pigments found in many animal tissues. The terms apply to many partially characterized lipopigments. In fact lipopigments isolated from normal brain have different densities to those found in patients with Batten disease. Their ultrastructural appearance is also distinct. The pigment isolated from normal brain is called lipofuscin and that from Batten brains, ceroid (Palmer *et al.* 1989). Lipofuscin normally accumulates in neurons with age, although in very variable amounts, and is regarded as a normal wear and tear substance. The chemical nature of these pigments is not

TABLE 10.2
Main types of neuronal ceroid–lipofuscinosis (NCL)

	Infantile (Santavuori–Hagberg) NCL1	Late infantile (Jansky–Bielschowski) NCL2	Juvenile (Spielmeyer–Vogt) NCL3	Late infantile variant NCL5	Adult (Kufs) NCL4
Age of onset	8–18 mo	18 mo–4 y	4–7 y	5–7 y	Occasionally early
Early features	Autism, deterioration	Deterioration	Visual failure	Deterioration, ataxia	Behavioural/cognitive
Later manifestations					
Deterioration	Rapid	Rapid	Less rapid, with psychiatric overtones	Variable	Slow
Epilepsy	Often absent	Prominent[1]	Present, late	Present	Present in some
Myoclonus	Early	Marked	Late	May be present	Possible
Acquired microcephaly	Marked	Absent or minimal	Absent	Absent	Absent
Ataxia	Present	Marked	Marked	Marked	Some cases
Extrapyramidal signs	Present	Present	Marked (dysarthria)	Variable	Marked (not all)
Visual deficit	Inconspicuous	Present, late	Early, marked	Present	Absent
Neurophysiology					
EEG[2]	'Vanishing EEG'	SW, SlW	SW, SlW	SW, SlW	SW, IPS in some
ERG	Extinguished	Extinguished	Extinguished	Extinguished	Normal
VEP	Abolished	Giant	Extinguished	Giant	Normal
Vacuolated lymphocytes	Absent	Absent	Present	Absent	Absent
Major cytosome type	Granular	Curvilinear	Fingerprints	Fingerprints, less curvilinear	Granular
Course duration	Rapid, death <5 y	Rapid, death 5–15 y	Intermediate, death 15–30 y	Death 10–15 y	Slow
Biopsy diagnosis	Lymphocytes, urinary sediment, skin, conjunctiva	Idem	Idem	Idem	Idem; rectal biopsy may be required
[3]Prenatal diagnosis	AFC, ChV, DNA linkage	AFC, ChV, SUc	AFC, ChV, SUc DNA linkage	—	—

[1]May simulate Lennox–Gastaut syndrome.
[2]SW = spike–wave complexes; SlW = slow waves; IPS = intermittent photic stimulation positive.
[3]AFC = amniotic fluid cells; ChV = chorionic villus biopsy; SUc = subunit c in cultured amniotic fluid cells.

established and their mechanism of formation remains a mystery. Although ceroid accumulates mainly in lysosome-like structures that give a positive acid phoshatase reaction, they are not classified as a lysosomal disease as no deficiency of lysosomal enzymes has yet been demonstrated, with the exception of the infantile type (see below). Ceroid–lipofuscin accumulation may be the end-stage of various pathological conditions in which these inert lipopigments are formed and stored in residual lysosomal bodies. A major component of the pigment stored in infantile and juvenile ceroid–lipofuscinosis comprises subunit c of the respiratory chain enzyme ATP-synthase (Hall *et al.* 1991).

The heterogeneity of the ceroid–lipofuscinoses is confirmed by the fact that different genes, located on different chromosomes are responsible, and the two currently known mutant proteins belong to different families of protein.

The term neuronal ceroid–lipofuscinosis (NCL) is not entirely accurate as ceroid–lipofuscin is also found in many extraneural tissues, which is the basis for diagnosis of NCL. In addition, the NCLs are not a single disease. Five subtypes and rare atypical forms are recognized (Santavuori 1988; Goebel 1992, 1995) (Table 10.2). Almost all forms of NCL are inherited as autosomal recessive traits. The NCLs are a panethnic group of

diseases; however, local variations are marked. The infantile form, which is very rare in most countries, is frequent in Finland, with an incidence of 7.7 per 100,000 live births, and the juvenile form in common in Germany.

INFANTILE NCL (SANTAVUORI–HALTIA–HAGBERG DISEASE, NCL1)
This form is due to a mutant gene on chromosome 1 (1p33–p35) that codes for the enzyme palmitoyl protein thioesterase, a lysosomal enzyme whose function is still unknown (Vesa *et al.* 1995). The early development of affected infants is normal. From 6 to 12 months of age, mental deterioration and ataxia are the main features. Anxiety and autistic-like features may be prominent; together with the abnormal stereotypic hand movements ('knitting movements'), they may wrongly suggest the diagnosis of Rett syndrome. Myoclonic jerks appear during the second year of life and there is progressive microcephaly. Macular and retinal degeneration and optic atrophy are frequent, and the ERG is always extinguished, except perhaps in the first few months of the illness. The EEG shows progressive slowing and loss of amplitude leading to an isoelectric tracing during the third year of life (Santavuori *et al.* 1973, Santavuori 1988).

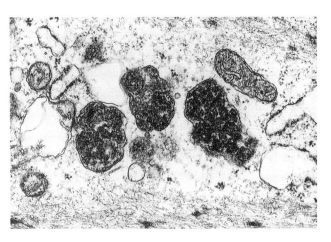

Fig. 10.5. Infantile neuronal ceroid–lipofuscinosis. Three electron-dense granular inclusions within a sweat gland cell. (Courtesy Dr M-L. Arsenio-Nunes, Hôpital de la Salpétrière, Paris.)

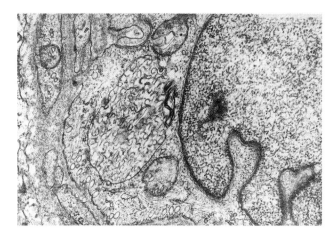

Fig. 10.6. Late infantile neuronal ceroid–lipofuscinosis. Skin biopsy: inclusion containing curvilinear profiles. (Courtesy Dr M-L. Arsenio-Nunes, Hôpital de la Salpétrière, Paris.)

The disease produces an extraordinary degree of brain atrophy. This is well demonstrated by MRI that shows, in addition, hypodensity of the thalami, a peripheral ring of increased T_2 signal and a reversal of the normal white–grey contrast in late stages (Vanhanen *et al.* 1995). Surviving neurons, as well as a number of extraneural cells contain large amounts of ceroid with a homogeneous, finely granular internal structure (Fig. 10.5). Death occurs following variable periods of vegetative state. In a few cases, a picture reminiscent of the Lennox–Gastaut syndrome is seen at onset of the disease (Santavuori 1988).

LATE INFANTILE NCL (JANSKY–BIELSCHOWSKY DISEASE, NCL2)

The mutant gene for this form has not yet been mapped, and there is a suggestion that the disease could be genetically heterogeneous. Linkage to chromosome 11 may be present in some families. The onset is between 18 months and 4 years of age. Brett and Lake (1997) found a mean age at first symptom of 22 months. The first symptom is an abnormality of developmental progress. Epilepsy is the prominent feature but usually begins after 30 months of age, soon followed by dementia and ataxia. Seizures are often myoclonic in type and may be associated with erratic and intention myoclonus. Children become bedridden by 3½–6 years of age. Visual failure is usually late after age 6 years. There is macular and retinal degeneration and optic atrophy but these usually appear by 3–4 years of age, and at onset even the ERG may be normal.

The neurophysiological picture is characteristic. The EEG shows, in addition to multifocal spikes and slow background rhythm, a peculiar response to photic stimulation at a low rate, each flash producing a spike in the posterior scalp regions (Harden and Pampiglione 1982). The ERG is extinguished. Visual evoked potentials (VEPs) and somatosensory evoked responses are also very large, although VEPs may become abolished at a late stage.

Brain atrophy is less marked than in the infantile type. No vacuolated lymphocytes are found. Skin or conjunctival biopsy (Arsenio-Nunes *et al.* 1981) shows cytosomes predominantly containing curvilinear profiles (Fig. 10.6). Death occurs between 6 and 15 years of age.

A variant of the late infantile type (NCL5) has been described (Santavuori *et al.* 1982, Autti *et al.* 1992, Wisniewski *et al.* 1993). The gene has been mapped to chromosome 13q31–q32. The onset is around 5 years of age with mental deterioration, ataxia or failing vision. Epileptic manifestations and EEG abnormalities are observed after 7–8 years and the course is slower than in the late infantile type. Most cytosomes are of the 'fingerprint' type (containing linear, curved patterns reminiscent of fingerprints) but the neurophysiological features are similar to those of the late infantile type.

JUVENILE NCL (SPIELMEYER–VOGT–SJÖGREN DISEASE, NCL3)

In this form, whose gene is located to chromosome 16 (Gardiner 1993) and codes for a novel protein, the onset is between 4 and 7 years. It is marked by failing vision that begins with hemeralopia and leads to very low acuity in about two years. Deterioration is initially absent or mild but behavioural disturbances may be prominent, often leading to a misdiagnosis of a psychiatric condition. A special type of dysarthria with precipitate and indistinct emission becomes obvious by 10–15 years of age. Neurological signs develop slowly and include extrapyramidal manifestations (tremor and rigidity) and slight cerebellar and pyramidal signs. Myoclonic seizures are common but generalized and partial seizures may also supervene.

Ophthalmological examination reveals macular degeneration with pigment aggregates, present from 10 years onward.

The EEG may show pseudoperiodic bursts of high-amplitude slow waves or a low-amplitude, rather featureless tracing (Harden and Pampiglione 1982). The ERG and VEPs are decreased or abolished early in the course. Neuroimaging shows mild to moderate atrophy. Extensive calcification is present pathologically and may be apparent on CT (Bruun *et al.* 1991).

Vacuolated lymphocytes are usually present, and ultrastructural examination of the skin and conjunctiva, lymphocytes and

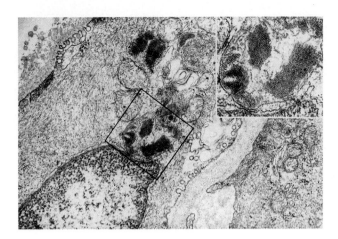

Fig. 10.7. Juvenile neuronal ceroid–lipofuscinosis. 'Fingerprint' inclusions within an endothelial cell of a skin capillary. Insert shows detail of inclusion with closely packed membranes. (Courtesy Dr M-L. Arsenio-Nunes, Hôpital de la Salpétrière, Paris.)

tonsillar tissue (Goebel 1995) shows a predominance of finger-print profiles (Fig. 10.7). A rare subtype is clinically similar but with homogeneously granular cytosomes (Lake *et al.* 1996). This variant does not map to the *NCL3* locus. An early juvenile variant has its onset between 3 and 5 years of age (Lake and Cavanagh 1978). The inclusions are both fingerprint and curvilinear profiles. This form probably maps to chromosome 15.

Death occurs between 15 and 30 years of age.

ADULT NCL (KUFS DISEASE, NCL4)

Despite its denomination, adult NCL may have its onset in childhood or adolescence and the first symptoms may appear as early as 3 years of age (Libert *et al.* 1982, Berkovic *et al.* 1988). They develop insidiously and consist mainly of mental and behavioural disturbances. A mild dementia is evident eventually. Late in the course extrapyramidal signs may appear, especially facial dyskinesia. There are no ophthalmological abnormalities or visual failure. Some patients may develop myoclonic seizures. Berkovic *et al.* (1988) separate two types: one of progressive myoclonic epilepsy and neuropsychiatric changes, and one of dementia and motor cerebellar and extrapyramidal manifestations. The EEG may show a remarkable response to photic stimulation, with high-amplitude spikes synchronous to flashes at low rhythm of repetition (Barthez-Carpentier *et al.* 1991).

Most reported cases have been sporadic, probably autosomal recessive in inheritance. In rare families, a dominant inheritance is likely.

Cytosomes containing granular osmiophilic inclusions can be found but they may be difficult to find in nonneural tissues.

ATYPICAL TYPES OF NCL

Such types may account for 10–20 per cent of cases in some series (Dyken and Wisniewski 1995, Goebel 1995). Several classifications have been proposed, some containing as many as 15 different types (Dyken and Wisniewski 1995) but none has been generally accepted (Goebel 1995). Whether some of the minor

forms are actually different entities or only 'variants' of more classic forms remains to be established.

Several cases of congenital NCL (Norman–Wood type) have been reported (Barohn *et al.* 1992, Dyken and Wisniewski 1995); however, these were only pathological cases and the interpretation of the histological findings as ceroid–lipofuscinosis has been questioned (Goebel 1995). The authenticity of the protracted type is better established (Libert *et al.* 1982). The onset is marked by visual difficulties with the slow development of seizures and dementia. The predominance of curvilinear profiles and visual failure separate these cases from the adult form. A pigment variant (Goebel *et al.* 1995) begins in childhood, also has a protracted course but differs by the appearance of the storage product. Chronic infantile (Dyken and Wisniewski 1995) and childhood (Edathodu *et al.* 1984) cases, and isolated cases with chorea, spinocerebellar signs, neuropathy and a slow progression (Wisniewski *et al.* 1993) have been described. A few cases associated with osteopetrosis are on record (Takahashi *et al.* 1990) and may have a prenatal onset (Fitch *et al.* 1973, Ambler *et al.* 1983).

DIAGNOSIS OF NCL

The diagnosis of NCL may be difficult in the less usual types. Neurophysiological features, especially an abnormal ERG and a peculiar response of the EEG to slow light stimulation (1–3 Hz), are of value in late infantile and some 'adult' forms. Brain atrophy on CT is usually present early but may not be found in the first year of illness.

Abnormal dolichol excretion in urine is found in infantile, late infantile and juvenile NCL but is nonspecific.

Demonstration of the characteristic inclusions in lymphocytes, skin, conjunctiva or other extraneural tissues is the ultimate diagnostic test. No type of inclusion is completely specific for one form, although there is usually one predominant type. Biopsy of extraneural tissue is occasionally negative. In such cases, rectal biopsy may show inclusion-containing neurons (Barthez-Carpentier *et al.* 1991). Molecular biology diagnosis is possible in NCL types 1 and 3.

Prenatal diagnosis is established in the infantile, and possible in the late infantile and juvenile forms of NCL. It can be made on the morphological appearance of inclusions in amniotic fluid cells or chorionic villus biopsies (Chow *et al.* 1993), on the presence of subunit C of mitochondrial ATPase in NCL2 and 3, combined with DNA linkage in NCL1 and 3 (Goebel *et al.* 1995). Direct gene diagnosis is possible in types 1 and 3. Detection of carriers is possible in selected cases of NCL1 (Goebel 1995).

TREATMENT

Antioxidant treatment with vitamins E and C and selenium has been proposed (Santavuori *et al.* 1985) but the results are controversial.

Anticonvulsant treatment is essential in most types. Sodium valproate and/or clonazepam are often effective but antiepileptic treatment should be individualized and seizures may be totally refractory.

Supportive care to the patients and families helps lessen the impact of these devastating diseases.

HEREDODEGENERATIVE DISEASES WITH DIFFUSE CNS INVOLVEMENT

A few degenerative disorders involve most parts of both the cerebrum and cerebellum or brainstem structures, without any evidence of storage or specific lesion. They are of proven or likely genetic origin but their mechanism is undetermined. The peripheral nervous system is also affected in the two main conditions of this group, neuroaxonal dystrophy and neuronal, intranuclear inclusion disease.

NEUROAXONAL DYSTROPHY (SEITELBERGER DISEASE)

This disease is transmitted as an autosomal recessive trait. Axonal swellings, known as spheroids, formed by branched tubular structures and bundles of filaments with mitochondria, are present in nerve fibres, especially at presynaptic endings. The spheroids are widespread throughout the CNS and are especially numerous in the posterior horns of the spinal cord, Goll and Burdach nuclei, and pallidum, which also contain excess ferric pigment and fat. Smaller bodies with a similar ultrastructure (eosinophilic bodies) are found in the cortex. There is associated diffuse gliosis of the white matter of the centrum semi-ovale and degeneration of several long tracts of certain systems (*e.g.* pyramidal, spinocerebellar) (Aicardi and Castelein 1979). A disturbance of retrograde axonal transport may be the cause of the disease.

The *infantile form* has its onset between 14 and 18 months of age with difficulties of ambulation. Progress stops and, after a period of stagnation of weeks to months, frank deterioration appears. Rapidly, there is hypotonia so marked as to suggest the diagnosis of a neuromuscular disease (Aicardi and Castelein 1979). However, pyramidal tract signs appear early even though deep tendon reflexes may be weak or absent. The disease slowly progresses to severe dementia accompanied by increasing spasticity that evolves into decorticate rigidity. Optic atrophy with nystagmus is present in 70 per cent of cases by 3 years of age. Ultimately, slow abnormal movements may appear and death supervenes by 5–10 years. Seizures are unusual and late. The CSF is normal and no specific biochemical marker is known. CT scan and MRI often show cerebellar atrophy but no abnormality of density of the white matter. Increased T_2 signal in the cerebellum was found in four of five cases studied by Tanabe *et al.* (1993) and calcification of the basal ganglia was present in one of these patients. A neurophysiological syndrome, very suggestive of neuroaxonal dystrophy, is virtually constant. It includes: (1) typical EMG signs of denervation, especially in distal muscles, with normal sensory and motor conduction velocities; (2) high-amplitude, fast (18–24 Hz) activity in waking and sleep EEG after 18–30 months of age; (3) absent or abnormal visual and somaesthetic evoked potentials after at least a few months course. A similar picture was found in eight patients by Ramaekers *et al.* (1987), although one of these had a quite atypical presentation.

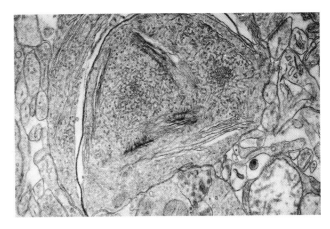

Fig. 10.8. Neuroaxonal dystrophy. Spheroid body in cortical biopsy from right frontal lobe. Branched tubular structures and bunches of nerve filaments in a neuronal process.

Pathological confirmation of the diagnosis can be obtained from peripheral biopsies, especially of the skin or conjunctiva (Arsenio-Nunes *et al.* 1981) (Fig. 10.8) but also of nerves and muscle (Kimura and Sasaki 1988). Brain biopsy is no longer justified. The mere presence of spheroids in nervous structures is not specific. Spheroids are also present in the brain of patients with Hallervorden–Spatz disease (see p. 340) and in various ill-defined chronic nonprogressive neurological disorders that have been reported as early infantile neuroaxonal dystrophies but are clinically totally distinct and most of which have no known genetic basis (Aicardi and Castelein 1979). Therefore, the typical clinical criteria are as important for the diagnosis of infantile neuroaxonal dystrophy as are the pathological lesions because neither alone is conclusive. However, atypical cases do occur and the progressive loss of skills may be masked by other presenting problems such as ataxia, toe-walking or visual deficits, and the neurophysiological features may not be apparent early. Some cases may have quite different features such as pontine atrophy with calcification of the basal ganglia (Ramaekers *et al.* 1987) or diencephalic signs (Nagashima *et al.* 1985). Familial cases of neuroaxonal dystrophy asociated with a *deficit in alpha-*N*-acetyl-galactosaminidase* have been reported (Schindler *et al.* 1989, De Jong *et al.* 1994). The clinical features were at variance with those of the common type (*e.g.* by the presence of myoclonus) and the deficit has not been found in several other cases.

The nosological situation of the forms of neuroaxonal dystrophy with onset in the first months of life is unclear. Such infants may have seizures, including infantile spasms (Wakai *et al.* 1994) and congenital hypertonia with basal ganglia calcification (Venkatesh *et al.* 1994). Congenital neuroaxonal dystrophy associated with storage of lipopigments has been reported in a few patients with the severe type of osteopetrosis with neurological disease (Jagadha *et al.* 1988).

Rare cases of *juvenile neuroaxonal dystrophy* are on record (Dorfman *et al.* 1978). They present in late childhood or adolescence with progressive myoclonic epilepsy usually with retinal degeneration. The late form is probably unrelated to the infantile type. Its diagnosis by rectal and skin biopsy may be possible (Schwendemann *et al.* 1987).

Only supportive treatment is available for any form of neuroaxonal dystrophy and prenatal diagnosis is not possible.

NEURONAL INTRANUCLEAR INCLUSION DISEASE

A progressive neurological disorder of unknown cause which occurs in children and adults, neuronal intranuclear inclusion disease is apparently transmitted as an autosomal recessive trait. Only 10 cases have been reported in children (Goutières *et al.* 1990). The disease begins between 2 and 12 years of age with behavioural disturbances, learning difficulties and extrapyramidal disorder. Cerebellar signs and parkinsonian rigidity develop progressively (Sloane *et al.* 1994). Dysarthria, temper tantrums and oculogyric crises are of diagnostic importance as is the frequent involvement of anterior horn cells in the spinal cord (Patel *et al.* 1985). Autonomic involvement is possible (Schuffler *et al.* 1978). Characteristic eosinophilic inclusions are widespread in the central and peripheral nervous system and also involve the myenteric plexus. Diagnosis by rectal biopsy is feasible (Goutières *et al.* 1990). Only symptomatic treatment is available.

OTHER DIFFUSE HEREDODEGENERATIVE DISORDERS OF THE CNS

A number of reports in the literature deal with cases of heredo-degenerative CNS diseases that have been observed only occasionally and whose clinical features and nosology are therefore uncertain. Examples of such disorders include the cases of *micro-cephaly, congenital cataracts, mental retardation, choreoathetosis and hypotonia* reported in three sibs by Tomiwa *et al.* (1987) and a case of *mental retardation, seizures, anterior horn cell involvement and neuropathy* with accumulation of phosphorylated neurofil-aments described by Wiley *et al.* (1987) and Lee *et al.* (1989). Towfighi *et al.* (1975) and Martin *et al.* (1977) have reported two patients with an *encephalopathy with lamellar residual bodies* characterized clinically by early seizures, loss of acquired mile-stones starting at about 1 year of age; progressive microcephaly, optic atrophy, cerebellar and pyramidal tract signs and retinal degeneration may be a part (Nishimura *et al.* 1987). In adult patients, a syndrome of *palatal myoclonus and progressive ataxia* has been observed (Leger *et al.* 1986, Howard *et al.* 1993, Malandrini *et al.* 1996b). I have seen a similar condition with onset in early childhood in one patient who later also developed brain atrophy and progressive diplegia. Ashwal *et al.* (1984) presented a case of a progressive degenerative condition with onset in early childhood of seizures, choreoathetosis, ataxia, spas-ticity and mild mental retardation, complicated at age 13 by a rapidly progressive peripheral nervous system involvement and without evidence of ceroid–lipofuscinosis or sphingolipid metabolism disturbance. Exceptional cases of polyglucosan storage disease in children are on record (De León *et al.* 1996).

In many cases of rare degenerative diseases, only a diagnosis of progressive disorder is possible, and even that may be extremely difficult in slowly evolving conditions. Even brain biopsy—

which is seldom if ever indicated—and post-mortem examina-tion may not permit a diagnosis to be made. It is therefore of great importance to establish databases as a help to the diagnosis of such rare disorders and also as a tool for better delineation of syndromes and diseases (Tomiwa *et al.* 1987).

HEREDODEGENERATIVE DISORDERS WITH PREDOMINANT INVOLVEMENT OF THE BASAL GANGLIA

These include conditions in which there is anatomical or functional evidence or both of involvement of the basal structures responsible for the control of movement. Such involvement may be limited to the 'extrapyramidal system' or be associated with more diffuse damage or dysfunction. *Movement disorders* are the predominant feature of such cases. A few conditions in which there is no definite pathological evidence of basal ganglia involve-ment but which are characterized by abnormalities of movement (*viz.* tics, Tourette syndrome, and mirror movements) are included in this section even though they may not be heredo-degenerative.

CHOREAS

This group contains two main degenerative conditions, Huntington chorea and benign hereditary chorea. Chorea may also be a feature of several disorders, some of them treatable (Table 10.3).

HUNTINGTON CHOREA

Huntington chorea is a genetic, dominantly inherited disease characterized by extrapyramidal features (choreiform movements or rigidity) and progressive dementia. The disorder is due to the expansion of a CAG repeat within the coding region of a gene mapping to the distal end of chromosome 4p. The gene product (huntingtin) is a novel protein of unknown function. Control individuals have less than 30 repeats; patients have 36–121 triplets (mean 44) (Kremer *et al.* 1994). As expected with this genetic mechanism, there is anticipation (progressively earlier appearance with successive generations) and sex bias in trans-mission. The length of trinucleotide repeat increases dramatically, with transmission in about one-third of cases. The disorder is of paternal origin in 70–90 per cent of cases. The length of the trinucleotide expansion is positively correlated to an earlier age of onset and a greater severity of the disease (Ashizawa *et al.* 1994, Illarioshkin *et al.* 1994, Xuereb *et al.* 1996). Huntington chorea is a rare disease in childhood although the incidence in the general population is 1 in 24,000 persons and the prevalence rate is 7.61 per 100,000 (Walker *et al.* 1981). The frequency of heterozygotes may be 1 in 5000 persons. However, cases with onset below the age of 20 years account for only 5–10 per cent of the total number.

From a pathological viewpoint there is gross atrophy of the striatum, especially the caudate nucleus, resulting in the disap-pearance of the normal bulge of the head of the caudate into the frontal ventricular horns. The frontal cortex is also atrophic.

TABLE 10.3
Main causes of chorea

Cause	References
Acquired disorders	
Sydenham (rheumatic) chorea	Nausieda (1986)
Lupus erythematosus	Bruyn and Padberg (1984b)
Chorea and lupus anticoagulant	Okseter and Sirnes (1988)
Lymphoblastic leukaemia	Schiff and Ortega (1992)
Tumours of basal ganglia	Krauss et al. (1992)
Hormonal contraception	Leys et al. (1987), Nausieda (1986)
Encephalitis involving the basal ganglia	Peters et al. (1979), Leber et al. (1995)
Epstein–Barr virus infection	Connelly and De Witt (1994)
Infantile chorea as a sequel of bronchopulmonary dysplasia	Hadders-Algra et al. (1994)
Behçet syndrome	Bussone et al. (1982)
Multiple sclerosis	Chapter 12
Bilateral infantile striatal necrosis	Mito et al. (1986)
Following cardiac surgery with hypothermia	Robinson et al. (1988)
Chronic subdural haematoma	Bae et al. (1980)
Thyroiditis	Cohn et al. (1971)
Thyrotoxicosis*	Shahar et al. (1988, Pozzan et al. (1992)
Idiopathic hypoparathyroidism*	McKinney (1962)
Splenorenal shunt	Yokota et al. (1988)
Polycythaemia and cyanotic heart disease*	Edwards et al. (1975)
Essential polycythaemia	Bruyn and Padberg (1984b)
Lithium toxicity*	Walevski and Radwan (1986)
Methylphenidate* hydrochloride toxicity	Weiner et al. (1978)
Cyclosporine toxicity	Combarros et al. (1993)
Phenobarbitone toxicity	Wiznitzer and Younkin (1984)
Phenothiazine therapy*	Singer and Wong (1970)
Alcohol toxicity*	Mullin et al. (1970)
Amphetamine toxicity*	Leys et al. (1985)
Phenytoin toxicity	Harrison et al. (1993)
Carbon monoxide toxicity	Sawada et al. (1980)
Withdrawal of fentanyl	Bergman et al. (1991)
Central pontine myelinolysis	Brunner et al. (1990)
Moyamoya disease	Chapter 15
Metabolic and congenital causes	
Wilson disease	Chapter 9
Huntington chorea	See text
Gangliosidosis types 1 and 2	Chapter 9
Progressive chorea without dementia	See text
Familial benign chorea with intention tremor	See text
Glutaric aciduria type I*	Chapter 9
Choreoacanthocytosis	Spencer et al. (1987)
Leigh disease	Chapter 9
Propionic and methylmalonic acidaemias	Chapter 9
Other organic acids	Chapter 9
Pallidoluysian–dentatonigral degeneration	Warner et al. (1995)
Mitochondrial encephalomyopathies	Aicardi et al. (1985)
Dihydropteridine reductase deficiency (hyperphenylalaninaemia type IV)	Chapter 9
Homocystinuria	Hagberg et al. (1979)
Tuberous sclerosis	Evans and Jankovic (1983)
Holoprosencephaly	Louis et al. (1995)
Ataxia, chorea, seizures and dementia	Farmer et al. (1989)
Ataxia–telangiectasia	Chapter 4
Mastocytosis	Iriarte et al. (1988)
Sulfite oxidase deficiency	Shih et al. (1977)

*May be chronic or persist after an acute onset.

There is neuronal depletion affecting mainly the small neurons that are mainly GABA-ergic and also contain substance P and enkephalins. The large neurons that mainly contain somatostatin or neuropeptide Y are involved only in advanced cases. The lipofuscin content of the striatum is increased and dense, and degenerating mitochondria are present in some cases. The reduction in cell number is associated with reduced GABA content and acetylcholine synthesis as judged from the low content of acetylcholine transferase. The concentration of somatostatin and peptide Y is also decreased (Beal et al. 1988). However, administration of substances that increase GABA concentration has not been useful. Dopamine concentration within the striatum is normal but administration of L-dopa increases the choreiform movements. Subpopulations of projection neurons (whose axons terminate outside the striatum) are preferentially affected (Albin et al. 1990a,b). There is early loss of enkephalinergic neurons projecting to the external globus pallidus and substance P-containing neurons projecting to the pars reticulata of the substantia nigra, while substance P-containing neurons that project to the internal globus pallidus and pars compacta of the substantia nigra are involved late in the disease.

Rarely does the disease appear in a child of a preclinically affected parent. The age of onset in 46 childhood cases reviewed by Osborne et al. (1982) was between 3 and 9 years. The most common manifestation in children is rigidity, although mental deterioration can precede extrapyramidal features. Indeed, neuropsychological studies in preclinical adult cases indicate early involvement of frontal lobe function (Jason et al. 1988, Foroud et al. 1995), but study of at-risk children has no predictive value (Catona et al. 1985). In Osborne's series, the rigid, juvenile variant of Huntington disease resembled the classical Westphal variant observed in adults, with rigidity in 26 of 46 patients, choreic movements in nine and mixed rigidity and chorea in three. Choreic movements are similar to those of Sydenham chorea although they may affect more the trunk and proximal part of limbs. Dysarthria is an early and prominent symptom and cerebellar signs can be a feature. Oculomotor apraxia is often conspicuous (Lasker et al. 1987). Seizures occur in one half of childhood cases, and myoclonic attacks are not rare (Osborne et al. 1982). A myoclonic form has been described (Garrel et al. 1978). The course is rapidly progressive, the average duration of the illness being eight years. There is no biochemical marker for the condition so the diagnosis depends on clinical features and family history. CT scan and MRI demonstrate ventricular dilatation with atrophy of the head of the caudate (Bamford et al. 1989) (Fig. 10.9). Increased signal in the striatum may be present in the rigid forms (Lenti and Bianchini 1993). MRI changes may be a late sign, and localized hypometabolism as shown by positron emission tomography (PET) using deoxyglucose is more sensitive (Berent et al. 1988).

The differential diagnosis (Folstein et al. 1986) includes drug-induced and spontaneous dystonia and abnormal movements, Hallervorden–Spatz disease, Wilson disease, dystonic lipidosis, Lesch–Nyhan syndrome, Sydenham chorea and choreoacanthocytosis in young adults or even in young adolescents

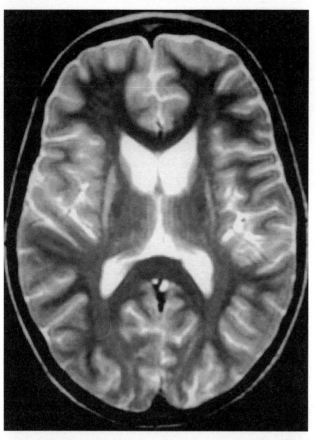

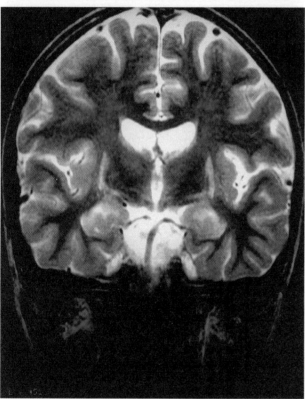

Fig. 10.9. Huntington chorea. 4-year-old girl with seizures, myoclonia and developmental deterioration. Axial *(top)* and coronal *(bottom)* T₂-weighted MRI scans show atrophy of the caudate with resulting enlargement of the frontal horns and high signal from external putamina. (Courtesy Dr F. Goutières, Hôpital des Enfants Malades, Paris.)

(Hardie *et al.* 1991, Orrell *et al.* 1995). The last of these conditions features both tics and choreic movements, a peripheral neuropathy with amyotrophy of the lower limbs and mental disturbances. Acanthocytes are present in blood. Some cases of hereditary chorea without dementia may be observed in patients with an expanded CAG repeat, suggesting that the phenotypic variation in Huntington disease may be wide (MacMillan *et al.* 1993, Britton *et al.* 1995). Such cases may complicate the diagnosis, as may a newly reported syndrome of striatothalamic degeneration (Gieron *et al.* 1995). This syndrome features onset in the first year of life, developmental regression, choreiform movements, hypotonia and swallowing difficulties. There is progressive atrophy of the head of the caudate and abnormal signal from the lenticular nuclei. Pathologically, there is atrophy of the thalamus and the striate. The DNA is normal.

Preclinical and even prenatal diagnosis of Huntington disease using DNA probes is possible. This may raise ethical problems but permit an informed decision regarding parenthood.

No effective treatment has yet been devised (Furtado and Suchowersky 1995). Haloperidol may alleviate the abnormal movements. Levodopa has been used with some success in the hypokinetic–rigid form (Jongen *et al.* 1980). Diazepam, tetrabenazine, sodium valproate and carbamazepine may be of some help.

BENIGN HEREDITARY CHOREAS

Not all chronic choreas lead to dementia and early death. Benign forms without mental deterioration have been known for several years (Nutting *et al.* 1969). They may be sporadic but most commonly they are familial diseases usually transmitted as a dominant trait with variability in expression within the same pedigree (Schady and Meara 1988). The choreic movements are isolated without associated weakness. Recessive inheritance is rare (Nutting *et al.* 1969). In some cases, the choreic movements tend to decrease with age so that the diagnosis may not be obvious in an affected parent. However, progression occurs in some patients (Schady and Meara 1988). Fisher *et al.* (1979) reported in one family a condition described as 'inverted chorea' in which the lower limbs were first and more severely affected. In some families, there may be associated axial dystonia (Schady and Meara 1988), tremor or sensorineural hearing loss (Wheeler *et al.* 1993). The term benign may not be appropriate for all cases, especially those in which associated signs develop (Fisher *et al.* 1979). The recent finding that an expansion of CAG repeat similar to that in Huntington chorea may be present in apparently benign cases of chorea (MacMillan *et al.* 1993, Britton *et al.* 1995) is worrying. These are mainly associated with relatively small expansions (36–39 repeats) that may remain asymptomatic but be transmitted in a more severe form to the following generation. The diagnosis rests on the family history and absence of mental deterioration. Atypical forms may raise nosological problems with disorders presenting with dystonia or familial tremor. Dantrolene has been used in one case. Generally, no treatment is advisable and the disorder tends to become less conspicuous with the passing of time.

DYSTONIAS

The term dystonia is used in three distinct ways. First, it is employed to describe a pattern of sustained disturbed muscle contractions causing abnormal postures, frequently associated with involuntary movements that have two main distinctive features: they are typically torsional which may result in postural deformities and pain, and they are repetitive in character. Second, dystonia is applied to a disease of undetermined aetiology which can be sporadic or hereditary. Third, the term has been used to describe a group of diseases of known causes, featuring the abnormal movements mentioned above (secondary dystonia) (Calne and Lang 1988, Fahn 1988).

CLASSICAL TORSION DYSTONIA (DYSTONIA MUSCULORUM DEFORMANS)

Idiopathic torsion dystonia has no known pathology. A functional disorder of the basal ganglia is suggested by the finding of abnormalities in the distribution and metabolism of neurotransmitters (Hornykiewicz *et al.* 1986, Wolfson *et al.* 1988, Dejong *et al.* 1989) which include a decrease in norepinephrine and dopamine as well as the peptidergic neurotransmitter somatostatin (Wolfson *et al.* 1988). The genetics of torsion dystonia have been largely clarified. The condition is heterogeneous. Most cases are dominantly inherited with a reduced penetrance and the occurrence of many incomplete forms among relatives of affected patients. A gene has been mapped to chromosome 9q34 (*DYT-1* gene) both in Ashkenazi Jews (Kramer *et al.* 1990) and in non-Jewish patients (Ozelius *et al.* 1989). Whereas linkage to 9q34 is regularly found in Jewish families (Warner *et al.* 1993, Bressman *et al.* 1994a), it is not present in 45 per cent of non-Jewish patients (Bressman *et al.* 1994b). The problem is complicated by the frequency of partial and atypical forms and of apparently sporadic cases (Marsden and Harrison 1974). In a recent British study of 107 patients, 58 were familial cases without evidence of heterogeneity, and an estimated 85 per cent showed genetic inheritance 'due to an autosomal dominant gene with about 40 per cent penetrance and highly variable expression, possibly reflecting environmental influences' (Fletcher *et al.* 1990). The estimated risk for first-degree relatives was 21 per cent, and 75 per cent of the gene carriers had developed signs before age 30 years. X-linked forms occur in the Philippine island of Panay (Kupke *et al.* 1990a,b) and seem to be linked to Xq21. Clinical differences in some ethnic groups (*e.g.* Swedes and French Canadians) suggest further heterogeneity (Warner *et al.* 1993). 'Sporadic' focal dystonia was recently shown to be a dominantly inherited genetic disease with low penetrance and mapped to chromosome 18p in German patients (Leube *et al.* 1997).

The *clinical features* are variable. Onset is usually after 5 years of age but may be earlier, even in the first year of life in rare cases (Mostofsky *et al.* 1996). The dystonia may be focal, segmental, multifocal or generalized depending on the extent of the territory involved by dystonic contractures. In 25 of the 42 patients of Marsden and Harrison (1974) onset occurred before the age of 15 years. In these patients, the first difficulties were with the lower limb, usually unilaterally. However, Angelini *et al.*

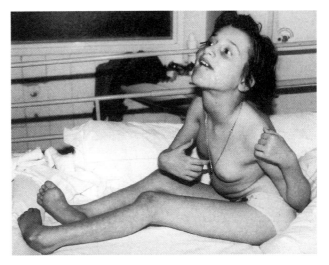

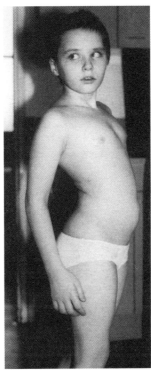

Fig. 10.10. Dystonia musculorum deformans. *(Above)* Severe form in 8-year-old girl. Note inverted feet, spinal deformity, dystonic posture of right hand and retrocollis. This patient also had marked involvement of pharyngeal and laryngeal muscles and ceaseless tongue thrusts. *(Left)* Initial manifestations in 7-year-old girl. Note prominent lordosis.

(1989) found an equal frequency of upper-limb onset in prepubertal patients. The typical early picture is inversion of the foot with plantar flexion. In most cases the disturbance in gait is bizarre and intermittent so that a misdiagnosis of hysteria is virtually always made. In fact, the dystonia is highly task-selective. Some children may walk normally backwards, while the contracture appears prominent in forward ambulation. Emotion and stress increase the dystonia. Eventually, the affected limb or limbs assume a more or less permanently abnormal posture with superimposed fluctuations that also affect the rest of the body. Lordosis is frequent and lateral incurvation of the trunk with torsion along its vertical axis commonly occurs (Fig. 10.10). The face remains unaffected in most cases, and speech and swallowing are disturbed in a minority of patients. In Marsden and Harrison's series, the dystonia became generalized in 50 per cent of

TABLE 10.4
Causes of secondary dystonia, including hemidystonia

Cause	References
Traumatic, infectious and vascular causes	
Prenatal/perinatal damage (athetoid cerebral palsy)	Chapter 8
Prenatal/perinatal delayed-onset type	Grimes *et al.* (1982), Saint Hilaire *et al.* (1991)
Infarction of basal ganglia	Dusser *et al.* (1986)
Arteriovenous malformations	Friedman *et al.* (1986)
Tumours of basal ganglia	Narbona *et al.* (1984)
Trauma (secondary vascular lesions)	Brett *et al.* (1981)
Traumatic dystonia	Jankovic (1994)
Hypoxic or toxic (cyanide) injury	Bhatt *et al.* (1993)
Peripheral injury (?reflex)	Jankovic (1994)
Thalamotomy	Pettigrew and Jankovic (1985)
AIDS encephalopathy	Nath *et al.* (1987)
Viral disease, *e.g.* varicella	Gollomp and Fahn (1987)
Drug-induced dystonia (including anticonvulsant drugs, phenothiazine)	Aguglia *et al.* (1987), Singer (1986), Moss *et al.* (1994)
Wasp sting (vascular mechanism)	Romano *et al.* (1989)
Metabolic causes	
Wilson disease	Chapter 9
GM1 gangliosidosis	Goldman *et al.* (1981)
GM2 gangliosidosis	Specola *et al.* (1990)
Sulfatidosis (metachromatic leukodystrophy)	Lang *et al.* (1985)
Ceroid–lipofuscinosis	Karpati *et al.* (1977)
Fucosidosis	Gordon *et al.* (1995)
Lesch–Nyhan syndrome	Chapter 8
Homocystinuria	Hagberg *et al.* (1979)
Methylmalonic and propionic acidurias	Hagberg *et al.* (1979)
Glutaric aciduria type I	Chapter 9
D-glyceric acidaemia	Hagberg *et al.* (1979)
Malignant hyperphenylalaninaemia	Chapter 9
2-oxyglutaric aciduria	Kohlschütter *et al.* (1982)
Sulfite-oxidase deficiency	Shih *et al.* (1977)
Triose-phosphate isomerase (TPI) deficiency	Poll-Thé *et al.* (1985)
Leigh syndrome	Chapter 9
Mitochondrial encephalomyopathy	Chapter 9
Heredodegenerative causes	
Calcification of the basal ganglia	Callender (1995)
Hallervorden–Spatz disease	Dooling *et al.* (1974)
Huntington disease	See text
Idiopathic torsion dystonia–parkinsonism	Dobyns *et al.* (1993)
Ataxia–telangiectasia	Chapter 4
Ataxia–oculomotor apraxia	Aicardi *et al.* (1988)
Neuroacanthocytosis	Hardie *et al.* (1991)
Neuronal inclusion disease	Goutières *et al.* (1990)
Dystonic lipidosis	Karpati *et al.* (1977)
Pelizaeus–Merzbacher disease	Boulloche and Aicardi (1986)
Dystonia with striatal lucencies	Novotny *et al.* (1986)
Machado–Joseph disease	Giunti *et al.* (1995)
Olivopontocerebellar atrophy	Berciano (1982)
Dentatorubral pallidoluysian atrophy	Warner *et al.* (1995)
Dystonic familial paraplegia	Brown (1975)
Neuroaxonal dystrophy (infantile type)	Aicardi and Castelein (1979)
Familial (progressive) striatal necrosis	Miyoshi *et al.* (1969)

childhood-onset cases but in as many as 15 of the 19 with onset before 11 years of age. Visceral dystonia with respiratory difficulties has been observed (Corbin *et al.* 1987). Although the movement disturbance is such that it may prevent any kind of movement and threaten life, intellectual function always remains intact.

A late-onset form occurs in adolescents and young adults. In such cases the dystonia tends to remain localized or to have a limited extension. The neck (paroxysmal torticollis) and the upper limbs are more commonly involved in patients presenting after 15 years. Dystonia narrowly limited to one muscle group has been reported (Goldman and Ahlskog 1993, Stojanovic *et al.* 1995). Writer's cramp is an uncommon mode of onset (Rosenbaum and Jankovic 1988), but other task-specific (*e.g.* playing an instrument) localized dystonias can be also a first manifestation (Rosenbaum and Jankovic 1988, Stojanovic *et al.* 1995). The late-onset forms usually run a more benign course and tend to remain segmental even though fluctuations and exacerbations are possible. The ultimate outcome of childhood cases is rather poor as almost a half of the early-onset patients of Marsden and Harrison (1974) were bedridden or wheelchair-dependent by 35 years of age, whereas only three of the late-onset cases were nonambulatory. The course is usually but not always progressive and some fluctuation in intensity may occur, especially in late-onset forms. Sudden exacerbations of the symptoms, known as status dystonicus, are rare but life-threatening events requiring emergency treatment.

Variants of classical torsion dystonia include paradoxical dystonia (Fahn 1989) in which dystonia is made worse by repetition of movement. Powell and Staunton (1981) reported a family in which torsion dystonia, athetosis, ataxia and spasticity were present in different members. Forms with onset in infancy may be genetically different from classsical torsion dystonia (Mostofsky *et al.* 1996).

No laboratory examination is useful in classical dystonia except those that rule out other diseases especially those with symptomatic dystonia. These may include complex investigations, including skin or muscle biopsy.

Differential diagnoses are listed in Table 10.4. Imaging gives normal results, while PET scan for identification of dopamine receptors is still in an experimental stage. The most important differential diagnosis is Wilson disease because it is a treatable condition. Hysteria is the most common misdiagnosis. Drug-induced dystonia, which can result from a variety of psychotropic or anticonvulsant drugs, is an important consideration and may be associated with other dyskinetic phenomena (Singer 1986, Sechi *et al.* 1988). Transient dystonic phenomena may occur in infants without apparent cause (Willemse 1986, Crouchman 1987, Angelini *et al.* 1988). Delayed dystonia, in children with previous perinatal lesions in the basal ganglia, may appear at up to 5–10 years of age (Saint-Hilaire *et al.* 1991). The presence of abnormal imaging is diagnostic. Bizarre attitudes reminiscent of dystonia may occur with hiatus hernia (Sutcliffe 1969) and are known as Sandifer syndrome. This is an important consideration as surgical treatment of reflux is curative.

TABLE 10.5
Treatments available for dystonia in order of preference*

1. *Levodopa* should be tried in all cases for 1–3 months as a diagnostic test for dopa-responsive dystonia (dose 25–300 mg/d)
2. *Benzhexol (Artane)* (anticholinergic agent) starting with 2–4 mg/d, slowly increasing (2.5 mg every 2 weeks) up to 30–80 mg/d or to tolerance
3. *Tetrabenazine* (dopamine depleting agent) 50–200 mg/d
4. *Baclofen* (GABA$_B$ receptor antagonist) 40–120 mg/d
5. *Clonazepam* (or other benzodiazepine)
6. Combined tetrabenazine, benzhexol and haloperidol or primozide (for resistant cases and status dystonicus)
7. Carbamazepine or sodium valproate, usually in association with other agents
8. Botulinum toxin in specific muscle groups for release of contractures
9. Thalamotomy (risk of speech disturbances when bilateral)
10. Status dystonicus may require curarization, assisted ventilation and intrathecal baclofen

*Multiple treatment schemes are used depending on preferences of individual clinicians. Except for the systematic use of L-dopa, no scheme is universally accepted.

Therapy for idiopathic torsion dystonia (Table 10.5) is often disappointing. A trial of L-dopa is always indicated as dopa-sensitive dystonia may be indistinguishable (Fletcher *et al.* 1993). Moreover, even a few cases of symptomatic dystonia respond to L-dopa (Fletcher *et al.* 1993). High-dosage anticholinergic therapy with doses of up to 70 mg/d progressively reached by 2.5 mg increases every two weeks (Marsden 1984, Burke *et al.* 1986) has given promising results but usually at the cost of some degree of drug-induced parkinsonism and sometimes of psychosis. Baclofen or tetrabenazine (Jankovic and Orman 1988) may partially control dystonia as well as other abnormal movements. Baclofen, clonazepam, haloperidol, carbamazepine and sodium valproate may be of some help (Pranzatelli 1996). Biopterines should be added in case of partial results with L-dopa (Segawa and Nomura 1993). Botulinum toxin has only rarely been used in young patients for partial dystonia (Seiff *et al.* 1989) but seems promising. Surgical treatment by stereotaxic thalamotomy usually produces some benefit, unfortunately often transient. Disturbances of speech are frequent following bilateral operation that is, as a rule, necessary to induce improvement (Tasker *et al.* 1988). It has been suggested that pallidoansotomy might not produce speech disorder (Iacono *et al.* 1996). Some authors have suggested that unilateral symptomatic dystonia is the best indication for surgery (Andrew *et al.* 1983, Nardocci *et al.* 1996). There is no consensus as to the value of thalamotomy but I have observed spectacular results in two patients with only partial recurrence. Emergency treatment of episodes of status dystonicus may require combined therapy with trihexyphenidyl, tetrabenazine and haloperidol, or intravenous baclofen. Paralysis and artificial ventilation may be required (Marsden *et al.* 1984).

DOPA-RESPONSIVE DYSTONIA, DOPA-SENSITIVE
DYSTONIA (HEREDITARY PROGRESSIVE DYSTONIA WITH
MARKED DIURNAL FLUCTUATIONS, SEGAWA DISEASE)
Segawa *et al.* (1976) first described a type of idiopathic dystonia

with a typical clinical presentation but with a remarkable degree of fluctuation of the symptoms in relation to the sleep–waking cycle. Affected patients were not dystonic on awakening from night sleep or a nap, but dystonic symptoms reappeared after 30–40 minutes and continued to increase throughout the day. The dystonia had its onset usually before the age of 5 years in one lower limb with secondary generalization. Involvement of axial muscles was rare. The response to L-dopa at low dosages was dramatic with restoration of a completely normal motility. Similar cases have been reported since (De Yebenes *et al.* 1988, Segawa and Nomura 1993). Untreated patients may develop parkinsonism in adolescence or adulthood. Remarkably, affected patients remain completely sensitive to the same doses for many years and 'on–off' phenomenon does not develop. Late treatment is effective; in a remarkable family, all manifestations were abolished even after 36–52 years of untreated course (Harwood *et al.* 1994).

It has become apparent, however, that dystonia amenable to successful treatment with L-dopa may present in a less characteristic manner, that diurnal fluctuation may not be prominent and that atypical forms with only mild dystonia or even spasticity may be present (Deonna 1986, Fink *et al.* 1988a, Fahn 1989, Kaiser and Ziegler 1992, Chutorian *et al.* 1994, Gordon 1996). The term *dopa-responsive dystonia* has been coined to designate these cases (Nygaard 1995). The degree of dopa-sensitivity may be variable: some patients may respond only to relatively high doses, and a long time (up to 14 months) may be required for a full effect (Rondot and Ziegler 1983), although a very rapid effect, in a matter of days, is the norm.

Dopa-responsive dystonia is transmitted as a dominant trait with a relatively low penetrance. The gene of both fluctuating forms (Ichinose *et al.* 1994) and of most other dopa-responsive types maps to chromosome 14q (Tanaka *et al.* 1995) and codes for the enzyme GTP cyclohydrolase 1 which is involved in the synthesis of the biopterins.

Several different mutations of this gene have been described in both Japanese and European cases (Ichinose *et al.* 1994, Bandmann *et al.* 1996). In a few cases, a different, recessive defect involving the enzyme thyroxine-hydroxylase has been found (Lüdecke *et al.* 1996). Other recessive defects involving the enzyme 6-pyruvoyl-tetrahydrobiopterin synthase and, in exceptional cases, 6-GTP hydrolase have been recently reported (Hyland *et al.* 1997), so dopa-sensitive dystonia now appears to be a syndrome with several causes. All defects hamper the synthesis of dopamine, which appears to be the critical abnormality in all cases. On the other hand, there is no pathological abnormality in the basal ganglia (Rajput *et al.* 1994) and the dopamine uptake by the basal ganglia is normal (Snow *et al.* 1993), thus explaining the complete response to L-dopa whose synthesis from dopamine is considerably reduced. The expression of the molecular defect may vary with different clinical presentations and various degrees of dopa sensitivity even within the same family (Bandmann *et al.* 1996). The diagnosis of dopa-responsive dystonia should be considered in all cases of dystonia regardless of clinical features, including cases of apparent dystonic cerebral palsy, as the onset may be as early as 1 year of age, and a therapeutic trial is indicated when any doubt exists. Some atypical presentations, particularly features reminiscent of spastic diplegia, are important to recognize; brisk tendon reflexes and a pseudo-Babinski sign ('striate toe') have been repeatedly reported (Fink *et al.* 1988b, Chutorian *et al.* 1994).

Treatment with L-dopa, often combined with an inhibitor of peripheral catabolism, is usually with small doses (50–250 mg/d) and effective in as little as one or two days. Given the existence of atypical responses, a trial of larger doses, up to 750 mg/d for one to three months is advised.

INFANTILE AND JUVENILE PARKINSONISM
The relationship of dopa-responsive dystonia to the rare cases of *infantile (< 10 years) or juvenile (< 20 years) Parkinson disease* is still being discussed. Most cases of parkinsonism in children are secondary to other disorders such as infections, drug toxicity or Wilson disease (Pranzatelli *et al.* 1994). Rare cases of transient parkinsonism subsequent to episodes of hypoxia have been recorded (Straussberg *et al.* 1993). Primary dominant infantile Parkinson disease is exceptional (Dwork *et al.* 1993). Although response to L-dopa may be excellent, it may wear off secondarily. The dopamine uptake by the basal ganglia is decreased (Snow *et al.* 1993), and degeneration of the striatum is present in such cases (Calne *et al.* 1993). *Dystonia–parkinsonism* in children and adolescents is probably only one presentation of dopa-responsive dystonia (Chutorian *et al.* 1994). The differentiation can probably be helped by PET scanning, which is normal in dopa-responsive dystonia but abnormal in early Parkinson disease (Calne *et al.* 1993, Turjanski *et al.* 1993). Dystonia–parkinsonism also appears to be a metabolic disorder due to reduced synthesis of dopamine without degeneration in the striatum. A rapid-onset form of dystonia–parkinsonism, not linked to the *DYT-1* gene and with dominant autosomal transmission, has been observed in two families (Dobyns *et al.* 1993, Brashear *et al.* 1996). A family with parkinsonism, amyotrophy, disinhibition and dementia with linkage to chromsome 17 is on record (Lynch *et al.* 1994).

OTHER GENETIC DYSTONIAS
Myoclonic dystonia (Obeso *et al.* 1983, Fahn 1989) accounts for less than 3 per cent of the cases of dystonia. It presents with a mixture of fast movements of myoclonic type superimposed on the slow, twisting, dystonic movements. *Alcohol-sensitive myoclonic dystonia* (Quinn 1996, Kyllerman *et al.* 1990, 1993) is probably more closely related to essential myoclonus than to dystonia and does not map to chromosome 9q. Myoclonus is often the earliest feature and may remain the only manifestation; in only rare cases is dystonia an early and prominent feature (Kyllerman *et al.* 1993).

Progressive dystonia with bilateral putaminal hypodensities (Leber disease and dystonia)
Dystonia with typical clinical presentation may be associated with bilateral putaminal lucencies (Berkovic *et al.* 1987). This disorder occurs in the same families as cases of optic atrophy of the Leber type. Either dystonia or optic atrophy can be the presenting feature, and different members of the same family may have either anomaly or both (Marsden *et al.* 1986, Novotny *et al.* 1986). The inheritance may be mitochondrial in type as in Leber disease, although it is not known whether the disorder has the same origin in a mitochondrial DNA point mutation. One such case has been associated with partial cytochrome *b* deficiency (Nigro *et al.* 1990). The main causes of basal ganglia hypodensities are shown in Table 10.6.

OTHER ATYPICAL FORMS OF DYSTONIA
A few cases of dystonia of undetermined cause but with calcification of the basal ganglia are on record (Larsen *et al.* 1985). The nosological situation of these familial cases is uncertain. The same applies to cases of dystonia secondary to peripheral trauma (Fletcher *et al.* 1991, Goldman and Ahlskog 1993, Jankovic 1994), sometimes in association with signs of sympathetic dystrophy (Bhatia *et al.* 1993), or to head trauma (Lee *et al.* 1994). Whether such cases represent idiopathic dystonia triggered by trauma or are secondary or psychogenic in origin (Fahn and Williams 1988) is undecided. Blepharospasm (Elston *et al.* 1989) and hemifacial spasm (Ronen *et al.* 1986) rarely occur in children. Most reported cases of hemifacial spasm in childhood (Al Shahwan *et al.* 1995) seem to represent epileptic phenomena (Chapters 16, 21).

HALLERVORDEN–SPATZ DISEASE
Hallervorden–Spatz *syndrome* is defined pathologically by: (1) the presence of a rusty brown ferrocalcic pigment in the pallidum and substantia nigra; (2) symmetrical destruction of the pallidum and the pars reticulata of the substantia nigra; and (3) the presence of spheroids in the basal ganglia and to a lesser extent in the cortex (Dooling *et al.* 1974). This pathological syndrome is not specific and may be seen with fixed encephalopathies (Aicardi and Castelein 1979). Hallervorden–Spatz *disease*, on the other hand, designates a progressive heredodegenerative, recessively transmitted disorder that has the above-mentioned pathological features.

The onset is usually in infancy or early childhood, but adolescent onset is not rare (Dooling *et al.* 1974, Angelini *et al.* 1992). In typical cases, initial development is slow from age 18 months to 2 years. Bilateral pyramidal tract signs are present and, together with the slow course, often suggest a nonprogressive disease. At 7–10 years, more typical manifestations including progressive dystonia, rigidity and pyramidal tract signs appear. Oromandibular involvement is prominent (Savoiardo *et al.* 1993). Mental deterioration is of variable importance. Choreoathetosis is present in at least 50 per cent of cases. A pigmentary retinopathy with extinguished ERG is found in at least one-third of patients. In some cases acanthocytes are present in peripheral blood (Malandrini *et al.* 1996a). Swaiman *et al.* (1983) found sea-blue histiocytes in one case in which a large amount of ceroid–lipofuscin was present in the brain. CT scan may show high-density images in the pallidum (Tennison *et al.* 1988) (Fig. 10.11a). However, hypodensities in the same region have been reported (Dooling *et al.* 1980). MRI findings are highly suggestive: signal from both pallida is very low as a result of the

TABLE 10.6
Lucencies in the basal ganglia

Cause	References
Acute conditions	
Unilateral lucencies	
Arterial infarcts (lacunae) involve the lenticular nucleus and internal capsule, less commonly the thalamus	Brett *et al.* (1981)
Infections: bacterial abcesses, viral diseases	
Coxsackievirus A9	Roden *et al.* (1975)
Echovirus 25	Peters *et al.* (1979)
Varicella-zoster virus	Eda *et al.* (1983)
Trauma	Horowitz and Niparko (1994)
Haemolytic–uraemic syndrome	Barnett *et al.* (1995)
Bilateral lucencies	
Trauma	Brett *et al.* (1981)
Haemolytic–uraemic syndrome	Barnett *et al.* (1995)
Infantile striatal bilateral necrosis	Goutières and Aicardi (1982)
Toxic causes, predominantly pallidal	
Carbon monoxide	Sawada *et al.* (1980)
Methanol	Ley and Gali (1983)
Disulfiram	Mahajan *et al.* (1997)
Metabolic causes, predominantly pallidal	
Methylmalonic and propionic acidaemia	Korf *et al.* (1986)
Sulfite oxidase deficiency	Personal case
Infections (SSPE*); may also be unilateral	Colamaria *et al.* (1988)
Chronic conditions	
Unilateral lucencies	
Tumours	Narbona *et al.* (1984)
Vascular malformations	Chuang (1989)
Bilateral lucencies	
Holotopistic striatal necrosis	Miyoshi *et al.* (1969)
Dystonia with Leber optic atrophy (predominantly striatal)	Novotny *et al.* (1986)
Infantile bilateral striatal necrosis, chronic stage	Mito *et al.* (1986)
Wilson disease (mainly striatal)	Walshe (1986)
Mitochondrial encephalomyopathy (MELAS** and related conditions)	Chapter 9
Leigh disease (pallidal, striatal, thalamic)	Hall and Gardner-Medwin (1978); Chapter 9
Sequelae of neonatal hypoxia	Aicardi *et al.* (1985)

*SSPE = subacute sclerosing panencephalitis.
**MELAS = mitochondrial encephalopathy with lactic acidosis and stroke-like episodes.

paramagnetic effect of iron (Fig. 10.11b). High signal appears in the central areas of the pallidum attributed to necrotic tissue, giving rise with the peripheral hypodensity to the 'eye-of-the-tiger' sign (Schaffert *et al.* 1989, Savoiardo *et al.* 1993, Østergaard *et al.* 1995) (Fig. 10.11c). This sign may be difficult to evaluate because of the normally low T_1 signal of the area and may be missing at the onset. Hypobetalipoproteinaemia may be present in association with acanthocytosis and retinitis pigmentosa, and this association has been reported as a distinct syndrome (*h*ypobetalipoproteinaemia, *a*canthocytosis, *r*etinitis *p*igmentosa or HARP syndrome). It probably represents only an especially characteristic form (Higgins *et al.* 1992, Orrell *et al.* 1995). Forms revealed by optic atrophy have been described (Casteels *et al.* 1994). Acanthocytosis is also present in neuroacanthocytosis and in McLeod syndrome, but in the latter is rarely symptomatic (Witt *et al.* 1992). Attempts at detecting excessive amounts of ^{59}Fe in the basal ganglia after administration of a tracer dose have been

difficult to interpret (Rutledge *et al.* 1987), so the diagnosis is essentially based on clinical and imaging findings. The outcome is poor, the patients being rapidly severely crippled. No treatment is available except that of dystonia and rigidity.

LEIGH SYNDROME AND RELATED CONDITIONS

Cases of chronic extrapyramidal syndromes, at times associated with pyramidal tract signs and signs of brainstem involvement, occur with Leigh syndrome (Chapter 9) and are usually associated with lucencies of the basal ganglia on CT scan (Hall and Gardner-Medwin 1978). The relationship of Leigh syndrome with acute cases of *bilateral striatal necrosis in infants* is not clear (Chapter 11). Some may be of viral origin (Hattori *et al.* 1983) and be only transient (Kimura *et al.* 1988). On the other hand, chronic hypodense lesions of the striatum can represent a specific genetic condition of unknown origin (Leuzzi *et al.* 1988) termed familial *holotopistic striatal necrosis* by Miyoshi *et al.* (1969). The

341

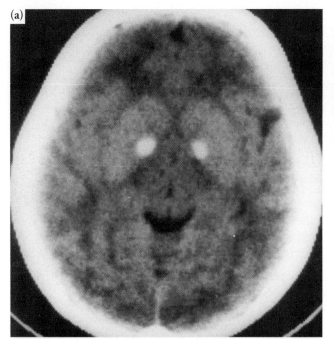

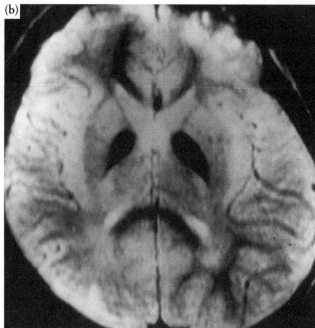

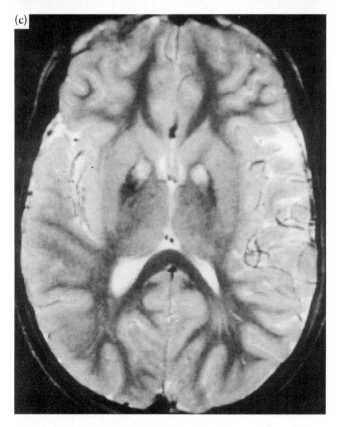

Fig. 10.11. Hallervorden–Spatz disease. *(a)* CT scan showing spontaneous opacities of both pallida. *(b)* MRI scan (1.5 T) showing marked hyposignal from pallida, probably due to their high iron content. *(c)* MRI scan of another patient shows, in centre of dark pallida, symmetrical areas of high T$_2$ signal, the so-called 'eye of the tiger' sign. These areas may be due to necrosis and may be absent—as illustrated in *(b)*—especially in early stages of the disease.

hypodensities in the basal ganglia usually found in these cases are suggestive of mitochondrial disorder. Psychiatric symptoms may be a feature (Richfield *et al.* 1987). The differential diagnosis of these 'holes' in the central nuclei is shown in Table 10.6.

DEGENERATIVE DISORDERS WITH CALCIFICATION OF THE BASAL GANGLIA

Idiopathic calcification of the basal ganglia is still commonly termed Fahr disease although it results from a collection of different disorders that have little in common (Flint and Goldstein 1992). Table 10.7 indicates the main causes of the highly heterogeneous group of basal ganglia calcification disorders. From a pathological viewpoint, idiopathic cases are characterized by the presence of calcium within capillary walls, in the media of larger vessels or lying free in brain tissue. The calcification frequently extends beyond the limits of the basal ganglia, especially to the

TABLE 10.7
Main causes of calcification of the basal ganglia in infancy and childhood*

Cause	References†
Inflammatory causes	
Cytomegalovirus infection	
Toxoplasmosis	
Tuberculomas (solitary or multiple)	
Neurocysticercosis	
Polioencephalitis in immunodepressed patients	Davis *et al.* (1977)
HIV infection	Belman *et al.* (1986)
Encephalitis in Cree Indians	Black *et al.* (1988b)
Tumours and dysplasias	
Calcified astrocytoma of basal ganglia	
Subependymal astrocytoma	
Tuberous sclerosis	
Vascular and hypoxic causes	
Arteriovenous malformations of basal ganglia	
Calcified infarct	
Hypoxic–ischaemic encephalopathy	Bamford *et al.* (1988), Ansari *et al.* (1990)
Symmetrical thalamic degeneration in infancy	Abuelo *et al.* (1981), Di Mario and Clancy (1989)
Endocrine disorders	
Hypoparathyroidism	
Pseudo- and pseudopseudohypoparathyroidism	
Hyperparathyroidism	
Toxic disorders	
Carbon monoxide poisoning	Sawada *et al.* (1980)
Lead poisoning	
Hypervitaminosis D	
X-ray therapy of leukaemia or tumours with and without methotrexate	
Long-term therapy with acetazolamide	Katsumori *et al.* (1990)
Metabolic and heredodegenerative diseases	
Mitochondrial encephalomyopathy (MELAS and related diseases)	
Cockayne syndrome and related syndromes	
Calcification of basal ganglia with leukodystrophy and CSF lymphocytosis	
Familial calcification of basal ganglia	
Neuroaxonal dystrophy	Ramaekers *et al.* (1987)
Hallervorden–Spatz disease[1]	Savoiardo *et al.* (1993)
Dystonia–basal ganglia calcification syndrome	Larsen *et al.* (1985)
Biopterin deficiency	Woody *et al.* (1989)
Biotinidase deficiency	Schulz *et al.* (1988)
Carbonic anhydrase II deficiency	Ohlsson *et al.* (1986)
Microcephaly with calcification of basal ganglia	Baraitser *et al.* (1983)
Trichothiodystrophy	Happle *et al.* (1984)
Retinopathy with calcification of basal ganglia	Hammerstein *et al.* (1982)
Prenatal cerebral calcification, Coats disease, dysmorphism and movement disorder	Tolmie *et al.* (1988)
Miscellaneous	
Down syndrome	Takashima and Becker (1985)
Familial amentia with familial calcification of choroid plexus and raised CSF protein[2]	Lott *et al.* (1979)
CDG syndrome[3]	Stibler and Jaeken (1990)
Lupus erythematosus	Nordstrom *et al.* (1985)
Lethal arthrogryposis with calcification	Illune *et al.* (1988)

*Calcification of the basal ganglia may be associated with calcification of the dentate nuclei. The latter may occasionally be isolated (Koller and Klawans 1980). It may also occur with eosinophilic granuloma (Adornato *et al.* 1980) and in central neurofibromatosis (Van Tassel *et al.* 1987).

†References given only for unusual causes.

[1]May not be true calcification but rather iron storage.

[2]Calcification mainly in choroid plexuses.

[3]Diffuse calcification of white matter.

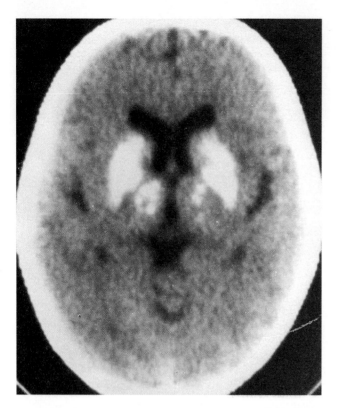

Fig. 10.12. Idiopathic calcification of basal nuclei in 10-year-old girl with progressive extrapyramidal rigidity and dystonia and mental deterioration. (By permission of Adis Health Science Press, Sydney.)

dentate nuclei but also to the white matter, cortex and brainstem (Fig. 10.12). Associated neuronal lesions are highly variable depending on aetiology. *Mitochondrial diseases* are a prominent cause and should be systematically sought. Calcification should be distinguished from high signal in T_1-weighted sequences that may be seen in chronic liver disease (Pujol *et al.* 1993) and as a result of manganese toxicity in children receiving prolonged parenteral nutrition (Mirowitz *et al.* 1991).

HYPOPARATHYROIDISM AND
PSEUDOHYPOPARATHYROIDISM
Primary hypoparathyroidism is usually transmitted as an X-linked condition (Patten *et al.* 1990). Attacks of tetany with epileptic seizures and carpopedal and laryngeal spasms are major acute manifestations and can be precipitated by hyperpnoea. Mental retardation or psychosis is present in 60 per cent of cases, extrapyramidal signs in 30 per cent and signs of intracranial hypertension in 25–30 per cent. Cataracts and skin lesions are common. Chvostek sign is nonspecific, and the diagnosis rests on demonstration of low calcium and high phosphorus levels. Punctate calcification may also involve the white matter especially in the frontal lobes (Fig. 10.12). In *pseudoparahypothyroidism*, similar manifestations are associated with obesity, a moon-shaped facies, mental retardation, short metacarpals (especially the third and fourth) and impaired sense of taste and smell. Calcification is present in one-third of cases. This condition, also known as Albright hereditary osteodystrophy, is dominantly inherited. The

condition is more common in females and is caused by an inability of the renal tubule to respond to parathyroid hormone as a result of reduced expression or function of the alpha subunit of a stimulatory G protein of adenylate cyclase which is necessary for the action of parathyroid and other hormones that use cyclic AMP as an intracellular second messenger (Patten *et al.* 1990). The same morphological syndrome without abnormality of calcium/phosphorus metabolism is known as pseudopseudohypoparathyroidism but is also a part of Albright osteodystrophy as shown by the occurrence of cases both with and without calcium/phosphorus disturbances in the same kindreds.

IDIOPATHIC CALCIFICATION OF THE BASAL GANGLIA
A few families are on record with striopallidodentate calcification unassociated with any abnormality of the parathyroid or kidney or any dysmorphism. Such calcification may remain asymptomatic for many years and only give rise to extrapyramidal symptoms and signs in adulthood (Laxova *et al.* 1985). The disease can be recessively (Ellie *et al.* 1989, Manyam *et al.* 1992) or dominantly (Kobari *et al.* 1997) inherited. No mitochondrial abnormality has been found. Martinelli *et al.* (1993) found a possible deficit in vitamin D_3 25-hydroxylase.

OSTEOPETROSIS, RENAL ACIDOSIS AND CEREBRAL
CALCIFICATION (CARBONIC ANHYDRASE II DEFICIENCY:
MARBLE BONES–MARBLE BRAIN DISEASE)
This is a rare autosomal recessive disease characterized by mental retardation and somatic growth delay, dense bones, antimongoloid eye slant and a small mandible (Ohlsson *et al.* 1986). The disorder was first reported from the Middle East (Al Rajeh *et al.* 1988) but is also observed in Europeans (Sly *et al.* 1985) in whom it is mainly manifested by fractures. The degree of brain calcification is impressive.

OTHER DISORDERS WITH BASAL GANGLIA
CALCIFICATION
These are dealt with in various chapters. A special mention should be made of brain calcification in children with AIDS because this is now a common disease that can mimic any progressive CNS disorder and in which basal ganglia calcification is present in 20–30 per cent of cases (Belman *et al.* 1986). Nonfamilial calcification of the basal ganglia is frequent in Down syndrome (Takashima and Becker 1985). Physiological calcification of the basal ganglia is so rare in children—it occurred in only 0.03 per cent of 18,000 paediatric CTs reported by Kendall and Cavanagh (1986)—that it can be considered abnormal in virtually all cases. It is frequent following CNS irradiation for leukaemia or other malignancies. Isolated calcification of the cerebellum may occur in type 2 neurofibromatosis (Chapter 4).

TARDIVE DYSKINESIA
Tardive dyskinesia is observed only in children receiving or having received neuroleptic drugs, especially phenothiazines, butyrophenones or diphenylbutylpiperidine (Gualtieri *et al.* 1984, Singer 1986). The incidence is poorly known. Several types can

occur. Tardive dyskinesia proper usually appears in children who have been receiving high doses of these medications for months or years, or with an increase in dosage. However, even low doses for short periods have uncommonly been responsible. The most usual type of movement is orofacial dyskinesia with stereotypic protrusion of the tongue, lip smacking or chewing motions. The intensity is variable.

Other types of dyskinesia may be observed such as dystonic or choreic movements. The abnormal movements can improve following discontinuation of the responsible drug over a period of several months but are permanent in about one third of patients.

Various types of dyskinesia may supervene on withdrawal of neuroleptics. These do not usually include orofacial movements, and they tend to disappear in a few weeks or months.

The mechanisms of tardive dyskinesia are imperfectly understood. Supersensitivity of dopamine receptors induced by the medication plays a major role. However, why only some patients are affected is unexplained.

Treatment of tardive dyskinesia is unsatisfactory. Drugs used in the treatment of movement disorders such as tetrabenazine or clonidine are rarely effective. Clozapine may be more efficacious but can induce agranulocytosis (Lieberman *et al.* 1991). Limitation of the use of neuroleptics in children is strongly advised.

TICS AND GILLES DE LA TOURETTE SYNDROME

Tics are involuntary, purposeless contractions of functionally related groups of skeletal muscles, involuntary noises or involuntary utterance of words. Motor tics are brief, rapid, sudden, unexpected, repetitive and stereotypic. Although they can be voluntarily suppressed for variable periods of time, they cannot be resisted indefinitely. They often predominate on facial muscles. Typical movements include eye blinking, contraction of neck or shoulder muscles, sniffing or snorting. Tics are probably caused by some disturbance of the motor system, especially the basal ganglia (Singer 1994), with a compulsory component. Psychic disturbances that are frequently associated may be in part secondary to the social inconvenience of the abnormal movements (Fahn 1982, Jankovic and Fahn 1986). Vocal tics are less common and may be of more serious significance than simple motor tics. Isolated transient tics are very common and usually disappear in a few months. Chronic motor tics and multiple chronic tics are less common and tend to persist.

Tourette syndrome (Chapter 28) is defined by four criteria: (1) multiple motor tics; (2) one or more vocal tics; (3) age of onset <21 years; (4) duration >1 year (Kurlan *et al.* 1986). There is probably a continuum between multiple chronic tics and Tourette syndrome which appear to be genetically related (Pauls and Leckman 1986). Coprolalia and echolalia are often lacking in otherwise typical cases, and there is a tendency to diagnose Tourette syndrome when multiple motor and vocal tics occur in a patient (Comings and Comings 1985, Park *et al.* 1993). Tourette syndrome is often familial (Kurlan *et al.* 1986) and has been reported in monozygotic twins. No pathological basis is known (Haber *et al.* 1986), although decreased volume of the basal ganglia on MRI has been reported (Singer *et al.* 1993). Boys are affected three to four times more often than girls. Marked emotional overtones, which are almost always present, may well be secondary features. Attention deficit disorder and obsessive–compulsive traits are present in 50 per cent of patients (Golden 1990). The onset of tics, whether simple or multiple, is between 5 and 10 years. Tourette syndrome may last for life but complete remissions are possible. Treatment is discussed in Chapter 28.

Several abnormal movement disorders that seem related to tics but also include echopraxia and suggestibility have been reported from Maine as 'jumping Frenchmen of Maine' (Saint-Hilaire *et al.* 1986) and from other parts of the world as 'latah' or 'myriachit' (Andermann and Andermann 1986a).

MIRROR MOVEMENTS

Mirror movements are involuntary, symmetrical, identical movements associated with a voluntary movement carried out by the contralateral limb in particular finger motions. They may be congenital and familial, following a dominant mendelian pattern (Rasmussen 1993), and are not associated with any brain pathology. In some cases, cervical abnormalities such as Klippel–Feil syndrome may be associated. They may occur with cervical spina bifida, so an X-ray of the spinal cord should be obtained (Rasmussen 1993). They may be associated with Kallmann syndrome (Schwankhaus *et al.* 1989; see Chapter 21). Mirror movements may also occur in patients with childhood hemiparesis (Cohen *et al.* 1991). The mechanism of mirror movement is unclear. The abnormal movements tend to decrease with age but they often persist into adulthood.

HEREDITARY TREMOR AND MYOCLONUS (ESSENTIAL TREMOR AND MYOCLONUS)

ESSENTIAL TREMOR

Essential tremor is a relatively common disorder usually transmitted as an autosomal dominant character (Lou and Jankovic 1991, Bain *et al.* 1994). Sporadic cases are known to occur. The tremor may appear as early as 5 years of age. Shuddering attacks in young children may be the first manifestation of the condition (Vanasse *et al.* 1976). In nine of 42 cases (26 of which were isolated) reported by Critchley (1972), onset was before 20 years of age. The abnormal movements are rhythmical and oscillatory. They are absent at rest and increase with action and maintenance of postures. In adults, they are suppressed or considerably improved by alcohol ingestion. Although the syndrome is progressive at onset, it later stabilizes. Neurological examination is normal as is neurodevelopmental progress. Diagnosis is easy if familial cases are known. Otherwise, physiological tremor and rare cases of symptomatic tremor (Gordon *et al.* 1992) have to be excluded. Treatment is not needed in many cases. If necessary, propanolol is the first choice drug. Primidone is also effective (Seyfert *et al.* 1988, Lou and Jankovic 1991). Clonazepam may be useful in some cases.

Familial trembling of the chin is a benign condition (Alsager *et al.* 1991) that may be socially disabling. Although treatment with botulinum toxin has been used (Gordon *et al.* 1993), no treatment is usually indicated.

ESSENTIAL MYOCLONUS

Essential myoclonus (paramyoclonus multiplex) is characterized by brief, shock-like muscle contractions that may be more or less widespread and constitute the sole neurological abnormality. Aetiology is unknown but familial cases with dominant inheritance are frequent.

The disorder usually has its onset after 5–7 years of age. Muscles of the trunk are more commonly affected than those of the limbs (Bressman and Fahn 1986), but any territory can be involved. It appears that several neurophysiological mechanisms may be at play (Hallett *et al.* 1979). Ballistic overflow myoclonus (Hallettt *et al.* 1977) induced by rapid ballistic movements is one model of idiopathic intention myoclonus. Tremor and myoclonus may be difficult to distinguish. Indeed, their coexistence in different members of the same family has been reported (Korten *et al.* 1974). Cases of essential myoclonus with onset in early infancy have been observed (E. Fernandez, personal communication 1997).

Acquired postinfectious myoclonus is very similar to the essential type but appears acutely following a febrile disease of possible viral origin (Bhatia *et al.* 1992). Similar cases following group A beta-haemolytic *Streptococcus* infections have been reported (Di Fazio *et al.* 1997).

Palatal myoclonus may be symptomatic of a brainstem lesion, although this is exceptional in children, or idiopathic (Deuschl *et al.* 1994). The term 'tremor' is more correct as the movement is typically periodic. Symptomatic myoclonus may be associated with obscure degenerative diseases (Sperling and Herman 1985, Howard *et al.* 1993, Malandrini *et al.* 1996b). The idiopathic type occurs in isolation, often revealed by audible clicks in the ears. It disappears after a variable duration and seems entirely benign (Boulloche and Aicardi 1984, Corbin and Williams 1987, Yokota *et al.* 1990).

The *treatment* of myoclonus may be difficult. Clonazepam is often effective. According to Obeso *et al.* (1989), a combination of clonazepam, piracetam, mysoline and sodium valproate gives good results in crippling forms. Some cases may respond to 5-hydroxytryptophan.

THE PROGRESSIVE MYOCLONIC EPILEPSIES

Progressive myoclonic epilepsies with known metabolic defects have been considered in Chapter 9. This paragraph deals with the so-called 'degenerative' types (Marseille Consensus Group 1990, Berkovic *et al.* 1993) and Lafora disease. Both disorders combine generalized tonic–clonic or massive myoclonic jerks, localized myoclonus which may be spontaneous but is often induced by external stimuli such as touch, action or intention, and various degrees of neurological and mental deterioration. Mitochondrial disorders, however, can produce a similar clinical picture

TABLE 10.8
Diseases featuring progressive myoclonic epilepsy (PME)

Diseases in which PME syndrome is pure or in forefront of clinical picture
Lafora disease
Unverricht–Lundborg syndrome*
Sialidosis (types I and II)
Juvenile neuroaxonal dystrophy
Juvenile Gaucher disease (type III) (Nishimura *et al.* 1980)
Myoclonic epilepsy with ragged red fibres (MERRF)
PME with lipomas (Ekbom syndrome)** (Berkovic *et al.* 1993)
PME with deafness (May–White syndrome)** (Berkovic *et al.* 1993)
PME with renal failure** (Berkovic *et al.* 1993)
Hereditary dentatorubral–pallidoluysian degeneration

Diseases in which PME is atypical or associated with other manifestations
Neuronal ceroid–lipofuscinosis
   Early type (Santavuori–Hagberg disease)
   Late infantile type (Jansky–Bielschowsky disease)
   Juvenile type (Spielmeyer–Vogt disease)
Poliodystrophies with or without lactic acidosis and/or mitochondrial abnormalities
Huntington chorea (myoclonic variant) (Garrel *et al.* 1978)
Hallervorden–Spatz disease
Biopterin deficiency (Chapter 9)
Mitochondrial encephalomyopathy with lactic acidosis and stroke-like episodes (MELAS)

Diseases in which PME is overshadowed by other manifestations
Nonketotic hyperglycinaemia
D-glyceric aciduria
Biopterin deficiency
Menkes disease
Krabbe disease
Tay–Sachs disease
Sandhoff disease
Niemann–Pick C disease

Unless indicated, see text for references.
*The same (or a very similar) disorder is referred to as Ramsay Hunt syndrome in some publications (Genton *et al.* 1990).
**These syndromes may be related to the mitochondrial diseases.

(Fukuhara *et al.* 1980, Berkovic *et al.* 1993). The main disorders featuring myoclonus and myoclonic epilepsy are shown in Table 10.8. Before accepting the diagnosis of idiopathic progressive myoclonic epilepsy one should always first exclude the diagnosis of myoclonic encephalomyopathy with ragged red fibres (MERRF), if necessary by muscle biopsy and by searching for the mitochondrial DNA mutation.

LAFORA DISEASE

Lafora disease is the best defined type of myoclonus epilepsy with a detectable storage. Lafora (amyloid) bodies are found within neurons throughout the neuraxis, especially in the substantia nigra, dentate nucleus, reticular substance and hippocampus. They are also present in muscle and liver, and in sweat gland ducts in the skin thus permitting diagnosis by skin biopsy (Carpenter and Karpati 1981). Biochemically, Lafora bodies consist of a glucose polymer chemically related to glycogen in association with protein. The basic metabolic defect is unknown. The disease is inherited as an autosomal recessive trait and has recently been mapped to chromosome 6q23–q25.

The onset of *clinical manifestations* is between 6 and 19 years and is marked in 80 per cent of cases by epileptic seizures, mainly myoclonic, clonic or tonic–clonic in type. Partial seizures with visual symptoms are associated in half the cases (Roger *et al.* 1983). Erratic, fragmentary myoclonic jerks and massive myoclonias are constantly associated and are exaggerated by movement and intention. Mental retardation is often rapidly progressive but may be absent for several years. Pyramidal, extrapyramidal and cerebellar signs appear after a variable delay.

The EEG initially shows discharges of polyspike–wave complexes. Background rhythm then deteriorates.

Death occurs, on average, 5–6 years after onset. Skin biopsy is the best diagnostic method. Liver and muscle biopsy can also reveal the polyglucosan storage.

No therapy is available, except symptomatic treatment of epilepsy.

UNVERRICHT–LUNDBORG DISEASE (BALTIC MYOCLONUS, RAMSAY HUNT SYNDROME)

This disorder is the best example of the degenerative myoclonic epilepsies. It is transmitted as an autosomal recessive condition (Norio and Koskiniemi 1979). It is apparent that cases reported as Baltic myoclonus by some groups and as Ramsay Hunt syndrome by others (Roger *et al.* 1987) in fact represent the same disease. The pathology is limited to the cerebellum with loss of Purkinje cells and sometimes of neurons in deep cerebellar nuclei and inferior olive (Friede 1989). Onset of the clinical manifestations occurs between 6 and 16 years with tonic–clonic seizures in 50 per cent of cases and myoclonic seizures in the other half (Koskiniemi *et al.* 1974a). The myoclonus disappears during sleep or rest and is induced by external stimuli but mainly by maintenance of posture or intended movement. Its intensity increases progressively and it becomes totally incapacitating in adulthood. Epileptic seizures are seldom severe and include generalized tonic–clonic fits, often occurring on awakening, and massive myoclonic jerks very similar to those in Janz syndrome (Chapter 16). Absences or drop-attacks are observed in a minority of patients. Intelligence is relatively preserved but in most cases there is a slow and mild deterioration. Kyllerman *et al.* (1991) reported the occurrence of 'cascades' of seizures and myoclonic jerks. Neurological signs such as intention tremor tend to appear after a few years but pyramidal tract signs are seen in only one-third of cases (Berkovic *et al.* 1993). Cerebellar signs are very difficult to assess because of the intention myoclonus. The EEG seems to show variable slowing of background activity with superimposed paroxysmal activity (Koskiniemi *et al.* 1974b). In some cases the background rhythm remains normal for many years aside from paroxysmal abnormalities identical to those in the primary generalized epilepsies. Runs of spikes appear at the vertex during REM sleep. Such differences are considered to be of nosological significance by some investigators who prefer to separate a subgroup of Mediterranean myoclonus (Genton *et al.* 1990) from the Baltic form that corresponds to the original description of Unverricht. However, both types are linked to the same locus on chromosome 21 (Malafosse *et al.* 1992, Cochius

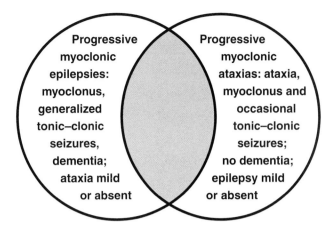

Fig. 10.13. Nosological relationships between progressive myoclonic epilepsies and ataxias (after Marsden *et al.* 1990). Note overlap between the two groups. The term 'Ramsay Hunt syndrome' is applied to either group by different authors.

et al. 1993), and the same mutation has been found in both Finnish and Italian cases (Lehesjoki *et al.* 1997). Giant somaesthetic evoked potentials are present in all cases, indicating a cortical-type myoclonus (Hallett *et al.* 1979, Shibasaki *et al.* 1986). The treatment is that of intention myoclonus, and the use of polytherapy with sodium valproate, primidone, clonazepam and 5-hydroxytryptophan and/or piracetam may be effective (Obeso *et al.* 1989). Phenytoin may aggravate incapacity and is contraindicated. The prognosis is poor from a functional standpoint, but with modern treatment the disease is rarely life-threatening. The term Ramsay Hunt syndrome remains controversial. For some investigators it designates a disorder identical with or similar to Unverricht–Lundborg disease. For other authors (Lance 1986, Marsden *et al.* 1990) it applies to a progressive ataxia associated with intention myoclonus, with or without epilepsy but accompanied by cerebellar signs (Fig. 10.13).

OTHER RARE DEGENERATIVE MYOCLONIC EPILEPSIES

The reader is referred to the reviews by Berkovic *et al.* (1993) and the Marseille Consensus Group (1990) for details. At least some of the rare syndromes classically described, *e.g.* myoclonic epilepsy and deafness (May–White syndrome) and myoclonic epilepsy with lipomas (Ekbom syndrome) should now be classified among the mitochondrial disorders. The nosological situation of myoclonic epilepsy associated with Friedreich ataxia (Ziegler *et al.* 1974) is uncertain. The syndrome of myoclonic epilepsy with renal failure (Andermann *et al.* 1986b) has been described so far in only two families. A unique syndrome of severe course has been reported by Logigian *et al.* (1986).

HEREDITARY DENTATORUBRAL–PALLIDOLUYSIAN ATROPHY

This disorder shares features of both the myoclonic epilepsies and other movement disorders of extrapyramidal origin. Pathologically, there is atrophy of the dentatorubral efferent system as in

TABLE 10.9
Metabolic and acquired disturbances encountered in patients with a clinical picture of spinocerebellar degeneration

Disorder	References
Disorders of proven metabolic nature for which a reliable diagnosis is feasible	
Adrenomyeloneuropathy	Chapter 9; Maris *et al.* (1995)
GM1 gangliosidosis	Goldman *et al.* (1981)
GM2 gangliosidosis	Specola *et al.* (1990)
Abetalipoproteinaemia	Illingworth *et al.* (1980)
Vitamin E deficiency	Stumpf *et al.* (1987), Ben Hamida *et al.* (1993), Gotoda *et al.* (1995)
Variant of HGPRT deficiency	Page *et al.* (1987)
Variant of hyperglycinaemia	Bank and Morrow (1972)
Mevalonic aciduria	Hoffmann *et al.* (1993)
Cholestanolosis	Kuriyama *et al.* (1991)
Refsum disease	Chapter 21
Defects found in patients with spinocerebellar degeneration, the significance of which is not yet clear	
Pyruvate dehydrogenase complex deficiency	Robinson *et al.* (1988)
Glutamate dehydrogenase deficiency	Plaitakis *et al.* (1984)
Mitochondrial malic enzyme deficiency	Stumpf *et al.* (1982)
Other disorders that may produce a similar clinical picture	
Alpers disease (late forms)	Harding *et al.* (1995)
Human lymphotropic virus types 1 and 2 infection	Salazar-Grueso *et al.* (1990)
Langerhans histiocytosis	Goldberg-Stern *et al.* (1995)
Pelizaeus–Merzbacher disease and some other slowly progressive leukodystrophies	See text
Some cases of ataxic diplegia and sequelae of cardiac arrest	Lance (1986)
Creutzfeld–Jakob disease, Gerstmann–Sträussler–Scheinker disease and other prion diseases	Chapter 11
Ataxia–telangiectasia	Chapter 4
Ataxia–oculomotor apraxia	Aicardi *et al.* (1988)

Ramsay Hunt syndrome, associated with pallidoluysian non-specific atrophy (Iizuka *et al.* 1984). The clinical features include myoclonus, tonic–clonic seizures, choreoathetosis, cerebellar signs and dementia. Onset is usually in adulthood. Childhood cases are on record (Minami *et al.* 1994); they usually present with myoclonic epilepsy and dementia. The disorder is usually dominantly inherited with anticipation. Occasional sporadic cases occur. The disease seems uncommon outside Japan, although cases have been reported in Europeans (Warner *et al.* 1995). The disease is due to an expansion of a CAG trinucleotide repeat on chromosome 12. Early-onset forms are associated with longer repeats and are usually severe (Ikeuchi *et al.* 1995).

HEREDODEGENERATIVE DISEASES OF CEREBELLUM, BRAINSTEM AND SPINAL CORD (SPINOCEREBELLAR DEGENERATIONS AND RELATED CONDITIONS)

The term spinocerebellar degeneration designates a broad category of diseases that are characterized by untimely death of cells in certain systems or structures as a consequence of some essential defect of 'vital endurance' known as 'abiotrophy'. This premature failure of specific cellular systems or pathways may be the result of a defect in energy metabolism of the neurons or be due to abnormalities in structural proteins. Although many

molecular genetic abnormalities have been discovered in the past few years, little is currently known about the gene products and their role. None of the proposed metabolic defects has been confirmed. However, glutamate dehydrogenase deficiency has been repeatedly found in adult cases (Plaitakis *et al.* 1984) although its significance remains obscure. It is essential to remember that cases of so-called atypical spinocerebellar degeneration can belong to completely different diseases with demonstrable metabolic defect that permit a more precise diagnosis, genetic counselling and sometimes prenatal diagnosis (Tables 10.9, 10.10). This applies especially to some forms of leukodystrophies, to adrenoleukodystrophies and to deficits in hexosaminidases.

Because of the absence of biochemical markers, many systems of classification of the spinocerebellar degenerations have been proposed. Pathological classification (Table 10.10) is not convincing because the lesions associated with the same genetic defect are variable and even the pathological findings in several cases of the same family may not be identical. Thus cases of olivopontocerebellar atrophy can coexist in the same pedigree with cases that do not involve the olivary nuclei (Sequeiros and Suite 1986), and cases from the same family have been classified under different subgroups (Konigsmark and Weiner 1970). To avoid such difficulties, Harding (1981a,b,c, 1993) proposed a scheme based on clinical and genetic data which is convenient for classification of the common types (Table 10.11). Progress in molecular genetics, by permitting determination of genotypes,

TABLE 10.10
Spinocerebellar degeneration: pathological data

Main location of pathological findings	Disorder	Subtypes
Cerebellum and inferior olivary nucleus	Cerebello-olivary atrophy (adults)	With hypogonadism (Matthews–Rundle syndrome)
Brainstem and cerebellum	Olivopontocerebellar atrophy	Menzel type (centripetal); Déjerine–Thomas type (centrifugal); with retinal degeneration
Spinal cord	Familial spastic paraplegia; familial spastic ataxia; isolated involvement of posterior columns (Biemond syndrome)	Pure forms; complicated forms
Spinal cord and peripheral sensory nerves	Friedreich ataxia	
Peripheral nerves	Hereditary sensory and motor/sensory neuropathies	

TABLE 10.11
Classification of the hereditary spinocerebellar ataxias*

Autosomal recessive ataxias

Friedreich ataxia (FA) and variants due to mutation of the FA gene on chromosome 9

Early-onset ataxia with retained deep tendon reflexes. Probably a heterogeneous group including very early and later onset forms. Some cases may be atypical forms of FA

Other rare forms with associated features, *e.g.* hypogonadism, cataracts, retinopathy, deafness or myoclonus

Autosomal dominant cerebellar ataxias (ADCAs)

ADCA1: Mostly in adults but childhood cases exist. Many cases in this group were previously classified as olivopontocerebellar atrophies (OPCAs). Signs variably include optic atrophy, cranial nerve deficits, pyramidal and extrapyramidal signs, peripheral neuropathy, sometimes dementia. Subdivided into several spinocerebellar atrophies (SCAs):
    SCA1
    SCA2
    SCA3/Machado–Joseph disease
    SCA4
    SCA5
    SCA6
ADCA2: Previously classified as OPCA3, associated with retinal (macular) degeneration
ADCA3: Isolated cerebellar involvement

X-linked cerebellar ataxias

*Adapted from Harding (1993).

will eventually lead to a completely new classification (Rosenberg 1995). Currently, Harding's scheme is useful and takes into account the clinical presentation of the conditions. In this classification, Friedreich ataxia stands out as a clearly defined entity inherited according to an autosomal recessive pattern, even though dominant forms which should be classified differently had

been described earlier. More recently, linkage studies have established that the dominant forms of spinocerebellar degeneration are not all linked to the same chromosome and should therefore be regarded as a heterogeneous group (Zoghbi *et al.* 1988). It now seems clear that the spinocerebellar degenerations comprise a large number of unrelated diseases which are grouped only for convenience although they have different modes of inheritance (Farlow *et al.* 1987). It is impossible, in many cases, to decide whether one is dealing with a single condition with different clinical presentations or with separate disorders that share some common clinical and pathological features. For practical purposes atypical cases should suggest other diagnoses (Table 10.10). Transmissible diseases such as result from slow viruses (HTLV1 and 2) and unconventional agents or prions (Hsiao and Prusiner 1990) may also produce slowly progressive disorders mimicking spinocerebellar degenerations although they are rare in children. Rare cases of paraneoplasic ataxia are on record (Topçu *et al.* 1992).

RECESSIVELY TRANSMITTED ATAXIAS
FRIEDREICH ATAXIA
Friedreich ataxia is the best delineated and most common spinocerebellar degeneration. The gene frequency is 1 per 110 persons in England (Harding 1981a), and about 1 in 10,000 persons are clinically affected in Sweden.

The gene for Friedreich ataxia has recently been isolated. It includes a repeat GAA sequence in intron 1 that is expanded in affected persons (120–1700 repeats). The normal gene product is a protein of unknown function termed frataxin. Ninety-four per cent of patients with typical Friedreich ataxia are homozygous for the GAA expansion, although the length of the repeat is usually unequal on each of the pair of chromosomes (Dürr *et al.* 1996a). A few have only one expanded sequence, but a point mutation at the homologous locus has been demonstrated in several such cases (Campuzano *et al.* 1996). Large expansions are correlated with an early onset, a more rapid course and the presence of cardiomyopathy (Dürr *et al.* 1996a). The main pathological lesion is a dying-back neuropathy that affects neurons of the long ascending and descending tracks of the spinal cord and the large sensory fibres of peripheral nerves, and posterior root ganglia (Ouvrier *et al.* 1982, Saïd *et al.* 1986). Loss of nerve fibres has also been documented in the optic pathways but the cerebellum itself is largely unaffected. The heart is enlarged and in most cases there is hypertrophic cardiomyopathy with necrosis of fibres and fibrosis mainly involving the left ventricle. The criteria for the diagnosis of Friedreich ataxia include an onset before 25 years of age (usually before 16 years), an autosomal recessive inheritance and the combined involvement of large sensory fibres in peripheral nerve, cerebellar tracts, pyramidal tracts and posterior columns. Allegedly dominant cases appear to be cases of hereditary motor and sensory neuropathy with skeletal deformities and sensory loss, but some cases may be impossible to classify.

The *clinical manifestations* of Friedreich ataxia have been determined in 115 patients from 90 families by Harding (1981a).

TABLE 10.12
Signs and symptoms of Friedreich ataxia

Sign or symptom	Frequency
Onset before 20 years of age (mean age 10.5 ± 7.4 y)	100%
Progressive ataxia	100%
Dysarthria	100%
Abolished deep tendon reflexes	100%*
Extensor plantar response	>90%
Disturbances of deep sensation	>90%
Cardiomyopathy	60–90%
Weakness + amyotrophy of lower limbs	50–80%
Skeletal deformities (scoliosis and/or pes cavus)	90%
Optic atrophy	15–30%
Nystagmus	20–50%
Motor conduction velocity	Slightly decreased (in most cases)
Sensory conduction velocity	Slightly decreased (in most cases)
Sensory evoked potential	Absent or markedly reduced (always)
Visual evoked potential	Diminished, delayed (in 60%)
Diabetes mellitus	10–25%

Data from Harding (1981b).
*Reflexes may be retained at onset (Salih *et al.* 1990). An important negative finding from this study was that—despite reported associations in the literature—in no case was either dementia or a CT scan finding of cerebellar atrophy a feature of Friedreich ataxia.

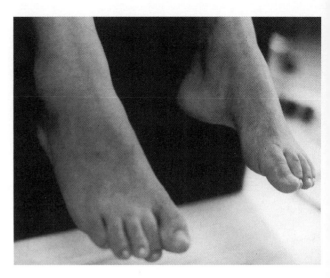

Fig. 10.14. Friedreich ataxia: typical pes cavus.

The main features are shown in Table 10.12. The onset is mostly between 5 and 16 years with a few cases manifesting between 2 and 5 years. Progressive ataxia of lower limbs with gait disturbance is the main presenting manifestation, whereas involvement of upper limbs with resulting clumsiness is seen early in only 25 per cent of cases. Scoliosis, tremor and cardiac symptoms are rarely the first manifestation, but they eventually develop especially in those with early onset. Pes cavus is also an early sign (Fig. 10.14). Examination shows absent deep tendon reflexes (70–95 per cent of cases). Dysarthria, pyramidal tract signs in the legs, and loss of joint-position and vibration sense may appear later but are constant findings. Nystagmus is infrequent (20 per cent of cases), and slow broken pursuit eye movements are present in 12 per cent of cases (Harding 1981a). Optic atrophy is not rare but deafness occurs in only 10 per cent of patients. Distal wasting is present in almost half the cases. Intelligence is consistently unaffected.

Cardiac involvement is found by ECG in two-thirds of cases or even more when echocardiography is systematically performed (Morvan *et al.* 1992). T-wave changes and abnormalities of the ST segment are early signs but cardiac failure is seldom a presenting feature (Tsao *et al.* 1992). Progressive cardiac failure or arrhythmia with atrial fibrillation eventually develops, and over half the patients die of cardiac failure (Leone *et al.* 1988).

The neurological course is relentlessly progressive. On average, in Harding's series, patients were unable to walk by 25 years of age after a median duration of 15.5 years.

Diabetes mellitus is a further complication in 10 per cent of patients (Finocchiaro *et al.* 1988). It tends to be associated with optic atrophy, and diabetic coma is sometimes the cause of death.

Atypical forms include mild cases that seem to be linked to the same locus on chromosome 9 (Keats *et al.* 1989), cases with preserved deep tendon reflexes (Palau *et al.* 1995), and late forms with onset in early adulthood (Berciano *et al.* 1993, Klockgether *et al.* 1993, De Michele *et al.* 1994). Recent work taking advantage of possible detection of the mutant gene suggests that the clinical picture is more variable than previously thought (Palau *et al.* 1995). Twenty-five per cent of patients in one large series (Dürr *et al.* 1996a) had one or more atypical feature (onset after 25 years, retained or even brisk tendon reflexes or absence of Babinski sign).

The *diagnosis* of Friedreich ataxia is based on clinical findings. CT scan is regularly normal thus excluding tumour or hydrocephalus. MRI shows the absence of cerebellar atrophy and a small cervical spinal cord (Wüllner *et al.* 1993). Motor and sensory nerve conduction velocities are normal or mildly slowed but the evoked sensory nerve potential is absent or considerably reduced in amplitude (Ouvrier *et al.* 1982). Visual evoked responses are abnormal in two-thirds of patients (Pinto *et al.* 1988), and colour vision is impaired in 40 per cent of cases even though the ERG is normal.

Friedreich ataxia is usually a fairly stereotyped disease easy to differentiate from other spinocerebellar degenerations described below (De Michele *et al.* 1996), although incomplete forms are not rare at onset (Berciano *et al.* 1997). Ataxia–telangiectasia (Chapter 4) has an earlier onset. Cutaneous manifestations and repeated infections are suggestive. The recently described condition of ataxia–ocular motor apraxia (Aicardi *et al.* 1988) has characteristic eye-movement findings. The so-called intermediate forms between Friedreich ataxia and the heredodegenerative motor and sensory neuropathies can usually be classified into either type. The Roussy–Lévy syndrome is not a *forme fruste* of Friedreich ataxia but a variant of the heredodegenerative hyper-

TABLE 10.13
Early spastic ataxias: frequency of signs and symptoms in three series

Signs/symptoms	Ataxia with retained deep reflexes (Harding 1981b)	Charlevoix–Saguenay disease (Bouchard et al. 1978)	Spastic ataxia (Hogan and Bauman 1977)
Onset before age 20 years	20/20	14/14	5/5
Progressive ataxia	20/20	14/14	5/5
Dysarthria	20/20	14/14	5/5
Extensor plantar responses	19/20	14/14	4/5
Spasticity of lower limbs	12/20	14/14	2/5
Deep tendon reflexes present or exaggerated	20/20	14/14	5/5
Decreased deep sensation	11/20	14/14	3/5
Skeletal deformities	12/20	12/14	3/5
Weakness and amyotrophy	6/20	Frequent[1]	0/5
Nystagmus or abnormal ocular movements	8/20	14/14	5/5
Mental deterioration	0/20	0	3/5
Optic atrophy	0/20	0[2]	4/5
Cardiomyopathy	0/20	0	0/5
Motor conduction velocity normal	6/6	100%[3]	—
Sensory evoked potential decreased	2/6	14/14	—
Cerebellar atrophy	5/9[4]	2/2[5]	—

[1]In lower limbs.
[2]Myelin striae radiating from the papilla are characteristic.
[3]Not reported in this paper (personal communication).
[4]CT scan.
[5]Pneumoencephalography.

trophic neuropathies (Lapresle 1982). The neural forms of hereditary motor and sensory neuropathy constitute by far the most common area of misdiagnosis. It is important not to diagnose them as Friedreich ataxia as their prognosis is much more favourable (Chapter 22). Primary or secondary vitamin E deficiency may closely simulate Friedreich ataxia (Stumpf *et al.* 1987, Ben Hamida *et al.* 1993) and these are treatable (Chapter 21).

No *treatment* is known for Friedreich ataxia except for remedial exercises and the maintenance of as high a degree of activity as possible. Surgery may prolong the ability to walk. Various trials such as amantadine (Peterson *et al.* 1988) or the ketogenic diet have not been conclusive.

OTHER RECESSIVELY TRANSMITTED SPINOCEREBELLAR ATAXIAS
Early onset ataxia with retained deep tendon reflexes
Harding (1981b), in her study of 200 patients with progressive ataxia, found 20 cases of early-onset ataxia apparently transmitted as an autosomal recessive character (Table 10.13). Fourteen similar cases with a mean age of onset of 15.9 ± 6.0 years and a strong male predominance (11/14) were reported by Klockgether *et al.* (1991). The disorder was marked by a progressive ataxia, especially of gait, developing during the first two decades of life. There was marked to moderate dysarthria and pyramidal tract signs. Knee jerks were present but ankle jerks were absent in some patients. No patient had optic atrophy, cardiomegaly, no

diabetes mellitus or severe skeletal deformities but some had pes cavus or mild scoliosis. Nerve conduction velocities and sensory evoked potentials were mildly reduced in two patients. Cerebellar atrophy was shown by CT scan in five of nine studied patients. There was no marked muscular weakness or wasting. The prognosis seems more favourable than in Friedreich ataxia, and ambulation is maintained on average 10 years longer. A recent study (Filla et al. 1990) indicates that this group is probably heterogeneous with both very early (<3 years) and later onsets. Moreover, some patients have evidence of corticospinal tract involvement or electrical evidence of motor and/or sensory neuropathy. Some cases have been shown to result from a Friedreich mutation (Dürr *et al.* 1996a) so the nosological situation of this group is not yet clear.

The condition reported by Harding is difficult to separate clearly from the childhood-onset cases described by Hogan and Bauman (1977) as *familial spastic ataxia* (Table 10.13) which appeared to be recessively inherited. However, some of the latter patients had optic atrophy and the course was more heterogeneous. A similar case associated with episodes of dystonia is on record (Graff-Radford 1986). In some genetic isolates, clusters of cases of spastic ataxia have been reported. The Charlevoix–Saguenay type in Quebec is characterized by an abnormal fundus and marked distal wasting (Bouchard *et al.* 1978) (Table 10.13). The Troyer syndrome (Cross and McKusick 1967) is closer to spastic paraplegia.

Behr syndrome

Behr syndrome or complicated optic atrophy is characterized by early optic atrophy associated with pes cavus, ataxia and spasticity with a slow progression (Horoupian *et al.* 1979, Marzan and Barron 1994). A neuropathy may be present. Occasional cases with pseudo-dominant inheritance are on record (Thomas *et al.* 1984). This disorder may be simulated by 3-methylglutaconic aciduria (Costeff *et al.* 1989).

Other rare forms

Rare diseases such as '*dégénerescence systématisée optico-cochléo-dentelée*'(Ferrer *et al.* 1987) or recessive spastic ataxia with corneal dystrophy, cataracts, macular degeneration and oval vertically tilted discs (Mousa *et al.* 1986) may belong to the spinocerebellar degeneration group.

Ataxia–oculomotor apraxia is a rare syndrome that closely resembles ataxia–telangiectasia but without evidence of extra-neurological involvement (Aicardi *et al.* 1988, Gascon *et al.* 1995). Unlike ataxia–telangiectasia, it is not associated with a raised alpha-fetoprotein level, chromosomal abnormalities or increased radiosensitivity of cultured fibroblasts (Hannan *et al.* 1994).

A familial association of cerebellar ataxia, posterior column dysfunction and sea-blue histiocytes in the bone marrow has been reported (Swaiman *et al.* 1975). Posterior column dysfunction associated with deafness, hypotonia, small stature and moderate delay has also been described (Koletzko *et al.* 1987, Thomson *et al.* 1990). Optic atrophy and myoclonus is on record (Senanayake 1992).

Various syndromes combine cerebellar ataxia with extra-neurological dysfunction. These include cases associated with renal disease, a syndrome of idiopathic diabetes insipidus and ataxia (Birnbaum *et al.* 1989), cases of ataxia and hypogonadism with hyper- or hyposecretion of gonadotrophins and various other features (Fok *et al.* 1989, De Michele *et al.* 1990, Toscano *et al.* 1995) and cases with osteosclerosis (Charrow *et al.* 1991). Some of the cases of ataxia with visceral involvement in children (Kawahara *et al.* 1988) probably belong to the carbohydrate-deficient glycoprotein (CDG) syndrome (Chapter 9).

AUTOSOMAL DOMINANT CEREBELLAR ATAXIA (ADCA)

ADCA forms a group of diseases (see Table 10.11) manifested by ataxia and other neurological features which are seen mostly in adults, with some early-onset cases. Pathologically, there is a progressive cerebellar atrophy and, in most cases, involvement of the spinal cord. In many cases the inferior olives and the intrinsic brainstem nuclei are involved in the degenerative process. Such cases are traditionally grouped under the heading of olivoponto-cerebellar atrophy (OPCA). However, the concept of OPCA is a purely pathological one and is therefore impossible to combine with the clinical and genetic classification used in this chapter. Moreover, it includes a number of heterogeneous diseases with diverse causes, and the distribution of lesions may vary within the same entity.

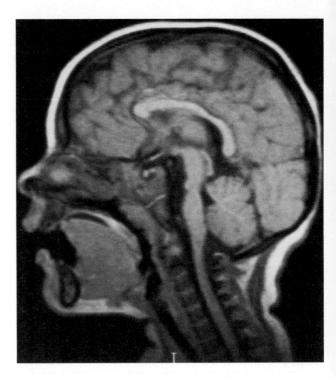

Fig. 10.15. Pontocerebellar atrophy in 2-year-old girl with mental retardation, atypical retinitis pigmentosa and ataxia. The brainstem is abnormally thin and there is no protrusion of the pons. The cerebellar vermis is relatively small.

ADCA observed in childhood includes two main forms, ADCA1 and 2 (Hammans 1996).

AUTOSOMAL DOMINANT CEREBELLAR ATAXIA TYPE 1 (ADCA1)

This disorder is common in adults but only rare cases occur in children. The clinical manifestations include progressive ataxia and a variety of associated abnormalities such as ophthalmo-paresis, optic atrophy, a rigid–akinetic syndrome, cranial nerve deficits, and loss of position and vibration sense (Genis *et al.* 1995, Bürk *et al.* 1996). Mild mental deterioration may occur. Peripheral neuropathy is possible (Bennett *et al.* 1984). The onset is usually between 20 and 40 years of age but the phenomenon of anticipation occurs in this condition so paediatric cases are seen. ADCA1 includes several genetically distinct entities (spinocerebellar ataxia or SCA types 1–6) whose clinical presentation is very similar (Rosenberg 1995).

In most cases, MRI shows marked cerebellar atrophy involving primarily the vermis, and brainstem atrophy particularly of the pons whose normal bulge is no longer visible (Wüllner *et al.* 1993) (Fig. 10.15).

Spinocerebellar ataxia type 1

This disease is due to an expansion of an unstable CAG repeat on chromosome 6p22–p23 (Giunti *et al.* 1994). SCA1 has been observed in children aged 12 years or more. Along with SCA3 it seems to be the most usual type of ADCA1 in Western European countries (Dürr *et al.* 1996c).

TABLE 10.14
TABLE 10.14
Congenital ataxias and cerebellar atrophies*

Disorder	Characteristic features	Genetics	References
Olivopontocerebellar hypoplasia (OPCH)**			
OPCH type 1	Anterior horn cell, involvement of spinal cord	AR	Goutières *et al.* (1977)
OPCH type 2	Microcephaly, movement disorder	AR	Barth (1993)
Carbohydrate-deficient glycoprotein syndrome CDG type 1	Dysmorphism, systemic involvement, stroke-like episodes, neuropathy	AR	Pavone *et al.* (1996)
Progressive encephalopathy with oedema, hypsarrhythmia and optic atrophy (PEHO syndrome)	Infantile spasms, peripheral oedema, dysmorphism	AR	Haltia and Somer (1993)
Cerebellar atrophies***			
Marinesco–Sjögren syndrome	Cataracts, muscle disease	AR	Superneau *et al.* (1987)
Norman's atrophy of granule cells	Microcephaly, mental retardation	AR?	Pascual-Castroviejo *et al.* (1994)
Infantile-onset spinocerebellar ataxia (IOSCA)	Sensory neuropathy, deafness, athetosis, epilepsy	AR	Koskinen *et al.* (1994)
With demyelination	Diffuse involvement	AR?	Chatkupt *et al.* (1993)
With deafness, loss of vision and quadriplegia	Diffuse involvement	XL?	Arts *et al.* (1993)
With retinopathy and hypogonadism	Normal intelligence	AR	Abs *et al.* (1990), Erdem *et al.* (1994)

*Differentiation between atrophy and hypoplasia may be artificial in some cases, and most disorders are slowly, if at all, progressive.
**Usually referred to as atrophies, the term hypoplasia is more exact.
***This is a confused group of rare disorders with various modes of inheritance, many of which are represented by very few or single cases.

Spinocerebellar ataxia types 2, 3 and 4
The loci for these forms have been mapped respectively to chromosomes 12q, 14q and 16q (Dubourg *et al.* 1995, Rosenberg 1995, Nechiporuk *et al.* 1996). The locus for SCA3 appears to be the same as that of Machado–Joseph disease (Dürr *et al.* 1996c). It is also an expanded CAG repeat (Tuite *et al.* 1995). *Machado–Joseph disease* is uncommon in children. The clinical presentation is variable. Some cases present mainly as parkinsonism, others as ophthalmoplegia with extrapyramidal features, some with cerebellar ataxia with or without peripheral neuropathy (Coutinho *et al.* 1982, Giunti *et al.* 1995, Matilla *et al.* 1995). The disease is not limited to persons originating from the Azores Islands, as was originally thought.

AUTOSOMAL DOMINANT CEREBELLAR ATAXIA TYPE 2 (ADCA2)
This condition was previously described as OPCA3. The picture in adults is that of a progressive cerebellar ataxia with macular degeneration. The latter may long be isolated. Anticipation can be observed in affected lineages, and a very early onset (from age 6 months) may occur (Benomar *et al.* 1994, Enevoldson *et al.* 1994). Such cases run a rapidly fatal course. Infants born to clinically unaffected parents may develop the disease, and in about 10 per cent of cases infants or children become symptomatic

before the affected parents (Enevoldson *et al.* 1994, Gouw *et al.* 1994). The gene maps to 3p12–p21.1 (Benomar *et al.* 1995).

AUTOSOMAL DOMINANT CEREBELLAR ATAXIA TYPE 3 (ADCA3)
This is a purely cerebellar degeneration of adults. A few families with early onset are on record (Frontali *et al.* 1992).

X-LINKED SPINOCEREBELLAR ATAXIA
Only a handful of cases with X-linked transmission are on record, mostly in adult patients (Spira *et al.* 1979). In a few families, X-linked cerebellar degeneration had its onset in infancy (Malamud and Cohen 1958) or in adolescence (Carter and Sukavajana 1956). The distinction between these rare forms of spinocerebellar ataxia and cerebellar parenchymal ataxia is hardly possible in cases without post-mortem examination. Indeed, cases with and without brainstem and spinal involvement may occur in the same lineage.

CEREBELLAR HYPOPLASIA OR ATROPHY OF CONGENITAL OR EARLY INFANTILE ONSET
This section includes heterogeneous conditions of undetermined mechanism and nosologic situation. The main types are delineated in Table 10.14. Some are probably real degenerative

disorders of prenatal onset (Barth 1993); others may be developmental disorders, at least some of which are genetically transmitted, and are usually regarded as hypoplasia (Gadisseux *et al.* 1984). Some may be due to chromosomal abnormalities (Arts *et al.* 1995). Most cases are associated with other neurological or dysmorphic features and with developmental retardation and are thus difficult to recognize at onset.

PONTOCEREBELLAR HYPOPLASIA OF PRENATAL ONSET
One of the most important conditions in this group, the carbohydrate-deficient glycoprotein (CDG) syndrome (Harding *et al.* 1988) has been described in Chapter 9.

Two forms, not associated with known metabolic defects, are currently distinguished.

Autosomal recessive pontocerebellar hypoplasia with anterior horn cell disease (type 1 or amyotrophic cerebellar hypoplasia) is described in Chapter 20. It has a lethal outcome (Goutières *et al.* 1977).

Autosomal recessive pontocerebellar hypoplasia with microcephaly and dyskinesia (Barth–Brun OPCA or type 2) is characterized by severe developmental retardation, abnormal choreoathetotic movements and progressive microcephaly. CT or MRI scans show marked hypoplasia of the posterior fossa structures. The outcome is very poor (Albrecht *et al.* 1993, Barth *et al.* 1995).

A further type of cerebellar hypoplasia or atrophy has been reported from Finland (Koskinen *et al.* 1994) as *i*nfantile-*o*nset *s*pino-*c*erebellar *a*taxia or IOSCA. It includes deafness, axonal peripheral sensory neuropathy and primary hypergonadotrophic hypogonadism in females.

PEHO syndrome (*p*eripheral o*e*dema, *h*ypsarrhythmia and *o*ptic atropy) is a recessive disorder reported from Finland (Salonen *et al.* 1991), although cases have been observed elsewhere. The main features are seizures of early onset, mild dysmorphism, peripheral oedema and regression from 3–5 months of age. Optic atrophy develops towards the end of the first year (Haltia and Somer 1993).

Rare forms of cerebellar hypoplasia also featuring cerebral hypomyelination (Chatkupt *et al.* 1993) or progressive weakness, deafness and loss of vision with a fatal outcome (Arts *et al.* 1993) are difficult to classify. *Dentato-olivary dysplasia* (Harding and Boyd 1991) is marked mainly by seizures and severe retardation (Chapter 3).

NONPROGRESSIVE OR VERY SLOWLY PROGRESSIVE ATAXIAS OF CONGENITAL OR EARLY ONSET
This group consists of a heterogeneous collection of disorders, some of them imperfectly distinguished.

Marinesco–Sjögren syndrome includes cerebellar atrophy predominantly involving the vermis, with early onset of slowly progressive ataxia, cataracts, mild mental retardation and the late development of a peculiar myopathy (Herva *et al.* 1987, Sewry *et al.* 1988). *Gillespie syndrome* comprises the association of vermal atrophy and aniridia or iris hypoplasia (Crawfurd *et al.* 1979). Both syndromes are recessively inherited. Cases with dominant transmission and associated retinopathy (Dooley *et al.*

1992) and others with recessive inheritance and retinal atrophy (Ferri *et al.* 1996) have been reported.

OTHER DISORDERS FEATURING CONGENITAL CEREBELLAR HYPOPLASIA OR ATROPHY
Cases of congenital ataxia with associated renal diseases such as nephronophthisis (Keuth *et al.* 1996) or with a complex association of nephropathy, retinitis pigmentosa and skeletal abnormalities (Mainzer *et al.* 1970) and immunodeficiency (Berthet *et al.* 1994) or with hypogonadism (Toscano *et al.* 1995) have been reported.

Atrophy of the granular layer is marked by seizures, microcephaly, mental retardation and only inconstantly ataxia or choreoathetosis. Chou *et al.* (1987) reported 18 cases, two of which also had degeneration of the granule cells in the dentate gyrus. Pascual-Castroviejo *et al.* (1994) confirmed that the condition was usually transmitted as an autosomal recessive character. Their 14 patients could be classified into a severe group with microcephaly, severe mental retardation and often early death, and less severe cases presenting as congenital ataxia. Some of these cases are not progressive and are indistinguishable from those of recessively inherited congenital cerebellar hypoplasia (Kornberg and Shield 1991, Guzzetta *et al.* 1993). The cases of familial cerebellar degeneration of early onset reported by Harding and Brett (1995) involve mainly the Purkinje cells and the visual pathways. The group of *familial congenital hypoplasias* is still imperfectly classified (Al Shahwan *et al.* 1995). Such cases probably account for the known genetic risk of familial recurrence in patients with ataxic cerebral palsy.

Cases of dominant cerebellar hypoplasia (Tomiwa *et al.* 1987, Rivier and Echenne 1992, Chatkupt *et al.* 1993, Imamura *et al.* 1993) as well as X-linked forms (Fenichel and Phillips 1989) may also be observed.

Other rare cases such as X-linked recessive ataxia with dementia (Farlow *et al.* 1987) or dominantly inherited cases of cerebellar atrophy with mild ataxia and upbeating nystagmus (Furman *et al.* 1985) have been reported. Whether they are progressive diseases is not established. Linkage to chromosome Xq has been recently established in such a case (Illarioshkin *et al.* 1996).

FAMILIAL SPASTIC PARAPLEGIA
Patients with familial spastic paraplegia form a heterogeneous group from the clinical and genetic points of view. Linkage to chromosomes 1, 2p, 8q and 14q (Dürr *et al.* 1996b; Fink *et al.* 1996a,b) and X has been reported. X-linked cases are genetically heterogeneous. One form (SPG2) is allelic to Pelizaeus–Merzbacher disease (Saugier-Veber *et al.* 1994, Cambi *et al.* 1996). Another type (SPG1) is related to the MASA syndrome (Chapter 7). Two broad groups are recognized.

PURE SPASTIC PARAPLEGIA (STRÜMPELL–LORRAIN TYPE)
This disease is characterized pathologically by degeneration of the pyramidal tract and of the posterior columns below the cervical level and clinically by bilateral spasticity beginning and predominating in the lower limbs. Involvement of the upper limbs

is unusual, but deep tendon reflexes in the arms are often exaggerated (Polo *et al*. 1993). Vesical disturbances occur in 20 per cent of cases but are often late. Sensory disturbances are mild, affecting only vibration but not position sense. Pure spastic paraplegia is a fairly common condition: 104 cases have been reviewed by Holmes and Shaywitz (1977). Harding (1981c) in her study of 22 families separated type I cases, with onset below 35 years of age, and type II cases, where the apparent onset occurred after 35 years. She found a dominant inheritance in 19 families and a recessive mode in only three. The disease was dominantly inherited in seven of nine families studied by Polo *et al*. (1993). Although 40 per cent of Harding's patients had symptoms by 5 years of age, there is no doubt that mild cases are common and go easily unrecognized. Of the 41 patients of Behan and Maia (1974) only seven had sought medical advice, and it is a common experience to discover the disease in one apparently healthy parent of affected children, so that actual examination of both parents is essential for diagnosis. The uncommon recessive forms may have an earlier onset than dominant cases. The children are ofen slow to walk, clumsy, fall frequently and tend to walk on tiptoes. In rare cases, mild cerebellar symptoms and signs are present (Behan and Maia 1974) and mild impairment of vibration and position sense may be seen. Motor and sensory nerve conduction velocities are normal. The course of dominant forms is slow and may remain stationary until late in adulthood. Recessive forms may run a faster course. It is usually easy to exclude a tumour or syrinx, and only a few cases will require myelography or MRI. The most difficult differential diagnosis is with spastic diplegic cerebral palsy (Chapter 8), and familial spastic paraplegia should be suspected in all cases especially when there is no history of preterm birth or other pre- or perinatal abnormalities. However, I have seen cases with abrupt deterioration diagnosed as myelitis, and marked fluctuations of signs, in some cases on the occasion of respiratory infections. Treatable conditions such as spinal compression, lesions of the parasagittal motor strip, adrenomyeloneuropathy and hyperargininaemia (Brockstedt *et al*. 1990) should be ruled out. HTLV-1 virus infection may produce a very similar syndrome and this disorder has been reported in three members of a family indicating the possibility of vertical transmission (Salazar-Grueso *et al*. 1990).

Treatment is based on physiotherapy.

Complicated Spastic Paraplegia
Hereditary spastic paraplegia can occur in association with many different symptoms and signs, thus producing a number of syndromes whose description is often based on only a few cases or a single family. These syndromes have been mainly described in adults but onset often occurs in childhood or even infancy (Appleton *et al*. 1991). Their inheritance is usually autosomal recessive but dominant cases are known and X-linked inheritance has been mentioned (Appleton *et al*. 1991). They include hereditary spastic paraplegia with ocular and extrapyramidal symptoms, the so-called Ferguson–Critchley syndrome (Brown 1975); cases of paraplegia associated with dystonia (Gilman and Romanul 1975); familial spastic paraplegia with amyotrophy, oligophrenia

and central retinal degeneration or Kjellin syndrome (Kjellin 1975); paraplegia and deafness (Wells and Jankovic 1986); paraplegia with palmoplantar keratosis (Dyck *et al*. 1988); paraplegia with disordered pigmentation; and paraplegia with isolated mental retardation (Nicolaides *et al*. 1993). A complex syndrome featuring optic atrophy, abnormal choreic movements, mild mental retardation and sometimes ataxia in addition to spastic paraplegia was recognized by Costeff *et al*. (1989). This has been shown to be associated with 3-methylglutaconic aciduria. Paraplegia can also be associated with a sensory neuropathy involving either the small fibres and responsible for trophic lesions (Cavanagh *et al*. 1979), or the large fibres without trophic damage (Schady and Smith 1994, Thomas *et al*. 1994).

The complicated forms tend to run a faster course than pure paraplegia (Appleton *et al*. 1991).

X-Linked Paraplegia Type 2
This is a mild form of Pelizaeus–Merzbacher disease due to mutations involving the *PLP* gene. All transitional forms with the full-fledged Pelizaeus leukodystrophy can be observed, and cases of both conditions can occur in the same pedigree. MRI demonstrates a moderate deficiency of myelin in the temporo-occipital lobe (Boespflug-Tanguy *et al*. 1996). Most patients have a complicated form of spastic paraplegia while simple type is rare (Saugier-Veber *et al*. 1994). The mothers of affected boys may have mild symptoms of CNS involvement.

MULTLIPLE SYSTEM ATROPHY
The multisystem atrophy group of conditions share common features with some of the spinocerebellar degeneration group which, in fact, can affect other systems within and without the nervous system. Most of the disorders in this group affect adults. Machado–Joseph disease is clearly related to type 3 spinocerebellar ataxia (see p. 353).

Multisystem degenerations with retinal degeneration (Nishimura *et al*. 1987) or with ataxia and deafness (Koletzko *et al*. 1987) have occurred in childhood. Wilhelmsen–Lynch disease, featuring familial parkinsonism, amyotrophy and dementia has been observed in adolescents in a few families (Lynch *et al*. 1994).

CURRENTLY UNCLASSIFIABLE HEREDODEGENERATIVE DISORDERS

PROGRESSIVE CNS DEGENERATION WITH OPHTHALMOPLEGIA AND CHOREOATHETOSIS
A few of these syndromes have suggestive diagnostic features. A progressive disorder of infantile CNS degeneration with ophthalmoplegia and choreoathetosis was reported in eight children from Canada by Holmes and Logan (1980) and in 11 children from Finland, where the disease seems common, by Kallic *et al*. (1983), under the name of O-HAHA syndrome (*o*phthalmoplegia, *h*ypoacusis, *a*taxia, *h*ypotonia and *a*thetosis). This syndrome has now been reclassified among the spinocerebellar ataxias and renamed *i*nfantile *o*nset *s*pino-*c*erebellar *a*taxia (IOSCA). The disease begins early in infancy with

developmental delay. Onset of choreoathetosis is before the end of the first year of life, and ophthalmoplegia and sensorineural deafness are apparent by 3–4 years of age. Optic atrophy, hypotonia, areflexia due to a sensory neuropathy, dysmorphic facial features, and marked growth and mental retardation become progressively manifest. An autosomal recessive inheritance seems likely. Nerve conduction velocities were normal, but changes indicative of slight chronic neurogenic lesion were found by EMG.

PSEUDOXANTHOMA ELASTICUM

This is a multisystem hereditary disorder characterized by skin photosensitivity, peculiar loosening of the skin, angioid streaks of the retina, and multiple DNA anomalies. Neurological manifestations include spasticity, choreoathetosis, ataxia, deafness and progressive intellectual deterioration, sometimes with psychiatric disturbances (Mimaki *et al.* 1986, Demaerel *et al.* 1992).

AXONAL DEVELOPMENT DISORDERS

A disorder of axonal development, necrotizing myopathy, cardiomyopathy and cataracts has been recently recognized (Lyon *et al.* 1990). It includes extreme hypoplasia of the corpus callosum and overall reduction in the axons of the white matter with absence of pyramidal tracts. This disorder and similar cases previously reported (Guazzi *et al.* 1974) may be due to an abnormal extension of the normal phenomenon of axonal elimination during development. The cases of two siblings described by Curatolo *et al.* (1993) share many of these features, although the authors regard them as a different syndrome. Lynch *et al.* (1992) reported two brothers with arrested maturation of cerebral neurons, axons and myelin. Additional features included clouding of the cornea, macrogyria and abnormal cortical architecture.

RETT SYNDROME

Rett syndrome is a characteristic cluster of clinical manifestations that includes early psychomotor regression with autistic features, loss of purposeful use of the hands which is replaced by stereotypic activity, ataxia and apraxia of gait, and acquired microcephaly (Hagberg *et al.* 1983). The syndrome is observed almost exclusively in girls, with very few exceptions (Zoghbi 1988, Hagberg 1993).

Rett syndrome now appears to be a developmental rather than a degenerative disorder (Naidu 1997). Structural brain abnormalities are mild, including a small brain with densely packed neurons and a decrease in cell processes. It is not, in a vast majority of cases, an hereditary condition even though the exclusive involvement of girls suggests a genetic origin. A dominant mutation or a chromosomal accident involving the X chromosome has been proposed but other mechanisms are possible. The prevalence of Rett syndrome in Sweden and in Western Scotland is 1 in 10,000 to 1 in 15,000 girls (Hagberg 1993). No biochemical, chromosomal or other laboratory marker has yet been found.

The course of Rett syndrome is remarkable. The disorder initially presents as a progressive condition with a more or less

TABLE 10.15
Diagnostic criteria for Rett syndrome*

Necessary criteria
Apparently normal prenatal and perinatal period
Apparently normal psychomotor development through the first 6 months[1]
Normal head circumference at birth
Deceleration of head growth between ages 5 months and 4 years
Loss of acquired purposeful hand skills between ages 6 and 30 months, temporally associated with communication dysfunction and social withdrawal
Development of severely impaired expressive and receptive language, and presence of severe psychomotor retardation
Stereotypic hand movements such as hand wringing/squeezing, clapping/tapping, mouthing and 'washing'/rubbing automatisms appearing after loss of purposeful hand use
Mouthing and buccal stereotypies (tooth grinding)
Appearance of gait apraxia and truncal apraxia/ataxia between 1 and 4 years of age
Diagnosis tentative until 2–5 years of age[2]

Supportive criteria
Breathing dysfunction
EEG abnormalities
Seizures
Spasticity often associated with development of muscle wasting and dystonia
Peripheral vasomotor disturbances
Kyphoscoliosis
Growth retardation
Hypotrophic small feet

Exclusion criteria
Evidence of intrauterine growth retardation
Organomegaly or other signs of storage disease
Retinopathy or optic atrophy
Microcephaly at birth
Evidence of perinatally acquired brain damage
Existence of identifiable progressive disorder
Acquired neurological disorders due to infection or trauma

*From the Rett Syndrome Diagnostic Criteria Work Group (1988).
[1]Development may appear slightly slow from birth.
[2]Early diagnosis may be possible (<1 year in some cases).

rapid deterioration with loss of previously acquired skills. It accounts for a significant proportion (up to 30 per cent) of the cases of apparently progressive encephalopathy of obscure origin in girls (Goutières and Aicardi 1985).

Because of the prominent psychiatric featurees, Rett syndrome is described in Chapter 29. Table 10.15 shows the internationally accepted criteria for the diagnosis (Rett Syndrome Diagnostic Criteria Work Group 1988, Trevathan and Naidu 1988).

The course of Rett syndrome can be divided into four stages (Table 10.16).

The onset of clinical manifestations is between 6 months and 3 years, most cases becoming manifest before 18 months of age. Initial development may be entirely normal but affected girls are often somewhat hypotonic from birth and have a mildly slowed development. Acquisition of purposeful use of the hands is a prerequisite for the diagnosis, and loss of hand use is a major feature. It is often rapid over a few weeks and may be 'explosive' in a few days.

TABLE 10.16
Rett syndrome: staging*

Stage	Clinical features
Early onset deceleration stage	
Onset 6–18 months	Developmental stagnation
Duration: months	Deceleration of head growth
	Disinterest in play
	Hypotonia
Rapid 'destructive' stage	
Onset: 1–3 years	Rapid regression with irritability
Duration: weeks to months	Loss of purposeful hand use
	Hand stereotypies
	Autistic manifestations
	Loss of language
Pseudostationary stage	
Onset: 2–10 years	Severe mental retardation
Duration: years	Improvement of autistic features
	Seizures
	Hand stereotypies
	Ataxia/apraxia
	Scoliosis
	Respiratory disturbances
Late motor deterioration	
Onset: after 10 years	Combined upper and lower
Duration: years	motor neuron signs
	Progressive scoliosis
	Decreasing mobility, eventually
	wheelchair-dependent
	Trophic disturbances of feet and hands
	Reduced seizure frequency

*Adapted from Hagberg and Witt-Engerström (1986).

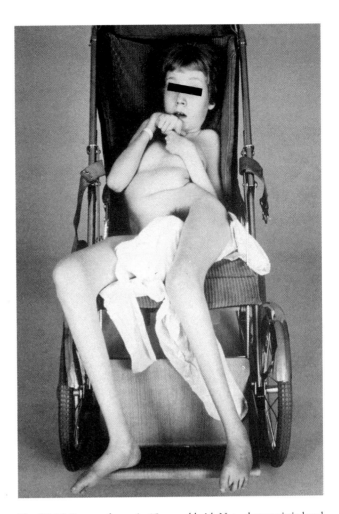

Fig. 10.16. Rett syndrome in 15-year-old girl. Note characteristic hand stereotypies, marked scoliosis and atrophy of lower limbs. (Courtesy Prof. B. Hagberg, Östrasjukhuset, Göteborg.)

The third stage of the disease is marked by the slow appearance of neurological signs such as pyramidal tract signs. Epileptic seizures appear in two-thirds to three-quarters of cases at this stage. They are often preceded by EEG abnormalities that include paroxysmal features (spikes or spike–waves) often posteriorly located, bursts of slow spike–waves especially during sleep, and a progressive slowing and deterioration of background tracing (Niedermeyer *et al.* 1986, Glaze *et al.* 1987).

Hyperventilation with intervening respiratory pauses is a frequent finding and it may be responsible for episodes of syncope often mistaken for epileptic seizures.

Between two-thirds and three-quarters of patients do not acquire independent ambulation, and with the progression of the fourth stage of the disease, ambulation is ultimately lost in most patients (Hagberg and Witt-Engerström 1986). Growth failure is present in most cases (Fig. 10.16).

No consistent laboratory feature has been found. The hyper-ammonaemia initially reported is found only in rare cases and usually due to external factors such as sodium valproate therapy. Abnormalities of neurotransmitters seem to be inconsistent. MRI shows a diminished cerebral volume, predominantly at the expense of white matter, reduced volume of the caudate and midbrain and a normal gyration (Reiss *et al.* 1993).

Kyphoscoliosis is one of the major complications of the syndrome.

The main differential diagnosis is with the autistic syndromes (Chapter 26). The infantile type of ceroid–lipofuscinosis with the 'knitting hand movements' described by Santavuori may resemble Rett syndrome but is very rare outside Finland (Santavuori *et al.* 1973, Santavuori 1988). Ornithine transcarbamylase deficiency has also been mistaken for Rett syndrome. Angelman syndrome may resemble Rett syndrome because of the jerky ataxia observed in both conditions in addition to autistic features, mental retardation and seizures. Chromosomal studies permit differentiation in difficult cases.

Treatment of Rett syndrome is unsatisfactory. Bromocriptine and naloxone have been tried without convincing results. Physical therapy and careful attention to details of everyday life are essential. Stimulation should be provided to affected girls who respond well following the early period of withdrawal. Orthopaedic management to avoid or limit the development of scoliosis is a major part of the care of Rett patients.

Atypical forms may be quite frequent (Goutières and Aicardi 1985) but the lack of a reliable marker should prevent definite inclusion in many cases. Hagberg and Skjeldal (1994) recognize 'formes frustes' with mild but typical features, an infantile onset variant in which seizures—often infantile spasms—are the first manifestation in the first year of life, a congenital form, late childhood regression and preserved speech variants. The possible coexistence of Rett syndrome and mental retardation in siblings suggests the possibility of a wide spectrum of manifestations, but confirmation by a definitive test is needed.

REFERENCES

Abs, R., van Vleyman, E., Parizel, P.M., *et al.* (1996) 'Congenital cerebellar hypoplasia and hypogonadotropic hypogonadism.' *Journal of the Neurological Sciences*, **98**, 259–265.

Abuelo, D.N., Barsel-Bowers, G., Tutschka, B.G., *et al.* (1981) 'Symmetrical infantile thalamic degeneration in two sibs.' *Journal of Medical Genetics*, **18**, 448–450.

Adornato, B.T., Eil, C., Head, G.L., Loriaux, D.L. (1980) 'Cerebellar involvement in multifocal eosinophilic granuloma: demonstration by computerized tomographic scanning.' *Annals of Neurology*, **7**, 125–129.

Aguglia, J., Zappia, M., Quattrone, A. (1987) 'Carbamazepine-induced nonepileptic myoclonus in a child with benign epilepsy.' *Epilepsia*, **28**, 515–518.

Aicardi, J., Castelein, P. (1979) 'Infantile neuroaxonal dystrophy.' *Brain*, **102**, 727–748.

—— Goutières, F. (1984) 'A progressive familial encephalopathy in infancy with calcifications of the basal ganglia and chronic cerebrospinal fluid lymphocytosis.' *Annals of Neurology*, **15**, 49–54.

—— Gordon, N., Hagberg, B. (1985) 'Holes in the brain.' *Developmental Medicine and Child Neurology*, **27**, 249–260.

—— Barbosa, C., Andermann, E., *et al.* (1988) 'Ataxia–ocular motor apraxia: a syndrome mimicking ataxia–telangiectasia.' *Annals of Neurology*, **24**, 497–502.

Albin, R.L., Reiner, A., Anderson, K.D., *et al.* (1990a) 'Striatal and nigral neuron subpopulations in rigid Huntington's disease: implications for the functional anatomy of chorea and rigidity–akinesia.' *Annals of Neurology*, **27**, 357–365.

—— Young, A.B., Penney, J.B., *et al.* (1990b) 'Abnormalities of striatal projection neurons and *N*-methyl-D-aspartate receptors in presymptomatic Huntington's disease.' *New England Journal of Medicine*, **322**, 1293–1298.

Albrecht, S., Schneider, M.C., Belmont, J., Armstrong, D.L. (1993) 'Fatal infantile encephalopathy with olivopontocerebellar hypoplasia and micrencephaly. Report of three siblings.' *Acta Neuropathologica*, **85**, 394–399.

Al Rajeh, S., El Mouzan, M.I., Ahlberg, A., Ozaksoy, D. (1988) 'The syndrome of osteopetrosis, renal acidosis and cerebral calcifications in two sisters.' *Neuropediatrics*, **19**, 162–165.

Alsager, D.E., Bowen, P., Bamforth, J.S. (1991) 'Trembling chin—a report of this inheritable dominant character in a four-generation Canadian family.' *Clinical Genetics*, **40**, 186–189.

Al Shahwan, S.A., Bruyn, G.W., Al Deeb, S.M. (1995) 'Non-progressive familial congenital cerebellar hypoplasia.' *Journal of the Neurological Sciences*, **128**, 71–77.

Ambler, M.W., Trice, J., Grauerholz, J., O'Shea, P.A. (1983) 'Infantile osteopetrosis and neuronal storage disease.' *Neurology*, **33**, 437–441.

American Academy of Pediatrics Committee on Genetics (1994) 'Prenatal genetic diagnosis for pediatricians.' *Pediatrics*, **93**, 1010–1015.

Andermann, E., Andermann, F., Carpenter, S., *et al.* (1986) 'Action myoclonus–renal failure syndrome: a previously unrecognized neurological disorder unmasked by advances in nephrology.' *In*: Fahn, S., Marsden, C.D., Van Woert, M. (Eds.) *Advances in Neurology, Vol. 43. Myoclonus.* New York: Raven Press, pp. 87–103.

Andermann, F., Andermann, E. (1986) 'Excessive startle syndromes: startle disease, jumping, startle epilepsy.' *In*: Fahn, S., Marsden, C.D., Van Woert, M. (Eds.) *Advances in Neurology, Vol. 43. Myoclonus.* New York: Raven Press, pp. 321–338.

Andrew, J., Fowler, C.J., Harrison, M.J.G. (1983) 'Stereotaxic thalamotomy in 55 cases of dystonia.' *Brain*, **106**, 981–1000.

Angelini, L., Rumi, V., Lamperti, E., Nardocci, N. (1988) 'Transient paroxysmal dystonia.' *Neuropediatrics*, **19**, 171–174.

—— Nardocci, N., Rumi, V., Lamperti, E. (1989) 'Idiopathic dystonia with onset in childhood.' *Journal of Neurology*, **236**, 319–321.

—— —— —— *et al.* (1992) 'Hallervorden–Spatz disease: clinical and MRI study of 11 cases diagnosed in life.' *Journal of Neurology*, **239**, 417–425.

Ansari, M.Q., Chincanchan, C.A., Armstrong, D.L. (1990) 'Brain calcification in hypoxic–ischemic lesions: an autopsy review.' *Pediatric Neurology*, **6**, 94–101.

Antonarakis, S.E. (1989) 'Diagnosis of genetic disorders at the DNA level.' *New England Journal of Medicine*, **320**, 153–163.

Apkarian, P., Koestveld-Baart, J.C., Barth, P.G. (1993) 'Visual evoked potential characteristics and early diagnosis of Pelizaeus–Merzbacher disease.' *Archives of Neurology*, **50**, 981–985.

Appleton, R.E., Farrell, K., Dunn, H.G. (1991) '"Pure" and "complicated" forms of hereditary spastic paraplegia presenting in childhood.' *Developmental Medicine and Child Neurology*, **33**, 304–312.

Arsenio-Nunes, M.L., Goutiéres, F., Aicardi, J. (1981) 'An ultramicroscopic study of skin and conjunctival biopsies in chronic neurological disorders of childhood.' *Annals of Neurology*, **9**, 163–173.

Arts, W.F.M., Loonen, M.C.B., Sengers, R.C.A., Slooff, J.L. (1993) 'X-linked ataxia, weakness, deafness, and loss of vision in early childhood with a fatal course.' *Annals of Neurology*, **33**, 535–539.

—— Hofstee, Y., Drejer, G.F., *et al.* (1995) 'Cerebellar and brainstem hypoplasia in a child with a partial monosomy for the short arm of chromosome 5 and partial trisomy for the short arm of chromosome 10.' *Neuropediatrics*, **26**, 41–44.

Ashizawa, T., Wong, L-J.C., Richards, C.S., *et al.* (1994) 'CAG repeat size and clinical presentation in Huntington's disease.' *Neurology*, **44**, 1137–1143.

Ashwal, S., Thrasher, T.V., Rice, D.R., Wenger, D.A. (1984) 'A new form of sea-blue histiocytosis associated with progressive anterior horn cell and axonal degeneration.' *Annals of Neurology*, **16**, 184–192.

Autti, T., Raininko, R., Launes, J., *et al.* (1992) 'Jansky–Bielschowsky variant disease: CT, MRI, and SPECT findings.' *Pediatric Neurology*, **8**, 121–126.

Bae, S.H., Vates, T.S., Kenton, E.J. (1980) 'Generalized chorea associated with chronic subdural hematomas.' *Annals of Neurology*, **8**, 449–450.

Bain, P.G., Findley, L.J., Thompson, P.D., *et al.* (1994) 'A study of hereditary essential tremor.' *Brain*, **117**, 805–823.

Bamford, J., Bodansky, H., Bradey, N., Currie, S., Barnett, D. (1988) 'Rapid development of basal ganglia hyperdensity caused by anoxia.' *Journal of Neurology, Neurosurgery, and Psychiatry*, **51**, 1364–1372.

Bamford, K.A., Caine, E.D., Kido, D.K., *et al.* (1989) 'Clinical–pathologic correlation in Huntington's disease: a neuropsychological and computed tomography study.' *Neurology*, **39**, 796–801.

Bandmann, O., Nygaard, T.G., Surtees, R., *et al.* (1996) 'Dopa-responsive dystonia in British patients: new mutations of the GTP-cyclohydrolase I gene and evidence for genetic heterogeneity.' *Human Molecular Genetics*, **5**, 403–406.

Bank, W.J., Morrow, G. (1972) 'A familial spinal cord disorder with hyperglycinemia.' *Archives of Neurology*, **27**, 136–139.

Baraitser, M., Brett, E.M., Piesowicz, A.T. (1983) 'Microcephaly and intracranial calcification in two brothers.' *Journal of Medical Genetics*, **20**, 210–212.

Barnett, N.D., Kaplan, A.M., Bernes, S.M., Cohen, M.L. (1995) 'Hemolytic uremic syndrome with particular involvement of basal ganglia and favorable outcome.' *Pediatric Neurology*, **12**, 155–158.

Barohn, R.J., Dowd, D.C., Kagan-Hallet, K.S. (1992) 'Congenital ceroid–lipofuscinosis.' *Pediatric Neurology*, **8**, 54–59.

Barth, P.G. (1991) 'Inherited progressive disorders of the fetal brain: a field in need of recognition.' *In*: Fukuyama, Y., Suzuki, Y., Kamoshita, S., Casaer, P. (Eds.) *Fetal and Perinatal Neurology.* Basel: Karger, pp. 299–313.

—— (1993) 'Pontocerebellar hypoplasias. An overview of a group of inherited neurodegenerative disorders with fetal onset.' *Brain and Development*, **15**, 411–422.

—— Vrensen, G.J.F.M., Uylings, H.B.M., *et al.* (1990) 'Inherited syndrome of microcephaly, dyskinesia and pontocerebellar hypoplasia: a systemic atrophy with early onset.' *Journal of the Neurological Sciences*, **97**, 25–42.

—— Blennow, G., Lenard, H.G., *et al.* (1995) 'The syndrome of autosomal recessive pontocerebellar hypoplasia, microcephaly, and extrapyramidal dyskinesia (pontocerebellar hypoplasia type 2): compiled data from 10 pedigrees.' *Neurology*, **45**, 311–317.

Barthez-Carpentier, M.A., Billard, C., Maheut, J., *et al.* (1991) 'A case of childhood Kuf's disease.' *Journal of Neurology, Neurosurgery, and Psychiatry*, **54**, 655–657.

Beal, M.F., Mazurek, M.F., Ellison, D.W., *et al.* (1988) 'Somatostatin and neuropeptide Y concentration in pathologically graded cases of Huntington's disease.' *Annals of Neurology*, **23**, 562–569.

Behan, W.M.H., Maia, M. (1974) 'Strümpell's familial spastic paraplegia: genetics and neuropathology.' *Journal of Neurology, Neurosurgery, and Psychiatry*, **37**, 8–20.

Belec, L., Gray, F., Louarn, F., *et al.* (1988) 'Leucodystrophie orthochromatique pigmentaire. Maladie de van Bogaert et Nyssen.' *Revue Neurologique*, **144**, 347–357.

Belman, A.L., Lantos, G., Horoupian, D., *et al.* (1986) 'AIDS calcification of the basal ganglia in infants and children.' *Neurology*, **36**, 1192–1199.

Ben Hamida, M., Belal, S., Sirugo, A., *et al.* (1993) 'Friedreich's ataxia phenotype not linked to chromosome 9 and associated with selective autosomal recessive vitamin E deficiency in two inbred Tunisian families.' *Neurology*, **43**, 2179–2183.

Bennett, R.H., Ludvigson, P., De León, G., Berry, G. (1984) 'Large-fiber sensory neuronopathy in autosomal dominant spinocerebellar degeneration.' *Archives of Neurology*, **41**, 175–178.

Benomar, A., Le Guern, E., Dürr, A., *et al.* (1994) 'Autosomal-dominant cerebellar ataxia with retinal degeneration (ADCA type II) is genetically different from ADCA type I.' *Annals of Neurology*, **35**, 439–444.

—— Krols, L., Stevanin, G., *et al.* (1995) 'The gene for autosomal dominant cerebellar ataxia with pigmentary macular dystrophy maps to chromosome 3p12–p21.1.' *Nature Genetics*, **10**, 84–88.

Berciano, J. (1982) 'Olivopontocerebellar atrophy.' *Journal of the Neurological Sciences*, **53**, 253–272.

—— Combarros, O., Calleja, J., *et al.* (1993) 'Friedreich's ataxia presenting with pure sensory ataxia: a long-term follow-up study of two patients.' *Journal of Neurology*, **240**, 177–180.

—— —— De Castro, M., Palau, F. (1997) 'Intronic GAA triplet repeat expansion in Friedreich's ataxia presenting with pure sensory ataxia.' *Journal of Neurology*, **244**, 390–391. *(Letter.)*

Berent, S., Giordani, B., Lehtinen, S., *et al.* (1988) 'Positron emission tomographic scan investigations of Huntington's disease: cerebral metabolic correlates of cognitive function.' *Annals of Neurology*, **23**, 541–546.

Bergman, I., Steeves, M., Burckart, G., Thompson, A. (1991) 'Reversible neurologic abnormalities associated with prolonged intravenous midazolam and fentanyl administration.' *Journal of Pediatrics*, **119**, 644–649.

Berkovic, S.F., Karpati, G., Carpenter, S., Lang, A.E. (1987) 'Progressive dystonia with bilateral putaminal hypodensities.' *Archives of Neurology*, **44**, 1184–1187.

—— Carpenter, S., Andermann, F., *et al.* (1988) 'Kufs' disease: a critical reappraisal.' *Brain*, **111**, 27–62.

—— Cochius, J., Andermann, E., Andermann, F. (1993) 'Progressive myoclonus epilepsies: clinical and genetic aspects.' *Epilepsia*, **34**, Suppl. 3, S19–S30.

Berthet, F., Caduff, R., Schaad, U.B., *et al.* (1994) 'A syndrome of primary combined immunodeficiency with microcephaly, cerebellar hypoplasia, growth failure and progessive pancytopenia.' *European Journal of Pediatrics*, **153**, 333–338.

Bhatia, K., Thompson, P.D., Marsden, C.D. (1992) '"Isolated" postinfectious myoclonus.' *Journal of Neurology, Neurosurgery, and Psychiatry*, **55**, 1089–1091.

—— Bhatt, M.H., Marsden, C.D. (1993) 'The causalgia–dystonia syndrome.' *Brain*, **116**, 843–851.

Bhatt, M.H., Obeso, J.A., Marsden, C.D. (1993) 'Time course of postanoxic akinetic–rigid and dystonic syndromes.' *Neurology*, **43**, 314–317.

Biary, N., Koller, W. (1987) 'Kinetic predominant essential tremor: successful treatment with clonazepam.' *Neurology*, **37**, 471–474.

Bicknese, A.R., May, W., Hickey, W.F., Dodson, W.E. (1992) 'Early childhood hepatocerebral degeneration misdiagnosed as valproate hepatotoxicity.' *Annals of Neurology*, **32**, 767–775.

Billard, C, Dulac, O., Boulloche, J., *et al.* (1989) 'Encephalopathy with calcifications of the basal ganglia in children: a reappraisal of Fahr's syndrome with respect to 14 new cases.' *Neuropediatrics*, **20**, 12–19.

Birnbaum, D.C., Shields, D., Lippe, B., *et al.* (1989) 'Idiopathic central diabetes insipidus followed by progressive spastic cerebellar ataxia.' *Archives of Neurology*, **46**, 1001–1003.

Black, D.N., Booth, F., Watters, G.V., *et al.* (1988a) 'Leucoencephalopathy among native Indian infants in Northern Quebec and Manitoba.' *Annals of Neurology*, **24**, 490–496.

—— Watters, G.V., Andermann, E., *et al.* (1988b) 'Encephalitis among Cree children in Northern Quebec.' *Annals of Neurology*, **24**, 483–489.

Boespflug-Tanguy, O., Mimault, C., Melki, J., *et al.* (1994) 'Genetic homogeneity of Pelizaeus–Merzbacher disease: tight linkage to the proteolipoprotein locus in 16 affected families.' *American Journal of Human Genetics*, **55**, 461–467.

—— —— Giraud, G., *et al.* (1996) 'The Pelizaeus–Merzbacher disease and X-linked dysmyelinating disease.' *In:* Arzimanoglou, A., Goutières, F. (Eds.) *Trends in Child Neurology.* Paris: John Libbey, pp. 189–193.

Boltshauser, E., Wilson, J. (1976) 'Value of brain biopsy in neurodegenerative disease in childhood.' *Archives of Disease in Childhood*, **51**, 264–268.

—— Sternlin, M., Boesch, C., *et al.* (1991) 'Magnetic resonance imaging in infantile encephalopathy with cerebral calcification and leukodystrophy.' *Neuropediatrics*, **22**, 33–35.

Borrett, D., Becker, L.E. (1985) 'Alexander's disease: a disease of astrocytes.' *Brain*, **108**, 367–385.

Bouchard, J.P., Barbeau, A., Bouchard, R., Bouchard, R.W. (1978) 'Autosomal recessive spastic ataxia of Charlevoix–Saguenay.' *Canadian Journal of Neurological Sciences*, **5**, 61–69.

Boulloche, J., Aicardi, J. (1984) 'Syndrome de myoclonies du voile spontanément régressif chez l'enfant.' *Archives Françaises de Pédiatrie*, **41**, 645–647.

—— (1986) 'Pelizaeus–Merzbacher disease: clinical and nosological study.' *Journal of Child Neurology*, **1**, 233–239.

Bourgeois, M., Goutières, F., Chrétien, D., *et al.* (1992) 'Deficiency in complex II of the respiratory chain, presenting as a leukodystrophy in two sisters with Leigh syndrome.' *Brain and Development*, **14**, 404–408.

Boustany, R-M.N., Fleischnick, E., Alper, C.A., *et al.* (1987) 'The autosomal dominant form of "pure" familial spastic paraplegia: clinical findings and linkage analysis of a large pedigree.' *Neurology*, **37**, 910–915.

Boyd, S.G., Harden, A., Egger, J., Pampiglione, G. (1986) 'Progressive neuronal degeneration of childhood with liver disease ("Alpers' disease"): characteristic neurophysiological features.' *Neuropediatrics*, **17**, 75–80.

Brashear, A., Farlow, M.R., Butler, I.J., *et al.* (1996) 'Variable phenotype of rapid-onset dystonia–parkinsonism.' *Movement Disorders*, **11**, 151–156.

Bressman, S., Fahn, S. (1986) 'Essential myoclonus.' *In:* Fahn, S., Marsden, C.D., Van Woert, M. (Eds.) *Advances in Neurology, Vol. 43. Myoclonus.* New York: Raven Press, pp. 287–294.

—— De León, D., Kramer, P.L., *et al.* (1994a) 'Dystonia in Ashkenazi Jews: clinical characterization of a founder mutation.' *Annals of Neurology*, **36**, 771–777.

—— Heiman, G.A., Nygaard, T.G., *et al.* (1994b) 'A study of idiopathic torsion dystonia in a non-Jewish family: evidence for genetic heterogeneity.' *Neurology*, **44**, 283–287.

Brett, E.M., Lake, B.D. (1975) 'A reassessment of the rectal approach to neuropathology in childhood: a review of 507 biopsies over an 11-year period.' *Archives of Disease in Childhood*, **50**, 753–762.

—— —— (1997) 'Progressive neurometabolic diseases.' *In:* Brett, E.M. (Ed.) *Pediatric Neurology, 3rd Edn.* London: Churchill Livingstone, pp. 143–199.

—— Hoare, B.D., Sheehy, M.P., Marsden, C.D. (1981) 'Progressive hemidystonia due to focal basal ganglia lesion after mild head trauma.' *Journal of Neurology, Neurosurgery, and Psychiatry*, **44**, 460. *(Letter.)*

Brismar, J., Ozand, P.T. (1994) 'CT and MR of the brain in the diagnosis of organic acidemias. Experiences from 107 patients.' *Brain and Development*, **16** (Suppl.), 104–124.

Britton, J.W., Uitti, R.J., Ahlskog, J.E., *et al.* (1995) 'Hereditary late-onset chorea without significant dementia: genetic evidence for substantial phenotypic variations in Huntington disease.' *Neurology*, **45**, 443–447.

Brockstedt, M., Smit, L.M.E., de Grauw, A.J.C., *et al.* (1990) 'A new case of hyperargininaemia: neurological and biochemical findings prior to and during dietary treatment.' *European Journal of Pediatrics*, **149**, 341–343.

Brown, J.W. (1975) 'Hereditary spastic paraplegia with ocular extrapyramidal symptoms (Ferguson–Critchley syndrome).' *In:* Vinken, P.J., Bruyn, G.W. (Eds.) *Handbook of Clinical Neurology. Vol. 22. System Disorders and Atrophies, Part II.* Amsterdam: North Holland, pp. 433–443.

Brunner, J.E., Redmond, J.M., Haggar, A.M., *et al.* (1990) 'Central pontine myelinolysis and pontine lesion after rapid correction of hyponatremia: a prospective magnetic resonance imaging study.' *Annals of Neurology*, **27**, 61–66.

Bruun, I., Reske-Nielsen, E., Oster, S. (1991) 'Juvenile ceroid–lipofuscinosis and calcifications of the CNS.' *Acta Neurologica Scandinavica*, **83**, 1–8.

Bruyn, G.W., Padberg, G. (1984a) 'Chorea and systemic lupus erythematosus.' *European Neurology*, **23**, 278–290.

—— —— (1984b) 'Chorea and polycythaemia.' *European Neurology*, **23**, 26–33.

—— Bots, G.T.A.M., Went, L.N., Klinkhamer, P.J.J.M. (1992) 'Hereditary spastic dystonia with Leber's hereditary optic neuropathy: neuropathological findings.' *Journal of the Neurological Sciences*, **113**, 55–61.

Bürk, K., Abele, M., Fetter, M., *et al.* (1996) 'Autosomal dominant cerebellar ataxia type I. Clinical features and MRI in families with SCA1, SCA2 and SCA3.' *Brain*, **119**, 1497–1505.

Burke, R.E., Fahn, S., Marsden, C.D. (1986) 'Torsion dystonia: a double blind, prospective trial of high-dosage trihexyphenidyl.' *Neurology*, **36**, 160–164.

Bussone, L.A., Mantia, L., Boiardi, A., Giovannini, P. (1982) 'Chorea in Behçet syndrome.' *Journal of Neurology*, **227**, 89–92.

Callender, J.S. (1995) 'Non-progressive familial idiopathic intracranial calcification: a family report.' *Journal of Neurology, Neurosurgery, and Psychiatry*, **59**, 432–434.

Calne, D.B., Lang, A.E. (1988) 'Secondary dystonia.' *In:* Fahn, S., Marsden, C.D., Calne, D.B. (Eds.) *Advances in Neurology, Vol. 50. Dystonia 2.* New York: Raven Press, pp. 9–33.

—— Nygaard, T.G., Snow, B.J. (1993) 'The distinction between early onset idiopathic (juvenile Parkinson disease) and dopa-responsive dystonia (hereditary progressive dystonia, Segawa disease).' *In:* Segawa, M. (Ed.) *Hereditary Progressive Dystonia.* New York: Parthenon, pp. 215–225.

Cambi, F., Tang, X-M., Cordray, P., *et al.* (1996) 'Refined genetic mapping and proteolipid protein mutation analysis in X-linked pure hereditary spastic paraplegia.' *Neurology*, **46**, 1112–1117.

Campuzano, V., Montermini, L., Molto, M.D., *et al.* (1996) 'Friedreich's ataxia: autosomal recessive disease caused by intronic GAA triplet repeat expansion.' *Science*, **271**, 1423–1427.

Carango, P., Funanage, V.L., Quirós, R.E., *et al.* (1995) 'Overexpression of DM20 messenger RNA in two brothers with Pelizaeus–Merzbacher disease.' *Annals of Neurology*, **38**, 610–617.

Cardenas-Mera, N., Campos-Castello, J., Lucas, F., Carreaga Maldonado, J. (1995) 'Progressive familial encephalopathy in infancy with calcifications of the basal ganglia and cerebrospinal fluid lymphocytosis.' *Acta Neuropediatrica*, **1**, 207–213.

Carpenter, S., Karpati, G. (1981) 'Sweat gland duct cells in Lafora disease: diagnosis by skin biopsy.' *Neurology*, **31**, 1564–1568.

Carter, H.R., Sukavajana, C. (1956) 'Familial cerebello-olivary degeneration with late development of rigidity and dementia.' *Neurology*, **6**, 876–884.

Cassidy, S., Sheehan, N.C., Farrell, D.F., *et al.* (1987) 'Connatal Pelizaeus–Merzbacher disease: an autosomal recessive form.' *Pediatric Neurology*, **3**, 300–305.

Casteels, I., Spilleers, W., Swinnen, T., *et al.* (1994) 'Optic atrophy as the presenting sign in Hallervorden–Spatz disease.' *Neuropediatrics*, **25**, 265–267.

Catona, M.C., Lazarini, A.M., McCormack, M.K. (1985) 'A psychometric study of children at-risk for Huntington disease.' *Clinical Genetics*, **28**, 307–316.

Cavanagh, N.P.C., Eames, R.A., Galvin, R.J., *et al.* (1979) 'Hereditary sensory neuropathy with spastic paraplegia.' *Brain*, **102**, 79–94.

Charrow, J., Poznanski, A.K., Unger, F.M., Robinow, M. (1991) 'Autosomal recessive cerebellar hypoplasia and endosteal sclerosis: a newly recognized syndrome.' *American Journal of Medical Genetics*, **41**, 464–468.

Chatkupt, S., Wolansky, L.J., Jotkowitz, A., Cook, S.D. (1993) 'A new syndrome of autosomal dominant spinocerebellar degeneration and cerebral hypomyelination.' *American Journal of Human Genetics*, **53** (Suppl.), 415. *(Abstract.)*

Chou, S.M., Mizuno, Y., Rothner, A.D. (1987) 'Congenital granuloprival hypoplasia of cerebellar and hippocampal cortex.' *Journal of Child Neurology*, **2**, 279–286.

Chow, C.W., Borg, J., Billson, V.R., Lake, B.D. (1993) 'Fetal tissue involvement in the late infantile type of neuronal ceroid lipofuscinosis.' *Prenatal Diagnosis*, **13**, 833–841.

Chuang, S. (1989) 'Vascular diseases of the brain in children.' *In:* Edwards, M.S.B., Hoffman, H.J. (Eds.) *Cerebral Vascular Disease in Children and Adolescents.* Baltimore: Williams & Wilkins, pp. 69–93.

Chutorian, A.M., Nygaard, T.G., Waran, S. (1994) 'Dopa-responsive dystonia.' *International Pediatrics*, **9** (Suppl.), 49–54.

Cleaver, J.E., Volpe, J.P.G., Charles, W.C., Thomas, G.H. (1994) 'Prenatal diagnosis of xeroderma pigmentosum and Cockayne syndrome.' *Prenatal Diagnosis*, **14**, 921–928.

Cochius, J.L., Figlewicz, D.A., Kälviäinen, R., *et al.* (1993) 'Unverricht–Lundborg disease: absence of nonallelic genetic heterogeneity.' *Annals of Neurology*, **34**, 739–741.

Cohen, L.G., Meer, J., Tarkka, I., *et al.* (1991) 'Congenital mirror movements. Abnormal organization of motor pathways in two patients.' *Brain*, **114**, 381–403.

Cohn, D.F., Herishanu, Y., Streiffer, M. (1971) 'Subacute thyroiditis complicated by chorea minor.' *Bulletin of the Los Angeles Neurological Society*, **36**, 58–60.

Colamaria, V., Plouin, P., Dulac, O., *et al.* (1988) 'Kojewnikow's epilepsia partialis continua: two cases associated with striatal necrosis.' *Neurophysiologie Clinique*, **18**, 525–530.

Combarros, O., Fábrega, E., Polo, J.M., Berciano, J. (1993) 'Cyclosporine-induced chorea after liver transplantation for Wilson's disease.' *Annals of Neurology*, **33**, 108–109. *(Letter.)*

Comings, D.E., Comings, B.G. (1985) 'Tourette syndrome: clinical and psychological aspects of 250 cases.' *American Journal of Human Genetics*, **37**, 435–450.

Connelly, K.P., De Witt, L.D. (1994) 'Neurologic complications of infectious mononucleosis.' *Pediatric Neurology*, **10**, 180–184.

Corbin, D.O.C., Williams, A.C. (1987) 'Palatal myoclonus influenced by head posture.' *Journal of Neurology, Neurosurgery, and Psychiatry*, **50**, 366. *(Letter.)*

—— —— Johnson, A.P. (1987) 'Dystonia complicated by respiratory obstruction.' *Journal of Neurology, Neurosurgery, and Psychiatry*, **50**, 1707. *(Letter.)*

Costeff, H., Gadoth, N., Apter, N., *et al.* (1989) 'A familial syndrome of infantile optic atrophy, movement disorder and spastic paraplegia.' *Neurology*, **39**, 595–597.

Coutinho, P., Guimaraes, A., Scaravilli, F. (1982) 'The pathology of Machado–Joseph disease. Report of a possible homozygous case.' *Acta Neuropathologica*, **58**, 48–54.

Crawfurd, M.d'A., Harcourt, R.B., Shaw, P.A. (1979) 'Non-progressive cerebellar ataxia, aplasia of pupillary zone of iris, and mental subnormality (Gillespie's syndrome) affecting 3 members of a non-consanguineous family in 2 generations.' *Journal of Medical Genetics*, **16**, 373–378.

Critchley, E. (1972) 'Clinical manifestations of essential tremor.' *Journal of Neurology, Neurosurgery, and Psychiatry*, **35**, 365–372.

Cross, H.E., McKusick, V.A. (1967) 'The Troyer syndrome. A recessive form of spastic paraplegia with distal muscle wasting.' *Archives of Neurology*, **16**, 473–485.

Crouchman, M. (1987) 'Environmentally induced transient motor signs in infancy.' *Developmental Medicine and Child Neurology*, **29**, 685–688.

Curatolo, P., Cilio, M.R., Del Giudice, E., *et al.* (1993) 'Familial white matter hypoplasia, agenesis of the corpus callosum, mental retardation and growth deficiency: a new distinctive syndrome.' *Neuropediatrics*, **24**, 77–82.

Dabbagh, O., Swaiman, K.F. (1988) 'Cockayne syndrome: MRI correlates of hypomyelination.' *Pediatric Neurology*, **4**, 113–116.

Davis, L.E., Bodian, D., Price, D., *et al.* (1977) 'Chronic progressive poliomyelitis secondary to vaccination of an inmunodeficient child.' *New England Journal of Medicine*, **297**, 241–245.

Dejong, A.P.M.J., Haan, E.A., Manson, J.I., *et al.* (1989) 'Kinetic study of catecholamine metabolism in hereditary progressive dystonia.' *Neuropediatrics*, **20**, 3–11.

De Jong, J., van den Berg, C., Wijburg, H., *et al.* (1994) 'Alpha-*N*-acetyl-galactosaminidase deficiency with mild clinical manifestations and difficult biochemical diagnosis.' *Journal of Pediatrics*, **125**, 385–391.

De León, G.A., Crawford, S.E., Stack, C., *et al.* (1996) 'Amylaceous (polyglucosan) bodies in familial cerebral atrophy of early onset.' *Journal of Child Neurology*, **11**, 58–62.

Demaerel, P., Kendall, B.E., Kingsley, D. (1992) 'Cranial CT and MRI in diseases with DNA repair defects.' *Neuroradiology*, **34**, 117–121.

De Michele, G., Filla, A., D'Armiento, F.P., *et al.* (1990) 'Cerebellar ataxia and hypogonadism. A clinicopathological report.' *Clinical Neurology and Neurosurgery*, **92**, 67–70.

—— —— Cavalcanti, F., *et al.* (1994) 'Late onset Friedreich's disease: clinical features and mapping of mutation to the FRDA locus.' *Journal of Neurology, Neurosurgery, and Psychiatry*, **57**, 977–979.

—— Di Maio, L., Filla, A., *et al.* (1996) 'Childhood onset of Friedreich ataxia: a clinical and genetic study of 36 cases.' *Neuropediatrics*, **27**, 3–7.

Deonna, T. (1986) 'DOPA-sensitive progressive dystonia of childhood with fluctuations of symptoms—Segawa's syndrome and possible variants. Results of a collaborative study of the European Federation of Child Neurology.' *Neuropediatrics*, **17**, 81–85.

Deuschl, G., Toro, C., Valls-Solé, J., *et al.* (1994) 'Symptomatic and essential palatal tremor. 1. Clinical, physiological and MRI analysis.' *Brain*, **117**, 775–788.

De Yebenes, J.G., Moskowitz, C., Fahn, S., Saint-Hilaire, M.H. (1988) 'Long-term treatment with levodopa in a family with autosomal dominant torsion dystonia.' *In:* Fahn, S. (Ed.) *Advances in Neurology, Vol. 50. Dystonia 2.* New York: Raven Press, pp. 101–111.

Di Fazio, M.P., Patterson, F., Morales, J., Davis, R. (1997) 'Acute myoclonus secondary to group A, β-haemolytic *Streptococcus* infection: a PANDAS variant.' *Annals of Neurology*, **42**, 51. *(Abstract.)*

Di Mario, F.J., Clancy, R. (1989) 'Symmetrical thalamic degeneration with calcification of infancy.' *American Journal of Diseases of Children*, **143**, 1056–1060.

Dobyns, W.B., Ozelius, L.J., Kramer, P.L., *et al.* (1993) 'Rapid-onset dystonia–parkinsonism.' *Neurology*, **43**, 2596–2602.

Dooley, J.M., LaRoche, G.R., Tremblay, F., Riding, M. (1992) 'Autosomal recessive cerebellar hypoplasia and tapeto-retinal degeneration: a new syndrome.' *Pediatric Neurology*, **8**, 232–234.

Dooling, E.C., Schoene, W.C., Richardson, E.P. (1974) 'Hallervorden–Spatz syndrome.' *Archives of Neurology*, **30**, 70–83.

—— Richardson, E.P., Davis, K.R. (1980) 'Computed tomography in Hallervorden–Spatz disease.' *Neurology*, **30**, 1128–1130.

Dorfman, L.J., Pedley, T.A., Tharp, B.R., Scheithauer, B.W. (1978) 'Juvenile neuroaxonal dystrophy: clinical, electrophysiological and neuropathological features.' *Annals of Neurology*, **3**, 419–428.

Dubourg, O., Dürr, A., Cancel, G., *et al.* (1995) 'Analysis of the SCA1 CAG repeat in a large number of families with dominant ataxia: clinical and molecular correlations.' *Annals of Neurology*, **37**, 176–180.

Dürr, A., Cossee, M., Agid, Y., *et al.* (1996a) 'Clinical and genetic abnormalities in patients with Friedreich's ataxia.' *New England Journal of Medicine*, **335**, 1169–1175.

—— Davoine, C-S., Paternotte, C., *et al.* (1996b) 'Phenotype of autosomal dominant spastic paraplegia linked to chromosome 2.' *Brain*, **119**, 1487–1496.

—— Stevanin, G., Cancel G., *et al.* (1996c) 'Spinocerebellar ataxia 3 and Machado–Joseph disease: clinical, molecular, and neuropathological features.' *Annals of Neurology*, **39**, 490–499.

Dusser, A., Goutières, F., Aicardi, J. (1986) 'Ischemic strokes in children.' *Journal of Child Neurology*, **1**, 131–136.

Dwork, A.J., Balmaceda, C., Fazzini, E.A., *et al.* (1993) 'Dominantly inherited early-onset parkinsonism: neuropathology of a new form.' *Neurology*, **43**, 69–74.

Dyck, P.J., Litchy, W.J., Gosselin, S. (1988) 'Dominantly inherited spastic paraplegia and multifocal palmoplantar keratosis.' *Revue Neurologique*, **144**, 421–424.

Dyken, P., Wisniewski, K. (1995) 'Classification of the neuronal ceroid lipofuscinoses: expansion of the atypical forms.' *American Journal of Medical Genetics*, **57**, 150–154

Eda, I., Takashima, S., Takeshita, K. (1983) 'Acute hemiplegia with lacunar infarct after varicella infection in childhood.' *Brain and Development*, **5**, 494–499.

Edathodu, A.K., Dyken, P.R., Trefz, J.I., Kelloes, C.L. (1984) 'Two new forms of neuronal ceroid–lipofuscinosis: expanded clinical, morphologic, and biochemical classification.' *Neurology*, **34** (Suppl.1), 150. *(Abstract.)*

Edwards, P.D., Prosser, R., Wells, E.C. (1975) 'Chorea, polycythaemia, and cyanotic heart disease.' *Journal of Neurology, Neurosurgery, and Psychiatry*, **38**, 729–739.

Ellie, E., Julien, J., Ferrer, X. (1989) 'Familial idiopathic striopallidodendate calcifications.' *Neurology*, **39**, 381–385.

Elston, J.S., Granje, F.C., Lees, A.J. (1989) 'The relationship between eye-winking tics, frequent eye-blinking and blepharospasm.' *Journal of Neurology, Neurosurgery, and Psychiatry*, **52**, 477–480.

Enevoldson, T.P., Sanders, M.D., Harding, A.E. (1994) 'Autosomal dominant cerebellar ataxia with pigmentary macular dystrophy. A clinical and genetic study of eight families.' *Brain*, **117**, 445–460.

Erdem, E., Kiratli, H., Erbas, T., *et al.* (1994) 'Cerebellar ataxia associated with hypogonadotropic hypogonadism and chorioretinopathy: a poorly recognized association.' *Clinical Neurology and Neurosurgery*, **96**, 86–91.

Evans, B.K., Jankovic, J. (1983) 'Tuberous sclerosis and chorea.' *Annals of Neurology*, **13**, 106–107.

Fahn, S. (1982) 'The clinical spectrum of motor tics.' *In:* Friedhoff, A.J., Chase, T.N. (Eds.) *Advances in Neurology, Vol. 35. Gilles de la Tourette Syndrome.* New York: Raven Press, pp. 341–344.

—— (1988) 'Concept and classification of dystonia.' *In:* Fahn, S. (Ed.) *Advances in Neurology, Vol. 50. Dystonia 2.* New York: Raven Press, pp. 1–8.

—— (1989) 'Clinical variants of idiopathic torsion dystonia.' *Journal of Neurology, Neurosurgery, and Psychiatry*, **52** (Suppl.), S96–S100.

—— Williams, D.T. (1988) 'Psychogenic dystonia.' *In:* Fahn, S. (Ed.) *Advances in Neurology, Vol. 50. Dystonia 2.* New York: Raven Press, pp. 431–455.

Farlow, M.R., Demyer, W., Dlovhy, S.R., Hodes, M.E. (1987) 'X-linked recessive inheritance of ataxia and adult-onset dementia.' *Neurology*, **37**, 602–607.

Farmer, T.W., Wingfield, M.S., Lynch, S.A., *et al.* (1989) 'Ataxia, chorea, seizures and dementia—pathologic features of a newly defined familial disorder.' *Archives of Neurology*, **46**, 774–779.

Fenichel, G.M., Phillips, J.A. (1989) 'Familial aplasia of the cerebellar vermis. Possible X-linked dominant inheritance.' *Archives of Neurology*, **46**, 582–583.

Ferrer, I., Campistol, J., Tobeña, L., *et al.* (1987) 'Dégénérescence systématisée optico-cochléo-dentelée.' *Journal of Neurology*, **234**, 416–420.

Ferri, R., Azan, G., Del Gracco, S., *et al.* (1996) 'Congenital cerebellar ataxia, mental retardation, and atrophic retinal lesions in two brothers.' *Journal of Neurology, Neurosurgery, and Psychiatry*, **61**, 424–425. *(Letter.)*

Filla, A., De Michele, G., Cavalcanti, F., *et al.* (1990) 'Clinical and genetic heterogeneity in early onset cerebellar ataxia with retained tendon reflexes.' *Journal of Neurology, Neurosurgery, and Psychiatry*, **53**, 667–670.

Fink, J.K., Barton, N., Cohen, W., *et al.* (1988a) 'Dystonia with marked diurnal variation associated with biopterin deficiency.' *Neurology*, **38**, 707–711.

—— Filling-Katz, M.R., Barton, N.W., *et al.* (1988b) 'Treatable dystonia presenting as spastic cerebral palsy.' *Pediatrics*, **82**, 137–138. *(Letter.)*

—— Heiman-Patterson, T., for the Hereditary Spastic Paraplegia Working Group (1996a) 'Hereditary spastic paraplegia: advances in genetic research.' *Neurology*, **46**, 1507–1514.

—— Jones, S.M., Sharp, G.B., *et al.* (1996b) 'Hereditary spastic paraplegia linked to chromosome 15q: analysis of candidate genes.' *Neurology*, **46**, 835–836.

Finocchiaro, G., Baio, G., Micossi, P., *et al.* (1988) 'Glucose metabolism alterations in Friedreich's ataxia.' *Neurology*, **38**, 1292–1296.

Fisher, M., Sargent, J., Drachman, D. (1979) 'Familial inverted choreoathetosis.' *Neurology*, **29**, 1627–1631.

Fitch, N., Carpenter, S., Lachance, R.C. (1973) 'Prenatal axonal dystrophy and osteopetrosis.' *Archives of Pathology*, **95**, 298–301.

Fletcher, N.A., Harding, A.E., Marsden, C.D. (1990) 'A genetic study of torsion dystonia in the United Kingdom.' *Brain*, **113**, 379–395.

—— —— —— (1991) 'The relationship between trauma and idiopathic torsion dystonia.' *Journal of Neurology, Neurosurgery, and Psychiatry*, **54**, 713–717.

—— Thompson, P.D., Scadding, J.W., Marsden, C.D. (1993) 'Successful treatment of childhod onset symptomatic dystonia with levodopa.' *Journal of Neurology, Neurosurgery, and Psychiatry*, **56**, 865–867.

Flint, J., Goldstein, L.H. (1992) 'Familial calcification of the basal ganglia: a case report and review of the literature.' *Psychological Medicine*, **22**, 581–595.

Fok, A.C.K., Wong, M.C., Cheah, J.S. (1989) 'Syndrome of cerebellar ataxia with hypogonadotrophic hypogonadism: evidence for pituitary gonadotrophin deficiency.' *Journal of Neurology, Neurosurgery, and Psychiatry*, **52**, 407–409.

Folstein, S.E., Leigh, R.J., Parhad, I.M., Folstein, M.F. (1986) 'The diagnosis of Huntington's disease.' *Neurology*, **36**, 1279–1283.

Foroud, T., Siemers, E., Kleindorfer, D., *et al.* (1995) 'Cognitive scores in carriers of Huntington's disease gene compared to noncarriers.' *Annals of Neurology*, **37**, 657–664.

Franco, A., Colamaria, V., Dulac, O., *et al.* (1994) 'Mal di Alpers: studio electroclinico e anatomopatologico in due fratelli afferiti da epilessia parziale continua.' *In:* Atti (Vol. 1) *XVI Congresso Nazionale Società Italiana di Neuropsichiatria Infantile Brescia, 21–24 Sept. 1994*, pp. 201–203.

Friede, R.L. (1989) *Developmental Pathology, 2nd Edn.* Berlin: Springer Verlag.

Friedman, D.I., Jankovic, J., Rolak, L.A. (1986) 'Arteriovenous malformation presenting as hemidystonia.' *Neurology*, **36**, 1590–1593.

Frontali, M., Spadaro, M., Giunti, P., *et al.* (1992) 'Autosomal dominant pure cerebellar ataxia. Neurological and genetic study.' *Brain*, **115**, 1647–1654.

Fryns, J.P., Bulcke, J., Verdu, P., *et al.* (1991) 'Apparent late-onset Cockayne syndrome and interstitial deletion of the long arm of chromosome 10 (del (10) (q11.23q21.2)).' *American Journal of Medical Genetics*, **40**, 343–344.

Fukuhara, N., Tokiguchi, S., Shirakawa, K., Tsubaki, T. (1980) 'Myoclonus epilepsy associated with ragged-red fibres: disease entity or a syndrome?' *Journal of the Neurological Sciences*, **47**, 117–133

Furman, J.M., Baloh, R.W., Chugani, H., *et al.* (1985) 'Infantile cerebellar atrophy.' *Annals of Neurology*, **17**, 399–402.

Furtado, S., Suchowersky, O. (1995) 'Huntington's disease: recent advances in diagnosis and management.' *Canadian Journal of the Neurological Sciences*, **22**, 5–12.

Gabreëls, F.J.M., Prick, M.J.J., Trijbels, J.M.F., *et al.* (1984) 'Defects in citric acid cycle and the electron transport chain in progressive poliodystrophy.' *Acta Neurologica Scandinavica*, **70**, 145–154.

Gadisseux, J.F., Rodriguez, J., Lyon, G. (1984) 'Pontoneocerebellar hypoplasia—a probable consequence of prenatal destruction of the pontine nuclei and a possible role of phenytoin intoxication.' *Clinical Neuropathology*, **3**, 160–167.

Gardiner, R.M. (1993) 'Genetic analysis of Batten disease.' *Journal of Inherited Metabolic Disease*, **16**, 787–790.

Garrel, S., Joannard, A., Feuerstein, C., Serre, F. (1978) 'Formes myocloniques de la chorée de Huntington.' *Revue d'Electroencéphalographie et de Neurophysiologie Clinique*, **8**, 123–128.

Gascon, G.G., Abdo, N., Sigut, D., *et al.* (1995) 'Ataxia–oculomotor apraxia syndrome.' *Journal of Child Neurology*, **10**, 118–122.

Genis, D., Matilla, T., Volpini, V., *et al.* (1995) 'Clinical, neuropathologic, and genetic studies of a large spinocerebellar ataxia type I (SCA1) kindred: (CAG)$_n$ expansion and early premonitory signs and symptoms.' *Neurology*, **45**, 24–30.

Genton, P., Michelucci, R., Tassinari, C.A., Roger, J. (1990) 'The Ramsay Hunt syndrome revisited: Mediterranean myoclonus versus mitochondrial encephalomyopathy with ragged-red fibers and Baltic myoclonus.' *Acta Neurologica Scandinavica*, **81**, 8–15.

Gieron, M.A., Gilbert-Barness, E., Vonsattel, J.P., Korthals, J.R. (1995) 'Infantile progressive striato–thalamic degeneration in two siblings: a new syndrome.' *Pediatric Neurology*, **12**, 260–263.

Gilman, S., Romanul, F.C.A. (1975) 'Hereditary dystonic paraplegia with amyotrophy and mental deficiency: clinical and neuropathological characteristics.' *In:* Vinken, P.J., Bruyn, G.W. (Eds.) *Handbook of Clinical Neurology. Vol. 22. System Disorders and Atrophies, Part II*. Amsterdam: North Holland, pp. 445–465.

Giunti, P., Sweeney, M.G., Spadaro, M., *et al.* (1994) 'The trinucleotide repeat expansion on chromosome 6p (SCA1) in autosomal dominant cerebellar ataxias.' *Brain*, **117**, 645–649.

—— Harding, A.E. (1995) 'Detection of the Machado–Joseph disease/spinocerebellar ataxia three trinucleotide repeat expansion in families with autosomal dominant motor disorders, including the Drew family of Walworth.' *Brain*, **118**, 1077–1085.

Glaze, D.G., Frost, J.D., Zoghbi, H.Y., Percy, A.K. (1987) 'Rett's syndrome: correlation of electroencephalographic characteristics with clinical staging.' *Archives of Neurology*, **44**, 1053–1056.

Goebel, H. (1992) 'Neuronal ceroid–lipofuscinoses: the current status.' *Brain and Development*, **14**, 203–211.

—— (1995) 'The neuronal ceroid–lipofuscinoses.' *Journal of Child Neurology*, **16**, 424–437.

—— Bode, G., Caesar, R., Kohlschütter, A. (1981) 'Bulbar palsy with Rosenthal fiber formation in the medulla of a 15-year-old girl. Localized form of Alexander's disease?' *Neuropediatrics*, **12**, 382–391.

—— Vesa, J., Reitter, B., *et al.* (1995) 'Prenatal diagnosis of infantile neuronal ceroid–lipofuscinosis: a combined electron microscopic and molecular genetic approach.' *Brain and Development*, **17**, 83–88.

Goldberg-Stern, H., Weitz, R., Zaizov, R., *et al.* (1995) 'Progressive spinocerebellar degeneration "plus" associated with Langerhans histiocytosis: a new paraneoplastic syndrome?' *Journal of Neurology, Neurosurgery, and Psychiatry*, **58**, 180–183.

Golden, G.S. (1990) 'Tourette syndrome: recent advances.' *Neurologic Clinics*, **8**, 705–714.

Goldman, J.E., Katz, D., Rapin, I., *et al.* (1981) 'Chronic GM1-gangliosidosis presenting as dystonia: I. Clinical and pathological features.' *Annals of Neurology*, **9**, 465–475.

Goldman, S., Ahlskog, J.E. (1993) 'Posttraumatic cervical dystonia.' *Mayo Clinic Proceedings*, **68**, 443–448.

Gollomp, S.M., Fahn, S. (1987) 'Transient dystonia as a complication of varicella.' *Journal of Neurology, Neurosurgery, and Psychiatry*, **50**, 1228–1229.

Gordon, B.A., Gordon, K.E., Seo, H.C., *et al.* (1995) 'Fucosidosis with dystonia.' *Neuropediatrics*, **26**, 325–327.

Gordon, K., Masotti, R., Waddell, W. (1992) 'Tremorogenic toxic encephalopathy: a role of mycotoxins in the production of CNS disease in humans?' *Annals of Neurology*, **32**, 453. (Abstract.)

—— Cadera, W., Hinton, G. (1993) 'Successful treatment of hereditary trembling chin with botulinum toxin.' *Journal of Child Neurology*, **8**, 154–156.

Gordon, N. (1996) 'Dopa-responsive dystonia: a widening spectrum.' *Developmental Medicine and Child Neurology*, **38**, 554–559.

Gotoda, T., Arita, M., Arai, H., *et al.* (1995) 'Adult-onset spinocerebellar dysfunction caused by a mutation in the gene for the α-tocopheral transfer protein.' *New England Journal of Medicine*, **333**, 1313–1318.

Goutières, F., Aicardi, J. (1982) 'Acute neurological dysfunction associated with destructive lesions in the basal ganglia in children.' *Annals of Neurology*, **12**, 328–332.

—— —— (1985) 'Rett syndrome: clinical presentation and laboratory investigations in 12 further French patients.' *Brain and Development*, **7**, 305–306.

—— —— Farkas, E. (1977) 'Anterior horn cell disease associated with pontocerebellar hypoplasia in infants.' *Journal of Neurology, Neurosurgery, and Psychiatry*, **40**, 370–378.

—— Mikol, J., Aicardi, J. (1990) 'Neuronal intranuclear inclusion disease in a child: diagnosis by rectal biopsy.' *Annals of Neurology*, **27**, 103–106.

—— Boulloche, J., Bourgeois, H., Aicardi, J. (1996) 'Leucoencephalopahy, megalencephaly and mild clinical course. A recently individualized familial leukodystrophy. Report on five new cases.' *Journal of Child Neurology*, **11**, 439–443.

Gouw, L.G., Digre, K.B., Harris, C.P., *et al.* (1994) 'Autosomal dominant cerebellar ataxia with retinal degeneration: clinical, neuropathologic, and genetic analysis of a large kindred.' *Neurology*, **44**, 1441–1447.

Graff-Radford, N.R. (1986) 'A recessively inherited ataxia with episodes of dystonia.' *Journal of Neurology, Neurosurgery, and Psychiatry*, **49**, 591–594.

Grimes, J.D., Hassan, M.N., Quarrington, A.M., D'Alton, J. (1982) 'Delayed-onset posthemiplegic dystonia: CT demonstration of basal ganglia pathology.' *Neurology*, **32**, 1033–1035.

Grunnet, M.L., Zimmerman, A.W., Lewis, R.A. (1983) 'Ultrastructure and electrodiagnosis of peripheral neuropathy in Cockayne's syndrome.' *Neurology*, **33**, 1606–1609.

Gualtieri, C.T., Quade, D., Hicks, R.E., *et al.* (1984) 'Tardive dyskinesia and other clinical consequences of neuroleptic treatment in children and adolescents.' *American Journal of Psychiatry*, **141**, 20–23.

Guazzi, G.C., Stoppolini, G., Ventruto, V., Di Iorio, G. (1974) 'Immaturité corticale avec agénésie des grandes commissures interhémisphériques et hypoplasie des voies optico-pyramidales chez trois enfants issus d'une même famille.' *Acta Neurologica*, **39**, 659–674.

Guzzetta, F., Mercuri, E., Bonanno, S., *et al.* (1993) 'Autosomal recessive congenital cerebellar atrophy. A clinical and neuropsychological study.' *Brain and Development*, **15**, 439–445.

Haber, S.N., Kowall, N.W., Vonsattel, J.P., *et al.* (1986) 'Gilles de la Tourette's syndrome. A postmortem neuropathological and immunohistochemical study.' *Journal of the Neurological Sciences*, **75**, 225–241.

Hadders-Algra, M., Bos, A.F., Martijn, A., Prechtl, H.F.R. (1994) 'Infantile chorea in an infant with severe bronchopulmonary dysplasia: an EMG study.' *Developmental Medicine and Child Neurology*, **36**, 177–182.

Haenggeli, C-A., Engel, E., Pizzolato, G-P. (1989) 'Connatal Pelizaeus–Merzbacher disease.' *Developmental Medicine and Child Neurology*, **31**, 803–815.

Hagberg, B. (1993) *Rett Syndrome—Clinical and Biological Aspects. Clinics in Developmental Medicine No. 127*. London: Mac Keith Press.

—— Skjeldal, O.H. (1994) 'Rett variants: a suggested model for inclusion criteria.' *Pediatric Neurology*, **11**, 5–11.

—— Witt-Engerström, I. (1986) 'Rett syndrome: a suggested staging system for describing impairment profile with increasing age towards adolescence.' *American Journal of Medical Genetics*, **24**, Suppl. 1, 47–59.

—— Kyllerman, M., Steen, G. (1979) 'Dyskinesia and dystonia in neurometabolic disorders.' *Neuropädiatrie*, **19**, 305–320.

—— Aicardi, J., Dias, K., Ramos, O. (1983) 'A progressive syndrome of autism, dementia, ataxia and loss of purposeful hand use in girls: Rett syndrome: report of 35 cases.' *Annals of Neurology*, **14**, 471–479.

Hall, K., Gardner-Medwin, D. (1978) 'CT scan appearances in Leigh's disease (subacute necrotizing encephalomyelopathy).' *Neuroradiology*, **16**, 48–50.

Hall, N.A., Lake, B.D., Dewji, N.N., Parick, A.D. (1991) 'Liposomal storage of subunit C of mitochondrial ATP synthase in Batten's disease (ceroid–lipofuscinosis).' *Biochemical Journal*, **275**, 269–272.

Hallett, M., Chadwick, D., Marsden, C.D. (1977) 'Ballistic overflow movement myoclonus. A form of essential myoclonus.' *Brain*, **100**, 299–312.

—— —— (1979) 'Cortical reflex myoclonus.' *Neurology*, **29**, 1107–1125.

Haltia, M., Somer, M. (1993) 'Infantile cerebello-optic atrophy. Neuropathology of the progressive encephalopathy syndrome with edema, hypsarrhythmia and optic atrophy (the PEHO syndrome).' *Acta Neuropathologica*, **85**, 241–247.

Hammans, S.R. (1996) 'The inherited ataxias and the new genetics.' *Journal of Neurology, Neurosurgery, and Psychiatry*, **61**, 327–332.

Hammerstein, W., Bischof, G., Keck, E. (1982) 'A tapetoretinal degeneration with symmetrical calcifications of the basal ganglia.' *European Neurology*, **21**, 249–255.

Hanefeld, F., Holzbach, U., Kruse, B., *et al.* (1993) 'Diffuse white matter disease in three children: an encephalopathy with unique features on magnetic resonance imaging and proton magnetic resonance spectroscopy.' *Neuropediatrics*, **24**, 244–248.

Hannan, M.A., Sigut, D., Waghray, M., Gascon, G.G. (1994) 'Ataxia–ocular motor apraxia syndrome: an investigation of cellular radiosensitivity of patients and their families.' *Journal of Medical Genetics*, **31**, 953–956.

Happle, R., Traupe, H., Gröbe, H., Bonsmann, G. (1984) 'The Tay syndrome (congenital ichthyosis with trichothiodystrophy).' *European Journal of Pediatrics*, **141**, 147–152.

Harbord, M.G., Harden, A., Harding, B., *et al.* (1990) 'Megalencephaly and dysmyelination, spasticity, ataxia, seizures and distinctive neurophysiological findings in two siblings.' *Neuropediatrics*, **21**, 164–168.

Harden, A.E., Pampiglione, G. (1982) 'Neurophysiological studies (EEG/EG/VEP/SEP) in 88 children with so-called ceroid lipofuscinosis.' *In:* Armstrong, D., Koppang, N., Ridder, J.H. (Eds.) *Ceroid-lipofuscinosis (Batten's Disease).* Amsterdam: Elsevier, pp. 61–70.

Hardie, R.J., Pullon, H.W.M., Harding, A.E., *et al.* (1991) 'Neuroacanthocytosis. A clinical, haematological and pathological study of 19 cases.' *Brain*, **114**, 13–49.

Harding, A.E. (1981a) 'Early onset cerebellar ataxia with retained tendon reflexes: a clinical and genetic study of a disorder distinct from Friedreich's ataxia.' *Journal of Neurology, Neurosurgery, and Psychiatry*, **44**, 503–508.

—— (1981b) 'Friedreich's ataxia: a clinical and genetic study of 90 families with an analysis of early diagnostic criteria and intrafamilial clustering of clinical features.' *Brain*, **104**, 589–620.

—— (1981c) 'Hereditary "pure" spastic paraplegia: a clinical and genetic study of 22 families.' *Journal of Neurology, Neurosurgery, and Psychiatry*, **44**, 871–883.

—— (1993) 'Clinical features and classification of inherited ataxias.' *In:* Harding, A.E., Deufel, T. (Eds.) *Advances in Neurology, Vol. 61. Inherited Ataxias.* New York: Raven Press, pp. 1–14.

Harding, B.N. (1990) 'Progressive neuronal degeneration of childhood with liver disease (Alpers–Huttenlocher syndrome): a personal view.' *Journal of Child Neurology*, **5**, 273–287.

—— Boyd, S.G. (1991) 'Intractable seizures from infancy can be associated with dentato-olivary dysphasia.' *Journal of the Neurological Sciences*, **104**, 157–165.

—— Brett, E.M. (1995) 'Familial cerebellar degeneration of early onset.' *Journal of Neurology, Neurosurgery, and Psychiatry*, **54**, 469.

—— Dunger, D.B., Grant, D.B., Erdohazi, M. (1988) 'Familial olivopontocerebellar atrophy with neonatal onset: a recessively inherited syndrome with systemic and biochemical abnormalities.' *Journal of Neurology, Neurosurgery, and Psychiatry*, **51**, 385–390.

—— Alsanjari, N., Smith, S.J.M., *et al.* (1995) 'Progressive neuronal degeneration of childhood with liver disease (Alpers' disease) presenting in young adults.' *Journal of Neurology, Neurosurgery, and Psychiatry*, **58**, 320–325.

Harrison, M.B., Lyons, G.R., Landow, E.R. (1993) 'Phenytoin and dyskinesias: a report of two cases and review of the literature.' *Movement Disorders*, **8**, 19–27.

Harwood, G., Hierons, R., Fletcher, N.A., Marsden, C.D. (1994) 'Lessons from a remarkable family with dopa-responsive dystonia.' *Journal of Neurology, Neurosurgery, and Psychiatry*, **57**, 460–463.

Hattori, H., Kawamori, J., Takao, T., *et al.* (1983) 'Computed tomography in postinfluenzal encephalitis.' *Brain and Development*, **5**, 564–567.

Herva, R., Von Wendt, L., Von Wendt, G., *et al.* (1987) 'A syndrome with juvenile cataract, cerebellar atrophy, mental retardation and myopathy.' *Neuropediatrics*, **18**, 164–169.

Hess, D.C., Fisher, A.Q., Yagmai, F., *et al.* (1990) 'Comparative neuroimaging with pathologic correlates in Alexander's disease.' *Journal of Child Neurology*, **5**, 248–252.

Higgins, J.J., Patterson, M.C., Papadopoulos, N.M., *et al.* (1992) 'Hypoprebetalipoproteinemia, acanthocytosis, retinitis pigmentosa, and pallidal degeneration (HARP syndrome).' *Neurology*, **42**, 194–198.

Hoffmann, G.F., Charpentier, C., Mayatepek, E., Mancini, J., *et al.* (1993) 'Clinical and biochemical phenotype in 11 patients with mevalonic aciduria.' *Pediatrics*, **91**, 915–921.

Hogan, G.R., Bauman, M.L. (1977) 'Familial spastic ataxia: occurrence in childhood.' *Neurology*, **27**, 520–526.

Holland, I.M., Kendall, B.E. (1980) 'Computed tomography in Alexander's disease.' *Neuroradiology*, **20**, 103–106.

Holmes, G., Logan, W.J. (1980) 'A syndrome of infantile CNS degeneration.' *American Journal of Diseases of Children*, **134**, 262–266.

—— Shaywitz, B.A. (1977) 'Strümpell's pure familial spastic paraplegia: case study and review of the literature.' *Journal of Neurology, Neurosurgery, and Psychiatry*, **40**, 1003–1008.

Hooft, C., Deloore, G., van Bogaert, I., Guazzi, G.C. (1965) 'Sudanophilic leukodystrohy with meningeal angiomatosis in two brothers: infantile form of diffuse sclerosis with meningeal angiomatosis.' *Journal of the Neurological Sciences*, **2**, 30–51.

Hornykiewicz, O., Kish, S.J., Becker, L.E., *et al.* (1986) 'Brain neurotransmitters in dystonia musculorum deformans.' *New England Journal of Medicine*, **315**, 347–353.

Horoupian, D.S., Zucker, D.K., Moshe, S., Peterson, H.C. (1979) 'Behr syndrome: a clinicopathologic report.' *Neurology*, **29**, 323–327.

Horowitz, I.N., Niparko, N.A. (1994) 'Vertebral artery dissection with bilateral hemiparesis.' *Pediatric Neurology*, **11**, 252–254.

Howard, R.S., Greenwood, R., Gawler, J., *et al.* (1993) 'A familial disorder associated with palatal myoclonus, other brainstem signs, tetraparesis, ataxia and Rosenthal fibre formation.' *Journal of Neurology, Neurosurgery, and Psychiatry*, **56**, 977–981.

Hsiao, K., Prusiner, S.B. (1990) 'Inherited human prion disease.' *Neurology*, **40**, 1820–1827.

Hutchinson, M., O'Riordan, J., Javed, M., *et al.* (1995) 'Familial hemiplegic migraine and autosomal dominant arteriopathy with leukoencephalopathy (CADASIL).' *Annals of Neurology*, **38**, 817–824.

Huygen, P.L.M., Verhagen, W.I.M., Renier, W.O. (1992) 'Oculomotor and vestibular anomalies in Pelizaeus–Merzbacher disease: a study on a kindred with 2 affected and 3 normal males, 3 obligate and 8 possible carriers.' *Journal of the Neurological Sciences*, **113**, 17–25.

Hyland, K., Fryburg, J.S., Wilson, W.G., *et al.* (1997) 'Oral phenylalanine loading in dopa-responsive dystonia: a possible diagnostic test.' *Neurology*, **48**, 1290–1297.

Iacono, R.P., Kuniyoshi, S.M., Lonser, R.R., *et al.* (1996) 'Simultaneous bilateral pallidoansotomy for idiopathic dystonia musculorum deformans.' *Pediatric Neurology*, **14**, 145–148.

Ichinose, H., Ohye, T., Takahashi, E-i., *et al.* (1994) 'Hereditary progressive dystonia with marked diurnal fluctuation caused by mutations in the GTP cyclohydrolase I gene.' *Nature Genetics*, **8**, 236–242.

Iizuka, R., Hirayama, K., Maehara, K. (1984) 'Dentato-rubro-pallido-luysian atrophy: a clinicopathological study.' *Journal of Neurology, Neurosurgery, and Psychiatry*, **47**, 1288–1298.

Ikeuchi, T., Koide, R., Tanaka, H., *et al.* (1995) 'Dentatorubral pallidoluysian atrophy: clinical features are closely related to unstable expansions of trinucleotide (CAG) repeat.' *Annals of Neurology*, **37**, 769–775.

Illarioshkin, S.N., Igarashi, S., Onodera, O., *et al.* (1994) 'Trinucleotide repeat length and rate of progression of Huntington's disease.' *Annals of Neurology*, **36**, 630–635.

—— Tanaka, H., Markova, E.D., *et al.* (1996) 'X-linked non-progressive congenital cerebellar hypoplasia: clinical description and mapping to chromosome Xq.' *Annals of Neurology*, **40**, 75–83.

Illingworth, D.R., Connor, W.E., Miller, R.G. (1980) 'Abetalipoproteinaemia: report of two cases and review of therapy.' *Archives of Neurology*, **37**, 659–662.

Illune, N., Reske-Nielsen, E., Skovby, F., *et al.* (1988) 'Lethal autosomal recessive arthrogryposis multiplex congenita with whistling face and calcifications of the nervous system.' *Neuropediatrics*, **19**, 186–192.

Imamura, S., Tachi, N., Oya, K. (1993) 'Dominantly inherited early-onset non-progressive cerebellar ataxia syndrome.' *Brain and Development*, **15**, 372–376.

Iriarte, L.M., Mateu, J., Cruz, G., Escudero, J. (1988) 'Chorea: a new manifestation of mastocytosis.' *Journal of Neurology, Neurosurgery, and Psychiatry*, **51**, 1457–1458. *(Letter.)*

Jagadha, V., Halliday, W.C., Becker, L.E., Hinton, D. (1988) 'The association of infantile osteopetrosis and neuronal storage disease in two brothers.' *Acta Neuropathologica*, **75**, 233–240.

Jankovic, J. (1994) 'Post-traumatic movement disorders: central peripheral mechanisms.' *Neurology*, **44**, 2006–2014.

—— Fahn, S. (1986) 'The phenomenology of tics.' *Movement Disorders*, **1**, 17–26.

—— Orman, J. (1988) 'Tetrabenazine therapy of dystonia, chorea, tics, and other dyskinesias.' *Neurology*, **38**, 391–394.

Janota, I. (1974) 'Spongy degeneration of grey matter in three children: neuropathological report.' *Archives of Disease in Childhood*, **49**, 571–575.

Jason, G.W., Pajurkova, E.M., Suchowersky, O., *et al.* (1988) 'Presymptomatic neuropsychological impairment in Huntington's disease.' *Archives of Neurology*, **45**, 769–773.

Jongen, P.J.H., Renier, W.O., Gabreëls, F.J.M. (1980) 'Seven cases of Huntington disease in childhood and levodopa induced improvement in the hypokinetic–rigid form.' *Clinical Neurology and Neurosurgery*, **82**, 251–261.

Kaiser, R., Ziegler, G. (1992) 'Hereditary progressive dystonia with diurnal fluctuation (Segawa's syndrome)—an unusual case.' *Neuropediatrics*, **23**, 268–271.

Kallio, A-K. (1983) 'A new syndrome with ophthalmoplegia, hypacusis, ataxia, hypotonia and athetosis (O-HAHA syndrome).' *Neuropediatrics*, **14**, 118. *(Abstract.)*

Karpati, G., Carpenter, S., Wolfe, L.S., Andermann, F. (1977) 'Juvenile dystonic lipidosis: an unusual form of neurovisceral storage disease.' *Neurology*, **27**, 32–42.

Katsumori, H., Imaizumi, T., Izumi, T., *et al.* (1990) 'Basal ganglia calcification in an epileptic child who had long been treated with acetazolamide.' *Brain and Development*, **12**, 355–356. *(Abstract.)*

Kawahara, H., Tomita, Y., Takashima, S., *et al.* (1988) 'Neurophysiological and neuropathological studies in two children with unusual form of multiple system degeneration: evidence for cerebellar and brainstem involvement.' *Brain and Development*, **10**, 312–318.

Kaye, E.M., Doll, R.F., Natowicz, M.R., Smith, F.I. (1994) 'Pelizaeus–Merzbacher disease presenting as spinal muscular atrophy: clinical and molecular studies.' *Annals of Neurology*, **36**, 916–919.

Keats, B.J.B., Ward, L.J., Shaw, J., *et al.* (1989) '"Acadian" and "classical" forms of Friedreich ataxia are most probably caused by mutations at the same locus.' *American Journal of Medical Genetics*, **33**, 266–268.

Kendall, B., Cavanagh, N. (1986) 'Intracranial calcification in paediatric computed tomography.' *Neuroradiology*, **28**, 324–330.

—— Boyd, S.G., Egger, J., Harding, B.N. (1987) 'Progressive neuronal degeneration of childhood with liver disease.' *Neuroradiology*, **29**, 174–180.

Keuth, B., Alon, U., Fuchshuber, A., *et al.* (1996) 'Aplasia of the cerebellar vermis associated with chronic renal disease. A report of six cases and a review of the literature.' *European Journal of Pediatrics*, **155**, 963–967.

Kimura, S., Sasaki, Y. (1988) 'Ultrastructural muscle pathology in infantile neuroaxonal dystrophy.' *Brain and Development*, **10**, 327–329.

—— Keiji, K., Kanaya, A. (1988) 'A case of transient hypodensity of the caudatum and putamen.' *Brain and Development*, **10**, 191–192.

Kjellin, K.G. (1975) 'Hereditary spastic paraplegia and retinal degeneration (Kjellin syndrome and Barnard–Scholz syndrome).' *In:* Vinken, P.J., Bruyn, G.W. (Eds.) *Handbook of Clinical Neurology. Vol. 22. System Disorders and Atrophies, Part II.* Amsterdam: North Holland, pp. 467–473.

Klockgether, T., Petersen, D., Grodd, W., Dichgans, J. (1991) 'Early onset cerebellar ataxia with retained tendon reflexes. Clinical, electrophysiological and MRI observations in comparison with Friedreich's ataxia.' *Brain*, **114**, 1559–1573.

—— Chamberlain, S., Wüllner, U., *et al.* (1993) 'Late-onset Friedreich's ataxia. Molecular genetics, clinical neurophysiology, and magnetic resonance imaging.' *Archives of Neurology*, **50**, 803–806.

Kobari, M., Nogawa, S., Sugimoto, Y., Fukuuchi, Y. (1997) 'Familial idiopathic brain calcification with autosomal dominant inheritance.' *Neurology*, **48**, 645–649.

Kohlschütter, A., Behbehani, A., Langenbeck, U., *et al.* (1982) 'A familial progressive neurodegenerative disease with 2-oxoglutaric aciduria.' *European Journal of Pediatrics*, **138**, 32–37.

Koletzko, S., Koletzko, B., Lamprecht, A., Lenard, H.G. (1987) 'Ataxia–deafness–retardation syndrome in three sisters.' *Neuropediatrics*, **18**, 18–21.

Koller, W.C., Klawans, H.L. (1980) 'Cerebellar calcification on computerized tomography.' *Annals of Neurology*, **7**, 193–194.

Konigsmark, B., Weiner, R.L. (1970) 'The olivopontocerebellar atrophies: a review.' *Medicine*, **49**, 227–241.

Korf, B., Wallman, J.K., Levy, H.L. (1986) 'Bilateral lucency of the globus pallidus complicating methylmalonic acidemia.' *Annals of Neurology*, **20**, 364–366.

Kornberg, A.J., Shield, L.K. (1991) 'An extended phenotype of an early-onset inherited nonprogressive cerebellar ataxia syndrome.' *Journal of Child Neurology*, **6**, 20–23.

Korten, J.J., Notermans, S.L.H., Frenken, C.W.G.M., *et al.* (1974) 'Familial essential myoclonus.' *Brain*, **97**, 131–138.

Koskinen, T., Santavuori, P., Sainio, K., *et al.* (1994) 'Infantile onset spinocerebellar ataxia with sensory neuropathy: a new inherited disease.' *Journal of Neurological Sciences*, **121**, 50–56.

Koskiniemi, M., Donner, M., Majuri, H., *et al.* (1974a) 'Progressive myoclonus epilepsy—a clinical and histopathological study.' *Acta Neurologica Scandinavica*, **50**, 307–332.

—— Toivakka, E., Donner, M. (1974b) 'Progressive myoclonus epilepsy—electroencephalographical findings.' *Acta Neurologica Scandinavica*, **50**, 333–359.

Kramer, P.L., De León, D., Ozelius, L., *et al.* (1990) 'Dystonia gene in Ashkenazi Jewish population is located on chromosome 9q32–34.' *Annals of Neurology*, **27**, 114–120.

Krauss, J.K., Nobbe, F., Wakhloo, A.K., *et al.* (1992) 'Movement disorders in astrocytomas of the basal ganglia and the thalamus.' *Journal of Neurology, Neurosurgery, and Psychiatry*, **55**, 1162–1167.

Kremer, B., Goldberg, P., Andrew, S.E., *et al.* (1994) 'A worldwide study of the Huntington's disease mutation. The sensitivity and specificity of measuring CAG repeats.' *New England Journal of Medicine*, **330**, 1401–1406.

Kupke, K.G., Lee, L.V., Müller, U. (1990a) 'Assignment of the X-linked torsion dystonia gene to Xq21 by linkage analysis.' *Neurology*, **40**, 1438–1442.

—— Lee, L.V., Viterbo, G.H., *et al.* (1990b) 'X-linked recessive torsion dystonia in the Philippines.' *American Journal of Medical Genetics*, **36**, 237–242.

Kuriyama, M., Fujiyama, J., Yoshidome, H., *et al.* (1991) 'Cerebrotendinous xanthomatosis: clinical and biochemical evaluation of eight patients and review of the literature.' *Journal of the Neurological Sciences*, **102**, 225–232.

Kurlan, R., Behr, J., Medved, L., *et al.* (1986) 'Familial Tourette's syndrome: report of a large pedigree and potential for linkage analysis.' *Neurology*, **36**, 772–776.

Kyllerman, M., Forsgren, L., Sanner, G., *et al.* (1990) 'Alcohol-responsive myoclonic dystonia in a large family: dominant inheritance and phenotypic variation.' *Movement Disorders*, **5**, 270–279.

—— Sommerfelt, K., Hedström, A., *et al.* (1991) 'Clinical and neurophysiological development of Unverricht–Lundborg disease in four Swedish siblings.' *Epilepsia*, **32**, 900–909.

—— Sanner, G., Forsgren, L., *et al.* (1993) 'Early onset dystonia decreasing with development. Case report of two children with familial myoclonic dystonia.' *Brain and Development*, **15**, 295–298.

Labrune, P., Lacroix, C., Goutières, F., *et al.* (1996) 'Extensive brain calcifications, leukodystrophy, and formation of parenchymal cysts: a new progressive disorder due to diffuse cerebral microangiopathy.' *Neurology*, **46**, 1297–1301.

Lake, B.D., Cavanagh, N.P.C. (1978) 'Early-juvenile Batten's disease—a recognizable sub-group distinct from other forms of Batten's disease.' *Journal of the Neurological Sciences*, **36**, 265–271.

—— Brett, E.M., Boyd, S.G. (1996) 'A form of juvenile Batten disease with granular osmiophilic deposits.' *Neuropediatrics*, **27**, 265–269.

Lance, J.W. (1986) 'Action myoclonus, Ramsay Hunt syndrome, and other cerebellar myoclonic syndromes.' *In:* Fahn, S., Marsden, C.D., Van Woert, M. (Eds.) *Advances in Neurology, Vol. 43. Myoclonus.* New York: Raven Press, pp. 33–55.

Lang, A.E., Clark, J.T.E., Resch, L., *et al.* (1985) 'Progressive long-standing pure dystonia: a new phenotype of juvenile metachromatic leukodystrophy.' *Neurology*, **35**, Suppl. 1, 194.

Lapresle, J. (1982) 'La dystasie aréfléxique héréditaire de Roussy–Lévy.' *Revue Neurologique*, **138**, 967–978.

Larsen, T.A., Dunn, H.G., Jan, J.E., Calne, D.B. (1985) 'Dystonia and calcification of the basal ganglia.' *Neurology*, **35**, 533–537.

Lasker, A.G., Zee, D.S., Hain, T.C., *et al.* (1987) 'Saccades in Huntington disease: initiation defects and distractability.' *Neurology*, **37**, 364–370.

Laxova, R., Brown, E.S., Hogan, K., *et al.* (1985) 'An X-linked recessive basal ganglia disorder with mental retardation.' *American Journal of Medical Genetics*, **21**, 681–689.

Leber, S.M., Brunberg, J.A., Pavkovic, I.M. (1995) 'Infarction of basal ganglia associated with California encephalitis virus.' *Pediatric Neurology*, **12**, 346–349.

Lebon, P., Badoual, J., Ponsot, G., *et al.* (1988) 'Intrathecal synthesis of interferon-alpha in infants with progressive familial encephalopathy.' *Journal of the Neurological Sciences*, **84**, 201–208.

Lee, M.S., Rinne, J.O., Ceballos-Baumann, A., *et al.* (1994) 'Dystonia after head trauma.' *Neurology*, **44**, 1374–1378.

Lee, S., Park, Y.D., Yen, S-H.C., *et al.* (1989) 'A study of infantile motor neuron disease with neurofilament and ubiquitin immunocytochemistry.' *Neuropediatrics*, **20**, 107–111.

Leech, R.W., Brumback, R.A., Miller, R.H., *et al.* (1985) 'Cockayne syndrome: clinicopathologic and tissue culture studies of affected siblings.' *Journal of Neuropathology and Experimental Neurology*, **44**, 507–519.

Leger, J.M., Duyckaerts, C., Brunet, P. (1986) 'Syndrome of palatal myoclonus and progressive ataxia: report of a case.' *Neurology*, **36**, 1409–1410.

Lehesjoki, A-E., Carelli, V., Posar, A., *et al.* (1997) 'Familial Unverricht–Lundberg disease: a clinical, neurophysiologic, and genetic study.' *Epilepsia*, **38**, 637–641.

Lehmann, A.R. (1982) 'Three complementation groups in Cockayne syndrome.' *Mutation Research*, **106**, 347–356.

Lenti, C., Bianchini, E. (1993) 'Neuropsychological and neuroradiological study of a case of early-onset Huntington's chorea.' *Developmental Medicine and Child Neurology*, **35**, 1007–1010.

Leone, M., Rocca, W.A., Rosso, M.G., *et al.* (1988) 'Friedreich's disease: survival analysis in an Italian population.' *Neurology*, **38**, 1433–1438.

Leube, B., Hendgen, T., Kessler, K.R., *et al.* (1997) 'Sporadic focal dystonia in Northwest Germany: molecular basis on chromosome 18p.' *Annals of Neurology*, **42**, 111–114.

Leuzzi, V., Favatà, I., Seri, S. (1988) 'Bilateral striatal lesions.' *Developmental Medicine and Child Neurology*, **30**, 252–257.

Ley, C.O., Gali, F.G. (1983) 'Parkinsonian syndrome after methanol intoxication.' *European Neurology*, **22**, 405–409.

Leys, D., Bourgeois, P., Destée, A., Petit, H. (1985) 'Syndrome choréique et état psychotique aigus provoqués par une substance amphétaminique.' *Revue Neurologique*, **141**, 499–500.

—— Destée, A., Petit, H., Warot, P. (1987) 'Chorea associated with oral contraception.' *Journal of Neurology*, **235**, 46–48.

Libert, J., Martin, J.J., Ceuterick, C. (1982) 'Protracted and atypical forms of ceroid–lipofuscinosis.' *In:* Armstrong, B., Koppang, N., Rider, J.A. (Eds.) *Ceroid-lipofuscinosis (Batten's Disease).* Amsterdam: Elsevier, pp. 45–57.

Lieberman, J.A., Saltz, B.L., Johns, C.A., *et al.* (1991) 'The effects of clozapine on tardive dyskinesia.' *British Journal of Psychiatry*, **158**, 503–510.

Logigian, E.L., Kolodny, E.H., Griffith, J.F., *et al.* (1986) 'Myoclonus epilepsy in two brothers: clinical features and neuropathology of a unique syndrome.' *Brain*, **109**, 411–429.

Lossos, A., Cooperman, H., Soffer, D., *et al.* (1995) 'Hereditary leukoencephalopathy and palmoplantar keratoderma: a new disorder with increased skin collagen content.' *Neurology*, **45**, 331–337.

Lott, I.T., Williams, R.S., Schnur, J.A., Hier, D.B. (1979) 'Familial amentia, unusual ventricular calcifications, and increased cerebrospinal fluid protein.' *Neurology*, **29**, 1571–1577.

Lou, J.S, Jankovic, J. (1991) 'Essential tremor: clinical correlates in 350 patients.' *Neurology*, **41**, 234–238.

Louis, E.D., Lynch, T., Cargan, A.L., Fahn, S. (1995) 'Generalized chorea in an infant with semilobar holoprosencephaly.' *Pediatric Neurology*, **13**, 355–357.

Lüdecke, B., Knappskog, P.M., Clayton, P.T., *et al.* (1996) 'Recessively inherited L-DOPA-responsive parkinsonism in infancy caused by a point mutation (L205P) in the tyrosine-hydroxylase gene.' *Human Molecular Genetics*, **5**, 1023–1028.

Lynch, B.J., Becich, M.J., Torack, R.M., Rust, R.S. (1992) 'Arrested maturation of cerebral neurons, axons and myelin: a new familial syndrome of newborns.' *Neuropediatrics*, **23**, 180–187.

Lynch, T., Sano, M., Marder, K.S., *et al.* (1994) 'Clinical characteristics of a family with chromosome 17-linked disinhibition–dementia–parkinsonism–amyotrophy complex.' *Neurology*, **44**, 1878–1884.

Lyon, G., Arita, F., Le Galloudec, E., *et al.* (1990) 'A disorder of axonal development, necrotizing myopathy, cardiomyopathy and cataracts: a new familial disease.' *Annals of Neurology*, **27**, 193–191.

—— Adams, R.D., Kolodny, E.H. (1996) *Neurology of Hereditary Metabolic Diseases of Children, 2nd Edn.* New York: McGraw Hill.

MacMillan, J.C., Morrison, P.J., Nevin, N.C., *et al.* (1993) 'Identification of an expanded CAG repeat in the Huntington's disease gene (IT15) in a family reported to have benign hereditary chorea.' *Journal of Medical Genetics*, **30**, 1012–1013.

Mahajan, P., Lieh-Lai, M.W., Sarnaik, A., Kottamasu, S.R. (1997) 'Basal ganglia infarction in a child with disulfiram poisoning.' *Pediatrics*, **99**, 605–608.

Mainzer, F., Saldino, R.F., Ozonoff, M.B., Minaghi, H. (1970) 'Familial nephropathy associated with retinitis pigmentosa, cerebellar ataxia and skeletal abnormaliities.' *American Journal of Medicine*, **49**, 556–562.

Malafosse, A., Lehesjoki, A.E., Genton, P., *et al.* (1991) 'Identical genetic locus for Baltic and Mediterranean myoclonus.' *Lancet*, **339**, 1080–1081.

Malamud, N., Cohen, P. (1958) 'Unusual form of cerebellar ataxia with sex-linked inheritance.' *Neurology*, **8**, 261–266.

Malandrini, A., Fabrizi, G.M., Bartalucci, P., *et al.* (1996a) 'Clinicopathological study of familial late infantile Hallervorden–Spatz disease: a particular form of neuroacanthocytosis.' *Child's Nervous System*, **12**, 155–160.

—— Scarpini, C., Palmeri, S., *et al.* (1996b) 'Palatal myoclonus and unusual MRI findings in a patient with membranous lipodystrophy.' *Brain and Development*, **18**, 59–63.

Manuelidis, E.E., Rorke, L.B. (1989) 'Transmission of Alpers' disease (chronic progressive encephalopathy) produces experimental Creutzfeldt–Jakob disease in hamsters.' *Neurology*, **39**, 615–621.

Manyam, B.V., Bhatt, M.H., Moore, W.D., *et al.* (1992) 'Bilateral striato-pallidodentate calcinosis: cerebral spinal fluid, imaging, and electrophysiological studies.' *Annals of Neurology*, **31**, 379–384.

Maris, T., Androulidakis, E.J., Tzagournissakis, M., *et al.* (1995) 'X-linked adrenoleukodystrophy presenting as neurologically pure familial spastic paraparesis.' *Neurology*, **45**, 1101–1104.

Marsden, C.D., Harrison, M.J.G. (1974) 'Idiopathic torsion dystonia (DMD). A review of 42 patients.' *Brain*, **97**, 793–810.

—— Marion, M-H., Quinn, N. (1984) 'The treatment of severe dystonia in children and adults.' *Journal of Neurology, Neurosurgery, and Psychiatry*, **47**, 1166–1173.

—— Lang, A.E., Quinn, N.P., *et al.* (1986) 'Familial dystonia and visual failure with striatal CT lucencies.' *Journal of Neurology, Neurosurgery, and Psychiatry*, **49**, 500–509.

—— Harding, A.E., Obeso, J.A., Lu, C-S. (1990) 'Progressive myoclonic ataxia (the Ramsay Hunt syndrome).' *Archives of Neurology*, **47**, 1121–1125.

Marseille Consensus Group (1990) 'Classification of progressive myoclonus epilepsies and related disorders.' *Annals of Neurology*, **28**, 113–116.

Martin, J.J., Ceuterick, C. (1978) 'Morphological study of skin biopsy specimens: a contribution to the diagnosis of metabolic disorders with involvement of the nervous system.' *Journal of Neurology, Neurosurgery, and Psychiatry*, **41**, 232–248.

—— Martin, L., Ceuterick, C.M. (1977) 'Encephalopathy associated with lamellar residual bodies in astrocytes (Towfighi, Grover and Gonatas 1975): a new observation.' *Neuropädiatrie*, **8**, 181–189.

—— Ceuterick, C.M., Leroy, J.G., *et al.* (1984) 'The Wiedemann–Rautenstrauch or neonatal progeroid syndrome. Neuropathological study of a case.' *Neuropediatrics*, **15**, 43–48.

Martinelli, P., Giuliani, S., Ippoliti, M., *et al.* (1993) 'Familial idiopathic strio-pallido-dentate calcifications with late onset extrapyramidal syndrome.' *Movement Disorders*, **8**, 220–222.

Marzan, K.A.B., Barron, T.F. (1994) 'MRI abnormalities in Behr syndrome.' *Pediatric Neurology*, **10**, 247–248.

Matilla, T., McCall, A., Subramony, S.H., Zoghbi, H.Y. (1995) 'Molecular and clinical correlations in spinocerebellar ataxia type 3 and Machado–Joseph disease.' *Annals of Neurology*, **38**, 68–72.

Matsuyama, H., Watanabe, I., Mihm, M.C., Richardson, E.P. (1978) 'Dermatoleukodystrophy with neuroaxonal spheroids.' *Archives of Neurology*, **35**, 329–336.

McKinney, A.S. (1962) 'Idiopathic hypoparathyroidism presenting as chorea.' *Neurology*, **12**, 485–491.

Mimaki, T., Itoh, N., Abe, J., *et al.* (1986) 'Neurological manifestations in xeroderma pigmentosum.' *Annals of Neurology*, **20**, 70–75.

Minami, T., Otsuka, M., Ichiya, Y., *et al.* (1994) 'Different patterns of [18F] dopa uptake in siblings with hereditary dentato-rubro-pallido-luysian atrophy.' *Brain and Development*, **16**, 335–338.

Mirowitz, S.A., Westrich, T.J., Hirsch, J.D. (1991) 'Hyperintense basal ganglia on T1-weighted MR images in patients receiving parenteral nutrition.' *Radiology*, **181**, 117–120.

Mito, T., Tanaka, T., Becker, L.E., *et al.* (1986) 'Infantile bilateral striatalnecrosis. Clinicopathological classification.' *Archives of Neurology*, **43**, 677–680.

Miyoshi, K., Matsuoka, T., Mizushima, S. (1969) 'Familial holotopistic striatal necrosis.' *Acta Neuropathologica*, **13**, 240–249.

Morvan, D., Komajda, M., Doan, L.D., *et al.* (1992) 'Cardiomyopathy in Friedreich's ataxia: a Doppler-echocardiographic study.' *European Heart Journal*, **13**, 1393–1398.

Moss, W., Ojukwu, C., Chiriboga, C.A. (1994) 'Phenytoin-induced movement disorder. Unilateral presentation in a child and response to diphenhydramine.' *Clinical Pediatrics*, **33**, 634–638.

Mostofsky, S.H., Blasco, P.A., Butler, I.J., Dobyns, W.B. (1996) 'Autosomal dominant torsion dystonia with onset in infancy.' *Pediatric Neurology*, **15**, 245–248.

Mousa, A.R.A-M., Al-Din, A.S.M., Al-Nassar, K.E., *et al.* (1986) 'Autosomally inherited recessive spastic ataxia, macular corneal dystrophy, congenital cataracts, myopia and vertically oval temporally tilted discs. Report of a Bedouin family—a new syndrome.' *Journal of the Neurological Sciences*, **76**, 105–121.

Mullin, P.J., Kershaw, P.W., Bolt, J.M.W. (1970) 'Choreoathetotic movement disorder in alcoholism.' *British Medical Journal*, **4**, 278–281.

Nagashima, K., Suzuki, S., Ichikawa, E., *et al.* (1985) 'Infantile neuroaxonal dystrophy: peri-natal onset with symptoms of diencephalic syndrome.' *Neurology*, **35**, 735–738.

Naidu, S. (1997) 'Rett syndrome: a disorder affecting early brain growth.' *Annals of Neurology*, **42**, 3–10.

—— Thirumalai, S., Hosain, S., *et al.* (1993) 'Leukodystrophies of unknown etiology.' *Annals of Neurology*, **34**, 465. (*Abstract*.)

Nance, M.A., Berry, S.A. (1992) 'Cockayne syndrome: review of 140 cases.' *American Journal of Medical Genetics*, **42**, 68–84.

Narbona, J., Obeso, J.A., Martinez-Lage, J.M., Marsden, C.D. (1984) 'Hemidystonia secondary to localised basal ganglia tumour.' *Journal of Neurology, Neurosurgery, and Psychiatry*, **47**, 704–709.

Nardocci, N., Zorzi, G., Grisoli, M., *et al.* (1996) 'Acquired hemidystonia in childhood: a clinical and neuroradiological study of thirteen patients.' *Pediatric Neurology*, **15**, 108–113.

Nath, A., Jankovic, J., Pettigrew, L.C. (1987) 'Movement disorders and AIDS.' *Neurology*, **37**, 37–42.

Nausieda, P.A. (1986) 'Sydenham's chorea, chorea gravidarum and contraceptive-induced chorea.' *In:* Vinken, P.J., Bruyn, G.W., Klawans, H.L. (Eds.) *Handbook of Clinical Neurology. Vol. 49. Extrapyramidal Disorders.* Amsterdam: Elsevier, pp. 359–367.

Nechiporuk, A., Lopes-Cendes, I., Nechiporuk, T., *et al.* (1996) 'Genetic mapping of the spinocerebellar ataxia type 2 gene on human chromosome 12.' *Neurology*, **46**, 1731–1735.

Nezu, A. (1995) 'Neurophysiological study in Pelizaeus–Merzbacher disease.' *Brain and Development*, **17**, 175–181.

—— Kimura, S., Uehara, S., *et al.* (1996) 'Pelizaeus–Merzbacher-like disease: female case report.' *Brain and Development*, **18**, 114–118.

Nicolaides, P., Baraitser, M., Brett, E.M. (1993) 'Two siblings with mental retardation and progressive spasticity.' *Clinical Genetics*, **43**, 312–314.

Niedermeyer, E., Rett, A., Renner, H. (1986) 'Rett syndrome and the electroencephalogram.' *American Journal of Medical Genetics*, **24**, Suppl. 1, 195–199.

Nigro, M.A., Martens, M.E., Awerbuch, G.I., *et al.* (1990) 'Partial cytochrome-b deficiency and generalized dystonia.' *Pediatric Neurology*, **6**, 407–410.

Nishimura, N., Mito, T., Takashima, S., *et al.* (1987) 'Multiple system atrophy with retinal degeneration in a young child.' *Neuropediatrics*, **18**, 91–95.

Nishimura, R., Omos-Lau, N., Ajmone-Marsan, C., Barranger, J.A. (1980) 'Electroencephalographic findings in Gaucher disease.' *Neurology*, **30**, 152–159.

Nordstrom, D.M., West, S.G., Andersen, P.A. (1985) 'Basal ganglia calcifications in central nervous system lupus erythematosus.' *Arthritis and Rheumatism*, **28**, 1412–1416.

Norio, R., Koskiniemi, M.L. (1979) 'Progressive myoclonus epilepsy: genetic and nosological aspects with special reference to 107 Finnish patients.' *Clinical Genetics*, **15**, 382–398.

Norman, R.M., Tingey, A.H., Valentine, J.C., Danby, T.A. (1962) 'Sudanophilic leucodystrophy in a pachygyric brain.' *Journal of Neurology, Neurosurgery, and Psychiatry*, **25**, 363–369.

Novotny, E.J., Singh, G., Wallace, D.C., *et al.* (1986) 'Leber's disease and dystonia: a mitochondrial disease.' *Neurology*, **36**, 1053–1060.

Nutting, P.A., Cole, B.R., Schimke, R.N. (1969) 'Benign, recessively inherited choreo-athetosis of early onset.' *Journal of Medical Genetics*, **6**, 408–410.

Nygaard, T.G. (1995) 'Dopa-responsive dystonia.' *Current Opinion in Neurology*, **8**, 310–313.

Obeso, J.A., Rothwell, J.C., Thompson, P.D., Marsden, C.D. (1983) 'Myoclonic dystonia.' *Neurology*, **33**, 825–830.

—— Artieda, J., Rothwell, J.C., *et al.* (1989) 'The treatment of severe action myoclonus.' *Brain*, **112**, 765–777.

Ohlsson, A., Cumming, W.A., Paul, A., Sly, W.S. (1986) 'Carbonic anhydrase II deficiency syndrome: recessive osteopetrosis with renal tubular acidosis and cerebral calcification.' *Pediatrics*, **77**, 371–381.

Okseter, K., Sirnes, K. (1988) 'Chorea and lupus anticoagulant.' *Acta Neurologica Scandinavica*, **78**, 206–209.

Orrell, R.W., Amrolia, P.J., Heald, A., *et al.* (1995) 'Acanthocytosis, retinitis pigmentosa, and pallidal degeneration: a report of three patients, including the second reported case with hypoprebetalipoproteinemia (HARP syndrome).' *Neurology*, **45**, 487–492.

Osborne, J.P., Munson, P., Burman, D. (1982) 'Huntington's chorea. Report of 3 cases and review of the literature.' *Archives of Disease in Childhood*, **57**, 99–103.

Østergaard, J.R., Christensen, T., Hansen, K.N. (1995) '*In vivo* diagnosis of Hallervorden–Spatz disease.' *Developmental Medicine and Child Neurology*, **37**, 827–833.

Ouvrier, R.A., McLeod, J.G., Conchin, T.E. (1982) 'Friedreich's ataxia—early detection and progression of peripheral nerve abnormalities.' *Journal of the Neurological Sciences*, **55**, 137–145.

Ozelius, L., Kramer, P.L., Moskowitz, C., *et al.* (1989) 'Human gene for torsion dystonia located on chromosome 9q32–q34.' *Cytogenetic and Cell Genetics*, **51**, 1056. (*Abstract*.)

Page, T., Nyhan, W.L., Morena de Vega, V. (1987) 'Syndrome of mild mental retardation, spastic gait and skeletal malformations in a family with partial deficiency of hypoxanthine–guanine phosphoribosyltranferase.' *Pediatrics*, **79**, 713–717.

Palau, F., De Michele, G., Vilchez, J.J., *et al.* (1995) 'Early-onset ataxia with cardiomyopathy and retained tendon reflexes maps to the Friedeich's ataxia locus on chromosome 9q.' *Annals of Neurology*, **37**, 359–362.

Palmer, D.N., Martinus, R.D., Cooper, S.M., *et al.* (1989) 'Ovine ceroid–lipofuscinosis. The major lipopigment protein and the lipid-binding subunit of mitochondrial ATP synthase have the same NH$_2$-terminal sequence.' *Journal of Biological Chemistry*, **264**, 5736–5740.

Park, S., Como, P.G., Cui, L., Kurlan, R. (1993) 'The early course of the Tourette's syndrome clinical spectrum.' *Neurology*, **43**, 1712–1715.

Pascual-Castroviejo, I., Guttierez, M., Morales, C., *et al.* (1994) 'Primary degeneration of the granular layer of the cerebellum. A study of 14 patients and review of the literature.' *Neuropediatrics*, **25**, 183–190.

Patten, J.L., Johns, D.R., Valle, D., *et al.* (1990) 'Mutation of the gene encoding the stimulatory G protein of adenylate cyclase in Albright's hereditary osteodystrophy.' *New England Journal of Medicine*, **322**, 1412–1419.

Pauls, D.S., Leckman, J.F. (1986) 'The inheritance of Gilles de la Tourette syndrome and associated behaviors.' *New England Journal of Medicine*, **315**, 993–997.

Pavone, L., Fiumara, A., Barone, R., *et al.* (1996) 'Olivopontocerebellar atrophy leading to recognition of carbohydrate-deficient glycoprotein syndrome type I.' *Journal of Neurology*, **243**, 700–705.

Penner, M.W., Li, K.C., Gebarski, S.S., Allen, R.J. (1987) 'MR imaging of Pelizaeus–Merzbacher disease.' *Journal of Computer Assisted Tomography*, **11**, 591–593.

Peters, A.C.B., Vielvoye, G.J., Versteeg, J., *et al.* (1979) 'Echo 25 focal encephalitis and subacute hemichorea.' *Neurology*, **29**, 676–681.

Peterson, P.L., Saad, J., Nigro, M.A. (1988) 'The treatment of Friedreich's ataxia with amantadine hydrochloride.' *Neurology*, **38**, 1478–1480.

Pettigrew, L.C., Jankovic, J. (1985) 'Hemidystonia: a report of 20 patients and a review of the literature.' *Journal of Neurology, Neurosurgery, and Psychiatry*, **48**, 650–657.

Pinto, F., Amantini, A., De Scisciolo, G., *et al.* (1988) 'Visual involvement in Friedreich's ataxia: PERG and VEP study.' *European Neurology*, **28**, 246–251.

Plaitakis, A., Berl, S., Yahr, M.D. (1984) 'Neurological disorders associated with deficiency of glutamate dehydrogenase.' *Annals of Neurology*, **15**, 144–153.

Poll-Thé, B.T., Aicardi, J., Girot, R., Rosa, R. (1985) 'Neurological findings in triose-phosphate isomerase deficiency.' *Annals of Neurology*, **17**, 439–443.

Polo, J.M., Calleja, J., Combarros, O., Berciano, J. (1993) 'Hereditary "pure" spastic paraplegia: a study of nine families.' *Journal of Neurology, Neurosurgery, and Psychiatry*, **56**, 175–181.

Powell, F., Staunton, H. (1981) 'Benign familial motor genotypia.' *In:* Huber, A, Klein, D. (Eds.) *Neurogenetics and Neuro-ophthalmology.* Amsterdam: Elsevier, pp. 189–192.

Pozzan, G.B., Battistella, P.A., Rigon, F., *et al.* (1992) 'Hyperthyroid-induced chorea in an adolescent girl.' *Brain and Development*, **14**, 126–127.

Pranzatelli, M.R. (1996) 'Antidyskinetic drug therapy for pediatric movement disorders.' *Journal of Child Neurology*, **11**, 355–369.

—— Mott, S.H., Pavlakis, S.G., *et al.* (1994) 'Clinical spectrum of secondary parkinsonism in childhood: a reversible disorder.' *Pediatric Neurology*, **10**, 131–140.

Pratt, V.M., Naidu, S., Dlouhy, S.R., *et al.* (1995) 'A novel mutation in exon 3 of the proteolipid protein gene in Pelizaeus–Merzbacher disease.' *Neurology*, **45**, 394–395.

Prick, M.J.J., Gabreëls, F.J.M., Renier, W.O., *et al.* (1981) 'Progressive infantile poliodystrophy: association with disturbed pyruvate oxidation in muscle and liver.' *Archives of Neurology*, **38**, 767–772.

—— —— —— *et al.* (1982) 'Progressive infantile poliodystrophy (Alpers' disease) with a defect in citric acid cycle activity in liver and fibroblasts.' *Neuropediatrics*, **13**, 108–111.

Pridmore, C.L., Baraitser, M., Harding, B., *et al.* (1993) 'Alexander's disease: clues to diagnosis.' *Journal of Child Neurology*, **8**, 134–144.

Pujol, A., Pujol, J., Graus, F., *et al.* (1993) 'Hyperintense globus pallidus on T1-weighted MRI in cirrhotic patients is associated with severity of liver failure.' *Neurology*, **43**, 65–69.

Quinn, N.P. (1996) 'Essential myoclonus and myoclonic dystonia.' *Movement Disorders*, **11**, 119–124.

Rajput, A.H., Gibb, W.R.G., Zhong, X.H., *et al.* (1994) 'Dopa-responsive dystonia: pathological and biochemical observations in a case.' *Annals of Neurology*, **35**, 396–402.

Ramaekers, V.T., Lake, B.D., Harding, B., *et al.* (1987) 'Diagnostic difficulties in infantile neuroaxonal dystrophy. A clinicopathological study of eight cases.' *Neuropediatrics*, **18**, 170–175.

Rasmussen, P. (1993) 'Persistent mirror movements: a clinical study of 17 children, adolescents and young adults.' *Developmental Medicine and Child Neurology*, **35**, 699–707.

Razavi-Encha, F., Larroche, J-C., Gaillard, D. (1988) 'Infantile familial encephalopathy with cerebral calcifications and leukodystrophy.' *Neuropediatrics*, **19**, 72–79.

Reiss, A.L., Faruque, F., Naidu, S., *et al.* (1993) 'Neuroanatomy of Rett syndrome: a volumetric imaging study.' *Annals of Neurology*, **34**, 227–234.

Renier, W.O., Gabreëls, F.J.M., Hustinx, T.W.J., *et al.* (1981) 'Connatal Pelizaeus–Merzbacher disease with congenital stridor in two maternal cousins.' *Acta Neuropathologica*, **54**, 11–17.

Rett Syndrome Diagnostic Criteria Work Group (1988) 'Diagnostic criteria for Rett syndrome.' *Annals of Neurology*, **23**, 425–428.

Richfield, E.K., Twyman, R., Berent, S. (1987) 'Neurological syndrome following bilateral damage to the head of the caudate nuclei.' *Annals of Neurology*, **22**, 768–771.

Rivier, F., Echenne, B. (1992) 'Dominantly inherited hypoplasia of the vermis.' *Neuropediatrics*, **23**, 206–208.

Robinson, R.O., Samuels, M., Pohl, K.R.E. (1988) 'Choreic syndrome after cardiac surgery.' *Archives of Disease in Childhood*, **63**, 1466–1469.

Roden, V.J., Cantor, H.E., O'Connor, D.M., *et al.* (1975) 'Acute hemiplegia of childhood associated with Coxsackie type A9 viral infection.' *Journal of Pediatrics*, **86**, 56–58.

Roger, J., Pellissier, J.F., Bureau, M., *et al.* (1983) 'Le diagnostic précoce de la maladie de Lafora. Importance des manifestations paroxystiques visuelles et intérêt de la biopsie cutanée.' *Revue Neurologique*, **139**, 115–124.

—— Genton, P., Bureau, M., *et al.* (1987) 'Dyssynergia cerebellaris myoclonica (Ramsay Hunt syndrome) associated with epilepsy. A study of 32 cases.' *Neuropediatrics*, **18**, 117. *(Abstract.)*

Romano, J.T., Riggs, J.E., Bodensteiner, J.B., Gutmann, L. (1989) 'Wasp sting-associated occlusion of the supraclinoid internal carotid artery: implications regarding the pathogenesis of moyamoya syndrome.' *Archives of Neurology*, **46**, 607–608.

Rondot, P., Ziegler, M. (1983) 'Dystonia—L-dopa responsive or juvenile parkinsonism?' *Journal of Neural Transmission*, Suppl. 19, 273–281.

Ronen, G., Donat, J.R., Hill, A. (1986) 'Hemifacial spasm in children.' *Canadian Journal of the Neurological Sciences*, **13**, 342–343.

Rosenbaum, F., Jankovic, J. (1988) 'Focal task-specific tremor and dystonia: categorization of occupational movement disorders.' *Neurology*, **38**, 522–527.

Rosenberg, R.N. (1995) 'Autosomal dominant cerebellar phenotypes: the genotype has settled the issue.' *Neurology*, **45**, 1–5.

Russo, L.S., Aron, A., Anderson, P.J. (1976) 'Alexander's disease: a report and reappraisal.' *Neurology*, **26**, 607–614.

Rutledge, J.N., Hilal, S.K., Silver, A.S. (1987) 'Study of movement disorders and brain iron by magnetic resonance.' *American Journal of Neuroradiology*, **8**, 397–412.

Sabatino, G., Domizio, S., Verrotti, A., *et al.* (1994) 'Fetal encephalopathy with cerebral calcifications: a case report.' *Child's Nervous System*, **10**, 195–197.

Said, G., Marion, M.H., Selva, J., Jamet, C. (1986) 'Hypotrophic and dying-back nerve fibers in Friedreich's ataxia.' *Neurology*, **36**, 1292–1299.

Saint-Hilaire, H.H., Saint-Hilaire, J.M., Granger, L. (1986) 'Jumping Frenchmen of Maine.' *Neurology*, **36**, 1269–1271.

Saint-Hilaire, M.H., Burke, R.E., Bressman, S.B., *et al.* (1991) 'Delayed-onset dystonia due to perinatal or early childhood asphyxia.' *Neurology*, **41**, 216–222.

Salazar-Grueso, E.F., Holzer, T.J., Gutierrez, R.A., *et al.* (1990) 'Familial spastic paraparesis syndrome associated with HTLV-I infection.' *New England Journal of Medicine*, **323**, 732–737.

Salih, M.A.M., Ahlsten, G., Stalberg, E., *et al.* (1990) 'Friedreich ataxia in 13 children: presentation and evolution with neurophysiologic, electrocardiographic and echocardiographic features.' *Journal of Child Neurology*, **5**, 321–326.

Salonen, R., Somer, M., Haltia, M., *et al.* (1991) 'Progressive encephalopathy with edema, hypsarrhythmia, and optic atrophy (PEHO syndrome).' *Clinical Genetics*, **39**, 287–293.

Santavuori, P. (1988) 'Neuronal ceroid–lipofuscinoses in childhood.' *Brain and Development*, **10**, 80–83.

—— Haltia, M., Rapola, J., Raitta, C. (1973) 'Infantile type of so-called ceroid–lipofuscinosis. Part I. A clinical study of 15 patients.' *Journal of the Neurological Sciences*, **18**, 257–267.

—— Rapola, J., Sainio, K., Raitta, C. (1982) 'A variant of Jansky–Bielschowsky disease.' *Neuropediatrics*, **13**, 135–141.

—— Westermarck, T., Rapola, J., *et al.* (1985) 'Antioxidant treatment in Spielmeyer–Sjögren's disease.' *Acta Neurologica Scandinavica*, **71**, 136–145.

—— Rapola, J., Nuutila, A., *et al.* (1991) 'The spectrum of Jansky–Bielschowsky disease.' *Neuropediatrics*, **22**, 92–96.

Saugier-Veber, P., Munnich, A., Bonneau, D., *et al.* (1994) 'X-linked spastic paraplegia and Pelizaeus–Merzbacher disease are allelic disorders at the proteolipid protein locus.' *Nature Genetics*, **6**, 257–262.

Savoiardo, M., Halliday, W.C., Nardocci, N., *et al.* (1993) 'Hallervorden–Spatz disease: MR and pathologic findings.' *American Journal of Neuroradiology*, **14**, 155–162.

Sawada, Y., Takahashi, M., Ohashi, N., *et al.* (1980) 'Computerised tomography as an indication of long-term outcome after acute carbon monoxide poisoning.' *Lancet*, **1**, 783–784.

Schady, W., Meara, R.J. (1988) 'Hereditary progressive chorea without dementia.' *Journal of Neurology, Neurosurgery, and Psychiatry*, **51**, 295–297.

—— Smith, C.M.L. (1994) 'Sensory neuropathy in hereditary spastic paraplegia.' *Journal of Neurology, Neurosurgery, and Psychiatry*, **57**, 693–698.

Schaffert, D.A., Johnsen, S.D., Johnson, P.C., Drayer, B.P. (1989) 'Magnetic resonance imaging in pathologically proven Hallervorden–Spatz disease.' *Neurology*, **39**, 440–442.

Scheffer, I.E., Baraitser, M., Wilson, J., *et al.* (1991) 'Pelizaeus–Merzbacher disease: classical or connatal?' *Neuropediatrics*, **22**, 71–78.

Schiff, D.E., Ortega, J.A. (1992) 'Chorea, eosinophilia, and lupus anticoagulant associated with acute lymphoblastic leukemia.' *Pediatric Neurology*, **8**, 466–468.

Schiffmann, R., Trapp, B.D., Moller, J.R., *et al.* (1992) 'Childhood ataxia with diffuse CNS hypomyelination.' *Annals of Neurology*, **32**, 484. *(Abstract.)*

Schindler, D., Bishop, D.F., Wolfe, D.E., *et al.* (1989) 'Neuroaxonal dystrophy due to lysosomal α-*N*-acetylgalactosaminidase deficiency.' *New England Journal of Medicine*, **320**, 1735–1740.

Schuffler, M.D., Bird, T.D., Sumi, A., Cook, A. (1978) 'A familial neuronal disease presenting as intestinal pseudo-obstruction.' *Gastroenterology*, **75**, 889–898.

Schulz, P.E., Weiner, S.P., Belmont, J.W., Fishman, M.A. (1988) 'Basal ganglia calcifications in a case of biotinidase deficiency.' *Neurology*, **38**, 1326–1328.

Schwankhaus, J.D., Currie, J., Jaffe, M.J., *et al.* (1989) 'Neurologic findings in men with isolated hypogonadotrophic hypogonadism.' *Neurology*, **39**, 223–226.

Schwendemann, G., Arendt, G., Noth, J., *et al.* (1987) 'Diagnosis of juvenile–adult form of neuroaxonal dystrophy by electron microscopy of rectum and skin biopsy.' *Journal of Neurology, Neurosurgery, and Psychiatry,* **50,** 818–821.

Sechi, G.P., Piras, M.R., Rosati, G., *et al.* (1988) 'Phenobarbital-induced buccolingual dyskinesia in oral apraxia.' *European Neurology,* **28,** 139–141.

Segawa, M., Nomura, Y. (1993) 'Hereditary progressive dystonia with marked diurnal fluctuation.' *In:* Segawa, M. (Ed.) *Hereditary Progressive Dystonia.* New York: Parthenon, pp. 3–19.

—— Hosaka, A., Miyagawa, F., *et al.* (1976) 'Hereditary progressive dystonia with marked diurnal fluctuations.' *Advances in Neurology, Vol. 14.* New York: Raven Presss, pp. 215–233.

Seiff, S.R., Freeman, L.N., Bluestone, D.L., Berg, B.O. (1989) 'Use of botulinum toxin to treat blepharospasm in a 16-year-old with a dystonic syndrome.' *Pediatric Neurology,* **5,** 121–123.

Seiser, A., Jellinger, K., Brainin, M. (1990) 'Pigmentary type of orthochromatic leukodystrophy with early onset and protracted course.' *Neuropediatrics,* **21,** 48–52.

Senanayake, N. (1992) 'A syndrome of early onset spinocerebellar ataxia with optic atrophy, internuclear ophthalmoplegia, dementia, and startle myoclonus in a Sri Lankan family.' *Journal of Neurology,* **239,** 293–294.

Sequeiros, J., Suite, N.M.D.A. (1986) 'Spinopontine atrophy disputed as a separate entity: the first description of Machado–Joseph disease.' *Neurology,* **36,** 1048. *(Letter.)*

Sewry, C.A., Voit, T., Dubowitz, V. (1988) 'Myopathy with unique ultrastructural feature in Marinesco–Sjögren syndrome.' *Annals of Neurology,* **24,** 576–580.

Seyfert, S., Honé, A., Holl, G. (1988) 'Primidone and esssential tremor.' *Journal of Neurology,* **235,** 168–170.

Shahar, E., Shapiro, M.S., Shenkman, L. (1988) 'Hyperthyroid-induced chorea. Case report and review of the literature.' *Israel Journal of Medical Science,* **24,** 264–266.

Shapira, Y., Cederbaum, S.D., Cancilla, P.A., *et al.* (1975) 'Familial poliodystrophy, mitochondrial myopathy, and lactate acidemia.' *Neurology,* **25,** 614–621.

Shih, V.E., Abroms, I.F., Johnson, J.L., *et al.* (1977) 'Sulfite oxidase deficiency. Biochemical and clinical investigations of a hereditary metabolic disorder in sulfur metabolism.' *New England Journal of Medicine,* **297,** 1022–1028.

Shibasaki, H., Yamashita, Y., Tobimatsu, S., Neshige, R. (1986) 'Electroencephalographic correlates of myoclonus.' *In:* Fahn, S., Marsden, C.D., Van Woert, M. (Eds.) *Advances in Neurology, Vol. 45. Myoclonus.* New York: Raven Press, pp. 357–372.

Shimomura, C., Matsui, A., Choh, H., *et al.* (1988) 'Magnetic resonance imaging in Pelizaeus–Merzbacher disease.' *Pediatric Neurology,* **4,** 124–125.

Silverstein, A.M., Hirsch, D.K., Trobe, J.D., Gebarski, S.S. (1989) 'MR imaging of the brain in five members of a family with Pelizaeus–Merzbacher disease.' *American Journal of Neuroradiology,* **11,** 495–499.

Singer, H.S. (1986) 'Tardive dyskinesia: a concern for the pediatrician.' *Pediatrics,* **77,** 553–556.

—— (1994) 'Neurobiological issues in Tourette syndrome.' *Brain and Development,* **16,** 353–364.

—— Reiss, A.L., Brown, J.E., *et al.* (1993) 'Volumetric MRI changes in basal ganglia of children with Tourette's syndrome.' *Neurology,* **43,** 950–956.

Singer, K., Wong, M. (1970) 'Severe persistent chorea with phenothiazine therapy.' *Postgraduate Medical Journal,* **46,** 633–634.

Singh, B., Jamil, A., al-Shahwan, S.A., *et al.* (1993) 'Choroido-cerebral calcification syndrome with retardation.' *Neurology,* **43,** 2387–2389.

Singhal, B.S., Gursahani, R.D., Udani, V.P., Biniwale, A. (1996) 'Megalencephalic leukodystrophy in an Asian Indian ethnic group.' *Pediatric Neurology,* **14,** 291–296.

Sloane, A.E., Becker, L.E., Ang, L.C., *et al.* (1994) 'Neuronal intranuclear hyaline inclusion disease with progressive cerebellar ataxia.' *Pediatric Neurology,* **10,** 61–66.

Sly, W.S., Whyte, M.P., Sundaram, V., *et al.* (1985) 'Carbonic anhydrase II deficiency in 12 families with the autosomal recessive syndrome of osteopetrosis with renal tubular acidosis and cerebral calcification.' *New England Journal of Medicine,* **313,** 139–145.

Small, S.L., Fukui, M.B., Bramblett, G.T., Eidelman, B.H. (1996) 'Immunosuppression-induced leukoencephalopathy from tacrolimus (FK506).' *Annals of Neurology,* **40,** 575–580.

Snow, B.J., Nygaard, T.G., Takahashi, H., Calne, D.B. (1993) 'Positron emission tomographic studies of dopa-responsive dystonia and early-onset idopathic parkinsonism.' *Annals of Neurology,* **34,** 733–738.

Specola, N., Vanier, M.T., Goutières, F., *et al.* (1990) 'The juvenile and chronic forms of GM2 gangliosidosis: clinical and enzymatic heterogeneity.' *Neurology,* **40,** 145–150.

Spencer, S.E., Walker, F.O., Moore, S.A. (1987) 'Chorea–amyotrophy with chronic hemolytic anemia: a variant of chorea–amyotrophy with acanthocytosis.' *Neurology,* **37,** 645–649.

Spira, P.J., McLeod, J.G., Evans, W.A. (1979) 'A spinocerebellar degeneration with X-linked inheritance.' *Brain,* **102,** 27–41.

Stibler, H., Jaeken, J. (1990) 'Carbohydrate deficient serum transferrin in a new systemic hereditary syndrome.' *Archives of Disease in Childhood,* **65,** 107–111.

Stojanovic, M., Cvetkovic, D., Kostic, V.S. (1995) 'A genetic study of idiopathic focal dystonias.' *Journal of Neurology,* **242,** 508–511.

Straussberg, R., Shahar, E., Gat, R., Brand, N. (1993) 'Delayed Parkinsonism associated with hypotension in a child undergoing open-heart surgery.' *Developmental Medicine and Child Neurology,* **35,** 1011–1014.

Stumpf, D.A., Parks, J.K., Eguren, L.A., Haas, R. (1982) 'Friedreich ataxia. III: Mitochondrial malic enzyme deficiency.' *Neurology,* **32,** 221–227.

—— Sokol, R., Bettis, D., *et al.* (1987) 'Friedreich's disease: V. Variant form with vitamin E deficiency and normal fat absorption.' *Neurology,* **37,** 68–74.

Sugama, S., Kusano, K. (1995) 'A sporadic case of very slow progressive leukodystrophy involving the cerebellar peduncles.' *Brain and Development,* **17,** 280–282.

Sugita, K., Kakinuma, H., Okajima, Y., *et al.* (1995) 'Clinical and MRI findings in a case of D-2 hydroxyglutaric aciduria.' *Brain and Development,* **17,** 139–141.

Superneau, D.W., Wertelecki, W., Zellweger, H., Bastian, F. (1987) 'Myopathy in Marinesco–Sjögren syndrome.' *European Neurology,* **26,** 8–16.

Sutcliffe, J. (1969) 'Torsion spasms and abnormal postures in children with hiatus hernia. Sandifer's syndrome.' *Progress in Pediatric Radiology,* **2,** 190–197.

Swaiman, K.F., Garg, A.P., Lockman, L.A. (1975) 'Sea-blue histiocyte and posterior column dysfunction: a familial disorder.' *Neurology,* **25,** 1084–1087.

—— Smith, S.A., Trock, G.L., Siddiqui, A.R. (1983) 'Sea-blue histiocytes, lymphocytic cytosomes, movement disorder and ^{59}Fe-uptake in basal ganglia: Hallervorden–Spatz disease or ceroid storage disease with abnormal isotope scan?' *Neurology,* **33,** 301–305.

Takahashi, K., Naito, M., Yamamura, F., *et al.* (1990) 'Infantile osteopetrosis complicating neuronal ceroid lipofuscinosis.' *Pathology, Research and Practice,* **186,** 697–706.

Takashima, S., Becker, L.E. (1985) 'Basal ganglia calcification in Down's syndrome.' *Journal of Neurology, Neurosurgery, and Psychiatry,* **48,** 61–64.

Tanabe, Y., Iai, M., Ishii, M., *et al.* (1993) 'The use of magnetic resonance imaging in diagnosing infantile neuroaxonal dystrophy.' *Neurology,* **43,** 110–113.

Tanaka, H., Endo, K., Tsuji, S., *et al.* (1995) 'The gene for hereditary progressive dystonia with marked diurnal fluctuation maps to chromosome 14q.' *Annals of Neurology,* **37,** 405–408.

Tasker, R.R., Doorly, T., Yamashiro, K. (1988) 'Thalamotomy in generalized dystonia.' *In:* Fahn, S. (Ed.) *Advances in Neurology, Vol. 50. Dystonia II.* New York: Raven Press, pp. 615–631.

Tennison, M.B., Bouldin, T.W., Whaley, R.A. (1988) 'Mineralization of the basal ganglia detected by CT in Hallervorden–Spatz syndrome.' *Neurology,* **38,** 154–155.

Thomas, P.K., Workman, J.M., Thage, O. (1984) 'Behr's syndrome—a family exhibiting pseudodominant inheritance.' *Journal of the Neurological Sciences,* **64,** 137–148.

—— Mista, V.P., Kino, R.H.M., *et al.* (1994) 'Autosomal recessive hereditary sensory neuropathy with spastic paraplegia.' *Brain,* **117,** 651–659.

Thomson, A., MacKenzie, J., Rosenbloom, L. (1990) 'Two siblings with a previosly undescribed dorsal column degeneration syndrome.' *Developmental Medicine and Child Neurology,* **32,** 168–171.

Tolmie, J.L., Browne, B.H., McGettrick, P.M., Stephenson, J.B.P. (1988) 'A familial syndrome with Coats' reaction retinal angiomas, hair and nail defects and intracranial calcification.' *Eye,* **2,** 297–303.

—— Shillito, P., Hughes-Benzie, R., Stephenson, J.B.P. (1995) 'The Aicardi–Goutières syndrome (familial, early onset encephalopathy with calcifications of the basal ganglia and chronic cerebrospinal fluid lymphocytosis).' *Journal of Medical Genetics,* **32,** 881–884.

Tomiwa, K., Baraitser, M., Brett, E.M., Wilson, J. (1987) 'The use of computerised database for the diagnosis of a rare neurological syndrome.' *Neuropediatrics*, **18**, 231–234.

Topçu, M., Gucuyener, K., Topaloglu, H., *et al.* (1992) 'Paraneoplastic syndrome manifesting as chronic cerebellar ataxia in a child with Hodgkin disease.' *Journal of Pediatrics*, **120**, 275–277.

Torillo, H.V. (1990) 'Cockayne syndrome type II.' *In:* Bruyse, M.L. (Ed.) *Birth Defects Encyclopedia*. Dover, MA: Blackwell Scientific, pp. 421–422.

Torreman, M., Smit, L.M.E., van der Valk, P., *et al.* (1993) 'A case of macrocephaly, hydrocephalus megacerebellum, white matter abnormalities and Rosenthal fibres.' *Developmental Medicine and Child Neurology*, **35**, 732–736.

Toscano, A., Fazio, M.C., Vita, G., *et al.* (1995) 'Early-onset cerebellar ataxia, myoclonus and hypogonadism in a case of mitochondrial complex III deficiency treated with vitamins K_3 and C.' *Journal of Neurology*, **242**, 203–209.

Towfighi, J., Grover, W., Gonatas, N.N. (1975) 'Mental retardation, hypotonia and generalised seizures associated with astrocytic "residual" bodies. An ultrastructual study.' *Human Pathology*, **6**, 667–680.

Trevathan, E., Naidu, S. (1988) 'The clinical recognition and differential diagnosis of Rett syndrome.' *Journal of Child Neurology*, **3** (Suppl.), S5–S16.

Tsao, C.Y., Lo, W.D., Craenen, J. (1992) 'Congestive heart failure and cardiac thrombus as first presentation of Friedreich ataxia.' *Pediatric Neurology*, **8**, 313–314.

Tuite, P.J., Rogaeva, E.A., St George-Hyslop, P.H., Lang, A.E. (1995) 'Dopa-responsive parkinsonism phenotype of Machado–Joseph disease: confirmation of 14q CAG expansion.' *Annals of Neurology*, **38**, 684–687.

Turjanski, N., Bhatia, K., Burn, D.J., *et al.* (1993) 'Comparison of striatal ^{18}F-dopa uptake in adult-onset dystonia–parkinsonism, Parkinson's disease and dopa-responsive dystonia.' *Neurology*, **43**, 1563–1568.

Uziel, G., Garavaglia, B., Ciceri, E., *et al.* (1995) 'Riboflavin-responsive glutaric aciduria type II presenting as a leukodystrophy.' *Pediatric Neurology*, **13**, 333–335.

Vanasse, M., Bédard, M., Andermann, F. (1976) 'Shuddering attacks in children: an early clinical manifestation of essential tremor.' *Neurology*, **26**, 1027–1030.

Van der Knaap, M.S., Valk, J. (1989) 'The reflection of histology in MR imaging of Pelizaeus–Merzbacher disease.' *American Journal of Neuroradiology*, **10**, 99–103.

—— van der Grond, J., Luyten, P.R., *et al.* (1992) '[1]H and ^{31}P magnetic resonance spectroscopy of the brain in degenerative cerebral disorders.' *Annals of Neurology*, **31**, 202–211.

—— Barth, P.G., Stroink, H., *et al.* (1995) 'Leukoencephalopathy with swelling and a discrepantly mild clinical course in eight children.' *Annals of Neurology*, **37**, 324–334.

—— —— Gabreëls, F.J.M., *et al.* (1997) 'A new leukoencephalopathy with vanishing white matter.' *Neurology*, **48**, 845–855.

Vanhanen, S.L., Raininko, R., Santavuori, P., *et al.* (1995) 'MRI evaluation of the brain in infantile neuronal ceroid–lipofuscinosis. Part I: Postmortem MRI with histopathologic correlation.' *Journal of Child Neurology*, **10**, 438–443.

Van Tassel, P., Yeakley, J.W., Lee, K.F. (1987) 'Cerebellar calcification in central neurofibromatosis: CT in two cases.' *American Journal of Neuroradiology*, **8**, 913–915.

Venkatesh, S., Coulter, D.L., Kemper, T.D. (1994) 'Neuroaxonal dystrophy at birth with hypertonicity and basal ganglia mineralization.' *Journal of Child Neurology*, **9**, 74–76.

Wakai, S., Asanuma, H., Hayasaka, H., *et al.* (1994) 'Ictal video–EEG analysis of infantile neuroaxonal dystrophy.' *Epilepsia*, **35**, 823–826.

Walevski, A., Radwan, M. (1986) 'Choreoathetosis as toxic effect of lithium treatment.' *European Neurology*, **25**, 412–415.

Walker, D.A., Harper, P.S., Wells, C.E.C., *et al.* (1981) 'Huntington's chorea in South Wales—a genetic and epidemiological study.' *Clinical Genetics*, **19**, 213–221.

Walshe, J.M. (1986) 'Wilson's disease.' *In:* Vinken, P.J., Bruyn, G.W., Klawans, H.L. (Eds.) *Handbook of Clinical Neurology. Vol. 49. Extrapyramidal Disorders*. Amsterdam: Elsevier, pp. 223–238.

Wang, P.J., Young, C., Liu, H.M., *et al.* (1995) 'Neurophysiologic studies and MRI in Pelizaeus–Merzbacher disease: comparison of classic and connatal forms.' *Pediatric Neurology*, **12**, 47–53.

Warner, T.T., Fletcher, N.A., Davis, M.B., *et al.* (1993) 'Linkage analysis in British and French families with idiopathic torsion dystonia.' *Brain*, **116**, 739–744.

—— Williams, L.D., Walker, R.W.H., *et al.* (1995) 'A clinical and molecular genetic study of dentatorubropallidoluysian atrophy in four European families.' *Annals of Neurology*, **37**, 452–459.

Watanabe, I., Patel, V., Goebel, H.H., *et al.* (1973) 'Early lesion of Pelizaeus–Merzbacher disease: electron microscopic and biochemical study.' *Journal of Neuropathology and Experimental Neurology*, **32**, 313–333.

Watanabe, K., Negoro, T., Maehara, M., *et al.* (1990) 'Moyamoya disease presenting with chorea.' *Pediatric Neurology*, **6**, 40–42.

Weiner, W.J., Nausieda, P.A., Klawans, H.L. (1978) 'Methylphenidate-induced chorea: case report and pharmacologic implications.' *Neurology*, **28**, 1041–1044.

Wells, C.R., Jankovic, J. (1986) 'Familial spastic paraparesis and deafness: a new X-linked neurodegenerative disorder.' *Archives of Neurology*, **43**, 943–946.

Wheeler, P.G., Weaver, D.D., Dobyns, W.B. (1993) 'Benign hereditary chorea.' *Pediatric Neurology*, **9**, 337–340.

Wiley, C.A., Love, S., Skoglund, R.R., Lampert, P.W. (1987) 'Infantile neurodegenerative disease with neuronal accumulation of phosphorylated neurofilaments.' *Acta Neuropathologica*, **72**, 369–376.

Willemse, J. (1986) 'Benign idiopathic dystonia with onset in the first year of life.' *Developmental Medicine and Child Neurology*, **28**, 355–360.

Wilson, J., Manners, B.T.B., Robins, D.G., Erdohazi, M. (1981) 'Persistent hiccup as a presenting feature of Alexander's leucodystrophy.' *Developmental Medicine and Child Neurology*, **23**, 660–661. *(Letter.)*

Wisniewski, K.E., Kida, E., Connell, F., *et al.* (1993) 'New subform of the late infantile form of neuronal ceroid lipofuscinosis.' *Neuropediatrics*, **24**, 155–163.

Witt, T.N., Danek, A., Reiter, M., *et al.* (1992) 'McLeod syndrome: a distinct form of neuroacanthocytosis. Report of two cases and literature review with emphasis on neuromuscular manifestations.' *Journal of Neurology*, **239**, 302–306.

Wiznitzer, M., Younkin, D. (1984) 'Phenobarbital-induced dyskinesia in a neurologically impaired child.' *Neurology*, **34**, 1600–1601.

Wolfson, L.I., Sharpless, N.S., Thal, L.J. (1988) 'Diminished levels of ventricular fluid norepinephrine metabolite and somatostatin in childhood-onset dystonia.' *In:* Fahn, S., Marsden, C.D., Calne, D.B. (Eds.) *Advances in Neurology, Vol. 50. Dystonia II*. New York: Raven Press, pp. 177–181.

Woody, R.C., Brewster, M.A., Glasier, C. (1989) 'Progressive intracranial calcification in dihydropteridine reductase deficiency prior to folinic acid therapy.' *Neurology*, **39**, 673–675.

Wüllner, U., Klockgether, T., Petersen, D., *et al.* (1993) 'Magnetic resonance imaging in hereditary and idiopathic ataxia.' *Neurology*, **43**, 318–325.

Xuereb, J.H., MacMillan, J.C., Snell, R., *et al.* (1996) 'Neuropathological diagnosis and CAG repeat expansion in Huntington's disease.' *Journal of Neurology, Neurosurgery, and Psychiatry*, **60**, 78–81.

Yokota, T., Tsuchiya, K., Umetani, K., *et al.* (1988) 'Choreoathetoid movements associated with a splenorenal shunt.' *Journal of Neurology*, **235**, 487–488.

—— Hirashima, F., Ito, Y., *et al.* (1990) 'Idiopathic palatal myoclonus.' *Acta Neurologica Scandinavica*, **81**, 239–242.

Zafeiriou, D.I., Koletzko, B., Mueller-Felber, W., *et al.* (1995) 'Deficiency in complex IV (cytochrome c oxidase) of the respiratory chain, presenting as a leukodystrophy in two siblings with Leigh syndrome.' *Brain and Development*, **17**, 117–121.

Ziegler, D.K., Van Speybroech, N.W., Seitz, E.F. (1974) 'Myoclonic epilepsia partialis continua and Friedreich ataxia.' *Archives of Neurology*, **31**, 308–311.

Zoghbi, H. (1988) 'Genetic aspects of Rett syndrome.' *Journal of Child Neurology*, **3** (Suppl.), S76–S78.

—— Pollack, M.S., Lyons, L.A., *et al.* (1988) 'Spinocerebellar ataxia: variable age of onset and linkage to human leukocyte antigen in a large kindred.' *Annals of Neurology*, **23**, 580–584.

PART V

POSTNATAL EXTRINSIC AGGRESSIONS

11
INFECTIOUS DISEASES

Infections of the CNS remain common life-threatening conditions with great potential for permanent damage in survivors despite the great advances that have taken place during recent decades in health care and in the development of antibacterial and antiviral agents. These infections pose a difficult diagnostic problem as they must be recognized in their earliest stage when many types of meningitis and encephalitis are clinically indistinguishable. Their diagnosis therefore requires close cooperation between clinicians and several specialists, not only for bacteriological and viral isolation but also for investigative procedures such as radiology, biochemistry and the like, which are often required for optimal management.

ACUTE BACTERIAL MENINGITIS

Purulent meningitides are still the cause of a high mortality and morbidity especially among newborn infants. Several factors contribute toward this disappointing situation: the difficulty of an early diagnosis because of the nonspecific character of the symptoms; the relative ineffectiveness of available antibiotics against many gram-negative enteric bacilli; the emergence of resistant strains of common pathogens such as *Haemophilus influenzae* and *Streptococcus pneumoniae*; and the weakness of the immunological defenses of the newborn infant. Newly developed antibiotics and prophylaxis, especially by specific immunization, offer hope of better results in the future. Currently, early diagnosis and instigation of treatment, careful monitoring of its efficacy and rapid detection of emerging complications give the best chances of an optimal outcome. The role of the child neurologist is thus important whenever the course of bacterial meningitis does not conform to the usual scheme.

EPIDEMIOLOGY
The incidence of purulent meningitis depends on age and on other poorly known factors. In children over 2 months of age, it varies with the country and with socioeconomic conditions (Fortnum and Davis 1993). Estimates for the frequency of the three main types of meningitis in France are of the order of 35–40 per 100,000 per year (Carrère *et al.* 1984).

Most cases are due to *H. influenzae*, *Neisseria meningitidis* and *Str. pneumoniae*. Seventy per cent of cases occur before age 5 years. The respective frequency of the three main pathogens in childhood varies considerably with the part of the world and time of study. In the early 1980s *N. meningitidis* was the most frequently

isolated organism in France and the UK (Marshall 1983), whereas by the end of the decade *H. influenzae* was more common (Tudor-Williams *et al.* 1989), accounting for 45 per cent of cases, as against 39 per cent for meningococcal and 16 per cent for streptococcal infections (Livartowski *et al.* 1989). The introduction of the *H. influenzae* conjugate vaccine is rapidly changing the situation and the frequency of *H. influenzae* meningitis is declining significantly (Peltola *et al.* 1992, Tunkel 1993, Vadheim *et al.* 1993). *Str. pneumoniae* is now the most common cause of meningitis, raising new therapeutic problems.

PATHOLOGY AND PATHOPHYSIOLOGY
Whatever the age of occurrence, most cases of bacterial meningitis progress through four stages. First, there is infection of the respiratory tract, followed by bacteraemia from the respiratory focus, seeding of the meninges by blood-borne organisms, and finally inflammation of the meninges and brain. Little is known of the way in which bacteria attach to and penetrate the mucosal surface or enter the blood stream and escape destruction by host defense mechanisms. The same applies to the manner in which pathogens penetrate into the CSF and survive in the fluid and brain tissue (McGee and Kaiser 1985, Baraff *et al.* 1993b). For some organisms, specific surface components such as the K1 polysaccharide antigen of *Escherichia coli* are essential for attachment to mucosal surfaces and are responsible for special virulence. Group B but not group A or C meningococci have antigenic similarities with the K1 antigen and with certain polysialosylglycopeptides of the human brain.

The size of the inoculum of bacteria in the blood has been shown to be important in producing meningitis in experimental animals, and this may also be the case in humans (Moxon *et al.* 1974). The mechanisms whereby bacteria, once inside the CNS, incite inflammation and cause tissue damage are multiple. With *N. meningitidis* and *H. influenzae*, the initiating factor is endotoxin, a lipopolysaccharide component of gram-negative bacteria. With *Str. pneumoniae*, a similar role is played by other cell-wall components, especially teichoic acid and peptidoglycans (Lambert 1994). After a time-lag of a few hours, proinflammatory cytokines including tumour-necrosis factor (Bazzoni and Beutler 1996) and interleukins 1, 6 and 8 are induced. These and other factors from macrophages and platelets mediate inflammation and tissue injury (Sáez-Llorens *et al.* 1990, Saukkonen 1990). The situation is made worse by the fact that neutrophils, which are major agents of defense against bacteria, can produce proinflammatory factors including reactive oxygen species, after adhesion, migration and degranulation (Ashwal *et al.* 1992, Quagliarello and Scheld 1992). Vascular congestion and increased vessel permeability result with cytotoxic and vasogenic brain oedema and increased intracranial pressure (ICP). The CSF volume increases during the first two or three days of disease (Ashwal *et al.* 1992). The levels of endotoxin (Mertsola *et al.* 1991) and of other cytokines (Arditi *et al.* 1989) are correlated to the severity of the disorder (Dulkerian *et al.* 1995). Vasculitis is a frequent complication and can lead to infarction in 2–19 per cent of cases. Cerebral blood flow is decreased by 30–70 per cent in 30 per cent of patients (Ashwal *et al.* 1992) but autoregulation of blood flow is generally maintained (Ashwal *et al.* 1990). An increased release of cytokines can be produced by bacterial lysis following antibiotic therapy (Arditi *et al.* 1989). Administration of dexamethasone before that of antibiotics can prevent this untoward effect in experimental animals (see below).

Penetration of bacteria is much less commonly directly from foci into the underlying brain parenchyma, from osteomyelitis of the skull or spine, or through fractures or congenital defects in the skull. In the last case, infection may recur. Penetrating head injuries following wounds of the upper eyelid or of the temporal squama region by sharp objects can produce an acute or chronic meningitis that may be due to unusual organisms (Thomas and Whittet 1991). Such wounds should be treated with antibiotics in 'meningitic' doses until penetration can be excluded.

The fundamental pathological change is an inflammation of the leptomeninges with initial hyperaemia, followed by migration of polymorphonuclear cells into the subarachnoid space. The leptomeningeal exudate rapidly increases and extends into the Virchow–Robin spaces along the penetrating vessels. Neutrophils then degenerate and are removed by macrophages. Fibroblasts may be seen later and may participate in the organization of the meningeal exudate and lead to fibrosis of the arachnoid.

Involvement of vessels is important in the mechanism and complications of leptomeningitis. Adventitial connective tissue is infiltrated by inflammatory cells which also appear beneath the arterial intima. Such changes can produce stenosis or obliteration of involved vessels. A similar process occurs in veins more frequently than in arteries. Resulting areas of brain softening, which may be haemorrhagic, frequently result. Necrosis may be limited to one vascular territory or difffusely involve a large portion or the whole of the cerebral cortex (Dodge and Swartz 1965).

Brain swelling is often present and, in isolation or in association with acute obstructive hydrocephalus due to purulent cisternal exudate, can be responsible for intracranial hypertension. This in turn can impede cerebral perfusion (Minns *et al.* 1989), setting the stage for a vicious circle.

Organization of the meningeal exudate may lead to chronic hydrocephalus, especially in young infants. Hydrocephalus can also result from aqueductal stenosis that may supervene as a consequence of ventriculitis. The latter is extremely common in neonates, being found in as many as 92 per cent of autopsy cases (Berman and Banker 1966), but exists also in a lower proportion of older children (around 10 per cent).

BACTERIAL MENINGITIS IN INFANTS AND CHILDREN
CLINICAL MANIFESTATIONS AND DIAGNOSIS
The importance of an early diagnosis is axiomatic (Stutman and Marks 1987). Late diagnosis remains frequent, however, because meningitis is relatively rare in a general practice, compared with the frequency of common, mostly viral, febrile diseases. In fact, especially with *H. influenzae* infection, meningitis is often preceded for a few days by fever so that it may be impossible to determine its actual onset. As a result, 33–40 per cent of patients have received antibiotics prior to diagnosis (Kaplan *et al.* 1986). The mode of onset is an important prognostic feature: a progressive onset merging with previous disease often predicts a favourable outcome, while a fulminating onset is of ominous significance (Radetsky 1992, Kilpi *et al.* 1993).

Moderate fever, headache, vomiting and nausea, and some disturbance of consciousness (more commonly mild stupor than coma) should suggest the diagnosis. Stiffness of the neck and sometimes also of the back and Kernig's sign make lumbar puncture imperative. In very early cases, mild irritability and change in mood together with reluctance to flex the neck may be the only features. The occurrence of a generalized seizure is possible especially in children under 4 years of age. In 43 cases of bacterial meningitis found among 169,849 liveborn infants, Wiswell *et al.* (1995) considered that the diagnosis would have been delayed for want of suggestive symptoms and signs in 16 (37 per cent), had not systematic lumbar puncture been performed because of sepsis. Carraccio *et al.* (1995) also found cases of meningitis in febrile patients without neurological symptoms. In children under 18 months of age meningeal signs may be absent, so lumbar puncture should be performed if the child does not revert to a completely normal state soon after the seizure. Although systematic lumbar puncture, in the case of a febrile convulsion, only rarely reveals meningitis (Rutter and Smales 1977), it is prudent to perform it in infants under 1 year of age and, at any age, if the slightest doubt persists. Green *et al.* (1993) found that 23 per cent of 503 children with meningitis had seizures, but most were in addition obtunded or comatose and only eight had a normal level of consciousness. They reviewed 2780 published cases, of which only 1.7 per cent had isolated seizures and only seven had no meningeal signs.

Atypical onset, such as acute cerebellar ataxia (Yabek 1973), is uncommonly observed.

LABORATORY DIAGNOSIS
Examination of the CSF is the essential step. If bacterial meningitis is not immediately confirmed, further tests should be systematically planned. Although concern has arisen regarding the potential risks of lumbar puncture in the case of meningitis with high ICP (Klein *et al.* 1986), it is the experience of this writer that the balance of risks strongly favours the performance of an early lumbar puncture in suspicious cases. However, the risk of death by herniation in meningitis was thought to be between 4.3 (Rennick *et al.* 1993) and 6 per cent (Wright *et al.* 1993, Lambert 1994), and lumbar puncture is felt to precipitate coning although

this clearly may occur spontaneously. It therefore seems reasonable to defer lumbar puncture when the level of consciousness is severely depressed, when there are dilated pupils, ophthalmoparesis or papilloedema. CT scan is of doubtful value in detecting oedema or increased ICP (Pike *et al.* 1990, Heyderman *et al.* 1992), although it may show compression of the ambient cistern suggestive of temporal herniation. MRI (Lebel *et al.* 1989b) is not indicated. Mellor (1992) advise deferring lumbar puncture to at least 30 minutes following seizures as these are known to produce a transient increase in ICP. Administration of mannitol before lumbar puncture is indicated in doubtful cases. It has been shown to effectively reduce ICP and increase cerebral perfusion pressure and blood flow velocity (Goh and Minns 1993). Another contraindication to lumbar puncture is the need for urgent treatment of shock (Lambert 1994). This applies especially to meningococcal disease, whose diagnosis can be made by blood culture and which has highly suggestive clinical signs in the form of purpura.

'Blind' treatment of meningitis is unsound, however, because of the frequency of diagnostic errors and the usefulness of accurate bacteriological diagnosis, especially with the increasing frequency of antibiotic-resistant organisms.

Should lumbar puncture be delayed, the causes of delay should be managed as expeditiously as feasible. Cultures of blood and urine should be taken, and antimicrobial drugs should be given in doses large enough for treatment of meningitis. CSF obtained later will often be sterile but biochemical study and a search for bacterial antigens may provide evidence for or against meningitis.

Characteristically, the CSF is under increased pressure and cloudy. In some children, however, the fluid may initially be clear and contain only a few cells or be altogether normal with a negative culture but subsequently demonstrate a positive culture when re-examined 8–72 hours later (Teele *et al.* 1981). Cultures may be positive for pathogenic bacteria in the presence of normal cytological and chemistry findings, if puncture is done after bacterial invasion but before the inflammatory response (Onorato *et al.* 1980). If clinical suspicion persists, repeat puncture is indicated within 6–12 hours.

The cells present in CSF usually number between 1000 and 10,000/mm^3. Organisms may be seen intracellularly and extracellularly in smears. Initially, polymorphonuclear leukocytes predominate or are seen exclusively. Gram stains are positive in 25 per cent of cases, depending on the concentration of pathogens in the CSF (La Scolea and Dryja 1984). Staining with acridine orange may be positive in some patients with a negative Gram stain (Kleiman *et al.* 1984), especially if partially treated.

Cultures on blood agar or chocolate agar plate and in broth should always be obtained, even when the fluid is clear. Counting the number of colony-forming units (CFUs) gives an idea of the concentration of organisms in the CSF and is important for therapeutic purposes. It has been shown that an increase in the number of CFUs from 10^5 to 10^7/mL can be associated with a marked increase in the resistance of certain bacteria to antibiotics (Denis *et al.* 1981, Feldman *et al.* 1982). It is possible to isolate

an organism and determine its sensitivity to antibiotics in 90 per cent of cases of bacterial meningitis (Bohr *et al.* 1983).

A raised protein level (>0.4 g/L) is usual, and local production of immunoglobulins can be demonstrated (Maida and Horvatits 1986). CSF glucose is usually depressed but this is dependent on the blood concentration. The CSF–blood glucose ratio is reduced well below the normal value of 0.66. Blood and CSF glucose levels should therefore be determined simultaneously (Donald *et al.* 1983). A normal glucose level is found in up to 20 per cent of cases (Lambert 1994) and does not exclude the diagnosis.

A rapid diagnosis can be made by countercurrent immunoelectrophoresis of the CSF, blood and urine for group B streptococci, K1 strains of *E. coli*, *H. influenzae* type b, *N. meningitidis* groups A, B, C, Y and W 135, *S. pneumoniae*, *Listeria monocytogenes*, *Klebsiella pneumoniae* and *Pseudomonas aeruginosa* (Feigin *et al.* 1976). For the major pathogens, the method is sensitive and can detect nonviable bacteria. It is especially useful for the diagnosis of partially treated meningitis. In such cases, direct examination and culture are often negative and the CSF contains both polymorphonuclear cells and lymphocytes so the distinction from aseptic or tuberculous meningitis can be difficult. However, in most cases the cytological and biochemical characteristics of the CSF are not markedly modified except for the increased frequency of negative cultures (Kaplan *et al.* 1986, Talan *et al.* 1988). The polymerase chain reaction test has been used for the diagnosis of meningococcal (Ni *et al.* 1992) and *H. influenzae* meningitides. Finding a high lactate level in the CSF has been found useful by some investigators in pyogenic and tuberculous meningitis, but the test does not contribute significantly to the management of children with suspected meningitis (Rutledge *et al.* 1981). Determination of lysozyme level (Gerbaut and Mallet 1988) and of lactic dehydrogenase and glutamic-oxaloacetic transaminase are of little clinical interest.

Latex particle agglutination can be used for the detection of the three common pathogens and group B streptococci. The test is highly sensitive but nonspecific agglutination may occur (Feigin *et al.* 1992). Presence of interleukin 6 in CSF reliably identifies purulent meningitis. Tumour necrosis factor is highly specific for bacterial meningitis (Dulkerian *et al.* 1995).

Difficulties in the interpretation of CSF findings may arise in the case of blood contamination of the sample. Both protein level and cell count are elevated (Rubenstein and Yogev 1985). Sequential cell counts help in differentiating traumatic haemorrhage from that due to associated bleeding.

In patients with meningitis but no bacteria grown from the CSF or other body fluids, the physician must consider other causes of the *aseptic meningitis syndrome*. Many aseptic meningitides are due to viral infections but other causes are possible (Table 11.1). Such children should have a skin test for tuberculosis, and exclusion of other possibly treatable causes is a major consideration. Careful clinical, neuroradiological and laboratory examinations should be considered, as applicable to the individual child.

TABLE 11.1
Causes of the 'aseptic meningitis syndrome'

Infectious causes

Bacteria: *Actinomyces* spp., *Borrelia burgdorferi* (Lyme disease), *Brucella melitensis*, *Leptospira* spp., *Mycoplasma pneumoniae* and *M. hominis*, *Mycobacterium tuberculosis*, atypical mycobacteria, *Nocardia* spp., *Rickettsia rickettsii* (Rocky Mountain spotted fever), *Treponema pallidum*. Bacterial endocarditis, brain abscess and parameningeal suppuration, partially treated meningitis, sinus thrombophlebitis, children with systemic infection[1]

Viruses: Arboviruses, arenaviruses (lymphocytic choriomeningitis), enteroviruses, herpes viruses (including cytomegalovirus and Epstein–Barr virus), human immunodeficiency virus, paramyxoviruses (measles, influenza), live viral vaccines[2]

Fungi: *Blastomyces dermatidis*, *Candida* spp., *Coccidioides immitis*, *Cryptococcus neoformans*, *Histoplasma capsulatum*, *Sporotrichum schenkii*

Protozoa: Amoebae (*Naegleria* spp.), *Plasmodium falciparum*, *Toxoplasma gondii*, visceral larva migrans

Cestodes: Cysticercosis

Noninfectious causes

Malignancies: leukaemia, lymphoma, metastatic brain tumours

Granulomatous disease: sarcoidosis, Langerhans histiocytosis

Collagen and vascular diseases: lupus erythematosus, panarteritis, other vasculitides

Trauma following lumbar puncture, subarachnoid haemorrhage, postoperative meningitis

Toxic causes: intrathecal contrast media, anaesthetics, systemic toxicity (lead, mercury), catheters[3]

Drug induced meningitis (azathioprine, cytosine-arabinoside, isoniazid, nonsteroidal anti-inflammatory drugs, penicillin, cephalosporins[4])

Immunological causes: high-dose immunoglobulins, OKT3 therapy (Chapter 12)

Status epilepticus

Unknown mechanism

Multiple sclerosis; Schilder disease; uveomeningitis syndromes (Behçet, Harada–Vogt–Koyanagy); Kawasaki disease; Mollaret meningitis; meningitis following heart transplant

---

[1]Carraccio *et al.* (1995).
[2]Rare complication, mainly with poliomyelitis vaccine, measles vaccine.
[3]A similar syndrome may occur with dermoid tumours as a result of chemical meningitis due to rupture of cyst (Erdem *et al.* 1994).
[4]Mainly in patients with collagen vascular disorders but also in healthy persons (Gordon *et al.* 1990, Creel *et al.* 1993, River *et al.* 1994, Creel and Hurtt 1995).

Other laboratory procedures

Blood cultures are positive in 80–90 per cent of cases of meningitis. Occasionally blood cultures are positive at the same time as CSF cultures are negative and thus give useful guidelines for therapy. *Nose and throat cultures* are neither sensitive nor specific. Urine cultures and Gram-stained smears of skin lesions may provide clues to the identity of pathogens, the latter immediately. Bacteriological study of the middle ear fluid obtained by aspiration in the case of associated otitis media may show the same organism as is present in the CSF but this is inconstant, and even when the same bacterium is found in both sites, it is not uncommonly of a different strain.

Blood cell counts and tests of inflammatory response should be performed. There is usually a high white cell count, and the C-reactive protein is present in the CSF in 80–100 per cent of patients with purulent meningitis but in only 10–15 per cent

of those with aseptic meningitis. A raised C-reactive protein in the serum is found 12 hours after bacterial but not aseptic meningitis (Hansson *et al.* 1993).

NEUROIMAGING

Imaging methods are mainly useful for the diagnosis of complications (Klein *et al.* 1986). Riordan *et al.* (1993) list the following indications for CT scanning: prolonged depressed consciousness, prolonged partial or late seizures, focal neurological abnormalities, enlarging head circumference, evidence of continuing infection, and recurrence of symptoms and signs. Some investigators regard CT as potentially useful before lumbar puncture (Archer 1993). MRI with or without gadolinium (Lebel *et al.* 1989b) does not appear to be superior to CT and is therefore not indicated.

COMPLICATIONS OF ACUTE BACTERIAL MENINGITIS

Vasculitis is a component of the pathological complex of purulent meningitis. It can cause thrombosis of veins or of small or occasionally large arteries with secondary cortical or more extensive necrosis (Taft *et al.* 1986). The location of ischaemic foci is variable, from localized well-defined softenings to diffuse necrotic lesions that may be responsible for multicystic encephalomalacia. Ischaemic lesions can be found in the absence of vascular thrombosis. They are the main cause of the neurological and cognitive sequelae of purulent meningitis. The inflammatory disruption of small vascular walls within the CNS can permit organisms to invade the parenchyma, producing small foci of septic necrosis. It seems likely that such foci give rise to the cerebral abscesses that in rare cases complicate bacterial meningitis. Vasculitis also plays a prominent role in the genesis of subdural effusions that seem to be related to thrombophlebitis of the bridging veins.

Seizures, which occur in 30–40 per cent of children with *H. influenzae* and *Str. pneumoniae* meningitides, may be simple febrile seizures, especially when they are generalized and occur early in the course. Focal seizures are due to localized involvement of the hemispheres, usually as a result of vasculitis. In some cases status epilepticus occurs and requires emergency treatment (Chapter 16).

Focal cerebral signs such as hemiplegia or monoplegia are also a consequence of phlebitis or arteritis. Involvement of the cranial nerves as they cross the inflamed leptomeningeal spaces may lead to paralysis that mainly affects the IIIrd and VIth nerves, less commonly the facial nerve. Such palsies usually remit following cure of the meningitis. Opsoclonus has been reported (Rivner *et al.* 1982).

Neuroimaging procedures permit a good assessment of the type and location of the responsible lesions. They usually present as areas of hypodensity that can be located in an arterial territory or they may be more diffuse. Such lesions may be partly haemorrhagic. They frequently take up contrast (Diebler and Dulac 1987, Kaplan and Fishman 1988, Heyderman *et al.* 1992) (Fig. 11.1).

Spinal cord infarction is an uncommon complication also related to vascular involvement. Exceptionally it has been seen

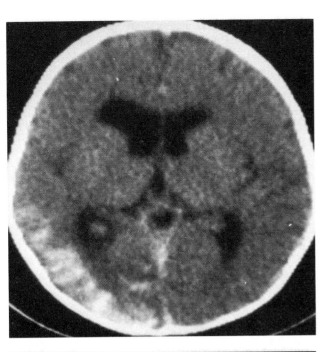

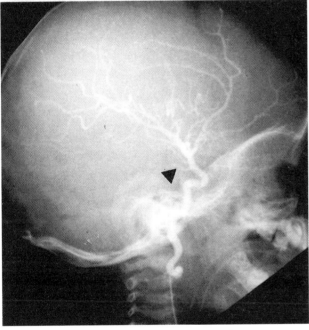

Fig. 11.1. Acute pneumococcal meningitis. *(Top)* CT scan showing contrast enhancement of posterior cortex characteristic of a recent infarct. *(Bottom)* Angiography of right carotid artery showing interruption of right posterior communicating artery *(arrowed)* without opacification of basilar artery or posterior cerebral artery. (14-month-old boy who developed left-sided status epilepticus and mild hemiparesis on third day of disease.)

as a presenting feature (Boothman *et al.* 1988). The appearance of bilateral sensory or motor deficit in the course of bacterial meningitis should suggest spinal cord infarction (Glista *et al.* 1980). The paralysis may resolve with time. Other unusual neurological abnormalities include movement disorders (Burstein and Breningstall 1986), hypothalamic dysfunction and central diabetes insipidus (Greger *et al.* 1986).

Subdural effusions have been increasingly recognized especially in *H. influenzae* meningitis. Most effusions are located over the frontoparietal region bilaterally. The subdural fluid is rarely bloody but has a disproportionately high albumin to globulin ratio (Rabe *et al.* 1968). The clinical importance of subdural effusions remains controversial. The introduction of CT scan has shown that they are very common and usually of limited thickness and volume. Persistent or recurring fever, focal neurological signs and persistently positive CSF cultures are probably more closely related to cortical damage than to the presence of an effusion (Syrogiannopoulos *et al.* 1986, Snedeker *et al.* 1990). Large effusions with enlargement of the head or signs of increased ICP are rare but necessitate drainage. This can be accomplished by tapping through the fontanelle. If the collection reforms rapidly, drainage through a subdural catheter can be used. Most subdural collections resolve spontaneously.

Snedeker *et al.* (1990) found that patients with effusion were more likely to have neurological abnormalities and seizures during the acute illness, but that hearing loss, seizures and developmental delay were not more frequent at follow-up. They concluded that specific invasive therapy was not indicated in most cases.

Intracranial hypertension of a severe degree is a serious complication of bacterial meningitis and can be due to at least two different mechanisms: altered CSF absorption and cerebral oedema.

Acute hydrocephalus is caused by increased resistance to the circulation and resorption of CSF, as a result of the presence of thick leptomeningeal exudate in the basal cisterns or the cerebral convexity in the vicinity of the granulations of Pacchioni, or consequent to ventriculitis with obstruction of the aqueduct. It is usually transient but can lead to late hydrocephalus if extensive meningeal fibrosis develops, especially when treatment has been late or ill-adapted (Snyder 1984).

Cerebral oedema probably results from several mechanisms. These include cytotoxic oedema precipitated by infection, vasogenic oedema due to increased capillary permeability related to the inflammatory response to infection, and interstitial oedema from disturbance to CSF resorption by the normal route. Inappropriate secretion of antidiuretic hormone (Kaplan and Feigin 1978) can occur with acute bacterial meningitis and lead to hyponatraemia and hypotonic extracellular fluid which can exacerbate the cerebral oedema. However, arginine-vasopressin concentrations in blood normalize when children with meningitis are given adequate maintenance and replacement fluid therapy, indicating that high levels are a response to dehydration (Powell *et al.* 1990). Therefore, adequate maintenance and replacement fluids should be administered to maintain hydration and avoid vascular collapse (Lambert 1994).

The clinical manifestations of high ICP may not be obvious. They include an increase in or reappearance of disturbances of the level of consciousness, headache and vomiting, tense fontanelle and split sutures. Papilloedema is rare. CT scan may show the absence of subdural effusion or other space-occupying lesions and diffuse hypodensity of the brain parenchyma. MRI has been

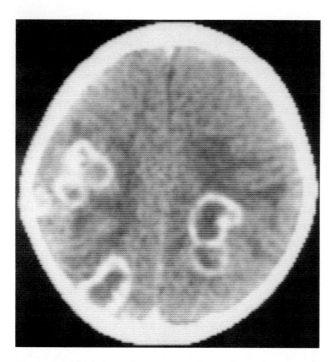

Fig. 11.2. Multiple brain abscesses in newborn infant with *Morganella* (formerly *Proteus*) *morganii* meningitis (CT scan). Several cavities lined by a ring of enhancement are present in both cerebral hemispheres. The abscesses are surrounded by oedema of the white matter. (Courtesy Prof. F. Brunelle, Hôpital des Enfants Malades, Paris.)

used to try to assess directly the brain water content (Lebel *et al.* 1989b). Monitoring of ICP may be a necessary part of treatment in cases of marked or sustained intracranial hypertension (Goiten *et al.* 1983, Minns *et al.* 1989). The head should be raised to approximately 30° to combat ICP. More aggressive measures are described in Chapter 14. Intracranial hypertension is associated with reduced brain perfusion and reduced cerebral blood flow velocity (McMenamin and Volpe 1984), so even moderate episodes of systemic hypotension can have serious consequences and should be avoided (Kaplan and Fishman 1988).

The development of a *brain abscess* is rare in the course of meningitis with the notable exception of neonatal meningitis due to *Proteus* spp. (Renier *et al.* 1988) (Fig. 11.2) and to *Citrobacter diversus* (Foreman *et al.* 1984, Kline *et al.* 1988). In older children, CT scan is indicated only if complications develop or if the course is prolonged or otherwise abnormal (Naidu *et al.* 1982).

Ventriculitis is almost constant in neonatal meningitis but is relatively uncommon in older children. When ventriculitis is associated with stenosis of the sylvian aqueduct, the infection becomes localized (pyocephalus) and may behave as a cerebral abscess. In most cases, ventriculitis is diagnosed because of persistence of positive CSF cultures with or without clinical signs. Ultrasonography and CT scan may allow identification of ventriculitis. The ventricles are usually dilated and there is a thick hyperdense (on CT scan) or hyperechogenic edging around the ventricular cavities (Diebler and Dulac 1987). Ventriculitis may respond to massive doses of parenteral antibiotics but local

treatment and drainage may become necessary. If not rapidly treated, hydrocephalus is prone to develop in survivors.

Subdural empyema is rare (Jacobson and Farmer 1981). It is often marked by the persistence of fever and infective symptoms and signs in association with focal signs such as convulsions and hemiplegia. The diagnosis is easily made by neuroimaging that shows a pericerebral collection with a thick, contrast-enhancing border.

Other septic complications are the result of concurrent bacteraemia. They include septic arthritis, pericarditis, pneumonia, endophthalmitis and hypopyon (Kaplan and Fishman 1988). Arthritis appearing after five to seven days of antibiotic therapy is probably mediated by an immune mechanism and frequently responds to anti-inflammatory agents (Rush *et al.* 1986). Gastrointestinal bleeding, anaemia and disseminated intravascular coagulation can be observed in severe cases, especially but not exclusively with meningococcal meningitis.

Fever is prolonged for 10 days or longer in 13 per cent of patients and recurs secondarily in 16 per cent (Lin *et al.* 1984). Fever may be due to the persistence of foci of inflammation, superficial thrombophlebitis from intravenous infusions, nosocomial infections, or septic or aseptic abscesses. More commonly, no cause is found. In such cases, lumbar puncture is indicated. If the child appears well and CSF values are approaching normal, antimicrobial therapy can generally be discontinued at the usual time.

SEQUELAE OF BACTERIAL MENINGITIS
Sensorineural hearing loss of a severe to profound degree occurs in about 10 per cent of children with meningitis and is bilateral in 4 per cent. Hearing loss is thought to result from labyrinthitis, presumably due to extension of infection from the subarachnoid space through the cochlear aqueduct (Kaplan *et al.* 1981, Eavey *et al.* 1985). The risk of deafness is increased if the CSF glucose concentration on admission is less than 1.1 mmol/L (20 mg/dL) (Dodge *et al.* 1984), if seizures occur before admission and if sterilization of the CSF is delayed (Schaad *et al.* 1990). Deafness appears to set in early in the course of meningitis. It is difficult to detect clinically. Therefore systematic assessment of hearing should be performed before hospital discharge by evoked response audiometry (Vienny *et al.* 1984, Cohen *et al.* 1988). Repeat examination is recommended after discharge if the results of the initial examination are abnormal. Early evoked responses may be transiently abnormal in approximately 20 per cent of cases, with recovery in one or two months (Vienny *et al.* 1984). The occurrence of deafness is not correlated to the age of the patient or the duration of illness before hospitalization. Thus it is unlikely to be prevented by an early diagnosis.

Deafness is frequently present in children with ataxia but occurs in its absence in most patients. *Ataxia* seems to be of vestibular origin although cerebellar dysfunction may be operative in some cases (Kaplan *et al.* 1981). Virtually all patients are able to compensate for balance deficits in a few weeks or months.

Blindness following purulent meningitis is rare. It may be due to intraocular pathology or optic neuritis, or be of cortical origin.

In the latter case it is only exceptionally lasting (Swartz and Dodge 1965, Thun-Hohenstein *et al.* 1992).

Chronic hydrocephalus is uncommon following childhood meningitis. It is due to meningeal fibrosis of the basal cisterns or of the brain convexity or to stenosis of the aqueduct of Sylvius by granular ependymitis. Chronic hydrocephalus may follow early obstructive hydrocephalus. More commonly it develops insidiously and may not be recognized for weeks or months. Therefore systematic ultrasound examination of the CNS is indicated following neonatal meningitis, as ventricular dilatation may occur long before any increase in head circumference. Management is by an external drain in early cases, later by insertion of a shunt.

Neurological sequelae include hemiplegia, quadriplegia and permanent seizure disorders (Marks *et al.* 1992) which can be isolated but are more often associated with mental retardation of variable severity. Such sequelae are the consequence of parenchymal changes resulting from the direct and toxic action of the organisms, vasculitis, and perhaps hypoxia and increased ICP. Permanent sequelae were found in only 4 per cent of children in studies by Pomeroy *et al.* (1990) and Taylor *et al.* (1990), in contrast with a much higher rate for transient neurological complications, which were found in approximately 30 per cent of patients and which may last up to several months.

Severe *mental deficits* are relatively uncommon in children with treated meningitis but some degree of impairment may be present. Taylor *et al.* (1984) studied 24 children who had recovered from meningitis six to eight years previously. Twenty-four siblings served as controls. The mean IQ of all children was within the normal range but children with meningitis scored significantly lower in performance IQ (94 *vs* 103) and full scale IQ (97 *vs* 104) than the controls. In another study (Feigin and Dodge, quoted by Klein *et al.* 1986), the mean IQ for a group of 235 patients was 94 ± 23 with a range of 33–150. When compared to control children, a significantly higher proportion of children who had recovered from meningitis had IQ scores < 80. Taylor *et al.* (1990) found that more children in the meningitis group than in the controls were in a special programme class or received tutoring at school and more family help with homework. However, there is some discrepancy between the results of various studies (Bohr *et al.* 1983a, Smith 1988, Davies 1989). Feldman and Michaels (1986) reported that the academic achievements of children tested 10–12 years after recovering from *H. influenzae* meningitis did not differ from their siblings' and there was no specific pattern of learning disabilities, attentional deficits or behaviour problems. Baraff *et al.* (1993a) reviewed the outcome in 4920 children with meningitis in 45 published reports after 1955. Of these children, 1602 had been enrolled in 19 prospective studies from developed countries and were investigated for sequelae after discharge. Deafness was found in 10.5 per cent of them and was bilateral and profound in 5.1 per cent. 42 per cent had learning difficulties or mental retardation, 3.5 per cent had spasticity or paresis and 16.4 per cent had at least one major adverse outcome including intellectual sequelae, neurological deficits, seizures or deafness. No sequelae were observed in 83.6 per cent. In the remaining 3318 cases, only 73.9 per cent had no sequelae and the mortality rate was 8.1 per cent as against 4.8 per cent in the first group. Grimwood *et al.* (1995) studied 158 survivors of meningitis incurred between 1983 and 1986 (74 per cent with *H. influenzae* b disease): 11 of 130 followed up for over six years (8.5 per cent) were found to have major deficits (IQ < 70, seizures, hydrocephalus, spasticity, blindness or profound deafness), while 24 (18.5 per cent) had minor deficits (school difficulties, behaviour problems or mild hearing loss) as compared to 10.8 per cent of control children. However, an unusually high proportion of these patients had had a complicated course (coma in 18.2 per cent, seizures in 32 per cent, paresis or marked hypotonia in 10.7 per cent).

MANAGEMENT OF ACUTE BACTERIAL MENINGITIS
ANTIBACTERIAL CHEMOTHERAPY
The aim of chemotherapy is to select an antimicrobial agent to which the organisms are susceptible, and which reaches the CSF in concentrations sufficient to kill the pathogens. Inhibition of growth is not enough, as bacterial concentrations may often be optimal at 10–30 times the minimum inhibitory concentration (Quagliarello and Scheld 1997). This can be achieved, in most cases, with adequate plasma concentration; direct instillation of the drug into the ventricles is only rarely indicated (Feigin *et al.* 1992).

The initial choice of antibiotic depends on the causative organism (Table 11.2). However, treatment must be started without delay and so without a complete bacteriological diagnosis. Selection of a drug will depend on the frequency of particular pathogens, therefore largely on age. The treatment will be modified as the results of bacterial examination, including determination of the minimal inhibitory concentration of specific antibiotics against the responsible organism (Table 11.3), become available. Care should be taken to test *H. influenzae* strains for the production of beta-lactamase. All antibiotics should be given by the intravenous route with the exception of chloramphenicol.

For infants over 2 months and children, the third-generation cephalosporins tend to be preferred over the classical combination of ampicillin and chloramphenicol, though the latter continues to be effective and relatively safe in most cases. Selection of a particular cephalosporin must be based on personal experience and dosing schedules (Marks *et al.* 1986, Rodriguez *et al.* 1986, Hart *et al.* 1993).

After identification of the responsible organism, the appropriate antibiotic as listed in Table 11.2 should be given.

H. influenzae strains resistant to both chloramphenicol and ampicillin obviously demand the use of the cephalosporins. Such strains are increasingly found (Klass and Klein 1992). Penicillin G or ampicillin are usually satisfactory for most strains of *N. meningitidis* and of *Str. pneumoniae*. Chloramphenicol is often active against penicillin-tolerant strains of *Str. pneumoniae*. This drug should not be used in case of shock with liver and renal impairment unless serum levels are carefully monitored and not allowed to rise above 50 μg/mL (Robinson and Roberts 1990).

TABLE 11.2
Antibiotic therapy for acute bacterial meningitis (children >2 months)

Organism	Current regimen	Classical regimen
Haemophilus influnzae	Cefotaxime Ceftriaxone Ceftazidime	Ampicillin and chloramphenicol
Neisseria meningitidis	Penicillin G or 3rd generation cephalosporins*	Penicillin G
Streptococcus pneumoniae	Penicillin G Chloramphenicol 3rd generation cephalosporins* Vancomycin Rifampicin	Penicillin G
Group B streptococcus	Penicillin G Ampicillin 3rd generation cephalosporins*	Penicillin G
Listeria monocytogenes	Ampicillin and aminoglycoside**	Ampicillin
Group D streptococcus	Ampicillin and aminoglycoside**	Ampicillin
Escherichia coli	Ampicillin and cephalosporin*	Ampicillin and aminoglycoside
Pseudomonas aeruginosa	Ticarcillin Ceftazidime Piperacillin Aminoglycoside	—
Proteus mirabilis	Ampicillin and aminoglycosides Carbenicillin Ticarcillin	Ampicillin and aminoglycoside
Staphylococcus aureus	Methicillin Nafcillin	Penicillin G
Pasteurella spp.	Ampicillin Penicillin, chloramphenicol	—
Citrobacter spp.	Ampicillin and aminoglycoside. (Sensitivities required)	—
Klebsiella pneumoniae	Aminoglycosides, polymyxin. (Sensitivities required)	Ampicillin and aminoglycoside
Yersinia pestis	Chloramphenicol, gentamicin Tetracyclines	—
Unknown	Cephalosporin and ampicillin, methicillin or nafcillin if question of staphylococcal infection	Ampicillin, chloramphenicol, aminoglycosides

*Cephalosporins (especially ceftazidime or ceftriaxone) are usually preferred because they are effective against most common bacteria.
**Ototoxicity and renal toxicity.

However, third-generation cephalosporins have proved to be superior to chloramphenicol (Peltola *et al.* 1989). Ceftriaxone has the added advantage of once-a-day administration. Biliary pseudolithiasis has been demonstrated by ultrasound study to be present in more than half of patients having received ceftriaxone for several days. Clinical manifestations were present in some of these children but the outcome was regularly favourable (Schaad *et al.* 1988). Ceftriaxone, however, may be more effective, and hearing loss may be less frequent than with cefuroxime (Schaad *et al.* 1990), so the latter is not recommended (American Academy of Pediatrics 1988a). When no organism is isolated, third-generation cephalosporins or a combination of ampicillin and chloramphenicol are usually effective. Ampicillin is the first choice drug for *L. monocytogenes* (Klein *et al.* 1986). Cefotaxime and ceftriaxone are effective in meningitides caused by *H. influenzae*, *N. meningitidis* and most strains of *Str. pneumoniae*. However, cases of pneumococcal meningitis resistant to third-generation cephalosporins and sometimes also to penicillin are now increasingly reported (John 1994, Leggiadro 1994, Muñoz *et al.* 1995), which is of particular concern given its present frequency. Vancomycin is effective against resistant strains of *Str. pneumoniae* (Viladrich *et al.* 1991, Friedland and McCracken 1994) and also against methicillin- and cephalosporin-resistant staphylococci, and is indicated in such cases even though it is potentially ototoxic and nephrotoxic. Rifampicin (Peters *et al.* 1994) may also be effective for such cases, particularly when given in conjunction with ceftriaxone (Quagliarello and Scheld 1997). This combination or that of vancomycin and ceftriaxone now tends to be preferred as initial treatment, given the frequency of resistant *Str. pneumoniae*.

The duration of antibiotic therapy is dependent on clinical response, age and causative organism. Seven days of treatment suffice for meningococcal meningitis. Children with meningitis due to *H. influenzae* type b or *Str. pneumoniae* are traditionally

TABLE 11.3
Minimal bactericidal concentrations against common meningeal pathogens and CSF concentrations of main antibiotics*

Antibiotic	Visual MIC[1] (mg/mL)				Dose (kg/day)	CSF concentrations (mg/mL)	
	H. influenzae	S. pneumoniae	N. meningitidis	E. coli		Early[2]	Late[2]
Penicillin	0.25–1.0	0.01–0.03	0.01–0.06		250,000 U	0.8 (1–2)	0.3 (1–2)
Ampicillin	0.5–3.1	0.03–1.56	1.0	3.12–6.25	400 mg	3.4 (0–50)	1.9 (0–40)
Chloramphenicol	2.0–8.0	0.5–12.5	2.0–8.0	1.56–>100	100 mg	6.0–13.0	3.0–10.0
Cefotaxime	0.04	0.04	0.02	0.5	200 mg	2.2–3.7	0.8 (0–3.3)
Cefuroxime	0.03–0.6	0.02–0.16	0.02–1.0	>50	200 mg	6.4 (1.1–18.8)	3.6 (0.5–4.1)
Ceftazidime	0.8	0.4	0.04	0.6	150 mg	9.3	5.1
Ceftriaxone	<0.03	<0.03	<0.001	0.25	100 mg	4.6 (0.9–9.1)	2.0 (0.6–5.5)

*Modified from Kaplan and Fishman (1988).
[1]MIC = minimum inhibitory concentration.
[2]Early = first 1–2 days of illness; late = 7–10 days.

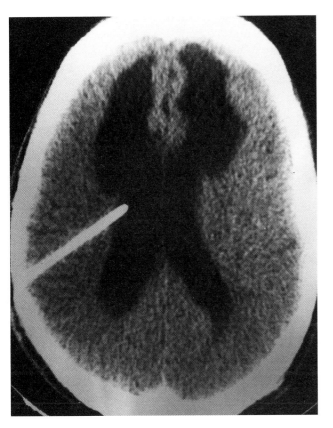

Fig. 11.3. So-called 'puncture porencephaly'. 18-year-old adolescent who developed acute hydrocephalus at age 4 months as a result of meningitis. Several ventricular taps through the anterior fontanelle were performed. Successive radiological examinations (initially pneumoencephalography and later CT scan) demonstrated the appearance of cavities alongside the needle tracts, indicating the danger of ventricular puncture, especially when CSF pressure is elevated.

treated for at least 10 days or until afebrile for five full days, although seven-day treatment has been found to be no less effective and to be attended by no more complications or sequelae than 10- to 14-day treatment (Lin et al. 1984, Jadavji et al. 1986). In meningitides that are difficult to sterilize, ventriculitis should be suspected. If confirmed by ventricular fluid study, antibodies should be instilled into the ventricular CSF via a

reservoir or by direct puncture (Bayston et al. 1987). However, the latter, especially when repeated in the face of increased ICP, may lead to the formation of puncture porencephalies (Fig. 11.3).

MONITORING OF TREATMENT
Patients with meningococcal and pneumococcal meningitis whose disease runs a smooth, uncomplicated course do not need a control lumbar puncture and the same possibly applies to *H. influenzae* meningitis. In the latter, however, a repeat lumbar puncture at 36–48 hours of treatment is helpful as there is a correlation between delayed CSF sterilization and the occurrence of sequelae and hearing loss (Lebel and McCracken 1989, Schaad et al. 1990). 'End of treatment' lumbar puncture is useless in regular cases of childhood meningitis as the cell and chemical composition of the CSF is extremely variable (Schaad et al. 1981, Durack and Spanos 1982).

ADJUVANT AND SUPPORTIVE TREATMENT
Corticosteroids have been recommended by some investigators for the treatment of increased ICP on the basis of experimental data (Syrogiannopoulos et al. 1987). Lebel et al. (1988) found that dexamethasone therapy was associated with a lower frequency of hearing loss in patients treated with steroids in addition to cephalosporins. Interpretation of this result may not be simple as patients who developed deafness were predominantly receiving cefuroxime which is less active than ceftriaxone or cefotaxime (Schaad et al. 1990). Girgis et al. (1989) found a lower mortality rate in children receiving dexamethasone in addition to antibiotics. A placebo-controlled double-blind trial showed an advantage for cefotaxime plus dexamethasone given 15–30 minutes before antibiotics over cefotaxime in the treatment of 101 children with bacterial meningitis aged 6 weeks to 3 years, but did not reduce the incidence of deafness (Odio et al. 1991). In over three-quarters of these cases *H. influenzae* b was the infecting organism. Dexamethasone (0.4 mg/kg given twice daily, 10 minutes before cefotaxime) reduced the incidence of deafness in patients with *H. influenzae* meningitis (Schaad et al. 1993). In children with pneumococcal meningitis, administration of 0.15 mg/kg of dexamethasone every six hours for four days was associated with a reduction of fever duration and with a decrease

in the frequency of septic shock and 'cerebrovascular' instability in those who had received dexamethasone before antibiotics (Kennedy *et al.* 1991). However, Wald *et al.* (1995) in a comparative trial involving 143 patients (69 receiving 0.15 mg/kg dexamethasone every six hours for four days, plus ceftriaxone; 74 receiving ceftriaxone plus placebo) did not find any significant difference in mortality or sequelae. Prober (1995) and Prasad and Haines (1995) concluded that dexamethasone was indicated for children with *H. influenzae* meningitis but not for pneumococcal disease. It seems that dexamethasone therapy probably reduces the likelihood of deafness without adverse effects in *H. influenzae* cases and individual consideration of dexamethasone for bacterial meningitis in patients 2 months of age and older is recommended (American Academy of Pediatrics 1990).

Contrary to previous advice, fluid restriction is not indicated for patients with meningitis, and sufficient amounts of fluids are essential for the prevention of shock.

Convulsions should be treated with intravenous diazepam or lorazepam. If unsuccessful, benzodiazepines should be replaced by phenytoin in doses adequate for treatment of status epilepticus (Chapter 16). Preventive treatment is used in some centres. My personal practice is to use prophylactic phenobarbitone systematically from the time of diagnosis and to discontinue the drug after 7–10 days. At regular doses (4 mg/kg/d) no disturbance of consciousness attributable to the drug is observed. Treatment of high ICP is described in Chapter 14. Hyperventilation may be dangerous as it can decrease cerebral blood flow dangerously (Ashwal *et al.* 1990, Minns 1991).

PECULIARITIES OF THE MAIN TYPES OF ACUTE BACTERIAL MENINGITIS

H. influenzae type b meningitis is primarily a disease of infants and preschool children. More than 95 per cent of cases occur before age 2 years. Considerable variations in incidence exist between different countries and even within the same country, and immunization with conjugate vaccine has considerably decreased its frequency.

Symptoms of upper respiratory tract infection, including otitis media, frequently precede the onset of meningitis, which is thus less abrupt than that of meningococcal or pneumococcal meningitides. This is a cause for both delayed correct treatment and the 'blind' administration of antibiotics with resulting sterile CSF. A sparse petechial rash may be present (Marshall 1983). Purpura fulminans is on record (Jacobs *et al.* 1983).

Subdural effusions occur in 15 per cent of patients but are of limited clinical significance.

The mortality rate is 3–4 per cent but sequelae occur in 9–20 per cent of children. Hearing loss is a major problem, occurring in approximately 10 per cent of cases. Although it was initially thought that hearing loss was more common with ampicillin therapy, this has not been confirmed. Some recovery can occur up to six months after the acute attack (Roeser *et al.* 1975).

Anaemia is commoner and more severe in patients with *H. influenzae* disease than in other meningitides (Kaplan and Oski 1980).

The outcome is poorer in cases complicated for more than three days by persistent seizures, deep coma and pretreatment symptoms.

The attack rate in household contacts is higher than in non-exposed children (Glode *et al.* 1980). However, chemoprophylaxis for day-care centre contacts is not generally recommended because of conflicting evidence. If given, rifampicin should be used at a dose of 20 mg/kg/d for four days.

Primary prevention can be obtained through the use of polyribosylribitol vaccine (Harrison *et al.* 1989). The vaccine is safe and efficacious for children over 2 years of age, but no protection has been demonstrated for children under 18 months who are at a much greater risk. Conjugate vaccine resulting from coupling a protein carrier to a polysaccharide confers T-cell-dependent characteristics to an otherwise cell-independent antigen. The *H. influenzae* type b diphtheria toxoid conjugate vaccine has been recommended for all children at 18 months of age (American Academy of Pediatrics 1988b, Granoff *et al.* 1989) and has been shown to be effective from 15 months of age (Madore *et al.* 1990) and even in newborn infants (Vadheim *et al.* 1993, Kurikka *et al.* 1995). Currently, type b conjugate vaccine is administered at 2 and 4 months of age (American Academy of Pediatrics 1996).

Meningococcal infection is a common cause of meningitis in most Western countries. *N. meningitidis* belonging to groups A, B, C, D, X, Y, Z and W135 has been identified as a cause. The corresponding antigens can be found in the blood, CSF and urine of infected patients. Epidemics are most often caused by group A and group C organisms, while group B and others are mostly responsible for sporadic cases (Marshall 1983).

The onset of clinical symptoms is usually abrupt. In some cases, a fulminating disease can develop in a few hours. A rash that may be petechial, maculopapular or morbilliform is present in 50–75 per cent of cases (Swartz and Dodge 1965). Bacteria can be found in petechial lesions. A rapid extension of the skin lesion may be of ominous significance as it often heralds intravascular coagulation leading to purpura fulminans, as a consequence of tissue sensitization responsible for a Schwartzmann phenomenon. This is due to the endotoxin of the organism which also induces shock, bilateral adrenal haemorrhage and other bacterial emboli which may be prominent in the lungs.

Pericarditis, arthritis and eye involvement are infrequent. Eye lesions include hypopyon and panophthalmitis (Edwards and Baker 1981).

Specific treatment is mainly with penicillin G because up to two-thirds of group B strains are sulfonamide-resistant. However, meningococci resistant to both sulfonamides and penicillin are now encountered so cephalosporins may be indicated. Careful monitoring is important for early detection and treatment of shock which must be vigorous and has precedence over performing lumbar puncture in very ill patients. Corticosteroids are of uncertain value.

Chronic meningococcaemia is rare and is marked by fever, fleeting rashes, joint pain or effusion. Spontaneous remission is possible. Meningeal involvement is rare in such cases. Meningococcal meningitis may manifest as progressive hydrocephalus with mild fever and variable CSF pleocytosis (personal case). This form was formerly known as 'posterior basilar meningitis' and is now rare (Diebler and Dulac 1987).

Recurrent meningococcal meningitis is seen in patients with IgG2 subclass deficiency (Bass *et al.* 1983) and in patients with acquired or genetic deficiency of the complement system (Ross and Densen 1984) especially the C5–C9 terminal fraction (Davis *et al.* 1983, Ross and Densen 1984). Meningitis associated with such complement deficiency is often mild and due to uncommon serogroups (Fijen *et al.* 1989).

The risk of developing the disease for household contacts is about 1000 times the endemic attack rate. Rifampicin prophylaxis is therefore recommended for household, day-care centre and nursery school contacts of a patient with meningococcal meningitis. A total dose of 20 mg/kg/d in one or two divided doses up to 600 mg/d is adequate. Polysaccharide vaccines against type A and C meningococci are available for children 3 months to 5 years of age (Lepow and Gold 1983).

Other members of the *Neisseria* family, *e.g. N. catarrhalis* (Feigin *et al.* 1969), *N. subflava* (Lewin and Hughes 1966) and *N. gonorrhea* can produce septicaemia, meningitis and purpura fulminans.

Pneumococcal meningitis is becoming prominent in children under 10 years of age because of the decreasing incidence of *H. influenzae* meningitis. Most cases are due to bacteraemia but direct extension, from a septic focus in the ears, or following a skull fracture with CSF leak, or due to a congenital defect in the cribriform plate or the roof of the inner ear, is possible. In the latter cases, recurrent meningitis is frequent and the causal organisms often appear to be unusual strains. When associated with ear infection, organisms isolated from the middle ear are not always the same as those from the CSF. The risk of pneumococcal meningitis is particularly high in children with sickle cell disease, especially those under 5 years (Nottidge 1983), as a result of functional asplenia in such patients. The same applies to children whose spleen has been removed, and regular prophylactic administration of oral penicillin V is recommended for them. In overwhelming infection, the CSF may contain less than 75 cells/mm³ and more than 10 organisms per high power field on first examination.

Pneumococcal meningitis has the highest mortality and complication rate of the three common bacterial meningitides of childhood. Convulsions occur in up to 44 per cent of patients and coma is frequent. Hearing loss is seen in more than 20 per cent of cases. Ataxia was found in 17 of 93 patients by Bohr *et al.* (1984). Hydrocephalus is also more frequent than in other meningitides and this may be related to the greater thickness and abundance of purulent exudate as compared with that produced by other pathogens.

Penicillin is the antibiotic of choice but chloramphenicol should be used for patients allergic to penicillin.

The increasing frequency of strains resistant to both penicillin and cephalosporins is of concern. The use of vancomycin is justified in such cases (Viladrich *et al.* 1991). Quagliarello and Scheld

(1997) considered the possible use of the drug as a first-line treatment for 48 hours, pending determination of drug-sensitivity of the isolated strain. Combined use of third-generation cephalosporins and vancomycin or rifampicin (Friedland and McCracken 1994) or imipenem and cilastatin (Asensi *et al.* 1993) is being investigated. Early repeat lumbar puncture is essential when dealing with beta-lactam-resistant pneumococci (Kleiman *et al.* 1993). Sensitivity tests should guide the treatment in patients with resistant or relatively resistant strains.

Staphylococcal meningitis is often due to secondary invasion of the CNS as a result of wounds, surgery or nearby infections. *S. aureus* is generally the cause of such cases. *S. epidermidis* is a common pathogen in patients with ventriculoperitoneal or ventriculo-atrial shunts (Chapter 7).

BACTERIAL MENINGITIS IN NEWBORN INFANTS

Meningitis in the first 28 days of life differs in many ways from that in older children (Davies and Rudd 1994). The causal bacteria are not the same, and the characteristics of the neonatal brain as well as the immature mechanisms of defense against infection result in a different picture and outcome.

In newborn infants weighing >2500 g, a frequency of 0.37 per 1000 has been found (Klein *et al.* 1986). In infants <2500 g, this rises to 1.36 per 1000 births. The age-specific incidence is higher in the first month of life than in any subsequent period, at 99.5 per 100,000 per year (Schlech *et al.* 1985). Boys are more commonly affected than girls, especially with gram-negative infections.

In newborn infants and those under 3–4 months of age, diagnostic difficulties are often considerable. The major early features are changes in consciousness and behaviour. Meningitis should be thought of in any unwell infant who is drowsy or irritable. In 50 per cent of cases, there is anorexia or vomiting. Low-grade fever and other systemic manifestations such as jaundice or respiratory distress are common but nonspecific. Convulsions, usually focal in type, are a clear indication to perform lumbar puncture. Meningeal signs are rare, and a full or bulging fontanelle is present in less than one-third of patients (Davies and Rudd 1994).

Not infrequently, symptoms and signs of sepsis, without any feature suggestive of meningeal involvement, dominate the clinical picture. CSF study is thus mandatory in every case of suspected serious neonatal infection.

A history of prolonged rupture of the membranes, maternal fever or difficult obstetrical manipulations should enhance the suspicion of meningitis. Such is also the case when colonization of the maternal genital tract by group B streptococcus or *L. monocytogenes* is known to be present.

Interpretation of the results of lumbar puncture may be difficult in neonates because of the characteristics of the CSF at this age (Rodriguez *et al.* 1990). In one study, Bonadio (1992) found that 31 per cent of infants under 8 weeks old had more than 10 white blood cells per mm³ of CSF and that only 10 per cent had no white blood cells. A majority of the white cells were polymorphs. The protein level was on average 0.44 g/L in preterm infants, and figures as high as 1.5 g/L are known to occur. Low glucose levels are frequent in neonates and especially in infants aged between 4 and 8 weeks. In addition, traumatic lumbar puncture is frequent in this age group, and up to 4 per cent of newborn babies with meningitis, especially preterm infants, may have a normal CSF at the first examination. This emphasizes the need for repeat lumbar puncture 6–12 hours after the first tap in case of doubt (this also applies to older patients).

Up to 30 per cent of neonates with group B streptococcal meningitis may have less than 30 white blood cells/mm³, while the same is rare with *E. coli* meningitis. However, Klein *et al.* (1986) reported that fewer than 1 per cent of patients had completely normal CSF (including cell count, protein and sugar).

Finally, lumbar puncture may be dangerous and temporarily contraindicated in sick newborn infants because flexion of the trunk during holding may produce hypoxaemia (Eldadah *et al.* 1987, Weiss *et al.* 1991).

Meningitis in the neonatal period can be due to a wide range of infecting organisms. The most common pathogens are group B beta-haemolytic streptococcus, and *E. coli*, especially K1-positive strains. Other causes include *Morganella morganii* (formerly *Proteus morganii*) and *Citrobacter diversus*, which in most cases are responsible for the occurrence of brain abscesses; *L. monocytogenes* (Bortolussi and Seeliger 1990, Kessler and Dajani 1990); *Pseudomonas aeruginosa* or *Ps. cepacia* (Darby 1976); *Flavobacterium meningosepticum*; *Klebsiella* spp.; *Enterobacter* spp.; and other rare organisms.

Meningitis caused by group B streptococci may involve any of the group B subtypes (Ia, Ib, II or III). Most cases are caused by the subtype III organism. Approximately 25–35 per cent of pregnant women are colonized vaginally or rectally by group B streptococci. Vertical transmission from mother to infant is one important cause of septicaemia and meningitis. However, spread of the pathogen may also be horizontal from the hands of nursery personnel.

Strains of *E. coli* containing K1 capsular polysaccharide antigen cause 75 per cent of *E. coli* neonatal meningitis, and the disease is more severe than that due to non-K1 strains. Infants acquire the pathogen from their mother in most cases although 10–15 per cent are born to K1-negative mothers (Klein *et al.* 1986).

Meningitis due to *M. morganii* or *C. diversus* is associated with brain abscesses, often multiple, in about 75 per cent of cases. These are often paucisymptomatic but are clearly shown by CT scanning (see Fig. 11.2), which demonstrates multiple hypodensities surrounded by enhancing rims. Neuroimaging procedures are clearly indicated for all patients infected with these organisms. In general, CT scan or ultrasonography should be performed in most if not all cases of neonatal meningitis (Han *et al.* 1985, Hung 1986) (see also p. 378).

The *clinical manifestations* of neonatal meningitis are quite variable and often nonspecific. Two distinct syndromes can be tentatively described. *Early-onset disease* manifests within 48 hours of birth with signs of sepsis and pulmonary disease. Meningeal signs are often totally lacking. This syndrome occurs

with type I group B streptococcus and *L. monocytogenes* infections (Larsson *et al.* 1979). *Late-onset disease* occurs at the end of the first week of life in term babies and the clinical features are more clearly meningitic (Baker *et al.* 1973). Late-onset syndrome occurs with type III streptococcus and may also occur with *Proteus*, *Citrobacter* or *Pseudomonas* infection (Marshall 1983).

Neonatal meningitis is often associated with complications of pregnancy and labour, and with maternal infections especially of the urinary tract. Septicaemia is present in about 60 per cent of cases.

The *outcome of neonatal meningitis* is far worse than that of later cases. Mortality is still around 24–30 per cent although it has significantly decreased in the past three decades (Wald *et al.* 1986, Davies and Rudd 1994). It is higher for low-birthweight infants and for those with early onset of the disease in the first week of life. The frequency of cognitive sequelae is high. From 30 to 50 per cent of infants are left with intellectual or neurological complications or both. Hydrocephalus remains common. The EEG may have predictive value as very slow tracings are of unfavourable prognostic significance (Chequer *et al.* 1992).

The *initial empirical treatment regimen* for neonatal meningitis usually combines ampicillin or amoxycillin and an aminoglycoside, or a cephalosporin (cefotaxime or ceftazidime). Ceftazidime may be prefered for the low-birthweight infant in whom nosocomial *Pseudomonas* infection is possible. However, the cephalosporins are not efficacious against *L. monocytogenes*. An optimal combination before determination of the causal organism may be cefotaxime, penicillin and gentamicin (Gandy and Rennie 1990). For *E. coli* meningitis, the combination of a third-generation cephalosporin with ampicillin is logical, although actual superiority over standard treatment with ampicillin and an aminoglycoside has not been demonstrated (McCracken *et al.* 1984). Chloramphenicol can be associated with shock (the grey baby syndrome) so that small doses not in excess of 25 mg/kg/d should be used for preterm infants and term infants in the first week of life. Blood level determination is desirable.

Group B streptococcal meningitis is effectively treated with penicillin or ampicillin (Pyati *et al.* 1983). *Listeria* meningitis responds to ampicillin alone or in combination with aminoglycosides but not to cephalosporins (Kessler and Dajani 1990). Ventriculitis is a frequent complication.

Compartmentalization of the cerebral ventricles, especially at the level of the foramen of Monro may lead to localized hydrocephalus (Kalsbeck *et al.* 1980) although diffuse hydrocephalus due to cisternal blockage is much more frequent.

In newborn infants with brain abscesses, especially due to *Proteus* or *Citrobacter* spp., drug treatment is often sufficient. Puncture of the larger cavities is indicated when they are large and/or produce increased ICP.

Prophylactic therapy of early-onset neonatal group B streptococcal disease has been proposed with selective chemotherapy (Boyer and Gotoff 1986) but the indications remain in dispute.

In infants 28 days to 3 months of age, there is overlap between the organisms responsible for neonatal meningitis and those of childhood meningitis that become increasingly prevalent in older

TABLE 11.4
Antibiotics for treatment of meningitis

Drug	Newborn infants		Older infants (≥ 28 days) and children	
	Total dose (mg/kg/d)	No. of daily doses	Total dose (mg/kg/d)	No. of daily doses
Ampicillin	100–200	2–4	200–300	4
Penicillin G	100,000–200,000[1]	3–4	150–240,000[1]	4–6
Methicillin	100–200	2–4	100–200	2–4
Nafcillin	100–200	2–4	100–200	2–4
Ticarcillin	150–300	2–4	300	4
Piperacillin	200–300	3	—	—
Vancomycin	20–40	2–4	40–60	4
Tobramycin	4–6	2–3	3–5	3
Chloramphenicol[2]	25–50	1–2	75–100	4
Gentamicin	5–7.5	2	4–5	2–3
Kanamycin	15–30	2–3	15	2
Amikacin	15–30	2–3	15	2
Cefotaxime	100–150	2–4	200	4
Ceftriaxone	50–100	2[3]	80–100	1–2[4]
Ceftazidime	60–90	2–3	125–150	3
Cefuroxime	60–120	2–4	240	3
Moxalactam	100–200	2	200	3–4

[1]U/kg.
[2]Optimal dosage should be based on determination of serum concentrations, especially in low-birthweight infants.
[3]One dose/day may be used.
[4]For the first day, two 80 mg/kg doses 12 hours apart is recommended (American Academy of Pediatrics 1988).

babies (Baumgartner *et al.* 1983). However, the pathogens of childhood meningitis are occasionally the cause of neonatal disease.

RARE CAUSES OF ACUTE BACTERIAL MENINGITIS

Rare causes of *acute purulent meningitis* include *Bacillus* spp. (Feder *et al.* 1988a), *Pasteurella multocida* (Kolyvas *et al.* 1978), *Yersinia pestis* (Mann *et al.* 1982), *Salmonella* spp. (Appelbaum and Scragg 1977), *Acinetobacter* (previously *Mimae*) spp. (Graber *et al.* 1965), *Serratia marcescens* (Campbell *et al.* 1992), anaerobic organisms (Law and Aronoff 1992), nonanthrax *Bacillus* (Weisse *et al.* 1991) and *Pseudomonas pseudomallei*, the agent of melioidosis which is common in some tropical countries (Visudhipan *et al.* 1990). This bacterium may also be the cause of brain abscess and empyema. Treatment is shown in Table 11.4.

Unhanand *et al.* (1993) reviewed 98 cases of meningitis due to gram-negative bacilli both in neonates and in infants. A predisposing factor such as neural tube defect or urinary tract anomaly was present in 25 per cent of cases. *E. coli* organisms accounted for 53 per cent of cases, *Klebsiella/Enterobacter* for 16 per cent, *Salmonellae* for 9 per cent and rare organisms for the rest.

In patients with ventriculoatrial and ventriculoperitoneal shunts, unusual organisms such as diphtheroids may be found (Everett *et al.* 1976, Berke *et al.* 1981).

Dual infection with both viral and bacterial invaders is rare (Hutchinson *et al.* 1977).

Meningitis in patients with a shunt has been reviewed in Chapter 7. The commonest organisms are *S. epidermidis* and *S. aureus*. Enteric bacilli are responsible for about 10 per cent of cases

(Hirsch and Hoppe-Hirsch 1988). Rare organisms are sometimes isolated from patients with meningitis complicating a shunt procedure (Arisoy *et al.* 1993).

RECURRENT BACTERIAL MENINGITIS

Recurrent purulent meningitis usually occurs in children with an underlying surgical or medical disorder facilitating infection of the nervous system (Table 11.5). *S. pneumoniae* is responsible in about three-quarters of cases, with *S. aureus*, *Pseudomonas* spp., *Klebsiella* spp. and *H. influenzae* accounting for only a minority. The clinical manifestations are often relatively mild, but severe cases can occur (Holguin and Manotas 1988).

Traumatic leaks resulting from fractures of the skull base are the most common cause of recurrent meningitis. Approximately 1 per cent of cases of head injury requiring hospitalization develop CSF fistulae that become a source of infection in 10–24 per cent. Infection is usually an early event but may be delayed for months or even years; it may occur even in the absence of CSF rhinorrhoea or otorrhoea. Nontraumatic fistulae that represent congenital defects of the skull bones are often difficult to detect and necessitate careful radiological survey (Steele *et al.* 1985), otological examination, and isotopic examination with radioiodinated albumin or technetium injected intrathecally. *Congenital dermal sinuses* are an important cause. In all cases of recurrent meningitis, careful examination of the lumbosacral area (Schwartz and Balentine 1978) and the cervico-occipital midline is mandatory. Occipital sinuses may be especially difficult to detect, and shaving of the region is imperative as the external orifice may be pinpoint. CT scan of the head may show a dermoid cyst of the posterior fossa (Fig. 11.4). Sphenoidal and basioccipital meningoceles (Hemphill *et al.* 1982) may also be difficult to

TABLE 11.5
Causes of recurrent bacterial meningitis

Cause	References
Surgical causes	
Post-traumatic fistulae following fractures of the cribriform plate, petrous pyramids, frontal, ethmoidal or sphenoidal sinuses	Wilson *et al.* (1990, 1991)
Nontraumatic fistulae	Ommaya (1976), Steele *et al.* (1985)
Congenital dehiscence of the cribriform plate	
Defects of the foot plate of the stapes	
Defects of the middle ear	
Congenital defects of the tegmen tympani	
Mondini syndrome	
Congenital dermal sinus with or without intraspinal or intracranial dermoid cyst (lumbosacral, cervico-occipital)	Chapter 3; Schwartz and Balentine (1978)
Craniopharyngioma and other intracranial dermoid or epidermoid cysts	Kitai *et al.* (1992)
Myelomeningoceles and meningoencephaloceles including occult forms such as sphenoidal or basioccipital meningoencephaloceles or neurenteric cysts	Chapter 3; Hemphill *et al.* (1982)
Shunt-treated hydrocephalus	Hirsch and Hoppe-Hirsch (1988)
Nonsurgical causes	
Congenital agammaglobulinaemia (or hypogammaglobulinaemia)	Bass *et al.* (1983)
Deficiency of the terminal components of complement (C5–C9)	Davis *et al.* (1983)
Splenectomy in infancy	
Mixed immunological deficiency	
Sickle cell anaemia	Nottidge (1983)
Unknown causes	
Pneumococci are the most common pathogens in post-traumatic cases, in children with congenital defects of nose and ear, and following splenectomy; gram-negative bacteria and staphylococci are common with dermal sinuses and neural tube defects; *S. epidermidis* in patients with shunt; and meningococci in children with complement deficiency	

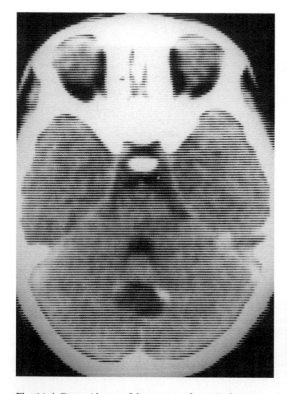 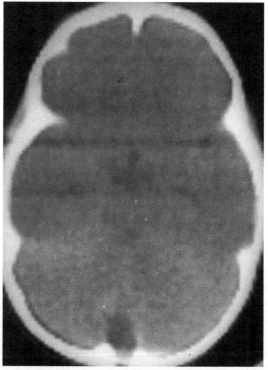

Fig. 11.4. Dermoid cysts of the posterior fossa. *(Left)* CT scan shows hypodense area lined by thin ring of contrast enhancement. *(Right)* CT scan of another patient shows hole in occipital squama. Both patients had recurrent chemical meningitis.

recognize, emphasizing the necessity for a careful neuroradiological examination.

Treatment of recurrent meningitis is directed primarily against respiratory pathogens in the case of CSF fistulae and against enteric organisms in cases of dermal sinus. Pneumococcal vaccine may be useful for some patients. Prophylactic antibiotics are used by some clinicians but may favour the emergence of resistant bacteria. There is a consensus that surgical correction of fistulae lasting more than 4–6 weeks and surgical intervention for chronic otitis, sinusitis or mastoiditis should be performed. Dermoid tracts need total removal.

SUBACUTE OR CHRONIC AND GRANULOMATOUS BACTERIAL MENINGITIS

TUBERCULOUS MENINGITIS

Meningitis caused by *Mycobacterium tuberculosis* is a major cause of childhood death and neurological disability in developing countries. Although, strictly speaking, it is spontaneously an acute disorder with a mean duration without treatment of 20–30 days, it is currently a chronic process as it is virtually always treated at some stage. In industrialized countries, tuberculous meningitis is still observed. Because its frequency has considerably diminished, its diagnosis is often missed, as doctors and bacteriologists are no longer considering it as a priority. The mortality rate and incidence of sequelae are much higher when treatment is not started until the child is in coma or presenting focal neurological signs (Bateman *et al.* 1983).

PATHOLOGY AND PATHOGENESIS

Most cases are now caused by the human type of *Mycobacteria*. Because of the widespread pasteurization of milk, the bovine type is responsible for less than 5 per cent of cases. Exceptional cases have been observed following BCG immunization of immunodeficient and even of normal children (Tardieu *et al.* 1988). Tuberculous meningitis due to atypical *Mycobacteria* has been reported in the last three decades.

Involvement of the meninges is probably secondary to ulceration of a small parenchymal tuberculoma in the cortex, itself associated with widespread haematogenous dissemination of *Mycobacteria* in the early stages of tuberculous infection. Miliary pulmonary tuberculosis is often associated. However, meningitis may rarely be caused by dissemination from other visceral foci or by extension of spinal or cranial osteitis. Although BCG vaccination is an effective preventive measure (Udani 1991), approximately 20 per cent of children with tuberculous meningitis have been immunized. Because of partial immunity, they tend to develop atypical forms with encephalitic symptomatology and prolonged course.

At autopsy, an opaque and gelatinous exudate fills the basal cisterns. Small superficial tuberculomas are frequently found. Hydrocephalus is present in most autopsied cases, and ischaemic lesions, in particular of the basal ganglia, are extremely frequent in childhood cases.

TABLE 11.6
Clinical features at presentation of children with tuberculous meningitis*

Nuchal rigidity	77%
Apathy	72%
Fever	47%
Vomiting	30%
Drowsiness	23%
Headache	21%
Coma	14%
Papilloedema	9%
Convulsions	9%
Facial palsy	9%
VIth nerve palsy	9%
IIIrd nerve palsy	9%
Hemiparesis	5%
VIIIth nerve involvement	2%
Diabetes insipidus	2%

*Data from Idriss *et al.* (1976).

Large *tuberculomas* are still relatively common in Asiatic and African countries and may be supratentorial or involve the brainstem (Dastur and Desai 1965). Vasculitis with frequent thrombosis particularly affects the internal carotid artery and sylvian vessels whereas the posterior circulation is relatively preserved. A *tuberculous encephalopathy* has been described in some cases of tuberculous meningitis (Udani and Dastur 1970). The condition is characterized by oedema and, less frequently, perivascular myelin loss with vasculitis of capillary and small vessels. This might result from an allergic reaction to proteins liberated from lysed tubercle bacilli in partially immune children and can occur with little or no evidence of meningitis.

In partially immune patients, localized forms are common and are apt to produce a wide variety of lesions, including localized meningitis of the posterior fossa with cerebellar signs and hydrocephalus, chiasmatic involvement with visual deficits (Silverman *et al.* 1995) or brainstem damage with alternate syndromes (Udani 1991).

CLINICAL MANIFESTATIONS

The clinical manifestations of tuberculous meningitis are extremely variable (Table 11.6) so that the diagnosis may be very difficult. Virtually any neurological picture can be seen. Fifty to 60 per cent of cases are in children less than 3 years of age, although there is a tendency for cases to occur later as the age of primary tuberculous infection tends to increase in most countries.

The most common clinical form corresponds to *caseous meningitis*. Onset may be precipitated by any condition that lowers general resistance, particularly measles. It is customary to describe three successive stages in the untreated disease, which inexorably progresses to death in three to four weeks. The prodromal stage is seen in 60 per cent of cases and usually lasts two to three weeks. It is marked by apathy, irritability, disturbances of sleep, vomiting and abdominal pain. At this stage, there are no neurological manifestations. Onset of the disease proper is usually marked by a moderate fever although 10–20 per cent of patients in large series are afebrile. Headache is uncommonly complained of by children under 3 years but abdominal pain is present in 15 per cent of cases. Apathy, irritability and photophobia rapidly set in. Mental changes are present in 80 per cent of patients and focal neurological signs in approximately one-third of cases (Waeker and O'Connor 1990, Curless and Mitchell 1991, Davis *et al.* 1993). Meningeal signs appear, and paralysis of cranial nerves III, IV, VI and VII is frequently present at this second stage. Hemiplegia and movement disorders due to frequent involvement of the basal ganglia are often observed (Gelabert and Castro-Gago 1988). During the third stage, stupor and coma replace apathy. Symptoms and signs of increased ICP are obvious. The pupils are fixed, respiration is irregular and signs of decerebration with tonic extensor spasms develop. Hydrocephalus is present in a majority of patients at this stage.

Atypical manifestations are common. A febrile convulsion may occur at onset. Focal neurological deficits preceding the classical meningeal irritation have been reported in all large series and include field defects, aphasia, hemiparesis, monoparesis and abnormal movements. Isolated high fever, severe convulsions and features mimicking intracranial tumours may be observed (Udani and Bhat 1974).

In the rarer serous forms seen mainly in children partially immunized by BCG, symptoms include headache, crying, vomiting and sometimes seizures. Children remain conscious, and febrile and meningeal signs are not obvious. The CSF may be normal or show only mild lymphocytosis and mildly increased protein (Udani and Bhat 1974). Recovery is the rule and may even occur in the absence of treatment.

A *spinal form* of tuberculous meningitis may manifest as fever and meningeal signs rapidly followed by paraplegia, with secondary intracranial spread. Such cases are apt to be mistaken for acute viral meningomyelitis.

Tuberculous encephalopathy (Udani and Dastur 1970) is characterized by convulsions and coma. The CSF is usually normal or shows only a mild increase of protein and cells. A diffuse encephalopathy may develop in a child already treated for tuberculous meningitis.

In rare cases, the disease evolves without CSF abnormalities being present (serous form) in children with primary tuberculosis and symptoms of meningeal irritation.

DIAGNOSIS
The diagnosis classically rests on CSF changes, a history of exposure to persons with pulmonary tuberculosis, often an asymptomatic older relative, and a positive tuberculin skin test in association with a compatible clinical picture. However, skin anergy is present in 10–40 per cent of cases (Doerr *et al.* 1995). A positive test may be difficult to interpret in patients immunized with BCG vaccine but who nevertheless develop tuberculous meningitis (Udani 1991). Miliary tuberculosis of the lungs or primary complex are present in well over half the patients and are an important diagnostic clue. Retinal tubercles are also of great value.

The *CSF findings* although fundamental are not always unequivocal. The fluid may be crystal-clear or have a ground-glass appearance. It contains 10–400 cells/mm³, which are lymphocytes in over 85 per cent of cases. In one series, however, the CSF contained fewer than 10 cells/mm³ in three of 32 cases (Ponsot *et al.* 1980). Polymorphonuclear leukocytes may outnumber lymphocytes in the early stages; and occasionally, transient, spontaneously disappearing, polymorphonuclear pleocytosis may occur during later stages (Teoh *et al.* 1986). Repetition of lumbar puncture may be helpful in such cases for distinguishing partially treated acute bacterial meningitis from tuberculous meningitis (Feigin and Shackelford 1973). CSF protein is always raised, often to 200 mg/dL or more, and glucose is always lowered, in 80 per cent of cases to below 1.5 mmol/L (Lambert 1994). Chloride is usually low. Direct visualization of acid-fast organisms is uncommon.

Culture of CSF is positive in 12–57 per cent of cases and results are available only after weeks; hence, treatment should often be started on indirect evidence, and a significant proportion of the cases of tuberculous meningitis remain unproved (Traub *et al.* 1984). Rapid diagnosis using enzyme-linked immunosorbent assay (ELISA) (Sada *et al.* 1983), latex particle agglutination of mycobacterial antigens (Krambovitis *et al.* 1984), adenosine deaminase activity of CSF (Ribera *et al.* 1987) or radioactive bromide partition between CSF and serum (Coovadia *et al.* 1986) has been reported. Recent results favour the ELISA, but none of these techniques has yet gained widespread acceptance because of discrepant results or the need for sophisticated equipment. Diagnosis by polymerase chain reaction (Shankar *et al.* 1991, Lin *et al.* 1995, Smith *et al.* 1996) can be obtained rapidly and seems reliable but is often not available where tuberculous meningitis is common.

Although CT is not a recommended technique of diagnosis, it is assuming increasing importance as many children with tuberculous meningitis are now receiving such examinations before lumbar puncture. Findings vary with the stage at which examination is performed. Meningeal enhancement is present in two-thirds of the patients (Kingsley *et al.* 1987, Teoh and Humphries 1991). CT is of diagnostic importance as it excludes other conditions such as cerebral abscess which may mimic tuberculous meningitis (Fig. 11.5). Enhancement usually persists for months even when the course is favourable. Hydrocephalus may be present from stage I but increases in degree and frequency in later stages. Infarction is more common in children than in older patients. It involves especially the central grey matter (Teoh and Humphries 1991). Multiple hypodensities in the central grey matter or in the territory of the anterior or middle cerebral arteries on CT scan are characteristic. MRI gives similar results (Kumar *et al.* 1993) showing parenchymal enhancement with gadolinium and brainstem damage (Offenbacher *et al.* 1991).

Pathological studies have emphasized the frequency of vasculitis (Poltera 1977), which may also be demonstrated by angiography. An angiographic pattern of moyamoya syndrome may obtain (Mathew *et al.* 1970). Angiography has now largely been superceded by MR techniques.

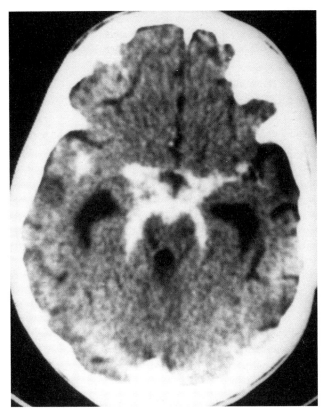

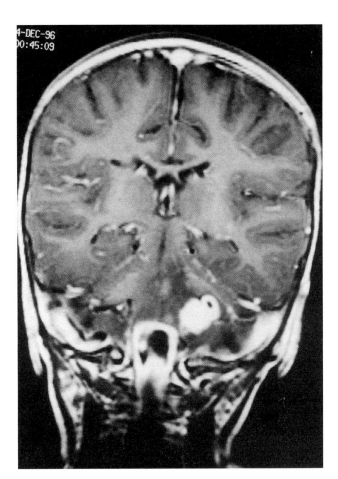

Fig. 11.6. Tuberculoma developed in left peripeduncular cistern and left temporal lobe. (Courtesy Dr Kling Chong, Great Ormond Street Hospital, London.)

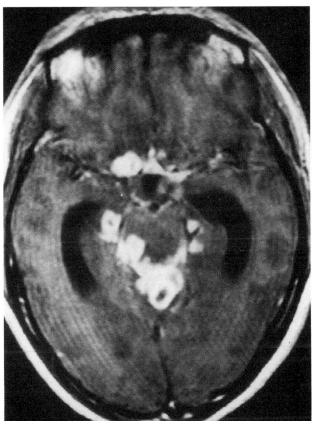

Fig. 11.5. Tuberculous meningitis. *(Top)* Enhanced CT scan shows ventricular dilatation and intense contrast enhancement in prepeduncular and ambient cisterns and in the sylvian fissure, indicating arachnoiditis. *(Bottom)* MRI scan with gadolinium enhancement shows arachnoiditis in peripeduncular and preoptic cisterns. Note ventricular dilatation.

Tuberculomas may be seen initially. Paradoxical increase in size (Chambers *et al.* 1984) or appearance during therapy (Lees *et al.* 1980, Teoh *et al.* 1988) may be observed. Brainstem tuberculomas are still frequently observed in developing countries (Talamás *et al.* 1989). A tuberculoma appears on CT or MRI scan as a round mass sometimes with a necrotic, clear centre (ring lesion). They may be polycystic in contour and behave as space-occupying lesions. Occasionally they may be poorly limited and surrounded by extensive oedema. Calcification is common (Fig. 11.6).

Oedema and signs of diffuse encephalopathy may also be detected (Trautman *et al.* 1986). The finding of an entirely normal scan (with contrast enhancement) in a drowsy patient virtually excludes a diagnosis of tuberculous meningitis.

DIFFERENTIAL DIAGNOSIS

The differential diagnosis of tuberculous meningitis includes a large part of the neurological pathology of childhood, in particular other lymphocytic meningitides and aseptic meningitis. Neoplastic meningitis that occurs in cases of metastatic tumours, especially germinomas, ependymomas, choroid plexus tumours, medulloblastomas and sarcomas, may mimic tuberculous meningitis. The CSF in such cases contains lymphocytes or shows a mixed pleocytosis, protein is raised and hypoglycorrhachia is frequent. The diagnosis is usually made by CT scan. Malignant cells may be demonstrated in the fluid. The diagnosis of partially treated bacterial meningitis is easily ruled out on CSF features. In case of doubt repeat study settles the issue. The diagnoses of viral meningoencephalitis or myelitis should not be accepted without reservation. In some cases, antituberculous drug treatment should be started and discontinued later. Emond and McKendrick (1973) have described 'transient aseptic meningitis' and recovery without treatment. Tuberculomas can occur in the absence of meningeal involvement as a first CNS manifestation as well as during the course of meningitis (Dastur and Desai 1965).

TREATMENT

The optimal treatment for tuberculous meningitis has not been completely determined. Pyrazinamide (35 mg/kg/d), isoniazid (10 mg/kg/d orally up to 300 mg/d) and rifampicin (10–20 mg/kg/d orally up to 600 mg/d) are the basic chemicals used. Pyrazinamide concentration in CSF is 75–110 per cent of that in blood, and that of isoniazid is approximately equal, whereas rifampicin penetrates poorly uninflamed meninges. The administration of streptomycin (20 mg/kg/d) is recommended as a fourth agent by some investigators but the ototoxicity limits the duration of its use to the initial two months of treatment. Ethionamide, at a dose of 15–20 mg/kg/d, reaches high concentration in the CSF and, for that reason, is preferred to ethambutol. Ethionamide can produce optic neuritis so visual acuity should be monitored. Isoniazid can induce a peripheral neuropathy and vitamin B_6 should be administered. Resistance to either of these antibiotics can develop when they are given alone. Administration of several drugs largely prevents the emergence of resistant strains (Iseman 1993). Determination of the sensitivity of the organism, if cultured, should be obtained and treatment adjusted accordingly.

Although the value of adjunctive corticosteroid treatment is not demonstrated, these drugs are often used for a period of one to three months in an effort to prevent meningeal fibrosis and vasculitis and to limit the degree of intracranial hypertension. Girgis et al. (1991) found a fatality rate of 43 per cent in patients treated with dexamethasone and of 59 per cent without. The frequency of sequelae was also higher in the latter group. Isoniazid and rifampicin are potentially hepatotoxic so regular monitoring of transaminases is recommended.

Total duration of treatment is usually 18 months. However, short-term treatment (for six months) may give similar results (Alarcón et al. 1990). Jacobs et al. (1992) indicate that an intensive short course of treatment including pyrazinamide is more efficacious than long-term therapy without it. They advise two months teatment with isoniazid, rifampicin, pyrazinamide and streptomycin, followed by four months of two-drug treatment and the use of dexamethasone at 0.3–0.5 mg/kg/d for one week, followed by prednisolone at 2 mg/kg/d for three to four weeks.

Indications for surgical treatment include high ICP, and especially hydrocephalus which often requires the placement of a shunt (Bullock and Van Dellen 1982).

General management includes the correction of hyponatraemia and other electrolyte disturbances and that of alkalosis.

PROGNOSIS

Despite the availability of antituberculous chemotherapy, the mortality rates remains high at 20–38 per cent (Kingsley et al. 1987, Alarcón et al. 1990). Intercurrent infection is responsible for about half the deaths. Severe sequelae occur in 35–53 per cent of cases (Delage and Dusseault 1979). Sequelae include cranial nerve palsies, decerebration, hemiparesis or monoparesis, epilepsy and intellectual deficits. Visual loss is a frequent problem and occurs in about a quarter of the patients (Silverman et al. 1995). It usually starts six to eight weeks after onset but may supervene later. Treatment with antituberculous drugs does not always impede progressive deterioration, and resistant strains are increasingly common. Surgical decompression may or may not be effective (Kingsley et al. 1987). Most sequelae are the result of infarction and hydrocephalus.

Tuberculomas usually run a favourable course with chemotherapy and only rarely require surgical treatment when associated with meningitis. Paraplegia may be due to infarction of the spinal cord or to chronic adhesive arachnoiditis. Damage to the hypothalamus frequently causes precocious puberty (Olinsky 1970), diabetes insipidus, and less commonly a ravenous appetite or disturbed sleep patterns (Kingsley et al. 1987). Important prognostic factors include the stage of the disease at onset of treatment and the delay between onset and initiation of therapy (Delage and Dusseault 1979, Bateman et al. 1983). Most patients treated during stage I recover fully, whereas late treated stage III patients have a very high mortality or severe sequelae.

OTHER GRANULOMATOUS OR CHRONIC MENINGITIDES

Chronic meningitis is a syndrome characterized by various combinations of fever, headache, lethargy, confusion, stiff neck and vomiting, along with pleocytosis which fails to improve over four weeks (Swartz 1987). The main causes of this syndrome are infective and are shown in Table 11.1 (p. 376).

A majority of the cases demonstrate a lymphocytic or mononuclear CSF pleocytosis. Many of the causes of chronic lymphocytic meningitis are described in the next sections. They include such important conditions as Lyme disease, neurobrucellosis and *Cryptococcus neoformans* meningitis. Chronic polymorphonuclear pleocytosis is also caused by infectious agents such as *Nocardia*, *Actinomyces* and *Arachnia* spp. and a number of fungi (Peacock et al. 1984, Héron et al. 1990).

INTRACRANIAL ABSCESS AND EMPYEMA

CEREBRAL ABSCESS

Brain abscesses consist of localized suppuration within the brain substance.

The responsible organisms gain access to the brain most commonly by the haematogenous route from a distant focus or as a consequence of sepsis. Extension of a nearby focus such as otitis or sinusitis is less common and occurs either by direct contiguity or as a result of septic thrombophlebitis of bridging veins. Direct penetration through a skull wound is uncommon.

The initial stage of an abscess is septic encephalitis or cerebritis, which consists of an oedematous area with softening and congestion of the brain. The centre becomes liquefied thus forming the abscess cavity, while the wall, initially thin, becomes a thick, firm capsule. Initially composed of inflammatory granulation tissue, the capsule becomes fibrous. A marked oedema surrounds the abscess and is responsible in part for the high ICP that is prominent in cases of brain abscess.

The most common causal organisms in large series are *Streptococcus* spp., including *Str. pneumoniae, Staphylococcus, Bacteroides* and *Haemophilus* (Hirsch *et al.* 1983). Brook (1992, 1995) found anaerobic organisms to be predominant in abscesses caused by otitis, teeth infection or sinusitis, while *S. aureus, Str. pneumoniae* and *Str. viridans* were common in cases of cardiac disease. In immunodepressed patients, enteric bacilli, *Pseudomonas* spp., yeasts, fungi and *Mycobacteria* could be found. *Toxoplasma gondii* has become a common cause of abscess in immunodepressed patients (see p. 413). Rare cases due to *Nocardia* (Adaïr *et al.* 1987), melioidosis (Pelekanos and Appleton 1989) or tuberculosis (Henrickson and Weisse 1992) are on record. Several pathogens are often associated. Negative culture is found in up to 50 per cent of cases (Hirsch *et al.* 1983), especially in patients who received antibiotics before operation.

One major predisposing factor is *cyanotic congenital heart disease* with a right-to-left shunt, found in 20 per cent of cases (Tekkök and Erbengi 1992). In such cases, abscesses are exceptionally seen before 2–3 years of age. The absence of a pulmonary filter probably allows access to the brain during bacteraemic episodes and previous small brain lesions (ischaemic?) may be necessary for an abscess to occur. Otitis and sinusitis are now the second most common cause at our institution (Hirsch *et al.* 1983). Closed head trauma and cystic fibrosis (Fischer *et al.* 1979) are less frequent predisposing causes.

Those abscesses that result from bacteraemia are mainly located in the central regions of the hemispheres; they commonly form at the border between white and grey matter and tend to develop towards the ventricular cavity, into which they occasionally rupture. Abscesses from focal infections are more often frontal and temporal. Cerebellar abscesses are almost always due to propagation from a septic mastoid focus. Brainstem abscesses are uncommon. Lesions in the central grey matter may be observed and raise special treatment problems. Multiple location is not exceptional (Ersahin *et al.* 1994) and was present in four of 34 cases seen at our institution (Hirsch *et al.* 1983).

The occurrence of brain abscess in infants under 6 months of age is infrequent. Most such cases occur in the neonatal period and are associated with purulent meningitis and infection due to *Proteus* or *Citrobacter* (Hirsch *et al.* 1983, Renier *et al.* 1988).

CLINICAL MANIFESTATIONS
The clinical manifestations of brain abscess consist of a triad of intracranial hypertension, sepsis and focal neurological features

TABLE 11.7
Symptoms and signs of brain abscess—frequency of occurrence in three series

Feature	Percentage in series		
	Fischer et al. (1981) (N=94)	Eggerding (1981)* (N=66)	Hirsch et al. (1983) (N=34)
Headache and vomiting	72[1]	50	53
Neurological manifestations	59	36	45[2]
Seizures	36	29	29
Fever	39	24	62
Papilloedema	—	54	70

*Quoted in Marshall (1983).
[1]Headache only (49% had vomiting).
[2]'Focal signs' (56% had 'impairment of consciousness').

(Table 11.7). Chronic abscesses may present as a slow-growing tumour.

Fever is inconstant as is polymorphonuclear leucocytosis. It is not uncommon for abscesses to manifest initially by isolated symptoms or signs such as fever and loss of weight, persistent vomiting, convulsive seizures or rapid enlargement of the head in infants. Cerebellar abscesses give rise to nystagmus, vertigo, cerebellar ataxia and signs of increased ICP. Infection of the ear is constantly present. Although lumbar puncture is contraindicated it is often performed in the early stage and may show sterile pleocytosis with mostly polymorphonuclear cells in two-thirds of cases. A low CSF glucose is present in 30 per cent of cases.

DIAGNOSIS
The diagnosis of brain abscess is now confirmed by CT scan or MRI (Fig. 11.7). Among other investigations, the EEG may be useful as it shows a good correlation between the location of the abscess and that of a focus of slow delta waves. Angiography and isotopic brain scan are now obsolete. At the initial stage, neuroimaging may show only localized ill-defined hypodensity with a mass effect. Later, a rim of contrast enhancement appears and becomes thicker with the passing of time. Contrast infusion is mandatory with CT scan but initially may be difficult to interpret. Massive oedema surrounds the ring-lesion. Multiple abscesses and multilocular abscesses are clearly visualized. Differential diagnosis includes cavitated brain tumours, tuberculomas, focal ischaemic lesions, intracerebral cysts and Schilder disease (Chapter 12).

MANAGEMENT
Antibiotic therapy is the mainstay of the treatment of brain abscess. Initial treatment conventionally used intravenous chloramphenicol, ampicillin and methicillin, at times in association with an aminoglycoside. Third-generation cephalosporins and metronidazole are now widely used. Subsequent therapy is guided by antibiotic sensitivity when available but many specimens are negative on culture. Antibiotics should be maintained for four to five weeks and the patients carefully monitored by repeated CT scans.

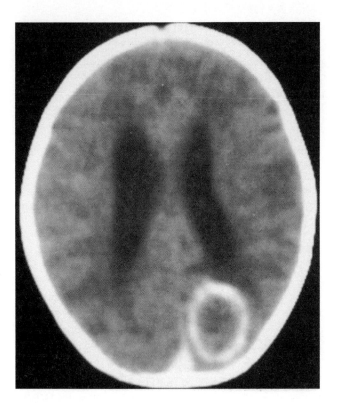

Fig. 11.7. Brain abscess in left occipital lobe of 2-month-old infant with gram-negative sepsis. (Courtesy Prof. F. Brunelle, Hôpital des Enfants Malades, Paris.)

Follow-up scans often continue to demonstrate ring enhancement for several weeks, with or without surgical puncture.

Antibiotic treatment can certainly achieve a complete cure of brain abscess (Rosenblum *et al.* 1980, Petit *et al.* 1983). Disappearance of the capsule on CT scan should be verified.

If antibiotic therapy is not rapidly—or systematically—effective, surgical drainage by tapping through a burr-hole is performed. Systematic puncture has the advantage of rapid decompression and permits isolation of the responsible organism. Removal of the capsule is not generally advised and is limited to patients in whom a residual cavity or large persistent hyperintensity is present on late scans.

The mortality rate of brain abscess is now around 10 per cent. Sequelae include epilepsy, which is still common (30–40 per cent of cases) and usually of partial type; localized neurological deficits; hydrocephalus; and mental retardation, although this mainly occurs in conjunction with abscesses associated with congenital heart disease and may be directly related to the cardiopathy rather than the abscess (Hirsch *et al.* 1983). The onset of epilepsy is, on average, 3.3 years following abscess (range 1–15 years) and does not seem to be related to the mode of surgical therapy (Legg *et al.* 1973).

Neonatal abscesses are associated with meningitis in most cases. Organisms of the *Citrobacter* (Graham and Band 1981) and *Proteus* (Renier *et al.* 1988) spp. are overwhelmingly predominant. In a series of 30 cases from our institution (Renier *et al.* 1988), *P. mirabilis* was found in 27 patients, *E. coli* and *Serratia*

marcescens accounting for the remaining three. Onset is within the first month of life, usually within 10 days, and is marked by seizures in two-thirds of patients. Sepsis was present in 18 of our cases, hydrocephalus developed in 15, and multiple abscesses in 18. Treatment is by puncture of the abscesses and antibiotic therapy, the usual combination being cefotaxime and gentamicin. Outcome is poor, with mental retardation being present in over two-thirds of the patients. Residual epilepsy occurs in over half the cases.

SUBDURAL EMPYEMA
Subdural abscess results from sepsis, from direct extension of infection from a focus of sinusitis or mastoiditis (Brock and Bleck 1992, Skelton *et al.* 1992) or from bacterial contamination of a subdural effusion in meningitis or of a post-traumatic subdural haematoma. Subdural empyema may be associated with brain abscess. Most lesions are located on the convexity of the brain, commonly in the frontal region. These appear on neuroimaging as thin lens-shaped lesions with enhancement of the inner membrane. They are sometimes multiloculated. Empyemas are not infrequently localized to the interhemispheric fissure giving rise to the same type of image which may extend along the whole length of the fissure or remain limited to a small portion thereof (Weisberg 1986).

Symptoms and signs are identical to those in brain abscess. The mortality rate is 10–20 per cent. Treatment usually combines antibiotics, bearing in mind that the most common organisms found are nonhaemolytic streptococci and anaerobic organisms (Miller *et al.* 1987), and surgical evacuation, although the latter may not always be necessary (Leys *et al.* 1986). A poor prognosis is associated with a low level of consciousness at admission and with a large collection of pus (Mauser *et al.* 1987).

EPIDURAL ABSCESS
Epidural abscesses can affect the head and the spinal canal. They develop from infection of structures contiguous to the brain or spinal cord (Smith and Hendrick 1983).

Spinal epidural abscesses are uncommon. Infection remains limited to the dorsal aspect of the cord except in its lowermost portion where the epidural space completely surrounds the cord. Staphylococci are the predominating causal organisms. Backache is the first manifestation, followed by radicular pain and spinal cord compression. The condition may be indistinguishable from transverse myelitis and should be thought of in all cases suggesting this diagnosis. Gadolinium-enhanced MRI allows an early diagnosis by showing increased signal in the epidural space and posterior compression of the cord (Teman 1992), demanding immediate surgery. Lumbar puncture is dangerous because it may result in contamination of the subarachnoid space. If performed, it should be done carefully under X-ray guidance with a large-gauge needle and frequent aspiration. The issue of pus confirms the diagnosis of epidural abscess and permits determination of the pathogen. Immediate treatment by laminectomy at the level of the block is mandatory. If an acute abscess is found the area is drained and packed open and closed secondarily. If the abscess is chronic and consists primarily of granulation tissue, the spinal cord is fully decompressed and the wound closed. Ideally, operation should be performed before paraplegia sets in to avoid sequelae. It seems that cord damage is more extensive than can be accounted for by mechanical compression alone and may be due to impairment of cord vascularization.

In rare cases, epiduritis has been secondary to infection of a dermal sinus (Baker *et al.* 1975). Atypical mycobacteria may be a cause in immunodepressed patients (Shope *et al.* 1994).

INTRAMEDULLARY ABSCESS

Intramedullary abscess is a rare condition but is relatively common in young people (DiTullio 1977). It may be due to suppuration of a dermoid cyst associated with a dermal sinus. Chronic abscesses represent one quarter of cases. Intramedullary abscess is a cause of medullary compression, acute or chronic.

INFECTION AND INFLAMMATION OF THE VERTEBRAE AND DISC SPACE

Vertebral osteomyelitis is often associated with a limp or other walking difficulties. Neurological deficit in the lower limb was present in 19 per cent of cases in one series (Correa *et al.* 1993).

Discitis is an imperfectly understood condition. Staphylococci, gram-negative bacteria and diphtheroids may be the cause but in many cases no organism is found and the infectious nature is not certain.

A stiff back, and back, hip and abdominal pain may all be present. On examination, extension of the spine is markedly restricted. X-rays of the spine show narrowing of the disk-space in 80 per cent of cases (Jansen *et al.* 1993). Radionuclide uptake is increased at the level of the lesion.

The condition should be distinguished from vertebral tuberculosis.

Treatment is by immobilization. The usefulness of antibiotics has not been demonstrated.

NONSUPPURATIVE BACTERIAL INFECTIONS

SPIROCHAETAL INFECTIONS

SYPHILIS

Congenital syphilis has been studied in Chapter 1. In older children, syphilitic meningitis is exceptional yet is important to diagnose because of the effectiveness of therapy. Classical meningeal signs may be associated with other neurological signs including cranial nerve paralysis, hemiplegia and hypoacousia (Marcus 1982, Dodge 1987). The presence of interstitial keratitis is characteristic.

Tertiary congenital syphilis is rare. Juvenile paresis is the most common form beginning 5–20 years after infection. Mental deterioration is the initial symptom. Neurological signs set in later and include spasticity in half the cases and cerebellar signs in a quarter. Seizures occur in 30 per cent of cases and optic atrophy in 10–15 per cent. Deafness and multiple cranial nerve deficits may be present. Juvenile paresis should be distinguished from the

much more frequent progressive metabolic or degenerative diseases.

Diagnosis of syphilis is easily confirmed by the VDRL test or by the rapid plasma reagin test which is equally reliable and gives immediate results. More specific techniques (Bromberg *et al.* 1993) are now available (see also Chapter 1). However, cases of maternal infection acquired late in pregnancy may be associated with negative serological tests at birth (Dorfman and Glaser 1990, Stoll *et al.* 1993). These should be repeated in case of doubt.

In the CSF, there is lymphocytic pleocytosis, increased protein and at times a low glucose level. Oligoclonal globulins are present. Treatment is with penicillin G for all stages of neurosyphilis.

LEPTOSPIROSIS

Leptospirosis can be caused by several serotypes of the *Leptospira interrogans* complex (icterohaemorrhagiae, canicola, pomona, grippotyphosa). Signs of meningeal irritation occur in about 10 per cent of patients. CSF pleocytosis may persist for several weeks but the outcome is uniformly favourable. Encephalitic manifestations are exceptional.

Diagnosis can be made by isolation of the responsible organism.

BORRELIOSIS (LYME DISEASE)

Lyme disease is caused by a spirochaete, *Borrelia burgdorferi*, that can be isolated with difficulty from blood, skin lesions and CSF. It is transmitted from animal reservoirs to man by tick vectors of the *Ixodes* genus. The same organism is responsible for a meningoneuritis known in Europe as the Garin–Bujadoux–Bannwarth syndrome (Sindic *et al.* 1987, Steere 1989, Hansen and Lebech 1992). However, there are antigenic differences between European and American *Borrelia*, and the European strain may represent a different species referred to as *B. garini* (Stanek *et al.* 1985). Borreliosis usually occurs from spring to autumn and follows the bite of a tick which goes unnoticed in half the cases.

The disease can be divided into three stages. The first stage is characterized by localized *erythema chronicum migrans* located in the area of the tick bite that extends centrifugally. Minor constitutional symptoms may be present.

The second stage of disseminated infection may feature systemic symptoms and is associated with blood-borne dissemination and the appearance of an antibody response. Neurological involvement occurs within weeks or months in 5–15 per cent of patients. In Europe, the first sign may be radicular pain which is followed by the development of pleocytosois in the CSF often without meningeal signs. In 80 per cent of children, neuroborreliosis manifests as *facial palsy* which may be the only abnormality or as *aseptic meningitis* (Christen *et al.* 1993, Bingham *et al.* 1995). Facial palsy is unilateral in most cases (Hansen and Lebech 1992); bilateral involvement 8–15 days apart is highly suggestive of borreliosis (Angerer *et al.* 1993). In American Lyme disease, meningeal signs are frequently observed but radiculitis is uncommon (Williams *et al.* 1990, Belman *et al.* 1993). The peripheral neuritis (Bannwarth syndrome) is usually asymmetrical, motor, sensory or mixed and involves the limbs or trunk (Pachner and Steere 1985, Hansen and Lebech 1992, Christen *et al.* 1993). Rare manifestations include other cranial neuropathies, ataxia, symmetrical neuropathy of the Guillain–Barré type or, rarely, focal encephalitis (Christen *et al.* 1993, Bingham *et al.* 1995) or transverse myelitis (Linssen *et al.* 1991). Pleocytosis is present in 95 per cent of children and the CSF protein is raised. However, oligoclonal banding is found only in one-third of cases. The meningeal reaction is apt to become chronic, and Lyme disease is, with mumps, a major cause of prolonged abacterial meningitis, accounting for 11.7 per cent of cases in the experience of Christen *et al.* (1993). Cardiac and articular problems may occur as late manifestations of the second stage.

The third stage of persistent infection may be observed in untreated patients from one to many years after the initial infection. Chronic arthritis is a common feature but *B. burgdorferi* may cause late syndromes of both the central and peripheral nervous system in adults and, less frequently, in children. The spectrum of these abnormalities is wide with progressive encephalomyelitis as the prominent involvement (Finkel 1988, Kollikowski *et al.* 1988, Halperin *et al.* 1989, Pachner *et al.* 1989) but its exact limits are not yet determined. In particular, the role of neuroborreliosis in the syndrome of cognitive deficits and disturbances of mood, sleep and appetite (Ackerman *et al.* 1988) is still in dispute. CNS manifestations have been reported in childhood (Feder *et al.* 1988b). Subtle neurological manifestations such as paraesthesiae, radicular pain or memory changes may occur (Wokke *et al.* 1987). Abnormal MRI findings in the form of punctate or larger areas of increased T_2 signal in the white matter that may simulate multiple sclerosis are found in such cases (Belman *et al.* 1992). Atypical cases can masquerade as brainstem tumour (Curless *et al.* 1996).

The *diagnosis* of Lyme disease rests on the history, clinical manifestations and laboratory demonstration of *Borrelia* infection. A history of tick bite is frequently missing, and erythema migrans occurs in only 67 per cent of cases (Williams *et al.* 1990). Three-quarters of cases occur from June to October. Serological diagnosis, most commonly using the ELISA test, is not always reliable as many commercial tests are not standardized and as seronegativity is the rule at onset of the disease and can occur even later in proven cases. Positive results are frequent in endemic areas but are not always related to current neurological disease (Halperin *et al.* 1989). Moreover, cross-reaction may occur with Epstein–Barr and varicella-zoster viruses. The presence of IgM antibodies to *B. burgdorferi* is a more reliable criterion (Christen *et al.* 1993). Immunoblot testing is recommended for confirmation of diagnosis (Golightly 1997) but is not available everywhere. The polymerase chain reaction is useful when positive, as the reported rate for false positives is only 3 per cent, although in 54–60 per cent of tested cases it proved inconclusive (Pachner and Delaney 1993, Golightly 1997). Recently, detection of specific *B. burgdorferi* antigen in the absence of antibodies has been found to be relatively common and specific (Coyle *et al.* 1995).

Treatment includes doxycycline (100 mg twice daily), penicillin G or amoxicillin for early disease (Karlsson *et al.* 1994). In later stages intravenously administered penicillin G, 500,000 units/kg to a maximum of 12 megaunits over 10 days is recommended (Weber and Pfister 1994). Ceftriaxone or cefotaxime for 14 days are also effective. Treatment is indicated for all patients with neurological abnormalities and is usually sufficient for facial palsy (Wormser 1997), although Steere (1989) did not advise it for patients with facial palsy alone and no CSF abnormalities. Vaccination is being studied (Wormser 1997).

BRUCELLOSIS

Involvement of the CNS in systemic brucellosis is rare. Meningitis may occur. The diagnosis is relatively easy using the classical agglutination tests in systemic forms. Localized forms of the disease (Pascual *et al.* 1988) are more difficult to diagnose. The clinical presentation of brucellosis localized to the nervous system is diverse. Meningoencephalitis with a lymphocytic pleocytosis of the CSF, polyradiculoneuritis and diffuse CNS involvement featuring myelitis with associated cranial nerve abnormalities or a cerebellar syndrome have been reported (Shakir *et al.* 1987, Bahemuka *et al.* 1988, Al Deeb *et al.* 1989). Serological test (ELISA) confirms the diagnosis. Treatment with cotrimoxazole and tetracycline for eight weeks has been successful in adult patients. Rifampicin is also effective (Shakir *et al.* 1987).

The prognosis is favourable except in patients with diffuse involvement in whom significant disability may persist.

OTHER BACTERIAL INFECTIONS
MYCOPLASMA INFECTIONS

Mycoplasma pneumoniae may produce neurological disease in up to 7 per cent of infected subjects, and half of the cases are in children. The mechanisms of involvement of the CNS are complex with both direct invasion (Abramovitz *et al.* 1987) and indirect affectation by toxins or immunological disturbances. Clinical manifestations can include meningitis (Al-Mateen *et al.* 1988), transverse myelitis (Francis *et al.* 1988, Mills and Schoolfield 1992), cranial neuritis and Guillain–Barré syndrome (Fernandez *et al.* 1993).

Encephalitis is commonly associated with *M. pneumoniae* infection (Lehtokski-Lehtiniemi and Koskiniemi 1989, Fernandez *et al.* 1993, Thomas *et al.* 1993) and is discussed below.

The diagnosis rests on elevation of the complement fixation titres for *M. pneumoniae* that starts about a week after onset of infection and persists for several years.

The disease may be severe with residua in about one third of cases and a mortality rate close to 10 per cent. Antimicrobial therapy is not effective.

LISTERIA MONOCYTOGENES INFECTION

This can produce a rhombencephalitis with formation of multiple abscesses. It is observed mainly in adults and in immunodepressed patients including children (Frith *et al.* 1987). Vigorous antibiotic treatment is imperative (see Table 11.3, p. 381).

TABLE 11.8
Major rickettsial diseases

Type	Vector	Responsible rickettsia	Place of occurrence
Typhus fever	Louse	*R. prowazekii*	Ubiquitous*
Murine typhus		*R. typhi*	Ubiquitous*
Scrub typhus		*R. tsutsugamushi*	Australia, India, Japan
Q fever		*Coxiella burnetii*	Ubiquitous
Rickettsialpox	Mouse mite	*R. akari*	Ubiquitous
Trench fever	Louse	*Rochimalaea quintana*	Ubiquitous
Rocky Mountain spotted fever	Ticks	*R. rickettsii*	Eastern and western USA

*Strongly associated with poor living conditions.

CAT-SCRATCH DISEASE

This is caused by two proteobacteria, *Afipia felis* and *Rochalimaea henselae* (Adal *et al.* 1994). Neurological involvement is infrequent. Encephalopathy is the most frequent manifestation (Carithers and Margileth 1991, Revol *et al.* 1992) but spinal cord or root involvement and status epilepticus may occur (Lewis and Tucker 1986). Cerebral arteritis (Selby and Walker 1979) and optic neuropathy (Sweeney and Drance 1970) are also on record. CSF pleocytosis is uncommon and protein is usually normal. Diagnosis is by demonstration of induration greater than 5 mm with the cat-scratch disease antigen. Rarely, lymph node biopsy is necessary to confirm the diagnosis. Treatment with gentamicin or trimethoprim-sulfamethoxazole is effective.

OTHER RARE CAUSES OF CNS INVOLVEMENT ASSOCIATED WITH BACTERIAL INFECTION

These include *Legionella* infection, which has been associated with convulsions, encephalopathy and peripheral neuropathy (Heath *et al.* 1986).

Whipple disease has a purely neurological form (Louis *et al.* 1996) of which ataxia, mental deterioration, hypersomnia, hyperphagia, seizures, ophthalmoplegia and nystagmus are the major features. Imaging may be normal or show multiple lesions. Neurological manifestations may also occur along with gastrointestinal and rheumatological symptoms and signs.

Bacilliform bodies are visible by electron microscopy. These have been shown to be microorganisms, based on their morphological features and antibiotic sensitivity. They have been identified as *Tropheryma whippleii*.

Chloramphenicol and trimethoprim sulfamethoxasole can arrest the course of the disease. Although usually a disorder of adults, Whipple disease has been observed in children (Barakat *et al.* 1973).

RICKETTSIAL INFECTIONS

Rickettsiae are dealt with briefly in this paragraph for convenience even though they are not conventional bacterial agents. Rickettsial disorders, with the exception of Rocky Mountain spotted fever which is frequent in the eastern United States and is responsible for a meningoencephalitic picture (Bell and Lascari 1970), are rare

in Western countries and virtually absent in Western Europe. Table 11.8 lists the main rickettsial disorders.

VIRUS INFECTIONS

Viral infections of the CNS induce a wide spectrum of disease from the most benign to lethal conditions. The frequency of viral diseases is certainly very high but no accurate data on the incidence of CNS involvement in individual virus infections or the overall incidence of viral infections in the causation of CNS disease are available. This is in part due to the fact that many viral CNS infections are so mild and transient that no precise investigations are performed. As a result, the frequency of viral disease of the CNS is probably underestimated. A clue to the viral aetiology of CNS disease may be their frequent occurrence in epidemics. In individual patients, information about past history of immunization, of contact with known infections and of similar illnesses among contacts may help to orientate the diagnosis.

The mechanisms of CNS involvement by viruses are complex. In most cases, the viruses are carried from their original portal of entry, which is specific to each group and their original place of multiplication (*e.g.* lymphoid tissue), to the CNS by haematogeneous dissemination. The characteristics of viruses and hosts that determine penetration into the CNS have been studied extensively (see Gonzales-Scarano and Tyler 1987) and are still being actively explored.

The treatment of CNS viral infections remains unsatisfactory in spite of recent progress. The main drugs active against viruses are shown in Table 11.9. Some of these drugs such as acyclovir and vidarabine are of proven efficacy while others are still in the experimental stage.

Two main types of CNS viral infections are commonly encountered.

Viral meningitis is due to haematogeneous spread of the virus, often through the choroid plexus. Some viruses grow in the choroid plexus and this may explain the ease with which echoviruses and coxsackie viruses can be isolated from the CSF.

Encephalitis or encephalomyelitis results from direct or indirect involvement of the brain tissue proper by viruses. Indeed, in a

TABLE 11.9
Main antiviral drugs for neurological disorders*

Drug	Virus	Route	Dose (mg/kg)	Frequency of administration	Toxicity
Acyclovir	Herpes viruses	i.v.	5–16	t.i.d.	Renal
Vidarabine	Herpes simplex	i.v.	15–30	Once/day	CNS
Ganciclovir	Cytomegalovirus	i.v.	2.5	t.i.d.	Bone marrow
Phosphonoformate	Cytomegalovirus	i.v.	Under study	t.i.d.	Renal
Amantadine	Influenza A	Oral	2.2–4.4	b.i.d.	CNS
Rimantadine	Influenza A	Oral	3.3	b.i.d.	CNS
Ribavirine	Myxoviruses	Oral, i.v.	Under study	Once/day	Anaemia
AZT** Didanosine**	Retroviruses, HIV-1	i.v.		180mg/m^2/d	Anaemia, renal
Stavudine**	HIV-1	i.v.		2mg/kg/d	
Zalcitobine**	HIV-1	i.v.	Under study		

*Modified from Balfour and Englund (1989).
**Several reverse-transcriptase inhibitors and protease inhibitors are being tested. Combination therapy is becoming increasingly used.

majority of cases of encephalitis, there is no direct invasion by viruses, the inflammatory lesions that characterize encephalitis being the result of an indirect effect of the pathogenic agent which is thought to be in most cases an immunoallergic reaction. A similar mechanism seems to be at play in neurological disease caused by some nonviral agents, especially *Mycoplasma pneumoniae*; these are therefore studied in this section. In some of the acute neurological disorders observed in the course of a proven or suspected viral infection, no inflammatory manifestations are found in the brain or meninges. These are termed *acute parainfectious encephalopathies* because they may be difficult or impossible to distinguish from cases of true inflammatory CNS involvement; these cases will also be considered in this section.

Any classification of the CNS syndromes associated with viral infection is difficult and, to some extent, arbitrary. Many viruses can produce the whole gamut of aseptic meningitis, postinfectious encephalitis, primary encephalitis and acute encephalopathy (Boos and Esiri 1986). Also, it is often difficult to decide in a particular case of virus infection whether meningeal involvement is isolated or associated with parenchymal disease; and the actual presence of encephalitis in the sense of an inflammatory process within the brain itself, in association with lymphocytic meningitis, is uncertain with many viral infections such as influenza A or B, adenovirus, varicella-zoster (Leis and Butler 1987), mumps (Levitt *et al.* 1970) or enteroviruses (Kaiser *et al.* 1989).

In this section I shall adopt the simple classification of cases of CNS viral infection into two groups that will be dealt with in succession: (1) cases of viral (aseptic) meningitis; (2) cases of clinically related encephalitis and CNS disorders ('encephalitic illnesses'). Some special syndromes with specific clinical features or lesions such as paralytic poliomyelitis or the vascular complications of varicella-zoster infection will be dealt with separately. Such a classification may have some practical merit as it is based on clinical data and is applicable in the many cases in which no aetiological agent or mechanism is established.

VIRAL (ASEPTIC) MENINGITIS
CLINICAL FEATURES
The clinical features of viral aseptic meningitis do not differ from those in other types of aseptic meningitis (see Table 11.1, p. 376). The onset is usually acute with fever, headache, vomiting and neck stiffness. In the CSF, there is predominantly lymphocytic pleocytosis with little or no elevation in protein and normal levels of glucose in the vast majority of patients. An increased level of gammaglobulins and the presence of oligoclonal banding may be of value for determination of the cause. During the first 12–48 hours of the illness, polymorphonuclear leukocytes may predominate. In such cases, repeat lumbar puncture will show a rapid shift to lymphocytosis (Feigin and Shackelford 1973). Brief episodes of obtundation or delirium may occur in a few patients but convulsions are unusual. Neurological examination is negative except for neck and back stiffness. The EEG often shows mild to moderate diffuse slowing. It is difficult to determine whether this is the result of the causal disease or of meningitis itself, as several of the diseases that generate lymphocytic meningitis, for example measles, may be associated with EEG slowing.

Many mild forms probably occur. They may be discovered fortuitously, *e.g.* when a lumbar puncture is systematically performed following a febrile seizure.

Associated clinical features may help discover the cause of an aseptic meningitis and should be carefully sought. The presence of maculopapular or petechial rash, of parotitis, or of hepatosplenomegaly may be of value.

The course of most viral meningitides is benign. Complications may be the result of diffusion of the infection to neighbouring structures, for example the VIIIth nerve or labyrinth with resulting hearing loss. Inappropriate secretion of antidiuretic hormone has been reported in up to 64 per cent of children with viral meningitis (Fajardo *et al.* 1989). However, clinical manifestations such as seizures are not seen.

Specific Features in Relation to Causal Agent

Mumps

Mumps is the most frequently identified cause of viral aseptic meningitis. A full-blown clinical picture of leptomeningitis is encountered in 0.5–2 per cent of patients with mumps (Marshall 1983). However, pleocytosis has been observed in 56 per cent of those with parotitis (Russell and Donald 1958). Parotitis was absent in up to one-third or 47 per cent of cases in some series (Levitt *et al.* 1970), and in such cases the diagnosis can only be made by serology or virus isolation. Symptoms of meningitis have their onset from eight days before to 20 days after the appearance of parotitis. A high fever often occurs concomitantly.

The CSF shows lymphocytic pleocytosis often of marked intensity with several hundreds of cells/mm^3. The glucose content may be reduced (Wilfert 1969). Although the course is usually benign, pleocytosis may last for up to several months and there is protracted persistence of specific intrathecally produced oligoclonal IgG (Vandvik *et al.* 1978a). Production of interferon alpha occurs intrathecally in cases of mumps meningitis, reflecting the replication of the virus within the CSF (Tardieu *et al.* 1986), whose presence is also responsible for the persistent oligoclonal pattern.

Complications are uncommon. Vertigo and optic nerve atrophy have been occasionally reported (*e.g.* Wilfert 1969). Meningoencephalitis or myelitis may occur and occasionally become chronic (Ito *et al.* 1991). The occurrence of multifocal epileptic seizures has been recorded (Parain and Boulloche 1988). Hearing loss is the most common severe sequela (Hall and Richards 1987). Ataxia and opsoclonus (Ichiba *et al.* 1988) and vestibular neuritis (Thömke and Hopf 1992) are on record. Hydrocephalus (Yanofsky *et al.* 1981, Lahat *et al.* 1993) has been rarely reported.

Enteroviruses

These have consisted of three types of poliovirus, 30 types of coxsackie viruses and 34 types of echoviruses. More recent isolates are simply assigned an enterovirus number, carrying on from enterovirus 68 without further subdivision. These viruses enter the body via the gastrointestinal tract, replicate there and induce a viraemia that may lead to infection of the CNS. The organisms can be isolated from the CSF and also from blood, stool and oropharynx.

Infection can occur at any age, including the first weeks of life (Kaplan *et al.* 1983).

Enterorivuses commonly associated with aseptic meningitis are coxsackie B1–5 and coxsackie A7, 9 and 25, echoviruses 4, 6, 9, 11, 14, 16, 18, 20 and 30, as well as polioviruses. *Acute epidemic conjunctivitis* due to enterovirus 70 can be complicated by meningitis, cranial nerve palsy or limb involvement or both. Severe pain and fasciculations are common (Wadia *et al.* 1983, Chopra *et al.* 1986).

Group A coxsackie virus meningitis may be associated with or preceded by herpangina, respiratory infections and parotitis. In group B disease, pleurodynia (Bornholm disease or epidemic myalgia) or diarrhoea may occur. Myocarditis and encephalitis may complicate meningitis, especially in young infants (Kaplan *et al.* 1983).

With echovirus infections both sporadic and epidemic infections may occur. A maculopapular rash is common, especially in echovirus 4, 9 and 16 infections. Rashes sometimes occur also in coxsackie A9 and A23 disease.

In all enterovirus meningitides including poliovirus meningitis, virus can be isolated from the CSF and from other sources. Because of the vast number of strains, serological diagnosis is impractical. The diagnosis should rest on isolation of the responsible virus later confirmed by homologous seroconversion. The polymerase chain reaction test might permit precise diagnosis more frequently (Schlesinger *et al.* 1994).

Sequelae of enteroviral meningitis have been reported (Kaplan *et al.* 1983). It is likely that sequelae are the result of encephalitic involvement, concomitant with meningitis. They are especially common in neonatal enteroviral meningitides which also feature fever, poor feeding, diarrhoea, hepatomegaly and rashes. Paralytic poliomyelitis is discussed later in this chapter.

It is clear that a sharp distinction betwen 'pure' enteroviral meningitis and meningoencephalitis cannot be made. Intrathecal synthesis of virus-specific oligoclonal antibodies in patients with enterovirus infection, including apparently pure meningitis, has been reported (Kaiser *et al.* 1989), reflecting the artificial nature of too strict a delimitation of viral-induced neurological syndromes. Cases difficult to classify also include those of patients with enterovirus meningitis associated with features of focal cerebral involvement as demonstrated by clinical and neuroradiological signs (Roden *et al.* 1975, Chahlub *et al.* 1977). The nature of cerebral affectation in such cases remains undetermined.

Herpes virus infection

Several members of the herpes virus group cause lymphocytic meningitis. *Herpes simplex virus (HSV) type 2* (Nahmias *et al.* 1982) is more often responsible than type 1 which mainly causes encephalitis. However, mild cases of HSV-1 infection can manifest only by meningeal irritation (Whitley *et al.* 1982), and patients recover in 7–14 days. Herpes virus 6 infection, the agent of exanthema subitum, can produce both an acute encephalopathy (Asano *et al.* 1992, Jones *et al.* 1994) and, more commonly, febrile convulsions (Barone *et al.* 1995, Bertolani *et al.* 1996).

Varicella-zoster virus

Varicella-zoster virus can cause aseptic meningitis as well as more complex involvement of the CNS, described in a later section. Pre-eruptive neurological manifestations may occur (Tsolia *et al.* 1995).

Epstein–Barr virus

Epstein–Barr virus is also the agent of both aseptic meningitis and several other CNS complications (Connelly and DeWitt 1994). Meningitis may herald several other nervous complications such as infectious polyneuritis (the Guillain–Barré syndrome), encephalomyelitis or cranial nerve involvement (De Simone and Snyder 1978, Beg 1981). About one-third of patients with infectious mononucleosis have ≥5 cells/mm³ on examination of CSF and these may persist for months often after complete clinical recovery (Pejme 1964). Recovery may be delayed for several weeks or months. However, the *chronic fatigue syndrome* does not appear to be specifically associated with Epstein–Barr virus infection (Marshall *et al.* 1991). Rare cases of cytomegalovirus infection in nonimmunodepressed patients are on record. In one such case CMV infection presented as a transverse myelitis (Miles *et al.* 1993).

Adenovirus infections

Adenoviruses may cause aseptic meningitis. Certain strains are responsible for an encephalitis that may be quite severe (Kim and Gohd 1983). Myelitis is possible (Linssen *et al.* 1991).

Lymphocytic choriomeningitis

This is a benign infection of the meninges caused by an arena virus. Infection with the virus is frequent but often inapparent (Adair *et al.* 1953). In some patients, an initial phase is marked by influenza-like symptoms, myalgia, malaise and photophobia. After one to three weeks, definite meningeal irritation sets in. During the convalescent period, arthralgias are common. The disease subsides spontaneously without sequelae, although posterior fossa arachnoiditis has been reported in one case (Green *et al.* 1949). Rarely do encephalitis or neural complications supervene (Adair *et al.* 1953). The CSF shows a marked lymphocytic pleocytosis that may be as high as 6000 cells/mm³. Sugar concentration remains normal and protein is only mildly elevated.

Other and undetermined viruses

These are probably the cause of the many cases—indeed a majority—in which no pathogenic organism can be isolated. This is easily understandable as the number of possible viral agents is very high and as the disease is most often benign so that complex investigations are not undertaken or pursued. An acute encephalopathy associated with rotavirus infection has been described (Keidan *et al.* 1992).

ENCEPHALITIS AND MENINGOENCEPHALITIS

Encephalitis is an inflammatory process involving the brain. In most cases the meninges are also affected, and myelitis may be part of the process, hence the terms meningoencephalitis and encephalomyelitis that apply to the same spectrum of diseases. Encephalitides can be acute or chronic. The two types will be described separately as they pose completely different problems. Acute encephalitides are a major cause of acute neurological disease in childhood and have to be distinguished from a number of other infectious and metabolic processes that require immediate diagnosis. Subacute and chronic encephalitides raise the issue of degenerative or other slowly evolving disorders.

ACUTE ENCEPHALITIS

Acute encephalitides are the most common cause of acute nonsuppurative neurological disease in children. Several other conditions produce an 'encephalitic illness' or 'acute encephalo-

TABLE 11.10
Main causes of acute encephalitis in a series of 412 children*

Viruses	% of cases of known origin	
Measles, mumps, rubella group	30.4	
Measles		12.8
Mumps		16.0
Rubella		1.6
Herpes viruses	24.1	
Varicella-zoster		15.4
Herpes simplex		6.4
Cytomegalovirus		1.3
Epstein–Barr virus		1.0
Respiratory viruses	18.3	
Influenza, parainfluenza and respiratory syncytial		9.6
Adenovirus		8.7
Enterovirus group	9.7	
Enteroviruses		7.7
Others		2.0
Mycoplasma pneumoniae	13.1	
Other known cause including immunization	3.9	
Unknown agent	32.0	

*Data from Koskiniemi and Vaheri (1989). No distinction made between primary and postinfectious encephalitides.

pathy', require different therapy and have different outcomes so that an accurate diagnosis is necessary.

Aetiology

The vast majority of cases of acute encephalitis are caused by viruses (Table 11.10). However, some bacteria can be responsible. *Mycoplasma pneumoniae* is of particular importance and was implicated in 13.1 per cent of cases in Finland (Koskiniemi *et al.* 1991, Rantala *et al.* 1991). Other bacteria such as *Legionella*, *Campylobacter jejuni* (Nasralla *et al.* 1993) and *Bordetella pertussis* are rarely a cause, but in as many as a third of cases no responsible agent can be identified. The incidence of encephalitis varies greatly in different countries and in different seasons of the year. This is due to the seasonal variation in incidence of common viral infections and to the geographical restriction of some agents such as the arboviruses to specific regions.

The relationship between the occurrence of encephalitis and viral or bacterial infections is complex and several mechanisms are at play in different cases. Two major mechanisms are recognized. The first mechanism is operative in the *primary encephalitides* in which the virus is present in the CNS and actually replicates within neurons, glial cells or macrophages. A second mechanism seems to involve an immunoallergic response similar to what is observed in experimental allergic encephalitis (Johnson 1982) and applies to the *postinfectious meningoencephalitides*.

A distinction between the various mechanisms responsible for encephalitis-like illnesses can be made on a pathological basis in at least some of the autopsied cases (Johnson 1982). The presence of inflammatory infiltrates, round cells of glial nodules, neuronal necrosis, and sometimes intranuclear inclusions or perivenous demyelination allows separation of primary and postinfectious cases, and the absence of inflammatory signs excludes the diagnosis of encephalitis. In clinical practice, however, a distinction between primary and postinfection encephalitis, or even between encephalitis and parainfectious encephalopathies, is often impossible, and it is clearly impossible to ascribe many of the published cases of encephalitis to one of the specific mechanisms. For example, considerable doubts surround the very existence of encephalitis, in a restricted, pathological sense, as a complication of influenza (Hawkins *et al.* 1987), parainfluenza virus infections (McCarthy *et al.* 1990), hepatitis A (Hodges 1987), enterovirus or adenovirus infections (Kim and Gohd 1983) and many other viral infections, if only cases of perivenous encephalitis are accepted. Still, such infections undoubtedly can and do give rise to encephalitis-like illnesses. Very few criteria allow allocation of a particular case to one mechanism. For example, isolation of a virus from the CSF, which has been used by some authors (Kennedy *et al.* 1987) to separate 'true' viral encephalitis from other related syndromes, is unreliable because the presence of virus in the CSF may be associated with several different mechanisms and pathological findings. Conversely, pathologically demonstrated encephalitic inflammation is common without the presence of a virus in the CSF. Even intrathecal synthesis of specific antibodies directed against certain viruses such as mumps virus (Vandvik *et al.* 1978a) and evidence of intrathecal viral replication as shown by the presence of interferon alpha in the CSF (Dussaix *et al.* 1985, Tardieu *et al.* 1986, Lebon *et al.* 1988) are not sufficient to allow distinction between encephalitis and purely meningeal disease.

I shall consider successively: (i) the clinical features of the syndrome of acute meningoencephalitis and its differential diagnosis and management; (ii) the special features of the common types of encephalitis and of clinically related encephalitis-like CNS disease; and (iii) some atypical aspects of encephalitis or acute encephalopathies of infectious origin.

Clinical features

The major clinical manifestations of encephalitis are deteriorating consciousness with confusion, drowsiness or coma, altered behaviour, convulsions and a variety of neurological signs. These usually appear acutely but there may be a prodromal phase with memory and behavioural disturbances. Neurological manifestations referable to any part of the CNS involve mostly the cerebral hemispheres (hemiplegia, aphasia) but may affect the brainstem or cerebellum, with ataxia, present in 58 per cent of cases in one series (Rantala *et al.* 1991), or the spinal cord with a picture of acute myelitis. Additional signs can include involvement of the cranial nerves of the hypothalamus with lethargy (Howard and Lees 1987) and of the basal ganglia with rigidity or abnormal movements (Gollomp and Fahn 1987, Donovan and Lenn 1989).

An abnormal EEG is virtually always present, the most common manifestation being generalized or predominantly unilateral slowing. Less commonly, periodic discharges may be seen especially with certain types or aetiologies such as HSV infection or subacute sclerosing panencephalitis (see below), but occasionally with other types (Hemachudha and Kocen 1986). The CSF is usually abnormal with a pleocytosis consisting of lymphocytes and mononuclear cells, an elevated protein level and a normal glucose level. The CSF cell count varies from a few to several hundred in most cases with a majority of mononuclear cells although polymorphonuclear cells may predominate in very acute cases with necrotic lesions. In such cases red blood cells may also be present. The protein content is increased; an oligoclonal pattern and/or an elevated immunoglobulin level is sometimes found. CSF sugar is sometimes lowered. However, the CSF remains normal in a high proportion of cases (Rautonen *et al.* 1991).

Neuroimaging features may to a certain extent help distinguish some forms of encephalitis such as herpes simplex encephalitis. CT and even MRI scans may be normal in patients with postinfectious meningoencephalitis but often CT shows multiple areas of low density and contrast enhancement while MRI shows increased signal on T_2-weighted images (Kesselring *et al.* 1990). Abnormalities involve mainly the white matter in postinfectious encephalitis but also the cortical grey matter in primary encephalitides. Exceptions to that general rule are not rare.

The time course of acute encephalitis may be fulminating. In many cases, however, new symptoms and signs appear over a few days to weeks. This is an important diagnostic feature, as in many other acute encephalopathies the full picture is abruptly completed.

Differential diagnosis

The differential diagnosis of meningoencephalitis includes a large number of encephalopathies and other disorders marked by disturbances of consciousness that may arise with pathology outside the CNS (Table 11.11). Because the clinical features are not specific, special attention should be given to disorders that require immediate effective therapy, especially bacterial meningitis, tuberculous meningitis and brain abscesses. Lumbar puncture is needed to exclude meningitis; however, it may be dangerous in the face of high ICP which is not excluded by the absence of papilloedema. In case of doubt, a CT scan is indicated. In some patients, the diagnosis of tuberculosis or even of bacterial meningitis may remain a possibility even after CSF study. Exclusion of cerebral abscess may be difficult in the early stage of bacterial cerebritis. Contrast enhancement is important as it may demonstate the peripheral round-ring image suggestive of suppuration. The CT appearance of tuberculous meningitis is characteristic. Treatment with antibiotics and/or antituberculous agents may have to be started in dubious cases together with that of herpes simplex encephalitis, until the diagnosis is clarified. Cerebral thrombophlebitis usually produces characteristic CT images (Chapter 15). Occasionally, an acute arterial thrombosis mimics an encephalitic process. Cryptogenic status epilepticus may be accompanied by pleocytosis (Chapter 16). Acute metabolic diseases should also be excluded. Therefore, blood sugar, serum electrolytes, blood ammonia level and, in selected cases, amino acid and organic acid profiles should be obtained. These will help

TABLE 11.11
Differential diagnosis of the acute encephalitides

Intracranial infections
Bacterial meningitis
Tuberculous meningitis
Brain abscess
Cerebral malaria

Para-infectious encephalopathies
Reye syndrome
Haemorrhagic shock and encephalopathy
Toxic shock syndrome

Metabolic disorders
Fluid, electrolyte and acid-base disorders
Inherited metabolic diseases
    Amino acid and organic acids
    Urea cycle disorders
    Lactic acidosis

Hypoxic–ischaemic injuries
Vascular collapse and shock of various causes
Cardiorespiratory arrest
Near-miss sudden infant death syndrome*

Vascular diseases
Stroke of embolic or thrombotic origin
Haemorrhage from vascular malformations
Venous thrombosis

Toxic injuries
Endogenous (diabetes, uraemia, liver failure)
Exogenous (drugs or household agents)

Seizure disorders
Status epilepticus
Hemiconvulsions–hemiplegia syndrome

Increased intracranial pressure
Tumours
Haematomas
Acute hydrocephalus
Lead poisoning

*May be associated with status epilepticus.

to rule out Reye syndrome or an intermittent and/or late mani-festing form of aminoaciduria or organic aciduria. In some patients examination of urine for toxic substances may be useful, although the course of intoxication is generally much faster and there are no focal neurological signs or meningeal involvement. Lead intoxication can simulate encephalitis, but CSF shows high protein with only a few or no cells and other features of lead toxicity are present.

Management

The general management of acute encephalitis is the same as that of other acute encephalopathies and is a paediatric emer-gency. Priority must be given to ensuring a patent airway and maintaining adequate circulation.

A complete assessment of the child is then in order (Table 11.12). Neurological examination is essential in establishing the correct diagnosis, evaluating prognosis and planning therapy.

A majority of children with acute encephalopathy do not require assisted ventilation or high-technology care. Critically ill children with a very depressed level of consciousness are best treated in intensive care units and this applies particularly to those with evidence of high ICP (Brown and Steers 1986, Tasker *et al.* 1988a). Maintenance of an adequate cardiac output is essential and may require large quantities of fluid rather than the tradi-tional limitation often advised in case of CNS disease. Monitoring of respiration, blood pressure and body temperature and efforts at controlling hyperthermia and seizures are essential. When available, EEG monitoring is extremely useful in detecting subclinical seizure activity and evaluating the degree of brain dysfunction (Tasker *et al.* 1988b). Monitoring of ICP is not generally required in acute encephalitis but may be essential in some related conditions such as Reye syndrome (see below). Treatment of high ICP is discussed in Chapter 14. Osmotic agents and, in some cases, corticosteroids may be needed. The risks of hyperventilation that may decrease the blood flow to the brain have been underlined (Ashwal *et al.* 1990). Extensive craniectomy may be lifesaving for patients with intractable brain swelling (Schwab *et al.* 1997).

Primary encephalitides

Primary encephalitides are characterized by the presence of viruses and their replication in target-cells within the CNS. Although a large number of viruses can induce a primary encephalitis, the most common agent in Western Europe is the herpes simplex virus. Enteroviruses can also produce a primary encephalitis. In other parts of the world including North America, however, *arboviruses* are important causal agents.

In infants older than 6 months and children, primary en-cephalitis is most often caused by *HSV type 1*. The frequency at all ages seems to be 1 in 200,000 to 1 in 400,000 persons per year in Western countries and represents about 10 per cent of all severe viral CNS infections. Thirty-one per cent of cases occur in patients below 20 years of age and 12 per cent in those between 6 months and 10 years (Whitley *et al.* 1982).

Most cases are due to reactivation of a latent virus but cases associated with primary infection may occur, especially in neonates and young infants. Latent HSV-1 can persist in the trigeminal ganglia (Johnson 1982) and lead to recurrent cuta-neous or mucosal infections by means of dendritic spread. The virus may occasionally spread along meningeal branches and this might give it access to the brain. Entry into the CNS might also be from the nasal mucosa through the cribriform plate to involve the parenchymal cells of the olfactory bulb (Johnson 1982).

From a pathological viewpoint, HSV encephalitis is charac-terized by the frankly necrotic nature of the lesions which are often haemorrhagic with gross softening, and in severe cases, loss of all neural and glial elements. Damage predominates in the orbital and mesial temporal regions of the cerebral hemispheres although it is usually widespread and may extend to the brain-stem (Duarte *et al.* 1994). Intranuclear eosinophilic inclusions (Cowdry type A bodies) are recognized in neurons, oligoglial cells and astrocytes.

The *clinical symptoms* of encephalitis are preceded in 60 per cent of cases by prodromal symptoms that may be purely systemic

400

TABLE 11.12
Assessment and emergency management of the child with acute encephalopathy

History

Past medical history (early development, seizures)

History of acute event, especially presence of a prodromal illness and recent history of infectious disease and immunization

General physical examination

Vital signs (respiratory rate, blood pressure, temperature)

Skin and mucous membranes (exanthema, herpes)

Visceral examination

Status of peripheral circulation

Neurological examination

Level of consciousness using paediatric modifications of the Glasgow Coma Scale (Chapter 13)

Ocular responses (Chapter 13) including corneal reflex, pupillary responses, oculocephalic reflex (doll's eye manoeuvre), oculovestibular response

Motor asymmetry; response to noxious stimulation (appropriate withdrawal, decorticate or decerebrate posturing)

Signs of increased intracranial pressure (Chapter 14), especially examination of the fundi

Laboratory investigations

Blood gases, urea, electrolytes, creatinine, sugar

Full blood count

Labstix on urine (sugar, ketone bodies, organic acids)   } In all cases

Chest X-ray

CT scan

Blood biochemistry: liver enzymes, ammonia, calcium, clotting factors

More complete metabolic investigations (lactic acid, amino acids, organic acids) in selected cases (preserve blood and CSF)

EEG when available without delaying therapy; ideally polygraphic recording

CSF examination. Lumbar puncture should be deferred when patient deeply unconscious, evidence of high intracranial pressure or unstable vital conditions

Toxicology in urine

Immediate therapeutic measures

Ensure safe i.v. access (using large veins if necessary)

Ensure adequate airway

Maintain adequate blood pressure with i.v. fluids and pressor agents (*e.g.* dopamine) if necessary

Lowering of very high temperature

Intensive care treatment often required, especially when assisted ventilation is required.

---

such as fever and malaise, but are sometimes more suggestive when disturbances of memory or behaviour are prominent. The prodromal phase often lasts a few days, with increasing affectation of consciousness and a high fever. The full-blown picture includes the symptoms common to all cases of encephalitis, *i.e.* lethargy, obtundation or coma and convulsive seizures. These are particularly frequent and often repeated in cases of HSV infection, and they are almost always focal, reflecting the gross asymmetry of lesions that is apparent pathologically. Unilateral status epilepticus is not rare. Increased ICP is frequent, and papilloedema is present in 15 per cent of cases. Hemiplegia often develops, and aphasia may be a prominent and initial finding in older children and adolescents. Changes pointing to focal necrosis of the temporobasal structures such as anosmia, olfactory hallucinations and disordered behaviour may be in the forefront (Whitley *et al.* 1981). In many cases, however, clinical features are uncharacteristic but HSV is always thought of because of its frequency (Rose *et al.* 1992). In infants and young children, febrile seizures, usually partial, are often the dominant symptom and may remain isolated for several days. Such cases may pose particularly difficult diagnostic problems. Millner and Puchhammer-Stöckl (1993) reported five cases presenting as 'complicated febrile convulsions' among 151 cases of HSV

encephalitis diagnosed by the polymerase chain reaction. In three of these the CSF contained no cells, and in only one was the MR image suggestive of the diagnosis.

In some patients the disease appears more progressively. Aphasia or sensory abnormalities precede the more severe neurological signs by several days.

A bilateral opercular syndrome, reminiscent of the Foix–Chavany–Marie syndrome caused by vascular lesions in adults, may occur as a result of the predominant basal involvement (Rantala *et al.* 1991).

Atypical forms with only mild encephalitic involvement and spontaneously favourable outcome in the absence of therapy are rare (Marton *et al.* 1995), and where there is doubt treatment is always indicated. Focal forms with pseudotumoural features are on record (Counsell *et al.* 1994).

Certain *EEG and laboratory features* are of diagnostic value. Contrary to the diffuse slow waves that are seen in other meningoencephalitides, the tracings in HSV cases are usually very asymmetrical and often exhibit clear foci of spikes on an abnormally slow background. Low amplitude in one or more regions, especially over the temporal lobe, is not unusual. Periodic complexes one to three seconds apart are frequent in the same area but are often only transient (Mizrahi and Tharp 1982). The

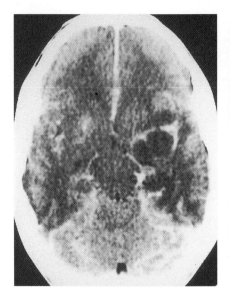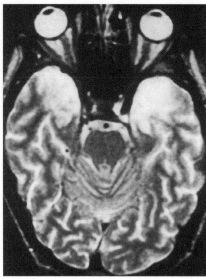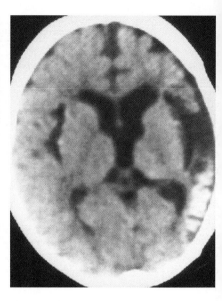

Fig. 11.8. Herpes simplex encephalitis. *(Left)* CT scan showing extensive necrosis and haemorrhage in left temporal lobe. Note also diffuse brain oedema and smaller lesion in right temporal lobe. *(Centre)* MRI of another patient showing bilateral high T_2 signal from both temporal lobes. *(Right)* CT scan of another patient at a late stage showing enlargement of sylvian fissure and areas of calcification in left temporal cortex. (Courtesy Prof. M. Tardieu, Hôpital Bicêtre, Paris, and Dr Kling Chong, Great Ormond Street Hospital, London.)

periodic complexes occur most commonly between the second and fifteenth day of the disease and are rarely seen thereafter (Schauseil-Zipf *et al.* 1982). They are not specific, however, and may occur with encephalitis caused by *M. pneumoniae* (Hulihan *et al.* 1992) or Epstein–Barr virus.

CT scan shows decreased attenuation predominating in the temporal lobes, usually asymmetrically. Contrast enhancement often appears at the periphery or within the lesions (Dutt and Johnson 1982). Isolated parietal or occipital lesions are uncommon (Bergey *et al.* 1982). Small haemorrhages frequently appear within the oedematous density. CT scans may remain normal during the first days of the disease (Greenberg *et al.* 1981) but this has no prognostic significance. MRI may show early abnormalities in the form of increased signal in T_2-weighted images unilaterally or predominantly unilaterally, even when CT scan is still normal (Kapur *et al.* 1994), and may thus help make an early diagnosis (Fig. 11.8).

During the course of the illness, there may be an initial increase in the extent of abnormalities (Koskiniemi and Ketonen 1981). Later on, atrophy of the parenchyma with a marked perisylvian and temporal predominance progressively appears and will persist, and calcification may develop. Total disappearance of CT abnormalities is rare in infants but may be seen in older patients.

The *CSF* may be normal in 20–25 per cent of patients. In most cases it is under increased pressure and contains an excess number of cells, usually lymphocytes, with less than 50 mononuclear cells/mm³ in about a quarter of cases (Whitley *et al.* 1982). The CSF is frequently haemorrhagic or xanthochromic because of the necrotic and haemorrhagic character of the lesions.

Establishing definitively the herpetic origin of a case of acute encephalitis may be difficult. Isolation of virus from CSF is virtually always negative. Demonstration of a fourfold rise of

antibody titre against HSV-1 infection in the CSF is significant but requires 10–14 days to appear (Koskiniemi *et al.* 1984), although more sensitive tests may enable the diagnosis to be established earlier than 10 days in some patients. The antibodies initially belong to the IgM class and later switch to IgG type. They are associated with the presence of an oligoclonal protein pattern in the CSF (Mathiesen *et al.* 1988). The antibodies and the oligoclonal pattern persist for years following an attack of herpes encephalitis (Tardieu and Lapresle 1980) reflecting the persistence of HSV within the CNS. The presence of interferon alpha in serum and CSF, although nonspecific, is suggestive in conjunction with a consistent clinical picture (Lebon *et al.* 1988). Rapid diagnosis can now be achieved by demonstration of viral DNA in the CSF by polymerase chain reaction. This method has been shown to be highly specific and 75 per cent sensitive (Boerman *et al.* 1989, Anderson *et al.* 1993, Troendle-Atkins *et al.* 1993, Koskiniemi *et al.* 1996) and may be effective even when the CSF is otherwise normal (Millner and Puchhammer-Stöckl 1993).

When the clinical and/or neuroimaging features are suggestive of HSV encephalitis, treatment (see below) should be started immediately. Brain biopsy is indicated when another diagnosis that may require a different therapy is suspected rather than for confirmation of the diagnosis. Such diagnoses include especially brain abscess or granulomatous meningitis (Whitley *et al.* 1989). Other conditions that may mimic HSV encephalitis such as paraneoplasic limbic encephalitis or MELAS (Johns *et al.* 1993) are rare in children and not amenable to effective therapy. The procedure is not devoid of risk, and attempted isolation of virus from brain tissue is not uncommonly negative because of sampling error or technical problems in patients with typical HSV encephalitis.

I believe that a reasonably safe diagnosis can be made without recourse to brain biopsy in most cases if advantage is taken of the recent laboratory advances.

The *treatment* of herpes encephalitis is with cytosine arabinoside (acyclovir). Vidarabine (adenosine arabinoside) was the first effective agent but is inferior to cytarabine (Sköldenberg *et al.* 1984) which is also easier to administer. Acyclovir inhibits the viral DNA polymerase. The doses used are 10–15 mg/kg every eight hours instilled intravenously over one hour for 14 days. In the series of Sköldenberg *et al.*, mortality with such treatment was 19 per cent, and 14 per cent of patients were left with significant sequelae. Fifty-six per cent of patients were cured without residua. This is in contrast to a mortality of 70–80 per cent before therapy was available. In series of children, the efficacy seems as great as in adults (for a review, see Kohl and James 1985), although no controlled study has been reported. However, infants less than 12–18 months of age have an unfavourable outlook, and severe neurological, behavioural and epileptic sequelae are frequent.

Resistant strains (Crumpacker *et al.* 1982) are occasionally encountered, and the problem of resistance to antiviral agents may be a growing one (Hirsch and Schooley 1989). Increased dosage (30 mg/kg/d or 500 mg/m^2 t.i.d.) for 15 days and increased duration of therapy may be tried in such cases.

Administration of corticosteroids together with antiviral drugs has been used to reduce oedema but the possibility of diminishing the host resistance exists and it is not recommended (Wood *et al.* 1994).

Relapses following apparently successful treatment of herpes encephalitis occur uncommonly. They are rarely associated with the persistence of virus despite adequate treatment. Other relapses may be an immunoallergic response of obscure origin and are associated with extensive demyelination (Barthez *et al.* 1987, Pike *et al.* 1991, Rautonen *et al.* 1991). Relapses are frequently marked by recurrent fever and the occurrence of abnormal movements of choreoathetotic or ballistic type (Barthez *et al.* 1987, Shanks *et al.* 1991, Wang *et al.* 1994). The prognosis is exceedingly poor.

The mortality rate is high in infants, and sequelae persist in approximately half the cases. Sequelae include hemiplegia (Rautonen *et al.* 1991), bilateral opercular syndrome (van der Poel *et al.* 1995) and severe epilepsy which, in infants, may manifest as infantile spasms. Behavioural sequelae are frequent. Aphasia, which may be global or more specialized, is common because of the frequent temporal location of the lesions.

Atypical forms of HSV encephalitis have been reported. Brainstem encephalitis with involvement of cranial nerves has been shown to result from herpes infection in some cases (Duarte *et al.* 1994). Acute myelitis due to HSV is also on record (Wiley *et al.* 1987). The latter is seen mainly with type 2 virus infection. Type 2 virus causes most neonatal HSV infections. These include encephalitis, associated with disseminated viral infection in two-thirds of cases (Chapter 2). Encephalitis due to HSV-2 infection is more severe than type 1 disease (Corey *et al.* 1988) and may lead to diffuse encephalomalacia. In the neonate, the presence of a multifocal periodic pattern on the EEG, together with inflam-matory CSF, is highly suggestive of herpetic encephalitis and may be present before any abnormal image is visible on CT or MRI. In older patients, cases of severe temporal lobe epilepsy have been attributed to smouldering HSV-2 infection (Cornford and McCormick 1997).

• *Rabies* is rare in industrialized countries. The virus is in the saliva of infected mammals and is transmitted to man through a bite or skin abrasion and occasionally through intact skin or mucous membranes. A history of animal bite is absent in many cases (Fishbein and Robinson 1993). The virus reaches the CNS via peripheral nerves. Characteristic viral inclusions (Negri bodies) are found in the neurons, especially in the pyramidal cells of the hippocampus.

The incubation period lasts from 10 days to eight months. A brief premonitory period of fever and malaise precedes a second phase of excitement during which hyperacusis and hydrophobia with pharyngeal spasms are the most striking manifestations. A third, paralytic, phase may be seen if the patient survives the second phase or, on occasion, from onset. Death is constant once neurological signs have appeared.

Prevention is now with human diploid cell vaccine (Fishbein and Robinson 1993). Rabies is unique in that the long incubation period allows the induction of active as well as passive immunity prior to the onset of the illness. A combination of rabies immune serum (40 IU/kg for equine antirabies serum, 20 IU/kg for human rabies immune globulins) and human diploid cell vaccine has proved very effective. The recommended procedure for prevention of the disease in the exposed child has been detailed (American Academy of Pediatrics 1982b). Passive immunization with hyperimmune antirabies serum is administered for all severe exposures as well as for all bites of animals suspected of rabies.

• *Varicella-zoster virus* can cause both postinfectious encephalitis and primary encephalitis. The latter occurs principally in patients with immunosuppression (Gilden *et al.* 1988). Vasculitis due to the varicella-zoster virus is described below. Acute myelitis has been reported (Gilden *et al.* 1994). Treatment with acyclovir may be effective.

• *Enterovirus encephalitis.* Encephalitis and/or meningoencephalitis-like illnesses caused by enteroviruses are of uncertain mechanism. Their pathology is poorly known. As indicated above, they usually occur in association with signs of diffuse systemic involvement and are mainly encountered in the first three months of life. Diagnosis is by isolation of virus from the CSF with secondary confirmation by a rise in antibodies directed against the particular strain found (Tardieu 1986). Polymerase chain reaction may help make an early diagnosis (Schlesinger *et al.* 1994).

• *Arbovirus (tick-borne) encephalitides.* Arboviruses are RNA viruses transmitted between susceptible vertebrate hosts by blood-sucking arthropods (Rehle 1989). These agents play a significant pathogenic role in many parts of the world including South-east

TABLE 11.13
Main arbovirus (tick-borne) encephalitides

Name	Distribution	Vector	Reference
Japanese B	China, Korea, Taiwan, Eastern Siberia, South-east Asia	Mosquito	Monath (1988)
California encephalitis	North America	Mosquito	Johnson *et al.* (1968)
Eastern equine encephalitis	Americas	Mosquito	Monath (1990), Deresiewicz *et al.* (1997)
Western equine encephalitis	Americas	Mosquito	Monath (1990)
Saint Louis encephalitis	Americas	Mosquito	Monath and Tsai (1987)
Murray Valley encephalitis	Eastern Australia, New Guinea	Mosquito	Whitley (1990)
Russian spring–summer encephalitis	Siberia, Eastern Europe	Tick	Günther *et al.* (1997)
Powassan virus	Canada	Tick	Clarke and Casals (1965)

TABLE 11.14
Relative frequency of the occurrence of encephalitis in the course of various viral infections*

Virus disease	Frequency of encephalitis
Measles	1:1000
Mumps	1:2000
Chickenpox	1:10,000
Epstein–Barr virus	1:10,000
Rubella	1:20,000
Adenovirus	< 1:1,000,000
Influenza A	< 1:1,000,000
Parainfluenza	< 1:1,000,000

*After Miller *et al.* (1956).

Asia (Monath 1988), North America, Russia/Siberia and recently Eastern Europe and Scandinavia (Günther *et al.* 1997), where it has become one of the commonest causes of encephalitis.

Table 11.13 lists some of the main members of the group. Infection with arboviruses is often asymptomatic or produces only a mild nonspecific disease; less commonly it results in serious neurological disease. Involvement of the cervical spinal roots with paralysis of the shoulders and scapular girdle was a presenting feature in some of the Russian and Scandinavian cases (Günther *et al.* 1997). Diagnosis rests on a significant antibody rise that may take several weeks to occur. The virus can be isolated from blood or nervous tissue but not from CSF. The clinical features and CSF changes, when CNS affectation is present, are nonspecific. Aseptic meningitis, cranial nerve involvement or severe encephalitic symptoms may all be present. Infants and children of all ages can be affected. Sequelae are more common in younger patients.

• Rare cases of primary encephalitis may be due to *M. pneumoniae* infection (Abramovitz *et al.* 1987).

Postinfectious encephalitis (acute disseminated encephalomyelitis)
The clinical picture of acute encephalitis often occurs in the course of childhood exanthematous diseases and immunizations. In most pathologically verified cases of postinfectious encephalitides there is demyelination and no virus can be isolated from the CNS.

The incidence of postinfectious encephalitis, also referred to as parainfectious encephalitis and acute disseminated encephalomyelitis (ADEM), is imperfectly known but is probably higher than that of the primary encephalitides. Measles is the most common cause; thus, the incidence of encephalitis will depend upon the incidence of measles and immunization against measles in any population. Cases of postinfectious encephalitis following measles immunization have occurred but their frequency is considerably lower than that of encephalitis following wild measles (Landrigan and Witte 1973). An estimate of the frequency of various causes is given in Table 11.14. The incidence with measles may vary from one epidemic to another (Miller *et al.* 1956). In fact, the precise frequency of postinfectious encephalitis can only

be estimated as in many cases no data are available on the pathology and mechanism of an acute encephalitic picture. Thus, in mumps, meningitis is very common but evidence of perivenous encephalitis is present in only a very few cases (Johnson 1982). In a number of cases, the disease that precedes the onset of encephalitis is not diagnosed and, even in retrospect, no virus can be identified. The diagnosis of viral infection is then inferred from the clinical manifestations and course of the premonitory illness.

The *pathology* of postinfectious encephalitis is distinctive. Numerous foci of perivenous demyelination are present. Axis cylinders are usually better preserved than myelin. Cuffing of veins and venules by mononuclear cells is prominent, and microglial cells and macrophages are seen in the demyelinated areas. This pathological picture is very much like that of experimental allergic encephalitis.

Except in rare cases (ter Meulen *et al.* 1972), no virus can be isolated from the CNS, no nucleocapsids are visible by electron microscopy, and there is no secretion of interferon alpha in the CSF (Lebon *et al.* 1988).

It is generally thought that the disease is caused by an immune response induced by the viral illness either because stimulation of B lymphocytes by a viral agent induces a polyclonal antibody secretion, one or several antibodies being able to recognize an antigenic structure within the CNS, or because there exist antigenic structures common to neural tissue and viral proteins (Gendelman *et al.* 1984, Tardieu *et al.* 1984, Sharpe and Fields 1985). T lymphocytes may also play a role, *e.g.* in the production of various lymphokines.

The *clinical manifestations* are those already described for all types of encephalomyelitis. In a majority of cases, the onset is abrupt with disturbances of consciousness and seizures (Miller *et al.* 1956) that occur in 60 per cent of cases and are often inaugural. These symptoms appear on average six days (up to 21 days) after the occurrence of an upper respiratory tract infection or an exanthematous disease, in most cases in a child over the age of 2 years. Various neurological signs may be seen, including hemiparesis, extrapyramidal signs, ataxia, facial palsy, nystagmus and cranial nerve involvement (Kennard and Swash 1981, Marks *et al.* 1988).

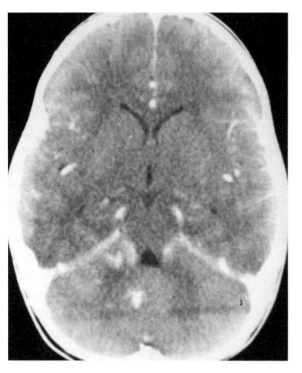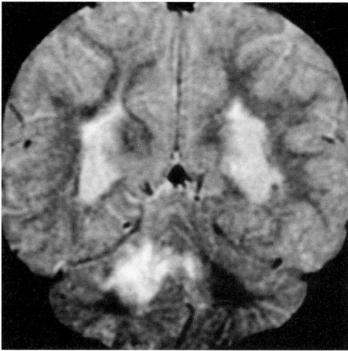

Fig. 11.9. Acute parainfectious encephalitis. *(Left)* CT scan showing small areas of contrast enhancement in posterior fossa. *(Right)* MRI, T$_2$-weighted spin–echo sequence showing more extensive zone of intense signal from right cerebellar hemisphere and bilateral intense signal from supratentorial hemispheric white matter. (4-year-old girl with cerebellar ataxia of sudden onset lasting for several weeks associated with mild stupor that disappeared in a few days. All clinical and imaging abnormalities disappeared eventually.)

The EEG shows, from onset, a slow background rhythm. Electrical discharges and spikes may be seen but periodic complexes are not found except in very occasional cases (Hemachuda and Kocen 1986).

CSF examination shows, in a majority of patients, a moderate pleocytosis and a mild increase of protein. On electrophoresis, the protein pattern is polyclonal, suggestive of a transudate in 70 per cent of cases. Evidence of intrathecal antibody synthesis with a polyclonal pattern is found in 30 per cent of patients.

The course is variable from case to case and depends on the causal agent (see below). The death rate is low. In over three-quarters of cases the duration is brief (Miller *et al.* 1956) with recovery in less than two weeks. However, during the first few days, it is usual to notice the appearance of new neurological symptoms or signs and this is important for differentiating post-infectious encephalitis from cases of acute encephalopathy of obscure origin in which the clinical manifestations are more explosive and no new manifestations appear after the first 24–48 hours (Lyon *et al.* 1961).

CT imaging occasionally discloses areas of oedematous density in the white matter (Saito *et al.* 1980) (Fig. 11.9). In most cases, CT scan remains normal throughout the course. In the late stages, progressive cerebral atrophy may appear and is of unfavourable significance (Diebler and Dulac 1987).

MRI is usually more informative and shows disseminated areas of increased signal on T$_2$-weighted sequences. They usually involve predominantly the white matter (Kesselring *et al.* 1990, Kimura *et al.* 1992). Some of the lesions occasionally enhance

with gadolinium contrast (Fujii *et al.* 1992). Marked swelling, particularly of the cerebellum, may be prominent (Hurst and Mehta 1988).

Lesions of the spinal cord may be visible (Marks *et al.* 1988). The pathological correlates of these images are imperfectly known. Residual images can persist for years and probably correspond to gliosis.

The clinical picture of postinfectious encephalitis may be different in a minority of patients. In these *subacute and often prolonged forms*, the onset is much less abrupt and disturbances of consciousness are less profound, with lethargy or obtundation rather than coma. New neurological manifestations may occur over a period of several weeks or even one to three months. These may include evidence of myelitic involvement with sphincter disturbances or paraparesis, behaviour disturbances, optic neuritis, epilepsy and hemiparesis. A recurrent course has occasionally been reported (Kamio *et al.* 1982, Gutowski *et al.* 1993). When such manifestations occur following a minor infection that may have been forgotten, the clinical features may suggest the diagnosis of possible multiple sclerosis. Some of these patients respond much more readily to steroids than those with the usual form of acute postinfectious encephalitis (Pasternak *et al.* 1980) and may become steroid-dependent with recurrences appearing with each attempt to discontinue or decrease steroid therapy. In other children, the disorder can be multiphasic in the absence of steroid therapy (Khan *et al.* 1995). Multiple recurrences sometimes occur (Monteiro and Correia 1991, Gutowski *et al.* 1993) so the diagnosis of multiple sclerosis is often

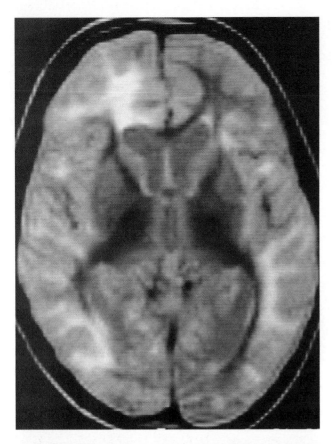

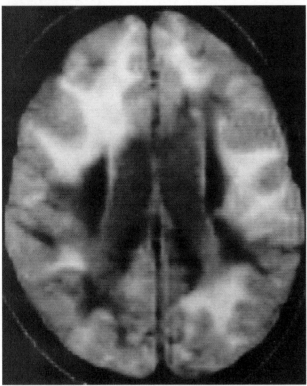

Fig. 11.10. Acute disseminated encephalomyelitis. T₂-weighted MRI sequences (axial cuts) showing multiple areas of high signal from both white and grey matter. 9-year-old boy with acute appearance of lethargy and neurological signs, responding to steroid therapy. Normal CT scan. Brain biopsy showed demyelination and perivenous inflammatory infiltrates. (Courtesy Dr C. Haenggeli, Hôpital Cantonal, Geneva.)

considered. However, recurrences often tend to occur at intervals of less than one month, MRI abnormalities usually do not have the periventricular distribution seen in multiple sclerosis, and oligoclonal banding in CSF is rather uncommon (Fig. 11.10).

In other atypical cases, subtle manifestations, sometimes of a psychiatric character, have been attributed to postinfectious encephalitis (DeLong *et al.* 1984, Johnsen *et al.* 1989) on the basis of disseminated white matter images. The patients described reverted to normal after courses that could last several months. Some cases may masquerade as progressive degenerative disorders (Garg and Kleiman 1994).

Another variant of postinfectious encephalitis is *acute haemorrhagic leukoencephalitis*. This is a fulminating disease which is characterized by the rapid evolution of focal neurological symptoms and signs, especially hemiplegia, accompanied by confusion, coma and fever. The CSF is xanthochromic in 20 per cent of cases and shows a polymorphonuclear pleocytosis. A striking leukocytosis is often present in the peripheral blood. A biphasic course is possible. The demyelinating lesions are haemorrhagic, due to a necrotizing angiitis of venules and capillaries. CT and MRI may help to make the diagnosis by showing the presence of large areas of hypodensity sometimes with a haemorrhagic component (Watson *et al.* 1984, Huang *et al.* 1988).

The treatment of postinfectious encephalitis is mainly that of all acute encephalitic illnesses (see above). The value of steroid treatment remains uncertain, although its immediate effectiveness may be spectacular in some cases (Pasternak *et al.* 1980). Intravenous immunoglobulins have been used in a few cases (Kleiman and Brunquell 1995).

• *Measles* encephalitis has it onset six to eight days after commencement of the rash (Johnson *et al.* 1984). Although of variable intensity, the disease is often severe with a 10 per cent mortality and frequent sequelae that include seizures and mental retardation. Learning difficulties and behavioural disturbances are common in children who had an apparently complete recovery.

Acute perivenous leukoencephalitis is not the only neurological complication of measles. Replication of measles virus within the CNS occurs with subacute sclerosing panencephalitis and the delayed acute form. Myelitis is not infrequent.

• *Chickenpox* encephalitis is usually mild and often presents as an acute cerebellar ataxia (Horowitz *et al.* 1991, Gieron-Korthals *et al.* 1994). This is observed in 34 per cent of patients with varicella encephalitis versus 10–15 per cent in measles or rubella encephalitis (Miller *et al.* 1956). An early pre-eruptive onset of encephalitis has been reported in a few cases (Maguire and Meissner 1985). Seizures and coma are uncommon. Myelitis and aseptic meningitis are rare (Johnson *et al.* 1984). Acute cerebellar swelling has been observed (Hurst and Mehta 1988). Varicella may also induce Reye syndrome (see below).

• *Rubella* encephalomyelitis tends to be a severe illness with a mortality of about 20 per cent. Associated arterial thrombosis has been noted (Connolly *et al.* 1975, and personal case).

• *Postvaccinal encephalitis* has now disappeared. Encephalitis may rarely follow Epstein–Barr virus infection or influenza (Hawkins *et al.* 1987). Not infrequently the responsible virus is not determined.

• *Postinfectious encephalitis of nonviral origin.* Cases of postinfectious encephalitis may be associated with nonviral infections, especially with *M. pneumoniae* and *B. burgdorferi* (Fisher *et al.* 1983, Den Heijer *et al.* 1986, Koskiniemi *et al.* 1991). The clinical presentation is indistinguishable from that of viral cases.

Acute encephalopathies of obscure origin in relation to virus infections

Acute encephalopathies without pathological evidence of inflammation in the CNS are uncommon. Such cases have been studied in detail by Lyon *et al.* (1961) under the name of 'acute encephalopathies of obscure origin'. Lyon *et al.* showed the clinical and aetiological heterogeneity of these conditions. More recently, several syndromes of CNS disease not associated with an abnormal CSF and not accompanied pathologically by inflammatory lesions of the brain have been reported. Such syndromes occur in close temporal relationship to a defined or an undetermined viral infection and are probably a consequence of such an infection. Among these conditons, Reye syndrome has aroused considerable interest (Crocker 1979). Other, perhaps less well defined syndromes may also be observed such as the syndrome of haemorrhagic shock and encephalopathy (Levin *et al.* 1983) as well as nonsyndromic cases.

Clearly, these acute parainfectious, noninflammatory encephalopathies form a heterogeneous group with diverse mechanisms. Some cases may be represented by episodes of status epilepticus or accidental complications of epileptic seizures as a result of choking on food or inhalation. Others may be the consequence of shock or circulatory failure in the course of a severe viral infection (Lyon *et al.* 1961). Still other cases are yet unexplained.

In a majority of cases, acute encephalopathies appear as a secondary event in the course of a definite or probable viral disorder. Their onset is marked by a rapid change in consciousness often in association with repeated vomiting. Convulsions are frequent.

The CSF remains normal throughout the course of the illness which is monophasic without the appearance of new signs and symptoms after the first few hours or days.

Progressive recovery of neurological functions in nonfatal cases may be rapid or extend over weeks or months.

• *Reye syndrome* is the best studied type of noninflammatory postviral acute encephalopathy. It is characterized pathologically by an acute encephalopathy with brain oedema, associated with microvesicular fatty degeneration of the liver and sometimes the kidneys (De Vivo and Keating).

The aetiology of the condition is multiple but in most cases there is a clear association with a viral illness, especially varicella (Hurwitz *et al.* 1982) and influenza B (Norman *et al.* 1968). Other viruses have also been implicated: the condition occurs most commonly following a respiratory disease (60–70 per cent of cases), varicella (20–30 per cent of cases) and gastrointestinal illnesses with diarrhoea (5–15 per cent of cases) (American Academy of Pediatrics 1982a). The association of the syndrome with the use of salicylates for treatment of the fever accompanying the antecedent illnesses has been established by epidemiological studies (*Lancet* 1987). Whether the dramatic decrease in frequency observed in the past few years is related to diminished use of aspirin has not been established (Hall *et al.* 1988). The role of undetected metabolic defects in causation of the syndrome is probably important (Greene *et al.* 1988).

The *pathology* of Reye syndrome includes liver abnormalities in the form of microvesicular steatosis unassociated with necrosis. Similar changes are often found in the kidneys and occasionally in the myocardium. On electron microscopy, the most striking abnormalities are seen in mitochondria which are swollen and pleomorphic (Partin *et al.* 1971). Cerebral oedema is constant and is apparently the usual cause of death.

Clinical manifestations appear after the symptoms of the premonitory disease have subsided and in the absence of fever. Initial symptoms include repeated vomiting with progressive deterioration of consciousness to stupor and coma over a few hours. Convulsions may occur and changes in muscle tone in the form of opisthotonus or decorticate or decerebrate rigidity are frequent. Central neurogenic hyperventilation can be seen in late stages. The liver is enlarged in about half the cases. The clinical picture is conspicuous by the absence of focal signs and of icterus and by the normal CSF.

Clinical manifestations of high ICP are in the forefront and may include papilloedema and signs such as mydriasis and decerebrate attitude that indicate brainstem dysfunction. The CSF pressure is high but it may be safer to measure it by an intracranial strain gauge than by lumbar puncture which may be dangerous in such critically ill patients.

Elevated transaminases (aspartate transaminase and alanine transaminase) are an early biological feature. Hyperammonaemia is almost constant but may be transient and is relatively late. Bilirubin is below 50 mmol/L (3 mg/dL). Hypoglycaemia is present in about half the cases, especially in infants (Glasgow 1984). A prolonged prothrombin time and an elevated creatine-kinase level are inconstant features.

Serum concentrations of alanine, glutamine, lysine and alpha-amino-*N*-butyrate are elevated, whereas citrulline and arginosuccinic acid levels are usually markedly depressed. Serum levels of short-chain fatty acids are quite high (Trauner *et al.* 1975).

The course of Reye syndrome is severe but the case fatality rate for children has regularly decreased over the years from 50–60 per cent in the early 1970s to less than 30 per cent in the early '80s (Glasgow 1984).

In fact, global figures are of limited significance because mortality and morbidity depend on the severity of the disease and on the stage at which treatment is started. The staging system of Lovejoy *et al.* (1974) is widely used. Stages I and II are characterized by absence or only mild depression of consciousness and are associated with a favourable outcome, with less than 10 per

TABLE 11.15
Inborn errors of metabolism that may produce a Reye-like picture

Systemic carnitine deficiency
Muscle carnitine deficiency
Late-onset glutaric aciduria type II
Medium-chain acyl-CoA dehydrogenase deficiency (MCAD)
Long-chain acyl-CoA dehydrogenase deficiency (LCAD)
ETF dehydrogenase deficiency ⎫
Multiple dehydrogenase deficiency ⎬ Glutaric aciduria type 2

cent mortality and no sequelae in survivors. Stages III and IV are marked by progressively more profound coma with symptoms and signs of increasing CNS dysfunction. EEG staging (Aoki and Lombroso 1973) includes five stages and is also correlated to the prognosis.

Residual neurological abnormalities are present in 30 per cent of patients with severe disease (Benjamin *et al.* 1982).

The *pathogenesis* of Reye syndrome remains enigmatic (DeLong and Glick 1982). Most hypotheses are based on the presence of biochemical and pathological changes indicative of mitochondrial dysfunction. Direct mitochondrial involvement by a virus is conceivable but no virus has ever been isolated from the liver or brain (Trauner *et al.* 1988). Another possibility would be the decompensation of a latent innate metabolic abnormality by the viral aggression. A third possibility would be the action of a cofactor to the viral infection. The factor most commonly suspected has been aspirin.

The *differential diagnosis* of Reye syndrome includes the other neurological complications of viral disorders as described above. A more important problem is posed by intoxications with various substances that may produce a similar clinical picture. These include alcohol intoxication, salicylate toxicity and valproic acid or valproate toxicity (Chapter 23). Intoxication with hypoglycine is caused by the absorption of 'bush tea' containing this substance in Jamaica (Tanaka *et al.* 1976), and a toxin of *Aspergillus flavus* has been associated with cases of Reye syndrome in Thailand (Olson *et al.* 1971).

Several innate errors of metabolism (Table 11.15) including hereditary fructose intolerance, deficit of glycogen synthetase, and especially disorders of the beta-oxidation of long-, medium- and short-chain fatty acids, can give rise to a picture which is indistinguishable from Reye syndrome (Stumpf *et al.* 1985, Greene *et al.* 1988). A history of a previous similar accident in a sibling or, in a milder form, in the child her/himself, should make one reluctant to accept a diagnosis of Reye syndrome.

Finally, other acute postviral encephalopathies without clinical or even pathological evidence of liver involvement (see above) may be related to Reye syndrome. Indeed cases are on record of Reye syndrome without marked fatty liver (Glasgow *et al.* 1972).

The *treatment* of Reye syndrome is, in the first place, symptomatic. Careful attention to metabolic and physiological disturbances including hypoglycaemia, correction of electrolyte imbalance and bleeding diathesis may suffice in many early cases.

In more severe cases, an aggressive therapeutic approach seems justified given the high mortality rate. Intensive care, mechanical ventilation, correction of metabolic abnormalities and treatment of intracranial hypertension are essential. Exchange transfusion and peritoneal dialysis have been advocated but their value has not been established.

Control of intracranial hypertension is one of the critical and controversial issues in the management of Reye syndrome. High pressure should be reduced using mannitol (Chapter 15) or hyperventilation to maintain arterial pCO_2 at about 25 mmHg (Trauner 1986). Barbiturate therapy is proposed by some (Shaywitz *et al.* 1986) but not by others (Trauner 1986). Steroid treatment is not indicated.

The *prognosis* depends on staging of the clinical and EEG findings and on certain biochemical data, especially the blood ammonia level. A high ammonia level is associated with a poor prognosis (Fitzgerald *et al.* 1982).

• *Haemorrhagic shock and encephalopathy* is thought to be due to sepsis but the aetiology is unknown (Whittington *et al.* 1985, Levin *et al.* 1988). A defect in the synthesis or reuptake of protease inhibitors (alpha-2-antitrypsin and alpha-2-macroglobulin) could be involved and these changes can be used to assist the diagnosis (Jardine and Bratton 1995). Most affected children are under 1 year of age. The onset is abrupt with unresponsiveness, fever and convulsions. Fever of 39.5° to over 40.1°C is a constant feature. The skin is mottled, and oozing of blood occurs at all puncture sites as a result of intravascular coagulopathy. Profound hypotension is the rule (Chaves-Carballo *et al.* 1990, Bacon and Hall 1992). Corrigan (1990) has emphasized the diagnostic importance of hyperpyrexia which may also be of aetiological significance. The EEG may be of diagnostic importance by showing runs of paroxysmal discharges, rapidly changing in amplitude, rate and morphology often with shifting focal distribution, which have been termed 'electrical storms' (Harden *et al.* 1991). MRI may show haemorrhages and areas of ischaemia (Glauser *et al.* 1992).

The course is often fatal and neurological sequelae are present in survivors, although complete recovery has been documented (Bonham *et al.* 1992). The CSF is normal. Treatment is symptomatic. Plasmapheresis has been proposed (Roth *et al.* 1987).

• *Dengue* is due to a specific virus with three major serotypes. The illness is common in South-east Asia but is also encountered in other parts of the world. The usual clinical presentation is with high fever with two consecutive peaks a few days apart, associated with myalgia, cephalalgia and malaise. The CSF is usually normal. Severe forms can present as an acute encephalopathy with coma, convulsions and a high mortality rate or as a haemorrhagic disease with skin and digestive tract bleeding and shock (Hendarto and Hadinegoro 1990, Hayes and Gubler 1992).

• Acute encephalopathies of uncertain mechanism have also been reported in other viral infections, particularly *herpes virus*

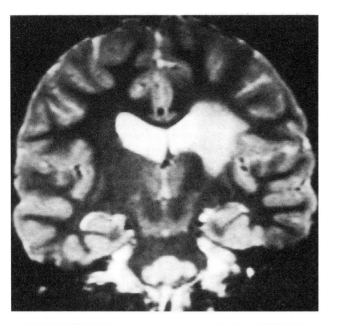

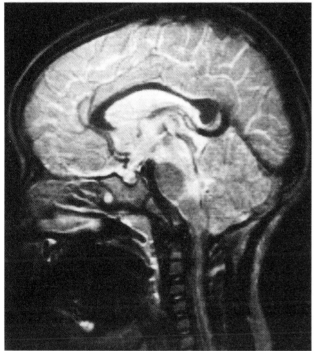

Fig. 11.11. Brainstem encephalitis. *(Top)* T$_2$-weighted MRI showing high signal in the pes pedunculi. Note another large lesion in white matter of left hemisphere. *(Bottom)* T$_2$-weighted sagittal cut of another child (4-year-old girl with stupor and multiple cranial nerve palsies) shows intense signal from cerebral peduncles and dorsal aspect of pons. A repeat MRI scan 2 months later was completely normal.

6 infections (Asano *et al.* 1992, 1994). Hall *et al.* (1994) found that 21 of 160 infants and young children with herpes virus 6 infection had seizures often occurring late in the course of fever, often prolonged or recurrent and more severe on average than usual febrile seizures. *Rotavirus infections* have also been associated with encephalopathic manifestations (Keidan *et al.* 1992). Similar manifestations with seizures and disturbances of consciousness may be a complication of diarrhoeal disease due to

Shigella spp. infection (Mulligan *et al.* 1992) and of *C. jejuni* enteritis (Nasralla *et al.* 1993).

• *Toxic shock syndrome.* A form of toxic shock syndrome may be related to influenza virus infection (MacDonald *et al.*. 1987). Most cases are due to staphylococcal toxins (Chesney *et al.* 1982) from a local focus of infection.

Brainstem and cerebellar encephalitis
The brainstem may be involved radiologically in cases of acute disseminated encephalitis. Localized brainstem involvement is uncommon and may occur both with primary encephalitides (Kaplan and Kovelevski 1978, North *et al.* 1993, Duarte *et al.* 1994) and, less rarely, with the postinfectious type.

The clinical presentation consists of fever, systemic symptoms and aseptic meningitis, in association with symptoms and signs of brainstem dysfunction. Involvement of ocular motor nerves and lower facial pairs is prominent and may be associated with obtundation and signs of involvement of the long tracts with resulting pyramidal and cerebellar manifestations. Cranial nerve involvement and ataxia may mimic the Miller Fisher syndrome (Chapter 21) that has been considered by some authors to be a form of brainstem encephalitis.

CT scan is usually unrevealing although medullary enlargement has been evidenced by pneumoencephalography and is visible on CT. MRI is able to demonstrate increased signal in the cerebral peduncles, pons, cerebellum and medulla (Ormerod *et al.* 1986, Hosoda *et al.* 1987) and may be of great value in distinguishing encephalitis from brainstem tumour, abscesses or other neurosurgical problems (Fig. 11.11).

Predominant involvement of the cerebellum is frequently observed with the varicella virus and occasionally with mumps (Cohen *et al.* 1992). Marked swelling of the cerebellum with consequent obstructive hydrocephalus has been reported in varicella virus infection (Hurst and Mehta 1988), in Epstein–Barr virus infection and with undetermined viral agents (Roulet Perez *et al.* 1993) and may run a fatal course. Severe cerebellar atrophy with persistent cerebellar signs may follow the acute attack (Hayakawa and Katoh 1995). The possibility of *L. monocytogenes* rhombencephalitis should always be kept in mind as antibiotic treatment is effective (Frith *et al.* 1987).

CHRONIC ENCEPHALITIDES
Although most of the chronic encephalitides of children are primary encephalitides with presence of the responsible viruses in the CNS, they have not been described in the preceding paragraphs dedicated to acute encephalitides and encephalitis-like diseases that have a fairly uniform and quite different clinical presentation. They form a heterogeneous group that includes well-defined types (subacute sclerosing panencephalitis, human immunodeficiency virus encephalopathy, rubella panencephalitis, prion diseases) and poorly understood cases that are possibly not directly due to virus infection. The mechanisms of chronic viral encephalitis are complex. The study of relationships between host and virus is beyond the scope of this book.

SUBACUTE SCLEROSING PANENCEPHALITIS (SSPE)

SSPE is by far the most common of the chronic encephalitides. The disease is caused by the measles virus. Its pathogenesis is unclear and involves an altered host response to infection with measles virus. SSPE occurs preferentially following measles occurring during the first two years of life. No general immunological deficiency is present in SSPE patients but specific response to measles infection may be abnormal. The synthesis of the M (assembly) viral protein is abnormal in cases of SSPE. However, multiple viral mutations rather than host factors seem to cause the defective expression of measles virus gene. Although strains of SSPE measles virus can code for the M protein, the conformation of the protein is defective and it is unable to bind to nucleocapsids (Hirano *et al.* 1993).

On neuropathological examination, the brain usually appears normal. The white matter may be firm and granular. Microscopically, there is vascular cuffing by mononuclear cells, neuronal loss and marked fibrillary glial proliferation. Intranuclear inclusion bodies are seen in most cases in neurons and oligodendrocytes. By electron microscopy, they are shown to be made of packed nucleocapsids with the characteristics of those of the measles agent.

The risk of developing SSPE is 4.0 per 100,000 cases of natural measles, whereas the risk after vaccinal measles is only 0.4 per 100,000. The risk is particularly high if measles is contracted before 2 years of age (Miller *et al.* 1992). The incidence of SSPE has sharply declined in Western countries since 1970 apparently as a result of measles immunization. The median interval between measles and SSPE is eight years.

The first stage of the illness is of insidious onset and progresses slowly in typical cases. It is marked in two-thirds of cases by personality changes and a subtle intellectual deterioration with an aphasic–apractic–agnostic predominance. Often, such children are regarded as suffering from psychological problems and referred to psychiatric clinics. In a quarter of patients neurological signs or seizures that may be atonic, myoclonic or even partial (Kornberg *et al.* 1991) are the first manifestations.

Involuntary movements usually appear within two to three months and are characteristic of the second stage. The movements may be myoclonic jerks. More often, they are more complex, involving in succession several segments in a repetitive pattern. Onset of each movement is abrupt but the duration is longer than that of a common myoclonic jerk, often lasting several seconds. Abnormal movements recur periodically although the intervals between two jerks are not equal and may vary from day to day in the same patient. The movements are usually bilateral, but strictly unilateral jerks may occur. They are absent during sleep and may disappear and reappear without apparent reason. In some patients, they may be replaced or preceded by periodic manifestations more typical of epilepsy, in particular by atonic seizures with head nods or complete falls or rarely by typical myoclonias. Generalized epileptic seizures, absence-like fits (Andermann 1967) or partial seizures (Kornberg *et al.* 1991) are uncommon.

In the third stage, extrapyramidal or pyramidal dysfunction or both become prominent. Extrapyramidal dyskinesias may

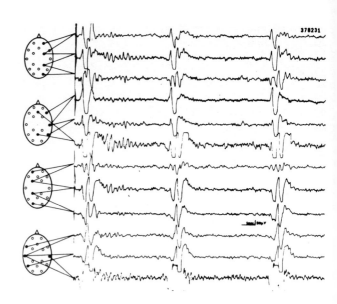

Fig. 11.12. Subacute sclerosing panencephalitis: pseudo-periodic EEG complexes. Note that the complexes are identical in any given lead.

appear, and parkinsonian rigidity is frequent. Dementia is severe and the child is bedridden.

In the terminal stage, progressive unresponsiveness, with increasing hypotonia and decerebrate rigidity, is associated with increasing swallowing and respiratory difficulties and with autonomic dysfunction.

The median duration of the disease is about 12 months and the course is usually regularly progressive. Subacute forms, lethal in as little as six weeks, are occasionally seen (Nihei *et al.* 1977). Contrariwise, long periods of arrested progression may occur. Periods of spontaneous remission may last up to several years (Risk and Haddad 1979).

Ophthalmic manifestations consist mainly of choroidoretinitis which preferentially involves the macular area and may be associated with pallor of the disc. These may appear months or even years before the classical manifestations (Robb and Watters 1970). Cortical blindness is uncommon, but optic atrophy is frequent. Papilloedema can be observed with transient increases of ICP. The ERG is normal but visual evoked potentials are impaired.

Characteristic EEG abnormalities can be observed before any clinical manifestation (Wulff 1982). Paroxysmal EEG complexes typically are formed of high-voltage slow waves recurring periodically at the time of clinical jerks (Fig. 11.12). They are usually identical in shape in any given lead. They may occur in the absence of clinical manifestations and are seen at some stage in about 80 per cent of patients. In some cases bursts of spike–wave activity may replace the typical complexes. Background tracings may be initially normal but become progressively slower while the amplitude diminishes.

The CSF contains no cells and the total protein is normal or slightly elevated. Gammaglobulins, mainly IgG, are always considerably raised, up to 50–60 per cent of total protein, and an oligoclonal pattern is constant. Specific antibodies against measles are present in a high titre. They are also considerably elevated in the serum.

The diagnosis is easy in typical cases. Cases with lateralizing or focal features may pose diagnostic problems. Spastic hemiplegia and unilateral spasms may occur. Some cases present with cortical blindness or hemianopia and may be confusing. Occasionally, signs of intracranial hypertension in association with focal features may wrongly suggest a tumour (Glowacki *et al.* 1967).

CT scan is usually normal in the weeks following onset. Diffuse swelling with ventricular compression may be seen. Focal hypodense areas are rare. Later, cerebral atrophy sets in and the white matter takes a hypodense appearance. MRI shows increased signal on T_2-weighted sequences which may later disappear (Brismar *et al.* 1996).

Despite multiple attempts, no satisfactory therapy has been developed. Isoprinosine seems to be able to induce remission in some cases (Durant *et al.* 1982). A combination of intraventricular interferon and isoprinosine was reported to increase the rate of remissions from 5–10 per cent to 45 per cent (Yalaz *et al.* 1992, Gascon *et al.* 1993), but late recurrences may occur after several years of remission (Anlar *et al.* 1997). Cimetidine has been tried by Anlar *et al.* (1993). Controlled trials are currently being run. Symptomatic treatment with carbamazepine may in part control the abnormal movements. Rapidly evolving forms may lead to death in only a few weeks.

PROGRESSIVE RUBELLA PANENCEPHALITIS
A few children with congenital rubella (Townsend *et al.* 1975) and an occasional patient with acquired rubella (Lebon and Lyon 1974) have developed a fatal panencephalitis with prominent cerebellar involvement about 10 years after initial infection. Insidiously progressive dementia is the first manifestation, followed by ataxia and myoclonic seizures. CSF examination shows mononuclear pleocytosis and increased protein with massively raised IgG globulins. Rubella virus has been isolated from the brain and leukocytes. Oligoclonal virus-specific antibodies are found in the CNS (Vandvik *et al.* 1978b). Pathologically, inflammatory infiltrates and astrocytosis are prominent (Townsend *et al.* 1982). The course is fatal in several years. No treatment is known.

OTHER UNCOMMON CHRONIC ENCEPHALITIDES
These can result from mumps (Ito *et al.* 1991), and a few cases of progressive cytomegalovirus disease in nonimmunodepressed infants (Riikonen 1993) are on record.

A syndrome of *chronic encephalitis with CSF pleocytosis* and in some cases calcification of the basal ganglia has been reported among Indian children from Northern Quebec (Black *et al.* 1988a,b) but its viral origin is uncertain.

PROTRACTED CHRONIC ENCEPHALITIS OF UNKNOWN ORIGIN
In rare cases, a protracted disorder with repeated emergence of new neurological manifestations over several weeks, associated with prominent clinical and/or EEG paroxysmal abnormalities

is observed following a viral infection. In such cases, long-lasting cognitive or behavioural changes are often prominent (DeLong *et al.* 1984, Lee *et al.* 1988). The course may extend over several months and abnormal movements are often a major feature (Sébire *et al.* 1992, Haimi-Cohen *et al.* 1996). CSF and CT scan remain consistently normal. Total or subtotal recovery is possible. The mechanism of such cases is uncertain. Lee *et al.* (1988) regarded them as cases of limbic encephalitis but their relationship to a virus infection is not established. Similar cases have been regarded, without definite evidence, as unusual and prolonged forms of partial complex status epilepticus (Mikati *et al.* 1985).

HUMAN IMMUNODEFICIENCY VIRUS (HIV) INFECTION
HIV type 1 is a retrovirus which is responsible for the acquired immunodeficiency syndrome (AIDS), a severe acquired immunodeficiency that results in multiple infections with opportunistic microorganisms. The immunologic deficit is associated with viral infection of cell populations of the immune system, essentially T4 lymphocytes and macrophages. HIV infection and disease have been recognized in paediatric patients since 1983. HIV infection in infants and children may involve a wide spectrum of clinical diseases in multiple systems. Approximately 80 per cent of paediatric cases are due to vertical infection, 20 per cent to transfusion or other blood products and about 1 per cent to sexual contact in adolescents.

It seems that a majority of vertically transmitted HIV infections are acquired during the birth process rather than prenatally, although this can occur (Oxtoby 1990). Duliège *et al.* (1995) have shown that the firstborn of twin sets was more likely to become infected and that caesarian section reduced the frequency of transmission suggesting that most cases were acquired during passage through the birth canal. Rupture of the membranes more than four hours before birth seems to be associated with a higher risk of transmission to the baby than later rupture, again favouring an intrapartum contamination (Chapter 1). The rate of transmission is between 15 and 20 per cent in Western countries and of the order of 30 per cent in Africa (European Collaborative Study 1991, 1994; Husson *et al.* 1995). The transmission rate is higher with preterm birth and when infection of mothers is severe with confirmed AIDS (Abrams *et al.* 1995, Peckham and Gibb 1995), and the severity of HIV infection in the infant is greater in such cases. Infants born to mothers with AIDS at the time of birth more often develop symptoms and die before 18 months of age than other infected infants (Duliège *et al.* 1992, Tovo *et al.* 1992, Blanche *et al.* 1994, Abrams *et al.* 1995).

Approximately 26 per cent of infected children become symptomatic in the first year of life, and 40 per cent by 4 years (European Collaborative Group 1994, Grubman *et al.* 1995); 70 per cent are alive at 6 years and 50 per cent at 9 years (Tovo *et al.* 1992). The risk of acquired encephalopathy is higher in infants with AIDS than in those of asymptomatic HIV infection (Lobato *et al.* 1995), and greater in AIDS-defining conditions (Belman *et al.* 1996).

HIV is a neurotropic virus although productive infection in the CNS is probably limited to macrophages and microglia.

Brain involvement can occur soon after infection as infected microglia has been identified as early as seven days after transfusion of infected blood. The mechanism of neurological disease probably involves indirect effects such as expression by macrophages of cytokines or toxicity of virus products for neurons (Epstein and Gendelman 1993).

Pathological findings (Sharer *et al.* 1986) include diminished brain weight for age. Inflammatory cell infiltrates consisting of microglia, lymphocytes, plasma cells and, especially, multinucleated giant cells are distributed throughout the brain but are more prominent in the deep structures, including the basal ganglia and brainstem. Prominent inflammatory changes and calcification of small or medium-sized vessels are present, especially in the deep brain structures. These may explain the occurrence of ischaemic infarcts and strokes in children with AIDS (Park *et al.* 1988, Frank *et al.* 1989). The spinal cord only rarely shows the vacuolar myelopathy which is frequent in adults (Dickson *et al.* 1989).

The *clinical manifestations* of involvement of the CNS by HIV-1 may appear between 1 month of age and adolescence. *Encephalopathy* is a prominent manifestation (Lobato *et al.* 1995). In the severe forms of early onset, it features loss of acquired milestones, impaired brain growth with increasing microcephaly and the progressive development of neurological signs, especially involving the pyramidal tracts bilaterally. Abnormal tone and reflexes are present and ataxia may occur in older children (Belman *et al.* 1985; European Collaborative Study 1990; Belman 1990, 1992; Duliège *et al.* 1992). The clinical picture is reminiscent of that of the leukodystrophies. However, systemic manifestations of HIV-1 infection, especially pulmonary infections, are usually present as there is a rough parallelism between the neurological features and the severity of immunodepression (European Collaborative Group 1991, Duliège *et al.* 1992). In a few patients, the neurological features may appear in isolation so the diagnosis of AIDS should always be considered in progressive neurological disorders in infancy and childhood.

Neurological symptoms and signs may appear at a later age. They may present as spastic diplegia in children aged 2–5 years (Belman 1990, 1992). Some children develop progressive dementia in later childhood. Isolated hearing loss may occur in a small percentage of children (Grubman *et al.* 1995).

More subtle abnormalities include absence of developmental progress and/or behavioural disturbances such as attention deficit disorder, found in 12 per cent of patients (Gay *et al.* 1995, Grubman *et al.* 1995). Sixty-seven per cent of 133 survivors had normal school achievement at a mean age of 9.5 years, 54 per cent had abnormal visuospatial and time orientation tests; and 44 per cent had speech or language delay or articulation disorders (Tardieu *et al.* 1995).

CT imaging of symptomatic children shows brain atrophy in over three-quarters of cases, and increased white matter attenuation and calcification of the basal ganglia in approximately a quarter (Belman *et al.* 1986, De Carli *et al.* 1993) (Fig. 11.13). MRI shows high signal from the white matter and cortical atrophy in most (Chamberlain *et al.* 1991, Pavlakis *et al.* 1995).

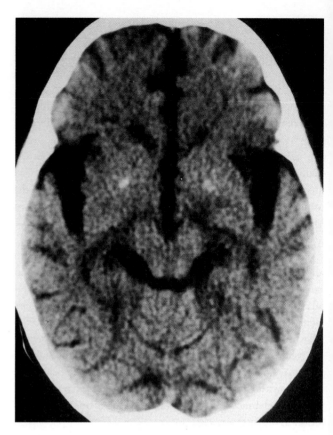

Fig. 11.13. Congenital encephalopathy due to HIV-1. Note massive brain atrophy and calcification of the basal nuclei. (Courtesy Dr Kling Chong, Great Ormond Street Hospital, London.)

The signs and symptoms point to a disorder predominating on the subcortical white matter which is in agreement with neuropathological findings and clinical symptoms suggestive of 'subcortical dementia'.

The CSF is most often normal but may contain a mild excess of lymphocytes associated with a modest, often transient, elevation of protein. Chronic aseptic meningitis has been reported infrequently (Tardieu *et al.* 1987). Gammaglobulins may be increased and there is often evidence of intrathecal synthesis of HIV-specific antibodies.

The *diagnosis* is made by demonstrating HIV antigens or antibodies to virus antigens in serum or CSF or by culture of the virus. The latter is impractical in many centres and is often negative in neonates. Antibodies may be undetectable even in the presence of HIV antigens; their presence is difficult to interpret in infants as maternally derived antibodies may persist until age 18 months. Early detection of HIV infection in newborn infants can be achieved by serological testing for immune-complex-dissociated HIV p24 antigen. Polymerase chain reaction for the detection of proviral DNA (Husson *et al.* 1990) may be useful.

The *course of the disease* is invariably fatal but the duration may extend into adolescence. The persistence of HIV-1 antigenaemia is correlated with a high fatality rate, whereas persistent inability to detect free antigen is associated with a significantly lower mortality and slower deterioration rate.

Opportunistic infections of the CNS are less common than in adults but may occur. In children, bacterial infections caused by common pathogens are common (Krasinski *et al.* 1988). Toxoplasmosis, cryptococcal meningoencephalitis, infection with atypical mycobacteria (Shope *et al.* 1994) and aspergillosis (Kline *et al.* 1994) may also occur. Certain children have recently been shown to be unusually sensitive to atypical mycobacteria as a result of a mutation of their interferon-gamma-receptor gene (Newport *et al.* 1996). A related mutation may be associated with fatal Bacille Calmette–Guérin infection (Jouanguy *et al.* 1996). Rare cases of disseminated viral infection in children with AIDS are on record (Vandersteenhoven *et al.* 1992, Herrold and Hahn 1994).

Treatment of HIV encephalopathy is currently unsatisfactory although there is a trend towards a lengthening of the infection-free period and a decrease of severity of neurological complications. Azidothymidine (AZT) via continuous intravenous infusion for several months may improve the neurodevelopmental state and decrease the mortality rate (Blanche *et al.* 1993). It seems to be partly effective against encephalopathy (Pizzo *et al.* 1988).Other drugs (dideoxycytidine and dideoxyadenosine) are being tested. Immunoglobulin therapy has been found effective in the prevention of bacterial infections (Spector *et al.* 1994). Combined therapy with multiple agents has significantly improved results (Collier *et al.* 1996, Kline *et al.* 1996, Luzuriaga *et al.* 1997). Ribavirin has been disappointing. Treatment of infectious complications of AIDS has been reviewed extensively by Glatt *et al.* (1988). Some degree of prevention of maternally transmitted infection seems possible with AZT or other agents (Connor *et al.* 1994, *Lancet* 1994, Abrams *et al.* 1995, Duliège *et al.* 1995, Corey and Holmes 1996, Sperling *et al.* 1996).

HUMAN T LYMPHOCYTE VIRUS (HTLV) INFECTION
HTLV-1 has been shown to be the agent of pure spastic paraplegia observed mainly in warm countries (tropical spastic paraplegia) and in Southern Japan (HTLV-1-associated myelopathy). The disorder is usually manifest only in adults (Shibasaki *et al.* 1988) although infection is probably early in life (Van Dyke *et al.* 1995), possibly through human milk. Rare cases have been reported in children as young as 6 or 7 years of age (Roman 1988, Gessain and Gout 1992), and occasional familial cases are on record (Mori *et al.* 1987). Pathologically, there are chronic inflammatory signs in the spinal cord, and the virus has been shown to be present locally (Höllsberg and Hafler 1993, Kuroda *et al.* 1994, Lehky *et al.* 1995). In about half the cases, MRI of the brain may show disseminated lesions (Gessain and Gout 1992). Optic atrophy and cerebellar signs are found in some patients and may occasionally be prominent (Kira *et al.* 1993). An almost identical disorder can result from nutritional and toxic factors, particularly the consumption of insufficiently dried cassava (Howlett *et al.* 1990). HTLV-2 virus infection in adult patients may produce the related clinical picture of tropical ataxic neuropathy (Harrington *et al.* 1993), a disorder which can also result from dietary deficiencies and, possibly, from toxic factors.

Treatment with anabolic steroids has been proposed.

NONCONVENTIONAL AGENTS (PRION DISEASES)
Diseases attributed to 'slow viruses' or prions are increasingly observed in adults (Prusiner and Hsiao 1994). They include Creutzfeld–Jakob disease, Gerstmann–Sträussler–Scheinker disease (Brown *et al.* 1994b) and fatal familial insomnia (Medori *et al.* 1992). Pathologically they are characterized by a spongiform encephalopathy with the presence in some cases of amyloid plaques. They present clinically with slowly progressive disturbances, mainly dementia, myoclonus and cerebellar signs. In about 15 per cent of cases, these diseases are inherited as dominant genetic conditions but they may also be transmitted experimentally to animals or accidentally to humans. Most appear to occur sporadically. Cases of Creutzfeld–Jakob disease have been reported in children who became infected through treatment of dwarfism with human extractive growth hormone (Billette de Villemeur *et al.* 1996). The disorder was marked initially by cerebellar signs followed by deterioration and myoclonus, leading to death in a few months (Brown *et al.* 1994b). Exceptional cases have been observed in adolescents following accidental intracerebral inoculation of the agent through improperly sterilized EEG depth electrodes. Iatrogenic cases run a faster course than the classical types and show cerebellar involvement pathologically (Brown *et al.* 1994a, Deslys *et al.* 1994). A new type of prion disease of probable bovine origin (bovine spongiform encephalopathy) has been recently observed in humans in the UK with features and age of occurrence similar to those of Creutzfeld–Jakob disease due to growth hormone inoculation (Will *et al.* 1996, Epstein and Brown 1997). A new CSF marker for prion diseases (14-3-3 protein) has been identified (Hsich *et al.* 1996). The mechanism of prion diseases remains imperfectly understood (Collinge 1996).

MENINGOENCEPHALITIS IN IMMUNODEPRESSED CHILDREN
Patients with congenital or acquired immunodeficiency are prone to acquire certain viral infections or to respond by an unusual disorder to common viral pathogens.

DELAYED TYPE OF ACUTE MEASLES ENCEPHALITIS
Acute delayed measles encephalitis is observed mainly in immunocompromised patients (Murphy and Yunis 1976) although it occasionally occurs in children with apparently normal immune mechanisms. Contrary to what occurs in the usual postinfectious encephalomyelitides, the measles virus is present in large quantities within the brain and nucleocapsids are seen by electron microscopy in the nuclei of glial cells and neurons. The inflammatory reaction is variable but often inconspicuous (Lacroix *et al.* 1995).

The disease occurs two to six months following measles or contact with cases of measles. Epileptic seizures are often a prominent symptom and *epilepsia partialis continua* is the first manifestation in many cases (Aicardi *et al.* 1977, Luna *et al.* 1990, Barthez-Carpentier *et al.* 1992). Progressive deterioration with obtundation and coma rapidly appears, and focal signs, especially hemiplegia, are common. New neurological signs continue to appear for variable durations. In some patients, a retinopathy is present (Haltia *et al.* 1977).

The diagnosis may be difficult as CSF may be normal or show only slight changes. In a majority of cases, there is intrathecal synthesis of specific anti-measles antibodies and a high titre of antibodies against measles virus in the serum and CSF. In the most severely depressed children, however, the antibody titre may be mildly elevated or normal (Aicardi *et al.* 1977).

CT scan usually gives normal images. Hypodense images in the central grey matter have been reported (Colamaria *et al.* 1989b). MRI may show areas of intense signal in T_2-weighted sequences (Barthez-Carpentier *et al.* 1992). The EEG may show slowing of the basal activity with repetitive slow-wave complexes at a rate of about 1 Hz (Aicardi *et al.* 1977, Colamaria *et al.* 1989b).

The course of the illness is usually fatal. Arrest of the disease may occur but the rare survivors are left with severe sequelae (Mustafa *et al.* 1993).

The rare occurrence of acute delayed encephalitis in patients without overt immunosuppression is poorly understood. A deficit of specific defences against the measles virus has been postulated (Lyon *et al.* 1977).

CHRONIC ENTEROVIRUS INFECTION IN CHILDREN WITH X-LINKED HYPOGAMMAGLOBULINAEMIA

Children with X-linked hypogammaglobulinaemia (Bruton disease) often suffer viral CNS infections in addition to bacterial complications (purulent meningitis).

The most common such infections are caused by echoviruses and by coxsackie B3 virus (Cooper *et al.* 1983). The clinical picture may be that of a *chronic lymphocytic meningitis* with variable features of brain involvement such as disturbances of consciousness and focal seizures or neurological deficits. The course is chronic and often fatal. Treatment by intrathecal and intraventricular injection of gammaglobulins may be successful (Erlendsson *et al.* 1985) but must be continued indefinitely and failures occur (Johnson *et al.* 1985). Patients with Bruton disease may also suffer from a *chronic progressive encephalopathy* characterized by seizures often myoclonic in type and progressive motor and intellectual deterioration, very similar to the encephalopathy of AIDS. In most such cases, examination of the CSF gives normal results. The EEG may show a repetitive pattern reminiscent of that observed in subacute sclerosing panencephalitis, or a periodic myoclonic pattern (Colamaria *et al.* 1989a). Optic atrophy has been reported (Lyon *et al.* 1980). The course seems to be regularly fatal. Thirteen cases have been reported recently by Rudge *et al.* (1996), seven in association with X-linked hypogammaglobulinaemia. Eight presented as a pure encephalopathy, four with both encephalitis and myelitis, and one as a pure myelopathy. Three patients had a pigmentary retinopathy, two had sensorineural hearing loss, and three also had features of dermatomyositis. CSF pleocytosis was present in nine cases and brain atrophy in eight.

Although the disease resembles a viral illness, no pathogen has been isolated so far. No treatment is available.

OTHER INFECTIONS IN IMMUNOSUPPRESSED CHILDREN
Cytomegalovirus (CMV) infection
CMV infection may cause a nodular encephalitis which has been responsible for neurological complications in adults with AIDS (Masdeu *et al.* 1988, Vinters *et al.* 1989). In children, this complication is only rarely observed with AIDS but cases of progressive CNS disease occur in children with other diseases that cause immunodepression. Cases of CMV encephalitis in children are infrequent. Riikonen (1993) has reported aggravation of congenital CMV disease following treatment of infantile spasms with ACTH or steroids. Treatment of progressive CMV encephalitis with ganciclovir and foscarnet may be effective (Masdeu *et al.* 1988, Bamborschke *et al.* 1992).

Poliovirus infection
Poliovirus in immunodepressed patients can induce a typical picture of paralytic poliomyelitis. This has been reported in X-linked hypogammaglobulinaemia (Wright *et al.* 1977) and in T-cell disorders. An exceptional patient may develop a more diffuse disease with encephalitic involvement and calcification of the thalami following immunization with live, attenuated virus (Davis *et al.* 1977; and one personal case).

Varicella-zoster infection
Disseminated encephalomyelitis due to varicella-zoster infection has been reported in adults and children with immunodepression (Carmack *et al.* 1993, Herrold and Hahn 1994).

Human papovavirus infection
Progressive multifocal leukoencephalopathy caused by human papovaviruses (JC virus and exceptionally SV40 virus) is mainly encountered in adults with underlying diseases such as lymphoma, AIDS and other illnesses causing immunosuppression (Willoughby *et al.* 1980). Only a handful of cases are on record in adolescents (Redfearn *et al.* 1993).

Epstein–Barr virus (EBV) infection
EBV infection may be responsible for a severe and often fatal illness in certain families in which a special sensitivity to EBV appears to be transmitted as an X-linked character. This disease is known as the *X-linked lymphoproliferative syndrome* (Grierson and Purtilo 1987) and variably features fatal infectious mononucleosis, malignant lymphoma, acquired hypo- or agammaglobulinaemia, virus-associated haemophagocytic syndrome (Wilson *et al.* 1981) or associations of several of these features (Pagano 1992). It might be due to unregulated cytotoxic lymphocytic responses to EBV. A similar syndrome of mono- or polyclonal lymphocyte proliferation may occur in immunosuppressed patients, especially in transplant recipients (Randhawa *et al.* 1992). It may improve with diminution of immunosuppressive therapy.

Subacute focal adenovirus encephalitis
This disorder (Chou *et al.* 1973) has not been reported in children. Fatal encephalitis may occur in receivers of transplants (Davis *et al.* 1988).

Nonviral infections

Nonviral infections are also prone to occur in immunodepressed children with malignant diseases or immunosuppression due to therapy or to disease.

NONINFECTIOUS NEUROLOGICAL DISORDERS THAT CAN MIMIC INFECTION IN IMMUNODEPRESSED PATIENTS

Many of the neurological manifestations that occur in cases of severe combined immunodeficiency (*e.g.* in adenosine deaminase deficiency) are of infectious origin. However, immunodeficiency due to *purine nucleoside phosphorylase (PNP) deficiency* is associated with spastic tetraparesis and mental retardation that seem to be a direct consequence of the metabolic defect (Simmonds *et al.* 1987). Recently, the case of dysequilibrium–diplegia syndrome reported by Graham-Pole *et al.* (1975) has been shown to be a case of PNP deficiency (Chapter 10).

VIRUS INFECTIONS WITH SPECIAL CHARACTERISTICS

This section deals with some special problems including paralytic poliomyelitis, vascular involvement in varicella-zoster infection and cases of acute focal encephalitis.

PARALYTIC POLIOMYELITIS

With widespread immunization, poliomyelitis has become a preventable disease and only rare sporadic cases are encountered in industrialized countries. However, the disease remains prevalent in some third world countries and clusters of imported cases may still be observed.

Infection by polioviruses is most often inapparent or associated with a mild nonspecific febrile illness. Lymphocytic meningitis is also possible and the paralytic form of the disease is uncommon. This is, at least in part, related to the presence in the host of specific virus receptors without which the virus is unable to enter neural cells.

The *pathological lesions* involve the anterior horn cells, the motor and sensory cranial nuclei of the medulla, the reticular formation, the cerebellar vermis and, to a lesser extent, the thalamus and layers III and V of the motor cortex. Neurons undergo degenerative changes accompanied by an initially polymorphonuclear reaction which later becomes mononuclear.

The *clinical manifestations* appear after an incubation period of 3–35 days. Initial symptoms consist of headache, vomiting and fever, followed, within two to five days, by signs of meningeal irritation and severe pain in the lower back and limbs. Paralysis appears during the first two days of the major illness. The common spinal poliomyelitis is characterized by asymmetrical flaccid paralysis involving the legs, arms and/or trunk with absent tendon reflexes. Urinary retention is present at onset in 20–30 per cent of cases. The bulbar form is rarely isolated as at least the cervical cord is involved in 90 per cent of cases. All cranially innervated muscles may be affected. In addition, respiratory failure and hypertension may result from involvement of the brainstem reticular substance. Encephalitic signs may be associated but they may also be due to respiratory insufficiency consequent upon paralysis of diaphragmatic and intercostal muscles.

Examination of the CSF shows 30–200 cells/mm^3. Initially, these are predominantly polymorphonuclear cells, followed after five to seven days by a lymphocytic pleocytosis. The protein content rises late, reaching a maximum about the 25th day of illness.

A recent report (Kibe *et al.* 1996) described swelling of the spinal cord with an abnormal signal from its central part in one case.

Before clinical onset the virus can be isolated from the stools and oropharynx as early as 19 days and as late as three months after the first clinical features (mean five weeks). Typing of the virus shows one of the three types of poliovirus. Serological diagnosis is made by demonstration of an elevation of the titre of neutralizing or complement-fixing antibodies.

The *prognosis* of paralytic poliomyelitis depends on the extent of involvement. Recovery in some affected muscles is frequent for up to one year or more but muscles still totally paralysed after one month usually remain so definitively. A progressive motor neuron disease (*post-polio syndrome*) resembling amyotrophic sclerosis is sometimes observed in adults 20 or more years after an acute attack (Dalakas 1986).

Cases of *paralytic poliomyelitis due to live vaccine* may occur in immunocompromised patients receiving the vaccine or in contacts (Nkowane *et al.* 1987, Sen *et al.* 1989). Such cases may have an atypical presentation. Although a majority of the cases of postvaccinal poliomyelitis have been in immunocompetent children, defective immunity should be systematically looked for (Groom *et al.* 1994). Rare cases of poliomyelitis in vaccinated nonimmunodepressed children are on record (Dussaix *et al.* 1987).

The diagnosis is easy provided the disease is kept in mind. Guillain–Barré syndrome differs in its mode of onset, the symmetrical distribution of weakness and CSF characteristics. Rare cases of paralytic disease due to other viruses have been recorded (Kyllerman *et al.* 1993) as well as cases of intoxication by chemicals or insect bites (Gear 1981). A syndrome of acute peripheral paralysis closely resembling poliomyelitis (*Hopkins syndrome*) has been reported following acute asthmatic attacks or asthmatic status epilepticus (Mizuno *et al.* 1995). Various viruses have been isolated from such cases (Nihei *et al.* 1987, Shahar *et al.* 1991, Kyllerman *et al.* 1993).

VASCULITIS CAUSED BY VARICELLA-ZOSTER VIRUS INFECTION

Nervous system syndromes associated with varicella-zoster infections include varicella myositis, zoster radiculopathy, zoster myelitis (Rosenfeld *et al.* 1993, Gilden *et al.* 1994, Herrold and Hahn 1994), cranial neuropathy including Ramsay Hunt syndrome, and meningoencephalitis (MacKendall and Klawans 1978). A distinctive syndrome of herpes zoster ophthalmicus followed by ipsilateral cerebral angiitis and consequent contralateral hemiplegia has been described in adults and has been recorded with infantile zoster ophthalmicus following intrauterine chickenpox (Leis and Butler 1987). A closely related syndrome of delayed hemiparesis following chickenpox is on record (Kamholz and Tremblay 1985, Ichiyama *et al.* 1990). The mechanism of angiitis is unclear but the presence of the virus in the CNS has been demonstrated. Some of the adult patients were immunocompromised. Disseminated infarcts have been reported in some cases (Tsolia *et al.* 1995) although usually only large brain arteries are involved (Amlie-Lefond *et al.* 1995). Involvement of the basal ganglia (Silverstein and Brunberg 1995) and lateral medullary syndrome (Kovacs *et al.* 1993) have been reported.

ACUTE FOCAL ENCEPHALITIS
Acute focal encephalitis affecting a limited territory during infection with coxsackie A9 (Roden *et al.* 1975, Chahlub *et al.* 1977) and echovirus 25 (Peters *et al.* 1979) can produce acute hemiplegia or hemichorea. Lacunar lesion in the central grey matter or internal capsule may result from vascular infarction or focal cerebritis.

DISORDERS OF PRESUMED VIRAL CAUSE
BEHÇET SYNDROME
Behçet syndrome is rare in children but has been reported in infants as young as 2 months (Ammann *et al.* 1985). A transient form has been observed in babies born to affected mothers (Lewis and Priestley 1986). The disease features recurrent ulcerations of the mouth and genitalia, skin lesions often resembling erythema nodosum, anterior uveitis, keratitis, hypopyon and, less commonly, retinal involvement that in some cases may be isolated. CNS involvement is present in up to 25 per cent of patients and may rarely precede the oculocutaneous manifestations. Neurological manifestations may indicate involvement of the cerebral hemispheres, spinal cord, cerebellum or brainstem (Nakamura *et al.* 1994). Pseudotumour cerebri with or without sinus thrombosis may be observed (Shakir *et al.* 1990). MRI may show disseminated areas of intense signal in T_2 sequences (Wechsler *et al.* 1993). The brainstem is consistently involved. Perivenous infiltrates with or without thrombosis are frequent (Wechsler *et al.* 1992). The disease may present as a cerebrovascular disease (Iragui and Maravi 1986) or as a chronic brainstem encephalitis (Iseki *et al.* 1988). The diagnosis may be helped by the cutaneous sensitivity to mechanical trauma (pathergy). Many Oriental patients belong to the HLA B5 group. The prognosis is guarded although the disorder is not usually fatal (Rakover *et al.* 1989), and recurrences are not rare. Treatment with immosuppressant drugs has been used with some measure of success (O'Duffy *et al.* 1984, Yazici *et al.* 1990).

MOLLARET MENINGITIS
Mollaret meningitis is a multirecurrent mononuclear meningitis of undetermined, but not necessarily single, cause. Attacks of aseptic meningitis recur at irregular intervals for months or years. Large mononuclear cells are present in the earliest stages of an attack preceding lymphocytic pleocytosis (Stoppe *et al.* 1987). Viral infections (Graham 1987, Picard *et al.* 1993) are sometimes demonstrated. In some patients, an epidermoid cyst has been

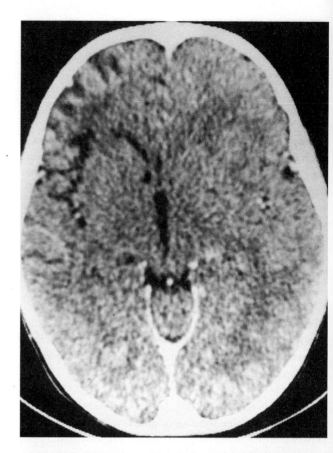

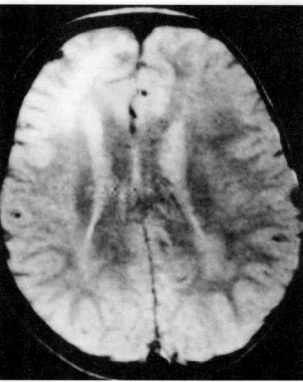

Fig. 11.14. Rasmussen encephalitis. 3½-year-old girl with left partial motor seizures and left-sided choreoathetotic movements and weakness for one year. Right frontal biopsy showed glial nodules and perivascular cuffing. *(Top)* CT scan showing atrophy of right hemisphere, especially anteriorly. *(Bottom)* MRI scan, T_2-weighted sequence. Intense signal from right frontal cortex and subcortical white matter.

found to be the cause and such an aetiology should always be carefully excluded (De Chadarévian and Becker 1988).

HARADA–VOGT–KOYANAGY DISEASE
Harada–Vogt–Koyanagy disease is a rare cause of uveomeningitis that may simulate multiple sclerosis. Bilateral posterior uveitis with retinal detachment may accompany or precede disseminated neurological signs. Auditory loss and areas of skin and hair depigmentation often appear. The course is subacute but neurological recovery within months with auditory and visual sequelae is the rule (Gruich *et al.* 1995).

LETHARGIC (EPIDEMIC) ENCEPHALITIS
Lethargic (epidemic) encephalitis which occurred in a major epidemic in the 1920s is now rare. Howard and Lees (1987) have established diagnostic criteria (somnolence, akinetic mutism, ophthalmoplegia, basal ganglia involvement, oculogyric crises) that are satisfied in an occasional patient. Parkinsonism, sometimes only transient, may supervene (Mellon *et al.* 1991).

RASMUSSEN ENCEPHALITIS
Rasmussen encephalitis is an inflammatory condition of the brain that involves particularly the frontal and temporal lobes in a predominantly or exclusively unilateral distribution (Fig. 11.14) and manifests clinically as focal seizures and often as *epilepsia partialis continua* (Gupta *et al.* 1984). Reports of detection of cytomegalovirus and Epstein–Barr virus in the brain (Walter and Renella 1989, Jay *et al.* 1995) await confirmation.

CHRONIC FATIGUE SYNDROME
The chronic fatigue syndrome, also known as Akureyri disease, neuromyasthenia or postviral fatigue syndrome (Behan *et al.* 1985, Marshall *et al.* 1991), is a poorly defined syndrome of myalgia, fatigue and, at times, paraesthesiae and muscle fasciculations, which follows a presumed viral infection and can persist for weeks and months. Biochemical study of such cases has been negative (Byrne and Trounce 1987). The disorder occurs often in epidemics in hospitals or other institutions and may be of nonorganic origin in some cases.

INFANTILE BILATERAL STRIATAL NECROSIS (IBSN)
IBSN is an acute neurological disorder marked by fever and often CSF pleocytosis, obtundation and sometimes seizures, followed within a few days by the appearance of extrapyramidal rigidity and dystonia, exacerbated intermittently in stereotyped attacks of paroxysmal tonic contractions, usually in flexion, with facial grimacing and protracted monotonous whining. CT and MRI show bilateral hypodensities involving predominantly the putamina in a symmetrical manner (Fig. 11.15). Considerable oedematous swelling initially extends into the neighbouring white matter but progressively disappears. The clinical abnormalities tend to decrease over weeks or months and may even disappear (Fujita *et al.* 1994), and no recurrences have been reported. Extrapyramidal sequelae persist in most cases (Goutières and Aicardi 1982, Rosemberg *et al.* 1992) but mild cases with

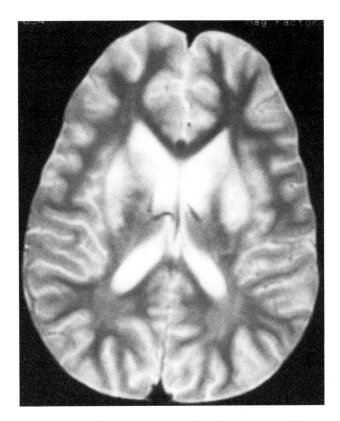

Fig. 11.15. Acute bilateral striatal necrosis. T$_2$-weighted MRI showing low signal from the basal ganglia extending into surrounding white matter. 4-year-old child with acute onset of fever, disturbances of consciousness and convulsions with subsequent development of rigidity and dystonia. Pleocytosis in CSF and negative metabolic studies. (Courtesy Dr Arzimanoglou, Hôpital Robert Debré, Paris.)

full recovery occur (Kim *et al.* 1995). The nature of this syndrome is unclear. The acute onset, fever and association, in some cases, with evidence of *M. pneumoniae* infection (Larsen and Crisp 1992, Saitoh *et al.* 1993) suggest an infectious process, and a relationship to encephalitis lethargica has been discussed (Al-Mateen *et al.* 1988). Alternatively, a metabolic abnormality such as mitochondrial disorder or organic aciduria, decompensated by an intercurrent disease, might be responsible. De Meirleir *et al.* (1995) have reported IBSN of a less acute form in a child with a mutation in the mitochondrial *ATPase 6* gene. Acute bilateral infarction of the striatum may be seen following trauma (Brett 1991) or spontaneously (Bogousslavsky *et al.* 1988) but the clinical picture differs by the absence of inflammatory features. Cases with similar imaging features but with a chronic course and often a familial transmission are discussed in Chapter 10 (see Mito *et al.* 1986, Roig *et al.* 1993) and may represent mitochondrial disorders.

A possibly related syndrome features *acute symmetrical thalamic necrosis* (Yagishita *et al.* 1995, Mizuguchi 1997) following an acute, apparently viral disorder such as influenza, acute diarrhoeal disease or herpes virus 6 infection (Oki *et al.* 1995). Affected infants develop a sudden quadriplegia and are left with severe sequelae including persistent vegetative state. Leigh disease and other mitochondrial abnormalities were excluded. The syndrome has been mainly reported from Japan but non-Japanese cases are on record (Wang and Huang 1993, Cusmai *et al.* 1994, Pedro Vieira 1995; and personal case).

MYCOTIC INFECTIONS OF THE NERVOUS SYSTEM

Mycotic infections of the nervous system produce granulomatous meningitis or abscesses. In a majority of cases, mycotic infections occur as opportunistic infections in patients with a primary disorder that diminishes resistance or requires antibiotic therapy.

CANDIDA INFECTIONS
Candida albicans can invade the meninges from the bloodstream in cases of disseminated candidiasis. Such cases occur mostly in young infants who receive prolonged antibiotic treatment or suffer immunosuppression. Small preterm infants with congenital anomalies, receiving total parenteral nutrition, and patients with shunted hydrocephalus are candidates for the development of generalized *Candida* infections (Feigin and Cherry 1987).

Widespread microabscesses in the brain are more common than gross abscess formation. Vascular invasion with granulomatous vasculitis and thrombi formation with resultant necrosis and haemorrhages is not rare (Roessmann and Friede 1967).

Because of the debility of most patients, the clinical manifestations of candidiasis of the CNS easily escape recognition, and a high index of suspicion should be kept for all infants with predisposing factors. The course of the illness is usually subacute. Mild fever and irritability may be present but the disease may be almost asymptomatic (Lenoir *et al.* 1990). CSF study inconstantly shows pleocytosis, raised protein and low glucose levels. Culture of the CSF is occasionally positive. Some patients present with hydrocephalus caused by basilar blockage (Héron *et al.* 1990). Neurological manifestations such as hemiparesis and cranial nerve palsies may occur (Coker and Beltran 1988). CT scan may show ventricular dilatation, sometimes with periventricular enhancement.

Diagnosis is often made only shortly before death as there are few suggestive signs and the organism is difficult to culture. Yet, in infants with risk factors, even a single colony of yeast in the CSF should not be considered a contaminant and treatment should be considered even without positive identification (Faix 1984).

Treatment with amphotericin B and 5-fluorocytosine is effective if given relatively early (Chesney *et al.* 1978).

CRYPTOCOCCUS NEOFORMANS INFECTION
Cryptococosis is a systemic fungal infection whose frequency has escalated in recent years as the number of immunosuppressed patients has increased. CNS involvement is the most serious complication. The organism produces a granulomatous arachnoiditis that may cause hydrocephalus, cranial nerve palsies and vasculitis of large vessels. The disease may also occur in previously well children (Tjia *et al.* 1985).

Headache is the main symptom. Fever is only inconstantly present. Disturbances of consciousness eventually develop. Cranial nerve involvement, especially of the VIth nerve, and papilloedema are commonly seen. Impairment of consciousness and areflexia, probably due to spinal arachnoiditis, signify a poor prognosis.

The diagnosis of cryptococcosis is difficult, especially in immunosuppressed patients. The CSF usually shows moderate lymphocytic pleocytosis, increased protein and low sugar. India ink staining demonstrates yeasts in only 60 per cent of patients with positive culture. Cultures may take many days to yield growth and may be initially negative in up to 25 per cent of cases. Demonstration of the presence of antigen in the CSF is both reliable and specific. However, patients with immunosuppres-sion have positive cultures and antigen tests but these are often negative in nonimmunocompromised patients (Berlin and Pincus 1989). An oligoclonal IgG and IgM response in CSF is usually found (La Mantia *et al.* 1987). The CSF may be normal in some cases, hence the need to repeat lumbar puncture and to culture large amounts of fluid. CT scan may show cerebral oedema, hydrocephalus and occasionally mass lesions (Fujita *et al.* 1981).

Untreated CNS cryptococcocis is regularly fatal. Treatment with amphotericin B, 1 mg/kg/d, in association with 5-fluorocytosine, 150 mg/kg/d, in divided doses, is effective but late recurrences are possible. Monitoring of blood levels is necessary (Como and Dismukes 1993). It is effective in the prevention of relapses (Powderly *et al.* 1992). Ketoconazole is used for the treatment of non-CNS cryptococcocis but does not cross the blood–brain barrier. Sequelae in late-treated cases may include blindness, deafness and chronic hydrocephalus.

OTHER MYCOTIC INFECTIONS
HISTOPLASMOSIS AND COCCIDIOIDOSIS
CNS infections caused by *Coccidioides immitis* and by *Histoplasma capsulatum* are rare in Western Europe. The latter is common in some regions of the Americas. CNS infection occurs as part of a disseminated infection usually with pulmonary manifestations. Clinical features include headaches, low-grade fever, weight loss and minimal meningeal signs. Hydrocephalus occasionally results (Plouffe and Fass 1980). The diagnosis is suggested by the presence of pulmonary lesions and can be confirmed by the detection of antibodies against the organisms (Wheat *et al.* 1986). Amphotericin is effective. Fluconazole has been shown to be active (Rivera *et al.* 1992).

MUCORMYCOSIS
Mucormycosis is a rare fungal infection that usually occurs in diabetic or immunosuppressed patients. It is caused by *Phycomycetes* of the genera *Mucor*, *Absidia* and *Rhizopus* that invade the base of the brain from the paranasal cavities, causing arterial and/or venous thrombosis and consequent infarction (Cuadrado *et al.* 1988, Washburn *et al.* 1988, Galetta *et al.* 1990). Treatment is with amphotericin B and debridement. Removal of the eye may be necessary. Hyperbaric oxygen is being tried.

TABLE 11.16
Some protozoan and parasitic infestations of the CNS

Disease (organism)	Main clinical features	Treatment	References
Amoebiasis (*Naegleria*)	Meningoencephalitis	Amphotericin B, miconazole, rifampin	Lowichik and Ruff (1995a), Barnett *et al.* (1996)
Amoebiasis (*Entamoeba histolytica*)	Brain abscess secondary to hepatic and pulmonary involvement	Emetine, chloroquine, metronidazole	Schmutzhard *et al.* (1986)
Visceral larva migrans (*Toxocara canis* or *T. cati*)	Encephalopathy, seizures, optic neuritis, myelitis	None	Arpino *et al.* (1990), Fortenberry *et al.* (1991)
African trypanosomiasis (*T. gambiense* or *T. rhodesiense*)	Convulsions, disturbed consciousness, sometimes focal deficits (hemiplegia), spastic diplegia, choreoathetosis	Tryparsamide	Bittencourt *et al.* (1988)
Schistosomiasis (*S. japonicum, S. mansoni, S. hematobium*)	Transverse myelitis, granuloma of spinal cord, radiculitis, encephalopathy	Niridazole, praziquantel, metrafonate, oxamniquine	Bittencourt *et al.* (1988), Boyce (1990), Haribhai *et al.* (1991)
Trichinosis (*T. spiralis*)	Fever, myalgia, encephalopathy, focal signs, papilloedema	Thiabendazole, corticosteroids	Fröscher *et al.* (1988), Fourestié *et al.* (1993)

OTHER MYCOTIC INFECTIONS OF THE CNS
These include aspergillosis (Walsh *et al.* 1985) and blastomycosis, which mainly cause brain abscess, and sporotrichosis (Fetter *et al.* 1967).

PROTOZOAN AND PARASITIC INFESTATION OF THE CNS

With the exception of toxoplasmosis and, to a certain extent, of cysticercosis, protozoan or parasitic involvement of the CSF is rare in industrialized countries. Malaria is, however, of increasing importance because mass travel to infested countries has developed enormously and because preventive treatment is not always taken or effective. Table 11.16 lists some features of some parasitic and protozoan diseases and refers the reader to recent literature.

MALARIA

Malaria is caused by four species of the genus *Plasmodium: P. vivax, P. falciparum, P. malariae* and *P. ovale*. Cerebral malaria is a severe complication of *P. falciparum* infestation, with an average mortality rate of 37 per cent (Bittencourt *et al.* 1988). At least 1,000,000 children are estimated to die from malaria annually in Africa alone (Zucker and Campbell 1993) and cerebral involvement is a major cause of death. Cerebral malaria is defined by three criteria: disturbances of consciousness with inability to localize pain; presence of *P. falciparum* parasitaemia; and absence of other causes of encephalopathy. Acute organic mental syndrome, movement disorders and personality changes also occur (Phillips and Solomon 1990). Focal signs are rare and transient. Cerebellar ataxia has been reported (Senanayake 1987). Seizures are common, occurring in up to 80 per cent of cases, and may be seen with any form of malaria. Febrile convulsions are a frequent presentation, often followed by coma, and if the latter persists for more than six hours cerebral involvement should be diagnosed. Status epilepticus is present in 10–20 per cent of cases. Simple febrile seizures without cerebral involvement are mainly due to benign malaria. Hypoglycaemia is present in 30 per cent of patients and is of severe prognostic significance (Molyneux *et al.* 1989). Evidence of increased ICP is conflicting. It was not seen in Thailand (Looareesuwan *et al.* 1983) but was significant in African cases (Newton *et al.* 1994) and may require therapy. Residual disability is present in about 20 per cent of survivors.

Treatment should be started without definite proof in case of doubt in any person who may have been exposed in the past two months. Parenteral quinine is recommended in most countries because of the frequency of chloroquine-resistant strains. Chloroquine remains used in uncomplicated malaria. Quinine is best administered intravenously. Combined therapy with pyrimethamine and sulfadoxine can be useful as it increases the rate of parasite clearance. Continuous infusion of quinidine gluconate has been recently advocated, sometimes in association with exchange transfusion (Miller *et al.* 1989). The latter, however, may not give better results than quinidine alone (Saddler *et al.* 1990). Corticosteroids were strongly recommended in the past but their use has no definite pathophysiological basis and is now controversial (Hoffman *et al.* 1988). The frequent occurrence of resistant organisms has also modified recommendations for prophylaxis and treatment for countries with a high proportion of resistant plasmodia. Recent advices of prophylaxis and treatment have been published (Krogstad and Herwaldt 1988, White *et al.* 1988, White 1996). Newly developed drugs such as artemether seem promising but may have significant toxicity (Taylor *et al.* 1993). Artemisine derivatives clear parasites more rapidly than quinine and can be administered once a day instead of in three divided doses. Artemether is as effective as quinine for severe malaria (Boele van Hensbroek *et al.* 1996) but its possible neurotoxicity is a cause of concern (Boele van Hensbroek *et al.* 1996, Hoffman 1996).

ACQUIRED TOXOPLASMOSIS

Infestation by *T. gondii* is rare in nonimmunodepressed persons. A few cases of acquired *Toxoplasma* encephalitis are on record (Cottrell 1986) as well as an occasional case of toxoplasmic myelitis (Mehren *et al.* 1988). Couvreur and Desmonts (1988) have reviewed extensively the literature on acquired toxoplasmosis.

NEUROCYSTICERCOSIS

Infestation by the encysted form of *Taenia solium* may occur within brain parenchyma or the basilar cisterns, causing inflammation, oedema and residual calcification. The disease is common in countries with inadequate sanitation but is also encountered in Western countries like the USA (Scharf 1988) and France. In these countries, neurocysticercosis usually presents as a single lesion which is primarily responsible for seizures, usually of focal type (Mitchell and Crawford 1988). In countries of heavy infestation, multiple lesions are frequent (Lowichik and Ruff 1995a). Such cases feature signs of increased ICP in addition to seizures (Bittencourt *et al.* 1988, Wadia *et al.* 1988). Hydrocephalus caused by racemose cysticercus in the basal cistern or the ventricular system may occur.

CT scan in the unifocal form shows at the acute stage a punctiform or ring enhancement surrounded by a focal area of oedema (Fig. 11.16). In the multifocal form, disseminated cystic areas may be seen, with diffuse brain oedema, and later multiple foci of calcification are present (Lopez-Hernandez and Garaizar 1982, Mitchell and Crawford 1988, Wadia *et al.* 1988).

Antibodies against cysticercus can help make the diagnosis (Corona *et al.* 1986).

Cases of unifocal cysticercosis in nonendemic countries usually require only anticonvulsant treatment (Scharf 1988). For severe cases, praziquantel and albendazole are both effective but their respective indications are still controversial (Alarcón *et al.* 1989, Medina *et al.* 1993, Kramer 1995). Albendazole (15 mg/kg/d for eight or 30 days) has proved effective in 85 per cent of cases, and superior to praziquantel (50 mg/kg/d for eight or 15 days) (Sotelo *et al.* 1990).

ECHINOCOCCOSIS

Endemic echinococcosis is common in sheep-raising countries where it is a common cause of intracranial hypertension (Lowichik and Ruff 1995b).

The usual form of echinococcosis is *cerebral hydatid cyst* which often reaches considerable dimensions. Due to their slow growth the cysts are relatively well-tolerated for long periods. Clinical features are mainly symptoms and signs of intracranial hypertension, while focal neurological deficits are rare.

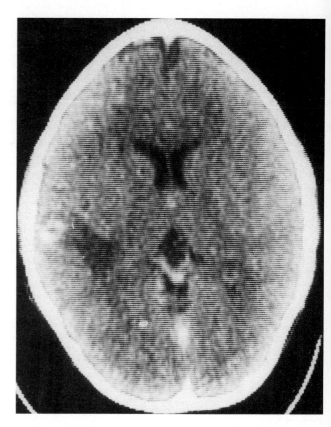

Fig. 11.16. Cerebral cysticercosis. Enhanced CT scan showing annular lesion in right parietal lobe (left side of figure) with adjacent oedema. The diagnosis was verified at surgery in this 11-year-old boy who presented with partial motor seizures.

On CT scan, the cysts appear as round or oval masses with a smooth border and a content of CSF density. In the rare multivesicular type, the image may appear heterogeneous (Sharma and Abraham 1983).

Alveolar echinococcosis is rare (Weber *et al.* 1988). Multiple cerebral localizations are usually fatal.

EOSINOPHILIC MENINGITIS

Parasitic or protozoan diseases are the most common cause of eosinophilic meningitis (Woods *et al.* 1993). However, a high proportion of eosinophilic cells (more than 4 per cent) may also be present in some cases of *C. albicans* meningitis, syphilitic meningitis, lymphocytic choriomeningitis and postoperative meningitis (personal data, unpublished), and as a late reaction to the presence of plastic material such as shunts (Kennedy and Singer 1988, Vinchon *et al.* 1992).

Angiostrongylus cantonensis is a common cause of eosinophilic meningitis in Polynesia and may cause a syndrome of radiculomyeloencephalitis (Scemama *et al.* 1988, Clouston *et al.* 1990). In Southeastern Asia, *Gnathostoma spinigerum* may also be responsible. In this case, subarachnoid haemorrhage may be associated (Schmutzhard *et al.* 1988). Other parasites (*Paragonimus westermani* and *P. cysticerci*) may be the cause (Jaroonvesama 1988).

TOXI-INFECTIONS

TETANUS

Tetanus is the result of the action of a soluble exotoxin of *Clostridium tetani*, tetanospasmin, which binds to specific receptors on the neuronal cell membrane. It is taken up by nerve terminals and is transported via retrograde axonal transport to the corresponding cell bodies and surrounding presynaptic terminals. The toxin prevents the release of inhibitory neurotransmitters from the presynaptic terminals thus producing uncontrolled firing, with consequent muscle spasms.

The spores of *C. tetani* are introduced through a wound or, rarely, a focus of anaerobic infection such as otitis media. The spores germinate and multiply and release their toxins. Isolation of *C. tetani* is successful in only 30 per cent of cases, and no responsible wound is apparent in 7–30 per cent (Crone and Reder 1992).

The *clinical manifestations* are due to both the central and peripheral actions of the toxin on the release of acetylcholine in the motor plate. Symptoms appear between three and 14 days after injury. Shorter incubations are associated with the most severe forms.

The first manifestation is usually trismus, often associated with neck and back stiffness, salivary stasis and dysphagia. Retraction of the angles of the mouth results in the classical '*risus sardonicus*' appearance.

Subsequently, rigidity becomes generalized and tetanic spasms develop, often precipitated by sensory stimuli. Consciousness is preserved. Sudden respiratory failure due to prolonged spasms, airway blockage or bronchopneumonia accounts for most fatalities.

In some cases tetanus remains localized around the infected wound, in the form of a spasm limited to neighbouring muscles.

Cephalic tetanus is consecutive to *C. tetani* otitis or a facial wound. Some degree of trismus is present. Often facial palsy and occasionally paralysis of other cranial nerves are seen. All forms of localized tetanus may secondarily become generalized.

Treatment of tetanus demands maintenance of a free airway and adequate ventilation. The use of sedatives, especially benzodiazepines, is helpful. If adequate ventilation cannot be maintained because of the spasms, neuromuscular blockade is indicated. At the same time, antibiotic treatment (usually with penicillin G) is given to eradicate the organisms, and neutralization of any as yet unbound toxin is achieved with antitoxin.

Despite such measures, the mortality of tetanus is still high. Recovery in survivors is slow with frequent sleep disturbances.

The best prophylaxis of tetanus is immunization with tetanus toxoid. However, severe tetanus may occur in immunized patients (Crone and Reder 1992). A booster dose is administered in case of a wound, especially if sustained in the countryside and/or deep and tortuous in character. In unvaccinated patients or in those with uncertain state of immunity, antitoxin and toxoid are both indicated.

Neonatal tetanus due to infection of the umbilical scar remains a major cause of neonatal mortality in some third world countries. It appears between the third and 15th days of life (Simental *et al.* 1993). The first symptom is usually failure to suck and nurse as a result of trismus. Generalized muscular rigidity and spasms then develop.

Treatment is difficult. Mechanical ventilation and neuromuscular blockade are effective but rarely available in countries where neonatal tetanus is frequent. Antitoxin (30,000 to 40,000 U), antibiotic treatment and sedatives are always used. Pyridoxine may lower the mortality (Godel 1977), which remains however around 25 per cent (Daud *et al.* 1981).

DIPHTHERIA

Diphtheria is a rare disease in developed countries. It is caused by infection with *Corynebacterium diphtheriae* that establishes on the mucous membranes of the throat and nasopharynx and produces a toxin that blocks the incorporation of amino acids into polypeptide chains.

Neurological manifestations present as one of two forms: local paralyses and polyneuropathy. Local paralyses appear four to five weeks following throat infection and consist primarily of paralysis of the soft palate and paralysis of accomodation. Oculomotor and pharyngeal paralyses are possible. Sensorimotor polyneuropathy occurs several weeks following infection and involves symmetrically all four limbs with abolition of the deep tendon reflexes. Deep sensation is more involved than motor functions because the toxin induces a segmental demyelination that predominates on the posterior roots (Solders *et al.* 1989). Cardiac involvement may occur and the neurological picture may closely resemble the Guillain–Barré syndrome.

The course is usually towards complete spontaneous cure. There is no specific treatment of diphtheritic paralyses but these are preventable by standard antitoxin therapy.

BOTULISM

Botulism is caused by the powerful toxin produced by *Clostridium botulinum*. The toxin is a simple protein that blocks acetylcholine release by impairing the influx of calcium normally associated with depolarization and produces a myasthenia-like syndrome. Three forms of botulism are known. The common type is due to ingestion of the toxin preformed in improperly sterilized preserves or canned foods. Rarely the toxin is produced as a result of a wound infection by *C. botulinum*. The third form is known as *infantile botulism*. In this type, *C. botulinum* toxin, produced by organisms in the digestive tract, is absorbed through the intestinal wall. Several toxins are known. Types A, B, E and F are usually responsible for clinical disease.

Symptoms appear within hours after ingestion of contaminated food. The major features are blurring of vision as a result of paralysis of the ciliary muscles and dilated pupils unreactive to light. Diffuse paralysis with areflexia, respiratory difficulties, dryness of the mucous membranes and bladder distension are all common. Such signs in the presence of fully preserved consciousness are highly characteristic. The diagnosis can be confirmed by EMG and repetitive stimulation of the motor nerves and by finding the toxin in the serum (Hagenah and Müller-Jensen 1978).

Infantile botulism has been recognized mainly in the USA during the past 15 years but also in Europe. It occurs in infants under 6 months of age (average 3–4 months) but may affect neonates (Thilo *et al.* 1993) and is characterized by a prodromal phase of constipation with progressive development over four or five days of the complete picture of hypotonia, areflexia, poor sucking, ptosis and paralysis of other cranial nerves and of the limbs (Thompson *et al.* 1980, Schreiner *et al.* 1991). Respiratory difficulty is frequent, and ventilatory support is necessary for most patients. Administration of aminoglycoside antibiotics may precipitate respiratory difficulties (L'Hommedieu *et al.* 1979, Long *et al.* 1985). Decreased salivation, tearing and bladder distension may occur. Changes in skin colour and fluctuations of cardio-respiratory rates are sometimes seen. Otitis media and aspiration pneumonia were seen in 32 per cent of patients in one large series (Long *et al.* 1985). Onset of the disease often follows the introduction of solid food in breast-fed babies, and ingestion of honey may be a risk factor. A mild form may be marked only by hypotonia and poor feeding (Thompson *et al.* 1980). Moreover, asymptomatic carriers are known to exist. It is thus difficult to attribute other syndromes, such as the sudden infant death syndrome, to botulism on the sole basis of isolation of *C. botulinum* from the stools (Sonnabend *et al.* 1985).

Differential diagnosis includes neonatal myasthenia, sepsis, viral CNS infections and various causes of disordered neuromuscular transmission (Swift 1981). The toxin is not present in the blood except in very rare cases (Paton *et al.* 1983). The electromyogram shows brief, low-amplitude potentials and an incremental response to fast (25–30 Hz) repetitive nerve stimulation characteristic of a presynaptic block (Guttierez *et al.* 1994). The response to slow (2–5 Hz) stimulation is more variable, with increased, normal or decreased responses (Cornblath *et al.* 1983).

Recovery takes place over a period of several weeks but some weakness may persist for months. Relapses may occur (Glauser *et al.* 1990). It is of note that large quantities of toxin are secreted for months but tolerance develops for unknown reasons.

Treatment involves both respiratory and nutritional supportive care.

OTHER TOXI-INFECTIONS

Some other bacterial infections may act on the CNS through neurotoxins. *Shigella* infection is associated with a higher incidence of convulsions than explained by associated fever (Ashkenazi *et al.* 1987). Infection by *E. coli* O157:H7 seems to be a frequent cause of the haemolytic–uraemic syndrome (Boyce *et al.* 1995). The toxic effects of *Bordetella pertussis* are discussed in Chapter 12.

REFERENCES

Abramovitz, P., Schvartzman, P., Harel, D., *et al.* (1987) 'Direct invasion of the central nervous system by *Mycoplasma pneumoniae*: a report of two cases.' *Journal of Infectious Diseases*, **155**, 482–487.
Abrams, E.J., Matheson, P.B., Thomas, P.A., *et al.* (1995) 'Neonatal predictors of infection status and early death among 332 infants at risk of HIV-1 infection monitored prospectively from birth.' *Pediatrics*, **96**, 451–458.
Ackerman, R., Rehse-Kupper, B., Gollmer, E., Schmidt, R. (1988) 'Chronic neurologic manifestations of erythema migrans borreliosis.' *Annals of the New York Academy of Sciences*, **539**, 16–23.
Adair, C.V., Gauld, R.L., Smadel, J.E. (1953) 'Aseptic meningitis, a disease of diverse etiology: clinical and etiologic studies on 854 cases.' *Annals of Internal Medicine*, **39**, 675–704.
Adair, J.C., Beck, A.C., Apfelbaum, R.I., Baringer, J.R. (1987) 'Nocardial cerebral abscess in the acquired immunodeficiency syndrome.' *Archives of Neurology*, **44**, 548–550.
Adal, K.A., Cockerell, C.J., Petri, W.A. (1994) 'Cat scratch disease, bacillary angiomatosis, and other infections due to *Rochalimaea*.' *New England Journal of Medicine*, **330**, 1509–1515.
Aicardi, J., Goutières, F., Arsenio-Nunes, M.L., Lebon, P. (1977) 'Acute measles encephalitis in children with immunosuppression.' *Pediatrics*, **55**, 232–239.
Alarcón, F., Escalante, L., Duenas, G., *et al.* (1989) 'Neurocysticercosis: short course of treatment with albendazole.' *Archives of Neurology*, **46**, 1231–1236.
—— Pérez, Y., *et al.* (1990) 'Tuberculous meningitis. Short course of chemotherapy.' *Archives of Neurology*, **47**, 1313–1317.
Al Deeb, S.M., Yaqub, B.A., Sharif, H.S., Phadke, J.G. (1989) 'Neurobrucellosis: clinical characteristics, diagnosis, and outcome.' *Neurology*, **39**, 498–501.
Al-Mateen, M., Gibbs, M., Dietrich, R., *et al.* (1988) 'Encephalitis lethargica-like illness in a girl with mycoplasma infection.' *Neurology*, **38**, 1155–1158.
American Academy of Pediatrics (1982a) 'Special report. Aspirin and Reye syndrome.' *Pediatrics*, **69**, 810–812.
—— Committee on Infectious Diseases (1982b) 'Rabies.' *In: Report of the Committee on Infectious Diseases.* Evanston, IL: American Academy of Pediatrics, p. 212.
—— Committee on Infectious Diseases (1988a) 'Treatment of bacterial meningitis.' *Pediatrics*, **81**, 904–907.
—— Committee on Infectious Diseases (1988b) '*Haemophilus influenzae* type b conjugate vaccine.' *Pediatrics*, **81**, 908–911.
—— Committee on Infectious Diseases (1990) 'Dexamethazone therapy for bacterial meningitis in infants and children.' *Pediatrics*, **86**, 130–133.
—— Committee on Infectious Diseases (1996) 'Recommended childhood immunization schedule.' *Pediatrics*, **97**, 143.
Amlie-Lefond, C., Kleinschmidt-DeMasters, B.K., Mahalingam, R., *et al.* (1995) 'The vasculopathy of varicella-zoster virus encephalitis.' *Annals of Neurology*, **37**, 784–790.
Ammann, A.J., Johnson, A., Fyfe, G.A., *et al.* (1985) 'Behçet syndrome.' *Journal of Pediatrics*, **107**, 41–43.
Andermann, F. (1967) 'Absence attacks and diffuse neuronal disease.' *Neurology*, **17**, 205–212.
Anderson, N.E., Powell, K.F., Croxson, M.C. (1993) 'A polymerase chain reaction assay of cerebrospinal fluid in patients with suspected herpes simplex encephalitis.' *Journal of Neurology, Neurosurgery, and Psychiatry*, **56**, 520–525.
Anlar, B., Gücüyener, K., Imir, T., *et al.* (1993) 'Cimetidine as an immunomodulator in subacute sclerosing panencephalitis: a double blind, placebo-controlled study.' *Pediatric Infectious Disease Journal*, **12**, 578–581.
—— Yalaz, K., Öktem, F., Köse, G. (1997) 'Long-term follow-up of patients with subacute sclerosing panencephalitis treated with intraventricular α-interferon.' *Neurology*, **48**, 526–528.
Angerer, M., Pfadenhauer, K., Stöhr, M. (1993) 'Prognosis of facial palsy in *Borrelia burgdorferi* meningopolyradiculoneuritis.' *Journal of Neurology*, **240**, 319–321.
Aoki, Y., Lombroso, C.T. (1973) 'Prognostic value of electroencephalography in Reye's syndrome.' *Neurology*, **23**, 333–338.
Appelbaum, P.C., Scragg, J. (1977) '*Salmonella* meningitis in infants.' *Lancet*, **1**, 1052–1053. *(Letter.)*
Archer, B.D. (1993) 'Computed tomography before lumbar puncture in acute meningitis: a review of the risks and benefits.' *Canadian Medical Association Journal*, **148**, 961–965.
Arditi, M., Herold, B.C., Yogev, R. (1989) 'Cefuroxime treatment failure and *Haemophilus influenzae* meningitis: case report and review of literature.' *Pediatrics*, **84**, 132–135.
Arisoy, E.S., Demmler, G.J., Dunne, W.M. (1993) '*Corynebacterium xerosis* ventriculoperitoneal shunt infection in an infant: report of a case and review of the literature.' *Pediatric Infectious Disease Journal*, **12**, 536–538.
Arpino, C., Gattinara, G.C., Piergili, D., Curatolo, P. (1990) 'Toxocara infection and epilepsy in children: a case–control study.' *Epilepsia*, **31**, 33–36.

Asano, Y., Yoshikawa, T., Kajita, Y., *et al.* (1992) 'Fatal encephalitis/encephalopathy in primary human herpesvirus-6 infection.' *Archives of Disease in Childhood*, **67**, 1484–1485.

—— Yoshikawa, T., Suga, S., *et al.* (1994) 'Clinical features of infants with primary human herpesvirus 6 infection (exanthem subitum, roseola infantum).' *Pediatrics*, **93**, 104–108.

Asensi, F., Otero, M.C, Pérez-Tamarit, D., *et al.* (1993) 'Risk/benefit in the treatment of children with imipenem–cilastatin for meningitis caused by penicillin-resistant pneumococcus.' *Journal of Chemotherapy*, **5**, 133–134.

Ashkenazi, S., Dinari, G., Zevulunov, A., Nitzan, M. (1987) 'Convulsions in childhood shigellosis. Clinical and laboratory features in 153 children.' *American Journal of Diseases of Children*, **141**, 208–210.

Ashwal, S., Stringer, W., Tomasi, L., *et al.* (1990) 'Cerebral blood flow and carbon dioxide reactivity in children with bacterial meningitis.' *Journal of Pediatrics*, **117**, 523–530.

—— Tomasi, L., Schneider, S., *et al.* (1992) 'Bacterial meningitis in children: pathophysiology and treatment.' *Neurology*, **42**, 739–748.

Bacon, C.J., Hall, S.M. (1992) 'Haemorrhagic shock encephalopathy syndrome in the British Isles.' *Archives of Disease in Childhood*, **67**, 985–993.

Bahemuka, M., Shemena, A.R., Panayiotopoulos, C.P., *et al.* (1988) 'Neurological syndromes of brucellosis.' *Journal of Neurology, Neurosurgery, and Psychiatry*, **51**, 1017–1021.

Baker, A.S., Ojemann, R.G., Swartz, M.N., Richardson, E.P. (1975) 'Spinal epidural abscess.' *New England Journal of Medicine*, **293**, 463–468.

Baker, C.J., Barrett, F.F., Gordon, F.C., Yow, M.D. (1973) 'Suppurative meningitis due to streptococci of Lancefield group B: a study of 33 infants.' *Journal of Pediatrics*, **82**, 724–729.

Balfour, H.H., Englund, J.A. (1989) 'Antiviral drugs in pediatrics.' *American Journal of Diseases of Children*, **143**, 1307–1316.

Bamborschke, S., Wullen, T., Huber, M., *et al.* (1992) 'Early diagnosis and successful treatment of acute cytomegalovirus encephalitis in a renal transplant recipient.' *Journal of Neurology*, **239**, 205–208.

Baraff, L.J., Lee, S.I., Schriger, D.L. (1993a) 'Outcomes of bacterial meningitis in children: a meta-analysis.' *Pediatric Infectious Disease Journal*, **12**, 389–394.

—— Oslund, S., Prather, M. (1993b) 'Effect of antibiotic therapy and etiologic microorganism on the risk of bacterial meningitis in children with occult bacteremia.' *Pediatrics*, **92**, 140–143.

Barakat, A.Y., Bitar, J., Nassar, V.H. (1973) 'Whipple's disease in a seven-year old child: report of a case.' *American Journal of Proctology*, **24**, 312–315.

Barnett, N.D.P., Kaplan, A.N., Hopkin, R.J., *et al.* (1996) 'Primary amoebic meningoencephalitis with *Naegleria fowleri*: clinical review.' *Pediatric Neurology*, **15**, 230–234.

Barone, S.R., Kaplan, M.H., Krilov, L.R. (1995) 'Human herpesvirus-6 infection in children with first febrile seizures.' *Journal of Pediatrics*, **127**, 95–97.

Barthez, M.A., Billard, C., Santini, J.J., *et al.* (1987) 'Relapse of herpes simplex encephalitis.' *Neuropediatrics*, **18**, 3–7.

Barthez-Carpentier, M.A., Billard, C., Maheut, J., *et al.* (1992) 'Acute measles encephalitis of the delayed type: neuroradiological and immunological findings.' *European Neurology*, **32**, 235–237.

Bass, J.L., Nuss, R., Mehta, K.A., *et al.* (1983) 'Recurrent meningococcemia associated with IgG2-subclass deficiency.' *New England Journal of Medicine*, **309**, 430. *(Letter.)*

Bateman, D.E., Newman, P.K., Foster, J.B. (1983) 'A retrospective survey of proven cases of tuberculous meningitis in the Northern region 1970–1980.' *Journal of the Royal College of Physicians*, **17**, 106–110.

Baumgartner, E.T., Augustine, A., Steele, R.W. (1983) 'Bacterial meningitis in older neonates.' *American Journal of Diseases of Children*, **137**, 1052–1054.

Bayston, R., Hart, C.A., Barnicoat, M. (1987) 'Intraventricular vancomycin in the treatment of ventriculitis associated with cerebrospinal fluid shunting and drainage.' *Journal of Neurology, Neurosurgery, and Psychiatry*, **50**, 1419–1423.

Bazzoni, F., Beutler B. (1996) 'The tumor necrosis factor ligand and receptor families.' *New England Journal of Medicine*, **334**, 1717–1725.

Beg, J.A. (1981) 'Bilateral sensorineural hearing loss as a complication of infectious mononucleosis.' *Archives of Otolaryngology*, **107**, 620–622.

Behan, P.O., Behan, W.M.H., Bell, E.J. (1985) 'The postviral fatigue syndrome—an analysis of the findings in 50 cases.' *Journal of Infection*, **10**, 211–222.

Bell, W.E., Lascari, A.D. (1970) 'Rocky Mountain spotted fever. Neurological symptoms in the acute phase.' *Neurology*, **20**, 841–847.

Belman, A.L. (1990) 'Neurological syndromes associated with symptomatic human immunodeficiency virus infection in infants and children.' *In:* Kozlowski, P.B., Snider, D.A., Vietze, P.M., Wisniwski, H.M. (Eds.) *Brain in Pediatric AIDS*. Basel: Karger, pp. 112–121.

—— (1992) 'Acquired immunodeficiency syndrome and the child's central nervous system.' *Pediatric Clinics of North America*, **39**, 691–714.

—— Ultmann, M.H., Horoupian, D., *et al.* (1985) 'Neurological complications in infants and children with acquired immune deficiency syndrome.' *Annals of Neurology*, **18**, 560–566.

—— Lantos, G., Horoupian, D., *et al.* (1986) 'AIDS calcification of the basal ganglia in infants and children.' *Neurology*, **36**, 1192–1199.

—— Coyle, P.K., Roque, C., Cantos, E. (1992) 'MRI findings in children infected by *Borrelia burgdorferi*.' *Pediatric Neurology*, **8**, 428–431.

—— Iyer, M., Coyle, P.K., Dattwyler, R. (1993) 'Neurologic manifestations in children with North American Lyme disease.' *Neurology*, **43**, 2609–2614.

—— Muenz, L.R., Marcus, J.C., *et al.* (1996) 'Neurologic status of human immunodeficiency virus 1-infected infants and their controls: a prospective study from birth to 2 years.' *Pediatrics*, **98**, 1109–1118.

Benjamin, P.Y., Levisohn, M., Drotar, D., Hanson, E.E. (1982) 'Intellectual and emotional sequelae of Reye's syndrome.' *Critical Care Medicine*, **10**, 583–587.

Bergey, G.K., Coyle, P.K., Krumholz, A., Niedermeyer, E. (1982) 'Herpes simplex encephalitis with occipital localization.' *Archives of Neurology*, **39**, 312–313.

Berke, E., Collins, W.F., Von Graevenitz, A., Bia, F.J. (1981) 'Fulminant postsurgical *Bacillus cereus* meningitis: case report.' *Journal of Neurosurgery*, **55**, 637–639.

Berlin, L., Pincus, J.H. (1989) 'Cryptococcal meningitis: false negative antigen test results and cultures in nonimmunosuppressed patients.' *Archives of Neurology*, **46**, 1312–1316.

Berman, P.H., Banker, B.Q. (1966) 'Neonatal meningitis. A clinical and pathological study of 29 cases.' *Pediatrics*, **38**, 6–24.

Bertolani, M.F., Portolani, M., Marotti, F., *et al.* (1996) 'A study of childhood febrile convulsions with particular reference to HHV-6 infection: pathogenic considerations.' *Child's Nervous System*, **12**, 534–539.

Billette de Villemeur, T., Deslys, J-P., Pradel, A., *et al.* (1996) 'Creutzfeldt–Jakob disease from contaminated growth hormone extracts in France.' *Neurology*, **47**, 690–695.

Bingham, P.M., Galetta, S.L., Athreya, B., Sladky, J. (1995) 'Neurologic manifestations in children with Lyme disease.' *Pediatrics*, **96**, 1053–1056.

Bittencourt, P.R.M., Garcia, C.M., Lorenzana, P. (1988) 'Epilepsy and parasitosis of the central nervous system.' *In:* Pedley, T.A., Meldrum, B.S. (Eds.) *Recent Advances in Epilepsy, Vol.4*. Edinburgh: Churchill Livingstone, pp. 123–159.

Black, D.N., Booth, F., Watters, G.V., *et al.* (1988a) 'Leukoencephalopathy among native Indian infants in Northern Quebec and Manitoba.' *Annals of Neurology*, **24**, 490–496.

—— Watters, G.V., Andermann, E., *et al.* (1988b) 'Encephalitis among Cree children in Northern Quebec.' *Annals of Neurology*, **24**, 483–489.

Blanche, S., Calvez, T., Rouzioux, C., *et al.* (1993) 'Randomized study of two doses of didanosine in children infected with human immunodeficiency virus.' *Journal of Pediatrics*, **122**, 966–973.

—— Mayaux, M-J., Rouzioux, C., *et al.* (1994) 'Relation of the course of HIV infection in children to the severity of the disease in their mothers at delivery.' *New England Journal of Medicine*, **330**, 308–312.

Boele van Hensbroek, M., Onyiorah, E., Jaffar, S., *et al.* (1996) 'A trial of artemether or quinine in children with cerebral malaria.' *New England Journal of Medicine*, **335**, 69–75.

Boerman, R.H., Peters, A.C.B., Verheij, M., *et al.* (1988) 'Immunofluorescence detection of herpes simplex virus type I antigen in cerebrospinal fluid cells of experimentally infected mice.' *Journal of the Neurological Sciences*, **87**, 245–254.

—— Arnoldus, E.P.J., Raap, A.K., *et al.* (1989) 'Polymerase chain reaction and viral culture techniques to detect HSV in small volumes of cerebrospinal fluid. An experimental mouse encephalitis study.' *Journal of Virological Methods*, **25**, 189–198.

Bogousslavsky, J., Regli, F., Uske, A. (1988) 'Thalamic infarcts: clinical syndromes, etiology and prognosis.' *Neurology*, **38**, 837–848.

Bohr, V., Hansen, B., Kjersem, H., *et al.* (1983a) 'Sequelae from bacterial meningitis and their relation to the clinical condition during acute illness, based on 667 questionnaire returns. Part II of a three-part series.' *Journal of Infection*, **7**, 102–111.

—— Rasmussen, N., Hansen, B., *et al.* (1983b) '875 cases of bacterial meningitis: diagnostic procedures and the impact of preadmission antibiotic therapy. Part III of a three-part series.' *Journal of Infection,* **7**, 193–202.

—— Paulson, O.B., Rasmussen, N. (1984) 'Pneumococcal meningitis. Late neurologic sequelae and features of prognostic impact.' *Archives of Neurology,* **41**, 1045–1049.

Bonadio, W.A. (1992) 'The cerebrospinal fluid: physiologic aspects and alterations associated with bacterial meningitis.' *Pediatric Infectious Disease Journal,* **11**, 423–432.

Bonham, J.R., Meeks, A., Levin, M., *et al.* (1992) 'Complete recovery from hemorrhagic shock and encephalopathy.' *Journal of Pediatrics,* **120**, 440–443.

Boos, J., Esiri, M. (1986) *Viral Encephalitis: Pathology, Diagnosis and Management.* Oxford: Blackwell.

Boothman, B.R., Bamford, J.M., Parsons, M.R. (1988) 'Paraplegia as a presenting feature of meningococcal meningitis.' *Journal of Neurology, Neurosurgery, and Psychiatry,* **51**, 1241. *(Letter.)*

Bortolussi, R., Seeliger, H.P.R. (1990) 'Listeriosis.' *In:* Remington, J.S., Klein, J.O. (Eds.) *Infectious Diseases of the Fetus and Newborn Infant, 3rd Edn.* Philadelphia: W.B. Saunders, pp. 812–833.

Boyce, T.G. (1990) 'Acute transverse myelitis in a 6-year-old girl with schistosomiasis.' *Pediatric Infectious Disease Journal,* **9**, 279–284.

—— Swerdlow, D.L., Griffin, P.M. (1995) '*Escherichia coli* O157:H7 and the hemolytic–uremic syndrome.' *New England Journal of Medicine,* **333**, 364–368.

Boyer, K.M., Gotoff, S.P. (1986) 'Prevention of early-onset neonatal group B streptococcal disease with selective intrapartum chemoprophylaxis.' *New England Journal of Medicine,* **314**, 1665–1669.

Brett, E.M. (1991) *Paediatric Neurology, 2nd Edn.* Edinburgh: Churchill Livingstone.

Brismar, J., Gascon, G.G., Von Steyern, K.V., Bohlega, S. (1996) 'Subacute sclerosing panencephalitis: evaluation with CT and MR.' *American Journal of Neuroradiology,* **17**, 761–772.

Brock, D.G., Bleck, T.P. (1992) 'Extra-axial suppurations of the central nervous system.' *Seminars in Neurology,* **12**, 263–272.

Bromberg, K., Rawstron, S., Tannis, G. (1993) 'Diagnosis of congenital syphilis by combining *Treponema pallidum*-specific IgM detection with immunofluorescent antigen detection for *T. pallidum*.' *Journal of Infectious Disease,* **168**, 238–242.

Brook, I. (1992) 'Aerobic and anaerobic bacteriology of intracranial abscesses.' *Pediatric Neurology,* **8**, 210–214.

—— (1995) 'Brain abscess in children: microbiology and management.' *Journal of Child Neurology,* **10**, 283–288.

Brown, J.K., Steers, C. (1986) 'Strategies in the management of children with acute encephalopathies.' *In:* Gordon, N., McKinlay, I. (Eds.) *Neurologically Handicapped Children. Treatment and Management. Vol. 2.* Oxford: Blackwell, pp. 219–293.

Brown, P., Cervenáková, L., Goldforb, L.G., *et al.* (1994a) 'Iatrogenic Creutzfeld–Jakob disease: an example of the interplay between ancient genes and modern medicine.' *Neurology,* **44**, 291–293.

—— Gibbs, C.J., Rodgers-Johnson, P., *et al.* (1994b) 'Human spongiform encephalopathy: the National Institutes of Health series of 300 cases of experimentally transmitted disease.' *Annals of Neurology,* **35**, 513–529.

Bullock, M.R., Van Dellen, J.R. (1982) 'The role of cerebrospinal fluid shunting in tuberculous meningitis.' *Surgical Neurology,* **18**, 274–277.

Burstein, L., Breningstall, G.N. (1986) 'Movement disorders in bacterial meningitis.' *Journal of Pediatrics,* **109**, 260–264.

Byrne, E., Trounce, I. (1987) 'Chronic fatigue and myalgia syndrome: mitochondrial and glycolytic studies in skeletal muscle.' *Journal of Neurology, Neurosurgery, and Psychiatry,* **50**, 743–746.

Campbell, J.R., Diacovo, T., Baker, C.J. (1992) '*Serratia marcescens* meningitis in neonates.' *Pediatric Infectious Disease Journal,* **11**, 881–886.

Carithers, H.A., Margileth, A.M. (1991) 'Cat-scratch disease. Acute encephalopathy and other neurologic manifestations.' *American Journal of Diseases of Children,* **145**, 98–101.

Carmack, M.A., Twiss, J., Enzmann, D.R., *et al.* (1993) 'Multifocal leukoencephalitis caused by varicella-zoster virus in a child with leukemia: successful treatment with acyclovir.' *Pediatric Infectious Disease Journal,* **12**, 402–406.

Carraccio, C., Blotny, K., Fisher, M.C. (1995) 'Cerebrospinal fluid analysis in systemically ill children without central nervous system disease.' *Pediatrics,* **96**, 48–51.

Carrère, C., Parra, J.P., Bouvet, E. (1984) *Epidémiologie des Méningites Purulentes. Publication de la Sous-Direction des Actions Sanitaires.* France: Ministère de la Santé.

Chahlub, E.G., De Vivo, D.C., Siegal, B.A. (1977) 'Coxsackie A9 focal encephalitis associated with acute infantile hemiplegia and porencephaly.' *Neurology,* **27**, 574–579.

Chamberlain, M.C., Nichols, S.L., Chase, C.H. (1991) 'Pediatric AIDS: comparative cranial MRI and CT scans.' *Pediatric Neurology,* **7**, 357–362.

Chambers, S.T., Hendrickse, W.A., Ricord, C., *et al.* (1984) 'Paradoxical expansion of intracranial tuberculoma during chemotherapy.' *Lancet,* **2**, 181–184.

Chaves-Carballo, E., Montes, J.E., Nelson, W.B., Chrenka, B.A. (1990) 'Hemorrhagic shock and encephalopathy—clinical definition of a catastrophic syndrome in infants.' *American Journal of Diseases of Children,* **144**, 1079–1082.

Chequer, R.S., Tharp, B.R., Dreimane, D., *et al.* (1992) 'Prognostic value of EEG in neonatal meningitis: retrospective study of 29 infants.' *Pediatric Neurology,* **8**, 417–422.

Chesney, P.J., Justman, R.A., Bogdanowicz, W.M. (1978) '*Candida* meningitis in newborn infants. A review and report of combined amphotericin B-5 flucytosine therapy.' *Johns Hopkins Medical Journal,* **142**, 155–158.

—— Crass, B.A., Polyak, M.B. (1982) 'Toxic shock syndrome. Management and long-term sequelae.' *Annals of Internal Medicine,* **96**, 847–851.

Chopra, J.S., Shawney, I.M.S., Dhand, U.K., *et al.* (1986) 'Neurological complications of acute haemorrhagic conjunctivitis.' *Journal of the Neurological Sciences,* **73**, 177–191.

Chou, S.M., Roos, R., Burrell, R., *et al.* (1973) 'Subacute focal adenovirus encephalitis.' *Journal of Neuropathology and Experimental Neurology,* **32**, 34–50.

Christen, H.J., Hanefeld, F., Eiffert, H., Thomssen, R. (1993) 'Epidemiology and clinical manifestations of Lyme borreliosis in childhood. A prospective multicentre study with special regard to neuroborreliosis.' *Acta Paediatrica,* Suppl. 386, 1–75.

Clarke, D.H., Casals, J. (1965) 'Arboviruses group B.' *In:* Horsfall, F.L., Tamm, I. (Eds.) *Viral and Rickettsial Infections of Man, 4th Edn.* Philadelphia: J.B. Lippincott, pp. 606–625.

Clouston, P.D., Corbett, A.J., Pryor, D.S., Garrick, R. (1990) 'Eosinophilic meningitis: cause of a chronic pain syndrome.' *Journal of Neurology, Neurosurgery, and Psychiatry,* **53**, 778–781.

Cohen, B.A., Schenk, V.A., Sweeney, D.B. (1988) 'Meningitis-related hearing loss evaluated with evoked potentials.' *Pediatric Neurology,* **4**, 18–22.

Cohen, H.A., Ashkenazi, A., Nussinovitch, M., *et al.* (1992) 'Mumps-associated acute cerebellar ataxia.' *American Journal of Diseases of Children,* **146**, 930–931.

Coker, S.B., Beltran, R.S. (1988) '*Candida* meningitis: clinical and radiographic diagnosis.' *Pediatric Neurology,* **4**, 317–319.

Colamaria, V., Marradi, P., Boner, A., *et al.* (1989a) 'Progressive myoclonic encephalopathy in X-linked hypogamma-globulinemia. Case report, review of the literature and its relationship with progressive encephalopathy in children with A.I.D.S.' *Neuropediatrics,* **20**, 223–229.

—— —— Merlin, D., *et al.* (1989b) 'Acute measles encephalitis of the delayed type in an immunosuppressed child.' *Brain and Development,* **11**, 322–326.

Collier, A.C., Coombs, R.W., Schoenfeld, D.A., *et al.* (1996) 'Treatment of human immunodeficiency virus infection with Saquinavir, Zidovudine and Zalcitabine.' *New England Journal of Medicine,* **334**, 1011–1017.

Collinge, C. (1996) 'New diagnostic tests for prion diseases.' *New England Journal of Medicine,* **335**, 963–965.

Como, J.A., Dismukes, W.E. (1993) 'Oral azole drugs as systemic antifungal therapy.' *New England Journal of Medicine,* **330**, 263–272.

Connelly, K.P., De Witt, L.D. (1994) 'Neurologic complications of infectious mononucleosis.' *Pediatric Neurology,* **10**, 181–184.

Connolly, J.H., Hutchinson, W.M., Allen, I.V., *et al.* (1975) 'Carotid artery thrombosis, encephalitis, myelitis and optic neuritis associated with rubella virus infections.' *Brain,* **98**, 583–594.

Connor, E.M., Sperling, R.S., Gelber, R., *et al.* (1994) 'Reduction of maternal–infant transmission of human immunodeficiency virus type 1 with zidovudine treatment.' *New England Journal of Medicine,* **331**, 1173–1180.

Cooper, J.B., Pratt, W.R., English, B.K., Sharer, W.T. (1983) 'Coxsackievirus B3 producing fatal meningoencephalitis in a patient with X-linked agamma-globulinemia.' *American Journal of Diseases of Children,* **137**, 82–83.

Coovadia, Y.M., Dawood, A., Ellis, M.E., *et al.* (1986) 'Evaluation of adenosine deaminase activity and antibody to *Mycobacterium tuberculosis* antigen 5 in cerebrospinal fluid and the radioactive bromide partition test for the early diagnosis of tuberculous meningitis.' *Archives of Disease in Childhood*, **61**, 428–435.

Corey, L., Holmes, K.K. (1996) 'Therapy for human immunodeficiency virus infection—what have we learned?' *New England Journal of Medicine*, **335**, 1142–1144.

—— Whitley, R.J., Stone, E.F., Mohan, K. (1988) 'Difference between herpes simplex virus type 1 and type 2 neonatal encephalitis in neurological outcome.' *Lancet*, **1**, 1–4.

Cornblath, D.R., Sladky, J.T., Sumner, A.J. (1983) 'Clinical electrophysiology of infantile botulism.' *Muscle and Nerve*, **6**, 448–452.

Cornford, M.E., McCormick, G.F. (1997) 'Adult-onset temporal lobe epilepsy associated with smoldering herpes simplex 2 infection.' *Neurology*, **48**, 425–430.

Corona, T., Pascoe, D., González-Baranco, D., *et al.* (1986) 'Anticysticercous antibodies in serum and cerebrospinal fluid in patients with cerebral cysticercosis.' *Journal of Neurology, Neurosurgery, and Psychiatry*, **49**, 1044–1049.

Correa, A.G., Edwards, M.S., Baker, C.J. (1993) 'Vertebral osteomyelitis in children.' *Pediatric Infectious Disease Journal*, **12**, 228–233.

Corrigan, J.J. (1990) 'The 'H' in hemorrhagic shock and encephalopathy syndrome should be 'hyperpyrexia'.' *American Journal of Diseases of Children*, **144**, 1077.

Cottrell, A.J. (1986) 'Acquired toxoplasma encephalitis.' *Archives of Disease in Childhood*, **61**, 84–85.

Counsell, C.E., Taylor, R., Whittle, I.R. (1994) 'Focal necrotising herpes simplex encephalitis: a report of two cases with good clinical and neuro-psychological outcomes.' *Journal of Neurology, Neurosurgery, and Psychiatry*, **57**, 1115–1117.

Couvreur, J., Desmonts, G. (1988) 'Acquired and congenital toxoplasmosis.' *In:* Vinken, P.J., Bruyn, G.W., Klawans, H.L. (Eds.) *Handbook of Clinical Neurology. Revised Series. Vol. 8. Microbial Disease.* Amsterdam: Elsevier, pp. 351–363.

Coyle, P.K., Schutzer, S.E., Deng, Z., *et al.* (1995) 'Detection of *Borrelia burgdorferi*-specific antigen in antibody-negative cerebrospinal fluid in neurologic Lyme disease.' *Neurology*, **45**, 2010–2015.

Creel, G.B., Hurtt, M. (1995) 'Cephalosporin-induced recurrent aseptic meningitis.' *Annals of Neurology*, **37**, 815–817.

—— Sullivan, T., Hurtt, M. (1993) 'Cryptogenic aseptic meningitis due to cephalosporin allergy.' *Neurology*, **43**, Suppl. 2, A253. *(Abstract.)*

Crocker, J.F.S. (Ed.) (1979) *Reye's Syndrome II.* New York: Grune & Stratton.

Crone, N.E., Reder, A.T. (1992) 'Severe tetanus in immunized patients with high anti-tetanus titers.' *Neurology*, **42**, 761–764.

Crumpacker, C.S., Schnipper, L.E., Marlowe, S.I., *et al.* (1982) 'Resistance to antiviral drugs of herpes simplex virus isolated from a patient treated with acyclovir.' *New England Journal of Medicine*, **306**, 343–346.

Cuadrado, L.M., Guerrero, A., Lopez Garcia Asenjo, L.G., *et al.* (1988) 'Cerebral mucormycosis in two cases of acquired immunodeficiency syndrome.' *Archives of Neurology*, **45**, 109–111.

Curless, R.G., Mitchell, C.D. (1991) 'Central nervous system tuberculosis in children.' *Pediatric Neurology*, **7**, 270–274.

—— Schatz, N.J., Bowen, B.C., *et al.* (1996) 'Lyme neuroborreliosis masquerading as a brainstem tumor in a 15-year-old.' *Pediatric Neurology*, **15**, 258–260.

Cusmai, R., Bertini, E., Di Capua, M., *et al.* (1994) 'Bilateral, reversible, selective thalamic involvement demonstrated by brain MR and acute severe neurological dysfunction with favorable outcome.' *Neuropediatrics*, **25**, 44–47.

Dalakas, M.C. (1986) 'New neuromuscular symptoms in patients with old poliomyelitis: a three-year follow-up study.' *European Neurology*, **25**, 381–387.

Darby, C.P. (1976) 'Treating *Pseudomonas cepacia* meningitis with trimethoprim-sulfamethoxazole.' *American Journal of Diseases of Children*, **130**, 1365–1366.

Dastur, H.M., Desai, A.D. (1965) 'A comparative study of brain tuberculomas and gliomas based on 107 case records of each.' *Brain*, **88**, 375–396.

Daud, S., Mohammad, T., Ahmad, A. (1981) 'Tetanus neonatorum.' *Journal of Tropical Pediatrics*, **27**, 308–311.

Davies, P.A. (1989) 'Long-term effects of meningitis.' *Developmental Medicine and Child Neurology*, **31**, 398–400.

—— Rudd, P.T. (1994) *Neonatal Meningitis. Clinics in Developmental Medicine No. 132.* London: Mac Keith Press.

Davis, C.A., Shurin, S.B., Pate, K., Congeni, B.C. (1983) 'Neutrophil function

in a patient with meningococcal meningitis and C7 deficiency.' *American Journal of Diseases of Children*, **137**, 404–406.

Davis, D., Henslee, P.J., Markesbery, W.R. (1988) 'Fatal adenovirus meningoencephalitis in a bone marrow transplant patient.' *Annals of Neurology*, **23**, 385–389.

Davis, L.E., Bodian, D., Price, D., *et al.* (1977) 'Chronic progressive poliomyelitis secondary to vaccination of an immunodeficient child.' *New England Journal of Medicine*, **297**, 241–245.

—— Rastogi, K.R., Lambert, L.C., Skipper, B.J. (1993) 'Tuberculous meningitis in the southwest United States: a community-based study.' *Neurology*, **43**, 1775–1778.

DeCarli, C., Civitello, L.A., Brouwers, P., Pizzo, P.A. (1993) 'The prevalence of computed tomographic abnormalities of the cerebrum in 100 consecutive children symptomatic with the human immune deficiency virus.' *Annals of Neurology*, **34**, 198–205.

De Chadarévian, J-P., Becker, W.J. (1988) 'Mollaret's recurrent aseptic meningitis: relationship to epidermoid cysts. Light microscopic and ultrastructural cytological studies of the cerebrospinal fluid.' *Journal of Neuropathology and Experimental Neurology*, **39**, 661–669.

Delage, G., Dusseault, M. (1979) 'Tuberculous meningitis in children: a retrospective study of 79 patients, with an analysis of prognostic factors.' *Canadian Medical Association Journal*, **120**, 305–309.

DeLong, G.R., Glick, T.H. (1982) 'Encephalopathy of Reye's syndrome: a review of pathogenetic hypotheses.' *Pediatrics*, **69**, 53–63.

—— Bean, S.C., Brown, F.R. (1984) 'Acquired reversible autistic syndrome in acute encephalopathic illness in children.' *Archives of Neurology*, **38**, 191–194.

De Meirleir, L., Seneca, S., Lissens, W., *et al.* (1995) 'Bilateral striatal necrosis with a novel point mutation in the mitochondrial ATPase 6 gene.' *Pediatric Neurology*, **13**, 242–246.

Den Heijer, J.C., Peters, A.C.B., Van Gemert, G.W. (1986) 'Post-infectious meningoencephalitis complicating *Mycoplasma pneumoniae* in a child.' *Journal of Neurology, Neurosurgery, and Psychiatry*, **49**, 600–602.

Denis, F., Cadoz, M., Diop Mar, I., Saulnier, M. (1981) 'Bacterial antigen concentrations in cerebrospinal fluid and prognosis of purulent meningitis.' *Lancet*, **1**, 1361. *(Letter.)*

Deresiewicz, R.L., Thaler, S.J., Hsu, L., Zamani, A.A. (1997) 'Clinical and neuroradiographic manifestations of Eastern equine encephalitis.' *New England Journal of Medicine*, **336**, 1867–1874.

DeSimone, P.A., Snyder, D. (1978) 'Hypoglossal nerve palsy in infectious mononucleosis.' *Neurology*, **28**, 844–847.

Deslys, J-P., Lasmézas, C., Dormont, D. (1994) 'Selection of specific strains in iatrogenic Creutzfeld–Jakob disease.' *Lancet*, **343**, 848–849. *(Letter.)*

De Vivo, C.D., Keating, J.P. (1976) 'Reye's syndrome.' *Advances in Pediatrics*, **22**, 175–229.

Dickson, D.W., Belman, A.L., Kim, T.S., *et al.* (1989) 'Spinal cord pathology in pediatric acquired immunodeficiency syndrome.' *Neurology*, **39**, 227–235.

Diebler, C., Dulac, O. (1987) *Pediatric Neurology and Neuroradiology.* Berlin: Springer Verlag.

DiTullio, M.V. (1977) 'Intramedullary spinal abscess: a case report with review of 53 previously described cases.' *Surgical Neurology*, **7**, 351–357.

Dodge, P.R. (1987) 'Neurosyphilis.' *In:* Feigin, R.D., Cherry, J.D. (Eds.) *Textbook of Pediatric Infectious Diseases, 2nd Edn.* Philadelphia: W.B. Saunders, pp. 466–467.

—— Swartz, M.N. (1965) 'Bacterial meningitis—a review of selected aspects. II. Special neurologic problems, postmeningitic complications and clinicopathological correlations.' *New England Journal of Medicine*, **272**, 954–960, 1003–1010.

—— Davis, H., Feigin, R.D., *et al.* (1984) 'Prospective evaluation of hearing impairment as a sequela of acute bacterial meningitis.' *New England Journal of Medicine*, **311**, 869–874.

Doerr, C.A., Starke, J.R., Ong, L.T. (1995) 'Clinical and public health aspects of tuberculous meningitis in children.' *Journal of Pediatrics*, **127**, 27–33.

Donald, P.R., Malan, C., Van der Walt, A. (1983) 'Simultaneous determination of cerebrospinal fluid glucose and blood glucose concentrations in the diagnosis of bacterial meningitis.' *Journal of Pediatrics*, **103**, 413–416.

Donovan, M.K., Lenn, N.J. (1989) 'Postinfectious encephalomyelitis with localized basal ganglia involvement.' *Pediatric Neurology*, **5**, 311–313.

Dorfman, D.H., Glaser, J.H. (1990) 'Congenital syphilis presenting in infants after the newborn period.' *New England Journal of Medicine*, **323**, 1299–1302.

Duarte, J., Argente, P., Gutierrez, P., *et al.* (1994) 'Herpes simplex brainstem encephalitis with a relapsing course.' *Journal of Neurology*, **241**, 401–403.

Duliège, A-M., Messiah, A., Blanche, S., *et al.* (1992) 'Natural history of human immunodeficiency virus type I infection in children: prognostic value of laboratory tests on the bimodal progression of the disease.' *Pediatric Infectious Disease Journal*, **11**, 630–635.

—— Amos, C.I., Felton, S., *et al.* (1995) 'Birth order, delivery route, and concordance in the transmission of human immunodeficiency virus type 1 from mothers to twins.' *Journal of Pediatrics*, **126**, 625–632.

Dulkerian, S.J., Kilpatrick, L., Costarino, A.T., *et al.* (1995) 'Cytokine elevations in infants with bacterial and aseptic meningitis.' *Journal of Pediatrics*, **126**, 872–876.

Durack, C.K., Spanos, A. (1982) 'End-of-treatment spinal tap in bacterial meningitis.' *Journal of the American Medical Association*, **248**, 75–78.

Durant, R.H., Dyken, P.R., Swift, A.V. (1982) 'The influence of inosiplex treatment on the neurological disability of subacute sclerosing panencephalitis patients.' *Journal of Pediatrics*, **101**, 288–293.

Dussaix, E., Lebon, P., Ponsot, G., *et al.* (1985) 'Intrathecal synthesis of different alpha-interferons in patients with various neurological diseases.' *Acta Neurologica Scandinavica*, **71**, 504–509.

—— Huault, G., Landrieu, P., *et al.* (1987) 'Paralytic poliomyelitis in vaccinated children.' *Neuropediatrics*, **18**, 153–154.

Dutt, M.K., Johnson, I.D.A. (1982) 'Computed tomography and EEG in herpes simplex encephalitis.' *Archives of Neurology*, **39**, 99–102.

Eavey, R.D., Gao, Y.Z., Schuknecht, H.F., Gonzalez-Pineda, M. (1985) 'Otologic features of bacterial meningitis of childhood.' *Journal of Pediatrics*, **106**, 402–407.

Edwards, M.S., Baker, C.J. (1981) 'Complications and sequelae of meningococcal infections in children.' *Journal of Pediatrics*, **99**, 540–545.

Eldadah, M., Frenkel, L.D., Hiatt, I.M., Hegyi, T. (1987) 'Evaluation of routine lumbar punctures in newborn infants with respiratory distress syndrome.' *Pediatric Infectious Disease Journal*, **6**, 243–245.

Emond, R.T.D., McKendrick, G.D.W. (1973) 'Tuberculosis as a cause of transient aseptic meningitis.' *Lancet*, **2**, 234–236.

Epstein, L.G., Brown, P. (1997) 'Bovine spongiform encephalopathy and a new variant of Creutzfeldt–Jakob disease.' *Neurology*, **48**, 569–571.

—— Gendelman, H.E. (1993) 'Human immunodeficiency virus type 1 infection of the nervous system: pathogenetic mechanisms.' *Annals of Neurology*, **33**, 429–436.

Erdem, G., Topçu, M., Topaloglu, H., *et al.* (1994) 'Dermoid tumor with persistently low CSF glucose and unusual CT and MRI findings.' *Pediatric Neurology*, **10**, 75–77.

Erlendsson, K., Swatz, T., Dwyer, J.M. (1985) 'Successful reversal of echovirus encephalitis in X-linked hypogammaglobulinemia by intraventricular administration of immunoglobulin.' *New England Journal of Medicine*, **312**, 351–353.

Ersahin, Y., Mutluer, S., Güzelbag, E. (1994) 'Brain abscess in infants and children.' *Child's Nervous System*, **10**, 185–189.

European Collaborative Group (1994) 'Natural history of vertically acquired human immunodeficiency virus-1 infection.' *Pediatrics*, **94**, 815–819.

European Collaborative Study (1990) 'Neurologic signs in young children with human immunodeficiency virus infection.' *Pediatric Infectious Disease Journal*, **9**, 402–406.

—— (1991) 'Children born to women with HIV-1 infection: natural history and risk of transmission.' *Lancet*, **337**, 253–260.

Everett, E.D., Eickhoff, T.C., Simon, R.H. (1976) 'Cerebrospinal fluid shunt infections with anaerobic diphtheroids (*Propionibacterium* species).' *Journal of Neurosurgery*, **44**, 580–584.

Faix, R.G. (1984) 'Systemic *Candida* infections in infants in intensive care nurseries: high incidence of central nervous system involvement.' *Journal of Pediatrics*, **105**, 616–622.

Fajardo, J.E., Stafford, E.M., Bass, J.W., *et al.* (1989) 'Inappropriate antidiuretic hormone in children with viral meningitis.' *Pediatric Neurology*, **5**, 37–40.

Feder, H.M., Garibaldi, R.A., Nurse, B.A., Kurker, R. (1988a) '*Bacillus* species isolates from cerebrospinal fluid in patients without shunts.' *Pediatrics*, **82**, 909–913.

—— Zalneraitis, E.L., Reik, L. (1988b) 'Lyme disease: acute focal meningoencephalitis in a child.' *Pediatrics*, **82**, 931–934.

Feigin, R.D., Cherry, J.D. (Eds.) (1987) *Textbook of Pediatric Infectious Diseases, 2nd Edn.* Philadelphia: W.B. Saunders.

—— Shackelford, P.G. (1973) 'Value of repeat lumbar puncture in the differential diagnosis of meningitis.' *New England Journal of Medicine*, **289**, 571–574.

—— Joaquin, V.S., Middelkamp, J.N. (1969) 'Purpura fulminans associated with *Neisseria catarrhalis* septicemia and meningitis.' *Pediatrics*, **44**, 120–123.

—— Wong, M., Shackelford, P.G., *et al.* (1976) 'Countercurrent immunoelectrophoresis of urine as well as of CSF and blood for diagnosis of bacterial meningitis.' *Journal of Pediatrics*, **89**, 773–775.

—— McCracken, G.H., Klein, J.O. (1992) 'Diagnosis and management of meningitis.' *Pediatric Infectious Disease Journal*, **11**, 785–814.

Feldman, H., Michaels, R.H. (1986) 'Academic achievement 10 to 12 years after *Haemophilus influenzae* meningitis.' *Pediatric Research*, **20**, 309A. *(Abstract.)*

Feldman, W.E., Ginsburg, C.M., McCracken, G.H., *et al.* (1982) 'Relation of concentrations of *Haemophilus influenzae* type b in cerebrospinal fluid to late sequelae of patients with meningitis.' *Journal of Pediatrics*, **100**, 209–212.

Fernandez, C.V., Bortolussi, R., Gordon, K., *et al.* (1993) '*Mycoplasma pneumoniae* infection associated with central nervous system complications.' *Journal of Child Neurology*, **8**, 27–31.

Fetter, B.F., Klinworth, G.K., Hendry, W.S. (1967) *Mycoses of the Central Nervous System.* Baltimore: Williams & Wilkins.

Fijen, C.A.P., Kuijper, E.J., Hannema, A.J., *et al.* (1989) 'Complement deficiencies in patients over 10 years old with meningococcal disease due to uncommon serogroups.' *Lancet*, **2**, 585–588.

Finkel, M.F. (1988) 'Lyme disease and its neurological complications.' *Archives of Neurology*, **45**, 99–104.

Fischer, E.G., Schwachman, H., Wepsic, J.G. (1979) 'Brain abscess and cystic fibrosis.' *Journal of Pediatrics*, **95**, 385–388.

—— McLennan, J.E., Suzuki, Y. (1981) 'Cerebral abscess in children.' *American Journal of Diseases of Children*, **135**, 746–749.

Fishbein, D.B., Robinson, L.E. (1993) 'Rabies.' *New England Journal of Medicine*, **329**, 1632–1638.

Fisher, R.S., Clark, A.W., Wolinsky, J.S., *et al.* (1983) 'Postinfectious leukoencephalitis complicating *Mycoplasma pneumoniae* infection.' *Archives of Neurology*, **40**, 109–113.

Fitzgerald, J.F., Clark, J.H., Angelides, A.G., Wyllie, R. (1982) 'The prognostic significance of peak ammonia levels in Reye syndrome.' *Pediatrics*, **70**, 997–1000.

Foreman, S.D., Smith, E.E., Ryan, N.J., Hogan, G.R. (1984) 'Neonatal *Citrobacter* meningitis: pathogenesis of cerebral abscess formation.' *Annals of Neurology*, **16**, 655–659.

Fortenbery, J.D., Kenney, R.D., Younger, J. (1991) 'Visceral larva migrans producing static encephalopathy in an infant.' *Pediatric Infantious Disease Journal*, **10**, 403–406.

Fortnum, H.M., Davis, A.C. (1993) 'Epidemiology of bacterial meningitis.' *Archives of Disease in Childhood*, **68**, 763–767.

Fourestié, V., Douceron, H., Brugières, P., *et al.* (1993) 'Neurotrichinosis. A cerebrovascular disease associated with myocardial injury and hypereosinophilia.' *Brain*, **116**, 603–616.

Francis, D.A., Brown, A., Miller, D.H., *et al.* (1988) 'MRI appearances of the CNS manifestations of *Mycoplasma pneumoniae*: a report of two cases.' *Journal of Neurology*, **235**, 441–443.

Frank, Y., Lim, W., Kahn, E., *et al.* (1989) 'Multiple ischemic infarcts in a child with AIDS, varicella zoster infection, and cerebral vasculitis.' *Pediatric Neurology*, **5**, 64–67.

Friedland, I.R., McCracken, G.H. (1994) 'Management of infections caused by antibiotic-resistant *Streptococcus pneumoniae*.' *New England Journal of Medicine*, **331**, 377–382.

Frith, R.W., Buchanan, P.R., Glasgow, G.L. (1987) '*Listeria monocytogenes* infection with rhombencephalitis.' *Journal of Neurology, Neurosurgery, and Psychiatry*, **50**, 1383–1384.

Fröscher, W., Gullotta, F., Saathoff, M., Tackmann, W. (1988) 'Chronic trichinosis. Clinical, bioptic, serological and electromyographic observations.' *European Neurology*, **28**, 221–226.

Fujii, Y., Kuriyama, M., Konishi, Y., Sudo, M. (1992) 'MRI and SPECT in influenzal encephalitis.' *Pediatric Neurology*, **8**, 133–136.

Fujita, K., Takeuchi, Y., Nishimura, A., *et al.* (1994) 'Serial MRI in infantile bilateral striatal necrosis.' *Pediatric Neurology*, **10**, 157–160.

Fujita, N.K., Reynard, M., Sapico, F., *et al.* (1981) 'Cryptococcal intracerebral mass lesions. The role of computed tomography and nonsurgical management.' *Annals of Internal Medicine*, **94**, 382–388.

Galetta, S.L., Wulc, A.E., Goldberg, H.I., *et al.* (1990) 'Rhinocerebral mucormycosis: management and survival after carotid occlusion.' *Annals of Neurology*, **28**, 103–107.

Gandy, G., Rennie, J. (1990) 'Antibiotic treatment of suspected neonatal meningitis.' *Archives of Disease in Childhood*, **65**, 1–2.

Garg, B.P., Kleiman, M.B. (1994) 'Acute disseminated encephalomyelitis presenting as a neurodegenerative disease in infancy.' *Pediatric Neurology*, **11**, 57–58.

Gascon, G., Yamani, S., Crowell, J., *et al.* (1993) 'Combined oral isoprinosine–intraventricular α-interferon therapy for subacute sclerosing panencephalitis.' *Brain and Development*, **15**, 346–355.

Gay, C.L., Armstrong, F.D., Cohen, D., *et al.* (1995) 'The effects of HIV on cognitive and motor development in children born to HIV-seropositive women with no reported drug use: birth to 24 months.' *Pediatrics*, **96**, 1078–1082.

Gear, J.H.S. (1984) 'Nonpolio causes of polio-like paralytic syndromes.' *Review of Infectious Diseases*, **6**, Suppl. 2, S379–S384.

Gelabert, M., Castro-Gago, M. (1988) 'Hydrocephalus and tuberculous meningitis in children. Report on 26 cases.' *Child's Nervous System*, **4**, 268–270.

Gendelman, H.E., Wolinsky, J.S., Johnson, R.T., *et al.* (1984) 'Measles encephalomyelitis: lack of evidence of viral invasion of the central nervous system and quantitative study of the nature of demyelination.' *Annals of Neurology*, **15**, 353–360.

Gerbaut, L., Mallet, E. (1988) 'Le lysozyme du liquide céphalo-rachidien au cours des méningites de l'enfant—intérêt dans l'orientation du diagnostic.' *Archives Françaises de Pédiatrie*, **45**, 799–8O3.

Gessain, A., Gout, O. (1992) 'Chronic myelopathy associated with human T-lymphotropic virus type 1 (HTLV-1).' *Annals of Internal Medicine*, **117**, 933–946.

Gieron-Korthals, M.A., Westberry, K.R., Emmanuel, P.J. (1994) 'Acute childhood ataxia: 10-year experience.' *Journal of Child Neurology*, **9**, 381–384.

Gilden, D.H., Beinlich, B.R., Rubinstien, E.M., *et al.* (1994) 'Varicella-zoster virus myelitis: an expanding spectrum.' *Neurology*, **44**, 1818–1823.

Girgis, N.I., Mikhail, I.A., Farrag, I., *et al.* (1989) 'Dexamethasone treatment for bacterial meningitis in children and adults.' *Pediatric Infectious Disease Journal*, **8**, 848–851.

—— Farid, Z., Kilpatrick, M.E., *et al.* (1991) 'Dexamethasone adjunctive treatment for tuberculous meningitis.' *Pediatric Infectious Disease Journal*, **10**, 179–183.

Glauser, T.A., Pachter, L.M., Zimmerman, R.A. (1992) 'Abnormal magnetic resonance images in hemorrhagic shock and encephalopathy syndrome.' *Journal of Child Neurology*, 7, 371–374.

Glasgow, A.M., Cotton, R.B., Bourgeois, C.H., *et al.* (1972) 'Reye's syndrome. II. Occurrence in the absence of severe fatty infiltration of the liver.' *American Journal of Diseases of Children*, **124**, 834–836.

Glasgow, J.F.T. (1984) 'Clinical features and prognosis of Reye's syndrome.' *Archives of Disease in Childhood*, **59**, 230–235.

Glatt, A.E., Chirgwin, K., Landesman, S.H. (1988) 'Treatment of infections associated with human immunodeficiency virus.' *New England Journal of Medicine*, **318**, 1439–1448.

Glauser, T.A., Maguire, H.C., Sladky, J.T. (1990) 'Relapse of infant botulism.' *Annals of Neurology*, **28**, 187–189.

Glista, G.C., Sullivan, T.D., Brumlik, J. (1980) 'Spinal cord involvement in acute bacterial meningitis.' *Journal of the American Medical Association*, **243**, 1362–1363.

Glode, M.P., Daum, R.S., Goldman, D.H., *et al.* (1980) '*Haemophilus infuenzae* type b meningitis. A contagious disease of children.' *British Medical Journal*, **280**, 899–901.

Glowacki, J., Guazzi, G.C., van Bogaert, L. (1967) 'Pseudo-tumoral presentation of certain cases of subacute sclerosing panencephalitis.' *Journal of the Neurological Sciences*, **4**, 199–215.

Godel, J.C. (1982) 'Trial of pyridoxine therapy for tetanus neonatorum.' *Journal of Infectious Diseases*, **145**, 547–549.

Goh, D., Minns, R.A. (1993) 'Cerebral blood flow velocity monitoring in pyogenic meningitis.' *Archives of Disease in Childhood*, **68**, 111–119.

Goiten, K.J., Amit, Y., Mussaffi, H. (1983) 'Intracranial pressure in central nervous system infections and cerebral ischaemia of infancy.' *Archives of Disease in Childhood*, **58**, 184–186.

Golightly, H.G. (1997) 'Lyme borreliosis: laboratory considerations.' *Seminars in Neurology*, **17**, 11–17.

Gollomp, S.M., Fahn, S. (1987) 'Transient dystonia as a complication of varicella.' *Journal of Neurology, Neurosurgery, and Psychiatry*, **50**, 1228–1229.

Gonzalez-Scarano, F., Tyler, K.L. (1987) 'Molecular pathogenesis of neurotropic viral infections.' *Annals of Neurology*, **22**, 565–574.

Gordon, M.F., Allon, M., Coyle, P.K. (1990) 'Drug-induced meningitis.' *Neurology*, **40**, 163–164.

Goutières, F., Aicardi, J. (1982) 'Acute neurological dysfunction associated with destructive lesions of the basal ganglia in children.' *Annals of Neurology*, **12**, 328–333.

Graber, C.D., Higgins, L.S., Davis, J.S. (1965) 'Seldom-encountered agents of bacterial meningitis.' *Journal of the American Medical Association*, **192**, 956–960.

Graham, D.R., Band, J.D. (1981) '*Citrobacter diversus* brain abscess and meningitis in neonates.' *Journal of the American Medical Association*, **245**, 1923–1925.

Graham, P.S. (1987) 'Mollaret's meningitis associated with acute Epstein–Barr virus mononucleosis.' *Archives of Neurology*, **44**, 1204–1205.

Graham-Pole, J., Ferguson, A., Gibson, A.A.M., Stephenson, J.B.P. (1975) 'Familial dysequilibrium–diplegia with T-lymphocyte deficiency.' *Archives of Disease in Childhood*, **50**, 927–932.

Granoff, D.M., Chacko, A., Lottenbach, K.R., Sheetz, K.E. (1989) 'Immunogenicity of *Haemophilus influenzae* type b polysaccharide–outer membrane protein conjugate vaccine in patients who acquired *Haemophilus* despite previous vaccination with type b polysaccharide vaccine.' *Journal of Pediatrics*, **114**, 925–933.

Green, S.M., Rothrock, S.G., Clem, K.J., *et al.* (1993) 'Can seizures be the sole manifestation of meningitis in febrile children?' *Pediatrics*, **92**, 527–534.

Green, W.R., Sweet, L.K., Prichard, R.W. (1949) 'Acute lymphocytic choriomeningitis: a study of 21 cases.' *Journal of Pediatrics*, **35**, 688–691.

Greenberg, S.B., Taber, L., Septimus, E., *et al.* (1981) 'Computerized tomography in brain biopsy-proven herpes simplex encephalitis. Early normal results.' *Archives of Neurology*, **38**, 58–59.

Greene, C.L., Blitzer, M.G., Shapira, E. (1988) 'Inborn errors of metabolism and Reye syndrome: differential diagnosis.' *Journal of Pediatrics*, **113**, 156–159.

Greger, N.G., Kirkland, R.T., Clayton, G.W., Kirkland, J.L. (1986) 'Central diabetes insipidus. 22 years' experience.' *American Journal of Diseases of Children*, **140**, 551–554.

Grierson, H., Purtilo, D.T. (1987) 'Epstein–Barr virus infections in males with the X-linked lymphoproliferative syndrome.' *Annals of Internal Medicine*, **106**, 538–545.

Grimwood, K., Anderson, V.A., Bond, L., *et al.* (1995) 'Adverse outcomes of bacterial meningitis in school-age survivors.' *Pediatrics*, **95**, 646–656.

Groom, S.N., Clewley, J., Litton, P.A., Brown, D.W. (1994) 'Vaccine-associated poliomyelitis.' *Lancet*, **343**, 609–610. *(Letter.)*

Grubman, S., Gross, E., Lerner-Weiss, N., *et al.* (1995) 'Older children and adolescents living with perinatally acquired human immunodeficiency virus infection.' *Pediatrics*, **95**, 657–663.

Gruich, M.J., Evans, O.B., Storey, J.M., *et al.* (1995) 'Vogt–Koyanagi–Harada syndrome in a 4-year-old child.' *Pediatric Neurology*, **13**, 50–51.

Günther, G., Haglund, M., Lindquist, L., *et al.* (1997) 'Tick-borne encephalitis in Sweden in relation to aseptic meningo-encephalitis of other etiology: a prospective study of clinical course and outcome.' *Journal of Neurology*, **244**, 230–238.

Gupta, P.C., Rapin, I., Houroupian, D.S., *et al.* (1984) 'Smouldering encephalitis in children.' *Neuropediatrics*, **15**, 191–197.

Gutowski, N.J., Davenport, R.J., Heron, J.R., *et al.* (1993) 'Benign relapsing meningo-encephalomyelitis.' *Journal of Neurology, Neurosurgery, and Psychiatry*, **56**, 568–569. *(Letter.)*

Guttierez, A.R., Bodensteiner, J., Gutmann, L. (1994) 'Electrodiagnosis of infantile botulism.' *Journal of Child Neurology*, **9**, 362–366.

Hagenah, H., Müller-Jensen, A. (1978) 'Botulism: clinical neurophysiological findings.' *Journal of Neurology*, **217**, 159–171.

Haimi-Cohen, Y., Soen, G., Amir, J., *et al.* (1996) 'Coma with abnormal movements and prolonged cognitive disturbances: a new subset of acute encephalopathy.' *Neuropediatrics*, **27**, 270–272.

Hall, C.B., Long, C.E., Schnabel, K.C., *et al.* (1994) 'Human herpesvirus-6 infection in children. A prospective study of complications and reactivation.' *New England Journal of Medicine*, **331**, 432–438.

Hall, R., Richards, H. (1987) 'Hearing loss due to mumps.' *Archives of Disease in Childhood*, **62**, 189–191.

Hall, S.M., Plaster, P.A., Glasgow, J.F.T., Hancock, P. (1988) 'Preadmission antipyretics in Reye's syndrome.' *Archives of Disease in Childhood*, **63**, 857–866.

427

Halperin, J.J., Luft, B.J., Anand, A.K., *et al.* (1989) 'Lyme neuroborreliosis: central nervous system manifestations.' *Neurology*, **39**, 753–759.

Haltia, M., Paetau, A., Vaheri, A. (1977) 'Fatal measles encephalopathy with retinopathy during toxic chemotherapy.' *Journal of the Neurological Sciences*, **32**, 323–330.

Han, B.K., Babcock, D.S., McAdams, L. (1985) 'Bacterial meningitis in infants: sonographic findings.' *Radiology*, **154**, 645–650.

Hansen, K., Lebech, A-M. (1992) 'The clinical and epidemiological profile of Lyme neuroborreliosis in Denmark 1985–1990. A prospective study of 187 patients with *Borrelia burgdorferi* specific intrathecal antibody production.' *Brain*, **115**, 399–423.

Hansson, L-O., Axelsson, G., Linné, T., *et al.* (1993) 'Serum C-reactive protein in the differential diagnosis of acute meningitis.' *Scandinavian Journal of Infectious Diseases*, **25**, 625–630.

Harden, A., Boyd, S.G., Cole, G., Levin, M. (1991) 'EEG features and their evolution in the acute phase of haemorrhagic shock and encephalopathy syndrome.' *Neuropediatrics*, **22**, 194–197.

Haribhai, H.C., Bhigjee, A.I., Bill, P.L., *et al.* (1991) 'Spinal cord schistosomiasis. A clinical, laboratory and radiological study, with a note on therapeutic aspects.' *Brain*, **114**, 709–726.

Harrington, W.J., Sheremata, W., Hjelle, B., *et al.* (1993) 'Spastic ataxia associated with human T-cell lymphotrophic virus type II infection.' *Annals of Neurology*, **33**, 411–414.

Harrison, L.H., Broome, C.V., Hightower, A.W., and the *Haemophilus* Vaccine Efficacy Study Group (1989) '*Haemophilus influenzae* type b polysaccharide vaccine: an efficacy study.' *Pediatrics*, **84**, 255–261.

Hart, C.A., Cuevas, L.E., Marzouk, O., *et al.* (1993) 'Management of bacterial meningitis.' *Journal of Antimicrobial Chemotherapy*, **32**, Suppl. A, 49–59.

Hawkins, S.A., Lyttle, J.A., Connolly, J.H. (1987) 'Two cases of influenza B encephalitis.' *Journal of Neurology, Neurosurgery, and Psychiatry*, **50**, 1236–1237.

Hayakawa, H., Katoh, T. (1995) 'Severe cerebellar atrophy following acute cerebellitis.' *Pediatric Neurology*, **12**, 159–161.

Hayes, E.B., Gubler, D.J. (1992) 'Dengue and dengue hemorrhagic fever.' *Pediatric Infectious Disease Journal*, **11**, 311–317.

Heath, P.D., Booth, L., Leigh, P.N., Turner, A.M. (1986) '*Legionella* brainstem encephalopathy and peripheral neuropathy without preceding pneumonia.' *Journal of Neurology, Neurosurgery, and Psychiatry*, **49**, 216–218.

Hemachudha, N.S., Kocen, R.S. (1986) 'Unusual EEG pattern in rubella encephalitis.' *Journal of Neurology, Neurosurgery, and Psychiatry*, **49**, 458–459. *(Letter.)*

Hemphill, M., Freeman, J.M., Martinez, C.R., *et al.* (1982) 'A new treatable source of recurrent meningitis: basioccipital meningocele.' *Pediatrics*, **70**, 941–943.

Hendarto, S.K., Hadinegoro, S. (1990) 'Current knowledge of pathogenesis and management of dengue encephalopathy.' *In: Proceedings of the Fifth International Child Neurology Congress, Tokyo*, pp. 610–611.

Henrickson, M., Weisse, M.E. (1992) 'Tuberculous brain abscess in a three-year-old South Pacific Islander.' *Pediatric Infectious Disease Journal*, **11**, 488–491.

Héron, B., Texier, J.L., Boespflug, O., *et al.* (1990) 'Hydrocéphalie aiguë révélatrice d'une méningite à *Candida* à l'âge de deux mois.' *Archives Françaises de Pédiatrie*, **47**, 279–281.

Herrold, J.D., Hahn, J.S. (1994) 'Disseminated multifocal herpes zoster leukoencephalitis and subcortical hemorrhage in an immunosuppressed child.' *Journal of Child Neurology*, **9**, 56–58.

Heyderman, R.S., Robb, S.A., Kendall, B.E., Levin, M. (1992) 'Does computed tomography have a role in the evaluation of complicated acute bacterial meningitis in childhood?' *Developmental Medicine and Child Neurology*, **34**, 870–875.

Hirano, A., Ayata, M., Wang, A.H., Wong, T.C. (1993) 'Functional analysis of matrix proteins expressed from cloned genes of measles virus variants that cause subacute sclerosing panencephalitis reveals a common defect in nucleocapsid binding.' *Journal of Virology*, **67**, 1848–1853.

Hirsch, J.F., Hoppe-Hirsch, E. (1988) 'Shunts and shunt problems in childhood.' *In: Symon, L. (Ed.) Advances and Technical Standards in Neurosurgery, Vol. 16*. Wien: Springer, pp. 177–196.

—— Roux, F.X., Sainte-Rose, C., *et al.* (1983) 'Brian abscess in childhood. A study of 34 cases treated by puncture and antibiotics.' *Child's Brain*, **10**, 251–265.

Hirsch, M.S., Schooley, R.T. (1989) 'Resistance to antiviral drugs: the end of the innocence.' *New England Journal of Medicine*, **320**, 313–314.

Hodges, J.R. (1987) 'Hepatitis A and meningo-encephalitis.' *Journal of Neurology*, **234**, 364.

Hoffman, S.L. (1996) 'Artemether in severe malaria—still too many deaths.' *New England Journal of Medicine*, **335**, 124–126.

—— Rustama, D., Punjabi, N.H., *et al.* (1988) 'High-dose dexamethasone in quinine-treated patients with cerebral malaria: a double-blind placebo-controlled trial.' *Journal of Infectious Diseases*, **158**, 325–331.

Holguin, J., Manotas, R. (1988) 'Recurrent purulent meningitis.' *International Pediatrics*, **3**, 175–183.

Höllsberg, P., Hafler, D.A. (1993) 'Pathogenesis of diseases induced by human lymphotropic virus type 1 infection.' *New England Journal of Medicine*, **328**, 1173–1182.

Horowitz, M.B., Pang, D., Hirsch, W. (1991) 'Acute cerebellitis: case report and review.' *Pediatric Neurosurgery*, **17**, 142–145.

Hosoda, K., Tamaki, N., Masumura, M., Matsumoto, S. (1987) 'Magnetic resonance images of brainstem encephalitis: case report.' *Journal of Neurosurgery*, **66**, 283–285.

Howard, R.S., Lees, A.J. (1987) 'Encephalitis lethargica: a report of four recent cases.' *Brain*, **110**, 19–33.

Howlett, W.P., Brubaker, G.R., Mlingi, N., Rosling, H. (1990) 'Konzo, an epidemic upper motor neuron disease studied in Tanzania.' *Brain*, **113**, 223–235.

Hsich, G., Kenney, K., Gibbs, C.J., *et al.* (1996) 'The 14-3-3 brain protein in cerebrospinal fluid as a marker for transmissible spongiform encephalopathies.' *New England Journal of Medicine*, **335**, 924–930.

Huang, C.C., Chu, N.S., Chen, T.J. (1988) 'Acute haemorrhagic leucoencephalitis with a prolonged clinical course.' *Journal of Neurology, Neurosurgery, and Psychiatry*, **51**, 870–874.

Hulihan, J.F., Bebin, E.M., Westmoreland, B.F. (1992) 'Bilateral periodic lateralized epileptiform discharges in *Mycoplasma* encephalitis.' *Pediatric Neurology*, **8**, 292–294.

Hung, K.L. (1986) 'Cranial ultrasound in the detection of postmeningitic complications in the neonate.' *Brain and Development*, **8**, 31–36.

Hurst, D.L., Mehta, S. (1988) 'Acute cerebellar swelling in varicella encephalitis.' *Pediatric Neurology*, **4**, 122–123.

Hurwitz, E.S., Nelson, B., Davis, C., *et al.* (1982) 'National surveillance for Reye syndrome. A five-year review.' *Pediatrics*, **70**, 895–900.

Husson, R.N., Comeau, A.M., Hoff, R. (1990) 'Diagnosis of human immunodeficiency virus infection in infants and children.' *Pediatrics*, **86**, 1–10.

—— Lan, Y., Kojima, E., *et al.* (1995) 'Vertical transmission of human immunodeficiency virus type 1: autologous neutralizing antibody, virus load, and virus phenotype.' *Journal of Pediatrics*, **126**, 865–871.

Hutchinson, D.N., Hesling, A.G., Darling, W.M. (1977) 'Simultaneous bacterial and viral infections of meninges.' *Lancet*, **1**, 371. *(Letter.)*

Ichiba, N., Miyake, Y., Sato, K., *et al.* (1988) 'Mumps-induced opsoclonus–myoclonus and ataxia.' *Pediatric Neurology*, **4**, 224–227.

Ichiyama, T., Houdou, S., Kisa, T., *et al.* (1990) 'Varicella with delayed hemiplegia.' *Pediatric Neurology*, **6**, 279–281.

Idriss, Z.H., Sinno, A.A., Kronfol, N.M. (1976) 'Tuberculous meningitis in childhood. Forty-three cases.' *American Journal of Diseases of Children*, **130**, 364–367.

Iragui, V.J., Maravi, E. (1986) 'Behçet syndrome' presenting as cerebrovascular disease.' *Journal of Neurology, Neurosurgery, and Psychiatry*, **49**, 838–840.

Iseki, E., Iwabuchi, K., Yagishita, S., *et al.* (1988) 'Two necropsy cases of chronic encephalomyelitis: variants of neuro-Behçet's syndrome.' *Journal of Neurology, Neurosurgery, and Psychiatry*, **51**, 1084-1087.

Iseman, M.D. (1993) 'Treatment of multidrug-resistant tuberculosis.' *New England Journal of Medicine*, **329**, 784–791.

Ito, M., Go, T., Okuno, T., Mikawa, H. (1991) 'Chronic mumps virus encephalitis.' *Pediatric Neurology*, **7**, 467–470.

Jacobs, R.F., Hsi, S., Wilson, C.B., *et al.* (1983) 'Apparent meningococcemia: clinical features of disease due to *Haemophilus influenzae* and *Neisseria meningitidis*.' *Pediatrics*, **72**, 469–472.

—— Sunakorn, P., Chotpitayasunonah, T., *et al.* (1992) 'Intensive short course chemotherapy for tuberculous meningitis.' *Pediatric Infectious Disease Journal*, **11**, 194–198.

Jacobson, P.L., Farmer, T.W. (1981) 'Subdural empyema complicating meningitis in infants: improved prognosis.' *Neurology*, **31**, 190–193.

Jadavji, T., Biggar, W.D., Gold, R., Prober, C.G. (1986) 'Sequelae of acute bacterial meningitis in children treated for seven days.' *Pediatrics*, **78**, 21–25.

Jansen, B.R.H., Hart, W., Schreuder, O. (1993) 'Discitis in childhood. 12–35-year follow-up of 35 patients.' *Acta Orthopaedica Scandinavica*, **64**, 33–36.

Jardine, D.S., Bratton, S.L. (1995) 'Using characteristic changes in laboratory values to assist in the diagnosis of hemorrhagic shock and encephalopathy syndrome.' *Pediatrics*, **96**, 1126–1131.

Jaroonvesama, N. (1988) 'Differential diagnosis of eosinophilic meningitis.' *Parasitology Today*, **4**, 262–266.

Jay, V., Becker, L.E., Otsubo, H., *et al.* (1995) 'Chronic encephalitis and epilepsy (Rasmussen's encephalitis): detection of cytomegalovirus and herpes simplex virus 1 by the polymerase chain reaction and in situ hybridization.' *Neurology*, **45**, 108–117.

John, C.C. (1994) 'Treatment failure with use of a third-generation cephalosporin for penicillin-resistant pneumococcal meningitis: case report and review.' *Clinics in Infectious Diseases*, **18**, 188–193.

Johns, D.R., Stein, A.G., Wityk, R. (1993) 'MELAS syndrome masquerading as herpes simplex encephalitis.' *Neurology*, **43**, 2471–2473.

Johnsen, S.D., Sidell, A.D., Bird, R. (1989) 'Subtle encephalomyelitis in children: a variant of acute disseminated encephalomyelitis.' *Journal of Child Neurology*, **4**, 214–217.

Johnson, K.P., Lepow, M.L., Johnson, R.T. (1968) 'California encephalitis. I. Clinical and epidemiological studies.' *Neurology*, **18**, 250–254.

Johnson, P.R., Edwards, K.M., Wright, P.F. (1985) 'Failure of intraventricular gammaglobulin to eradicate echovirus encephalitis in a patient with X-linked hypogammaglobulinemia.' *New England Journal of Medicine*, **313**, 1546–1547.

Johnson, R.T. (1982) *Viral Infections of the Nervous System.* New York: Raven Press.

—— Griffin, D.E., Hirsch, R.L., *et al.* (1984) 'Measles encephalomyelitis—clinical and immunologic studies.' *New England Journal of Medicine*, **310**, 137–141.

Jones, C.M.V., Dunn, H.G., Thomas, E.E., *et al.* (1994) 'Acute encephalopathy and status epilepticus associated with human herpes virus 6 infection.' *Developmental Medicine and Child Neurology*, **36**, 646–650.

Jouanguy, E., Altare, F., Lamhamedi, S., *et al.* (1996) 'Interferon-γ-receptor deficiency in an infant with fatal Bacille Calmette–Guérin infection.' *New England Journal of Medicine*, **335**, 1956–1961.

Kaiser, R., Dörries, R., Martin, R., *et al.* (1989) 'Intrathecal synthesis of virus-specific oligoclonal antibodies in patients with enterovirus infection of the central nervous system.' *Journal of Neurology*, **236**, 395–399.

Kalsbeck, J.E., De Souza, A.L., Kleiman, M.B., *et al.* (1980) 'Compartmentalization of the cerebral ventricles as a sequel of neonatal meningitis.' *Journal of Neurosurgery*, **52**, 547–552.

Kamholz, J., Tremblay, G. (1985) 'Chickenpox with delayed contralateral hemiparesis caused by cerebral angiitis.' *Annals of Neurology*, **18**, 358–360.

Kamio, M., Tahira, K., Ono, J., Ikehara, C. (1982) 'Acute relapsing disseminated encephalomyelitis: case report and clinical study of 24 patients in previous reports.' *Journal of the Japanese Pediatric Society*, **86**, 559–566.

Kaplan, A.M., Kovelevski, J.T. (1978) 'Saint-Louis encephalitis with particular involvement of the brain stem.' *Archives of Neurology*, **35**, 45–46.

Kaplan, K.M., Oski, F.A. (1980) 'Anemia with *Haemophilus influenzae* meningitis.' *Pediatrics*, **65**, 1101–1104.

Kaplan, M.H., Klein, W.S., McPhee, J., Harper, R. (1983) 'Group B coxsackie virus infections in infants younger than three months of age: a serious childhood illness.' *Reviews of Infectious Diseases*, **5**, 1019–1032.

Kaplan, S.L., Feigin, R.D. (1978) 'The syndrome of inappropriate secretion of antidiuretic hormone in children with bacterial meningitis.' *Journal of Pediatrics*, **92**, 758–761.

—— Fishman, M.A. (1988) 'Update on bacterial meningitis.' *Journal of Child Neurology*, **3**, 82–93.

—— Goddard, J., Van Kleek, M., *et al.* (1981) 'Ataxia and deafness in children due to bacterial meningitis.' *Pediatrics*, **68**, 8–13.

—— Smith, E.O'B., Wills, C., Feigin, R.D. (1986) 'Association between preadmission oral antibiotic therapy and cerebrospinal fluid findings and sequelae caused by *Haemophilus influenzae* type B meningitis.' *Pediatric Infectious Disease Journal*, **5**, 626–632.

Kapur, N., Barker, S., Burrows, E.H., *et al.* (1994) 'Herpes simplex encephalitis: long term magnetic resonance imaging and neuropsychological profile.' *Journal of Neurology, Neurosurgery, and Psychiatry*, **57**, 1334–1342.

Karlsson, M., Hammers-Berggren, S., Lindquist, L., *et al.* (1994) 'Comparison of intravenous penicillin G and oral doxycycline for treatment of Lyme neuroborreliosis.' *Neurology*, **44**, 1203–1207.

Keidan, I., Shif, I., Keren, G., Passwell, J.H. (1992) 'Rotavirus encephalopathy: evidence of central nervous system involvement during rotavirus infection.' *Pediatric Infectious Disease Journal*, **11**, 773–775.

Kennard, C., Swash, M. (1981) 'Acute viral encephalitis. Its diagnosis and outcome.' *Brain*, **104**, 129–148.

Kennedy, C.R., Singer, H.S. (1988) 'Eosinophilia of the cerebrospinal fluid: late reaction to a silastic shunt.' *Developmental Medicine and Child Neurology*, **30**, 386–390.

—— Duffy, S.W., Smith, R., Robinson, R.O. (1987) 'Clinical predictors of outcome in encephalitis.' *Archives of Disease in Childhood*, **62**, 1156–1162.

Kennedy, W.A., Hoyt, M.J., McCracken, G.H. (1991) 'The role of corticosteroid therapy in children with pneumococcal meningitis.' *American Journal of Diseases of Children*, **145**, 1374–1378.

Kesselring, J., Miller, D.H., Robb, S.A., *et al.* (1990) 'Acute disseminated encephalomyelitis. MRI findings and the distinction from multiple sclerosis.' *Brain*, **113**, 291–302.

Kessler, S.L., Dajani, A.S. (1990) '*Listeria* meningitis in infants and children.' *Pediatric Infectious Disease Journal*, **9**, 61–63.

Khan, S., Yaqub, B.A., Poser, C.M., *et al.* (1995) 'Multiphasic disseminated encephalomyelitis presenting as alternating hemiplegia.' *Journal of Neurology, Neurosurgery, and Psychiatry*, **58**, 467–470.

Kibe, T., Fujimoto, S., Ishikawa, T., *et al.* (1996) 'Serial MRI findings of benign poliomyelitis.' *Brain and Development*, **18**, 147–149.

Kilpi, T., Anttila, M., Kallio, M.J.T., Peltola, H. (1993) 'Length of prediagnostic history related to the course and sequelae of childhood bacterial meningitis.' *Pediatric Infectious Disease Journal*, **12**, 184–188.

Kim, J.S., Choi, I.S., Lee, M.C. (1995) 'Reversible parkinsonism and dystonia following probable *Mycoplasma pneumoniae* infection.' *Movement Disorders*, **10**, 510–512.

Kim, K.S., Gohd, R.S. (1983) 'Acute encephalopathy in twins due to adenovirus type 7 infection.' *Archives of Neurology*, **40**, 58–59.

Kimura, S., Unayama, T., Mori, T. (1992) 'The natural history of acute disseminated leuko-encephalitis. A serial magnetic resonance imaging study.' *Neuropediatrics*, **23**, 192–195.

Kingsley, D.P.E., Hendrickse, W.A., Kendall, B.E., *et al.* (1987) 'Tuberculous meningitis: role of CT in management and prognosis.' *Journal of Neurology, Neurosurgery, and Psychiatry*, **50**, 30–36.

Kira, J-i., Goto, I., Otsuka, M., Ichiya, Y. (1993) 'Chronic progressive spinocerebellar syndrome associated with antibodies to human T-lymphotropic virus type I: clinico-virological and magnetic resonance imaging studies.' *Journal of the Neurologic Sciences*, **115**, 111–116.

Kitai, I., Navas, L., Rohlicek, C., *et al.* (1992) 'Recurrent aseptic meningitis secondary to an intracranial cyst: a case report and review of clinical features and imaging modalities.' *Pediatric Infectious Disease Journal*, **11**, 671–675.

Klass, P.E., Klein, J.O. (1992) 'Therapy of bacterial sepsis, meningitis and otitis media in infants and children: 1992 poll of directors of programs in pediatric infectious diseases.' *Pediatric Infectious Disease Journal*, **11**, 702–705.

Kleiman, M., Brunquell, P. (1995) 'Acute disseminated encephalomyelitis: response to intravenous immunoglobulin.' *Journal of Child Neurology*, **10**, 481–483.

—— Reynolds, J.K., Watts, N.H., *et al.* (1984) 'Superiority of acridine orange stain versus Gram stain in partially treated bacterial meningitis.' *Journal of Pediatrics*, **104**, 401–404.

—— Weinberg, G.A., Reynolds, J.K., Allen, S.D. (1993) 'Meningitis with beta-lactam-resistant *Streptococcus pneumoniae*: the need for early repeat lumbar puncture.' *Pediatric Infectious Disease Journal*, **12**, 782–784.

Klein, J.O., Feigin, R.D., McCracken, G.H. (1986) 'Report of the Task Force on Diagnosis and Management of Meningitis.' *Pediatrics*, **78**, 959–982.

Kline, M., Mason, E.O., Kaplan, S.L. (1988) 'Characterization of *Citrobacter diversus* strains causing neonatal meningitis.' *Journal of Infectious Diseases*, **157**, 101–105.

—— Fletcher, C.V., Federici, M.E., *et al.* (1996) 'Combination therapy with stavudine and didanosine in children with advanced human immunodeficiency virus infection: pharmacokinetic properties, safety, and immunologic and virologic effects.' *Pediatrics*, **97**, 886–890.

Kohl, S., James, A.R. (1985) 'Herpes simplex virus encephalitis during childhood: importance of brain biopsy diagnosis.' *Journal of Pediatrics*, **107**, 212–215.

Kolyvas, E., Sorger, S., Marks, M., Pai, C.H. (1978) '*Pasteurella ureae* meningoencephalitis.' *Journal of Pediatrics*, **92**, 81–82.

Kornberg, A.J., Harvey, A.S., Shield, L.K. (1991) 'Subacute sclerosing panencephalitis presenting as simple partial seizures.' *Journal of Child Neurology*, **6**, 146–149.

Koskiniemi, M., Ketonen, L. (1981) 'Herpes simplex virus encephalitis: progression of lesion shown by CT.' *Journal of Neurology*, **225**, 9–14.

—— Vaheri, A. (1989) 'Effect of measles, mumps, rubella vaccination on pattern of encephalitis in children.' *Lancet*, **1**, 31–34.

—— —— Taskinen, E. (1984) 'Cerebrospinal fluid alterations in herpes simplex encephalitis.' *Reviews of Infectious Diseases*, **6**, 608–618.

—— Rautonen, J., Lehtokoski-Lehtiniemi, E., Vaheri, A. (1991) 'Epidemiology of encephalitis in children: a 20-year survey.' *Annals of Neurology*, **29**, 492–497.

—— Piiparinen, H., Mannonen, L., *et al.* (1996) 'Herpes encephalitis is a disease of middle aged and elderly people: polymerase chain reaction for detection of herpes simplex virus in the CSF of 516 patients with encephalitis.' *Journal of Neurology, Neurosurgery, and Psychiatry*, **60**, 174–178.

Kovacs, S.O., Kuban, K., Strand, R. (1993) 'Lateral medullary syndrome following varicella infection.' *American Journal of Diseases of Children*, **147**, 823–825.

Krambovitis, E., McIlmurray, M.B., Lock, P.E., *et al.* (1984) 'Rapid diagnosis of tuberculosis meningitis by latex particle agglutination.' *Lancet*, **2**, 1229–1231.

Kramer, L.D. (1995) 'Medical treatment of cysticercosis—ineffective.' *Archives of Neurology*, **52**, 101–102.

Krasinski, K., Borkowsky, W., Bonk, S., *et al.* (1988) 'Bacterial infections in human immunodeficiency virus-infected children.' *Pediatric Infectious Disease Journal*, **7**, 323–328.

Krogstad, D.J., Herwaldt, B.L. (1988) 'Chemoprophylaxis and treatment of Malaria.' *New England Journal of Medicine*, **319**, 1538–1540.

Krüger, H., Kohlhepp, W., König, S. (1990) 'Follow-up of antibiotically treated and untreated neuroborreliosis.' *Acta Neurologica Scandinavica*, **82**, 59–67.

Kumar, A., Montanera, W., Willinsky, R., *et al.* (1993) 'MR features of tuberculous arachnoiditis.' *Journal of Computer Assisted Tomography*, **17**, 127–130.

Kurikka, S, Käyhty, H., Peltola, H., *et al.* (1995) 'Neonatal immunization: response to *Haemophilus influenzae* type b–tetanus toxoid conjugate vaccine.' *Pediatrics*, **95**, 815–822.

Kuroda, Y., Matsui, M., Kikuchi, M., *et al.* (1994) 'In situ demonstration of the HTLV-1 genome in the spinal cord of a patient with HTLV-1-associated myelopathy.' *Neurology*, **44**, 2295–2299.

Kyllerman, M.G., Herner, C., Bergström, T.B., Ekholm, S.E. (1993) 'PCR diagnosis of primary herpesvirus type I in poliomyelitis-like paralysis and respiratory tract disease.' *Pediatric Neurology*, **9**, 227–229.

Lacroix, C., Blanche, S., Dussaix, E., Tardieu, M. (1995) 'Acute necrotizing measles encephalitis in a child with AIDS.' *Journal of Neurology*, **242**, 249–251. *(Letter.)*

Lahat, E., Aladjem, M., Schiffer, J., Starinsky, R. (1993) 'Hydrocephalus due to bilateral obstruction of the foramen of Monro: a 'possible' late complication of mumps encephalitis.' *Clinical Neurology and Neurosurgery*, **95**, 151–154.

La Mantia, L., Salmaggi, A., Tajoli, L., *et al.* (1987) 'Cryptococcal meningo-encephalitis: intrathecal immunological response.' *Journal of Neurology*, **233**, 362–366.

Lambert, H.P. (1994) 'Meningitis.' *Journal of Neurology, Neurosurgery, and Psychiatry*, **57**, 405–415.

Lancet (1987) 'Reye's syndrome and aspirin: epidemiological associations and inborn errors of metabolism.' *Lancet*, **2**, 429–431. *(Editorial.)*

—— (1994) 'Zidovudine for mother, fetus, and child: hope or poison?' *Lancet*, **344**, 207–209.

Landrigan, P.J., Witte, J.J. (1973) 'Neurologic disorders following live measles-virus vaccination.' *Journal of the American Medical Association*, **223**, 1459–1462.

Larsen, P.D., Crisp, D. (1992) 'Acute bilateral striatal necrosis associated with *Mycoplasma pneumoniae* infection.' *Pediatric Neurology*, **8**, 363. *(Abstract.)*

Larsson, S., Cronberg, S., Winblad, S. (1979) 'Listeriosis during pregnancy and neonatal period in Sweden 1958–1974.' *Acta Paediatrica Scandinavica*, **68**, 485–493.

La Scolea, L.J., Dryja, D. (1984) 'Quantitation of bacteria in cerebrospinal fluid and blood of children with meningitis and its diagnostic significance.' *Journal of Clinical Microbiology*, **19**, 187–190.

Law, D.A., Aronoff, S.C. (1992) 'Anaerobic meningitis in children: case report and review of the literature.' *Pediatric Infectious Disease Journal*, **11**, 968–971.

Lebel, M.H., McCracken, G.H. (1989) 'Delayed cerebrospinal fluid steriliza-tion and adverse outcome of bacterial meningitis in infants and children.' *Pediatrics*, **83**, 161–167.

—— Freij, B.J., Syrogiannopoulos, G.A., *et al.* (1988) 'Dexamethasone therapy for bacterial meningitis: results of two double-blind, placebo controlled trials.' *New England Journal of Medicine*, **319**, 964–971.

—— Hoyt, J., Waagner, D.C., *et al.* (1989) 'Magnetic resonance imaging and dexamethasone therapy for bacterial meningitis.' *American Journal of Diseases of Children*, **143**, 301–306.

Lebon, P., Lyon, G. (1974) 'Non-congenital rubella encephalitis.' *Lancet*, **2**, 468.

—— Boutin, B., Dulac, O., *et al.* (1988) 'Interferon γ in acute and subacute encephalitis.' *British Medical Journal*, **296**, 9–11.

Lee, W.L., Dooling, E.C., Mikati, M.A., De Long, G.R. (1988) 'Limbic encephalopathy presenting as prolonged complex partial status epilepticus: a new entity?' *Annals of Neurology*, **24**, 359. *(Abstract.)*

Lees, A.J., MacLeod, A.F., Marshall, J. (1980) 'Cerebral tuberculomas developing during treatment of tuberculous meningitis.' *Lancet*, **1**, 1208–1211.

Legg, N.J., Gupta, P.C., Scott, D.F. (1973) 'Epilepsy following cerebral abscess.' *Brain*, **96**, 259–268.

Leggiadro, R.J. (1994) 'Penicillin—and cephalosporin—resistant *Streptococcus pneumoniae*: an emerging microbial threat.' *Pediatrics*, **93**, 500–503.

Lehky, T.J., Fox, C.H., Koenig, S., *et al.* (1995) 'Detection of human T-lymphotropic virus type I (HTLV-1) tax RNA in the central nervous system of HTLV-1-associated myelopathy/tropical spastic paraparesis patients by in situ hybridization.' *Annals of Neurology*, **37**, 167–175.

Lehtokoski-Lehtiniemi, E., Koskiniemi, M-L. (1989) '*Mycoplasma pneumoniae* encephalitis: a severe entity in children.' *Pediatric Infectious Disease Journal*, **8**, 651–652.

Leis, A.A., Butler, I.J. (1987) 'Infantile herpes zoster ophthalmicus and acute hemiparesis following intrauterine chickenpox.' *Neurology*, **37**, 1537–1538.

Lenoir, P., De Meirleir, L., Bougatef, A., *et al.* (1990) 'Unexpected diagnosis of *Candida albicans* meningitis in a premature neonate.' *Pediatric Neurology*, **5**, 370–372.

Lepow, M.I., Gold, R. (1983) 'Meningococcal A and other polysaccharide vaccines. A five-year report.' *New England Journal of Medicine*, **308**, 1158–1160.

Levin, M., Hjelm, M., Kay, J.D.S., *et al.* (1983) 'Haemorrhagic shock and encephalopathy: a new syndrome with a high mortality in young children.' *Lancet*, **2**, 64–67.

—— Pincott, J.R., Hjelm, M., *et al.* (1988) 'Hemorrhagic shock and encephalopathy: clinical, pathologic and biochemical picture.' *Journal of Pediatrics*, **114**, 194–203.

Levitt, L.P., Rich, T.A., Kinde, S.W., *et al.* (1970) 'Central nervous system mumps. A review of 64 cases.' *Neurology*, **20**, 829–834.

Lewin, R.A., Hughes, W.T. (1966) '*Neisseria subflava* as a cause of meningitis and septicemia in children.' *Journal of the American Medical Association*, **195**, 821–826.

Lewis, D.W., Tucker, S.H. (1986) 'Central nervous system involvement in cat scratch disease.' *Pediatrics*, **77**, 714–721.

Lewis, M.A., Priestley, B.L. (1986) 'Transient neonatal Behçet's disease.' *Archives of Disease in Childhood*, **61**, 805–806.

Leys, D., Destee, A., Petit, H., Warot, P. (1986) 'Management of subdural intracranial empyemas should not always require surgery.' *Journal of Neurology, Neurosurgery, and Psychiatry*, **49**, 635–639.

L'Hommedieu, C., Stough, R., Brown, L., *et al.* (1979) 'Potentiation of neuromuscular weakness in infantile botulism by aminoglycosides.' *Journal of Pediatrics*, **95**, 1065–1070.

Lin, J-J., Harn, H-J., Hsu, Y-D., *et al.* (1995) 'Rapid diagnosis of tuberculous meningitis by polymerase chain reaction assay of cerebrospinal fluid.' *Journal of Neurology*, **242**, 147–152.

Lin, T.Y., Nelson, J.D., McCracken, G.H. (1984) 'Fever during treatment for bacterial meningitis.' *Pediatric Infectious Disease Journal*, **3**, 319–332.

Linssen, W.H.J.P., Gabreëls, F.J.M., Wevers, R.A. (1991) 'Infective acute transverse myelopathy. Report of two cases.' *Neuropediatrics*, **22**, 107–109.

Livartowski, A., Guyot, C., Dabernat, H., *et al.* (1989) 'Épidémiologie des méningites à *Haemophilus influenzae* type b dans deux départements français.' *Archives Françaises de Pédiatrie*, **46**, 175–179.

Long, S., Gajewski, J.L., Brown, L.W., Gilligan, P.H. (1985) 'Clinical, laboratory and environmental features of infant botulism in South Eastern Pennsylvania.' *Pediatrics*, **75**, 945–951.

Looareesuwan, S., Warrell, D.A., White, N.J., *et al.* (1983) 'Do patients with cerebral malaria have cerebral oedema? A computed tomography study.' *Lancet*, **1**, 434–437.

Lobato, M.N., Caldwell, M.B., Ng, P., *et al.* (1995) 'Encephalopathy in children with perinatally acquired human immunodeficiency virus infection.' *Journal of Pediatrics*, **126**, 710–715.

Lopez-Hernandez, A., Garaizar, C. (1982) 'Childhood cerebral cysticercosis: clinical features and computed tomographic findings in 89 Mexican children.' *Canadian Journal of Neurological Sciences*, **9**, 401–407.

Louis, E.D., Lynch, T., Kaufmann, P., *et al.* (1996) 'Diagnostic guidelines in central nervous system Whipple's disease.' *Annals of Neurology*, **40**, 561–568.

Lovejoy, F.J., Smith, A.L., Bresnan, M.J., *et al.* (1974) 'Clinical staging in Reye's syndrome.' *American Journal of Diseases of Children*, **128**, 36–41.

Lowichik, A., Ruff, A.J. (1995a) 'Parasitic infections of the central nervous system in children. Part II: Disseminated infections.' *Journal of Child Neurology*, **10**, 77–87.

—— —— (1995b) 'Parasitic infections of the central nervous system in children. Part III: Space-occupying lesions.' *Journal of Child Neurology*, **10**, 177–190.

Luna, D., Williams, C., Dulac, O., *et al.* (1990) 'L'encéphalite aiguë retardée de la rougeole.' *Archives Françaises de Pédiatrie*, **47**, 339–344.

Luzuriaga, K., Bryson, Y., Krogstad, P., *et al.* (1997) 'Combination treatment with zidovudine, didanosine, and nevirapine in infants with human immunodeficiency virus type 1 infection.' *New England Journal of Medicine*, **336**, 1343–349.

Lyon, G., Dodge, P.R., Adams, R.D. (1961) 'The acute encephalopathies of obscure origin in infants and children.' *Brain*, **84**, 680–708.

—— Griscelli, C., Fernandez-Alvarez, E., *et al.* (1980) 'Chronic progressive encephalitis in children with X-linked hypogammaglobulinemia.' *Neuropädiatrie*, **11**, 57–71.

—— Ponsot, G., Lebon, P. (1977) 'Acute measles encephalitis of the delayed type.' *Annals of Neurology*, **2**, 322–327.

MacDonald, K.L., Osterholm, M.T., Hedberg, C.W., *et al.* (1987) 'Toxic shock syndrome. A newly recognized complication of influenza and influenzalike illness.' *Journal of the American Medical Association*, **257**, 1053–1058.

MacKendall, R.R., Klawans, H. (1978) 'Nervous system complications of varicella-zoster virus.' *In:* Vinken, P.J., Bruyn, G.W. (Eds.) *Handbook of Clinical Neurology. Vol. 34. Infections of the Nervous System. Part II.* Amsterdam: North Holland, pp. 161–183.

Madore, D.V., Johnson, C.L., Phipps, D.C., *et al.* (1990) 'Safety and immunogenicity of *Haemophilus influenzae* type b oligosaccharide–CRM197 conjugate vaccine in infants aged 15 to 23 months.' *Pediatrics*, **86**, 527–534.

Maguire, J.F., Meissner, H.C. (1985) 'Onset of encephalitis early in the course of varicella infection.' *Pediatric Infectious Disease Journal*, **4**, 699–701.

Maida, E., Horvatits, E. (1986) 'Cerebrospinal fluid alterations in bacterial meningitis.' *European Neurology*, **25**, 110–116.

Mann, J.M., Shandler, L., Cushing, A.H. (1982) 'Pediatric plague.' *Pediatrics*, **69**, 762–767.

Marcus, J.C. (1982) 'Congenital neurosyphilis: a reappraisal.' *Neuropediatrics*, **13**, 195–199.

Marks, D.A., Kim, J., Spencer, D.D., *et al.* (1992) 'Characteristics of intractable seizures following meningitis and encephalitis.' *Neurology*, **42**, 1513–1518.

Marks, W.A., Stutman, H.R., Marks, M.I., *et al.* (1986) 'Cefuroxime versus ampicillin plus chloramphenicol in childhood bacterial meningitis: a multicenter randomized controlled trial.' *Journal of Pediatrics*, **109**, 123–130.

—— Bodensteiner, J.B., Bobele, G.B., *et al.* (1988) 'Parainflammatory leukoencephalomyelitis: clinical and magnetic resonance imaging findings.' *Journal of Child Neurology*, **3**, 205–213.

Marshall, G.S., Gesser, R.M., Yamanishi, K., Starr, S.E. (1991) 'Chronic fatigue in children: clinical features, Epstein–Barr virus and human herpesvirus 6 serology and long term follow-up.' *Pediatric Infectious Disease Journal*, **10**, 287–290.

Marshall, W.C. (1983) 'Infections of the nervous system.' *In:* Brett, E.M. (Ed.) *Paediatric Neurology.* Edinburgh: Churchill Livingstone, pp. 508–567.

Marton, R., Gotlieb-Stematsky, T., Klein, C., *et al.* (1995) 'Mild form of acute herpes simplex encephalitis in childhood.' *Brain and Development*, **17**, 360–361.

Masdeu, J.C., Small, C.B., Weiss, L., *et al.* (1988) 'Multifocal cytomegalovirus encephalitis in AIDS.' *Annals of Neurology*, **23**, 97–99.

Mathew, N.T., Abraham, J., Chandy, J. (1970) 'Cerebral angiographic features in tuberculous meningitis.' *Neurology*, **20**, 1015–1023.

Mathiesen, T., Linde, A., Olding-Stenkvist, E., Wahren, B. (1988) 'Specific IgG subclass reactivity in herpes simplex encephalitis.' *Journal of Neurology*, **235**, 400–406.

Mauser, H.W., Van Houwelingen, H.C., Tulleken, C.A.F. (1987) 'Factors affecting the outcome in subdural empyema.' *Journal of Neurology, Neurosurgery, and Psychiatry*, **50**, 1136–1141.

McCarthy, V.P., Zimmerman, A.W., Miller, C.A. (1990) 'Central nervous system manifestations of parainfluenza virus type 3 infections in childhood.' *Pediatric Neurology*, **6**, 197–201.

McCracken, G.H., Threlkeld, N., Mize, S., *et al.* (1984) 'Moxalactam therapy for neonatal meningitis due to gram-negative enteric bacilli. A prospective controlled evaluation.' *Journal of the American Medical Association*, **252**, 1427–1432.

McGee, Z.A., Kaiser, A.B. (1985) 'Acute meningitis.' *In:* Mandell, G.L., Douglas, R.G., Bennett, J.E. (Eds.) *Principles and Practice of Infectious Diseases, 2nd Edn.* New York: John Wiley, pp. 560–573.

McMenamin, J.B., Volpe, J.J. (1984) 'Bacterial meningitis in infancy: effects on intracranial pressure and cerebral blood flow velocity.' *Neurology*, **34**, 500–504.

Marks, D.A., Kim, J., Spencer, D.D., *et al.* (1992) 'Characteristics of intractable seizures following meningitis and encephalitis.' *Neurology*, **42**, 1513–1518.

Medina, M., Genton, P., Montoya, M.C., *et al.* (1993) 'Effect of anticysticercal treatment on the prognosis of epilepsy in cysticercosis: a pilot trial.' *Epilepsia*, **34**, 1024–1027.

Medori, R., Tritschler, H.J., LeBlanc, A., *et al.* (1992) 'Fatal familial insomnia, a prion disease with a mutation at codon 178 of the prion protein gene.' *New England Journal of Medicine*, **326**, 444–449.

Mehren, M., Burns, P.J., Mamani, F. *et al.* (1988) 'Toxoplasmic myelitis mimicking intramedullary spinal cord tumor.' *Neurology*, **38**, 1648–1650.

Mellon, A.F., Appleton, R.E., Gardner-Medwin, D., Aynsley-Green, A. (1991) 'Encephalitis lethargica-like illness in a five-year-old.' *Developmental Medicine and Child Neurology*, **33**, 158–161.

Mellor, D.H. (1992) 'The place of computed tomography and lumbar puncture in suspected bacterial meningitis.' *Archives of Disease in Childhood*, **67**, 1417–1419.

Mertsola, J., Kennedy, W.A., Waagner, D., *et al.* (1991) 'Endotoxin concentrations in cerebrospinal fluid correlate with clinical severity and neurologic outcome of *Haemophilus influenzae* type b meningitis.' *American Journal of Diseases of Children*, **145**, 1099–1103.

Mikati, M.A., Lee, W.L., DeLong, G.R. (1985) 'Protracted epileptiform encephalopathy: an unusual form of partial complex status epilepticus.' *Epilepsia*, **26**, 563–571.

Miles, C., Hoffman, W., Lai, C-W., Freeman, J.W. (1993) 'Cytomegalovirus-associated transverse myelitis.' *Neurology*, **43**, 2143–2145.

Miller, C., Farrington, C.P., Harbert, K. (1992) 'The epidemiology of subacute sclerosing panencephalitis in England and Wales 1970–1989.' *International Journal of Epidemiology*, **21**, 998–1006.

Miller, E.S., Dias, P.S., Uttley, D. (1987) 'Management of subdural empyema: a series of 24 cases.' *Journal of Neurology, Neurosurgery, and Psychiatry*, **50**, 1415–1418.

Miller, H.G., Stanton, J.B., Gibbons, J.L. (1956) 'Para-infectious encephalomyelitis and related syndromes.' *Quarterly Journal of Medicine*, **25**, 427–505.

Miller, K.D., Greenberg, A.E., Campbell, C.C. (1989) 'Treatment of severe malaria in the United States with a continuous infusion of quinidine gluconate and exchange transfusion.' *New England Journal of Medicine*, **321**, 65–70.

Millner, M.M., Puchhammer-Stöckl, E. (1993) 'Herpes simplex virus encephalitis and febrile convulsions: contribution of polymerase chain reaction and magnetic resonance imaging.' *Annals of Neurology*, **34**, 503. *(Abstract.)*

Mills, R.W., Schoolfield, L. (1992) 'Acute transverse myelitis associated with *Mycoplasma pneumoniae* infection: a case report and review of the literature.' *Pediatric Infectious Disease Journal*, **11**, 228–231.

Minns, R.A. (Ed.) (1991) *Problems of Intracranial Pressure in Childhood. Clinics in Developmental Medicine No. 113/114.* London: Mac Keith Press.

—— Engleman, H.M., Stirling, H. (1989) 'Cerebrospinal fluid pressure in pyogenic meningitis.' *Archives of Disease in Childhood*, **64**, 814–820.

Mitchell, W.G., Crawford, T.O. (1988) 'Intraparenchymal cerebral cysticercosis in children: diagnosis and treatment.' *Pediatrics*, **82**, 76–82.

Mito, T., Tanaka, T., Becker, L.E., *et al.* (1986) 'Infantile bilateral striatal necrosis. Clinicopathological classification.' *Archives of Neurology*, **43**, 677–680.

Mizrahi, E., Tharp, B.R. (1982) 'A characteristic EEG pattern in neonatal herpes simplex encephalitis.' *Neurology*, **32**, 1215–1220.

Mizuguchi, M. (1997) 'Acute necrotizing encephalopathy of childhood: a novel form of acute encephalopathy prevalent in Japan and Taiwan.' *Brain and Development*, **19**, 81–92.

Mizuno, Y., Komori, S., Shigetomo, R., et al. (1995) 'Poliomyelitis-like illness after acute asthma (Hopkins syndrome): a histological study of biopsied muscle in a case.' *Brain and Development*, **17**, 126–129.

Molyneux, M.E., Taylor, T.E., Wirima, J.J., Borgstein, A. (1989) 'Clinical features and prognostic indicators in paediatric cerebral malaria: a study of 131 comatose Malawian children.' *Quarterly Journal of Medicine*, **71**, 441–459.

Monath, T.P. (1988) 'Japanese encephalitis—a plague of the Orient.' *New England Journal of Medicine*, **319**, 641–643.

—— (1990) 'Alphaviruses (Eastern, Western and Venezuelian equine encephalitis).' *In:* Mandell, G.L., Douglas, R.G., Bennett, J.E. (Eds.) *Principles and Practice of Infectious Diseases, 3rd Edn.* New York: Churchill Livingstone, pp. 1241–1242.

—— Tsai, T.-F. (1987) 'Saint-Louis encephalitis: lessons from the last decade.' *American Journal of Tropical Medicine and Hygiene*, **37** (Suppl.), 405–595.

Monteiro, L.M., Correia, M. (1991) 'Benign relapsing meningo-myelitis.' *Journal of Neurology, Neurosurgery, and Psychiatry*, **54**, 939–940.

Mori, M., Ban, N., Kinoshita, K. (1987) 'Familial occurrence of HTLV-1-associated myelopathy.' *Annals of Neurology*, **23**, 100. (Letter.)

Moxon, E.R., Smith, A.L., Averill, D.L., Smith, D.H. (1974) '*Haemophilus influenzae* meningitis in infant rats after intranasal inoculation.' *Journal of Infectious Diseases*, **129**, 154–162.

Mulligan, K., Nelson, S., Friedman, H.S., Andrews, P.I. (1992) 'Shigellosis-associated encephalopathy.' *Pediatric Infectious Disease Journal*, **11**, 889–890.

Muñoz, M., Valderrabanos, E.S., Diaz, E., et al. (1995) 'Appearance of resistance to beta-lactam antibiotics during therapy for *Streptococcus pneumoniae* meningitis.' *Journal of Pediatrics*, **127**, 98–99.

Murphy, J.V., Yunis, E.G. (1976) 'Encephalopathy following measles infection in children with chronic illness.' *Journal of Pediatrics*, **88**, 937–942.

Mustafa, M.M., Weitman, S.D., Winick, N.J., et al. (1993) 'Subacute measles encephalitis in the young immunocompromised host: report of two cases diagnosed by polymerase chain reaction and treated with ribavirin and review of the literature.' *Clinical Infectious Diseases*, **16**, 654–660.

Nagai, T., Yagishita, A., Tsuchiya, Y., et al. (1993) 'Symmetrical thalamic lesions on CT in influenza A virus infection presenting with or without Reye syndrome.' *Brain and Development*, **15**, 67–74.

Nahmias, A.J., Whitley, R.J., Visintine, A.N., et al. (1982) 'Herpes simplex virus encephalitis: laboratory evaluation and their diagnostic significance.' *Journal of Infectious Diseases*, **145**, 829–836.

Naidu, S., Glista, G., Fine, M., et al. (1982) 'Serial CT scans in *Haemophilus influenzae* meningitis of childhood.' *Developmental Medicine and Child Neurology*, **24**, 69–76.

Nakamura, Y., Takahashi, M., Ueyama, K., et al. (1994) 'Magnetic resonance imaging and brain-stem auditory evoked potentials in neuro-Behçet's disease.' *Journal of Neurology*, **241**, 481–486.

Nasralla, C.A.W., Pay, N., Goodpasture, H.C., et al. (1993) 'Post-infectious encephalopathy in a child following *Campylobacter jejuni* enteritis.' *American Journal of Neuroradiology*, **14**, 1042–1044.

Newport, M.J., Huxley, C.M., Huston, S., et al. (1996) 'A mutation in the interferon-γ-receptor gene and susceptibility to mycobacterial infection.' *New England Journal of Medicine*, **335**, 1941–1949.

Newton, C.R.J.C., Peshu, N., Kendall, B., et al. (1994) 'Brain swelling and ischaemia in Kenyans with cerebral malaria.' *Archives of Disease in Childhood*, **70**, 281–287.

Ni, H., Knight, A.I., Cartwright, K., et al. (1992) 'Polymerase chain reaction for diagnosis of meningococcal meningitis.' *Lancet*, **340**, 1432–1434.

Nihei, K., Kamoshita, S., Mizutani, H., et al. (1977) 'Atypical subacute sclerosing panencephalitis.' *Acta Neuropathologica*, **38**, 163–166.

—— Naitoh, H., Ikeda, K. (1987) 'Poliomyelitis-like syndrome following asthmatic attack (Hopkins syndrome).' *Pediatric Neurology*, **3**, 166–168.

Nkowane, B.H., Wassilak, S.G.F., Orenstein, W.A., et al. (1987) 'Vaccine associated paralytic poliomyelitis. United States: 1973 through 1984.' *Journal of the American Medical Association*, **257**, 1335–1340.

Norman, M.G., Lowden, J.A., Hill, D.E., Bannatyne, R.M. (1968) 'Encephalopathy and fatty degeneration of the viscera in children. II. Report of a case with isolation of influenza B virus.' *Canadian Medical Association Journal*, **99**, 549–554.

North, K., de Silva, L., Procopis, P. (1993) 'Brain-stem encephalitis caused by Epstein–Barr virus.' *Journal of Child Neurology*, **8**, 40–42.

Nottidge, V.A. (1983) 'Pneumococcal meningitis in sickle cell disease in childhood.' *American Journal of Diseases of Children*, **137**, 29–31.

Odio, C.M., Faingezicht, I., Paris, M., et al. (1991) 'The beneficial effects of early dexamethasone administration in infants and children with bacterial meningitis.' *New England Journal of Medicine*, **324**, 1526–1531.

O'Duffy, J.D., Robertson, D.M., Golstein, N.P. (1984) 'Chlorambucil in the treatment of uveitis and meningoencephalitis of Behçet's disease.' *American Journal of Medicine*, **76**, 75–84.

Offenbacher, H., Fazekas, F., Schmidt, R., et al. (1991) 'MRI in tuberculous meningoencephalitis: report of four cases and review of the neuroimaging literature.' *Journal of Neurology*, **238**, 340–344.

Oki, J., Yoshida, H., Tokumitsu, A., et al. (1995) 'Serial neuroimages of acute necrotizing encephalopathy associated with human herpesvirus 6 infection.' *Brain and Development*, **17**, 356–359.

Olinsky, A. (1970) 'Precocious sexual development following tuberculous meningitis. Case report.' *South African Medical Journal*, **44**, 1189–1190.

Olson, L.C., Bourgeois, C.H., Cotton, R.B., et al. (1971) 'Encephalopathy and fatty degeneration of the viscera in Northeastern Thailand. Clinical syndrome and epidemiology.' *Pediatrics*, **47**, 707–716.

Ommaya, A.K. (1976) 'Spinal fluid fistulae.' *Clinical Neurosurgery*, **23**, 363–392.

Onorato, I.M., Wormser, G.P., Nicholas, P. (1980) '"Normal" CSF in bacterial meningitis.' *Journal of the American Medical Association*, **24**, 1469–1471.

Ormerod, I.E.C., Bronstein, A., Rudge, P., et al. (1986) 'Magnetic resonance imaging in clinically isolated lesions of the brain stem.' *Journal of Neurology, Neurosurgery, and Psychiatry*, **49**, 737–743.

Oxtoby, M.J. (1990) 'Perinatally acquired human immunodeficiency virus infection.' *Pediatric Infectious Disease Journal*, **9**, 609–619.

Pachner, A.R., Delaney, E. (1993) 'The polymerase chain reaction in the diagnosis of Lyme neuroborreliosis.' *Annals of Neurology*, **34**, 544–550.

—— Steere, A.L. (1985) 'The triad of neurologic manifestations of Lyme disease: meningitis, cranial neuritis and radiculoneuritis.' *Neurology*, **35**, 47–53.

—— Duray, P., Steere, A.C. (1989) 'Central nervous system manifestations of Lyme disease.' *Archives of Neurology*, **46**, 790–795.

Pagano, J.S. (1992) 'Epstein–Barr virus: culprit or consort?' *New England Journal of Medicine*, **327**, 1750–1752.

Parain, D., Boulloche, J. (1988) 'Crises épileptiques multifocales post-ourliennes.' *Neurophysiologie Clinique*, **18**, 187–191.

Park, Y.D., Belman, A.L., Dickson, D.W., et al. (1988) 'Stroke in pediatric acquired immunodeficiency syndrome.' *Annals of Neurology*, **24**, 359–360. (Abstract.)

Partin, J.C., Schubert, W.K., Partin, J.S. (1971) 'Mitochondrial ultrastructure in Reye's syndrome.' *New England Journal of Medicine*, **285**, 1339–1343.

Pascual, J., Combarros, O., Polo, J.M., Berciano, J. (1988) 'Localised CNS brucellosis: report of 7 cases.' *Acta Neurologica Scandinavica*, **78**, 282–289.

Pasternak, J.F., De Vivo, D.C., Prensky, A.L. (1980) 'Steroid-responsive encephalomyelitis in childhood.' *Neurology*, **30**, 481–486.

Paton, J.C., Lawrence, A.J., Steven, I.M. (1983) 'Quantities of *Clostridium botulinum* organisms and toxin in feces and presence of *Clostridium botulinum* toxin in the serum of an infant with botulism.' *Journal of Clinical Microbiology*, **17**, 13–15.

Pavlakis, S.G., Lu, D., Frank, Y., et al. (1995) 'Magnetic resonance spectroscopy in childhood AIDS encephalopathy.' *Pediatric Neurology*, **12**, 277–282.

Peacock, J.E., McGinnis, M.R., Cohen, M.S. (1984) 'Persistent neutrophilic meningitis: report of four cases and review of literature.' *Medicine*, **63**, 379–395.

Peckham, C., Gibb, D. (1995) 'Mother-to-child transmission of the human immunodeficiency virus.' *New England Journal of Medicine*, **333**, 298–302.

Pedro Vieira, J., Lobo Antunes, M., Levy Gomes, A. (1995) 'Acute infantile thalamic necrosis.' *Developmental Medicine and Child Neurology*, **37**, 1010–1012.

Pejme, J. (1964) 'Infectious mononucleosis.' *Acta Medica Scandinavica*, Suppl. 413, 51–63.

Pelekanos, J.T., Appleton, D.B. (1989) 'Melioidosis with multiple cerebral abscesses.' *Pediatric Neurology*, **5**, 48–52.

Peltola, H., Anttila, M., Renkonen, O.V., and the Finnish Study Group (1989) 'Randomised comparison of chloramphenicol, ampicillin cefotaxime and ceftriaxone for childhood bacterial meningitis.' *Lancet*, **1**, 1280–1287.

—— Kilpi, T., Anttila, M. (1992) 'Rapid disappearance of *Haemophilus influenzae* type b meningitis after routine childhood immunisation with conjugate vaccines.' *Lancet*, **340**, 592–594.

Peters, A.C.B., Vielvoye, G.J., Versteeg, J., *et al.* (1979) 'ECHO 25 focal encephalitis and subacute hemichorea.' *Neurology*, **29**, 676–681.

Peters, M.J., Pizer, B.L., Millar, M. (1994) 'Rifampicin in pneumococcal meningoencephalitis.' *Archives of Disease in Childhood*, **71**, 77–79.

Petit, H., Rousseaux, M., Lesoin, F., *et al.* (1983) 'Primauté du traitement médical des abcès cérébraux (19 cas).' *Revue Neurologique*, **139**, 575–581.

Phillips, R.E., Solomon, T. (1990) 'Cerebral malaria in children.' *Lancet*, **336**, 1355–1360.

Picard, F.J., Dekaban, G.A., Silva, J., Rice, G.P.A. (1993) 'Mollaret's meningitis associated with herpes simplex type 2 infection.' *Neurology*, **43**, 1722–1727.

Pike, M.G., Wong, P.K.H., Bencivenga, R., *et al.* (1990) 'Electrophysiologic studies, computed tomography, and neurologic outcome in acute bacterial meningitis.' *Journal of Pediatrics*, **116**, 702–706.

—— Kennedy, C.R., Neville, B.G.R., Levin, M. (1991) 'Herpes simplex encephalitis with relapse.' *Archives of Disease in Childhood*, **66**, 1242–1244.

Pizzo, P.A., Eddy, J., Falloon, J., *et al.* (1988) 'Effect of continuous intravenous infusion of zidovudine (AZT) in children with symptomatic HIV infection.' *New England Journal of Medicine*, **319**, 889–896.

Plouffe, J.F., Fass, R.J. (1980) 'Histoplasma meningitis: diagnostic value of cerebrospinal fluid serology.' *Annals of Internal Medicine*, **92**, 189–191.

Poltera, A.A. (1977) 'Thrombogenic intracranial vasculitis in tuberculous meningitis. A 20-year post-mortem study.' *Acta Neurologica Belgica*, **77**, 12–24.

Pomeroy, S.L., Holmes, S.J., Dodge, P.R., Feigin, R.D. (1990) 'Seizures and other neurologic sequelae of bacterial meningitis in children.' *New England Journal of Medicine*, **323**, 1651–1657.

Ponsot, G., Brette, C., Auberge, C., *et al.* (1980) 'La méningite tuberculeuse de l'enfant à l'époque de l'izoniazide. A propos de trente-deux observations.' *Revue de Pédiatrie*, **16**, 95–106.

Powderly, W.G., Saag, M.S., Cloud, G.A., *et al.* (1992) 'A controlled study of fluconazole or amphotericin B to prevent relapse of cryptococcal meningitis in patients with acquired immunodeficiency syndrome. The NAIAD AIDS Clinical Trials Group and Mycoses Study Group.' *New England Journal of Medicine*, **326**, 793–798.

Powell, K.R., Sugarman, L.I., Eskenazi, A.E., *et al.* (1990) 'Normalization of plasma arginine vasopressin concentrations when children with meningitis are given maintenance plus replacement fluid therapy.' *Journal of Pediatrics*, **117**, 515–522.

Prasad, K., Haines, T. (1995) 'Dexamethasone treatment for acute bacterial meningitis: how srong is the evidence for routine use?' *Journal of Neurology, Neurosurgery, and Psychiatry*, **59**, 31–37.

Prober, C.G. (1995) 'The role of steroids in the management of children with bacterial meningitis.' *Pediatrics*, **95**, 29–31.

Prusiner, S.B., Hsiao, K.K. (1994) 'Human prion diseases.' *Annals of Neurology*, **35**, 385–395.

Pyati, S.P., Pildes, R.S., Jacobs, N.M., *et al.* (1983) 'Penicillin in infants weighing two kilograms or less with early-onset group B streptococcal disease.' *New England Journal of Medicine*, **308**, 1383–1389.

Quagliariello, V.J., Scheld, W.M. (1992) 'Bacterial meningitis: pathogenesis, pathophysiology, and progress.' *New England Journal of Medicine*, **327**, 864–872.

—— —— (1997) 'Treatment of bacterial meningitis.' *New England Journal of Medicine*, **336**, 708–716.

Rabe, E.F., Flynn, R.E., Dodge, P.R. (1968) 'Subdural collections of fluids in infants and children: a study of 62 patients with special reference to factors influencing prognosis and efficacy of various forms of therapy.' *Neurology*, **18**, 559–570.

Radetsky, M. (1992) 'Duration of symptoms and outcome in bacterial meningitis: an analysis of causation and the implication of a delay in a diagnosis.' *Pediatric Infectious Disease Journal*, **11**, 694–698.

Rakover, Y., Adar, H., Tal, I., *et al.* (1989) 'Behçet disease: long-term follow-up of three children and review of the literature.' *Pediatrics*, **83**, 986–992.

Randhawa, P.S., Jaffe, R., Demetris, A.J., *et al.* (1992) 'Expression of Epstein–Barr virus-encoded small RNA (by the EBER-1 gene) in liver specimens from transplant recipients with post-transplantation lymphoproliferative disease.' *New England Journal of Medicine*, **327**, 1710–1714.

Rantala, H., Uhari, M., Uhari, M., *et al.* (1991) 'Outcome after childhood encephalitis.' *Developmental Medicine and Child Neurology*, **33**, 858–867.

Rautonen, J., Koskiniemi, M., Vaheri, A. (1991) 'Prognostic factors in childhood acute encephalitis.' *Pediatric Infectious Disease Journal*, **10**, 441–446.

Redfearn, A., Pennie, R.A., Mahony, J.B., Dent, P.B. (1993) 'Progressive multifocal leukoencephalopathy in a child with immunodeficiency and hyperimmunoglobulinemia M.' *Pediatric Infectious Disease Journal*, **12**, 399–401.

Rehle, T.M. (1989) 'Classification, distribution and importance of arboviruses.' *Tropical Medicine and Parasitology*, **40**, 391–395.

Renier, D., Flandin, C., Hirsch, E., Hirsch, J-F. (1988) 'Brain abscesses in neonates. A study of 30 cases.' *Journal of Neurosurgery*, **69**, 877–882.

Rennick, G., Shann, F., de Campo, J. (1993) 'Cerebral herniation during bacterial meningitis in children.' *British Medical Journal*, **306**, 953–955.

Revol, A., Vighetto, A., Jouvet, A., *et al.* (1992) 'Encephalitis in cat scratch disease with persistent dementia.' *Journal of Neurology, Neurosurgery, and Psychiatry*, **55**, 133–185.

Ribera, E., Martinez-Vazquez, J.M., Ocaña, I., *et al.* (1987) 'Activity of adenosine deaminase in cerebrospinal fluid for the diagnosis and follow-up of tuberculous meningitis in adults.' *Journal of Infectious Diseases*, **155**, 603–607.

Riikonen, R. (1978) 'Cytomegalovirus infection and infantile spasms.' *Developmental Medicine and Child Neurology*, **20**, 570–579.

—— (1993) 'Infantile spasms: infectious disorders.' *Neuropediatrics*, **24**, 274–280.

Riordan, F.A.I., Thomson, A.P.I., Sills, J.A, Hart, C.A. (1993) 'Does computed tomography have a role in the evaluation of complicated acute bacterial meningitis in childhood?' *Developmental Medicine and Child Neurology*, **35**, 275–276. *(Letter.)*

Risk, W.S., Haddad, F.S. (1979) 'The variable natural history of subacute sclerosing panencephalitis.' *Archives of Neurology*, **36**, 610–614.

River, Y., Averbuch-Heller, L., Weinberger, M., *et al.* (1994) 'Antibiotic-induced meningitis.' *Journal of Neurology, Neurosurgery, and Psychiatry*, **57**, 705–708.

Rivera, I.V., Curless, R.G., Indacochea, F.J., Scott, G.B. (1992) 'Chronic progressive CNS histoplasmosis presenting in childhood: response to fluconazole therapy.' *Pediatric Neurology*, **8**, 151–153.

Rivner, M.H., Jay, W.M., Green, J.B., Dyken P.R. (1982) 'Opsoclonus in *Haemophilus influenzae* meningitis.' *Neurology*, **32**, 661–663.

Robb, R.M., Watters, G.V. (1970) 'Ophthalmic manifestations of subacute sclerosing panencephalitis.' *Archives of Ophthalmology*, **83**, 426–435.

Robinson, R.O., Roberts, H. (1990) 'Acute bacterial meningitis. I: Diagnosis.' *Developmental Medicine and Child Neurology*, **32**, 83–86.

Roden, V.J., Cantor, H.E., O'Connor, D.M., *et al.* (1975) 'Acute hemiplegia of childhood associated with Coxsackie A9 viral infection.' *Journal of Pediatrics*, **86**, 56–58.

Rodriguez, A.F., Kaplan, S.L., Mason, E.O. (1990) 'Cerebrospinal fluid values in the very low birth weight infant.' *Journal of Pediatrics*, **116**, 971–974.

Rodriguez, W.J., Puig, J.R., Khan, W.N., *et al.* (1986) 'Ceftazidime *vs.* standard therapy for pediatric meningitis: therapeutic, pharmacologic and epidemiologic observations.' *Pediatric Infectious Disease Journal*, **5**, 408–415.

Roeser, R.J., Campbell, J.C., Dalty, D.D. (1975) 'Recovery of auditory function following meningitic deafness.' *Journal of Speech and Hearing Disorders*, **40**, 405–411.

Roessmann, U., Friede, R.L. (1967) 'Candidal infection of the brain.' *Archives of Pathology*, **84**, 495–498.

Roig, M., Calopa, M., Rovira, A., *et al.* (1993) 'Bilateral striatal lesions in childhood.' *Pediatric Neurology*, **9**, 349–358.

Roman, G.C. (1988) 'The neuroepidemiology of tropical spastic paraparesis.' *Annals of Neurology*, **23** (Suppl.), S113–S120.

Rose, J.W., Stroop, W.G., Matsuo, F., Henke, J. (1992) 'Atypical herpes simplex encephalitis: clinical, virologic, and neuropathologic evaluation.' *Neurology*, **42**, 1809–1812.

Rosemberg, S., Amaral, L.C., Kliemann, S.E., Arita, F.N. (1992) 'Acute encephalopathy with bilateral striatal necrosis. A distinctive clinicopathological condition.' *Neuropediatrics*, **23**, 310–315.

Rosenblum, M., Hoff, J.T., Norman, D., *et al.* (1980) 'Nonoperative treatment of brain abscesses in selected high-risk patients.' *Journal of Neurosurgery*, **52**, 217–225.

Rosenfeld, J., Taylor, C.L., Atlas, S.W. (1993) 'Myelitis following chickenpox: a case report.' *Neurology*, **43**, 1834–1836.

Ross, S.C., Densen, P. (1984) 'Complement deficiency states and infection: epidemiology, pathogenesis and consequences of Neisserial and other infections in an immune deficiency.' *Medicine*, **63**, 243–273.

Roth, B., Younossi-Hartenstein, A., Schröder R., *et al.* (1987) 'Haemorrhagic shock–encephalopathy syndrome. Plasmapheresis as a therapeutic approach.' *European Journal of Pediatrics*, **146**, 83–85.

Roulet Perez, E., Maeder, P., Cotting, J., *et al.* (1993) 'Acute fatal parainfectious cerebellar swelling in two children. A rare or an overlooked situation?' *Neuropediatrics*, **24**, 346–351.

Rubenstein, J.S., Yogev, R. (1985) 'What represents pleocytosis in blood-contaminated ("traumatic tap") cerebrospinal fluid in children?' *Journal of Pediatrics*, **107**, 249–251.

Rudge, P., Webster, A.D.B., Revesz, T., *et al.* (1996) 'Encephalomyelitis in primary hypogammaglobulinaemia.' *Brain*, **119**, 1–15.

Rush, P.J., Shore, A., Inman, R., *et al.* (1986) 'Arthritis associated with *Haemophilus influenzae* meningitis: septic or reactive?' *Journal of Pediatrics*, **109**, 412–415.

Russell, R.R., Donald, J.C. (1958) 'The neurological complications of mumps.' *British Medical Journal*, **2**, 27–34.

Rutledge, J., Benjamin, D., Hood, L., Smith, A. (1981) 'Is the CSF lactate measurement useful in the management of children with suspected bacterial meningitis?' *Journal of Pediatrics*, **98**, 20–24.

Rutter, N., Smales, O.R.C. (1977) 'Role of routine investigations in children presenting with their first febrile convulsion.' *Archives of Disease in Childhood*, **52**, 188–191.

Sada, E., Ruiz-Palacios, G.M., López-Vidal, Y., Ponce de León, S. (1983) 'Detection of mycobacterial antigens in cerebrospinal fluid of patients with tuberculosis meningitis by enzyme-linked immunosorbent assay.' *Lancet*, **2**, 651–652.

Saddler, M., Barry, M., Ternouth, I., Emmanuel, J. (1990) 'Treatment of severe malaria by exchange transfusion.' *New England Journal of Medicine*, **322**, 58. *(Letter.)*

Saez-Llorens, X., Ramilo, O., Mustafa, M.M., *et al.* (1990) 'Molecular pathophysiology of bacterial meningitis: current concepts and therapeutic implications.' *Journal of Pediatrics*, **116**, 671–684.

Saitoh, S., Wada, T., Narita, M., *et al.* (1993) '*Mycoplasma pneumoniae* infection may cause striatal lesions leading to acute neurologic dysfunction.' *Neurology*, **43**, 2150–2151.

Saukkonen, K., Sande, S., Cioffe, C. (1990) 'The role of cytokines in the generation of inflammation and tissue damage in experimental gram-positive meningitis.' *Journal of Experimental Medicine*, **171**, 439–448.

Saito, H., Endo, M., Takase, S., Itahara, K. (1980) 'Acute disseminated encephalomyelitis after influenza vaccination.' *Archives of Neurology*, **37**, 564–566.

Scemama, M., Chiron, C., Georges, P., Dulac, O. (1988) 'Radiculomyeloencéphalite à *Angiostrongylus cantonensis* chez l'enfant.' *Archives Françaises de Pédiatrie*, **45**, 417–419.

Schaad, U.B., Nelson, J.D., McCracken, G.H. (1981) 'Recrudescence and relapse in bacterial meningitis of childhood.' *Pediatrics*, **67**, 188–195.

—— Wedgwood-Krucko, J., Tschaeppeler, H. (1988) 'Reversible ceftriaxone-associated biliary pseudolithiasis in children.' *Lancet*, **2**, 1411–1413.

—— Suter, S., Gianella-Borradori, A., *et al.* (1990) 'A comparison of ceftriaxone and cefuroxime for the treatment of bacterial meningitis in children.' *New England Journal of Medicine*, **322**, 141–147.

—— Lips, U., Gnehm, H.E., *et al.* (1993) 'Dexamethasone therapy for bacterial meningitis in children.' *Lancet*, **342**, 457–461.

Scharf, D. (1988) 'Neurocysticercosis. Two hundred thirty-eight cases from a California hospital.' *Archives of Neurology*, **45**, 777–780.

Schauseil-Zipf, U., Harden, A., Hoare, R., *et al.* (1982) 'Early diagnosis of Herpes simplex encephalitis in childhood.' *European Journal of Pediatrics*, **138**, 154–161.

Schlech, W.F., Ward, J.I., Band, J.D., *et al.* (1985) 'Bacterial meningitis in the United States, 1978 thru 1981. The National Bacterial Meningitis Surveillance Study.' *Journal of the American Medical Association*, **253**, 1749–1754.

Schlesinger, Y., Sawyer, M.H., Storch, G.A. (1994) 'Enteroviral meningitis in infancy: potential role for polymerase chain reaction in patient management.' *Pediatrics*, **94**, 157–162.

Schmutzhard, E., Mayr, U., Rumpl, E., *et al.* (1986) 'Secondary cerebral amebiasis due to infection with *Entamoeba histolytica*. A case report with computer tomographic findings.' *European Neurology*, **25**, 161–165.

—— Boongird, P., Vejjajiva, A. (1988) 'Eosinophilic meningitis and radiculomyelitis in Thailand, caused by CNS invasion of *Gnathostoma spinigerum* and *Angiostrongylus cantonensis*.' *Journal of Neurology, Neurosurgery, and Psychiatry*, **51**, 80–87.

Schreiner, M.S., Field, E., Ruddy, R. (1991) 'Infant botulism: a review of 12 years' experience at the Children's Hospital of Philadelphia.' *Pediatrics*, **87**, 159–165.

Schwab, S., Jünger, E., Spranger, M., *et al.* (1997) 'Craniectomy: an aggressive treatment approach in severe encephalitis.' *Neurology*, **48**, 412–417.

Schwartz, J.F., Balentine, J.D. (1978) 'Recurrent meningitis due to an intracranial epidermoid.' *Neurology*, **28**, 124–129.

Sébire, G., Devictor, D., Huault, G., *et al.* (1992) 'Coma associated with intense bursts of abnormal movements and long-lasting cognitive disturb-

ances: an acute encephalopathy of obscure origin.' *Journal of Pediatrics*, **121**, 845–851.

Selby, G., Walker, G.L. (1979) 'Cerebral arteritis in cat scratch disease.' *Neurology*, **29**, 1413–1418.

Sen, S., Sharma, D., Singh, D., *et al.* (1989) 'Poliomyelitis in vaccinated children.' *Indian Journal of Pediatrics*, **26**, 423–429.

Senanayake, N. (1987) 'Delayed cerebellar ataxia: a new complication of falciparum malaria?' *British Medical Journal*, **294**, 1253–1254.

Shahar, E.M., Hwang, P.A., Niesen, C.E., Murphy, E.G. (1991) 'Poliomyelitis-like paralysis during recovery from acute bronchial asthma: possible etiology and risk factors.' *Pediatrics*, **88**, 276–279.

Shakir, R.A., Al-Din, A.S.N., Araj, G.F., *et al.* (1987) 'Clinical categories of neurobrucellosis: a report on 19 cases.' *Brain*, **110**, 213–223.

—— Sulaiman, K., Kahn, R.A., Rudwan, M. (1990) 'Neurological presentation of neuro-Behçet's syndrome: clinical categories.' *European Neurology*, **30**, 249–253.

Shankar, P., Manjunath, N., Mohan, K.K., *et al.* (1991) 'Rapid diagnosis of tuberculous meningitis by polymerase chain reaction.' *Lancet*, **337**, 5–7.

Shanks, D.E., Blasco, P.A., Chason, D.P. (1991) 'Movement disorder following herpes simplex encephalitis.' *Developmental Medicine and Child Neurology*, **33**, 348–352.

Sharer, L.R., Epstein, L.G., Cho, E-S., *et al.* (1986) 'Pathologic features of AIDS encephalopathy in children. Evidence for LAV/HTLV III infection of brain.' *Human Pathology*, **17**, 271–284.

Sharma, A., Abraham, J. (1983) 'Multiple giant hydatid cysts of the brain.' *Journal of Neurosurgery*, **57**, 413–415.

Sharpe, A.H., Fields, B.N. (1985) 'Pathogenesis of viral infections. Basic concepts derived from the reovirus model.' *New England Journal of Medicine*, **312**, 486–497.

Shaywitz, B.A., Lister, G., Duncan, C.C. (1986) 'What is the best treatment for Reye's syndrome?' *Archives of Neurology*, **43**, 730–731.

Shibasaki, H., Endo, C., Kuroda, Y., *et al.* (1988) 'Clinical picture of HTLV-1 associated myelopathy.' *Journal of the Neurological Sciences*, **87**, 15–24.

Shope, T.R., Garrett, A.L., Waecker, N.J. (1994) '*Mycobacterium bovis* spinal epidural abscess in a 6-year-old boy with leukemia.' *Pediatrics*, **93**, 835–837.

Silverman, I.E., Liu, G.T., Bilaniuk, L.T., *et al.* (1995) 'Tuberculous meningitis with blindness and perichiasmal involvement on MRI.' *Pediatric Neurology*, **12**, 65–67.

Silverstein, F.S., Brunberg, J.A. (1995) 'Postvaricella basal ganglia infarction in children.' *American Journal of Neuroradiology*, **16**, 449–452.

Simental, P.S., Parra, M.M., Valdéz, J.M., *et al.* (1993) 'Neonatal tetanus experience at the National Institute of Pediatrics in Mexico City.' *Pediatric Infectious Disease Journal*, **12**, 722–725.

Simmonds, H.A., Fairbanks, L.D., Morris, G.S., *et al.* (1987) 'Central nervous system dysfunction and erythrocyte guanosine triphosphate depletion in purine nucleoside phosphorylase deficiency.' *Archives of Disease in Childhood*, **62**, 385–391.

Sindic, C.J.M., Depré, A., Bigaignon, G., *et al.* (1987) 'Lymphocytic meningoradiculitis and encephalomyelitis due to *Borrelia burgdorferi*: a clinical and serological study of 18 cases.' *Journal of Neurology, Neurosurgery, and Psychiatry*, **50**, 1565–1571.

Skelton, R., Maixner, W., Isaacs, D. (1992) 'Sinusitis-induced subdural empyema.' *Archives of Disease in Childhood*, **67**, 1478–1480.

Sköldenberg, B., Forsgren, M., Alestig, K., *et al.* (1984) 'Acyclovir versus vidarabine in herpes simplex encephalitis. Randomised multicentre study in consecutive Swedish patients.' *Lancet*, **2**, 707–711.

Smith, A.L. (1988) 'Neurologic sequelae of meningitis.' *New England Journal of Medicine*, **319**, 1012–1014.

Smith, H.P., Hendrick, E.B. (1983) 'Subdural empyema and epidural abscess in children.' *Journal of Neurosurgery*, **58**, 392–397.

Smith, K.C., Starke, J.R., Eisenach, K., *et al.* (1996) 'Detection of *Mycobacterium tuberculosis* in clinical specimens from children using a polymerase chain reaction.' *Pediatrics*, **97**, 155–160.

Snedeker, J.D., Kaplan, S.L., Dodge, P.R., *et al.* (1990) 'Subdural effusion and its relationship with neurologic sequelae of bacterial meningitis in infancy: a prospective study.' *Pediatrics*, **86**, 163–170.

Snyder, R.D. (1984) 'Ventriculomegaly in childhood bacterial meningitis.' *Neuropediatrics*, **15**, 136–138.

Solders, G., Nennesmo, I., Persson, A. (1989) 'Diphtheritic neuropathy, an analysis based on muscle and nerve biopsy and repeated neurophysiological and autonomic function tests.' *Journal of Neurology, Neurosurgery, and Psychiatry*, **52**, 876–880.

Sonnabend, O., Sonnabend, W.F.F., Krech, U., et al. (1985) 'Continuous microbiological and pathological study of 70 sudden and unexpected infant deaths: toxigenic intestinal *Clostridium botulinum* infection in 9 cases of sudden infant death syndrome.' *Lancet*, **1**, 237–241.

Sotelo, J., del Brutto, O.H., Penagos, P., et al. (1990) 'Comparison of therapeutic regimen of anticysticercal drugs for parenchymal brain cysticercosis.' *Journal of Neurology*, **237**, 69–72.

Spector, S.A., Gelber, R.D., McGrath, N., et al. (1994) 'A controlled trial of intravenous immune globulin for the prevention of serious bacterial infections in children receiving zidovudine for advanced human immunodeficiency virus infection.' *New England Journal of Medicine*, **331**, 1181–1187.

Sperling, R.G., Shapiro, D.E., Coombs, R.W., et al. (1996) 'Maternal viral load, zidovudine treatment, and the risk of transmission of human immunodeficiency virus type 1 from mother to infant.' *New England Journal of Medicine*, **335**, 1621–1629.

Stanek, G., Wewalka, G., Groh, V., et al. (1985) 'Differences between Lyme disease and European arthropod-born *Borrelia* infections.' *Lancet*, **1**, 401. *(Letter.)*

Steele, R.W., McConnell, J.R., Jacobs, R.F., Mawk, J.R. (1985) 'Recurrent bacterial meningitis: coronal thin-section cranial computed tomography to delineate anatomic defects.' *Pediatrics*, **76**, 950–953.

Steere, A.C. (1989) 'Lyme disease.' *New England Journal of Medicine*, **321**, 586–596.

Stoll, B.J., Lee, F.K., Larsen, S., et al. (1993) 'Clinical and serologic evaluation of neonates for congenital syphilis: a continuing diagnostic dilemma.' *Journal of Infectious Diseases*, **167**, 1093–1099.

Stoppe, G., Stark, E., Patzold, U. (1987) 'Mollaret's meningitis: CSF-immunocytological examinations.' *Journal of Neurology*, **234**, 103–106.

Stumpf, D.A., Parker, W.D., Angelini, C. (1985) 'Carnitine deficiency, organic acidemias, and Reye's syndrome.' *Neurology*, **35**, 1041–1045.

Stutman, H.R., Marks, M.I. (1987) 'Bacterial meningitis in children: diagnosis and therapy: a review of recent developments.' *Clinical Pediatrics*, **26**, 431–438.

Swartz, M.N. (1987) '"Chronic meningitis". Many causes to consider.' *New England Journal of Medicine*, **317**, 957–959.

—— Dodge, P.R. (1965) 'Bacterial meningitis—a review of selected aspects. I. General clinical features, special problems and unusual meningeal reactions mimicking bacterial meningitis.' *New England Journal of Medicine*, **272**, 725–731, 779–787, 842–848, 898–902.

Sweeney, V.P., Drance, S.M. (1970) 'Optic neuritis and compressive neuropathy associated with cat scratch disease.' *Canadian Medical Association Journal*, **103**, 1380–1381.

Swift, T.R. (1981) 'Disorders of neuromuscular transmission other than myasthenia gravis.' *Muscle and Nerve*, **4**, 334–353.

Syrogiannopoulos, G.A., Nelson, J.D., McCracken, G.H. (1986) 'Subdural collections of fluid in acute bacterial meningitis: a review of 136 cases.' *Pediatric Infectious Disease Journal*, **5**, 343–352.

—— Olsen, K.D., Reisch, J.S., McCracken, G.H. (1987) 'Dexamethasone in the treatment of experimental *Haemophilus influenzae* type b meningitis.' *Journal of Infectious Diseases*, **155**, 213–219.

Taft, T.A., Chusid, M.J., Sty, J.R. (1986) 'Cerebral infarction in *Haemophilus influenzae* type b meningitis.' *Clinical Pediatrics*, **25**, 177–180.

Talamás, O., Del Brutto, O.H., Garcia-Ramos, G. (1989) 'Brain-stem tuberculoma. An analysis of 11 patients.' *Archives of Neurology*, **46**, 529–535.

Talan, A.D., Hoffman, J.R., Yoshikawa, T.T., Overturf, G.D. (1988) 'Role of empiric parenteral antibiotics prior to lumbar puncture in suspected bacterial meningitis: state of the art.' *Reviews of Infectious Diseases*, **10**, 365–376.

Tanaka, K., Kean, E.A., Johnson, B. (1976) 'Jamaican vomiting sickness.' *New England Journal of Medicine*, **295**, 461–467.

Tardieu, M., Lapresle, J. (1980) 'Persistance d'une atteinte inflammatoire herpétique du système nerveux central, quatre ans après une encéphalite aiguë.' *Revue Neurologique*, **136**, 67–69.

—— Powers, M.L., Hafler, D.A., et al. (1984) 'Autoimmunity following viral infection: demonstration of monoclonal antibodies against normal tissue following infection of mice with reovirus and demonstration of shared antigenicity between virus and lymphocytes.' *European Journal of Immunology*, **14**, 561–565.

—— Dussaix, E., Lebon, P., Landrieu, P. (1986) 'Etude prospective de 59 méningites virales de l'enfant. Diagnostic clinique et virologique. Epidémiologie et physiopathologie.' *Archives Françaises de Pédiatrie*, **43**, 9–14.

—— Blanche, S., Rouzioux, C., et al. (1987) 'Atteintes du système nerveux au cours des infections à HIV 1 du nourrisson.' *Archives Françaises de Pédiatrie*, **44**, 495–499.

—— Truffot-Pernot, C., Carrière, J.P., et al. (1988) 'Tuberculous meningitis due to BCG in two previously healthy children.' *Lancet*, **1**, 440–441.

—— Mayaux, M-J., Seibel, N., et al. (1995) 'Cognitive assessment of school-age children infected with maternally transmitted human immunodeficiency virus type 1.' *Journal of Pediatrics*, **126**, 375–379.

Tasker, R.C., Boyd, S., Harden, A., Matthew, D.J. (1988a) 'Monitoring in non-traumatic coma. Part II: Electroencephalography.' *Archives of Disease in Childhood*, **63**, 895–899.

—— Matthew, D.J., Helms, P., et al. (1988b) 'Monitoring in non-traumatic coma. Part I: Invasive intracranial measurements.' *Archives of Disease in Childhood*, **63**, 888–894.

Taylor, H.G., Michaels, R.N., Masur, P.M., et al. (1984) 'Intellectual, neuropsychological and achievement outcomes of children six to eight years after recovery from *Haemophilus influenzae* meningitis.' *Pediatrics*, **74**, 198–205.

—— Mills, E.I., Ciampi, A. et al. (1990) 'The sequelae of *Haemophilus influenzae* meningitis in school-age children.' *New England Journal of Medicine*, **323**, 1657–1663.

Taylor, T.E., Wills, B.A., Kazembe, P., et al. (1993) 'Rapid coma resolution with artemether in Malawian children with cerebral malaria.' *Lancet*, **341**, 661–662.

Teele, D.W., Dashefsky, B., Rakusan, T. (1981) 'Meningitis after lumbar puncture in children with bacteremia.' *New England Journal of Medicine*, **305**, 1079–1081.

Tekkök, I.H., Erbengi, A. (1992) 'Management of brain abscess in children: review of 130 cases over a period of 21 years.' *Child's Nervous System*, **8**, 411–416.

Teman, A.J. (1992) 'Spinal epidural abscess. Early detection with gadolinium magnetic resonance imaging.' *Archives of Neurology*, **49**, 743–746.

Teoh, R., Humphries, M. (1991) 'Tuberculous meningitis.' In: Lambert, H.P. (Ed.) *Infections of the Central Nervous System*. Philadelphia: B.C. Decker, pp. 189–206.

—— O'Mahony, G., Yeung, V.T.F. (1986) 'Polymorphonuclear pleocytosis in the cerebrospnal fluid during chemotherapy for tuberculous meningitis.' *Journal of Neurology*, **233**, 237–241.

—— Poon, W., Humphries, M.J., O'Mahony, G.O. (1988) 'Suprasellar tuberculoma developing during treatment of tuberculous meningitis requiring urgent surgical decompression.' *Journal of Neurology*, **235**, 321–322.

—— Humphries, M.J., Hoare, R.D., O'Mahony, G. (1989) 'Clinical correlation of CT changes in 64 Chinese patients with tuberculous meningitis.' *Journal of Neurology*, **236**, 48–51.

Ter Meulen, V., Müller, D., Käckell, Y. (1972) 'Isolation of infectious measles virus in measles encephalitis.' *Lancet*, **2**, 1172–1175.

Thilo, E.H., Townsend, S.F., Deacon, J. (1993) 'Infant botulism at 1 week of age: report of two cases.' *Pediatrics*, **92**, 151–153.

Thomas, M., Whittet, H. (1991) 'Atypical meningitis complicating a penetrating head injury.' *Journal of Neurology, Neurosurgery, and Psychiatry*, **54**, 92–93. *(Letter.)*

Thomas, N.H., Collins, J.E., Robb, S.A., Robinson, R.O. (1993) '*Mycoplasma pneumoniae* infection and neurological disease.' *Archives of Disease in Childhood*, **69**, 573–576.

Thömke, F., Hopf, H.C. (1992) 'Unilateral vestibular paralysis as the sole manifestation of mumps.' *Journal of Neurology, Neurosurgery, and Psychiatry*, **55**, 858–859. *(Letter.)*

Thompson, J.A., Glasgow, L.A., Warpinski, J.R., Olson, C. (1980) 'Infant botulism: clinical spectrum and epidemiology.' *Pediatrics*, **66**, 936–942.

Thun-Hohenstein, L., Schmitt, B., Steinlin, H., et al. (1992) 'Cortical visual impairment following bacterial meningitis: magnetic resonance imaging and visual evoked potentials findings in two cases.' *European Journal of Pediatrics*, **15**, 779–782.

Tjia, T.L., Yeow, Y.K., Tan, C.B. (1985) 'Cryptococcal meningitis.' *Journal of Neurology, Neurosurgery, and Psychiatry*, **48**, 853–858.

Tovo, P.A., de Martino, M., Gabiano, C., et al. (1992) 'Prognostic factors and survival in children with perinatal HIV-1 infection.' *Lancet*, **339**, 1249–1253.

Townsend, J.J., Baringer, J.R., Wolinsky, J.S., et al. (1975) 'Progressive rubella panencephalitis. Late onset after congenital rubella.' *New England Journal of Medicine*, **292**, 990–993.

—— Stroop, W.G., Baringer, J.R., et al. (1982) 'Neuropathology of progressive rubella panencephalitis after childhood rubella.' *Neurology*, **32**, 185–190.

Traub, M., Colchester, A.C.F., Kingsley, D.P.E., Swash, M. (1984) 'Tuberculosis of the central nervous system.' *Quarterly Journal of Medicine*, **53**, 81–100.

Trauner, D.A. (1986) 'What is the best treatment for Reye's syndrome?' *Archives of Neurology*, **43**, 729.

—— Nyhan, W.L., Sweetman, L. (1975) 'Short-chain organic acidemia and Reye's syndrome.' *Neurology*, **25**, 296–300.

—— Horvath, E., Davis, L.E. (1988) 'Inhibition of fatty acid beta oxidation by influenza B virus and salicylic acid in mice: implications for Reye's syndrome.' *Neurology*, **38**, 239–241.

Trautmann, M., Kluge, W., Otto, H.S., Loddenkemper, R. (1986) 'Computed tomography in CNS tuberculosis.' *European Neurology*, **25**, 91–97.

Troendle-Atkins, J., Demmler, G.J., Buffone, G.J. (1993) 'Rapid diagnosis of herpes simplex virus encephalitis by using the polymerase chain reaction.' *Journal of Pediatrics*, **123**, 376–380.

Tsolia, M., Skardoutsou, A., Tsolas, G., *et al.* (1995) 'Pre-eruptive neurologic manifestations associated with multiple cerebral infarcts in varicella.' *Pediatric Neurology*, **12**, 165–168.

Tudor-Williams, G., Frankland, J., Isaacs, D., *et al.* (1989) '*Haemophilus influenzae* type b disease in the Oxford region.' *Archives of Disease in Childhood*, **64**, 517–519.

Tunkel, A.R. (1993) 'Bacterial meningitis: non-antibiotic modes of therapy.' *Current Opinion on Infectious Diseases*, **6**, 638–643.

Udani, P.M. (1991) 'BCG vaccination and neurotuberculosis.' *In:* Fukuyama, Y., Kamoshita, S., Ohtsuka, C., Suzuki, Y. (Eds.) *Modern Perspectives in Child Neurology.* Tokyo: Japanese Society of Child Neurology, pp. 103–140.

—— Bhat, S. (1974) 'Tuberculosis of central nervous system. Part II. Clinical aspects.' *Indian Pediatrics*, **11**, 7–19.

—— Dastur, D.K. (1970) 'Tuberculous encephalopathy with and without meningitis. Clinical features and pathological correlations.' *Journal of the Neurological Sciences*, **10**, 543–551.

Unhanand, M., Mustafa, M.M., McCracken, G.H., Nelson, J.D. (1993) 'Gram-negative enteric bacillary meningitis: a twenty-one-year experience.' *Journal of Pediatrics*, **122**, 15–21.

Vadheim, C.M., Greenberg, D.P., Partridge, S., *et al.* (1993) 'Effectiveness and safety of an *Haemophilus influenzae* type b conjugate vaccine (PRP-T) in young infants.' *Pediatrics*, **92**, 272–279.

Van der Poel, J.C., Haenggeli, C.A., Overweg-Plandsoen, W.C.G. (1995) 'Operculum syndrome: unusual feature of herpes simplex encephalitis.' *Pediatric Neurology*, **12**, 246–249.

Vandersteenhoven, J.J., Dbaibo, G., Boyko, O.B., *et al.* (1992) 'Progressive multifocal leukoencephalopathy in pediatric acquired immunodeficiency syndrome.' *Pediatric Infectious Disease Journal*, **11**, 232–237.

Vandvik, B., Norrby, E., Steen-Johnsen, J., Stensvold, K. (1978a) 'Mumps meningitis: prolonged pleocytosis and occurrence of mumps virus-specific oligoclonal IgG in the cerebrospinal fluid.' *European Neurology*, **17**, 13–22.

—— Weil, M.L., Grandien, M., Norrby, E. (1978b) 'Progressive rubella panencephalitis: synthesis of oligoclonal virus-specific IgG antibodies and homogeneous free light chains in the central nervous system.' *Acta Neurologica Scandinavica*, **57**, 53–64.

Van Dyke, R.B., Heneine, W., Perrin, M.E., *et al.* (1995) 'Mother-to-child transmission of human T-lymphotropic virus type II.' *Journal of Pediatrics*, **127**, 924–928.

Vienny, H., Despland, P.A., Lütschug, J., *et al.* (1984) 'Early diagnosis and evolution of deafness in childhood bacterial meningitis: a study using brainstem auditory evoked potentials.' *Pediatrics*, **73**, 579–586.

Viladrich, P.F., Gudiol, F., Liñares, J., *et al.* (1991) 'Evaluation of vancomycin for therapy of adult pneumococcal meningitis.' *Antimicrobial Agents and Chemotherapy*, **35**, 2467–2472.

Vinchon, M., Vallée, L., Prin, L., *et al.* (1992) 'Cerebro-spinal fluid eosinophilia in shunt infections.' *Neuropediatrics*, **23**, 235–240.

Vinters, H.V., Kwok, M.K., Ho, H.W., *et al.* (1989) 'Cytomegalovirus in the nervous system of patients with the acquired immune deficiency syndrome.' *Brain*, **112**, 245–268.

Visudhiphan, P., Chiemchanya, S., Dheandhanoo, D. (1990) 'Central nervous system melioidosis in children.' *Pediatric Infectious Disease Journal*, **9**, 658–661.

Wadia, N.H., Wadia, P.N., Katrak, S.M., Misra, V.P. (1983) 'A study of the neurological disorder associated with acute haemorrhagic conjunctivitis due to enterovirus 70.' *Journal of Neurology, Neurosurgery, and Psychiatry*, **46**, 599–610.

—— Desai, S., Bhatt, M. (1988) 'Disseminated cysticercosis: new observations including CT scan findings and experience with treatment by praziquantel.' *Brain*, **111**, 597–614.

Waecker, N.J., O'Connor, J.D. (1990) 'Central nervous system tuberculosis in children: a review of 30 cases.' *Pediatric Infectious Disease Journal*, **9**, 539–543.

Wald, E.R., Bergman, I., Taylor, G., *et al.* (1986) 'Long-term outcome of group B streptococcal meningitis.' *Pediatrics*, **77**, 217–221.

—— Kaplan, S.L., Mason, E.O., *et al.* (1995) 'Dexamethasone therapy for children with bacterial meningitis.' *Pediatrics*, **95**, 21–28.

Walsh, T.J., Hier, D.B., Caplan, L.R. (1985) 'Aspergillosis of the central nervous system: clinicopathological analysis of 17 patients.' *Annals of Neurology*, **18**, 574–582.

Walter, G.F., Renella, R.R. (1989) 'Epstein–Barr virus in brain and Rasmussen's encephalitis.' *Lancet*, **1**, 279–280. *(Letter.)*

Wang, H.S., Huang, S.C. (1993) 'Infantile panthalamic infarction with a striking sonographic finding: "the bright thalamus".' *Neuroradiology*, **35**, 92–96.

—— Kuo, M.F., Huang, S.C., Chou, M.L. (1994) 'Choreoathetosis as an initial sign of relapsing of herpes simplex encephalitis.' *Pediatric Neurology*, **11**, 341–345.

Washburn, R.G., Kennedy, D.W., Begley, M.G., *et al.* (1988) 'Chronic fungal sinusitis in apparently normal hosts.' *Medicine*, **67**, 231–247.

Watson, R.T., Ballinger, W.E., Quisling, R.G. (1984) 'Acute hemorrhagic leukoencephalitis: diagnosis by computed tomography.' *Annals of Neurology*, **15**, 611–612.

Weber, K., Pfister, H-W. (1994) 'Clinical management of Lyme borreliosis.' *Lancet*, **343**, 1017–1020.

Weber, M., Vespignani, H., Jacquier, P., *et al.* (1988) 'Manifestations neurologiques de l'echinococcose alvéolaire.' *Revue Neurologique*, **144**, 104–112.

Wechsler, B., Vidailhet, M., Piette, J.C., *et al.* (1992) 'Cerebral venous thrombosis in Behçet's disease: clinical study and long-term follow-up of 25 cases.' *Neurology*, **42**, 614–618.

—— Dell Isola, B., Vidailhet, M., *et al.* (1993) 'MRI in 31 patients with Behçet's disease and neurological involvement: prospective study with clinical correlation.' *Journal of Neuroradiology, Neurosurgery, and Psychiatry*, **56**, 793–798.

Weisberg, L. (1986) 'Subdural empyema: clinical and computed tomographic correlations.' *Archives of Neurology*, **43**, 497–500.

Weiss, M.G., Ionides, S.P., Anderson, C.L. (1991) 'Meningitis in premature infants with respiratory distress: role of admission lumbar puncture.' *Journal of Pediatrics*, **119**, 973–975.

Weisse, M.E., Bass, J.W., Jarrett, R.V., Vincent, J.M. (1991) 'Nonanthrax *Bacillus* infections of the central nervous system.' *Pediatric Infectious Disease Journal*, **10**, 243–246.

Wheat, L.J., Kohler, R.B., Tewari, R.P. (1986) 'Diagnosis of disseminated histoplasmosis by detection of *Histoplasma capsulatum* antigen in serum and urine specimens.' *New England Journal of Medicine*, **315**, 83–88.

White, N.J. (1996) 'The treatment of malaria.' *New England Journal of Medicine*, **335**, 800–806.

—— Miller, K.D., Churchill, F.C., *et al.* (1988) 'Chloroquine treatment of severe malaria in children. Pharmacokinetics, toxicity and new dosage recommendations.' *New England Journal of Medicine*, **319**, 1493–1500.

Whitley, R.J. (1990) 'Viral encephalitis.' *New England Journal of Medicine*, **323**, 242–250.

—— Soong, S-J., Hirsch, M.S. (1981) 'Herpes simplex encephalitis. Vidarabine therapy and diagnostic problems.' *New England Journal of Medicine*, **304**, 313–318.

—— —— Linneman, C., *et al.* (1982) 'Herpes simplex encephalitis: clinical assessment.' *Journal of the American Medical Association*, **247**, 317–320.

—— Cobbs, C.G., Alford, C.A., *et al.* (1989) 'Diseases that mimic herpes simplex encephalitis. Diagnosis, presentation, and outcome.' *Journal of the American Medical Association*, **262**, 234–239.

Whittington, L.K., Roscelli, J.D., Parry, W.H. (1985) 'Hemorrhagic shock and encephalopathy: further description of a new syndrome.' *Journal of Pediatrics*, **106**, 599–602.

Wiley, C.A., Van Patten, P.D., Carpenter, P.M., *et al.* (1987) 'Acute ascending necrotizing myelopathy caused by herpes simplex virus type 2.' *Neurology*, **37**, 1791–1794.

Wilfert, C.M. (1969) 'Mumps meningoencephalitis with low cerebrospinal fluid glucose, prolonged pleocytosis and elevation of protein.' *New England Journal of Medicine*, **280**, 855–859.

Will, R.G., Ironside, J.W., Zeidler, M., *et al.* (1996) 'A new variant of Creutzfeld–Jakob disease in the UK.' *Lancet*, **347**, 921–925.

Williams, C.L., Strobino, B., Lee, A., *et al.* (1990) 'Lyme disease in childhood: clinical and epidemiologic features of ninety cases.' *Pediatric Infectious*

Disease Journal, **9**, 10–14.

Willoughby, E., Price, R.W., Padgett, B.L., *et al.* (1980) 'Progressive multifocal leukoencephalopathy (PML): *in vitro* cell-mediated immune response to mitogens and JC virus.' *Neurology*, **30**, 256–262.

Wilson, E.R., Malluh, A., Stagno, S., Crist, W.M. (1981) 'Fatal Epstein–Barr virus-associated hemophagocytic syndrome.' *Journal of Pediatrics*, **98**, 260–262.

Wilson, N.W., Copeland, B., Bastian, J.F. (1990–1991) 'Posttraumatic meningitis in adolescents and children.' *Pediatric Neurosurgery*, **16**, 17–20.

Wiswell, T.E., Baumgart, S., Gannon, C.M., Spitzer, A.R. (1995) 'No lumbar puncture in the evaluation for early neonatal sepsis: will meningitis be missed?' *Pediatrics*, **95**, 803–806.

Wokke, J.H.H., Van Gijn, J., Elderson, A., Stanek, G. (1987) 'Chronic forms of *Borrelia burgdorferi* infection of the nervous system.' *Neurology*, **37**, 1031–1034.

Wood, M.J., Johnson, R.W., McKendrick, M.W., *et al.* (1994) 'A randomized trial of acyclovir for 7 days or 21 days with and without prednisolone for treatment of acute herpes zoster.' *New England Journal of Medicine*, **330**, 896–900.

Woods, C.R., Englund, J., Black, M. (1993) 'Congenital toxoplasmosis presenting with eosinophilic meningitis.' *Pediatric Infectious Disease Journal*, **12**, 347–348.

Wormser, G.P. (1997) 'Treatment and prevention of Lyme disease with emphasis on antimicrobial therapy for neuroborreliosis and vaccination.' *Seminars in Neurology*, **17**, 45–52.

Wright, P.F., Hatch, M.H., Kasselberg, A.G., *et al.* (1977) 'Vaccine-associated poliomyelitis in a child with sex-linked agammaglobulinemia.' *Journal of Pediatrics*, **91**, 408–412.

Wright, P.W., Avery, W.G., Ardill, W.D., McLarty, J.W. (1993) 'Initial clinical assessment of the comatose patient: cerebral malaria *vs.* meningitis.' *Pediatric Infectious Disease Journal*, **12**, 37–41.

Wulff, C.H. (1982) 'Subacute sclerosing panencephalitis: serial electroencephalographic studies.' *Journal of Neurology, Neurosurgery, and Psychiatry*, **45**, 418–421.

Yabek, S.M. (1973) 'Meningococcal meningitis presenting as acute cerebellar ataxia.' *Pediatrics*, **52**, 718–720.

Yagishita, A., Nakano, I., Ushioda, T., *et al.* (1995) 'Acute encephalopathy with bilateral thalamotegmental involvement in infants and children: imaging and pathology findings.' *American Journal of Neuroradiology*, **16**, 439–447.

Yalaz, K., Anlar, B., Oktem, F., *et al.* (1992) 'Intraventricular interferon and oral inosiplex in the treatment of subacute sclerosing panencephalitis.' *Neurology*, **42**, 488–491.

Yanofsky, C.S., Hanson, P.A., Lepow, M. (1981) 'Parainfectious acute obstructive hydrocephalus.' *Annals of Neurology*, **10**, 62–63.

Yazici, H., Pazarli, H., Barnes, C.G., *et al.* (1990) 'A controlled trial of azathioprine in Behçet's syndrome.' *New England Journal of Medicine*, **322**, 281–285.

Zucker, J.R., Campbell, C.C. (1993) 'Malaria. Principles of prevention and treatment.' *Infectious Diseases Clinics of North America*, **7**, 547–567.

12

PARAINFECTIOUS AND OTHER INFLAMMATORY DISORDERS OF IMMUNOLOGICAL ORIGIN

The diseases considered in this chapter are characterized pathologically by an inflammatory reaction of the brain and/or spinal cord that induces the appearance of perivascular and/or intraparenchymal lymphomononuclear and oligoglial infiltrates, with or without associated perivascular demyelination. The inflammatory reaction appears to result from an immunological response to various antigens, some of which may be of foreign—*e.g.* viral or bacterial—origin. However, the antigens, if any, responsible for the immune response often remain unknown and the factors that trigger the response remain obscure. In at least some cases, the immune response seems to be directed against components of the CNS of the host, an autoimmune process. This can be due to several mechanisms: some pathogens may share antigens with CNS cell membranes and the latter therefore become the target of an immune response; viral or other aggressors may produce alterations in the chemical and antigenic properties of host cells so that they are identified as foreign proteins by the immunological surveillance system; or the immunological system itself may be functioning abnormally and react against normal host components.

In all such cases, the result is that the immunological response itself, rather than the agent that originates it, is responsible for most of the harm produced, and therefore treatment may have to be directed against the response rather than against the initial cause which is often beyond reach.

Several groups of disorders can be included among the inflammatory conditions of immunological origin. I will consider in succession: (1) rheumatic diseases; (2) demyelinating conditions, including multiple sclerosis; (3) cerebellar ataxias of unknown origin and the myoclonic encephalopathy of Kinsbourne; (4) virus-induced and familial haemophagocytic syndromes and related proliferative disorders; (5) neurological complications of immunization and serotherapy as well as other rare causes of CNS damage of allergic origin

The postinfectious encephalitides belong to the group of disorders studied in this chapter. They have been described in Chapter 11, however, because their clinical presentation and circumstances of occurrence make it difficult to dissociate them from the primary encephalitides and other neurological complications of viral infections.

RHEUMATIC DISEASES

The rheumatic diseases include a series of disorders characterized by diffuse inflammatory changes in connective tissue. The exact nature of these disorders and their mutual relationships remain uncertain but CNS involvement is a feature of many of them. Sigal (1987) extensively reviewed the neurological features of this group of diseases.

SYDENHAM CHOREA (ST VITUS DANCE)
Sydenham chorea is the major neurological manifestation of rheumatic fever. Most cases of chorea are preceded by a streptococcal infection or by other manifestations of rheumatic fever. The incidence of chorea has recently increased in several countries including the USA. This increase is thought to be due to the emergence of certain serological types of group A streptococci (Hosier *et al.* 1987). Chorea tends to be a late feature of rheumatic disease so that serological evidence of streptococcal infection is absent in about a quarter of the cases. Rheumatic heart disease often develops insidiously in patients with chorea.

Little is known of the pathology of chorea. Mild perivascular infiltrates have been inconstantly found in the brain without specific localization to the basal ganglia. No Aschoff bodies have been found in the brain.

The clinical manifestations are striking but they now tend to be misinterpreted because the disease has become rare (Nausieda *et al.* 1980) and many physicians have not seen a single case.

The onset is usually after 3 years of age and the condition is somewhat more common in girls. Most cases used to occur in underprivileged children from ethnic minorities but cases are now often observed in middle-class children (Hosier *et al.* 1987).

The disease appears insidiously. The behaviour of the child changes and s/he becomes fidgety and clumsy. Involuntary movements are of various types. Some are myoclonic-like: most resemble purposeful movements but they occur abruptly and in an unpredictable sequence. Facial movements are especially prominent but all four limbs are affected and movements of the trunk and hips are responsible for the 'dancing' appearance that is at the origin of the name of the disease. Brief myoclonic jerks of the proximal limbs are often associated with more complex distal movements.

In the fully fledged disease, continuous abnormal motions during wakefulness impair coordination and make writing, feeding or dressing difficult or impossible. A dysarthric, explosive speech is often present and chewing or swallowing may be affected in the most severe cases. Involuntary movements are characterized by bursts of EMG activity lasting more than 100 ms, occurring asynchronously in antagonist muscles. Exaggerated voluntary movements may be produced with EMG bursts lasting longer than normal (Hallett and Kaufman 1981).

Predominance of the abnormal movements on one side of the body is not infrequent and true hemichorea occurs in 15–20 per cent of cases. Sustained muscle contraction is often impossible. Severe hypotonia is usually present. In some cases (paralytic chorea), the hypotonia and weakness are so marked as to prevent the occurrence of choreic movements. However, power is not totally lost but initiation of movement is difficult, motor spontaneity is lacking and the grip waxes and wanes abruptly. Severe behaviour disturbances may be observed and may last for months.

Neuroimaging studies are usually normal. In some cases, transiently increased T_2 signal may be present in the head of the caudate and putamen (Heye *et al.* 1993, Traill *et al.* 1995). PET scan has shown increased glucose metabolism in the basal ganglia (Weindl *et al.* 1993).

Usually, deep tendon reflexes are normal and the plantar responses flexor. Emotional lability is frequently present. Severe forms are rare and may feature extremely intense movements with hemiballismus (Konagaya and Konagaya 1992). Encephalitic syndromes are sometimes observed (Munn *et al.* 1982).

Most patients recover completely in two to three months but a longer course is possible and late recurrences may occur. Complications are rare, although the occurrence of papilloedema has been reported (Chun *et al.* 1961). Convalescent children may develop choreic reactions to a variety of drugs (Nausieda *et al.* 1983).

Chorea gravidarum and chorea induced by oral contraceptives appear to be closely related to Sydenham chorea and often occur as recurrences of a previous choreic episode. However, they may also supervene spontaneously or with other previous insults to the basal ganglia (Nausieda *et al.* 1979, Nausieda 1986).

The differential diagnosis of Sydenham chorea includes simple tics or habit spasms as well as other causes of chorea (see Chapter 10). Unlike chorea, simple tics tend to involve repeatedly the same muscle groups. The multiple tics of Tourette syndrome may raise a difficult diagnostic problem, the more so as tics may follow a streptococcal infection and progressively merge into Sydenham chorea (Kerbeshian *et al.* 1990). Antineuronal antibodies may play a role at the origin of tics and Tourette syndrome (Kiessling *et al.* 1993). Choreic movements induced by neuro-

leptic drugs may be a problem as they may have been administered at an early stage because of behaviour disorders or incipient abnormal movements.

Treatment is classically with haloperidol, 0.5–1 mg twice daily for two to six months with progressive discontinuation (Shenker *et al.* 1973). Carbamazepine may be effective (Roig *et al.* 1988) and sodium valproate (Dhanaraj *et al.* 1985) is also a possibility. Both agents avoid the risk of tardive dyskinesia. Penicillin prophylaxis is indicated even in case of negative throat culture.

LUPUS ERYTHEMATOSUS
Neurological complications occur in 25–75 per cent of patients with systemic lupus erythematosus (SLE) and may often be the presenting features.

Pathologically, diffuse perivascular infiltration with round cells and multiple ischaemic lesions due to intimal proliferation of the small cerebral arteries are found. However, true vasculitis with presence of inflammatory cells within the vessel's walls is not frequent, and emboli from a Libman–Saks endocarditis and lesions of thrombotic, thrombocytopenic purpura (Devinsky *et al.* 1988) also have to be considered in the genesis of CNS damage. Brain-reactive antibodies may be a cause of the neurological features in SLE, and immunoglobulins adherent to neurons have been observed in post-mortem material in cases of SLE with neurological manifestations. Antibodies to ribosomal P proteins are present in the majority of patients with psychosis or depression (Bonfa *et al.* 1987). The circulating antiphospholipid antibodies commonly present in lupus patients may play a role in the genesis of vascular thrombosis and coagulation cascade and thus contribute to brain damage (Van Dam 1991, Seaman *et al.* 1995).

The *clinical manifestations* can be seen at any age. The majority of cases are in girls in the second decade of life. However, 22 per cent of cases occurred in the first decade in one large series (Lehman *et al.* 1989). Psychiatric disorders and seizures are the most common symptoms and were present in 40 and 48 per cent respectively in two large recent series (Parikh *et al.* 1995, Steinlin *et al.* 1995a). They include severe depression, disturbances of concentration or behaviour, and often frank psychosis.

An organic psychosis, probably due to toxic encephalopathy in which brain lesions, electrolyte disturbances and, in rare cases, steroid therapy may all play a role, may feature delirium, depression, delusions or hallucinations. This syndrome may appear during acute exacerbations of the disease and subside with improvement of systemic manifestations (Futrell *et al.* 1992). Headache was present in 22–64 per cent of children and is often migraine-like. Neurological symptoms and signs include focal or more commonly generalized seizures, focal neurological deficits such as hemiplegia or diplegia resulting from ischaemic cerebral events, stupor or coma, spastic quadriplegia, cranial nerve dysfunction, especially of the IIIrd and VIth pairs, and optic neuritis (Hackett *et al.* 1974). Such manifestations were present in 16 of 37 children with SLE and, in the vast majority, could be noted at the time of diagnosis (Yancey *et al.* 1981). They may occur up to several months before the other manifestations (Tola *et al.* 1992, Steinlin *et al.* 1995a).

Acute myelopathy (Provenzale and Bouldin 1992) can be the first manifestation of the disease (Linssen *et al.* 1988) and can simulate multiple sclerosis in juvenile patients (Oppenheimer and Hoffbrand 1986). Chorea or hemichorea may occur in 1–28 per cent of patients with SLE, especially in young patients (Parikh *et al.* 1995), and can precede systemic manifestations by several months or years (Bruyn and Padberg 1984). Contrary to previous belief it does not seem to herald a poor outcome.

CSF examination may show a mild pleocytosis and mild to moderate increase in protein. CT scan is usually normal but may show areas of infarction and haemorrhage. In the late stages, evidence of cerebral atrophy and calcification of the basal ganglia may be seen (Falko *et al.* 1979, Carette *et al.* 1982). MRI may show lesions in cases with normal CT scans and neurological disease (Stimmler *et al.* 1993). However, findings are often negative, and a normal image in a young girl with encephalopathy is suggestive of systemic lupus.

The *diagnosis* of SLE may be difficult as neurological disease may be present long before serological confirmation of the diagnosis is possible (Falko *et al.* 1979). Antinuclear antibodies are present in almost every patient but are also found in some patients with dermatomyositis and in most of those with rheumatoid arthritis and chronic active hepatitis. Antibodies against DNA are much more specific and are found in 86 per cent of patients (Yancey *et al.* 1981). Antibodies against ribonucleoprotein and sm antigen may also help make the diagnosis. The LE cell test is rarely positive in the absence of a positive test for antinuclear antibodies.

The *treatment* of SLE is based on the use of steroids and immunosuppressant drugs. Plasmapheresis has been used in some instances. The use of steroids may be complicated by psychotic symptoms. These however are more often a consequence of the disease itself and are not an indication to discontinue the drug. The outcome of neurological manifestations of lupus is favourable. In two recent large series (Parikh *et al.* 1995, Steilin *et al.* 1995) the mortality rate was under 4 per cent, and functional recovery, including from ischaemic accidents, is remarkably good.

Neurological complications have been exceptionally reported in infants with *neonatal lupus erythematosus*, a rare condition that consists of facial skin lesions, heart block and the passive transfer of antibodies against the Ro/SSA antigen and, occasionally, the La/SSB antigen (Watson *et al.* 1984, Telang *et al.* 1993). Myelopathy in one such case is on record and has also been reported in *infantile lupus* associated with deficiency of complement components (Kaye *et al.* 1987). Vasculopathy involving the thalami and basal ganglia has been shown by colour Doppler studies (Cabañas *et al.* 1996). Its significance is unclear.

SLE may be associated with the presence of antiphospholipid antibodies and anticardiolipin antibodies (lupus anticoagulant) which may also be detected in some asymptomatic persons (primary antiphospholipid syndrome (Rumi *et al.* 1993, Seaman *et al.* 1995) or in patients with disorders other than SLE. The presence of antiphospholipid antibodies has been associated with arterial and venous thrombotic phenomena, myelopathy, optic neuritis, amaurosis fugax, unilateral paraesthesia, transient ischaemic events and chorea (Levine and Welch 1987, Seaman *et al.* 1995). The last of these associations is of particular interest in adolescents because the clinical picture is indistinguishable from that of chorea minor. Yet, treatment is distinct as anticoagulants and not corticosteroids are indicated and effective (Økseter and Siernes 1988).

A disorder with manifestations similar to those of SLE occurs in some children who receive anticonvulsant drugs, especially phenytoin, ethosuximide and carbamazepine (Singsen *et al.* 1976, Hess 1988). The clinical manifestations may disappear after discontinuation of the responsible drug but steroid treatment may be needed. Twenty per cent of children receiving anticonvulsants have been found to have a positive antinuclear antibody test but only a few develop a clinical lupus-like syndrome.

POLYARTERITIS NODOSA (PERIARTERITIS NODOSA)

Polyarteritis nodosa is characterized pathologically by necrosis and acute inflammation of medium- and small-sized arteries that may affect both the central and the peripheral nervous system. Obliteration and aneurysm formation may result in infarction due to ischaemia or in haemorrhage.

Cerebral oedema, seizures and focal deficits are the usual central manifestations (Ford and Siekert 1965, Sigal 1987), while multiple mononeuropathy (mononeuritis multiplex) is the characteristic feature of peripheral involvement. Cranial nerve involvement is common. Ozen *et al.* (1992) found severe myalgia to be the first symptom in over three-quarters of affected children. Peripheral nerve involvement in the form of mononeuritis multiplex and encephalitic symptoms were less common. Relapses of the neuropathy are common. The diagnosis can be confirmed by renal biopsy or muscle biopsy, although sampling errors are frequent with the latter technique. Angiographic demonstration of peripheral aneurysms, especially in liver and kidney, is of diagnostic value.

Treatment is with corticosteroids combined with immunosuppressant drugs (Ettlinger *et al.* 1979). However, a complete remission was obtained in only 13 per cent of patients in one series (Ozen *et al.* 1992).

Cases of infantile periarteritis nodosa with marked involvement of the coronary arteries have been reported. Such cases do not differ significantly from those of Kawasaki disease (see below).

Other vasculitides are uncommon in childhood (see also Chapter 15). Wegener granulomatosis involves small- and medium-size arteries and veins. Granulomatous lesions in the upper respiratory tract and lungs are the hallmark of the disease but the nervous system may be affected with neuropathy, cranial nerve palsies and seizures (Rottem *et al.* 1993).

RHEUMATOID ARTHRITIS

Rheumatoid arthritis can be accompanied by a symmetrical sensorimotor neuropathy (Pallis and Scott 1965) or by an encephalopathy with disturbances of consciousness, marked slowing of the EEG and, occasionally, neurological signs suggestive of intra-cranial hypertension such as decorticate rigidity (Jan *et al.* 1972). The possible role of salicylate toxicity has been considered. About 6 per cent of patients with rheumatoid arthritis develop an acute encephalopathy which is usually spontaneously reversible.

A *c*hronic *i*nfantile, *n*eurological, *c*utaneous and *a*rticular (CINCA) inflammatory disease with onset by a skin rash in early infancy, arthritis of the knees, ankles, elbows, wrists and hands, chronic aseptic meningitis, headaches, seizures and sometimes optic atrophy, deafness and hoarseness has been reported (Prieur and Griscelli 1981, Yarom *et al.* 1985, Prieur *et al.* 1987). Mental retardation is common. Except for three families, the disease is sporadic and of unknown cause. Cerebral atrophy and sometimes areas of softening of probable vascular origin are present on CT scan.

SCHOENLEIN–HENOCH PURPURA

Anaphylactoid purpura is characterized pathologically by a gen-eralized small-vessel vasculitis of the hypersensitivity type and can occur at any age, including infancy. Neurological manifestations occur in 2–7 per cent of cases. Headache, changes in conscious-ness or behaviour and seizures are the usual manifestations and account for 25–50 per cent of the neurological complications of Schoenlein–Henoch disease (Belman *et al.* 1985). Less frequent anomalies include focal deficits that may be hemiplegia, para-paresis, quadriplegia, cortical blindness or polyneuropathy (Ritter *et al.* 1983). Mononeuropathy and brachial plexopathy have been recorded (Belman *et al.* 1985). Some complications probably result from hypertension or renal involvement, but neurological symptoms may occur in the absence of any systemic disturbance and are probably caused by cerebral vasculitis.

KAWASAKI DISEASE

This disease, also known as mucocutaneous lymph node syn-drome, is a disorder of obscure origin although various pathogens such as *Rickettsia*, *Propionibacterium acnes*, *Streptococcus sanguis* and others have been incriminated. An abnormal immune re-sponse to staphylococcal toxin (Leung *et al.* 1993) or parvovirus B19 (Sissons 1993, Nigro *et al.* 1994) has been proposed. Criteria for diagnosis of Kawasaki disease include a fever lasting five days or more, conjunctival injection, inflammation of respiratory mucous membranes, cutaneous abnormalities, in particular desquamation of the digital extremities, cervical adenitis, and the absence of a known cause to explain these features.

Kawasaki disease is complicated in 10–50 per cent of cases by the occurrence of coronary artery aneurysms that may be responsible for death. The condition occurs in many parts of the world outside Japan and accounts for the cases of infantile periarteritis nodosa published before its description. About 25 per cent of the patients have aseptic meningitis with a mononuclear CSF pleocytosis of 25–100 cells/mm^3 (Bell *et al.* 1983). Hemi-plegia, epilepsy and myositis have also been reported (Laxer *et al.* 1984). The incidence of neurological complications in a large series (Terasawa *et al.* 1983) was 1.1 per cent. CT scan changes may include diffuse or localized widening of sulci which appears to be reversible. Facial nerve paralysis of lower motor neuron type has occurred in several patients (Terasawa *et al.* 1983).

Prevention of the development of coronary artery disease using high-dose intravenous globulin (400 mg/kg/d for four days) in combination with aspirin (3–10 mg/kg/d) is currently recommended for all cases (Bierman and Gersony 1987). However, uncertainties remain regarding the dose, schedule and indications for such treatment.

HAEMOLYTIC–URAEMIC SYNDROME

This condition has been associated with toxin-producing *Escherichia coli* especially *E. coli* O157:H7 (Boyce *et al.* 1995) and with *Shigella dysenteriae* infection (Ashkenazi 1993). The presence of thrombocytopenia, haemolytic anaemia and azotaemia defines the syndrome. Two patterns of thrombi are encountered. In one, they form a loose fibrin meshwork. In the other, they appear as a coarse granular aggregation of eosinophilic material in the arterioles, capillaries and venules. Such abnormalities are not limited to the kidney and may be seen in the CNS. They may be responsible for small or large areas of infarction.

Neurological symptoms occur in 30–50 per cent of cases (Bale *et al.* 1980, Sheth *et al.* 1986). They consist of seizures, disturbances of consciousness such as stupor, hallucinations or coma, and focal deficits including extrapyramidal signs (Barnett *et al.* 1995). They may occur in the absence of renal insufficiency and hypertension. Haemorrhagic infarction may occur and may be responsible for sequelae (Crisp *et al.* 1981). CSF protein is often raised in patients who have a poor outcome (Bale *et al.* 1980).

CT scan and MRI (Sherwood and Wagle 1991) often show abnormal areas of ischaemic infarction and, sometimes, of haemorrhagic infarction. Involvement of the basal ganglia has been reported in patients who presented clinically with intractable seizures and intermittent decerebrate posturing. Even in such severe cases, a satisfactory recovery remains possible but sequelae persist in 10–20 per cent of patients (Barnett *et al.* 1995).

COGAN SYNDROME

This syndrome is rare in childhood (Kundell and Ochs 1980). The major features are interstitial keratitis and deafness. Involve-ment of the aortic sigmoids and skin is common, and seizures, focal neurological deficits and behavioural disturbances may occur (Vollertsen *et al.* 1986). Treatment with steroids, if given early, may prevent the development of deafness and is effective in controlling the inflammatory reaction. The mechanism is unknown.

OTHER INFLAMMATORY DISORDERS OF PRESUMED IMMUNOLOGICAL MECHANISM

Neurological symptoms and signs may occur in the course of diseases of obscure mechanism such as Hashimoto thyroiditis (Shaw *et al.* 1991), familial Mediterranean fever (Gedalia and Zamir 1993), and Sjögren syndrome (Ohtsuka *et al.* 1995). Cases of aseptic meningitis have been reported in recipients of cardiac transplants (Adair *et al.* 1991) and in other patients in whom immunosuppression had been induced with OKT3, a monoclonal antibody of murine origin directed against T-cell surface molecules. A case of encephalopathy with quadriparesis and impaired consciousness due to OKT3 has been observed in a renal transplant recipient (Coleman and Norman 1990), and transient hemiparesis is on record (Osterman *et al.* 1993). Neurological abnormalities disappear with discontinuation of OKT3 therapy. Rare cases of aseptic meningitis with a benign course have been reported in patients receiving high-dose intravenous immunoglobulin therapy (Watson *et al.* 1991).

DEMYELINATING DISEASES

Demyelinating CNS diseases include multiple sclerosis, optic neuritis, acute transverse myelitis, acute disseminated encephalomyelitis and some rare conditions such as Schilder disease. Acute disseminated encephalomyelitis has been dealt with in Chapter 11.

MULTIPLE SCLEROSIS (MS)
MS is one of the major neurological problems in adult neurology. It is, however, rare in children under 10 years and uncommon in adolescents. In a recent study of 4632 cases of MS, only 125, or 2.7 per cent, had their onset before 16 years of age. The mean age at onset in this group was 13 years, and in only eight patients did the disorder manifest before age 11 years (Duquette *et al.* 1987). According to Hanefeld *et al.* (1991), 176 cases in patients under 18 years of age were published between 1980 and 1990, and cases may occur even in infants (Bye 1985; Cole *et al.* 1995a,b). Girls are more commonly affected than boys, especially among those younger than 12 years (Hanefeld *et al.* 1991). Very early onset under 3 years of age has been reported (Bye *et al.* 1985, Hanefeld *et al.* 1991, Cole *et al.* 1995a). The disease is characterized by the successive occurrence of foci of demyelination disseminated in various areas of the CNS white matter, including the periventricular region, spinal cord, brainstem, cerebellum and optic nerve.

From a diagnostic point of view, the essential feature of MS is the dissemination of lesions in both time and space.

The *aetiology* of MS remains unknown in spite of an enormous amount of investigation. Two main possibilities are usually considered. One is an infection of oligodendrocytes by an agent capable of persisting locally in a hidden, perhaps genomic, form and which may become activated at intervals for unknown reasons. A second possibility is the induction, by one or several undetermined mechanisms, of an altered functioning of the immune system, resulting in a noxious effect on the CNS of the patient. These two mechanisms are not mutually exclusive (ffrench-Constant 1994, Hohlfeld 1997).

It is widely held that MS is probably initiated by exposure to an aetiological agent, possibly a virus, in early life, as suggested by the fact that persons migrating from a high-incidence to a low-incidence area before age 15 years develop the disease with approximately the same frequency as if they had stayed in their place of origin, and *vice versa*, whereas the reverse applies for people who migrate in infancy.

High-incidence areas generally correspond to temperate and cold climates (Poser 1994).

Genetic factors are also operative as MS is 10–20 times more frequent in relatives of patients than in the general population. HLA groups DRw2, HLA-A3 and HLA B7 are more frequent in patients with MS than in control persons from the same populations (Visscher *et al.* 1979). This suggests that genes controlling the immune response, which are known to be linked to the HLA genes, are in some way involved in the pathogenesis of the disease.

Recent data suggest that the activity of the immune system in human beings is modulated by a network of regulatory controls mediated, in part, through inducer and suppressor T-cells. Abnormalities of circulating T-cell subsets have been demonstrated in both adults and children with multiple sclerosis (Hauser *et al.* 1983, Rose *et al.* 1988, Olsson 1992, Hohlfeld 1997). Loss of T-suppressor/cytotoxic cells with an increase in the ratio of inducer to suppressor cells (T4:T5) has been found during attacks. Other anomalies affect the production of immunoglobulins in the CSF, which in a majority of adults and children with MS are elevated and/or demonstrate oligoclonal banding. The pathogenetic significance of this finding remains obscure and the same applies to the finding of antibodies (especially against measles virus) in the CSF and blood. Such antibodies are generally regarded as indicating an abnormal modulation of the immune response rather than being specifically directed against a particular viral agent (Martin *et al.* 1992).

PATHOLOGY
Multiple lesions (plaques) are formed of round areas of greyish gelatinous appearance, scattered in the white matter. Within the plaques, which are generally located around small vessels, there is destruction of the myelin sheath with relative preservation of axons. In recent plaques oedema and inflammatory cells can be seen and neutral lipids that represent myelin breakdown products are present. Old lesions are mostly gliotic with astrocytic proliferation (McDonald *et al.* 1992).

Efforts to identify a virus or other infectious agents in brain of MS patients have so far been unsuccessful even though an occasional positive report has appeared.

CLINICAL FEATURES
MS can present in several different manners, from acute forms leading to death in only a few weeks to a completely asymptomatic disease incidentally discovered at autopsy. The two most common forms in adults are the relapsing–remitting and the chronic progressive forms (Koopmans *et al.* 1989a,b). The latter is rare in childhood. In the series of Duquette *et al.* (1987), 56 per cent of patients had a relapsing–remitting course, 22 per cent had a progressive type and another 22 per cent had a mixed form. All the 14 children studied by Guilhoto *et al.* (1995) had a relapsing–remitting form. A majority of the progressive forms are preceded by several years of relapsing–remitting course. Only

four of the 28 patients of Cole and Stuart (1995) had primary progressive MS, and only two of 23 children with a relapsing–remitting form developed secondarily progressive disease. In one such patient seen by me, the presentation was very similar to that in adults, with myelopathy progressing unremittingly and few progressive additional new manifestations. This is in conformity with the experience of others (Boutin *et al.* 1988a). In the classical relapsing–remitting form, the diagnosis can only be made retrospectively as dissemination in time is a major criterion. Oriental patients tend to present preferentially with optic neuritis and myelitis and may have an immunologically distinct disease (Kira *et al.* 1996).

The main features of the first manifestation of MS in children are shown in Table 12.1. The symptoms and signs are generally similar to those in adults, with visual impairment, sensory manifestations and ataxia in the forefront. Vestibular symptoms are less common in children and adolescents than in adults (Haslam 1987). In the series of Hanefeld *et al.* (1991), ataxia and general manifestations were more prominent whereas optic atrophy was not a feature. However, ophthalmological features were present in 16 of 17 children reported by Steinlin *et al.* (1995b), and 12 of them had optic neuritis. Abnormal eye movements are frequent because of the frequency of brainstem lesions (Barnes and McDonald 1992).

Several studies (Bye *et al.* 1985, Hanefeld *et al.* 1991, Sindern *et al.* 1992, Bauer and Hanefeld 1993) emphasized the relative frequency of systemic manifestations such as fever and vomiting and that of encephalopathic presentation, especially in cases of very early onset. This seems to be uncommon, however, in series that do not originate from tertiary referral centres (Cole and Stuart 1995, Cole *et al.* 1995).

The progression of the disease is unpredictable (Bauer and Hanefeld 1993). Some children may have only one attack during childhood with relapses occurring after many years, whereas in others repeated episodes accumulate within a few months. Hanefeld *et al.* (1991) computed a mortality rate of 10 per cent in five years in 71 paediatric cases. Cole and Stuart, on the contrary, found the course of their patients more benign than in adults.

LABORATORY FINDINGS

These are also largely identical to those in adults especially regarding the presence of oligoclonal banding, which was present in 85 per cent of the cases of Boutin *et al.* (1988a). In children, however, pleocytosis is often more marked than in older patients, with 50–100 lymphocytes/mm^3 (Bye *et al.* 1985, Sindern *et al.* 1992).

Evoked potential studies are frequently abnormal. An increase in the latency of the P100 potential of the visual evoked response is frequent and attests to the presence of an infraclinical lesion when there is no clinical evidence of optic neuritis. The same applies to the central components of the somatosensory evoked response. Increased interwave latency (I–III or III–V) is also frequent as well as a decrease in amplitude of wave V of the brainstem auditory evoked response.

TABLE 12.1
First manifestation of multiple sclerosis in 125 childhood cases*

Pure sensory disturbances	26%
Optic neuritis	14%
Diplopia	11%
Pure motor disturbances	11%
Blurred vision	6%
Cerebellar ataxia	5%
Sensorimotor disturbances	5%
Myelitis	3%
Vestibular disturbances	2%
Sphincter disturbances	1%
Unclassified/not known	6%

*From Duquette *et al.* (1987).

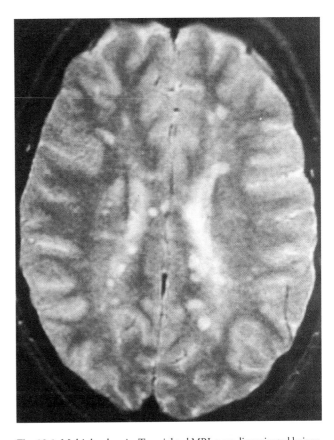

Fig. 12.1. Multiple sclerosis. T$_2$-weighted MRI: note disseminated lesions, giving an intense signal, with predominant periventricular involvement (adolescent girl with several episodes of neurological symptoms). (Courtesy Dr Kling Chong, Great Ormond Street Hospital, London.)

Myelin basic protein is elevated in most children with acute exacerbations of MS but is frequently normal in quiescent periods (Cohen *et al.* 1980).

NEUROIMAGING

Neuroimaging techniques have considerably improved the ease of diagnosis of MS as they show the dispersal of lesions better than other methods including evoked potential studies.

CT scan may show areas of low density and/or of contrast enhancement in 50–66 per cent of patients. The use of double-dose contrast enhancement has been recommended in adults. MRI is clearly more sensitive than CT scan, and MRI abnormalities can be demonstrated in 70 to over 90 per cent of patients with definite or possible MS (Ormerod *et al.* 1987, Paty *et al.* 1988, Millner *et al.* 1990). In most patients, several areas of increased signal appear on T_2-weighted sequences (Fig. 12.1). These areas are of variable size and may be located in the cerebellum, brainstem, spinal cord and hemispheral white matter. In the latter case, their periventricular location is suggestive (Ormerod *et al.* 1984, Isaac *et al.* 1988, Miller *et al.* 1989, Willoughby *et al.* 1989) but the images are not specific as they have been reported in adults with vascular disorders (Ormerod *et al.* 1984), in patients with other inflammatory conditions, including HTLV-1 infection (Jacobson *et al.* 1990), in patients with Lyme disease (Chapter 11) and, occasionally, in subjects without evidence of neurological disease (Baker *et al.* 1985). In addition to its diagnostic value, MRI also indicates that new lesions frequently appear over a period of a few months in asymptomatic patients (Ormerod *et al.* 1987) thus posing the problem of definition of an attack (Millner *et al.* 1990). MRI following gadolinium enhancement enables recent lesions that take up the product, indicating impairment of the blood–brain barrier with consequent oedema, to be distinguished from old plaques that do not enhance and are probably mainly gliotic (Miller *et al.* 1988b). Lesions of the optic nerve can also be detected by MRI (Miller *et al.* 1988a, Koopmans *et al.* 1989c). MRI in children seems to give similar results (Golden and Woody 1987, Haas *et al.* 1987, Millner *et al.* 1990).

MS IN CHILDREN UNDER 10 YEARS OF AGE

MS in this age group, and especially in infants or children under 5 years, may have unusual features clinically and from the viewpoint of imaging. Seizures have been reported to occur more frequently than in adults, and acute encephalopathic states with diminished consciousness, seizures and pyramidal tract signs may occur (Bye *et al.* 1985, Shaw and Alvord 1987, Cole *et al.* 1995a). Mental deterioration can be seen early in young patients (Bye *et al.* 1985).

In some cases diagnosed as MS, large lesions of the white matter (Maeda *et al.* 1989), atypical butterfly-like enhancement and ring enhancement have been reported (Ishiara *et al.* 1984, Morimoto *et al.* 1985). Some of these cases were also clinically atypical and the diagnosis of MS may not be demonstrated. However, a similar appearance has been described in adult patients (Vliegenthart *et al.* 1985). An association between certain mitochondrial mutations responsible for Leber hereditary optic neuropathy (especially the nt11778 mutation) and the development of an MS-like disease with prominent early optic nerve disease has been reported (Chalmers and Harding 1996, Funalot *et al.* 1996), especially in women. The significance of this association remains to be explored.

DIAGNOSIS

The diagnosis of MS is particularly difficult in children and should be accepted only reluctantly in patients under age 10.

It is customary to use diagnostic criteria and to separate cases of definite, probable and possible MS (Poser *et al.* 1983). Clinically, definite cases are characterized by the occurrence of two attacks and clinical evidence of two separate lesions, or two attacks and clinical evidence of one lesion plus paraclinical evidence of another separate lesion. The two attacks must involve different parts of the CNS, must be separated by a period of at least one month and must last a minimum of 24 hours. Laboratory-supported definite MS consists of two attacks plus either clinical or paraclinical evidence of one lesion plus IgG oligoclonal banding in CSF, or of one attack plus clinical evidence of two separate lesions, or one attack plus clinical evidence of one lesion and paraclinical evidence of another lesion.

DIFFERENTIAL DIAGNOSIS

The differential diagnosis of MS includes a large number of clinically fluctuating neurological diseases such as recurrent hemiplegias due to moyamoya disease or to lupus erythematosus or to coagulation disorders (Chapter 15). Protracted forms of acute disseminated encephalomyelitis following a nonspecific infection may pose a very difficult problem (Khan *et al.* 1995). In acute disseminated encephalomyelitis (ADEM) there is often widespread CNS disturbance with coma or drowsiness, seizures and multifocal neurological signs. In contrast, MS usually presents as a monosymptomatic syndrome such as optic neuritis or a subacute myelopathy. However, ADEM may also present in this way with some differences such as bilateral rather than unilateral optic neuritis or severe myelopathy rather than partial involvement. The presence on MRI of large symmetrical areas of high signal and of involvement of the grey matter also favours ADEM (Kesselring *et al.* 1990, Poser 1994, Tsai and Hung 1996). The diagnosis may be especially difficult in patients treated with corticosteroids who relapse on discontinuing therapy. Such recurrences should be distinguished from true relapses of MS.

The diagnosis of optic neuritis in relation to MS is discussed below as is its relationship to Schilder disease. Some metabolic conditions such as recurrent ataxia with lactic acidosis and Leigh disease (Powell *et al.* 1990) and diseases due to posterior fossa or cervical spinal lesions may also raise diagnostic problems. In many cases, the diagnosis of MS can only be made after months or years and it is even more difficult to exclude.

TREATMENT

No definite therapy of MS is available. Evaluation of any form of treatment is very difficult because of the remitting nature of the disease, and many therapies that had been highly praised initially have since been completely abandoned (McFarlin 1983). The existence of benign forms of the disorder makes evaluation even more problematic (Thompson *et al.* 1986). Corticosteroids or ACTH increase the rate of recovery from relapses but do not affect the long-term course of the disease (Milligan *et al.* 1987). High-dose intravenous corticosteroid treatment seems to be more effective but should often be followed by a slowly tapered course of oral therapy (Troiano *et al.* 1987). Interferon-beta significantly decreases the frequency of attacks, especially severe ones (IFNB 1995), but its long-term efficacy is still to be assessed.

Conventional immunosuppressant therapy may be effective but it is poorly tolerated and the benefits are not sufficiently clear to offset the balance in its favour. A number of novel immunotherapies are being tested and some have given encouraging preliminary results (Hohlfeld 1997). Hyperbaric oxygen and various forms of dietary therapy have not proved effective.

NEUROMYELITIS OPTICA (DEVIC DISEASE)
Neuromyelitis optica is characterized by the occurrence, simultaneously or in rapid sucession, of optic neuritis and transverse myelitis. The optic neuritis is often bilateral and presents as neuropapillitis. The transverse myelitis is responsible for paraplegia of sudden onset. It is likely that Devic disease is, in most cases, a form of MS (Haslam 1987, Steinlin *et al.* 1995b). However, pathological lesions sometimes have a necrotic character with occasional cavitation of the spinal cord that is demonstrable by MRI which usually also indicates the absence of brainstem and other cerebral lesions (Mandler *et al.* 1993). O'Riordan *et al.* (1996) also considered Devic disease as different from MS. Such cases are probably different from disseminated sclerosis. Thus neuromyelitis optica is probably a syndrome with several unknown causes.

SCHILDER MYELINOCLASTIC DIFFUSE SCLEROSIS
This rare entity, also known as encephalitis periaxialis diffusa, is an acquired subacute or chronic white matter disease of unknown origin. The disease causes large demyelinating lesions of the hemispheric cerebral white matter with relative sparing of the axons and sparing of subcortical U-fibres (Mehler and Rabinowich 1988). The histological characteristics of brain tissue are identical to those of multiple sclerosis. At least one, and more commonly two or more roughly symmetrical bilateral plaques of large dimensions (more than 3×2 cm) are present in the centrum ovale and can be demonstrated by brain imaging. Cavitation may occur.

The disease is observed mostly in children between 5 and 14 years of age. Focal neurological signs, especially hemiplegia, were the first clinical manifestation in four of five personally observed patients and in the majority of cases from the literature (Barth *et al.* 1989). Behavioural deterioration, cerebellar symptoms, progressive clumsiness, impaired vision, headaches, lethargy and personality changes are other presenting features. On examination, focal neurological deficits may include hemiplegia, aphasia, disturbances of swallowing, ataxia and bilateral pyramidal tract signs with pseudobulbar features (Kepes 1993, Afifi *et al.* 1994). Papilloedema may be found (Konkol *et al.* 1987, Mehler and Rabinowich 1988). The CSF may contain excess cells but seems to be more often normal.

CT scan shows the large plaques that present as areas of hypodensity with peripheral enhancement after contrast infusion, often with a mass effect (Fig. 12.2). Contrary to what obtains in adrenoleukodystrophy, the lesions are located in the frontal rather

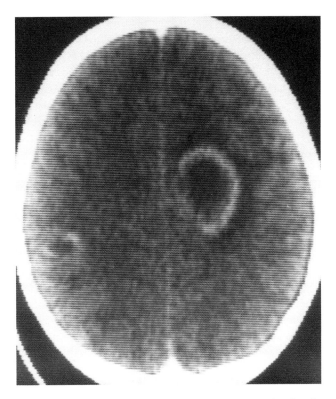

Fig. 12.2. Schilder disease. 11-year-old boy who presented with right hemiplegia of recent onset, headache and papilloedema. CT shows ring images in left central region and smaller lesion in opposite parietal area. Stereotaxic puncture yielded only yellow fluid with some necrotic debris. Clinical symptoms disappeared rapidly on steroid therapy. Repeat CT scan was normal but MRI showed persistence of small area of increased signal on T₂-weighted sequences.

than the parieto-occipital lobes in most cases. MRI shows an intense signal in T₂-weighted sequences.

Brain lesions in Schilder disease are extremely sensitive to steroids, which produce a rapid decrease in their size and disappearance of contrast enhancement. Hyperintense images on MRI appear to persist for prolonged periods (several years). T₁-weighted sequences show the persistence of focal loss of myelin.

The course of the disease is imperfectly known. With steroid treatment, improvement is obtained over weeks or months but sequelae may persist. Recurrences may occur (Harpey *et al.* 1983, Konkol *et al.* 1987) but the long-term prognosis is not known. No recurrences were observed in our five patients followed up for up to nine years and in most of the cases of Kepes (1993).

The diagnosis rests largely on neuroimaging techniques (Mehler and Rabinowich 1989). Cerebral abscess is an essential consideration as ring images may be identical to those in Schilder disease. Aspiration of the mass is then necessary, but if it is negative, the diagnosis of Schilder disease should be thought of and broad surgical approach avoided. Exclusion of adrenoleukodystrophy by determination of very-long-chain fatty acid plasma level is an absolute requirement. Other criteria include the absence of other types of lesions demonstrable on the basis of clinical and laboratory study, the absence of involvement of the peripheral nervous system, and histological features identical to those in multiple sclerosis (Poser *et al.* 1986). Such criteria exclude the diagnoses of genetic myelin disorders, multifocal tumours and vascular accidents.

The relationship of Schilder disease to MS remains unclear. Whilst transitional forms with small satellite plaques in addition to the large ones have been described (Poser *et al.* 1986), the age of occurrence, clinical features and course, and the absence of IgG oligoclonal CSF banding in most cases of Schilder disease distinguish the two conditions.

The same applies to *Baló concentric sclerosis* which does not appear to have been recognized in children but can be diagnosed in some cases on radiological and biopsy features and also responds to steroids (Garbern *et al.* 1986).

OPTIC NEURITIS

Optic neuritis consists of involvement of the nerve by inflammation, degeneration or demyelination resulting in impaired function (Riikonen *et al.* 1988a). Optic neuritis is often an early symptom of MS and it has been suggested that both disorders have the same aetiology. However, only some children who suffer from optic neuritis later develop MS. Only six of the 39 children with idiopathic optic neuritis studied by Kriss *et al.* (1988) developed MS during a mean follow-up of 8.8 years, while none of 17 children studied by Parkin *et al.* (1984) did so over a period of 18 years. This is in contrast with the experience of Riikonen *et al.* (1988a) who observed the development of MS in 12 of their 21 children. This discrepancy remains unexplained. The higher incidence in recent series may reflect the improvement of diagnostic methods for MS such as MRI.

A number of viral infections such as measles, varicella and mumps (Kline *et al.* 1982, Purvin *et al.* 1988) can also induce optic neuritis, either in isolation or associated with other manifestations of disseminated encephalomyelitis. Optic neuritis may also follow immunization with live vaccines (Riikonen 1989) and has been reported in Miller Fisher syndrome (Toshniwal 1987).

Clinical Features

Sudden monocular or binocular reduction of visual activity is the major manifestation. It may be preceded by headaches or painful eye movements (Riikonen *et al.* 1988a). Initially, there is blurred vision with progression within a few days to partial or complete blindness. Bilateral involvement is present in about 75 per cent of children and occurs either simultaneously or sequentially. The neuritis may be retrobulbar in which case fundoscopic examination is normal. In children, however, a swollen optic disc (neuropapillitis) is seen in three-quarters of cases during the acute phase (Kriss *et al.* 1988). In some cases, vasculitic changes such as retinal exudates, local vessel tortuosity or sheathing of veins may be seen (Riikonen *et al.* 1988a). Visual field examination reveals central scotomas, and visual evoked responses are delayed, a finding that persists for several years even when recovery seems complete. Involvement of the optic chiasm can produce unusual field cuts (Newman *et al.* 1991).

Most patients recover normal or useful vision despite the frequent persistence of optic atrophy, but colour vision and stereoscopic vision may remain impaired. Persistent severe loss of vision is rare (Purvin *et al.* 1988).

Diagnosis

It is essential to exclude other causes of acute impairment of vision, in particular compression of the optic nerve which may closely mimic unilateral optic neuritis (Chapter 18). Malingering and hysteria can be excluded, when necessary, by testing the visual evoked response. Papilloedema is not accompanied by early loss of vision and is therefore readily excluded when fundoscopic manifestations of neuropapillitis include severe disc swelling with haemorrhages. MRI may demonstrate demyelinating lesions in one or both optic nerves (Miller *et al.* 1988a, Jacobs *et al.* 1991).

The occurrence of optic neuritis raises the possibility of its being the first manifestation of MS. The risk of the child developing MS is greater in the case of a unilateral neuritis and seems very small in bilateral cases (Parkin *et al.* 1984). CSF studies often show pleocytosis and intrathecal IgG production of oligoclonal antibodies (Riikonen *et al.* 1988a,b). Lymphocyte subsets in blood and CSF do not differ between children who develop MS and those who do not (Riikonen and von Willebrandt 1988c). Pleocytosis may be more frequent in patients who later develop MS but may also occur in other cases. Therefore lumbar puncture is not of great help. However, the presence of free, kappalight chains in CSF appears to be correlated with the existence of hyperintense areas suggestive of MS (Rudick *et al.* 1986). MRI is indicated in all cases. Areas of abnormal signal were found in 71 per cent of cases in one series (Riikonen *et al.* 1988b). Although such images are not specific for MS and may occur, in particular, with encephalomyelitis, they are suggestive when present in periventricular location (Ormerod *et al.* 1986). Their association with IgG oligoclonal bands in CSF and HLA Dr 2 group is indicative of a high risk of developing disseminated disease (Jacobs *et al.* 1986).

No treatment is of proven value. Corticosteroids, especially in the form of methylprednisolone (1 g/d for three days in adults, followed by prednisone 1 mg/kg/d for two weeks), have been advised (Beck *et al.* 1992, 1993).

ACUTE TRANSVERSE MYELITIS

Transverse myelitis is an acute disorder characterized by signs of lesions in motor and sensory tracts on both sides of the spinal cord. Patients with a history of neurological disease or with evidence of lesions outside the spinal cord are excluded from this diagnosis.

Several neuropathological processes may affect the spinal cord and give rise to this syndrome. These include postinfectious myelitis, multiple sclerosis, vascular insufficiency, direct viral infection, X-irradiation and vascular malformations. Only idiopathic and postinfectious cases are considered here. In such cases, the lesion may be necrotic and cavitated. More commonly, there is inflammation and demyelination especially in a perivenous distribution.

The cause of most cases remains unknown. Transverse myelitis often follows a viral infection, and a long list of viruses have been associated with the syndrome including cytomegalovirus, herpes simplex virus, hepatitis A virus (Breningstall and Belani 1995) and adenoviruses (Linssen *et al.* 1991). Other infectious agents have been occasionally implicated, for example that causing Lyme disease (Rousseau *et al.* 1986, Linssen *et al.* 1991), *Mycoplasma pneumoniae* (Dewez *et al.* 1992, Logigian *et al.* 1994) and typhoid vaccine (Breningstall and Belani 1995). One-third to one-half of cases seem to be related to a viral infection, often an exanthematous disease. A cell-mediated immune response is a likely mechanism in many cases, as suggested by the observation that the lymphocytes of seven of 10 patients with transverse myelitis responded to bovine myelin basic protein and to human peripheral nerve myelin P2 protein (Abramsky and Teitelbaum 1977).

CLINICAL FEATURES
Most cases occur in patients over 5 years of age (Berman *et al.* 1981). However, I have observed transverse myelitis in infants as young as 5 months. Onset is preceded by evidence of acute infection in 60 per cent of children (Paine and Byers 1953). The onset may be hyperacute and is then marked by pain and the abrupt development of paraplegia with sphincter paralysis and marked sensory disturbances. Another mode of onset is more progressive over two or three days or even a week or more. In such cases, paraesthesiae may be an initial manifestation, although weakness and urinary retention are generally the most prominent features (Ropper and Poskanzer 1978). Back pain is present in 60 per cent of patients. Fever is common, and meningeal signs with neck stiffness are found in 30 per cent of cases.

Weakness is initially flaccid but evidence of pyramidal involvement gradually appears. Paraplegia is the usual presentation but more extensive paralysis may occur in cases of cervical affectation. Gross sensory disturbances are almost always present but a clear-cut level is often not easily defined. Pain sensation may be more impaired than position sense. In 80 per cent of cases the sensory and motor level is thoracic, and in another 10 per cent it is cervical (Berman *et al.* 1981). Involvement of respiratory muscles occurs in up to 20 per cent of cases (Ponsot and Arthuis 1981). In rare cases the Brown–Sequard syndrome is found.

Pleocytosis is found in about a quarter of the patients and an increased protein level in a quarter to a half.

DIAGNOSIS
The diagnosis of acute transverse myelitis may be difficult. Exclusion of cord compression by a neoplasm or an abscess is an absolute requirement, so the use of myelography or preferably of MRI of the cord is always indicated. In some patients with transverse myelitis moderate swelling of the cord may be present and an intraspinal area of increased signal on T_2-weighted MRI or gadolinium enhancement (Sanders *et al.* 1990) is possible (Miller *et al.* 1987). Scanning of the head may be of interest as intracranial abnormalities are sometimes detected in patients with only clinical signs of cord involvement (Campi *et al.* 1995). The significance of such images is, however, uncertain. Other causes of the transverse myelitis syndrome such as lupus erythematosus,

meningitis, schistosomiasis, spontaneous or post-traumatic occlusive vascular disease (Linssen *et al.* 1990) should be excluded as far as possible. In cases with an apoplectic onset, the possibility of a vascular malformation of the spinal cord should always be kept in mind (Chapter 15). In all cases, epiduritis must be ruled out. Polyradiculoneuritis in young patients may be difficult to distinguish from transverse myelopathy because sensory disturbances and sphincter dysfunction are not always easy to appreciate in such instances.

COURSE AND PROGNOSIS
In large series of both adults and children (Ropper and Poskanzer 1978, Berman *et al.* 1981, Ponsot and Arthuis 1981, Dunne *et al.* 1986), approximately 60 per cent of the patients made a good recovery that was rapid or extended over several months. Only 10–20 per cent of patients fail to improve significantly. The development of MS following transverse myelitis is observed in less than 10 per cent of adult patients and is exceptional in children. A normal MR scan is of considerable help in excluding MS. The most important prognostic factor is the mode of onset (Ropper and Poskanzer 1978). A large majority of patients with catastrophic onset of pain and paralysis are left with sequelae, whereas the reverse applies to those with a progressive onset (Dunne *et al.* 1986).

Treatment is purely symptomatic. Corticosteroids are not generally considered effective. However, high-dose pulses of methylprednisolone are often used in an attempt to reduce the frequent cord swelling.

ACUTE MYELOPATHIES OF OBSCURE ORIGIN
Other forms of myelopathy are exceptional in children. The vascular myelopathy associated with AIDS is virtually limited to adults (Rosenblum *et al.* 1989), and HTLV-1-associated progressive myelopathy (Link *et al.* 1989) has only rarely been reported in children. HTLV-1 may be associated with the presence of disseminated areas of intense signal on T_2-weighted MRI scans, thus mimicking MS (Newton *et al.* 1987).

CNS DEMYELINATING DISEASE ASSOCIATED WITH DEMYELINATING PERIPHERAL NEUROPATHY
The association of central demyelination with peripheral demyelinating neuropathy is unusual.

Some patients with combined demyelination present mainly as cases of polyneuropathy which may be preceded or accompanied by optic neuropathy (Toshniwal 1987) or by obtundation, seizures and other signs of CNS involvement (Mendell *et al.* 1987, Pakalnis *et al.* 1988, Uncini *et al.* 1988, Willis and Van den Bergh 1988).

In other patients the CNS manifestations may be in the forefront of the clinical picture while the neuropathy is more or less evident clinically (Amit *et al.* 1986, Rubin *et al.* 1987, Thomas *et al.* 1987). Such patients may present with manifestations suggestive of MS or encephalomyelitis and chronic or relapsing polyneuropathy.

NEUROLOGICAL INVOLVEMENT IN THE HAEMOPHAGOCYTIC SYNDROMES, SARCOIDOSIS AND RELATED PROLIFERATIVE DISORDERS

The exact nosological situation of the disorders considered in this section is still in doubt and their aetiologies are multiple. Some of them, at least, represent an abnormal response of the histiocytic system or of blood cell precursors, or both, to various aggressions especially of viral nature. Others are clearly malignant in nature but are mentioned here for convenience as they share many features with the reactive types. A genetic predisposition is probably present in most cases (Risdall *et al.* 1979).

FAMILIAL AND VIRUS-ASSOCIATED ERYTHROPHAGOCYTIC LYMPHOHISTIOCYTOSIS

These disorders are characterized pathologically by an infiltration of multiple tissues with lymphocytes and haemophagocytic histiocytes of benign appearance. The proliferation also involves the meninges and the brain in the form of disseminated infiltrates (Martin and Cras 1985). Infiltration can extend to affect nerve roots and peripheral nerves.

Some of the cases of lymphohistiocytosis are familial, apparently transmitted as a recessive character (Rettwitz *et al.* 1983, Henter *et al.* 1993). Other cases occur in a sporadic manner in apparent relationship with a viral infection in children and adults who were either previously healthy or immunosuppressed (Risdall *et al.* 1979, Wilson *et al.* 1981). Even in previously healthy patients, impaired natural killer activity of lymphocytes has been demonstrated (Perez *et al.* 1984).

Both familial and virus-associated forms are characterized by hepatosplenomegaly, pancytopenia and intractable fever. Approximately 30 per cent of patients demonstrate CNS abnormalities and lymphocytic meningitis. Neuroimaging may show disseminated areas of abnormal signal with contrast enhancement.

The familial form has an early onset, usually during the first semester of life. High levels of triglycerides and other lipid abnormalities are found (Ansbacher *et al.* 1983).

The course is severe, ending in death in most cases. Rapid neurological deterioration with progressive brain atrophy is on record (Rettwitz *et al.* 1983).

Involvement of the peripheral nervous system has been the main neurological finding in rare cases (Boutin *et al.* 1988b). Treatment with epipodophyllotoxin, steroids, intrathecal methotrexate and cranial irradiation may induce remissions (mostly temporary) (Fischer *et al.* 1985).

LYMPHOMATOID GRANULOMATOSIS

Lymphomatoid granulomatosis is a rare disease which has the characteristics both of an inflammatory process and of a lymphoproliferative disorder (Katzenstein *et al.* 1979). The disease affects the lungs, skin and CNS and occurs mostly in adults, although I have observed cases in children and adolescents. Mental confusion, ataxia, hemiparesis and seizures occur in 20–30 per cent of cases (Hogan *et al.* 1981, Rimsza *et al.* 1993). Spinal cord involvement may occur (Herderscheê *et al.* 1988). Treatment with steroids and cytotoxic drugs can be completed by surgical excision of solitary CNS lesions as medical treatment across the blood–brain barrier is of limited efficacy (Schmidt *et al.* 1984).

SARCOIDOSIS

Sarcoidosis is a granulomatous inflammatory disease of unknown aetiology that may affect any part of the central and peripheral nervous system as well as muscles (Scott 1993). The disorder, especially its neurological manifestations, is uncommon in children, although McGovern and Merritt (1956) collected 13 cases. Pathologically, sarcoidosis is characterized by the presence of non-necrotizing granulomas with giant cells and epithelioid cells in the absence of demonstrable microorganisms or other agents. The granulomas usually involve many tissues, especially lymph nodes, lungs, skin, bone and eye. In the CNS, granulomas have a predilection for the basal meninges, the floor of the third and fourth ventricles and the hypothalamus.

Active sarcoidosis is associated with immunological abnormalities (Daniele *et al.* 1980). The capacity of peripheral blood lymphocytes to participate in cellular immune reactions is decreased, while the systemic humoral immune response is activated, as reflected by production of antibodies with a wide variety of specificities.

In children, *Heerfordt syndrome* is the most common manifestation of sarcoidosis (McGovern and Merritt 1956). This consists of uveitis and less commonly optic neuritis associated with swelling of the parotid gland and facial nerve palsy. Cranial neuropathy, which is the commonest feature of CNS sarcoidosis in adults, papilloedema and diabetes insipidus are rare in children. Spinal cord involvement has been reported (Rubinstein *et al.* 1984). Isolated CNS sarcoidosis is rare (Lee *et al.* 1989). CSF examination may show mononuclear pleocytosis, blood–brain barrier damage and a decreased CSF/serum glucose ratio. CT scan may demonstrate hydrocephalus with enhancement of the basilar meninges (Kendall and Tatler 1978). Intrathecal production of oligoclonal IgM and IgG has been reported (Kinnman and Link 1984).

The diagnosis rests on the demonstration of associated lesions, especially hilar lymphoid enlargement on chest X-ray, negative PPD skin test, positive Kveim test, hypercalcaemia, radioactive gallium scanning and deficiency in angiotensin-conversion enzyme (Chapelon *et al.* 1990, Scott 1993).

The course of the disorder is slow and partial, or complete remission may supervene.

LANGERHANS HISTIOCYTOSIS (HISTIOCYTOSIS X)

This multisystemic disease of unknown cause is characterized by proliferation of mononucleated phagocytes with characteristic inclusions. Involvement of the CNS is uncommon except for hypothalamic histiocytic, or sometimes purely hypophyseal, infiltration responsible for diabetes insipidus (Schmitt *et al.* 1993, Egeler and D'Angio 1995). This is often part of Hand–Schuller–Christian disease with multiple skull lacunae, exophthalmia and possible involvement of the optic chiasm (Goodman *et al.* 1979).

Localized areas of pseudotumoural infiltration in the extradural or subdural spaces are often an extension of the granulomatous lesions of the membranous bones of the skull with compression of the cranial nerves. Localized, isolated or multiple parenchymal lesions are rare (Barthez Carpentier *et al.* 1991). Progressive cerebellar ataxia, often associated with pyramidal tract signs and cognitive deterioration, may occur. In such cases CT or MRI scans usually show bilateral symmetrical areas of low density or abnormal signal in the central cerebellar white matter and, occasionally, in the basal ganglia (Poe *et al.* 1994). In rare cases there is only diffuse cerebellar atrophy that has been regarded as a paraneoplastic phenomenon (Goldberg-Stern *et al.* 1995). Abnormal images may precede cerebellar symptoms by months or even years. The outcome of CNS involvement is relatively favourable in the case of mass lesions, which often respond to prednisone, vinblastine and methotrexate, but outcome is poor for cerebellar degeneration which is also little influenced by irradiation.

Involvement of the CNS has been observed in non-Langerhans histiocytosis (Foucar *et al.* 1979) and in systemic mastocytosis, marked by headache, dizziness, seizures and alterations in cognitive function (Korenblat *et al.* 1984). Parenchymal lesions have also been reported in a few cases of *juvenile xanthogranuloma*, a form of non-Langerhans histiocytosis (Botella-Estreda *et al.* 1993). The situation of cases of diabetes insipidus with infundibuloneurohypophysitis (Imura *et al.* 1993) is not clear

OPSOCLONUS–MYOCLONUS SYNDROME AND SOME FORMS OF ACUTE OR SUBACUTE CEREBELLAR ATAXIA

Myoclonic encephalopathy of Kinsbourne and acute/subacute cerebellar ataxia, although clinically and aetiologically distinct, share some clinical features and may be observed under similar circumstances. Thus, both syndromes can be observed following acute viral infections, *e.g.* with enteroviruses (Kuban *et al.* 1983) or Epstein–Barr virus (Sheth *et al.* 1995), and cerebellar ataxia has been occasionally reported as a presenting manifestation of neuroblastoma (Koh *et al.* 1994), although this tumour is more commonly associated with the opsoclonus–myoclonus syndrome (Lemerle *et al.* 1969). An immunoallergic mechanism is likely for both syndromes, although cases of opsoclonus–myoclonus have occurred as a result of hydrocephalus (Shetty and Rosman 1972) or of acute intoxications (Garcin *et al.* 1965), and cerebellar ataxia may have multiple causes (Chapter 10). Table 12.2 indicates the major causes of acute ataxia.

ACUTE AND SUBACUTE CEREBELLAR ATAXIA
This condition is characterized by the sudden or rapid onset of ataxia, usually following a specific (*e.g.* varicella) or nonspecific infectious illness.

It is likely that in some cases, a direct viral infection of the CNS is responsible for the clinical picture, even though there has been no direct demonstration of the presence of a virus in cerebellar cells. Several viruses have been isolated from the CSF

TABLE 12.2
Major causes of acute ataxia*

Cause	Reference
Infectious and parainfectious cerebellar ataxia	
Viral infections (varicella, measles, mumps, herpes simplex, Epstein–Barr virus, coxsackie and echovirus, poliomyelitis)	See text
Bacterial infections	
Mycoplasma pneumoniae	Behan *et al.* (1986)
Legionella pneumophila	Nigro *et al.* (1983)
Toxic causes	
Benzodiazepines	Chapter 16
Phenytoin, barbiturates, carbamazepine*	Chapter 16
Antihistamine drugs	Chapter 13
Vitamin A	Chapter 23
Methotrexate	Chapter 14
Piperazine ('worm wobble')	Chapter 13
Acute ataxia revealing structural lesion of the posterior fossa	
Posterior fossa tumour	Chapter 14
Chiari I anomaly and other anomalies of the cervico-occipital region	Chapter 3
Vascular causes	
Basilar migraine**	Lapkin and Golden (1978)
Basilar artery thrombosis or emboli	Echenne *et al.* (1983)
Cryptogenic ataxia	
Possibly related to unnoticed infections	See text
Ataxia due to peripheral nerve involvement	Chapter 21
Miller Fisher syndrome	
Other neuropathies	
Ataxia following an acute neurological disease	
Multiple sclerosis	See text
Head trauma	Chapter 13
Heat stroke	Chapter 13
Acute purulent meningitis	Chapter 11
Cerebellar abscess	Chapter 11
Pseudoataxia due to nonconvulsive epileptic activity**	Bennett *et al.* (1982)
Nonconvulsive status epilepticus	Chapter 16
Periods of uncontrolled activity in Lennox–Gastaut syndrome and myoclonic epilepsies	Guerrini *et al.* (1993)

*Excluding intermittent ataxias that are dealt with in Table 17.3 (p. 644).
In most cases of acute ataxia, it is difficult to distinguish between cerebellar, sensory or other (vestibular) causes, and additional signs of CNS involvement may be present.
**May be recurrent.

or extraneural sites including polioviruses (Arthuis *et al.* 1960), echovirus 9 (McAllister *et al.* 1959) and coxsackie B virus (Kuban *et al.* 1983) but they may have induced ataxia through an indirect mechanism similar to what occurs in postinfectious encephalomyelitis. Such is probably the causal mechanism for cases of acute ataxia following chickenpox (Johnson and Milbourn 1970), mumps (Koskiniemi *et al.* 1983), varicella immunization (Sunaga *et al.* 1995) or other exanthematous diseases of childhood and for the rare cases of ataxia that may be the initial feature of MS.

Acute cerebellar ataxia is the most common parainfectious CNS disease in children. It may occur at any age, most commonly during the second year of life. In one series (Connolly *et al.* 1988), 26 per cent of cases were associated with chicken pox, 52 per cent with other presumably viral illness and 3 per cent with immunizations. The clinical picture is marked by severe truncal ataxia and gait disturbance. Tremor of the extremities or head is less common. Nystagmus is present in 45 per cent of patients (Weiss and Carter 1959). CSF pleocytosis is found in a quarter of the cases and late increase in CSF protein has been observed (Weiss and Carter 1959).

Most patients recover spontaneously in a few weeks to six months. However, a residual cerebellar syndrome may persist in a quarter to a third of the patients, and persistence of an incapacitating ataxia may be seen. In such cases, CT scan may demonstrate residual cerebellar atrophy. Areas of altered signal in the cerebellum, sometimes with contrast enhancement, may be observed in the early stage of the illness and may persist for several months, although they are uncommon. Acute cerebellar swelling demonstrated by neuroimaging with symptoms and signs of high intracranial pressure may occur following varicella (Hurst and Mehta 1988) or undetermined, probably viral infections (Roulet Perez *et al.* 1993) and may be fatal in rare cases.

Acute cerebellar ataxia should not be confused with posterior fossa or other tumours. Acute labyrinthitis is difficult to separate from cerebellar ataxia. Nausea, intense vertigo and abnormal tests of labyrinthine function permit the diagnosis (Eviatar and Eviatar 1977). The course of acute vestibular ataxia is often briefer than that of cerebellar ataxia and recovery is the rule. The most common differential diagnosis is from drug or other intoxications which account for up to one-third of cases of acute ataxia. Ataxia may also follow heat stroke (Freedman and Schental 1953), and a reversible although prolonged ataxic syndrome can be seen in severe epilepsies during periods of intense seizure activity (Bennett *et al.* 1982).

OPSOCLONUS–MYOCLONUS SYNDROME (MYOCLONIC ENCEPHALOPATHY OF KINSBOURNE)

The syndrome of myoclonic encephalopathy is observed mostly in infants and children under 3 years of age.

The disorder may follow an infectious illness of established or presumed viral origin such as poliomyelitis (Arthuis *et al.* 1960) or other enterovirus infections (Kuban *et al.* 1983, Sheth *et al.* 1995). Mumps-induced cases have been reported (Ichiba *et al.* 1988). In a high proportion of cases, the syndrome is associated with a neuroblastoma which is often occult. The tumour is often thoracic in location but may be found in any situation, including the pelvis. It may be very small and difficult to detect, hence the necessity in every case of repeated complete investigation including rectal examination, careful palpation and ultrasound and CT or MRI scan of the abdomen and pelvis, and repeated determinations of urinary vanillyl-mandelic and homovanillic acids as the levels of these compounds may be only mildly and intermittently raised (Mitchell and Snodgrass 1990) or (in one-third of cases) remain normal (Engle *et al.* 1995). MRI and metaiodobenzylguanidine radionuclide scans are more effective

in the detection of neuroblastoma and may further increase the proportion of cases due to sympathetic tumours. Neuroblastoma is not excluded by the presence of an acute infectious disease preceding the syndrome (Kuban *et al.* 1983). Hammer *et al.* (1995) found a neuroblastoma in seven of 11 patients with this syndrome. The frequency of sympathetic tumours may even be higher, as cases are known in which a spontaneously regressive tumour has been responsible for the syndrome (Engle *et al.* 1995).

The clinical picture is distinctive (Pampiglione and Maia 1972, Boltshauser *et al.* 1979) and unlike that seen in any other condition. The most remarkable feature is the presence of chaotic, rapid, irregular eye movements that can be in the horizontal or oblique planes and occur in sudden bursts frequently precipitated by changing fixation. The opsoclonus is associated with violent jerking of the limbs on attempted movements. This remarkable association of eye and limb jerking has been termed 'dancing eyes, dancing feet syndrome' (Dyken and Kolár 1968). The clinical myoclonus is unassociated with any paroxysmal EEG abnormality.

The condition is self-limiting in most cases even when associated with a neuroblastoma.

Its time relation to the opsoclonus–myoclonus is variable. It is often the first manifestation of the tumour that should be strongly suspected in all cases. It may disappear with successful treatment of the neuroblastoma. However, in most cases, the movement disorder follows its own course irrespective of the course of the tumour.

Initially, the movements are extremely intense and the child in panic. Progressively, and especially with steroid therapy, the intensity of jerking diminishes and the opsoclonus often disappears, followed by the myoclonus of limbs. The course is often prolonged, lasting months or even years, with recurrences precipitated by intercurrent respiratory infections or decreases in the dose of steroids (Pohl *et al.* 1996). The myoclonus and any associated ataxia eventually disappear, but a majority of affected children are left with mental retardation, motor difficulties and speech disturbances (Boltshauser *et al.* 1979).

Neuroblastomas associated with Kinsbourne syndrome have a better prognosis for survival than neuroblastoma in general, suggesting that the neurological manifestations in these children may result from an unknown, perhaps autoimmune factor which is also effective in checking the growth of the tumour (Altman and Baehner 1976). Anti-CNS antibodies may play a role in the genesis of this syndrome (Pliopys *et al.* 1989, Fisher *et al.* 1994).

Other factors of favourable prognosis include a thoracic location of the tumour, histological features with a greater differentiation toward ganglioneuroma, and the presence of a single copy of the *N-myc* proto-oncogen in tumour cells (Koh *et al.* 1994).

Corticosteroid treatment is often dramatically effective. After initial treatment with about 1 mg/kg/d of prednisone, the lowest possible dosage should be attained by slowly decreasing the dose. Long-term treatment is often required, and recurrences may necessitate temporary increases of dosage during months or even years (Pohl *et al.* 1996).

TABLE 12.3
Immunoallergic complications of immunizations

Immunization	Neurological complication	Reference
Influenza	Guillain–Barré syndrome	Schonberger *et al.* (1981)
	Encephalitis/encephalomyelitis	Yahr and Lobo-Antunes (1972)
	Acute transverse myelitis	Wells (1971)
	Optic neuritis	Bienfang *et al.* (1977)
	Brachial plexus neuropathy	Weintraub and Chia (1977)
	Cranial neuropathies	Yahr and Lobo-Antunes (1972)
Rabies	Encephalomyelitis	Hemachuda *et al.* (1987, 1988)
	Acute transverse myelitis	Hemachuda *et al.* (1987)
	Guillain–Barré syndrome	Hemachuda *et al.* (1987)
	Optic neuritis	Hemachuda *et al.* (1987)
Rubella	Acute transverse myelitis	Holt *et al.* 1976
Measles	Encephalopathy/encephalitis	Miller *et al.* (1993)
	Acute cerebellar ataxia	Trump and White (1967)
Diphtheria–tetanus–pertussis	Guillain–Barré syndrome	Pollard and Selby (1978)
	Brachial plexus neuropathy	Fenichel (1994)
	Acute transverse myelitis	Fenichel (1994)

Treatment with intravenous gammaglobulin is effective in many cases of postinfectious acute cerebellar ataxia or opsoclonus (Otten *et al.* 1996), including cases associated with a neuroblastoma (Sugie *et al.* 1992, Petruzzi and De Alarcon 1995), but often only temporarily, and is rarely sufficient to enable avoidance of corticosteroids. Removal of the neuroblastoma is indicated in all cases.

NEUROLOGICAL COMPLICATIONS OF IMMUNIZATIONS

The neurological complications of immunizations undoubtedly have different causes and mechanisms, including direct action of attenuated pathogens or of their toxins. Immunoallergic mechanisms are probably most important, and for convenience all complications will be dealt with in this section.

COMPLICATIONS OF PROBABLE IMMUNOALLERGIC MECHANISM

Complications probably due to an immunoallergic mechanism can involve the central or the peripheral nervous system or both. They include encephalopathy, encephalitis, encephalomyelitis or polyradiculoneuritis (the Guillain–Barré syndrome), brachial plexus neuropathy, acute transverse myelitis, cranial neuropathies and optic neuritis (Peter 1992, Fenichel 1994). The terms encephalopathy and encephalitis are often used synonymously to refer to any combination of alteration of behaviour or consciousness, convulsions and focal neurological deficits. Encephalitis is the preferred term when inflammatory features such as CSF pleocytosis are present.

These disorders do not differ clinically from similar diseases that occur following viral infections or apparently spontaneously (Chapters 11, 12). Complications of probable immunoallergic mechanism have followed immunization against influenza, rabies, smallpox, yellow fever, and rarely rubella, measles (Table 12.3)

and Japanese B encephalitis (Ohtaki *et al.* 1992). Neurological complications following mumps immunization are extremely rare (Fenichel 1994). No pathologically confirmed case of immunoallergic complication is on record following the use of diphtheria–tetanus–pertussis vaccine. Cases of encephalopathy without inflammatory features are described below. The overall frequency of such neurological complication is extremely low and should not deter the use of vaccines.

COMPLICATIONS DUE TO THE DIRECT ACTION OF A VACCINE PATHOGEN OR TO TOXIC MECHANISMS

Complications that represent direct infections by live, attenuated vaccines are quite rare. They are more variable in type and clinical presentation than immunoallergic complications. Therefore, they are described individually for each vaccine. This section also describes the complications of pertussis immunization, as a toxic mechanism appears more probable than an immunoallergic pathogenesis, although the latter has not been totally excluded.

MUMPS, MEASLES AND RUBELLA

Rare cases of acute encephalopathy have occurred following live-virus *measles immunization* but a cause-and-effect relationship between the neurological disorder and immunization is far from proven. The frequency of convulsions following measles vaccine, including febrile convulsions, is much lower than following the wild disease (Landrigan and Witte 1973). Seizures were observed in 1.9 per cent of vaccine recipients as against an incidence of 7.7 per cent in patients with the wild disease. The incidence of encephalitis was observed 15–35 days following immunization in 1:11,000 to 1:100,000 doses (D. Miller *et al.* 1993). The outcome is usually good.

Subacute sclerosing panencephalitis (SSPE) following live-virus immunization has been reported, but epidemiological studies have established that such cases are much rarer than cases following natural measles (0.14:100,000 doses of vaccine as opposed to 4:100,000 following the natural disease). Administration of vaccine following natural measles does not increase the incidence of SSPE (Miller *et al.* 1992). It is probable that immunization is responsible for the marked fall in incidence of SSPE over the past decade.

Rubella vaccination is rarely associated with immunoallergic complications. Two syndromes of pain in the upper limbs with paraesthesiae 2–35 days after immunization and of pain in the lower limbs for 2–14 days occurring 29–70 days after vaccination, have been reported (Schaffner *et al.* 1974). They are probably the result of a mixture of arthritis and neuritis.

Transmission of the rubella virus to the fetus following immunization of pregnant women can occur (Modlin *et al.* 1975), hence the need for vaccination of prepubertal girls. Seizures rarely follow administration of mumps–measles–rubella vaccine (E. Miller *et al.* 1993). Meningitis has been reported following mumps vaccine (Sugiura and Yamada 1991).

POLIO VACCINE
The inactivated (Salk) polio vaccine has an excellent safety record and is effective. Administration of the oral live attenuated virus vaccine has been associated with the occurrence of paralytic poliomyelitis in some recipients or their close contacts. Fifteen per cent of these cases were in immunodeficient children (Ruuskanen *et al.* 1980). In such patients the disease is often atypical and incubation may be longer than the one-month incubation observed in healthy recipients. Live vaccine is contraindicated for immunodepressed children or their contacts (Querfurth and Swanson 1990). Rantala *et al.* (1994) found no relationship between the occurrence of Guillain–Barré syndrome and the administration of oral polio vaccine.

DIPHTHERIA–TETANUS–PERTUSSIS (DTP) VACCINE
Neurological complications following triple immunization for diphtheria, tetanus and pertussis can be attributed almost entirely to the pertussis component (Cody *et al.* 1981, Miller *et al.* 1981, Cherry *et al.* 1988). Occasional cases of immunoallergic complication of DTP vaccine or one of its components have been reported (Fenichel 1994) but the relationship of such accidents with the vaccine is unproved.

Convulsions and hypotonic–hyporesponsive episodes appear to bear a clear relationship to the pertussis component of the DTP vaccine (Baraff *et al.* 1988, Fenichel 1988), although Pollock and Morris (1983) found that hypotonic–hyporesponsive episodes also occurred following diphtheria–tetanus vaccine without the pertussis component, and the frequency of convulsions in their study did not differ following administration of either DT or DTP vaccine. An association between febrile convulsions and DTP administration has been found (Miller *et al.* 1981, Shields *et al.* 1988) and was confirmed by the change of distribution of febrile seizures in Denmark following a change in DTP schedule. Shields *et al.* (1988) estimated that a maximum of 5.9 per cent of febrile convulsions occurring before age 2 years were associated

with DTP immunization. Approximately 10 per cent of seizures following DTP are afebrile (Blumberg *et al.* 1993).

Hypotonic–hyporesponsive episodes may occur on average 12 hours after immunization, may last from a few minutes to four hours and do not leave residua. In the series of Blumberg *et al.* (1993) seizures or hypotonic–hyporesponsive episodes occurred in 1 in 1750 immunizations, persistant crying in 1:100 and fever >40.5°C in 1:330. Bulging of the fontanelle has been observed also after DT vaccine administration (Gross *et al.* 1989).

Encephalopathy characterized by repeated convulsions, coma and death or sequelae is the major neurological complication attributed to the pertussis vaccine. However, the clinical picture is nonspecific and many reported cases are undoubtedly mere coincidences. A national study of cases of acute encephalopathy in the United Kingdom (D. Miller *et al.* 1981, 1993) indicated that acute encephalopathy attributable to the vaccine occurred in 1 in 140,000 immunizations (range 1:44,000–1:360,000 at 5% confidence limits) and that permanent damage occurred in 1 of 310,000 cases (range 1:54,000 to 1:5,000,000). Even these small figures have been contested (Cherry *et al.* 1988, Shields *et al.* 1988). The available evidence seems to indicate that there is a rare association between DTP vaccine and serious neurological disease but that the occurrence of permanent brain damage, although possible, has not been convincingly demonstrated. It seems reasonable to conclude that pertussis vaccine encephalopathy, although quite rare, does exist and is marked by status epilepticus, coma and, rarely, focal neurological deficits which occur within 72 hours, and especially within 12–24 hours of administration of the vaccine (Aicardi and Chevrie 1975). Cases of brief convulsions or cases with onset after 48 hours are unlikely to represent complications of immunization (Menkes and Kinsbourne 1990). The occurrence of a severe seizure disorder beginning within 24 hours of immunization was noted in 1:106,000 patients in a retrospective study (Walker *et al.* 1988). Most of those cases probably represent cases of severe myoclonic epilepsy (Chapter 16) whose onset is generally at this age.

Pertussis vaccine encephalopathy is probably caused by a direct toxic effect, rather than being immune-mediated. Novel cell-free vaccines may avoid the occurrence of such complications as they are free of endotoxin and other noninactivated toxins (for review, see Menkes and Kinsbourne 1990).

Other neurological complications, including infantile spasms, have been attributed to pertussis immunization. There is good evidence that the occurrence of infantile spasms after DTP immunization is coincidental (Miller *et al.* 1981), and changes in the immunization programmes in Denmark (Melchior 1977) and in Japan (Tsuchiya *et al.* 1978) did not alter the frequency or age of occurrence of West syndrome.

The *complications of pertussis* itself are probably only in part of toxic origin. It is interesting to compare them with the complications of the vaccine. Some of the noxious effects of pertussis on the CNS are related to toxins produced by the organism. Hypoxia and increased venous pressure due to intense cough probably play an important role in the genesis of cerebral complications. Brain lesions are mostly of an hypoxic type. In addition, diffuse petechiae and, sometimes, subdural or spinal epidural haematomas may be present.

The clinical picture of pertussis encephalopathy includes convulsions and coma, and sometimes hemiplegia which often appears at the peak of the paroxysmal cough (Zellweger 1959). Severe sequelae are not uncommon.

The frequency of neurological complications of whooping cough is poorly known but currently they appear to be rare. They are especially observed in young infants and are one of the reasons that militate in favour of pertussis immunization. The latter is possibly contraindicated for infants with a prior history of seizures or with a history of severe reaction to previous injections of pertussis vaccine (American Academy of Pediatrics 1984). The Academy's Committee on Infectious Diseases currently recommends deferral of DTP immunization in children with convulsions or other neurological symptoms until the physician is certain that they do not suffer from a progressive neurological disease. The solution to the problem will be the development of acellular nontoxic vaccines.

OTHER IMMUNIZATIONS
Influenza vaccination was associated with the development of a Guillain–Barré-like syndrome in the USA (Fenichel 1994), appearing 5–16 weeks after administration.

Sunaga *et al.* (1995) have reported cerebellar ataxia following varicella vaccination.

Complications of rabies immunization are rare with the use of current human diploid cell vaccines but are common when old vaccines are used. They present as encephalitis or aseptic meningitis, transverse myelitis or Guillain–Barré syndrome (Hemachuda *et al.* 1987, 1988, Fenichel 1994).

Smallpox vaccination as a cause of neurological complications is now of only historical interest.

OTHER NEUROLOGICAL ACCIDENTS OF ALLERGIC ORIGIN

NEUROLOGICAL FEATURES OF SERUM SICKNESS
Injection of therapeutic serum can produce neurological manifestations. Certain sera have been blamed more frequently than others. Tetanus antitoxin is most often causal but this may well result from its more frequent use.

Symptoms usually appear 5–12 days after administration of the serum. Brachial plexus neuropathy is the most usual manifestation (Chapter 21). Symptoms of meningeal irritation may be associated, and systemic features, including fever, pruritus, urticaria and vomiting are frequently present. In other cases, the picture is one of polyneuritis. In occasional patients cerebral manifestations such as headache, confusion, papilloedema and focal deficits are found (Ford 1952).

The prognosis is generally good with recovery over weeks or months. The cerebral symptoms disappear in a matter of days or at most of weeks.

Serum sickness has become rare as the use of animal sera has all but disappeared.

OTHER ACCIDENTS OF ALLERGIC ORIGIN
Allergic reactions involving the nervous system can occur following a variety of precipitating injuries. Wasp and bee stings as well as other insect bites can induce central or peripheral lesions.

Central system reactions consist of brain oedema sometimes with associated haemorrhagic phenomena (Means *et al.* 1973). In rare cases major destructive lesions of the brain have been observed.

Peripheral nervous system involvement may present as Guillain–Barré syndrome or in association with spinal cord disorder (Van Antwerpen *et al.* 1988).

REFERENCES

Abramsky, O., Teitelbaum, D. (1977) 'The autoimmune features of acute transverse myelopathy.' *Annals of Neurology*, **2**, 36–40.

Adair, J.C., Woodley, S.L., O'Connell, J.B., *et al.* (1991) 'Aseptic meningitis following cardiac transplantation: clinical characteristics and relationship to immunosuppressive regimen.' *Neurology*, **41**, 249–252.

Afifi, A.K., Bell, W.E., Menezes, A.H., Moore, S.A. (1994) 'Myelinoclastic diffuse sclerosis (Schilder's disease): report of a case and review of the literature.' *Journal of Child Neurology*, **9**, 398–403.

Aicardi, J., Chevrie, J.J. (1975) 'Accidents neurologiques consécutifs à la vaccination contre la coqueluche.' *Archives Françaises de Pédiatrie*, **32**, 309–318.

Altman, A.J., Baehner, R.L. (1976) 'Favorable prognosis for survival in children with coincident opso-myoclonus and neuroblastoma.' *Cancer*, **37**, 846–852.

American Academy of Pediatrics Committee on Infectious Diseases (1984) 'Pertussis vaccine.' *Pediatrics*, **74**, 303–305.

Amit, R., Shapira, Y., Blank, A., Aker, M. (1986) 'Acute severe central and peripheral nervous system combined demyelination.' *Pediatric Neurology*, **2**, 47–50.

Ansbacher, L.E., Singsen, B.H., Hosler, M.W., *et al.* (1983) 'Familial erythrophagocytic lymphohistiocytosis: an association with serum lipid abnormalities.' *Journal of Pediatrics*, **102**, 270–273.

Arthuis, M., Lyon, G., Thieffry, S. (1960) 'La forme ataxique de la maladie de Heine-Medin.' *Revue Neurologique*, **103**, 329–340.

Ashkenazi, S. (1993) 'Role of bacterial cytotoxins in hemolytic uremic syndrome and thrombotic thrombocytopenic purpura.' *Annual Review of Medicine*, **44**, 11–18.

Baker, H.L., Berquist, T.H., Kispert, D.B., *et al.* (1985) 'Magnetic resonance imaging in a routine clinical setting.' *Mayo Clinic Proceedings*, **60**, 75–90.

Bale, J.F., Brasher, C., Siegler, R.L. (1980) 'Central nervous system manifestations of hemolytic–uremic syndrome: relationship to metabolic alterations and prognosis.' *American Journal of Diseases of Children*, **134**, 869–872.

Baraff, L.J., Shields, W.D., Beckwith, L., *et al.* (1988) 'Infants and children with convulsions and hypotonic–hyporesponsive episodes following diphtheria–tetanus–pertussis immunization: follow-up evaluation.' *Pediatrics*, **81**, 789–794.

Barnes, D., McDonald, W.I. (1992) 'The ocular manifestations of multiple sclerosis. 2. Abnormalities of eye movement.' *Journal of Neurology, Neurosurgery, and Psychiatry*, **55**, 863–868.

Barnett, N.D.P., Kaplan, A.M., Bernes, S.M., Cohen, M.L. (1995) 'Hemolytic uremic syndrome with particular involvement of basal ganglia and favorable outcome.' *Pediatric Neurology*, **12**, 155–158.

Barth, P.G., Derix, M.M.A., De Krom, M.C.T.F.M., *et al.* (1989) 'Schilder's diffuse sclerosis: case study with three years' follow-up and neuro-imaging.' *Neuropediatrics*, **20**, 230–233.

Barthez Carpentier, M.A., Maheut, J., Grangepont, M-C., *et al.* (1991) 'Disseminated cerebral histiocytosis X responding to vinblastine therapy: a case report.' *Brain and Development*, **13**, 193–195.

Bauer, H.J., Hanefeld, F.A. (1993) *Multiple Sclerosis: Its Impact from Childhood to Old Age*. Philadelphia: W.B. Saunders.

Beck, R.W., Cleary, P.A., Anderson, M.M., *et al.* (1992) 'A randomized, controlled trial of corticosteroids in the treatment of acute optic neuritis.' *New England Journal of Medicine*, **326**, 581–588.

—— —— Trobe, J.D., *et al.* (1993) 'The effect of corticosteroids for acute optic neuritis on the subsequent development of multiple sclerosis.' *New England Journal of Medicine*, **329**, 1764–1769.

Behan, P.O., Feldman, R.G., Segerra, J.M., Draper, I.T. (1986) 'Neurological aspects of mycoplasmal infection.' *Acta Neurologica Scandinavica*, **74**, 314–322.

Bell, D.M., Morens, D.M., Holman, R.C., *et al.* (1983) 'Kawasaki syndrome in the United States 1976 to 1980.' *American Journal of Diseases of Children*, **137**, 211–214.

Belman, A.L., Leicher, C.R., Moshé, S.L., Mezey, A.P. (1985) 'Neurologic manifestations of Schoenlein–Henoch purpura: report of three cases and review of the literature.' *Pediatrics*, **75**, 687–692.

Bennett, H.S., Selman, J.E., Rapin, I., Rose, A. (1982) 'Nonconvulsive epileptiform activity appearing as ataxia.' *American Journal of Diseases of Children*, **136**, 30–32.

Berman, M., Feldman, S., Alter, M., *et al.* (1981) 'Acute transverse myelitis: incidence and etiologic considerations.' *Neurology*, **31**, 966–971.

Bienfang, D.C., Kantrowitz, F.G., Noble, J.L., Raynor, A.M. (1977) 'Ocular abnormalities after influenza immunization.' *Archives of Ophthalmology*, **95**, 1649. *(Letter.)*

Bierman, F.Z., Gersony, W.M. (1987) 'Kawasaki disease: clinical perspective.' *Journal of Pediatrics*, **111**, 789–793.

Blumberg, D.A., Lewis, K., Mink, C.M., *et al.* (1993) 'Severe reactions associated with diphtheria–tetanus–pertussis vaccine: detailed study of children with seizures, hypotonic–hyporesponsive episodes, high fevers, and persistent crying.' *Pediatrics*, **91**, 1158–1165.

Boltshauser, E., Deonna, T., Hirt, H.R. (1979) 'Myoclonic encephalopathy of infants or "dancing eyes syndrome".' *Helvetica Paediatrica Acta*, **34**, 119–133.

Bonfa, E., Golombek, S.J., Kaufman, L.D., *et al.* (1987) 'Association between lupus psychosis and anti-ribosomal P protein antibodies.' *New England Journal of Medicine*, **317**, 265–271.

Botella-Estrada, R., Sanmartín, O., Grau, M., *et al.* (1993) 'Juvenile xanthogranuloma with central nervous system involvement.' *Pediatric Dermatology*, **10**, 64–68.

Boutin, B., Esquivel, E., Mayer, M., *et al.* (1988a) 'Multiple sclerosis in children: report of clinical and paraclinical features of 19 cases.' *Neuropediatrics*, **19**, 118–123.

—— Routon, M.C., Rocchiccioli, F., *et al.* (1988b) 'Peripheral neuropathy associated with erythrophagocytic lymphohistiocytosis.' *Journal of Neurology, Neurosurgery, and Psychiatry*, **51**, 291–294.

Boyce, T.G., Swerdlow, D.L., Griffin, P.M. (1995) '*Escherichia coli* O157:H7 and the hemolytic–uremic syndrome.' *New England Journal of Medicine*, **333**, 364–368.

Breningstall, G.N., Belani, K.K. (1995) 'Acute transverse myelitis and brainstem encephalitis associated with hepatitis A infection.' *Pediatric Neurology*, **12**, 169–171.

Bruyn, G.W., Padberg, G. (1984) 'Chorea and systemic lupus erythematosus.' *European Neurology*, **23**, 278–290.

Bye, A.M.E., Kendall, B., Wilson, J. (1985) 'Multiple sclerosis in childhood. A new look.' *Developmental Medicine and Child Neurology*, **27**, 215–222.

Cabañas, F., Pellicer, A., Valverde, E., *et al.* (1996) 'Central nervous system vasculopathy in neonatal lupus erythematosus.' *Pediatric Neurology*, **15**, 124–126.

Campi, A., Filippi, M., Comi, G., *et al.* (1995) 'Acute transverse myelopathy: spinal and cranial MR study with clinical follow-up.' *American Journal of Neuroradiology*, **16**, 115–123.

Carette, S., Urowitz, M.B., Grossman, H., Louis, E.L. (1982) 'Cranial computerized tomography in systemic lupus erythematosus.' *Journal of Rheumatology*, **9**, 855–859.

Chalmers, R.H., Harding, A.E. (1996) 'A case-control study of Leber's hereditary optic neuropathy.' *Brain*, **119**, 1481–1486.

Chapelon, C., Ziza, J.M., Piette, J.C., *et al.* (1990) 'Neurosarcoidosis: signs, course and treatment in 35 confirmed cases.' *Medicine*, **65**, 261–276.

Cherry, J.D., Brunell, P.A., Golden, G.S., Karzon, D.T. (1988) 'Report of the Task Force on Pertussis and Pertussis Immunization—1988.' *Pediatrics*, **81**, Suppl. 6, 939–984.

Chun, R.W.M., Smith, N.J., Forster, F.M. (1961) 'Papilledema in Sydenham's chorea.' *American Journal of Diseases of Children*, **101**, 641–644.

Cody, C.L., Baraff, L.J., Cherry, J.D., *et al.* (1981) 'Nature and rates of adverse reactions associated with DTP and DT immunizations in infants and children.' *Pediatrics*, **68**, 650–660.

Cohen, S.R., Brooks, B.R., Herndon, R.M., McKhann, G. (1980) 'A diagnostic index of active demyelination: myelin basic protein in cerebrospinal fluid.' *Annals of Neurology*, **8**, 25–31.

Cole, G.F., Stuart, C.A. (1995) 'A long perspective on childhood multiple sclerosis.' *Developmental Medicine and Child Neurology*, **37**, 661–666.

—— Auchterlonie, L.A., Best, P.V. (1995) 'Very early onset multiple sclerosis.' *Developmental Medicine and Child Neurology*, **37**, 667–672.

Coleman, A.E., Norman, D.J. (1990) 'OKT3 encephalopathy.' *Annals of Neurology*, **28**, 837–838.

Connolly, A.M., Rust, R.S., Dodson, W.E., Prensky, A.L. (1988) 'Presentation and outcome of acute cerebellar ataxia in childhood.' *Annals of Neurology*, **24**, 340A.

Crisp, D.E., Siegler, R.L., Bale, J.F., Thompson, J.A. (1981) 'Hemorrhagic cerebral infarction in the hemolytic–uremic syndrome.' *Journal of Pediatrics*, **99**, 273–276.

Daniele, R.P., Dauber, J.H., Rossman, M.D. (1980) 'Immunologic abnormalities in sarcoidosis.' *Annals of Internal Medicine*, **92**, 406–416.

Devinsky, O., Petito, C.K., Alonso, D.R. (1988) 'Clinical and neuropathological findings in systemic lupus erythematosus: the role of vasculitis, heart emboli, and thrombotic, thrombocytopenic purpura.' *Annals of Neurology*, **23**, 380–384.

Dewez, P., North, K., de Silva, L., *et al.* (1992) 'Fever and spastic quadriparesis caused by *Mycoplasma pneumoniae*.' *Pediatric Infectious Disease Journal*, **11**, 129–130.

Dhanaraj, M., Radhakrishnan, A.R., Srinivas, K., Sayeed, Z.A. (1985) 'Sodium valproate in Sydenham's chorea.' *Neurology*, **35**, 114–115.

Dunne, K., Hopkins, I.J., Shield, L.K. (1986) 'Acute transverse myelopathy in childhood.' *Developmental Medicine and Child Neurology*, **28**, 198–204.

Duquette, P., Murray, T.J., Pleines, J., *et al.* (1987) 'Multiple sclerosis in childhood: clinical profile in 125 patients.' *Journal of Pediatrics*, **111**, 359–363.

Dyken, P., Kolár, O. (1968) 'Dancing eyes, dancing feet: infantile polymyoclonia.' *Brain*, **91**, 305–320.

Echenne, B., Gras, M., Astruc, J., *et al.* (1983) 'Vertebrobasilar arterial occlusion in childhood—report of a case and review of the literature.' *Brain and Development*, **5**, 577–581.

Egeler, R.M., D'Angio, G.J. (1995) 'Langerhans cell histiocytosis.' *Journal of Pediatrics*, **127**, 1–11.

Engle, E.C., Schaefer, P.W., Hedley-Whyte, E.T., *et al.* (1995) 'A 29-month-old girl with worsening ataxia, nystagmus, and subsequent opsoclonus and myoclonus (Case Records of the Massachusetts General Hospital 27-1995).' *New England Journal of Medicine*, **339**, 579–586.

Ettlinger, R.E., Nelson, A.M., Burke, E.C., Lie, J.T. (1979) 'Polyarteritis nodosa in childhood. A clinical pathologic study.' *Arthritis and Rheumatism*, **22**, 820–825.

Eviatar, L., Eviatar, A. (1977) 'Vertigo in children: differential diagnosis and treatment.' *Pediatrics*, **59**, 833–838.

Falko, J.M., Williams, J.C., Harvey, D.G., *et al.* (1979) 'Hyperlipoproteinemia and multifocal neurological dysfunction in systemic lupus erythematosus.' *Journal of Pediatrics*, **95**, 523–529.

Fenichel, G.M. (1988) 'Pertussis: the disease and the vaccine.' *Pediatric Neurology*, **4**, 201–206.

—— (1994) 'Neurological complications of immunization.' *International Pediatrics*, **9**, Suppl. 1, 44–48.

ffrench-Constant, C. (1994) 'Pathogenesis of multiple sclerosis.' *Lancet*, **343**, 271–275.

Fischer, A., Virelizier, J.L., Arenzana-Seisdedos, F., *et al.* (1985) 'Treatment of four patients with erythrophagocytic lymphohistiocytosis by a combination of epipodophyllotoxin, steroids, intrathecal methotrexate, and cranial irradiation.' *Pediatrics*, **76**, 263–268.

Fisher, P.G., Wechsler, D.S., Singer, A.S. (1994) 'Anti-Hu antibody in a neuroblastoma-associated paraneoplastic syndrome.' *Pediatric Neurology*, **10**, 309–312.

Ford, F.R. (1952) *Diseases of the Nervous System in Infancy, Childhood and Adolescence, 3rd Edn.* Springfield: C.C Thomas.

Ford, R.G., Siekert, R.G. (1965) 'Central nervous system manifestations of periarteritis nodosa.' *Neurology*, **15**, 114–122.

Foucar, E., Rosai, J., Dorfman, R.F. (1979) 'The ophthalmologic manifestations of sinus histiocytosis with massive lymphadenopathy.' *American Journal of Ophthalmology*, **87**, 354–367.

Freedman, D., Schenthal, J. (1953) 'A parenchymatous cerebellar syndrome following protracted high body temperature.' *Neurology*, **3**, 513–517.

Funalot, B., Ranoux, D., Mas, J-L., *et al.* (1996) 'Brainstem involvement in Leber's hereditary optic neuropathy: association with the 14 484 mitochondrial DNA mutation.' *Journal of Neurology, Neurosurgery, and Psychiatry*, **61**, 533–534. *(Letter.)*

Futrell, N., Schultz, L.R., Millikan, C. (1992) 'Central nervous system disease in patients with systemic lupus erythematosus.' *Neurology*, **42**, 1649–1657.

Garbern, J., Spence, A.M., Alvord, E.C. (1986) 'Baló's concentric demyelination diagnosed premortem.' *Neurology*, **36**, 1610–1614.

Garcin, R., Ginsbourg, M., Godlewski, S., Emile, J. (1965) 'Intoxication par le DDT, syndrome méningo-encéphalique régressif avec décharges cloniques diffuses et mouvements désordonnés "en salves" des globes oculaires.' *Revue Neurologique*, **113**, 559–565.

Gedalia, A., Zamir, S. (1993) 'Neurologic manifestations in familial Mediterranean fever.' *Pediatric Neurology*, **9**, 303–305.

Goldberg-Stern, H., Weitz, R., Zaizov, R., *et al.* (1995) 'Progressive spinocerebellar degeneration "plus" associated with Langerhans cell histiocytosis: a new paraneoplastic syndrome?' *Journal of Neurology, Neurosurgery, and Psychiatry*, **58**, 180–183.

Golden, G.S., Woody, R.C. (1987) 'The role of nuclear magnetic resonance imaging in the diagnosis of MS in childhood.' *Neurology*, **37**, 689–693.

Goodman, R.H., Post, K.D., Molitch, M.E., *et al.* (1979) 'Eosinophilic granuloma mimicking a pituitary tumour.' *Neurosurgery*, **5**, 723–725.

Gross, T.P., Milstien, J.B., Kuritsky, J.N. (1989) 'Bulging fontanelle after immunization with diphtheria–tetanus–pertussis vaccine and diphtheria–tetanus vaccine.' *Journal of Pediatrics*, **114**, 423–425.

Guerrini, R., Dravet, C., Genton, P., *et al.* (1993) 'Epileptic negative myoclonus.' *Neurology*, **43**, 1078–1083.

Guilhoto, L.M.deF.F., Osório, C.A.M., Machado, L.R., *et al.* (1995) 'Pediatric multiple sclerosis. Report of 14 cases.' *Brain and Development*, **17**, 9–12.

Haas, G., Schroth, G., Krägeloh-Mann, I., Buchwald-Saal, M. (1987) 'Magnetic resonance imaging of the brain of children with multiple sclerosis.' *Developmental Medicine and Child Neurology*, **29**, 586–591.

Hackett, E.R., Martinez, R.D., Larson, P.F., Paddison, R.M. (1974) 'Optic neuritis in systemic lupus erythematosus.' *Archives of Neurology*, **31**, 9–11.

Hallett, M., Kaufman, C. (1981) 'Physiological observations in Sydenham's chorea.' *Journal of Neurology, Neurosurgery, and Psychiatry*, **44**, 829–832.

Hammer, M.S., Larsen, M.B., Stack, C.V. (1995) 'Outcome of children with opsoclonus–myoclonus regardless of etiology.' *Pediatric Neurology*, **13**, 21–24.

Hanefeld, F., Bauer, H.J., Christen, H.J., *et al.* (1991) 'Multiple sclerosis in childhood: report of 15 cases.' *Brain and Development*, **13**, 410–416.

Harpey, J.P., Renault, J.F., Foncin, J.F., *et al.* (1983) 'Démyélinisation aiguë pseudotumorale à poussées régressives.' *Archives Françaises de Pédiatrie*, **40**, 407–409.

Haslam, R.H.A. (1987) 'Multiple sclerosis: experience at the Hospital for Sick Children.' *International Pediatrics*, **2**, 163–167.

Hauser, S.L., Reinherz, E.L., Hoban, C.J., *et al.* (1983) 'Immunoregulatory T-cells and lymphocytotoxic antibodies in active multiple sclerosis: weekly analysis over a six-month period.' *Annals of Neurology*, **13**, 418–425.

Hemachuda, T., Phanuphak, P., Johnson, R.T., *et al.* (1987) 'Neurologic complications of Semple-type rabies vaccine: clinical and immunologic studies.' *Neurology*, **37**, 550–556.

—— Griffin, D.E., Johnson, R.T., Giffels, J.J. (1988) 'Immunologic studies of patients with chronic encephalitis induced by post-exposure Semple rabies vaccine.' *Neurology*, **38**, 42–44.

Henter, J-I., Ehrnst, A., Andersson, J., Elinder, G. (1993) 'Familial hemophagocytic lymphohistiocytosis and viral infections.' *Acta Paediatrica*, **82**, 369–372.

Herderscheê, D., Troost, D., de Visser, M., Neve, A.J. (1988) 'Lymphomatoid granulomatosis: clinical and histopathological report of a patient presenting with spinal cord involvement.' *Journal of Neurology*, **235**, 432–434.

Hess, E. (1988) 'Drug-related lupus.' *New England Journal of Medicine*, **318**, 1460–1462.

Heye, N., Jergas, M., Hötzinger, H., *et al.* (1993) 'Sydenham chorea: clinical, EEG, MRI and SPECT findings in the early stage of the disease.' *Journal of Neurology*, **240**, 121–123.

Hogan, P.J., Greenberg, M.K., McCarty, G.E. (1981) 'Neurologic complications of lymphomatoid granulomatosis.' *Neurology*, **31**, 619–620.

Hohlfeld, R. (1997) 'Biotechnological agents for the immunotherapy of multiple sclerosis. Principles, problems and perspectives.' *Brain*, **120**, 865–916.

Holt, S., Hudgkins, D., Krishnan, K.R., Critchley, E.M.R. (1976) 'Diffuse myelitis associated with rubella vaccination.' *British Medical Journal*, **2**, 1037–1038.

Hosier, D.M., Craenen, J.M., Teske, D.W., Wheller, J.J. (1987) 'Resurgence of acute rheumatic fever.' *American Journal of Diseases of Children*, **141**, 730–733.

Hurst, D.L., Mehta, S. (1988) 'Acute cerebellar swelling in varicella encephalitis.' *Pediatric Neurology*, **4**, 122–123.

Ichiba, N., Miyake, Y., Sato, K., *et al.* (1988) 'Mumps-induced opsoclonus–myoclonus and ataxia.' *Pediatric Neurology*, **4**, 224–227.

Imura, H., Nakao, K., Shimatsu, A., *et al.* (1993) 'Lymphocytic infundibuloneurohypophysitis as a cause of central diabetes insipidus.' *New England Journal of Medicine*, **329**, 683–689.

IFNB Multiple Sclerosis Study Group and the University of British Columbia MS/MRI Analysis Group (1995) 'Interferon beta-1b in the treatment of multiple sclerosis: final outcome of the randomized controlled trial.' *Neurology*, **45**, 1277–1285.

Isaac, C., Genton, M., Jardine, C., *et al.* (1988) 'Multiple sclerosis: a serial study using MRI in relapsing patients.' *Neurology*, **38**, 1511–1515.

Ishihara, O., Yamaguchi, Y., Matsuishi, T., *et al.* (1984) 'Multiple ring enhancement in a case of acute reversible demyelinating disease in childhood suggestive of acute multiple sclerosis.' *Brain and Development*, **6**, 401–406.

Jacobs, L., Kinkel, P.R., Kinkel, W.R. (1986) 'Silent brain lesions in patients with isolated idiopathic optic neuritis—a clinical and nuclear magnetic resonance imaging study.' *Archives of Neurology*, **43**, 452–455.

—— Munschauer, F.E., Kaba, S.E. (1991) 'Clinical and magnetic resonance imaging in optic neuritis.' *Neurology*, **41**, 15–19.

Jacobson, S., Gupta, A., Mattson, D., *et al.* (1990) 'Immunological studies in tropical spastic paraparesis.' *Annals of Neurology*, **27**, 149–156.

Jan, J.E., Hill, R.H., Low, M.D. (1972) 'Cerebral complications in juvenile rheumatoid arthritis.' *Canadian Medical Association Journal*, **107**, 623–625.

Johnson, R., Milbourn, P.E. (1970) 'Central nervous system manifestations of chickenpox.' *Canadian Medical Association Journal*, **102**, 831–833.

Katzenstein, A-L.A., Carrington, C.B., Liebow, A.A. (1979) 'Lymphomatoid granulomatosis. A clinicopathologic study of 152 cases.' *Cancer*, **43**, 360–373.

Kaye, E.M., Butler, I.J., Conley, S. (1987) 'Myelopathy in neonatal and infantile lupus erythematosus.' *Journal of Neurology, Neurosurgery, and Psychiatry*, **50**, 923–926.

Kendall, B.E., Tatler, G.L.V. (1978) 'Radiological findings in neurosarcoidosis.' *British Journal of Radiology*, **51**, 81–92.

Kepes, J.J. (1993) 'Large focal tumor-like demyelinating lesions of the brain: intermediate entity between multiple sclerosis and acute disseminated encephalomyelitis? A study of 31 patients.' *Annals of Neurology*, **33**, 18–27.

Kerbeshian, J., Burd, L., Pettit, R. (1990) 'A possible post-streptococcal movement disorder with chorea and tics.' *Developmental Medicine and Child Neurology*, **32**, 642–644.

Kesselring, J., Miller, D.H., Robb, S.A., *et al.* (1990) 'Acute disseminated encephalomyelitis: MRI findings and the distinction from multiple sclerosis.' *Brain*, **113**, 291–302.

Khan, S., Yaqub, B.A., Poser, C.M., *et al.* (1995) 'Multiphasic disseminated encephalomyelitis presenting as alternating hemiplegia.' *Journal of Neurology, Neurosurgery, and Psychiatry*, **58**, 467–470.

Kiessling, L.S., Marcotte, A.C., Culpepper, L. (1993) 'Antineuronal antibodies in movement disorders.' *Pediatrics*, **92**, 39–43.

Kinnman, J., Link, H. (1984) 'Intrathecal production of oligoclonal IgM and IgG in CNS sarcoidosis.' *Acta Neurologica Scandinavica*, **69**, 97–106.

Kira, J-i., Kanai, T., Nishimura, Y., *et al.* (1996) 'Western versus Asian types of multiple sclerosis: immunogenetically and clinically distinct disorders.' *Annals of Neurology*, **40**, 569–574.

Kline, L.B., Margulies, S.L., Joong, S. (1982) 'Optic neuritis and myelitis following rubella vaccination.' *Archives of Neurology*, **39**, 443–444.

Koh, P.S., Raffensperger, J.G., Berry, S., *et al.* (1994) 'Long-term outcome in children with opsoclonus–myoclonus and ataxia and coincident neuroblastoma.' *Journal of Pediatrics*, **125**, 712–716.

Konagaya, M., Konagaya, Y. (1992) 'MRI in hemiballism due to Sydenham's chorea.' *Journal of Neurology, Neurosurgery, and Psychiatry*, **55**, 238–239. *(Letter.)*

Konkol, R.J., Bousounis, D., Kuban, K.C. (1987) 'Schilder's disease: additional aspects and a therapeutic option.' *Neuropediatrics*, **18**, 149–152.

Koopmans, R.A., Li, D.K.B., Grochowski, E., *et al.* (1989a) 'Benign versus chronic progressive multiple sclerosis: magnetic resonance imaging features.' *Annals of Neurology*, **25**, 74–81.

—— —— Oger, J.J.F., *et al.* (1989b) 'Chronic progressive multiple sclerosis: serial magnetic resonance brain imaging over six months.' *Annals of Neurology*, **26**, 248–256.

—— —— —— *et al.* (1989c) 'The lesion of multiple sclerosis: imaging of acute and chronic stages.' *Neurology*, **39**, 959–963.

Korenblat, P., Wedner, H., Whyte, M., *et al.* (1984) 'Systemic mastocytosis.' *Archives of Internal Medicine*, **144**, 2249–2253.

Koskiniemi, M., Donner, M., Pettay, O. (1983) 'Clinical appearance and outcome in mumps encephalitis in children.' *Acta Paediatrica Scandinavica*, **72**, 603–609.

Kriss, A., Francis, D.A., Cuendet, F., *et al.* (1988) 'Recovery after optic neuritis in childhood.' *Journal of Neurology, Neurosurgery, and Psychiatry*, **51**, 1253–1258.

Kuban, K.C., Ephros, M.A., Freeman, R.L., *et al.* (1983) 'Syndrome of opso-clonus–myoclonus caused by Coxsackie B3 infection.' *Annals of Neurology*, **13**, 69–71.

Kundell, S.P., Ochs, H.D. (1980) 'Cogan syndrome in childhood.' *Journal of Pediatrics*, **97**, 96–98.

Landrigan, P.J., Witte, J.J. (1973) 'Neurologic disorders following live measles-virus vaccination.' *Journal of the American Medical Association*, **223**, 1459–1462.

Lapkin, M., Golden, G. (1978) 'Basilar artery migraine: a review of 30 cases.' *American Journal of Diseases of Children*, **132**, 278–281.

Laxer, R.M., Dunn, H.G., Flodmark, O. (1984) 'Acute hemiplegia in Kawasaki disease and infantile polyarteritis nodosa.' *Developmental Medicine and Child Neurology*, **26**, 814–818.

Lee, S.C., Spencer, J., Rumberg, J., Dickson, D.W. (1989) 'Isolated central nervous system granulomatosis resembling sarcoidosis.' *Journal of Neurology*, **236**, 356–358.

Lehman, T.J.A., McCurdy, D.K., Bernstein, B.H., *et al.* (1989) 'Systemic lupus erythematosus in the first decade of life.' *Pediatrics*, **83**, 235–239.

Lemerle, J., Lemerle, M., Aicardi, J., *et al.* (1969) 'Trois cas d'association à un neuroblastome d'un syndrome opso-myoclonique.' *Archives Françaises de Pédiatrie*, **26**, 547–558.

Leung, D.Y.M., Meissner, H.C., Fulton, D.R., *et al.* (1993) 'Toxic shock syndrome toxin-secreting *Staphylococcus aureus* in Kawasaki syndrome.' *Lancet*, **343**, 1260–1261.

Levine, S.R., Welch, K.M.A. (1987) 'The spectrum of neurologic disease associated with antiphospholipid antibodies. Lupus anticoagulans and anticardiolipin antibodies.' *Archives of Neurology*, **44**, 876–883.

Link, H., Cruz, M., Gessain, A., *et al.* (1989) 'Chronic progressive myelopathy associated with HTLV-1: oligoclonal IgG and anti-HTLV-1 IgG antibodies in cerebrospinal fluid and serum.' *Neurology*, **39**, 1566–1572.

Linssen, W.H.J.P., Fiselier, T.J.W., Gabreëls, F.J., *et al.* (1988) 'Acute transverse myelopathy as the initial manifestation of probable systemic lupus erythe-matosus in a child.' *Neuropediatrics*, **19**, 212–215.

—— Praamstra, P., Gabreëls, F.J.M., Rotteveel, J.J. (1990) 'Vascular insuffi-ciency of the cervical cord due to hyperextension of the spine.' *Pediatric Neurology*, **6**, 123–125.

—— Gabreëls, F.J.M., Wevers, R.A. (1991) 'Infective acute transverse myelo-pathy. Report of two cases.' *Neuropediatrics*, **22**, 107–109.

Logigian, E.L., Murray, M.B., Adams, R.D., Rordorf, G.A. (1994) 'A 19-year-old man with rapidly progressive lower-extremity weakness and dysesthesias after a respiratory tract infection (Case Records of the Massachusetts General Hospital, Case 42-1994).' *New England Journal of Medicine*, **331**, 1437–1444.

Maeda, Y., Kitamoto, I., Kurokawa, T., *et al.* (1989) 'Infantile multiple sclerosis with extensive white matter lesions.' *Pediatric Neurology*, **5**, 317–319.

Mandler, R.N., Davis, L.E., Jeffery, D.R., Kornfeld, M. (1993) 'Devic's neuro-myelitis optica: a clinicopathological study of 8 patients.' *Annals of Neurology*, **34**, 162–168.

Martin, J.J., Cras, P. (1985) 'Familial erythrophagocytic lymphohistiocytosis: a neuropathologic study.' *Acta Neuropathologica*, **66**, 140–144.

Martin, R., McFarland, H.F., McFarlin, D. (1992) 'Immunological aspects of demyelinating diseases.' *Annual Review of Immunology*, **10**, 153–187.

McAllister, R.M., Hummeler, K., Coriell, L.L. (1959) 'Acute cerebellar ataxia. Report of a case with isolation of type 9 ECHO virus from the cerebro-spinal fluid.' *New England Journal of Medicine*, **261**, 1159–1162.

McDonald, W.I., Miller, D.H., Barnes, D. (1992) 'The pathological evolution of multiple sclerosis.' *Neuropathology and Applied Neurobiology*, **18**, 319–334.

McFarlin, D.E. (1983) 'Treatment of multiple sclerosis.' *New England Journal of Medicine*, **308**, 215–217.

McGovern, J.P., Merritt, D.H. (1956) 'Sarcoidosis in childhood.' *Advances in Pediatrics*, **8**, 97–135.

Means, E.D., Barron, K.D., Van Dyne, B.J. (1973) 'Nervous system lesions after sting by a yellow jacket. A case report.' *Neurology*, **23**, 881–890.

Mehler, M.F., Rabinowich, L. (1988) 'Inflammatory myelinoclastic diffuse sclerosis.' *Annals of Neurology*, **23**, 413–415.

—— —— (1989) 'Inflammatory myelinoclastic diffuse sclerosis (Schilder's disease): neuroradiologic findings.' *American Journal of Neuroradiology*, **10**, 176–180.

Melchior, J.C. (1977) 'Infantile spasms and early immunization against whooping cough: Danish survey from 1970 to 1975.' *Archives of Disease in Childhood*, **52**, 134–137.

Mendell, J.R., Kolkin, S., Kissel, J.T., *et al.* (1987) 'Evidence for central nervous system demyelination in chronic inflammatory demyelinating polyradiculo-neuropathy.' *Neurology*, **37**, 1291–1294.

Menkes, J.H., Kinsbourne, M. (1990) 'Workshop on neurologic complications of pertussis and pertussis vaccination.' *Neuropediatrics*, **21**, 121–126.

Miller, C., Farrington, C.P., Harbert, K. (1992) 'The epidemiology of subacute sclerosing panencephalitis in England and Wales 1970–1989.' *International Journal of Epidemiology*, **21**, 998–1006.

Miller, D.H., McDonald, W.I., Blumhardt, L.D., *et al.* (1987) 'Magnetic resonance imaging in isolated noncompressive spinal cord syndromes.' *Annals of Neurology*, **22**, 714–723.

—— Newton, M.R., Van der Poel, J.C., *et al.* (1988a) 'Magnetic resonance imaging of the optic nerve in optic neuritis.' *Neurology*, **38**, 175–179.

—— Rudge, P., Johnson, G., *et al.* (1988b) 'Serial gadolinium enhanced magnetic resonance imaging in multiple sclerosis.' *Brain*, **111**, 927–939.

—— Ormerod, I.E.C., Rudge, P., *et al.* (1989) 'The early risk of multiple sclerosis following isolated acute syndromes of the brainstem and spinal cord.' *Annals of Neurology*, **26**, 635–639.

Miller, D.L., Ross, E.M., Alderslade, R., *et al.* (1981) 'Pertussis immunisation and serious acute neurological illness in children.' *British Medical Journal*, **282**, 1595–1599.

—— Madge, N., Diamond, J., *et al.* (1993) 'Pertussis immunisation and serious acute neurological illness in children.' *British Medical Journal*, **307**, 1171–1176.

Miller, E., Goldacre, M., Pugh, S., *et al.* (1993) 'Risk of aseptic meningitis after measles, mumps, and rubella vaccine in UK children.' *Lancet*, **341**, 979–982.

Milligan, N.M., Newcombe, R., Compston, D.A.S. (1987) 'A double-blind controlled trial of high dose methylprednisolone in patients with multiple sclerosis. 1. Clinical effects.' *Journal of Neurology, Neurosurgery, and Psychi-atry*, **50**, 511–516.

Millner, M.M., Ebner, F., Justich, E., Urban, C. (1990) 'Multiple sclerosis in childhood: contribution of serial MRI to earlier diagnosis.' *Developmental Medicine and Child Neurology*, **32**, 769–777.

Mitchell, W.G., Snodgrass, S.R. (1990) 'Opsoclonus–ataxia due to childhood neural crest tumors: a chronic neurologic syndrome.' *Journal of Child Neurology*, **5**, 153–158 + *erratum*, 266.

Moake, J.L. (1994) 'Haemolytic–uraemic syndrome: basic science.' *Lancet*, **343**, 393–397.

Modlin, J.F., Brandling-Bennett, D., Witte, J.J., *et al.* (1975) 'A review of five years experience with rubella vaccine in the United States.' *Pediatrics*, **55**, 20–29.

Morimoto, T., Nagao, H., Sano, N., *et al.* (1985) 'A case of multiple sclerosis with multi-ring-like and butterfly-like enhancement on computerized tomography.' *Brain and Development*, **7**, 43–45.

Munn, R., Farrell, K., Cimolai, N. (1992) 'Acute encephalomyelitis: extending the neurological manifestations of acute rheumatic fever?' *Neuropediatrics*, **23**, 196–198.

Nausieda, P.A. (1986) 'Sydenham's chorea, chorea gravidarum and contra-ceptive-induced chorea.' *In:* Vinken, P.J., Bruyn, G.W. (Eds.) *Handbook of Clinical Neurology. Revised Series, Vol. 5. Extrapyramidal Disorders.* Amsterdam: North Holland, pp. 359–367.

—— Koller, W., Weiner, W., Klawans, H.L. (1979) 'Chorea induced by oral contraceptives.' *Neurology*, **29**, 1605–1609.

—— Grossman, B.J., Koller, W.C., *et al.* (1980) 'Sydenham chorea: an update.' *Neurology*, **30**, 331–334.

—— Bieliauskas, L.A., Bacon, L.D., *et al.* (1983) 'Chronic dopaminergic sensitivity after Sydenham's chorea.' *Neurology*, **33**, 750–754.

Newman, N.J., Lessell, S., Winterkorn, J.M.S. (1991) 'Optic chiasmal neuritis.' *Neurology*, **41**, 1203–1210.

Newton, M., Cruikshank, E.K., Miller, D., *et al.* (1987) 'Antibody to human T-lymphotropic virus type I in West-Indian-born UK residents with spastic paraparesis.' *Lancet*, **1**, 415–416.

Nigro, G., Castellani Pastoris, M., Mazzotti Fantasia, M., Midulla, M. (1983) 'Acute cerebellar ataxia in pediatric legionellosis.' *Pediatrics*, **72**, 847–849.

—— Zerbini, M., Krzysztofiak, A., *et al.* (1994) 'Active or recent parvovirus B19 infection in children with Kawasaki disease.' *Lancet*, **343**, 1260–1261.

Ohtaki, E., Murakami, Y., Komori, H., *et al.* (1992) 'Acute disseminated encephalomyelitis after Japanese B encephalitis vaccination.' *Pediatric Neurology*, **8**, 137–139.

Ohtsuka, T., Saito, Y., Hasegawa, M., *et al.* (1995) 'Central nervous system disease in a child with primary Sjögren syndrome.' *Journal of Pediatrics*, **127**, 961–963.

Økseter, K., Sirnes, K. (1988) 'Chorea and lupus anticoagulant: a case report.' *Acta Neurologica Scandinavica*, **78**, 206–209.

Olsson, T. (1992) 'Immunology of multiple sclerosis.' *Current Opinion in Neurology and Neurosurgery*, **5**, 195–202.

Oppenheimer, S., Hoffbrand, B.I. (1986) 'Optic neuritis and myelopathy in systemic lupus erythematosus.' *Canadian Journal of Neurological Science*, **13**, 129–132.

O'Riordan, J.I., Gallagher, H.L., Thompson, A.J., *et al.* (1996) 'Clinical, CSF, and MRI findings in Devic's neuromyelitis optica.' *Journal of Neurology, Neurosurgery, and Psychiatry*, **60**, 382–387.

Ormerod, I.E.C., Roberts, R.C., Du Boulay, E.P.G.H., *et al.* (1984) 'NMR in multiple sclerosis and cerebral vascular disease.' *Lancet*, **2**, 1334–1335.

—— McDonald, W.I., Du Boulay, E., *et al.* (1986) 'Disseminated lesions at presentation in patients with optic neuritis.' *Journal of Neurology, Neurosurgery, and Psychiatry*, **49**, 124–127.

—— Miller, D.H., McDonald, W.I., *et al.* (1987) 'The role of NMR imaging in the assessment of multiple sclerosis and isolated neurological lesions. A quantitative study.' *Brain*, **110**, 1579–1616.

Osterman, J.D., Trauner, D.A., Reznik, V.M., Lemire, J. (1993) 'Transient hemiparesis associated with monoclonal CD3 antibody (OKT3) therapy.' *Pediatric Neurology*, **9**, 482–484.

Otten, A., Vermeulen, M., Bossuyt, P.M.M., Otten, A. (1996) 'Intravenous immunoglobulin treatment in neurological diseases.' *Journal of Neurology, Neurosurgery, and Psychiatry*, **60**, 359–361.

Ozen, S., Besbas, N., Saatsi, U., Bakkaloglu, A. (1992) 'Diagnostic criteria for polyarteritis nodosa in childhood.' *Journal of Pediatrics*, **120**, 206–209.

Paine, R.S., Byers, R.K. (1953) 'Transverse myelopathy in childhood.' *American Journal of Diseases of Children*, **85**, 151–163.

Pakalnis, A., Drake, M.E., Barohn, J., *et al.* (1988) 'Evoked potentials in chronic inflammatory demyelinating polyneuropathy.' *Archives of Neurology*, **45**, 1014–1016.

Pallis, C.A., Scott, J.T. (1965) 'Peripheral neuropathy in rheumatoid arthritis.' *British Medical Journal*, **1**, 1141–1147.

Pampiglione, G., Maia, M. (1972) 'Syndrome of rapid irregular movements of eyes and limbs in childhood.' *British Medical Journal*, **1**, 469–473.

Parikh, S., Swaiman, K.F., Kim, Y. (1995) 'Neurologic characteristics of childhood lupus erythematosus.' *Pediatric Neurology*, **13**, 198–201.

Parkin, P., Hierons, R., McDonald, W.I. (1984) 'Bilateral optic neuritis: a long-term follow-up.' *Brain*, **107**, 951–964.

Paty, D.W., Oger, J.J.F., Kastrukoff, L.F., *et al.* (1988) 'MRI in the diagnosis of MS: a prospective study with comparison of clinical evaluation, evoked potentials, oligoclonal banding, and CT.' *Neurology*, **38**, 180–185.

Perez, N., Virelizier, J.L., Arenzana-Seisdedos, F., Fisher, A. (1984) 'Impaired natural killer activity in lymphohistiocytosis syndrome.' *Journal of Pediatrics*, **104**, 569–573.

Peter, G. (1992) 'Childhood immunizations.' *New England Journal of Medicine*, **327**, 1794–1800.

Petruzzi, M.J., de Alarcon, P.A. (1995) 'Neuroblastoma-associated opsoclonus–myoclonus treated with intravenously administered immune globulin G.' *Journal of Pediatrics*, **127**, 328–329.

Pliopys, A.V., Greaves, A., Yoshida, W. (1989) 'Anti-CNS antibodies in childhood neurologic disease.' *Neuropediatrics*, **20**, 93–102.

Poe, L.B., Dubowy, R.L., Hochhauser, L., *et al.* (1994) 'Demyelinating and gliotic cerebellar lesions in Langerhans cell histiocytosis.' *American Journal of Neuroradiology*, **15**, 1921–1928.

Pohl, K.R.E., Pritchard, J., Wilson, J. (1996) 'Neurological sequelae of the dancing eye syndrome.' *European Journal of Pediatrics*, **155**, 237–244.

Pollard, J.D., Selby, G. (1978) 'Relapsing polyneuropathy due to tetanus toxoid.' *Journal of the Neurological Sciences*, **37**, 113–125.

Pollock, T.M., Morris, J. (1983) 'A 7-year survey of disorders attributed to vaccination in North-west Thames region.' *Lancet*, **1**, 753–757.

Ponsot, G., Arthuis, M. (1981) 'Myélopathies aiguës de l'enfant. Aspects cliniques et évolutifs, facteurs de pronostic. A propos de 88 cas.' *In: Journées Parisiennes de Pédiatrie*. Paris: Flammarion Médecine-Science, pp. 253–265.

Poser, C.M. (1994) 'The epidemiology of multiple sclerosis: a general overview.' *Annals of Neurology*, **36**, Suppl. 2, S180–S193.

—— Paty, D.W., Scheinberg, L., *et al.* (1983) 'New diagnostic criteria for multiple sclerosis: guidelines for research protocols.' *Annals of Neurology*, **13**, 227–231.

—— Goutières, F., Carpentier, M.A., Aicardi, J. (1986) 'Schilder's myelino-clastic diffuse sclerosis.' *Pediatrics*, **77**, 107–112.

Powell, B.R., Kennaway, N.G., Rhead, W.J., *et al.* (1990) 'Juvenile multiple sclerosis-like episodes associated with a defect of mitochondrial beta oxidation.' *Neurology*, **40**, 487–491.

Prieur, A.M., Griscelli, C. (1981) 'Arthropathy with rash, chronic meningitis, eye lesions and mental retardation.' *Journal of Pediatrics*, **99**, 79–83.

—— Griscelli, C., Lampert, F., *et al.* (1987) 'A chronic infantile, neurological cutaneous and articular (CINCA) syndrome. A specific entity analyzed in 30 patients.' *Scandinavican Journal of Rheumatology*, Suppl. 66, 57–68.

Provenzale, J., Bouldin, T.W. (1992) 'Lupus-related myelopathy: report of three cases and review of the literature.' *Journal of Neurology, Neurosurgery, and Psychiatry*, **55**, 830–835.

Purvin, V., Hrisolamos, N., Dunn, D. (1988) 'Varicella optic neuritis.' *Neurology*, **38**, 501–503.

Querfurth, H., Swanson, P.D. (1990) 'Vaccine-associated paralytic polio-myelitis. Regional case series and review.' *Archives of Neurology*, **47**, 541–547.

Rantala, H., Cherry, J.D., Shields, W.D., Uhari, M. (1994) 'Epidemiology of Guillain–Barré syndrome in children: relationship of oral polio vaccine administration to occurrence.' *Journal of Pediatrics*, **124**, 220–223.

Rettwitz, W., Sauer, D., Burow, H.M., *et al.* (1983) 'Neurological and neuropathological findings in familial erythrophagocytic lymphohistiocytosis.' *Brain and Development*, **5**, 322–327.

Riikonen, R. (1989) 'The role of infection and vaccination in the genesis of optic neuritis and multiple sclerosis in children.' *Acta Neurologica Scandinavica*, **80**, 425–431.

—— Von Willebrandt, E. (1988) 'Lymphocyte subclasses and function in patients with optic neuritis in childhood with special reference to multiple sclerosis.' *Acta Neurologica Scandinavica*, **78**, 58–64.

—— Donner, M., Erkkilä, H. (1988a) 'Optic neuritis in children and its relationship to multiple sclerosis: a clinical study of 21 children.' *Developmental Medicine and Child Neurology*, **30**, 349–359.

—— Ketonen, L., Sipponen, J. (1988b) 'Magnetic resonance imaging, evoked responses and cerebrospinal fluid findings in a follow-up study of children with optic neuritis.' *Acta Neurologica Scandinavica*, **77**, 44–49.

Rimsza, L.M., Rimsza, M.E., Gilbert-Barness, E. (1993) 'Special feature. Lymphomatoid granulomatosis.' *American Journal of Diseases of Children*, **147**, 693–694.

Risdall, R.J., McKenna, R.W., Nesbit, M.E., *et al.* (1979) 'Virus-associated hemophagocytic syndrome: a benign histiocytic proliferation distinct from malignant histiocytosis.' *Cancer*, **44**, 993–1002.

Ritter, F.J., Seay, A.R., Lahey, M.E. (1983) 'Peripheral mononeuropathy complicating anaphylactoid purpura.' *Journal of Pediatrics*, **103**, 77–78.

Roig, M., Monsterrat, L., Gallart, A. (1988) 'Carbamazepine: an alternative drug for the treatment of nonhereditary chorea.' *Pediatrics*, **82**, 492–495.

Ropper, A.H., Poskanzer, D.C. (1978) 'The prognosis of acute and subacute transverse myelopathy based on early signs and symptoms.' *Annals of Neurology*, **4**, 51–59.

Rose, L.M., Ginsberg, A.H., Rothstein, T.L., *et al.* (1988) 'Fluctuations of CD4+ T-cell subsets in remitting–relapsing multiple sclerosis.' *Annals of Neurology*, **24**, 192–199.

Rosenblum, M., Scheck, A.C., Cronin, K., *et al.* (1989) 'Dissociation of AIDS-related vacuolar myelopathy and productive HIV-1 infection of the spinal cord.' *Neurology*, **39**, 892–896.

Rottem, M., Fauci, A.S., Hallahan, C.W., *et al.* (1993) 'Wegener granulomatosis in children and adolescents: clinical presentation and outcome.' *Journal of Pediatrics*, **122**, 26–31.

Roulet Perez, E., Maeder, P., Cotting, J., *et al.* (1993) 'Acute fatal parainfectious cerebellar swelling in two children. A rare or an overlooked situation?' *Neuropediatrics*, **24**, 346–351.

Rousseau, J.J., Lust, C., Zangerle, P.F., Bigaignon, G. (1986) 'Acute transverse myelitis as presenting neurological feature of Lyme disease.' *Lancet*, **2**, 1222–1223. *(Letter.)*

Rubin, M., Karpati, G., Carpenter, S. (1987) 'Combined central and peripheral myelinopathy.' *Neurology*, **37**, 1287–1290.

Rubinstein, I., Hiss, J., Baum, G.L. (1984) 'Intramedullary spinal cord sarcoidosis.' *Surgical Neurology*, **21**, 272–274.

Rudick, R.A., Jacobs, L., Kinkel, P.R., Kinkel, W.R. (1986) 'Isolated idiopathic optic neuritis. Analysis of free K-light chains in cerebrospinal fluid and correlation with nuclear magnetic resonance findings.' *Archives of Neurology*, **43**, 456–458.

Rumi, V., Angelini, L., Scaioli, V., *et al.* (1993) 'Primary antiphospholipid syndrome and neurologic events.' *Pediatric Neurology*, **9**, 473–475.

Ruuskanen, O., Salmi, T.T., Stenvik, M., Lapinleimu, K. (1980) 'Inactivated poliovaccine: adverse reactions and antibody responses.' *Acta Paediatrica Scandinavica*, **69**, 397–401.

Sanders, K.A., Khandji, A.G., Mohr, J.P. (1990) 'Gadolinium-MRI in acute transverse myelopathy.' *Neurology*, **40**, 1614–1616.

Schaffner, W., Fleet, W.F., Kilroy, A.W., *et al.* (1974) 'Polyneuropathy following rubella immunization. A follow-up study and review of the problem.' *American Journal of Diseases of Children*, **127**, 684–688.

Schmidt, B.J., Meagher-Villemure, K., Del Carpio, J. (1984) 'Lymphomatoid granulomatosis with isolated involvement of the brain.' *Annals of Neurology*, **15**, 478–481.

Schmitt, S., Wichmann, W., Martin, E., *et al.* (1993) 'Pituitary stalk thickening with diabetes insipidus preceding typical manifestations of Langerhans cell histiocytosis in children.' *European Journal of Pediatrics*, **152**, 399–401.

Schonberger, L.B., Hurwitz, E.S., Katona, P., *et al.* (1981) 'Guillain–Barré syndrome: its epidemiology and associations with influenza vaccination.' *Annals of Neurology*, **9** (Suppl.), 31–38.

Scott, T.F. (1993) 'Neurosarcoidosis: progress and clinical aspects.' *Neurology*, **43**, 8–12.

Seaman, D.E., Londino, A.V., Kwoh, C.K., *et al.* (1995) 'Antiphospholipid antibodies in pediatric systemic lupus erythematosus.' *Pediatrics*, **96**, 1040–1045.

Shaw, C.M., Alvord, E.C. (1987) 'Multiple sclerosis beginning in infancy.' *Journal of Child Neurology*, **2**, 252–256.

Shaw, P.J., Walls, T.J., Newman, P.K., *et al.* (1991) 'Hashimoto's encephalopathy: a steroid-responsive disorder associated with high anti-thyroid antibody titers—report of 5 cases.' *Neurology*, **41**, 228–233.

Shenker, D.M., Grossman, H.J., Klawans, H.L. (1973) 'Treatment of Sydenham's chorea with haloperidol.' *Developmental Medicine and Child Neurology*, **15**, 19–24.

Sherwood, J.W., Wagle, W.A. (1991) 'Hemolytic uremic syndrome: MR findings of CNS complications.' *American Journal of Neuroradiology*, **12**, 703–704.

Sheth, K.J., Swick, H.M., Haworth, N. (1986) 'Neurologic involvement in hemolytic–uremic syndrome.' *Annals of Neurology*, **19**, 90–93.

Sheth, R.D., Horwitz, S.J., Aronoff, S., *et al.* (1995) 'Opsoclonus myoclonus syndrome secondary to Epstein–Barr virus infection.' *Journal of Child Neurology*, **10**, 297–299.

Shetty, T., Rosman, N.P. (1972) 'Opsoclonus in hydrocephalus.' *Archives of Ophthalmology*, **88**, 585–588.

Shields, W.D., Nielsen, C., Buch, D., *et al.* (1988) 'Relationship of pertussis immunization to the onset of neurologic disorders: a retrospective epidemiologic study.' *Journal of Pediatrics*, **113**, 801–805.

Sigal, L.H. (1987) 'The neurologic presentation of vasculitic and rheumatologic syndromes. A review.' *Medicine*, **66**, 157–180.

Sindern, E., Haas, J., Stark, E., Wurster, U. (1992) 'Early onset of MS under the age of 16: clinical and paraclinical features.' *Acta Neurologica Scandinavica*, **86**, 280–284.

Singsen, B.H., Fishman, L., Hanson, J. (1976) 'Antinuclear antibodies and lupus-like syndromes in children receiving anticonvulsants.' *Pediatrics*, **57**, 529–534.

Sissons, J.G.P. (1993) 'Superantigens and infectious disease.' *Lancet*, **341**, 1627–1629.

Steinlin, M.I., Blaser, S.I., Gilday, D.L., *et al.* (1995a) 'Neurologic manifestations of pediatric systemic lupus erythematosus.' *Pediatric Neurology*, **13**, 191–197.

—— —— MacGregor, D.L., Buncic, J.R. (1995b) 'Eye problems in children with multiple sclerosis.' *Pediatric Neurology*, **12**, 207–212.

Stimmler, M.M., Coletti, P.M., Quismorio, F.P. (1993) 'Magnetic resonance imaging of the brain in neuropsychiatric systemic lupus erythematosus.' *Seminars in Arthritis and Rheumatology*, **22**, 335–349.

Sugiura, A., Yamada, A. (1991) 'Aseptic meningitis as a complication of mumps vaccination.' *Pediatric Infectious Disease Journal*, **10**, 209–213.

Sugie, H., Sugie, Y., Akimoto, H., *et al.* (1992) 'High-dose i.v. human immunoglobulin in a case with infantile opsoclonus polymyoclonia syndrome.' *Acta Paediatrica*, **81**, 371–372.

Sunaga, Y., Hikima, A., Otsuka, T., Morikawa, A. (1995) 'Acute cerebellar ataxia with abnormal MRI lesions after varicella vaccination.' *Paediatric Neurology*, **13**, 340–342.

Telang, G., Leong, K.K., Koblenzer, P., Tunnesen, W.W. (1993) 'Picture of the month: Neonatal lupus erythematosus.' *American Journal of Diseases of Children*, **147**, 903–904.

Terasawa, K., Ichinose, E., Matsuishi, T., Kato, H. (1983) 'Neurological complications in Kawasaki disease.' *Brain and Development*, **5**, 371–374.

Thomas, P.K., Walker, P.H., Rudge, P., *et al.* (1987) 'Chronic demyelinating peripheral neuropathy associated with multifocal central nervous system demyelination.' *Brain*, **110**, 53–76.

Thompson, A.J., Hutchinson, M., Brazil, J., *et al.* (1986) 'A clinical and laboratory study of benign multiple sclerosis.' *Quarterly Journal of Medicine*, **58**, 69–80.

Tola, M.R., Granieri, E., Caniatti, L., *et al.* (1992) 'Systemic lupus erythematosus presenting with neurological disorders.' *Journal of Neurology*, **239**, 61–64.

Toshniwal, P. (1987) 'Demyelinating optic neuropathy with Miller–Fisher syndrome.' *Journal of Neurology*, **234**, 353–358.

Traill, Z. Pike, M., Byrne, J. (1995) 'Sydenham's chorea: a case showing reversible striatal abnormalities on CT and MRI.' *Developmental Medicine and Child Neurology*, **37**, 270–273.

Troiano, R., Cook, S.D., Dowling, P.C. (1987) 'Steroid therapy in multiple sclerosis: point of view.' *Archives of Neurology*, **44**, 803–807.

Trump, R.C., White, T.R. (1967) 'Cerebellar ataxia presumed due to live, attenuated measles virus vaccine.' *Journal of the American Medical Association*, **199**, 129–130.

Tsai, M-L., Hung, K-L. (1996) 'Multiphasic disseminated encephalomyelitis mimicking multiple sclerosis.' *Brain and Development*, **18**, 412–414.

Tsuchiya, S., Kagawa, K., Fukuyama, Y. (1978) 'Critical evaluation of the role of immunization as an etiological factor in infantile spasms.' *Brain and Development*, **3**, 171–172. *(Abstract.)*

Uncini, A., Treviso, M., Basciani, M., *et al.* (1988) 'Associated central and peripheral demyelination: an electrophysiological study.' *Journal of Neurology*, **235**, 238–240.

Van Antwerpen, C.L., Gospe, S.M., Wade, N. (1988) 'Myeloradiculopathy associated with wasp sting.' *Pediatric Neurology*, **4**, 379–380.

Van Dam, A.P. (1991) 'Diagnosis and pathogenesis of CNS lupus.' *Rheumatology International*, **11**, 1–11.

Visscher, B.R., Myers, L.W., Ellison, G.W., *et al.* (1979) 'HLA types and immunity in multiple sclerosis.' *Neurology*, **29**, 1561–1565.

Vliegenthart, W.E., Sanders, E.A.C.M., Bruyn, G.W., Vielvoye, G.J. (1985) 'An unusual CT scan appearance in multiple sclerosis.' *Journal of the Neurological Sciences*, **71**, 129–134.

Vollertsen, R.S., McDonald, T.J., Younge, B.R., *et al.* (1986) 'Cogan's syndrome: 18 cases and a review of the literature.' *Mayo Clinic Proceedings*, **61**, 344–361.

Walker, A.M., Jick, H., Perera, D.R., *et al.* (1988) 'Neurologic events following diphtheria–tetanus–pertussis immunization.' *Pediatrics*, **81**, 345–349.

Watson, J.D.G., Gibson, J., Joshua, D., Kronenberg, H. (1991) 'Aseptic meningitis associated with high dose intravenous immunoglobulin therapy.' *Journal of Neurology, Neurosurgery, and Psychiatry*, **54**, 275–276.

Watson, R.M., Lane, A.T., Barnett, N.K., *et al.* (1984) 'Neonatal lupus erythematosus: a clinical, serological and immunogenetic study with review of the literature.' *Medicine*, **63**, 362–378.

Weindl, A., Kuwert, T., Leenders, K.L., *et al.* (1993) 'Increased striatal glucose consumption in Sydenham's chorea.' *Movement Disorders*, **8**, 437–444.

Weintraub, M.I., Chia, D.T.S. (1977) 'Paralytic brachial neuritis after swine flu vaccination.' *Archives of Neurology*, **34**, 518. *(Letter.)*

Weiss, S., Carter, S. (1959) 'Course and prognosis of acute cerebellar ataxia in children.' *Neurology*, **9**, 711–721.

Wells, C.E.C. (1971) 'A neurological note on vaccination against influenza.' *British Medical Journal*, **3**, 755–756.

Willis, J., Van den Bergh, P. (1988) 'Cerebral involvement in children with acute and relapsing inflammatory polyneuropathy.' *Journal of Child Neurology*, **3**, 200–204.

Willoughby, E.N., Grochowski, E., Li, D.K.B., *et al.* (1989) 'Serial magnetic resonance scanning in multiple sclerosis: a second prospective study in relapsing patients.' *Annals of Neurology*, **25**, 43–49.

Wilson, E.R., Malluh, A., Stagno, S., Crist, W.M. (1981) 'Fatal Epstein–Barr virus-associated hemophagocytic syndrome.' *Journal of Pediatrics*, **98**, 260–262.

Yahr, M.D., Lobo-Antunes, J. (1972) 'Relapsing encephalomyelitis following the use of influenza vaccine.' *Archives of Neurology*, **27**, 182–183.

Yancey, C.L., Doughty, R.A., Athreya, B.H.L. (1981) 'Central nervous system involvement in childhood systemic lupus erythematosus.' *Arthritis and Rheumatism*, **24**, 1389–1395.

Yarom, A., Rennebohm, R.M., Levinson, J.E. (1985) 'Infantile multisystem inflammatory disease: a specific syndrome?' *Journal of Pediatrics*, **106**, 390–396.

Zellweger, H. (1959) 'Pertussis encephalopathy.' *Archives of Pediatrics*, **76**, 381–386.

13
ACCIDENTAL AND NONACCIDENTAL INJURIES BY PHYSICAL AGENTS AND TOXIC AGENTS

Accidents of all types are the most frequent cause of death and significant impairment and disability in children and adolescents between 5 and 19 years of age. They account for 8.5–56.8 per cent of deaths of all causes depending on age. Prevention of accidents is therefore a major public health problem, and proper organization of emergency rooms is important for taking appropriate care of such patients.

A better knowledge of the causes, circumstances of occurrence and outcome of accidents in children is essential for adequate preventive measures. All types of accidents are more common in boys than in girls by a factor of around 3:1 to 4:1. In addition, accidents are not distributed haphazardly. They are more frequent in lower socioeconomic levels, due to crowding and unfavourable material circumstances. They also affect certain children more than others, and the psychological profile of 'repeaters' has been studied as such children and their families have particular needs (Schor 1987).

Age is a significant factor. Adolescents have an overall higher frequency of accidents than younger patients and are especially exposed to traffic accidents and to accidents related to athletics and sports.

Accidents involving motor vehicles have increased in frequency. In a majority, the child is a pedestrian and is hit by a moving car. Such accidents occur mainly between 7 and 11 years of age and are often severe (Rivara and Barber 1985). Less commonly, the child or infant is a passenger in a car involved in an accident. The consequences of such traumas can be attenuated by appropriate restraints (Agran *et al.* 1985, Bull and Stroup 1985). Bicycle-related injuries are common and wearing a helmet can prevent some of their complications (Selbst *et al.* 1987).

Home accidents are the commonest, but head trauma less frequently results. Most common falls from beds, cots, dressing tables and the like only rarely result in serious head injuries (Kravitz *et al.* 1969, Helfer *et al.* 1977). On the other hand, burns, ingestion of toxic products and similar accidents occur mainly in the home, although injuries to preschool children in day-care centres are becoming more frequent (Chang *et al.* 1989, Kopjar and Wickizer 1996) with the increasing use of these facilities.

HEAD INJURIES

Head injuries account for approximately one-third of accidental deaths in children. The annual incidence of head trauma is around 2–3 per 1000 population. Approximately 5 per cent of these are severe with a Glasgow coma score of 8 or less, 5–10 per cent are moderate (Glasgow coma score of 9–12), and 85–90 per cent are minor (Miller 1992). The number of children admitted to hospitals for head injuries has increased dramatically over the past 50 years. Head trauma was responsible for 3.6 per cent of hospital admissions in the USA (North 1976) and for 13.9 per cent in Newcastle-upon-Tyne (Craft *et al.* 1972). In the UK, between 2000 and 3000 per million population are admitted to hospital each year because of head injury. A 15–20 per cent reduction in mortality following severe injuries has been obtained with modern management without increase in residual problems (Miller 1992). Accidental head injury mainly results from falls from various heights and motor vehicle accidents.

This section deals only with postnatal brain injury and its medical treatment. More detailed information on management can be found elsewhere (Jennett and Teasdale 1981, Miller 1992).

PHYSIOPATHOLOGY AND PATHOLOGY OF HEAD INJURY
Head injury produces brain damage through both direct and indirect effects of trauma.

DIRECT EFFECTS OF TRAUMA
Head trauma generates physical forces that act upon the brain through acceleration–deceleration (linear or rotary) and deformation. Brain damage that results from the action of these forces comes from compression, shearing or tearing occurring alone or successively.

Low-velocity impacts such as result from falls, car accidents or direct blows on the head produce linear skull fractures and/or intracranial injuries by an acceleration or deceleration mechanism, depending on whether the head is fixed or mobile at the time of accident. Approximately three-quarters of skull fractures are linear.

High-velocity impacts, such as missile injuries, are responsible for depressed and comminuted fractures and for penetrating brain injuries.

Compression injuries occur when the head is compressed between two surfaces, and result in bursting fractures with suture diastasis and often involvement of the skull base. As there is no concussion, rotation or shearing, the child may be conscious even after severe injury.

Laceration of the brain is usually associated with penetrating trauma or depressed skull fracture.

Contusion of the brain presents as areas of gross or petechial haemorrhage with associated tearing of nerve fibres and cellular damage surrounded by oedema. Contusions more often result from contrecoup than from coup mechanism and are then localized preferentially to the frontal region in relation to the roof or the orbits and to the temporal poles, due to the irregular osseous middle fossa on which the brain gets bruised when propelled forwards. Occipital pole lesions may occur with backward projection of the brain mass. MRI studies show that lesions are exclusively frontal or involve the frontal lobe in 80 per cent of cases. In the remaining 20 per cent, the lesions predominate in the temporal lobes. Cortical or corticosubcortical contusions are very frequent with severe head trauma, as indicated by MRI which shows such lesions in most severe cases (Jenkins *et al.* 1986) and twice as often as CT scanning.

Shearing injury results from distortion of the brain that moves differentially in relation to the skull (Adams *et al.* 1977, 1982, 1984) with consequent disruption of axons in the white matter and shearing of vessels with resulting haemorrhages. The severity is variable. Pathologically, numerous retraction balls are visible at the ends of interrupted fibres. Secondary degeneration ensues with detectable atrophy when enough fibres are disrupted. Capillaries can be involved with resulting macro- or microscopic haemorrhages. Such lesions mainly involve the subcortical or deep white matter and the corpus callosum and are visible on MRI scans (Jenkins *et al.* 1986, Gentry *et al.* 1988) and sometimes on CT scans. In one study (Mendelsohn *et al.* 1992), haemorrhagic lesions of the corpus callosum were found in 26 per cent of cases. Contrary to what obtains in adults, they were not associated with a particularly severe outcome, an unusual incidence of low coma scores, brainstem insult or intraventricular haemorrhage. This type of lesion may be associated with immediate loss of consciousness and signs of decerebration and autonomic dysfunction (Blumbergs *et al.* 1989). Such features have been classically attributed to primary brainstem injury (in contrast with secondary brainstem lesions that are due to high intracranial pressure (ICP) and herniation and distortion of the brain). However, shearing injury of the white matter appears to be the basis for the so-called 'primary brainstem injury' which is only a part of diffuse damage and does not occur in isolation (Adams *et al.* 1977). Indeed, brainstem lesions are rare on MRI scans (Jenkins *et al.* 1986). Plum and Saper (1983) have adduced evidence to the effect that brainstem arousal mechanisms are being suppressed in such cases, as a consequence of diffuse hemispheric damage, by a mechanism akin to that of spinal shock, 'suprareticular

shock'. Similar distortion can lead to *rupture of the bridging veins* between brain and the dural sinuses with consequent subdural bleeding.

Concussion produces no or only minor pathological lesions. It is characterized clinically by a brief loss of consciousness and often by anterograde amnesia. Subtle axonal changes have been shown to occur in minor head trauma (Povlishok *et al.* 1983), as well as chromatolysis of neurons in the upper brainstem and mitochondrial changes that could be responsible for the changes in energy metabolism following head injury.

INDIRECT EFFECTS OF TRAUMA—SECONDARY LESIONS
A substantial part of the mortality and morbidity of head injury is not due to immediate brain damage but to secondary consequences of trauma.

Ischaemic brain damage is present in about 90 per cent of fatal cases (Lewelt *et al.* 1980, Graham *et al.* 1989b). Ischaemic brain damage may result from direct stretching and consequent thrombosis of blood vessels, from reduced perfusion pressure due to shock and visceral damage, or to increased ICP, or from vasospasm. Ischaemia may be generalized as seen in cases complicated by status epilepticus or shock, or localized. Chest injury and systemic haemorrhage are major factors of hypoxic–ischaemic damage. The pathological lesions produced by ischaemia may involve preferentially the boundaries between the territories of the major brain arteries or be more diffuse (Graham *et al.* 1987, 1989a).

The effects of any general circulatory disturbance may be considerably increased by the loss of cerebral autoregulation that prevents drops in systemic blood pressure being transmitted to the brain. There is, however, some disagreement on this point. Some authors (Lewelt *et al.* 1980, Bruce *et al.* 1981, Obrist *et al.* 1984) think that autoregulation is impaired in patients with severe head injury, while others (*e.g.* Muizelaar *et al.* 1989b) have found mostly a normal autoregulation.

Other vascular effects of head injury include changes in the distribution of blood between parenchymal and meningeal compartments and an increase in blood volume and blood flow (Bruce *et al.* 1981, Obrist *et al.* 1984, Muizelaar *et al.* 1989a). Children with head injuries are especially prone to exhibit a response different from that in adults with maximum vasodilatation of the white matter and massive increase in white matter blood flow (Chan *et al.* 1992). This causes a severe rise of ICP but is different from cerebral oedema. In some cases, however, oedema may be present and initiate a vicious circle by producing ischaemic damage which, in turn, will increase oedema and can lead to further ischaemia and to mass displacements of the brain with herniation if localized. Prevention of these secondary consequences is the major aim of management as these are in part preventable, whereas immediate traumatic lesions are already acquired at the time the child is brought to the hospital.

Macroscopic stroke is probably due to direct stretching of vessels, especially the perforating branches of the middle cerebral artery with resulting infarction in the territory of the basal ganglia (Maki *et al.* 1988).

Early intracranial haemorrhage is another preventable consequence of head injury. Haemorrhages occur exceptionally in isolation following head trauma (Kang *et al.* 1989). In most cases they are associated with other lesions.

Extradural haematomas in children are usually of venous rather than arterial origin and result from tearing of dural veins. Haemorrhage is often sufficient to produce shock and thus aggravate the primary lesions.

Acute subdural haematomas may also be an early cause of additional brain damage by compressing the brain. They are generally a consequence of rupture of the bridging veins as they cross the subdural space to drain into the venous sinuses. They are bilateral in over 80 per cent of cases. During the acute stage they are formed of pure blood which may clot. Later, the collection becomes encapsulated by a thin membrane that may become thick with the passing of time and even calcify.

Posterior fossa subdural haemorrhage is rare after the neonatal period (Vielvoye *et al.* 1982; see also Chapter 2). Traumatic extradural haematoma of the posterior fossa has been reviewed by Pozzati *et al.* (1989). Nonsurgical treatment has been proposed (Kawakami *et al.* 1990).

Subarachnoid haemorrhage is frequent and, except in rare cases, is not associated with clinical manifestations. It may, however, lead to meningeal fibrosis and eventual post-traumatic hydrocephalus (Oi and Matsumoto 1987). Subarachnoid haemorrhage is frequently associated with subdural haematoma (Aicardi and Goutières 1971).

Intracerebral haemorrhages are rarely isolated. They are frequently seen on CT scans as a manifestation of contusion but are generally of small size. In rare cases large haemorrhagic contusions can be responsible for oedema with secondary deterioration, especially when bilateral (Statham *et al.* 1989).

EARLY CLINICAL MANIFESTATIONS OF CLOSED HEAD INJURY

The clinical presentation of patients with head injury is extremely variable depending on the significance of the trauma and the presence or absence of brain damage. I shall consider separately trivial, mild and severe head injuries because the problems they pose are distinct. In all cases, even mild ones, it should be remembered that trauma may involve any part of the body in addition to the head, therefore a general examination is mandatory.

MINOR HEAD INJURY

Trivial head traumas represent the vast majority of cases and most commonly are the consequence of a fall or a direct blow to the head. There are no immediate symptoms beyond crying and, perhaps, immediate vomiting. Consciousness is at no point impaired. In an occasional child or adolescent, trivial head trauma can trigger a migrainous attack with throbbing headache and vomiting which may last for several hours. In adolescent patients, confusional migraine may be observed (Haas and Lourie 1988).

Except in such rare cases, the clinical problem raised by trivial head injuries is that of the need for further evaluation (see below). In rare cases, early post-traumatic symptoms such as described under mild head injury may occur.

MILD HEAD INJURY

Mild head injury is defined by the occurrence of a brief immediate loss of consciousness which is often followed by a period of *post-traumatic amnesia*. This is an anterograde amnesia with absence of fixation of memories that may last from a few minutes to several hours. Retrograde amnesia is sometimes associated. Any loss of consciousness often lasts only seconds to minutes and the Glasgow coma score is between 13 and 15 (Alexander 1995). Some children are listless or somnolent for a few hours. Vomiting, pallor and irritability are common and may be observed even in children who did not lose consciousness. Any loss of consciousness in such patients is immediate and no secondary loss of consciousness is ever observed, a point that must be made clear by precise questioning of witnesses. Fourteen to 33 per cent of patients have associated skull fractures.

The problem raised by mild head injury is to determine the risk of complications and the need for further assessment and hospitalization. A skull X-ray is usually obtained for such children. Rosenthal and Bergman (1989) found that only six of 52 children with mild head trauma and skull fracture had intracranial complications, including five with epidural haematoma. None of 306 children without fracture developed intracranial problems. These authors estimate the risk of intracranial complication in patients with mild trauma to be of the order of 1 in 5000 to 1 in 6000 cases. Leonidas *et al.* (1982) found a lower incidence of fractures (4.2 per cent), and the presence of a fracture had no effect on the prognosis. They proposed limiting the indications for X-rays to children of less than 1 year and those with unconsciousness lasting more than five minutes, palpable haematoma, skull depression, blood in the middle ear or CSF nasal discharge. Such indications clearly exclude children with trivial head trauma. On the other hand, most doctors think an X-ray is systematically indicated for children with loss of consciousness, however brief. CT scan using bone windows is diagnostically superior and may be more cost-efficient than simple skull X-rays (Stein *et al.* 1991). CT scan may show areas of mixed density, traces of blood on brain surface and in the ventricles and variable swelling. Normal or mildly abnormal CT scans are good predictors of ultimate outcome as well as duration of post-traumatic amnesia (Ruijs *et al.* 1993, 1994). Davis *et al.* (1995) used CT scanning in 400 paediatric patients with mild head injury (Glasgow coma score 13–15). Only four had to be readmitted within one month because of delayed complications, including one intracranial haematoma. They regarded CT as an effective triage method for such cases.

EEG tracings taken after injury may reveal focal or generalized abnormalities, usually of the slow wave type. Such anomalies tend to be transient. There is a good correlation between the degree of EEG abnormalities and the severity of the concussion (Mizrahi and Kellaway 1984). Ruijs *et al.* (1994) found that normal EEGs and those with only a small proportion of theta rhythms were of favourable prognostic significance.

There is no agreement regarding the criteria for hospitalization of children with mild head trauma. Practice in the USA varies widely. Forty-four per cent of paediatricians questioned by Dershewitz *et al.* (1983) systematically hospitalized all children who had had a loss of consciousness. Among others, the commonest reasons for hospitalization were abnormal vital signs, skull fracture, suspicion of child abuse, unreliable caretaker at home, vomiting and change in the level of consciousness. There is clearly a need to determine more rational rules as the effectiveness of present policy is, at best, doubtful.

COURSE OF MILD AND MINOR HEAD INJURIES
Neurological manifestations are uncommon following mild trauma. Mueller *et al.* (1993) have reported the occurrence of transient bilateral internuclear ophthalmoplegia.

Epileptic seizures are present in 5–10 per cent of patients and occur within two hours of the trauma in almost all cases (Snoek *et al.* 1984) and, in one-fifth, take the form of partial or generalized status epilepticus. Even when repeated, they are usually of favourable prognosis both immediately and at longer term (Jennett 1973, Grand 1974). Early post-traumatic seizures in children are much more common than in adult patients following mild head injury. They do not indicate the presence of intracranial haematoma.

Delayed deterioration may be observed within a few minutes to a few hours (generally within 60 minutes) after head trauma. The onset of deterioration is acute or subacute and marked by loss of consciousness with or without focal neurological signs. Initial vomiting is almost constant. The signs and symptoms end quickly or even abruptly after a short period not exceeding 12 hours and usually lasting only 30–120 minutes. Convulsions may appear in some of these children before recovery (Oka *et al.* 1977, Snoek *et al.* 1984).

Some children may present with delayed focal neurological manifestations without loss of consciousness. Such manifestations include *post-traumatic blindness*, hemianopia, hemiparesis, aphasia or brainstem signs and may be related to migraine or to the mechanism of the spreading depression of Leão (Oka *et al.* 1977, Kaye and Herskowitz 1986, Haas and Lourie 1988).

SEVERE HEAD INJURY
In severe head injuries, consciousness is lost more profoundly and for longer periods than in minor injuries. The greatest neurological deficit is as a rule present immediately following trauma. In the largest series of children reported (Hendrick *et al.* 1964), consciousness was impaired at the time of admission to hospital in 34 per cent. Focal neurological signs may indicate localized brain contusion. Children with the clinical picture of severe brain injury may follow one of several courses.

Some will die without regaining consciousness (Graham *et al.* 1989a). Generalized ischaemic damage is almost universally present in fatal cases. Death is potentially avoidable in some of these cases. Sharples *et al.* (1990) found that delay of proper treatment, failure to diagnose haematomas and aspiration of fluids or other respiratory problems were preventable causes and computed

that avoiding these could have decreased the mortality of children with head trauma in North England from 5.3 per 100,000 (observed figure) to 3.9 per 100,000.

Survivors may either regain consciousness and recover, often completely although transient sequelae are not unusual, or remain severely impaired with prolonged disturbances of consciousness without further deterioration. This is associated with diffuse white matter damage as a result of shearing injury. In the most severe cases, coma or apallic state now termed persistent vegetative state (Kennard and Illingworth 1995) (see below) may last months or years. There is, however, a continuum of axonal damage varying from functional abnormalities alone to severe and widespread axonal injury, and some children may not remain permanently unconscious (Blumbergs *et al.* 1989). Patients with focal lesions in addition to diffuse injury fare worse than those with diffuse injury only (Filley *et al.* 1987). The prognosis is uniformly poor after two years (Mahoney *et al.* 1983). The age of the patient at the time of injury is an important prognostic factor. Children over 6 years of age have better cognitive and motor function and less brain atrophy than younger patients (Kriel *et al.* 1989).

Secondary deterioration is frequent, beginning several minutes to hours following head injury. In the series of Hendrick *et al.* (1964) almost 50 per cent of the children who died were conscious on admission. Such a course in children is much more frequently associated with *brain swelling* than with intracranial bleeding contrary to what occurs in adults (Bruce *et al.* 1981, Snoek *et al.* 1984). With aggressive therapy, patients with head injuries who 'talk and die' (Bowers and Marshall 1980) have become rare, although some mortality still persists. The syndrome of secondary diffuse brain swelling has a favourable outcome in 75–82 per cent of cases in recent series (Berger *et al.* 1985, Kalff *et al.* 1989) but higher mortality figures for acute brain swelling have been reported (Sganzerla *et al.* 1989). The exact mechanism of the syndrome as well as the nature of the swelling shown by CT scan remain in dispute. An increase in blood volume may not be sufficient to account for such an abnormality (Snoek *et al.* 1984). In fact, Muizelaar *et al.* (1989a) found little evidence of hyperaemia, and Sharples *et al.* (1995a,b) found evidence of hyperaemia in only 7 per cent of 151 physiological measures in 21 children. These investigators demonstrated an inverse relationship between brain cerebral blood flow and increased ICP and that the cerebral perfusion pressure, PaO_2 and $PaCO_2$ and cerebral metabolic rate ($CMRO_2$) were normal except in the four childen who died. In some cases, unilateral or focal swelling with similar CT attenuation characteristics has been observed (Waga *et al.* 1979).

The treatment of the syndrome of diffuse acute brain swelling is still controversial, at least with regard to the necessity of monitoring ICP, the use of antihypertensive treatment and brain 'protection' with phenobarbitone (Ward *et al.* 1985) or other agents (see Minns 1991).

EXAMINATION AND MANAGEMENT OF PATIENTS WITH HEAD INJURY
Examination of those patients with both mild and severe head

TABLE 13.1
Paediatric Glasgow coma scale*

Eye opening (E)	
Spontaneous	4
To speech	3
To pain	2
None	1
Best verbal response (V)	
Oriented	5
Words	4
Inappropriate words	3
Vocal sounds	3
Cries	2
None	1
Best motor response (M)	
Obeys commands	6
Localizes pain	5
Withdraws	4
Abnormal flexion to pain	3
Abnormal extension to pain	2
None	1

*Simpson and Reilly (1982).
Coma score = E + V + M.
In children, the normal score is 9 before age
6 months, 11 between 6 and 12 months, 12
from 1 to 2 years, 13 from 2 to 5 years, and
14 above 5 years.

trauma should be rapid but comprehensive and include a general examination and a search for associated visceral lesions. Examination is performed in parallel with emergency treatment. Repeated determinations of the level of consciousness are essential. This enables a score to be established allowing comparison between successive examinations. The Glasgow coma scale (Teasdale and Jennett 1974) has been adapted for children (Simpson and Reilly 1982) and is widely used (Table 13.1). A low score (< 8) corresponds to coma and is often used to define severe head injury. Other scales are available. In general, there is more interobserver agreement using the scales with fewer categories than with the more complex ones (see Newton *et al.* 1995).

Brainstem signs, such as pupillary size, response to light, extent and symmetry of voluntary and reflex movements, and eye response to vestibular stimulation, are also important.

Radiographic examination of the skull contributes little to initial assessment of brain-injured children. CT scan on the other hand is essential (Johnson and Lee 1992, White and Likavec 1992). The most common finding is diffuse cerebral swelling with obliteration or narrowing of lateral and third ventricles and peri-mesencephalic cisterns, while attenuation values are higher than on follow-up scans (Bruce *et al.* 1981). CT can also demonstrate the presence of an intracranial haematoma or of brain contusions characterized by small, often multiple areas of blood density with surrounding hypodense areas of oedema. The CT scan may rapidly change over a short period, and repeat examination should be performed if the clinical situation is modified. In addition, CT can give information on the possible existence of lesions of the base of the skull and cervical spine (Kaiser *et al.*

1981). MRI is more sensitive than CT. It may be especially valuable for detection of smaller lesions or haematomas, which may be isodense on CT scan or too close to the inner table to be visualized, and of brainstem or corpus callosum haemorrhages (Sklar *et al.* 1992). The predictive value of EEG during coma seems to be mainly for short-term prognosis (Dusser *et al.* 1989). A slow monotonous pattern is associated with a higher mortality and a longer coma but not with a worse long-term prognosis.

Studies of evoked potentials following head injury have indicated that absent somaesthetic evoked responses are associated with a poor prognosis (De Meirleir and Taylor 1987). Abnormal visual evoked responses are less reliable, with both false positives and false negatives, athough they may be useful when measurement of somaesthetic evoked potentials is not possible (Taylor and Farrell 1989). Such studies, however, should be deferred until after the initial examination and emergency therapeutic measures.

Following initial assessment, resuscitation and more complete evaluation are indicated. Careful monitoring of vital signs is essential, as the clinical condition of children with head trauma can change rapidly and emergency decisions may have to be made at very short notice.

Maintenance of an adequate airway often requires intubation and artificial ventilation. Shock must be vigorously treated since the injured brain is highly susceptible to episodes of systemic hypotension because of marginal perfusion pressure due to increased vascular resistance resulting from brain oedema (Sharples *et al.* 1995a). Particular care should be given to maintenance of an adequate fluid and electrolyte balance. Although both cerebral salt-wasting and excess antidiuretic hormone secretion can produce hyponatraemia and may be difficult to distinguish (Sivakumar *et al.* 1994), hypovolaemia is the major danger. Measurement of central venous pressure may help make the diagnosis and indicate appropriate therapy. Seizures should be controlled with intravenous benzodiazepines or phenytoin as they increase ICP and cerebral metabolism (Brown and Hussain 1991). The treatment of increased ICP is outlined in Chapter 14. Continous monitoring of ICP is indicated in severe cases (Leggate and Minns 1991), and every effort should be made to maintain an adequate perfusion pressure. Mannitol is usually the most effective agent. Hyperventilation is effective but can potentially reduce cerebral blood flow, so PCO_2 should be closely monitored. Steroids have no proven value (Hall 1992), and the effectiveness and safety of barbiturates and hypothermia remain to be established. In addition, therapeutic measures aiming to reduce the cerebral metabolic rate for oxygen ($CMRO_2$) need to be specific for brain and it should not be assumed that measures that decrease whole-body energy expenditure will have the same effect on the brain (Matthews *et al.* 1995).

The value of monitoring ICP has been questioned (Berger *et al.* 1985). With aggressive therapy, most patients conscious on admission should survive (Bruce *et al.* 1981). Intensive care has clearly decreased the overall mortality of head trauma. Although it may have increased the proportion of children left with some disability (West *et al.* 1989), this is not confirmed in most recent studies (see Miller 1992).

464

DELAYED MANIFESTATIONS OF CLOSED HEAD INJURY

This section deals with complications of head injury which occur in the weeks or months following head trauma and include mainly chronic subdural haematoma and post-traumatic hydrocephalus. For convenience, the clinical features of more acute haematomas will be also described in this section even though they are often early events.

HAEMATOMAS
Haematomas are less common in children than in adults.

Extradural haematomas
Extradural haematomas are localized collections of blood between the skull and the dura and occur in about 1 per cent of head traumas in childhood (Hendrick *et al.* 1964). The bleeding may originate from the meningeal artery or its branches, or from torn dural veins. It may arise from an undetermined source (Mazza *et al.* 1982, Choux *et al.* 1986). Arterial bleeding results in rapid progression of the symptoms and is often associated with brain oedema that increases the risk of acute intracranial hypertension. When bleeding arises from veins, the progression of symptoms is slower, a feature more common in children than in adults. In children even a mild or trivial injury can be responsible for an epidural haematoma. Approximately half the cases occur in children under 2 years of age (Matson 1969).

The typical sequence of clinical features seen in adults with extradural haematoma, which includes initial loss of consciousness, recovery and subsequent rapid deterioration, is rare in children. More commonly, there is no initial unconsciousness. After a variable interval of minutes to days, which tends to be longer in younger patients, a progressive deterioration with loss of consciousness and neurological signs appears. Vomiting, papilloedema, hemiparesis, IIIrd nerve palsy and retinal haemorrhages are the most frequent manifestations (Choux *et al.* 1986). A dilated fixed pupil on the side of the haematoma is present in 90 per cent of cases. A skull fracture is found in less than half the cases. Decerebrate rigidity follows in the absence of treatment along with hypertension and bradycardia. Anaemia and collapse may be prominent in infants (Motte *et al.* 1985). Atypical clinical symptoms such as chorea (Adler and Winston 1984) occasionally occur.

CT scan characteristically evidences a convex area of increased density located immediately beneath the inner skull table (Fig. 13.1). In infants, this frequently communicates with an extracranial haematoma. Parenchymal lesions are often associated.

Epidural haematomas are occasionally found in the posterior fossa (Pozzati *et al.* 1989). They are usually associated with a fracture of the occipital squama crossing the lateral sinus. Signs of posterior fossa involvement such as cerebellar ataxia and nystagmus are only inconstantly present. CT scanning has permitted an earlier diagnosis of these lesions thus improving their prognosis.

Treatment of extradural haemorrhage is operative evacuation of the collection. Conservative treatment has been proposed for

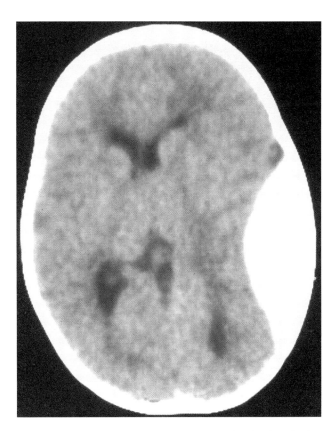

Fig. 13.1. Left extradural haematoma in a 9-month-old girl involved in a traffic accident. There is marked shift of the midline toward the side opposite the haematoma and some degree of oedema and compression of the left lateral ventricle.

cases with mild symptoms, seen early, with intact consciousness and in which there is no evidence of fracture crossing a meningeal artery or a venous sinus (Lahat *et al.* 1994).

Chronic subdural haematoma
Chronic subdural haematomas have a characteristic clinical presentation. They follow recognized and unrecognized head trauma and there is no difference between so-called idiopathic and clearly traumatic cases with regard to age, sex or clinical manifestations.

The *pathophysiology* of subdural haematoma is incompletely understood. The collections are bilateral in more than 85 per cent of cases and are located in the frontoparietal region. Bleeding probably originates from bridging veins but the mechanism that is responsible for the organization and chronicity is uncertain. The membrane that surrounds the haematoma starts forming at the interface between the dura and arachnoid (Friede 1989) and ultimately envelops the clot. Albumin leakage from the thin-walled, abnormally permeable blood vessels of the outer membrane into the subdural pocket may increase the osmotic pressure and cause influx of water (Rabe *et al.* 1968). Some exchange with CSF must exist as the protein composition of the collections at a late stage includes proteins characteristic of CSF such as prealbumin. Subdural collections act as space-occupying lesions and produce increased ICP. They may be responsible for hydrocephalus as

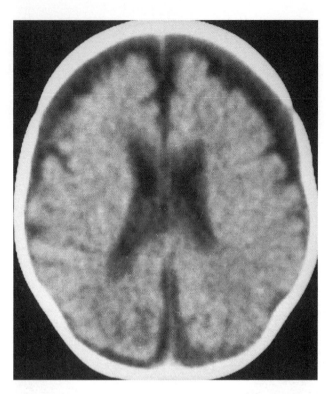

Fig. 13.2. Chronic subdural haematoma. CT scan of 7-month-old infant who presented with vomiting, hypotonia and tense fontanelle. Note anterior and symmetrical location of effusion, whose most superficial part is of higher density than CSF. Note also widening of interhemispheric fissure.

CT shows anterior enlargement of the pericerebral spaces (Fig. 13.2). The density of the collection is initially increased, then decreases to approximate, in the late stage, that of the CSF. At an intermediate stage the collection may be isodense to the brain, but medial displacement of the cortical sulci or cortical veins after enhancement and the presence of small, laterally compressed ventricles is suggestive (Kim *et al.* 1978). Parenchymal lesions in the form of haemorrhages or multiple areas of oedematous density are often present, and some degree of diffuse brain atrophy is seen in many cases and correlates with a less favourable outcome. A frequent appearance which is suggestive of the battered baby syndrome is that of *interhemispheric subdural haematoma*, usually located to the posterior third of the interhemispheric fissure (Zimmerman *et al.* 1979, 1982).

The *diagnosis* of subdural haematoma is now generally made by CT examination. Subdural tap remains an excellent means of confirmation of the diagnosis. It should be performed at the lateral angle of the fontanelle or through the enlarged coronal suture to avoid puncturing the sagittal sinus. Aspiration should never be used as it may induce rebleeding into the haematoma pouch.

Treatment consists of evacuation of the collection. This can be achieved by simple bilateral tapping on alternate sides but probably should not be prolonged for more than a few days. The aim is to relieve increased pressure, not to dry up the collection if normal pressure can be achieved. In cases in which the collection re-forms under increased pressure for more than a few days, shunting of the subdural collection to the peritoneal cavity (Kotwica and Brzezinski 1991) appears preferable as it allows for progressive disappearance of the haematoma, membranes and hypervascularity while avoiding the occurrence of peaks of pressure (Aoki 1990). Removal of the membranes is no longer recommended.

The *prognosis* of chronic subdural haematoma best correlates to the presence or absence of underlying brain damage. Occurrence of status epilepticus and of a slow EEG are indicators of a poor mental outcome (Aicardi and Goutières 1971), which is the case in about half the patients. However, increased ICP plays an aggravating role and may diminish cortical perfusion. The mode of evacuation of the collection was not found to correlate with the outcome (Rabe *et al.* 1968), and in a recent series (Aoki 1990) only 57 per cent of children showed normal development and 13 per cent were severely retarded. In the series of Kotwica and Brzezinski (1991) the recovery rate was 80 per cent with a mortality rate of only 3 per cent.

Acute subdural haematomas
Acute subdural haematomas are located between the dura and the cerebral mantle. They belong to two different types. Isolated acute haematomas often occur without loss of consciousness following minor trauma and without evidence of brain contusion. They are mainly seen in infants under 1 year of age. They often present with tonic or tonic–clonic generalized convulsions associated with retinal haemorrhages without signs of neurological deficit (Aoki and Masuzawa 1984). Their course is usually benign following removal of the blood.

a result of the compression of the underlying subarachnoid space, although associated subarachnoid bleeding may more commonly be the cause. Sequelae may be the consequence of brain compression but seem mainly to depend on the presence of accompanying brain damage (Aicardi and Goutières 1971).

Following evacuation, subdural collections tend to reform rapidly. This is probably due to initial enlargement of the skull and the discrepancy between skull and brain leaving a dead space where fluid tends to accumulate.

Chronic subdural haematomas occur mainly in infants 2–9 months of age. *Presenting manifestations* include convulsions, vomiting, lethargy or irritability and fever. Many such infants present with failure to thrive, with frequent episodes of vomiting that may be projectile. Enlargement of the head may be the initial feature.

On examination the head is enlarged with a square appearance. The anterior fontanelle is tense or bulging and the eyes may show a 'setting sun' sign. Retinal or preretinal haemorrhage are present in at least half the cases. Retinal haemorrhages have been ascribed to vigorous shaking of the infant (Caffey 1974, Duhaime *et al.* 1987). They are strongly suggestive of nonaccidental injury. Focal neurological features are uncommon but hemiparesis may occur. The CSF is bloody or has an increased level of protein in most cases studied (Aicardi and Goutières 1971). However, lumbar puncture can be dispensed with and CT scan is the examination of choice.

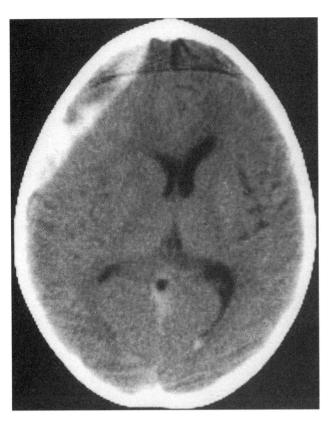

Fig. 13.3. Unilateral subacute subdural haematoma in 6-year-old girl: CT scan. Pronounced shift of midline structures to the left. The collection has mixed density with areas of high attenuation due to the presence of fresh blood and areas of lower attenuation corresponding to older, modified blood. (Courtesy Dr D. Renier, Prof. J-F. Hirsch, Hôpital des Enfants Malades, Paris.)

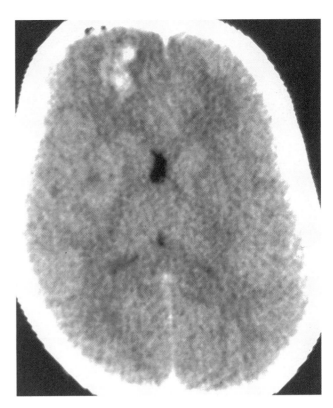

Fig. 13.4. Right frontal contusion in 3½-year-old boy, a few hours after trauma. Unenhanced CT scan shows haemorrhagic area surrounded by hypodensity due to oedema. Anterior midline is shifted to the left. (Courtesy Dr D. Renier, Prof. J-F. Hirsch, Hôpital des Enfants Malades, Paris.)

A more severe picture obtains in cases of acute *subdural haematoma associated with brain contusion*. Signs and symptoms of increased ICP, seizures, often amounting to status epilepticus, and focal neurological deficit may evolve quickly. Skull fractures may be associated (Gutierrez and Raimondi 1975). Acute subdural haematomas present on CT scan as collections of blood density which are more often unilateral than bilateral (Fig. 13.3). Depending on the date of the CT scan in relation to injury and to the presence of anaemia that decreases blood density, subdural haematomas may be isodense to the brain and can thus be missed (Smith *et al.* 1981). In unilateral cases, marked shift of the midline is frequent, reflecting the presence of brain oedema or contusion rather than the effect of the haematoma itself which is usually of small volume. Such lesions are highly suggestive of nonaccidental head injuries.

The prognosis of such complicated acute subdural haematomas is determined principally by the extent of associated parenchymal damage, and treatment is mainly directed at oedema and increased ICP, even though evacuation of the collection may be of some help.

Acute subdural haematomas of the posterior fossa are very rare in infants (Vielvoye *et al.* 1982) past the neonatal period in which most cases occur (Deonna and Oberson 1974, Hernansanz *et al.* 1984).

Intraparenchymal haemorrhages
Intraparenchymal haemorrhages are rarely of large size, but small petechial haemorrhages are often visible on CT scan in the white matter, corpus callosum or cerebral cortex (Fig. 13.4). Haemorrhages in the brainstem probably result from increase in the anteroposterior diameter of the brainstem as a consequence of lateral compression by temporal herniation with stretching of central vessels. Large parenchymal haemorrhages are sometimes present in cases of extensive brain contusion (Statham *et al.* 1989). Contrecoup contusion with a combination of oedema and haemorrhage is frequently present in the frontal and/or anterior temporal regions (Fig. 13.5). *Traumatic intracerebellar haematoma* with progressive loss of consciousness, bilateral VIth nerve palsy and other signs of high ICP has been reported only exceptionally in paediatric patients (Pozzati *et al.* 1982). Late hydrocephalus may develop.

POST-TRAUMATIC HYDROCEPHALUS
Hydrocephalus developed following head trauma in 2.8 per cent of 428 children who had had either brain contusion or acute subdural haematoma and were initially comatose (Oi and Matsumoto 1987). Twenty per cent of these children had a skull fracture, and 12 per cent had intracranial haematomas. Haematohydrocephalus was an early occurrence as was hydrocephalus associated with massive brain oedema. The majority of cases,

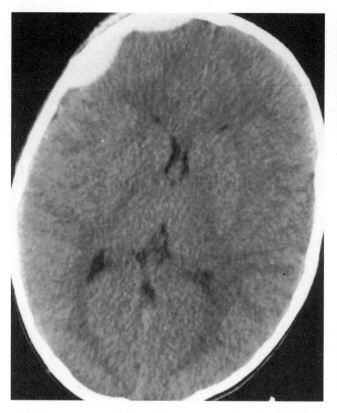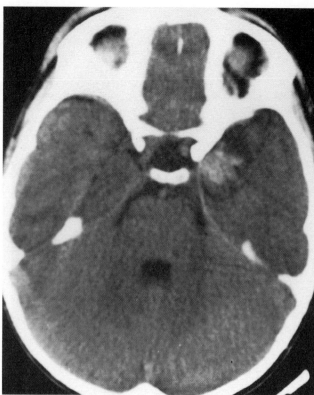

Fig. 13.5. Head trauma in 5-year-old girl who was hit by a car. *(Left)* Extradural haematoma of right frontal region. *(Right)* Contrecoup lesion in left temporal lobe with haemorrhage and oedema due to impact of temporal lobe against sphenoidal ridge. (Courtesy Dr M-A. Barthez-Carpentier, Prof. J.J. Santini, Hôpital de Clocheville, Tours.)

however, were subacute or chronic hydrocephalus, occasionally unilateral. The interval between trauma and onset of symptoms suggestive of hydrocephalus is generally several weeks or months. Delayed ventricular enlargement is common after a head injury resulting in low Glasgow coma score and prolonged coma, whereas an early enlargement is more common in a head injury with subarachnoid or intraventricular haemorrhage (Meyers *et al.* 1983). Hydrocephalus is probably due to subarachnoid space obliteration by posthaemorrhagic fibrosis.

Treatment is usually by ventriculoperitoneal shunting. In some cases distinction between post-traumatic atrophy and hydrocephalus is difficult and pressure measurements may be required.

OTHER DELAYED MANIFESTATIONS
Dizziness occurs in 50 per cent of children, even after mild trauma (Eviatar *et al.* 1986). Persistent ataxia and/or vertigo is commonly of vestibular origin and usually subsides within days (Chapter 19).

Stroke is a rare early complication of head trauma. It may follow both mild and severe injuries. Clinical manifestations usually become apparent after a free interval of 6–12 hours but immediate or late cases (one to two weeks after trauma) are on record (Schneider *et al.* 1972). Although any vascular territory can be involved, the basal nuclei appear to be especially fragile (Brett *et al.* 1981, Maki *et al.* 1988).

Mutism is an unusual complication of head injury (Levin *et al.* 1983). Children with head trauma may remain mute for variable periods despite recovery of consciousness and nonverbal communication. In about half the 37 patients of Levin *et al.*, areas of oedematous density were present either diffusely or in the putaminocapsular area.

Excessive daytime sleepiness is not uncommon after head trauma, especially in adolescents. It may be associated with sleep apnoea or resemble closely narcolepsy (Guilleminault *et al.* 1983). Sleepiness may persist months to years and its duration correlates with the severity of the initial injury. Methylphenidate may prevent excessive somnolence.

Haemorrhage in the basal ganglia occurs in about 3 per cent of severe closed head injuries in adults and has been observed in children (Katz *et al.* 1989). Hemiparesis contralateral to the lesion is a constant feature and muteness is frequent. CT scan shows localized haemorrhage, sometimes followed by cavitation. The outcome is favourable when haemorrhage occurs in isolation.

Isolated intracerebral haemorrhage may also involve other brain areas, especially the frontal lobe (Kang *et al.* 1989), and is usually of good prognosis.

LATE COMPLICATIONS AND SEQUELAE OF HEAD INJURY
Mental retardation, behavioural and motor deficits, and epilepsy

are the major sequelae of head injury. Post-traumatic epilepsy is considered below.

COGNITIVE AND BEHAVIOURAL SEQUELAE

These are common after moderate to severe head trauma. Minor and mild injuries do not seem to be associated with sequelae (Bijur *et al.* 1990). These are especially frequent following severe injury with coma, and there is a clear relationship between the duration of coma and the presence of sequelae (Mahoney *et al.* 1983, Filley *et al.* 1987). A period of coma exceeding one week in duration is associated with an increased incidence of cognitive deficits, while coma of less than a week is not (Jennett and Teasdale 1977, Chadwick 1985). A rapid return to normality is often observed after head injury. A significant part of post-traumatic dysfunction in children appears to be reactive in origin and therefore preventable by a correct psychological management during recovery. Memory impairment may persist following coma lasting more than 24 hours. Kalff *et al.* (1989), in a series composed exclusively of children with severe injuries, found that only 6.6 per cent of their patients with coma had severe disability and this was the case of 3.3 per cent of the whole series. Attention deficit is especially common (Kaufmann *et al.* 1993).

However, closer scrutiny of children with head injury has indicated that behavioural difficulties and school failure are more common in children who have had head trauma than in the general population (Chadwick 1985, Ewing-Cobbs *et al.* 1989). In a study by Fuld and Fisher (1977), persistent intellectual changes documented on standardized tests were not always apparent to parents and physicians, and recovery of intellectual abilities lagged behind the disappearance of neurological abnormalities. Even an apparently normal neuropsychological profile does not preclude the appearance of permanent changes in behaviour and personality (Miner *et al.* 1986). Also disturbing is the result of a study by Costeff *et al.* (1988), who found that even moderate and relatively common traumatic injury may be associated with detectable late cognitive deficits, which can be demonstrated by specific testing. Wrightson *et al.* (1995) compared 78 children with mild head trauma not requiring hospitalization and 86 control children who had incurred other forms of injury and found that the former scored less than controls on reading and solving a visual puzzle.

Behaviour and personality changes are also present in many children but some of them, at least, may be secondary to stress on impaired perceptual and cognitive difficulties. There are indications that behavioural problems in such patients were often present before the accident, which aggravated rather than created the problem (Costeff 1988). Klonoff *et al.* (1993) found that the IQ in the postacute phase was a reliable predictor of outcome. They reported that subjective sequelae, observed in 31 per cent of 159 children followed for 23 years, were clearly related to the extent of head injury and a low IQ.

Knowledge of such difficulties is important when measures to help these children are considered and for prevention of secondary psychosocial difficulties. The need for rehabilitation after severe head injury was assessed by Scott-Jupp *et al.* (1992) who found that 18 of 43 children had persistent neurological impairment and 15 needed special educational support.

POST-TRAUMATIC HEADACHES AND POSTCONCUSSION SUBJECTIVE SYNDROME

Headache is much less frequent in children than in adults as a sequel to head injury (Barlow 1984). Dillon and Leopold (1961) found that personality changes and psychological phenomena were the outstanding postconcussion symptoms. Behavioural changes included increased aggressiveness, withdrawal and antisocial behaviour. Sleep disturbances are extremely common (Guilleminault *et al.* 1983). Headache is often only a minor complaint in children.

NEUROLOGICAL SEQUELAE

Neurological deficits may persist as a result of vascular damage or of diffuse or localized traumatic brain damage. Hemiparesis, hemianopia, dyspraxia or other specialized deficits are possible. Such sequelae are usually the consequence of severe brain injury and are associated with CT evidence of brain atrophy with ventricular dilatation and enlargement of the sulci, with cavitation of the white matter or with chronic subdural hydroma. Postural and intentional tremor (Johnson and Hall 1992), also termed volitional dyskinesia, due to injury to the superior cerebellar peduncle may appear in children several weeks or months after injury (Arnould *et al.* 1966). It is characterized by unilateral abnormal movements and tremor, especially of the upper limbs on attempts to maintain a posture or on attempted movements. Johnson and Hall observed it in 45 per cent of 289 children with severe head injury. The tremor subsided in up to 50 per cent of patients.

Sensory deficits, especially optic atrophy, may occur, especially as a result of hydrocephalus or haematoma (Gerber *et al.* 1992).

POST-TRAUMATIC EPILEPSY

Post-traumatic epilepsy refers here only to late-onset seizures. These tend to develop in the first two years following trauma, 50 per cent appearing within the first year. The likelihood of late seizures is increased by the incidence of early seizures and the presence of an acute haematoma and a depressed skull fracture (Jennett 1973). Prevention of early post-traumatic seizures can be achieved by administration of phenytoin (Temkin *et al.* 1990) or carbamazepine (Glötzner *et al.* 1983) but is not effective beyond the first weeks after trauma and does not prevent the development of late post-traumatic epilepsy. The possible preventive effect of lipid peroxidation inhibitors such as methylprednisolone and vitamin E (Willmore 1990) and free-radical scavengers (Muizelaar *et al.* 1993) is being studied.

SKULL FRACTURES

Skull fractures are a frequent consequence of head trauma. They are commonly associated with brain injury, although the latter is not the direct result of the fracture. Fractures may have specific complications and may raise diagnostic and therapeutic problems.

Most skull fractures in children are linear. They are mostly asymptomatic. In infants they should be differentiated from disunited spheno-occipital, metopic or mendosal sutures of from wormian bones. Most linear fractures heal uneventfully in three or four months and require no treatment.

Growing skull fractures are seen mainly in children under 3 years of age with nonaccidental trauma. They are associated with the presence of a leptomeningeal cyst that develops because of unrecognized dural laceration at the time of trauma. The arachnoid herniates through the dural tear into the fracture separation. Fluid accumulates in the hernia forming a cyst whose pulsations induce erosion of the bone and widening of the fracture (Kingsley *et al.* 1978). Most growing fractures are located in the parietal region. CT scan shows that cavitation of the brain parenchyma underlies the fracture thus permitting unattenuated transmission of CSF pulsations to the skull (Lye *et al.* 1981, Scarfo *et al.* 1989). Skull X-rays show an irregular bony defect with scalloped margins. Neurological manifestations may include focal seizures and deficits related to the brain cavitated lesions.

Treatment by excision of the meningeal cyst and repair of the dural defect enables healing of the defects.

Basal skull fractures should be suspected when there is bleeding from the nasopharynx, the middle ear, postauricular ecchymoses (Battle's sign) or periorbital ecchymoses ('racoon eyes'). Fractures of the cribriform plate may be accompanied by rhinorrhoea which is associated with a high risk of infection. CSF rhinorrhoea is usually transient, disappearing in 70 per cent of cases within one week and in a majority of the remaining cases within six months. Anosmia is a frequent accompaniment. Rhinorrhoea that persists more than 10 days is an indication for surgical repair. Prophylactic administration of antibiotics (ampicillin) does not reduce the incidence of meningitis and may change the flora to gram-negative organisms (Ignelzi and Van der Ark 1975), so it is preferable to watch the patients closely and to treat infection early.

Other complications of basal skull fractures include injuries to cranial nerve, especially the facial nerve which usually recovers spontaneously. Labyrinthine disturbances are due to haemorrhage or to perilymphatic fistula. Vertigo, positional nystagmus, episodic vertigo, ataxia and hearing loss are uncommon (Healy *et al.* 1978, Healy 1982).

CSF otorrhoea is rare and generally transient. Demonstration of basal fractures by X-ray often requires specially angled views or tomography. CT scan of the base using a bone window is more precise. Such examinations are only justified if required for therapy, that is in a minority of cases.

Children with basal fractures associated with CSF rhinorrhoea, Battle's sign or haemotympanum should be hospitalized. A pneumocele may develop in rare cases and will require antibiotic treatment.

Depressed or comminuted fractures are mainly the consequence of high velocity (missile) injuries or of compound trauma. They often require surgical treatment to remove bone within the cranial cavity.

INTRACRANIAL VASCULAR INJURY

Traumatic lesions of the major brain vessels are uncommon. Dissection and thrombosis of the carotid or vertebral artery as a result of cervical trauma is considered in Chapter 15, and injury to the perforating artery with thrombosis of the basal ganglia has been referred to above (p. 461).

Traumatic aneurysm of the carotid artery is a very unusual lesion (Endo *et al.* 1980). *Carotid–cavernous fistulae* are generally the consequence of fracture of the sphenoid bone which lacerates the internal carotid artery as it passes through the cavernous sinus. They are marked clinically by unilateral pulsating exophthalmos, an intracranial bruit and paralysis of the VIth or IIIrd cranial nerves (Hosobuchi 1989). Definitive diagnosis is by angiography, which also provides information on the size and precise location of the fistula. Treatment is by surgery or embolization, but 5 per cent of fistulae will disappear spontaneously so that indications are limited to long-standing cases or those with unacceptable cosmetic consequences or an intolerable bruit.

NONACCIDENTAL HEAD INJURIES

Nonaccidental head injuries are but one part of the wide domain of child abuse which also includes emotional abuse, neglect and sexual abuse as well as other non-neurological physical injuries and less obvious forms of aggression such as the Munchausen syndrome by proxy. Nonaccidental head injuries are the commonest type of head injury in children under 2 years of age. Billmire and Myers (1985) found that in children under 2 years, 64 per cent of all head injuries, excluding uncomplicated skull fractures, and 95 per cent of serious head injuries were of nonaccidental cause.

INCIDENCE, RISK FACTORS, AND PSYCHOSOCIAL FACTORS AND MECHANISMS

The actual incidence of child abuse is unknown. In the United States in 1974, 200,000 cases were reported, 2000 children having been murdered (Solomons 1979). Most authorities regard such figures as a low estimate and accept much higher figures of the order of one million cases per year. In the United Kingdom, Mac Keith (1974) estimated that there would be approximately 400 cases of chronic brain damage each year in the UK as a result of child abuse. Hahn *et al.* (1988) considered that the head injuries in 4.4 per cent of 318 children were the result of abuse, whereas Duhaime *et al.* (1992) found a much higher prevalence of 24 per cent in 100 carefully studied children.

Child abuse occurs at all socioeconomic and educational levels. It is more often reported in lower socioeconomic groups. The parents are the most common offenders but step-parents, custodians, boyfriends and baby-sitters have been found to abuse childen. Sixty to 90 per cent of abusers have a history of having been abused themselves. Frequently, there is one child in the family who is the scapegoat and is abused, while the siblings may be well-treated.

Fewer than 10 per cent of abusers are severely emotionally disturbed (Solomons 1979). Most abusers have no severe psychopathology but succumb under the stresses and strains of living and rearing children in difficult socioeconomic circumstances. Their way of responding to stresses is in part conditioned by their own personal experience and they often perpetuate through the generations a cycle of violence. Most of them have difficulties controlling their immediate impulses and respond violently to breakdown of the family group as a whole.

Some children may be more vulnerable than others. These include low-birthweight infants and infants with developmental disability. For preterm infants, impaired maternal–infant bonding is thought to be an important factor. Impaired bonding may occur because of abnormally low responsiveness of the infant as a result of immaturity and perhaps because of separation from the mother during the first hours of life, although it is clear that perfectly normal bonding usually occurs later in such cases (Klaus and Kennel 1976). Term low-birthweight infants, however, were not found to run a higher risk of child abuse than normal-weight controls (Leventhal *et al.* 1987).

Children with developmental disabilities before abuse seem to be at special risk (Glaser and Bentovim 1979), including children with cerebral palsy (Diamond and Jaudes 1983).

Prevention of child abuse is clearly a major public health problem. Individual action by the doctor is important, but primary prevention by acting upon socioeconomic factors and providing guidance and support for at-risk parents-to-be, and secondary prevention by intervention in families in which one or several children have been abused or are seen as being under threat of abuse, are likely to be in the long run the most effective measures against a major threat to children (Dubowitz 1989).

CLINICAL MANIFESTATIONS AND DIAGNOSIS
Head injuries due to nonaccidental trauma are often severe. Nineteen of 29 children with nonaccidental head injury studied by Hobbs (1984) died as a result of the trauma. In addition, recurrences are likely to occur if the diagnosis is missed. A high index of suspicion is therefore essential, and nonaccidental injury should be suspected in all children with severe traumatic brain lesions such as subdural haematomas. Proof of the diagnosis, however, may be difficult or impossible to provide.

A major reason for suspecting nonaccidental trauma is the discrepancy between the severity of injury and the history of trauma given by the parents or custodians (O'Doherty 1982). Falls from heights of less than one meter are only exceptionally the cause of multiple, complex, depressed or growing skull fractures (Helfer *et al.* 1977), and certain locations such as the occipital bone are virtually pathognomonic of abuse (Hobbs 1984). Kravitz *et al.* (1969) found only three skull fractures and one subdural haemorrhage among 330 falls of children younger than 2 years old who fell from couches, dressing tables and cots, and fewer than 10 per cent had evidence of minor concussion. Cardiac massage in infants is only exceptionally associated with rib fractures, which are frequent in abused infants (Feldman and Brewer 1984), and only exceptionally with the appearance of retinal haemorrhage (Odom *et al.* 1997).

The presence of multiple fractures, especially metaphysal injuries that give rise to characteristic X-ray images, is also very

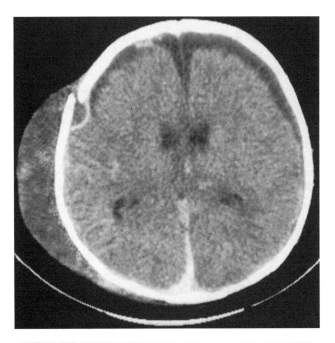

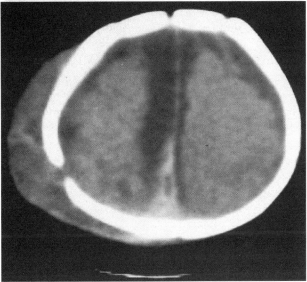

Fig. 13.6. Nonaccidental injury. Unenhanced CT scans showing subdural haematoma in posterior third of interhemispheric fissure. *(Top)* Lower cut showing, in addition, skull fracture, massive effusion under scalp, small extradural effusion and some bleeding in posterior half of right hemisphere. There is also an anterior subdural effusion. *(Bottom)* Higher slice indicating bleeding within the falx cerebri.

suggestive (Kleiman 1987). Likewise multiple cutaneous lesions such as bites, cigarette burns and ecchymoses are strong evidence of abuse. Subgaleal haemorrhage is highly suggestive of the child being pulled or shaken by the hair. Parasagittal subdural haematoma (see above) is also suggestive of a nonaccidental origin (Zimmermann *et al.* 1979, 1982) (Fig. 13.6). Dental lesions, laceration of tongue frenulum and eye abnormalities are also frequently caused by abuse. Retinal and preretinal haemorrhages have been considered to be a feature of the *whiplash shaken baby syndrome* and are often found in association with subdural haematoma (Caffey 1974, Lambert *et al.* 1986, Hadley *et al.* 1989). They are not pathognomonic, however, and some authors have expressed doubts about the possibility of producing severe intracranial injury by shaking only, without actual impact, again stressing that major, if untold, trauma is necessary to produce severe brain damage (Duhaime *et al.* 1987). Shaking is thought to produce shearing injury but a mixed mechanism is probably at play in many cases (Zepp *et al.* 1992).

Most affected children are generally unwell, irritable or too quiet. Some may be pale and shocked or have cyanotic attacks or tachycardia (Brown and Minns 1993), so that even with such atypical presentations, brain injury should be suspected.

The diagnosis rests on a conjunction of features rather than on isolated symptoms which rarely constitute adequate evidence of child abuse (Brown and Minns 1993).

The differential diagnosis includes unintentional trauma and benign subdural collections (Chapter 7). Osseous disorders associated with multiple metaphyseal lesions such as scurvy may simulate the battered child syndrome. Osteogenesis imperfecta, especially in its less severe forms (mild type I and type IV) may pose difficult diagnostic problems (Paterson and McAllion 1989, Taitz 1991). The presence of many wormian bones, osteopenia, joint laxity and blue sclera are useful, but not infallible, clues. Biochemical analysis of type I collagen can be very helpful as 87 per cent of patients have a demonstrable abnormality of procollagen (Gahagan and Rimsza 1991). A similar problem may arise with copper deficiency in preterm infants (Shaw 1988) and in cases of Menkes disease (Chapter 9). Haematological diseases such as idiopathic thrombocytopenic purpura can also resemble the syndrome when associated with bone lesions. Retinal scarring is highly suggestive of child abuse.

Many children with nonaccidental trauma have also been abused in other manners. Therefore a low height and especially a low weight is an indication of possible neglect and abuse. A special problem is posed by the *Meadow syndrome (Munchausen syndrome by proxy)* (Meadow 1982, 1991; Rosenberg 1987) in which the child is abused in various manners by a parent—usually the mother. Munchausen syndrome is the term that designates individuals who purposely and needlessly subject themselves to potentially painful and life-threatening procedures or treatments. Some parents involve their progeny in this form of child abuse by submittting them to similar procedures and hiding these manoeuvres from physicians. In Meadow syndrome, the parent submits the child to a form of abuse by fabricating or producing signs or symptoms so that the child becomes involved in hospital investigations and procedures, often over a long period. Meadow syndrome may be initiated by poisoning but other forms are known, involving, for example, suffocation or strangulation to produce 'pseudoepileptic' attacks (Stephenson 1990).

Neurological manifestations usually include lethargy, coma and seizures which may be fictitious or be actually induced by various aggressions. Involved mothers are usually of good educational level, have an interest in medical matters, are cooperative with medical and nursing staff and seem proud of the unusual nature of their children's illnesses. They do not leave the child

alone but exhibit an unusual detachment while recounting horrible stories (Guandolo 1985).

The diagnosis may be extremely difficult, especially as mothers take their offspring to another doctor or hospital as soon as doubts begin to arise. Psychological sequelae may be severe (McGuire and Feldman 1989). Recurrences may occur in 8–25 per cent of cases (Alexander *et al.* 1990).

PROGNOSIS

The prognosis of child abuse is guarded, not only because of the residual brain damage caused by trauma but also, in part, as a result of psychological deprivation, malnutrition and general neglect. Great difficulty may be found in separating nonaccidental suffocation from sudden infant death syndrome (Brown and Minns 1993). The IQ of abused children is below 70 in 25 per cent of cases as compared with a frequency of 3 per cent in the general population (Sandgrund *et al.* 1974).

Emotional consequences are frequent in abused children (Friedman 1976), and, when adults, such children tend to reproduce the behaviour of their parents towards their own children. There is evidence that even nonabused siblings of battered infants may have unsatisfactory mental and emotional development.

The mortality rate of child abuse may be high. Elmer and Gregg (1967) found that eight of 52 children with multiple bone injuries had died. Thirty per cent of the abused children had signs of CNS damage and 57 per cent had an IQ of 80 or below. Bonnier *et al.* (1995) have emphasized the late effects of whiplash injury that include arrest of brain and skull growth with increasingly obvious psychomotor delay as the children grow older.

SPINAL CORD INJURY

Injuries to the spinal cord are generally the result of indirect trauma involving hyperflexion or hyperextension of the neck or vertical compression of the spine by falls on the head or buttocks. Most cases result from traffic accidents, diving, skiing or horseback riding accidents, and falls from windows or other elevated locations. Relatively minor trauma, such as that often suffered during somersaulting exercise, may produce spinal cord injury. This is due to vascular insufficiency of the cord resulting from hyperextension of the spine (Linssen *et al.* 1990). The most common sites of spinal injury are C1–C2, C5–C6 and D12–L1. Dislocations are frequent in cervical cord injuries, as are compression fractures in dorsolumbar insults. It is not uncommon for the spinal cord to be injured without any bone lesion (Hadley *et al.* 1988). Hamilton and Myles (1992) reviewed 174 paediatric cases. Fracture of the vertebral body or the posterior elements was present in over half the cases, while subluxation without fracture was seen in only 2 per cent. Thirteen per cent had major injury to the spinal cord without any radiological abnormality. Injury to the cervical spine with epidural spinal haemorrhage and bruising of the cervicomedullary junction are not rare with nonaccidental whiplash injury (Hadley *et al.* 1988).

Pathological lesions include swelling of the cord with multiple punctate haemorrhages, major haemorrhages extending over

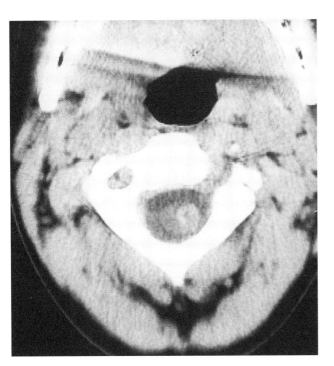

Fig. 13.7. Haematomyelia in 11-year-old boy who sustained a cervical trauma and developed a left hemiplegia that eventually disappeared. Note rounded area of high attenuation in left half of spinal cord at C2 level.

TABLE 13.2
Neurological features of the commonest spinal cord injuries

Transverse lesions
  C1–C2
    Complete quadriplegia
    Respiratory paralysis
  C5–C6
    Quadriplegia
    Preservation of diaphragmatic movements
    Sensory level at upper thoracic level with preservation of sensation over lateral aspects of the arm
  T12–L1
    Paraplegia
    Sensory level at inguinal folds
    Loss of sphincter control

Unilateral or predominantly unilateral lesions
  Brown–Sequard syndrome
    Unilateral paralysis ipsilateral to affected side
    Unilateral disturbances of deep sensation
    Disturbances of position and vibration sense ipsilateral to paralysis
    Unilateral (contralateral to lesion) disturbances of superficial (pain and thermal) sensation
    Incomplete forms frequent
  Spinal hemiplegia
    Either purely motor, respecting the face, or
    Associated with sensory deficits

Central cord lesions
  Involvement of upper limbs greater than that of lower limbs (lesion affects the more medial segment of corticospinal tract)
  Lower motor neuron involvement of upper limbs
  Disturbances in pain and thermal sensation below the level of the lesion

Anterior spinal syndrome
  Paraplegia
  Loss of pain and thermal sensation
  Preservation of deep sensation
  May be due to lesion of the anterior spinal artery

several segments in the central part of the cord (haematomyelia) (Fig. 13.7), and direct trauma by bone or intervertebral disc material. With concussion of the spinal cord, there is no gross pathological abnormality despite early paraplegia. Spinal epidural and subdural haematomas may compress the cord and necessitate urgent evacuation. They may occur following lumbar puncture or other minor trauma in children with clotting disorders (Dulac *et al.* 1975). Cavitation may occur at a late stage and often involves cord segments above the original site of trauma (Shannon *et al.* 1981, Schurch *et al.* 1993). Such late post-traumatic syringomyelia is sometimes associated with increasing neurological deficit, although the mechanism of this complication is unknown. Drainage of the cavity may then be indicated.

Minor trauma to the spinal cord may result in infarction of the cord. Choi *et al.* (1986) found this to occur in 8 per cent of children with spinal injury. In such cases, symptoms appear after a latent period of two hours to four days and tend to persist. Occlusion of the anterior spinal artery is sometimes demonstrated by angiography.

The *clinical features* of spinal cord injury vary with the location of the trauma and the structures affected, and with the severity of the insult. Topographical syndromes of spinal cord involvement are indicated in Table 13.2.

Concussion of the spinal cord produces transient neurological deficits of unclear mechanism. Loss of function may be complete or partial but signs of recovery appear within hours or a few days. Recovery is often complete but in more severe cases there may be only partial recovery with persisting physical signs or symptoms or cord dysfunction.

In *severe cord injury* there occurs a period of *spinal shock* below the injured segment. It is characterized by complete loss of motor, sensory and sphincter functions with complete areflexia lasting two to six weeks. Gradually, a muscular response to stimuli in the involved territory appears and spasticity with extensor plantar reflexes, mass flexion reflexes and increased deep tendon reflexes follows. Extensor reflexes ultimately appear and become the dominant reflex activity.

The final picture may be one of purely reflex activity in the most severe cases, with variable degrees of preserved function in patients with less extensive damage. Three-quarters of the patients of Hamilton and Myles (1992) with physiologically incomplete spinal cord deficit improved significantly and more than half made a complete recovery, whereas a similar improvement was seen in only 10 per cent of those with physiologically complete section.

Radiological investigations are important in cases of spinal cord trauma. Fracture or dislocation are often present but special views may be necessary to demonstrate them. The patients, however, should be manipulated with the utmost care to avoid provoking damage or increasing any previous insult. CT or MRI scans are usually required to determine the presence or absence of a block and the extent to which nervous structures have been compromised by the trauma. They are also indicated in cases of anterior spinal artery syndrome with preservation of posterior column function or when there is progression of symptoms and signs. Pending such examination, temporary immobilization of the spine should be maintained. CT gives a good picture of bone lesions and is easy to perform in most centres. MRI is often not possible as an emergency examination. It provides considerable information about the cord itself: acute haemorrhage and syrinx give a low signal in T_1-weighted sequences, whereas oedema and punctate haemorrhages are well demonstrated on T_2-weighted images (Davis 1995). Late imaging studies may show cavitation of the spinal cord which may be progressive whether due to accidental or surgical trauma (Avrahami *et al.* 1989).

Treatment of spinal cord injury includes postural treatment and prevention of movement especially in cervical injuries (Sonntag and Hadley 1988). Skeletal traction may be indicated. High-dose methylprednisolone (30 mg/kg bolus followed by 5.4 mg/kg/h for 23 hours) is being evaluated comparatively and appears promising (Bracken *et al.* 1990, 1992; Young 1992). Although GM1 ganglioside has seemed encouraging, there is serious doubt about its efficacy and innocuity. Surgical treatment is indicated in the case of suspected block, in wounds in which imaging shows bony fragments in the spinal canal, in cases in which deficit is shown to increase, and in cases of dislocation of the spine that cannot be reduced by traction.

The outlook for spinal cord function depends on the extent of the injury. Recovery may extend over 6–12 months. The outlook for recovery is better in patients with central cord injuries than in those with transverse lesions (Schneider *et al.* 1954).

Special problems arise in children with congenital abnormalities of the spine, especially those with atlantoaxoidal instability as a consequence of Down syndrome (Chaudry *et al.* 1987, Pueschel *et al.* 1987, Davidson 1988, Pueschel 1988) or of congenital or acquired abnormalities of the cervico-occipital articulation or of the odontoid (Greenberg 1968, Hukuda *et al.* 1980). Such childen are prone to develop quadriparesis or other deficits such as spinal hemiplegia following minor trauma (Chapter 6).

INJURIES BY OTHER PHYSICAL AGENTS

ACUTE ACCIDENTAL HYPOXIA AND ISCHAEMIA
CAUSES AND GENERAL CLINICAL FEATURES
Hypoxia and ischaemia often occur together but hypoxia may occur alone under certain circumstances such as carbon monoxide poisoning or near-drowning whilst ischaemia may be an isolated phenomenon in certain paroxysmal arrhythmias with circulatory compromise. Partial ischaemia also occurs in various circumstances such as acute dehydration, hypovolaemic shock, haemorrhagic shock and apparently life-threatening events (near-miss sudden death) (Aubourg *et al.* 1985, Constantinou *et al.* 1989). This section will consider acute hypoxia resulting from cardiac or cardiorespiratory arrest and carbon monoxide intoxication.

Pathology and pathophysiology
Cerebral function requires the maintenance of an adequate supply of oxygen and substrates, mainly glucose. Eighty-five per cent of glucose utilized by the brain is oxidized to CO_2 through the Krebs cycle or after conversion to alpha-amino acids. A constant oxygen supply is necessary to maintain these reactions. Only 10 per cent of the glucose used by the brain is metabolized through the glycolytic pathway with production of lactate.

Pathological lesions of hypoxia consist initially of astrocytic swelling and extracellular oedema of the white matter. The most affected areas include the border zones between arterial territories in the cerbral cortex, the hippocampus, the caudate nuclei and the cerebellar Purkinje cells (Brierley *et al.* 1971).

Clinical features
Acute hypoxia is most frequently the result of cardiac arrest or sudden hypotension but may be unassociated with ischaemia. However, prolonged hypoxia inevitably leads to bradycardia and cardiac arrest, and hypoxic damage cannot be dissociated from that due to ischaemia. Consciousness is lost within seconds of cerebral circulatory failure. Irreversible damage with cell death is already apparent in sensitive areas such as the hippocampus after four minutes, and 10 minutes is believed to be the limit of brain viability.

Loss of consciousness is sometimes preceded by sensations of visual loss or light-headedness and is rapidly followed by convulsions and the appearance of decerebrate rigidity. Coma follows episodes of hypoxia–ischaemia that last longer than one or two minutes. *Coma* is defined as a state of unresponsiveness in which patients are not aware of their surroundings, usually lie with eyes closed and have no sleep–wake cycles.

Myoclonic status epilepticus often develops within a day or two of the onset of hypoxic coma. The myoclonus is typically of small amplitude, irregular, asynchronous, and predominantly involving the face. The EEG may show generalized periodic complexes of spikes and waves or may not display paroxysmal anomalies. Shorvon (1994) proposed the term 'myoclonic status epilepticus in coma' for such cases, which are highly suggestive of sequelae of acute hypoxic damage and usually run a fatal course. It is important to study brainstem function: normal vestibular responses, maintenance of spontaneous respiration and intact doll's eye movements and pupillary reactions indicate a relatively good prognosis for recovery (Plum and Posner 1980). If the coma lasts for more than 24 hours permanent neurological impairment will be present in over 80 per cent of patients (Levy *et al.* 1985), although outcome may be slightly better in children. Neurological outcome remains poor for patients with out-of-hospital cardiac arrest (Roine *et al.* 1989).

The EEG is always altered from mild slowing to flat tracing, and the latter is never associated with full recovery (Pampiglione *et al.* 1978). Theta–delta slowing and burst–suppression represent intermediate stages. Burst–suppression is consistently associated with a poor outcome, but lesser abnormalities are generally not useful in predicting the prognosis (Kuroiwa and Celesia 1980). Alpha-coma, the finding of predominantly alpha-frequency rhythms in the EEGs of unconscious patients is generally due to hypoxia resulting from cardiac arrest. The prognosis of alpha-coma in hypoxic patients is poor, although it may not be very different from that of other severe EEG patterns (Austin *et al.* 1988). 'Theta pattern' coma has a similarly dismal prognosis (Synek and Synek 1984). In children, the various types of rhythmic coma (alpha, beta, theta and spindle coma) have a less gloomy outcome than in adults (Horton *et al.* 1990). Alpha-coma may also be caused by head trauma, drug intoxication and brainstem vascular accidents (Tomassen and Kamphuisen 1986).

CT often shows areas of oedematous density (Fitch *et al.* 1985) that may evolve into cavitation and atrophy and may enhance following contrast injection (Aubourg *et al.* 1985). Such late changes indicate a poor prognosis.

The course of acute hypoxia of whatever cause can be complicated by the appearance of two delayed syndromes of neurological deterioration. *Delayed post-hypoxic encephalopathy* is characterized by the reappearance of lethargy and coma following recovery from the initial coma. The lucid interval may last from 24 hours up to 25 days (Zagami *et al.* 1993). Coma is accompanied by rigidity and spasticity and the course is not infrequently lethal. This syndrome is observed following carbon monoxide intoxication in which it was seen in 12 per cent of cases (Zagami *et al.* 1993) and is also associated with white matter involvement (Weinberger *et al.* 1994) and near-drowning.

Delayed posthypoxic action and intention myoclonus (Lance–Adams syndrome) usually follows severe hypoxia consequent on cardiac arrest. Myoclonic jerks involve all voluntary muscles and appear on intended movement and are not associated with EEG paroxysms. The myoclonus begins during the recovery phase of an acute hypoxic–ischaemic encephalopathy and is lifelong (Witte *et al.* 1988).

Hypoxia is the most common cause of nontraumatic coma. Other causes include meningitis, encephalitis and metabolic encephalopathies (Table 13.3). Posthypoxic coma has a poorer outcome than coma of other causes (Margolis and Shaywitz 1980). Increased ICP lasting more than 48 hours and coma lasting longer than two weeks are indicators of poor prognosis. Seizures and myoclonus have no specific prognostic value but status epilepticus or myoclonicus is a predictor of poor outcome in adults (Krumholz *et al.* 1988). In infants under 1 year of age (Tardieu *et al.* 1987) sequelae may be minor, with mild mental retardation or attention deficit, or major with profound retardation and seizures. Seshia *et al.* (1977, 1983) also found that disability was more likely in children who had been comatose more than four days and in those with deep coma. Kriel *et al.* (1994) studied 25 children with a period of unconsciousness ≥24 hours. Eleven remained in chronic vegetative state, five died, only seven regained some language skills (all had unconsciousness lasting <60 days), and four walked (unconsciousness of <30 days). One patient developed chorea.

In very severe cases of coma of whatever cause, the course may be towards a *persistent vegetative state* (PVS). The term refers to a state of wakefulness without cognition. Affected persons are lacking awareness of self and environment and are unable to

TABLE 13.3
Causes of nontraumatic coma in 104 children*

Cause	n	
Cardiorespiratory arrest	21	
Purulent meningitis	17	
Epilepsy	16	
Poisoning	15	
Barbiturates		5
Alcohol		4
Other		6
Encephalitis	8	
Cerebrovascular accidents	7	
Thrombosis		2
Intracranial haemorrhage		5
Hypoxia–ischaemia**	6	
Hepatic encephalopathy	5	
Gastroenteritis	4	
Others	3	
Unknown	2	
Total	104	

*Data from Seshia *et al.* (1983).
**Without cardiorespiratory arrest.

communicate with others. Sleep–wake cycles are preserved as well as hypothalamic and brainstem autonomic functions (Multisociety Task Force 1994, American Academy of Neurology 1995). The condition should be distinguished from the locked-in syndrome in which awareness is preserved despite complete paralysis, respecting only the extraocular movements (Plum and Posner 1980). The prognosis of PVS is poor, although survival can be very long with good nursing care. Heindl and Laub (1996) found that 84 per cent of 82 children and adolescents with post-traumatic and 56 per cent of 45 with posthypoxic PVS recovered some degree of consciousness but only a few became independent in everyday life. PVS is probably less frequent than in adults in whom it occurs in over 10 per cent of patients with nontraumatic coma (Campbell 1984). Although PVS may be observed with all causes of coma, head trauma and hypoxic–ischaemic encephalopahty, especially after cardiac arrest, are the most frequent aetiologies. The prognosis is poor but significant recovery can be observed until three months of PVS.

Brain death is important to recognize for legal purposes and for organ donation. The usual criteria for brain death are applicable to children (Moshe and Alvarez 1986). Guidelines for the determination of brain death in infants have been published (Ashwal and Schneider 1989) (Table 13.4).

The *treatment* of hypoxic–ischaemic encephalopathy is basically the symptomatic treatment of comatose patients (Bates 1993; Chapters 11, 14). Vital signs should be closely monitored and maintained within reasonably normal values to be a useful guide of treatment (Nussbaum and Galant 1983). Lowering of the ICP allows satisfactory cerebral perfusion (Chapter 14). Steroid treatment for patients admitted following cardiac arrest has not affected the outcome and has therefore no role in the treatment of global brain ischaemia (Grafton and Longstreth 1988). Barbiturate coma has no demonstrated value in the treatment of

TABLE 13.4
Guidelines for the determination of brain death in children*

History: determine the cause of coma to eliminate reversible conditions

Physical examination criteria:

    Coma and apnoea

    Absence of brainstem function:

- Fully dilated pupils in midposition
- Absence of doll's eye and caloric-induced eye movements
- Absence of movement of bulbar musculature, and of corneal, gag, cough, sucking and rooting reflexes
- Absence of respiratory effort with standardized testing for apnoea

    Flaccid tone and absence of spontaneous or induced movements excluding activity mediated at spinal cord level

    Examination should remain consistent for brain death throughout the predetermined period of observation

    Observation period varies with age:

- 7 days to 2 months: two examinations and EEGs 48 hours apart
- 2 months to 1 year: two examinations and EEGs 24 hours apart and/or one examination and an initial EEG showing electrocerebral silence combined with a radionuclide angiogram showing no cerebral blood flow
- Over 1 year: two examinations 12–24 hours apart. EEG and isotope angiography optional

*Ashwal and Schneider (1989).

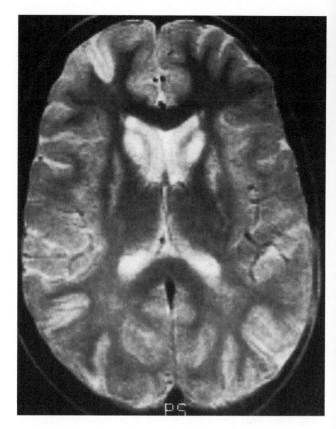

Fig. 13.8. Carbon monoxide poisoning in 11-year-old girl due to faulty heating apparatus. She demonstrated typical two-stage course with secondary deterioration but eventually regained consciousness. She was left with bilateral rigidity and significant loss of intellectual abilities. T_2-weighted MRI scan shows bilateral intense signal from heads of caudate nuclei. Note also two small areas of abnormal signal in right frontal and both parieto-occipital regions.

cardiac arrest (Dearden 1985, Nussbaum and Maggi 1988). Hypothermia as well as resuscitation measures have been reviewed (Conn *et al.* 1979, Frewen *et al.* 1985). Prevention of accidents that can generate acute hypoxia is obviously essential. Prevention of drowning is by educating parents and children about the dangers of water. Other accidents such as choking can be prevented or treated by simple measures (American Academy of Pediatrics 1986).

NEAR-DROWNING

Near-drowning is one of the most common causes of hypoxic accidents, accounting for about 10 per cent of accidental deaths in children (Orlowski 1987, Shaw and Briede 1989). In addition to acute asphyxia, drowning is associated with inhalation of water. In freshwater drowning, fluid enters the circulatory system and haemolysis, hyponatraemia and hypoproteinaemia develop. Ventricular fibrillation is a frequent terminal event.

In saltwater drowning, a different sequence of events is observed. Saltwater is highly irritating for the alveolar membrane because of its hypertonic concentration and induces massive pulmonary oedema. Because of the large quantities of fluid that are drawn from the vascular sector, hypovolaemic shock and hypotension may be seen.

The prognosis is difficult to establish. The overall survival rate is 75–93 per cent, and survival with intact CNS is 58–90 per cent (Shaw and Griede 1989). All patients awake in the emergency room and 90 per cent of those arousable have a normal neurological outcome, whereas this is the case for only 32–55 per cent of those comatose on admission. Initial elevated blood glucose levels are highly predictive of death or PVS (Ashwal *et al.* 1990). Noonan *et al.* (1996) proposed that the prognosis of freshwater near-drowning can be determined by 18 hours and that prolonga-

tion of hospitalization is unnecessary if the child is well after this delay. Quan *et al.* (1990) recently reported that 32 per cent of patients with cardiopulmonary arrest following submersion could be salvaged with prehospital care. Patients with submersion lasting more than nine minutes and those who needed more than 25 minutes of cardiopulmonary resuscitation died or remained severely impaired.

CARBON MONOXIDE POISONING

Carbon monoxide poisoning causes hypoxia both by combining haemoglobin to form carboxyhaemoglobin that dissociates less than haemoglobin thus reducing delivery of oxygen to the tissues and by interfering with the function of cytochrome (Crocker and Walker 1985). Mild intoxication results in headaches, vomiting, sweating and dyspnoea. Severe intoxication results in coma, retinal haemorrhages, convulsions and cardiac irregularities. Poisoning is caused generally by malfunctioning household heating equipment or car exhaust. A delayed posthypoxic encephalopathy is observed in some severe cases (Zagami *et al.* 1993). CT scan often shows a diffuse leukoencephalopathy with extensive demyelination (Fig. 13.8) and/or destructive lesions in the globus pallidus bilaterally in the form of hypodense areas that initially may enhance following injection of contrast (Vieregge et al. 1989).

Residual deficits are frequent after acute CO poisoning and include extrapyramidal manifestations such as choreoathetosis, bradykinesia and tremor, cognitive manifestations such as dementia, dysphasia and dyspraxia, convulsions and peripheral neuropathy (Snyder 1970, Davous et al. 1986).

Treatment consists of removal of the patient from the CO atmosphere, supportive treatment and hyperbaric oxygen (Cregler and Mark 1986).

BURNS AND OTHER INJURIES

BURN ENCEPHALOPATHY
Neurological manifestations occur in 5 per cent (Mohnot et al. 1982) to 14 per cent (Antoon et al. 1972) of burned children. This encephalopathy may begin 48 hours to several weeks after the burn. Only severe burns (30 per cent or more of body surface) are associated with neurological symptoms. These include lethargy or coma, generalized or partial seizures, and sometimes hallucinations and personality changes. In three of 13 children reported by Mohnot et al. (1982) a relapsing course was observed, and in one child there was temporary enlargement of the cerebral ventricles on CT scan. The course is usually favourable and 11 of these children improved to normal. Although neurological disturbances may be seen in children with minor burns and do not have a recognizable cause (Warlow and Hinton 1969), in most cases the encephalopathy can be attributed to hypoxia, hypovolaemia, sepsis or hyponatraemia. Several factors are usually operative. Cortical venous thrombosis was the cause of focal seizures in one child (Antoon et al. 1972). Brain swelling has been found in lethal cases. Hypertension and hypercalcaemia are possible causes. Central pontine myelinolysis has been reported (Winkelman and Galloway 1992). Polyneuropathy is a possible complication of extensive burns (Marquez et al. 1993).

ELECTRICAL INJURIES
Electrical injuries can be produced by household outlets, wires or appliances or by lightning (Silversides 1964, Kotagal et al. 1982, Hawkes and Thorpe 1992). Electrical injuries may be immediately fatal as a result of cardiorespiratory arrest. Prolonged coma may follow the injury and is attributed to cerebral oedema. Temporary paralysis may be observed secondarily and last up to five days (Panse 1970).

Late sequelae include hemiplegia, paraplegia or other focal deficits (Silversides 1964). Long-term memory and behavioural disturbances may last for several months (Kotagal et al. 1982).

Treatment of severe electrical injuries includes removal of the child from the electrical contact in the safest and most expeditious way, respiratory assistance and cardiac massage when necessary.

HEAT-STROKE
Heat-stroke results from prolonged exposure to sunshine, excessive clothing or wrapping, or from intense physical activity under thermal conditions that do not permit elimination of the heat load. Heat-stroke can also be determined pharmacologically, especially following the use of neuroleptic drugs. This malignant neuroleptic syndrome shares many features with malignant hyperthermia induced by anaesthetic agents (Chapter 22) (Moore et al. 1986, Araki et al. 1988, Brower et al. 1989). In drug-induced hyperthermia, heat production results from abnormal muscle contractures (Martin and Swash 1987, Araki et al. 1988), whereas in sunstroke the source of heat is exogenous. In both cases, there is breakdown of the heat-regulating mechanism with extreme elevation of body temperature. The onset of sunstroke is sudden with loss of sweating rapidly followed by loss of consciousness, cyanosis, hyperthermia and often seizures (Malamud et al. 1946). Spinal cord lesions have rarely been found (Delgado et al. 1985).

Treatment of sunstroke involves removal of the patient from the sun, physical means of reducing temperature with ice-packs and fanning, and the administration of intravenous fluids.

Sequelae in the form of cerebellar syndrome may occur (Lefkowitz et al. 1983).

POISONING

Accidental poisoning is common in toddlers and young children 1–4 years of age who ingest chemicals and drugs left within their reach.

A second peak of frequency occurs in adolescents who use drugs for intentional poisoning. About 2000 children die each year from poisoning in the USA, and 6–9 per cent of urban children between 1 and 4 years of age have a clinically significant episode of poisoning. Twenty-five per cent of these children have repeat episodes that may reflect a propensity of the child to such behaviour or to carelessness or unfavourable sociopsychological conditions in the home.

Poisoning is a major diagnostic consideration in any child who presents with disturbances of consciousness, abnormal behaviour, convulsions, involuntary movements or autonomic disturbances, especially when such symptoms appear abruptly. Meadow syndrome (Munchausen by proxy) should be thought of, especially in cases of recurrent episodes compatible with poisoning (Lorber et al. 1980).

Most cases of poisoning are caused by drugs or by common household products such as insecticides, herbicides, and products containing alcohol or hydrocarbons. In adolescents, however, substance abuse has become a significant cause of intoxication, and any unexplained acute change in behaviour in this age range should raise the suspicion of substance abuse.

When faced with such clinical pictures, toxicological analysis is indicated, but careful questioning of the parents or caretakers is always in order as blind routine investigations are of necessity negative in many cases. Moreover, the analysis usually requires several hours, so results are rarely available in time to guide initial treatment. Careful clinical examination with special attention to state of consciousness, eye movements and pupillary abnormalities may bring about important diagnostic clues.

The list of prescription drugs and other chemicals that can produce poisoning is extremely long. Only a few of the most

TABLE 13.5
Poisoning with some drugs: main characteristics and causes

Drug	Neurological manifestations	Non-neurological features
Amphetamines	Depressed consciousness, delirium, agitation, mydriasis, hyperreflexia, choreiform syndrome	Cardiac arrhythmia, hyperpyrexia, hypertension, sweating, tachycardia
Anticonvulsants	See Chapter 16	
Antidepressants (tricyclic)	Agitation, muscle rigidity, seizures, coma, mydriasis	Sweating, tachycardia, hyperpyrexia, vomiting
Antihistamines	Depressed consciousness, hallucinations, tremulousness, mydriasis, convulsions	Dry mouth, urinary retention, hypotension
Barbiturates	Ataxia, coma, absent tendon reflexes, miosis, respiratory depression	Hypothermia, hypotension
Lithium	Nausea, drowsiness, dysarthria, tremor, ataxia	Vomiting, cardiac arrhythmias
Methadone	Depressed consciousness, respiratory depression, miosis	Faecal and urinary retention, hypotension
Phenothiazines	Dystonia, extrapyramidal signs, lethargy	Hypotension
Piperazine	Ataxia and hypotonia	Vomiting, diarrhoea
Salicylates	Depressed consciousness, convulsions, tinnitus	Hyperventilation, hyperpyrexia, hypoglycaemia, metabolic acidosis
Theophylline	Seizures, depressed consciousness	

important causes of poisoning will be considered in this section. The reader is referred to specialized texts for complete information.

PRESCRIPTION DRUGS

A partial list of drugs commonly involved in poisoning, whether accidental or intentional, appears in Table 13.5. A few details are given on some selected agents (see also Mitchell *et al.* 1988).

BARBITURATES

Barbiturates are general depressants. Clinical symptoms include coma, absent deep tendon reflexes and respiratory disturbances. Hypoxia, hypotension and pulmonary complications are frequent. Intoxication is accidental in young children but usually intentional in adolescents, especially in epileptic patients who have easy access to the drug. For that reason, it may be preferable to use anticonvulsant drugs with a greater margin of safety whenever possible.

The diagnosis is easily confirmed by rapid screening tests.

Treatment obeys the general principles of the therapy of poisoning, that is, prevention of further absorption by gastric lavage, supportive care, especially intubation and assisted ventilation, and promotion of elimination by alkalinization of urine. Haemodialysis or peritoneal dialysis are used in the most severe cases (Bismuth 1983). No antidote is known.

PHENOTHIAZINES AND BUTYROPHENONES

These agents can produce depression of consciousness, seizures and hypotension when an overdose is absorbed. Dystonic movements are the most characteristic manifestation (Knight and Roberts 1986). They involve particularly the posterior neck muscles, face and eyes and result in attacks of opisthotonus,

facial and oral dystonia, trismus and oculogyric crises. Prochlorperazine and haloperidol are particularly apt to induce abnormal movements. The onset of symptoms is often delayed for up to 24 hours following administration and the symptoms may fluctuate or appear intermittently.

The diagnosis should be considered in all children with abnormal movements and can be confirmed by a positive urine test. A similar clinical picture is caused by *metoclopramide poisoning* (Low and Goel 1980, Leopold 1984).

Treatment with diphenylhydramine (2 mg/kg) is often dramatically effective.

TRICYCLIC ANTIDEPRESSANTS

Tricyclic antidepressants are one of the major causes of drug toxicity and account for 25 per cent of serious drug toxicity in the USA (Braden *et al.* 1986). Coma, hypotension and anticholinergic effects including dilated pupils, tachycardia, urinary retention and flushing are the usual features. Seizures are frequent and may be repeated to produce status epilepticus. Myocardial depression may also occur and electrocardiographic monitoring is indicated.

PIPERAZINE

Piperazine is a frequently used vermifuge that can induce neurotoxic effects with overdosage and, less commonly, after normal therapeutic doses. Cerebellar ataxia and hypotonia appear a few hours to two days after ingestion and disappear rapidly and completely in all cases. The main problem raised by this 'worm wobble' is to differentiate it from other more severe causes of tremor and cerebellar symptoms (Parsons 1971). True epileptic seizures may also occur (Yohai and Barnett 1989).

478

THEOPHYLLINE AND AMINOPHYLLINE

These agents are used for the treatment of apnoea in newborn infants and of asthma and other pulmonary diseases in older children. In both cases, they may induce epileptic seizures (Gal *et al.* 1980). Seizures usually occur with high serum levels but have been reported with levels within the accepted therapeutic range (Yarnell and Chu 1975). Prolonged status epilepticus precipitated by theophylline/aminophylline may produce neurological sequelae such as hemiplegia and partial epilepsy. Therapeutic agents other than drugs may be responsible for neurotoxicity. Intravenous fat emulsion used for parenteral alimentation may produce a fat overload syndrome with multiple focal neurological deficits and focal seizures (Schulz *et al.* 1994).

HOUSEHOLD POISONS

Most cases of poisoning by household products occur in small children, generally as a result of ingestion. Poisoning rarely occurs after the use of sprays. In most cases the diagnosis is rapidly suspected because the child becomes sick and vomits. However, there are exceptions to this rule and the diagnosis of organophosphate or carbamate poisoning is often suspected late (Zwiener and Ginsburg 1988). A wide variety of products including herbicides, insecticides and cleaning products can be responsible.

Organophosphates and carbamates are chemical agents that inhibit the hydrolysis of the enzyme acetylcholinesterase at various sites within the central and peripheral nervous system. The resulting accumulation of acetylcholine produces stimulation then suppression of cholinergic neurotransmission.

The main clinical features are miosis, excessive salivation, muscle weakness and lethargy which are present in 54–73 per cent of cases, tachycardia and seizures (Zwiener and Ginsburg 1988). Opsoclonus has been observed (Pullicino and Aquilina (1989). Marked hypotonia may be the presenting feature in infants (Wagner and Orwick 1994). The correct diagnosis is often missed. Red blood cell and/or serum cholinesterase activity is less than 50 per cent of the lower limit of normal in most patients but may occasionally be normal. A secondary syndrome develops in many patients which includes profound muscular weakness that may affect the respiratory muscles and often dystonia (Senanayake and Karalliedde 1987). A polyneuropathy may be a later complication.

Treatment with atropine (0.02 mg/kg initial dose that can be repeated several times and increased up to 0.05 mg/kg) should be started before cholinesterase levels are available. Pralidoxime is given to patients with organophosphate poisoning but is unnecessary for those with carbamate poisoning.

Death and neurological sequelae are possible in severe cases (Michotte *et al.* 1989).

Not all poisons produce an acute clinical picture. In the past, chronic toxicity of foods, such as lathyrism, or of contaminants such as ergotism were responsible for major epidemics with prominent neurological manifestations. Some mycotoxins may play a role in the genesis of Reye-like syndrome in some parts of the world, *e.g.* aflatoxins (Chapter 11), and improperly prepared cassava may be responsible for some cases of tropical paraplegia (Chapter 23). Contaminated mussels containing dromoic acid have recently been responsible for severe—and even fatal—neurological toxicity. A toxic encephalopathy with marked tremor has been attributed to mycotoxins.

'SUBSTANCE' ABUSE

Substance abuse is an increasingly frequent problem in the industrialized countries and affects especially adolescents. It is estimated that more than 90 per cent of high school seniors in the USA have used alcohol one or more times and that 6 per cent are daily drinkers. About 6 per cent use marijuana daily (Kulberg 1986). Seventeen per cent of high school seniors had tried cocaine in 1986 as compared with 9 per cent in 1975 (Smith *et al.* 1989).

Alcohol intake may induce depression of the CNS following a phase of disturbed judgement, intellectual function and ataxia. With high doses, coma may result. Accidental ingestion of alcohol by young children may cause marked hypoglycaemia (MacLaren *et al.* 1970).

Marijuana intoxication produces an initial euphoria at low doses. With higher doses, responsiveness is decreased with a marked slowness of responses, and a dream-like state is observed. Depersonalization, sensory disturbances and disorientation may occur with very high doses. Hallucinations may supervene with mixed-drug use but seldom with marijuana alone.

Amphetamine abuse may be responsible for agitation, hyperreflexia, delirium, mania and, uncommonly, convulsions and severely disturbed consciousness. Signs of adrenergic stimulation such as diaphoresis, mydriasis and reflex bradycardia are often present.

Cocaine abuse can lead to cardiac arrhythmias and acute myocardial infarction. Neurological complications include cerebrovascular accidents and subarachnoid haemorrhage. Seizures are relatively common (Cregler and Mark 1986). Euphoria, mydriasis, headache and tachycardia are usual minor effects. Psychiatric complications include dysphoria, paranoid psychosis and severe depression. Psychiatric manifestations may be the presenting features of cocaine abuse. Passive exposure to cocaine ('crack') in young children has been associated with seizures, delirium, obtundation and ataxia (Mott *et al.* 1994).

Organic solvent abuse produces acute toxicity with euphoria. Chronic sequelae may persist following repeated use, with mental deterioration, tremor and ataxia (Hormes *et al.* 1986, Wiedmann *et al.* 1987). Brain atrophy, especially involving the white matter (Rosenberg *et al.* 1988), has been reported.

The *diagnosis* of substance abuse is often difficult. In the absence of a history obtained from friends or family, acute intoxication is easily mistaken for schizophrenia or manic psychosis. Associated features such as cardiac or vegetative disturbances and the state of pupils and of skin may be important clues.

Therapy is variable with the substance used. Supportive care is essential. Sedation and anticonvulsive treatment may be necessary and are effectively obtained with benzodiazepine drugs.

Basic treatment of addiction should always be attempted.

HEAVY METAL POISONING

LEAD POISONING

Plumbism remains a significant problem in childhood, even though the situation may differ between countries because measures to prevent exposure to lead have been implemented at different periods. Putty and paint pigments are the main hazards, but other sources are soft water conveyed in lead pipes, lead-glazed ceramic vessels, the burning of storage battery cases (Dolcourt *et al.* 1981), and atmospheric pollution due to automobile emissions or to the neighbourhood of smelting works and factories making batteries (Rutter 1980). Eye shadows containing lead sulfite applied in some third world countries to children were responsible for cases among immigrants to the United Kingdom.

Lead toxicity is mainly observed in toddlers of low socioeconomic status with pica, or perverted appetite, who ingest lead usually in the form of paint scrapings. Most absorbed lead is tightly bound to growing bone and some is deposited in the hair and nails. Only a small amount enters the brain where it is present mostly in the cortical and central grey matter. Almost all the absorbed lead is eventually excreted in the urine, and the levels of lead in blood and urine are an index of exposure to the toxin. Acceptable levels remain controversial. In the 1960s and '70s a blood level of 30–60 µg/dL was accepted but by 1985 this had decreased to 25 µg/dL, and the present recommendation of the American Academy of Pediatrics (1993) is ≤10 µg/dL. Even low levels below 10–25 µg/dL partially inhibit haem synthesis and may be responsible for cognitive and behavioural problems (Rutter 1980). Levels in excess of 70 µg/dL are an indication for immediate chelation (American Academy of Pediatrics 1993).

Lead inhibits numerous sulfhydryl enzymes and interferes with haem synthesis with resultant inhibition of delta-aminolevulinic acid dehydratase in erythrocytes, a sensitive index of subclinical lead poisoning. Inhibition of coproporphyrin oxidase provokes an increased excretion of coproporphyrin III.

The pathology of lead toxicity is characterized by widespread capillary damage with consequent interstitial brain oedema. Axonal damage is prominent in peripheral nerves whose myelin is not affected.

Clinical features

The early symptoms of lead poisoning are often vague and nonspecific. For several weeks, the child is irritable or apathic and pale, coordination may be poor, and recently acquired skills may regress. There is constipation and poor appetite. Iron deficiency anaemia is almost always present.

Acute encephalopathy is most common between 12 and 36 months of age. Sudden onset of repeated generalized convulsions and altered consciousness interrupts the vague symptoms of the premonitory period. There is evidence of increased ICP with a bulging fontanelle and separation of sutures more commonly than papilloedema. Nuchal rigidity is common. Cerebellar ataxia is occasionally present and optic neuritis is possible with sudden visual loss. A diagnosis of acute meningoencephalitis is frequently entertained. The CSF is generally abnormal with a pleocytosis of 10–60 mononuclear cells/mm3 and a marked elevation of pro-tein, often to 0.8–4 g/L. However, a history of pica, the presence of anaemia with basophilic stippling and the clinical history should lead to the suspicion of plumbism. Plain X-rays of the abdomen may show the presence of opaque material, and X-rays of the bones show dense lead lines at their growing ends. Renal function is frequently abnormal with glycosuria and generalized aminoaciduria. In rare cases, swelling of the cerebellum is prominent and the clinical features mimic those of a posterior fossa tumour (Perelman *et al.* 1993).

Sequelae are frequent, in the form of mental retardation, hemiplegia, quadriplegia and/or severe epilepsies. The mortality rate varies between 5 and 50 per cent.

Peripheral neuropathy is rare in children, whereas it is the commonest sign of toxicity in adults. Children with sickle-cell anaemia, however, may exhibit such a manifestation (Anku and Harris 1974).

Diagnosis

Confirmation of the diagnosis of lead poisoning is best obtained by determination of blood levels. Urine lead determinations may be less reliable than blood levels because of possible renal impairment. Increased coproporphyrin level may be more sensitive. In doubtful cases, a stimulation test with calcium disodium EDTA can be helpful if the excretion increases to greater than 500 mg/L. Determination of ALA dehydratase in erythrocytes is also helpful as the enzyme assay is rapid and requires little blood, and low levels correlate well with exposure to lead (Boeckx *et al.* 1977).

Lead toxicity may not be limited to acute encephalopathy and peripheral neuropathy. A low global IQ and impairment of fine motor coordination and visuomotor performance as well as behavioural disturbances have been noted in children with blood levels of over 10–30µg/dL, in those with increased lead content in hair or deciduous teeth and in those with elevation of free erythrocyte protoporphyrin. Severe epilepsy has also been attributed to subliminal lead intoxication (Fejerman *et al.* 1973). The exact significance of such findings is still in debate (Rutter 1980), and unfavourable socioeconomic factors usually associated with plumbism may be the cause of abnormal behaviour, rather than lead itself (Smith *et al.* 1983). Although a maximum acceptable level of ≤10 µg/dL is currently recommended (American Academy of Pediatrics 1993), the evidence for undesirable effects on cognition and fine motor control at such levels remains controversial (Needleman *et al.* 1990, Bellinger *et al.* 1991, Baghurst *et al.* 1992, Kimbrough *et al.* 1994, Bhattacharya *et al.* 1995, Lucas *et al.* 1996) because of the presence of many sociocultural confounding factors. Identification of children at risk remains difficult (Haan *et al.* 1996), and the indications for screening blood levels are still uncertain. They are currently being revised and universal screening is no longer recommended, although specific attention should be given to children of at-risk groups (Harvey 1997).

Treatment

Therapy of lead poisoning aims at reducing ICP and at removing lead from blood and tissues through increased excretion. Means of reducing ICP are detailed in Chapter 14. Chelation of lead should be started on an emergency basis without awaiting blood test results. Usually 75 mg/kg/d of EDTA (versene) is given in divided doses for five to seven consecutive days, by intravenous route if lead is present in the gastrointestinal tract. Concomitant use of dimercaprol (BAL), 3–5 mg/kg i.m. every four hours for three to five days, is advocated by Chisolm and Barltrop (1979). The indications for treatment of children with slightly elevated blood lead levels are still discussed. Treatment of all children with levels > 10 µg/dL was advised by the US Centers for Disease Control (1991) but is not universally accepted. Kimbrough *et al.* (1994) found the mean blood level of 490 children to be 6.9 µg/dL with 78 (16 per cent) having a level > 10 µg/dL, and favour treatment only for levels ≥ 20 µg/dL.

Supportive treatment and removal of lead in the intestine by small saline enemas is advised. Prevention of further lead absorption implies identification of the source of lead and its elimination.

MERCURY POISONING

Intoxication with metallic mercury is exceptional in children. Intoxication with organic mercury compounds has been responsible for outbreaks caused by ingestion of wheat treated with such components (Amin-Zaki *et al.* 1978) and for Minamata Bay disease, an encephalopathy caused by the consumption of fish contaminated by organic mercury from industrial plants in Japan (Kurland *et al.* 1960).

The neurological manifestations in children include visual impairment, tingling and other sensory disturbances, ataxia, tremor and mental deterioration.

Substantial degrees of recovery are possible if the intoxication is stopped.

It is likely that acrodynia or pink disease, a condition characterized by erythema of the hands and feet, profound hypotonia and weakness, extreme irritability and hyperaesthesia with arterial hypertension and autonomic changes was related to a mercury-induced neuropathy (Cheek 1953). The disorder has disappeared with the abandonment of calomel- and mercury-containing teething powders.

Fetal effects of methylmercury (Marsh *et al.* 1987) are considered in Chapter 1.

THALLIUM POISONING

This is caused by ingestion of thallium-containing insecticides. In nonfatal cases there is peripheral neuropathy affecting the lower limbs, cerebellar ataxia, depressed consciousness, seizures and, sometimes, retrobulbar optic neuropathy and cranial nerve palsies. Depilation is a suggestive feature. Mental retardation and ataxia are common sequelae. Treatment with Prussian blue has been advised (Stevens *et al.* 1974).

ARSENIC POISONING

This also results from ingestion of pesticides and rarely from contaminated well-water. Gastrointestinal symptoms are prominent

in the early stages. Neurological symptoms are those of a sensori-motor peripheral polyneuropathy. Treatment with dimercaprol and penicillamine is advised (Peterson and Rumack 1977).

MANGANESE POISONING

Manganese toxicity may be observed in patients with liver disease and in those receiving total parenteral nutrition. The clinical manifestations include extrapyramidal signs and symptoms. MRI shows high T_1 signal from the basal ganglia (Barron *et al.* 1994).

REFERENCES

Adams, J.H., Mitchell, D.E., Graham, D.I., Doyle, D. (1977) 'Diffuse brain damage of immediate impact type. Its relationship to "primary brain stem damage" in head injury.' *Brain*, **100**, 489–502.
—— Graham, G.I., Murray, L.S., Scott, G. (1982) 'Diffuse axonal injury due to nonmissile head injury in humans: an analysis of 45 cases.' *Annals of Neurology*, **12**, 557–563.
—— Doyle, D., Graham, D.I., *et al.* (1984) 'Diffuse axonal injury in head injuries caused by a fall.' *Lancet*, **2**, 1420–1422.
Adler, J.R., Winston, K.R. (1984) 'Chorea as a manifestation of epidural hematoma.' *Journal of Neurosurgery*, **60**, 856–857.
Agran, P.F., Dunkle, D.E., Winn, D.G. (1985) 'Motor vehicle accident trauma and restraint usage patterns in children less than 4 years of age.' *Pediatrics*, **76**, 382–386.
Aicardi, J., Goutières, F. (1971) 'Les épanchements sous-duraux du nourrisson.' *Archives Françaises de Pédiatrie*, **28**, 233–247.
Alexander, M.P. (1995) 'Mild traumatic brain injury: pathophysiology, natural history, and clinical management.' *Neurology*, **45**, 1253–1260.
Alexander, R., Smith, W., Stevenson, R. (1990) 'Serial Munchausen syndrome by proxy.' *Pediatrics*, **86**, 581–585.
American Academy of Neurology (1995) 'Practice parameters: assessment and management of patients in the persistent neurovegetative state. Report of the Quality Standards Subcommittee.' *Neurology*, **45**, 1015–1018.
American Academy of Pediatrics, Committee on Accident and Poison Prevention (1986) 'Revised first aid for the choking child.' *Pediatrics*, **78**, 177–178.
—— Committee on Environmental Health (1993) 'Lead poisoning: from screening to primary prevention.' *Pediatrics*, **92**, 176–183.
Amin-Zaki, L., Majeed, M.A., Clarkson, T.W., Greenwood, M.R. (1978) 'Methylmercury poisoning in Iraqi children: clinical observations.' *British Medical Journal*, **1**, 613–616.
Anku, V.D., Harris, J.W. (1974) 'Peripheral neuropathy and lead poisoning in a child with sickle-cell anemia.' *Journal of Pediatrics*, **85**, 337–340.
Antoon, A.Y., Volpe, J.J., Crawford, J.D. (1972) 'Burn encephalopathy in children.' *Pediatrics*, **50**, 609–616.
Aoki, N. (1990) 'Chronic subdural hematoma in infancy: clinical analysis of 30 cases in the CT era.' *Journal of Neurosurgery*, **73**, 201–202.
—— Masuzawa, H. (1984) 'Infantile acute subdural hematoma: clinical analysis of 26 cases.' *Journal of Neurosurgery*, **61**, 273–280.
Araki, M., Takagi, A., Higuchi, I., Sugita, H. (1988) 'Neuroleptic malignant syndrome: caffeine contracture of single muscle fibers and muscle pathology.' *Neurology*, **38**, 297–301.
Arnould, G., Lepoire, J., Tridon, P., *et al.* (1966) 'Dyskinésies volitionnelles d'attitude, séquelles de traumatismes graves du tronc cérébral chez l'enfant (à propos de 10 observations).' *Revue Neurologique*, **114**, 150–157.
Ashwal, S., Schneider, S. (1989) 'Brain death in the newborn.' *Pediatrics*, **84**, 429–437.
—— Tomasi, L., Thompson, J. (1990) 'Prognostic implications of hyperglycemia and reduced cerebral blood flow in children with near-drowning.' *Neurology*, **40**, 820–823.
Aubourg, P., Dulac, O., Plouin, P., Diebler, C. (1985) 'Infantile status epilepticus as a complication of 'near-miss' sudden infant death.' *Developmental Medicine and Child Neurology*, **27**, 40–48.
Austin, E.J., Wilkus, R.J., Longstreth, W.T. (1988) 'Etiology and prognosis of alpha coma.' *Neurology*, **38**, 773–777.
Avrahami, E., Tadmor, R., Cohn, D.F. (1989) 'Magnetic resonance imaging in patients with progressive myelopathy following spinal surgery.' *Journal of Neurology, Neurosurgery, and Psychiatry*, **52**, 176–181.

Baghurst, P.A., McMichael, A.J., Wigg, N.R., *et al.* (1992) 'Environmental exposure to lead and children's intelligence at the age of seven years. The Port Pirie cohort study.' *New England Journal of Medicine*, **327**, 1279–1284.

Barlow, C.F. (1984) 'Traumatic headache syndromes.' *In: Headaches and Migraine in Childhood. Clinics in Developmental Medicine No. 91.* London: Spastics International Medical Publications, pp. 181–197.

Barron, T.F., Devenyi, A.G., Mamourian, A.C. (1994) 'Symptomatic manganese neurotoxicity in a patient with chronic liver disease: correlation of clinical symptoms with MRI findings.' *Pediatric Neurology*, **10**, 145–148.

Bates, D. (1993) 'The management of medical coma.' *Journal of Neurology, Neurosurgery, and Psychiatry*, **56**, 589–598.

Bellinger, D., Sloman, J., Leviton, A., *et al.* (1991) 'Low-level lead exposure and children's cognitive function in the preschool years.' *Pediatrics*, **87**, 219–227.

Berger, M.S., Pitts, C.H., Lovely, M., *et al.* (1985) 'Outcome from severe head injury in children and adolescents.' *Journal of Neurosurgery*, **62**, 194–199.

Bhattacharya, A., Shukla, R., Dietrich, K., *et al.* (1995) 'Effect of early lead exposure on children's postural balance.' *Developmental Medicine and Child Neurology*, **37**, 861–878.

Bijur, P.E., Haslum, M., Golding, J. (1990) 'Cognitive and behavioral sequelae of mild head injury in children.' *Pediatrics*, **86**, 337–344.

Billmire, M.E., Myers, P.A. (1985) 'Serious head injury in infants: accident or abuse?' *Pediatrics*, **75**, 340–342.

Bismuth, C. (1983) 'Management of specific poisonings.' *In:* Tinker, J., Rapin, M. (Eds.) *Care of the Critically Ill Patient.* Berlin: Springer Verlag, pp. 811–839.

Blumbergs, P.C., Jones, N.G., North, J.B. (1989) 'Diffuse axonal injury in head trauma.' *Journal of Neurology, Neurosurgery, and Psychiatry*, **52**, 838–841.

Boeckx, R.L., Postl, B., Coodin, F.J. (1977) 'Gasoline sniffing and tetraethyl lead poisoning in children.' *Pediatrics*, **60**, 140–145.

Bonnier, C., Nassogne, M-C., Evrard, P. (1995) 'Outcome and prognosis of whiplash shaken infant syndrome: late consequences after a symptom-free interval.' *Developmental Medicine and Child Neurology*, **37**, 943–956.

Bowers, S.H., Marshall, L.F. (1980) 'Outcome of 200 consecutive cases of severe head injury treated in San Diego County: a prospective analysis.' *Neurosurgery*, **6**, 237–242.

Bracken, M.B., Shepard, M.J., Collins, W.F., *et al.* (1990) 'A randomized, controlled trial of methylprednisolone or naloxone in the treatment of acute spinal-cord injury. Results of the Second National Acute Spinal Cord Injury Study.' *New England Journal of Medicine*, **322**, 1405–1411.

—————— *et al.* (1992) 'Methylprednisolone or naloxone treatment after acute spinal cord injury: 1-year follow-up data.' *Journal of Neurosurgery*, **76**, 23–31.

Braden, N.J., Jackson, J.E., Walson, P.D. (1986) 'Tricyclic antidepressant overdose.' *Pediatric Clinics of North America*, **33**, 287–297.

Brett, E.M., Hoare, R.D., Sheehy, M.P., Marsden, C.D. (1981) 'Progressive hemi-dystonia due to focal basal ganglia lesion after mild head trauma.' *Journal of Neurology, Neurosurgery, and Psychiatry*, **44**, 460. *(Letter.)*

Brierley, J.B., Adams, J.H., Graham, D.I., Simpson, J.A. (1971) 'Neocortical death after cardiac arrest. A clinical, neurophysiological, and neuropathological report of two cases.' *Lancet*, **2**, 560–565.

Brower, R.D., Dreyer, C.F., Kent, T.A. (1989) 'Neuroleptic malignant syndrome in a child treated with metoclopramide for chemotherapy-related nausea.' *Journal of Child Neurology*, **4**, 230–232.

Brown, J.K., Hussain, I.H.M.I. (1991) 'Status epilepticus. II: Treatment.' *Developmental Medicine and Child Neurology*, **33**, 97–109.

—— Minns, R.A. (1993) 'Non-accidental head injury, with particular reference to whiplash shaking injury and medico-legal aspects.' *Developmental Medicine and Child Neurology*, **35**, 849–869.

Bruce, D.A., Alavi, A., Bilaniuk, L., *et al.* (1981) 'Diffuse cerebral swelling following head injuries in children: the syndrome of malignant brain edema.' *Journal of Neurosurgery*, **54**, 170–178.

Bull, M.J., Stroup, K.B. (1985) 'Premature infants in car seats.' *Pediatrics*, **75**, 336–339.

Caffey, J. (1974) 'The whiplash shaken infant syndrome. Manual shaking by the extremities with whiplash-induced intracranial and intraocular bleedings, linked with residual permanent brain damage and mental retardation.' *Pediatrics*, **54**, 396–403.

Campbell, A.G.M. (1984) 'Children in a persistent vegetative state.' *British Medical Journal*, **289**, 1022–1023.

Centers for Disease Control (1991) *Preventing Lead Poisoning in Young Children. A Statement of the Centers for Disease Control.* Atlanta, GA: Centers for Disease Control.

Chadwick, O. (1985) 'Psychological sequelae of head injury in children.' *Developmental Medicine and Child Neurology*, **27**, 72–75.

Chan, K-H., Miller, J.D., Dearden, N.M. (1992) 'Intracranial blood flow velocity after head injury: relationship to severity of injury, time, neurological status and outcome.' *Journal of Neurology, Neurosurgery, and Psychiatry*, **55**, 787–791.

Chang, A., Lugg, M.M., Nebedum, A. (1989) 'Injuries among preschool children enrolled in day-care centers.' *Pediatrics*, **83**, 272–277.

Chaudry, V., Sturgeon, C., Gates, A.J., Myers, G. (1987) 'Symptomatic atlanto-axial dislocation in Down's syndrome.' *Annals of Neurology*, **21**, 606–609.

Cheek, D.B. (1953) 'Pink disease (infantile acrodynia). A physiological approach. (An evaluation of adrenal function and the importance of water and electrolyte metabolism.)' *Journal of Pediatrics*, **42**, 239–260.

Chisolm, J.J., Barltrop, D. (1979) 'Recognition and management of children with increased lead absorption.' *Archives of Disease in Childhood*, **54**, 249–262.

Choi, J-U., Hoffman, H.J., Hendrick, E.B., *et al.* (1986) 'Traumatic infarction of the spinal cord in children.' *Journal of Neurosurgery*, **65**, 608–610.

Choux, M., Lena, G., Genitori, L. (1986) 'Intracranial haematomas.' *In:* Raimondi, A.J., Choux, M., di Rocco, C. (Eds.) *Head Injuries in the Newborn and Infant.* Heidelberg: Springer Verlag, pp. 203–216.

Conn, A.W., Edmonds, J.F., Barker, G.A. (1979) 'Cerebral resuscitation in near-drowning.' *Pediatric Clinics of North America*, **26** (3), 691–701.

Constantinou, J.E.C., Gillis, J., Ouvrier, R.A., Rahilly, P.M. (1989) 'Hypoxic-ischaemic encephalopathy after near miss sudden infant death syndrome.' *Archives of Disease in Childhood*, **64**, 703–708.

Costeff, H., Abraham, E., Brenner, T., *et al.* (1988) 'Late neuropsychologic status after childhood head trauma.' *Brain and Development*, **10**, 371–374.

Craft, A.W., Shaw, D.A., Cartlidge, N.E. (1972) 'Head injuries in children.' *British Medical Journal*, **4**, 200–203.

Cregler, L.L., Mark, H. (1986) 'Medical complications of cocaine abuse.' *New England Journal of Medicine*, **315**, 1495–1500.

Crocker, P.J., Walker, J.S. (1985) 'Pediatric carbon monoxide toxicity.' *Journal of Emergency Medicine*, **3**, 443–448.

Davidson, R.G. (1988) 'Atlantoaxial instability in individuals with Down syndrome: a fresh look at the evidence.' *Pediatrics*, **81**, 857–865.

Davis, P.C. (1995) 'Pediatric spinal diseases.' *In:* Faerber, E.N. (Ed.) *CNS Magnetic Resonance Imaging in Infants and Children. Clinics in Developmental Medicine No. 134.* London: Mac Keith Press, pp. 236–278.

Davis, R.L., Hughes, M., Gubler, K.D., *et al.* (1995) 'The use of cranial CT scans in the triage of pediatric patients with mild head injury.' *Pediatrics*, **95**, 345–349.

Davous, P., Rondot, P., Marion, M.H., Gueguen, B. (1986) 'Severe chorea after acute carbon monoxide poisoning.' *Journal of Neurology, Neurosurgery, and Psychiatry*, **49**, 206–208.

Dearden, N.M. (1985) 'Ischaemic brain.' *Lancet*, **2**, 255–259.

De Meirleir, L.J., Taylor, M.J. (1987) 'Prognostic utility of SEPs in comatose children.' *Pediatric Neurology*, **3**, 78–82.

Delgado, G., Tunon, T., Gallego, J., Villanueva, J.A. (1985) 'Spinal cord lesions in heat stroke.' *Journal of Neurology, Neurosurgery, and Psychiatry*, **48**, 1065–1067.

Deonna, T., Oberson, R. (1974) 'Acute subdural hematoma in the newborn.' *Neuropädiatrie*, **5**, 181–190.

Dershewitz, R.A., Kaye, B.A., Swisher, C.N. (1983) 'Treatment of children with posttraumatic transient loss of consciousness.' *Pediatrics*, **72**, 602–607.

Diamond, L.J., Jaudes, P.K. (1983) 'Child abuse in a cerebral-palsied population.' *Developmental Medicine and Child Neurology*, **25**, 169–174.

Dillon, H., Leopold, R.L. (1961) 'Children and the post-concussion syndrome.' *Journal of the American Medical Association*, **175**, 86–92.

Dolcourt, J.L., Finch, C., Coleman, G.D., *et al.* (1981) 'Hazard of lead exposure in the home from recycled automobile storage batteries.' *Pediatrics*, **68**, 225–230.

Dubowitz, H. (1989) 'Prevention of child maltreatment: what is known.' *Pediatrics*, **83**, 570–577.

Duhaime, A.C., Gennarelli, T.A., Thibault, L.E., *et al.* (1987) 'The shaken baby syndrome: a clinical, pathological and biomedical study.' *Journal of Neurosurgery*, **66**, 409–415.

—— Alario, A.J., Lewander, W.J., *et al.* (1992) 'Head injury in very young children: mechanisms, injury types, and ophthalmologic findings in 100 hospitalized patients younger than 2 years of age.' *Pediatrics*, **90**, 179–185.

Dulac, O., Aicardi, J., Jarriau, P. (1975) 'Hematome épidural intrarachidien après ponction lombaire.' *Archives Françaises de Pédiatrie*, **32**, 77–80.

Dusser, A., Navelet, Y., Devictor, D., Landrieu, P. (1989) 'Short- and long-term prognostic value of the electroencephalogram in children wIth severe head injury.' *Electroencephalography and Clinical Neurophysiology*, **73**, 85–93.

Elmer, E., Gregg, G. (1967) 'Developmental characteristics of abused children.' *Pediatrics*, **40**, 596–602.

Endo, S., Takaku, A., Aihara, H., Suzuki, J. (1980) 'Traumatic cerebral aneurysm associated with widening skull fracture. Report of two infancy cases.' *Child's Brain*, **6**, 131–139.

Eviatar, l., Bergtraum, M., Randez, R.M. (1986) 'Post-traumatic vertigo in children: a diagnostic approach.' *Pediatric Neurology*, **2**, 61–64.

Ewing-Cobbs, L., Miner, M.E., Fletcher, J.M., Levin, H.S. (1989) 'Intellectual, motor, and language sequelae following closed head injury in infants and preschoolers.' *Journal of Pediatric Psychology*, **14**, 531–547.

Fejerman, N., Gimenez, E.R., Vallejo, N.E., Medina, C.S. (1973) 'Lennox's syndrome and lead intoxication.' *Pediatrics*, **52**, 227–234.

Feldman, K.W., Brewer, D.K. (1984) 'Child abuse, cardiopulmonary resuscitation and rib fractures.' *Pediatrics*, **73**, 339–342.

Filley, C.M., Cranberg, L.D., Alexander, M.P., Hart, E.J. (1987) 'Neurobehavioral outcome after closed head injury in childhood and adolescence.' *Archives of Neurology*, **44**, 194–198.

Fitch, S.J., Gerald, B., Magill, H.L., Tonkin, I.L.D. (1985) 'Central nervous system hypoxia in children due to near drowning.' *Radiology*, **156**, 647–650.

Frewen, T.C., Sumabat, W.O., Han, V.K., *et al.* (1985) 'Cerebral resuscitation therapy in pediatric near-drowning.' *Journal of Pediatrics*, **106**, 615–617.

Friede, R. (1989) *Developmental Neuropathology*. Berlin: Springer.

Friedman, R. (1976) 'Child abuse: a review of the psychosocial research.' *In: Four Perspectives on the Status of Child Abuse and Neglect Research.* Washington, DC: National Center on Child Abuse and Neglect, DHEW, pp. 19–23.

Fuld, P.A., Fisher, P. (1977) 'Recovery of intellectual ability after closed head-injury.' *Developmental Medicine and Child Neurology*, **19**, 495–502.

Gahagan, S., Rimsza, M.E. (1991) 'Child abuse or osteogenesis imperfecta: how can we tell?' *Pediatrics*, **88**, 987–992.

Gal, P., Roop, C., Robinson, H., Erkan, V. (1980) 'Theophylline-induced seizures in accidentally overdosed neonates.' *Pediatrics*, **65**, 547–549.

Gentry, L.R., Godersky, J.C., Thompson, B. (1988) 'MR imaging of head trauma: review of the distribution and radiopathologic features of traumatic lesions.' *American Journal of Roentgenology*, **150**, 663–672.

Gerber, C.J., Neil-Dwyer, G., Kennedy, P. (1992) 'Posterior ischaemic optic neuropathy after a spontaneous extradural haematoma.' *Journal of Neurology, Neurosurgery, and Psychiatry*, **55**, 630. *(Letter.)*

Glaser, D., Bentovim, A. (1979) 'Abuse and risk to handicapped and chronically ill children.' *Child Abuse and Neglect*, **3**, 565–575.

Glötzner, F.L., Haubitz, I., Miltner, F., *et al.* (1983) 'Anfallsprophylaxe mit Carbamazepin nach schweren Schädelhirnverletzungen.' *Neurochirurgia*, **26**, 66–79.

Grafton, S.T., Longstreth, W.T. (1988) 'Steroids after cardiac arrest: a retrospective study with concurrent nonrandomized controls.' *Neurology*, **38**, 1315–1316.

Graham, D.I., Lawrence, H.E., Adams, J.H., *et al.* (1987) 'Brain damage in non-missile head injury secondary to high intracranial pressure.' *Neuropathology and Applied Neurobiology*, **13**, 209–217.

—— Ford, I., Hume Adams, J., *et al.* (1989a) 'Fatal head injury in children.' *Journal of Clinical Pathology*, **42**, 18–22.

—— —— —— *et al.* (1989b) 'Ischaemic brain damage is still common in fatal non-missile head injury.' *Journal of Neurology, Neurosurgery, and Psychiatry*, **52**, 346–350.

Grand, W. (1974) 'The significance of post-traumatic status epilepticus in childhood.' *Journal of Neurology, Neurosurgery, and Psychiatry*, **37**, 178–180.

Greenberg, A.D. (1968) 'Atlantoaxial dislocation.' *Brain*, **91**, 655–684.

Guandolo, V. (1985) 'Munchausen syndrome by proxy: an outpatient challenge.' *Pediatrics*, **75**, 526–530.

Guilleminault, C., Faull, K., Miles, L., Van der Hoed, J. (1983) 'Posttraumatic excessive daytime sleepiness: a review of 10 patients.' *Neurology*, **33**, 1584–89.

Gutierrez, F.A., Raimondi, A.J. (1975) 'Acute subdural hematoma in infancy and childhood.' *Child's Brain*, **1**, 269–290.

Haan, M.N., Gerson, M., Zishka, B.A. (1996) 'Identification of children at risk for lead poisoning: an evaluation of routine pediatric blood lead screening in an HMO-insured population.' *Pediatrics*, **97**, 79–83.

Haas, D.C., Lourie, H. (1988) 'Trauma-triggered migraine: an explanation for common neurological attack after mild head injury. Review of the literature.' *Journal of Neurosurgery*, **68**, 181–188.

Hadley, M.N., Zabramski, J.M., Browner, C.M., *et al.* (1988) 'Pediatric spinal trauma. Review of 122 cases of spinal cord and vertebral column injury.' *Journal of Neurosurgery*, **68**, 18–24.

—— Sonntag, V.K.H., Rekate, H.L., Murphy, A. (1989) 'The infant whiplash-shake injury syndrome: a clinical and pathological study.' *Neurosurgery*, **24**, 536–540.

Hahn, Y.S., Chyung, C., Barthel, M.J., *et al.* (1988) 'Head injuries in children under 36 months of age.' *Child's Nervous System*, **4**, 34–40.

Hall, E.D. (1992) 'The neuroprotective pharmacology of methylprednisolone.' *Journal of Neurosurgery*, **76**, 13–22.

Hamilton, M.G., Myles, S.T. (1992) 'Pediatric spinal injury: review of 174 hospital admissions.' *Journal of Neurosurgery*, **77**, 700–704.

Harvey, B. (1997) 'New lead screening guidelines from the Centers for Disease Control and Prevention: How will they affect pediatricians?' *Pediatrics*, **100**, 384–388.

Hawkes, C.H., Thorpe, J.W. (1992) 'Acute polyneuropathy due to lightning injury.' *Journal of Neurology, Neurosurgery, and Psychiatry*, **55**, 388–390.

Healy, G.B. (1982) 'Hearing loss and vertigo secondary to head injury.' *New England Journal of Medicine*, **306**, 1029–1031.

—— Friedman, J.M., Ditroia, J. (1978) 'Ataxia and hearing loss secondary to perilymphatic fistula.' *Pediatrics*, **61**, 238–241.

Heindl, U.T., Laub, M.C. (1996) 'Outcome of persistent vegetative state following hypoxic or traumatic brain injury in children and adolescents.' *Neuropediatrics*, **27**, 94–100.

Helfer, R.E., Slovis, T.L., Black, M. (1977) 'Injuries resulting when small children fall out of bed.' *Pediatrics*, **60**, 533–535.

Hendrick, E.B., Harwood-Nash, D.C.F., Hudson, A.R. (1964) 'Head injuries in children: a survey of 4465 consecutive cases at the Hospital for Sick Children, Toronto, Canada.' *Clinical Neurosurgery*, **11**, 46–65.

Hernansanz, J., Muñoz, F., Rodríguez, D., *et al.* (1984) 'Subdural hematomas of the posterior fossa in normal weight newborns.' *Journal of Neurosurgery*, **61**, 972–974.

Hobbs, C.J. (1984) 'Skull fractures and the diagnosis of abuse.' *Archives of Disease in Childhood*, **59**, 246–252.

Hormes, J.T., Filley, C.M., Rosenberg, N.L. (1986) 'Neurologic sequelae of chronic solvent vapor abuse.' *Neurology*, **36**, 698–702.

Horton, E.J., Goldie, W.D., Baram, T.Z. (1990) 'Rhythmic coma in children.' *Journal of Child Neurology*, **5**, 242–247.

Hosobuchi, Y. (1989) 'Carotid-cavernous fistulas.' *In:* Edwards, M.S.B., Hofman, H.H. (Eds.) *Cerebral Vascular Disease in Children and Adolescents.* Baltimore: Williams & Wilkins, pp. 215–228.

Hukuda, H., Ota, H., Okabe, N., Tazima, K. (1980) 'Traumatic atlantoaxial dislocation causing os odontoideum in infants.' *Spina*, **5**, 207–210.

Ignelzi, R.J., Van der Ark, G.D. (1975) 'Analysis of the treatment of basilar skull fractures with and without antibiotics.' *Journal of Neurosurgery*, **43**, 721–725.

Jenkins, A., Teasdale, G., Hadley, M.D.M., *et al.* (1986) 'Brain lesions detected by magnetic resonance imaging in mild and severe head injuries.' *Lancet*, **2**, 445–446.

Jennett, B. (1973) 'Trauma as a cause of epilepsy in childhood.' *Developmental Medicine and Child Neurology*, **15**, 56–62.

—— Teasdale, G. (1977) 'Aspects of coma after severe head injury.' *Lancet*, **1**, 878–881.

—— —— (1981) *Management of Head Injuries*. Philadelphia: F.A. Davis.

Johnson, M.H., Lee, S.H. (1992) 'Computed tomography of acute cerebral trauma.' *Radiologic Clinics of North America*, **30**, 325–352.

Johnson, S.L.J., Hall, D.M.B. (1992) 'Post-traumatic tremor in head injured children.' *Archives of Disease in Childhood*, **67**, 227–228.

Kaiser, M.C., Petterson, H., Harwood-Nash, D.C (1981) 'CT for trauma of the base of the skull and spine in children.' *Neuroradiology*, **22**, 27–31.

Kalff, R., Kocks, W., Pospiech, J., Grote, W. (1989) 'Clinical outcome after head injury in children.' *Child's Nervous System*, **5**, 156–159.

Kang, J.K., Park, C.K., Kim, M.C., *et al.* (1989) 'Traumatic isolated intracerebral hemorrhage in children.' *Child's Nervous System*, **5**, 303–306.

Katz, D.I., Alexander, M.P., Seliger, G.M., Bellas, D.N. (1989) 'Traumatic basal ganglia hemorrhage: clinicopathologic features and outcome.' *Neurology*, **39**, 897–904.

Kaufmann, P.M., Fletcher, J.M., Levin, H.S., *et al.* (1993) 'Attentional disturbance after pediatric closed head injury.' *Journal of Child Neurology*, **8**, 348–353.

Kawakami, Y., Tamiya, T., Tanimoto, T., *et al.* (1990) 'Nonsurgical treatment of posterior fossa epidural hematoma.' *Pediatric Neurology*, **6**, 112–118.

Kaye, E.M., Herskowitz, J. (1986) 'Transient post-traumatic cortical blindness: brief *v* prolonged syndromes in childhood.' *Journal of Child Neurology*, **1**, 206–210.

Kennard, C., Illingworth, R. (1995) 'Persistent vegetative state.' *Journal of Neurology, Neurosurgery, and Psychiatry*, **59**, 347–348.

Kim, K.S., Hemmati, M., Weinberg, P.E. (1978) 'Computerized tomography in isodense subdural hematoma.' *Radiology*, **128**, 71–74.

Kimbrough, R.D., LeVois, M., Webb, D.R. (1994) 'Management of children with slightly elevated blood lead level.' *Pediatrics*, **93**, 188–191.

Kingsley, D., Till, K., Hoare, R. (1978) 'Growing fractures of the skull.' *Journal of Neurology, Neurosurgery, and Psychiatry*, **41**, 312–318.

Klaus, H.M., Kennel, J.H. (1976) *Maternal Infant Bonding*. Saint Louis: C. Mosby.

Kleiman, P.K. (1987) *Diagnostic Imaging of Child Abuse*. Baltimore: Williams & Wilkins.

Klonoff, H., Clark, C., Klonoff, P.S. (1993) 'Long-term outcome of head injuries: a 23 year follow up study of children with head injuries.' *Journal of Neurology, Neurosurgery, and Psychiatry*, **56**, 410–415.

Knight, M.E., Roberts, R.J. (1986) 'Phenothiazine and butyrophenone intoxication in children.' *Pediatric Clinics of North America*, **33**, 299–309.

Kopjar, B., Wickizer, T. (1996) 'How safe are day care centers? Day care versus home injuries among children in Norway.' *Pediatrics*, **97**, 43–47.

Kotagal, S., Rawlings, C.A., Chen, S-c., *et al.* (1982) 'Neurologic, psychiatric and cardiovascular complications in children struck by lightning.' *Pediatrics*, **70**, 190–192.

Kotwica, Z., Brzezinski, J. (1991) 'Chronic subdural haematoma treated by burr-holes and closed system drainage: personal experience in 131 patients.' *British Journal of Neurosurgery*, **5**, 461–465.

Kravitz, H., Driessen, G., Gomberg, R., Korach, A. (1969) 'Accidental falls from elevated surfaces in infants from birth to one year of age.' *Pediatrics*, **44** (Suppl.), 869–876.

Kriel, R.L., Krach, L.E., Panser, L.A. (1989) 'Closed head injury: comparison of children younger and older than 6 years of age.' *Pediatric Neurology*, **5**, 296–300.

—— —— Luxenberg, M.G., *et al.* (1994) 'Outcome of severe anoxic/ischemic brain injury in children.' *Pediatric Neurology*, **10**, 207–212.

Krumholz, A., Stern, B.J., Weiss, H.D. (1988) 'Outcome from coma after cardiopulmonary resuscitation: relation to seizures and myoclonus.' *Neurology*, **38**, 401–405.

Kulberg, A. (1986) 'Substance abuse: clinical identification and management.' *Pediatric Clinics of North America*, **33**, 325–361.

Kurland, L.T., Faro, S.N., Siedler, H. (1960) 'Minamata disease. The outbreak of a neurologic disorder in Minamata, Japan, and its relationship to the ingestion of seafood contaminated by mercuric compounds.' *World Neurology*, **1**, 370–395.

Kuroiwa, Y., Celesia, G.G. (1980) 'Clinical significance of periodic EEG patterns.' *Archives of Neurology*, **37**, 15–20.

Lahat, E., Livne, M., Barr, J., *et al.* (1994) 'The management of epidural haematomas—surgical versus conservative treatment.' *European Journal of Pediatrics*, **153**, 198–201.

Lambert, S.R., Johnson, T.E., Hoyt, C.S. (1986) 'Optic nerve sheath and retinal hemorrhages associated with the shaken baby syndrome.' *Archives of Ophthalmology*, **104**, 1509–1512.

Lefkowitz, D., Ford, C.S., Rich, C., *et al.* (1983) 'Cerebellar syndrome following neuroleptic induced heat stroke.' *Journal of Neurology, Neurosurgery, and Psychiatry*, **46**, 183–185.

Leggate, J.R.S., Minns, R.A. (1991) 'Intracranial pressure monitoring—current methods.' *In:* Minns, R.A. (Ed.) *Problems of Intracranial Pressure in Childhood. Clinics in Developmental Medicine No. 113/114*. London: Mac Keith Press, pp. 123–140.

Leonidas, J.C., Ting, W., Binkiewicz, A., *et al.* (1982) 'Mild head trauma in children: when is a roentgenogram necessary?' *Pediatrics*, **69**, 139–143.

Leopold, N.A. (1984) 'Prolonged metoclopramide-induced dyskinetic reaction.' *Neurology*, **34**, 238–239.

Leventhal, J.M., Berg, A., Egerter, S.A. (1987) 'Is intrauterine growth retardation a risk factor for child abuse?' *Pediatrics*, **79**, 515–519.

Levin, H.S., Madison, C.F., Bailey, C.B., *et al.* (1983) 'Mutism after closed head injury.' *Archives of Neurology*, **40**, 601–606.

Levy, D.E., Caronna, J.J., Singer, B.H. (1985) 'Predicting outcome from hypoxic–ischemic coma.' *Journal of the American Medical Association*, **253**, 1420–1426.

Lewelt, W., Jenkins, L.W., Miller, J.D. (1980) 'Auroregulation of cerebral blood flow after experimental fluid percussion injury of the brain.' *Journal of Neurosurgery*, **53**, 500–511.

Linssen, W.H.J.P., Praamstra, P., Gabreëls, F.J.M., Rotteveel, J.J. (1990) 'Vascular insufficiency of the cervical cord due to hyperextension of the spina.' *Pediatric Neurology*, **6**, 123–125.

Lorber, J., Reckless, J.P.D., Watson, J.B.G. (1980) 'Nonaccidental poisoning: the clinical diagnosis.' *Archives of Disease in Childhood*, **55**, 643–646.

Low, L.C.K., Goel, K.M. (1980) 'Metoclopramide poisoning in children.' *Archives of Disease in Childhood*, **55**, 310–312.

Lucas, S.R., Sexton, M., Langenberg, P. (1996) 'Relationship between blood lead and nutritional factors in preschool children: a cross-sectional study.' *Pediatrics*, **97**, 74–78.

Lye, R.H., Occleshaw, J.V., Dutton, J. (1981) 'Growing fracture of the skull and the role of computerized tomography.' *Journal of Neurosurgery*, **55**, 470–472.

Mac Keith, R. (1974) 'Speculations on non-accidental injury as a cause of chronic brain disorder.' *Developmental Medicine and Child Neurology*, **16**, 216–218.

MacLaren, N.K., Valman, H.B., Levin, B. (1970) 'Alcohol-induced hypoglycaemia in childhood.' *British Medical Journal*, **1**, 278–280.

Mahoney, W.J., D'Souza, B.J., Haller, J.A., *et al.* (1983) 'Long-term outcome of children with severe head trauma and prolonged coma.' *Pediatrics*, **71**, 756–762.

Maki, Y., Akimoto, H., Enomoto, T. (1988) 'Injuries of basal ganglia following trauma in children.' *Child's Brain*, **7**, 113–123.

Malamud, N., Haymaker, W., Custer, R.P. (1946) 'Headstroke: a clinico-pathologic study of 125 fatal cases.' *Military Surgery*, **99**, 397–407.

Margolis, L.H., Shaywitz, B.A. (1980) 'The outcome of prolonged coma in childhood.' *Pediatrics*, **65**, 477–483.

Marquez, S., Turley, J.J.E., Peters, W.J. (1993) 'Neuropathy in burn patients.' *Brain*, **116**, 471–483.

Marsh, D.O., Clarkson, T.W., Cox, C., *et al.* (1987) 'Fetal methylmercury poisoning: relationship between concentration in single strands of maternal hair and child effects.' *Archives of Neurology*, **44**, 1017–1022.

Martin, D.T., Swash, M. (1987) 'Muscle pathology in the neuroleptic malignant syndrome.' *Journal of Neurology*, **235**, 120–121.

Matson, D.D. (1969) *Neurosurgery of Infancy and Childhood, 2nd Edn.* Springfield: C.C. Thomas.

Matthews, D.S.F., Matthews, J.N.S., Aynsley-Green, A., *et al.* (1995) 'Changes in cerebral oxygen consumption are independent of changes in body oxygen consumption after severe head injury in childhood.' *Journal of Neurology, Neurosurgery, and Psychiatry*, **59**, 359–367.

Mazza, C., Pasqualin, A., Feriotti, G., Da Pian, R. (1982) 'Traumatic extra-dural haematoma in children: experience with 62 cases.' *Acta Neurochirurgica*, **65**, 67–80.

McGuire, T.L., Feldman, K.W. (1989) 'Psychologic morbidity of children subjected to Munchausen syndrome by proxy.' *Pediatrics*, **83**, 289–292.

Meadow, R. (1982) 'Munchausen syndrome by proxy.' *Archives of Disease in Childhood*, **57**, 92–98.

—— (1985) 'Management of Munchausen syndrome by proxy.' *Archives of Disease in Childhood*, **60**, 385–393.

—— (1991) 'Neurological and developmental variants of Munchausen syndrome by proxy.' *Developmental Medicine and Child Neurology*, **33**, 270–272.

Mendelsohn, D.B., Levin, H.S., Harward, H., Bruce, D. (1992) 'Corpus callosum lesions after closed head injury in children: MRI, clinical features and outcome.' *Neuroradiology*, **34**, 384–388.

Meyers, C.A., Levin, H.S., Eisenberg, H.M., Guinto, F.C. (1983) 'Early versus late lateral ventricular enlargement following closed head injury.' *Journal of Neurology, Neurosurgery, and Psychiatry*, **46**, 1092–1097.

Michotte, A., Van Dijck, I., Maes, V., D'Haenen, H. (1989) 'Ataxia as the only delayed neurotoxic manifestation of organophosphate insecticide poisoning.' *European Neurology*, **29**, 23–26.

Miller, J.D. (1992) 'Head injury.' *Journal of Neurology, Neurosurgery, and Psychiatry*, **56**, 440–447.

Miner, M.E., Fletcher, J.M., Ewing-Cobbs, L. (1986) 'Recovery versus outcome after head injury in children.' *In:* Miner, M.E., Wagner, K.A. (Eds.) *Neurotrauma: Treatment, Rehabilitation and Related Issues.* Boston: Butterworths, pp. 233–240.

Minns, R.A. (Ed.) (1991) *Problems of Intracranial Pressure in Childhood. Clinics in Developmental Medicine No. 113/114.* London: Mac Keith Press.

Mitchell, A.A., Lacouture, P.G., Sheehan, J.E., *et al.* (1988) 'Adverse drug reactions in children leading to hospital admission.' *Pediatrics,* **82,** 24–29.

Mizrahi, E.M., Kellaway, P. (1984) 'Cerebral concussion in children: assessment of injury by electroencephalography.' *Pediatrics,* **73,** 419–425.

Mohnot, D., Snead, O.C., Benton, J.W. (1982) 'Burn encephalopathy in children.' *Annals of Neurology,* **12,** 42–47.

Moore, A., O'Donohoe, N.V., Monaghan, H. (1986) 'Neuroleptic malignant syndrome.' *Archives of Disease in Childhood,* **61,** 793–795.

Moshe, S.L., Alvarez, L.A. (1986) 'Diagnosis of brain death in children.' *Journal of Clinical Neurophysiology,* **3,** 239–249.

Mott, S.H., Packer, R.J., Soldin, S.J. (1994) 'Neurologic manifestations of cocaine exposure in childhood.' *Pediatrics,* **93,** 557–560.

Motte, J., Dulac, O., Rousseaux, P., Morville, P. (1985) 'L'hématome extra-dural chez l'enfant de moins d'un an.' *Archives Françaises de Pédiatrie,* **42,** 301–303.

Mueller, C., Koch, S., Toifl, K. (1993) 'Transient bilateral internuclear ophthalmoplegia after minor head-trauma.' *Developmental Medicine and Child Neurology,* **35,** 163–166.

Muizelaar, J.P., Marmarou, A., De Salles, A.F., *et al.* (1989a) 'Cerebral blood flow and metabolism in severely head-injured children. Part I. Relationship with GCS score, outcome, ICP, and PVI.' *Journal of Neurosurgery,* **71,** 63–71.

—— Ward, J.D., Marmarou, A., *et al.* (1989b) 'Cerebral blood flow and metabolism in severely head-injured children. Part II. Autoregulation.' *Journal of Neurosurgery,* **71,** 72–76.

—— Marmarou, A., Young, H.F., *et al.* (1993) 'Improving the outcome of severe head injury with the oxygen radical scavenger polyethylene glycol-conjugated superoxide dismutase: a Phase II trial.' *Journal of Neurosurgery,* **78,** 375–382.

Multi-society Task Force on PVS (1994) 'Medical aspects of the persistent vegetative state.' *New England Journal of Medicine,* **330,** 1499–1508; 1572–1579.

Needleman, H.L., Schell, A., Bellinger, D., *et al.* (1990) 'The long-term effects of exposure to low doses of lead in childhood. An 11 year follow-up report.' *New England Journal of Medicine,* **322,** 83–88.

Newton, C.R.J.C., Kirkham, F.J., Johnston, B., Marsh, K. (1995) 'Interobserver agreement of the assessment of coma scales and brainstem signs in non-traumatic coma.' *Developmental Medicine and Child Neurology,* **37,** 807–813.

Noonan, L., Howrey, R., Ginsburg, C.M. (1996) 'Freshwater submersion injuries in children: a retrospective review of seventy-five hospitalized patients.' *Pediatrics,* **98,** 368–371.

North, A.F. (1976) 'When should a child be in the hospital?' *Pediatrics,* **57,** 540–543.

Nussbaum, E., Galant, S.P. (1983) 'Intracranial pressure monitoring as a guide to prognosis in the nearly drowned, severely comatose child.' *Journal of Pediatrics,* **102,** 215–218.

—— Maggi, J.C. (1988) 'Pentobarbital therapy does not improve neurologic outcome in nearly drowned flaccid–comatose children.' *Pediatrics,* **81,** 630–634.

Obrist, W.D., Langfitt, T.W., Jaggi, J.L., *et al.* (1984) 'Cerebral blood flow and metabolism in comatose patients with acute head injury. Relationship to intacranial hypertension.' *Journal of Neurosurgery,* **61,** 241–253.

O'Doherty, N. (1982) *The Battered Child: Recognition in Primary Care.* London: Baillière Tindall.

Odom, A., Christ, E., Kerr, N., *et al.* (1997) 'Prevalence of retinal hemorrhages in pediatric patients after in-hospital cardiopulmonary resuscitation: a prospective study.' *Pediatrics electronic pages:* http://www.pediatrics.org.cgi/content/full/99/6/e3. (Abstract e3 in *Pediatrics,* **99,** 861–862.)

Oi, S., Matsumoto, S. (1987) 'Post-traumatic hydrocephalus in children. Pathophysiology and classification.' *Journal of Pediatric Neurosciences,* **3,** 133–147.

Oka, H., Kako, M., Matsushima, M., Ando, K. (1977) 'Traumatic spreading depression syndrome. Review of a particular type of head injury in 37 patients.' *Brain,* **100,** 287–298.

Orlowski, J.P. (1987) 'Drowning, near-drowning, and ice-water submersions.' *Pediatric Clinics of North America,* **34,** 75–92.

Pampiglione, G., Chaloner, J., Harden, A., O'Brien, J. (1978) 'Transitory ischemia/anoxia in young children and the prediction of quality of survival.' *Annals of the New York Academy of Sciences,* **315,** 281–291.

Panse, F. (1970) 'Electrical lesions of the nervous system.' *In:* Vinken, P.J., Bruyn, G.W. (Eds.) *Handbook of Clinical Neurology, Vol. 7.* Amsterdam: North-Holland, pp. 344–387.

Parsons, A.C. (1971) 'Piperazine neurotoxicity: "worm wobble".' *British Medical Journal,* **4,** 792.

Paterson, C.R., McAllion, S.J. (1989) 'Osteogenesis imperfecta in the differential diagnosis of child abuse.' *British Medical Journal,* **299,** 1451–1454.

Perelman, S., Hertz-Pannier, L., Hassan, M., Bourrillon, A. (1993) 'Lead encephalopathy mimicking a cerebellar tumor.' *Acta Paediatrica,* **82,** 423–425.

Peterson, R.G., Rumack, B.H. (1977) 'D-penicillamine therapy of acute arsenic poisoning.' *Journal of Pediatrics,* **91,** 661–666.

Plum, F., Posner, J.B. (1980) *The Diagnosis of Stupor and Coma.* Philadelphia: F.A. Davis.

—— Saper, C.B. (1983) 'Abnormal physiology in relation to arousal, newer concepts of autonomic dysfunction.' *In:* Villani, R., Papo, J., Giovanelli, M., *et al.* (Eds.) *Advances in Neurotraumatology.* Amsterdam: Excerpta Medica, pp. 67–73.

Povlishok, J.T., Becker, D.P., Cheng, C.L., Vaughan, G.W. (1983) 'Axonal changes in minor head injury.' *Journal of Neuropathology and Experimental Neurology,* **42,** 225–242.

Pozzati, E., Grossi, L., Padovani, R. (1982) 'Traumatic intracerebellar hematomas.' *Journal of Neurosurgery,* **56,** 691–694.

—— Tognetti, F., Cavallo, M., Acciarri, N. (1989) 'Extradural hematomas of the posterior cranial fossa. Observations on a series of 32 consecutive cases treated after the introduction of computed tomography scanning.' *Surgical Neurology,* **32,** 300–303.

Pueschel, S.M. (1988) 'Atlantoaxial instability and Down syndrome.' *Pediatrics,* **81,** 879–880.

—— Findley, T.W., Furia, J., *et al.* (1987) 'Atlantoaxoidal instability in persons with Down syndrome: roentgenographic, neurologic and somatosensory evoked potential studies.' *Journal of Pediatrics,* **110,** 515–521.

Pullicino, P., Aquilina, J. (1989) 'Opsoclonus in organophosphate poisoning.' *Archives of Neurology,* **46,** 704–705.

Quan, L., Wentz, K.R., Gore, E.J., Copass, M.K. (1990) 'Outcome and predictors of outcome in pediatric submersion victims receiving prehospital care in King County, Washington.' *Pediatrics,* **86,** 586–593.

Rabe, E.F., Flynn, R.E., Dodge, P.R. (1968) 'Subdural collection of fluid in infants and children.' *Neurology,* **18,** 559–570.

Rivara, F.P., Barber, M. (1985) 'Demographic analysis of childhood pedestrian injury.' *Pediatrics,* **76,** 375–381.

Roine, R.O., Somer, H., Kaste, M., *et al.* (1989) 'Neurologic outcome after out-of-hospital cardiac arrest.' *Archives of Neurology,* **46,** 753–756.

Rosenberg, D.A. (1987) 'Web of deceit: a literature review of Munchausen syndrome by proxy.' *Child Abuse and Neglect,* **11,** 547–563.

Rosenberg, N.L., Kleinschmidt-DeMasters, B.K., Davis, K.A., *et al.* (1988) 'Toluene abuse causes diffuse central nervous system white matter changes.' *Archives of Neurology,* **23,** 611–614.

Rosenthal, B.W., Bergman, I. (1989) 'Intracranial injury after moderate head trauma in children.' *Journal of Pediatrics,* **115,** 346–350.

Ruijs, M.B.M., Gabreëls, F.J.M., Keyser, A. (1993) 'The relation between neurological trauma parameters and long-term outcome in children with closed head injury.' *European Journal of Pediatrics,* **152,** 844–847.

—— —— Thijssen, H.O.M. (1994) 'The utility of electroencephalography and cerebral computed tomography in children with mild and moderately severe closed head injuries.' *Neuropediatrics,* **25,** 73–77.

Rutter, M. (1980) 'Raised lead levels and impaired cognitive/behavioural functioning: a review of the evidence.' *Developmental Medicine and Child Neurology,* **22,** Suppl. 42, 1–26.

Sandgrund, A., Gaines, R., Green, A. (1974) 'Child abuse and mental retardation: a problem of cause and effect.' *American Journal of Mental Deficiency,* **79,** 327–330.

Scarfo, G.B., Mariottini, A., Tomaccini, D., Palma, L. (1989) 'Growing skull fractures: progressive evolution of brain damage and effectiveness of surgical treatment.' *Child's Nervous System,* **5,** 163–167.

Schneider, R.C., Cherry, G., Pantek, H. (1954) 'The syndrome of acute central cervical spinal cord injury with special reference to the mechanism involved in hyperextension injuries of the cervical spine.' *Journal of Neurosurgery,* **11,** 546–592.

—— Gosh, H.H., Taren, J.A. (1972) 'Blood vessel trauma following head and neck injuries.' *Clinical Neurosurgery*, **19**, 314–354.

Schor, E.L. (1987) 'Unintentional injuries. Patterns within families.' *American Journal of Diseases of Children*, **141**, 1280–1284.

Schulz, P.E., Weiner, S.P., Haber, L.M., *et al.* (1994) 'Neurological complications from fat emulsion therapy.' *Annals of Neurology*, **35**, 628–630.

Schurch, B., Wichmann, W., Rossier, A.B. (1996) 'Post-traumatic syringomyelia (cystic myelopathy): a prospective study of 449 patients with spinal cord injury.' *Journal of Neurology, Neurosurgery, and Psychiatry*, **60**, 61–67.

Scott-Jupp, R., Marlow, N., Seddon, N., Rosenbloom, L. (1992) 'Rehabilitation and outcome after severe head injury.' *Archives of Disease in Childhood*, **67**, 222–226.

Selbst, S.M., Alexander, D., Ruddy, R. (1987) 'Bicycle-related injuries.' *American Journal of Diseases of Children*, **141**, 140–144.

Senanayake, N., Karalliedde, L. (1987) 'Neurotoxic effects of organophosphorus insecticides. An intermediate syndrome.' *New England Journal of Medicine*, **316**, 761–763.

Seshia, S.S., Seshia, M.M.K., Sachdeva, R.K. (1977) 'Coma in childhood.' *Developmental Medicine and Child Neurology*, **19**, 614–628.

—— Johnston, B., Kasian, G. (1983) 'Non-traumatic coma in childhood: clinical variables in prediction of outcome.' *Developmental Medicine and Child Neurology*, **25**, 493–501.

Sganzerla, E.P., Tomei, G., Guerra, P., *et al.* (1989) 'Clinicoradiological and therapeutic considerations in severe diffuse traumatic brain injury in children.' *Child's Nervous System*, **5**, 168–171.

Shannon, N., Symon, L., Logue, V., *et al.* (1981) 'Clinical features, investigation and treatment of post-traumatic syringomyelia.' *Journal of Neurology, Neurosurgery, and Psychiatry*, **44**, 35–42.

Sharples, P.M., Storey, A., Aynsley-Green, A., Eyre, J.A. (1990) 'Avoidable factors contributing to death of children with head injury.' *British Medical Journal*, **300**, 87–91.

—— Matthews, D.S.F., Eyre, J.A. (1995a) 'Cerebral blood flow and metabolism in children with severe head injuries. Part 2: cerebrovascular resistance and its determinants.' *Journal of Neurology, Neurosurgery, and Psychiatry*, **58**, 153–159.

—— Stuart, A.G., Matthews, D.S.F., *et al.* (1995b) 'Cerebral blood flow and metabolism in children with severe head injuries. Part 1: relation to age, Glasgow coma score, outcome, intracranial pressure, and time after injury.' *Journal of Neurology, Neurosurgery, and Psychiatry*, **58**, 145–152.

Shaw, J.C.L. (1988) 'Copper deficiency and non-accidental injury.' *Archives of Disease in Childhood*, **63**, 448–455.

Shaw, K.N., Briede, C.A. (1989) 'Submersion injuries: drowning and near-drowning.' *Emergency Medicine Clinics of North America*, **7**, 355–370.

Shorvon, S. (1994) *Status Epilepticus. Its Clinical Features and Treatment in Children and Adults*. Cambridge: Cambridge University Press.

Silversides, J. (1964) 'The neurological sequelae of electrical injury.' *Canadian Medical Association Journal*, **91**, 195–197.

Simpson, D., Reilly, P. (1982) 'Pediatric coma scale.' *Lancet*, **2**, 450. *(Letter.)*

Sivakumar, V., Rajshekhar, V., Chandy, M.J. (1994) 'Management of neurosurgical patients with hyponatremia and natriuresis.' *Neurosurgery*, **34**, 269–274.

Sklar, E.M.L., Quencer, R.M., Bowen, B.C., *et al.* (1992) 'Magnetic resonance applications in cerebral injury.' *Radiologic Clinics of North America*, **30**, 353–366.

Smith, D.E., Schwartz, R.H., Martin, D.M. (1989) 'Heavy cocaine use by adolescents.' *Pediatrics*, **83**, 539–542.

Smith, M., Delves, T., Lansdown, R., *et al.* (1983) 'The effects of lead exposure on urban children: the Institute of Child Health/Southampton Study.' *Developmental Medicine and Child Neurology*, **25**, Suppl. 47, 1–54.

Smith, W.P., Batnitzky, S., Renchagary, S.S. (1981) 'Acute isodense subdural hematomas: a problem in anemic patients.' *American Journal of Neuroradiology*, **2**, 37–40.

Snoek, J.W., Minderhould, J.M., Wilmink, J.T. (1984) 'Delayed deterioration following mild head injury in children.' *Brain*, **107**, 15–36.

Snyder, R.D. (1970) 'Carbon monoxide intoxication with peripheral neuropathy.' *Neurology*, **20**, 177–180.

Solomons, G. (1979) 'Child abuse and developmental disabilities.' *Developmental Medicine and Child Neurology*, **21**, 101–106.

Sonntag, V.K.H., Hadley, M.N. (1988) 'Nonoperative management of cervical spine injuries.' *Clinics in Neurosurgery*, **34**, 630–649.

Statham, P.F., Johnston, R.A., Macpherson, P. (1989) 'Delayed deterioration in patients with traumatic frontal contusions.' *Journal of Neurology, Neurosurgery, and Psychiatry*, **52**, 351–354.

Stein, S.C., O'Malley, K.F., Ross, S.E. (1991) 'Is routine computed tomography scanning too expensive for mild head injury?' *Annals of Emergency Medicine*, **20**, 1286–1289.

Stevens, W., van Peteghem, C., Heyndrickx, A., Barbier, F. (1974) 'Eleven cases of thallium intoxication treated with Prussian blue.' *International Journal of Clinical Pharmacology*, **10**, 1–22.

Synek, V.M., Synek, B.J.L. (1984) '"Theta pattern coma', a variant of alpha pattern coma.' *Clinical Electroencephalography*, **15**, 116–121.

Taitz, L.S. (1991) 'Child abuse and metabolic bone disease: are they often confused?' *British Medical Journal*, **302**, 1244.

Tardieu, M., Devictor, D., Wood, C., *et al.* (1987) 'Facteurs pronostiques au cours des hypoxies–ischémies cérébrales du nourrisson de moins de un an.' *Archives Françaises de Pédiatrie*, **44**, 833–838.

Taylor, M.J., Farrell, E.J. (1989) 'Comparison of the prognostic utility of VEPs and SEPs in comatose children.' *Pediatric Neurology*, **5**, 145–150.

Teasdale, G., Jennett, B. (1974) 'Assessment of coma and impaired consciousness. A practical scale.' *Lancet*, **2**, 81–84.

Temkin, N.R., Dikmen, S.S., Wilensky, A.J., *et al.* (1990) 'A randomized, double-blind study of phenytoin for the prevention of post-traumatic seizures.' *New England Journal of Medicine*, **323**, 497–502.

Tomassen, W., Kamphuisen, H.A.C. (1986) 'Alpha coma.' *Journal of the Neurological Sciences*, **76**, 1–11.

Vielvoye, G.J., Peters, A.C., Van Dulken, H. (1982) 'Acute infratentorial traumatic subdural hematoma associated with a torn tentorium cerebelli in a one year old boy.' *Neuroradiology*, **22**, 259–261.

Vieregge, P., Klostermann, W., Blümm, R.G., Borgis, K.J. (1989) 'Carbon monoxide poisoning: clinical, neurophysiological and brain imaging observations in acute disease and follow-up.' *Journal of Neurology*, **236**, 478–481.

Waga, S., Tochioi, H., Sakakura, M. (1979) 'Traumatic cerebral swelling developing within 30 minutes after injury.' *Surgical Neurology*, **11**, 191–193.

Wagner, S.L., Orwick, D.L. (1994) 'Chronic organophosphate exposure associated with transient hypertonia in an infant.' *Pediatrics*, **94**, 94–97.

Ward, J.D., Becker, D.P., Miller, J.D., *et al.* (1985) 'Failure of prophylactic barbiturate coma in the treatment of severe head injury.' *Journal of Neurosurgery*, **62**, 383–388.

Warlow, C.P., Hinton, P. (1969) 'Early neurological disturbances following relatively minor burns in children.' *Lancet*, **2**, 978–982.

Weinberger, L.M., Schmidley, J.W, Schafer, I.A., Raghavan, S. (1994) 'Delayed postanoxic demyelination and arylsulfatase-A pseudodeficiency.' *Neurology*, **44**, 152–154.

West, C.G.H., Kumar, R., Hall, E.L., *et al.* (1989) 'Do children with severe closed head injury benefit from intensive care?' *Journal of Neurology, Neurosurgery, and Psychiatry*, **52**, 1457–1458.

White, R.J., Likavec, M.J. (1992) 'The diagnosis and initial management of head injury.' *New England Journal of Medicine*, **327**, 1507–1511.

Wiedmann, K.D., Power, K.G., Lindsay Wilson, J.T., Hadley, D.M. (1987) 'Recovery from chronic solvent abuse.' *Journal of Neurology, Neurosurgery, and Psychiatry*, **50**, 1712–1713. *(Letter.)*

Willmore, L.J. (1990) 'Post-traumatic epilepsy: cellular mechanisms and implications for treatment.' *Epilepsia*, **31**, Suppl. 3, S67–S73.

Winkelman, M.D., Galloway, P.G. (1992) 'Central nervous system complications of thermal burns. A postmortem study of 139 patients.' *Medicine*, **71**, 271–283.

Witte, O.W., Niedermeyer, E., Arendt, G., Freund, H.J. (1988) 'Post-hypoxic action (intention) myoclonus: a clinico-electroencephalographic study.' *Journal of Neurology*, **235**, 214–218.

Wrightson, P., McGinn, V., Gronwall, D. (1995) 'Mild head injury in preschool children: evidence that it can be associated with a persisting cognitive defect.' *Journal of Neurology, Neurosurgery, and Psychiatry*, **59**, 375–380.

Yarnell, P.R., Chu, N-S. (1975) 'Focal seizures and aminophylline.' *Neurology*, **25**, 819–822.

Yohai, D., Barnett, S.H. (1989) 'Absence and atonic seizures induced by piperazine.' *Pediatric Neurology*, **5**, 393–394.

Young, W. (1992) 'Medical treatments of acute spinal cord injury.' *Journal of Neurology, Neurosurgery, and Psychiatry*, **55**, 635–639.

Zagami, A.S., Lethlean, A.K., Mellick, R. (1993) 'Delayed neurological deterioration following carbon monoxide poisoning: MRI findings.' *Journal of Neurology*, **240**, 113–116.

Zepp, F., Brühl, K., Zimmer, B., Schumacher, R. (1992) 'Battered child syndrome: cerebral ultrasound and CT findings after vigorous shaking.' *Neuropediatrics*, **23**, 188–191.

Zimmerman, R.A., Bilaniuk, L.T., Bruce, D., *et al.* (1979) 'Computed tomography of craniocerebral injury in the abused children.' *Radiology*, **130**, 687–690.

—— Russell, E.J., Yurberg, E., Leeds, N.E. (1982) 'Falx and interhemispheric fissure on axial CT: II. Recognition and differentiation of interhemispheric subarachnoid and subdural hemorrhage.' *American Journal of Neuroradiology*, **3**, 635–642.

Zwiener, R.J., Ginsburg, C.M. (1988) 'Organophosphate and carbamate poisoning in infants and children.' *Pediatrics*, **81**, 121–126.

PART VI

TUMOURS AND VASCULAR DISORDERS

14

TUMOURS OF THE CENTRAL NERVOUS SYSTEM AND OTHER SPACE-OCCUPYING LESIONS

BRAIN TUMOURS

FREQUENCY AND AETIOLOGICAL FACTORS

Tumours of the CNS are the second most common malignancy of childhood, following leukaemia. The overall population incidence of intracranial neoplasms varies between 1 and 5 per 100,000 in different series (see Walker *et al.* 1985). These tumours may be slightly less common in adolescents than in younger children (Gold and Gordis 1979, Diebler and Dulac 1987). However, the location varies with age. In infants, there is a predominance of supratentorial tumours, especially astrocytomas, over infratentorial neoplasms, mainly medulloblastomas and ependymomas in this age group. In children older than 4 years, infratentorial tumours, mostly cerebellar astrocytomas, medulloblastomas and ependymomas, are the most frequent. In children over 8 years of age, Harwood-Nash and Fitz (1976) found a slight majority of supratentorial tumours due to an increase in cerebellar astrocytomas. Overall, supratentorial tumours account for about half the cases (Table 14.1).

The reasons for the changing age distribution of supratentorial and infratentorial tumours, for the predominance of midline tumours and for the predominance of neuroectodermal neoplasms in childhood are poorly understood (Giuffré 1989).

Most tumours of the CNS occur in children without personal or familial predisposing conditions. Several surveys of the incidence of neoplasms in relatives have demonstrated a higher incidence of CNS tumours and of leukaemia but not of other malignancies (see Farwell and Flannery 1984). Cases of familial tumours of various histological types are on record (Battersby *et al.* 1986, Vieregge *et al.* 1987) and may be part of genetic syndromes of predisposition to malignant tumours, *e.g.* Li–Fraumeni syndrome (Santibáñez-Koref *et al.* 1991); neurofibromatosis; some syndromes of multifocal cell proliferation, *e.g.* Turcot syndrome of colonic polyposis and brain tumours (Mastronardi *et al.* 1991); and some immunodeficiency syndromes, *e.g.* Wiskott–Aldrich syndrome and ataxia–telangiectasia, which are genetically transmitted and in which the incidence of tumours is high.

Certain tumours—in particular retinoblastoma, a retinal neoplasm which usually develops in young children below 4 years of age and often metastasizes to the CNS—occur in patients who have a heritable predisposition to the tumour, as well as to a number of other cancers, especially osteosarcoma (Dryja *et al.* 1986, Friend *et al.* 1986). Retinoblastoma occurs in both hereditary (40 per cent of patients) and nonhereditary forms. The hereditary predisposition is determined by mutations at a locus within the q14 band of chromosome 13 (Sparkes *et al.* 1983). Patients with nonhereditary retinoblastoma have somatic mutations at the same genetic locus (Dryja *et al.* 1986). The gene for sensitivity to retinoblastoma normally functions as a dominant suppressor of tumour formation, and alterations or inactivation of both homologous alleles is the key element in the development of a retinoblastoma. This 'anti-oncogene' has also been implicated in the genesis of other cancers, *e.g.* osteosarcoma.

Such a model can apply to other familial (*e.g.* neurofibromatosis) or nonfamilial tumours. Its potential importance is considerable because: (1) detection of an abnormality at the specific locus can allow diagnosis of susceptibility to a tumour in the absence of clinical manifestations (Wiggs *et al.* 1988, Yandell *et al.* 1989); (2) it emphasizes the role of oncogenes in at least certain tumours (Slamon 1987) and establishes a link between chromosomal abnormalities and carcinogenesis. It is known that chromosomal abnormalities are frequently present in tumour cells (*e.g.* abnormalities of chromosome 22 in acoustic schwannomas) and may have a prognostic significance: the presence of clones with specific deletions in human cerebral astrocytomas has been associated with an unfavourable outcome (Kimmel *et al.* 1992). There is evidence that such abnormalities may be associated with transformation of normal proto-oncogenes into oncogenes which are altered or overexpressed versions of their normal proto-oncogene counterparts (Druker *et al.* 1989, Stanbridge 1992, Krontiris 1995). Such a mechanism is at play in Burkitt lymphoma where the primary event is excessive expression of the *c-myc* proto-oncogene, itself resulting from translocation of the *c-myc* gene locus from band 8q24 to chromosome 14. In the process, the *c-myc* gene is deregulated, becoming an oncogene.

TABLE 14.1
Location of brain gliomas in paediatric series*

Series	Total N	Location					
		Supratentorial		Cerebral		Infratentorial	
		n	(%)	n	(%)	n	(%)
Odom *et al.* (1956)	164	74	(45)	34	(21)	90	(55)
French (1959)	273	145	(53)	128	(47)		
Tönnis and Friedmann (1964)	457	228	(50)	105	(23)	229	(50)
Matson (1969)	750	332	(44)	118	(16)	418	(56)
Koos and Miller (1971)	670	337	(50)	189	(28)	333	(50)

*Modified from Koos and Miller (1971).

TABLE 14.2
Classification of brain tumours according to their degree of malignancy*

Grade	Prognosis	Intracerebral tumours	Extracerebral tumours
Grade 1: benign	Favourable with removal only	Gangliocytomas Plexus papillomas Cerebellar astrocytomas Haemangioblastomas Isomorphic pinealomas	Neurinomas Meningiomas Craniopharyngiomas Pituitary adenomas Ventricular ependymomas
Grade 2: semi-benign	Favourable, additional therapy required	Extraventricular ependymomas Isomorphic astrocytomas Anisomorphic pinealomas	Polymorphic pituitary adenomas
Grade 3: semi-malignant	Guarded, additional therapy required	Polymorphic gangliocytomas Polymorphic ependymomas Polymorphic plexus papillomas Polymorphic astrocytomas Polymorphic oligodendrogliomas Polymorphic pinealomas	Polymitotic meningiomas Polymitotic neurinomas
Grade 4: malignant	Poor, but improved with modern treatment	Glioblastomas Medulloblastomas Primitive neuroectodermal tumours (PNETs) Sarcomas	Meningeal sarcomas

*Modified from Zülch and Wechsler (1968).

Amplification of a nucleotide sequence that shares similarities with *c-myc* (*N-myc*) is associated with 20 per cent of neuroblastomas and is associated with rapid tumour progression and poor prognosis. Proto-oncogenes may normally code for growth factors or transcription factors (Druker *et al.* 1989). The role of oncogenes and of cell growth factors in the genesis of brain tumours and the role they play in certain genetically determined cancers is being studied (Whelan *et al.* 1989, Krontiris 1995, Rubnitz and Crist 1997). The proto-oncogene *RET* is closely associated with the occurrence of multiple endocrine neoplasias (Eng 1996). Considerable attention is also given to tumour-suppressor genes whose deletion or mutation can result in the occurrence of several types of malignancy (Stanbridge 1990), especially the *p53* tumour-suppressor gene (Levine 1992) whose absence in the germline is associated with half the cases of Li–Fraumeni syndrome. The genes for types 1 and 2 neurofibromatosis also probably act as tumour suppressors. The gene for NF1 codes for a protein termed neurofibromin which seems to act as a negative regulator of the $p21^{ras}$ oncogene thus preventing aberrant cellular transformation mediated by this oncogene. The gene for NF2 codes for a protein, termed merlin, that also has tumour-suppressive properties (MacCollin 1995). In both cases, the development of tumours may result from a somatic mutation occurring in persons already at severe disadvantage because they have a genetic defect involving an anti-oncogene. In addition to oncogenes and anti-oncogenes, genes of susceptibility to certain cancers (*e.g.* breast cancer) have been recognized and are important in the understanding of malignant processes and potentially in early detection of susceptible persons, which could lead to preventive measures. A possible role of viruses as a causal factor of some brain tumours is suggested by the presence of viral DNA sequences in some choroid plexus papillomas and ependymomas (Bergsagel *et al.* 1992).

GENERAL PATHOLOGY

Tumours of the CNS may have variable grades of malignancy, from very malignant tumours such as neuroblastomas or medulloblastomas to very indolent tumours, some of which may be considered as hamartomas (Russell and Rubinstein 1989). In such cases, the growth of the lesion is *pari passu* with that of the rest of the CNS (*e.g.* hamartomas of the tuber cinereum).

TABLE 14.3
Histological type of 670 paediatric CNS tumours*

Type of tumour	Number of cases		(%)
Neuroepithelial tumours	478		(71.3)
Medulloblastomas[1]	132		(19.7)
Gliomas	265		(39.6)
Cerebellar astrocytomas		115	
Supratentorial astrocytomas		71	
Oligodendrogliomas		10	
Glioblastomas		32	
Others		37	
Paragliomas	81		(12.1)
Ependymomas		61	
Others[2]		20	
Gangliocytomas		0	
Mesodermal tumours	57		(8.5)
Meningiomas		19	
Sarcomas		29	
Others		9	
Ectodermal tumours	68		(10.1)
Craniopharyngiomas		58	
Pituitary adenomas		10	
Congenital and embryonic tumours	9		(1.3)
Unclassified	58		(8.7)

*Data from Koos and Miller (1971).
[1]Including cerebellar medulloblastomas (120), pinealoblastomas and retino-blastomas.
[2]Including choroid plexus papillomas, pinealomas, neurinomas.

There is still much controversy regarding the classification of tumours according to their degree of evolution (Russell and Rubinstein 1989, Heffner 1994). A commonly accepted classification is given in Table 14.2. The histological types and distribution of locations of tumours in childhood series (Pollack 1994) are shown in Tables 14.3 and 14.4.

It is important to note that even malignant CNS tumours rarely metastasize outside the CNS and those which do often metastasize only after operation. Most CNS tumours tend to metastasize along CSF pathways rather than by blood dissemination (Chamberlain 1995). It is also essential to realize that the *clinical* significance of pathological grading may be different from its biological value. A benign tumour that is strategically located so as to be impossible to remove while interfering with essential neural function is 'malignant' for the patient even if histologically benign. Pathological diagnosis may be difficult; in particular, some tumours may consist of histologically different areas. However, Revesz *et al.* (1993) found stereotactic biopsy reliable for diagnosis and grading of adult gliomas.

CLINICAL MANIFESTATIONS
The clinical symptomatology of intracranial tumours is often atypical, with only minor clinical symptoms that may not be different from those in common benign illnesses of children. Therefore, the possibility of a brain neoplasm should always be kept in mind even if it materializes only rarely. Symptoms and signs of brain tumours can result either from increased intracranial pressure (ICP) or from focal effects of the tumour on neighbouring neural structures or from both. The symptoms and signs differ with the location of the tumour and, to a certain extent, its histological nature, these two factors being related (Table 14.4).

INTRACRANIAL HYPERTENSION
Headache due to intracranial hypertension may be intense and relieved by vomiting (Rossi 1989). More often, it is mild and intermittent but its persistence, especially if it occurs in the morning, must always attract the physician's attention. The headache of intracranial tumours, however, may be intermittent and may be relieved by usual analgesic agents. Two-thirds of the patients of Honig and Charney (1982) had headaches that awakened them at night or were present on arising, and these morning headaches characteristically tend to recur repeatedly. Moreover, the children are often less active and generally unwell.

Vomiting is one of the most constant signs of intracranial hypertension. It is usually but not always associated with headaches, even in the case of posterior fossa tumours. Vomiting due to increased pressure is usually unremarkable except by its repetition and persistence and by its frequent morning occurrence. Changes in behaviour and personality are commonly an early manifestation of ICP (Cohen and Duffner 1994). Irritability or lethargy are especially of concern when associated with vomiting and headache.

Papilloedema (Fig. 14.1) is absent in almost half the children with brain tumours (Till 1975), especially those with a rapid course such as medulloblastoma, and in those with supratentorial tumours. The presence of papilloedema makes an intracranial mass highly probable but its absence in no way excludes such a diagnosis. Papilloedema should be distinguished from pseudo-papilloedema, a congenital anomaly consisting of excessive glial proliferation at the disk margins, and from drusen of the optic nerve head which, in children, are usually buried within the disk and produce elevation of the nerve head (Chapter 18). In such cases there is no vascular congestion or vessel tortuosity. In difficult cases, fluorescein fundus angiography may be useful, as the increased capillary network and exudation of fluorescein out of the vessels with persistence of fluorescence at the disk margins seen with papilloedema are absent in congenital disc anomalies (Ammarkrud 1977). Papilloedema is, of course, not specific for brain tumours and can be present with increased ICP of other causes as well as in certain conditions unassociated with intracranial hypertension such as polyradiculoneuritis (Chapter 21) and optic neuritis. In the latter case it is associated with blindness or scotoma.

Less commonly, ICP may be associated with diplopia due to *paralysis of the VIth cranial nerve* which may be unilateral or bilateral and may fluctuate.

Raised ICP from tumours or from other causes is dangerous because it leads to reduction of cerebral blood flow when the point is reached at which perfusion pressure (the difference between mean arterial pressure and intracranial pressure) falls to below 40 mmHg. Reduced blood flow can be responsible for lethargy, coma, and a number of autonomic manifestations generally

TABLE 14.4
TABLE 14.4
Location and histological nature of brain tumours in children*

Location	Incidence (%)	Nature	%
Supratentorial	50.0		
Cerebral hemispheres	27.1	Low-grade astrocytoma	8–20
		Malignant glioma	6–12
		Ependymoma	2–5
		Mixed glioma	1–5
		Oligodendroglioma	1–2
		Ganglioglioma	1–5
		PNET	1–2
		Meningioma	0.5–2
		Other	1–3
Thalamus and basal ganglia	3.1	Astrocytoma	**
		Other + undetermined	**
Midline	18.9		
Chiasma and sella turcica	12.1	Craniopharyngioma	6–9
		Chiasmatic/hypothalamic glioma	4–8
		Pituitary adenomas	0.5–2.5
Pineal region	4.3	Germ-cell tumour	0.5–2
		Parenchymal tumour	0.5–2
		Low-grade glioma	1–2
Ventricular system	4.7	Choroid plexus tumour	1–2
		Meningioma	**
		Colloid cyst	**
Infratentorial	50.0		
Cerebellum + 4th ventricle	39.9	Medulloblastoma	20–25
		Astrocytoma	12–18
		Ependymoma	4–8
		Other	2–5
Brainstem	6.7	Malignant glioma	3–9
		Low-grade astrocytoma	3–6
		Other	2–5
Miscellaneous	3.4		

*Data from Koos and Miller (1971) and Pollack (1994).
**Proportion unknown as often no histology available or cases too rare.

attributed to brain herniation or 'coning'. Such manifestations may occur only transiently during the 'plateau waves' of ICP and disappear with decrease in pressure.

Mass movements of the brain as a result of asymmetrical or unequal expansion of one brain compartment due to the presence of a mass lesion can produce herniation of the cerebellar tonsils through the foramen magnum or of the uncus hippocampi through the tentorial opening. Both types of herniation may induce secondary brainstem dysfunction, most probably by stretching brainstem vessels. Brainstem dysfunction also occurs with global downward movement of the brain substance without lateral herniation. This central syndrome of rostrocaudal deterioration (Plum and Posner 1980) is more common than uncus herniation and reflects progressive bilateral impairment, involving in succession the diencephalon, the midbrain and upper pons, the lower pontine–upper medulla, and finally the medulla with eventual death. Brain displacements can be demonstrated by MRI, and correlations have been proposed between the magnitude of displacements and the patient's level of consciousness (Ropper 1989). The importance of lateral displacement of the

brainstem seems to be better correlated with clinical disturbances than purely downward movement (Reich *et al.* 1993). Fisher (1995) also questioned the importance of downward displacements and suggested that herniation is a late phenomenon and that the clinical phenomena attributed to herniation may remain reversible for relatively long periods.

Herniations also produce localized signs, especially compression of the IIIrd cranial nerve by the uncus against the tentorial edge with unilateral pupillary dilatation. Rarely, there is compression of the posterior cerebral artery with occipital infarction (Lindenberg 1955). Paralysis of the last cranial pairs may occur with foramen magnum herniation, which can also be responsible for neck stiffness in children with posterior fossa tumours. Stiffness may be paroxysmal and associated with a rigid extension of the body, the so-called cerebellar fit of Jackson. A lesser degree of chronic herniation may account for the torticollis which is seen in children with posterior fossa tumours, a sign that mainly occurs with hemispheral cerebellar tumours.

Symptoms and signs or very high ICP threatening brain perfusion, and those of herniation (which are associated) are an

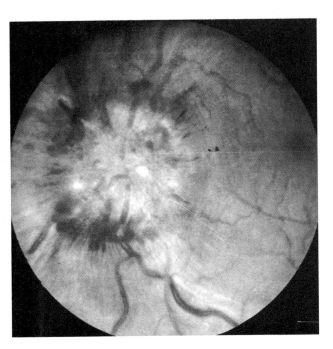

Fig. 14.1. Papilloedema in child with raised intracranial pressure. Optic nerve head protrudes above level of retina, and limits of disc are obscured by oedema and haemorrhage. (Courtesy Prof. J-L. Dufier, Hôpital des Enfants Malades, Paris.)

indication of imminent danger and require emergency treatment (see below).

FOCAL FEATURES

Focal neurological features of brain tumours occur in less than 15 per cent of cases and depend mainly on the location of the tumour. However, some focal signs are of no value in the presence of intracranial hypertension. This applies particularly to paralysis of the abducens nerve, as indicated above, and less commonly to paralysis of the IIIrd nerve. In general, compression of the ocular motor nerve by a herniated uncus produces only involvement of the pupillary fibres with unresponsive mydriasis (Kerr and Hollowell 1964). In rare cases there is complete paralysis of the IIIrd nerve with ptosis and extrinsic muscle deficit (Weiner and Porro 1965). Other false localizing signs include involvement of the IVth (Halpern and Gordon 1981), Vth and VIIth (Davie *et al.* 1992) nerves which is probably due to compression of the nerve fibres stretched over angular bony structures (O'Connell 1978).

Ataxia, which is a major manifestation of cerebellar tumours, may also occur with frontal lesions. In this case, there is often no nystagmus, dysmetria or adiadochokinesis and dysequilibrium is prominent.

DIAGNOSIS

The current diagnostic approach to a suspected brain tumour is primarily neuroimaging. Isotopic brain scan or ultrasound scan have only limited indications.

Plain X-rays of the skull often show widening of sutures, abnormal digital markings and rarefaction of the posterior clinoids and lamina dura in the pituitary fossa. Calcification may be seen in certain tumour types.

These signs are frequently absent, however, and CT scan is the major neuroradiological investigation. MRI is valuable to obtain further definition and is especially helpful in brainstem tumours and in small lesions located close to bony structures, but CT is usually sufficient for the diagnosis and is less expensive and more readily available than MRI. MRI is clearly superior to CT for the diagnosis of posterior fossa tumours because it is free from artefacts, and for certain midline tumours as images can be obtained in various planes, especially sagittal ones. Gadolinium-enhanced MRI is often superior to CT for demonstrating some lesions that may be otherwise difficult to diagnose (Dickman *et al.* 1989, Atlas 1991). MRI is also superior to CT scan for visualizing optic gliomas and CNS lymphomas (Zimmerman *et al.* 1992) and meningeal dissemination (River *et al.* 1996). Comparison between CT and MRI shows that MRI has a greater sensitivity and gives a better definition of the lesions but CT scan has more specificity (Sprung *et al.* 1989). CT should be performed with and without injection of iodine contrast substance except in patients with allergy to iodine. Unenhanced scans may fail to reveal existing tumours, and the presence and degree of enhancement provides information on the nature of the tumour.

Examination of the CSF is usually not essential for the diagnosis. In specific cases study of the CSF may be indicated for cytology, especially for the detection of meningeal spread and in cases of leukaemia, malignant meningeal tumours or melanomas. The presence of malignant cells in the CSF is not uncommon with malignant tumours such as medulloblastomas or ependymomas. However, false negative results are fairly common although false positives are rare (Glass *et al.* 1979). A search for markers (*e.g.* human chorionic gonadotropin or alphafetoprotein) for some types of embryonal tumours is sometimes useful (Edwards *et al.* 1985).

In most cases, the dangers of lumbar puncture probably outweigh the information that can be expected from its performance. How often a lumbar puncture produces or hastens the occurrence of transtentorial herniation is difficult to determine, and the literature presents conflicting opinions in this regard (for review, see Plum and Posner 1980). It is thus safer to refrain from performing lumbar puncture except in cases in which essential information can be expected, *e.g.* when it is necessary to exclude meningitis. The advent of CT scan has considerably simplified this problem and CT should be obtained before lumbar puncture when there is a suspicion of a mass lesion.

The differential diagnosis of brain tumours includes other intracranial mass lesions, hydrocephalus, intracranial haemorrhages and infections. Pseudotumour cerebri, lead encephalopathy and various types of brain oedema are described below.

TREATMENT: GENERAL CONSIDERATIONS

Surgery is generally the primary treatment for brain tumours. Total resection cannot be accomplished in many cases, however, but partial resection is useful to reduce the bulk of the tumour thus permitting destruction of the remaining malignant cells by irradiation and/or chemotherapy (Cohen and Duffner 1989, 1994).

Radiation therapy aims at achieving selective death of tumour cells with as little damage as possible to the surrounding brain. The principles of radiation therapy are beyond the scope of this book: they have been recently reviewed (Kun 1994). Attempts are currently being made at increasing the total dose of radiation delivered to neoplasms while minimizing damage to the surrounding CNS by modifying the schedule of delivery of irradiation. Hyperfractionation, with division of the daily dose into more than one treatment, separated by a minimum of six hours (a time shown to permit most cellular repair) may improve the results of treatment of highly malignant inaccessible tumours (Edwards *et al.* 1988a) and allows administration of a higher total dose. High energy irradiation with photon (X-ray or ^{60}Co), electron or neutron beams (Kun 1994) is variably used. Currently, heavy charged particles (protons and helium ions) and sensitizers to X-rays are being tested.

Chemotherapy (Brecher 1994) is increasingly used in the treatment of tumours. A number of new drugs are available and new treatment protocols are continuously being tried. The basic principles of chemotherapy have been reviewed (Shapiro and Shapiro 1986, Latimer *et al.* 1987, Sposto *et al.* 1989) but new developments are constantly taking place (Chastagner and Olive-Sommelet 1990).

Immunotherapy, using recombinant interferon and other lymphokine products including tumour necrosis factor and interleukin 2 (Allen and Hayes 1994) as well as molecular genetic treatment of cancers (Greenberg 1994) are under intensive investigation. The latter includes attempts at gene substitution to enhance resistance of patients and 'antisense therapy' blocking the expression of particular DNA sequences (Maria *et al.* 1997).

POSTERIOR FOSSA TUMOURS

MEDULLOBLASTOMA
Medulloblastoma accounts for 14–20 per cent of childhood intracranial tumours and is second only to cerebellar astrocytoma among posterior fossa tumours. Medulloblastoma is most frequent in the first decade of life and twice as common in boys as in girls. It has been reported in the neonatal period (Taboada *et al.* 1980).

The medulloblastoma is a malignant and rapidly growing tumour arising from undifferentiated neural cells. Its precise histological classification is difficult because of its primitive nature. It is often regarded as a primitive neuroectodermal tumour (PNET) (Rorke 1983) although this relationship is debated (McLendon and Burger 1987, Cohen and Duffner 1994). The tumour is poorly demarcated from normal tissue. It is very cellular and consists of small round cells without any definite pattern with frequent mitotic figures. Medulloblastomas usually arise from the cerebellar vermis in the region of the roof of the fourth ventricle. They extend toward the dorsum of the cerebellar vermis and into the lumen of the fourth ventricle thus producing hydrocephalus. Metastases along the CSF pathways are frequent, and imaging of the spinal canal is useful to determine the extent

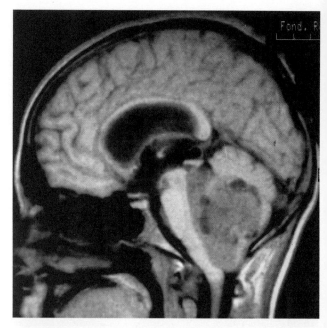

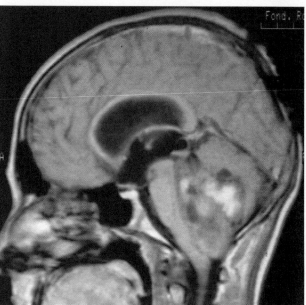

Fig. 14.2. Cerebellar medulloblastoma in 4-year-old boy: MRI, T_1-weighted sequences. *(Top)* Before gadolinium enhancement. Tumour is heterogeneous; brainstem is pushed forward and laminated. *(Bottom)* Gadolinium enhances dorsal part of tumour. (Courtesy Dr D. Renier, Prof J-F. Hirsch, Hôpital des Enfants Malades, Paris.)

of the tumour. Extraneural metastases may occur, especially following surgery (Kleinman *et al.* 1981) and involve preferentially bones and lymph nodes (Duffner and Cohen 1981).

The main *clinical features* are intracranial hypertension and ataxia. Ataxia is usually truncal or affects both lower limbs, with a tendency to fall backwards or forwards. Symptoms of raised ICP are prominent and may be isolated. The whole symptomatology develops rapidly in a few weeks and papilloedema is often lacking. Bilateral pyramidal tract signs may be present. Wasting is often marked. Occasionally, multiple cranial nerve involvement, spinal root pain or even paraplegia are seen early, indicating the presence of metastatic dissemination.

The imaging appearance of medulloblastoma on CT and MRI scans is highly suggestive. The tumour is median and rounded and has, on unenhanced scans, a slightly lower density than the surrounding parenchyma. The density increases homogeneously and markedly on contrast injection. In some cases, small cystic areas, haemorrhages or calcification are visible. Hydrocephalus is virtually constant (Fig. 14.2).

Therapy of medulloblastoma begins with removal of the tumour which should be as complete as possible because total excision followed by radiotherapy of the entire CNS is associated with better outlook than partial removal. Radiotherapy has a major role in extending survival rates. The use of high-energy sources and increased doses accounts for the recent marked increases in survival (Cohen and Duffner 1994). Recommended doses are currently 50–55 Gy to the posterior fossa and 35–40 Gy to the neuroaxis. Chemotherapy alone, with vincristine, cisplatin, nitrosurea or various combinations of alkylating agents such as CCNU, methotrexate, BCNU, cisplatin and prednisone appears to be effective and is indicated for children under 2 years of age, for those with partial excision and for those with brainstem involvement (Kretschmar *et al.* 1989, Packer *et al.* 1994), who can be recognized according to a set of radiological criteria, but not for all patients.

The *outlook* for children with medulloblastomas has improved during the past two decades. Approximately 75 per cent of children treated at major centres are alive by five years and 50 per cent by 10 years (Cohen and Duffner 1994), and adjuvant chemotherapy may increase this figure (Packer *et al.* 1988b). The quality of survival is not always satisfactory and many children are left with mental, behavioural and endocrinological sequelae apparently as a result of radiotherapy. Gross loss of IQ points is observed in 25 per cent of irradiated children less than 7 years old (Packer *et al.* 1989). Thus, the current trend is toward a limitation of the X-ray doses with increased use of chemotherapy.

CEREBELLAR ASTROCYTOMA

Cerebellar astrocytomas are about as frequent as medulloblastomas in children (Cohen and Duffner 1994). They are slowly growing tumours far more benign than astrocytomas of later life, even though exceptional cases of malignant cerebellar astrocytoma are on record (Kleinman *et al.* 1978, Alpers *et al.* 1982) as recurrences of operated astrocytomas. They may involve the vermis, the hemispheres or both locations simultaneously. Approximately half are purely midline tumours. About 80 per cent of cerebellar astrocytomas are cystic tumours with a mural nodule attached to one part of the cyst wall. Solid tumours are less common. There is no correlation between the macroscopic appearance of the tumour and the outcome (Garcia *et al.* 1989). From a microscopic point of view, cerebellar astrocytomas can be divided into a juvenile form, with microcysts, Rosenthal fibres and oligodendroglial fibres, and a diffuse type with high cell density necrosis and calcification (Russell and Rubinstein 1989).

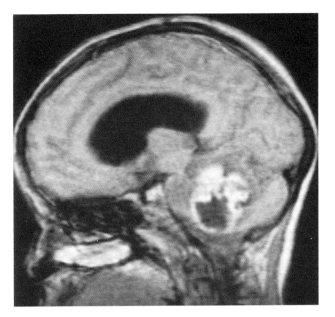

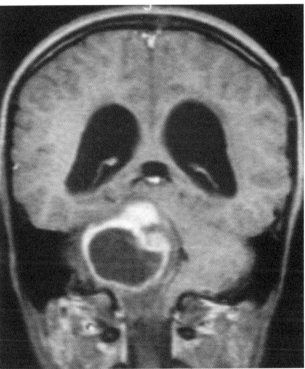

Fig. 14.3. Cystic cerebellar astrocytoma in 7-year-old boy: MRI, T_1-weighted sequences, gadolinium enhanced. *(Top)* Sagittal cut. Solid part of tumour takes up contrast and comprises more than half of tumour in this plane. *(Bottom)* Coronal cut. More classical aspect of a large tumour cyst with mural nodule. (Courtesy Dr D. Renier, Prof. J-F. Hirsch, Hôpital des Enfants Malades, Paris.)

The latter type seems to have a less favourable outcome than the juvenile type (Conway *et al.* 1991). Recurrences can occur with any type when removal has been incomplete (Shapiro and Katz 1983). Recurrences may occur very late and may not supervene even after incomplete removal (Austin and Alvord 1988). The long-term prognosis is usually excellent (Sgouros *et al.* 1995).

The *clinical features* of cerebellar astrocytomas are similar to those of medulloblastomas but the history is usually much longer and the child less ill. Unilateral or asymmetrical cerebellar signs are more common than with medulloblastomas because tumours may be hemispheric or extend asymmetrically to one hemisphere. A head tilt away from the lesion is commonly present. Papilloedema is frequent because of the long course and slow growth of the tumour.

CT and MRI scans (Fig. 14.3) usually show large masses, displacing and compressing the fourth ventricle. Low tumour density is mostly due to oedema. Contrast injection increases density and can delineate a dense nodule, several pericystic nodules or a large irregular tumour surrounded by several cysts. Calcification may be present. Hydrocephalus of a marked degree is the rule (Zimmerman *et al.* 1978).

Treatment is by surgical excision that can be total in many but not all cases. Total resection without further therapy will give a nearly 100 per cent five-year survival (Cohen and Duffner 1994). However, in a significant proportion of patients for whom resection had been reported as 'complete' by the neurosurgeon there was evidence of persistence of tumour tissue by MRI or CT within three days of surgery, so imaging control is required (Schneider *et al.* 1992). Recurrence is much more common after subtotal resection although even in such cases it does not necessarily occur (Austin and Alvord 1988, Garcia *et al.* 1989). Radiotherapy is not indicated in cases of confirmed complete removal. There is still debate about the indication for X-ray therapy with subtotal resection and this is currently being studied (Cohen and Duffner 1994). Seeding of CSF pathways has been reported even with histologically benign tumours but may respond to resection. X-ray treatment is clearly indicated in the uncommon cases of cerebellar glioblastoma (Chamberlain *et al.* 1990). Radiotherapy is not indicated in cases of incomplete removal. Late recurrences can be treated surgically. Postoperative MRI surveillance is essential for early detection of recurrences (Sutton *et al.* 1996).

POSTERIOR FOSSA EPENDYMOMA
Ependymomas most commonly arise from the region of the fourth ventricle. They account for 6–10 per cent of childhood tumours (Dohrman *et al.* 1976, Coulon and Till 1977) and 70 per cent are infratentorial.

Ependymomas of the fourth ventricle arise from the floor, the roof or the recesses of the cavity and obstruct CSF flow. They can extend into the cervical spinal canal and frequently metastasize along the CSF pathways. Malignant or anaplastic ependymomas may be difficult to distinguish from less aggressive types (Russell and Rubinstein 1989).

These are different from the very rare ependymoblastoma that arises from primitive cells. In one large series (Pierre-Kahn *et al.* 1983), 53 per cent of infratentorial ependymomas were malignant, as against 86 per cent of supratentorial ependymomas. With infratentorial ependymomas, meningeal seeding was mainly to the spinal canal and could occur with both benign and malignant tumours (15 per cent *vs* 50 per cent).

Ependymomas have a peak incidence in young children. Sixty per cent of cases occur under age 5. The clinical manifestations do not permit distinction from other posterior fossa tumours although palsies of cranial nerves and neck stiffness are more common with ependymomas.

CT scan shows a midline mass often filling the fourth ventricle and associated with hydrocephalus. Tumour density is usually lower than or similar to that of the brain. Cyst formation and calcification are common, often resulting in mixed attenuation. Enhancement is typically present. MRI better demonstrates extension of the tumour into the cerebellopontine angle, the cisterna magna and cervical spinal canal and is important to determine precisely the volume to irradiate (Cohen and Duffner 1994). Local recurrence, subarachnoid spread and ventricular seeding can be demonstrated by neuroimaging.

Spinal cord seeding is present in 9–15 per cent of cases, more commonly with malignant and infratentorial lesions. It can be detected by gadolinium-enhanced MRI and sometimes by CSF studies (Kovnar *et al.* 1991). However, most treatment failures are related to local recurrences with or without spinal recurrence, and isolated spinal recurrence is extremely rare (Healey *et al.* 1991).

Treatment includes as complete as possible resection, followed by radiotherapy. Resection is virtually always incomplete because the tumour penetrates the brainstem substance. Radiotherapy is therefore indicated but the outlook for ependymomas is poor despite the frequent histological benignity of the tumour. Spinal irradiation is clearly indicated with malignant posterior fossa tumours, in which the risk of seeding is high, and not indicated with low-grade supratentorial lesions. For other cases, the trend is not to give spinal irradiation when systematic gadolinium-enhanced imaging of the spine is normal because of the low incidence of preoperative seeding in a large study (Kovnar *et al.* 1991). Chemotherapy (Cohen and Duffner 1994) has no proven efficacy (Goldwein *et al.* 1990). The overall prognosis is poor. In the large series of Pierre-Kahn *et al.* (1983) the five-year survival rate was 39 per cent and recurrences occurred in 41 per cent of patients. Prognosis is especially poor for children under 2–3 years of age, and only 14 per cent of children under 5 years had a five-year survival (Lyons and Kelly 1991).

Complications of surgery for posterior fossa tumours are common. The development of postoperative hydrocephalus may require shunting that is not usually performed systematically. The syndrome of 'cerebellar mutism' is frequently observed following resection of large tumours (Asamoto *et al.* 1994, van Dongen *et al.* 1994), beginning between a few hours to nine days after operation and lasting from one to 20 weeks (Koh *et al.* 1997). Although recovery is constant, dysarthria may persist for some time after surgery.

Subependymomas are rare in children (Rea *et al.* 1983). They are variously interpreted as hamartomatous growths of subependymal cells or growth of astrocytes or oligoglia. They grow extremely slowly and are often discovered fortuitously as happened in two personal cases. Most are located in the floor of the fourth ventricle. They may occasionally be symptomatic (Scheithauer

1978, Kalfas and Hahn 1986) and then have a poor prognosis. They may also occur supratentorially.

OTHER TUMOURS OF THE CEREBELLUM AND FOURTH VENTRICLE

Cerebellar haemangioblastomas are rare in childhood. Approximately a quarter of the cases are an expression of the von Hippel–Lindau disease (Neumann *et al.* 1989). In such cases the tumour may be discovered at a preclinical stage. Angiography visualizes the solid part of these tumours, most of which are cystic with a single mural nodule. CT scan visualizes the cysts but visualization of the nodule may be possible only after enhancement. Solid tumours are rare and mimic meningiomas (Young and Richardson 1987). MRI with or without gadolinium enhancement gives a characteristic picture with a ring of increased signal surrounding the tumoural cyst (Guhl *et al.* 1987). The prognosis following resection is favourable for cystic tumours.

Dermoid cysts of the posterior fossa are generally midline tumours. They are often associated with a cutaneous fistula piercing the occipital squama. They rarely behave as tumours and are more commonly revealed by meningitis and have therefore been described in Chapter 11. Removal of the cyst and tract is the effective treatment (Berger and Wilson 1985). A shunt may be required when basilar block has resulted from repeated episodes of meningitis.

Cerebellar sarcomas are usually located to one cerebellar hemisphere (Naidich *et al.* 1977). They run a rapid and severe course. On CT scan they present as areas of spontaneously increased density with ill-defined limits which become denser after contrast injection.

Papilloma of the choroid plexus of the fourth ventricle is rare in children in whom most papillomas arise from the lateral ventricle (Pascual-Castroviejo *et al.* 1983).

Melanotic neuroectodermal tumours (progonomas) are rare tumours but occur mainly during the first year of life and are mostly located in the cerebellar vermis and the fourth ventricle. They are usually benign (Cohen *et al.* 1988).

Diffuse gangliocytoma of the cerebellum (Lhermitte–Duclos disease) presents as a diffuse increase in volume of several cerebellar lamellae, usually with a predominance on one cerebellar hemisphere. There is diffuse hypertrophy of both the white and grey matter (Marano *et al.* 1988). MRI gives highly suggestive images of localized lamellar hypertrophy with increased signal on T_2-weighted sequences (Kulkantrakorn *et al.* 1997). Lhermitte–Duclos disease is a feature of the Cowden syndrome of multiple hamartomas in one-third of cases (Vinchon *et al.* 1994).

Neurinoma (schwannoma) of the VIIIth cranial nerve and other tumours of the cerebellopontine angle

Neurinomas of the VIIIth nerve may be unilateral or bilateral. In the latter case, they are usually a component of type 2 neurofibromatosis (Chapter 4). They can be responsible for deafness often associated with facial paralysis and a contralateral cerebellar syndrome. The diagnosis rests on radiological demonstration of

the tumour which is most effectively realised by MRI scan. They may be multiple and may involve the Vth nerve.

Other tumours of the cerebellopontine angle include *epidermoid cysts* (De Souza *et al.* 1969), meningiomas and arachnoid cysts. According to Glasier *et al.* (1993) about 30 per cent of posterior fossa meningiomas show sarcomatous characteristics.

BRAINSTEM TUMOURS

In published series, tumours of the brainstem account for 6.7–16.1 per cent of all intracranial tumours in childhood and for 13.4–28.7 per cent of infratentorial tumours (Berger *et al.* 1983). Pilocytic or fibrillary astrocytomas and glioblastomas are the main histological types in series verified at autopsy or by biopsy. Xanthoastrocytomas, which despite the presence of increased cellularity, pleomorphism and necrosis behave in a benign fashion, are uncommon (Strom and Skullerud 1983, Cohen *et al.* 1986). Brainstem tumours may be entirely contained within the brainstem parenchyma that they infiltrate or they may have an outwardly growing portion that develops into the fourth ventricle or into the cisterns that surround the brainstem (Cohen *et al.* 1986, Stroink *et al.* 1986, Maria *et al.* 1993b). Meningeal seeding, especially spinal, is not rare (Packer *et al.* 1983).

The peak incidence of brainstem gliomas is between 5 and 9 years of age. The clinical presentation is usually with multiple palsies of the VIIth to XIIth cranial nerves and ocular motor palsies. Involvement of the nerves is initially unilateral but often later affects the contralateral side. Cranial nerve paralyses are associated with affectation of the long tracts with unilateral, pyramidal tract or cerebellar signs that eventually become bilateral and may be the first manifestation. Symptoms of increased ICP usually appear late, and papilloedema is often absent. However, vomiting, unassociated with evidence of increased ICP, is often present, probably as a result of direct involvement of brainstem centres, and irritability and emotional instability are common. Paroxysmal facial or nuchal itching may be the presenting sign (Summers and McDonald 1988). Exophytic gliomas developing posteriorly into the fourth ventricle can produce obstructive hydrocephalus (Stroink *et al.* 1986). They are relatively benign tumours, and surgical resection followed by X-ray therapy is indicated (Maria *et al.* 1993a,b). Another subset is represented by tumours of the quadrigeminal plate (Squires *et al.* 1994) and periaqueductal tumours (pencil tumours) that are revealed by hydrocephalus. MRI examination has shown these tumours to be a common cause of aqueductal stenosis (Raffel *et al.* 1989, Valentini *et al.* 1995). They are usually very slow growing or remain static for long periods, so no treatment is required beyond CSF shunting. Such lesions may occur with neurofibromatosis type 1 (Raffel *et al.* 1989). Brainstem tumours are frequent in this disease, mostly involve the medulla and are commonly static or slow growing so that aggressive treatment should be avoided except for CSF diversion when required and careful surveillance (Molloy *et al.* 1995). Other atypical presentations include failure to thrive (Cohen and Duffner 1994), acute hemiplegia, a syndrome of the cerebellopontine angle or psychiatric symptoms.

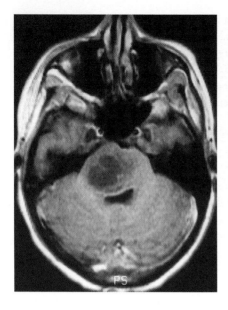
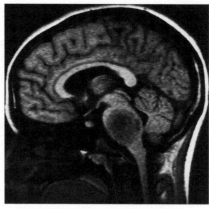
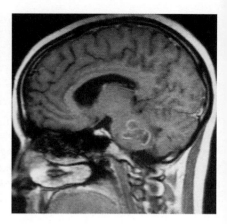

Fig. 14.4. Malignant brainstem astrocytoma. T_1-weighted MRI sequences. *(Left)* Axial cut showing enlarged pons with area of low signal predominating on right side. *(Centre)* Sagittal cut showing grossly enlarged brainstem with posteriorly dislocated fourth ventricle. *(Right)* Gadolinium-enhanced sagittal cut slightly to right of midline showing breakdown of blood–brain barrier. (Courtesy Prof. F. Brunelle, Hôpital des Enfants Malades, Paris.)

The *diagnosis* of brainstem tumour rests on CT or MRI. CT shows increase in the anteroposterior diameter of the brainstem with posterior displacement and compression of the fourth ventricle and of the interpeduncular and peripontine cisterns. The lateral and third ventricles are dilated in a quarter of the cases. In most cases, the density of the brainstem parenchyma is altered. Isodense tumours may appear only with enhancement and may have a more favourable outcome than hypodense tumours (Cohen and Duffner 1994). Conversely, hypodense lesions and ring enhancement are associated with a poor outlook and are mainly associated with malignant anaplastic or glioblastomatous tumours (Cohen *et al.* 1986, Stroink *et al.* 1986), although other authors have not found precise correlation between CT appearance and histological features (*e.g.* Berger *et al.* 1983). Outward expansion of the tumour seems to be more common with relatively benign gliomas. Calcification and cysts within the tumour have also been associated with a relatively benign prognosis (Cohen *et al.* 1986). MRI (Fig. 14.4) gives precise indications of the vertical extension of the tumour and better defines its exophytic expansion (Zimmerman *et al.* 1992), and has thus become the procedure of choice. Intraaxial tumours of the cervicomedullary junction constitute an interesting subset of brainstem gliomas of relatively benign prognosis (Epstein 1987). Robertson *et al.* (1994) studied 17 such cases (10 astrocytomas, one mixed glioma, four gangliogliomas and two anaplastic gangliogliomas). Clinical features included dysphonia, dysphagia, abnormal breathing, vomiting and quadriplegia in four children. Radical excision gave very good results with a 100 per cent survival rate for the 11 patients newly diagnosed.

The *differential diagnosis* of brainstem neoplasms may be difficult. It includes brainstem encephalitis that may give rise to swelling of the stem and changes in density or signal, multiple sclerosis, haematomas or vascular malformations, parasitic cysts and tuberculomas. The last of these should always be thought of in migrants from developing countries. Behçet disease has been responsible for midbrain mass (Kermode *et al.* 1989). Other mass lesions of that region such as enterogenic cysts (Van der Wal and Troost 1988) or epidermoid cysts are exceptional and their images are very different from those of gliomas.

The *treatment* of brainstem gliomas is based on radiotherapy with associated chemotherapy in some cases. The survival rate varies between 5 and 40 per cent (Berger *et al.* 1983, Cohen and Duffner 1994) and does not appear to be evenly distributed. Several authors have separated cases of brainstem tumours into two groups, one of which has a better long-term outlook for survival (Cohen *et al.* 1986, Stroink *et al.* 1986). CT appearance may help to make a prognosis (see above) but the histological appearance is poorly correlated with the outlook (Stroink *et al.* 1986), so that biopsy may not be indicated. However, experience suggests that stereotactic biopsy is helpful to predict the prognosis and guide therapy (Giunta *et al.* 1989). Drainage of a cystic tumour may be associated with rapid improvement, and some surgeons tend to operate on exophytic tumours (Pierre-Kahn *et al.* 1993, Pollack *et al.* 1993) in order to reduce their bulk and improve the efficiency of other therapies. Hyperfractionated radiotherapy is being tried in the treatment of brainstem gliomas (Packer *et al.* 1990). Doses of 60–72 Gy are currently recommended with this technique that may improve currently poor results (Cohen and Duffner 1994). The use of cisplatin as a radiosensitizer is currently being studied.

TUMOURS OF THE MIDLINE AND BASE OF THE BRAIN

Several pathologically diverse tumours arise from the midline region of the brain or from nearby structures such as cranial nerves, hypophysis, epiphysis and residua of the notochord. Craniopharyngioma is the most common midline tumour, followed by optic glioma. Most midline tumours may produce increased ICP through the development of hydrocephalus, visual impairment and endocrine and metabolic abnormalities.

CRANIOPHARYNGIOMA

Craniopharyngiomas arise from small cellular rests that are considered to represent remnants of the embryonic Rathke pouch. They represent about 50 per cent of midline tumours and 6–10 per cent of all tumours in infancy and childhood (Koos and Miller 1971, Richmond and Wilson 1980). They can develop either in the suprasellar region or in both suprasellar and intrasellar regions. Purely intrasellar craniopharyngiomas are rare in children. Large tumours are partly or completely cystic. The microscopic appearance is variable with squamous epithelium that may be thickened or degenerate with formation of microcysts. Calcification is a frequent and important feature of craniopharyngiomas. Craniopharyngiomas may manifest at any age from the neonatal period (Helmke *et al.* 1984) to adulthood.

The *clinical features* of craniopharyngioma are the result of endocrine abnormalities, increased ICP secondary to hydrocephalus, or interference with neighbouring structures, especially the optic pathways. Delayed growth resulting from growth hormone deficiency is a common feature (Richmond and Wilson 1980) although it is often found only in retrospect and may be absent in about half the cases. When hypothyroidism is present, excess weight gain, fatiguability and declining school performance are common. Diabetes insipidus results in excessive thirst and frequent urination. Less commonly, disturbances in fluid and electrolyte balance or abnormalities of autonomic function are present.

Symptoms and signs of increased pressure and visual disturbances are present at the time of diagnosis in a majority of patients and indeed are the most frequent initial manifestation in children (Cohen and Duffner 1994). They include visual complaints, blurred consciousness, vomiting, bitemporal hemianopia, nystagmus and optic atrophy (Keraly *et al.* 1986). Papilloedema is less common. Ataxia is occasionally observed (Richmond and Wilson 1980), wrongly suggesting the diagnosis of a posterior fossa tumour. Somnolence, apathy and change of mood are not infrequently present in patients without increased pressure. Unilateral loss of vision may supervene rapidly mimicking optic neuritis. Focal neurological signs are uncommon.

Skull X-rays regularly demonstrate erosion of the dorsum sellae or enlargement of the sella turcica or both. CT scan (Fig. 14.5) shows, in most cases, a cystic lesion which is suprasellar or intrasellar and suprasellar. The suprasellar expansion may be quite large, compressing the third ventricle and reaching the septum pellucidum or even the corpus callosum. Retrosellar expansions are less frequent. The density of the tumour before contrast injection is heterogeneous. Calcification is present in 80 per cent of cases. In rare cases, the tumour may be difficult to visualize (Volpe *et al.* 1978) or have an unusually dense appearance and extension (Nagasawa *et al.* 1980). MRI is more precise than CT scan, and medial sagittal cuts are particularly valuable for defining the relationship of the tumour to the optic nerve, chiasm, hypothalamus and brainstem, for the detection of small tumour remnants after surgery, and for exploration of the content of the sella turcica which is difficult to assess by CT because of the presence of bone artefacts.

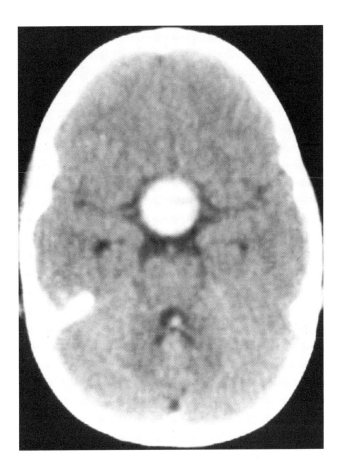

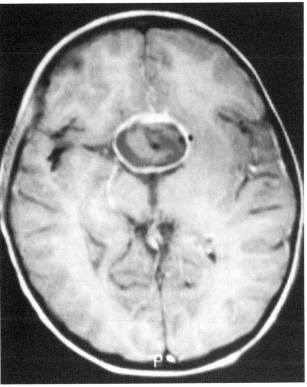

Fig. 14.5. Craniopharyngioma. *(Top)* Enhanced CT scan shows rounded cystic formation within prepeduncular cistern. Contrast is taken up strongly by capsule of cyst. *(Bottom)* T₁-weighted gadolinium-enhanced MRI shows that cyst wall takes up contrast, and content of cyst is heterogeneous. (Courtesy Prof. F. Brunelle, Hôpital des Enfants Malades, Paris.)

Endocrinological examination reveals a deficiency of growth hormone in approximately half the patients preoperatively (Newman *et al.* 1981). Gonadotropic hormones are also low in about 50 per cent of pubertal patients. Deficits in thyrotropin (TSH) and adrenocorticotropin (ACTH), and diabetes insipidus are less common in nonoperated patients but appear in most cases following operation (Fischer *et al.* 1985, Pierre-Kahn *et al.* 1988).

The diagnosis of craniopharyngioma is usually easy but is still often missed for surprisingly long periods. Once the diagnosis is suspected, other tumours of the region should be excluded (see below). Rarely does a craniopharyngioma produce the diencephalic cachexia syndrome.

Agreement is universal on the need for surgery but the extent of surgery remains controversial. Total removal is advocated by some surgeons and good results have been reported (Pierre-Kahn *et al.* 1988, Yasargil *et al.* 1990) but the mortality rate remains high (45.5 per cent) in retrochiasmatic craniopharyngiomas. Only partial removal is possible for many of the tumours. In such cases, postoperative irradiation combined with partial excision results in a dramatic reduction of the recurrence rate, from 75 to 30 per cent (Amacher 1980), and is generally advised (Fischer *et al.* 1985, Keraly *et al.* 1986, Pierre-Kahn *et al.* 1988, Fischer *et al.* 1990). In fact, the recurrence rate is not different from that obtained with attempted 'complete' removal and the operative risk is much lower (Regine and Kramer 1992, Rajan *et al.* 1993). The recommended dose for children is usually 50 Gy. Irradiation, however, may produce deafness, lowering of IQ levels, endocrinological disturbances and even neurological sequelae, although Cavazzuti *et al.* (1983) found that such sequelae were not common following X-ray treatment. It is probably best, for young children with only partial resection, to delay irradiation as much as possible, because of the high sensitivity of the young brain to ionizing agents.

Following surgical treatment, there is usually exacerbation of endocrine disturbances with the development of diabetes insipidus in three-quarters of the patients and frequent deficiency of TSH and ACTH. However, a paradoxical growth spurt following surgery has been reported (Cohen and Duffner 1994).

Such endocrine disturbances pose therapeutic problems which require special attention (Lyen and Crant 1982, Sorva *et al.* 1988). A variety of psychological deficits are often present (Cavazzuti *et al.* 1983, Fischer *et al.* 1985). Epilepsy is present in 11 per cent of patients (Pierre-Kahn *et al.* 1988) and may be intractable medically and require surgical treatment. In my experience, it has been related to frontal lobe lesions in most cases. The role of irradiation in the genesis of epilepsy and of cognitive deficits may be important. Patients not submitted to radiotherapy may have a higher mean IQ than those who were irradiated (Pierre-Kahn *et al.* 1988).

VISUAL PATHWAY GLIOMAS
Visual pathway tumours represent 3–5 per cent of primary intracranial neoplasms in children (Duffner and Cohen 1988). Approximately 26–36 per cent involve the prechiasmatic portion (optic nerves) and 64–74 per cent involve the chiasm

and tracts with or without involvement of the anterior third ventricle (Tenny *et al.* 1982). Ninety per cent of optic gliomas occur in children (Chutorian 1988). The tumours are typical pilocytic astrocytomas consisting of compact fibrillar areas with Rosenthal fibres and looser areas characterized by microcysts, or mixed astrocytomas and oligodendrogliomas (Rubinstein 1988). Malignant changes are exceptional.

From 14 to 36 per cent of visual pathway gliomas occur in children with neurofibromatosis type 1. The frequency of neurofibromatosis may be even higher in patients with isolated optic gliomas and may approach 100 per cent in the case of bilateral gliomas (Duffner and Cohen 1988, Packer *et al.* 1988a). Optic gliomas in children with NF1 tend to affect only the optic nerves more often than other optic nerve tumours. Isolated tumours of the optic nerve were found only in NF1 patients by Listernick *et al.* (1995). Screening systematically all patients with neurofibromatosis for optic gliomas will certainly increase the apparent frequency of these tumours. However, current recommendations based on symptomatic tumours may not be applicable to gliomas discovered by systematic investigation in patients with neurofibromatosis. According to some investigators, optic nerve gliomas that occur in patients with neurofibromatosis may differ from those in other patients in having a circumferential perineural growth in the subarachnoid space around the nerve which is relatively untouched or expanded but not invaded (Seiff *et al.* 1987).

The *clinical presentation* of optic pathway gliomas depends on the anatomical location of the lesion. Anterior lesions, confined to the optic nerve anterior to the chiasm, usually present with proptosis which is often a late sign and monocular visual loss developing over 6–12 months. This may easily be missed in children who adjust to gradual loss of vision (Appleton and Jan 1989). Papilloedema or optic atrophy are present on fundus examination.

In children with posterior lesions, involving the optic chiasm or extending further back along the optic radiations, loss of visual acuity is the common presentation. It is often asymmetrical or even unilateral and may be accompanied by nystagmus which is often pendular and should not be mistaken for congenital nystagmus. Sudden visual loss simulating optic neuritis may occur. Field cuts are variable. A symmetrical bitemporal hemianopia is less common than irregular, asymmetrical field defects or a central scotoma with contralateral impairment of the visual field. Fundoscopic examination generally shows optic atrophy, although papilloedema is occasionally noted. Papilloedema and nystagmus suggest chiasmatic involvement, whereas blurred discs with visual loss suggest an intraorbital lesion. With large lesions, there may be compression of the third ventricle with hydrocephalus, and involvement of the hypothalamus may give rise to diencephalic cachexia (Gunesson-Nordin *et al.* 1982, Davis *et al.* 1983) or to endocrine disturbances such as precocious puberty, diabetes insipidus or obesity. Comparison of groups of children with optic gliomas with and without NF1 has shown that precocious puberty was more common in NF1 patients whereas hydrocephalus was present only in non-neurofibromatosis patients (Listernick *et al.* 1995).

502

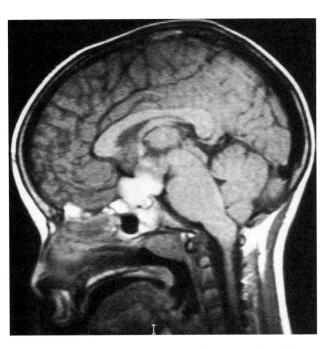

Fig. 14.6. Glioma of the optic chiasm. T₁-weighted MRI with gadolinium enhancement. The foremost part of the mass strongly takes up gadolinium. The tumour extends posteriorly into floor of third ventricle and upper brainstem. (Courtesy Prof. F. Brunelle, Hôpital des Enfants Malades, Paris.)

Plain skull films in the case of chiasmatic tumours usually show a J-shaped sella turcica, which is not a specific sign. Enlargement of the optic foramen to 6.5–7 mm in diameter and more than 3 mm greater than the contralateral foramen constitutes evidence of tumour within the optic canal. However, a widened canal and even a long tortuous optic nerve may not be associated with tumour, especially in patients with neurofibromatosis (Duffner and Cohen 1988).

CT and MRI are of primary importance for the diagnosis of gliomas of the optic pathway. High-resolution CT scan can detect even small tumours in the orbit but is less effective than MRI for assessment of intracranial extensions of optic gliomas (Fig. 14.6). The spontaneous density of chiasmatic tumours is close to that of the cerebral tissue, and homogeneous enhancement is usually obtained following injection of contrast. Tumoural cysts and calcification may be present. MRI visualizes small intracranial tumours extremely well, and multiplanar views are valuable to that effect. Intraorbital gliomas are readily identified on frontal cuts, and it has been reported that MRI could identify perineural arachnoidal gliomatosis characterized by a fusiform area of high signal intensity with a central core of lower intensity (Seiff *et al.* 1987) in patients with neurofibromatosis. Visual evoked potentials are apt to be more abnormal in patients with chiasmatic gliomas than in those with more anteriorly located tumours. However, false positives are common, limiting the usefulness of the technique (North 1997).

In neurofibromatosis, MRI often reveals areas of increased T₂ signal in the basal ganglia, geniculate bodies, optic radiations and noncontiguous areas of the CNS (Hashimoto *et al.* 1990).

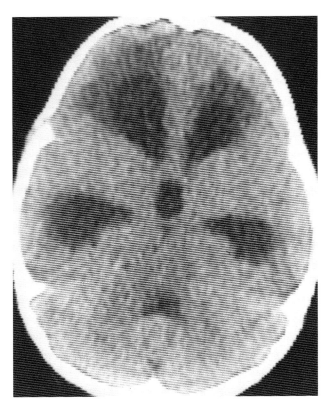

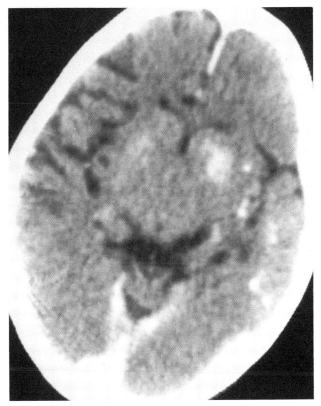

Fig. 14.7. Effect on brain of X-ray therapy given for treatment of brainstem tumour in 4-year-old girl with neurofibromatosis type I (optic glioma preceded occurrence of tumour). *(Top)* Brainstem glioma with hypodensity of brainstem, posterior dislocation of fourth ventricle and active hydrocephalus with transependymal CSF resorption around anterior ventricle horns. *(Bottom)* Following irradiation, there is disappearance of mass and hydrocephalus but marked atrophy and extensive calcification of basal nuclei and temporal cortex.

The significance of these areas remains unclear but they do not usually correspond to tumour extension (Chapter 4).

The course of optic gliomas is for the most part slow. However, they are tumours rather than hamartomas and some may have a rapid evolution which is difficult to predict. It seems that gliomas associated with NF1 tend to have a more favourable outcome. Listernick *et al.* (1995) found progression of the tumour in only two of 17 NF1 patients versus 12 of 19 children with glioma unassociated with NF1.

The *treatment* of optic pathway gliomas remains controversial. A surgical approach to unilateral anterior optic gliomas has given excellent results in terms of survival without the complications of X-ray therapy (Tenny *et al.* 1982, Chung and McCrary 1988). Some optic nerve tumours may be static (Hoyt and Baghdassarian 1986) and resection should be considered only after careful clinical and radiological follow-up if vision is severely compromised. Radiation therapy is widely used especially for the treatment of bilateral tumours and chiasmatic gliomas (Kalifa *et al.* 1981, Easley *et al.* 1988). Reduction in size of the tumour and improvement in vision undoubtedly occur (Chutorian 1988). However, the untoward effects of irradiation on the brain (Fig. 14.7) may be quite marked: over one-third of children with chiasmatic glioma who received radiation therapy had significant intellectual dysfunction, and endocrine effects are also frequent. For that reason, Packer *et al.* (1988c) elected to treat children under 5 years of age by chemotherapy with actinomycin D and vincristine and observed beneficial effects in over 80 per cent of cases. They concluded that chemotherapy can significantly delay the need for irradiation in young children. Other chemotherapeutic agents currently tried include carboplatin. In many patients, especially those with neurofibromatosis, a conservative attitude with careful follow-up is warranted.

The overall prognosis of optic pathway gliomas depends on the location and extension of the tumours. The prognosis for survival after excision in patients who have tumours confined to the optic nerve is uniformly excellent. The overall survival rate at 10 years is 60 per cent for patients with chiasmatic or optic nerve glioma whether or not associated with neurofibromatosis (Alvord and Lofton 1988). However, this may not apply to small gliomas detected by neuroradiological examination at a preclinical stage which may behave in an even more benign manner so the trend is towards a conservative approach.

HYPOTHALAMIC GLIOMAS

These tumours may be difficult to separate completely from large optic gliomas with posterior expansion (Davis *et al.* 1983). A majority are large tumours, mainly astrocytomas, in histologically verified cases. The most striking manifestation of hypothalamic gliomas is the diencephalic syndrome (Russell syndrome) which is characterized by the occurrence in an infant less than 3 years of age (average age of onset is 6 months) of emaciation without gastrointestinal abnormalities, euphoria and a hyperkinetic state. On examination marked cachexia is evident with lipoatrophy but with preservation of muscle bulk and stature. In most patients, a multidirectional nystagmus is present

TABLE 14.5
Pineal region tumours of children: histology*

Germ-cell tumours
  Two-cell type germinomas
    Seminomas
    Choriocarcinomas
  Teratomas
    Differentiated teratomas (dysgerminomas, embryonal carcinomas, yolk sac tumours, endodermal sinus tumours)
    Mixed intermediate teratomas
    Mixed undifferentiated teratomas
    Mixed trophoblastic teratomas
Pinealoblastomas
Pinealocytomas
Astrocytomas

*Adapted from Schulte *et al.* (1987) and Calaminus *et al.* (1994).
Cystic formations in the pineal region are common and are clinically indistinguishable from tumours.

and is the presenting feature in 43 per cent of patients.

The diencephalic syndrome of Russell is not limited to gliomas of the floor of the third ventricle. It is common with optic gliomas and is occasionally encountered with craniopharyngiomas and posterior fossa tumours (Burr *et al.* 1976). Conversely, other manifestations such as obesity, diabetes insipidus, hypogonadism and hydrocephalus are frequently encountered.

On CT or MRI scans, the tumours are clearly visible encroaching on the anterior third ventricle. The prognosis is poor, although occasional cases with long-term survival have been reported (Namba *et al.* 1985). Not infrequently, cachexia is replaced by obesity associated with short stature in infants who survive beyond the first few years of life. Irradiation is associated with two-year survival in over 90 per cent of cases, whereas death occurs before 1 year of age in virtually all untreated patients (Burr *et al.* 1976). In older patients a syndrome of emaciation reminiscent of anorexia nervosa has been reported (Chipkevitch 1994).

TUMOURS OF THE PINEAL REGION

Although tumours of the pineal region are classically considered to be rare in children, representing less than 2 per cent of all intracranial tumours (except in Japan where they account for 5–7 per cent), their actual frequency may be higher if they are correctly diagnosed (Schulte *et al.* 1987).

Concepts regarding these tumours have changed considerably over the past decade, and surgical approach with or without postoperative irradiation has become the accepted treatment. It has been reported that 36–50 per cent of pineal tumours are either benign or radioresistant (Hoffman *et al.* 1983) and surgical exploration is therefore recommended, especially as novel techniques have allowed better delineation of the tumours and improved surgical therapy.

Several different types of tumour are encountered in the pineal region (Table 14.5). Except for astrocytomas, pinealocytomas and perhaps a few differentiated teratomas, they are malignant tumours.

Germ-cell tumours are by far the most common pineal region tumours. They include germinomas and teratomas.

Germinomas are the most common tumour of the pineal region, accounting for one-third to one-half of cases (Hoffman *et al.* 1983, Packer *et al.* 1984, Edwards *et al.* 1988b, Calaminus *et al.* 1994). The typical two-cell type germinoma consists of a mixture of large clear cells and of small lymphocyte-like cells. The tumour is highly invasive and tumour cells are almost always present in the CSF (Schulte *et al.* 1987). However, distant metastases to the spine are rare (2–15 per cent) and seeding is mainly along the third and lateral ventricles producing a hyperintense rim around the ventricular cavities on enhanced CT scan. Extraneural metastases are rare (Lesoin *et al.* 1987). Invasion of the floor of the anterior third ventricle is common, even in the apparent absence of a pineal germinoma, the so-called ectopic germinoma. It may be that these ectopic tumours are the result of seeding from an undetectable pineal primary.

The predominant symptoms are related to the effects of increased ICP and hydrocephalus; these include headache, vomiting and lethargy (Jennings *et al.* 1985). Isosexual precocious puberty is a classical finding. Polyuria and polydypsia are relatively common (Sklar *et al.* 1981). The most prominent signs at presentation are associated with tectal compression (partial or complete Parinaud syndrome, signs of intracranial hypertension, ataxia and, sometimes, focal neurological dysfunction).

The neuroimaging features of germinoma are fairly distinctive (Fig. 14.8). The tumour presents as a round mass of slightly higher density than the brain, sometimes with small, spotty calcification. This should be distinguished from physiological pineal calcification, which is never present before age 4, and is found in 3 per cent of 5- to 8-year-olds, 12 per cent of 9- to 12-year-olds, and 19 per cent of 13- to 16-year-olds. After contrast, the density increases homogeneously. MRI shows well-defined lesions with homogeneous enhancement.

Human chorionic gonadotropin (HCG) may be found in the CSF in some cases of germinoma (Jordan *et al.* 1980, Edwards *et al.* 1985). AFP on the other hand is found only in cases of highly malignant tumours that belong to the general group of the teratomas (choriocarcinoma, endodermal sinus tumours, embryonal carcinoma). After completion of therapy, tumour markers may be predictive of recurrence before the presence of clinical or radiographic evidence (Edwards *et al.* 1985).

Therapy currently consists of surgical excision of the mass followed by irradiation which should be given systematically over the whole neural axis (Sano and Matsutani 1981, Schulte *et al.* 1987). Irradiation alone (Jooma and Kendall 1983) is now less commonly used. Doses used are commonly 50 Gy to the tumour bed, 40 Gy to the head and 35 Gy to the spine. Five-year survival may be as high as 50–80 per cent.

Teratomas present as heterogeneous masses with areas of calcification and of lipid density. Most of them are malignant. Tumour markers may be found in CSF (Eberts and Ransburg 1979, Jooma and Kendall 1983). AFP is found in cases of

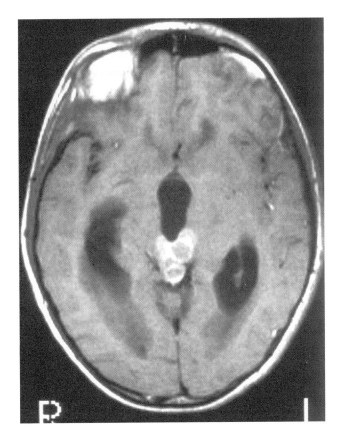

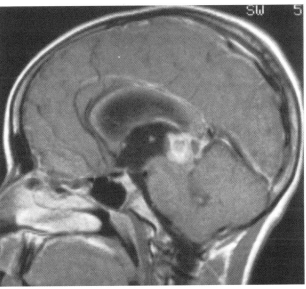

Fig. 14.8. Pineal germinoma in 12-year-old boy. MRI, T$_1$-weighted sequence, gadolinium enhanced. *(Top)* Axial cut. *(Bottom)* Sagittal cut demonstrating absence of flow void signal in aqueduct. Tumour is heterogeneous and causes marked obstructive hydrocephalus. (Courtesy Dr D. Renier, Prof. J-F. Hirsch, Hôpital des Enfants Malades, Paris.)

embryonal carcinoma, yolk sac tumours and sometimes in teratomas; HCG is present mainly in patients with choriocarcinoma, sometimes with seminoma, yolk sac tumours and teratomas (Calaminus *et al.* 1994). Combined treatment by surgery and irradiation is only moderately effective. Chemotherapy may somewhat improve the results (Dearnaley *et al.* 1990).

Parenchymatous tumours of the pineal body account for only a minority of pineal region tumours. *Pinealocytomas* are benign tumours. *Pinealoblastomas* are malignant and tend to metastasize along the CSF pathways especially to the walls of the ventricles.

Astrocytomas of the pineal region are benign tumours that run a slow course and may present as detectable masses or more rarely as small 'pencil gliomas' of the aqueduct with a picture of apparently pure aqueductal stenosis (Ho 1982). In most cases, astrocytomas present as isodense tumours of small to moderate size with some enhancement after contrast administration. Very small astrocytomas are best demonstrated by T_2-weighted sequences on MRI, which is particularly useful to detect small intrinsic tumours of the cerebral peduncles or quadrigeminal plate. Surgical resection is indicated for extrinsic astrocytomas.

Cysts of the pineal region, although they are not really tumours may present in the same manner. Many of them are fortuitously found on neuroradiological examination and are asymptomatic. No treatment is required but longitudinal follow-up is advised. Large symptomatic cysts should be resected (Vorkapic and Pendl 1987, Klein and Rubinstein 1989). Single or multiple cysts in the pineal region are common in Aicardi syndrome (Özek *et al.* 1995; see Chapter 3). Ectopic retinoblastoma may involve the pineal body. In association with bilateral ocular retinoblastoma, it is known as 'trilateral retinoblastoma' (Zimmerman *et al.* 1982, Pesin and Shields 1989).

OTHER TUMOURS OF THE THIRD VENTRICLE AND SELLAR REGION

Pituitary adenomas are rare in infancy and childhood and the majority of cases are seen in older children and adolescents (Mukai *et al.* 1986, Shalet 1986). The clinical features of adenoma include endocrine disturbances and visual defects. The various types encountered in adults (Martinez *et al.* 1980) can also occur in the paediatric age range. *Prolactin adenomas* are the most frequent type (Tyson *et al.* 1993). Patients have delayed growth and puberty and amenorrhoea. Endocrine investigations reveal a high level of prolactin with low levels of growth hormone, TSH and ACTH. *ACTH cell adenomas* are rare. Most cases of Cushing syndrome are caused by a microadenoma that may grow rapidly following adrenalectomy, resulting in the Nelson syndrome marked by melanodermia, asthenia and visual disturbances (Hopwood and Kenny 1977). *Growth hormone adenomas* are also quite rare in childhood. They may be associated with acromegaly or gigantism (Blumberg *et al.* 1989).

The radiological diagnosis of pituitary adenomas is based on sellar enlargement with erosion of sellar walls on plain films and on the presence of an intrasellar mass isodense to the brain and enhancing homogeneously after contrast on CT scan.

Suprasellar expansion is often observed in patients with prolactinomas, whereas growth hormone adenomas and especially ACTH adenomas usually remain intrasellar. MRI gives a better definition and even permits the diagnosis of microadenomas. Adenomas are typically hypodense on T_1-weighted sequences while their appearance is more variable on T_2-weighted images. A convex upper margin of the gland and an increased vertical diameter and surface of the pituitary image for age are characteristic (Konishi *et al.* 1990).

Therapy is mainly surgical but irradiation may be required if resection is incomplete. Bromocriptine, a dopamine antagonist inhibitor of the synthesis and release of prolactin, may dramatically reduce the size of large prolactinomas and may be a useful preoperative treatment (Dunne *et al.* 1987).

Hypothalamic hamartomas are ectopic masses of neuronal and glial tissue which may be small and pedunculated or sessile and relatively large. They arise from the region of the tuber cinereum or mamillary bodies and develop into the interpeduncular cistern. Their histological structure resembles that of grey matter with varying proportions of neurons, glia and fibre bundles (Russell and Rubinstein 1989). They do not behave as true tumours. Rather, they grow at approximately the same rate as the rest of the encephalon and never produce symptoms or signs of nerve tissue compression (Turjman *et al.* 1996).

Clinically, hypothalamic hamartomas may remain asymptomatic or they may be associated with precocious isosexual puberty of central origin, with a peculiar epileptic syndrome or with both. Precocious puberty is the most common clinical manifestation. Its central origin is demonstrated by the increased levels of gonadotropins. The epileptic syndrome associated with hamartomas has an early onset, usually before 2 years of age, and is characterized by the frequently repeated occurrence of attacks of laughter (Chapter 16). The CT appearance of hamartomas is characteristic with a well-limited rounded isodense mass surrounded by CSF in the interpeduncular cistern. On MRI the mass is clearly definable in multiplanar sequences. On T_2-weighted sequences it usually gives a more intense signal than the surrounding brain. Rare cases are part of the Pallister–Hall syndrome that also includes polydactyly and imperforate anus (Minns *et al.* 1994).

Resection of the hamartoma is often impossible or very difficult and it does not always result in disappearance of the epilepsy. It is therefore rarely advised even though medical treatment is only moderately effective. However, seizures may originate in the hamartomatous tissue and resection of pedunculated tumours may be effective. Callosotomy has been suggested for resistant seizures (Berkovic *et al.* 1988, Cascino *et al.* 1993).

Intracranial chordomas are generally located along the clivus (Eriksson *et al.* 1981, Wold and Laws 1983, Favre *et al.* 1994) and, when located anteriorly, may give rise to symptoms and signs similar to those of other parasellar tumours. Chordomas more posteriorly located produce palsies of the lower cranial nerve pairs. Plain skull X-rays are of value by showing destruction and deformation of the sella turcica and body of sphenoid bone. On CT, chordomas present as well-delineated masses with frequent calcification and contrast enhancement. Chondromas, developing from the spheno-occipital synchondrosis (Divitiis *et al.* 1979) are indistinguishable from chordomas, unless associated with Ollier disease (Diebler and Dulac 1987).

Colloid cyst of the third ventricle is very rare in children (Koos and Miller 1971). Papillomas of the choroid plexus have been reported (see below).

Paranasal sinus mucoceles are rare pseudotumoural lesions in children, presenting as dilated fluid-filled masses due to the accumulation of mucus and secretions within an occluded sinus cavity. All sinuses including the sphenoid sinus may be involved (Osborne *et al.* 1979). Mucoceles result from infection, trauma, congenital deformity of the ostium or cystic degeneration of the mucosa (Siegel *et al.* 1979). Mucoceles may present with ocular motor palsies, decrease in visual acuity and various eye signs. On CT scan they present as spontaneously dense areas with possible intracranial extensions (Perugini *et al.* 1982).

TUMOURS OF THE CEREBRAL HEMISPHERES

Tumours of the cerebral hemispheres are more common in younger than in older children. Their clinical manifestations are polymorphic with a high incidence of focal neurological symptoms and signs. Modern neuroimaging techniques have considerably facilitated the diagnosis of supratentorial tumours. However, the interpretation of images remains difficult in many cases as numerous lesions of different origins can give rise to similar radiological pictures. Most supratentorial tumours are gliomas.

GLIOMAS OF THE CEREBRAL HEMISPHERES

The *clinical presentation* of parenchymal supratentorial tumours depends more on the location of the tumour than on its histological nature. Signs of high ICP and focal neurological manifestations may occur in isolation or in various combinations. Headaches, nausea and vomiting may be the presenting manifestations in about 20 per cent of patients, mainly those with malignant tumours.

Epileptic seizures are the most common neurological manifestation, particularly in slowly growing, benign tumours such as low-grade astrocytomas and oligodendrogliomas. Seizures are mostly focal and partial complex seizures are most frequently observed (Table 14.6). In my experience, sensory seizures may be especially suspect. On the other hand, uncinate seizures may not be more likely than other types to be due to brain tumours (Howe and Gibson 1982). The occurrence of generalized seizures and of bilateral paroxysmal EEG abnormalities does not exclude the possibility of a tumour (Blume *et al.* 1982, Hirsch *et al.* 1989, Aicardi 1994). Long-standing seizures may be especially frequent in patients with brain tumours but the advent of CT scan and MRI has changed the situation and many cases are now recognized early.

Localized deficits are less frequently the presenting manifestation of supratentorial gliomas and are apt to be rather late features. However, hemiparesis, hemianopia and language disturbances may occasionally be the first clinical manifestation, especially with malignant neoplasms.

Low-grade astrocytomas (grades I and II) are the most frequent hemispheric tumours (Mercuri *et al.* 1981), accounting for 21 per cent of all supratentorial neoplasms in children. The CT scan appearance of benign astrocytomas is variable. In a majority of cases, the lesions are well-defined and regular in shape. They appear hypodense without contrast enhancement and their

TABLE 14.6
Clinical and EEG features of epilepsy revealing brain tumours in 48 children*

Feature	No. of patients with feature**	%	
Partial seizures		81	(39/48)
Partial motor	16		
Partial sensory	8		
Unilateral	7		
Partial complex	14		
Atypical	18		
Generalized seizures		33	(16/48)
Absences	1		
Infantile spasms	1		
Myotonic/atypical absences	4		
Tonic clonic	20		
Unclassified	10	20	(10/48)
Focal delta waves	22	49	(22/45)
Focal spikes on slow background rhythm	24	53	(24/45)
Focal/multifocal spikes	18	40	(18/45)
Bilateral synchronous paroxysms	13	29	(13/45)
Unremarkable	12	27	(12/45)

*From Aicardi (1994).
**Several types of seizures and of EEG abnormalities could occur in the same patient.

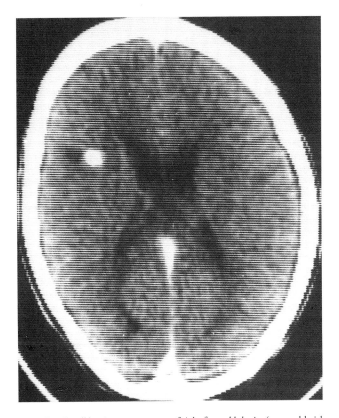

Fig. 14.9. Small benign astrocytoma of right frontal lobe in 4-year-old girl with intractable partial seizures. Several CT scans showed only what was thought to be atrophic enlargement of a sulcus. Eventually, calcification appeared. Limited resection of a small cystic astrocytoma with mural nodule led to complete disappearance of seizures, with no recurrence in seven years.

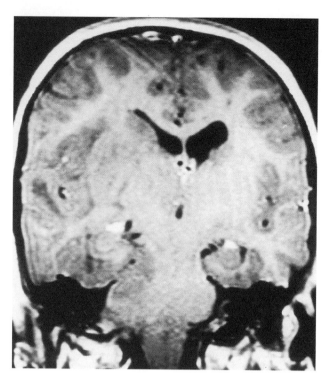

Fig. 14.10. High-grade cerebral astrocytoma. MRI coronal cut, T_1-weighted sequence shows considerable enlargement of right hemisphere with mass effect and midline shift toward the left side and compression of right ventricle. The limit between cortex and white matter is blurred on the right side and cortex is thickened in the temporal region. Note extension into brainstem. (Courtesy Dr Kling Chong, Great Ormond Street Hospital, London.)

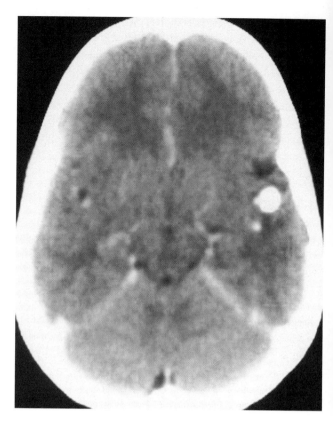

Fig. 14.11. Oligodendroglioma of left temporal lobe in 10-year-old boy with partial complex seizures. Calcification is associated with minimal area of hypodensity. (Courtesy Prof. F. Brunelle, Hôpital des Enfants Malades, Paris.)

density increases in a nonhomogeneous manner after contrast injection (Pedersen *et al.* 1981, Diebler and Dulac 1987). Many are cystic with only a small enhancing nodule (Fig. 14.9). Approximately 15 per cent of gliomas were not detected on CT scan and a wrong diagnosis of glioma was made in the face of a nonmalignant condition in a relatively old study (Kendall *et al.* 1979). MRI scans may be difficult to interpret as the peritumoural oedema can give an intense signal identical to that of the mass itself on T_2-weighted sequences. Gadolinium-enhanced MRI seems to be very effective in the detection of gliomas.

The prognosis of astrocytomas is clearly better in children than in adults (Mercuri *et al.* 1981, Laws *et al.* 1984). Radical excision is the preferred method. Irradiation may improve survival in the case of incomplete tumour removal but is associated with the complications of such therapy in children. It seems likely that the high proportion of incomplete removal reported by Gjerris (1978) has significantly decreased with modern technical advances (Hirsch *et al.* 1989).

High-grade astrocytomas (grade III–IV or anaplastic astrocytomas) and other malignant gliomas such as glioblastoma multiforme are uncommon in children, accounting for only 7–11 per cent of primary brain neoplasms in this age range (Dropcho *et al.* 1987). Seizures are the presenting feature in about one-third of patients but headache, hemiparesis and personality changes are more frequent. High-grade gliomas may

evolve from a low-grade lesion, not infrequently following irradiation of the lesion, or be observed several years after treatment of acute lymphocytic leukaemia (Hoppe-Hirsch *et al.* 1993). On imaging they are often irregular with finger-like configuration (Fig. 14.10). Contrast enhancement in a ring-like formation is almost constant in glioblastoma but may be absent in anaplastic astrocytomas (Chamberlain *et al.* 1988). Surgical treatment should be associated with irradiation and chemotherapy (Dropcho *et al.* 1987). The prognosis remains poor with an actuarial probability of survival of 32 per cent, three years after surgery. Metastases may occur (Duffner and Cohen 1981) but local invasion is the major problem.

Oligodendrogliomas are relatively rare tumours in childhood (21 per cent of all supratentorial tumours). Oligogliomas are slow-growing tumours with a strong tendency to calcify. Tice *et al.* (1993) studied 39 cases, 32 of which were located in the frontal lobe. The most common presenting symptoms are convulsive seizures that occur in 50–70 per cent of cases. The diagnosis is relatively easy by CT or MRI (Varma *et al.* 1983). Oligogliomas are usually hypointense on T_1 sequences and give a high signal in T_2 images. About 40 per cent are calcified and 60 per cent have well-defined margins (Fig. 14.11). They produce a mass effect in less than half and enhance with contrast in less than a quarter of the cases. They may produce thinning of the inner skull table. The latter sign only indicates a slowly enlarging lesion and can be seen with benign astrocytoma and with dysembryoplastic neuroepithelial tumours (Daumas-Duport *et al.* 1988).

The outcome following surgery is usually good, especially in young patients, and the tumours tend to remain stable for long periods even following only partial resection, although a poor outcome is associated with the presence of neurological deficit at the time of diagnosis and the presence of nuclear polymorphism of the tumour (Wilkinson *et al.* 1987) on histological examination. The prognosis of malignant oligogliomas is poor (Hoppe-Hirsch *et al.* 1993).

Ependymomas of the cerebral hemispheres represent 30–40 per cent of intracranial ependymomas in children. Malignant ependymomas are more common in a supratentorial location (Pierre-Kahn *et al.* 1983, Hoppe-Hirsch *et al.* 1993). In Pierre-Kahn's series, 86 per cent of supratentorial ependymomas were malignant. A majority of ependymomas are not located intraventricularly (see below). The main clinical manifestations are signs and symtoms of intracranial hypertension and focal deficits. Seizures are relatively uncommon. Neuroradiological appearance is nonspecific. Small multiple intratumoural calcification is frequent (Swartz *et al.* 1982).

Tumour recurrences or metastases are frequent. The latter are mainly intracranial, in contrast with the spinal metastases of posterior fossa ependymomas. The overall outcome is thus poor (Coulon and Till 1977, Pierre-Kahn *et al.* 1983).

Surgery is clearly the initial approach but it is rarely curative because complete excision may not be possible. However, surgery can be a definitive treatment for cystic astrocytomas and total removal of the mural nodule is likewise satisfactory. In the series of 43 children with benign astrocytomas and oligogliomas reported by Hirsch *et al.* (1989), the progression-free survival at 5 years was 95 per cent even though radiation had been given to only two patients. The role of radiation therapy in children is debated. It is clearly indicated for malignant tumours, but in benign astrocytoma of childhood no clear-cut advice can be given. Chemotherapy might improve the outcome of patients with high-grade gliomas (Sposto *et al.* 1989) but its role in the treatment of childhood astrocytomas is not yet defined.

OTHER TUMOURS OF THE CEREBRAL HEMISPHERES
Meningiomas are relatively rare in children, representing less than 2 per cent of intracranial tumours. Most meningiomas are found in the convexity of the brain, but a higher incidence of location within the lateral ventricles than in adults, with absence of dural attachment, an origin in the posterior fossa and cyst formation characterize meningiomas found in childhood (Cohen and Duffner 1994). Ferrante *et al.* (1989) reviewed 178 cases from the literature and added 19 cases of their own. Sixteen per cent were intraventricular, 90 per cent were supratentorial and 10 per cent arose from the fourth ventricle. Most meningiomas in childhood are of the fibroblastic type, consisting of spindles of prominent fibroglia. The syncytial and angioplastic types are much less common. Sarcomatous meningiomas are more frequent in children than in adults (Glasier *et al.* 1993, Cohen and Duffner 1994).

Increased ICP is responsible for most clinical manifestations but seizures may be the presenting feature in 8–31 per cent of cases. Intraventricular meningiomas are apt to present with signs of intermittent obstruction of CSF outflow tracts. Optic canal or orbital tumours produce central scotomas or variable field defects. They may be difficult to distinguish from gliomas of the optic pathway (Wilson *et al.* 1979). Hyperostosis or bone destruction favour the diagnosis of meningioma. CT scan clearly demonstrates most meningiomas especially after contrast enhancement. The CT picture, however, may be less characteristic in children than in adults (Ferrante *et al.* 1989). Large cystic formations are frequent, especially in children under 2 years of age. MRI shows a decreased T_1 and increased T_2 signal and usually demonstrates heterogeneity of the tumour due to tumour vascularity, cystic degeneration and calcification. It enables better delineation of the limits of the lesion and helps to indicate whether the tumour is intra- or extraaxial.

Therapy is basically surgical but radiation may play a role for patients in whom total removal is impossible, which is not infrequently the case in children because of size and location of the tumours. However, 18 of 22 patients in the series of Davidson and Hope (1989) were doing well up to 18 years after operation. Sarcomatous meningiomas show many mitotic figures and disorganized architecture. They have a strong tendency to local recurrence and can metastasize to the CNS or to remote tissues (Cohen and Duffner 1994).

Gangliogliomas and gangliocytomas are benign tumours of the cerebral hemispheres that are characterized histologically by the presence of both mature neuronal and glial cells. These tumours may be intermediate between cortical dysplasias and more aggressive tumours (Duchowny *et al.* 1989, 1996). Their outcome is benign when total removal is possible (Kalyan-Raman and Olivero 1987). Gangliogliomas are particularly apt to present as cases of isolated, intractable epilepsy, usually of a focal type (Demierre *et al.* 1986). In the series of Zentner *et al.* (1994), 84 per cent of tumours were in the temporal lobe and 92 per cent were revealed by epileptic seizures. They occur mainly in young children or even in neonates (Duchowny *et al.* 1989) without any sign of increased pressure. The diagnosis is often difficult. CT scan typically reveals hyperdense cortical lesions with gyriform or serpiginous outlines without marked mass effect. Most lesions are difficult to identify on T_1-weighted MRI sequences and may have low, intermediate or increased signal on T_2-weighted images (Sutton *et al.* 1983). Gangliocytomas differ from gangliogliomas that typically show cyst formation, calcification, contrast enhancement and mass effect (Hashimoto *et al.* 1993).

Surgical removal often results in the cure of epilepsy. The long-term prognosis is favourable.

Dysembryoplastic neuroepithelial tumours (Daumas-Duport *et al.* 1988) are probably related to gangliocytomas and gangliogliomas. Indeed both terms may well be used for the same lesions by different investigators. They include a mixture of neuronal and glial elements, both oligocytes and astrocytes, and appear to be of developmental origin. It is likely that a signficant proportion of the cases formerly diagnosed as low-grade oligoastrocytomas

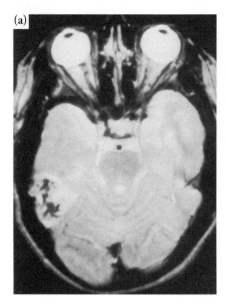

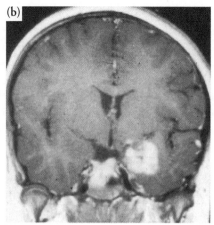

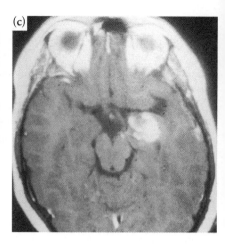

Fig. 14.12. Developmental neuroepithelial tumour (DNT). *(a)* T₂-weighted MRI showing large temporal lobe tumour with heterogeneous signal. Dark areas corresponded to calcification visible on CT scan. *(b,c)* DNT of left mesial temporal lobe seen on coronal *(b)* and axial *(c)* cuts. A mild mass effect is visible. (Courtesy Dr Kling Chong, Great Ormond Street Hospital, London.)

were in fact developmental neuroepithelial tumours. These tumours are located cortically but may involve the underlying white matter. They are often found in the temporal or frontal lobes of children and adolescents with chronic focal seizures of early onset. They are of mixed density on CT scan and only 18 per cent enhance after contrast infusion. A quarter of them are calcified, and one-third produce a focal cranial deformity as a result of erosion of the inner skull table. They give a mixed signal on MRI usually with hypodensity on T₁-weighted sequences and hyperdensity on T₂ images (Fig. 14.12). These lesions have little or no tendency to grow and usually remain stable on repeat examinations. They may be associated with some oedema of the white matter. However, a few mitoses can be seen (Raymond *et al.* 1994). Some of them develop in areas of cortical dysplasia (Prayson *et al.* 1993). Surgical removal, even if subtotal, seems to give good results without recurrences (Murphy *et al.* 1995). Irradiation is clearly contraindicated.

Primary cerebral neuroblastomas occur in the first decade in 81 per cent of cases and in 20 per cent before the age of 2 years. The clinical picture is that of hemispheric tumours in general. Survival following surgery and irradiation with or without chemotherapy reaches three years in 60 per cent of patients and exceeds five years in 30 per cent. Metastases along the cerebrospinal pathways are frequent and probably justify prophylactic spinal irradiation (Bennett and Rubinstein 1984).

Primitive neuroectodermal tumours (PNETs) are highly malignant neoplasms that occur mostly in children and young adults (Duffner *et al.* 1981). They consist of small undifferentiated cells without observable cytoplasm, and dark oval or irregular nuclei. Numerous mitotic figures and necrosis are often present. Occasional focal areas of differentiation toward neuronal or glial lines may often be recognized. By electron microscopy, the tumour cells have been reported to have similarities to the developing cortical plate of the fetus. PNETs are mainly hemispheric in location but they have similarities with medulloblastomas

which are sometimes regarded as being posterior fossa PNETs (Packer *et al.* 1985–1986).

Horten and Rubinstein (1976) have regarded PNETs as *cerebral neuroblastomas.* However, neuroblastomas are less malignant than PNETs, and histologically these neoplasms are not purely neuroblastic. Most PNETs have structural and/or numerical chromosomal abnormalities. Nerve growth factor receptors are demonstrated immunochemically in one-third of cases (Becker *et al.* 1990).

The clinical features of PNETs are those of malignant supratentorial tumours, with hypertension and focal deficits being more common than seizures. The course is usually very brief. CT scan may show cystic formation and extensive calcification (Duffner *et al.* 1981). Neoplastic meningitis may be the first manifestation (Jennings *et al.* 1993).

Treatment is with as complete a resection as possible, followed by irradiation and chemotherapy.

Intracranial metastases of extracranial tumours are rare in childhood. Wilms tumours, osteosarcoma, rhabdomyosarcoma and neuroblastoma are known occasionally to metastasize to the brain (Armstrong *et al.* 1982, Han *et al.* 1983, Graus *et al.* 1983).

Intracranial metastases have no distinctive features. They may be single or multiple and present as areas of hypodensity, which enhance following contrast injection, and surrounding oedema.

Diffuse gliomatosis (gliomatosis cerebri) is a rare neoplastic disorder involving large parts of the brain in a multicentric or diffuse overgrowth with cells of neuroglial lineage (Artigas *et al.* 1985). The disorder has been described in a newborn infant and was originally mistakenly diagnosed as lissencephaly (Barth *et al.* 1988). Jennings *et al.* (1995) reviewed 160 cases from the literature plus three of their own, involving primarily the centrum semi-ovale, the mesencephalon, brainstem and basal ganglia. Clinical features included corticospinal tract deficits in 58 per cent, dementia/mental retardation in 44 per cent, headache in 39

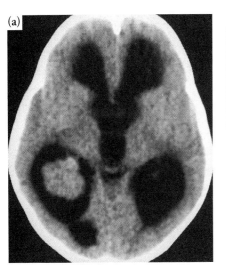 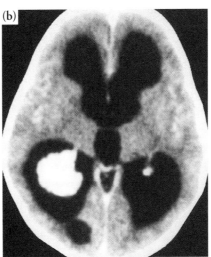 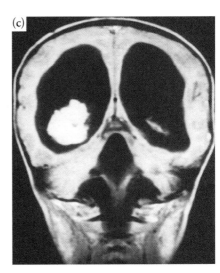

Fig. 14.13. Papilloma of right choroid plexus in 4-year-old boy with moderate psychomotor delay and large head. *(a,b)* CT scans before and after contrast injection. *(c)* MRI, coronal cut after gadolinium enhancement showing large papilloma in right ventricle and normal choroid plexus on left.

per cent, seizures in 38 per cent, cranial neuropathy in 37 per cent, raised intracranial pressure in 34 per cent and spinocerebellar deficit in 33 per cent.

Lipomas are space-occupying lesions of malformative origin which do not behave as tumours. The most frequent location of lipomas is the region of the corpus callosum. Lipomas are generally associated with total or partial agenesis of the callosal commissure (Gerber and Plotkin 1982). They may communicate through a narrow stalk with an extracranial lipoma in the region of the bregma (Kushnet and Goldman 1978). These should be distinguished from dermoid cysts of the anterior fontanelle (Saito *et al.* 1988), encephaloceles, haemangiomas, lipomas, lymphangiomas and sinus pericranii (extracranial varicoceles) by using preoperative MRI.

Lipomas of the corpus callosum may be asymptomatic. Epilepsy is the most frequent manifestation of symptomatic lesions. The diagnosis is readily made by demonstrating the presence of a mass of fat density, usually surrounded by 'eggshell' calcification. Lipomas, usually of small size and asymptomatic, may be found in other locations, notably in the pineal region.

INTRAVENTRICULAR TUMOURS

Tumours of different histological types can be located within the lateral ventricles. These include *intraventricular meningiomas*, which are more frequent in children than in adults (Cohen and Duffner 1994), *intraventricular neurocytomas*, also known as intraventricular oligodendrogliomas (Nishio *et al.* 1988), intraventricular cysts, ependymomas and, especially, papillomas of the choroid plexus (Pascual-Castroviejo *et al.* 1983). *Choroid plexus papillomas* arise from the epithelium of the plexus and are relatively common in infants as about 20 per cent of papillomas occur below 1 year of age (Koos and Miller 1971).

Papillomas are large, cauliflower-like tumours that present the structure of normal choroid plexus with a considerable degree of hyperplasia. Carcinomas of the choroid plexus are rare.

The usual manifestation of *choroid plexus papilloma* in infants is hydrocephalus (Chapter 7), which is generally rapidly evolving and may be accompanied by papilloedema, an uncommon finding in nontumoural hydrocephalus. The diagnosis is easy because papillomas present as large intraventricular masses with massive enhancement after contrast injection (Kendall *et al.* 1983) (Fig. 14.13). The hydrocephalus is thought to result from hypersecretion of CSF by the tumour but it may also be due to meningeal fibrosis resulting from haemorrhage from the tumour. The CSF frequently contains an excess of protein.

In rare cases, choroid plexus papilloma may mimic a degenerative CNS disorder. In older children, papillomas are often located in the temporal lobe and produce seizures rather than hydrocephalus. Calcification is sometimes present.

Excision of the papilloma is the treatment of choice. Total excision was achieved in 20 of 24 children with choroid plexus tumours (16 papillomas and eight carcinomas) reported by Lena *et al.* (1990). The overall mortality was 25 per cent, and five of 15 surviving papilloma patients had sequelae. In some cases, hydrocephalus persists following removal of the tumour and a shunt may be required. Radiation therapy is reserved for tumours having malignant histological patterns.

TUMOURS OF THE BASAL GANGLIA AND THALAMUS

These tumours represent 4–6 per cent of intracranial tumours in children. Most are astrocytomas of various grades, from benign pilocytic lesions to anaplastic astrocytomas and glioblastoma multiforme (Bernstein *et al.* 1984).

The most common clinical manifestation is progressive hemiparesis (Mayer *et al.* 1982), which may be associated with unilateral dystonia or intention tremor. Krauss *et al.* (1992) in a review of 225 cases in adults and children found only 20 with a movement disorder, most commonly tremor or dystonia. Seventy per cent of these patients had signs of corticospinal tract involvement. Homonymous hemianopia, nystagmus and

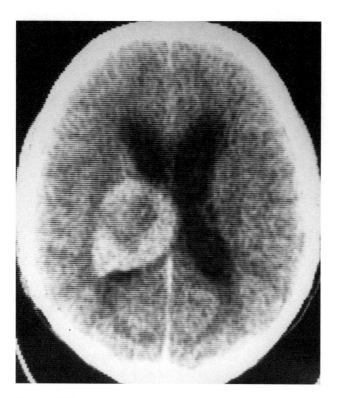

Fig. 14.14. Glioma of the thalamus in 11-year-old boy with mild left hemi-plegia, headache and vomiting for two months. Biopsy revealed a grade III astrocytoma with significant oligodendroglial component. (Courtesy Dr D. Renier, Prof. J-F. Hirsch, Hôpital des Enfants Malades, Paris.)

hearing loss may be observed. Sensory manifestations are exceptional.

The diagnosis is readily suggested by CT scan or MRI when the tumour is hypodense and when contrast enhancement is present (Fig. 14.14). The latter may occur in a ring-like manner. In some cases the tumour is infiltrating and its density does not differ, even after contrast injection, from that of the surrounding brain. In such cases recognition of the mass effect caused by the tumour is the only diagnostic criterion.

Complete surgical removal of tumours of the basal ganglia is not possible. Biopsy is advised by some authorities (see Bern-stein *et al.* 1984) who reserve irradiation for malignant tumours. Stereotactic biopsy is often used. Other authors (*e.g.* Mayer *et al.* 1982) advise irradiation of all basal ganglia tumours.

BRAIN TUMOURS IN INFANTS AND CHILDREN UNDER 2 YEARS OF AGE

These differ in location, pathology, clinical features and therapy from those of older children. The proportion of all childhood brain tumours occurring at this age may be at least 10 per cent (Cohen and Duffner 1994). A significant number of these are definite 'congenital' tumours, *i.e.* they produce symptoms within the first two weeks of life, or 'probably congenital' tumours, *i.e.* they are present or recognized within the first year of life (Fort and Rushing 1997).

In infants under 6 months of age, supratentorial tumours account for 70–75 per cent of all intracranial neoplasms. Cohen

and Duffner (1994) found that 30 per cent of children with brain tumours occurring under 2 years of age had ependymomas, 20 per cent medulloblastomas, 15 per cent astrocytomas, 8 per cent glioblastomas and 22 per cent an admixture of sarcomas, choroid plexus papillomas, pinealomas, primitive neuroectodermal tu-mours, gangliogliomas and teratomas. Wakai *et al.* (1984) in a review of congenital brain tumours found that 46.1 per cent were teratomas and 36.5 per cent were of neuroepithelial origin, fewer than 10 per cent being astrocytomas. Teratomas were much more frequent in Japanese series. The low incidence of dysontogenic tumours in the large series of Balestrini *et al.* (1994), in which 41 per cent of tumours were astrocytomas and 20 per cent medulloblastomas, is probably related to the fact that it included mostly children in the second year of life.

The clinical features of congenital and early-onset tumours are variable with the type and location of the tumour. Macro-crania, delayed milestones and behavioural disturbances are prominent (Galassi *et al.* 1989). In the case of congenital tumours, fetal death and preterm birth are very frequent (Wakai *et al.* 1984). Intracranial haemorrhage can be the presenting mani-festation. Vomiting, focal neurological signs, seizures and the diencephalic syndrome of emaciation (see p. 504) may also be early manifestations. Infantile spasms are an uncommon mani-festation (Asanuma *et al.* 1995).

The diagnosis may be delayed if it is not suggested by rela-tively trivial symptoms such as delayed milestones or vomiting. Tumours manifested by hemiplegia may be difficult to separate from congenital static hemiplegia so brain imaging is indicated if there is any doubt. CSF examination may be misleading as pleo-cytosis and increased protein are commonly found. CT scanning and MRI will, in most cases, readily permit the diagnosis.

The prognosis of congenital tumours is poor. Surgery is difficult because of the large size of many tumours. Surgical mortality was 17.4 per cent in 63 operated patients studied by Balestrini *et al.* (1994). Radiation is highly dangerous for the very young developing brain. Many tumours are malignant (Rubin-stein 1985) even though an occasional tumour of malignant ap-pearance may have a favourable outcome (Roosen *et al.* 1988). The survival rate at 5 years varies between 23 and 54 per cent, and the quality of life of the survivors is often poor. Chemother-apy appears to be effective, and results are as good as or better than those achieved with standard radiation therapy (Duffner and Cohen 1992, Duffner *et al.* 1993). However, the possible late effects of chemotherapy are as yet poorly known.

OUTCOME OF BRAIN TUMOURS IN CHILDREN

The results of recent advances in therapy have been impressive, especially for certain types of tumours that were regularly fatal a few years ago, such as medulloblastomas. An overall evaluation of the survival of children with brain tumours (Duffner *et al.* 1986) indicates that the global survival rate at five years is about 50 per cent. The worst prognosis is for children with brainstem tumours (18 per cent), whereas more than 90 per cent of children with cerebellar astrocytoma have a five-year survival and those with low-grade hemispheric astrocytoma a 71 per cent survival.

Medulloblastomas, high-grade astrocytomas and ependymomas have lower survival rates. Children under 2 years of age with tumours have a lower survival rate (36 per cent) than older children. These figures apply to an unselected group of patients, and results in individual institutions with a special interest and experience in the treatment of neoplasms should be better.

The quality of survival is one of the major concerns with current therapeutic approaches. In a prospective study of a small group of children (Duffner *et al.* 1988) most of the patients remained within the normal range of intelligence but their IQ scores declined over time. Learning disabilities were found in more than 90 per cent of children after irradiation and most required special educational services. Similar results, especially related to radiotherapy, have been reported by other investigators (Radcliffe *et al.* 1992, Garcia-Perez *et al.* 1993). In the series of Radcliffe *et al.*, there was an average loss of 27 IQ points in children treated under 7 years of age but no loss in children receiving therapy later. A young age at the time of radiation and adjuvant chemotherapy were risk factors associated with a decline in IQ (Packer *et al.* 1989). Radiotherapy for tumours is also associated with significant endocrinological complications (Avizonis *et al.* 1992, Cohen and Duffner 1994), mostly growth failure commonly caused by pituitary insufficiency but which may also result from irradiation of the spine. Thyroid and gonadal problems also occur. Finally, the risk of late development of second tumours, mostly meningiomas and gliomas, 2–40 years (average 20 years) after irradiation is small but real (Cohen and Duffner 1994).

NEUROLOGICAL MANIFESTATIONS OF LEUKAEMIAS AND LYMPHOMAS AND OF THEIR TREATMENT

Neurological manifestations frequently occur as an initial feature or as a late complication of leukaemias and lymphomas and can be their presenting manifestation (Aysun *et al.* 1994). Complex neurological pictures are often observed at various stages of these diseases and it has become extremely difficult to determine the cause of neurological manifestations as these may be due to the disease itself, to toxic complications of therapy, to viral or other opportunistic infections resulting from immunodepression, or to haemorrhagic accidents. Appropriate therapy, however, depends on a correct diagnosis of the nature of the neurological abnormality.

NEUROLOGICAL MANIFESTATIONS OF LEUKAEMIAS
COMPLICATIONS OF THE DISORDER
Complications of the leukaemic process may result from leukaemic infiltrations of the meninges, brain and cranial nerves or may be due to haemorrhage or infections.

Meningeal leukaemia may occur at any stage of the disease. One-third to one-half of children are in complete remission when neurological complications appear. Leukaemic infiltration primarily affects the arachnoid, and infiltration of the brain

tissue is found in less than 15 per cent of the children who die in a relapse (Price 1983). Presenting features of CNS leukaemia include headache, vomiting and papilloedema. Seizures occur in about 10 per cent of patients and the risk of seizure is considerably greater in children receiving methotrexate therapy (Ochs *et al.* 1984). Increased appetite and weight gain may occur in relation with hypothalamic infiltration (Greydanus *et al.* 1978). Cranial nerve palsies are frequently present. CT scan usually fails to demonstrate the leukaemic infiltrates (Curless 1980), but MRI with gadolinium enhancement may show the meningeal involvement.

The CSF shows an increased cell count and blast cells are usually recognized (Komp 1979). However, blast cells may be associated with a low CSF cell count (Mahmoud *et al.* 1993). The sugar content is low in about 50 per cent of affected children. Eosinophilic or basophilic meningitis has been recorded (Budka *et al.* 1976).

Large intracranial or paraspinal masses (granulocytic sarcomas or chloromas) are uncommon (Brown *et al.* 1989). They occur with myeloblastic leukaemia. This often affects the spinal canal and produces spinal and radicular compression. Retinal lesions including haemorrhages and white exudates sometimes with swelling of the disc occur in about 20 per cent of cases of leukaemia (Taylor 1990).

Prophylaxis of CNS involvement is part of the management of leukaemia and aims at preventing overt leukaemic infiltration of the nervous system.

A combination of radiotherapy in various doses and chemotherapy is used in most centres.

Intracranial haemorrhage is uncommon in acute lymphoblastic leukaemia but is a frequent cause of death in nonlymphoblastic types (Yamauchi and Umeda 1997). Subdural haematoma or subarachnoid haemorrhage usually indicates a poor prognosis. Sinus thrombosis (David *et al.* 1975) may present with seizures and symptoms of increased ICP. Cranial neuropathies resulting from leukaemic infiltration of the basilar meninges commonly involve the facial, abducens and auditory nerves. Epidural compression of the spinal cord may be an initial manifestation (Pui *et al.* 1985).

COMPLICATIONS MAINLY RELATED TO THERAPY
The effects of therapy of leukaemia on the nervous sytem, whether related to irradiation or to chemical toxicity, are a source of concern, and minimizing such effects is an important part of attempts to improve the treatment of leukaemia (Rowland *et al.* 1984). It is often difficult to separate toxicity mainly due to irradiation from the toxic effects of drugs (Hanefeld and Riehm 1980). In a somewhat arbitrary manner I will describe in succession the complications attributed primarily to irradiation, those due to chemical toxicity, and those that result from opportunistic infections facilitated by or due to therapeutically induced immunosuppression.

Complications mainly due to irradiation
These include a transient *syndrome of somnolence and apathy* that

may develop in 58–63 per cent of patients one or two months following completion of irradiation, with malaise, anorexia and vomiting (Hanefeld and Riehm 1980). The course is usually benign with resolution in 10–20 days. The EEG background frequencies decrease markedly during this syndrome, and learning disabilities and recurrent seizures seem to be more frequent in patients with the syndrome suggesting that somnolence may be an indicator of long-term neurological sequelae after cranial irradiation (Ch'ien *et al.* 1980). A similar syndrome may occur after irradiation of the spinal cord, appearing a few weeks to months after completion of treatment. The first symptom is often tingling in the back induced by neck flexion (Lhermitte sign). Paraesthesia may be a prominent feature but all symptoms abate after two to eight weeks. An acute intermittent confusional state may occur several years following completion of X-ray therapy (Hall *et al.* 1993) and is probably due to ischaemia from irradiation vasculopathy.

Necrotizing leukoencephalopathy is also due, at least in part, to irradiation, although the administration of methotrexate plays an important role in its genesis. Pathological lesions range from simple pallor of myelin to necrosis with cavitation. Numerous alterations of vessels with hyalinization and endothelial proliferation are present (Robain *et al.* 1984). Spinal involvement is usually absent although it has occasionally been reported (Ch'ien and Price 1982).

The clinical features include a change of behaviour with apathy, slurred speech and depressed mood, followed by akinesia and muteness.

Spastic and ataxic gait later becomes evident. CSF protein levels are often raised. The syndrome appears 2–12 months following completion of irradiation. Its mechanism is imperfectly understood. Both the dose of irradiation and that of methotrexate seem to play a role. However, similar CT findings have been found in patients receiving methotrexate who had not been irradiated (Peylan-Ramu *et al.* 1977) and in patients who had received radiotherapy and cytosine arabinoside (Fusner *et al.* 1977). The CT scan shows large, poorly-limited areas of hypodensity of the white matter bilaterally. Enhancement of the white matter is sometimes observed. Multiple areas of calcification mainly located at the junction of the white and grey matter appear secondarily.

A variable degree of atrophy is associated with the white matter lesions. Transient atrophy has been recorded following prophylactic CNS treatment of lymphoblastic leukaemia (Lund and Harsborg-Pedersen 1984).

Calcification of the basal ganglia, especially the putamen, commonly appears approximately one year after irradiation in many children, the majority of whom remain asymptomatic (Peylan-Ramu *et al.* 1978). Calcification in other deep cortical regions may also be asymptomatic (Price and Birdwell 1978). Calcification appears to result from a microangiopathy with secondary calcium deposition. The angiopathy also plays an important role as a cause of the white matter hypodense areas reflecting demyelination, necrosis and glial damage so often shown by CT or MRI examination of irradiated children

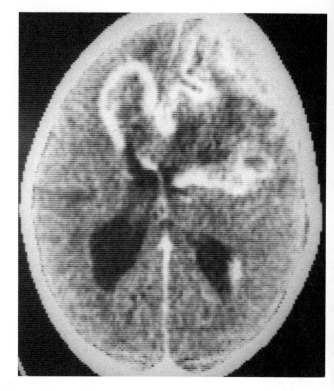

Fig. 14.15. Extensive glioblastoma multiforme in 9-year-old girl who had been treated for acute lymphocytic leukaemia at age 3 years and was subsequently retarded with a leukoencephalopathy due to methotrexate and X-irradiation. This is typical of a 'second tumour' probably induced by initial therapy.

(Constine *et al.* 1988). There is no established relationship between the extent of MRI abnormalities and clinical features, although the most severe lesions tend to be frequently associated with dementia. Brainstem demyelination in the form of multifocal areas or as central pontine myelinolysis has been reported (Lo Monaco *et al.* 1992). A leukoencephalopathy has also been observed in patients with malignancies receiving amphotericin B treatment (Walker and Rosenbloom 1992).

Cerebrovascular accidents can be related to radiotherapy. Mitchell *et al.* (1991) reported 11 cases occurring one to four years after completion of treatment. Seven patients had also received chemotherapy and five had repeated episodes. Cerebrovascular accidents may also result from disseminated intravascular coagulation, especially at onset of treatment of promyelocytic leukaemia (Packer *et al.* 1985). In such cases, the symptoms and signs are recurrent and fluctuating and the course is often lethal. Early anticoagulation may be effective in some cases. Packer *et al.* (1985) recognized four different syndromes in children treated for lymphoreticular malignancies and, less commonly, for solid tumours. These include, in addition to intravascular coagulation, acute neurological dysfunction in children treated for osteogenic sarcoma, acute hemiplegia in patients treated with L-asparaginase (see below) and a syndrome of impaired consciousness, seizures and focal neurological deficits produced by metastatic neuroblastoma compressing the torcular. The relationship of acute hemiplegia to irradiation is also suggested by reports of accelerated atherosclerosis following radiation therapy in adults and in children (Werner *et al.* 1988). Shuper *et al.* (1995) have reported 'complicated migraine-like' episodes in four irradiated children. Severe headache was associated with transient hemiparesis and/or aphasia. Angiography may exacerbate the symptoms.

Second tumours are well-recognized complications of irradiation (Ron *et al.* 1988). The development of tumours has been observed following irradiation for benign conditions such as tinea capitis (Anderson and Treip 1984). Meningiomas are frequent in adults (Mack and Wilson 1993) but rare in children. Glioblastoma multiforme is apt to develop in children with leukaemia treated with X-rays and methotrexate (Chung and McCrary 1986, Mulhern *et al.* 1986) (Fig. 14.15). Multiple primitive neuroectodermal tumours have been reported in the same circumstances (Barasch *et al.* 1988). Other complications of irradiation, especially of brain tumours or of extracranial tumours, include radionecrosis and postradiotherapy thrombosis of the carotid artery with development of deep anastomotic vessels mimicking moyamoya syndrome (Debrun *et al.* 1975).

Radionecrosis is a rare complication that usually becomes clinically manifest months to years following completion of the treatment, with a maximum frequency between one and three years. It occurs mainly following large doses of the order of 60 Gy or more. Pathologically, the lesions predominate in the white matter with characteristic vascular changes (endothelial proliferation and fibrinoid necrosis) that may lead to complete occlusion. The clinical manifestations include insidious and progressive deterioration, with dementia, focal neurological signs and seizures, and often death. They are often interpreted as indicating tumour relapse, an impression which is often also given by neuroradiological findings as neither CT nor MRI even with gadolinium enhancement can distinguish the mass effect of necrosis from that due to recurrence of a tumour. Excision of the lesion may be lifesaving (Cantini *et al.* 1989, Nelson *et al.* 1990) but is probably unnecessary in less severe cases (Woo *et al.* 1987). Radionecrosis has been reported following irradiation of extraneural tumours of the head or scalp (Vallée *et al.* 1984). A severe form of early delayed radiation-induced damage reported by Lampert and Davis (1964) manifested with rapidly progressive ataxia, focal motor signs, cranial neuropathies and nystagmus 13 weeks after X-ray treatment and was associated with plaques resembling those in multiple sclerosis. For severe radiation-induced injury, treatment with heparin and warfarin (Glantz *et al.* 1994) may improve the outcome.

A more benign syndrome featuring hallucinations progressing to seizures and areas of triangular hypodensity in watershed areas suggestive of infarcts has been described by Pihko *et al.* (1993). This syndrome regresses without sequelae.

Radiation-induced lesions of the peripheral nerves are much rarer than CNS damage. A few cases are on record mainly in adults (Lamy *et al.* 1991).

Complications mainly due to drug toxicity

All the drugs used in the treatment of cancer have significant toxicity.

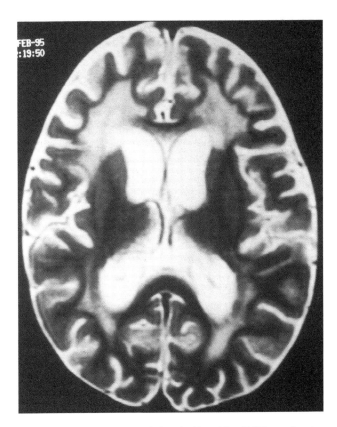

Fig. 14.16. Methotrexate encephalopathy. T_2-weighted MRI scan showing extensive leukoencephalopathy involving predominantly frontal and to a lesser extent occipital white matter. (Courtesy Dr Kling Chong, Great Ormond Street Hospital, London.)

High-dose administration of methotrexate by intraventricular route has been associated with reversible dementia in a nonirradiated child with myelogenic leukaemia (Pizzo *et al.* 1976). A variety of neurological manifestations, including cranial nerve palsies and focal and diffuse deficits, have been seen one or two weeks after intravenous administration for the treatment of osteogenic sarcoma (Fig. 14.16). Intrathecal methotrexate may be followed by a sudden paraplegia that may be transient or persistent (Gagliano and Costanzi 1976). A similar accident can be caused by intrathecal injection of vincristine (Bain *et al.* 1991) or of cytosine arabinoside (Lazarus *et al.* 1981, Özön *et al.* 1994). Both drugs given intrathecally more commonly induce arachnoiditis with signs of meningeal irritation, headache, vomiting and moderate pleocytosis (Hanefeld and Riehm 1980). Cerebellar degeneration may be induced by cytosine arabinoside (Winkelman and Hines 1983).

Vincristine toxicity includes a neuropathy (Chapter 21) and, rarely, an acute encephalopathic syndrome marked mainly by seizures that may be associated with cortical blindness (Byrd *et al.* 1981) and other neurological deficits. Hyponatraemia is frequently present and plays a role in the origin of seizures, but direct cerebral involvement seems likely in some cases. Cerebral blindness has also been reported during treatment with cyclosporin A in association with other manifestations of toxic encephalopathy

(Rubin and Kang 1987). Hypomagnesaemia appears to be a facilitating factor for the occurrence of a cyclosporin encephalopathy (Thompson *et al.* 1984).

L-asparaginase can produce thrombosis of the cerebral veins or dural sinuses that may be associated with either haemorrhage or infarction. This syndrome generally occurs after a few weeks of therapy, sometimes even after discontinuation of treatment. CT and MRI evidence of venous thrombosis may be apparent (Feinberg and Swenson 1988). The thrombogenic effect of the drug seems to be mediated through transient deficiencies of plasma proteins important for coagulation and fibrinolysis.

Carmustine therapy in high doses has been responsible for an acute encephalopathic syndrome (Burger *et al.* 1981). Cytosine arabinoside (Lazarus *et al.* 1981), intraventricular methotrexate (Boogerd *et al.* 1988) and cisplatin (Daugaard *et al.* 1987) can also produce delayed toxicity.

Cisplatin can cause a peripheral neuropathy (Chapter 21) and involvement of the auditory nerve (Schaefer *et al.* 1985).

Complications related to opportunistic infections

These include bacterial, viral, fungal and protozoan diseases that have been described in Chapter 11. In the series of Campbell *et al.* (1977) complicating infections were present in 21 of 438 children with leukaemia. Twelve were viral and nine bacterial in origin. Mumps was the most common, occurring in five patients, one of whom died. The subacute measles encephalitis seen in children with treated lymphatic malignancies is described in Chapter 11.

LATE EFFECTS OF THE TREATMENT OF LEUKAEMIAS ON COGNITIVE DEVELOPMENT

Prophylactic treatment of the CNS of patients with various types of leukaemia may produce cognitive deficits, which are particularly frequent in children who developed the early somnolence syndrome. Although many children function within the normal range, children who received treatment at a young age tend to perform below their matched controls, especially on tasks measuring quantitative, memory and motor skills, but not on language tasks. Their academic results are even poorer than their IQ would suggest and behavioural problems are common (Anderson *et al.* 1994, Jankovic *et al.* 1994, MacLean *et al.* 1995).

The mechanism of such deficits is probably multifactorial. Irradiation seems to play a prominant role but psychogenic factors are also probably operative to some extent.

NEUROLOGICAL MANIFESTATIONS OF LYMPHOMAS

NON-HODGKIN LYMPHOMAS

Involvement of the CNS is not uncommon (Franssila *et al.* 1987) and was observed in 25 per cent of 63 children at the time of diagnosis by Bergeron *et al.* (1989). Ten of these 16 patients had clinical manifestations, with frequent affectation of cranial nerves, including hypoacusis and sudden amaurosis. Seven of these children had an abnormal CSF. Six had asymptomatic meningitis. The characteristics of the CSF are similar to those in leukaemia.

Neuromeningeal relapses occurred in 19 children (30 per cent). A peripheral neuropathy is sometimes seen in patients with lymphomas and is of ominous prognostic significance. Involvement of the venous sinuses may occur (Ceyhan *et al.* 1994).

CNS involvement is much more frequent in lymphomas located in the cervical region than in those of abdominal or thoracic location. Small-cell (Burkitt) lymphomas seem to have a better prognosis than other types.

Primary lymphoma of the CNS is being recognized increasingly as a complication of the acquired immunodeficiency syndrome (AIDS). Lymphomas may be more common in children than opportunistic CNS infections (Epstein *et al.* 1988). They present as focal mass lesions, hyperdense before contrast with marked homogeneous enhancement, and give an intense signal on T_2-weighted MRI sequences. New lesions are apt to appear every few days. Two of the three children reported by Epstein *et al.* had large cell neoplasms, one a Burkitt-type lymphoma. These lesions, which may be mistaken for inflammatory lesions, are highly sensitive to steroid treatment, although recurrence is ultimately inevitable. The effects of lymphomas on the peripheral nervous system have been reviewed by Hughes *et al.* (1994).

HODGKIN DISEASE

Neurological complications of Hodgkin disease are uncommon in children (Sapozink and Kaplan 1983). They include intracerebral deposits that give rise to focal signs, basal meningeal involvement with cranial nerve palsies and spinal extradural deposits that can produce paraplegia. These are usually associated with CSF abnormalities, occasionally in the form of an eosinophilic meningitis (Patchell and Perry 1981).

Another type of neural involvement results from direct extension into the nervous system of visceral disease, producing compression of the brainstem, the brachial plexus and the spinal roots.

A polyneuropathy, due not to direct infiltration of the nerves but apparently to the remote effect of malignancy, has been reported in a child with Hodgkin disease (Kurczynski *et al.* 1980). Such paraneoplastic disorders which are common in adults are exceptional in children. A paraneoplastic cerebellar syndrome manifesting as chronic ataxia has been reported in one child (Topçu *et al.* 1992).

All lymphomas may be associated with the same opportunistic infections as leukaemias.

INTRACRANIAL CYSTS (EXCLUDING TUMOROUS AND PARASITIC CYSTS)

ARACHNOID CYSTS

Most intracranial cysts are arachnoid cysts. The term designates fluid-filled cavities that develop either within a duplication of the arachnoid membrane or between the arachnoid and the pia mater. Arachnoid cysts represent 1 per cent of space-occupying lesions (Hanieh *et al.* 1988), and 60–90 per cent of symptomatic lesions are recognized during childhood or adolescence (Harsh *et al.* 1986). Cysts may be an incidental finding in up to 5 per

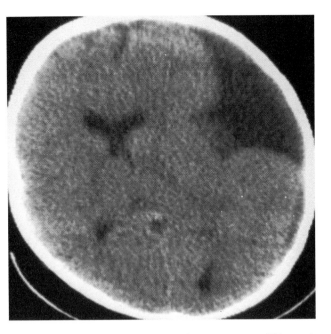

Fig. 14.17. Arachnoid cyst of the sylvian fissure in 10-year-old boy with large head from the first months of life and no other complaint. Note marked dislocation of ventricular system, which is of normal size.

cent of cases in autopsy studies (Naidich *et al.* 1985–1986). Arachnoid cysts are most usually malformations and only rarely follow arachnoiditis. Arachnoid cysts may or may not communicate with the subarachnoid space, whether located supratentorially or infratentorially.

SUPRATENTORIAL CYSTS

These are the most common type of intracranial cysts. Middle fossa (sylvian) arachnoid cysts have the highest frequency in most series, followed by suprasellar cysts and cysts of the cerebral convexity (Harsh *et al.* 1986, Diebler and Dulac 1987, Hanieh *et al.* 1988).

Middle fossa cysts are frequently asymptomatic and may be discovered incidentally on CT scans performed for various reasons (Fig. 14.17). Robertson *et al.* (1989) have proposed that hypoplasia or hypogenesis of the temporal lobe is the cause, although most authors consider that the temporal lobe is displaced rather than hypoplastic. When of moderate size and found in later childhood or adolescence these cysts do not require treatment. The only clinical manifestation is temporal bossing. Bilateral cysts of the temporal fossa have been reported in children with glutaric aciduria type I (Hald *et al.* 1991, Martinez-Lage *et al.* 1994). Such lesions are also reported as atrophy of the temporal lobe, a term that seems more appropriate than that of cyst, especially as no treatment is ever indicated in such cases. Symptomatic sylvian cysts can give rise to signs of increased pressure, especially headache and papilloedema, or to seizures, usually focal (Van der Meché and Braakman 1983), or become manifest as a result of haemorrhagic complications (Page *et al.* 1987). These include bleeding into the cyst which may render the cavity invisible on CT scan, and subdural haematoma with or without associated

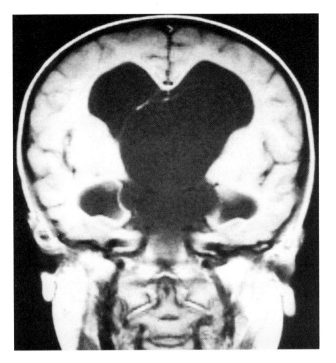

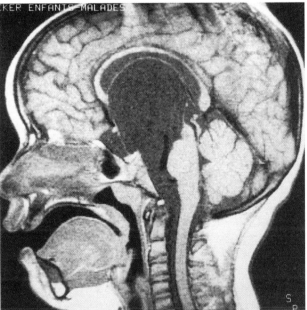

Fig. 14.18. Suprasellar arachnoid cyst. *(Top)* T₁-weighted MRI, frontal cut shows massive hydrocephalus of lateral ventricles. Third ventricle is entirely filled with a cyst, separated from lateral ventricle by a thin membrane, and with a fluid content slightly denser than CSF. *(Bottom)* Sagittal cut shows that the cyst extends upwards almost to the corpus callosum. (Courtesy Prof. F. Brunelle, Hôpital des Enfants Malades, Paris.)

intracystic haemorrhage. It seems likely that the 'juvenile relapsing subdural haematoma', characterized radiologically by bony changes similar to those of sylvian cysts, is a haematoma complicating a middle fossa cyst. Subdural haematoma may rarely be on the side opposite to the cyst.

Treatment of sylvian cyst is best performed by cystoperitoneal shunting. However, children with huge cysts and closed fontanelles are probably best left unoperated and carefully followed because the skull has accomodated both the cyst and the brain so that evacuation may be poorly tolerated.

Suprasellar cysts are manifested by hydrocephalus in 90 per cent of cases. Visual abnormalities and ataxia are observed in a quarter of the cases. In some patients they are responsible for a slow anteroposterior to-and-fro movement of the head at a rhythm of 2–3 Hz known as the *'bobble-head doll syndrome'*. Precocious puberty may be a feature. Partial hypopituitarism with especial involvement of corticotropin secretion is seen in 10 per cent of patients (Brauner *et al.* 1987).

The CT appearance is typical with a large rounded suprasellar image of fluid density obstucting the foramina of Monro with resulting hydrocephalus (Fig. 14.18). MRI scan may show that the cyst and the third ventricle are distinct cavities separated by a thin membrane. Treatment may be with shunting of the cyst. Opening of the cyst membrane by an endoscopic or open approach is also possible (Decq *et al.* 1996).

Arachnoid cysts of the convexity can produce focal signs and raised ICP. Interhemispheric cysts may be difficult to separate from dorsal cysts associated with agenesis of the corpus callosum. Cysts in this location are apt to be dysembryoplastic with cuboid or columnar epithelium rather than arachnoidal cells.

INFRATENTORIAL ARACHNOID CYSTS

Infratentorial arachnoid cysts are the second most frequent form of intracranial cysts after middle fossa cysts. Their histological structure is diverse and only a few are true arachnoid cysts (Friede 1989). In fact, there is some confusion regarding what should be considered as a posterior fossa arachnoid cyst, because other fluid collections are common in the posterior fossa. These include Dandy–Walker syndrome, megacisterna magna and even some cases of large but nonpathological cisterna magna (Chapter 3; see also Naidich *et al.* 1985–1986, Barkovich *et al.* 1989, Altman *et al.* 1992). Posterior fossa cysts are closed cavities that do not communicate with the fourth ventricle and are not associated with hypoplasia of the cerebellum. The most common clinical manifestations in infants and young children are macrocephaly and hydrocephalus, whereas typical posterior fossa syndrome is the presenting manifestation in older patients (Galassi *et al.* 1985, Harsh *et al.* 1986).The location of the cysts within the posterior fossa is variable. A majority are located behind the cerebellum, but some lesions may be supracerebellar, laterocerebellar or located to the cerebellopontine angle (Galassi *et al.* 1985).

Cysts of the incisura are often both infratentorial and supratentorial and are located anteriorly to the cerebellar vermis, posterior to the pineal region and above the quadrigeminal plate, extending above the roof of the third ventricle below the corpus callosum (Fig. 14.19). In addition to hydrocephalus, they may be associated with Parinaud syndrome or ataxia. Some mesencephalic and third ventricle cysts may be secondary to arachnoiditis caused by thalamic haemorrhage, or bacterial ventriculitis (Ramaeckers *et al.* 1994).

Treatment of posterior fossa cysts may be by direct operative approach (Hanieh *et al.* 1988). Derivation by cystoperitoneal

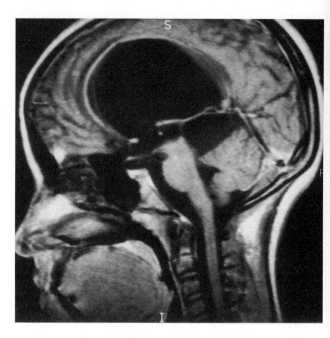

Fig. 14.19. Arachnoid cyst of the incisura with hydrocephalus due to aqueductal compression. The cystic quadrigeminal cistern also flattens the cerebellar vermis (T_1-weighted MRI).

shunting (Vaquero *et al.* 1981) seems to be the method of choice and leads in many cases to complete disappearance of the lesion.

OTHER INTRACRANIAL CYSTS

Ependymal cysts are rare. Their cavity is lined with an ependyma-like epithelium. They are rare, supratentorial, intracerebral or convexity lesions most often located within the frontal lobe (Friede and Yasargil 1977). They do not communicate with the ventricles and probably arise from displaced segments of the wall of the neural tube which correspond to the sites from which the tela choroidea forms. Ependymal cysts may be associated with complex brain malformations (Barth *et al.* 1984).

Huge cysts occupying the prepontine region but extending to the posterior and middle fossa have been reported (Yoshida *et al.* 1986). The lining epithelium in some cases was probably of respiratory origin.

Enterogenous cysts are also rare and generally found in the spine or posterior fossa. Rare instances of supratentorial enterogenous cysts are on record (Walls *et al.* 1986).

Cysts of the Rathke cleft develop in the suprasellar region and may be associated with endocrine or visual abnormalities or raised ICP (Rout *et al.* 1983).

The *empty sella syndrome* is in fact a misnomer as the sella is not completely empty but contains a remnant of pituitary tissue. Although not a cystic formation it is described here as the sella turcica is ballooned and may be mistakenly considered as harbouring a tumour or cyst. The aetiology of the condition is unknown as is its frequency in childhood. In some cases, the 'empty sella' is accompanied by visual or endocrine disturbances ranging from panhypopituitarism to precocious puberty (Shulman *et al.* 1986, Stanhope and Adlard 1987). Visual field defects have been reported (Costigan *et al.* 1984) and the condition may occur with microadenomas of the hypophysis. The syndrome may be seen in patients with pseudotumour cerebri, hydrocephalus and CSF rhinorrhoea. Empty sella in childhood may be less benign than in adults, and children with this condition require regular assessment.

PSEUDOTUMOUR CEREBRI (BENIGN INTRACRANIAL HYPERTENSION)

DEFINITION AND CAUSES
Benign intracranial hypertension is defined as a syndrome with raised ICP in the absence of a space-occupying lesion or apparent obstruction to the CSF pathways. Raised ICP can result from increased venous pressure, as in the superior vena cava syndrome or dural venous thrombosis, from increased resistance of arachnoid villi to resorption of CSF (usually of unknown cause), or from CSF hypersecretion perhaps related to endocrine abnormalities (Sørensen *et al.* 1986). Although it has been suggested that the same conditions can result in hydrocephalus if the skull is compliant, as in infants, or in pseudotumour if the compliance is less, other as yet undetermined factors are probably important. Particularly puzzling is the fact that, in a majority of cases, the ventricles are small rather than enlarged (Reid *et al.* 1980). Some investigators believe that brain swelling is a major factor and can be shown by CT scan (Rothwell *et al.* 1994) while others have been unable to demonstrate the presence of brain oedema by MRI (Connolly *et al.* 1992) or at post-mortem examination in two adult cases (Wall *et al.* 1995).

The main causes of pseudotumour cerebri are shown in Table 14.7. Venous factors, especially thrombosis of the lateral sinus as a result of otitis media, were the main cause of pseudotumour until recently. Currently, refeeding of malnourished children with nutritional deprivation or cystic fibrosis has emerged as an important cause in some tertiary care centres (Couch *et al.* 1985). However, a majority of the cases remain unexplained and some of the proposed aetiologies may, in fact, be the result of coincidences (Baker *et al.* 1989) as many of the supposed 'causes' were not more common in patients with hypertension than in controls. All large series show more frequent affectation of girls and the role of obesity, well known in adult women, is probably also important in adolescent girls who accounted for one-third of the cases reported by Babikian *et al.* (1994). Corticosteroid withdrawal is an interesting cause as it may throw some light on the mechanisms and has practical consequences on discontinuation of steroid treatment. A few familial cases are on record (Torlai *et al.* 1989).

CLINICAL FEATURES
Headache is the most common feature and often the sole complaint (Grant 1971). Diplopia due to VIth nerve palsy, vomiting, and loss of visual acuity or restriction of the visual field are present in 18–48 per cent of patients (Baker *et al.* 1989). Papilloedema sometimes with gross haemorrhages or at least some degree of blurring of the disc margins is present in almost

TABLE 14.7
Pseudotumour cerebri

Disorder	References
Ear infections (related to thrombosis of lateral sinus)	Grant (1971), Williams and Richardson (1988)
Vena cava and other venous thrombosis or obstruction	Sainte-Rose *et al.* (1984)
Refeeding of malnourished children	Couch *et al.* (1985)
Endocrine or metabolic dysfunction	
Addison disease	Donaldson (1981)
Corticosteroid therapy withdrawal	Neville and Wilson (1970)
Drug treatment of hypothyroidism with prostaglandin inhibitors	Van Dop *et al.* (1983)
Chronic hypocalcaemia (hypoparathyroidism)	Donaldson (1981) Sheldon *et al.* (1987)
Pseudohypoparathyroidism	Sheldon *et al.* (1987)
Vitamin D-deficient rickets	Cogan *et al.* (1978)
Chronic carbon dioxide retention	Austen *et al.* (1957)
Obesity	Babikian *et al.* (1994)
Iron deficiency anaemia	Stoebner *et al.* (1970)
Hyperthyroidism	Ono *et al.* (1987)
Growth hormone treatment	Malozowski *et al.* (1995)
Behçet syndrome	Shakir *et al.* (1990)
Exogenous drugs or toxins	
Antibiotics (tetracycline and minocycline)	Walters and Gubbay (1981), Lubetzki *et al.* (1988), Gardner *et al.* (1995)
Excess dose of vitamin A	Feldman and Schlezinger (1970)
Insecticide toxicity	Sanborn *et al.* (1979)
Nitrofurantoin	Mushet (1977)
Nalidixic acid	Deonna and Guignard (1970)
Praziquantel	Grogan and Narkun (1987)
Amiodarone	Van Zandijcke and Dewachter (1986)
Oral contraceptives	Soyza (1985)
Isotretinoin	Roytman *et al.* (1988)
Indomethacin	Konomi *et al.* (1978)
Diphtheria–tetanus–pertussis vaccine	Gross *et al.* (1989)
Idiopathic (may be familial)	Buchheit *et al.* (1969)

all cases in most series but only in less than 50 per cent in some studies. Other less common symptoms and signs may include facial palsy (Baker *et al.* 1989) occasionally bilateral (Selky *et al.* 1994), vertical strabismus or other ocular motor abnormalities, pupillary abnormalities, spinal and radicular pain (Macaya *et al.* 1988), facial pain (Hart and Carter 1982), tinnitus and ataxia (Round and Keane 1988). However, a majority of patients have remarkably few complaints despite evidence of marked intracranial hypertension.

Splaying of sutures is present in virtually all cases. A normal neuroimaging study must be obtained before considering the diagnosis of pseudotumour cerebri.

Visual loss is the main concern for patients with benign intracranial hypertension. It is observed in about 10 per cent of adults with the syndrome but is probably less common in children. Recent reports, however, have established that transient or permanent visual loss does occur in childhood (Baker *et al.* 1985, Lessell and Rosman 1986). Therefore, sequential perimetry and assessments of visual acuity are in order whenever possible (Wall and George 1987, Wall *et al.* 1995). For adults, study of contrast sensitivity seems to be a promising method more accurate for determination of prognosis than study of the visual evoked potentials (Verplanck *et al.* 1988). Such methods may be applicable at least to older children. Three of 39 children treated at Great Ormond Street Hospital, London, between 1984 and 1995 remain with a significant visual handicap at follow-up (M. Salman and F.J. Kirkham, personal communication 1996), clearly pointing to the need for continued investigation.

TREATMENT

In some patients spontaneous resolution of ICP may occur and in others treatment of the cause (Table 14.7) can lead to disappearance of symptoms and signs. Most patients, however, require nonspecific therapy but there is no agreement as to the most effective methods. Repeated lumbar punctures are often effective for up to a few days but cannot be indefinitely repeated. Steroid administration (dexamethasone, 0.1–0.25 mg/kg/d, or prednisone, 1 mg/kg/d) is commonly used although its value has not been fully assessed. Because of the frequency and severity of side-effects, many clinicians tend to use steroids only as a last resort. Acetazolamide (30–100 mg/kg/d) and furosemide (1–2 mg/kg t.i.d.) have been found useful in significantly lowering ICP (Schoeman 1994). Lumboperitoneal shunt may be necessary when vision appears threatened but often requires revision and may become infected. Optic nerve fenestration (Knight *et al.* 1986) is indicated when there is evidence of progressive optic neuropathy despite therapy.

CEREBRAL OEDEMA

DEFINITION AND CLINICAL FEATURES

Cerebral oedema is defined as an increase in brain volume due to an increase in its water content. Oedema is an important cause of ICP. However, localized oedema need not produce intracranial hypertension but may result in focal brain dysfunction.

The diagnosis of brain oedema may be difficult. The clinical manifestations are those of raised ICP, and differentiation of brain oedema from cerebral congestion, *i.e.* increase of cerebral blood volume, may be impossible. Increased blood volume may be caused by epileptic activity, vasoparalysis resulting from asphyxia, head injury, increase in CO_2 content of blood as a result of pulmonary or heart disease, venous obstruction, and the effects of drugs such as nitrites, chlorpromazine or halothane.

Cerebral oedema can often be detected by imaging. CT scanning may show diffuse or localized low attenuation as a result of high water content. On MRI, oedema often presents with intense signal on T_2-weighted spin–echo sequences (Barnes *et al.* 1987). Oedema may be an isolated finding, for example in patients with diabetic ketoacidosis (Rosenbloom *et al.* 1980, Franklin *et al.* 1982) or following unilateral or focal status epilepticus. It is frequently associated with other anomalies such as brain tumours or cerebral abscesses.

The symptoms and signs of cerebral oedema are often difficult to separate from those of its causal lesion. In some cases, oedema, especially of a diffuse type, is clearly the most important cause of the clinical signs, as for example in Reye syndrome, and, in such cases, oedema is the main target of therapy.

The presence of brain oedema, whether in association with other lesions or in isolation, has an important bearing on the management of patients and the understanding of the clinical picture.

TYPES OF BRAIN OEDEMA

Cerebral oedema can belong to several types depending on its location and pathogenesis, and each category of oedema is preferentially associated with certain causes (Crockard 1985).

Vasogenic oedema is the result of increased permeability of endothelium of capillaries of the blood–brain barrier, leading to the exudation of protein-rich plasma filtrate into the extracellular fluid. This type of oedema involves most markedly the cerebral white matter in a focal or generalized distribution. Vasogenic oedema is caused by inflammatory processes such as meningitis or abcesses, by focal lesions that produce an inflammatory response by various mechanisms, such as intracerebral haemorrhages, infarcts or tumours, and by disorders that primarily affect the cerebral vessels such as lead encephalopathy or hypertensive encephalopathy. Oedema that appears in the hours following head trauma probably belongs to this type (Chapter 13), as seems also to be the case with focal oedema following partial complex status epilepticus (Sammaritano *et al.* 1985), although, in both cases, more than one cause and one mechanism may be operative. Treatment with corticosteroids may be especially effective in this type of oedema.

Cytotoxic oedema often coexists with vasogenic oedema. In this type, cellular constituents of the brain, especially astrocytes but also neurons and endothelial cells, undergo rapid swelling as a consequence of dysfunction of the membranes and ionic pumps. The latter is usually due to energy failure and may lead to cellular death, in which case the oedema is irreversible. Hypoxia due to cardiac arrest or to any cause of hypoxic–ischaemic encephalopathy is the most frequent cause but various toxins and severe infectious processes, and increased ICP itself with decreasing cerebral blood flow, are possible causes. Other mechanisms include neuronal death following status epilepticus and infarction of arterial origin.

Hypoosmotic oedema is a consequence of osmotic dysequilibrium between a low osmolarity plasma compartment and the higher osmotic pressure of glial cells. Water accumulates within astrocytes. Such a type occurs with hyponatraemia whether iatrogenic or due to inappropriate ADH secretion, in patients with diabetes mellitus during treatment of ketoacidosis (Chapter 23) and with the dysequilibrium syndrome of patients undergoing dialysis for renal failure or other reasons.

Hydrostatic oedema results when increased intravascular pressure is transmitted to the capillary bed because of a lack of compensatory increase in the vascular resistance, with resulting outpouring of water into the extracellular space. Such an event

TABLE 14.8
Symptoms and signs of decompensation with raised intracranial pressure

Decreased level of consciousness (use modified coma scale)
Uni/bilateral hypertonia
    Decorticate posturing
    Decerebrate posturing
Uni/bilateral extensor plantar signs
Unilateral IIIrd nerve paralysis
Unilateral VIth nerve paralysis
Paralysis of upward gaze
Pupillary dilatation, unilateral, not or sluggishly reacting to light
Yawning, periodic respiration, spontaneous hyperventilation, shallow or irregular respiration

TABLE 14.9
Main causes of nontraumatic increased intracranial pressure (excluding intracranial mass lesions and hydrocephalus)

Cause	References
Primary intracranial diseases	
Infections	
Meningitis	
Encephalitis	Chapter 11
Reye syndrome	
Cerebrovascular diseases	
Bleeding secondary to vascular malformations	Chapter 15
Arterial strokes	
Sinus and venous thrombosis	
Epilepsy	
Transient with short seizures	Chapter 16
Prolonged (status epilepticus)	Brown and Hussain (1991)
Systemic diseases with cerebral involvement	
Diabetic ketoacidosis and coma	Chapter 23
Hypertensive encephalopathy	Chapter 15
Toxic agents	
Lead	
Ethyltin	Chapter 13
Hexachlorophane	
Renal disease	
Haemodialysis	Chapter 23
Haemolytic–uraemic syndrome	Hahn *et al.* (1989)
Hepatic encephalopathy	Chapter 23
Burns	Mohnot *et al.* (1982)
Hypoxic–ischaemic encephalopathy	
Cardiac arrest	Constantinou *et al.* (1989)
Near-drowning	Nussbaum and Maggi (1988)

occurs when the complex mechanisms of brain vascular auto-regulation fail as in cases of uncompensated hypertension, hypercapnia and, probably, in some cases of head trauma. Hydro-static oedema is usually diffuse in distribution and clearly does not respond to steroids.

Interstitial oedema is caused by the transependymal resorption of CSF from the ventricles into the extracellular space in patients with hydrocephalus. This type of oedema is clearly shown by CT scan or MRI, which demonstrate areas of decreased attenuation in a periventricular distribution, especially around the anterior and posterior horns of the ventricles.

Intramyelinic oedema is less common. It has been observed mainly following intoxication with triethyltin and hexachloro-phane (Goutières and Aicardi 1977). The oedema is located between myelin lamellae forming intramyelinic 'bubbles'. This type of oedema is always diffuse in distribution, involves mainly the white matter and may affect the spinal cord. It can produce very high pressure levels and may be lethal or leave residua, especially when the swollen spinal cord has been strangulated in its unextensible dural sheath with definitive paraplegia.

MANAGEMENT OF RAISED INTRACRANIAL PRESSURE

Raised ICP is a major problem in patients with brain tumours and other expansive lesions, but also in several acute pathological situations such as brain infections or ischaemia. It is responsible for many complications including mass displacements of the brain and herniation, so its early recognition and treatment are essential. Table 14.8 lists the symptoms and signs that herald impending life-threatening complications. These are usually attributed to herniation but high ICP with resulting decrease in cerebral blood flow may be responsible and regression of the symptoms with lowering of pressure can often be obtained.

In chronic situations such as brain tumours, treatment of the cause (removal of mass) is usually sufficient. In acute situations, however, treatment of the cause, although required, may not be sufficient. The most common causes of acutely raised ICP are shown in Table 14.9. For such cases, immediate lowering of ICP is often essential and may dramatically improve the outcome (see Minns 1991).

The goal of treatment is to reduce ICP to keep cerebral per-fusion pressure above 50 mmHg so that correct oxygenation of the brain is ensured. Cerebral perfusion pressure equals the dif-ference between median systemic pressure and ICP. Therefore maintenance of the systemic circulation is vital.

ICP can be determined in various manners but a single measure is of little value for correct management. For this reason, continuous ICP monitoring has gained increasing acceptance. It should be stressed, however, that it is certainly more important to treat urgently any underlying cause, such as meningitis, than to insert an ICP monitor (Kirkham 1991). Reversal of flow throughout diastole on Doppler study is usually seen when cerebral perfusion pressure approaches zero (Hassler *et al.* 1988), while EEG slowing and low amplitude are correlated with poor perfusion of the brain (Tasker *et al.* 1988).

The treatment of raised ICP, irrespective of its cause, includes meticulous avoidance of all factors, such as painful stimuli, which may transiently increase ICP. Crystalloid fluids should be re-stricted to approximately 60–70 per cent of the age-appropriate requirements and hypoosmolar fluids avoided. An adequate circulation must be quickly restored if necessary with volume expanders and vasopressor agents such as dopamine (10–20 µg/kg/min) and then maintained with lower doses (2 µg/kg/min) as required. Control of seizures which increase secondary deterioration (Constantinou *et al.* 1989) should be vigorously pursued.

It is probably reasonable to administer mannitol (0.25–2 g/kg in 20% solution) as a bolus over 10–15 minutes from the early stage of treatment. This agent is highly effective in reducing ICP; its peak action occurs within 30 minutes and its effect may last from two to six hours. Prolonged use may be associated with rebound intracranial hypertension and aggravation of vasogenic oedema (Kaufmann and Cardoso 1992) and the use of occasional small (0.25 g/kg) doses in response to acute rises of ICP tends to be preferred to regular doses without monitoring.

Hyperventilation produces cerebral vasoconstriction and decreases cerebral blood volume at least initially. The effect of prolonged hyperventilation is controversial as the vasoconstrictive effect may disappear and haemodynamics in the unconscious patient are often altered so that a decrease of CO_2 may be associated with increased cerebral blood flow (Kirkham 1991). Hyperventilation to obtain a PCO_2 of < 25 mmHg (3.3 kPa) may be associated with brain ischaemia although compensatory mechanisms reduce or suppress this effect.

Steroids are mainly useful for treatment of the perifocal oedema of tumours or abcesses. These agents do not appear to be effective in the prevention or improvement of oedema due to infections or ischaemia (Rogers 1987). Dexamethasone is commonly used. The drug is generally given intravenously at a dose of 0.1–0.25 mg per kg body weight initially and may be continued parenterally or orally in a total dose of 0.25–0.5 mg/kg/d in four divided doses. High-dose pulses may be more effective.

Barbiturate coma is not indicated, except perhaps in intractable cranial hypertension and in raised ICP due to status epilepticus (Lowenstein *et al.* 1988). The alleged protective effect of barbiturates on the brain has not been confirmed. Thiopentone is often used in doses of 3–5mg/kg over 10–20 minutes, followed by infusions of 1–2mg/kg at intervals of one or two hours. The agent seriously interferes with EEG monitoring of cerebral function.

Hypothermia is still used by some clinicians (Nussbaum and Maggi 1988) but its role is disputed.

CSF drainage is rarely advisable except in cases of pseudotumour cerebri in which it may be performed by repeated lumbar puncture. External diversion of CSF may be useful for certain neurosurgical patients but the high risk of infection limits the use of this method to specialized units.

Surgical decompression has probably only limited indications.

SPINAL CORD TUMOURS

Spinal cord tumours in childhood are five to ten times less common than brain tumours. Their initial signs are often relatively subtle and their symptoms may easily be disregarded as trivial complaints. Additionally, some spinal cord tumours may have atypical presentations such as acute spinal syndrome mimicking acute transverse myelitis (Chapter 12) or hydrocephalus. As a result, their diagnosis is often made late at a time when paraplegia and, not infrequently, irreparable damage has been produced.

Indeed, spinal cord compression is an even more serious emergency than raised ICP and this possibility must always be present in the mind of paediatricians, while the diagnoses of acute myelitis, of 'hysteria' or 'malingering' should never be accepted before cord compression has been clearly excluded.

Tumours can arise anywhere along the spinal cord. A majority are extradural and extramedullary lesions such as neuroblastomas that penetrate the spinal canal from the posterior mediastinum or the retroperitoneal region. Other tumours are extramedullary but intradural, such as neurofibromas developed on the roots after their emergence from the cord. Intramedullary tumours arise from within the cord. They are often associated with cyst formations and may mimic syringomyelia (Newman *et al.* 1981; see also Chapter 3). In addition to neoplasms, cord compression may result from leukaemic infiltration, lymphomas, arteriovenous malformations and congenital cysts (Pascual-Castraviejo 1990).

The clinical features of spinal cord compression include three groups of symptoms and signs: back pain and rigidity, signs of segmental spinal involvement, and signs resulting from interruption of long tracts within the spinal cord. The importance of back pain and, especially, of *spinal rigidity* as an early symptom of tumour of the cord has long been known. Pain may have a radicular distribution but is more often diffuse and is usually predominantly nocturnal. Rigidity is frequently associated with scoliosis. Segmental weakness, hyporeflexia, sensory disturbances and amyotrophy can result from involvement of the central grey matter or nerve roots. Segmental myoclonus is a rare presentation (Renault *et al.* 1995). Spasticity evolving into paraplegia, sphincter disturbances and sensory deficits result from long tract involvement. Disturbances of walking with claudication and stiffness may be present long before other symptoms. The presence of a definable sensory level, which may be difficult to demonstrate in young children, indicates the upper level of compression. Bilateral pyramidal tract signs are present with Babinski and Rossolimo* responses. Initial bladder symptoms are increased urgency followed by retention or incontinence. Sphincter disturbances, especially urinary retention, indicate urgent need for decompression.

The diagnosis of spinal cord tumour should be quickly confirmed because sudden aggravation with complete paraplegia due to compromised circulation in the anterior cerebral artery and its branches may occur at any time. One should be exceedingly suspicious of recurrent back pain and, in some patients, of recurrent abdominal pain (Eeg-Olofsson *et al.* 1981). Atypical presentations with paroxysmal attacks of arm pain or isolated abdominal discomfort simulating an irritable bowel syndrome (Robertson 1992) may delay recognition of a tumour.

Plain X-rays of the spine may be diagnostic by showing bone destruction, erosion of the spinal pedicles or of the posterior vertebral bodies and widening of both the anteroposterior and transverse diameters of the spinal canal.

*The Rossolimo sign is obtained by flicking the toes upwards. A positive response is active flexion of the toes and is indicative of pyramidal tract involvement. It is more reliable than the Babinski sign in infants and young children.

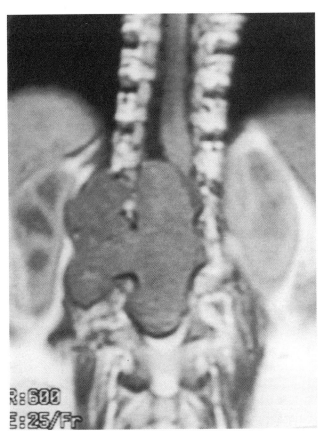

Fig. 14.20. Paraspinal neuroblastoma entering the spinal canal through intervertebral foramen and displacing and compressing the lower spinal cord and roots.

CSF protein is usually increased below the level of the block. However, there is a serious risk of damage to the cord by lumbar puncture at the site of compression possibly due to slight downward displacement of the cord.

Definitive diagnosis requires neuroradiological examination. Currently MRI is the technique of choice, when available. It clearly shows both intra- and extramedullary lesions and associated cystic formation, thus permitting separation of intramedullary tumours with associated cysts from syringomyelia (Williams *et al.* 1987). However, distinguishing a tumour from an area of increased signal due to myelitis can be difficult. Transverse cuts can be obtained allowing detailed studies of the zones of interest discovered with sagittal cuts. With gadolinium enhancement, MRI is as effective as metrizamide myelography for the diagnosis of metastases of brain tumours such as ependymomas or medullobastomas and avoids the reactions associated with the introduction of the contrast medium into the subarachnoid space. These are usually minor (headache, nausea and vomiting, radicular pain and hyperaesthesia) but may include in rare cases seizures (Junck and Marshall 1983) and minor status epilepticus (Obeid *et al.* 1988).

EXTRAMEDULLARY TUMOURS

Approximately half the extramedullary tumours are extradural in

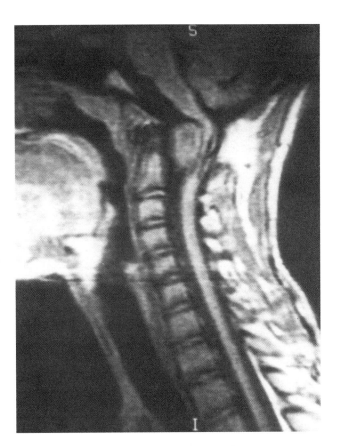

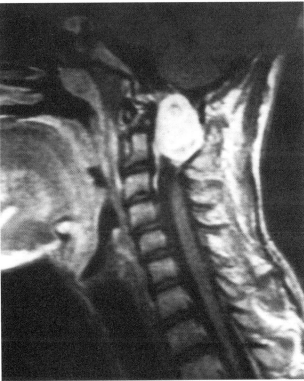

Fig. 14.21. Neurinoma of right C1 and C2 spinal roots. 12-year-old boy who presented with bilateral pyramidal tract signs in both lower limbs, predominantly on left side, and hemihypoaesthesia of right side of body up to base of neck. MRI scan, T₁-weighted sequences. *(Top)* Midline sagittal cut showing tumour compressing and dislocating spinal cord. *(Bottom)* Gadolinium-enhanced paramedian sagittal cut showing contrast take-up by tumour and marked erosion of surrounding bone.

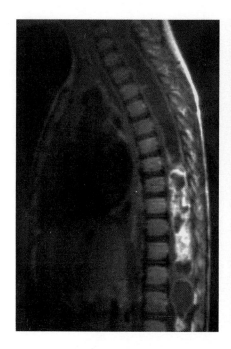
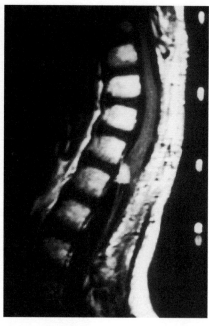

Fig. 14.22. Intramedullary tumour. *(Far left)* MRI, T_1-weighted sequence following gadolinium injection. Note extensive cavitation of spinal cord extending to conus medullaris, and solid area of tumour with mixed signal between upper and lower areas of cavitation. *(Left)* Ependymoma of lower spinal cord. Note enlargement of the lower cord and high T_2 signal. (Courtesy Dr Kling Chong, Great Ormond Street Hospital, London.)

origin, spreading from nearby bone or through intervertebral foramina. About a quarter are intradural. Neuroblastoma (Fig. 14.20) is the most frequent cause but other tumours of osseous or soft tissue origin such as rhabdomyosarcoma, Ewing sarcoma, aneurysmal cysts, metastases or histiocytosis X can be the cause of spinal compression. Intradural tumours account for approximately 25 per cent of cases, and meningiomas are the most common histological type (Levy *et al.* 1982) followed by schwannomas (Fig. 14.21). Metastases from intracranial tumours, especially ependymomas and medulloblastomas, are usually multiple and may be especially difficult to evidence.

The diagnosis of extradural tumours is often facilitated by the demonstration on plain X-ray films of a mass lesion in the cervical region or posterior mediastinum or by the discovery of the adrenal calcification of a neuroblastoma.

Extramedullary tumours tend to manifest initially with unilateral pain in segmental distribution often in association with paraesthesiae and weakness. Brown-Séquard syndrome is observed in a small proportion of children with extramedullary tumours. More commonly, there is only predominant weakness, spasticity and deep sensory loss on the side of the tumour, with more marked contralateral loss of pain and temperature sensation (Levy *et al.* 1982). Neurinomas are more common than meningiomas.

The treatment of extramedullary tumours depends on their nature. For extraspinal tumours with intraspinal extension, surgical removal of the intraspinal tumours should be done on an emergency basis, and later completed by surgical excision and/or other treatment of the extraspinal mass according to its nature. Intraspinal tumours should be treated by surgery (neurinomas) or irradiation and chemotherapy.

INTRAMEDULLARY TUMOURS
Intramedullary tumours are mainly represented by astrocytomas and ependymomas (Pascual-Castroviejo 1990) (Fig. 14.22). Haemangioblastomas (Roig *et al.* 1988) are rare and may be a part of the von Hippel–Lindau complex. These tumours are often cystic and commonly extend over considerable lengths in the cervicodorsal part of the cord. Some of them also involve the lower brainstem. They are frequently associated with cystic cavitation of the central cord, which may be difficult to differentiate from purely cystic intramedullary lesions. They can produce symmetrical weakness of the limbs and are often unassociated with pain. Intramedullary tumours often do not produce a clear-cut sensory level and some of them may be surprisingly well tolerated for long periods despite a considerable extension.

Some spinal tumours may present with the clinical manifestations of raised ICP without local signs (Gelabert *et al.* 1990, Rifkinson-Mann *et al.* 1990). Intracranial hypertension may result from meningeal fibrosis due to haemorrhage from the tumour or from decreased resorption of CSF because of its high protein content 'clogging' the arachnoid granulations. There are cases, however, in which papilloedema and raised pressure are not associated with ventricular dilatation. In two personal cases a tumoural basal arachnoiditis appeared to be responsible for the hydrocephalus and continued to be present years after successful treatment of spinal astrocytoma. An unusual case presenting with the features of spinal muscular atrophy is on record (Aysun *et al.* 1993).

In one infant (personal case), an intramedullary tumour involving the whole length of the cord simulated Werdnig–Hoffmann disease, but a Rossolimo sign was present.

The special features of intraaxial tumours of the cervicomedullary junction have been described earlier (p. 500).

Diagnosis of intramedullary tumours has been facilitated by MRI that allows separation of the cystic cavity from the solid part of the tumour (Williams *et al.* 1987).

Treatment of extended astrocytomas has been made possible by modern neurosurgical techniques (Epstein and Epstein 1982, Epstein 1987, Allen *et al.* 1994). If removal proves impossible, decompression and irradiation may afford fairly long symptomatic relief in 30–50 per cent of cases (Kopelson *et al.* 1980, Huddart *et al.* 1993). However, patients with malignant tumours such as glioblastomas do poorly (Kopelson and Linggood 1982).

OTHER SPINAL COMPRESSIONS

Compression of the cord may occur with epidural infections and with traumatic or spontaneous haematomas (Chapters 11, 13; Pascual-Castraviejo 1990).

Spinal arachnoid cysts can produce a slowly progressive myelopathy but, in some cases, symptoms can fluctuate with time and postural changes (Delodovici *et al.* 1994).

Spinal meningeal cysts (Richaud 1988, Delodovici *et al.* 1994) are a rare cause of cord compression which is accessible to effective treatment. Extradural meningeal cysts are diverticuli of the arachnoid through a dural opening, extending on the back of the cord in the extradural space (Naidich *et al.* 1983). Extradural cysts may be associated with acquired lymphoedema of the lower limbs and lower lid ectropion and distichiasis (double row of eyelashes) (Robinow *et al.* 1970) in a dominant syndrome.

Excessive growth of epidural fat has been reported in patients receiving corticosteroid therapy (Russell *et al.* 1984, Kaplan *et al.* 1989) and, exceptionally, in patients with hypothyroidism (Toshniwal and Glick 1987). This is a dangerous condition for which treatment is difficult (George *et al.* 1983).

Bony compression of the cord is occasionally seen in patients with thalassaemia or, rarely, with other types of haemolytic anaemia or myelosclerosis as a result of overgrowth of the bone marrow, encroaching on the spinal canal (Rutgers *et al.* 1979).

Other rare causes of spinal cord compression include chronic spinal arachnoiditis which is a low-grade inflammatory reaction that may follow trauma, shunt procedures or infections, or be idiopathic (Paisley *et al.* 1982), congenital intraspinal lipomas (Chapman 1982) or epidermoid tumours that can be a late consequence of lumbar puncture (MacDonald and Klump 1986).

REFERENCES

Aicardi, J. (1994) 'Epilepsy as a presenting manifestation of brain tumors and other selected brain disorders.' *In: Epilepsy in Children, 2nd Edn.* New York: Raven Press, pp. 334–353.

Allen, J.C., Hayes, R. (1994) 'Selected immunotherapy studies of the interferons and IL-2/LAK.' *In:* Cohen, M.E., Duffner, P.K. (Eds.) *Brain Tumors in Children, 2nd Edn.* New York: Raven Press, pp. 161–175.

Alpers, C.E., Davis, R.L., Wilson, C.B. (1982) 'Persistence and late malignant transformation of childhood cerebellar astrocytoma.' *Journal of Neurosurgery*, **57**, 548–551.

Altman, N.R., Naidich, T.P., Braffman, B.H. (1992) 'Posterior fossa malformations.' *American Journal of Neuroradiology*, **13**, 691–724.

Alvord, E.C., Lofton, S. (1988) 'Gliomas of the optic nerve or chiasm.' *Journal of Neurosurgery*, **68**, 85–98.

Amacher, A.L. (1980) 'Craniopharyngioma: the controversy regarding radiotherapy.' *Child's Brain*, **6**, 57–64.

Ammarkrud, N. (1977) 'The value of fluorescein fundus angiography in evaluating optic disc oedema.' *Acta Ophthalmologica*, **55**, 605–615.

Anderson, J.R., Treip, C.S. (1984) 'Radiation-induced intracranial neoplasms: a report of three possible cases.' *Cancer*, **53**, 426–429.

Anderson, V.A., Smibert, E., Ekert, H., Godber, T. (1994) 'Intellectual, educational and behavioural sequelae following cranial irradiation and chemotherapy.' *Archives of Disease in Childhood*, **70**, 476–483.

Appleton, R.E., Jan, J.E. (1989) 'Delayed diagnosis of optic nerve glioma: a preventable cause of visual loss.' *Pediatric Neurology*, **5**, 226–228.

Armstrong, E.A., Harwood-Nash, D.C.F., Ritz, C.R., *et al.* (1982) 'CT of neuroblastomas and ganglioneuromas in children.' *American Journal of Roentgenology*, **139**, 571–576.

Artigas, J., Cervos-Navarro, J., Iglesias, J.R., Ebhardt, G. (1985) 'Gliomatosis cerebri: clinical and histological findings. Review article.' *Clinical Neuropathology*, **4**, 135–148.

Asamoto, M., Ito, H., Suzuki, N., *et al.* (1994) 'Transient mutism after posterior fossa surgery.' *Child's Nervous System*, **10**, 275–278.

Asanuma, H., Wakai, S., Tanaka, T., Chiba, S. (1995) 'Brain tumors associated with infantile spasms.' *Pediatric Neurology*, **12**, 361–364.

Atlas, S.W. (1991) 'Intraaxial brain tumors.' *In:* Atlas, S.W. (Ed.) *Magnetic Resonance Imaging of the Brain and Spine.* New York: Raven Press, pp. 223–326.

Austen, F.K., Carmichael, M.W., Adams, R.D. (1957) 'Neurologic manifestations of chronic pulmonary insufficiency.' *New England Journal of Medicine*, **257**, 579–590.

Austin, E.J., Alvord, E.C. (1988) 'Recurrences of cerebellar astrocytomas: a violation of Collin's law.' *Journal of Neurosurgery*, **68**, 41–47.

Avizonis, V.N., Fuller, D.B., Thompson, J.W., *et al.* (1992) 'Late effects following central nervous system radiation in a pediatric population.' *Neuropediatrics*, **23**, 228–234.

Aysun, S., Cinbis, M., Özcan, O. (1993) 'Intramedullary astrocytoma presenting as spinal muscular atrophy.' *Journal of Child Neurology*, **8**, 354–356.

—— Topçu, M., Günay, M., Topaloglu, H. (1994) 'Neurologic features as initial presentations of childhood malignancies.' *Pediatric Neurology*, **10**, 40–43.

Babikian, P., Corbett, J., Bell, W. (1994) 'Idiopathic intracranial hypertension in children: the Iowa experience.' *Journal of Child Neurology*, **9**, 144–149.

Bain, P.G., Lantos, P.L., Djurovic, V., West, I. (1991) 'Intrathecal vincristine: a fatal chemotherapeutic error with devastating central nervous system effects.' *Journal of Neurology*, **238**, 230–234.

Baker, R.S., Carter, D., Hendrich, E.B. (1985) 'Visual loss in pseudotumor cerebri in children.' *Archives of Ophthalmology*, **103**, 1681–1686.

—— Baumann, R.J., Buncic, J.R. (1989) 'Idiopathic intracranial hypertension (pseudotumor cerebri) in pediatric patients.' *Pediatric Neurology*, **5**, 5–11.

Balestrini, M.R., Micheli, R., Giordano, L., *et al.* (1994) 'Brain tumors with symptomatic onset in the first two years of life.' *Child's Nervous System*, **10**, 104–110.

Barasch, E.S., Altieri, D., Decker, R.E., *et al.* (1988) 'Primitive neuroectodermal tumor presenting as a delayed sequela to cranial irradiation and intrathecal methotrexate.' *Pediatric Neurology*, **4**, 375–378.

Barkovich, A.J., Kjos, B.O., Norman, D., Edwards, M.S. (1989) 'Revised classification of posterior fossa cysts and cystlike malformations based on the results of multiplanar MR imaging.' *American Journal of Neuroradiology*, **10**, 977–988.

Barnes, D., McDonald, W.I., Johnson, G., *et al.* (1987) 'Quantitative nuclear magnetic resonance imaging: characterisation of experimental cerebral oedema.' *Journal of Neurology, Neurosurgery, and Psychiatry*, **50**, 125–133.

Barth, P.G., Uylings, H.B.M., Stam, F.C. (1984) 'Interhemispheral neuroepithelial (glioependymal) cysts, associated with agenesis of the corpus callosum and neocortical maldevelopment.' *Child's Brain*, **11**, 312–319.

—— Stam, F.C., Hack, W., Delemarre-Van de Waal, A.H. (1988) 'Gliomatosis cerebri in a newborn.' *Neuropediatrics*, **19**, 197–200.

Battersby, R.D.E., Ironside, J.W., Maltby, E.L. (1986) 'Inherited multiple meningiomas: a clinical, pathological and cytogenetic study of an affected family.' *Journal of Neurology, Neurosurgery, and Psychiatry*, **49**, 362–368.

Becker, D.L., Reddy, U.R., Pleasure, S., *et al.* (1990) 'Human central nervous system primitive neuroectodermal tumor expressing nerve growth factor receptors: CHP 707m.' *Annals of Neurology*, **28**, 136–145.

Bennett, J.P., Rubinstein, L.J. (1984) 'The biological behavior of primary cerebral neuroblastoma: a reappraisal of the clinical course in a series of 70 cases.' *Annals of Neurology*, **16**, 21–27.

Berger, M.S., Wilson, C.B. (1985) 'Epidermoid cysts of the posterior fossa.' *Journal of Neurosurgery*, **62**, 214–219.

—— Edwards, M.S.B., La Masters, D., *et al.* (1983) 'Pediatric brainstem tumors: radiographic, pathological and clinical correlations.' *Neurosurgery*, **12**, 298–302.

Bergeron, C., Patte, C., Caillaud, J.M., *et al.* (1989) 'Aspects cliniques, anatomopathologiques et résultats thérapeutiques de 63 lymphomes malins non Hodgkiniens ORL de l'enfant.' *Archives Françaises de Pédiatrie*, **46**, 583–587.

Bergsagel, D.J., Finegold, M.J., Butel, J.S., *et al.* (1992) 'DNA sequences similar to those of simian virus 40 in ependymomas and choroid plexus tumors of childhood.' *New England Journal of Medicine*, **326**, 988–993.

Berkovic, S.F., Andermann, F., Melanson, D., *et al.* (1988) 'Hypothalamic hamartomas and ictal laughter: evolution of a characteristic epileptic syndrome and diagnostic value of magnetic resonance imaging.' *Annals of Neurology*, **23**, 429–439.

Bernstein, M., Hoffman, H.J., Halliday, W.C., *et al.* (1984) 'Thalamic tumors in children. Long-term follow-up and treatment guidelines.' *Journal of Neurosurgery*, **61**, 649–656.

Blumberg, D.L., Sklar, C.A., David, R., *et al.* (1989) 'Acromegaly in an infant.' *Pediatrics*, **83**, 998–1002.

Blume, W.T., Girvin, J.P., Kaufmann, J.C.E. (1982) 'Childhood brain tumors presenting as chronic uncontrolled focal seizure disorders.' *Annals of Neurology*, **12**, 538–541.

Boogerd, W., van de Sande, J.J., Moffie, D. (1988) 'Acute fever and delayed leukoencephalopathy following low dose intraventricular methotrexate.' *Journal of Neurology, Neurosurgery, and Psychiatry*, **51**, 1277–1283.

Brauner, R., Pierre-Kahn, A., Nemedy-Sandor, E., *et al.* (1987) 'Pubertés précoces par kyste arachnoïdien supra-sellaire.' *Archives Françaises de Pédiatrie*, **44**, 889–893.

Brecher, M.L. (1994) 'Principles of chemotherapy.' *In:* Cohen, M.E., Duffner, P.K. (Eds.) *Brain Tumors in Children, 2nd Edn.* New York: Raven Press, pp. 117–146.

Brown, J.K., Hussain, I.H.M.I. (1991) 'Status epilepticus. I: Pathogenesis.' *Developmental Medicine and Child Neurology*, **33**, 3–17.

Brown, L.M., Daeschner, C., Timms, J., Crow, W. (1989) 'Granulocytic sarcoma in childhood acute myelogenous leukemia.' *Pediatric Neurology*, **5**, 173–178.

Buchheit, W.A., Burton, C., Haag, B., Shaw, D. (1969) 'Papilledema and idiopathic intracranial hypertension: report of a familial occurrence.' *New England Journal of Medicine*, **280**, 938–942.

Budka, H., Gusco, A., Jellinger, K. (1976) 'Intermittent meningitic reaction with severe basophilia and eosinophilia in CSF leukemia.' *Journal of the Neurological Sciences*, **28**, 459–468.

Burger, P.C., Kamenar, E., Schold, S.C., *et al.* (1981) 'Encephalomyelopathy following high-dose BCNU therapy.' *Cancer*, **48**, 1318–1327.

Burr, I.M., Slonim, A.E., Danish, R.K., *et al.* (1976) 'Diencephalic syndrome revisited.' *Journal of Pediatrics*, **88**, 439–443.

Byrd, R.L., Rohrbaugh, T.M., Raney, R.B., Norris, D.G. (1981) 'Transient cortical blindness secondary to vincristine therapy in childhood malignancies.' *Cancer*, **47**, 37–40.

Calaminus, G., Bamberg, M., Baranzelli, M.C., *et al.* (1994) 'Intracranial germ cell tumors: a comprehensive update of the European data.' *Neuropediatrics*, **25**, 26–32.

Campbell, R.H.A., Marshall, W.C., Chessells, J.M. (1977) 'Neurological complications of childhood leukaemia.' *Archives of Disease in Childhood*, **52**, 850–858.

Cantini, R., Giorgetti, W., Valleriani, A.M., *et al.* (1989) 'Radiation-induced cerebral lesions in childhood.' *Child's Nervous System*, **5**, 135–139.

Cascino, G.D., Andermann, F., Berkovic, S.F., *et al.* (1993) 'Gelastic seizures and hypothalamic hamartomas: evaluation of patients undergoing chronic intracranial EEG monitoring and outcome of surgical treatment.' *Neurology*, **43**, 747–750.

Cavazzuti, V., Fischer, E.G., Welch, K., *et al.* (1983) 'Neurological and psychophysiological sequelae following different treatments of craniopharyngioma in children.' *Journal of Neurosurgery*, **59**, 409–417.

Ceyhan, M., Erdem, G., Kaura, G., *et al.* (1994) 'Lymphoma with bilateral cavernous system involvement in early childhood.' *Pediatric Neurology*, **10**, 67–69.

Chamberlain, M.C. (1995) 'A review of leptomeningeal metastases in pediatrics.' *Journal of Child Neurology*, **10**, 191–199.

—— Murovic, J.A., Levin, V.A. (1988) 'Absence of contrast enhancement on CT brain scans of patients with supratentorial malignant gliomas.' *Neurology*, **38**, 1371–1374.

—— Silver, P., Levin, V.A. (1990) 'Poorly differentiated gliomas of the cerebellum. A study of 18 patients.' *Cancer*, **65**, 337–340.

Chapman, P.H. (1982) 'Congenital intraspinal lipomas: anatomic considerations and surgical treatment.' *Child's Brain*, **9**, 37–47.

Chastagner, P., Olive-Sommelet, D. (1990) 'La chimiothérapie des tumeurs cérébrales de l'enfant.' *Archives Françaises de Pédiatrie*, **47**, 147–154.

Ch'ien, L.T., Price, R.A. (1982) 'Severe leukomyelopathy in a patient with acute lymphocytic leukemia.' *Annals of Neurology*, **12**, 212. *(Abstract.)*

—— Aur, R.J.A., Stagner, S., *et al.* (1980) 'Long-term neurological implications of somnolence syndrome in children with acute lymphocytic leukemia.' *Annals of Neurology*, **8**, 273–277.

Chipkevitch, E. (1994) 'Brain tumors and anorexia nervosa syndrome.' *Brain and Development*, **16**, 175–179.

Chung, S.M., McCrary, J.A. (1988) 'Management of pregeniculate anterior visual pathway gliomas.' *Neurofibromatosis*, **1**, 240–247.

Chutorian, A.M. (1988) 'Optic gliomas in children.' *International Pediatrics*, **3**, 115–119.

Cogan, M.G., Covey, C.M., Arieff, A.I., *et al.* (1978) 'Central nervous system manifestations of hyperparathyroidism.' *American Journal of Medicine*, **65**, 963–970.

Cohen, B.H., Handler, M.S., De Vivo, D.C., *et al.* (1988) 'Central nervous system melanotic neuroectodermal tumor of infancy: value of chemotherapy in management.' *Neurology*, **38**, 163–164.

Cohen, M.E., Duffner, P.K. (1989) 'Treatment of CNS neoplasms in childhood by the Pediatric Oncology Group.' *Brain and Development*, **11**, 360–367.

—— —— (1994) *Brain Tumors in Children: Principles of Diagnosis and Treatment, 2nd Edn.* New York: Raven Press.

—— —— Heffner, R.R., *et al.* (1986) 'Prognostic factors in brainstem gliomas.' *Neurology*, **36**, 602–605.

Connolly, M.B., Farrell, K., Hill, A., Flodmark, O. (1992) 'Magnetic resonance imaging in pseudotumor cerebri.' *Developmental Medicine and Child Neurology*, **34**, 1091–1094.

Constantinou, J.E.C., Gillis, J., Ouvrier R.A., Rahilly, P.M. (1989) 'Hypoxic–ischaemic encephalopathy after near miss sudden infant death syndrome.' *Archives of Disease in Childhood*, **64**, 703–708.

Constine, L.S., Konski, A., Ekholm, S., *et al.* (1988) 'Adverse effects of brain irradiation correlated with MR and CT imaging.' *International Journal of Radiation, Oncology, Biology, Physics*, **15**, 319–330.

Conway, P.D., Oechler, H.W., Kun, L.E. Murray, K.J. (1991) 'Importance of histologic condition and treatment of pediatric cerebellar astrocytoma.' *Cancer*, **67**, 2772–2775.

Costigan, D.C., Daneman, D., Harwood-Nash, D., Holland, F.J. (1984) 'The 'empty sella' in childhood.' *Clinical Pediatrics*, **23**, 437–440.

Couch, R., Camfield, P.R., Tibbles, J.A.R. (1985) 'The changing picture of pseudotumor cerebri in children.' *Canadian Journal of Neurological Sciences*, **12**, 48–50.

Coulon, R.A., Till, K. (1977) 'Intracranial ependymomas in children. A review of 43 cases.' *Child's Brain*, **3**, 154–168.

Crockard, A. (1985) 'Brain swelling, brain oedema and the blood–brain barrier.' *In:* Crockard, A., Hayward, R., Hoff, J.T. (Eds.) *Neurosurgery. The Scientific Basis of Clinical Practice.* Oxford: Blackwell, pp. 333–349.

Curless, R.G. (1980) 'Cranial computerized tomography in childhood leukemia.' *Archives of Neurology*, **57**, 306–307.

Daugaard, G.K., Petrera, J., Trojaborg, W. (1987) 'Electrophysiological study of the peripheral and central neurotoxic effect of cis-platin.' *Acta Neurologica Scandinavica*, **76**, 86–93.

Daumas-Duport, C., Scheithauer, B.W., Chodkiewicz, J.P., *et al.* (1988) 'Dysembryoplastic neuroepithelial tumor: a surgically curable tumor of young patients with intractable partial seizures. Report of thirty-nine cases.' *Neurosurgery*, **23**, 545–556.

David, R.B., Hadield, M.G., Vines, F.S., Maurer, H.M. (1975) 'Dural sinus occlusion in leukemia.' *Pediatrics*, **56**, 793–796.

Davidson, G.S., Hope, J.K. (1989) 'Meningeal tumors of childhood.' *Cancer*, **63**, 1205–1210.

Davie, C., Kennedy, P., Katifi, H.A. (1992) 'Seventh nerve palsy as a false localising sign.' *Journal of Neurology, Neurosurgery, and Psychiatry*, **55**, 510–511. *(Letter.)*

Davis, P.C.M, Hoffman, J.C., Weidenheim, K.M. (1983) 'Large hypothalamic and optic chiasm gliomas in infants: difficulties in distinction.' *American Journal of Neuroradiology*, **5**, 579–585.

Dearnaley, D.P., A'Hern, R.P., Whittaker, S., Bloom, H.J.G. (1990) 'Pineal and CNS germ cell tumors: Royal Marsden Hospital experience 1962–1987.' *International Journal of Radiation Oncology and Biological Physics*, **18**, 773–781.

Debrun, G., Sauvegrain, J., Aicardi, J., Goutières, F. (1975) 'Moyamoya: a nonspecific radiological syndrome.' *Neuroradiology*, **8**, 241–244.

Decq, P., Brugières, P., Le Guerinel, C., et al. (1996) 'Percutaneous endoscopic treatment of suprasellar arachnoid cysts: ventriculocystostomy or ventriculocystocisternostomy? Technical note.' Journal of Neurosurgery, 84, 696–701.

Delodovici, L., Baruzzi, F., Bonaldi, G., et al. (1994) 'Spinal arachnoid cysts: neuroradiological findings, clinical presentation and outcome of 11 cases.' Journal of Neurology, 241, Suppl. 1, S2. (Abstract.)

Demierre, B., Stichnoth, F.A., Hori, A., Spoerri, O. (1986) 'Intracerebral ganglioglioma.' Journal of Neurosurgery, 65, 177–182.

Deonna, T., Guignard, J.P. (1974) 'Acute intracranial hypertension after nalidixic acid administration.' Archives of Disease in Childhood, 49, 743. (Letter.)

De Souza, C.E., De Souza, R., Da Costa, S., et al. (1969) 'Cerebellopontine angle epidermoid cysts: a report of 30 cases.' Journal of Neurology, Neurosurgery, and Psychiatry, 52, 986–990.

Dickman, C.A., Rekate, H.L., Bird, C.R., et al. (1989) 'Unenhanced and gadolinium-DTPA-enhanced MR imaging in postoperative evaluation in pediatric brain tumors.' Journal of Neurosurgery, 71, 49–53.

Diebler, C., Dulac, O. (1987) Pediatric Neurology and Neuroradiology. Berlin: Springer.

Divitiis, E., Spaziante, R., Cirillo, S., et al. (1979) 'Primary sellar chondromas.' Surgical Neurology, 11, 229–232.

Dohrmann, G.J., Farwell, J.R., Flannery, J.T. (1976) 'Ependymomas and ependymoblastomas in children.' Journal of Neurosurgery, 45, 273–283.

Donaldson, J.O. (1981) 'Pathogenesis of pseudotumor cerebri syndromes.' Neurology, 31, 877–880.

Dropcho, E.J., Wisoff, J.H., Walker, R.W., Allen, J.C. (1987) 'Supratentorial malignant gliomas in childhood: a review of fifty cases.' Annals of Neurology, 22, 355–364.

Druker, B.J., Mamon, A.J., Roberts, T.M. (1989) 'Oncogenes, growth and signal transduction.' New England Journal of Medicine, 321, 1383–1391.

Dryja, T.P., Rapaport, J.M., Joyce, J.M., Petersen, R.A. (1986) 'Molecular detection of deletions involving band q14 of chromosome 13 in retinoblastoma.' Proceedings of the National Academy of Sciences of the USA, 83, 7391–7394.

Duchowny, M.S., Resnick, T.J., Alvarez, L. (1989) 'Dysplastic gangliocytoma and intractable partial seizures in childhood.' Neurology, 39, 602–604.

—— Altman, N., Bruce, J. (1996) 'Dysplastic gangliocytoma of the cerebral hemisphere.' In: Guerrini, R., Andermann, F., Canapicchi, R., et al. (Eds.) Dysplasias of Cerebral Cortex and Epilepsy. Philadelphia: Lippincott–Raven, pp. 93–100.

Duffner, P.K., Cohen, M.E. (1981) 'Extraneural metastases in childhood brain tumors.' Annals of Neurology, 10, 261–265.

—— —— (1988) 'Isolated optic nerve gliomas in children with and without neurofibromatosis.' Neurofibromatosis, 1, 201–211.

—— —— (1992) 'Changes in the approach to central nervous system tumors in childhood.' Pediatric Clinics of North America, 39, 859–877.

—— —— Heffner, R.R., Freeman, A.I. (1981) 'Primitive neuroectodermal tumors of childhood: an approach to therapy.' Journal of Neurosurgery, 55, 376–381.

—— —— Myers, M.H., Heise, H.W. (1986) 'Survival of children with brain tumors: SEER program, 1973–1980.' Neurology, 36, 597–601.

—— —— Parker, M.S. (1988) 'Prospective intellectual testing in children with brain tumors.' Annals of Neurology, 23, 575–579.

—— Horowitz, M., Krischer, J. (1993) 'Postoperative chemotherapy and delayed radiotherapy in children less than 3 years of age with malignant brain tumors.' New England Journal of Medicine, 328, 1725–1731.

Dunne, J.W., Stewart-Wynne, E., Pullan, P.T. (1987) 'Abducens palsy after rapid shrinkage of a prolactinoma.' Journal of Neurology, Neurosurgery, and Psychiatry, 50, 496–498.

Easley, J.D., Scharf, L., Chou, L., Riccardi, J.M. (1988) 'Controversy in the management of optic pathway gliomas—29 patients treated with radiation therapy at Baylor College of Medicine from 1967 through 1987.' Neurofibromatosis, 1, 248–251.

Eberts, T.J., Ransburg, R.C. (1979) 'Primary intracranial endodermal sinus tumor: case report.' Journal of Neurosurgery, 50, 246–252.

Edwards, M.S.B., Davis, R.L., Laurent, J.P. (1985) 'Tumor markers and cytologic features of cerebrospinal fluid.' Cancer, 56, 1773–1777.

—— Gutin, P.H., Wara, W.M., Levin, V.A. (1988a) 'Brachytherapy for pediatric central nervous system tumors.' International Pediatrics, 3, 170–174.

—— Hudgins, R.J., Wilson, C.B., et al. (1988b) 'Pineal region tumors in children.' Journal of Neurosurgery, 68, 689–697.

Eeg-Olofsson, O., Carlsson, E., Jeppson, S. (1981) 'Recurrent abdominal pains as the first symptom of a spinal cord tumor.' Acta Paediatrica Scandinavica, 70, 595–597.

Eng, C. (1996) 'The RET proto-oncogene in multiple endocrine neoplasia type 2 and Hirschsprung's disease.' New England Journal of Medicine, 335, 943–951.

Epstein, F. (1987) 'Intra-axial tumors of the cervico-medullary junction in children.' Concepts in Pediatric Neurosurgery, 7, 117–133.

—— Epstein, N. (1982) 'Surgical treatment of spinal cord astrocytomas of childhood. A series of 19 patients.' Journal of Neurosurgery, 57, 682–685.

Epstein, L.G., Dicarlo, F.J., Joshi, V.V., et al. (1988) 'Primary lymphoma of the central nervous system in children with acquired immunodeficiency syndrome.' Pediatrics, 82, 355–363.

Eriksson, B., Gunterberg, B., Kindblom, L.L-G. (1981) 'Chordoma: a clinicopathological and prognostic study of a Swedish national series.' Acta Orthopaedica Scandinavica, 52, 49–58.

Farwell, J., Flannery, J.T. (1984) 'Cancer in relatives of children with central nervous system neoplasms.' New England Journal of Medicine, 311, 749–753.

Favre, J., Deruaz, J.P., Uske, A., De Tribolet, N. (1994) 'Skull base chordomas: presentation of six cases and review of the literature.' Journal of Clinical Neuroscience, 1, 7–18.

Feinberg, W.G., Swenson, M.R. (1988) 'Cerebrovascular complications of L-asparginase therapy.' Neurology, 38, 127–133.

Feldman, N.H., Schlezinger, N.S. (1970) 'Benign intracranial hypertension associated with hypervitaminosis A.' Archives of Neurology, 22, 1–7.

Ferrante, L., Acqui, M., Mastronardi, L., et al. (1989) 'Cerebral meningiomas in children.' Child's Nervous System, 5, 83–86.

Fischer, E.G., Welch, K., Belli, J.A., et al. (1985) 'Treatment results of craniopharyngiomas in children 1972–1981.' Journal of Neurosurgery, 62, 496–501.

—— —— Shillito, J., et al. (1990) 'Craniopharyngiomas in children. Long-term effects of conservative surgical procedures combined with radiation therapy.' Journal of Neurosurgery, 73, 534–540.

Fisher, C.M. (1995) 'Brain herniation: a revision of classical concepts.' Canadian Journal of Neurological Sciences, 22, 83–91.

Fort, D.W., Rushing, E.J. (1997) 'Congenital central nervous system tumors.' Journal of Child Neurology, 12, 157–164.

Franklin, B., Liu, J., Ginsberg-Fellner, F. (1982) 'Cerebral edema and ophthalmoplegia reversed by mannitol in a new case of insulin-dependent diabetes mellitus.' Pediatrics, 69, 87–90.

Franssila, K.O., Heiskala, M.K., Rapola, J. (1987) 'Non-Hodgkins's lymphomas in childhood. A clinicopathologic and epidemiologic study in Finland.' Cancer, 59, 1837–1846.

French, L.A. (1962) 'Some aspects of diagnosis and treatment of brain tumors in children.' In: Fields, W.S., Sharkey, P.C. (Eds.) The Biology and Treatment of Intracranial Tumors. Springfield, IL: C.C. Thomas, pp. 418–432.

Friede, R. (1989) Developmental Neuropathology, 2nd Edn. Berlin: Springer.

—— Yasargil, M.G. (1977) 'Supratentorial intracerebral epithelial (ependymal) cysts: review, case reports and fine structure.' Journal of Neurology, Neurosurgery, and Psychiatry, 40, 127–137.

Friend, S.H., Bernards, R., Rogelj, S., et al. (1986) 'A human DNA segment with properties of the gene that predisposes to retinoblastoma and osteosarcoma.' Nature, 323, 643–646.

Fusner, S.E., Poplack, D.G., Pizzo, P.A., Di Chiro, G. (1977) 'Leukoencephalopathy following chemotherapy for rhabdomyosarcoma: reversibility of cerebral changes demonstrated by computer tomography.' Journal of Pediatrics, 91, 77–79.

Gagliano, R.G., Costanzi, J.J. (1976) 'Paraplegia following intrathecal methotrexate.' Cancer, 37, 1663–1668.

Galassi, E., Tognetti, F., Franck, F., et al. (1985) 'Infratentorial arachnoid cysts.' Journal of Neurosurgery, 63, 210–217.

—— Godano, U., Cavallo, M., et al. (1989) 'Intracranial tumors during the 1st year of life.' Child's Nervous System, 5, 288–298.

Garcia, D.M., Latifi, A.R., Simpson, J.R., Picker, S. (1989) 'Astrocytomas of the cerebellum in children.' Journal of Neurosurgery, 71, 661–664.

Garcia-Perez, A., Narbona-Garcia, J., Sierrasesumaga, L., et al. (1993) 'Neuropsychological outcome of children after radiotherapy for intracranial tumours.' Developmental Medicine and Child Neurology, 35, 139–148.

Gardner, K., Cox, T., Digre, K.B. (1995) 'Idiopathic intracranial hypertension associated with tetracycline use in fraternal twins: case reports and review.' Neurology, 45, 6–10.

Gelabert, M., Bollar, A., Paseiro, M.J., Allut, A.G. (1990) 'Hydrocephalus and intraspinal tumor in childhood.' *Child's Nervous System*, **6**, 110–112.

George, W.E., Wilmot, M., Greenhouse, A., Hammeke, M. (1983) 'Medical management of steroid-induced epidural lipomatosis.' *New England Journal of Medicine*, **308**, 316–319.

Gerber, S.S., Plotkin, R. (1982) 'Lipoma of the corpus callosum.' *Journal of Neurosurgery*, **57**, 281–285.

Giuffré, R. (1989) 'Biological aspects of brain tumors in infancy and childhood.' *Child's Nervous System*, **5**, 55–59.

Giunta, F., Grasso, G., Marini, G., Zorzi, F. (1989) 'Brainstem expanding lesions: stereotactic diagnosis and therapeutical approach.' *Acta Neurochirurgica*, **46** (Suppl.), 86–89.

Gjerris, F. (1978) 'Clinical aspects and long-term prognosis in supratentorial tumors in infancy and childhood.' *Acta Neurologica Scandinavica*, **57**, 445–453.

Glantz, M.J., Burger, P.C., Friedman, A.H., *et al.* (1994) 'Treatment of radiation-induced nervous system injury with heparin and warfarin.' *Neurology*, **44**, 2020–2027.

Glasier, C.M., Husain, M.M., Chadduck, W., Boop, F.A. (1993) 'Meningiomas in children: MR and histopathologic findings.' *American Journal of Neuroradiology*, **14**, 237–241.

Glass, J.P., Melamed, M., Chernik, N.L., Posner, J.B. (1979) 'Malignant cells in cerebrospinal fluid (CSF): the meaning of a positive CSF cytology.' *Neurology*, **29**, 1369–1375.

Gold, E.B., Gordis, L. (1979) 'Patterns of incidence of brain tumors in children.' *Annals of Neurology*, **5**, 565–568.

Goldwein, J.W., Leahy, J.M., Packer, R.J., *et al.* (1990) 'Intracranial ependymomas in children.' *International Journal of Radiation, Oncology, Biology, Physics*, **19**, 1497–1502.

Gomori, J.M., Shaked, A. (1982) 'Radiation-induced meningiomas.' *Neuroradiology*, **23**, 211–212.

Goutières, F., Aicardi, J. (1977) 'Accidental percutaneous hexachlorophane intoxication in infants.' *British Medical Journal*, **2**, 663–665.

Grant, D.N. (1971) 'Benign intracranial hypertension: a review of 79 cases in infancy and childhood.' *Archives of Disease in Childhood*, **46**, 651–655.

Graus, F., Walker, R.W., Allen, J.C. (1983) 'Brain metastases in children.' *Journal of Pediatrics*, **103**, 558–561.

Greenberg, S.J. (1994) 'Advances in molecular genetic treatment of cancer.' *In:* Cohen, M.E., Duffner, P.K. (Eds.) *Brain Tumors in Children, 2nd Edn.* New York: Raven Press, pp. 147–160.

Greydanus, D., Burgert, O., Gilchrist, G.S. (1978) 'Hypothalamic syndrome in children with acute lymphocytic leukemia.' *Mayo Clinic Proceedings*, **53**, 217–220.

Grogan, W.A., Narkun, D.M. (1987) 'Pseudotumour cerebri with amiodarone.' *Journal of Neurology, Neurosurgery, and Psychiatry*, **50**, 651. *(Letter.)*

Gross, T.P., Milstein, J.B., Kuritzky, J.N. (1989) 'Bulging fontanelle after immunization with diphtheria–tetanus–pertussis vaccine and diphtheria–tetanus vaccine.' *Journal of Pediatrics*, **114**, 423–425.

Guhl, L., Mironov, A., Schroth, G. (1987) 'Contribution of MRI in the diagnosis of haemangioblastomas.' *Journal of Neurology*, **235**, 95–98.

Gunesson-Nordin, V., Blennow, G., Garwicz, G., *et al.* (1982) 'Gliomas of the anterior visual pathway in children. Tumour behaviour and effect of treatment.' *Neuropediatrics*, **13**, 82–87.

Hahn, J.S., Havens, P.L., Higgins, J.J., *et al.* (1989) 'Neurological complications of hemolytic–uremic syndrome.' *Journal of Child Neurology*, **4**, 108–113.

Hald, J.K., Nakstad, P.H., Skjeldal, O.H., Strømme, P. (1991) 'Bilateral arachnoid cysts of the temporal fossa in four children with glutaric aciduria type I.' *American Journal of Neuroradiology*, **12**, 407–409.

Hall, M., Keene, D., Hsu, E., *et al.* (1993) 'Acute confusional episode following cranial-axis radiation.' *Canadian Journal of Neurological Sciences*, **20**, Suppl. 2, S33. *(Abstract.)*

Halpern, J.R., Gordon, W.H. (1981) 'Trochlear nerve palsy as a false localizing sign.' *Annals of Ophthalmology*, **13**, 53–56.

Han, J.S., Zee, C-S., Ahmadi, J., *et al.* (1983) 'Intracranial metastatic Wilm's tumor in children: a report of 2 cases.' *Surgical Neurology*, **20**, 157–159.

Hanefeld, F., Riehm, H. (1980) 'Therapy of acute lymphoblastic leukaemia in childhood: effects on the nervous system.' *Neuropädiatrie*, **11**, 3–16.

Hanieh, A., Simpson, D.A., Worth, J.B. (1988) 'Arachnoid cysts: a critical survey of 41 cases.' *Child's Nervous System*, **4**, 92–96.

Harsh, G.R., Edwards, M.S.B., Wilson, C.B. (1986) 'Intracranial arachnoid cysts in children.' *Journal of Neurosurgery*, **64**, 835–842.

Hart, R.G., Carter, J.E. (1982) 'Pseudotumor cerebri and facial pain.' *Archives of Neurology*, **39**, 440–442.

Harwood-Nash, D.C., Fitz, C.R. (1976) 'Brain neoplasms.' *In: Neuroradiology in Infants and Children, Vol. 2.* St Louis: C.V. Mosby, pp. 668–788.

Hashimoto, T., Tayama, M., Miyazaki, M., *et al.* (1990) 'Cranial MR imaging in patients with von Recklinghausen's disease (neurofibromatosis type 1).' *Neuropediatrics*, **21**, 193–198.

Hashimoto, M., Fujimoto, K., Shinoda, S., Masuzawa, T. (1993) 'Magnetic resonance imaging of ganglion cell tumours.' *Neuroradiology*, **35**, 181–184.

Hassler, W., Steinmetz, H., Gawlowski, J. (1988) 'Transcranial Doppler ultrasonography in raised intracranial pressure and in intracranial circulatory arrest.' *Journal of Neurosurgery*, **68**, 745–751.

Healey, E.A., Barnes, P.D., Kupsky, W.J., *et al.* (1991) 'The prognostic significance of postoperative residual tumor in ependymoma.' *Neurosurgery*, **28**, 666–671.

Heffner, R.R. (1994) 'Principles of neuropathology.' *In:* Cohen, M.E., Duffner, P.K. (Eds.) *Brain Tumors in Children, 2nd Edn.* New York: Raven Press, pp. 51–78.

Helmke, K., Hausdorf, G., Moehrs, D., Laas, R. (1984) 'CCT and sonographic findings in congenital craniopharyngioma.' *Neuroradiology*, **26**, 523–526.

Hirsch, J.F., Sainte-Rose, C., Pierre-Kahn, A., *et al.* (1989) 'Benign astrocytic and oligodendrocytic tumors of the cerebral hemispheres in children.' *Journal of Neurosurgery*, **70**, 568–572.

Ho, K.L. (1982) 'Tumors of the cerebral aqueduct.' *Cancer*, **49**, 154–162.

Hoffman, H.J., Yoshida, M., Becker, L.F. (1983) 'Pineal region tumors in childhood.' *Concepts of Pediatric Neurosurgery*, **4**, 360–386.

Honig, P.J., Charney, E.B. (1982) 'Children with brain tumor headaches.' *American Journal of Diseases of Children*, **136**, 121–124.

Hoppe-Hirsch, E., Hirsch, J.F., Lellouch-Tubiana, A., *et al.* (1993) 'Malignant hemispheric tumors in childhood.' *Child's Nervous System*, **9**, 131–135.

Hopwood, N.J., Kenny, F.M. (1977) 'Incidence of Nelson's syndrome after adrenalectomy for Cushing's disease in children.' *American Journal of Diseases of Children*, **131**, 1353–1356.

Horten, B.C., Rubinstein, L.J. (1976) 'Primary cerebral neuroblastoma. A clinicopathological study of 35 cases.' *Brain*, **99**, 735–756.

Howe, J.G., Gibson, J.D. (1982) 'Uncinate seizures and tumors, a myth re-examined.' *Annals of Neurology*, **12**, 227.

Hoyt, W.A., Baghdassarian, S.A. (1986) 'Optic glioma of childhood.' *British Journal of Ophthalmology*, **53**, 793–798.

Huddart, R., Traish, D., Ashley, S., *et al.* (1993) 'Management of spinal astrocytoma with conservative surgery and radiotherapy.' *British Journal of Neurosurgery*, **7**, 473–481.

Hughes, R.A.C., Britton, T., Richards, M. (1994) 'Effects of lymphoma on the peripheral nervous system.' *Journal of the Royal Society of Medicine*, **87**, 526–530.

Jankovic, M., Browers, P., Valsecchi, M.G., *et al.* (1994) 'Association of 1800 cGy cranial irradiation with intellectual function in children with acute lymphoblastic leukaemia.' *Lancet*, **344**, 224–227.

Jennings, M.T., Gelman, R., Hochberg, F. (1985) 'Intracranial germ cell tumors: natural history and pathogenesis.' *Journal of Neurosurgery*, **63**, 155–167.

—— Slatkin, N., D'Angelo, M., *et al.* (1993) 'Neoplastic meningitis as the presentation of occult primitive neuroectodermal tumors.' *Journal of Child Neurology*, **8**, 306–312.

—— Frenchman, M., Shehab, T., *et al.* (1995) 'Gliomatosis cerebri presenting as intractable epilepsy during early childhood.' *Journal of Child Neurology*, **10**, 37–45.

Jooma, R., Kendall, B.E. (1983) 'Diagnosis and management of pineal tumors.' *Journal of Neurosurgery*, **58**, 654–655.

Jordan, R.M., Kendall, J.W., McClung, J., Kammer, H. (1980) 'Concentration of human chorionic gonadotropin in the cerebrospinal fluid of patients with germinal cell hypothalamic tumors.' *Pediatrics*, **65**, 121–124.

Junck, L., Marshall, W.H. (1983) 'Neurotoxicity of radiological contrast agents.' *Annals of Neurology*, **13**, 469–484.

Kalfas, I.H., Hahn, J.F. (1986) 'Symptomatic subependymoma in a 14-year-old girl, diagnosed by NMR scan.' *Child's Nervous System*, **2**, 44–46.

Kalifa, C., Ernest, C., Rodary, C., *et al.* (1981) 'Les gliomes du chiasma optique chez l'enfant: étude rétrospective de 57 cas traités par irradiation.' *Archives Françaises de Pédiatrie*, **38**, 309–313.

Kalyan-Raman, J.P., Olivero, W.C. (1987) 'Ganglioglioma: a correlative clinicopathological and radiological study of ten surgically treated cases with follow-up.' *Neurosurgery*, **20**, 428–433.

Kaplan, J.G., Barasch, E., Hirschfeld, A., *et al.* (1989) 'Spinal epidural lipomatosis: a serious complication of iatrogenic Cushing's syndrome.' *Neurology*, **39**, 1031–1034.

Kaufmann, A.M., Cardoso, E.R. (1992) 'Aggravation of vasogenic cerebral edema by multiple-dose mannitol.' *Journal of Neurosurgery*, **77**, 584–589.

Kendall, B.E., Jakubowski, J., Pullicino, P., Symon, A.L. (1979) 'Difficulties in diagnosis of supratentorial gliomas by CAT scan.' *Journal of Neurology, Neurosurgery, and Psychiatry*, **42**, 485–492.

—— Reide-Grosswasser, I., Valentine, A. (1983) 'Diagnosis of masses presenting within the ventricles on computed tomography.' *Neuroradiology*, **25**, 11–22.

Keraly, J.L., Hubier, F., Derome, P., *et al.* (1986) 'Évolution à moyen terme des craniopharyngiomes de l'enfant en fonction des choix thérapeutiques initiaux.' *Archives Françaises de Pédiatrie*, **43**, 593–599.

Kermode, A.G., Plant, G.T., MacManus, D.G., *et al.* (1989) 'Behçet's disease with slowly enlarging midbrain mass on MRI: resolution following steroid therapy.' *Neurology*, **39**, 1251–1252.

Kerr, F.W.L., Hollowell, O.W. (1964) 'Location of pupillomotor and accomodation fibres in the oculomotor nerve: experimental observations on paralytic mydriasis.' *Journal of Neurology, Neurosurgery, and Psychiatry*, **27**, 473–481.

Kimmel, D.W., O'Fallon, J.R., Scheithauer, B.W., *et al.* (1992) 'Prognostic value of cytogenetic analysis in human cerebral astrocytomas.' *Annals of Neurology*, **31**, 534–542.

Kirkham, F.J. (1991) 'Intracranial pressure and cerebral blood flow in non-traumatic coma in childhood.' *In:* Minns, R. (Ed.) *Problems of Intracranial Pressure in Childhood. Clinics in Developmental Medicine No. 113/114.* London: Mac Keith Press, pp. 283–348.

Klein, P., Rubinstein, L.J. (1989) 'Benign symptomatic glial cysts of the pineal gland: a report of seven cases and review of the literature.' *Journal of Neurology, Neurosurgery, and Psychiatry*, **52**, 991–995.

Kleinman, G.M., Schoene, W.C., Walse, T.M., Richardson, E.P. (1978) 'Malignant transformation of benign cerebellar astrocytoma.' *Journal of Neurosurgery*, **49**, 111–118.

—— Hochberg, F.H., Richardson, E.P. (1981) 'Systemic metastases from medulloblastoma: report of 2 cases and review of the literature.' *Cancer*, **48**, 2296–2309.

Knight, R.S.G., Fielder, A.R., Firth, J.L. (1986) 'Benign intracranial hypertension: visual loss and optic nerve sheath fenestration.' *Journal of Neurology, Neurosurgery, and Psychiatry*, **49**, 243–250.

Koh, S., Turkel, S.B., Baram, T.Z. (1997) 'Cerebellar mutism in children: report of six cases and potential mechanisms.' *Pediatric Neurology*, **16**, 218–219.

Komp, D.M. (1979) 'Diagnosis of CNS leukemia.' *American Journal of Pediatric Hematology and Oncology*, **1**, 31–35.

Konishi, Y., Kuriyama, M., Sudo, M., *et al.* (1990) 'Growth patterns of the normal pituitary gland and in pituitary adenoma.' *Developmental Medicine and Child Neurology*, **32**, 69–73.

Konomi, H., Imai, M., Nihei, K., *et al.* (1978) 'Indomethacin causing pseudotumor cerebri in Bartter's syndrome.' *New England Journal of Medicine*, **298**, 855. *(Letter.)*

Koos, W.T., Miller, M.H. (1971) *Intracranial Tumors of Infants and Children.* Saint Louis: C.V. Mosby.

Kopelson, G., Linggood, R.M. (1982) 'Intramedullary spinal cord astrocytoma versus glioblastoma: the prognostic importance of histologic grade.' *Cancer*, **50**, 732–735.

—— —— Kleinman, G.M., *et al.* (1980) 'Management of intramedullary spinal cord tumors.' *Radiology*, **135**, 473–479.

Kovnar, E., Kun, L., Burger, J., Krischer, J. (1991) 'Patterns of dissemination and recurrence in childhood ependymoma: preliminary results of Pediatric Oncology Group protocol, #8532.' *Annals of Neurology*, **30**, 457. *(Abstract.)*

Krauss, J.K., Nobbe, F., Wakhloo, A.K., *et al.* (1992) 'Movement disorders in astrocytomas of the basal ganglia and the thalamus.' *Journal of Neurology, Neurosurgery, and Psychiatry*, **55**, 1162–1167.

Kretschmar, C.S., Tarbell, N.J., Kupsky, W., *et al.* (1989) 'Pre-irradiation chemotherapy for infants and children with medulloblastoma: a preliminary report.' *Journal of Neurosurgery*, **71**, 820–825.

Krontiris, T.G. (1995) 'Oncogenes.' *New England Journal of Medicine*, **333**, 303–306.

Kulkantrakorn, K., Awwad, E.E., Levy, B., *et al.* (1997) 'MRI in Lhermitte–Duclos disease.' *Neurology*, **48**, 725–731.

Kun, L.L.E. (1994) 'Principles of radiation therapy.' *In:* Cohen, M.E., Duffner, P.K. (Eds.) *Brain Tumors in Children, 2nd Edn.* New York: Raven Press, pp. 95–115.

Kurczynski, T.W., Choudhury, A.A., Horwitz, S.J., *et al.* (1980) 'Remote effect of malignancy on the nervous system in children.' *Developmental Medicine and Child Neurology*, **22**, 205–222.

Kushnet, M.W., Goldman, R.L. (1978) 'Lipoma of the corpus callosum associated with a frontal bone defect.' *American Journal of Radiology*, **131**, 517–518.

Lampert, P.W., Davis, R.L. (1964) 'Delayed effects of radiation on the human central nervous system. "Early" and "late" delayed reactions.' *Neurology*, **14**, 912–917.

Lamy, C., Mas, J.L., Varet, B., *et al.* (1991) 'Postradiation lower motor neuron syndrome presenting as monomelic amyotrophy.' *Journal of Neurology, Neurosurgery, and Psychiatry*, **54**, 648–649.

Latimer, F.R., Alsaadi, A.A., Robbins, T.O. (1987) 'Cytogenetic studies of human brain tumors and their clinical significance.' *Journal of Neuro-oncology*, **4**, 287–291.

Laws, E.R., Taylor, W.F., Clifton, M.B., Okazaki, H. (1984) 'Neurosurgical management of low-grade astrocytoma of the cerebral hemispheres.' *Journal of Neurosurgery*, **61**, 665–673.

Lazarus, H.M., Herzig, R.H., Herzig, G.P., *et al.* (1981) 'Central nervous system toxicity of high-dose systemic cytosine arabinoside.' *Cancer*, **48**, 2577–2582.

Lena, G., Genitori, L., Molina, J., *et al.* (1990) 'Choroid plexus tumors in children: review of 24 cases.' *Acta Neurochirurgica*, **106**, 68–72.

Lesoin, F., Cama, A., Dhellemmes, P., *et al.* (1987) 'Extraneural metastasis of a pineal tumor: report of 3 cases and review of the literature.' *European Neurology*, **27**, 55–61.

Lessell, S., Rosman, N.P. (1986) 'Permanent visual impairment in childhood pseudotumor cerebri.' *Archives of Neurology*, **43**, 801–804.

Levine, A.J. (1992) 'The p53 tumor-suppressor gene.' *New England Journal of Medicine*, **326**, 1350–1352.

Levy, W.J., Bay, J., Dohn, D. (1982) 'Spinal cord meningioma.' *Journal of Neurosurgery*, **57**, 804–812.

Lindenberg, R. (1955) 'Compression of brain arteries as a pathogenetic factor for tissue necroses and their areas of predilection.' *Journal of Neuropathology and Experimental Neurology*, **14**, 223–243.

Listernick, R., Darling, C., Greenwald, M., *et al.* (1995) 'Optic pathway tumors in children: the effect of neurofibromatosis type 1 on clinical manifestations and natural history.' *Journal of Pediatrics*, **127**, 718–722.

LoMonaco, M., Milone, M., Batocchi, A.P., *et al.* (1992) 'Cisplatin neuropathy: clinical course and neurophysiological findings.' *Journal of Neurology*, **239**, 199–204.

Lowenstein, D.H., Aminoff, M.J., Simon, R.P. (1988) 'Barbiturate anesthesia in the treatment of status epilepticus. Clinical experience with 14 patients.' *Neurology*, **38**, 395–400.

Lubetzki, C., Sanson, M., Cohen, D., *et al.* (1988) 'Hypertension intracranienne bénigne et minocycline.' *Revue Neurologique*, **144**, 218–220.

Lund, E., Hamborg-Pedersen, B. (1984) 'Computed tomography of the brain following prophylactic treatment with irradiation therapy and intraspinal methotrexate in children with acute lymphoblastic leukemia.' *Neuroradiology*, **26**, 351–358.

Lyen, K.R., Grant, D.B. (1982) 'Endocrine function, morbidity and mortality after surgery for craniopharyngioma.' *Archives of Disease in Childhood*, **57**, 837–841.

Lyons, M.K., Kelly, P.J. (1991) 'Posterior fossa ependymomas: report of 30 cases and review of the literature.' *Neurosurgery*, **28**, 659–665.

Macaya, A., Roig, M., Fernandez, J.M., Boronat, M. (1988) 'Pseudotumor cerebri, spinal and radicular pain and hyporeflexia: a clinical variant of the Guillain–Barré syndrome?' *Pediatric Neurology*, **4**, 120–121.

MacCollin, M. (1995) 'CNS Young Investigator Award Lecture: Molecular analysis of the neurofibromatosis 2 tumor suppressor.' *Brain and Development*, **17**, 231–238.

MacDonald, J.V., Klump, T.E. (1986) 'Intraspinal epidermoid tumors caused by lumbar puncture.' *Archives of Neurology*, **43**, 936–939.

Mack, E.E., Wilson, C.B. (1993) 'Meningiomas induced by high-dose cranial irradiation.' *Journal of Neurosurgery*, **79**, 28–31.

MacLean, W.E., Noll, R.B., Stehbens, J.A., *et al.* (1995) 'Neuropsychological effects of cranial irradiation in young children with acute lymphoblastic leukemia 9 months after diagnosis.' *Archives of Neurology*, **52**, 156–160.

Mahmoud, H.H., Rivera, G.K., Hancock, H.L., *et al.* (1993) 'Low leucocyte counts with blast cells in cerebrospinal fluid of children with newly diagnosed acute lymphoblastic leukemia.' *New England Journal of Medicine*, **329**, 314–319.

Malozowski, S., Tanner, L.A., Wysowski, D.K., *et al.* (1995) 'Benign intracranial hypertension in children with growth hormone deficiency treated with growth hormone.' *Journal of Pediatrics*, **126**, 996–999.

Marano, S.R., Johnson, P.C., Spetzler, R.F. (1988) 'Recurrent Lhermitte–Duclos disease in a child. Case report.' *Journal of Neurosurgery*, **69**, 599–603.

Maria, B.L., Eskin, T.A., Quisling, R.G. (1993a) 'Brainstem and other malignant gliomas: II. Possible mechanisms of brain infiltration by tumor cells.' *Journal of Child Neurology*, **8**, 292–305.

—— Rehder, K., Eskin, T.A., *et al.* (1993b) 'Brainstem glioma: I. Pathology, clinical features, and therapy.' *Journal of Child Neurology*, **8**, 112–128.

—— Medina, C.D., Hoang, K.B.N., Phillips, I. (1997) 'Gene therapy for neurologic disease: benchtop discoveries to bedside applications. 2. The bedside.' *Journal of Child Neurology*, **12**, 77–84.

Martinez, A.J., Lee, A., Moossy, J., Maroon, J.C. (1980) 'Pituitary adenomas: clinicopathological and immunohistochemical study.' *Annals of Neurology*, **7**, 24–36.

Martinez-Lage, J.F., Casas, C., Fernández, M.A., *et al.* (1994) 'Macrocephaly, dystonia, and bilateral temporal arachnoid cysts: glutaric aciduria type 1.' *Child's Nervous System*, **10**, 198–203.

Mastronardi, L., Ferrante, L., Lunardi, P., *et al.* (1991) 'Association between neuroepithelial tumor and multiple intestinal polyposis (Turcot's syndrome): report of a case and critical analysis of the literature.' *Neurosurgery*, **28**, 449–452.

Matson, D.D. (1969) *Neurosurgery of Infancy and Childhood, 2nd Edn.* Springfield, IL: C.C. Thomas.

Mayer, M., Ponsot, G., Kalifa, C., *et al.* (1982) 'Tumeurs des noyaux gris centraux chez l'enfant. A propos de 38 observations.' *Archives Françaises de Pédiatrie*, **39**, 91–95.

McLendon, R., Burger, P.C. (1987) 'The primitive neuroepithelial tumor: a cautionary view.' *Journal of Pediatric Neuroscience*, **3**, 1–8.

Mercuri, S., Russo, A., Palma, L. (1981) 'Hemispheric supratentorial astrocytomas in children: long-term results in 29 cases.' *Journal of Neurosurgery*, **55**, 170–173.

Minns, R.A. (Ed.) (1991) *Problems of Intracranial Pressure in Childhood. Clinics in Developmental Medicine No. 113/114.* London: Mac Keith Press.

—— Stirling, H., Wu, F.C.W. (1994) 'Hypothalamic hamartoma with skeletal malformations, gelastic epilepsy and precocious puberty.' *Developmental Medicine and Child Neurology*, **36**, 173–176.

Mitchell, W.G., Fishman, L.S., Miller, J.H., *et al.* (1991) 'Stroke as a late sequela of cranial irradiation for childhood brain tumors.' *Journal of Child Neurology*, **6**, 128–133.

Mohnot, D., Snead, O.C., Benton, J.W. (1982) 'Burn encephalopathy in children.' *Annals of Neurology*, **12**, 42–47.

Molloy, P.T., Bilaniuk, L.T., Vaughan, S.N., *et al.* (1995) 'Brainstem tumors in patients with neurofibromatosis type 1: a distinct clinical entity.' *Neurology*, **45**, 1897–1962.

Mukai, K., Seljeskog, E.L., Dehner, L.P. (1986) 'Pituitary adenomas in patients under 20 years old. A clinicopathological study of 12 cases.' *Journal of Neuro-oncology*, **4**, 79–89.

Mulhern, R.K., Wasserman, A.L., Kovnar, E.H., *et al.* (1986) 'Serial neuropsychological studies of a child with acute lymphoblastic leukemia and subsequent glioblastoma multiforme.' *Neurology*, **36**, 1534–1538.

Murphy, M.A., Fabinyi, G.C.A., Berkovic, S.F., *et al.* (1995) 'Seizure outcome and pathological findings following temporal lobectomy in patients with complex partial seizures and foreign tissue lesions seen only on MRI.' *Journal of Clinical Neuroscience*, **1**, 38–41.

Mushet, G.R. (1977) 'Pseudotumor and nitrofurantoin therapy.' *Archives of Neurology*, **34**, 257. *(Letter.)*

Nagasawa, S., Handa, H., Yamashita, J., Kinuta, Y. (1980) 'Dense cystic craniopharyngioma with unusual extensions.' *Surgical Neurology*, **19**, 299–301.

Naidich, T.P., Lin, J-P., Leeds, N.E., *et al.* (1977) 'Primary tumors and other masses of the cerebellum and fourth ventricle: differential diagnosis by computed tomography.' *Neuroradiology*, **14**, 153–174.

—— McLone, D.G., Harwood-Nash, D.C. (1983) 'Arachnoid cysts, paravertebral meningoceles and perineural cysts.' *In:* Newton, T.H., Pott, D.G. (Eds.) *Modern Neuroradiology. Vol. 1. Computed Tomography of the Spine and Spinal Cord.* San Anselmo, CA: Clavaded Press, pp. 383–396.

—— McLone, D.G., Radkowski, M.A. (1985–1986) 'Intracranial arachnoid cysts.' *Pediatric Neurosciences*, **12**, 112–122.

Namba, S., Nishimoto, A., Yagu, Y. (1985) 'Diencephalic syndrome of emaciation (Russell's syndrome): long-term survival.' *Surgical Neurology*, **23**, 581–588.

Nelson, D.R., Yuh, W.T., Wen, B.C., *et al.* (1990) 'Cerebral necrosis simulating an intraparenchymal tumor.' *American Journal of Neuroradiology*, **11**, 211–212.

Neumann, H.P.H., Eggert, H.R., Weigel, K., *et al.* (1989) 'Hemangioblastomas of the central nervous system. A 10-year study with special reference to von Hippel–Lindau syndrome.' *Journal of Neurosurgery*, **70**, 24–30.

Neville, B.G.R., Wilson, J. (1970) 'Benign intracranial hypertension following corticosteroid withdrawal in childhood.' *British Medical Journal*, **3**, 544–556.

Newman, P.K., Terenity, T.R., Foster, J.B. (1981) 'Some observations on the pathogenesis of syringomyelia.' *Journal of Neurology, Neurosurgery, and Psychiatry*, **44**, 964–969.

Nishio, S., Tashima, T., Takeshita, I., Fukui, M. (1988) 'Intraventricular neurocytoma: clinicopathological features of 6 cases.' *Journal of Neurosurgery*, **68**, 665–670.

North, K. (1997) *Neurofibromatosis Type 1 in Children.* London: Mac Keith Press for the International Child Neurology Association.

Nussbaum, E., Maggi, J.C. (1988) 'Pentobarbital therapy does not improve neurologic outcome in nearly drowned, flaccid–comatose children.' *Pediatrics*, **81**, 630–634.

Obeid, T., Yaqub, B., Panayiotopoulos, C., *et al.* (1988) 'Absence status epilepticus with computed tomographic brain changes following metrizamide myelography.' *Annals of Neurology*, **24**, 582–584.

Ochs, J.J., Bowman, W.P., Pui, C-H., *et al.* (1984) 'Seizures in childhood lymphoblastic leukaemia patients.' *Lancet*, **2**, 1422–1424.

O'Connell, J.E.A. (1978) 'Trigeminal false localizing signs and their causation.' *Brain*, **101**, 119–142.

Odom, G.L., Davis, C.H., Woodhall, B. (1956) 'Brain tumors in children: clinical analysis of 164 cases.' *Pediatrics*, **18**, 856–868.

Ono, S., Morooka, S., Shimizu, N. (1987) 'Hyperthyroidism associated with papilledema and pyramidal tract involvement.' *Journal of Neurology*, **235**, 62–63.

Osborn, A.G., Johnson, L., Roberts, T.S. (1979) 'Sphenoidal mucoceles with intracranial extension.' *Journal of Computer Assisted Tomography*, **3**, 335–336.

Özek, E., Özek, M.M., Caliskan, M., *et al.* (1995) 'Multiple pineal cysts associated with an ependymal cyst presenting with infantile spasm.' *Child's Nervous System*, **11**, 246–249.

Özön, A., Topaloglu, H., Cila, A., *et al.* (1994) 'Acute ascending myelitis and encephalopathy after intrathecal cytosine arabinoside and methotrexate in an adolescent boy with acute lymphoblastic leukemia.' *Brain and Development*, **16**, 246–248.

Packer, R.J., Allen, J., Nielsen, S., *et al.* (1983) 'Brainstem glioma: clinical manifestations of meningeal gliomatosis.' *Annals of Neurology*, **14**, 177–182.

—— Sutton, L.N., Rosenstock, J.G., *et al.* (1984) 'Pineal region tumors of childhood.' *Pediatrics*, **74**, 97–102.

—— Rorke, L.B., Lange, B.J., *et al.* (1985) 'Cerebrovascular accidents in children with cancer.' *Pediatrics*, **76**, 194–201.

—— Sutton, L.N., D'Angio, G. (1985–1986) 'Management of children with primitive neuroectodermal tumors of the posterior fossa/medulloblastoma.' *Pediatric Neuroscience*, **12**, 272–282.

—— Bilaniuk, L.T., Cohen, B.H., *et al.* (1988a) 'Intracranial visual pathway gliomas in children with neurofibromatosis.' *Neurofibromatosis*, **1**, 212–222.

—— Siegel, K.R., Sutton, L.N., *et al.* (1988b) 'Efficacy of adjuvant chemotherapy for patients with poor-risk medulloblastoma: a preliminary report.' *Annals of Neurology*, **24**, 503–508.

—— Sutton, L.N., Bilaniuk, L.T., *et al.* (1988c) 'Treatment of chiasmatic/hypothalamic gliomas of childhood with chemotherapy: an update.' *Annals of Neurology*, **23**, 79–85.

—— —— Atkins, T.E., *et al.* (1989) 'A prospective study of cognitive function in children receiving whole-brain radiotherapy and chemotherapy: 2-year results.' *Journal of Neurosurgery*, **70**, 707–713.

—— Allen, J.C., Goldwein, J.L., *et al.* (1990) 'Hyperfractionated radiotherapy for children with brainstem gliomas: a pilot study using 7,200 cGy.' *Annals of Neurology*, **27**, 167–173.

—— Sutton, L.N., Elterman, R., *et al.* (1994) 'Outcome for children with medulloblastoma treated with radiation and cisplatin, CCNU, and vincristine chemotherapy.' *Journal of Neurosurgery*, **81**, 690–698.

Page, A., Paxton, R.M., Mohan, D. (1987) 'A reappraisal of the relationship between arachnoid cysts of the middle fossa and chronic subdural haematoma.' *Journal of Neurology, Neurosurgery, and Psychiatry*, **50**, 1001–1007.

Paisley, W.J., Ouvrier, R.A., Johnson, I., *et al.* (1982) 'Chronic spinal arachnoiditis in childhood.' *Developmental Medicine and Child Neurology*, **24**, 798–807.

Pascual-Castraviejo, I. (Ed.) (1990) *Spinal Tumors in Children and Adolescents.* New York: Raven Press.

—— Villarejo, F., Perez-Higueras, A., *et al.* (1983) 'Childhood choroid plexus neoplasms.' *European Journal of Pediatrics*, **140**, 51–56.

Patchell, R., Perry, M.C. (1981) 'Eosinophilic meningitis in Hodgkin disease.' *Neurology*, **31**, 887–888.

Pedersen, H., Gjerris, F., Klinken, L. (1981) 'Computed tomography of benign supratentorial astrocytomas of infancy and childhood.' *Neuroradiology*, **21**, 87–91.

Perugini, S., Pasquini, U., Menichelli, F., *et al.* (1982) 'Mucoceles in the paranasal sinuses involving the orbit: CT signs in 43 cases.' *Neuroradiology*, **23**, 133–139.

Pesin, S.R., Shields, J.A. (1989) 'Seven cases of trilateral retinoblastoma.' *American Journal of Ophthalmology*, **107**, 121–126.

Peylan-Ramu, N., Poplack, D.G., Blei, C.L., *et al.* (1977) 'Computer assisted tomography in methotrexate encephalopathy.' *Journal of Computer Assisted Tomography*, **1**, 216–221.

—— —— Pizzo, P.A., *et al.* (1978) 'Abnormal CT scans of the brain in asymptomatic children with acute lymphoblastic leukemia after prophylactic treatment of the central nervous system with radiation and intrathecal chemotherapy.' *New England Journal of Medicine*, **298**, 815–818.

Pierre-Kahn, A., Hirsch, J-F., Roux, F.X., *et al.* (1983) 'Intracranial ependymomas in childhood: survival and functional results in 47 cases.' *Child's Brain*, **10**, 145–156.

—— Brauner, R., Renier, C., *et al.* (1988) 'Traitement des craniopharyngiomes de l'enfant: analyse rétrospective de 50 observations.' *Archives Françaises de Pédiatrie*, **45**, 163–167.

—— Hirsch, J.F., Vinchon, M., *et al.* (1993) 'Surgical management of brainstem tumors in children: results and statistical analysis of 75 cases.' *Journal of Neurosurgery*, **79**, 845–852.

Pihko, H., Tyni, T., Virkola, K., *et al.* (1993) 'Transient ischemic cerebral lesions during induction chemotherapy for acute lymphoblastic leukemia.' *Journal of Pediatrics*, **123**, 718–724.

Pizzo, P.A., Bleyer, W.P., Poplack, D.G., Leventhal, B.G. (1976) 'Reversible dementia temporally associated with intraventricular therapy with methotrexate in a child with acute myelogenous leukemia.' *Journal of Pediatrics*, **88**, 131–133.

Plum, F., Posner, J.B. (1980) *The Diagnosis of Stupor and Coma, 3rd Edn.* Philadelphia: F.A. Davis.

Pollack, I.F. (1994) 'Current concepts: brain tumors in children.' *New England Journal of Medicine*, **331**, 1500–1507.

—— Hoffman, H.J., Humphreys, R.P., Becker, L. (1993) 'The long-term outcome after surgical treatment of dorsally exophytic brain-stem gliomas.' *Journal of Neurosurgery*, **78**, 859–863.

Prayson, R.A., Estes, M.L., Morris, H.H. (1993) 'Coexistence of neoplasia and cortical dysplasia in patients presenting with seizures.' *Epilepsia*, **34**, 609–615.

Price, R.A. (1983) 'The pathology of central nervous system leukemia.' *In:* Mastrangelo, R., Poplack, D.G., Riccardi, R. (Eds.) *Central Nervous System Leukemia.* Boston: Martinius Nijhoff, pp. 1–9.

—— Birdwell, D.A. (1978) 'The central nervous system in childhood leukemia. III: Mineralizing microangiopathy and dystrophic calcification.' *Cancer*, **42**, 717–728.

Pui, C-H., Dahl, G.V., Hustu, H.O., Murphy, S.B. (1985) 'Epidural spinal cord compression as the initial finding in childhood acute leukemia and non-Hodgkin lymphoma.' *Journal of Pediatrics*, **106**, 788–792.

Radcliffe, J., Packer, R.J., Atkins, T.E., *et al.* (1992) 'Three- and four-year cognitive outcome in children with noncortical brain tumors treated with whole-brain radiotherapy.' *Annals of Neurology*, **32**, 551–554.

Raffel, C., McComb, J.G., Bodner, S., Gilles, F.E. (1989) 'Benign brain stem lesions in pediatric patients with neurofibromatosis: case reports.' *Neurosurgery*, **25**, 959–964.

Rajan, B., Ashley, S., Gorman, C., *et al.* (1993) 'Craniopharyngioma—long-term results following limited surgery and radiotherapy.' *Radiotherapy and Oncology*, **26**, 1–10.

Ramaekers, V.T., Reul, J., Siller, V., Thron, A. (1994) 'Mesencephalic and third ventricle cysts: diagnosis and management in four cases.' *Journal of Neurology, Neurosurgery, and Psychiatry*, **57**, 1216–1220.

Raymond, A.A., Halpin, S.F.S., Alsanjari, N., *et al.* (1994) 'Dysembryoplastic neuroepithelial tumour. Features in 16 patients.' *Brain*, **117**, 461–475.

Rea, G.L., Akerson, R.D., Rockswold, G.L., Smith, S.A. (1983) 'Subependymoma in a 2¹/₂-year-old boy.' *Journal of Neurosurgery*, **59**, 1088–1091.

Regine, W.F., Kramer, S. (1992) 'Pediatric craniopharyngiomas: long-term results of combined treatment with surgery and radiation.' *International Journal of Radiation Oncology and Biological Physics*, **24**, 611–617.

Reich, J.B., Sierra, J., Camp, W., *et al.* (1993) 'Magnetic resonance imaging measurements and clinical changes accompanying transtentorial and foramen magnum brain herniation.' *Annals of Neurology*, **33**, 159–170.

Reid, A.C., Matheson, M.S., Teasdale, G. (1980) 'Volume of the ventricles in benign intracranial hypertension.' *Lancet*, **2**, 7–8.

Renault, F., Flores-Guevara, R., D'Allest, A.M. (1995) 'Segmental myoclonus in a child with spinal cord tumour.' *Developmental Medicine and Child Neurology*, **37**, 354–361.

Revesz, T., Scaravilli, F., Coutinho, L., *et al.* (1993) 'Reliability of histological diagnosis including grading in gliomas biopsied by image-guided stereotactic technique.' *Brain*, **116**, 781–793.

Richaud, J. (1988) 'Spinal meningeal malformations in children (without meningoceles or meningomyeloceles).' *Child's Nervous System*, **4**, 79–87.

Richmond, I.L., Wilson, C.B. (1980) 'Parasellar tumors in children. I: Clinical presentation, preoperative assessment, and differential diagnosis.' *Child's Brain*, **7**, 73–84.

Rifkinson-Mann, S., Wisoff, J.H., Epstein, F. (1990) 'The association of hydrocephalus with intramedullary spinal cord tumors: a series of 25 patients.' *Neurosurgery*, **27**, 749–754.

River, Y., Schwartz, A., Gomori, J.M., *et al.* (1996) 'Clinical significance of diffuse dural enhancement detected by magnetic resonance imaging.' *Journal of Neurosurgery*, **85**, 777–783.

Robain, O., Dulac, O., Dommergues, J.P., *et al.* (1984) 'Necrotising leucoencephalopathy complicating treatment of childhood leukaemia.' *Journal of Neurology, Neurosurgery, and Psychiatry*, **47**, 65–72.

Robertson, P.L. (1992) 'Atypical presentations of spinal cord tumors in children.' *Journal of Child Neurology*, **7**, 360–363.

—— Allen, J.C., Abbott, L.R., *et al.* (1994) 'Cervicomedullary tumors in children: a distinct subset of brainstem gliomas.' *Neurology*, **44**, 1798–1803.

Robertson, S.J., Wolpert, S.M., Runge, V.M. (1989) 'MR imaging of middle cranial fossa arachnoid cysts: temporal lobe agenesis syndrome revisited.' *American Journal of Neuroradiology*, **10**, 1007–1010.

Robinow, M., Johnson, G.F., Verhagen, A.D. (1970) 'Distichiasis lymphedema. A hereditary syndrome with multiple congenital defects.' *American Journal of Diseases of Children*, **119**, 343–347.

Rogers, M.C. (Ed.) *Textbook of Pediatric Intensive Care, Vol. 1.* Baltimore: Williams & Wilkins.

Roig, M., Ballesca, M., Navarro, C., *et al.* (1988) 'Congenital spinal cord haemangioblastoma: another cause of spinal cord section syndrome in the newborn.' *Journal of Neurology, Neurosurgery, and Psychiatry*, **51**, 1091–1093.

Ron, E., Modan, B., Brice, J.D., *et al.* (1988) 'Tumors of the brain and nervous system after radiotherapy in childhood.' *New England Journal of Medicine*, **319**, 1033–1039.

Roosen, N., Deckert, M., Nicola, N., *et al.* (1988) 'Congenital anaplastic astrocytoma with favorable prognosis. Case report.' *Journal of Neurosurgery*, **69**, 604–609.

Ropper, A.H. (1989) 'A preliminary MRI study of the geometry of brain displacement and level of consciousness with acute intracranial masses.' *Neurology*, **39**, 622–627.

Rorke, L.B. (1983) 'The cerebellar medulloblastoma and its relationship to primitive neuroectodermal tumors.' *Journal of Neuropathology and Experimental Neurology*, **42**, 1–15.

Rosenbloom, A.L., Riley, W.J., Weber, F.T., *et al.* (1980) 'Cerebral edema complicating diabetic ketoacidosis in childhood.' *Journal of Pediatrics*, **96**, 357–361.

Rossi, L. (1989) 'Headache in childhood.' *Child's Nervous System*, **5**, 129–134.

Rothwell, P.M., Gibson, R.J., Sellar, R.J. (1994) 'Computed tomographic evidence of cerebral swelling in benign intracranial hypertension.' *Journal of Neurology, Neurosurgery, and Psychiatry*, **57**, 1407–1409.

Round, R., Keane, J.R. (1988) 'The minor symptoms of increased intracranial pressure: 101 patients with benign intracranial hypertension.' *Neurology*, **38**, 1461–1464.

Rout, D., Das, L., Rao, V.R.K., Radhakrishnan, V.V. (1983) 'Symptomatic Rathke's cleft cysts.' *Surgical Neurology*, **19**, 42–45.

Rowland, J.A., Glidewell, O.J., Sibley, R.F., *et al.* (1984) 'Effects of different forms of central nervous system prophylaxis on neurophychologic function in childhood leukemia.' *Journal of Clinical Oncology*, **2**, 1317–1326.

531

Roytman, M., Frumkin, A., Bohn, T.G. (1988) 'Pseudotumor cerebri caused by isotretinoin.' *Cutis*, **5**, 399–400.

Rubin, A.M., Kang, H. (1987) 'Cerebral blindness and encephalopathy with cyclosporin A toxicity.' *Neurology*, **37**, 1072–1076.

Rubinstein, L.J. (1985) 'Embryonal central neuroepithelial tumors and their differentiating potential: a cytogenetic view of a complex neuro-oncological problem.' *Journal of Neurosurgery*, **62**, 795–805.

—— (1988) 'Pathological features of optic nerve and chiasmatic gliomas.' *Neurofibromatosis*, **1**, 152–158.

Rubnitz, J.E., Crist, W.M. (1997) 'Molecular genetics of childhood cancer.' *Pediatrics*, **100**, 101–108.

Russell, D.S., Rubinstein, L.J. (Eds.) (1989) *Pathology of Tumours of the Nervous System, 5th Edn.* London: Edward Arnold.

Russell, N.A., Belanger, G., Benoit, B.G., *et al.* (1984) 'Spinal epidural lipomatosis: a complication of glucocorticoid therapy.' *Canadian Journal of Neurological Science*, **11**, 383–386.

Rutgers, M.J., Van der Lugt, P.J., Van Turhout, J.M. (1979) 'Spinal cord compression by extramedullary hematopoietic tissue in pyruvate-kinase-deficiency-caused hemolytic anemia.' *Neurology*, **29**, 510–513.

Sainte-Rose, C., Lacombe, J., Pierre-Kahn, A., *et al.* (1984) 'Intracranial venous sinus hypertension: cause or consequence of hydrocephalus in infants.' *Journal of Neurosurgery*, **60**, 727–736.

Saito, M., Takagi, T., Ishikawa, T. (1988) 'Dermoid cyst of the anterior fontanel: advantage of MRI for the diagnosis.' *Brain and Development*, **10**, 252–255.

Sammaritano, M., Andermann, F., Melanson, D., *et al.* (1985) 'Prolonged focal cerebral edema associated with partial status epilepticus.' *Epilepsia*, **26**, 334–339.

Sanborn, G.E., Selhorst, J.B., Calabrese, V.P., Taylor, J.R. (1979) 'Pseudotumor cerebri and insecticide intoxication.' *Neurology*, **29**, 1222–1227.

Sano, K., Matsutani, M. (1981) 'Pinealoma (germinoma) treated by direct surgery and postoperative irradiation. A long-term follow-up.' *Child's Brain*, **8**, 81–97.

Santibáñez-Koref, M.F., Birch, J.M., Hartley, A.L., *et al.* (1991) 'p53 germline mutations in Li–Fraumeni syndrome.' *Lancet*, **338**, 1490–1491.

Sapozink, M.D., Kaplan, H.S. (1983) 'Intracranial Hodgkin's disease: a report of 12 cases and review of the literature.' *Cancer*, **52**, 1301–1307.

Schaefer, S.D., Post, J.D., Close, L.G., Wright, C.G. (1985) 'Ototoxicity of low- and moderate-dose cisplatin.' *Cancer*, **56**, 1934–1939.

Scheithauer, B.W. (1978) 'Symptomatic subependymoma. Report of 21 cases with review of the literature.' *Journal of Neurosurgery*, **49**, 689–696.

Schneider, J.H., Raffel, C., McComb, J.G. (1992) 'Benign cerebellar astrocytomas of childhood.' *Neurosurgery*, **30**, 58–63.

Schoeman, J.F. (1994) 'Childhood pseudotumor cerebri: clinical and intracranial pressure response in acetazolamide and furosemide treatment in a case series.' *Journal of Child Neurology*, **9**, 130–134.

Schulte, F.J., Herrmann, H.D., Müller, D., *et al.* (1987) 'Pineal region tumours of childhood.' *European Journal of Pediatrics*, **146**, 233–245.

Seiff, S.R., Brodsky, M.C., MacDonald, G., *et al.* (1987) 'Orbital optic glioma in neurofibromatosis. Magnetic resonance diagnosis of perineural arachnoidal gliomatosis.' *Archives of Ophthalmology*, **105**, 1689–1692.

Selky, A.K., Dobyns, W.B., Yee, R.D. (1994) 'Idiopathic intracranial hypertension and facial diplegia.' *Neurology*, **44**, 357.

Sgouros, S., Fineron, P.W., Hockley, A.D. (1995) 'Cerebellar astrocytoma of childhood: long-term follow-up.' *Child's Nervous System*, **11**, 89–96.

Shakir, R.A., Sulaiman, K., Kahn, R.A., Rudwan, M. (1990) 'Neurological presentation of neuro-Behçet's syndrome.' *European Neurology*, **30**, 249–253.

Shalet, S.M. (1986) 'Pituitary adenomas in childhood.' *Acta Endocrinologica*, **279** (Suppl.), 434–439.

Shapiro, K., Katz, M. (1983) 'The recurrent cerebellar astrocytoma.' *Child's Brain*, **10**, 168–176.

Shapiro, W.R., Shapiro, J.R. (1986) 'Principles of brain tumor chemotherapy.' *Seminars in Oncology*, **13**, 55–69.

Sheldon, R.S., Becker, W.J., Hanley, D.A., Culver, R.L. (1987) 'Hypoparathyroidism and pseudotumor cerebri: an infrequent clinical association.' *Canadian Journal of Neurological Science*, **14**, 622–625.

Shulman, D.I., Martinez, C.R., Bercu, B.B., Root, A.W. (1986) 'Hypothalamic–pituitary dysfunction in primary empty sella syndrome in childhood.' *Journal of Pediatrics*, **108**, 540–544.

Shuper, A., Packer, R.J., Vezina, L.G., *et al.* (1995) '"Complicated migraine-like episodes" in children following cranial irradiation and chemotherapy.' *Neurology*, **45**, 1837–1840.

Siegel, M.J., Shackelford, G.D., McAlister, W.H. (1979) 'Paranasal sinus mucoceles in children.' *Radiology*, **133**, 623–626.

Sklar, C.A., Grumbach, M.M., Kaplan, S.L. (1981) 'Hormonal and metabolic abnormalities associated with central nervous system germinoma in children and adolescents and the effect of therapy: report of 10 cases.' *Journal of Clinical Endocrinology and Metabolism*, **52**, 9–15.

Slamon, D.J. (1987) 'Proto-oncogenes and human cancers.' *New England Journal of Medicine*, **317**, 955–957.

Sørensen, P.S., Gjerris, F., Svenstup, B. (1986) 'Endocrine studies in patients with pseudotumor cerebri: estrogen levels in blood and cerebrospinal fluid.' *Archives of Neurology*, **43**, 902–906.

Sorva, R., Heiskanen, O., Perheentupa, J. (1988) 'Craniopharyngioma surgery in children: endocrine and visual outcome.' *Child's Nervous System*, **4**, 97–99.

Soysa, N.D. (1985) 'The oral contraceptive pill and benign intracranial hypertension.' *New Zealand Journal of Medicine*, **14**, 656–657.

Sparkes, R.S., Murphree, A.L., Lingua, R.W., *et al.* (1983) 'Gene for hereditary retinoblastoma assigned to human chromosome 13 by linkage to esterase D.' *Science*, **219**, 971–973.

Sposto, R., Ertel, I.J., Jenkin, R.D.T., *et al.* (1989) 'The effectiveness of chemotherapy for treatment of high grade astrocytoma in children: results of a randomized trial. A report from the Children's Cancer Study Group.' *Journal of Neurooncology*, **7**, 165–177.

Sprung, C., Baerwald, R., Henkes, H., Schörner, W. (1989) 'A comparative study of CT and MRI in midline tumors of childhood and adolescence.' *Child's Nervous System*, **5**, 102–106.

Squires, L.A., Allen, J.C., Abbott, R., Epstein, F.J. (1994) 'Focal tectal tumors: management and prognosis.' *Neurology*, **44**, 953–956.

Stanbridge, D. (1990) 'Human tumor suppressor genes.' *Annual Review of Genetics*, **24**, 615–657.

Stanhope, R., Adlard, P. (1987) 'Empty sella syndrome.' *Developmental Medicine and Child Neurology*, **29**, 397–404.

Stoebner, R., Kiser, R., Alperin, J.B. (1970) 'Iron deficiency anemia and papilledema. Rapid resolution with oral iron therapy.' *American Journal of Digestive Diseases*, **15**, 919–922.

Stroink, A.R., Hoffman, H.J., Hendrick, E.B., Humphreys, R.P. (1986) 'Diagnosis and management of pediatric brain-stem gliomas.' *Journal of Neurosurgery*, **65**, 745–750.

Strom, H.E., Skullerud, K. (1983) 'Pleomorphic xanthoastrocytoma: report of 5 cases.' *Clinical Neuropathology*, **2**, 188–191.

Summers, C.G., MacDonald, J.T. (1988) 'Paroxysmal facial itch: a presenting sign of childhood brainstem glioma.' *Journal of Child Neurology*, **3**, 189–192.

Sutton, L.N., Packer, R.J., Rorke, L.B., *et al.* (1983) 'Cerebral gangliogliomas during childhood.' *Neurosurgery*, **13**, 124–128.

—— Cnaan, A., Klatt, L., *et al.* (1996) 'Postoperative surveillance imaging in children with cerebellar astrocytomas.' *Journal of Neurosurgery*, **84**, 721–725.

Swartz, J.D., Zimmerman, R.A., Bilaniuk, L.T. (1982) 'Computed tomography of intracranial ependymomas.' *Radiology*, **143**, 97–101.

Taboada, D., Froufe, A., Alonso, A., *et al.* (1980) 'Congenital medulloblastoma. Report of 2 cases.' *Pediatric Radiology*, **9**, 5–10.

Tasker, R.C., Boyd, S., Harden, A., Matthew, D.J. (1988) 'Monitoring in non-traumatic coma. Part II: electroencephalography.' *Archives of Disease in Childhood*, **63**, 895–899.

Taylor, D. (1990) 'Leukemia.' *In:* Taylor, D. (Ed.) *Pediatric Ophthalmology.* Oxford: Blackwell, pp. 572–582.

Tenny, R.T., Lewis, E.R., Younge, B.R., Rush, J.A. (1982) 'The neurosurgical management of optic glioma. Results in 104 patients.' *Journal of Neurosurgery*, **57**, 452–458.

Thompson, C.B., June, C.H., Sullivan, K.M., Thomas, E.D. (1984) 'Association between cyclosporin neurotoxicity and hypomagnesaemia.' *Lancet*, **2**, 1116–1120.

Tice, H., Barnes, P.D., Goumnerova, L., *et al.* (1993) 'Pediatric and adolescent oligodendrogliomas.' *American Journal of Neuroradiology*, **14**, 1293–1300.

Till, K. (1975) *Paediatric Neurosurgery for Paediatricians and Neurosurgeons.* Oxford: Blackwell.

Tönnis, W., Friedmann, G. (1964) *Das Röntgenbild des Schädels bei intrakraniellen Drucksteigerung im Wachstumsalter.* Berlin: Springer Verlag.

Topçu, M., Gucuyener, K., Topaloglu, H., *et al.* (1992) 'Paraneoplastic syndrome manifesting as chronic cerebellar ataxia in a child with Hodgkin disease.' *Journal of Pediatrics*, **120**, 275–277.

Torlai, F., Galassi, G., Debbia, A., *et al.* (1989) 'Familial pseudotumor cerebri in male heterozygous twins.' *European Neurology*, **29**, 106–108.

Toshniwal, P.K., Glick, R.P. (1987) 'Spinal epidural lipomatosis: report of a case secondary to hypothyroidism and review of the literature.' *Journal of Neurology*, **234**, 172–176.

Turjman, F., Xavier, J.L., Froment, J.C., *et al.* (1996) 'Late MR follow-up of hypothalamic hamartomas.' *Child's Nervous System*, **12**, 63–68.

Tyson, D., Reggiardo, D., Sklar, C., David, R. (1993) 'Prolactin-secreting macroadenomas in adolescents. Response to bromocriptine therapy.' *American Journal of Diseases of Children*, **147**, 1057–1061.

Valentini, L., Solero, C.L., Lasio, G., *et al.* (1995) 'Triventricular hydrocephalus: review of 71 cases evaluated at the Istituto Neurologico "C. Besta", Milan, over the last 10 years.' *Child's Nervous System*, **11**, 170–172.

Vallée, B., Malhaire, J.P., Person, H., Colin, J. (1984) 'Delayed cerebral pseudotumoral radionecrosis following scalp-tumor irradiation. Case report and review of literature.' *Journal of Neurology*, **231**, 135–140.

Van der Meché, F.G.A., Braakman, R. (1983) 'Arachnoid cysts in the middle cranial fossa: cause and treatment of progressive and non-progressive symptoms.' *Journal of Neurology, Neurosurgery, and Psychiatry*, **46**, 1102–1107.

Van der Wal, A.C., Troost, D. (1988) 'Enterogenous cyst of the brainstem—a case report.' *Neuropediatrics*, **19**, 216–217.

van Dongen, H.R., Catsman-Berrevoets, C.E., van Mourik, M. (1994) 'The syndrome of 'cerebellar' mutism and subsequent dysarthria.' *Neurology*, **44**, 2040–2046.

Van Dop, C., Conte, F.A., Koch, T.K., *et al.* (1983) 'Pseudotumor cerebri associated with initiation of levothyroxine therapy for juvenile hypothyroidism.' *New England Journal of Medicine*, **308**, 1076–1080.

Van Zandijcke, M., Dewachter, A. (1986) 'Pseudotumor cerebri with amiodarone.' *Journal of Neurology, Neurosurgery, and Psychiatry*, **49**, 1463–1464.

Vaquero, J., Carillo, R., Cabezudo, J.M., *et al.* (1981) 'Arachnoid cysts of the posterior fossa.' *Surgical Neurology*, **16**, 117–121.

Varma, R.R., Crumrine, P.K., Bergman, I., *et al.* (1983) 'Childhood oligodendrogliomas presenting with seizures and low density lesions on computed tomography.' *Neurology*, **33**, 806–808.

Verplanck, M., Kaufman, D.I., Parsons, T., *et al.* (1988) 'Electrophysiology versus psychophysics in the detection of visual loss in pseudotumor cerebri.' *Neurology*, **38**, 1789–1792.

Vieregge, P., Gerhard, L., Nahser, H.C. (1987) 'Familial glioma: occurrence within the "familial cancer syndrome" and systemic malformations.' *Journal of Neurology*, **234**, 220–232.

Vinchon, M., Blond, S., Lejeune, J.P., *et al.* (1994) 'Association of Lhermitte–Duclos and Cowden disease: report of a new case and review of the literature.' *Journal of Neurology, Neurosurgery, and Psychiatry*, **57**, 699–704.

Volpe, B.T., Foley, K.M., Howieson, J. (1978) 'Normal CAT scans in craniopharyngioma.' *Annals of Neurology*, **3**, 87–89.

Vorkapic, P., Pendl, G. (1987) 'Microsurgery of pineal region lesions in children.' *Neuropediatrics*, **18**, 222–226.

Wakai, S., Arai, T., Nagai, M. (1984) 'Congenital brain tumors.' *Surgical Neurology*, **21**, 597–609.

Walker, A.E., Robins, M., Weinfeld, F. (1985) 'Epidemiology of brain tumors: the national survey of intracranial neoplasms.' *Neurology*, **35**, 219–226.

Walker, R.W., Rosenblum, M.K. (1992) 'Amphotericin B-associated leukoencephalopathy.' *Neurology*, **42**, 2005–2010.

Wall, M., George, D. (1987) 'Visual loss in pseudotumor cerebri. Incidence and defects related to visual field strategy.' *Archives of Neurology*, **44**, 170–175.

—— Dollar, J.D., Sadun, A.A., Kardon, R. (1995) 'Idiopathic intracranial hypertension. Lack of histologic evidence for cerebral edema.' *Archives of Neurology*, **52**, 141–145.

Walls, T.J., Purohit, D.P., Aji, W.S., *et al.* (1986) 'Multiple intracranial enterogenous cysts.' *Journal of Neurology, Neurosurgery, and Psychiatry*, **49**, 438–441.

Walters, B.N.J., Gubbay, S.S. (1981) 'Tetracycline and benign intracranial hypertension: report of five cases.' *British Medical Journal*, **282**, 19–20.

Weiner, L.P., Porro, R.S. (1965) 'Total third nerve paralysis: a case with hemorrhage in the oculomotor nerve in subdural hematoma.' *Neurology*, **15**, 87–90.

Werner, M.H., Burger, P.C., Heinz, E.R., *et al.* (1988) 'Intracranial atherosclerosis following radiotherapy.' *Neurology*, **38**, 1158–1160.

Whelan, H.T., Nelson, D.B., Strother, D., *et al.* (1989) 'Medulloblastoma cell line secretes platelet derived growth-factor.' *Pediatric Neurology*, **5**, 347–352.

Wiggs, J., Nordenskjöld, M., Yandell, D., *et al.* (1988) 'Prediction of the risk of hereditary retinoblastoma, using DNA polymorphisms within the retinoblastoma gene.' *New England Journal of Medicine*, **318**, 151–157.

Wilkinson, I.M.S., Anderson, J.R., Holmes, A.E. (1987) 'Oligodendroglioma: an analysis of 42 cases.' *Journal of Neurology, Neurosurgery, and Psychiatry*, **50**, 304–312.

Williams, A.L., Houghton, V.M., Pojunas, R.W., *et al.* (1987) 'Differentiation of intramedullary neoplasms and cysts by MR.' *American Journal of Roentgenology*, **149**, 159–164.

Williams, R.S., Richardson, E.P. (1988) 'MSG Case Records (Case 20-1988).' *New England Journal of Medicine*, **318**, 1322–1328.

Wilson, W.B., Gordon, M., Lehman, R.A.W. (1979) 'Meningiomas confined to the optic canal and foramina.' *Surgical Neurology*, **12**, 21–28.

Winkelman, M.D., Hines, J.D. (1983) 'Cerebellar degeneration caused by high-dose cytosine arabinoside: a clinicopathological study.' *Annals of Neurology*, **14**, 520–527.

Wold, L.E., Laws, E.R. (1983) 'Cranial chordomas in children and young adults.' *Journal of Neurosurgery*, **59**, 1043–1047.

Woo, E., Lam, K., Yu, L., *et al.* (1987) 'Cerebral radionecrosis: is surgery necessary?' *Journal of Neurology, Neurosurgery, and Psychiatry*, **50**, 1407–1414.

Yamauchi, K., Umeda, Y. (1997) 'Symptomatic intracranial haemorrhage in acute nonlymphoblastic leukaemia: analysis of CT and autopsy findings.' *Journal of Neurology*, **244**, 94–100.

Yandell, D.W., Campbell, T.P., Dayton, S.H., *et al.* (1989) 'Oncogenic point mutations in the human retinoblastoma gene: their application to genetic counselling.' *New England Journal of Medicine*, **321**, 1689–1695.

Yasargil, M.G., Curcic, M., Kis, M., *et al.* (1990) 'Total removal of craniopharyngiomas. Approaches and long-term results in 144 patients.' *Journal of Neurosurgery*, **73**, 3–11.

Yoshida, T., Nakatani, S., Shimizu, K., *et al.* (1986) 'Huge epithelium-lined cyst: report of two cases.' *Journal of Neurology, Neurosurgery, and Psychiatry*, **49**, 1458–1460.

Young, S., Richardson, A.E. (1987) 'Solid haemangioblastomas of the posterior fossa: radiological features and results of surgery.' *Journal of Neurology, Neurosurgery, and Psychiatry*, **50**, 155–158.

Zentner, J., Wolf, H.K., Ostertun, B., *et al.* (1994) 'Gangliogliomas: clinical, radiological and histopathological findings in 51 patients.' *Journal of Neurology, Neurosurgery, and Psychiatry*, **57**, 1497–1502.

Zimmerman, L.E., Burns, R.P., Wankum, G., *et al.* (1982) 'Trilateral retinoblastoma: ectopic intracranial retinoblastoma associated with bilateral retinoblastoma.' *Journal of Pediatric Ophthalmology and Strabismus*, **19**, 320–325.

Zimmerman, R.A., Bilaniuk, L.T., Bruno, L., Rosenstock, J. (1978) 'Computed tomography of cerebellar astrocytoma.' *American Journal of Roentgenology*, **130**, 929–933.

—— —— Packer, R., *et al.* (1985) 'Resistive NMR of brainstem gliomas.' *Neuroradiology*, **27**, 21–25.

—— —— Rebsamen, S. (1992) 'Magnetic resonance imaging of pediatric posterior fossa tumors.' *Pediatric Neurology*, **18**, 58–64.

Zülch, K.J., Wechsler, W. (1968) 'Pathology and classification of gliomas.' *In:* Krayenbuhl, H., Maspes, V.E., Sweet, W.H. (Eds.) *Progress in Neurological Surgery.* Basel: Karger, pp. 1–84.

15
CEREBROVASCULAR DISORDERS

This chapter considers the various disorders resulting from disease processes involving the blood vessels of the CNS. It covers vascular malformations including neurocutaneous syndromes with prominent vascular abnormalities and occlusive arterial and venous disease, as well as the general aspects of subarachnoid haemorrhage, acute hemiplegia and certain other stroke-like episodes which are described in more detail in Chapters 9 and 17.

The incidence of cerebrovascular disorders in childhood is poorly known because vascular malformations that are present from birth frequently become symptomatic only in adulthood. The annual incidence of strokes in children has been estimated at 2.52 cases per 100,000 in Rochester, Minnesota (Schoenberg *et al.* 1978), which, pro rata, equates to approximately half the incidence of brain tumours in children in the USA. Haemorrhagic strokes in that series were slighly more common (55 per cent) than ischaemic ones. Similar figures have been obtained in Sweden (Eeg-Olofsson and Ringheim 1983).

VASCULAR MALFORMATIONS OF THE CENTRAL NERVOUS SYSTEM

The vascular malformations of the CNS include aneurysms, arteriovenous malformations, vein of Galen malformations, and direct arteriovenous fistulae. Some neurocutaneous syndromes with a marked vascular component will also be described in this section. Angiomas in general are about three to ten times as common as aneurysms in children (Chuang 1989).

ARTERIOVENOUS MALFORMATIONS (AVMs)
This term applies to several types of vascular malformations from small cryptic lesions to huge anomalies of several centimetres in diameter. AVMs include three subtypes: true AVMs, cavernous angiomas and venous angiomas. The overall incidence of such malformations is difficult to know precisely. Approximately 10–20 per cent of AVMs are revealed by 20 years of age and up to 45 per cent by the third decade. The introduction of CT and MRI has enabled AVMs to be diagnosed before adulthood, especially cavernous angiomas that are usually not visualized by angiography.

PIAL AVMs PROPER
AVMs result from the failure of embryonic vessels to differentiate into arteries and veins. Increased blood flow through the direct shunts so created results in enlargement of the blood vessels.

The lesion has the classical 'bag of worms' appearance, the abnormal vessels being separated by compact glial tissue, presumably nonfunctional (McCormick 1984). Calcification in or about the vessels is present in a quarter of cases (Guazzo and Xuereb 1994). The malformations may extend from the cortical surface through the parenchyma to the ventricular cavity. About 80 per cent of AVMs are located in the supratentorial area (Humphreys 1989a, Kondziolka *et al.* 1992, Hladky *et al.* 1994), although the incidence of infratentorial lesions was as high as 40 per cent in one series (Humphreys 1989a) and as low as 10 per cent in another (Martin and Edwards 1989). An AVM may increase in size over the years (Waltimo 1973, Mendelow *et al.* 1987). Spontaneous regression has been occasionally observed (Omojola *et al.* 1982) and spontaneous thrombosis may occur (Guazzo and Xuereb 1994). An association of aneurysms and AVMs has been reported (Østergaard and Voldby 1984). The aneurysms may develop as a consequence of the haemodynamic stress of the AVM or represent another expression of a congenital vascular disorder. They are uncommon in children (Wilkins 1985).

AVMs can consist of only an arteriovenous fistula or, more often, comprise a central nidus with surrounding vessels. Micro-AVMs (Willinsky *et al.* 1990) with a nidus of less than 1 cm in diameter are usually revealed by an intracerebral haematoma and may be invisible on imaging. Multiple AVMs are rare in children. In infants they may account for up to 32 per cent of cases (Rodesch *et al.* 1995). AVMs are mostly sporadic but rare cases of familial AVMs are on record (Aberfeld and Rao 1981, Boyd *et al.* 1985, Allard *et al.* 1989. Yokoyama *et al.* 1991, Schievink *et al.* 1995, Larsen *et al.* 1997).

The mean age of onset of clinical manifestations is about 10 years. The presenting features include intracranial haemorrhage, epilepsy and focal deficits. Headache of a migrainous type is an uncommon manifestation in children (Stein and Mohr 1988). Hydrocephalus and high intracranial pressure (ICP) may occur occasionally, and cardiac failure is rare.

Haemorrhage is a more common feature of childhood than of adult AVMs. Celli *et al.* (1984) found haemorrhage to be the first manifestation in 73 per cent of children, as compared with 56 per cent in adults. Lasjaunias *et al.* (1995) recently reviewed 1017 vascular malformations in children from the literature and analyzed 179 personal cases including 102 pial AVMs. The first sign was intracranial bleeding in 50 per cent of these. The haemorrhage is often parenchymatous in children, probably because small deep lesions are more frequent and tend to bleed earlier than large AVMs, which are more often responsible for epilepsy or other symptoms. In the series of Celli *et al.*, the risk of bleeding from a known unruptured AVM was 32 per cent by ten years after diagnosis.

The clinical symptoms and signs are those of an isolated haemorrhage or the acute onset of focal cerebral deficits. Haemorrhage is generally intraparenchymal but blood can dissect into the subarachnoid space or the ventricular system. When massive, it gives rise to increased intracranial pressure (ICP) and can be fatal, especially when bleeding originates in the posterior fossa when the mortality rate can be as high as 57 per cent (Kondziolka *et al.* 1992). In some patients intermittent headache or transient motor deficit can precede the haemorrhage (Gerosa *et al.* 1980). Epilepsy occurs as a first feature in about 20 per cent of cases (Kelly *et al.* 1978, Murphy 1985). The seizures are commonly partial. Progressive neurological deficits include hemiplegia, hemidystonia, aphasia, hemianopia or ocular motor paralysis. Signs of cerebellar or brainstem involvement are common with AVMs of the brainstem and posterior fossa (Silber *et al.* 1987, Abe *et al.* 1989). Bruits in the head were found in only 25 per cent of AVM cases (Kelly *et al.* 1978). They are only uncommonly the revealing manifestation of AVMs. Rodesch *et al.* (1988) found this to be the case in three of 44 children with AVMs. Most bruits heard over the skull in children are innocent (Pruvost *et al.* 1989).

Some AVMs may present with progressive symptoms and signs such as increasing unilateral deficit, behavioural disturbances or progressive dementia. Such cases seem to result from vascular steal through high-flow malformations (Sheth and Bodensteiner 1995).

AVMs are almost always detectable on enhanced CT scans or on MRI (Norman 1984), and angiography is probably unnecessary when the CT is normal (Chuang 1989). On the other hand, angiography may be normal with small, partially thrombosed AVMs that can mimic small brain tumours (Abe *et al.* 1989).

On unenhanced scans, there is often an area of mixed attenuation with irregular density, and calcification in or around the malformation is not rare. Following contrast enhancement, the malformation and its draining veins become clearly visible in most cases (Fig. 15.1). An early draining vein may reveal the presence of a small AVM collapsed after haemorrhaging. There is usually no mass effect although some AVMs may bulge into the ventricular cavity. After an episode of bleeding, blood is usually visible in the subarachnoid space, thus rendering lumbar puncture unnecessary. Intraparenchymal haematomas are easily visible as well-limited areas of spontaneously homogeneous blood density. Resorption of a haematoma can produce ring-like contrast enhancement that may simulate a tumour (Diebler and Dulac 1987). The diagnostic specificity of CT is 60 per cent as compared with 75 per cent for angiography (Norman 1984, Chuang 1989). CT or MRI, however, can detect so-called cryptic lesions that are missed by angiography (Cohen *et al.* 1982). MRI is more specific than CT scan and, in rare instances, demonstrates that the lesions are multiple (Gomori *et al.* 1986, Lemme-Plaghos

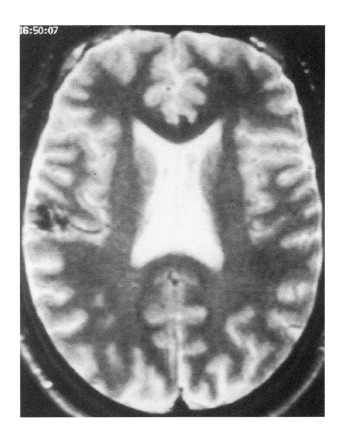

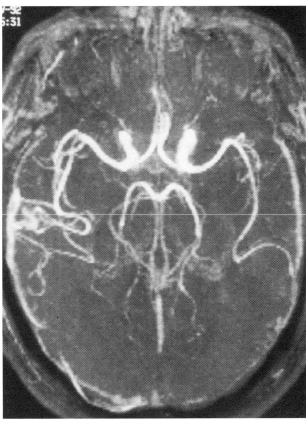

Fig. 15.1. Arteriovenous malformation involving the right hemisphere. *(Top)* T$_2$-weighted MR image showing the void signal due to rapid blood flow in the malformation and the drainage vein. *(Bottom)* MR angiography showing malformation and feeding vessels. (Courtesy Dr Kling Chong, Great Ormond Street Hospital, London.)

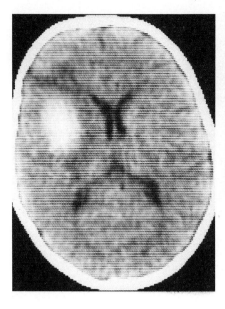
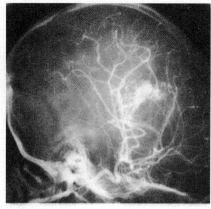
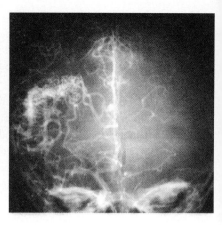

Fig. 15.2. Arteriovenous malformation involving the right central area in a 4-year-old girl. *(Left)* CT scan shows an intracerebral haematoma surrounded by oedema. *(Centre)* Right carotid angiography, lateral projection showing the malformation and its feeding vessels. There is early opacification of a draining vein that goes to the convexity of the hemisphere. *(Right)* Right carotid angiography, anteroposterior projection shows that the malformation extends as far as the ventricular body.

et al. 1986). Neuroimaging will also reveal brainstem haematomas (Howard 1986, Zimmerman *et al.* 1991).

Pial AVMs in infants are uncommon. Rodesch *et al.* (1995) reviewed 13 cases in neonates and 13 in infants. In this series, haemorrhage occurred in only four infants, whereas cardiac failure and epilepsy were present respectively in 14 and eight cases. Multiple lesions were found in eight patients.

Magnetic resonance angiography (MRA) is useful for the diagnosis of AVMs (Fisher *et al.* 1992, Koelfen *et al.* 1995). However, conventional angiography remains an essential examination for all patients with proved or suspected AVM. It provides vital information on the feeding and draining vessels (Fig. 15.2), the exact site of the AVM nidus and the size of arteriovenous communications. CT and MRI, on the other hand, show lesions suggesting hypoxia and hydrocephalus. The latter may be the presenting clinical manifestation of AVMs that bleed in a subclinical manner. Small vascular malformations, on the other hand, can cause massive, often fatal, bleeding (Margolis *et al.* 1961). Occult malformations can bleed repeatedly, even after angiographic demonstration of nonfilling (Ogilvy *et al.* 1988).

The course of AVMs is dominated by the risk of primary or recurrent haemorrhage as these may prove fatal or leave residua. The magnitude of haemorrhagic risk has been extensively studied mainly in series of adults or in mixed series of adults and children (Perret and Nishioka 1966, Drake 1979). The risk of rebleeding after a first stroke is approximately 2–3 per cent yearly with a possible decrease in incidence after the fourth year (Graf *et al.* 1983, Luessenhop and Rosa 1984, Jane *et al.* 1985, Wilkins 1985). In the series of Crawford *et al.* (1986) the risk 20 years after diagnosis was 42 per cent for haemorrhage, 29 per cent for death, 18 per cent for epilepsy and 27 per cent for major or minor neurological disability. In series of children, the risks seem even higher (So 1978, Celli *et al.* 1984, Fults and Kelly 1984). In So's series, 10 of 36 children were dead by six years after stroke and the rate of rebleeding was 25 per cent at five years. In 132 children reported by Kondziolka *et al.* (1992) the overall death rate was

25 per cent, but mortality decreased from 39 to 15 per cent following the introduction of CT scanning and subsequently improved management.

These figures justify aggressive treatment of AVMs. Two major therapeutic methods are currently available (Monaco *et al.* 1992, Hladky *et al.* 1994, Lasjaunias *et al.* 1995). *Embolization* is indicated for malformations fed by arteries large enough to be accessible to catheterization permitting selective occlusion (Beltramello *et al.* 1987). Hamilton and Spetzler (1994) propose that relatively small and superficial AVMs not located in critical areas are best treated by *excision*, while larger and less favourable cases benefit from presurgical embolization. In such cases multistage processes combining various techniques may have to be used. Lasjaunias *et al.* (1995) treated 56 children by complete embolization while in 21 cases a direct surgical approach was thought necessary. A combined approach is also advised by other investigators (Adelt *et al.* 1988, Heros *et al.* 1990).

For inaccessible lesions under 2.0 cm in diameter, proton-beam therapy or other stereotaxic methods (Loeffler *et al.* 1990, Steinberg *et al.* 1990) can be used for delivery of highly localized radiotherapy (Lunsford *et al.* 1990). With the 'gamma knife' (high energy gamma-beam), Steiner (1986) has reported obliteration in 35–50 per cent of cases at one year, 80–87 per cent at two years, and a rate of only 3 per cent for neurological sequelae due to photon therapy or rebleeding, in a series of 900 patients. Lateral lesions seem to respond better than deep malformations. The size of the lesion may not be an essential factor but malformations fed by a single pedicle are more favourable than those more diffusely vascularized (Kemeny *et al.* 1989). Radionecrosis seems infrequent following such therapy but has been reported (Statham *et al.* 1990) and may occur with helium ion therapy in as many as 9 per cent of the cases (Steinberg *et al.* 1990).

Epilepsy associated with AVMs may respond to surgery when feasible. Results, however, are not always good and epilepsy may even develop following surgical excision of an AVM (Murphy 1985).

DURAL AVMs

Dural AVMs are uncommon in children. They represented 11 per cent of all vascular malformations in one series (Garcia-Monaco *et al.* 1991b). Most dural AVMs have both external and internal carotid arterial supply. More than half of them are located in the occipital–suboccipital region. The tentorial artery branch of the internal carotid artery and the meningeal and occipital arteries from the external carotid system are the vessels most commonly involved (Albright *et al.* 1983, Batjer and Samson 1986, Humphreys 1989a). These AVMs usually drain into the transverse sinus or the torcular (Rosenbloom and Edwards 1989). It is generally accepted that dural AVMs are congenital in origin. However, Lasjaunias *et al.* (1984) have proposed that they could develop following sinus thrombosis.

Bruits are common and may be the only manifestation in adults and adolescents. Children may develop hydrocephalus, macrocephaly, distended scalp veins and cardiac failure as a result of high flow through the malformation (Rosenbloom and Edwards 1989), especially in the rare children with multiple fistulae (Garcia-Monaco *et al.* 1991b). Diagnosis of posterior fossa dural malformation may be easily missed if no angiography is performed as CT usually does not show them. MRI often demonstrates the abnormality (Grosssman *et al.* 1993). Dural AVMs located in the tentorium or around the foramen magnum usually drain into subarachnoidal veins, and 50–60 per cent of them haemorrhage (Pierot *et al.* 1992). Treatment is by embolization or a combination of embolization and surgery. Dural AVMs in the cavernous sinus are rare in children. They may produce proptosis, swelling of the eyelids and signs of increased ICP (Newton and Hoyt 1970).

Internal carotid–cavernous fistulae are almost always of traumatic origin. Fistulae can be occluded with an intravascular balloon preserving patency of the internal carotid artery (Hosobuchi 1989, Brosnahan *et al.* 1992). One case has been reported in a patient with Ehlers–Danlos syndrome (Schoolman and Kepes 1967). Spontaneous external carotid–cavernous sinus fistula is rare (Pang *et al.* 1981) and has also been reported with type IV Ehlers–Danlos syndrome (Schievink *et al.* 1991). Cerebral arteriovenous fistula can also occur in patients with the Klippel–Trenaunay syndrome (Oyesiku *et al.* 1988).

ANEURYSM (AVM) OF THE VEIN OF GALEN

Aneurysms of the vein of Galen are a special type of AVM resulting from abnormal communication between one or several cerebral arteries and the vein of Galen. Although dilatation of the vein of Galen, and sometimes of the straight sinus, is the most striking feature, it is secondary to the arteriovenous fistulae and often involves a persistent embryonal vein rather than the vein of Galen itself (Lasjaunias *et al.* 1989b). The most common clinical manifestation, cardiac failure, is due to high flow through the malformation after postnatal circulation is established. Less often the malformation or its draining veins may rupture, leading to intracranial haemorrhage. More commonly it is responsible for progressive hydrocephalus as a result of increased venous pressure or of compression of the sylvian aqueduct. In some cases, the blood steal through the malformation is such that ischaemia, sometimes with necrosis and calcification of the brain, occurs (Grossman *et al.* 1984). This was observed in a stillborn baby (personal case), indicating that occasionally establishment of a postnatal type of circulation may not be necessary for the blood to be diverted through the fistula away from brain parenchyma.

The clinical features of fistula of the vein of Galen depend upon the age of the patient and on the anatomical form of the malformation. Lasjaunias *et al.* (1989b) distinguish three types: a mural form in which arterial trunks open directly into the vein of Galen; a choroidal form characterized by multiple arteriovenous shunts located in the choroidal fissure and draining into the vein of Galen or an abnormal embryonal vein that dilates as a result of increased flow; and a parenchymal form in which multiple arteriovenous shunts are located within the parenchyma. Newborn infants characteristically have multiple choroidal fistulae that shunt more than 25 per cent of their cardiac output through the malformation, resulting in high-output cardiac failure. The head may be enlarged and the scalp veins are often distended. A loud continuous bruit is easily heard over the whole head. The diagnosis is best established by ultrasound examination which shows the dilated vein of Galen as a sonolucent area posterior to the third ventricle (Cubberley *et al.* 1982). Definitive diagnosis is established by CT and MRI scan and by angiography (Fig. 15.3). Antenatal diagnosis is possible with ultrasound (Monaco *et al.* 1992) and is of great importance for planning therapy. Caesarean section was performed in five of 18 cases of Rodesch *et al.* (1994) and four infants died shortly after birth. Eight of 12 patients who underwent embolization were normal on follow-up.

In neonates the prognosis is poor, most patients dying of heart failure. Subependymal haemorrhage may occur after attempt at shunting the hydrocephalus or spontaneously. Brain damage is often widespread (Norman and Becker 1974). Aneurysm of the vein of Galen is the most common extracardiac cause of heart failure in neonates and should be systematically looked for in such cases.

Infants between 1 and 15 months of age with galenic malformation usually have a smaller mural or parenchymal shunt. The most common feature in such cases is macrocrania due to hydrocephalus. Dilated scalp veins are present and subarachoid haemorrhage may occur (Diebler *et al.* 1981). The prognosis is guarded. In a few cases, spontaneous thrombosis has been observed (Diebler *et al.* 1981, Lasjaunias *et al.* 1989b).

Children and adults have relatively low flow fistulae and an angiomatous network supplying the vein of Galen. Haemorrhage, Parinaud syndrome, mental retardation and other features of arrested hydrocephalus are common. An occasional patient will present with a pseudodegenerative, progressive deterioration, apparently due to ischaemia resulting from steal by the fistula. Such patients may have extensive calcification in the brain (Chuang 1989).

CT and MRI with and without contrast will demonstrate the malformation, and angiography will allow for a detailed study of the feeding and draining vessels which is necessary for any form of treatment. CT in addition permits evaluation of the ventricular

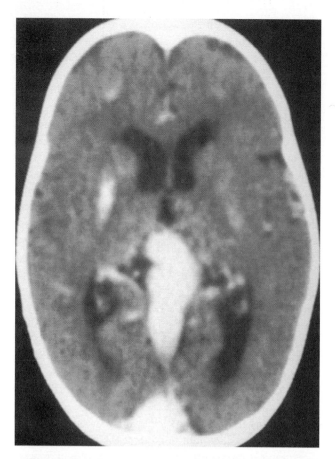

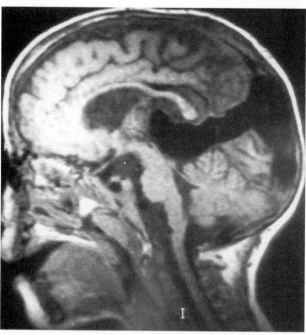

Fig. 15.3. Arteriovenous aneurysm of the vein of Galen. *(Top)* CT scan shows large venous drainage channel and abnormal veins draining the malformation. Note calcification of central grey matter indicative of hypoxia resulting from vascular steal through the malformation. *(Bottom)* T₁-weighted MRI, median sagittal cut showing marked dilatation of the ampulla of Galen draining into the sagittal sinus through an abnormal ascending venous trunk. Note 'void' appearance, indicating high flow within the venous channel, and moderate external hydrocephalus. (Courtesy Prof. F. Brunelle, Hôpital des Enfants Malades, Paris.)

system and parenchyma. MRI is useful for determining the exact topography, especially of venous drainage channels.

Treatment starts with anticongestive, cardiotonic drugs. Lasjaunias *et al.* (1989a) and Rodesch *et al.* (1994) prefer to defer attempts at curative treatment until the cardiac situation is stable, usually between 2 and 6 months of age. Reduction in the flow through the fistula is best performed. by interventional radiological techniques (Edwards *et al.* 1988, Hoffman 1989, Lasjaunias *et al.* 1991a). The best results are obtained in mural fistulae but embolization of other forms is sometimes possible. Garcia-Monaco *et al.* (1991a) reported complete exclusion of the malformation in 18 of 43 patients, and 13 of these were developmentally normal or only mildly retarded. Early shunting of hydrocephalus may be associated with subependymal haemorrhage or increased ventricular dilatation and should probably be deferred until after treatment of the malformation (Lasjaunias *et al.* 1989a). Surgical attack by transtentorial (Hoffman 1989) or other approaches can be used in older patients but is not indicated in most cases.

CAVERNOUS ANGIOMA

In cavernous angiomas of the brain, abnormal dilated blood vessels are clustered together so tightly that they are not separated by neural tissue. The vessels composing these lesions are usually but not always thin-walled and capacious. They are often calcified and contain haemosiderin deposits lying within the connective tissue that separates the vessels. They form well-limited masses in the parenchyma but may have a subarachnoid component (Rorke 1989, Weber *et al.* 1989).

The most common manifestation of cavernous angiomas is epilepsy, present in two-thirds of cases (Kattapong *et al.* 1995). Seizures may appear at any age from infancy to adulthood. The seizures are partial in type and are often difficult to control. Focal motor deficits, sometimes fluctuating, are a less common manifestation (Savoiardo *et al.* 1983, Simard *et al.* 1986, Vaquero *et al.* 1987, Requena *et al.* 1991). They are probably related to episodes of minor bleeding. Major bleeding is less common (Frima-Verhoeven *et al.* 1989). Headache and psychiatric manifestations are relatively common. Cavernous angiomas involve the brainstem in 15 per cent of cases (Zimmerman *et al.* 1991, Kattapong *et al.* 1995).

CT scan often shows small areas of calcification in about half the cases combined with changes in density varying from oedematous to haematoma-like. Enhancement may be only moderate and patchy. The MRI features of cavernous malformations are distinctive (Farmer *et al.* 1988, Zimmerman *et al.* 1991) and consist of well-defined lesions with a central focus of mixed signal intensity surrounded by a rim of void signal due to the paramagnetic effect of haemosiderin which becomes more evident on T₂-weighted images because of its long relaxation time (Fig. 15.4). Angiography is normal in most cases or reveals an avascular mass, and cavernous angiomas are the most common type of angiographically cryptic malformations (Becker *et al.* 1979).

Cavernous angiomas are not uncommonly multiple and can involve any area including the brainstem and cerebellum (Farmer

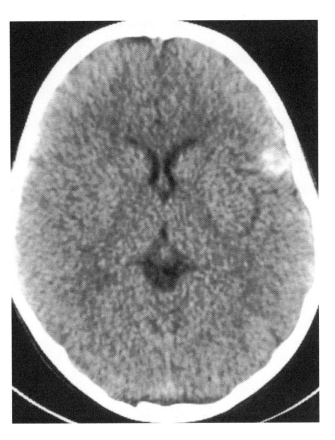

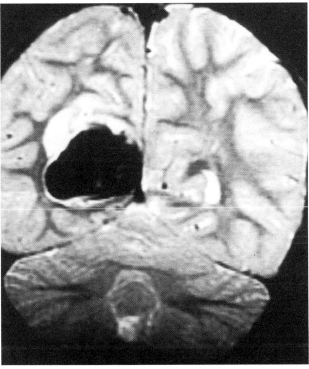

et al. 1988). Appearance of new lesions has been observed in some cases and the disorder may well be progressive (Kattapong *et al.* 1995). However, a more benign prognosis has been suggested (Churchyard *et al.* 1992). Multiple cutaneous and cavernous angiomas in infants may be part of a syndrome of neonatal miliary haemangiomatosis (Heudes *et al.* 1990) which includes CNS involvement in 30 per cent of cases.

Cavernous haemangiomas have a significant familial incidence especially when multiple lesions are present (Dobyns *et al.* 1987, Mason *et al.* 1988, Rigamonti *et al.* 1988). When families are investigated systematically with MRI, a dominant transmission is apparent (Steichen-Gersdorf *et al.* 1992) with almost complete penetrance. A gene, mapping to chromosome 7q, seems to be responsible (Dubovsky *et al.* 1995). Cavernomas may be a part of genetic syndromes featuring hepatic and retinal cavernous haemangiomas or limb reduction defects (Filling-Katz *et al.* 1992, Drigo *et al.* 1994) in addition to cerebral lesions.

The natural history of these lesions is poorly defined. Cavernous angiomas may enlarge (Farmer *et al.* 1988) and clinically they may mimic a tumour (Savoiardo *et al.* 1983). Operative treatment is recommended in patients with epilepsy and progressive focal deficit, provided the lesion is accessible, and gives excellent results. Fine-beam radiotherapy has also been used (Lance and Smee 1989). The attitude when facing a silent lesion is still uncertain, and surgery to eliminate the risk of massive haemorrhage is controversial for deep lesions (Mohr 1984, Tagle *et al.* 1986).

TELANGIECTASIAS
Capillary telangiectasias, like cavernous angiomas, consist of endothelium-lined sinusoidal channels of various sizes. They differ from cavernous angiomas by the absence of haemosiderin staining and the presence of normal intervening neural tissue (McCormick and Nofzinger 1966). They are predominantly located in the posterior fossa, especially the pons and medulla, less commonly the cerebellum (McCormick 1984). Both types of lesion sometimes occur together in the same patient so they may represent the same basic malformation at different evolutionary stages. Telangiectasias represent another type of cryptic vascular malformation. They may rarely rupture producing intracranial haematoma or subarachnoid haemorrhage (Howard 1986), especially in the brainstem and cerebellum (Erenberg *et al.* 1972, Bland *et al.* 1994).

VENOUS ANGIOMAS
These malformations have no arterial component. They consist of a radiating array of enlarged subcortical or periventricular veins that drain centripetally into a dilated venous trunk (Olson *et al.* 1984) (Fig. 15.5). These lesions constitute abnormalities of venous development and are better termed venous pseudoangiomas (Lasjaunias *et al.* 1991b). Venous angiomas are the most common of all intracranial vascular malformations. Sarwar and McCormick (1978) found they constituted 63 per cent of 165 vascular malformations in a study of 4069 consecutive autopsies. Garner *et al.* (1991) found 50 venous angiomas, 33 cavernomas

Fig. 15.4. *(Top)* Cavernous angioma in 6-year-old girl with right-sided focal motor seizures. Calcified lesion visible on unenhanced CT scan. There was minimal enhancement after contrast injection. (Courtesy Prof. F. Brunelle, Hôpital des Enfants Malades, Paris.)

(Bottom) Characteristic MR image of central low signal surrounded by a ring of high T_2-signal corresponding to haemosiderin deposited around the angioma by small haemorrhages. (Courtesy Dr Kling Chong, Great Ormond Street Hospital, London.)

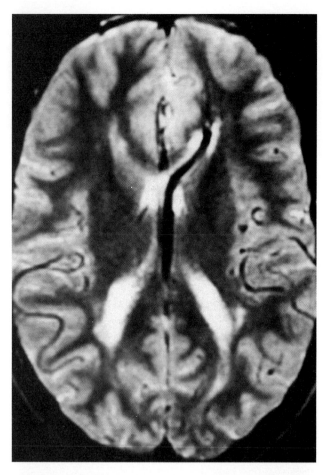

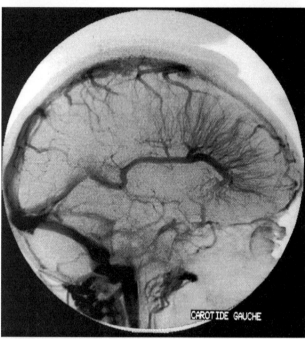

Fig. 15.5. So-called venous angioma of the left frontal region. *(Top)* MRI scan shows a large vessel, as indicated by a 'void' signal, running from the left frontal horn to the midline and back to the region of the vein of Galen. *(Bottom)* Digitalized angiography shows the vessel to be a large vein emptying into the vein of Galen. Veins from the anterior left frontal lobe drain into the abnormal venous trunk instead of the sagittal sinus. This represents abnormal venous drainage rather than an angioma.

and 17 AVMs in an MRI study of 8200 subjects. They are mainly located to the cerebellum and the frontal lobe. They rarely cause bleeding (Saito and Kobayashi 1981) unless they are associated with a cavernous angioma or there is venous obstruction in their drainage system. Migraine-like headache is not uncommon, except, perhaps, when the lesion is located in the posterior fossa (Rothfus *et al.* 1984). The MRI appearance is highly suggestive with images of radiating vessels usually draining into an enlarged venous channel. They are frequently discovered incidentally, and surgical excision should be considered only for those venous malformations from which bleeding has occurred (Martin and Edwards 1989).

RARE CONGENITAL ANGIODYSPLASIAS
Multiple angiomas of the CNS infrequently accompany multiple peripheral and visceral angiomas (Holden and Alexander 1970). They may be complicated by heart failure, hydrocephalus or meningitis. They can be transmitted as a dominant trait (Leblanc *et al.* 1996).

In *diffuse meningocerebral angiodysplasia* the whole cerebral surface is covered by densely packed, dilated, tortuous vessels (Jellinger *et al.* 1966). The relationship of such cases with Sturge–Weber disease on the one hand and with the diffuse cerebromeningeal noncalcifying angiomatosis of Divry and van Bogaert (Arseni *et al.* 1973) is unclear.

A diffuse vascular dysplasia may be responsible for the cases of leukodystrophy with cyst formation recently reported by Labrune *et al.* (1996).

INTRACRANIAL ARTERIAL ANEURYSMS
Aneurysms are dilated segments of an artery with thinned walls. Most cerebral aneurysms occur at the crotch of arterial bifurcations. They arise, probably at the site of congenital structural defects in the arterial wall, as a result of multiple factors (haemodynamic, ageing, hypertension). The frequency of aneurysms in childhood is much lower than that of AVMs but they have a greater tendency to rupture so that in one series they were responsible for 40 per cent of spontaneous intracranial haemorrhage before age 20 years (Sedzimir and Robinson 1973) though rarely in prepubertal patients. A defect of collagen III may be an aetiological factor in some cases (Pope *et al.* 1981, Neil-Dwyer *et al.* 1983) but was not found to be a common cause in two large series (Kuivaniemi *et al.* 1993, Schievink *et al.* 1994a). Acquired factors, particularly arterial hypertension, play a role in their genesis and rupture, as shown by their occurrence in patients with coarctation of the aorta and other causes of hypertension (Freedom 1989). Aneurysms may be familial in 8 per cent of cases (Norrgård *et al.* 1987, Schievink *et al.* 1995, Wang *et al.* 1995). Aneurysms are present in 10 per cent of patients with polycystic kidney disease (Proesmans *et al.* 1982, Chapman *et al.* 1992, Gabow 1993). Association with Marfan syndrome and with multiple malformations has been reported (Ter Berg *et al.* 1986, 1987). Aneurysms may follow a closed head injury or surgical operation; traumatic aneurysms represent 14–39 per cent of paediatric aneurysms (Ventureyra and Higgins 1994).

In children and adolescents, aneurysms are most commonly located at the bifurcation of the internal carotid artery (Finney *et al.* 1976, Heiskanen and Vilkki 1981, Humphreys 1989b) but are frequently found in unusual locations, often more distally than in adults (Amacher and Drake 1975). Giant aneurysms are present in 75 per cent of cases (Heiskanen and Vilkki 1981, Yu *et al.* 1982, Zee *et al.* 1986), and the saccular type is less frequent than in adults. Meyer *et al.* (1989) found that 10 of 24 aneurysms in children and adolescents were in the vertebrobasilar circulation and that 13 were of the giant type.

Haemorrhagic stroke is the presenting manifestation in three-quarters of the cases and may occur as early as 5 months of age. It may be preceded by premonitory symptoms such as severe focal headache, meningeal signs, transient neurological deficits or cranial nerve palsies. Such pseudotumoural features were present in almost half the cases of Meyer *et al.* (1989). Seizures may also be the first clinical manifestation of aneurysms (Gerosa *et al.* 1980). Complex partial seizures (Tanaka *et al.* 1994) are common. All children suspected of intracranial haemorrhage should undergo a CT or MRI scan. This will localize the aneurysm in many cases and may demonstrate the presence of muliple lesions, while four-vessel angiography will inform the surgeon of the status of collateral circulation and of the circle of Willis.

Prenatal diagnosis of basilar artery aneurysm by ultrasound examination has been reported (Muszynski *et al.* 1994).

Treatment is usually by surgery. Some cases may benefit from embolization or unusual techniques such as wrapping.

The mortality rate of bleeding aneurysms is of the order of 25 per cent, and residual neurological disability is not rare (Humphreys 1989b). Results of elective surgery are quite favourable. Operation at the time of bleeding is much more hazardous because of the possibility of vascular spasm, and the best timing of surgery remains disputed (Heros *et al.* 1983, H.P. Adams *et al.* 1988).

Mycotic aneurysms are a classic complication of bacterial endocarditis. They can result from local invasion of intracranial vessels by adjacent infections, especially septic cavernous thrombophlebitis (Rout *et al.* 1984, Andrews *et al.* 1989). The most frequent aetiologic agent is *Staphylococcus aureus* (Abbassioun *et al.* 1985). Fungal infections are a rare cause (Ahuja *et al.* 1978). The cornerstone of treatment of mycotic aneurysms is the prolonged administration of antimicrobial drugs. Surgical therapy is controversial.

Fusiform aneurysms, also termed giant serpentine aneurysms (Segal and McLaurin 1977) or dolichoectasic cranial arteries (Nishizaki *et al.* 1986, Gautier *et al.* 1988), are a common form of giant aneurysm. Common sites of dolichoectasia include the bifurcation of the internal carotid artery and the vertebrobasilar artery that may be affected in as many as 53 per cent of cases (Peerless *et al.* 1989). Bleeding occurs in over one-third of cases but focal neurological deficits, sometimes fluctuating, or thrombosis are the most frequent manifestation and a significant proportion are asymptomatic. Surgical treatment for selected cases can give favourable results (Chang *et al.* 1986).

SPINAL VASCULAR MALFORMATIONS

The most common vascular malformations occurring in relation with the spinal cord are the AVMs. Telangiectasias, cavernous malformations and aneurysms are very rare. Spinal AVMs are uncommon in children but may be seen even in infants (Binder *et al.* 1982, Aminoff and Edwards 1989).

Clinical manifestations include subarachnoid haemorrhage, myelopathy and radiculopathy (El Mahdi *et al.* 1989). Symptoms may appear suddenly and may fluctuate with exercise, posture and temperature. Local pain is an important diagnostic cue in patients with subarachnoid haemorrhage, and in unexplained cases it is important to explore the cord. Cutaneous angioma is sometimes associated (Baraitser and Schieff 1990). The diagnosis rests on specialized neuroradiological explorations (Gueguen *et al.* 1987, Koenig *et al.* 1989). Treatment is by surgery or embolization. The outcome depends on the site and type of the lesions.

Acute or subacute myelopathy with ascending necrosis of the spinal cord (subacute necrotizing myelitis or Foix–Alajouanine syndrome) is actually the result of thrombosis and venous hypertension in patients with dural arteriovenous fistulae (Criscuolo *et al.* 1989, Hurst *et al.* 1995).

'SPONTANEOUS' SUBARACHNOID AND OTHER INTRACRANIAL HAEMORRHAGES

Not all cases of subarachnoid haemorrhage are explained by detectable vascular malformations. In one series, no lesion was found in as many as 31 per cent of cases (Hourihan *et al.* 1984). Whatever the aetiology, subarachnoid haemorrhage may interfere with vascularization of the brain, although this is mainly observed in cases of malformations and is uncommon in 'spontaneous' subarachnoid haemorrhage (Spetzler and Selman 1984).

'Spontaneous' intracranial haematomas are probably caused by small vascular malformations that are destroyed or collapsed by the haemorrhage they induced. It is therefore essential in cases of apparently spontaneous subarachnoid haemorrhage or haematoma to repeat angiography (or imaging) some time after the acute episode as a causal AVM may then have become detectable.

Such haematomas mainly affect the cerebral hemispheres but they occasionally occur in the cerebellum or brainstem. In the latter case, the clinical picture may simulate multiple sclerosis although a rapidly fatal course is more usual.

Intracranial haematomas show a variable appearance on MRI at various times because the methaemoglobin they contain is in different phases of chemical breakdown (Gomori *et al.* 1988). In 321 patients younger than 20 years reviewed by Sedzimir and Robinson (1973) the recurrence rate was 41 per cent and the mortality rate 28 per cent.

Repeated bleeding in the subarachnoid space can cause superficial haemosiderosis which is rare in children (Zwarts *et al.* 1988, Fearnley *et al.* 1995). Progressive neurological impairment is associated with repeatedly xanthochromic CSF. High-field MRI may show marginal zones of hypointensity (Gomori *et al.* 1985). Recurrent haemorrhage can be the result of a bleeding spinal haemangioma (Naranjo *et al.* 1987) which should be sought when no cranial lesion is found.

OTHER VASCULAR ANOMALIES

Variants of intracranial vessels are found in 15 per cent of MRA studies (Koelfen *et al.* 1995). Congenital absence of one (Afifi *et al.* 1987) or both carotid arteries (Teal *et al.* 1980, Schlenska 1986) is usually unaccompanied by clinical manifestations and this also applies to absence or hypoplasia of the vertebral arteries. Other abnormalities of the carotid artery such as cervical stenosis or buckling have been implicated as causal factors of acute acquired hemiplegia. However, such abnormalities are mostly coincidental findings. Various anomalies of the circle of Willis, such as direct origin of the posterior cerebral artery from the carotid artery, are not rare (Koelfen *et al.* 1995). Abnormalities of cervical or intracranial arteries may be associated with abnormalities of the aorta and other systemic vessels, facial angioma and cerebellar hypoplasia (Pascual-Castroviejo 1985, Goh and Lo 1993). Persistence of anastomotic arteries at the base of the brain, such as the trigeminal, acoustic and hypoglossal arteries, may occur as normal variants (Stern *et al.* 1978, Resche *et al.* 1980). Their association with saccular aneurysm or spontaneous subarachnoid haemorrhage has been reported (Waga *et al.* 1978) but may be coincidental.

Vascular steal from the CNS as a result of the stenosis of a subclavian artery (Borushok *et al.* 1974) is a rare occurrence. The same phenomenon may be observed following Blalock–Taussig type anastomoses (Kurlan *et al.* 1984).

Abnormalities of the veins or sinuses resulting in increased sinusal pressure and consequent hydrocephalus are rare. Affected children may have extensive collateral circulation. Angiography can show stenosis or absence of segments of sinuses, and reflux into veins after contrast injection into the sagittal sinus is prominent. Treatment by venous bypass graft from the transverse sinus to the jugular vein has been shown to control hydrocephalus (Sainte-Rose *et al.* 1984).

NEUROCUTANEOUS SYNDROMES WITH PROMINENT VASCULAR ANOMALIES

Several syndromes are characterized by the association of cutaneous abnormalities and vascular malformations of the CNS (see also Chapter 4).

STURGE–WEBER SYNDROME

Sturge–Weber syndrome is by far the most important of the disorders of this group. In its complete form it consists of a venous angioma of the leptomeninges, ipsilateral flat facial angiomatous naevus ('port-wine stain') (Fig. 15.6) and choroidal angioma. An identical pial angioma may be present in isolation or in association with choroidal angioma without facial naevus in up to 13 per cent of cases (Gomez and Bebin 1987; Roach 1992; Pascual-Castroviejo *et al.* 1993, 1995a). Such cases, for all practical purposes, should be regarded as belonging to the same syndrome. On the other hand, cases of facial naevus without CNS involvement with or without glaucoma are common (Roach 1992). The naevus flammeus almost always lies above the level of the palpebral fissure (Alexander 1972, Enjolras *et al.* 1985)

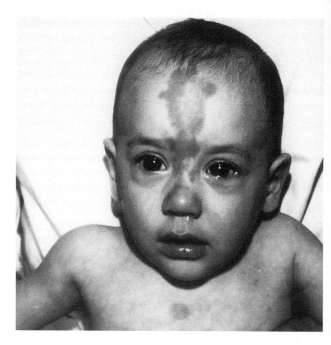

Fig. 15.6. 'Port wine' naevus in 17-month-old girl with Sturge–Weber syndrome. This girl had right-sided pial angioma with left-sided partial motor seizures as well as episodes of hemiplegia unassociated with convulsive seizures. CT scan showed cortical enhancement following a convulsive episode, which had disappeared on repeat CT scan three weeks later. The midline location of the naevus is unusual.

involving the upper eyelid or frontal region or both. Frontal lesions close to the midline are more commonly associated with anteriorly located pial lesions and more external frontal involvement with the more frequent occipitoparietal angiomas, but the correlation between the extent and location of the naevus and that of the pial angioma is poor. In a survey of 310 patients, Tallman *et al.* (1991) found neurological or ophthalmological involvement in 6 per cent of those with unilateral and 24 per cent of those with bilateral naevi in the territory of the first two divisions of the trigeminal nerve (only three patients had isolated involvement of the second division). These figures are likely to be underestimates as no imaging was performed. Sujansky and Conradi (1995) computed a frequency of between 8 and 33 per cent from a review of the literature. Some children have bilateral naevi with unilateral pial involvement (Gomez and Bebin 1987). Bilateral meningeal angiomas may coexist with either unilateral or bilateral facial naevi (Boltshauser *et al.* 1976). Pascual-Castroviejo *et al.* (1993) found 13 such cases in their 40 patients. In only three of these was the CNS angioma bilateral. Angiomas not uncommonly may extend beyond the face and involve the neck, trunk or limbs on one or both sides.

The intracranial angioma is limited to the pia mater that contains dilated and tortuous venules that may form several layers in the subarachnoid space but rarely enter the brain. The calcifications lie in the cortex underlying the angioma and subcortical white matter, tending to appear deeply at first and then extend toward the surface (Norman and Schoene 1977). Localized or unilateral brain atrophy is virtually constant. In one severe case, four-layer microgyria was found underlying the angioma, indicating a prenatal origin of cortical damage (Simonati *et al.* 1994).

Seizures are the major neurological manifestation of Sturge–Weber syndrome, occurring in 75–90 per cent of patients (Gilly *et al.* 1977, Gomez and Bebin 1987, Sujansky and Conradi 1995). They usually have their onset in the first months of life. They are generally partial motor in type and are often prolonged in episodes of status epilepticus. Generalized seizures and even myoclonic and atonic seizures or infantile spasms can occur (Chevrie *et al.* 1988, Arzimanoglou and Aicardi 1992). Many patients have frequent and repeated seizures (Oakes 1992) but some children have only an occasional fit, and approximately half the patients in one series responded well to drug therapy (Arzimanoglou and Aicardi 1992).

Hemiplegia occurs in at least one-third of cases and is localized to the side opposite the facial naevus except in a very few patients who probably have bilateral disease (Terdjman *et al.* 1990). Hemiplegia commonly first appears after an episode of seizures and may become more severe with the recurrence of fits. Hemianopia is virtually constant, isolated or in association with hemiparesis.

Transient hemiplegias not following an epileptic attack and sometimes accompanied by migraine-like headache are observed in many cases of Sturge–Weber syndrome (Gilly *et al.* 1977, Arzimanoglou and Aicardi 1992). These hemiplegic episodes are apparently not of epileptic nature and may be a consequence of vasomotor disturbances within and around the angioma (Terdjman *et al.* 1990).

Mental subnormality is present in about 40 per cent of the patients and in 75 per cent of those with seizures. It does not occur in patients without epilepsy and is more common and more severe in bilateral forms (Gomez and Bebin 1987, Sujansky and Conradi 1995). In many cases, there appears to be a definite regression of mental abilities parallel to the repetition and severity of the seizures.

Intracranial haemorrhage is not a feature of the Sturge–Weber syndrome. However, elevated spinal fluid protein is commonly found (Skoglund *et al.* 1978) and may correspond to minimal bleeding from the angioma. This interpretation is also consistent with the occasional occurrence of hydrocephalus (Fishman and Baram 1986, Diebler and Dulac 1987) as observed also in a personal case. Macrocephaly not due to hydrocephalus has also been reported.

Glaucoma is present in 30–48 per cent of Sturge–Weber patients (Sujansky and Conradi 1995) and 50 per cent of them have choroidal angioma that may sometimes be visible with the ophthalmoscope. The glaucoma may be the consequence of overproduction of aqueous fluid by the choroidal angioma or else exudate from the lesion may block the angle.

The *clinical diagnosis* of Sturge–Weber syndrome is usually straightforward. However, in mild cases and in very young infants it may be difficult to know whether a pial angioma is associated with a facial naevus that has been present from birth. EEG may be of value by showing reduced background amplitude or

paroxysmal abnormalities or both on the involved side, although this may be a late sign (Brenner and Sharbrough 1976). Generalized bisynchronous discharges can be present in patients with unilateral pial lesions (Chevrie *et al.* 1988).

Plain skull X-rays show the classical tram-like calcification most frequently in the parieto-occipital area. Although this has been occasionally detected in the neonatal period (Nellhaus *et al.* 1967), calcification on plain X-ray is often a late sign and may be absent even in adolescents. Angiography does not show the angioma but demonstrates lack of superficial cortical veins, non-filling of dural sinuses, and abnormal, tortuous veins that course toward the ventricle and vein of Galen system (Probst 1980).

CT scan is a much more powerful tool for the detection of calcium and can often show its presence in infants of only a few months of age or even in neonates. CT also clearly demonstrates atrophy of the brain, enlargement of the choroid plexus on the side of the pial angioma and abnormal veins draining into the deep venous circulation (Welch *et al.* 1980, Terdjman *et al.* 1990) (Fig. 15.7). Enhancement seen on CT scan does not represent opacification of the pial angioma but rather cortical injection similar to that occurring in postconvulsive hemiplegia, and it may disappear and reappear with the occurrence of seizures (Terdjman *et al.* 1990).

MRI does not show calcification well. With gadolinium enhancement, the pial angioma can be clearly made out (Elster and Chen 1990, Lipski *et al.* 1990, Sperner *et al.* 1990, Benedikt *et al.* 1993, Vogl *et al.* 1993). This may permit a preclinical diagnosis of the Sturge–Weber syndrome in patients with an apparently isolated facial naevus and indicate the extent of the angioma and the presence or absence of contralateral involvement (Fig. 15.8). Special techniques of 3D MRA may show a blush at the site of the angioma, and MRI may demonstrate advanced myelination at this locus.

Examination with PET or SPECT shows hypometabolism or marked underperfusion in the area of the pial angioma and may help to detect latent angioma (Chiron *et al.* 1989, Chugani *et al.* 1989).

The *differential diagnosis* includes other causes of cortical calcification and atrophy. The syndrome of cortical calcification, epilepsy and coeliac disease (Gobbi *et al.* 1988) may produce unilateral images, and vascular abnormalities in the form of foci of angiomatous venous dilatation were found in one case (Bye *et al.* 1993). Such foci were not found in another pathological case (Toti *et al.* 1996). There is usually no detectable atrophy associated with the calcification and no abnormalities of the veins or choroid plexus, but hypodensity of the white matter is often seen in the vicinity of calcified areas.

The neurological defects seen in the Sturge–Weber syndrome are probably the consequence of blood stagnation, hypoxaemia and impaired neuronal metabolism. The hypoxaemic effects are exaggerated by the increased metabolic rate resulting from epileptic seizures and probably also by vasomotor changes and thrombotic phenomena that take place in and about the pial lesion. Such a mechanism may explain the progressive aggravation of damage all too often observed in these patients. It would also

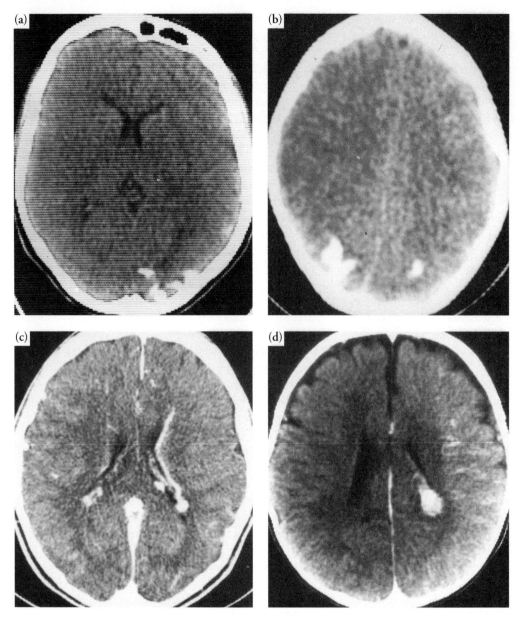

Fig. 15.7. Sturge–Weber syndrome: CT scans of four different patients. *(a)* Typical occipital calcification. *(b)* Bilateral calcification in a patient with a purely right-sided naevus. *(c)* Abnormal venous drainage along ventricular angle. *(d)* Enlarged choroid plexus and left parieto-occipital cortical enhancement a few days after an episode of status epilepticus. Enhancement had disappeared on repeat CT one month later.

account for the beneficial effect of early surgery, preventing this cascade of ill-effects.

A common embryological origin from the neural crest of the vascular bed of the leptomeninges and optic cup probably explains the Sturge–Weber association (Norman and Schoene 1977). The disease is sporadic and only a few, doubtful, familial cases are on record.

The natural course of Sturge–Weber syndrome depends on the presence, persistence and resistance to treatment of the seizures (Oakes 1992, Niijima *et al.* 1994). Onset of seizures before 1 year of age, a hypsarrhythmic EEG pattern, and the occurrence of episodes of status predict an unfavourable spontaneous outcome.

Treatment of patients with the Sturge–Weber syndrome is mainly directed against the seizures and an aggressive antiepileptic regimen should be established from the first seizure. Control can be obtained in about half the patients even in those with early-onset seizures (Arzimanoglou and Aicardi 1992). Arrest of status epilepticus (Chapter 16) is of utmost importance, as hemiplegia is often postconvulsive. In uncontrollable cases, especially in infants, occipital or parietal lobectomy or complete or functional hemispherectomy could render the patient seizure-free and probably prevent mental deterioration (Hoffman *et al.* 1979). Operation is indicated for uncontrollable seizures and, for hemispherectomy, only when fine hand movements are absent (Roach *et al.* 1994). Rappaport (1988) proposed callosotomy as

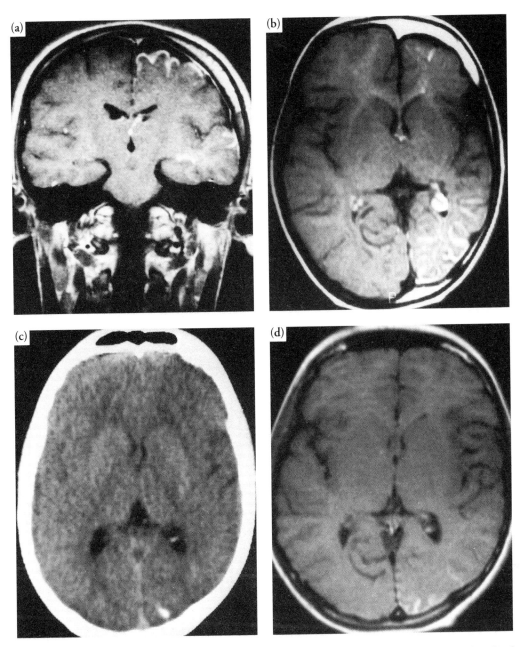

Fig. 15.8. Sturge–Weber syndrome. *(a)* Left-sided pial angioma involving the frontal and temporal lobe is clearly outlined following gadolinium enhancement in 6-year-old girl with left-sided facial angioma. *(b)* Left occipito-temporal angioma: gadolinium enhanced MRI. Note considerable atrophy of the whole hemisphere, angioma of the left choroid plexus glomus and marked increase in skull thickness. *(c)* CT scan of 14-year-old boy who suffered two attacks, at 20 and 26 months of age, of right focal motor seizures associated with headache and vomiting. The small left occipital calcification had not been present on CT scans performed at 26 and 48 months. *(d)* T$_1$-weighted MRI after gadolinium injection shows small pial angioma over the occipital pole. This is isolated pial angiomatosis as the child had no facial angioma.

an alternative to hemispherectomy. Local treatment of the port-wine stain is psychologically important and good results have been obtained with pulsed dye laser (Goldman *et al.* 1993).

SYNDROMES RELATED TO THE STURGE–WEBER SYNDROME
SYNDROME OF MACROCRANIA, FACIAL NAEVI AND ANOMALOUS VENOUS RETURN
In some cases of the Sturge–Weber syndrome, a macrocephaly can be present and may be related to hydrocephalus (Fishman and Baram 1986). This has been attributed to abnormal venous drainage with resulting intracranial hypertension. A *syndrome of bilateral facial naevi, macrocrania and anomalous venous return* through superficial veins (Shapiro and Shulman 1976, Orr *et al.* 1978) is probably different from the Sturge–Weber syndrome.

Children with *epilepsy and bilateral occipital calcification* may have an incomplete form of the Sturge–Weber syndrome.

TABLE 15.1

Neurocutaneous syndromes with prominent vascular components

Syndrome	Clinical features	Heredity*	References
Blue rubber bleb naevus syndrome	Subcutaneous and mucous angiomas. Gastrointestinal bleeding. Rare cases of multiple cavernous angiomas of the CNS	S or AD	Waybright et al. (1978), Satya-Murti et al. (1986), Moodley and Ramdial (1993)
Rendu–Osler–Weber disease	See text	AD	See text
Wyburn–Mason syndrome (Dechaume–Blanc–Bonnet syndrome)	Retinal arteriovenous angioma. Unilateral arteriovenous malformation extending from the retina along the visual pathways to cerebral peduncles and sometimes ipsilateral cerebellar hemisphere. Rupture frequent. Occasional facial (periorbital) involvement	S	Theron et al. (1974), Gomez (1994)
Klippel–Trenaunay syndrome	See text	S	See text
Cobb syndrome (cutaneomeningospinal angiomatosis)	Cutaneous flat angioma and myelopathy due to spinal cord angioma	Probably S	Baraitser and Shieff (1990)
Shapiro–Shulman syndrome	Bilateral facial naevi and abnormal venous drainage of the brain	Probably S	Shapiro and Shulman (1976)
Divry–van Bogaert syndrome	Noncalcifying leptomeningeal angioma with diffuse brain sclerosis, progressive neurological impairment and livedo reticularis	AR	Bussone et al. (1984)
Bannayan–Zonana syndrome	Macrocephaly, lipomatosis and cutaneous haemangiomas	AD	Higginbottom and Schulz (1982)
Familiar cavernous malformations of CNS and retina (Gass syndrome)	Cavernous angiomas of the brain, multiple in 50% of cases, retinal angiomas, occasional cutaneous involvement	AD	Dobyns et al. (1987)
Hereditary neurocutaneous angiomatosis	Cavernous angiomas of skin, cerebral or cerebellar arteriovenous malformations	AD	Zaremba et al. (1979), Leblanc et al. (1996)
Sneddon syndrome	Cutis marmorata associated with vascular occlusive disease that may affect the brain	AR?	Bruyn et al. (1987), Pettee et al. (1994), Lossos et al. (1995)
Cutis marmorata telangiectatica	Peculiar aspect of skin, various associations with hemihypertrophy, arterial occlusion	Probably S	Picascia and Esterly (1989), Baxter et al. (1993)
Riley–Smith syndrome	Macrocephaly, pseudopapilloedema and peripheral hemangiomas	AD	Hoover et al. (1989)

*AD = autosomal dominant; AR = autosomal recessive; S = sporadic.

However, Gobbi et al. (1988) have described a distinctive syndrome of occipital epilepsy with calcification different from that of the Sturge–Weber syndrome and sometimes associated with progressive mental and epileptic deterioration (Chapter 23). This syndrome may not be homogenous (Masson et al. 1988).

Several cases of *cyst of the posterior fossa with partial cerebellar agenesis in association with facial angiomas* have been reported (Mizuno et al. 1982, Hirsch et al. 1984, Reese et al. 1993). The angioma is variably flat or tuberous and lies in the territory of the first division of the trigeminal nerve. Some of these cases have been familial (Bordarier and Aicardi 1990). Pascual-Castroviejo (1985) and Goh and Lo (1993) have emphasized that the association of facial angioma—usually of capillary type and located, at least in part, in the territory of the first branch of the Vth cranial nerve—with diverse embryological abnormalities of the aortic arch and of extracranial and intracranial vessels, and with a variable degree of uni- or bilateral cerebellar hypoplasia, sometimes with a Dandy–Walker topography or with cortical dysplasia (Pascual-Castroviejo et al. 1995b), constitutes a distinct syndrome of vascular dysplasia. This syndrome predominates in girls and may be related to facial hemiatrophy and to the velocardiofacial syndrome (Strenge et al. 1996).

KLIPPEL–TRENAUNAY AND RELATED SYNDROMES
This unusual syndrome consists of angiomatous skin naevus, hypertrophy that is usually predominant in one limb or one side of the body but commonly involves both sides, and the presence of lymphangiomas or varicosities. The cutaneous naevus may be capillary or cavernous and often has irregular limits. It may be associated with verrucous or pigmentary naevi. It does not necessarily coincide with the hypertrophic territory. The lower limbs are usually more affected than the upper ones. Active arteriovenous fistulae may be present and require surgical treatment. The hypertrophy may be limited to one segment or involve a whole side including the trunk and face (Stickler 1987). Disproportionate enlargement of one or several digits may be present. Macrocephaly is common. Mental retardation sometimes occurs in patients with involvement of the head and face. Vascular abnormalities may be present in the brain (Oyesiku et al. 1988). Cerebral angiography and MRA demonstrate absence of deep venous drainage and dilatation of the superior petrosal and cavernous sinuses, and superior ophthalmic and facial veins, the route taken by venous blood when there is no jugular vein at the skull base (Gomez 1994). Hemimegalencephaly is frequent (Gomez 1994) and eye abnormalities are common. The disorder is

probably sporadic and only four familial cases have been reported out of almost 500 published cases. For patients with major involvement, various surgical techniques may bring about significant improvement.

Klippel–Trenaunay syndrome can be associated with Sturge–Weber syndrome (Williams and Elster 1992), although Gomez (1994) thinks the two conditions are different. Differentiation from the Proteus syndrome (Chapter 4) may pose a difficult problem.

RENDU–OSLER–WEBER SYNDROME
Hereditary haemorrhagic telangiectasia (Rendu–Osler–Weber syndrome) is a familial disorder, transmitted as an autosomal dominant trait, characterized by the presence of multiple dermal, mucosal and visceral telangiectasias associated with recurrent bleeding. Neurological involvement includes the complications of right-to-left shunt through pulmonary arteriovenous fistulae, *i.e.* brain abcess and thrombosis associated with polycythaemia, and the presence of vascular malformations of the brain such as angiomas, telangiectasias, aneurysms and arteriovenous fistulae (Román *et al.* 1978, Peery 1987, Porteous *et al.* 1992). Recurrent alternating hemiplegia has been reported (Myles *et al.* 1970).

The cutaneous lesions may be hard to discover and should be looked for carefully, especially when pulmonary arteriovenous fistulae are present.

VON HIPPEL–LINDAU DISEASE
The syndrome consists of the association of cerebellar or spinal haemangioma with retinal angioblastoma, cysts of the pancreas and renal carcinoma. The condition is transmitted as a dominant trait with a penetrance of 80–90 per cent. The gene has been mapped to chromosome 3p25–p26 and may act as a tumour suppressor gene (Latif *et al.* 1993).

The diagnosis is made in patients with more than one haemangioblastoma of the CNS or an isolated lesion in association with a visceral manifestation of the disease, or in patients with only one manifestation if there is a known family history (Huson *et al.* 1986). Neumann *et al.* (1992) found that 44 per cent of gene carriers had haemangioblastoma, multiple in 42 per cent, and 44 per cent of those with haemangioblastoma had retinal lesions. The retinal haemangioma has a characteristic appearance. About 20 per cent of patients with retinal angioma develop neurological complications, and 40 per cent of patients with cerebellar haemangioblastoma have von Hippel–Lindau disease (Huson *et al.* 1986). Polycythaemia is found in 10–20 per cent of patients with a cerebellar tumour. The disease manifests usually after 10 years of age by acute eye complications, *e.g.* haemorrhage, or by a posterior fossa syndrome. Pancreatic and renal cysts are asymptomatic and are detected by abdominal imaging in three-quarters of cases (Levine *et al.* 1982). Renal carcinomas and phaeochromocytomas (Atuk *et al.* 1979) should be detected early if conservative treatment is to be contemplated.

Patients and at-risk relatives should have annual ophthalmological assessment from 5 years of age, urinary vanillylmandelic acid (VMA) and noradrenaline estimation from 10 years, biennial brain imaging from 15 years and abdominal imaging from 20 years. The protocol should be extended to all patients presenting with cerebellar or retinal haemangioblastoma (Huson *et al.* 1986).

Treatment is purely surgical. The prognosis is dominated by the presence and size of tumours, both intracranial and intra-abdominal.

RARE NEUROCUTANEOUS SYNDROMES WITH PROMINENT VASCULAR COMPONENT
Neurocutaneous syndromes of which vascular abnormalities are an important part are listed in Table 15.1. Several of these are genetically determined. Cutaneous involvement may not be a major feature and neurological symptoms may be the presenting feature. In all cases of vascular abnormalities of the CNS it is important to make careful enquiries about possible other cases in the lineage. In cases with known genetic origin or where two cases of vascular malformation exist in the family, a thorough examination of all family members is in order. The exact nosological situation of several of these syndromes is unclear. The distinction between rare syndromes such as Riley–Smith, Bannayan–Zonana and Ruvalcaba–Myhre syndromes may well be artificial (Dvir *et al.* 1988). *Cutis marmorata telangiectatica* may be accompanied by neurological symptoms (Picascia and Esterly 1989, Pehr and Moroz 1993), and the occurrence of recurrent hemiplegias mimicking alternating hemiplegia has been reported (Baxter *et al.* 1993).

ARTERIAL OCCLUSIVE DISORDERS

MECHANISMS AND PATHOLOGY
Arterial occlusion can result from cerebral embolism or from thrombosis. Irrespective of the cause cerebral infarction results. When obstruction involves one of the larger cerebral arteries, infarction affects both the cortex and underlying white matter. In haemorrhagic infarction, the involved area is congested and stippled with petechial haemorrhages. In pale infarct, the tissue appears pale usually with a significant amount of swelling. In the centre of the infarcted region there is massive necrosis of all tissue components, while the damage becomes progressively less severe toward the periphery of the infarct. During the first hours of acute ischaemia, damage in this peripheral part (so-called 'penumbra') is reversible with reestablishment of blood flow. The area of penumbra is not shown by CT or standard MRI but gives a high signal with water-diffusion MRI technique. After a few hours polymorphonuclear infiltration is found, replaced within four or five days by mononuclear phagocytes. Eventually, astrocytes develop and lay down a fibre network with resulting retraction and sclerosis of cortical convolutions (ulegyria). The area of greatest damage may become cystic, leaving a cavity within the brain which is often improperly called 'porencephaly' (Chapter 3).

The vulnerability of the brain to even brief periods of ischaemia is well known. Swelling of brain tissue can increase the lesion by compressing capillaries, thus preventing revascularization from collateral sources, the 'no-reflow phenomenon' in

TABLE 15.2
Main syndromes of arterial occlusion

Artery involved	Area of ischaemia	Clinical features	References
Internal carotid artery (ICA)	Whole territory of MCA or only part of it. Rarely both territories of MCA and ACA	Hemiplegia, hemianopsia, aphasia if dominant hemisphere. Partial involvement with only incomplete hemiplegia is not rare	Meadows (1983)
Middle cerebral artery (MCA)	Convexity of hemispheres, except paramedial aspect and occipital lobe, insula, part of temporal lobe, internal capsule and basal ganglia, orbital aspect of frontal lobe	Hemiplegia with upper limb predominance. Hemianopsia. Aphasia if dominant hemisphere	Golden (1985), Van Dongen et al. (1985)
Anterior cerebral artery (ACA)	Mesial aspect of hemispheres. Paramedian part of their convexity. Anterior part of internal capsule and of basal ganglia	Hemiplegia predominating in lower limb	Golden (1985),
Anterior choroidal artery (AChA)	Optic tract, posterior limb of internal capsule, cerebral peduncle, pallidum, variable involvement of thalamus and caudate, lateral geniculate body	Hemiplegia, visual field defects, dysarthria, sometimes ataxia	Decroix et al. (1986), Helgason et al. (1986), Helgason (1988), Bogousslavsky et al. (1986)
Posterior cerebral artery (PCA)	Lower part of temporal lobe, posterior part of thalamus, subthalamic nuclei,	Homonymous hemianopia, ataxia, hemiparesis, vertigo, superior cerebellar peduncle, optic radiations, occipital lobe	Castaigne et al. (1973)
Basilar artery (BA)	Whole or part of PCA territory (uni- or bilateral). Brainstem nuclei and tracts. May involve cerebellar arteries	Variable manifestations—see text	Echenne et al. (1983)
Superior cerebellar artery (SCA)	Upper brainstem, superior cerebellar peduncles, dentate nucleus, upper cerebellar cortex	Vertigo, ataxia of limbs or trunk, tremor, pontine signs (cranial nerves VIII, VII, V)	Golden (1985)
Anterior inferior cerebellar artery (AICA)	Central brainstem, flocculus and adjacent part of cerebral hemisphere	Idem	Idem
Posterior inferior cerebellar artery (PICA) or vertebral artery and PICA	Roof nuclei of 4th ventricle, lateral medulla, lower aspect of cerebellum	Lateral medullary syndrome, vertigo, nystagmus, ipsilateral, ataxia, sensory loss, contralateral Horner syndrome	Barth et al. (1993), Gan and Noronha (1995)
Thalamostriate arteries and other penetrating branches	Caudate, putamen, internal capsule	Hemiplegia, motor sensory or mixed. No hemianopia. Language disturbances sometimes; possibility of bilateral signs	Kappelle et al. (1989), Garg and DeMyer (1995)
	Subcortical white matter of hemispheres or brainstem	Lacunar syndromes including: pure sensory or motor hemiplegia, ataxic hemiparesis*, mesencephalothalamic syndrome, abulia with IIIrd nerve palsy or paralysis of vertical gaze, crossed syndrome, locked-in syndrome, dementia	Kappelle et al. (1989), Katz et al. (1987) Moulin et al. (1995)

*Ataxic hemiplegia can also occur with mass lesions (Bendheim and Berg 1981). Responsible lesions typically are in the basis pontis but may also be in the internal capsule or in the corona radiata (Ichikawa et al. 1982, Helweg-Larsen et al. 1988).

which complex factors are implicated. In contrast with ischaemia within the infarcted territory, there is increased blood flow around the lesion, the so-called 'luxury perfusion' that is demonstrable by neuroimaging and brain scan. The role of lactic acid and of other abnormal metabolites in the sequence of events that lead to ischaemia and infarction has been extensively discussed (Plum 1983).

The causes of thrombosis or emboli are extremely variable (see below) but in many cases they remain undetermined.

CLINICAL AND RADIOLOGICAL FEATURES
In most cases the clinical features do not differ irrespective of whether the infarction results from thrombosis or embolism. In some cases, the aetiology or circumstances of occurrence suggest a particular mechanism. For example, the presence of bacterial endocarditis or valvular heart disease favours embolism, whereas a 'stuttering' onset of the clinical manifestations is more suggestive of thrombosis. A history of cervical trauma is suggestive of dissection of the carotid or vertebral arteries (Garg et al. 1993, Garg and DeMyer 1995). Essentially, occlusive vascular disease manifests itself by the sudden appearance of neurological deficit in the territory of one major cerebral vessel (Hilal et al. 1971a, Lanska et al. 1991). However, in the series of Abram et al. (1996), 23 per cent of idiopathic ischaemic strokes were preceded, usually

by about a week, by episodes of transient hemiplegia lasting from one to several hours. The anterior circulation is by far most commonly affected so that the typical picture of ischaemic stroke in children is that of *acute hemiplegia*, but cases of hemiplegia of vascular origin are distributed throughout childhood and adolescence whereas postconvulsive hemiplegias are concentrated in the first three years of life. Onset is at any age, most commonly before 6 years. Neonatal stroke is more common than previously thought, and onset is more often in the first month than at any other period; prenatal stroke is one of the possible causes of congenital hemiplegia (Lanska *et al.* 1991).

In one large series (Aicardi *et al.* 1969), 27 per cent of the cases of acquired hemiplegia in childhood were not preceded by convulsive seizures and most of these were thought to be due to vascular occlusions. Contrariwise, only occasional cases of demonstrated vascular occlusions are preceded by status epilepticus, although isolated fits may occur in up to 23 per cent of the cases of cerebral infarction in the territory of the middle cerebral artery (Gastaut *et al.* 1977) at onset of the hemiplegia. Fever may precede the onset of vascular hemiplegia although it is more common with postconvulsive cases. A search for prodromal features such as headache, cervical pain, ipsilateral Horner syndrome, and a history of transient ischaemic episodes preceding hemiplegia may help uncover particular causes such as dissection.

In all acquired hemiplegias, weakness is maximal immediately after onset and flaccidity is the rule (Isler 1984). Spasticity and pyramidal tract signs appear later. The degree of recovery is extremely variable. A substantial recovery can be expected to take place during the first two or three weeks and further slow progress may continue for several months. Involuntary movements of athetoid type or frank disturbances are rare. Dysphasia is present in right-sided hemiplegia when the cortex is affected. It has also been observed in some cases of infarcts restricted to the capsulo-putamino-caudate area (Ferro *et al.* 1982, Aram *et al.* 1983, Young *et al.* 1983, Dusser *et al.* 1986). The dysphasia tends to be mainly expressive in type in children under 8–10 years of age. In children younger than 5 years, aphasia is usually short-lived but patients tend to have learning difficulties later even though spoken language appears normal (Van Dongen *et al.* 1985). In fact, the presentation of aphasia in children is more variable than previously thought, and paraphasia and jargonaphasia may be observed (Cranberg *et al.* 1987). Fluent aphasia can be observed in children with posterior lesions.

The topography of the infarcts responsible for acquired hemiplegia is variable. Table 15.2 shows the arteries involved, the corresponding territories of infarction, and the main clinical features. However, the topography and extent of infarction depend on several factors in addition to the vessel involved, such as the quality of collateral and systemic circulation or individual anatomical variations. The location of infarct may also vary with the aetiology. Ischaemic strokes in the basal ganglia are more often idiopathic than superficial ones (Dusser *et al.* 1986, Kappelle *et al.* 1989).

Involvement of the posterior circulation is much rarer than that of the carotid arteries and their branches. Echenne *et al.*

(1983) reviewed 36 cases and only a few more cases have been added since. Many of the cases of vertebrobasilar occlusive diseases have been associated with trauma responsible for dissection (Katirji *et al.* 1985, Garg *et al.* 1993) which may also occur spontaneously (Sturzenegger 1995, Khurana *et al.* 1996), with cervical spine abnormalities (Singer *et al.* 1975, Ross *et al.* 1987, Phillips *et al.* 1988) or with vascular malformations (Randall *et al.* 1994), but all the causes of stroke can be found and idiopathic cases are frequent. More limited occlusions may affect only one cerebellar artery (Harbaugh *et al.* 1982, Chatkupt *et al.* 1987) with resulting cerebellar infarcts (Fig. 15.9). However, lateral medullary syndrome has been observed with vertebral artery thrombosis (Klein *et al.* 1976). Thalamic infarction may be due to proximal obstruction of one vertebral artery in the neck (Garg *et al.* 1993, Randall *et al.* 1994, Garg and DeMyer 1995, Garg and Edwards-Brown 1995). The clinical picture of vertebrobasilar occlusion includes vomiting, ataxia, tremor, hemiplegia, vertigo, ocular motor palsies, quadriplegia, dysarthria, nystagmus and lower cranial nerve involvement (Golden 1985, Lewis and Berman 1986, Mehler 1988). Disturbances of consciousness, opisthotonic attacks and respiratory disturbances have been reported (Echenne *et al.* 1983). Although some reports mention the occurrrence of tonic–clonic attacks, these are probably not true epileptic seizures (Ropper 1988). More limited infarcts can give rise to isolated ataxia and to abnormal ocular motility or to disturbances of consciousness and of language. Bilateral thalamic infarction can be due to a single thalamoperforate artery obstruction (Garg and DeMyer 1995). Dementia may follow strokes in the mesencephalon and diencephalon (Katz *et al.* 1987). Occlusive accidents in the posterior circulation are often preceded by repeated episodes of vertebrobasilar insufficiency, days, weeks or even months before the definitive attack. Compression of the vertebral artery by head rotation may be responsible for transient ischaemic attacks (Garg and Edwards-Brown 1995).

The *imaging appearance* of arterial occlusion is dependent both on the size of the infarct and on the delay between onset of stroke and examinations (Raybaud *et al.* 1985). CT and even MR scans obtained within the first 10–24 hours are normal but water diffusion MR can demonstrate extensive abnormal signal that may regress in part or totally (Warach *et al.* 1995). Later, there is an area of decreased attenuation with ill-defined borders which extends, becomes better defined and reaches its peak over the next few days. This low density area is accompanied by a variable mass effect that peaks in two to three days. Most infarcts do not enhance on contrast injection during the first week. In children, however, early enhancement is not uncommon even after 24–48 hours. Enhancement mostly involves the cortical grey matter and appears as an undulating ribbon following brain convolutions. Later, the infarct appears as a depressed, triangular scar (Fig. 15.10).

Small *lacunar infarcts* often do not enhance on contrast injection and may remain undetectable by CT scan (Zimmerman *et al.* 1983) but are usually visible on T_2-weighted MRI sequences (Inagaki *et al.* 1992). The largest lacunae, such as those that involve the putamen or pallidum, may sometimes take up contrast

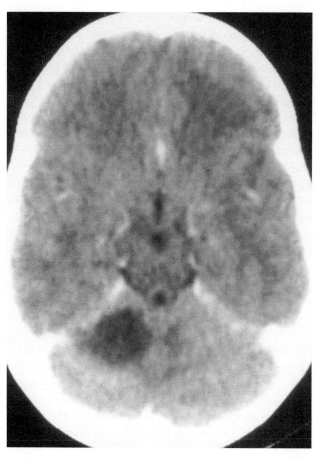

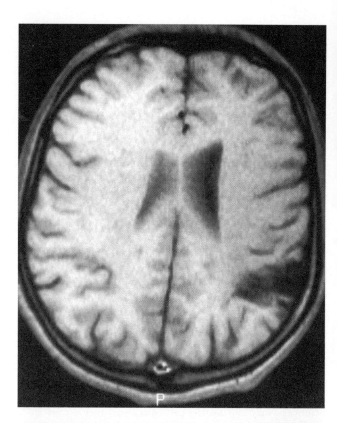

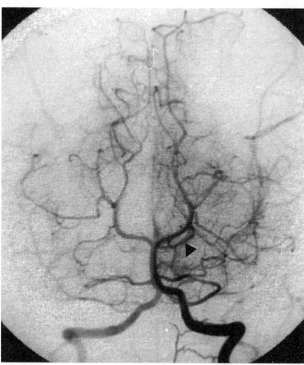

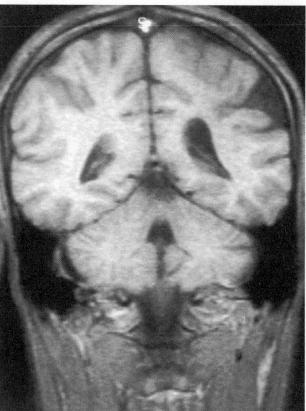

Fig. 15.9. Cerebellar infarct localized to the right hemisphere. *(Top)* CT scan shows area of hypodensity in right cerebellar hemisphere. *(Bottom)* Vertebral arteriography shows absence of injection of right superior cerebellar artery. *Arrow* indicates opposite superior cerebellar artery. (15-year-old boy with sudden appearance of right cerebellar syndrome that progressively subsided over the following months).

Fig. 15.10. Old infarct in a posterior branch of the left middle cerebral artery in 16-year-old boy who suddenly developed right hemiplegia at age 20 months in the course of a febrile illness. (There was minimal residual hemiparesis). T_1-weighted MRI scans show a triangular defect in the parietal cortex penetrating into the white matter. Note relatively small left hemisphere.

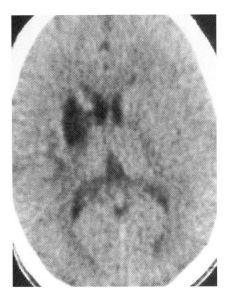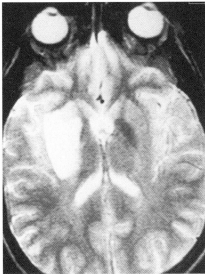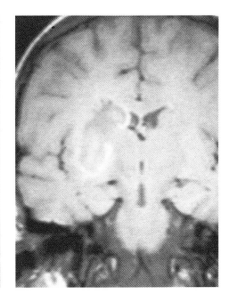

Fig. 15.11. Lacunar infarct in 14-year-old boy. *(Left)* CT scan showing lacuna in the right caudate nucleus and internal capsule. *(Centre)* MRI scan, T$_1$-weighted sequence showing large area of high signal probably corresponding to oedema. *(Right)* MRI scan, T$_2$-weighted sequence showing large area of low signal in right hemisphere, lined by high signal perhaps due to mild bleeding.

(Zimmerman *et al.* 1983). Haemorrhages within the infarcted area may appear during the first week of the course.

MRI reveals even small ischaemic areas giving a low-intensity signal in T$_1$-weighted sequences and an intense signal of probable oedematous nature in T$_2$-weighted sequences. Haemorrhage may be seen better on T$_1$-weighted MRI at the periphery of the infarct (Fig. 15.11).

Since the advent of modern neuroimaging, angiography is not required in most cases for diagnosis of infarction. Indeed, lacunar infarcts are generally unaccompanied by visible vascular abnormalities, because involved vessels are too small and too variable in appearance for angiography to permit a definite diagnosis (Kappelle *et al.* 1989). For patients with unexplained strokes, angiography is still indicated in my opinion to rule in or out intrinsic vascular disease such as fibromuscular dysplasia and dissection and to recognize cases with multiple vascular lesions of the moyamoya type. This is important for prognostic and therapeutic reasons. MRA may not be adequate for this purpose as it gives information on flow rather than on vascular structure. Reperfusion of thrombosed vessels may occur as early as two days after a stroke (Isler 1984), which may explain the frequency of normal angiograms in childhood strokes.

MRA is not precise enough to demonstrate subtle vascular abnormalities such as arterial stenosis or mural irregularities. New CT angiography (spiral CT) techniques are promising. Digital subtraction angiography by intravenous route may be sufficient for the detection of relatively large multiple lesions but precise analysis still requires the use of the arterial route. MRI examination can show dissection of neck and intracranial arteries as a cause of infarct (Zuber *et al.* 1993).

Transcranial and duplex/Doppler ultrasound examination is a noninvasive and valuable method allowing visualization of arterial anomalies and, with refined technique, assessment of

functional characteristics of circulation within a given vessel (Eljamel *et al.* 1990, Sturzenegger 1995).

DIFFERENTIAL DIAGNOSIS

Acquired vascular hemiplegia should be distinguished from the multiple other causes of acute hemiplegia. The differentiation from acute postconvulsive hemiplegia (HHE syndrome) that is only rarely due to vascular thrombosis (Chapters 8, 16) is usually easy. CT and MRI images are totally different as they show initially swelling and decreased density of a whole hemisphere without preferential involvement of any vascular territory, later followed by hemiatrophy of the brain (Gastaut *et al.* 1977, Kataoka *et al.* 1988). Hemiplegic migraine (Chapter 17) may be difficult to distinguish from arterial occlusion and may, in some cases, be the cause of a stroke. In cardiac patients, acquired hemiplegia may also result from venous thrombosis or from brain abcess, the latter only after 2–3 years of age (Tyler and Clark 1957, Kurlan and Griggs 1983). In case of doubt, it is reasonable to place all such children on antibiotic therapy which may be discontinued after one week if abcess is ruled out. Tumours, especially of the brainstem, may result in rapidly acquired hemiplegia (Chapter 14). In contrast, some infarcts develop progressively and mimic a mass lesion (Chatkupt *et al.* 1987). Epileptic seizures and other paroxysmal events can produce transient hemiplegia that is not usually difficult to distinguish from vascular hemiplegia, except at the very onset (Chapter 17). Haemorrhagic stroke has been discussed above (pp. 534–535). Transient ischaemic attacks are uncommon in children but can occur in patients with arterial stenosis of any cause or as a prodromal event in cases of dissection or thrombosis. They are marked by short-lived hemiplegia, hemianopia or hemisensory deficits. Acute but transitory attacks of hemiparesis that occur in children with insulin-dependent diabetes mellitus (MacDonald and Brown 1979,

TABLE 15.3
Main causes of arterial occlusion and stroke-like episodes in childhood

Cardiac diseases

Congenital heart disease	Tyler and Clark (1957), Freedom (1989)
Right-to-left shunts	Pellicer et al. (1992)
Rheumatic heart disease	Isler (1984)
Endocarditis	Salgado et al. (1989)
Myocarditis	Asinger et al. (1989)
Cardiac myxoma[1]	Carney (1985), Cerebral Embolism Task Force (1986)
Mitral valve prolapse[1]	Jackson et al. (1984)
Prosthetic valves	Riela and Roach (1993)
Conduction defects[1]	Ward et al. (1984), Atluru et al. (1985)
Disturbances of cardiac rhythm	Zapson et al. (1995)

Vascular dysplasias

Moyamoya syndrome, idiopathic[1]	Gordon and Isler (1989)
Moyamoya syndrome, acquired	Debrun et al. (1975)
Neurofibromatosis type 1[1]	Hilal et al. (1971b), Tomsik et al. (1976), Pellock et al. (1980)
Fibromuscular dysplasia[1]	Mettinger and Ericson (1982), Vles et al. (1990)
Williams syndrome[1]	Ardinger et al. (1994)
Vascular malformations	Kappelle et al. (1989)
Dissecting aneurysm	Chang et al. (1975), Nass et al. (1982), Lewis and Berman (1986), Patel et al. (1995)
Vascular spasm secondary to intracranial haemorrhage	Riela and Roach (1993)
Rendu–Osler disease[1]	Román et al. (1978)

Inflammatory vascular diseases

Panarteritis nodosa	Harvey and Alvord (1972)
Systemic lupus erythematosus	Chapter 12
Takayasu arteritis	Kohrman and Huttenlocher (1986)
Kawasaki disease	Lapointe et al. (1984)
Other vasculitides	Barron et al. (1993)
Schönlein–Henoch purpura	Belman et al. (1985)
Haemolytic–uraemic syndrome	Trevathan and Dooling (1987)
Other vascular diseases	Harvey and Alvord (1972)

Connective tissue disorders

Pseudoxanthoma elasticum[1]	Iqbal et al. (1978), Viljoen (1988)
Ehlers–Danlos (type IV)[1]	Pretorius and Butler (1983), North et al. (1995)
Defect in collagen III[1]	Pope et al. (1981)

Connective tissue disorders

Marfan syndrome[1]	Finney et al. (1976)
Mixed connective tissue disease	Graf et al. (1993)

Other vascular diseases

CADASIL (cerebral autosomal dominant arteriopathy with subcortical infarcts and leukoencephalopathy)	Chabriat et al. (1995b)
Idiopathic arterial calcification of infancy	Anderson et al. (1985)
Arterial hypertension	Wright and Mathews (1996)
Fabry disease[1,2]	Grewal (1994)
Sneddon syndrome[1]	Bruyn et al. (1987)
In association with lupus anticoagulant, anticardiolipin antibodies or antiphospholipid antibodies	Brey et al. (1990), Levine et al. (1990), Furie et al. (1994), Ravelli et al. (1994), Nuss et al. (1995)
Degos disease	Rosemberg et al. (1988)
Dissection of carotid, vertebral and intracranial arteries	
Traumatic	Mokri et al. (1988), Horowitz and Niparko (1994)
Spontaneous	Patel et al. (1995)
Familial	Schievink (1995)

Haematological diseases

Haemoglobinopathies (sickle cell disease)[1]	R.J. Adams et al. (1988), Adams (1995)
Polycythaemia[1]	Adamson et al. (1973), Riela and Roach (1993)
L-asparginase treatment of leukaemia	Priest et al. (1980)
Coagulopathies[1]	
Heparin cofactor II deficiency	Tran et al. (1985)
Protein C deficiency	Tarras et al. (1988), Dusser et al. (1988)
Antithrombin III deficiency	Vomberg et al. (1987)
Protein S deficiency	Natowicz and Kelley (1987), D'Angelo et al. (1993), Devilat et al. (1993), Simioni et al. (1994)
Plasminogen deficiency	Natowicz and Kelley (1987)
Resistance to activated protein C[1]	Svensson and Dahlbäck (1994), Ridker et al. (1995)
Iron deficiency anaemia	Hartfield et al. (1997)

Korobkin 1980) may represent a diagnostic challenge. CT scan does not demonstrate infarction and the hemiplegia resolves in 24–48 hours. Such attacks are different from the actual strokes that may occur in young diabetics during episodes of ketoacidosis. Occlusion of the posterior cerebral artery occurred in an 8-year-old diabetic girl with marked cerebral oedema as a result of improper treatment of ketoacidosis and was probably due to compression of the artery against the tentorial edge (personal case) (see also Chapter 17).

OUTCOME, PROGNOSIS AND THERAPY
The outcome of acquired occlusive disease depends in large part on the cause of the vascular disorder (see below). In general, the prognosis is poor or guarded if there is a detectable disorder of the brain vascular tree such as moyamoya disease or fibromuscular dysplasia or if there is a recognizable underlying metabolic or general cause to the occlusion, e.g. homocystinuria or vasculitis. If no such cause is present (i.e. in idiopathic arterial occlusion), the prognosis is relatively favourable, and recurrent vascular accidents occur only rarely (8–10 per cent) even after prolonged follow-up. However, Abram et al. (1996) encountered 16 recurrences in a series of 42 children with idiopathic stroke. Lacunar infarcts often have a favourable motor outcome (Dusser et al. 1986, Inagaki et al. 1992). In the series of Dusser et al., only five of 14 such patients had persisting weakness.

Most nonrecurrent vascular hemiplegias show significant motor improvement, and in one series total recovery occurred in over half the cases (Diebler and Dulac 1987). In less favourable

TABLE 15.3
(continued)

Metabolic diseases

Mitochondrial encephalomyopathy with stroke-like episodes (MELAS)[1,2]	Chapter 9
Dyslipoproteinaemia[1]	Glueck et al. (1982)
Sulfite oxidase deficiency[1]	Riela and Roach (1993)
Homocystinuria[1] (heterozygotes)	McCully (1969), Van Diemen-Steenvoorde et al. (1990), Clarke et al. (1991)
Propionic acidaemia[1]	Haas et al. (1995)
Menkes disease[1]	Chapter 9
Carbohydrate-deficient glycoprotein syndrome[1,2]	Jaeken and Carchon (1993)
Fabry disease[1,2]	Grewal (1994)
Ammonia cycle disorders[1]	Sperl et al. (1997)

Infectious diseases

Bacterial meningitides	Igarashi et al. 1984
Tuberculous meningitis	Leiguarda et al. (1988)
Viral disease	
Rubella	Connolly et al. (1975)
Herpes zoster	Hilt et al. (1983), Fukumoto et al. (1986), Leis and Butler (1987), Joy et al. (1989)
Varicella	Kamholz and Tremblay (1985), Caekebeke et al. (1990), Bodensteiner et al. (1992)
AIDS	Park et al. (1988)
Coxsackie A9	Chalhub et al. (1977)
Fungal disease, especially mucormycosis	Banker (1961)
Cervical infections	
Lymphadenopathy	Tagawa et al. (1985)
Cat scratch disease	Selby and Walker (1979)
Necrotizing fasciitis	Bush et al. (1984)
Amygdalitis, otitis media	Dusser et al. (1986)

Tumours

Direct invasion or compression by tumour, leukaemia (promyelocytic), distant cancer	Packer et al. (1985)
Disseminated intravascular coagulation	Packer et al. (1985)
L-asparaginase thrombosis	Barron et al. (1992)
Methotrexate-induced thrombosis	Hanefeld and Riehm (1980)

Trauma and toxic causes

Head injury including minor trauma	Isler (1984), Wanifuchi et al. (1988), Debehnke and Singer (1991)
Trauma to carotid artery	Pearl (1987), Schievink et al. (1994b), Patel et al. (1995)
Trauma to vertebral artery	Katirji et al. (1985), Garg and Edwards-Brown (1993)
Head rotation	Garg and Edwards-Brown (1995)
Catheterization of temporal artery	Prian et al. (1978)
X-irradiation (especially of brain tumours)	Beyer et al. (1986), Mitchell et al. (1991)
Traumatic fat embolism	Jacobson et al. (1986)
Nontraumatic fat embolism	McCarthy and Norenberg (1988), Horton et al. (1995)
Fat embolism from intravenous lipid infusion	Barson and Chiswick (1978)
Excessive use of nasal decongestants[2]	Montalban et al. (1989)
Cocaine abuse	Levine and Welch (1988), Mangiardi et al. (1988)
Phenylpropanolamine	Forman et al. (1989)
Wasp sting	Romano et al. (1989)
Solvent abuse	Parker et al. (1984)

Miscellaneous

Nephrotic syndrome	Igarashi et al. (1988)
Oral contraceptives	Longstreth and Swanson (1984)
Migraine[1,2]	Riikonen and Santavuori (1994)
Familial migraine linked to chromosome 19q12[1]	Chabriat et al. (1995a), Hutchinson et al. (1995)
Livedo reticularis	Baxter et al. (1993)

[1]Can be transmitted genetically (mendelian inheritance or otherwise).
[2]Mainly stroke-like episodes without demonstrable infarcts.

cases, the persistence of hemiplegia may be complicated by secondary dystonia (Demierre and Rondot 1983, Dusser et al. 1986). Intelligence is generally unaffected by arterial occlusive accidents except if they are multiple or recurrent or in the case of large infarcts occurring in young infants, especially in congenital heart disease. Epileptic seizures are uncommon. In one series (Aicardi et al. 1969), only two of 28 patients developed seizures and 25 were of normal intelligence. A poor outcome can be predicted if the hemiplegia persists after a month if the infarct is cortical rather than subcortical and with bilateral disease (Abram et al. 1996).

The acute treatment of stroke remains in dispute (see Miller 1993). Determination of the cause is essential in orientating therapy. Anticoagulation with heparin (especially low molecular weight heparin) followed by warfarin derivatives does not seem to increase the risk of haemorrhage within the infarcted area. Whether it is capable of limiting the volume of infarct when given early remains to be seen but it tends to be generally recommended in patients with arterial abnormalities or a thrombotic tendency. Aspirin treatment is generally indicated although few decisive data are available. Strepto/urokinase therapy has not been found to be effective in adult stroke. Anticoagulation may be indicated when there are vascular abnormalities such as dissection producing secondary embolic strokes (Khurana et al. 1996) or abnormal blood coagulation.

CAUSES OF ARTERIAL OCCLUSIVE DISEASE
Some children with arterial occlusion have a known predisposing

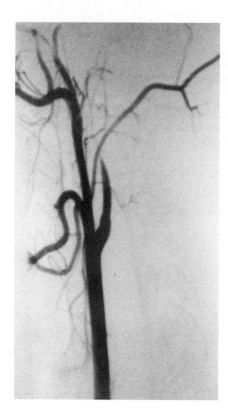
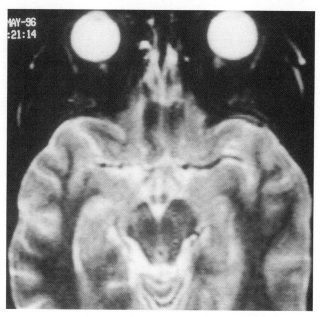

Fig. 15.12. Dissection of the internal carotid artery. *(Above)* MRI scan showing low turbulent flow in right middle cerebral artery. *(Left)* Conventional angiography shows typical progressive narrowing of right internal carotid. (Courtesy Dr Kling Chong, Great Ormond Street Hospital, London.)

condition such as cardiac disease, homocystinuria or sickle cell disease (Riela and Roach 1993). Stroke may also occur as a result of an acute infection or of trauma. The main causes are indicated in Table 15.3. The frequency of idiopathic stroke varies with the extent of the investigations performed. Recent work suggests that truly idiopathic strokes are uncommon when full investigation is carried out.

The possible role of antiphospholipid antibodies including lupus anticoagulant and anticardiolipin antibodies is still unclear. They probably play a role in the case of collagen disorders (Chapter 12). The *primary antiphospholipid syndrome* has been found in a significant number of children with cerebrovascular ischaemic events (Devilat *et al.* 1993, Tietjen *et al.* 1993, Angelini *et al.* 1994, Schöning *et al.* 1994) and even in infants (Roddy and Giang 1991) but its significance is variably appreciated (Rumi *et al.* 1993, Göbel 1994, Takanashi *et al.* 1995). Antiphospholipid antibodies should be part of the investigations for idiopathic stroke.

The role of coagulation disorders is probably less important in cases of arterial than in those of venous thrombosis. However, strokes of arterial origin have been reported with protein C and S deficiency (Devilat *et al.* 1993, van Kuijck *et al.* 1994, Schöning *et al.* 1994, Kennedy *et al.* 1995) and with resistance to activated protein C (Nowak-Göttl *et al.* 1996). High levels of triglycerides, low LDL (low density lipoprotein) cholesterol and depressed HDL (high density lipoprotein) cholesterol were found in one-third of the cases of Abram *et al.* (1996).

Idiopathic stroke can affect any arterial territory. Involvement of the internal capsule and lenticular nuclei has been said to be rare (Young *et al.* 1983) but in fact they are involved in approximately half the cases (Dusser *et al.* 1986). Angiography is usually normal in capsuloputaminal strokes. Dystonia is a common complication and may emerge long after the appearance of hemiplegia (Pettigrew and Jankovic 1985). Bilateral occlusion is exceptional (Tagawa *et al.* 1985, Shirane *et al.* 1992). An association with the human leukocyte antigen (HLA) B51 has been reported (Mintz *et al.* 1992). Hartfield *et al.* (1997) have suggested that iron deficiency anaemia may be a significant aetiological factor of stroke and reported six cases, three of them with arterial infarcts.

The role of *dissection of the arterial wall* (Fig. 15.12) as a cause of idiopathic stroke may well be important as shown by an increasing number of reports (see Sturzenegger 1995, Khurana *et al.* 1996). Moreover, stroke in such cases, which often results from embolism from the clot formed at the site of dissection, is potentially preventable by heparin treatment. None of 32 patients of Sturzenegger who received anticoagulant treatment subsequently deteriorated. Unilateral headache, transient ischaemic attacks and pain in the neck may be premonitory symptoms. Doppler and duplex sonography can confirm the clinical diagnosis by showing significant stenosis or occlusion. MRI can show a thickened vessel wall and/or a mural haematoma. Such signs and symptoms, in addition to an antecedent of trauma (often minor) should suggest this possibility. Recanalization is frequent.

MOYAMOYA DISEASE
Moyamoya disease is a slowly progressive stenosis and obliteration of the large vessels of the base of the brain. It affects mainly the supraclinoid segment of the internal carotid arteries and the initial portion of the middle or anterior cerebral arteries, less

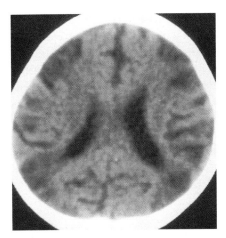
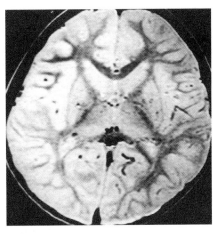
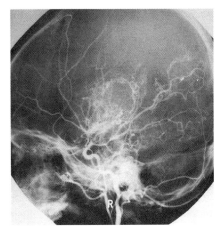
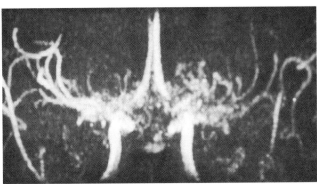

Fig. 15.13. Moyamoya disease in 5-year-old Korean girl with history of repeated strokes. *(Top left)* CT scan shows multiple cortical areas of infarction. *(Top centre)* MRI shows multiple vessels especially in region of basal ganglia. *(Top right)* Carotid angiography demonstrates occlusion of both anterior and middle cerebral arteries with extensive collateral network in region of basal ganglia and peripheral anastomoses between pial and meningeal circulations. *(Left)* MR angiography showing stenosis of both carotid arteries and extensive basal collaterals in the region of the basal ganglia. (Courtesy Dr Kling Chong, Great Ormond Street Hospital, London.)

commonly the posterior cerebral arteries. Inflammatory infiltration is absent but there is usually intimal thickening with severe stenosis. Because of the slow course, an extensive collateral circulation develops in the basal ganglia and multiple anastomoses form between the internal and external carotid arteries. This network produces a hazy appearance on angiography, termed moyamoya by Japanese investigators. The disease is common in Japan but occurs worldwide and affects boys more than girls in a ratio of 3:2 (Suzuki and Kodama 1983, Gordon and Isler 1989). Fifty per cent of patients are less than 10 years of age at onset. Bleeding is a rare manifestation before age 16. In most children, the onset is abrupt with seizures, hemiplegia, monoparesis or other localizations of stroke. Chorea may be the presenting manifestation (Watanabe *et al.* 1990). Multiple episodes are bound to occur on the same or contralateral side. Eventually, the patients are left with bilateral weakness, epilepsy and mental retardation. Transient ischaemic attacks with brief episodes of hemiplegia, dysaesthesia or hemianopia without loss of consciousness may occur repeatedly (Fukuyama and Umezu 1985). They may be precipitated by hyperpnoea, and overbreathing should not be requested in such patients during EEG (Allen *et al.* 1976). The reactivity of blood vessels to CO_2 is impaired (Tatemichi *et al.* 1988). After a few years, permanent weakness sets in. CT scan may show initially a single large infarction but multiple ischaemic areas are more characteristic (Takeuchi *et al.* 1982). Angiography is the definitive diagnostic test (Fukuyama and Umezu 1985) but MRI is sometimes capable of demonstrating the abnormal basal circulation (Watanabe *et al.* 1990) (Fig. 15.13).

Moyamoya is a syndrome rather than a single entity. The idiopathic form is sometimes familial and is most frequent in Japan (Kitahara *et al.* 1979). All causes of progressive obstruction of the arteries of the circle of Willis can be responsible for the development of moyamoya. These include sickle cell disease (Seeler *et al.* 1978, Vernant *et al.* 1988), neurofibromatosis with or without chiasmatic glioma (Beyer *et al.* 1986, Gordon and Isler 1989), chronic basilar meningitis, X-ray irradiation (Okuno *et al.* 1985), homocystinuria (Van Diemen-Steenvoorde *et al.* 1990) and Down syndrome (Fukuyama *et al.* 1992). In secondary forms, involvement of peripheral vessels is common and renovascular hypertension may be associated (Jansen *et al.* 1990).

Treatment of primary moyamoya is of limited efficacy. Intravenous calcium-channel blockers are effective acutely in increasing perfusion (McLean *et al.* 1985, Hosain *et al.* 1994). It is reasonable to use them chronically in conjunction with aspirin although the value of such therapy is unproved. Extracranial-to-intracranial bypass surgery (Takeuchi *et al.* 1982) seems unlikely to add much to the natural development of anastomoses but may prevent extension of damage. Angiomyosynangiosis is used for such cases especially in Japan. Encephaloduroarteriosynangiosis (laying the superficial temporal artery on the surface of the cerebral cortex to promote the formation of anastomoses between external and internal carotid circulation) may prevent the occurrence of new ischaemic accidents (Rooney *et al.* 1991, George *et al.* 1993, Ross *et al.* 1994). Inhalation of 100% O_2 in the event of transient ischaemic attacks prevents slowing of EEG tracings and seems to be clinically effective (Fujiwara *et al.* 1996).

FIBROMUSCULAR DYSPLASIA
Fibromuscular dysplasia of the internal carotid artery can produce transient ischaemic attacks and strokes (Llorens-Terol *et al.* 1983, Chiu *et al.* 1996). Angiography shows an irregularly narrowed vessel with a string-bead appearance. Intracranial involvement of the carotid artery is rare (Lemahieu and Marchau 1979). The disorder may be multifocal, especially involving the renal arteries, with resulting arterial hypertension. Neurofibromatosis type 1 may also affect the cervical or intracranial arteries as well as the renal arteries (Tomsik *et al.* 1976, Bolander *et al.* 1978). The anterior circulation is most affected. Angiography shows irregular narrowing of the carotid artery, extending into the bifurcation and origin of main branches. Stroke can also result from arterial hypertension without specific involvement of cerebral arteries (Pellok *et al.* 1980).

CARDIAC DISORDERS
Cardiac disorders are a major cause of acquired vascular hemiplegias, congenital cyanotic heart disease being the most common cause. Infarcts may occur spontaneously, especially in children under 2 years of age (Terplan 1976), and often appear following an attack of cyanosis and dyspnoea. Children with low haemoglobin concentrations are at particular risk for arterial accidents, whereas a high haematocrit is common in venous thrombosis (Tyler and Clark 1957). Hemiplegia not uncommonly appears following surgery as a result of air embolism or other complications (Terplan 1976, Furlan and Breuer 1984). It may also be the result of embolism due to bacterial endocarditis. About 90 per cent of vascular accidents occur in children with tetralogy of Fallot (Phornphutkul *et al.* 1973). About 20 per cent of the patients are left with mental retardation (Tyler and Clark 1957). Diffuse brain damage affecting either the grey or white matter is commonly found at autopsy of children who died with congenital cardiac disease (Bozoky *et al.* 1984). In patients with congenital left-to-right shunts, stroke may result from endocarditis, and this may also occur in children with rheumatic heart disease. The latter are exposed to embolism due to dysrhythmia. Mitral valve prolapse is a relatively common familial disorder (Greenwood 1984). It can be a rare cause of recurrent ischaemic attacks (Jackson *et al.* 1984). These may involve any territory, including retinal vessels, and are usually transient. Anticoagulation may be effective in the prevention of embolism for high-risk patients (Yatsu *et al.* 1988).

SICKLE CELL DISEASE
Hereditary haemoglobinopathies, especially sickle cell disease, are a common cause of neurological disorder in Black people. Neurological complications that usually become apparent before age 5 years occur in 20–30 per cent of patients and include headaches, seizures and behaviour disturbances. These are less common with sickle cell–haemoglobin C disease (Fabian and Peters 1984). Rarely, neurological symptoms appear in patients with sickle cell

trait, often at times of stress. Strokes occur in 10 per cent of patients and are recurrent if untreated in two-thirds of cases.

The major cerebral arteries are narrowed or obliterated due to intimal proliferation and fragmentation. Brain ischaemia apparently results mainly from occlusive disease of the large cerebral vessels (R.J. Adams *et al.* 1988). However, some involvement of microcirculation is also present, although not fully explained (Huttenlocher *et al.* 1994). Reduction in capillary flow possibly due to sickling is of less importance but may account for some of the neurological problems (R.J. Adams *et al.* 1988). The low blood flow is normalized by transfusions. Nontraumatic fat embolism is a possible cause of stroke in sickle cell patients (Horton *et al.* 1995).

Vascular occlusions occur mainly at the time of sickle cell crises. However, a significant proportion of infarctions remain silent (Adams 1995). When clinical stroke occurs, focal or generalized seizures are common. Hemiplegia or other focal neurological deficits are the main findings (Glauser *et al.* 1995). They may be transient or irreversible. Multiple lesions are the rule (Fig. 15.14) and eventually will result in dementia, epilepsy and pseudobulbar syndrome. Intracranial haemorrhage is uncommon in children (Van Hoff *et al.* 1985, Mallouh and Hamda 1986) but has a high mortality rate.

Sickle cell disease is a prime consideration in Black children with neurological symptoms even though these occur only uncommonly as a first manifestation. The diagnosis is confirmed by demonstration of the abnormal haemoglobin. The extent of brain damage is best evaluated by MRI scan that usually shows several areas of hypodensity or atrophy or both. There is a good correspondence between the results of MRI and the clinical evidence of ischaemic damage. Glauser *et al.* (1995) found that 12 of 13 patients with a normal MRI were neurologically intact and had no history of acute neurological event. Armstrong *et al.* (1996) identified MRI abnormalities in 17.9 per cent of 194 children. Those with silent infarcts on MRI performed significantly worse on cognitive tests than children without MRI anomaly. Those with a history of clinical stroke did worse than those with only MRI changes. Conventional angiography is not recommended. It shows stenosis often affecting several large or medium-size arteries so that the development of a moyamoya pattern is frequent (Seeler *et al.* 1978). MRA demonstrates the presence of stenosis or obstruction. Multiple aneurysms have been reported (Overby and Rothman 1985) but are not seen before 15 years of age (Van Hoff *et al.* 1985). Transcranial Doppler ultrasonography reliably shows high blood flow and increased velocity and correlates well with angiographic data (Adams 1995). An abnormal Doppler result may be predictive of the occurrence of stroke but this requires confirmation.

The *treatment* of vascular accidents in patients with known sickle cell disease is prevention. Sickle cell crises require prompt hydration, oxygen administration and packed red cell transfusion. Hyperventilation during EEG should be avoided as it may produce stroke (Allen *et al.* 1976), but apnoea has also been associated with stroke (Robertson *et al.* 1988). Recurrent strokes can be prevented by regular transfusions to maintain the level of

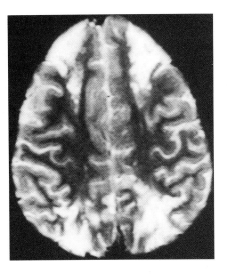

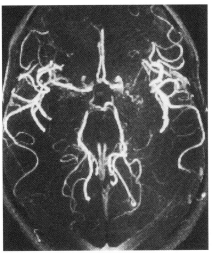

Fig. 15.14. Sickle-cell anaemia. *(Far left)* MRI scan, T_2-weighted sequence showing bilateral areas of ischaemia in both frontal and parietal areas. *(Left)* MR angiography showing abnormal flow in both middle cerebral arteries, predominantly on the left (right side of picture). Note development of collateral circulation. (Courtesy Dr F. Kirkham, Great Ormond Street Hospital, London.)

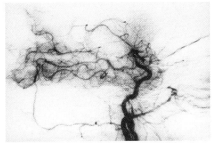

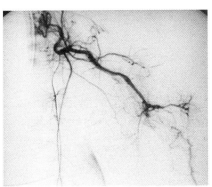

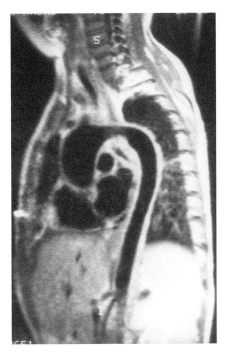

Fig. 15.15. Takayasu arteritis with thrombotic occlusion of right anterior cerebral artery (3-year-old girl with left hemiplegia of sudden onset). *(Far left, top)* Carotid angiogram showing thrombosis of distal carotid. *(Far left, bottom)* Angiogram of left subclavian artery showing thrombosis of humeral artery and development of multiple collateral channels. *(Left)* MRI scan of aorta showing marked dilatation of ascending aorta and gross thickening of aortic walls.

haemoglobin A above 60 per cent (Wilimas *et al.* 1980, Buchanan *et al.* 1983, Prohovnik *et al.* 1989, Pegelow *et al.* 1995). Intracranial haemorrhage associated with hypertension in overly transfused patients has been reported (Prohovnik *et al.* 1989), and a similar syndrome has been seen in thalassaemic patients after multiple blood transfusions (Wazi *et al.* 1978). The major problem is iron overload, in addition to the practical problem of repeated transfusions. The duration of treatment is not established but reccurrences have been observed on discontinuation of transfusions after three years and life-long therapy may be needed so there is a need for a safer and more practical prophylactic treatment.

INFECTIOUS VASCULITIS

Cases are on record of occlusion or strokes associated with cervical lymphadenopathy or chronic pharyngeal infections (Tagawa *et al.* 1985). Necrotizing fasciitis, secondary to dental infections (Bush *et al.* 1984) can lead to unilateral or even bilateral carotid occlusion. Vigorous antibiotic treatment is indicated. Vasculitis due to meningitis has been described in Chapter 11.

In the course of certain viral infections, an acute hemiplegia of arterial origin has been observed. Varicella-zoster virus is the major offender. The typical syndrome features the sudden appearance of hemiplegia contralateral to the side of herpes zoster ophthalmicus (Leis and Butler 1987, Joy *et al.* 1989). Direct spread of the virus to the adjacent carotid artery is postulated. In some cases, diffuse arteritis of probable viral origin has been observed. The same complication has been recorded with chicken pox (Kamholz and Tremblay 1985, Caekebeke *et al.* 1990, Bodensteiner *et al.* 1992).

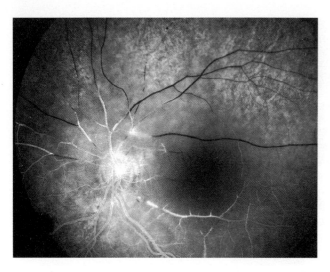

Fig. 15.16. Vasculitis of the CNS and retina. 15-year-old boy who suffered sudden loss of vision in the left eye following a four-month history of vertigo, unilateral left sensorineural deafness, ataxia, bilateral spasticity, and mental slowing with resulting school difficulties. MRI showed disseminated areas of intense signal on T_2-weighted sequences in both peripheral and periventricular locations. Fluorescein angiography shows multiple arterial occlusions that were also visible with the ophthalmoscope.

INFLAMMATORY VASCULITIDES

Takayasu arteritis may be of infectious origin and the relationship to tuberculosis has been stressed (Pantell and Goodman 1981), although its cause remains unknown. This is, in 90 per cent of cases, a disease of girls. Involvement of the brain occurs in 5–10 per cent of patients, usually resulting in acute hemiplegia. The disease rarely affects infants or young children (Kohrman and Huttenlocher 1986, Morales *et al.* 1991). The diagnosis may be suggested by absence of radial pulses or dilatation of the aorta visible on X-ray films of the chest. In one personal case, MRI clearly demonstrated thickening of the aortic wall in a 3-year-old girl (Fig. 15.15). Angiography and biopsy are necessary for firm diagnosis. Immunosuppressive treatment with prednisone is indicated during the acute, initial stage.

Inflammatory vasculitides of uncertain origin occur in Schoenlein–Henoch purpura, lupus erythematosus and panarteritis nodosa (Chapter 12). *Isolated angiitis of the CNS* has been reported in adults (Cupps *et al.* 1983, Koo and Massey 1988, Moore 1989) and uncommonly in children (Matsell *et al.* 1990, Barron *et al.* 1993). It is characterized by a variety of signs and symptoms of involvement of the brain and, sometimes, the spinal cord. Criteria for diagnosis include a clinical pattern of headaches and multifocal deficits, exclusion of systemic inflammation or infection, and vascular inflammation as shown by leptomeningeal/parenchymal biopsy (Moore 1989). Angiography shows multiple segmental narrowings of several arteries (Alhalabi and Moore 1994) but this finding alone is not specific. Some patients respond favourably to steroids alone (Craven and French 1985) or in combination with cyclophosphamide or azathioprine (Moore 1989, Barron *et al.* 1993). Attempts at treatment may also be justified in children with unexplained neurological disease even in the absence of angiographic anomalies (Vanderzant *et al.*

1988), even though demonstrated cases in children are rare (Fig. 15.16). Pathologically there is a necrotizing vascular inflammation with fibrinoid necrosis and monocytic infiltration. Granulomas may be prominent (Younger *et al.* 1988) but the spectrum of lesions is broad.

A somewhat similar clinical and radiological picture with a relatively benign course can result from the use of drugs such as cocaine, amphetamines and sympathomimetic agents (Le Coz *et al.* 1988).

TRAUMATIC HEMIPLEGIA

Direct cervical trauma and even mild or trivial trauma to the head and neck sustained during exercise and sports may induce thrombosis of the carotid artery, vertebral artery or intracranial vessels (Pitner 1966) due to stretching of the artery or dissection.

Trauma with long bone fracture can result in traumatic fat embolism that may provoke coma and/or focal neurological disturbances (Jacobson *et al.* 1986). Fat embolism may also complicate cardiopulmonary bypass surgery, pancreatitis, osteomyelitis and intravenous infusion of lipids.

Children who fall with a blunt object in their mouth can sustain injuries to the carotid artery in the tonsillar fossa. The onset of symptoms is often delayed for hours or days. Hemiparesis or other focal deficits may be transitory or persistent. Any child with a penetrating wound of the neck or trauma to the tonsillar fossa should be closely observed for neurological signs. However, the efficacy of preventive treatment, whether anticoagulation or surgery, has not been proved (Samson 1989).

Surgical trauma may result in hemiplegia: infarction of the anterior choroidal artery territory, the so-called 'manipulation' hemiplegia, is a rare complication of anterior temporal lobectomy (Helgason *et al.* 1987).

Traumatic carotid–jugular fistulae are a rare complication of trauma (Hosobuchi 1989). Iatrogenic trauma may cause cerebral thrombosis. This has been reported following temporal artery catheterization (Prian *et al.* 1978), and I have observed a few cases of cerebral infarction following catheterization for congenital cardiac disease.

X-irradiation of the brain may cause arterial stenosis and ischaemic accidents that may be transient or leave permanent residua. In some cases, anastomosis between the extracerebral and intracerebral arterial systems may be considered if the stenosis is limited to one segment with normal peripheral branches.

SPINAL ARTERIAL OCCLUSIONS

Spontaneous occlusions of spinal arteries leading to infarction of the spinal cord are uncommon. They are often the manifestation of an underlying vascular malformation.

Direct or indirect injuries to the spinal arteries are reviewed in Chapter 13. Spinal damage is a rare complication of surgery for the repair of coarctation of the aorta and may result in complete paraplegia or lesser degrees of weakness. It is related to the duration of aortic occlusion and to circulatory factors (Albert *et al.* 1969). Similar problems may occur with surgery of the sympathetic chain or vertebrae.

Paraplegia of vascular mechanism is a rare complication of catheterization of the umbilical artery or of injections of drugs into this vessel (Dulac and Aicardi 1975).

THROMBOSIS OF CEREBRAL VEINS AND DURAL SINUSES

The frequency of venous thrombosis is much lower than that of arterial stroke. Venous thrombosis occurs in variable circumstances (Table 15.4). Septic thrombosis may complicate otitis media and mastoiditis, infections of paranasal sinuses and facial infections. Although its frequency has decreased, it was still responsible for four of 15 cases of thrombosis in older children in one recent series (Barron *et al.* 1992). Aseptic or primary thrombosis is now more common than the septic form. It is a common complication of congenital cyanotic heart disease, in which it occurs preferentially in patients over 2–3 years of age with an haematocrit of more than 70 per cent and in association with dehydration. It may be difficult to distinguish from strokes of arterial origin. Alterations in haemodynamics such as dehydration (Aicardi and Goutières 1973), shock or heart failure, diabetic ketoacidosis and chronic debilitating conditions may be responsible. Haematological disorders such as leukaemia or thrombocytosis (Haan *et al.* 1988), or a hypercoagulable state such as results from the use of certain drugs especially 4-L-asparaginase (Priest *et al.* 1980, Barron *et al.* 1992) or from diseases such as the nephrotic syndrome (Igarashi *et al.* 1988), are important causes in older children. Lupus erythematosus may be a cause (Uziel *et al.* 1995), and the possible responsibility of antiphospholipid antibodies has been considered (Göbel 1994). Idiopathic cases occur (Konishi *et al.* 1987). Oral contraceptives, which are increasingly used by adolescent girls, may be a factor in some of these cases (Imai *et al.* 1982), and pregnancy is known to predispose to venous thrombosis. In neonates, sepsis plays a significant role (Barron *et al.* 1992) but many cases appear to be idiopathic (Wong *et al.* 1987, Shevell *et al.* 1989, Rivkin *et al.* 1992). Rarer causes include protein C or S deficiency (Koelman *et al.* 1992, Prats *et al.* 1992, Kennedy *et al.* 1995) which may, however, be secondary to the stroke and should be verified six months later (Dusser *et al.* 1988), and resistance to activated protein C resulting from a genetic mutation of factor V (Svensson and Dahlbäck 1994, Nowak-Göttl *et al.* 1996), which is the most frequent hereditary cause of venous thrombosis. It may also be a cause of arterial thrombosis in infants and even during late fetal life (Thorarensen *et al.* 1997). Dural sinus thrombosis complicating subclavian vein catheterization has been reported (Gebara *et al.* 1995).

The *clinical picture* of venous thrombosis is variable and nonspecific. In older children, headache, disturbances of consciousness, visual disturbances including papilloedema, and focal signs such as seizures, hemiparesis, hemianopia or aphasia should suggest the diagnosis when they complicate a febrile illness or another predisposing condition. Some cases, especially of isolated sinus thrombosis, present with isolated intracranial hypertension, the so-called pseudotumour cerebri (Chapter 14), whereas

TABLE 15.4
Main causes of dural sinus and cerebral venous thrombosis

Cause	References
Septic thrombosis	
Otitis media and mastoiditis	Southwick *et al.* (1986)
Paranasal sinuses	Lew *et al.* (1983)
Cutaneous infections (scalp or face)	Southwick *et al.* (1986)
Purulent meningitis	Swartz and Dodge (1965)
Metastatic infections	Southwick *et al.* (1986)
Sepsis in neonates	Barron *et al.* (1992)
Aseptic thrombosis	
Acute dehydration	Aicardi and Goutières (1973)
Cyanotic congenital heart disease	Tyler and Clark (1957)
Congestive heart failure	Towbin (1973)
Leukaemia and myeloproliferative disorders	Packer *et al.* (1985), Haan *et al.* (1988)
Haemolytic anaemia	Bousser *et al.* (1985)
Hereditary haemoglobinopathies	R.J. Adams *et al.* (1988)
Iron deficiency anaemia	Hartfield *et al.* (1997)
Resistance to activated protein C	Svensson and Dahlbäck (1994)
Protein C deficiency	Wintzen *et al.* (1985)
Protein S deficiency	Koelman *et al.* (1992)
Antithrombin III deficiency	Tarras *et al.* (1988)
Asparaginase therapy	Barron *et al.* (1992)
Disseminated intravascular coagulation	Packer *et al.* (1985)
Homocystinuria	Clarke *et al.* (1991)
Thrombocytosis	McDonald *et al.* (1989)
Polycythaemia	Adamson *et al.* (1973)
Nephrotic syndrome	Igarashi *et al.* (1988)
Lupus erythematosus	Uziel *et al.* (1995)
Pregnancy	Bousser *et al.* (1985)
Hormonal contraception	Buchanan and Brazinsky (1970), Dindar and Platts (1974)
Behçet syndrome	Bank and Weart (1984)
Ulcerative colitis	Wiznitzer and Masaryk (1991)
Diabetes mellitus	Bousser *et al.* (1985)
Trauma	Carrie and Jaffe (1954)
Catheterization	Newman *et al.* (1980), Gebara *et al.* (1995)
Cryptogenic	
Primary venous thrombosis in neonates	Barron *et al.* (1992), Rivkin *et al.* (1992)
Primary sinus thrombosis in adolescents and young adults	Barron *et al.* (1992)

convulsions and focal signs are usually present with cortical vein thrombosis that produces haemorrhagic infarcts. A dramatic picture of septic thrombosis with rigors and high spiking fever is now rare. When it involves the cavernous sinus, proptosis, ophthalmoplegia and papilloedema with high ICP may be associated (DiNubile *et al.* 1988). Thrombosis of the deep cerebral veins and straight sinus can produce profound disturbances of consciousness, dystonia and opisthotonus, seizures and ocular signs as a result of infarction of the thalami and deep grey and white structures.

In infants, and especially in neonates, dural sinus or cerebral vein thrombosis is mainly manifested by seizures and/or lethargy (Rivkin *et al.* 1992). Seizures were present in three of seven cases

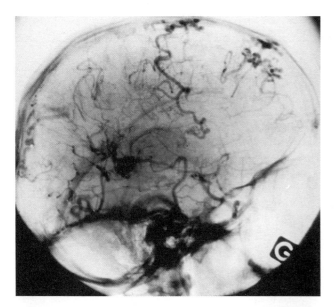

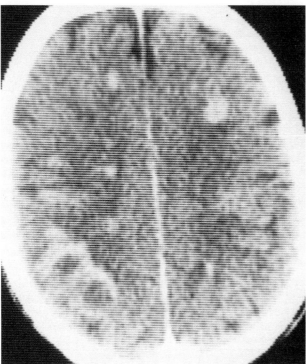

Fig. 15.17. Idiopathic thrombosis of the sagittal sinus in 13-year-old boy. *(Top)* Angiogram showing absence of opacification of sagittal sinus. Note stagnation of contrast in veins of hemispheral convexity. *(Bottom)* CT scan showing areas of hypodensity and haemorrhage in upper part of both hemispheres.

of Rivkin *et al.* and in 15 of 17 cases of Shevell *et al.* (1989). Paucisymptomatic cases are common and the diagnosis often goes unrecognized.

The CSF is often xanthochromic or haemorrhagic. The diagnosis has been made considerably easier by modern neuro-imaging techniques. Angiography best demonstrates obliteration or filling defects in the sinuses (McArdle *et al.* 1987) but has now been replaced by CT and MRI. CT can show areas of low density

and an abnormal visibility of the sinuses on unenhanced scans (Rao *et al.* 1981, Brant-Zawadzki *et al.* 1982, d'Avella *et al.* 1984). Multiple haemorrhagic areas are often present in the deep white matter bilaterally (Fig. 15.17). The empty delta sign is a filling defect within the posterior part of the sagittal sinus on contrast-enhanced scans. Although it may be mimicked by early division of the sagittal sinus, it is a fairly reliable sign (Virapongse *et al.* 1987), and CT has made angiography unnecessary in most cases. MRI is much more precise. Thrombosis suppresses the flow void that is normally seen in the main sinuses. The MRI findings pass through three successive stages: absence of flow void, with low signal in T_2-weighted sequences in the first one to five days, then increasing T_1 and T_2 signal from the sinuses between days six and 15, progressively returning to normal in three to four months; recanalization may occur (Grossman *et al.* 1993, Isensee *et al.* 1994, Perkin 1995).

A fluctuating course is not unusual. Evolution depends on the extent and location of parenchymal damage, which is usually haemorrhagic in type (Konishi *et al.* 1987). When parenchymal involvement is absent or modest the outcome is generally favourable. This was the case in the newborn infants studied by Shevell *et al.* (1989) and by Rivkin *et al.* (1992), but Barron *et al.* (1992) found sequelae only in neonates. Even extensive lesions involving the territory of the deep cerebral veins may regress without sequelae (Forsting *et al.* 1989), although such cases are usually severe and sometimes lethal. Cases due to disorders of coagulation may be associated with a severe clinical picture with extensive haemorrhage (Marciniak *et al.* 1985, Vieregge *et al.* 1989) and involvement of systemic veins (Igarashi *et al.* 1988, Prats *et al.* 1992).

The *treatment* of sinus and cerebral vein thrombosis is still disputed. Heparin treatment is usually not recommended because of the haemorrhagic character of venous infarction and the consequent risk of increasing the damage. No comparative study is available but some investigators have obtained satisfactory results (Isensee *et al.* 1994) with this therapy which tends to be increasingly used. Thrombolytic treatment with urokinase streptokinase is sometimes used (Isensee *et al.* 1994, Perkin 1995). Direct thrombolysis by injection in the sagittal sinus has been used in infants (Higashida *et al.* 1989). General treatment includes antibiotics for septic cases, control of seizures, and reduction of high ICP which may be obtained by the use of dexamethasone.

Thrombosis of the superior vena cava or of both jugular veins induced by indwelling catheters can result in intracranial hypertension or hydrocephalus that usually stabilizes spontaneously (Newman *et al.* 1980).

NEUROLOGICAL COMPLICATIONS OF ARTERIAL HYPERTENSION

Neurological symptoms are a frequent feature of high blood pressure in children and they may be the first manifestation of an unrecognized hypertension. Measurement of blood pressure should be systematic in all children with neurological problems.

HYPERTENSIVE ENCEPHALOPATHY

This disorder is characterized by multiple arteriolar dilatations with disturbance of the blood–brain barrier and consequent disseminated areas of oedema (Chester *et al.* 1978). Headache, seizures, disturbances of consciousness and cortical blindness or blurred vision are the main clinical features (Kandt *et al.* 1995, Wright and Mathews 1996). Hemiplegia, focal seizures, brainstem signs and symptoms suggestive of a mass lesion have been observed in some patients (Del Giudice and Aicardi 1979). Blindness and paraplegia have been recorded (Hulse *et al.* 1979). Papilloedema is often present and is of great diagnostic value especially when accompanied by stellate retinopathy and narrow, abnormal arteries. The EEG shows diffuse slow-wave activity sometimes alternating with episodes of seizure. Paroxysmal complexes reminiscent of those in herpes encephalitis have been reported (Del Giudice and Aicardi 1979). Neuroimaging may show widespread areas of diminished density in the white matter, mainly in the parietal and occipital areas of the hemispheres (Hauser *et al.* 1988, Kandt *et al.* 1995). MRI demonstates focal symmetrically increased signal intensity in white matter and cortex with occipital lobe involvement in each case on T_2-weighted sequences. Hypertensive encephalopathy requires emergency treatment with antihypertensive and anticonvulsant drugs. When high blood pressure is corrected there is clinical recovery, and complete resolution of the abnormal images is observed in a few weeks. The frequent affectation of the occipital cortex accounts for the visual manifestations such as cortical blindness. Renal disease, especially pyelonephritis, is the most common cause of hypertensive encephalopathy and should be systematically searched for. Hemiplegia may, in a few patients, be a manifestation of hypertension. In an occasional such case, CT scan has shown a 'fibre-splitting' haemorrhage of the internal capsule (Brett 1997).

FACIAL PARALYSIS AND HYPERTENSION

The association of facial palsy with hypertension is well recognized in children and adolescents. Facial palsy occurs only with severe hypertension and may be the presenting manifestation of high blood pressure (Siegler *et al.* 1991). Its onset usually co-incides with a rise in blood pressure whereas it tends to disappear when the pressure is lowered. Palsy may last weeks to months and may be recurrent. According to Brett (1997), 11 per cent of children with hypertension develop facial palsy and 11 per cent of peripheral lower facial palsies in children are caused by hypertension. Haemorrhage within the nerve sheath may be the cause of paralysis.

COMPLICATIONS OF HYPOTENSIVE TREATMENT

Hulse *et al.* (1979) reported severe neurological problems at the time of reduction of long-standing arterial hypertension in three children. All three patients developed optic nerve infarction with permanent loss of vision, and one child had, in addition, ischaemic transverse myelopathy. This serves to emphasize that lowering of blood pressure should be cautiously conducted in patients with established hypertensive disorder. Sudden reduction

of hypertension such as may occur in newborn infants with bronchopulmonary dysplasia (Abman 1984) following the use of captopril can produce seizures and focal neurological deficits (Perlman and Volpe 1989).

REFERENCES

Abbasioun, K., Amirjamshidi, A., Rahmat, H. (1985) 'Bilateral mycotic aneurysms of the intracavernous carotid artery.' *Neurosurgery*, **16**, 235–237.

Abe, M., Kjellberg, R.N., Adams, R.D. (1989) 'Clinical presentations of vascular malformations of the brain stem: comparison of angiographically positive and negative types.' *Journal of Neurology, Neurosurgery, and Psychiatry*, **52**, 167–175.

Aberfeld, D.C., Rao, K.R. (1981) 'Familial arteriovenous malformation of the brain.' *Neurology*, **31**, 184–187.

Abman, S.H. (1984) 'Systemic hypertension in infants with bronchopulmonary dysplasia.' *Journal of Pediatrics*, **104**, 928–931.

Abram, H.S., Knepper, L.E., Warty, V.S., Painter, M.J. (1996) 'Natural history, prognosis and lipid abnormalities of idiopathic ischemic childhood stroke.' *Journal of Child Neurology*, **11**, 276–282.

Adams, H.P., Kassell, N.F., Kongable, G.A., Torner, J.C. (1988) 'Intracranial operation within seven days of aneurysmal subarachnoid hemorrhage.' *Archives of Neurology*, **45**, 1065–1069.

Adams, R.J. (1995) 'Sickle cell disease and stroke.' *Journal of Child Neurology*, **10**, 75–76.

—— Nichols, F.T., McKie, V., *et al.* (1988) 'Cerebral infarction in sickle cell anemia: mechanism based on CT and MRI.' *Neurology*, **38**, 1012–1017.

Adamson, J.W., Stamatoyannopoulos, G., Kontras, S. (1973) 'Recessive familial erythrocytosis: aspect of narrow regulation in two families.' *Blood*, **41**, 641–651.

Adelt, D., Brückmann, H., Krenkel, W., *et al.* (1988) 'Combined neuro-radiological and neurosurgical treatment of intracerebral arteriovenous malformations.' *Journal of Neurology*, **235**, 355–358.

Afifi, A.K., Godersky, J.C., Menezes, A., *et al.* (1987) 'Cerebral hemiatrophy, hypoplasia of the internal carotid artery and intracranial aneurysm: a rare association occurring in an infant.' *Archives of Neurology*, **44**, 232–235.

Ahuja, G.K., Jian, N., Vijayaraghovan, M., Roy, S. (1978) 'Cerebral mycotic aneurysm of fungal origin.' *Journal of Neurosurgery*, **49**, 107–110.

Aicardi, J., Goutières, F. (1973) 'Les thromboses veineuses intracraniennes, complication des déshydratations aiguës du nourrisson.' *Archives Françaises de Pédiatrie*, **30**, 809–830.

—— Amsili, J., Chevrie, J.J. (1969) 'Acute hemiplegia in infancy and childhood.' *Developmental Medicine and Child Neurology*, **11**, 162–173.

Albert, M.L., Greer, W.E.R., Kantrowitz, W. (1969) 'Paraplegia secondary to hypotension and cardiac arrest in a patient who has had previous thoracic surgery.' *Neurology*, **19**, 915–918.

Albright, A.L., Latchaw, R.E., Price, R.A. (1983) 'Posterior dural arteriovenous malformations in infancy.' *Neurosurgery*, **13**, 129–135.

Alexander, G.L. (1972) 'Sturge–Weber syndrome.' *In:* Vinken, P.J., Bruyn, G.W. (Eds.) *Handbook of Clinical Neurology, Vol. 14. Phakomatoses.* Amsterdam: North Holland, pp. 223–240.

Alhalabi, M., Moore, P.M. (1994) 'Serial angiography in isolated angiitis of the central nervous system.' *Neurology*, **44**, 1221–1226.

Allard, J.C., Hochberg, P.H., Franklin, P.D., Carter, A.P. (1989) 'Magnetic resonance imaging in a family with hereditary cerebral arteriovenous malformations.' *Archives of Neurology*, **46**, 184–187.

Allen, J.P., Imbus, C.E., Powars, D.R., Haywood, L.J. (1976) 'Neurologic impairment induced by hyperventilation in children with sickle cell anemia.' *Pediatrics*, **58**, 124–126.

Amacher, A.L., Drake, C.G. (1975) 'Cerebral artery aneurysms in infancy, childhood and adolescence.' *Child's Brain*, **1**, 72–80.

Aminoff, M.S., Edwards, M.S.B. (1989) 'Spinal arteriovenous malformations.' *In:* Edwards, M.S.B., Hoffman, H.J. (Eds.) *Cerebral Vascular Disease in Children and Adolescents.* Baltimore: Williams & Wilkins, pp. 321–335.

Anderson, K.A., Burbach, J.A., Fenton, L.J., *et al.* (1985) 'Idiopathic arterial calcification of infancy in newborn siblings with unusual light and electron microscopic manifestations.' *Archives of Pathology and Laboratory Medicine*, **109**, 838–842.

Andrews, B.T., Hudgins, R.J., Edwards, M.S.B. (1989) 'Mycotic aneurysms in children.' *In:* Edwards, M.S.B., Hoffman, H.J. (Eds.) *Cerebral Vascular*

Disease in Children and Adolescents. Baltimore: Williams & Wilkins, pp. 275–282.

Angelini, L., Ravelli, A., Caporali, R., *et al.* (1994) 'High prevalence of antiphospholipid antibodies in children with idiopathic cerebral ischemia.' *Pediatrics*, **94**, 500–503.

Aram, D.M., Rose, D.F., Rekate, H.L., Whitaker, A.H. (1983) 'Acquired capsular/striatal aphasia in childhood.' *Archives of Neurology*, **40**, 614–617.

Ardinger, R.H., Goertz, K.K., Mattioli, L.F. (1994) 'Cerebrovascular stenoses with cerebral infarction in a child with Williams syndrome.' *American Journal of Medical Genetics*, **51**, 200–202.

Armstrong, F.D., Thompson, R.J., Wang, W., *et al.* (1996) 'Cognitive functioning and brain magnetic resonance imaging in children with sickle cell disease.' *Pediatrics*, **97**, 864–870.

Arseni, C., Nereantiu, F., Nicolescu, P. (1973) 'The infantile form of diffuse sclerosis with meningeal angiomatosis.' *Neurology*, **23**, 1297–1301.

Arzimanoglou, A., Aicardi, J. (1992) 'The epilepsy of Sturge–Weber syndrome: clinical features and treatment in 23 patients.' *Acta Neurologica Scandinavica*, **86**, Suppl. 140, 18–22.

Asinger, R.W., Dyken, M.L., Fisher, M., *et al.* (1989) 'Cardiogenic brain embolism. The second report of the Cerebral Embolism Task Force.' *Archives of Neurology*, **46**, 727–743.

Atluru, V.L., Epstien, L.G., Gootman, N. (1985) 'Childhood stroke and supraventricular tachycardia.' *Pediatric Neurology*, **1**, 54–56.

Atuk, N.O., McDonald, T., Wood, T., *et al.* (1979) 'Familial pheochromocytoma, hypercalcemia, and von Hippel–Lindau disease. A ten year study of a large family.' *Medicine*, **58**, 209–218.

Bank, I., Weart, C. (1984) 'Dural sinus thrombosis in Behçet's disease.' *Arthritis and Rheumatism*, **27**, 816–818.

Banker, B.Q. (1961) 'Cerebral vascular disease in infancy and childhood. I. Occlusive vascular diseases.' *Journal of Neuropathology and Experimental Neurology*, **20**, 127–140.

Baraitser, P., Shieff, C. (1990) 'Cutaneomeningospinal angiomatosis: the syndrome of Cobb. A case report.' *Neuropediatrics*, **21**, 160–161.

Barron, T.F., Gusnard, D.A., Zimmerman, R.A., Clancy, M.R. (1992) 'Cerebral venous thrombosis in neonates and children.' *Pediatric Neurology*, **8**, 112–116.

Barron, T.F., Ostrov, B.E., Zimmermann, R.A., Packer, R.J. (1993) 'Isolated angiitis of CNS: treatment with pulse cyclophosphamide.' *Pediatric Neurology*, **9**, 73–75.

Barson, A.J., Chiswick, M.L. (1978) 'Fat embolism in infancy after intravenous fat infusions.' *Archives of Disease in Childhood*, **53**, 218–223.

Barth, A., Bogousslavsky, J., Regli, F. (1993) 'The clinical and topographic spectrum of cerebellar infarcts: a clinical–magnetic resonance imaging correlation study.' *Annals of Neurology*, **33**, 451–456.

Batjer, H., Samson, D. (1986) 'Arteriovenous malformations of the posterior fossa. Clinical presentation, diagnostic evaluation and surgical treatment.' *Journal of Neurology*, **64**, 849–856.

Baxter, P., Gardner-Medwin, D., Green, S.H., Moss, C. (1993) 'Congenital livedo reticularis and recurrent stroke-like episodes.' *Developmental Medicine and Child Neurology*, **35**, 917–921.

Becker, D.H., Townsend, J.J., Kramer, R.A., Newton, T.H. (1979) 'Occult cerebrovascular malformations. A series of 18 histologically verified cases with negative angiography.' *Brain*, **102**, 249–287.

Belman, A.L., Leicher, C.R., Moshé, S.L., Mezey, A.P. (1985) 'Neurologic manifestations of Schoenlein–Henoch purpura: report of three cases and review of the literature.' *Pediatrics*, **75**, 687–692.

Beltramello, A., Benati, A., Maschio, A., Perini, S. (1987) 'Therapeutic angiography in infants and children.' *Journal of Pediatric Neurosciences*, **3**, 79–91.

Bendheim, P.E., Berg, B.O. (1981) 'Ataxic hemiparesis from a midbrain mass.' *Annals of Neurology*, **9**, 405–407.

Benedikt, R.A., Brown, D.C., Walker, R., *et al.* (1993) 'Sturge–Weber syndrome: cranial MR imaging with Gd-DTPA.' *American Journal of Neuroradiology*, **14**, 409–415.

Beyer, R.A., Paden, P., Sobel, D.F., Flynn, F.G. (1986) 'Moyamoya pattern of vascular occlusion after radiotherapy for glioma of the optic chiasm.' *Neurology*, **36**, 1173–1178.

Binder, B., Eng, G.D., Milhorat, T.H., Galioto, F. (1982) 'Spinal arteriovenous malformations in an infant: unusual symptomology and pathology.' *Developmental Medicine and Child Neurology*, **24**, 380–385.

Bland, L.I., Lapham, L.W., Ketonen, L., Okawara, S-H. (1994) 'Acute cerebellar hemorrhage secondary to capillary telangiectasia in an infant. A case report.' *Archives of Neurology*, **51**, 1151–1154.

Bodensteiner, J.B., Hille, M.R., Riggs, J.E. (1992) 'Clinical features of vascular thrombosis following varicella.' *American Journal of Diseases of Children*, **146**, 100–102.

Bogousslavsky, J., Regli, F., Delaloye, B., *et al.* (1986) 'Hémiataxie et déficit sensitif ipsilatéral. Infarctus du territoire de l'artère choroïdienne antérieure diaschisis cérébelleux croisé.' *Revue Neurologique*, **142**, 671–676.

Bolander, H., Hassler, O., Liléquiest, B., West, K.A. (1978) 'Cerebral aneurysm in an infant with fibromuscular hyperplasia of the renal arteries: case report.' *Journal of Neurosurgery*, **49**, 756–759.

Boltshauser, E., Wilson, J., Hoare, R.D. (1976) 'Sturge–Weber syndrome with bilateral intracranial calcification.' *Journal of Neurology, Neurosurgery, and Psychiatry*, **39**, 429–435.

Bordarier, C., Aicardi, J. (1990) 'Dandy–Walker syndrome and agenesis of the cerebellar vermis: diagnostic problems and genetic counselling.' *Developmental Medicine and Child Neurology*, **32**, 285–294.

Borushok, M.J., White, R.I., Oh, K.S., Dorst, J.P. (1974) 'Congenital subclavian steal.' *American Journal of Roentgenology*, **121**, 559–564.

Bousser, M.G., Chiras, J., Bories, J., Castaigne, P. (1985) 'Cerebral venous thrombosis: a review of 38 cases.' *Stroke*, **16**, 199–213.

Boyd, M.C., Steinbok, P., Paty, D.W. (1985) 'Familial arteriovenous malformations: report of four cases in one family.' *Journal of Neurosurgery*, **62**, 597–599.

Bozoky, B., Bara, D., Kertesz, E. (1984) 'Autopsy study of cerebral complications of congenital heart disease and cardiac surgery.' *Journal of Neurology*, **231**, 153–161.

Brant-Zawadzki, M., Chang, G.Y., McCarty, G.E. (1982) 'Computed tomography in dural sinus thrombosis.' *Archives of Neurology*, **39**, 446–447.

Brenner, R.P., Sharbrough, F.W. (1976) 'Electroencephalographic evaluation in Sturge–Weber syndrome.' *Neurology*, **26**, 629–632.

Brett, E.M. (1997) 'Vascular disorders of the nervous system in childhood.' *In:* Brett, E.M. (Ed.) *Paediatric Neurology, 3rd Edn.* Edinburgh: Churchill Livingstone, pp. 571–588.

Brey, R.L., Hart, R.G., Sherman, D.G., Tegeler, C.H. (1990) 'Antiphospholipid antibodies and cerebral ischemia in young people.' *Neurology*, **40**, 1190–1196.

Brosnahan, D., McFadzean, R.M., Teasdale, E. (1992) 'Neuro-ophthalmic features of carotid cavernous fistulas and their treatment by endoarterial balloon embolisation.' *Journal of Neurology, Neurosurgery, and Psychiatry*, **55**, 553–556.

Bruyn, R.P.M., Van der Veen, J.P.W., Donker, A.J.M. (1987) 'Sneddon's syndrome. Case report and literature review.' *Journal of Neurological Sciences*, **79**, 243–253.

Buchanan, D.S., Brazinsky, J.H. (1970) 'Dural sinus and cerebral venous thrombosis. Incidence in young women receiving oral contraceptives.' *Archives of Neurology*, **22**, 440–444.

Buchanan, G.R., Bowhan, W.P., Smith, S.J. (1983) 'Recurrent cerebral ischaemia during hypertransfusion therapy in sickle cell anemia.' *Journal of Pediatrics*, **103**, 921–923.

Bush, J.K., Givner, L.B., Whitaker, S.H., *et al.* (1984) 'Necrotizing fasciitis of the parapharyngeal space with carotid artery occlusion and acute hemiplegia.' *Pediatrics*, **73**, 343–347.

Bussone, G., Parati, E.A., Boiardi, A., *et al.* (1984) 'Divry–van Bogaert syndrome.' *Archives of Neurology*, **41**, 560–562.

Bye, A.M.E., Andermann, F., Robitaille, Y., *et al.* (1993) 'Cortical vascular abnormalities in the syndrome of celiac disease, epilepsy, bilateral occipital calcifications, and folate deficiency.' *Annals of Neurology*, **34**, 399–403.

Caekebeke, J.F.V., Peters, A.C.B., Vandvik, B., *et al.* (1990) 'Cerebral vasculopathy associated with primary varicella infection.' *Archives of Neurology*, **47**, 1033–1035.

Carney, J.A. (1985) 'Differences between nonfamilial and familial cardiac myxoma.' *American Journal of Surgical Pathology*, **9**, 53–55.

Carrie, A.W., Jaffe, F.A. (1954) 'Thrombosis of superior sagittal sinus caused by trauma without penetrating injury.' *Journal of Neurosurgery*, **11**, 173–182.

Castaigne, P., Lhermitte, F., Gautier, J.C., *et al.* (1973) 'Arterial occlusion in the vertebro-basilar system. A study of 44 patients with post-mortem data.' *Brain*, **96**, 133–154.

Celli, P., Ferrante, L., Palma, L. (1984) 'Cerebral arteriovenous malformations in children. Clinical features and outcome of treatment in children and adults.' *Surgical Neurology*, **22**, 43–49.

Cerebral Embolism Task Force (1986) 'Cardiogenic brain embolism.' *Archives of Neurology*, **43**, 71–84.

Chabriat, H., Tournier-Lasserve, E., Vahedi, K., *et al.* (1995a) 'Autosomal dominant migraine with MRI white-matter abnormalities mapping to the CADASIL locus.' *Neurology*, **45**, 1086–1091.

—— Vahedi, K., Iba-Zizen, M.T., *et al.* (1995b) 'Clinical spectrum of CADASIL: a study of 7 families.' *Lancet*, **346**, 934–939.

Chalhub, E.G., De Vivo, D.C., Siegel, B.A., *et al.* (1977) 'Coxsackie A9 focal encephalitis associated with acute infantile hemiplegia and porencephaly.' *Neurology*, **27**, 574–579.

Chang, H.S., Fukushima, T., Miyazaki, S., Tamagawa, T. (1986) 'Fusiform posterior cerebral artery aneurysm treated with excision and end-to-end anastomosis. Case report.' *Journal of Neurosurgery*, **64**, 501–504.

Chang, V., Rewcastle, N.B., Harwood-Nash, D.C. (1975) 'Bilateral dissecting aneurysm of the intracranial carotid arteries in an 8-year old boy.' *Neurology*, **25**, 573–579.

Chapman, A.B., Rubinstein, D., Hughes, R., *et al.* (1992) 'Intracranial aneurysms in autosomal dominant polycystic kidney disease.' *New England Journal of Medicine*, **327**, 916–920.

Chatkupt, S., Epstein, L.G., Rappaport, R., Koenigsberger, M.R. (1987) 'Cerebellar infarction in children.' *Pediatric Neurology*, **3**, 363–366.

Chester, E.M., Agamanolis, D.P., Banker, B.Q., Victor, M. (1978) 'Hypertensive encephalopathy: a clinicopathologic study of 20 cases.' *Neurology*, **28**, 928–939.

Chevrie, J.J., Specola, N., Aicardi, J. (1988) 'Secondary bilateral synchrony in unilateral pial angiomatosis: successful surgical treatment.' *Journal of Neurology, Neurosurgery, and Psychiatry*, **51**, 663–670.

Chiron, C., Raynaud, C., Tzourio, N., *et al.* (1989) 'Regional cerebral blood flow by SPECT imaging in Sturge–Weber disease: an aid for diagnosis.' *Journal of Neurology, Neurosurgery, and Psychiatry*, **52**, 1402–1409.

Chiu, N-C., DeLong, G.R., Heinz, R. (1996) 'Intracranial fibromuscular dysplasia in a 5-year-old child.' *Pediatric Neurology*, **14**, 262–264.

Chuang, S. (1989) 'Vascular diseases of the brain in children.' *In:* Edwards, M.S.B., Hoffman, H.J. (Eds.) *Cerebral Vascular Disease in Children and Adolescents*. Baltimore: Williams & Wilkins, pp. 69–93.

Chugani, H.T., Mazziotta, J.C., Phelps, M.E. (1989) 'Sturge–Weber syndrome: a study of cerebral glucose utilization with positron emission tomography.' *Journal of Pediatrics*, **114**, 244–253.

Churchyard, A., Khangure, M., Grainger, K. (1992) 'Cerebral cavernous angioma: a potentially benign condition? Successful treatment in 16 cases.' *Journal of Neurology, Neurosurgery, and Psychiatry*, **55**, 1040–1045.

Clarke, R., Daly, L., Robinson, K., *et al.* (1991) 'Hyperhomocysteinemia: an independent risk factor for vascular disease.' *New England Journal of Medicine*, **324**, 1149–1155.

Cohen, H.C.M., Tucker, W.S., Humphreys, R.P. (1982) 'Angiographically cryptic histologically verified cerebrovascular malformations.' *Neurosurgery*, **10**, 704–714.

Connolly, J.H., Hutchinson, W.M., Allen, I.V., *et al.* (1975) 'Carotid artery thrombosis, encephalitis, myelitis and optic neuritis associated with rubella virus infections.' *Brain*, **98**, 583–594.

Cranberg, L.D., Filley, C.M., Hart, E.J., Alexander, M.P. (1987) 'Acquired aphasia in childhood: clinical and CT investigations.' *Neurology*, **37**, 1165–1172.

Craven, R.S., French, J.K. (1985) 'Isolated angiitis of the central nervous system.' *Annals of Neurology*, **18**, 263–265.

Crawford, P.M., West, C.R., Chadwick, D.W., Shaw, M.D.M. (1986) 'Arteriovenous malformations of the brain: natural history in unoperated patients.' *Journal of Neurology, Neurosurgery, and Psychiatry*, **49**, 1–10.

Criscuolo, G.R., Oldfield, E.H., Doppman, J.L. (1989) 'Reversible acute and subacute myelopathy in patients with dural arteriovenous fistulas. Foix–Alajouanine syndrome reconsidered.' *Journal of Neurosurgery*, **70**, 354–359.

Cubberley, D.A., Jaffe, R.B., Nixon, G.W. (1982) 'Sonographic demonstration of Galenic arteriovenous malformation in the neonate.' *American Journal of Neuroradiology*, **3**, 435–439.

Cupps, T.R., Moore, P.M., Fauci, A.S. (1983) 'Isolated angiitis of the central nervous system. Prospective diagnostic and therapeutic experience.' *American Journal of Medicine*, **74**, 99–105.

D'Angelo, A., Della Valle, P., Crippa, L., *et al.* (1993) 'Autoimmune protein S deficiency in a boy with severe thromboembolic disease.' *New England Journal of Medicine*, **328**, 1753–1757.

D'Avella, D., Russo, A., Santoro, G. (1984) 'Diagnosis of superior sagittal sinus thrombosis by computed tomography.' *Journal of Neurosurgery*, **61**, 1129–1131.

Debehnke, D.J., Singer, J.I. (1991) 'Vertebrobasilar occlusion following minor trauma in an 8-year-old boy.' *American Journal of Emergency Medicine*, **9**, 49–51.

Debrun, G., Sauvegrain, J., Aicardi, J., Goutières, F. (1975) 'Moyamoya: a nonspecific radiological syndrome.' *Neuroradiology*, **8**, 241–244.

Decroix, J.P., Graveleau, P., Masson, M., Cambier, J. (1986) 'Infarction in the territory of the anterior choroidal artery. A clinical and computerized tomographic study of 16 cases.' *Brain*, **109**, 1071–1085.

Del Giudice, E., Aicardi, J. (1979) 'Atypical aspects of hypertensive encephalopathy in childhood.' *Neuropediatrics*, **10**, 150–157.

Demierre, B., Rondot, P. (1983) 'Dystonia caused by putamino-capsulo-caudate vascular lesions.' *Journal of Neurology, Neurosurgery, and Psychiatry*, **46**, 404–409.

Devilat, M., Toso, M., Morales, M. (1993) 'Childhood stroke associated with protein C or S deficiency and primary antiphospholipid syndrome.' *Pediatric Neurology*, **9**, 67–70.

Diebler, C., Dulac, O. (1987) *Pediatric Neurology and Neuroradiology.* Berlin: Springer Verlag.

—— —— Renier, D. (1981) 'Aneurysms of the vein of the Galen in infants aged 2 to 15 months. Diagnosis and natural evolution.' *Neuroradiology*, **21**, 185–197.

Dindar, F., Platts, M.E. (1974) 'Intracranial venous thrombosis complicating oral contraception.' *Canadian Medical Association Journal*, **111**, 545–548.

DiNubile, M.J. (1988) 'Septic thrombosis of the cavernous sinuses.' *Archives of Neurology*, **45**, 567–572.

Dobyns, W.B., Michels, V.V., Groover, R.V., *et al.* (1987) 'Familial cavernous malformations of the central nervous system and retina.' *Annals of Neurology*, **21**, 578–583.

Drake, C.G. (1979) 'Cerebral arteriovenous malformations: considerations for and experience with surgical treatment in 166 cases.' *Clinical Neurosurgery*, **26**, 145–208.

Drigo, P., Mammi, I., Battistella, P.A., *et al.* (1994) 'Familial cerebral, hepatic, and retinal cavernous angiomas: a new syndrome.' *Child's Nervous System*, **10**, 205–209.

Dubovsky, J., Zabramski, J.M., Kurth, J, *et al.* (1995) 'A gene responsible for cavernous malformations of the brain maps to chromosome 7q.' *Human Molecular Genetics*, **4**, 453–458.

Dulac, O., Aicardi, J.. (1975) 'Paraplégie compliquant le cathétérisme artériel ombilical.' *Archives Françaises de Pédiatrie*, **32**, 659–664.

Dusser, A., Goutières, F., Aicardi, J. (1986) 'Ischemic strokes in children.' *Journal of Child Neurology*, **1**, 131–136.

—— Boyer-Neumann, C., Wolf, M. (1988) 'Temporary protein C deficiency associated with cerebral arterial thrombosis in childhood.' *Journal of Pediatrics*, **113**, 849–851.

Dvir, M., Beer, S., Aladjem, M. (1988) 'Heredofamilial syndrome of mesodermal hamartomas, macrocephaly and pseudopapilledema.' *Pediatrics*, **81**, 287–290.

Echenne, B., Gras, M., Astruc, J., *et al.* (1983) 'Vertebrobasilar arterial occlusion in childhood. Report of a case and review of the literature.' *Brain and Development*, **5**, 577–581.

Edwards, M.S.B., Heishima, G., Higashida, R., Van Halbach, (1988) 'Management of vein of Galen malformations in the neonate.' *International Pediatrics*, **3**, 184–188.

Eeg-Olofsson, O., Ringheim, Y. (1983) 'Stroke in children: clinical characteristics and prognosis.' *Acta Paediatrica Scandinavica*, **72**, 391–396.

Eljamel, M.S.M., Humphrey, P.R.D., Shaw, M.D.M. (1990) 'Dissection of the cervical internal carotid artery. The role of Doppler/Duplex studies and conservative management.' *Journal of Neurology, Neurosurgery, and Psychiatry*, **53**, 379–383.

El Mahdi, M., Rudwan, M.A., Khaffaji, S.M., Jadallah, F.A. (1989) 'A giant spinal aneurysm with cord and root compression.' *Journal of Neurology, Neurosurgery, and Psychiatry*, **52**, 532–535.

Elster, A.D., Chen, M.Y.M. (1990) 'MR imaging of Sturge–Weber syndrome: role of gadopentetate dimeglumine and gradient echo techniques.' *American Journal of Neuroradiology*, **11**, 685–689.

Enjolras, O., Riche, M.C., Merland, J.J. (1985) 'Facial port-wine stains and Sturge–Weber syndrome.' *Pediatrics*, **76**, 48–51.

Erenberg, G., Rubin, R., Shulman, K. (1972) 'Cerebellar haematomas caused by angiomas in children.' *Journal of Neurology, Neurosurgery, and Psychiatry*, **35**, 304–310.

Fabian, R.H., Peters, B.H. (1984) 'Neurological complications of hemoglobin SC disease.' *Archives of Neurology*, **41**, 289–292.

Farmer, J-P., Cosgrove, G.R., Villemure, J-G., *et al.* (1988) 'Intracerebral cavernous angiomas.' *Neurology*, **38**, 1699–1704.

Fearnley, J.M., Stevens, J.M., Rudge, P. (1995) 'Superficial siderosis of the central nervous system.' *Brain*, **118**, 1051–1066.

Ferro, J.M., Martins, I.P., Castro-Caldas, F.P.A. (1982) 'Aphasia following right striato-insular infarction in a left-handed child: a clinico-radiological study.' *Developmental Medicine and Child Neurology*, **24**, 173–178.

Filling-Katz, M.R., Levin, S.W., Patronas, N.J., Katz, N.N.K. (1992) 'Terminal transverse limb defects associated with familial cavernous angiomatosis.' *American Journal of Medical Genetics*, **42**, 346–351.

Finney, H.L., Roberts, T.S., Anderson, R.E. (1976) 'Giant intracranial aneurysm associated with Marfan's syndrome.' *Journal of Neurosurgery*, **45**, 342–347.

Fisher, M., Sotak, C.H., Minematsu, K., Li, L. (1992) 'New magnetic resonance techniques for evaluating cerebrovascular disease.' *Annals of Neurology*, **32**, 115–122.

Fishman, M.A., Baram, T.Z. (1986) 'Megalencephaly due to impaired cerebral venous return in a Sturge–Weber variant syndrome.' *Journal of Child Neurology*, **1**, 115–118.

Forman, H.P., Levin, S., Stewart, B., *et al.* (1989) 'Cerebral vasculitis and hemorrhage in an adolescent taking diet pills containing phenylpropanolamine: case report and review of literature.' *Pediatrics*, **83**, 737–741.

Forsting, M., Krieger, D., Seier, U., Hacke, W. (1989) 'Reversible bilateral thalamic lesions caused by primary internal cerebral vein thrombosis: a case report.' *Journal of Neurology*, **236**, 484–486.

Freedom, R.M. (1989) 'Cerebral vascular disorders of cardiovascular origin in infants and children.' *In:* Edwards, B.S., Hoffman, H.J. (Eds.) *Cerebral Vascular Disease in Children and Adolescents.* Baltimore: Williams & Wilkins, pp. 423–428.

Friede, R.L. (1973) 'Cerebral infarcts complicating neonatal leptomeningitis. Acute and residual lesions.' *Acta Neuropathologica*, **23**, 245–253.

Frima-Verhoeven, P.A.W., Op de Coul, A.A.W., Pijssen, C.C., Maat, B. (1989) 'Intracranial cavernous angiomas: diagnosis and therapy.' *European Neurology*, **29**, 56–60.

Fujiwara, J., Nakahara, S., Enomoto, T., *et al.* (1996) 'The effectiveness of O_2 administration for transient ischemic attacks in moyamoya disease in children.' *Child's Nervous System*, **12**, 69–75.

Fukumoto, S., Kinjo, M., Hokamura, K., Tanaka, K. (1986) 'Subarachnoid hemorrhage and granulomatous angiitis of the basilar artery: demonstration of the varicella-zoster-virus in the basilar artery lesions.' *Stroke*, **17**, 1024–1028.

Fukuyama, Y., Umezu, R. (1985) 'Clinical and cerebral angiographic evolutions of idiopathic progressive occlusive disease of the circle of Willis ("Moyamoya" disease) in children.' *Brain and Development*, **7**, 21–37.

—— Osawa, M., Kanai, M. (1992) 'Moyamoya disease (syndrome) and the Down syndrome.' *Brain and Development*, **14**, 254–256.

Fults, D., Kelly, D.L. (1984) 'Natural history of arteriovenous malformations of the brain: a clinical study.' *Neurosurgery*, **15**, 658–662.

Furie, R., Ishikawa, T., Dhawan, V., Eidelberg, D. (1994) 'Alternating hemichorea in primary antiphospholipid syndrome: evidence for contralateral striatal hypermetabolism.' *Neurology*, **44**, 2197–2199.

Furlan, A.J., Breuer, A.C. (1984) 'Central nervous system complications of open heart surgery.' *Stroke*, **15**, 912–915.

Gabow, P.A. (1993) 'Autosomal dominant polycystic kidney disease.' *New England Journal of Medicine*, **329**, 332–342.

Gan, R., Noronha, A. (1995) 'The medullary vascular syndromes revisited.' *Journal of Neurology*, **242**, 195–202.

Garcia-Monaco, R., De Victor, D., Mann, C., *et al.* (1991a) 'Congestive cardiac manifestations from cerebrocranial arteriovenous shunts. Endovascular management in 30 children.' *Child's Nervous System*, **7**, 48–52.

—— Rodesch, G., Terbrugge, K., *et al.* (1991b) 'Multifocal dural arteriovenous shunts in children.' *Child's Nervous System*, **7**, 425–431.

Garg, B.P., DeMyer, W.E. (1995) 'Ischemic thalamic infarction in children: clinical presentation, etiology, and outcome.' *Pediatric Neurology*, **13**, 46–49.

—— Edwards-Brown, M.K. (1995) 'Vertebral artery compression due to head rotation in thalamic stroke.' *Pediatric Neurology*, **12**, 162–164.

—— Ottinger, C.J., Smith, R.R., Fishman, M.A. (1993) 'Strokes in children due to vertebral artery trauma.' *Neurology*, **43**, 2555–2558.

Garner, T.B., Curling, O.D., Kelly, D.L., Laster, D.W. (1991) 'The natural history of intracranial venous angiomas.' *Journal of Neurosurgery*, **75**, 715–722.

Gastaut, H., Pinsard, N., Gastaut, J.L., *et al.* (1977) 'Etude tomodensitométrique des accidents cérébraux responsables des hémiplégies aiguës de l'enfant.' *Revue Neurologique*, **133**, 595–607.

Gautier, J.C., Hauw, J.J., Awada, A., *et al.* (1988) 'Artères cérébrales dolichoectasiques: association aux aneurysmes de l'aorte abdominale.' *Revue Neurologique*, **144**, 437–446.

Gebara, B.M., Goetting, M.G., Wang, A-M. (1995) 'Dural sinus thrombosis complicating subclavian vein catheterization: treatment with local thrombolysis.' *Pediatrics*, **95**, 138–140.

George, B.D., Neville, B.G.R., Lumley, J.S.P. (1993) 'Transcranial revascularisation in childhood and adolescence.' *Developmental Medicine and Child Neurology*, **35**, 675–682.

Gerosa, M., Licata, C., Fiore, D.L., Iraci, G. (1980) 'Intracranial aneurysms of childhood and adolescence.' *Child's Brain*, **6**, 295–302.

Gilly, R., Lapras, C., Tommas, M. (1977) 'Maladie de Sturge–Weber–Krabbe. Réflexions à partir de 21 cas.' *Pédiatrie*, **32**, 45–64.

Glauser, T.A., Siegel, M.J., Lee, B.C.P., *et al.* (1995) 'Accuracy of neurologic examination and history in detecting evidence of MRI-diagnosed cerebral infarctions in children with sickle-cell hemoglobinopathy.' *Journal of Child Neurology*, **10**, 88–92.

Glueck, C.J., Daniels, S.R., Bates, S., *et al.* (1982) 'Pediatric victims of unexplained stroke and their families: familial lipid and lipoprotein abnormalities.' *Pediatrics*, **69**, 308–316.

Gobbi, G., Sorrenti, G., Santucci, M., *et al.* (1988) 'Epilepsy with bilateral occipital calcifications: a benign onset with progressive severity.' *Neurology*, **38**, 913–920.

Göbel, U. (1994) 'Inherited or acquired disorders of blood coagulation in children with neurovascular complications.' *Neuropediatrics*, **25**, 4–7.

Goh, W.H.S., Lo, R. (1993) 'A new 3C syndrome: cerebellar hypoplasia, cavernous haemangioma and coarctation of the aorta.' *Developmental Medicine and Child Neurology*, **35**, 637–641.

Golden, G.S. (1985) 'Stroke syndromes in childhood.' *Neurologic Clinics*, **3**, 59–75.

Goldman, M.P., Fitzpatrick, R.E., Ruiz-Esparza, J. (1993) 'Treatment of portwine stains (capillary malformation) with the flashlamp-pumped pulsed dye laser.' *Journal of Pediatrics*, **122**, 71–77.

Gomez, M.R. (1994) 'New observations in neurocutaneous angiomatosis.' *Acta Neuropediatrica*, **1**, 80–95.

—— Bebin, E.M. (1987) 'Sturge–Weber syndrome.' *In:* Gomez, M.R. (Ed.) *Neurocutaneous Diseases: a Practical Approach.* London: Butterworths, pp. 356–367.

Gomori, J.M., Grossman, R.I., Bilaniuk, L.T., *et al.* (1985) 'High-field MR imaging of superficial siderosis of the central nervous system.' *Journal of Computer Assisted Tomography*, **9**, 972–975.

—— Goldberg, H.I., *et al.* (1986) 'Occult cerebral vascular malformations: high-field MR imaging.' *Radiology*, **158**, 707–713.

—— Hackney, D.B., *et al.* (1988) 'Variable appearance of subacute intracranial hematomas on high-field spin-echo MR.' *American Journal of Roentgenology*, **150**, 171–178.

Gordon, N., Isler, W. (1989) 'Childhood moyamoya disease.' *Developmental Medicine and Child Neurology*, **31**, 103–107.

Graf, C.J., Perret, G.E., Torner, J.C. (1983) 'Bleeding from cerebral arteriovenous malformations as part of their natural history.' *Journal of Neurosurgery*, **58**, 331–337.

Graf, W.D., Milstein, J.M., Sherry, D.D. (1993) 'Stroke and mixed connective tissue disease.' *Journal of Child Neurology*, **8**, 256–259.

Greenwood, R.D. (1984) 'Mitral valve prolapse. Incidence and clinical course in a pediatric population.' *Clinical Pediatrics*, **23**, 318–320.

Grewal, R.P (1994) 'Stroke in Fabry's disease.' *Journal of Neurology*, **241**, 153–156.

Griesemer, D.A., Theodorou, A.A., Berg, R.A., Spera, T.D. (1994) 'Local fibrinolysis in cerebral venous thrombosis.' *Pediatric Neurology*, **10**, 78–80.

Grossman, R.J., Bruce, D.A., Zimmerman, R.A., *et al.* (1984) 'Vascular steal associated with vein of Galen aneurysm.' *Neuroradiology*, **26**, 381–386.

—— Novak, G., Patel, M., *et al.* (1993) 'MRI in neonatal dural sinus thrombosis.' *Pediatric Neurology*, **9**, 235–238.

Guazzo, E.P., Xuereb, J.H. (1994) 'Spontaneous thrombosis of an arteriovenous malformation.' *Journal of Neurology, Neurosurgery, and Psychiatry*, **57**, 1410–1412.

Gueguen, B., Merland, J.J., Riche, M.C., Rey, A. (1987) 'Vascular malformations of the spinal cord: intrathecal perimedullary arteriovenous fistulas fed by medullary arteries.' *Neurology*, **37**, 969–979.

Haan, J., Caekebeke, J.F.V., Van der Meer, F.J.M., Wintzen, A.R. (1988) 'Cerebral venous thrombosis as presenting sign of myeloproliferative disorders.' *Journal of Neurology, Neurosurgery, and Psychiatry*, **51**, 1219–1220.

Haas, R.H., Marsden, D.L., Capistrano-Estrada, S., *et al.* (1995) 'Acute basal ganglia infarction in propionic acidemia.' *Journal of Child Neurology*, **10**, 18–22.

Hamilton, M.G., Spetzler, R.F. (1994) 'The prospective application of a grading system for arteriovenous malformations.' *Neurosurgery*, **34**, 2–7.

Hanefeld, F., Riehm, H. (1980) 'Therapy of acute lymphoblastic leukaemia in childhood: effects on the nervous system.' *Neuropädiatrie*, **11**, 3–16.

Harbaugh, R.E., Saunders, R.L., Reeves, A.G. (1982) 'Pediatric cerebellar infarction: case report and review of the literature.' *Neurosurgery*, **10**, 593–596.

Hartfield, D.S., Lowry, N.S., Keene, D.L., Yager, J.Y. (1997) 'Iron deficiency: a cause of stroke in infants and children.' *Pediatric Neurology*, **16**, 50–53.

Harvey, F.H., Alvord, E.C. (1972) 'Juvenile cerebral arteriosclerosis and other cerebral arteriopathies of childhood. Six autopsied cases.' *Acta Neurologica Scandinavica*, **48**, 479–509.

Hauser, R.A., Lacey, M., Knight, M.R. (1988) 'Hypertensive encephalopathy: magnetic resonance imaging demonstration of reversible cortical and white matter lesions.' *Archives of Neurology*, **45**, 1078–1083.

Heiskanen, O., Vilkki, J. (1981) 'Intracranial arterial aneurysms in children and adolescents.' *Acta Neurochirurgica*, **59**, 55–63.

Helgason, C.M. (1988) 'A new view of anterior choroidal artery territory infarction.' *Journal of Neurology*, **235**, 387–391.

—— Caplan, L.R., Goodwin, J., Hedges, T. (1986) 'Anterior choroidal artery-territory infarction: report of cases and review.' *Archives of Neurology*, **43**, 681–686.

—— Bergen, D., Bleck, T., *et al.* (1987) 'Infarction after seizure focus resection. Manipulation hemiplegia revisited.' *Epilepsia*, **28**, 340–345.

Helweg-Larsen, S., Larsson, H., Henriksen, O., Sorensen, P.S. (1988) 'Ataxic hemiparesis: three different locations of lesions studied by MRI.' *Neurology*, **38**, 1322–1324.

Heros, R.C., Zervas, N.T., Varsos, V. (1983) 'Cerebral vasospasm after subarachnoid haemorrhage: an update.' *Annals of Neurology*, **14**, 599–608.

—— Korosue, K., Diebold, P.M. (1990) 'Surgical excision of cerebral arteriovenous malformations: late results.' *Neurosurgery*, **25**, 570–578.

Heudes, A.M., Boullie, M.C., Lauret, P., Mallet, E. (1990) 'Hemangiomatose néonatale miliaire.' *Archives Françaises de Pédiatrie*, **47**, 135–138.

Higashida, R.T., Helmer, E., Halbach, V.V., Hieshima, G.B. (1989) 'Direct thrombolytic therapy for superior sagittal sinus thrombosis.' *American Journal of Neuroradiology*, **10**, 54–56.

Higginbottom, M.C., Schultz, P. (1982) 'The Bannayan syndrome: an autosomal dominant disorder consisting of macrocephaly, lipomas, hemangiomas, and the risk for intracranial tumors.' *Pediatrics*, **69**, 632–634.

Hilal, S.K., Solomon, G.E., Gold, A.P., Carter, S. (1971a) 'Primary arterial occlusive disease in children. Part I: Acute acquired hemiplegia.' *Radiology*, **99**, 71–86.

—— —— —— —— (1971b) 'Primary arterial occlusive disease in children. Part II: Neurocutaneous syndromes.' *Radiology*, **99**, 87–94.

Hilt, D.C., Bucholz, D., Krumholz, A., *et al.* (1983) 'Herpes zoster ophthalmicus and delayed contralateral hemiparesis caused by cerebral angiitis: diagnosis and management approaches.' *Annals of Neurology*, **14**, 543–553.

Hirsch, J.F., Pierre-Kahn, A., Renier, D., *et al.* (1984) 'The Dandy–Walker malformation.' *Journal of Neurosurgery*, **61**, 515–522.

Hladky, J-P., Lejeune, J-P., Blond, S., *et al.* (1994) 'Cerebral arteriovenous malformations in children: report on 62 cases.' *Child's Nervous System*, **10**, 328–333.

Hoffman, H.J. (1989) 'Malformations of the vein of Galen.' *In:* Edwards, M.S.B., Hoffman, H.J. (Eds.) *Cerebral Vascular Disease in Children and Adolescents.* Baltimore: Williams & Wilkins, pp. 239–246.

—— Hendrick, E.B., Dennis, M., Armstrong, D. (1979) 'Hemispherectomy for Sturge–Weber syndrome.' *Child's Brain*, **5**, 233–248.

Holden, K.R., Alexander, F. (1970) 'Diffuse neonatal hemangiomatosis.' *Pediatrics*, **46**, 411–421.

Hoover, D.L., Robb, R.M., Petersen, R.A. (1989) 'Optic disc drusen and primary megalencephaly in children.' *Journal of Pediatric Ophthalmology and Strabismus*, **26**, 81–85.

Horowitz, I.N., Niparko, N.A. (1994) 'Vertebral artery dissection with bilateral hemiparesis.' *Pediatric Neurology*, **11**, 252–254.

Horton, D.P., Ferriero, D.M., Mentzer, W.C. (1995) 'Nontraumatic fat embolism syndrome in sickle cell anemia.' *Pediatric Neurology*, **12**, 77–80.

Hosain, S.A., Hughes, J.T., Forem, S.L., *et al.* (1994) 'Use of a calcium channel blocker (nicardipine HCl) in the treatment of childhood moyamoya disease.' *Journal of Child Neurology*, **9**, 378–380.

Hosobuchi, Y. (1989) 'Carotid–cavernous fistulas.' *In:* Edwards, M.S.B.,

Hoffman, H.J. (Eds.) *Cerebral Vascular Disease in Children and Adolescents.* Baltimore: Williams & Wilkins, pp. 215–228.

Hourihan, M., Gates, P.C., McAllister, V.L. (1984) 'Subarachnoid hemorrhage in childhood and adolescence.' *Journal of Neurosurgery*, **60**, 1163–1166.

Howard, R.S. (1986) 'Brainstem haematoma due to presumed cryptic telangiectasia.' *Journal of Neurology, Neurosurgery, and Psychiatry*, **49**, 1241–1245.

Hulse, J.A., Taylor, D.S., Dillon, M.J. (1979) 'Blindness and paraplegia in severe childhood hypertension.' *Lancet*, **2**, 553–556.

Humphreys, R.P. (1989a) 'Infratentorial arteriovenous malformations.' *In:* Edwards, M.S.D., Hoffman, H.J. (Eds.) *Cerebral Vascular Disease in Children and Adolescents.* Baltimore: Williams & Wilkins, pp. 309–320.

—— (1989b) 'Intracranial arterial aneurysms.' *In:* Edwards, M.S.B., Hoffman, H.J. (Eds.) *Cerebral Vascular Disease in Children and Adolescents.* Baltimore: Williams & Wilkins, pp. 247–254.

Hurst, R.W., Kenyon, L.C., Lavi, E., *et al.* (1995) 'Spinal dural arteriovenous fistula: the pathology of venous hypertensive myelopathy.' *Neurology*, **45**, 1309–1313.

Huson, S.M., Harper, P.S., Hourihan, M.D., *et al.* (1986) 'Cerebellar haemangioblastoma and von Hippel–Lindau disease.' *Brain*, **109**, 1297–1310.

Hutchinson, W., O'Riordan, M.D., Cole, G., *et al.* (1995) 'Familial hemiplegic migraine and autosomal dominant arteriopathy with leukoencephalopathy (CADASIL).' *Annals of Neurology*, **38**, 817–824.

Huttenlocher, P.R., Moohr, J.W., Johns, L., Brown, L.D. (1984) 'Cerebral blood flow in sickle cell cerebrovascular disease.' *Pediatrics*, **73**, 615–621.

Ichikawa, K., Tsutsumishita, A., Fujioka, A. (1982) 'Capsular ataxic hemiparesis. A case report.' *Archives of Neurology*, **39**, 585–586.

Igarashi, M., Gilmartin, R.C., Gerald, B., *et al.* (1984) 'Cerebral arteritis and bacterial meningitis.' *Archives of Neurology*, **41**, 531–535.

—— Roy, S., Stapleton, F.B. (1988) 'Cerebrovascular complications in children with nephrotic syndrome.' *Pediatric Neurology*, **4**, 362–365.

Imai, W.K., Everhart, F.R., Sanders, J.M. (1982) 'Cerebral venous sinus thrombosis: report of a case and review of the literature.' *Pediatrics*, **70**, 965–970.

Inagaki, M., Koeda, T., Takeshita, K. (1992) 'Prognosis and MRI after ischemic stroke of the basal ganglia.' *Pediatric Neurology*, **8**, 104–108.

Iqbal, A., Alter, M., Lee, S.H. (1978) 'Pseudoxanthoma elasticum: a review of neurological complications.' *Annals of Neurology*, **4**, 18–20.

Isensee, C., Reul, J., Thron, A. (1994) 'Magnetic resonance imaging of thrombosed dural sinuses.' *Stroke*, **25**, 29–34.

Isler, W. (1984) 'Stroke in children and adolescence.' *European Neurology*, **23**, 421–424.

Jackson, A.C., Boughner, D.R., Barnett, H.J.M. (1984) 'Mitral valve prolapse and cerebral ischemic events in young patients.' *Neurology*, **34**, 784–787.

Jacobson, D.M., Terrence, C.F., Reinmuth, O.M. (1986) 'The neurologic manifestations of fat embolism.' *Neurology*, **36**, 847–851.

Jaeken, J., Carchon, H. (1993) 'The carbohydrate-deficient glycoprotein syndromes: an overview.' *Journal of Inherited Metabolic Disease*, **16**, 813–820.

Jane, J.A., Kassell, N.F., Torner, J.C., Winn, H.R. (1985) 'The natural history of aneurysms and arteriovenous malformations.' *Journal of Neurosurgery*, **62**, 321–323.

Jansen, J.N., Donker, A.J.M., Luth, W.J., Smit, M.E. (1990) 'Moyamoya disease associated with renovascular hypertension.' *Neuropediatrics*, **21**, 44–47.

Jellinger, K., Kucsko, L., Seitelberger, F. (1966) 'Diffuse meningo-cerebrale Angiodysplasie mit hypoplasiogener Isthmusstenose bei einem Neugeborenen.' *Beitrag für Pathologische Anatomie*, **133**, 41–72.

Joy, J.L., Carlo, J.R., Vélez-Borrás, J.R. (1989) 'Cerebral infarction following herpes zoster: the enlarging clinical spectrum.' *Neurology*, **39**, 1640–1643.

Kamholz, J., Tremblay, G. (1985) 'Chickenpox with delayed contralateral hemiparesis caused by cerebral angiitis.' *Annals of Neurology*, **18**, 358–360.

Kandt, R.S., Caoili, A.Q., Lorentz, W.B., Elster, A.D. (1995) 'Hypertensive encephalopathy in children: neuroimaging and treatment.' *Journal of Child Neurology*, **10**, 236–239.

Kappelle, L.J., Willemse, J., Ramos, L.M.P., Van Gijn, J. (1989) 'Ischaemic stroke in the basal ganglia and internal capsule in childhood.' *Brain and Development*, **11**, 283–292.

Kataoka, K., Okuno, T., Mikawa, H., Hojo, H. (1988) 'Cranial computed tomographic and electroencephalographic abnormalities in children with post-convulsive hemiplegia.' *European Neurology*, **28**, 279–284.

Katirji, M.B., Reinmuth, O.M., Latchaw, R.E. (1985) 'Stroke due to vertebral artery injury.' *Archives of Neurology*, **42**, 242–248.

Kattapong, V.J., Hart, B.L., Davis, L.E. (1995) 'Familial cerebral cavernous angiomas: clinical and radiologic studies.' *Neurology*, **45**, 492–497.

Katz, D.I., Alexander, M.P., Mandell, A.M. (1987) 'Dementia following strokes in the mesencephalon and diencephalon.' *Archives of Neurology*, **44**, 1127–1133.

Kelly, J.J., Mellinger, J.F., Sundt, T.M. (1978) 'Intracranial arteriovenous malformations in childhood.' *Annals of Neurology*, **3**, 338–343.

Kemeny, A.A., Dias, P.S., Forster, D.M.C. (1989) 'Results of stereotactic radiosurgery of arteriovenous malformations: an analysis of 52 cases.' *Journal of Neurology, Neurosurgery, and Psychiatry*, **52**, 554–558.

Kennedy, C.R., Warner, G., Kai, M., Chisholm, M. (1995) 'Protein C deficiency and stroke in early life.' *Developmental Medicine and Child Neurology*, **37**, 723–730.

Khurana, D.S., Bonnemann, C.G., Dooling, E.C., *et al.* (1996) 'Vertebral artery dissection: issues in diagnosis and management.' *Pediatric Neurology*, **14**, 255–258.

Kitahara, T., Ariga, N., Yamaura, A., *et al.* (1979) 'Familial occurrence of moya-moya disease. Report of three Japanese families.' *Journal of Neurology, Neurosurgery, and Psychiatry*, **42**, 208–214.

Kᴇᴌᴌ, R.A., Snyder, R.D., Schwarz, H.J. (1976) 'Lateral medullary syndrome in a child. Arteriographic confirmation of vertebral artery occlusion.' *Journal of the American Medical Association*, **235**, 940–941.

Koelfen, W., Wentz, U., Freund, M., Schultze, C. (1995) 'Magnetic resonance angiography in 140 neuropediatric patients.' *Pediatric Neurology*, **12**, 31–38.

Koelman, J.H.T.M., Bakker, C.M., Plandsoen, W.C.G., *et al.* (1992) 'Hereditary protein S deficiency presenting with cerebral sinus thrombosis in an adolescent girl.' *Journal of Neurology*, **239**, 105–106.

Koenig, E., Thron, A., Schrader, V., Dichgans, J. (1989) 'Spinal arteriovenous malformations and fistulae: clinical, neuroradiological and neurophysiological findings.' *Journal of Neurology*, **236**, 260–266.

Kohrman, M.H., Huttenlocher, P.R. (1986) 'Takayasu arteritis: a treatable cause of stroke in infancy.' *Pediatric Neurology*, **2**, 154–158.

Kondziolka, D., Humphreys, R.P., Hoffman, H.J., *et al.* (1992) 'Arteriovenous malformations of the brain in children: a forty-year experience.' *Canadian Journal of Neurological Sciences*, **19**, 40–45.

Konishi, Y., Kuriyama, M., Sudo, M., *et al.* (1987) 'Superior sagittal thrombosis in infancy.' *Pediatric Neurology*, **3**, 222–225.

Koo, E.H., Massey, E.W. (1988) 'Granulomatous angiitis of the central nervous system: protean manifestations and response to treatment.' *Journal of Neurology, Neurosurgery, and Psychiatry*, **51**, 1126–1133.

Korobkin, R. (1980) 'Acute hemiparesis in juvenile insulin-dependent diabetes mellitus (JIDDM).' *Neurology*, **30**, 220–221.

Kuivaniemi, H., Prockop, D.J., Wu, Y., *et al.* (1993) 'Exclusion of mutations in the gene for type III collagen (COL3AI) as a common cause of intracranial aneurysms or cervical artery dissections. Results from sequence analysis of the coding sequences of type III collagen from 55 unrelated patients.' *Neurology*, **43**, 2652–2658.

Kurlan, R., Griggs, R.C. (1983) 'Cyanotic congenital heart disease with suspected stroke: should all patients receive antibiotics?' *Archives of Neurology*, **40**, 209–212.

Kurlan, R., Krall, R.L., Deweese, J.A. (1984) 'Vertebrobasilar ischemia after total repair of tetralogy of Fallot: significance of subclavian steal created by Blalock–Taussig anastomosis. Vertebrobasilar ischemia after correction of tetralogy of Fallot.' *Stroke*, **15**, 359–362.

Labrune, P., Lacroix, C., Goutières, F. *et al.* (1996) 'Extensive brain calcifications, leukodystrophy, and formation of parenchymal cysts: a new progressive disorder due to diffuse cerebral microangiopathy.' *Neurology*, **46**, 1297–1301.

Lance, J.W., Smee, R.I. (1989) 'Partial seizures with visual disturbance treated by radiotherapy of cavernous hemangioma.' *Annals of Neurology*, **26**, 782–785.

Lanska, M.J., Lanska, D.J., Horwitz, S.J., Aram, D.M. (1991) 'Presentation, clinical course, and outcome of childhood stroke.' *Pediatric Neurology*, **7**, 333–341.

Lapointe, J.S., Nugent, R.H., Graebn D.A. (1984) 'Cerebral infarction and regression of widespread aneurysms in Kawasaki's disease. Case report.' *Pediatric Radiology*, **14**, 1–5.

Larsen, P.D., Hellbusch, L.C., Lefkowitz, D.H., Schaefer, G.B. (1997) 'Cerebral arteriovenous malformation in three successive generations.' *Pediatric Neurology*, **17**, 74–76.

Lasjaunias, P., Lopez-Ibor, L., Abanou, A., Halimi, P. (1984) 'Radiological anatomy of the vascularization of cranial dural arteriovenous malformations.' *Anatomia Clinica*, **6**, 87–99.

——— Rodesch, G., Pruvost, P., *et al.* (1989a) 'Treatment of vein of Galen aneurysmal malformation.' *Journal of Neuosurgery*, **70**, 746–750.

——— ——— Ter Brugge, K., *et al.* (1989b) 'Vein of Galen aneurysmal malformations: report of 36 cases managed between 1982 and 1988.' *Acta Neurochirurgica*, **99**, 26–37.

——— Garcia-Monaco, R., Rodesch, G., *et al.* (1991a) 'Vein of Galen malformation. Endovascular management of 43 cases.' *Child's Nervous System*, **7**, 360–367.

——— Ter Brugge, K., Rodesch, G., *et al.* (1991b) 'True and false cerebral venous malformations (so-called venous angiomas and cavernous hemangiomas).' *Neuro-chirurgie*, **35**, 132–139.

——— Hui, F., Zerah, M., *et al.* (1995) 'Cerebral arteriovenous malformations in children. Management of 179 consecutive cases and review of the literature.' *Child's Nervous System*, **11**, 66–79.

Latif, F., Tory, K., Gnarra, J., *et al.* (1993) 'Identification of the von Hippel–Lindau disease tumor suppressor gene.' *Science*, **260**, 1317–1320.

Leblanc, R., Melanson, D., Wilkinson, R.D. (1996) 'Hereditary neurocutaneous angiomatosis. Report of four cases.' *Journal of Neurosurgery*, **85**, 1135–1142.

Le Coz, P., Woimant, F., Rougemont, D., *et al.* (1988) 'Angiopathies cérébrales bénignes et phenylpropanolamine.' *Revue Neurologique*, **144**, 295–300.

Leiguarda, R., Berthier, M., Starkstein, S., *et al.* (1988) 'Ischemic infarction in 28 children with tuberculous meningitis.' *Stroke*, **19**, 200–204.

Leis, A.A., Butler, I.J. (1987) 'Infantile herpes zoster ophthalmicus and acute hemiparesis following intrauterine chickenpox.' *Neurology*, **37**, 1537–1538.

Lemahieu, S.F., Marchau, M.M.B. (1979) 'Intracranial fibromuscular dysplasia and stroke in children.' *Neuroradiology*, **18**, 99–102.

Lemme-Plaghos, L., Kucharczyk, W., Brant-Zawadzki, M., *et al.* (1986) 'MRI of angiographically occult vascular malformations.' *American Journal of Roentgenology*, **146**, 1223–1228.

Levine, E., Collins, D.L., Horton, W.A., Schimke, R.N. (1982) 'CT screening of the abdomen in von Hippel–Lindau disease.' *American Journal of Roentgenology*, **139**, 505–510.

Levine, S.R., Welch, K.M.A. (1988) 'Cocaine and stroke.' *Stroke*, **19**, 779–783.

——— Deegan, M.J., Futrell, N., Welch, K.M.A. (1990) 'Cerebrovascular and neurologic disease associated with antiphospholipid antibodies: 48 cases.' *Neurology*, **40**, 1181–1189.

Lew, D., Southwick, F.S., Montgomery, W.W., *et al.* (1983) 'Sphenoid sinusitis: review of 30 cases.' *New England Journal of Medicine*, **309**, 1149–1154.

Lewis, D.W., Berman, P.H. (1986) 'Vertebral artery dissection and alternating hemiparesis in an adolescent.' *Pediatrics*, **78**, 610–613.

Lipski, S., Brunelle, F., Aicardi, J., *et al.* (1990) 'Gd-DOTA-enhanced MR imaging in two cases of Sturge–Weber syndrome.' *American Journal of Neuroradiology*, **11**, 690–692.

Llorens-Terol, J., Sole-Llenas, J., Tura, A. (1983) 'Stroke due to fibromuscular hyperplasia of the internal carotid artery.' *Acta Paediatrica Scandinavica*, **72**, 299–301.

Loeffler, I.S., Rossitch, E., Siddon, R., *et al.* (1990) 'Role of stereotactic radiosurgery with a linear accelerator in treatment of intracranial arteriovenous malformations and tumors in children.' *Pediatrics*, **85**, 774–782.

Longstreth, W.T., Swanson, P.D. (1984) 'Oral contraceptives and stroke.' *Stroke*, **15**, 747–750.

Lossos, A., Ben-Hur, T., Ben-Nariah, Z., *et al.* (1995) 'Familial Sneddon's syndrome.' *Journal of Neurology*, **242**, 164–168.

Luessenhop, A.J., Rosa, L. (1984) 'Cerebral arteriovenous malformations. Indications for and results of surgery, and the role of intravascular techniques.' *Journal of Neurosurgery*, **60**, 14–22.

Lunsford, L.D., Flickinger, J., Coffey, R.J. (1990) 'Stereotactic gamma knife radiosurgery. Initial North American experience in 207 patients.' *Archives of Neurology*, **47**, 169–175.

MacDonald, J.T., Brown, D.R. (1979) 'Acute hemiparesis in juvenile insulin-dependent diabetes mellitus (JIDDM).' *Neurology*, **29**, 893–896.

Mallouh, A.A., Hamda, J.A. (1986) 'Intracranial hemorrhage in patients with sickle cell anemia.' *American Journal of Diseases of Children*, **140**, 505–506.

Mangiardi, J.R., Daras, M., Geller, M.E., *et al.* (1988) 'Cocaine-related hemorrhage: report of nine cases and review.' *Acta Neurologica Scandinavica*, **77**, 177–180.

Marciniak, E., Wilson, H.D., Marlar, R.A. (1985) 'Neonatal purpura fulminans: a genetic disorder related to the absence of protein C in blood.' *Blood*, **65**, 15–20.

Margolis, G., Odom,G., Woodhall, B. (1961) 'Further experiences with small vascular malformations as a cause of massive cerebral bleeding.' *Journal of Neuropathology and Experimental Neurology*, **20**, 161–168.

Martin, N.A., Edwards, M.S.B. (1989) 'Supratentorial arteriovenous malformations.' *In:* Edwards, M.B.S., Hoffman, H.J. (Eds.) *Cerebral Vascular Disease in Children and Adolescents.* Baltimore: Williams & Wilkins, pp. 283–308.

Mason, I., Aase, J.M., Orrison, M.D., *et al.* (1988) 'Familial cavernous angiomas of the brain in an Hispanic family.' *Neurology,* **38,** 324–326.

Masson, G., Gallet, J.P., Cheron, F., *et al.* (1988) 'Epilepsies avec calcifications corticales bilatérales: discussion d'un déficit post-critique durable.' *Revue Neurologique,* **144,** 499–502.

Matsell, D.G., Keene, D.L., Jimenez, C., Humphreys, P. (1990) 'Isolated angiitis of the central nervous system in childhood.' *Canadian Journal of Neurological Sciences,* **17,** 151–154.

McArdle, C.B., Mirfakhraee, M., Amparo, E.G., Kulkarni, M.V. (1987) 'MR imaging of transverse/sigmoid dural sinus and jugular vein thrombosis.' *Journal of Computer Assisted Tomography,* **11,** 831–838.

McCarthy, M., Norenberg, M.D. (1988) 'Pontine hemorrhagic infarction in nontraumatic fat embolism.' *Neurology,* **38,** 1645–1647.

McCormick, W.F. (1984) 'Pathology of vascular malformations of the brain.' *In:* Wilson, C.B., Stein, B.M. (Eds.) *Intracranial Arteriovenous Malformations.* Baltimore: Williams & Wilkins, pp. 44–63.

—— Nofzinger, J.D. (1966) '"Cryptic" vascular malformations of the central nervous system.' *Journal of Neurosurgery,* **24,** 865–875.

McCully, K.S. (1969) 'Vascular pathology of homocysteinemia: implications for the pathogenesis of arteriosclerosis.' *American Journal of Pathology,* **56,** 111–128.

McDonald, T.D., Tatemichi, S.J., Kranzler, L., *et al.* (1989) 'Thrombosis of the superior sagittal sinus associated with essential thrombocytosis followed by MRI during anticoagulant therapy.' *Neurology,* **39,** 1554–1555.

McLean, M.J., Gebarski, S.S., Van der Spek, A.F.L., Goldstein, G.W. (1985) 'Response of moyamoya disease to Verapamil.' *Lancet,* **1,** 163–164.

Meadows, J.C. (1983) 'Clinical features of focal cerebral hemispheres infarction.' *In:* Russell, R.W. (Ed.) *Vascular Disease of the Central Nervous System, 2nd Edn.* Edinburgh: Churchill Livingstone, pp. 169–184.

Mehler, M.F. (1988) 'The neuro-ophthalmologic spectrum of the rostral basilar artery syndrome.' *Archives of Neurology,* **45,** 966–971.

Mendelow, A.D., Erfurth, A., Grossart, K., McPherson, P. (1987) 'Do cerebral arteriovenous malformations increase in size?' *Journal of Neurology, Neurosurgery, and Psychiatry,* **50,** 980–987.

Mettinger, K.L., Ericson, K. (1982) 'Fibromuscular dysplasia and the brain. Observations on angiographic, clinical and genetic characteristics.' *Stroke,* **13,** 46–52.

Meyer, F.B., Sundt, T.M., Fode, N.C., *et al.* (1989) 'Cerebral aneurysms in childhood and adolescence.' *Journal of Neurosurgery,* **70,** 420–425.

Miller, V.S. (1993) 'Pharmacologic management of neonatal cerebral ischemia and hemorrhage: old and new directions.' *Journal of Child Neurology,* **8,** 7–18.

Mintz, M., Epstein, L.G., Koenigsberger, M.R. (1992) 'Idiopathic childhood stroke is associated with human leucocyte antigen (HLA)-B51.' *Annals of Neurology,* **31,** 675–677.

Mitchell, W.G., Fishman, L.S., Miller, J.H., *et al.* (1991) 'Stroke as a late sequela of cranial irradiation for childhood brain tumors.' *Journal of Child Neurology,* **6,** 128–133.

Mizuno, Y., Kurokawa, T., Numagachi, Y., Goya, N. (1982) 'Facial hemangioma with cerebrovascular anomalies and cerebellar hypoplasia.' *Brain and Development,* **4,** 375–378.

Mohr, J.P. (1984) 'Neurological manifestations and factors related to therapeutic decision.' *In:* Wilson, C.B., Stein, B.A. (Eds.) *Intracerebral Arteriovenous Malformations.* Baltimore: Williams & Wilkins, pp. 1–8.

Mokri, B., Piepgras, D.G., Houser, O.W. (1988) 'Traumatic dissections of the extracranial internal carotid artery.' *Journal of Neurosurgery,* **68,** 189–197.

Monaco, R.D., Lasjaunias, P., Rodesch, G., *et al.* (1992) 'Cerebral arteriovenous malformations in newborns and infants: management of 92 patients.' *Pediatric Neurology,* **8,** 357. *(Abstract.)*

Montalban, J., Ibanez, L., Rodriguez, C., *et al.* (1989) 'Cerebral infarction after excessive use of nasal decongestants.' *Journal of Neurology, Neurosurgery, and Psychiatry,* **52,** 541–542.

Moodley, M., Ramdial, P. (1993) 'Blue rubber bleb nevus syndrome: case report and review of the literature.' *Pediatrics,* **92,** 160–162.

Moore, P.M. (1989) 'Diagnosis and management of isolated angiitis of the central nervous system.' *Neurology,* **39,** 167–173.

Morales, E., Pineda, C., Martínez-Lavín, M. (1991) 'Takayasu's arteritis in children.' *Journal of Rheumatology,* **18,** 1081–1084.

Moulin, T., Bogousslavsky, J., Chopard, J-L., *et al.* (1995) 'Vascular ataxic hemi-paresis: a re-evaluation.' *Journal of Neurology, Neurosurgery, and Psychiatry,* **58,** 422–427.

Murphy, M.J. (1985) 'Long-term follow-up of seizures associated with cerebral arteriovenous malformations. Results of therapy.' *Archives of Neurology,* **42,** 477–479.

Muszynski, C.A., Carpenter, R.J., Armstrong, D.L. (1994) 'Prenatal sonographic detection of basilar aneurysm.' *Pediatric Neurology,* **10,** 70–72.

Myles, S.J., Needham, C.W., Leblanc, F.E. (1970) 'Alternating hemiparesis associated with hereditary hemorrhagic telangiectasia.' *Canadian Medical Association Journal,* **103,** 509–511.

Naranjo, I.C., Rieger, J., Gonzalez, R.M., *et al.* (1987) 'Recurrent subarachnoid haemorrhage due to spinal haemangioma.' *Journal of Neurology, Neurosurgery, and Psychiatry,* **50,** 1722–1723.

Nass, R., Hays, A., Chutorian, A. (1982) 'Intracranial dissecting aneurysms in childhood.' *Stroke,* **13,** 204–207.

Natowicz, M., Kelley, R.I. (1987) 'Mendelian etiologies of stroke.' *Annals of Neurology,* **22,** 175–192.

Neil-Dwyer, G., Bartlett, J.R., Nicholls, A.C. (1983) 'Collagen deficiency and ruptured cerebral aneurysms: a clinical and biochemical study.' *Journal of Neurosurgery,* **59,** 16–20.

Nellhaus, G., Haberland, C., Hill, B.J. (1967) 'Sturge–Weber disease with bilateral intracranial calcifications at birth and unusual pathologic findings.' *Acta Neurologica Scandinavica,* **43,** 314–347.

Neumann, H.P.H., Eggert, H.R., Scheremet, R., *et al.* (1992) 'Central nervous system lesions in von Hippel–Lindau syndrome.' *Journal of Neurology, Neurosurgery, and Psychiatry,* **55,** 898–901.

Newman, L.J., Heitlinger, L., Hiesiger, E., *et al.* (1980) 'Communicating hydrocephalus following total parenteral nutrition.' *Journal of Pediatric Surgery,* **15,** 215–217.

Newton, T.H., Hoyt, W.F. (1970) 'Dural arteriovenous shunts in the region of the cavernous sinus.' *Neuroradiology,* **1,** 71–81.

Niijima, S.I., Arai, Y., Saitoh, M., *et al.* (1994) 'Clinical courses of 12 Sturge–Weber syndrome patients and evaluation of neurologic therapy.' *Paper presented at the joint ICNA–CNS Congress, San Francisco, October 1994.*

Nishizaki, T., Tamaki, N., Takeda, N., *et al.* (1986) 'Dolichoectatic basilar artery: a review of 23 cases.' *Stroke,* **17,** 1277–1281.

Norman, D. (1984) 'Computerized tomography of cerebrovascular malformations.' *In:* Wilson, C.B., Stein, B.M. (Eds.) *Intracranial Arteriovenous Malformations.* Baltimore: Williams & Wilkins, pp. 105–120.

Norman, M., Becker, L.E. (1974) 'Cerebral damage in neonates resulting from arteriovenous malformations of the vein of Galen.' *Journal of Neurology, Neurosurgery, and Psychiatry,* **37,** 252–258.

—— Schoene, W.C. (1977) 'Ultrastructure of Sturge–Weber disease.' *Acta Neuropathologica,* **37,** 199–205.

Norrgård, Ö., Ängquist, K-A., Fodstad, H., *et al.* (1987) 'Intracranial aneurysms and heredity.' *Neurosurgery,* **20,** 236–239.

North, K.N., Whiteman, D.A.H., Pepin, M.G., Byers, P.H. (1995) 'Cerebrovascular complications in Ehlers–Danlos syndrome type IV.' *Annals of Neurology,* **38,** 960–964.

Nowak-Göttl, U., Koch, H.G., Aschka, I., *et al.* (1996) 'Resistance to activated protein C (APCR) in children with venous or arterial thromboembolism.' *British Journal of Haematology,* **92,** 992–998.

Nuss, R., Hays, T., Manco-Johnson, M. (1995) 'Childhood thrombosis.' *Pediatrics,* **96,** 291–294.

Oakes, W.J. (1992) 'The natural history of patients with the Sturge–Weber syndrome.' *Pediatric Neurosurgery,* **18,** 287–290.

Ogilvy, C.S., Heros, R.C., Ojemann, R.G., New, P.F. (1988) 'Angiographically occult arteriovenous malformations.' *Journal of Neurosurgery,* **69,** 350–355.

Okuno, T., Prensky, A.L., Gado, M. (1985) 'The moyamoya syndrome associated with irradiation of an optic glioma in children: report of two cases and review of the literature.' *Pediatric Neurology,* **1,** 311–316.

Olson, E., Gilmor, R.L., Richmond, B. (1984) 'Cerebral venous angiomas.' *Radiology,* **151,** 97–104.

Omojola, M.F., Fox, A.J., Vinuela, F.V. (1982) 'Spontaneous regression of intracranial arteriovenous malformations: report of three cases.' *Journal of Neurosurgery,* **57,** 818–822.

Orr, L.S., Osher, R.H., Savino, P.J. (1978) 'The syndrome of facial nevi, anomalous cerebral venous return, and hydrocephalus.' *Annals of Neurology,* **3,** 316–318.

Østergaard, J.R., Voldby, B. (1983) 'Intracranial arterial aneurysms in children and adolescents.' *Journal of Neurosurgery,* **58,** 832–837.

567

Overby, M.C., Rothman, A.S. (1985) 'Multiple intracranial aneurysm in sickle cell anemia.' *Journal of Neurosurgery*, **62**, 430–434.

Oyesiku, N.M., Gahm, N.H., Goldman, R.L. (1988) 'Cerebral arteriovenous fistula in the Klippel–Trenaunay–Weber syndrome.' *Developmental Medicine and Child Neurology*, **30**, 245–251.

Packer, R.J., Rorke, L.B., Lange, B.J., *et al.* (1985) 'Cerebrovascular accidents in children with cancer.' *Pediatrics*, **76**, 194–201.

Pang, D., Kerber,C., Biglan, A.W. (1981) 'External carotid–cavernous sinus fistulas in infancy: case report and review of the literature.' *Neurosurgery*, **8**, 212–218.

Pantell, R.H., Goodman, B.W. (1981) 'Takayasu's arteritis: the relationship with tuberculosis.' *Pediatrics*, **67**, 84–88.

Park, Y.D., Belman, A.L., Dickson, D.W., *et al.* (1988) 'Stroke in pediatric acquired immunodeficiency syndrome.' *Annals of Neurology*, **24**, 359–360. (Abstract.)

Parker, M.J., Tarlow, M.J., Milne-Anderson, J. (1984) 'Glue sniffing and cerebral infarction.' *Archives of Disease in Childhood*, **59**, 675–677.

Pascual-Castroviejo, I. (1985) 'The association of extracranial and intracranial vascular malformations in children.' *Canadian Journal of Neurological Sciences*, **12**, 139–148.

—— Diaz-Gonzalez, C., García-Melian, R.M., *et al.* (1993) 'Sturge–Weber syndrome: study of 40 patients.' *Pediatric Neurology*, **9**, 283–288.

—— Pascual-Pascual, S-I., Viaño, J., *et al.* (1995a) 'Sturge–Weber syndrome without facial nevus.' *Neuropediatrics*, **26**, 220–222.

—— Viaño, J., Pascual-Pascual, S-I., Martinez, V. (1995b) 'Facial haemangioma, agenesis of the internal carotid artery and dysplasia of cerebral cortex: case report.' *Neuroradiology*, **37**, 692–695.

Patel, H., Smith, R.R., Garg, B.P. (1995) 'Spontaneous extracranial carotid artery dissection in children.' *Pediatric Neurology*, **13**, 55–60.

Pearl, P.L. (1987) 'Childhood stroke following intraoral trauma.' *Journal of Pediatrics*, **10**, 574–575.

Peerless, S.J., Nemoto, S., Drake, C.G. (1989) 'Giant intracranial aneurysms in children and adolescents.' *In:* Edwards, M.S.B., Hoffman, H.J. (Eds.) *Cerebral Vascular Disease in Children and Adolescents.* Baltimore: Williams & Wilkins, pp. 255–273.

Peery, W.H. (1987) 'Clinical spectrum of hereditary hemorrhagic telangiectasia (Osler–Weber–Rendu disease).' *American Journal of Medicine*, **82**, 989–997.

Pegelow, C.H., Adams, R.J., McVie, V., *et al.* (1995) 'Risk of recurrent stroke in patients with sickle cell disease treated with erythrocyte transfusions.' *Journal of Pediatrics*, **126**, 896–899.

Pehr, K., Moroz, B. (1993) 'Cutis marmorata telangiectatica congenita: long-term follow-up, review of the literature, and report of a case in conjunction with congenital hypothyroidism.' *Pediatric Dermatology*, **10**, 6–11.

Pellicer, A., Cabañas, F., Garcia-Alix, A., *et al.* (1992) 'Stroke in neonates with cardiac right-to-left shunt.' *Brain and Development*, **14**, 381–385.

Pellock, J.M., Kleinman, P.K., McDonald, B.M., Wixson, D. (1980) 'Childhood hypertensive stroke with neurofibromatosis.' *Neurology*, **30**, 650–659.

Perkin, G.D. (1995) 'Cerebral venous thrombosis: developments in imaging and treatment.' *Journal of Neurology, Neurosurgery, and Psychiatry*, **59**, 1–3. (Editorial.)

Perlman, J.M., Volpe, J.J. (1989) 'Neurologic complications of captopril treatment of neonatal hypertension.' *Pediatrics*, **83**, 47–52.

Perret, G., Nishioka, H. (1966) 'Report on the Cooperative Study of Intracranial Aneurysms and Subarachnoid Hemorrhage: Arteriovenous Malformations. An analysis of 545 cases of craniocerebral arteriovenous malformations and fistulae reported to the cooperative study.' *Journal of Neurosurgery*, **25**, 467–490.

Pettee, A.D., Wasserman, B.A., Adams, N.L., *et al.* (1994) 'Familial Sneddon's syndrome: clinical, hematologic, and radiographic findings in two brothers.' *Neurology*, **44**, 399–405.

Pettigrew, L.C., Jankovic, J. (1985) 'Hemidystonia: a report of 22 patients and a review of the literature.' *Journal of Neurology, Neurosurgery, and Psychiatry*, **48**, 650–657.

Phillips, P.C., Lorensten, K.J., Shropshire, L.C., Ahn, H.S. (1988) 'Congenital odontoid aplasia and posterior circulation stroke in childhood.' *Annals of Neurology*, **23**, 410–413.

Phornphutkul, C., Rosenthal, A., Nadas, A.S., Berenberg, W. (1973) 'Cerebrovascular accidents in infants and children with cyanotic congenital heart disease.' *American Journal of Cardiology*, **32**, 329–334.

Picascia, D.D., Esterly, N.B. (1989) 'Cutis marmorata telangiectatica congenita: report of 22 cases.' *Journal of the American Academy of Dermatology*, **20**, 1098–1104.

Pierot, L., Gobin, P., Cognard, C., *et al.* (1992) 'Fistules artérioveineuses durales intracraniennes. Aspects cliniques, explorations radiologiques et modalités thérapeutiques.' *Revue Neurologique*, **150**, 444–451.

Pitner, S.E. (1966) 'Carotid thrombosis due to intraoral trauma. An unusual complication of a common childhood accident.' *New England Journal of Medicine*, **274**, 764–767.

Plum, F. (1983) 'What causes infarction in ischemic brain? The Robert Wartenberg lecture.' *Neurology*, **33**, 222–233.

Pope, F.M., Nicholls, A.C., Narcisi, P., *et al.* (1981) 'Some patients with cerebral aneurysms are deficient in type III collagen.' *Lancet*, **1**, 973–975.

Porteous, M.E.M., Burn, J., Proctor, S.J. (1992) 'Hereditary haemorrhagic telangiectasia: a clinical analysis.' *Journal of Medical Genetics*, **29**, 527–530.

Prats, J.M., Garaizar, C., Zuazo, E., *et al.* (1992) 'Superior sagittal sinus thrombosis in a child with protein S deficiency.' *Neurology*, **42**, 2303–2305.

Pretorius, M.E., Butler, J.J. (1983) 'Neurologic manifestations of Ehlers–Danlos syndrome.' *Neurology*, **33**, 1087–1089.

Prian, G.W., Wright, G.B., Rumack, C.M., O'Meara, O.P. (1978) 'Apparent cerebral embolization after temporal artery catheterization.' *Journal of Pediatrics*, **93**, 115–118.

Priest, J.R., Ramsay, N.K.C., Latchaw, R.E., *et al.* (1980) 'Thrombotic and hemorrhagic strokes complicating early therapy for childhood acute lymphoblastic leukemia.' *Cancer*, **46**, 1548–1554.

Probst, F.P. (1980) 'Vascular morphology and angiographic flow pattern in Sturge–Weber angiomatosis: facts, thoughts and suggestions.' *Neuroradiology*, **20**, 75–78.

Proesmans, W., van Damme, B., Casaer, P., Marchal, G. (1982) 'Autosomal dominant polycystic kidney disease in the neonatal period: association with a cerebral arteriovenous malformation.' *Pediatrics*, **70**, 971–975.

Prohovnik, I., Pavlakis, S.G., Piomelli, S., *et al.* (1989) 'Cerebral hyperemia, stroke and transfusion in sickle cell disease.' *Neurology*, **39**, 344–348.

Pruvost, P., Lasjaunias, P., Rodesch, G., *et al.* (1989) 'Soufle pulsatile crânien bénin chez l'enfant: à propos de 6 cas.' *Archives Françaises de Pédiatrie*, **46**, 579–582.

Randall, J.M., Griffiths, P.D., Gardner-Medwin, D., Gholkar, A. (1994) 'Thalamic infarction in childhood due to extracranial vertebral artery abnormalities.' *Neuropediatrics*, **25**, 262–264.

Rao, K.C.V.G., Knipp, H.C., Wagner, E.J. (1981) 'Computed tomography findings in cerebral sinus and venous thrombosis.' *Radiology*, **140**, 391–398.

Rappaport, Z.H. (1988) 'Corpus callosum section in the treatment of intractable seizures in the Sturge–Weber syndrome.' *Child's Nervous System*, **4**, 231–232.

Ravelli, A., Martini, A., Burgio, G.R. (1994) 'Antiphospholipid antibodies in paediatrics.' *European Journal of Pediatrics*, **153**, 472–479.

Raybaud, C.A., Livet, M-O., Jiddane, M., Pinsard, N. (1985) 'Radiology of ischemic strokes in children.' *Neuroradiology*, **27**, 567–578.

Reese, V., Frieden, I.J., Paller, A.S., *et al.* (1993) 'Association of facial hemangiomas with Dandy–Walker and other posterior fossa malformations.' *Journal of Pediatrics*, **122**, 379–384.

Requena, I., Arias, M., López-Ibor, L., *et al.* (1991) 'Cavernomas of the central nervous system: clinical and neuroimaging manifestations in 47 patients.' *Journal of Neurology, Neurosurgery, and Psychiatry*, **54**, 590–594.

Resche, F., Resche-Perrin, I., Robert, R., *et al.* (1980) 'L'artère hypoglosse. Rapport d'un cas. Revue de la littérature.' *Journal of Neuroradiology*, **7**, 27–43.

Ridker, P.M., Hennekens, C.H., Lindpaintner, K., *et al.* (1995) 'Mutations in the gene coding for coagulation factor V and the risk of myocardial infarction, stroke and venous thrombosis in apparently healthy men.' *New England Journal of Medicine*, **332**, 912–917.

Riela, A.R., Roach, E.S. (1993) 'Etiology of stroke in children.' *Journal of Child Neurology*, **8**, 201–220.

Rigamonti, D., Hadley, M.N., Drayer, B.P., *et al.* (1988) 'Cerebral cavernous malformations: incidence and familial occurrence.' *New England Journal of Medicine*, **319**, 343–347.

Riikonen, R., Santavuori, P. (1994) 'Hereditary and acquired risk factors for childhood stroke.' *Neuropediatrics*, **25**, 227–233.

Rivkin, M.J., Anderson, M.L., Kaye, E.M. (1992) 'Neonatal idiopathic cerebral venous thrombosis: an unrecognized cause of transient seizures or lethargy.' *Annals of Neurology*, **32**, 51–56.

Roach, E.S. (1992) 'Neurocutaneous syndromes.' *Pediatric Clinics of North America*, **39**, 591–620.

—— Riela, A.R., Chugani, H.T., *et al.* (1994) 'Sturge–Weber syndrome: recommendations for surgery.' *Journal of Child Neurology*, **9**, 190–192.

Robertson, P.L., Aldrich, M.S., Hanash, S.M., Golstein, G.W. (1988) 'Stroke associated with obstructive sleep apnea in a child with sickle cell anemia.' *Annals of Neurology*, **23**, 614–616.

Roddy, S.M., Giang, D.W. (1991) 'Antiphospholipid antibodies and stroke in an infant.' *Pediatrics*, **87**, 933–935.

Rodesch, G., Lasjaunias, P., Ter Brugge, K., Burrows, P. (1988) 'Lésions vasculaires artérioveineuses intracrâniennes de l'enfant. Place des techniques endovasculaires à propos de 44 cas.' *Neurochirurgie*, **34**, 293–303.

—— Hui, F., Alvarez, H., *et al.* (1994) 'Prognosis of antenatally diagnosed vein of Galen aneurysmal malformations.' *Child's Nervous System*, **10**, 79–83.

—— Malherbe, V., Alvarez, H., *et al.* (1995) 'Nongalenic cerebral arteriovenous malformations in neonates and infants. Review of 26 consecutive cases (1982–1992).' *Child's Nervous System*, **11**, 231–241.

Román, G., Fisher, M., Perl, D.P., Poser, C.M. (1978) 'Neurological manifestations of hereditary hemorrhagic telangiectasia (Rendu–Osler–Weber disease): Report of 2 cases and review of the literature.' *Annals of Neurology*, **4**, 130–144.

Romano, J.T., Riggs, J.E., Bodensteiner, J.B., Gutmann, L. (1989) 'Wasp sting-associated occlusion of the supraclinoid internal carotid artery: implications regarding the pathogenesis of moyamoya syndrome.' *Archives of Neurology*, **46**, 607–608.

Rooney, C.M., Kaye, E.M., Scott, R.M., *et al.* (1991) 'Modified encephaloduroarteriosynangiosis as a surgical treatment of childhood moyamoya disease: report of five cases.' *Journal of Child Neurology*, **6**, 24–31.

Ropper, A.H. (1988) '"Convulsions" in basilar artery occlusion.' *Neurology*, **38**, 1500–1501.

Rorke, L.B. (1989) 'Pathology of cerebral vascular disease in children and adolescents.' *In:* Edwards, M.S.B., Hoffman, H.J. (Eds.) *Cerebral Vascular Diseases in Children and Adolescents.* Baltimore: Williams & Wilkins, pp. 95–136.

Rosemberg, S., Lopes, M.B.S., Sotto, M.N., Graudenz, M.S. (1988) 'Childhood Degos disease with prominent neurological symptoms: report of a clinicopathological case.' *Journal of Child Neurology*, **3**, 42–46.

Rosenbloom, S., Edwards, M.S.B. (1989) 'Dural arteriovenous malformations.' *In:* Edwards, M.S.B., Hoffman, H.J. (Eds.) *Cerebral Vascular Disease in Children and Adolescents.* Baltimore: Williams & Wilkins, pp. 343–365.

Ross, C.A., Curnes, J.T., Greenwood, R.S. (1987) 'Recurrent vertebrobasilar embolism in an infant with Klippel–Feil anomaly.' *Pediatric Neurology*, **3**, 181–183.

Ross, J.B., Shevell, M.I., Montes, J.L., *et al.* (1994) 'Encephaloduroarteriosynangiosis (EDAS) for the treatment of childhood moyamoya disease.' *Pediatric Neurology*, **10**, 199–204.

Rothfus, W.E., Albright, A.L., Casey, K.F., *et al.* (1984) 'Cerebellar venous angioma: "benign" entity?' *American Journal of Neuroradiology*, **5**, 61–66.

Rout, D., Sharma, A., Mohan, P.K., Rao, V.R.K. (1984) 'Bacterial aneurysms of the intracavernous carotid artery.' *Journal of Neurosurgery*, **60**, 1236–1242.

Rumi, V., Angelini, L., Scaioli, V., *et al.* (1993) 'Primary antiphospholipid syndrome and neurologic events.' *Pediatric Neurology*, **9**, 473–475.

Sainte-Rose, C., LaCombe, J., Pierre-Kahn, A., *et al.* (1984) 'Intracranial venous sinus hypertension: cause or consequence of hydrocephalus in infants?' *Journal of Neurosurgery*, **60**, 727–736.

Saito, Y., Kobayashi, N. (1981) 'Cerebral venous angiomas. Clinical evaluation and possible etiology.' *Radiology*, **139**, 87–94.

Salgado, A.N., Furlan, A.J., Keys, T.F., *et al.* (1989) 'Neurologic complications of endocarditis: a 12-year experience.' *Neurology*, **39**, 173–178.

Samson, D. (1989) 'Traumatic lesions of the cerebral vasculature.' *In:* Edwards, M.S.B., Hoffman, H.J. (Eds.) *Cerebral Vascular Disease in Children and Adolescents.* Baltimore: Williams & Wilkins, pp. 195–201.

Sarwar, M., McCormick, W.F. (1978) 'Intracerebral venous angioma: case report and review.' *Archives of Neurology*, **35**, 323–325.

Satya-Murti, S., Navada, S., Emmes, F. (1986) 'Central nervous system involvement in blue-rubber-bleb-nevus syndrome.' *Archives of Neurology*, **43**, 1184–1186.

Savoiardo, M., Strada, L., Passerini, A. (1983) 'Intracranial cavernous hemangioma: neuroradiological review of 36 operated cases.' *American Journal of Neuroradiology*, **4**, 945–950.

Schievink, W.I., Piepgras, D.G., Earnest, F., Gordon, H. (1991) 'Spontaneous carotid–cavernous fistulae in Ehlers–Danlos syndrome type IV.' *Journal of Neurosurgery*, **74**, 991–998.

—— Michels, V.V., Piepgras, D.G. (1994a) 'Neurovascular manifestations of heritable connective tissue disorders. A review.' *Stroke*, **25**, 889–903.

—— Mokri, B., Piepgras, D.G. (1994b) 'Spontaneous dissections of cervicocephalic arteries in childhood and adolescence.' *Neurology*, **44**, 1607–1612.

—— Schaid, D.J., Michels, V.V., Piepgras, D.G. (1995) 'Familial aneurysmal subarachnoid hemorrhage: a community-based study.' *Journal of Neurosurgery*, **83**, 426–429.

Schlenska, G.K. (1986) 'Absence of both internal carotid arteries.' *Journal of Neurology*, **233**, 263–266.

Schoenberg, B.S., Mellinger, J.F., Schoenberg, D.G. (1978) 'Cerebrovascular disease in infants and children: a study of incidence, clinical features and survival.' *Neurology*, **28**, 763–768.

Schöning, M., Klein, R., Krägeloh-Mann, I., *et al.* (1994) 'Antiphospholipid antibodies in cerebrovascular ischemia and stroke in childhood.' *Neuropediatrics*, **25**, 8–14.

Schoolman, A., Kepes, J.J. (1967) 'Bilateral spontaneous carotid–cavernous fistulae in Ehlers–Danlos syndrome.' *Journal of Neurosurgery*, **26**, 82–86.

Sedzimir, C.B., Robinson, J. (1973) 'Intracranial hemorrhage in children and adolescents.' *Journal of Neurosurgery*, **38**, 269–273.

Seeler, R.A., Royal, J.E., Powe, L., Goldberg, H.R. (1978) 'Moyamoya in children with sickle cell anemia and cerebrovascular occlusion.' *Journal of Pediatrics*, **93**, 808–810.

Segal, M.D., McLaurin, R.L. (1977) 'Giant serpentine aneurysm. Report of 2 cases.' *Journal of Neurosurgery*, **46**, 115–120.

Selby, G., Walker, G.L. (1979) 'Cerebral arteritis in cat scratch disease.' *Neurology*, **29**, 1413–1418.

Shapiro, U., Shulman, K. (1976) 'Facial nevi associated with anomalous venous return and hydrocephalus.' *Journal of Neurosurgery*, **45**, 20–25.

Sheth, R.D., Bodensteiner, J.B. (1995) 'Progressive neurologic impairment from an arteriovenous malformation vascular steal.' *Pediatric Neurology*, **13**, 352–354.

Shevell, M.I., Silver, K., O'Gorman, A.M., *et al.* (1989) 'Neonatal dural sinus thrombosis.' *Pediatric Neurology*, **5**, 161–165.

Shirane, R., Sato, S., Yoshimoto, T. (1992) 'Angiographic findings of ischemic stroke in children. '*Child's Nervous System*, **8**, 432–436.

Siegler, R.L., Brewer, E.D., Corneli, H.M., Thompson, J.A. (1991) 'Hypertension first seen as facial paralysis: case reports and review of the literature.' *Pediatrics*, **87**, 387–389.

Silber, M.H., Sandok, B.A., Earnest, F. (1987) 'Vascular malformations of the posterior fossa: clinical and radiologic features.' *Archives of Neurology*, **44**, 965–969.

Simard, J.M., Garcia-Bengochea, F., Ballinger, W.E., *et al.* (1986) 'Cavernous angioma: a review of 126 collected and 12 new clinical cases.' *Neurosurgery*, **18**, 162–172.

Simioni, P., Battistella, P.A., Drigo, P., *et al.* (1994) 'Childhood stroke associated with familial protein S deficiency.' *Brain and Development*, **16**, 241–245.

Simonati, A., Colamaria, V., Bricolo, A., *et al.* (1994) 'Microgyria associated with Sturge–Weber angiomatosis.' *Child's Nervous System*, **10**, 392–395.

Singer, W.D., Haller, J.S., Wolpert, S.M. (1975) 'Occlusive vertebrobasilar artery disease associated with cervical spine anomaly.' *American Journal of Diseases of Children*, **129**, 492–495.

Skoglund, R.R., Paa, D., Lewis, W.J. (1978) 'Elevated spinal-fluid protein in Sturge–Weber syndrome.' *Developmental Medicine and Child Neurology*, **20**, 99–102.

So, S.C. (1978) 'Cerebral arteriovenous malformations in children.' *Child's Brain*, **4**, 242–250.

Southwick, F.S., Richardson, E.P., Swartz, M.N. (1986) 'Septic thrombosis of the dural venous sinuses.' *Medicine*, **65**, 82–106.

Sperl, W., Felber, S., Skladal, D., Wermuth, B. (1997) 'Metabolic stroke in carbamyl phosphate synthetase deficiency.' *Neuropediatrics*, **28**, 229–234.

Sperner, J., Schmauser, I., Bittner, R., *et al.* (1990) 'MR-imaging findings in children with Sturge–Weber syndrome.' *Neuropediatrics*, **21**, 146–152.

Spetzler, R.F., Selman, W.R. (1984) 'Pathophysiology of cerebral ischemia accompanying arteriovenous malformations.' *In:* Wilson, C.B., Stein, B.M. (Eds.) *Intracranial Arteriovenous Malformations.* Baltimore: Williams & Wilkins, pp. 24–31.

Statham, P., Macpherson, P., Johnston, R., *et al.* (1990) 'Cerebral radiation necrosis complicating stereotactic radiosurgery for arteriovenous malformation.' *Journal of Neurology, Neurosurgery, and Psychiatry*, **53**, 476–479.

Steichen-Gersdorf, E., Felber, S., Fuchs, W., *et al.* (1992) 'Familial cavernous angiomas of the brain: observations in a four generation family.' *European Journal of Pediatrics*, **151**, 861–863.

Stein, B.M., Mohr, J.P. (1988) 'Vascular malformations of the brain.' *New England Journal of Medicine*, **319**, 368–370.

Steinberg, G.K., Fabrikant, J.I., Marks, M.P., *et al.* (1990) 'Stereotactic heavy-charged-particle Bragg-peak radiation for intracranial arteriovenous malformations.' *New England Journal of Medicine*, **323**, 96–101.

Steiner, L. (1986) 'Radiosurgery in cerebral arteriovenous malformations.' *In:* Flamm, E., Fein, J. (Eds.) *Textbook of Cerebrovascular Surgery, Vol. 4.* New York: Springer, pp. 1161–1215.

Stern, J., Correll, J.W., Bryan, N. (1978) 'Persistant hypoglossal artery and persistent trigeminal artery presenting with posterior fossa transient ischemic attacks. Report of two cases.' *Journal of Neurosurgery*, **49**, 614–619.

Stickler, G.R. (1987) 'Klippel–Trenaunay syndrome.' *In:* Gomez, M.R. (Eds.) *Neurocutaneous Diseases. A Practical Approach.* London: Butterworths, pp. 368–375.

Strenge, H., Cordes, P., Sticherling, M., Brossman, J. (1996) 'Hemifacial atrophy: a neurocutaneous disorder with coup de sabre deformity, telangiectatic naevus, aneurysmatic malformation of the internal carotid artery and crossed hemiatrophy.' *Journal of Neurology*, **243**, 658–660.

Sturzenegger, M. (1995) 'Spontaneous internal carotid artery dissection: early diagnosis and management in 44 patients.' *Journal of Neurology*, **242**, 231–238.

Sujansky, E., Conradi, S. (1995) 'Sturge–Weber syndrome: age of onset of seizures and glaucoma and the prognosis for affected children.' *Journal of Child Neurology*, **10**, 49–58.

Suzuki, J., Kodama, N. (1983) 'Moyamoya disease. A review.' *Stroke*, **14**, 104–109.

Svensson, P.J., Dahlbäck, B. (1994) 'Resistance to activated protein C as a basis for venous thrombosis.' *New England Journal of Medicine*, **330**, 517–522.

Swartz, M.N., Dodge, P.R. (1965) 'Bacterial meningitis—a review of selected aspects. I. General clinical features, special problems and unusual meningeal reactions mimicking bacterial meningitis.' *New England Journal of Medicine*, **272**, 779–787.

Tagawa, T., Mimaki, T., Yabuuchi, H., *et al.* (1985) 'Bilateral occlusions in the cervical portion of the internal carotid arteries in a child.' *Stroke*, **6**, 896–898.

Tagle, P., Huette, I., Mendez, J., Del Villar, S. (1986) 'Intracranial cavernous angioma: presentation and management.' *Journal of Neurosurgery*, **64**, 720–723.

Takanashi, J-i., Sugita, K., Miyazato, S., *et al.* (1995) 'Antiphospholipid antibody syndrome in childhood strokes.' *Pediatric Neurology*, **13**, 323–326.

Takeuchi, S., Kobayashi, K., Tsuchida, T. (1982) 'Computed tomography in moya moya disease.' *Journal of Computer Assisted Tomography*, **6**, 24–32.

Tallman, B., Tan, O.T., Morelli, J.G., *et al.* (1991) 'Location of port-wine stains and the likelihood of ophthalmic and/or central nervous system complications.' *Pediatrics*, **87**, 323–327.

Tan, O.T., Sherwood, K., Gilchrest, B.A. (1989) 'Treatment of children with port-wine stains using the flashlamp-pulse tunable dye laser.' *New England Journal of Medicine*, **320**, 416–421.

Tanaka, K., Hirayama, K., Hattori, H., *et al.* (1994) 'A case of cerebral aneurysm associated with complex partial seizures.' *Brain and Development*, **16**, 233–237.

Tarras, S., Gadia, C., Meister, L., *et al.* (1988) 'Homozygous protein C deficiency in a newborn. Clinicopathologic correlation.' *Archives of Neurology*, **45**, 214–216.

Tatemichi, T.K., Prohovnik, I., Mohr, J.P., *et al.* (1988) 'Reduced hypercapnic vasoreactivity in moya moya disease.' *Neurology*, **38**, 1575–1581.

Teal, J.S., Nasheedy, M.H., Hasso, A.N. (1980) 'Total agenesis of the internal carotid artery.' *American Journal of Neuroradiology*, **1**, 435–442.

Ter Berg, H.W.M., Bijlsma, J.B., Veiga Pires, J.A., *et al.* (1986) 'Familial association of intracranial aneurysms and multiple congenital anomalies.' *Archives of Neurology*, **43**, 30–33.

—— —— Willemse, J. (1987) 'Familial occurrence of intracranial aneurysms in childhood: a case report and review of the literature.' *Neuropediatrics*, **18**, 227–230.

Terdjman, P., Aicardi, J., Sainte-Rose, C., Brunelle, F. (1990) 'Neuroradiological findings in Sturge–Weber syndrome (SWS) and isolated pial angiomatosis.' *Neuropediatrics*, **22**, 115–120.

Terplan, K.L. (1976) 'Brain changes in newborns, infants and children with congenital heart disease in association with cardiac surgery. Additional observations.' *Journal of Neurology*, **212**, 225–236.

Theron, J., Newton, T.H., Hoyt, W.F. (1974) 'Unilateral retinocephalic vascular malformation.' *Neuroradiology*, **7**, 185–196.

Thorarensen, O., Ryan, S., Hunter, J., Younkin, D.P. (1997) 'Factor V Leiden mutation: an unrecognized cause of hemiplegic cerebral palsy, neonatal stroke, and placental thrombosis.' *Annals of Neurology*, **42**, 372–375.

Tietjen, G.E., Levine, S.R., Brown, E., *et al.* (1993) 'Factors that predict antiphospholipid immunoreactivity in young people with transient focal neurological events.' *Archives of Neurology*, **50**, 833–836.

Tomsik, T.A., Lukin, R.R., Chambers, A.A., Benton, C. (1976) 'Neurofibromatosis and intracranial arterial occlusive disease.' *Neuroradiology*, **11**, 229–234.

Toti, P., Balestri, P., Cano, M., *et al.* (1996) 'Celiac disease with cerebral calcium and silica deposits: X-ray spectroscopic findings, an autopsy study.' *Neurology*, **46**, 1088–1092.

Towbin, A. (1973) 'The syndrome of latent cerebral venous thrombosis: its frequency in relation to age and congestive heart failure.' *Stroke*, **4**, 419–430.

Tran, T.H., Marbet, G.A., Duckert, F. (1985) 'Association of hereditary heparin cofactor II deficiency with thrombosis.' *Lancet*, **2**, 413–414.

Trevathan, E., Dooling, E.C. (1987) 'Large thrombotic strokes in hemolytic–uremic syndrome.' *Journal of Pediatrics*, **111**, 863–866.

Tyler, H.R., Clark, D.B. (1957) 'Cerebro-vascular accidents in patients with congenital heart disease.' *Archives of Neurology and Psychiatry*, **77**, 483–489.

Uziel, Y., Laxer, R.M., Blaser, S., *et al.* (1995) 'Cerebral vein thrombosis in childhood systemic lupus erythematosus.' *Journal of Pediatrics*, **126**, 722–727.

Vanderzant, C., Bromberg, M., Macguire, A., McCune, W.J. (1988) 'Isolated small-vessel angiitis of the central nervous system.' *Archives of Neurology*, **45**, 683–687.

Van Diemen-Steenvoorde, R., Van Nieuwehuizen, O., De Klerk, J.B.C., Duran, M. (1990) 'Quasi-moyamoya disease and heterozygosity for homocystinuria in a five-year old girl.' *Neuropediatrics*, **21**, 110–112.

Van Dongen, H.R., Loonen, C.B., Van Dongen, K.J. (1985) 'Anatomical basis for acquired fluent aphasia in children.' *Annals of Neurology*, **17**, 306–309.

Van Hoff, J., Ritchey, A.K., Shaywitz, B.A. (1985) 'Intracranial hemorrhage in children with sickle cell disease.' *American Journal of Diseases of Children*, **139**, 1120–1123.

van Kuijck, M.A.P., Rotteveel, J.J., van Oostrom, C.G., Novakova, I. (1994) 'Neurological complications in children with protein C deficiency.' *Neuropediatrics*, **25**, 16–19.

Vaquero, J., Salazar, J., Martínez, R., *et al.* (1987) 'Cavernomas of the central nervous system: clinical syndromes, CT scan diagnosis, and prognosis after surgical treatment in 25 cases.' *Acta Neurochirurgica*, **85**, 29–33.

Ventureyra, E.C.G., Higgins, M.J. (1994) 'Traumatic intracranial aneurysms in childhood and adolescence. Case reports and review of the literature.' *Child's Nervous System*, **10**, 361–379.

Vernant, J.C., Delaporte, J.M., Buisson, G., *et al.* (1988) 'Complications cérébro-vasculaires de la drépanocytose.' *Revue Neurologique*, **144**, 465–473.

Vieregge, P., Schwieder, G., Kömpf, D. (1989) 'Cerebral venous thrombosis in hereditary protein C deficiency.' *Journal of Neurology, Neurosurgery, and Psychiatry*, **52**, 135–137. *(Letter.)*

Viljoen, D.L. (1988) 'Pseudoxanthoma elasticum (Grönblad–Strandberg syndrome).' *Journal of Medical Genetics*, **25**, 488–490.

Virapongse, C., Cazenave, C., Quisling, R., *et al.* (1987) 'The empty delta sign: frequency and significance in 76 cases of dural sinus thrombosis.' *Radiology*, **162**, 779–785.

Vles, J.S.H., Hendriks, J.J.E., Lodder, J., Janevski, B. (1990) 'Multiple vertebro-basilar infarctions from fibromuscular dysplasia related dissecting aneurysm of the vertebral artery in a child.' *Neuropediatrics*, **21**, 104–105.

Vogl, T.J., Stemmler, J., Bergman, C., *et al.* (1993) 'MR and MR angiography of Sturge–Weber syndrome.' *American Journal of Neuroradiology*, **14**, 417–425.

Vomberg, P.P., Breedeerveld, C., Fleury, P., Arts, W.F.M. (1987) 'Cerebral thromboembolism due to antithrombin III deficiency in two children.' *Neuropediatrics*, **18**, 42–44.

Waga, S., Okada, M., Kojima, T. (1978) 'Saccular aneurysm associated with absences of the left cervical carotid arteries.' *Neurosurgery*, **3**, 208–212.

Waltimo, O. (1973) 'The change in size of intracranial arteriovenous malformations.' *Journal of the Neurological Sciences*, **19**, 21–27.

Wang, P.S., Longstreth, W.T., Koepsell, T.D. (1995) 'Subarachnoid hemorrhage and family history. A population-based case–control study.' *Archives of Neurology*, **52**, 202–204.

Wanifuchi, H., Kagawa, M., Takeshita, M., *et al.* (1988) 'Ischemic stroke in infancy, childhood and adolescence.' *Child's Nervous System*, **4**, 361–364.

Warach, S., Gaa, J., Siewert, B., *et al.* (1995) 'Acute human stroke studied by whole brain echo planar diffusion-weighted magnetic resonance imaging.' *Annals of Neurology*, **37**, 231–241.

Ward, D.E., Ho, S.Y., Shinebourne, E.A. (1984) 'Familial atrial standstill and inexcitability in childhood.' *American Journal of Cardiology*, **53**, 965–967.

Watanabe, K., Negoro, T., Maehara, M., *et al.* (1990) 'Moyamoya disease presenting with chorea.' *Pediatric Neurology*, **6**, 40–42.

Waybright, E.A., Selhorst, J.B., Rosenblum, W.I., Suter, C.G. (1978) 'Blue-rubber-bleb nevus syndrome with CNS involvement and thrombosis of a vein of Galen malformation.' *Annals of Neurology*, **3**, 464–467.

Wazi, P., Na-Nakorn, S., Poutrakal, P. (1978) 'A syndrome of hypertension, convulsion and cerebral haemorrhage in thalassaemic patients after multiple blood transfusions.' *Lancet*, **1**, 602–604.

Weber, M., Vespignani, H., Bracard, S., *et al.* (1989) 'Les angiomes caverneux intracérébraux.' *Revue Neurologique*, **145**, 429–436.

Welch, K., Naheedy, M.H., Abroms, I.F., Strand, R. (1980) 'Computer tomography of Sturge–Weber syndrome in infants.' *Journal of Computer Assisted Tomography*, **4**, 33–36.

Wilkins, R.H. (1985) 'Natural history of intracranial vascular malformations: a review.' *Neurosurgery*, **16**, 421–430.

Wilimas, J., Goff, J.R., Anderson, H.R., *et al.* (1980) 'Efficacy of transfusion therapy for one to two years in patients with sickle cell disease and cerebrovascular accidents.' *Journal of Pediatrics*, **96**, 205–208.

Williams, D.M., Elster, A.D. (1992) 'Cranial CT and MR in the Klippel–Trenaunay–Weber syndrome.' *American Journal of Neuroradiology*, **13**, 291–294.

Willinsky, R., Lasjaunias, P., Ter Brugge, K., Burrows, P. (1990) 'Multiple cerebral arteriovenous malformations (AVMs). Review of our experience from 203 patients with cerebral vascular lesions.' *Neuroradiology*, **32**, 207–210.

Wintzen, A.R., Broekmans, A.W., Bertina, R.M., *et al.* (1985) 'Cerebral haemorrhagic infarction in young patients with hereditary protein C deficiency: evidence for "spontaneous" cerebral venous thrombosis.' *British Medical Journal*, **290**, 350–352.

Wiznitzer, M., Masaryk, T.J. (1991) 'Cerebrovascular abnormalities in pediatric stroke: assessment using parenchymal and angiographic magnetic resonance imaging.' *Annals of Neurology*, **29**, 585–589.

Wong, V.K., Le Mesurier, J., Franceschini, R., *et al.* (1987) 'Cerebral venous thrombosis as a cause of neonatal seizures.' *Pediatric Neurology*, **3**, 235–237.

Wright, R.R., Mathews, K.D. (1996) 'Hypertensive encephalopathy in childhood.' *Journal of Child Neurology*, **11**, 193–196.

Yatsu, F.M., Hart, R.G., Mohr, J.P., Grotta, J.C. (1988) 'Anticoagulation of embolic strokes of cardiac origin: an update.' *Neurology*, **38**, 314–316.

Yokoyama, K., Asano, Y., Murakawa, T., *et al.* (1991) 'Familial occurrence of arteriovenous malformation of the brain.' *Journal of Neurosurgery*, **74**, 585–589.

Young, R.S., Coulter, D.L., Allen, R.J. (1983) 'Capsular stroke as a cause of hemiplegia in infancy.' *Neurology*, **33**, 1044–1046.

Younger, D.S., Hays, A.P., Brust, J.C.M., Rowland, L.P. (1988) 'Granulomatous angiitis of the brain: an inflammatory reaction of diverse etiology.' *Archives of Neurology*, **45**, 514–518.

Yu, I.L., Moseley, I.F., Pullicino, P., McDonald, W.I. (1982) 'The clinical picture of ectasia of the intracerebral arteries.' *Journal of Neurology, Neurosurgery, and Psychiatry*, **45**, 29–36.

Zapson, D.S., Riviello, J.J., Bagwell, S. (1995) 'Supraventricular tachycardia leading to stroke in childhood.' *Journal of Child Neurology*, **10**, 239–241.

Zaremba, J., Stepien, M., Jelowicka, M., Ostrowska, D.N. (1979) 'Hereditary neurocutaneous angioma: a new genetic entity?' *Journal of Medical Genetics*, **16**, 443–447.

Zee, C.S., Segall, H.D., McComb, J.G., *et al.* (1986) 'Intracranial arterial aneurysms in childhood: more recent considerations.' *Journal of Child Neurology*, **1**, 99–114.

Zimmerman, R.A., Bilaniuk, L.T., Packer, R.J., *et al.* (1983) 'Computed tomographic–arteriographic correlates in acute basal ganglionic infarction of childhood.' *Neuroradiology*, **24**, 241–248.

Zimmerman, R.S., Spetzler, R.F., Lee, K.S., *et al.* (1991) 'Cavernous malformations of the brain stem.' *Journal of Neurosurgery*, **75**, 32–39.

Zuber, M., Meary, E., Meder, J-F., Mas, J-L. (1993) 'Magnetic resonance imaging and dynamic CT scan in cerebral artery dissections.' *Stroke*, **25**, 576–581.

Zwarts, M.J., Begeer, J.A., Le Coultre, R. (1988) 'Unexplained chronic subarachnoid bleeding and a slowly progressive neurological syndrome.' *Journal of Neurology, Neurosurgery, and Psychiatry*, **51**, 148–150. *(Letter.)*

PART VII

PAROXYSMAL DISORDERS

Paroxysmal phenomena represent the single most common neurological problem in childhood. Evidence from general practice suggests a lifetime prevalence of about 20 per 1000 for single or repeated paroxysmal attacks and of 17 per 1000 for recurrent seizures (Goodridge and Shorvon 1983). Ross *et al.* (1980) and Ross and Peckham (1983) found that 6.7 per cent of a national British cohort had experienced at least one episode of altered consciousness. However, paroxysmal disorders form a highly heterogeneous group of conditions with completely different mechanisms, causes, outcome and management, and epileptic attacks represent only one portion of all paroxysmal episodes. In the series referred to above, epilepsy was thought to account for 4.1 per cent of cases, while febrile convulsions, breath-holding attacks, faints or other paroxysmal events accounted for the remaining 2.6 per cent.

Whatever the figures, the essential fact is that acute transient loss of consciousness with or without other manifestations is not necessarily due to epilepsy and differentiation of epileptic seizures from attacks of other origin may be difficult. Jeavons (1983) has indicated that 30 per cent of patients referred to his epilepsy clinic did not have epilepsy, an experience shared by many investigators (see Stephenson 1990).

The main reason for misdiagnosis of nonepileptic events as epilepsy is that paroxysmal attacks are brief and usually witnessed only by parents or caregivers and that, between attacks, most such children have no abnormal clinical manifestations or signs. All too often, physicians attempt to determine the nature of an *ictal* event by studying interictal *status*, whether clinically or by laboratory examination, rather than trying to gather the maximum of descriptive information about the event itself. This is, clearly, a logical error, as there is no *necessary* relationship between, say, the presence of abnormal EEG potentials, and the nature of the event. Thus a child with a rolandic spike focus may have had a syncope or faint, even though the presence of EEG paroxysms increases the probability of a diagnosis of epilepsy. As emphasized by Stephenson (1990), detailed description of the clinical event is all-important and 'the diagnosis is as good as the history'. No amount of interictal information, technical or otherwise, will replace a missing description.

In this part, I will study separately seizures of epileptic mechanism (Chapter 16) and nonepileptic events (Chapter 17), but in real life the distinction may be extremely delicate. To quote Stephenson, 'the term epileptic seizure refers to sudden change in the electrical activity of the brain, usually accompanied by subjective or objective changes in behaviour. Non-epileptic seizures are sudden changes in objective or subjective behaviour which do not have at their root an independent sudden change in the electrical activity of the brain.' However, the changes in electrical activity during attacks are only seldom actually demonstrated in the individual patient and are therefore surmised rather than observed. Moreover, the origin of a 'nonepileptic' change in behaviour, *e.g.* a tonic motor discharge during an hypoxic attack, may well also originate from some sort of abnormal brain activity such as a discharge of tonigenic neurons liberated from inhibition by higher (cortical) structures. What distinguishes such an activity from some epileptic seizures such as tonic spasms is difficult to establish in electrophysiological terms, in the absence of an ictal EEG record.

Even though the distinction between epileptic and nonepileptic events may be theoretically and practically difficult, in general, experienced clinicians can recognize the epileptic 'flavour' of an attack by observing a seizure and even by history.

REFERENCES

Goodridge, D.M.G., Shorvon, S.D. (1983) 'Epileptic seizures in a population of 6000.' *British Medical Journal,* **287**, 641–647.
Jeavons, P.M. (1983) 'Non-epileptic attacks in childhood.' *In:* Rose, F.C. (Ed.) *Research Progress in Epilepsy.* London: Pitman, pp. 224–230.
Ross, E.M., Peckham, C.S. (1983) 'Seizure disorder in the National Child Development Study.' *In:* Rose, F.C. (Ed.) *Research Progress in Epilepsy.* London: Pitman, pp. 46–59.
—— West, P.B., Butler, N.R. (1980) 'Epilepsy in childhood: findings from the National Child Development Study.' *British Medical Journal,* **1**, 207–210.
Stephenson, J.B.P. (1990) *Fits and Faints. Clinics in Developmental Medicine No. 109.* London: Mac Keith Press.

16
EPILEPSY AND OTHER SEIZURE DISORDERS

INTRODUCTION, OVERVIEW AND DEFINITIONS

DEFINITIONS (see Aicardi 1994a)

Epileptic seizures are transient *clinical* events that result from abnormal and excessive activity of synchronized, more or less extensive populations of cerebral neurons. This abnormal activity results in paroxysmal *disorganization* of one or several brain functions, manifested by positive, excitatory phenomena (motor, sensory, psychic) or negative phenomena (such as loss of awareness or muscle tone), or by a mixture of the two.

The EEG events that underlie the seizure constitute the *epileptic discharge* which, in some cases, may remain without clinical expression or have only subtle clinical consequences, so-called subclinical seizure (Gastaut 1973). The seizure discharge and/or the clinical seizure may remain localized or express bilaterally over most of the cortical surface—so-called 'generalized seizure'. Contrary to common practice, I will use the term seizure in its etymological sense (from 'to seize') and apply it to both epileptic and nonepileptic events (Stephenson 1990).

Epileptic seizures may occur as a result of intercurrent events such as fever, hypoglycaemia, acute CNS infections and the like, or recur spontaneously without known precipitant. In the former case, they are termed *occasional seizures*, whereas in the latter, they constitute *epilepsy*. Epilepsy is therefore the repetition of apparently spontaneous epileptic seizures, but repetition may be variably defined. It is a chronic condition in which epileptic seizures tend to occur repeatedly as a result of either structural brain damage or of an intrinsic functional propensity to have seizures. Epilepsy may be more than the repetition of seizures (Aicardi 1997, Beckung and Uvebrant 1997). Subclinical epileptic activity when prolonged can probably disorganize many brain functions and be responsible for lasting cognitive and behavioural disturbances (Beckung and Uvebrant 1997, Deonna *et al.* 1997).

Convulsions are attacks of involuntary muscle contractions either sustained (tonic convulsions) or interrupted (clonic convulsions). In principle, convulsions may be either epileptic or nonepileptic in nature. However, the term is traditionally used to designate *occasional epileptic seizures*, such as febrile seizures, on the one hand because occasional seizures are almost exclusively marked by motor phenomena, and on the other because the

term has come to convey the idea of benignity and avoids the use of the dreaded word epilepsy. Epilepsy and occasional seizures will be considered in different sections of this chapter.

MECHANISMS OF EPILEPTIC SEIZURES

The epileptic discharge, which is the basic electrophysiological feature of epileptic seizure, typically consists of rhythmical and high-amplitude oscillations of electrical potential that can usually be recorded from the scalp on the EEG but may, in some cases, remain undetectable even on the surface of the brain, depending on the volume of brain involved, its geometry and the manner of propagation (Bancaud and Talairach 1975). It is the most direct evidence of the abnormal, excessive neuronal activity postulated by Hughlings Jackson as the origin of epilepsy. The scalp or cortical epileptic discharge is related both to the abnormal behaviour of individual neurons and to the excessive synchronization of a large cellular population. As shown schematically in Figure 16.1, the EEG spikes correspond to the summation of field potentials that are themselves the direct consequence of intracellular events. The most remarkable of these, in seizures of focal origin, is an enormous increase in the size of membrane depolarization induced by excitatory postsynaptic potentials, the *paroxysmal depolarization shift*. This corresponds to a spike on the interictal EEG record and is followed by prolonged increased after-polarization. When a seizure occurs, this hyperpolarization disappears so that repetitive bursting goes unchecked. This, in turn, recruits neighbouring neurons that discharge synchronously.

In generalized seizures, different mechanisms may be operative, but in the case of convulsive attacks, all involve sustained membrane depolarization. The mechanism of nonconvulsive seizures such as absences, on the other hand, involves a succession of excitatory and inhibitory potentials (Snead 1995). The EEG slow wave apparently reflects GABA-mediated increased inhibition which, together with enhanced excitation, helps to produce and maintain a state of epileptic hypersynchrony. Low-threshold calcium currents in reticular thalamic pacemaker neurons seem to be responsible for driving the hypersynchronous spike-and-wave discharge of absence epilepsy. Gloor and Fariello (1988) postulate that primary generalized epilepsy is characterized by a diffusely hyperexcitable cortex so that an epileptic discharge can be triggered by excitation of the thalamic reticular system induced

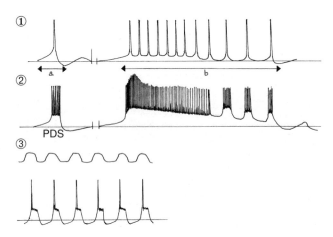

Fig. 16.1. Schematic representation of relationship between EEG discharges and cortical intracellular events in partial or secondarily generalized seizure.

1. EEG: *(a)* interictal spikes; *(b)* seizure discharge with tonic followed by clonic phases.

2. Intracellular events: paroxysmal depolarization shift (PDS) corresponds to EEG spike *(a)*. Transition to seizure is marked by failure to develop inhibitory potential thus allowing persistent depolarization and discharge.

3. In generalized spike–wave discharges, strong inhibitory potentials, probably of thalamic origin, follow each spike and correspond to the slow component. The oscillation in the thalamocortical circuit prevents continuous cortical neuron discharge.

by the thalamocortical input, and thus both the cortex and subcortical structure are necessary for its genesis.

Detailed study of the mechanisms responsible for the generation of epileptic discharge is beyond the scope of this book (for a review, see Schwartzkroin 1994).

The enhanced excitability of the brain may conceivably result from genetically determined chemical imbalance between excitatory and inhibitory neurotransmitters, from inbuilt subtle changes in cortical circuitry, or from the action of a localized lesion. In this regard, the possible influence of abnormally discharging neurons on the rest of the brain has attracted considerable attention. Focal subclinical stimulation of neuronal groups becomes increasingly effective with properly repeated stimulations and eventually may result in generalized seizures (Moshé and Ludvig 1988). The relevance of this 'kindling' phenomenon for human epilepsy, however, is still undetermined, although it may be a factor in the emergence of secondary foci (Morrell 1989).

Decreased inhibitory mechanisms are thought to play an important role in epilepsy, and the main cortical inhibitory neurotransmitter, gamma-aminobutyric acid (GABA), has been extensively studied. The GABA hypothesis has been at the origin of major therapeutic efforts and of the development of important antiepileptic drugs such as sodium valproate and vigabatrin.

Current research is also directed to the study of excitatory neurotransmitters such as glutamate and aspartate, an excess of which could account for the local or generalized enhanced cortical excitability (Meldrum 1985, Meldrum and Porter 1986, Spencer 1988). Changes in the receptors of both excitatory

(glutamate and aspartate) and inhibitory (GABA) neurotransmitters probably play a major role in the modulation of cortical excitability, and their differential rate of maturation with age may explain the changing susceptibility to epilepsy at various ages (Moshé 1987, Johnston 1996, Holmes 1997).

Whatever the mechanisms involved, brain maturation plays a critical role in the susceptibility to seizures and in their clinical expression. The morphological, electrophysiological and biochemical bases of brain maturation in relation to seizures are being actively explored (Holmes 1997).

PATHOLOGY

The pathology of epilepsy is extremely diverse, and seizures may occur in patients with almost any pathological process, from brain malformations and tumours to acquired traumatic or vascular lesions.

Two major types of pathological abnormalities are found in the brains of children with epilepsy: developmental cortical malformations, and acquired lesions, the commonest one being hippocampal (or mesial temporal) sclerosis.

Degenerative diseases, tumours and vascular abnormalities are less frequent findings.

The interpretation of some of the lesions found in the brain of epileptic patients, especially mesial temporal sclerosis, is difficult.

Mesial temporal sclerosis consists of neuronal loss in the CA1 and CA3–CA4 sectors of the hippocampus and in the dentate gyrus (Fig. 16.2). There is resulting gliosis and atrophy and, in patients with epilepsies dating back to infancy or early childhood, especially those that follow prolonged febrile seizures (Sagar and Oxbury 1987, Spencer 1988, Sutula *et al.* 1989, Mathern *et al.* 1996), sprouting of the mossy fibres is prominent and results in new synaptic contacts being established. Whether the repetition or prolongation of epileptic seizures can be responsible for such damage is still disputed (Corsellis and Bruton 1983, Babb *et al.* 1984, Babb and Brown 1987, Bruton 1988, Liu *et al.* 1995). There is experimental (Meldrum 1983) and clinical (Aicardi and Chevrie 1983) evidence that prolonged seizure activity is indeed capable of inducing brain damage, even in the absence of systemic disturbances (Meldrum 1978). Excessive release of excitatory amino acids at the synapses has been shown to produce excitotoxic hippocampal damage in experimental conditions (Fisher and Magistretti 1991, McDonald *et al.* 1991, Lipton and Rosenberg 1994). Nerve-cell death due to excessive activation (burst firing) probably results because of increase in intracellular calcium entry through NMDA receptors and some AMPA receptors, when the capacity of calcium-buffering proteins in postsynaptic cells is limited. This is the case in the CA1 and CA3 sectors of the hippocampus (Holthausen 1994).

Mesial temporal sclerosis affects both temporal lobes in about one-third of cases, and this may account for some surgical failures. The frequency of bilateral involvement varies with the aetiology, from 22 per cent in cases following febrile convulsions to 75 per cent for those following encephalitis or meningitis (Marks *et al.* 1995).

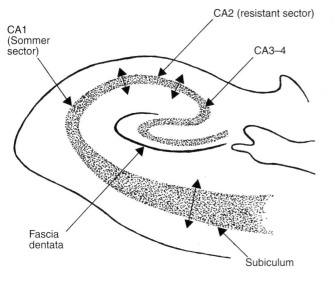

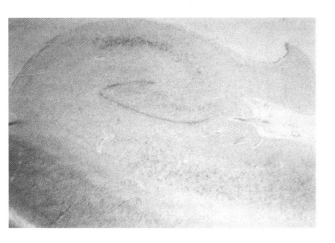

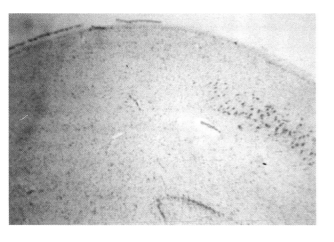

Fig. 16.2. Lesion of the CA1 sector (Sommer or fragile sector) in a case of epileptic encephalopathy. *(Top)* Schematic distribution of Ammon horn sectors. *(Centre)* Total disappearance of pyramidal cells in CA1 sector; moderate involvement of CA3–4; preservation of fascia dentata (dentate gyrus) and subiculum. *(Bottom)* Higher magnification of same specimen demonstrating abrupt disappearance of pyramidal cells at CA1–CA2 junction. (Courtesy Dr O. Robain, Hôpital Saint Vincent de Paul, Paris.)

More marked abnormalities include *migration disorders*. These may be diffuse, with a continuum of severity from lissencephaly, usually associated with infantile spasms, to laminar subcortical heterotopias (for reviews, see Aicardi 1991, Guerrini *et al.* 1996a), or localized. The latter include subcortical heterotopias, hemimegalencephaly (Vigevano and Di Rocco 1990), bilateral opercular polymicrogyria (Becker *et al.* 1989) and focal dysplasia which may affect any cortical area and be uni- or bilateral (Palmini *et al.* 1991). In some cases, giant cells that closely resemble those in cases of tuberous sclerosis are present in the dysplastic areas. Such cases have been termed 'formes frustes' of tuberous sclerosis but are unrelated to that disease either genetically (there is no family history of tuberous sclerosis) or clinically, as no other sign of the disease is present.

An interesting point about migration disorders is that they may tend to be multifocal. In 100 adult patients studied by Sisodiya *et al.* (1995), 27 were thought to have further areas of cortical abnormality when systematically examined by high-resolution MRI, a fact that may also account for some surgical failures.

Mesial temporal sclerosis in children may be associated with other lesions of developmental origin. Such dual pathology (Cendes *et al.* 1995) may render a surgical decision more difficult. It may also help to explain why, in all series, 20–30 per cent of patients continue to have seizures after surgery, possibly because the real culprit was left in place.

In a significant proportion of patients with epilepsy, the brain appears morphologically intact, even following frequently repeated attacks. Meencke and Janz (1984) and Meencke (1985) have drawn attention to the frequent presence of minor cortical anomalies in the brains of patients with apparently 'idiopathic' epilepsy. Such anomalies include excess cellularity of the molecular layer, and the presence of too many ectopic neurons in the superficial white matter (Chapter 3). These are not specific but are significantly more common in epileptic brains. Meencke and Veith (1992) believe that such minor cortical dysplasias may represent an anatomical substrate for idiopathic epilepsies as they may alter the cortical circuitry with consequent changes in excitability. This concept is debated (Lyon and Gastaut 1985). Similar changes have been reported in resected temporal lobes from patients with partial epilepsy (Hardiman *et al.* 1988, Kuzniecky *et al.* 1991) and in cases of infantile spasms (Meencke and Veith 1992), suggesting that widespread abnormality in cortical development might be of significance also in other forms of epilepsy.

AETIOLOGY OF SEIZURE DISORDERS

Occasional epileptic seizures as defined above can be provoked by a host of aggressors (Table 16.1). They almost always present as generalized convulsive seizures (Fig. 16.3). Precipitating factors include acute structural brain damage or metabolic dysfunction, *e.g.* convulsions due to meningitis, encephalitis, brain trauma or vascular accidents, hypoglycaemia and the like. Such conditions are capable of inducing seizure discharges in normal brains without any special proneness to seizures. These episodes have been

TABLE 16.1
Main causes of occasional epileptic seizures

Cause	References
Fever due to extracranial infections (febrile convulsions)	See text
Intracranial infections	
Bacterial	
Meningitis, brain abcess, empyema	Chapter 11
Septic venous thrombosis	Chapters 2, 11, 15
Viral: viral meningitis, encephalitis	Chapter 11
Fungal or parasitic	Chapter 11
Parainfectious encephalopathies	
Reye syndrome	Chapter 11
Other acute encephalopathies of obscure origin	Lyon *et al.* (1961)
Haemorrhagic shock	Harden *et al.* (1991)
Metabolic disturbances	
Hypocalcaemia and hypomagnesaemia	
Hypoglycaemia	
Hyponatraemia	Chapters 2, 23
Inappropriate secretion of ADH	
Water intoxication	
Inadequate rehydratation	
Hypernatraemia	Chapter 23
Consequence of vascular collapse due to dehydration	
Consequence of rapid correction of sodium levels	
Inborn errors of metabolism (especially during episodes of decompensation)	Chapter 9
Intoxications	
Endogenous	
Uraemia, renal dialysis	Chapter 23
Hepatic encephalopathy	Chapter 23
Diabetic ketoacidosis	Greene *et al.* (1990)
Hypertensive encephalopathy	Del Giudice and Aicardi (1979)
Renal disease	
Acute nephritis (may be paucisymptomatic)	Del Giudice and Aicardi (1979)
Haemolytic–uraemic syndrome	Chapter 23
Head trauma	
Early epileptic seizures	Chapter 13
Extradural/subdural haematoma	See text
Brain contusion	Chapter 13
Acute cerebral hypoxia	
Cardiac arrest	Aubourg *et al.* (1985)
Drowning	Chapter 13
Acute vascular collapse	Chapter 13
Cerebrovascular accidents	Chapter 15
Arterial occlusion (thrombosis or embolism)	Chapter 15
Venous thrombosis	Chapter 15
Haemorrhage from vascular malformations	Murphy (1985)
Burn encephalopathy	Mohnot *et al.* (1982)

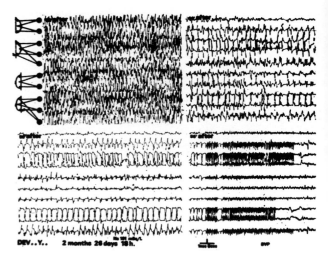

Fig. 16.3. Generalized epileptic seizure (in 2-month-old infant with hypernatraemia). Tonic discharge *(top left)*, followed by clonic discharge *(top right, continued bottom left)*. Trace at *bottom right* was recorded at slow paper speed and shows termination of seizure.

The EEG features of this seizure are slightly atypical, *e.g.* the rhythm of the tonic discharge is not the same over both hemispheres. This is common in infants, in whom typical generalized seizures are rare.

However, there is not an absolute opposition between the two groups of occasional seizures from an aetiological viewpoint. Structural lesions precipitate seizures more frequently in patients with a family history of epilepsy than in the general population (Andermann and Straszak 1982), and the same may apply to other causes, *e.g.* acute meningitis.

The same concepts apply to *epilepsies* that can also be due exclusively to genetic factors, or exclusively to chronic brain damage, congenital or acquired, or to various proportions of both (Berkovic *et al.* 1987). *Genetic factors* are of predominant importance in those epilepsies that are not associated with neurological abnormalities (idiopathic epilepsies) but may also play a role in epilepsies associated with demonstrable brain damage (Ottman 1989).

The *mode of inheritance* is variable with the type of epilepsy, and known genetic data will be indicated for each epileptic syndrome. Only a very small proportion of the cases (1–2 per cent) can be attributed to single-locus traits such as tuberous sclerosis or to metabolic errors. Epilepsy syndromes with a monogenic dominant transmission (Berkovic and Scheffer 1997) include benign neonatal convulsions (Leppert *et al.* 1989), benign infantile seizures (Vigevano *et al.* 1992, Echenne *et al.* 1994), and familial frontal (Scheffer *et al.* 1995a) and familial temporal lobe epilepsy (Berkovic *et al.* 1996). In rare cases such as Northern epilepsy, observed in Finland, a monogenic autosomal recessive inheritance is at play (Tahvanainen *et al.* 1994). In a majority of cases, the mode of genetic transmission is unknown or only suspected. Although dominant inheritance has been suggested for epilepsies with 3 Hz spike–wave activity and possibly applies to some forms of photosensitive epilepsy (Doose and Waltz 1993, Bianchi *et al.* 1995), polygenic inheritance now appears more probable (Andermann and Straszak 1982, Anderson and Hauser

termed 'symptomatic seizures' by Annegers *et al.* (1988). Other epileptic seizures are precipitated by events that do not result in seizures in the average person, the most common example being febrile seizures. In these cases, a special predisposition to seizures, present in only a minority of the population, should exist, which renders the individual susceptible to the action of specific stimuli.

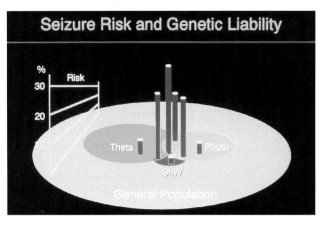

Fig. 16.4. Seizure risk and genetic liability. Each inner circle represents the fraction of the general population that exhibits one of the EEG features indicated. (Theta = abnormal theta rhythm; Photo = photosensitivity; ShW = sharp waves.) These features seem to be genetically determined. The risk of seizures associated with each of these features is indicated by a column (scale on left of figure). The risk of seizure increases markedly in patients with two or three EEG abnormalities (intersection of circles), suggesting a multifactorial inheritance of seizure liability. (Courtesy Prof. H. Doose, Kiel, Germany.)

TABLE 16.2
Aetiological factors of epilepsies due to brain damage

Prenatal factors

Dysgenetic (brain malformations, phakomatoses)
Infections (toxoplasmosis, cytomegalovirus, rubella, etc.)
Consequences of some metabolic disorders (maternal diabetes, maternal phenylketonuria) and some rare disorders such as Kohlschütter syndrome (Musumeci *et al.* 1995)
Haemorrhages (rare, due to platelet isoimmunization, etc.)
Vascular malformations, esp. cavernomas

Perinatal factors

Infections (purulent meningitis, viral encephalitis, brain abcess)
Haemorrhage (intraparenchymal, subdural, subarachnoid, intraventricular)
Stroke
Hypoxic–ischaemic encephalopathy
Metabolic or toxic (hypocalcaemia, hypoglycaemia, hyponatraemia)

Postnatal factors

Infections and parasitic lesions, *e.g.* cysticercosis (Del Brutto *et al.* 1992)
Postnatal hypoxia (near-drowning, cardiac arrest)
Trauma
Consequences of prolonged convulsive seizures (convulsive status epilepticus, hemiconvulsions–hemiplegia–epilepsy syndrome)

1991). Even in juvenile myoclonic epilepsy for which a dominant gene has been indicted (Greenberg *et al.* 1988), at least one secondary gene appears to be operative (Delgado-Escueta *et al.* 1994).

Doose and Baier (1987) have adduced evidence that certain EEG traits (*e.g.* photosensitivity or spontaneous spike–wave paroxysms) can be inherited independently and that the combination of such EEG traits (and probably of other factors) may account for the inherited propensity to various forms of epilepsy (Fig. 16.4). The problems associated with the study of the genetic factors in the epilepsies have been extensively reviewed (Bird

1987, Doose and Baier 1987, Anderson and Hauser 1991, Ottman *et al.* 1991).

Application of the new techniques of DNA analysis is being intensively investigated. Rapid progress is being made in the molecular genetics of childhood epilepsy (for reviews, see Malafosse *et al.* 1992, Berkovic and Scheffer 1997).

Brain damage is a major aetiological factor in partial or generalized epilepsies associated with clinical evidence of neuro-developmental defects. Modern techniques of neuroimaging have indicated that many cases of apparently cryptogenic epilepsy were in fact associated with abnormal intracranial processes (for reviews, see Aicardi 1990a, 1994c). The term 'brain-damaged' is used for cases in which lesions produce clinical or gross radio-logical signs, cognitive impairment and/or definite neuroimaging abnormalities. Clearly, microscopical lesions, not detectable during life, play a considerable, albeit imprecise, role in the genesis of epilepsies. Many such lesions are now recognizable by MRI, and developmental cortical abnormalities are a major cause of cryptogenic epilepsies. The main aetiological factors of brain damage associated with epilepsy are shown in Table 16.2.

CLASSIFICATION OF EPILEPTIC SEIZURES

A classification of epileptic seizures has been adopted by the International League Against Epilepsy: the 1981 revision of this Classification appears in Table 16.3. This classification is based on the distinction between *partial seizures* in which the first clinical symptoms indicate 'activation of an anatomico-functional system of neurons limited to a part of a single hemisphere', and *generalized seizures* in which the first electroclinical changes indicate involvement of both hemispheres. This classification applies only to epileptic *seizures* and a different classification system has been proposed for the *epilepsies* (see below).

The distinction between these two categories of seizures is somewhat artificial as the concept of seizures involving homogeneously the whole cortex is untenable, and as differentiation of secondarily generalized seizures of focal origin from generalized attacks may be impossible. However, it is practically important because treatment may not be the same and only partial seizures are amenable to surgical resective treatment.

Epileptic seizures are the clinical manifestations of a host of brain diseases and have very little specificity. They constitute the major element in the delineation of epileptic syndromes, and the various types of seizures wil be described with the syndromes to which they belong.

EPILEPSY SYNDROMES

To date, only a few epileptic disease entities have been identified. In the past few years, emphasis has been placed on *epilepsy syndromes*, defined as clusters of signs and symptoms associated in a nonfortuitous manner, and they have been incorporated into the new International Classification of Epilepsies and Epileptic Syndromes (Table 16.4). The International Classification, however, also uses as criteria the topographic origin of epilepsy ('localization-related' versus generalized epilepsies) and the cause

TABLE 16.3

Clinical seizure type	EEG seizure type
Partial seizures	
Simple partial seizures	Local contralateral discharge starting over the corresponding area of cortical representation (not always recorded on scalp)
With motor signs	
Focal motor with march (jacksonian)	
Focal motor without march	
Versive	
Postural	
Phonatory (vocalization or arrest of speech)	
With somatosensory or special sensory symptoms	
Somatosensory	
Visual	
Auditory	
Olfactory	
Gustatory	
Vertiginous	
With autonomic symptoms	
With psychic symptoms	
Dysphasic	
Dysmnesic (déjà vu, jamais vu)	
Cognitive	
Affective	
Experiential (complex) hallucinations	
Complex partial seizures	Unilateral or often bilateral discharge diffuse or focal over frontal and/or temporal regions
Simple partial onset followed by impairment of consciousness	
With simple partial features	
With automatisms	
With impairment of consciousness from onset	
Impairment of consciousness only	
With automatisms	
Partial seizures evolving to secondarily generalized seizures	
Simple partial seizures	
Complex partial seizures	
Simple partial seizures evolving to complex partial seizures	
Generalized seizures (convulsive or nonconvulsive)	
Absence seizures	Bursts of symmetrical rhythmic 3 Hz spike–waves
Impairment of consciousness only	
With mild clonic components	
With atonic components	
With tonic components	
With automatisms	
With autonomic components	
Atypical absence seizures	Variable discharges, irregular spike–wave complexes, fast activity; bilateral, may be asymmetrical
With changes in tone more pronounced	
Onset/cessation not abrupt	
Myoclonic seizures	Polyspike and wave or spike and wave or sharp and slow wave
Clonic seizures	Fast activity (> 10 Hz) and slow waves
Tonic seizures	Low voltage fast activity or fast (10 Hz rhythm)
Tonic–clonic seizures	10 Hz rhythm progressively slowed and intermingled with slow wave during clonic phase
Atonic seizures	As in tonic seizures
Unclassified seizures	

*Modified from the Commission on Classification (1981) of the International League Against Epilepsy.

TABLE 16.4
Classification of epilepsies and epileptic syndromes*

Localization-related (focal, local, partial) epilepsies and epileptic syndromes

Idiopathic (with age-related onset)

Benign childhood epilepsy with centrotemporal spikes

Childhood epilepsy with occipital paroxysms

Primary reading epilepsy

Symptomatic

Chronic progressive epilepsia partialis continua of childhood (Kojewnikow syndrome)

Syndromes characterized by seizures with specific modes of precipitation (include partial seizures following acquired lesions, usually involving tactile or propioceptive stimuli; partial seizures precipitated by sudden arousal or startle epilepsy)

Temporal lobe epilepsies

Frontal lobe epilepsies

Parietal lobe epilepsies

Occipital lobe epilepsies

Cryptogenic[1]

Generalized epilepsies and syndromes

Idiopathic (with age-related onset)

Benign neonatal familial convulsions

Benign neonatal convulsions

Benign myoclonic epilepsy in infancy

Childhood absence epilepsy (pyknolepsy)

Juvenile absence epilepsy

Juvenile myoclonic epilepsy (impulsive petit mal[2])

Epilepsy with grand mal seizures on awakening

Other generalized epilepsies (not defined above)

Epilepsies with seizures precipitated by specific modes of activation

Cryptogenic or symptomatic

West syndrome (infantile spasms, Blitz–Nick–Salaam Krämpfe)

Lennox–Gastaut syndrome

Epilepsy with myoclonic–astatic seizures[3]

Epilepsy with myoclonic absences

Symptomatic

Nonspecific aetiology

Early myoclonic encephalopathy

Early infantile epileptic encephalopathy with suppression–burst EEG

Other symptomatic generalized epilepsies not defined above

Specific syndromes (including diseases in which seizures are a presenting or predominant feature)

Epilepsies and epileptic syndromes undetermined whether focal or generalized

With both generalized and focal seizures

Neonatal seizures

Severe myoclonic epilepsy in infancy

Epilepsy with continuous spike–waves during slow-wave sleep

Acquired epileptic aphasia (Landau–Kleffner syndrome)

Other undetermined epilepsies not defined above

Without unequivocal generalized or focal features

Special syndromes

Situation-related seizures

Febrile convulsions

Isolated seizures or isolated status epilepticus

Seizures occurring only when there is an acute metabolic or toxic event

---

*Commission on Classification (1989).

[1]Cryptogenic epilepsies are defined as 'presumed to be symptomatic and the aetiology is unknown'; differs from symptomatic epilepsies only by the lack of aetiological evidence. Etymologically, cryptogenic signifies that the cause is unknown, which also applies to so-called idiopathic epilepsies.

[2]The term 'petit mal' would be better abandoned altogether.

[3]Probably identical with some myoclonic epilepsies. Criteria of definition different (see text).

of the disorder (symptomatic, cryptogenic and 'idiopathic' epilepsies. It is the contention of this writer that it is not possible to combine the concept of epileptic syndrome in a single classification with the other two categories of criteria.

Moreover, the present classification includes some disputable concepts. Thus, epilepsy syndromes are often regarded as cryptogenic on the basis of their unfavourable course rather than of any evidence pointing to brain damage. Likewise, the attribution of some syndromes to 'localization-related epilepsies' or 'generalized' epilepsy is arbitrary (*e.g.* neonatal seizures are 'generalized' when benign but undetermined when their diagnosis is not confirmed). Indeed, generalized seizures are uncommon in the neonatal period. Despite these serious deficiencies, the classification is presented in Table 16.4 because the reader is likely to be repeatedly exposed to it.

Delineating epilepsy syndromes permits a greater precision of diagnosis and prognosis than simply classifying seizure types, while dispensing with unverifiable assumptions on the symptomatic *vs* cryptogenic or local *vs* generalized character of the epilepsy of a particular patient (Aicardi 1994a). Epilepsy syndromes, however, are heterogeneous as the link between the components of a particular syndrome may be topographical, aetiological or not understood. More importantly, their specificity is variable. Some syndromes, *e.g.* benign rolandic epilepsy, are extremely well defined, whereas others, such as awakening grand mal, clearly include heterogeneous cases related only through the circumstances of occurrence of a common type of seizure. Because the concept of syndrome is an entirely pragmatic one and because agreement on what constitutes a particular syndrome may be difficult to reach, only well-defined and generally accepted syndromes are of value (Aicardi 1994b, Duchowny and Harvey 1996, Watanabe 1996). Multiplication of the number of poorly vindicated subgroups or squeezing atypical cases into generally accepted syndromes are two dangers that can defeat the whole aim of delineating epileptic syndromes, which is to help in diagnosis, prognosis and management, not to define entities. As a result, a variable proportion of cases of childhood epilepsy are better left unclassified.

The age of onset of epilepsy is critically important for classification and diagnosis, and epilepsies of infancy and later childhood will be studied successively.

EPILEPSY SYNDROMES OF INFANCY AND EARLY CHILDHOOD
INFANTILE SPASMS AND RELATED SYNDROMES
Infantile spasms are both a type of seizure and a syndrome with multiple causes. The classical syndrome, also known as West syndrome, has three major components: the spasms, the EEG tracing of *hypsarrhythmia* that accompanies the seizures in a typical or modified form, and the presence of mental deterioration or retardation. One of the elements of the triad may be absent (commonly the hypsarrhythmia) (Jeavons and Livet 1992), and additional features such as partial seizures, marked asymmetries and focal neurological signs may coexist. Such cases are not considered as West syndrome by some investigators.

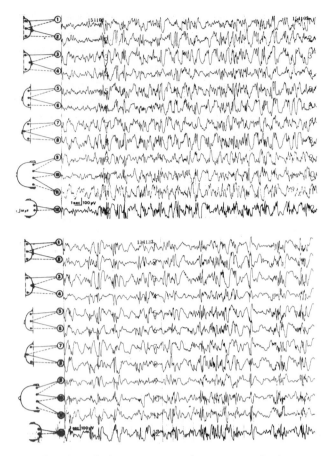

Fig. 16.5. Hypsarrhythmia in patient with cryptogenic infantile spasms. *(Top)* Waking EEG with high-amplitude slow waves irregularly interspersed with sharp waves arising multifocally. *(Bottom)* Sleeping record showing synchronization of multiple spikes separated by intervals of low-amplitude tracing.

Although *epileptic spasms* can occur outside the infantile period, they are most often observed in the first year of life as a major component of the infantile spasms syndrome or West syndrome. In later childhood, spasms are a possible mechanism of epileptic falls (Egli *et al.* 1985, Ikeno *et al.* 1985). The spasms are sudden, usually bilateral tonic contractions of the muscles of the neck, trunk and extremities which may be flexor, extensor or mixed (Hrachovy and Frost 1989). The intense abrupt contraction lasts less than two seconds but may be followed by a less intense contraction and/or by behavioural arrest lasting about 10 s. The spasms are sometimes isolated but characteristically occur in series of a few units to more than 100 individual jerks 5–30 s apart. The repetitive character of the spasms is an important diagnostic clue, especially as the individual spasms may have a very limited expression such as slight head nodding, elevation of the eyeballs or shrugging of the shoulders, which are all too often discounted as colic, Moro reflex or other benign phenomena. Clinical variants, especially unilateral spasms, are relatively common (Shewmon 1994).

The ictal EEG manifestations of epileptic spasms generally consist of a generalized high-amplitude slow wave coinciding with the clinical event, often with superimposed fast activity (Vigevano

et al. 1993). The latter may appear in isolation (Donat and Wright 1991c, Shewmon 1994). Other patterns have been reported (Hrachovy and Frost 1989) but appear to be rare.

The onset of West syndrome is virtually always during the first year of life with a peak frequency between 4 and 10 months of age, although spasms may begin shortly after birth. Asymmetrical and even unilateral spasms may occur and are usually associated with contralateral EEG activity, suggesting a cortical generator to infantile spasms (Donat and Wright 1991a,c; Gaily *et al.* 1995), and with damage to the same side. Other types of seizure frequently precede or accompany the spasms (Lombroso 1983a, Donat and Wright 1991b, Carrazana *et al.* 1993, Plouin and Dulac 1994).

Developmental retardation is present before the onset of the spasms in 68–85 per cent of cases (Matsumoto *et al.* 1981, Riikonen 1982, Hrachovy and Frost 1989). Such figures are minimal estimates as mild degrees of mental delay are difficult to identify retrospectively. In previously well infants, a definite *behavioural regression* is observed, the infants losing interest in their surroundings sometimes to the point of appearing blind and deaf. Deterioration may seem to be the first manifestation of the syndrome when the spasms are delayed or escape recognition, and West syndrome should be thought of in any infant who regresses developmentally during the first year of life. With the subsidence of attacks, the infant's development usually improves although resumption of mental functioning may lag for several weeks after cessation of seizures.

Autistic features are common at the onset of West syndrome and may persist as a sequela in a high proportion of patients (Riikonen and Amnell 1981, Chugani *et al.* 1996). Guzzetta *et al.* (1993) have clearly separated the manifestations of the acute phase, mainly including disturbances of awareness and communication, from the cognitive sequelae.

Hypsarrhythmia (Fig. 16.5) is the most remarkable EEG pattern associated with infantile spasms. It is characterized by a chaotic succession of very high amplitude slow waves interspersed at random with multifocal asynchronous spikes and sharp waves. During slow sleep, bursts of polyspikes separated by stretches of poorly active tracings are typically present (Lombroso 1983a). Modified hypsarrhythmia with preservation of some background rhythm, localizing features or synchronous spike–wave activity, is found in up to 40 per cent of cases (Jeavons and Livet 1992). Unilateral hypsarrhythmia is rare. Several other EEG patterns can be associated with infantile spasms, and only 60 per cent of patients were reported to have true or modified hypsarrhythmia (Dalla Bernardina and Watanabe 1994). Some infants may have nonparoxysmal EEG for a brief period at onset of the disorder or late in the course despite persistence of the clinical spasms.

The *diagnosis* of infantile spasms is easy if the repetitive character of the spasms and the associated phenomena are given due attention. However, only 12 per cent of primary care physicians made the correct diagnosis in one series (Bellman *et al.* 1983), whereas 15 per cent made a diagnosis of colic. *Benign myoclonus of early infancy* may closely mimic infantile spasms but the EEG

TABLE 16.5
Main causes of infantile spasms

Cause	References
Neurocutaneous syndromes	
Tuberous sclerosis	Chapter 4
Neurofibromatosis	Chapter 4
Sturge–Weber syndrome	Chapter 15
Incontinentia pigmenti	Chapter 4
Ito disease	Pascual-Castroviejo *et al.* (1988), Ogino *et al.* (1994)
Linear naevus syndrome	Chapter 4
Brain malformations	
Aicardi syndrome	Chapter 3
Agyria–pachygyria	Chapter 3
Congenital perisylvian syndrome	Kuzniecky *et al.* (1994)
Holoprosencephaly	Chapter 3
Hemimegalencephaly	Chapter 3, Vigevano and Di Rocco (1990)
Heterotopias, cortical dysplasias and other migration disorders	Aicardi (1994a), Palm *et al.* (1986), Robain and Vinters (1994)
Down syndrome	Guerrini *et al.* (1998)
Fragile X chromosome	Rugtveit (1986)
Metabolic and degenerative diseases	
Phenylketonuria	Chapter 9
Nonketotic hyperglycinaemia	Chapter 9
Hyperornithinaemia–hyperammonaemia–homocitrullinaemia (HHH syndrome)	Chapter 9
Leigh disease	Santorelli *et al.* (1993)
Pyridoxine dependency	Bankier *et al.* (1983)
Degenerative diseases of unknown cause (poliodystrophy, leukodystrophy)	Aicardi (1994a)
Mitochondrial disorders	Koo *et al.* (1993)
Biotinidase deficiency	Kalayci *et al.* (1994)
Carbohydrate-deficient glycoprotein (CDG) syndrome type IV	Stibler *et al.* (1993)
PEHO syndrome (progressive encephalopathy with oedema, hypsarrhythmia and optic atrophy)	Salonen *et al.* (1991), Somer and Sainio (1993)
X-linked infantile spasms	Claes *et al.* (1997)
Infectious disorders	
Fetal infections especially cytomegalovirus	Riikonen (1993)
Toxic	
Sequelae of neonatal hypoglycaemia	Aicardi (1994a), Ohtahara *et al.* (1993)
Lithium toxicity	Lombroso (1983b)
Hypoxic–ischaemic encephalopathy	
Prenatal, perinatal or postnatal	Aicardi (1994a)
Cerebral infarcts	Alvarez *et al.* (1987)
Near-drowning	Hrachovy *et al.* (1987)
Cardiac surgery with hypothermia	du Plessis *et al.* (1994)
Trauma and haemorrhage	Chapter 13
Brain tumours (rarely)	Ruggieri *et al.* (1989)
Neonatal haemangiomatosis	McShane *et al.* (1990)

is normal (Lombroso and Fejerman 1977, Dravet *et al.* 1986). The phenomenon seems related to tics or 'gratification phenomena'. Other forms of epilepsy, especially cryptogenic myoclonic epilepsy, are also erroneously diagnosed as infantile spasms, although the prognosis is more favourable. The same may apply to early-onset cases of the Lennox–Gastaut syndrome, and the high frequency of infantile spasms with onset after age 1 year in some series probably results from failure to separate such cases from real West syndrome. Seizures can occur in series in both syndromes (Donat and Wright 1991a).

The main causes of West syndrome are listed in Table 16.5. An important distinction is between *symptomatic* and *cryptogenic* spasms (Jeavons and Livet 1992). Cryptogenic cases are variably defined as those for which no cause can be identified or those that, in addition, have developed normally before the onset of attacks (Lombroso 1983a). With the latter definition, cryptogenic spasms account for only 10–15 per cent of cases, but these are much more likely than symptomatic cases to run a favourable course. Some investigators (Dulac *et al.* 1986, Vigevano *et al.* 1993) describe an idiopathic group of infantile spasms with a good prognosis and peculiar clinical and EEG features. However, Haga *et al.* (1995) were unable to differentiate aetiological groups on the basis of clinical or EEG (ictal or interictal) features. Brain dysgenesis and neurocutaneous syndromes (mainly tuberous sclerosis) are the most common identified causes of infantile spasms (Vigevano *et al.* 1994a). Gross malformations include lissencephaly, pachygyria, diffuse subcortical heterotopias and agenesis of the corpus callosum, especially Aicardi syndrome (Chapter 3). Tuberous sclerosis accounts for 10–20 per cent of cases. Focal cortical dysplasias (Chugani *et al.* 1990, 1996; Robain and Vinters 1994) may be the single most important cause of infantile spasms (van Bogaert *et al.* 1993). Chronic acquired lesions account for a majority of remaining symptomatic cases (Cowan and Hudson 1991). Metabolic diseases are rarely causative: one such is the PEHO syndrome of peripheral oedema, hypsarrhythmia and optic atrophy (Chapter 10). From a pathological point of view, a majority of autopsied cases of infantile spasms are due to prenatal factors (Meencke and Gerhard 1985, Jellinger 1987). Meencke and Gerhard found no detectable pathology in only 11 per cent of 107 cases. Most cases are related to diffuse lesions but unilateral lesions, in particular cystic softenings in the middle artery territory (so-called porencephalic cysts) (Palm *et al.* 1988), may be responsible for infantile spasms that are not necessarily of poor prognosis (Alvarez *et al.* 1987, Cusmai *et al.* 1988).

The *treatment* of West syndrome is difficult. Most conventional anticonvulsant drugs are ineffective. Corticosteroids and ACTH are considered most efficacious but the modalities of treatment have been extremely variable so that comparisons are impossible. One controlled comparative study between ACTH and corticosteroids did not reveal any superiority of one product over the other (Hrachovy *et al.* 1983). High-dose ACTH (150 IU/kg/d) was not found more effective than low dosage (20 IU/kg/d) in another study (Hrachovy *et al.* 1994). A more recent and larger study strongly favours high-dose ACTH (Baram et al. 1996), which produced remission in 13 of 15 infants as against four of 14 receiving prednisone. However, it seems that some cases may respond selectively to either agent, and various protocols are being proposed (Schlumberger and Dulac 1994). Heiskala et al. (1996) propose individualizing ACTH therapy, starting with a dose of 3 IU/kg/d and progressively increasing to a maximum of 12 IU/kg/d if no response is obtained. They noted that most cryptogenic cases responded to the smallest dose, whereas symptomatic cases required higher doses. This method limits dose-related side-effects. Corticosteroids obviate the need for injection and shorten hospitalization, but ACTH is to be preferred if its superiority is confirmed. The mode of action of both agents is unknown. Doses of ACTH used vary between 10 and 240 IU/kg/d and those of hydrocortisone between 10 and 25 mg/kg/d for durations of two weeks to many months (Aicardi 1994a). My own practice is to use hormonal treatment for short periods of the order of four to six weeks.

ACTH or steroid therapy seems to control the spasms in 50–70 per cent of cases and normalizes or improves the EEG in a slightly lower proportion. Relapses occur in 20–35 per cent of patients. The long-term effect of therapy, if any, is less striking (Glaze et al. 1988), and a near-normal mental development can be expected in only about 50 per cent of patients with cryptogenic spasms or only 10–20 per cent of all cases. The prognosis depends on aetiology, and better results are obtained in cryptogenic (or idiopathic) cases with a completely normal development before the spasms. The occurrence of previous seizures, of neurological signs and of major MRI abnormalities are predictors of a poor outcome. Koo et al. (1993) found an average developmental quotient of 71 in 17 cryptogenic and of 48 in 40 symptomatic cases. Fifty-one per cent of patients had other seizures and these were significantly associated with a symptomatic aetiology and a poor cognitive outcome. Ohtsuka et al. (1994) found that 56 per cent of 109 patients were ultimately seizure-free and 21 per cent had a normal development; however, about half the infants had relapses, 34 per cent of which occurred within six months of discontinuing treatment.

Epileptic seizures persist in approximately half the patients. They commonly present with the characteristics of the Lennox–Gastaut syndrome but partial seizures are also observed.

Side-effects of ACTH or corticosteroids are frequent (Riikonen and Donner 1980), perhaps less so with non-depot preparations (Kusse et al. 1993), and for that reason we formerly reserved these agents for cryptogenic cases in which it may improve long-term outlook. However, Hrachovy and Frost (1989) did not find any difference in response between cryptogenic and symptomatic spasms, and therefore advise systematic long-term treatment in all cases. It is, in fact, difficult to deny the alleged benefits of ACTH therapy to severely diseased infants. In addition, the good effect of ACTH/steroids on spasms and EEG anomalies are well established.

In addition to the classical side-effects of corticosteroids, brain shrinkage is usually observed (Glaze et al. 1986, Konishi et al. 1992). Therefore neuroimaging assessment of patients is best performed before starting treatment.

The benzodiazepines, especially nitrazepam, are sometimes effective against clinical spasms (Chamberlain 1996) but their effect on the EEG abnormalities is limited. One comparative study found no difference between nitrazepam and hormonal treatment (Dreifuss et al. 1986) but most authors regard this treatment as less active than steroids.

Sodium valproate in high doses (100–200 mg/kg/d) has given good results to some investigators (Siemes et al. 1988, Prats et al. 1991, Ohtsuka et al. 1994), with control of the spasms in 40–65 per cent of cases and improvement in mental outcome.

Vigabatrin appears to control the spasms in 50–60 per cent of patients (Chiron et al. 1991, Snead and Chiron 1994, Aicardi et al. 1996). A comparative study with ACTH (Vigevano and Cilio 1997) showed vigabatrin to be slightly less effective but better tolerated than ACTH. Its action is rapid in less than a week, and the side-effects are much less than with steroids, even with the very high doses (100–150 mg/kg) that seem to be necessary. At this stage, it appears reasonable to start treatment with vigabatrin and to switch to hormonal therapy if the attacks are not controlled within a week. Some investigators have found the drug particularly effective in the treatment of symptomatic forms (Chiron et al. 1991). Vigabatrin seems highly effective in spasms due to tuberous sclerosis and is probably the drug of choice in such cases (Chiron et al. 1990, Aicardi et al. 1996).

Other forms of treatment for infantile spasms have been with high-dose pyridoxal phosphate (Ohtsuka et al. 1994) with a response rate of 10–29 per cent (Pietz et al. 1993), and immunoglobulin therapy (Arizumi et al. 1987, Echenne et al. 1991). Surgical resection of localized brain areas of cortical dysplasia thought to be responsible for the spasms has been performed in a few patients (Chugani et al. 1990, Shields et al. 1992, Chugani and Pinard 1994) and may be indicated in selected resistant cases. Delimitation of the abnormal cortex is usually by MRI but some cases may be detectable only by positron emission tomography (PET—Chugani et al. 1990, 1996), or by single photon emission computed tomography (SPECT—Miyazaki et al. 1994). However, transient PET abnormalities, especially during the period of active hypsarrhythmia, have been found by Watanabe et al. (1994), and the relationship between PET anomalies and the causes and outcome of the syndrome is currently unclear (Watanabe 1996). 'Uncapping' of cystic softenings has also been reported to be an effective treatment (Palm et al. 1988). Results of these trials await confirmation. Identification, and possible preventive treatment, of infants with neonatal difficulties at-risk of developing infantile spasms has been attempted (Walther et al. 1987, Watanabe et al. 1987a).

Syndromes closely related to infantile spasms (Table 16.6) include neonatal myoclonic encephalopathy (Aicardi 1990b), Ohtahara syndrome or early infantile epileptic encephalopathy (EIEE) (Ohtahara et al. 1987) and the syndrome of periodic spasms described by Gobbi et al. (1987). All these syndromes are of lesional or metabolic origin and share a very poor prognosis. The separation between EIEE and neonatal myoclonic encephalopathy may be artificial (Lombroso 1990), and EIEE may be an early form of infantile spasms.

TABLE 16.6
Syndromes related to infantile spasms

Syndrome	Clinical features	EEG features	Aetiological factors
Neonatal myoclonic encephalopathy* (early myoclonic encephalopathy)	Erratic myoclonus and partial seizures from the first days of life. Infantile spasms appear secondarily. Severe course with death in first year in 50 per cent of cases	Suppression–burst pattern later evolving into atypical hypsarrhythmia	Unknown. Familial cases known
Glycine encephalopathy* (nonketotic hyperglycinaemia)	Same features, death within one month in 50 per cent of cases	Idem	Enzyme defect (Chapter 9)
Early infantile epileptic encephalopathy (Ohtahara syndrome)	Tonic spasms from the first days of life. Partial seizures sometimes	Idem	Brain malformations + unknown
Periodic lateralized spasms	Repetitive lateralized spasms often following a partial seizure	Asymmetrical slow complexes following a localized discharge with superimposed fast rhythms	Mainly brain malformations

*These two entities may be regarded as belonging to the same electroclinical syndrome.

Although neonatal myoclonic encephalopathy may be associated with metabolic disorders and be of genetic origin more often than early epileptic encephalopathy, both may result from the same causes: migration disorder has been shown to be a cause of myoclonic encephalopathy (du Plessis *et al.* 1993) and EIEE may occur with hyperglycinaemia.

Dentato-olivary dysplasia (Harding and Boyd 1991) is a rare cause of neonatal tonic seizures and possibly of infantile spasms. The prognosis is very poor and the diagnosis is possible only at autopsy. One familial case is known (Harding and Copp 1997).

LENNOX–GASTAUT SYNDROME
The Lennox–Gastaut syndrome (LGS) includes patients with epilepsies starting mainly between 1 and 7 years of age, who present with variable proportions of tonic, atonic and myoclonic seizures resulting in multiple falls and atypical absences, and whose interictal EEGs contain bilateral, though not necessarily symmetrical, slow (<2.5 Hz) spike–wave activity. The limits of the LGS are variably understood by different investigators who use diverse criteria for its definition (see Aicardi and Levy Gomes 1988; Aicardi 1994a, 1996) and for its separation from related syndromes such as the myoclonic epilepsies. Many investigators now accept the definition proposed by Beaumanoir and Dravet (1992), *i.e.* of a syndrome of multiple seizure types including tonic seizures, atypical absences, and episodes of tonic and non-convulsive status epilepticus with slow spike–waves, spikes and bursts of 10–20 Hz spikes during sleep.

Many cases of LGS are probably related to diffuse or multi-focal brain lesions although several aspects of the pathology remain obscure (Roger and Gambarelli-Dubois 1988). Boniver *et al.* (1987) recognized an idiopathic type of LGS. Renier (1988) found poor dendritic arborization and disturbed synaptic devel-

opment restricted to the deeper cortical layers despite absence of gross pathological lesions.

The *seizures* of the LGS include 'core' seizures (myoatonic and tonic, atypical absences and episodes of nonconvulsive status epilepticus) that can be variably associated with less characteristic attacks such as tonic–clonic, partial or unilateral seizures.

Tonic seizures are encountered in 55–92 per cent of cases. Clinically, they are marked by body stiffening involving mainly the axial and proximal limb muscles, with extension more commonly than flexion of the trunk, the lower limbs and the arms. They may be limited to the trunk and neck with opening of the eyes and frequently apnoea. They sometimes consist only of eye opening with mild 'stretching' movements. Their duration does not exceed 30s and is often no more than 10s. Even in such cases, the contraction is clearly tonic, resulting in sustained clinical and electromyographic muscle activity (Aicardi and Levy Gomes 1988). The ictal EEG shows a generalized discharge of fast activity (≥10 Hz) of increasing or high amplitude (Erba and Browne 1983, Beaumanoir and Dravet 1992, Donat 1992), sometimes followed by a few spike–wave complexes. Tonic seizures are often nocturnal but their manifestations in sleep may be so mild as to go unnoticed (Aicardi and Levy Gomes 1988, Livingston 1988, Beaumanoir and Dravet 1992, Yaqub 1993).

Atonic seizures occur in 26–56 per cent of LGS patients. They consist of abrupt muscle relaxation and are a common cause of falls in such children, although tonic and myoclonic attacks can also result in falls. These represent a major practical problem as they often cause injuries not easily prevented by wearing a helmet. The mechanisms of falls are unclear, so the non-committal term of astatic seizure should be preferred. Most atonic seizures are associated with loss of consciousness and it is not clear whether they are purely atonic or are associated with tonic phenomena. Most have the same EEG concomitants as tonic seizures. Thus, they seem to differ from pure atonic seizures associated with bursts of spike–wave activity as observed in the myoatonic epilepsies (Oguni *et al.* 1993).

True myoclonic seizures may be seen in up to 28 per cent of cases and may also be associated with falls. The type of seizure observed depends on the age of onset of LGS. In cases of early onset, tonic seizures predominate, whereas myoclonic jerks and absence are more frequent in late-onset cases (Chevrie and Aicardi 1972, Aicardi 1996).

Atypical absences are present in 17–60 per cent of patients. Although their onset and termination may be more progressive than in typical absences (see below), they are marked by the same interruption of awareness and responsiveness with only mild motor components (stiffness, hypotonia, simple automatisms) and their recognition depends on the clinical context and the EEG concomitants. These are sometimes ictal slow spike–waves, difficult to distinguish from interictal spike–waves, but more often fast discharges similar to those associated with tonic seizures.

Episodes of *nonconvulsive status epilepticus* are frequent (Dravet *et al.* 1985, Beaumanoir *et al.* 1988) and may last several days or even weeks. They may be responsible for the alternation of good and bad periods with considerable changes in reaction time and mental activity (Erba and Browne 1983). The most common type is characterized by the alternation of tonic attacks and episodes of confused behaviour, often with erratic myoclonic activity of the face and upper limbs, and may last from hours to weeks.

The characteristic *interictal EEG* of patients with LGS is a diffuse slow spike–wave pattern, with slow blunted spikes followed by irregular 1–2 Hz slow waves of variable amplitude. The paroxysms occur in runs of several seconds, usually on a slow, irregular background tracing. They may be asymmetrical and are often unaccompanied by obvious clinical manifestations. They show little or no response to hyperventilation or photic stimulation but are activated during drowsiness and slow sleep (Aicardi and Levy Gomes 1988). During non-REM sleep, runs of 10 Hz rhythms of a few seconds duration characteristically occur and probably represent subclinical or minimal tonic seizures (Fig. 16.6). At the same stage, slow spike–wave complexes are frequently replaced by polyspike–wave complexes.

Mental retardation is present before onset of seizures in 20–60 per cent of cases (Aicardi 1994a). The proportion of retarded patients increases with the passing of time and about 90 per cent of patients are retarded five years after onset (Chevrie and Aicardi 1972, Furune *et al.* 1988). Clear loss of skills is observed in some patients.

The *causes* of LGS are multiple. Most cases are due to brain lesions and a genetic predisposition has not been found in reported series, except that of Boniver *et al.* (1987). The same brain insults that produce infantile spasms can be responsible for LGS. Brain malformations, however, are less common in LGS, and LGS has been only rarely recorded in the course of Aicardi syndrome or of lissencephaly. Focal cortical malformations are frequent, and cases of band heterotopia and of bilateral perisylvian

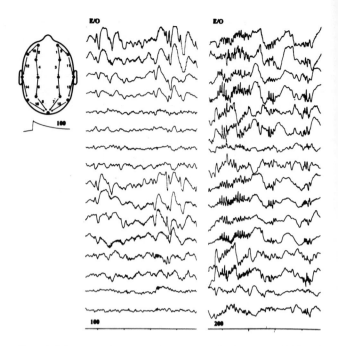

Fig. 16.6. Lennox–Gastaut syndrome. EEG findings in a child with multiple seizure types, but particularly tonic attacks and atypical absences. *(Left)* The portion of waking record shows sharp waves and slow components at around 2–2.5/s over the anterior half of the head. *(Right)* A burst of 10–12/s spiky components is seen during sleep associated with spontaneous eye opening. (Courtesy Dr S. Boyd, Great Ormond Street Hospital, London.)

syndromes are on record (Chapter 3). Tuberous sclerosis and less common neurocutaneous syndromes, such as linear naevus sebaceus (Kurokawa *et al.* 1981) and Ito hypomelanosis (personal cases) may be responsible. Metabolic diseases are exceptional, although LGS due to Leigh encephalomyelopathy has been recorded (Matsuishi *et al.* 1985). Rare cases of LGS secondary to brain tumours are known (Honda *et al.* 1985). The occurrence of LGS in patients with unilateral lesions has led to attempts at distinguishing 'true' LGS from bilateral secondary synchrony (Gastaut and Zifkin 1988). In fact, cases of bilateral secondary synchrony fulfil the usual criteria for the diagnosis of LGS, even though they may be important to recognize because of surgical possibilities. Studies with PET scan have recognized several metabolic patterns (focal, multifocal or diffuse) which may correspond to different mechanisms (Chugani *et al.* 1987, Iinuma *et al.* 1987, Theodore *et al.* 1987). Their practical significance is still unclear as the criteria for the diagnosis of LGS varied with the series (Dulac and N'Guyen 1993).

The *diagnosis* of LGS is not difficult if strict criteria are used. However, differentiation of LGS from some other syndromes associated with falls may be problematical (see Aicardi 1996 for discussion). A real problem may be posed by the rare cases of 'benign atypical epilepsy of children' (Aicardi and Levy Gomes 1992) or pseudo-Lennox syndrome (Doose and Baier 1989) in which repeated falls and diffuse paroxysmal EEG activity during sleep may suggest LGS. Such cases run a relatively benign course and it is important to recognize them.

The *prognosis* of LGS is poor. Approximately 80 per cent of patients continue to have seizures and, because of seizures or mental deterioration, only a very few patients are able to live independent lives. The outcome is especially poor for patients with brain damage, early onset of seizures, antecedents of infantile spasms, and mental retardation present before the initial seizures. Fewer than 10 per cent of patients have a normal intellectual level (Furune *et al.* 1988). It has proved difficult to distinguish such cases from those with less favourable outcome, although a later age of onset, a positive response to hyperventilation and a higher incidence of 3 Hz spike–wave complexes have some prognostic value (Aicardi and Levy Gomes 1988, 1992). Cases with such features were termed 'intermediate petit mal' but the separation of such a subgroup seems debatable as the criteria of diagnosis were similar to those of LGS in general.

The *treatment* of LGS is disappointing (see also p. 615). Among conventional antiepileptic drugs, combinations of sodium valproate and a benzodiazepine are least unsatisfactory (Aicardi 1996), but all such drugs may be worth a trial in individual patients. Vigabatrin has been used with some measure of success (Dulac and N'Guyen 1993). Lamotrigine seems efficacious especially against atonic seizures (Schlumberger *et al.* 1994) and is probably the best treatment now available, although felbamate may still be considered despite possible toxicity as it is often effective (Ritter *et al.* 1993). Topiramate is sometimes effective. The addition of a second drug may be necessary because some seizure types—especially tonic attacks—may not respond to lamotrigine and require addition of carbamazepine or phenytoin. Interestingly, combinations of drugs are often required as individual drugs may have a specific activity against only certain types of seizures. Because of the high rate of failure of drugs, other methods may be worth trying. The ketogenic diet has given good short-term effects despite practical difficulties (Schwartz *et al.* 1989a,b; Kinsman *et al.* 1992) because of unpalatability and side-effects. However, Kinsman *et al.* have been able to maintain the treatment for one or two years with control of seizures in half their patients. Interestingly, they claim that the diet can be withdrawn after two years without recurrence of the seizures. Steroids are used mainly to tide the patient over bad periods of very active epilepsy or status. Intravenous immunoglobulin has been advocated (Illum *et al.* 1990) but has not been properly tested. Thyrotropin-releasing hormone (Matsumoto *et al.* 1987) has been used mainly in Japan.

MYOCLONIC EPILEPSIES OF INFANCY AND EARLY CHILDHOOD

Epilepsies that consist mainly of true myoclonic seizures—*i.e.* seizures marked clinically by very brief shock-like muscle contractions and, electrically, by fast spike–wave or polyspike–wave complexes—occur in infancy and early childhood (Erba and Browne 1983, Aicardi 1994a, Aicardi 1996). Such epilepsies are often confused with LGS because of the frequent repetition of brief attacks that may produce multiple falls, the presence of spike–wave discharges in both groups, and the frequent association of mental subnormality or deterioration with the seizures.

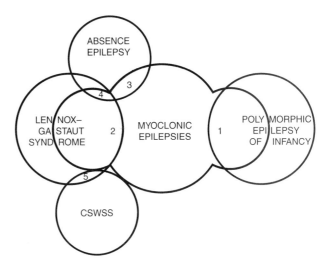

Fig. 16.7. Schematic representation of the relationships between cryptogenic myoclonic epilepsy and other epileptic syndromes in infancy (intersections between circles themselves have no quantitative significance).
1. Myoclonic form of polymorphic epilepsy of infancy (severe myoclonic epilepsy). Myoclonic forms are probably more common than nonmyoclonic ones.
2. 'Myoclonic variant' of Lennox–Gastaut syndrome (LGS) (intermediate forms between LGS and myoclonic epilepsy).
3. Myoclonic absence epilepsy.
4. Myoclonic absence epilepsy with secondary development of LGS.
5. Transitional forms between LGS and continuous spike-waves of slow sleep (CSWSS).
Doose myoclonic–astatic epilepsy is not shown because its criteria of definition differ from those used here and it probably corresponds in part to several of the syndromes shown.

However, the clinical and EEG manifestations of the myoclonic epilepsies differ from those of LGS, and the outlook for control of seizures and mental development may not be the same.

Myoclonic seizures consist of sudden, lightning-like muscle contractions that may involve the whole body (massive myoclonic attacks) or be limited to the upper limbs, the face or the eyelids. The jerks are usually symmetrical but may be unilateral or even localized to small muscle groups (Aicardi 1994a, 1996). Ictal EEG shows polyspike–wave paroxysms. Ictal electromyography demonstrates an extremely brief muscle contraction followed by a period of inactivity lasting 100–350ms. When this period is relatively long, muscle resolution may become clinically evident resulting in a myoatonic seizure (Oguni *et al.* 1994). Occasionally, only the atonic phase is detectable, the so-called 'negative myoclonus' (Guerrini *et al.* 1993). Clinically, atonia of variable intensity and duration often follows the myoclonic jerk. When generalized and long enough, it results in falls (*drop-attacks*) so the differentiation of atonic from myoclonic seizures may be impossible. Myoclonic–astatic epilepsy is thus only a variant of myoclonic epilepsy in which the atonic component is particularly obvious.

The nosology of the myoclonic epilepsies remains confused (Fig. 16.7). The International Classification identifies three major groups: *severe myoclonic epilepsy* (Dravet *et al.* 1985, 1992a), *benign myoclonic epilepsy* (Dravet *et al.* 1992a), and *myoclonic–astatic epilepsy* (Doose 1992) to which unclassifiable cases should be added.

Some investigators (*e.g.* Lombroso 1990) doubt that there is such a sharp separation between the various types of myoclonic epilepsy and think that there is a spectrum of myoclonic syndromes with all degrees of severity. The prediction of outcome would thus be impossible at the onset of clinical manifestations.

Benign myoclonic epilepsy according to Dravet *et al.* (1992a) is rare. It is characterized by the onset within the first two years of life of myoclonic seizures as the only form of attacks in otherwise neurodevelopmentally normal infants. The course is benign with a good response to therapy with sodium valproate or ethosuximide (Dulac *et al.* 1990, Gascon *et al.* 1992), although some affected children have learning difficulties or mild retardation. In fact, the benign prognosis of this form is far from constant and a number of patients end up with behavioural and mental difficulties. It is not clear whether benign myoclonic epilepsy should be limited to cases with only myoclonic seizures. Aicardi and Levy Gomes (1989) have reported on 19 young children, mainly boys with a high frequency of familial antecedents of seizures, who had infrequent tonic–clonic seizures and/or brief absences in addition to frequent myoclonic jerks and a relatively favourable outcome. Such cases suggest the existence of a spectrum of nonlesional, probably genetically determined, myoclonic epilepsies.

In some infants, the seizures are precipitated by sudden exteroceptive or proprioceptive stimuli. This 'touch' or reflex myoclonic epilepsy (Ricci *et al.* 1995) seems to have an excellent prognosis. Cases similar to benign myoclonic epilepsy may also occur in older children (Guerrini *et al.* 1994a).

Severe myoclonic epilepsy is characterized by the onset, usually between 4 and 10 months of age, of clonic seizures often unilateral and prolonged, precipitated by fever in 75 per cent of cases. Such seizures recur several times, at short intervals (usually less than two months). During the second or third year, other types of seizure appear including partial complex seizures, atypical absences, myoclonic jerks and episodes of nonconvulsive status. At the same time, slowing of mental development becomes evident. The EEG does not show slow spike–wave complexes but rather bursts of fast spike–wave complexes, often in association with multifocal spikes. Photosensitivity is present in 25 per cent of patients and self-precipitation of seizures is not rare. The long-term outcome is poor. The seizures persist mainly as grand mal attacks although myoclonic seizures tend to disappear. Mental retardation of variable degree is constant (Dravet *et al.* 1992b).

Similar cases with early onset of generalized or unilateral clonic seizures often precipitated by mild fevers, or even by hot baths, with rapid recurrence and secondary apparition of brief seizures of multiple types are not uncommon and usually herald a very severe course with intractable seizures and progressively increasing mental problems. The brief seizures, however, may not be prominent and may not always include myoclonic attacks, which, in any case, are seldom the most striking seizure form. Some investigators have described such cases as variants of severe myoclonic epilepsy (Ogino *et al.* 1989, Watanabe *et al.* 1989) or as epilepsy with hemi-grand mal and high-amplitude EEG slow

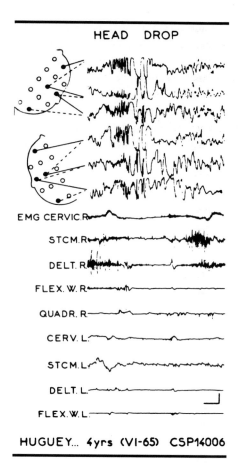

HEAD DROP

EMG CERVIC.R
STCM.R
DELT. R
FLEX. W. R
QUADR. R
CERV. L
STCM.L
DELT. L
FLEX.W.L

HUGUEY... 4yrs (VI-65) CSP14006

Fig. 16.8. Atonic seizure. EEG discharge starts with brief burst of fast rhythm, followed by a few spike–wave complexes and by slow waves. EMG trace shows disappearance of normal tonic activity during EEG discharge in posterior cervical muscles (CERVIC.R), sternomastoid (STCM.R) and deltoid (DELT.R) on right side. (Courtesy Dr J. Roger, Centre Saint Paul, Marseille.)

waves (Doose 1992). The course of such cases seems to be the same as for the typical form. The term *polymorphic epilepsy of infancy*, proposed by Cavazzuti (1980), seems appropriate to designate both the typical cases and the variants.

The *therapy* of severe myoclonic epilepsy is disappointing, although occasional cases of satisfactory outcome using large doses of sodium valproate have been reported (*e.g.* Hurst 1987). Lamotrigine (Schlumberger *et al.* 1994) and bromides (Oguni *et al.* 1994) have given some good results. Corticosteroids or ACTH may be temporarily useful.

The *myoclonic–astatic epilepsy* described by Doose (1985, 1992) is characterized clinically by the predominance of purely myoclonic and/or myoatonic seizures (Fig. 16.8); generalized tonic–clonic seizures, partial and, rarely, tonic attacks may also occur. The seizures may result in falls or produce only head drops and/or sagging at the knees when brief. The EEG shows fast (≥ 3 Hz) generalized spike–wave or polyspike–wave discharges of short duration (usually less than 4–5 s). Doose emphasized the presence of biparietal theta rhythms. In fact, the term myoclonic–astatic epilepsy applies to all the myoclonic epilepsies of nonlesional origin and includes the benign and the severe types of other authors (Doose 1992) as well as other unclassified myoclonic epilepsies. Some of the latter can also feature tonic seizures and atypical absences and have a severe outcome (Aicardi and Levy Gomes 1989, Aicardi 1996), and may be intermediate between LGS and the myoclonic epilepsies proper (Guerrini *et al.* 1994a).

The degenerative myoclonic epilepsies with a progressive course are studied in Chapter 10.

OTHER EPILEPSY SYNDROMES IN INFANCY AND EARLY CHILDHOOD

A large proportion of the seizures that occur in the first two years of life cannot be categorized into a recognized epileptic syndrome. A majority of such seizures are probably partial ones, even though their clinical manifestations may not obviously point to a focal origin. Features of partial seizures may include version of the head and eyes or focal tonic contraction, but seizures with generalized vasomotor phenomena or diffuse tonic changes may have a focal origin, as shown by the EEG. Most such seizures, especially partial attacks, are due to gross brain damage and their outlook is poor, both as to persistence of seizures and neurodevelopmental outcome (Chevrie and Aicardi 1977, 1979; Cavazzuti *et al.* 1984). Generalized seizures, which are rare in this age group, appear to have a better outlook in the absence of gross brain pathology (Chevrie and Aicardi 1978). More specific syndromes of *partial seizures in infancy* have been described (Dravet *et al.* 1989, Dulac 1995). A syndrome of partial migratory seizures in infancy with malignant outcome has been described (Coppola *et al.* 1995) but the criteria for its identification are not clear.

Distinctions between simple and complex partial seizures based on the state of consciousness are obviously very difficult in this age range (Acharya *et al.* 1997). Duchowny (1987, 1992) reported on 14 infants with complex partial seizures due to gross brain damage whose main ictal features were head version and body stiffening, very much like most cases of partial seizures of infants. Watanabe *et al.* (1987b) described as *benign complex partial epilepsy of infancy* the cases of nine infants with complex partial seizures that ran a favourable course. They later described a second group of seven children who developed secondarily generalized seizures with focal onset (Watanabe *et al.* 1993, Watanabe 1996). Such cases may be similar to those reported as benign infantile familial convulsions by Vigevano *et al.* (1992, 1994b) and by Echenne *et al.* (1994). The latter cases had a clearly genetic dominant inheritance and were also of focal origin. Benign familial epilepsy had long been recognized by Japanese investigators. It was also described in 23 Oriental patients in 11 families by Lee *et al.* (1993). Their patients had either generalized tonic–clonic or complex partial seizures that often occurred in clusters over a period of only a few weeks, sometimes following a benign diarrhoeal illness. Whether the 'benign' syndromes of infantile seizures belong to the same or several entities remains to be explored (Duchowny and Harvey 1996). The existence of infantile seizures with excellent prognosis is thus well-established, and their recognition is important as other seizures in this age group are usually of ominous significance. Rare cases of rolandic epilepsy may have their onset before age 2 years (Dulac *et al.* 1989).

EPILEPSY SYNDROMES OF LATER CHILDHOOD AND ADOLESCENCE

Several of the epileptic syndromes of infants and young children may persist or even have their onset later in life and there is no abrupt separation between the two age groups.

Most epileptic syndromes of later childhood and adolescence are unassociated with gross brain damage, and genetic factors probably play a prominent role at their origin. As a result, affected children are usually normal from both mental and neurological points of view and the prognosis is generally better than that of early-onset epilepsies in which brain lesions are the most common cause.

ABSENCE EPILEPSY (PETIT MAL EPILEPSY)

Typical absences are a well-defined type of seizures with a striking EEG correlate.

They are characterized by the sudden suppression or marked decrease of consciousness, with abolition of awareness, responsiveness and memory recording.

The International Classification recognizes two varieties of absences: typical and atypical absences. The latter are mainly observed in Lennox–Gastaut syndrome and some forms of polymorphic epilepsy. Typical absences can be simple or complex. *Simple typical absences* last 5–15 s in 90 per cent of cases (Penry *et al.* 1975) and do not involve motor phenomena, except for possible mild jerking of eyelids and minor changes in muscle tone. The onset and termination of the absence are abrupt: this is important to differentiate absences from complex partial seizures of limited expression. The same also applies to the lack of a postictal phase of impaired awareness and/or fatigue (Penry *et al.* 1975, Holmes *et al.* 1987). In *complex typical absences*, more marked motor components (increased or decreased muscle tone), simple automatisms (Penry *et al.* 1975) and autonomic phenomena accompany the loss of consciousness and the duration of the attack is often longer. The degree of consciousness impairment is variable depending on the epileptic syndrome of which the absences are a part (Panayiotopoulos *et al.* 1989b). The EEG in typical absences, whether simple or complex, shows rhythmical bursts of spike–wave complexes at a rhythm of 2.5–3.5Hz, with abrupt onset and termination, that are bilateral, synchronous and symmetrical (Fig. 16.9). Less ryhthmical discharges may be seen, especially during sleep, and some degree of asymmetry is present in 9 per cent of cases (Loiseau 1992). EEG variants are observed in some absence syndromes (Panayiotopoulos *et al.* 1989b, Panayiotopoulos 1998). The interictal records are often normal, but brief bursts of irregular spike–wave complexes are seen in 30 per cent of patients. Posterior 3Hz slow waves are present in 10–20 per cent of children with typical absences.

Hyperventilation is highly effective in precipitating typical absences and can be performed safely. A negative test makes the diagnosis of absences unlikely in an untreated child. About 10–20

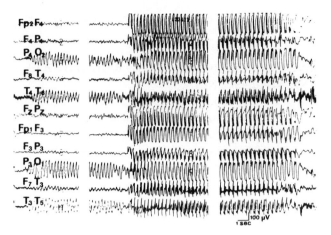

Fig. 16.9. Typical absence attack in a 6-year-old girl. The absence is preceded by a run of 3 Hz slow waves without spikes in the posterior leads over both sides.

per cent of children with absences may respond to light stimulation and these may be more likely to develop grand mal attacks. These may belong to different syndromes (Panayiotopoulos 1998).

Absences should be distinguished from inattention and daydreaming, from tics and from abnormal head movements. Distinction from complex partial seizures may be difficult. The brief duration of attacks, their frequent repetition and the lack of a postictal phase are all important features, but an EEG with ictal recording is necessary for final diagnosis. The differentiation from atypical absences rests on the EEG aspect and on the different history, often with other types of attacks in addition to absences. Absences due to frontal lobe damage result from posttraumatic atrophy or even from tumours (Ferrie *et al.* 1995).

The occurrence of typical absences as the predominant or exclusive type of seizure in a patient defines absence epilepsy. In fact, there are several syndromes of absence epilepsy. These include absence epilepsy of childhood, sometimes termed pyknolepsy, absence epilepsy of adolescence, myoclonic or clonic absences and some rarer syndromes.

Absence epilepsy of childhood (pyknolepsy) has its onset between the ages of 3 and 8 years, although rare cases can manifest as early as the first year of life (Aicardi 1995). It is more common in girls than in boys. The absences occur many times daily and constitute the first manifestation of epilepsy, although febrile convulsions may have taken place in infancy. Affected children are normal between the attacks and so is the interictal EEG, although brief bursts of spike–wave complexes without clinical absence may be recorded. The absences do not include prominent clonic or atonic phenomena but simple automatisms and complex absences are not rare (Loiseau and Duché 1995). The loss of consciousness is marked and the eyes open during the discharge (Panayiotopoulos 1994b, 1998).

In typical cases no neuroimaging study is useful, as there is no appreciable brain pathology, while a family history of seizures is frequent. A dominant mode of inheritance was suggested by Metrakos and Metrakos (1970), but polygenic inheritance appears more likely (Andermann 1982, Doose and Baier 1987). The occurrence of several cases of absence in the same lineage is not rare (Loiseau and Duché 1995). *Treatment* with sodium valproate or ethosuximide is usually effective. For more refractory cases, an association of both drugs may be effective. In some resistant cases, benzodiazepines (especially clobazam) or lamotrigine may control otherwise intractable attacks.

The outlook of childhood absence epilepsy is favourable. However, absences may persist in adulthood in a small proportion of cases, and generalized tonic–clonic seizures develop in about 10–30 per cent of patients followed into adulthood, though they are infrequent and easily treatable in most cases (Loiseau *et al.* 1983). This figure is probably excessive if strict criteria for the diagnosis of childhood absence epilepsy are used (Panayiotopoulos 1998). The socioprofessional outlook for absence patients is less favourable than that of benign partial epilepsy and such patients often fare less well than their mental level would normally allow (Loiseau *et al.* 1983).

Juvenile absence epilepsy occurs in patients beyond the age of 9–10 years, although the borderline between childhood and juvenile types is not clearly demarcated. Absences in adolescents are usually less frequently repeated than in children and often cluster in the hour following awakening. Loss of consciousness is less profound than in pyknolepsy (Panayiotopoulos *et al.* 1994b, Panayiotopoulos 1998). Other types of seizures, especially generalized tonic–clonic seizures, are associated in 90 per cent of cases, and in some youngsters myoclonic seizures are also present. In the latter cases the absences may be especially mild and often are limited to infraclinical discharges, so some investigators regard absences associated with juvenile myoclonic epilepsy as a distinct syndrome that may have its onset in early childhood and last into adulthood (Panayiotopoulos 1989a, 1998). The EEG of juvenile absences either is identical to that of childhood absences or may contain faster spike–wave activity (Janz 1994, Janz *et al.* 1994).

Juvenile absences, generalized tonic–clonic seizures on awakening and juvenile myoclonic epilepsy, often associated as a triad, constitute the group of *primary generalized epilepsy of adolescence* (see p. 592).

The genetics of absence epilepsy are poorly understood. Typical childhood absence epilepsy appears to be genetically unrelated to juvenile myoclonic epilepsy, and linkage to chromosome 6p has been excluded. The relationship of juvenile absence epilepsy with juvenile myoclonic epilepsy is still unclear (Janz 1994). Some cases of apparent childhood absence epilepsy may evolve to juvenile myoclonic epilepsy and are regarded as different from those of childhood absence epilepsy (Panayiotopoulos 1998). Photosensitive cases seem to be genetically distinct, often with a dominant inheritance. Some may be genetically related to juvenile myoclonic epilepsy (Bianchi *et al.* 1995).

Juvenile absences usually respond well to sodium valproate therapy but treatment needs to be maintained for long periods, probably indefinitely.

In the rare syndrome of *myoclonic absences (clonic absences)*, the intensity of the clonic jerking that affects the upper and

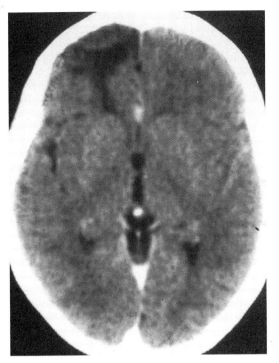

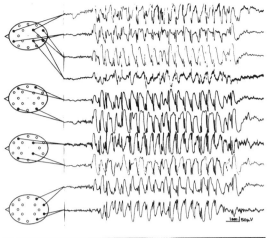

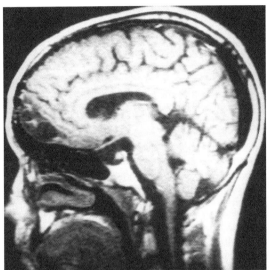

Fig. 16.10. Secondary bilateral synchrony in 15-year-old girl operated on at age 9 years for craniopharyngioma. Intractable epilepsy since operation with generalized tonic seizures (often starting with head turning to left side) and absence attacks, sometimes associated with head turning. *(Top right)* EEG showing absence with bilateral synchronous spike–wave activity. *(Above)* CT scan showing right frontal lesion. *(Bottom right)* Sagittal MRI showing anterior and inferior location of frontal lobe lesion. (Following removal of anterior frontal lobe, there was total disappearance of all seizures, persisting 19 months postoperatively.)

often the lower limbs is distinctive although the EEG expression is without specificity. The course is variable. Some cases develop mental retardation and may evolve to Lennox–Gastaut syndrome while others respond well to treatment and run a benign course (Manonmani and Wallace 1994, Tassinari *et al.* 1995). Some children develop tonic seizures.

Others less well-defined syndromes of absence epilepsy include cases of *absences preceded by generalized tonic–clonic seizures* other than febrile convulsions (Dieterich *et al.* 1985) that generally have an unfavourable outcome and *eyelid myoclonia with absences* (Panayiotopoulos 1998) which is essentially a form of myoclonic epilepsy (see below). Absences associated with brain damage are rare (Olsson 1990, Ferrie *et al.* 1995). They may be related either to diffuse lesions or to focal damage (Fig. 16.10), especially to the mediobasal frontal lobe. A focal component (clinical and/or EEG) may be present.

SYNDROMES WITH GENERALIZED TONIC–CLONIC SEIZURES
Generalized tonic–clonic seizures may be generalized from the start and are often a manifestation of idiopathic epilepsy. They may also represent the secondary generalization of a partial seizure

that is traditionally termed the 'aura' of the generalized attack. These two types may be difficult to separate clinically although their aetiological significance is different (Aicardi 1994a).

Generalized tonic–clonic seizures comprise a stereotyped succession of events, beginning with a tonic contraction of the entire musculature with respiratory blockade resulting in cyanosis, and loss of consciousness. After 10–30s, the tonic phase gives way to clonic jerks that progressively slow down and become increasingly violent. After 30–60s, muscular relaxation occurs. The patient remains unconscious for variable durations. Tongue-biting and urinary or, rarely, double incontinence are frequent manifestations but they are by no means specific and can be seen with nonepileptic seizures (Stephenson 1990, Aicardi 1994a). From the EEG viewpoint, generalized tonic–clonic seizures are characterized by the succession of a fast ($\geq 10\,Hz$) rhythm of increasing amplitude that becomes fragmented during the clonic phase converting to single spike–wave complexes. A flat tracing follows the clonic phase and is rapidly replaced by slow waves that progressively decrease to merge with interictal tracing.

Secondarily generalized tonic–clonic seizures can be of two varieties (Theodore *et al.* 1994). In some cases, the initial partial seizure is clinically manifest, with localized motor, sensory or other phenomena. In other cases, the seizure seems to be generalized from the start and only ictal EEG recordings demonstrate the existence of an initial, clinically silent, focal discharge. When no ictal records are available, the presence of a stable interictal spike focus—present in 20–40 per cent of patients with tonic–clonic seizures (Aicardi 1994a)—is indirect evidence for secondarily generalized attacks. Such seizures are usually the expression of a localized brain lesion but may also occur with nonlesional epilepsies.

Atypical tonic–clonic seizures are very common in childhood: the clonic phase may be extremely brief and the EEG activity is not always synchronous or symmetrical. In some children the tonic phase is too brief to be noted.

Generalized tonic–clonic seizures occur with a number of epileptic syndromes so they are not particularly helpful for classification and diagnosis. Indeed, when they occur in association with other seizures in the same patient, the latter are considered more characteristic.

Generalized tonic–clonic seizures on awakening (awakening grand mal) is considered as a form of primary generalized epilepsy. The diagnosis of this condition is easy when more specific manifestations of the triad (myoclonic attacks or juvenile absences) are present (Gastaut *et al.* 1973). When generalized seizures are the only manifestation, repeated attacks and a srict relation to awakening are necessary for the diagnosis. Janz (1994) states that the diagnosis should be accepted only if 90 per cent of seizures occur in the half-hour following awakening (Janz 1994). This syndrome may be due to the same gene(s) as juvenile myoclonic epilepsy, whereas that of primary generalized seizures randomly distributed is not (Greenberg *et al.* 1995).

In other cases, generalized tonic–clonic seizures may be a manifestation of either primary or secondarily generalized epilepsy, the seizures originating in one or several hemispheric foci. In primary grand mal, the EEG may show generalized spike–wave complexes, sometimes with a positive response to photic stimulation. Even in patients with typical bilateral paroxysms, lateralizing manifestations such as version or circling activity are sometimes present (Gastaut *et al.* 1986, Lancman *et al.* 1994).

Infrequent generalized afebrile seizures often succeed febrile seizures (Scheffer and Berkovic 1997), disappearing spontaneously before 9–10 years of age.

The overall prognosis of grand mal seizures of presumed nonlesional origin in children is favourable (Ehrhardt and Forsythe 1989).

SYNDROMES WITH MYOCLONIC SEIZURES
In children and adolescents the main myoclonic syndrome is juvenile myoclonic epilepsy.

Juvenile myoclonic epilepsy (myoclonic epilepsy of adolescence, Janz syndrome)
This is a well-defined epileptic syndrome that usually has its onset between 12 and 18 years of age (Delgado-Escueta and Enrile-Bacsal 1984, Janz 1989) but may occur outside this age range. The condition was sometimes termed 'myoclonic petit mal'

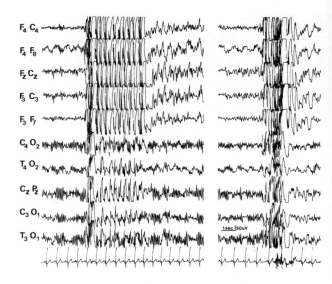

Fig. 16.11. Juvenile myoclonic epilepsy (Janz syndrome). Traces at left show fast (4 Hz) spike–wave discharge with initial polyspikes (no clinical correlate). Those at right show myoclonic jerk (note myographic artefact on ECG channel) and discharge of polyspike on EEG. (Reproduced by permission from Aicardi 1986.)

or 'impulsive petit mal' which is confusing as it is clearly different from absence epilepsy. It occurs in 5–11 per cent of adolescents with epilepsy.

The myoclonic jerks affect mainly the shoulders and arms, rarely the lower extremities. They may be asymmetrical and even unilateral (Genton *et al.* 1994, Janz 1994). Consciousness is usually preserved but the involuntary movements often result in the patient throwing out whatever s/he happens to be holding at the time.

The jerks occur mainly after awakening and may be single shocks or serial jerks that rarely amount to myoclonic status. Ninety per cent of patients have associated generalized tonic–clonic seizures. The latter may sometimes supervene following a series of jerks, a sequence referred to as clonic–tonic–clonic seizure (Delgado-Escueta and Enrile Bacsal 1984). Fifteen to 30 per cent of patients also have absence attacks.

The typical ictal EEG consists of a burst of spikes of high frequency followed by one or several slow waves (Fig. 16.11) (Janz 1994). Similar polyspike–wave complexes may be present interictally. Focal EEG features may be present in up to 20 per cent of cases (Panayiotopoulos 1994a). Sleep deprivation and often photic stimulation can trigger seizures.

About 80 per cent of patients respond well to sodium valproate therapy but treatment should be prolonged, probably indefinitely. In resistant cases, mysoline (Janz 1989) and the benzodiazepines are worth trying.

Genetic factors play a considerable role in the causation of this syndrome (Greenberg *et al.* 1988, Delgado-Escueta *et al.* 1989, Greenberg *et al.* 1995). A recessive inheritance has been postulated by Panayiotopoulos *et al.* (1989b) but a multifactorial transmission appears more probable. Linkage to the short arm of chromosome 6 (Greenberg and Delgado-Escueta 1993) remains debated (Whitehouse *et al.* 1993). Serratosa *et al.* (1996) recently reported definite linkage in a large pedigree. Juvenile myoclonic epilepsy may be genetically heterogeneous (Delgado-Escueta *et al.* 1994) and it is probable that at least a second gene is involved (Durner 1994).

Eyelid myoclonia with absences

This disorder is characterized by the very frequent occurrence of eyelid jerks with upwards deviation of the eyes, usually associated with a brief and mild loss of awareness (Jeavons 1982, Appleton *et al.* 1993, Panayiotopoulos 1998). The EEG shows discharges of polyspike–wave complexes of short duration (<6s) and there is marked photosensitivity. Treatment with sodium valproate is effective but has to be maintained into adulthood.

Other myoclonic syndromes

These include late cases similar to 'benign myoclonic' epilepsy of infancy but with a late onset up to 5–6 years of age (Guerrini *et al.* 1994a) and self-induced photomyoclonic seizures (see below).

Epilepsy Syndromes of Childhood with Partial Seizures

Partial epileptic seizures are defined as seizures that have their onset in a neuronal population limited to one part of a cerebral hemisphere (Fig. 16.12). Partial seizures in children are not necessarily indicative of the presence of a localized brain lesion: a majority of simple partial seizures in children are in fact idiopathic.

Partial seizures of lesional origin are caused mainly by dysplastic lesions (including developmental tumours) and by destructive lesions of pre-, peri- or postnatal origin. The extent of the causal lesion largely determines the outcome. Large lesions of prenatal origin may involve several lobes and raise formidable problems of treatment. However, even relatively small lesions may have a noxious effect on overall brain function and be responsible for behavioural and/or cognitive deterioration through poorly understood mechanisms. Early resection of lesions whenever possible may prevent a progressive course.

The International Classification of Epileptic Seizures recognizes two main categories of partial seizures depending on the presence or absence of impairment of consciousness. Consciousness is defined operationally as awareness and responsiveness (Commission on Classification 1981). Although this concept is highly debatable (Gloor 1986, Aicardi 1994a), this classification is now widely accepted. Seizures with impairment of awareness and/or responsiveness are termed *complex partial seizures*, those without impaired consciousness are termed *simple partial seizures*. Both forms can evolve into generalized seizures, and simple partial seizures can evolve into the complex form. It is especially common for simple partial seizures characterized by psychic and affective phenomena to evolve into the complex form, whilst this is rare in the case of simple partial seizures characterized by motor features. Both simple and complex partial seizures can occur in the same patient and be due to the same epileptic focus.

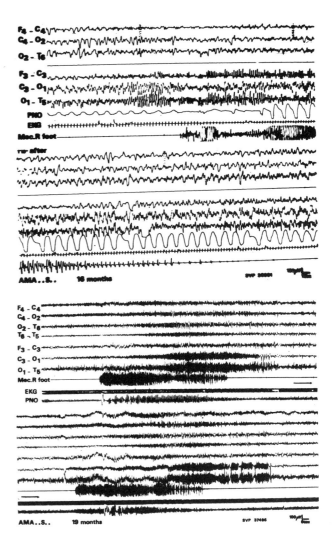

Fig. 16.12. Focal (or partial) epileptic seizure. *(Top)* Onset of spike discharge in left occipitotemporal region (O₁–T₅). Note secondary apnoea (PNO = pneumographic recording) and secondary onset of tonic followed by clonic activity in right lower limb (Mec. R foot = mechanographic recording of right foot movements). *(Bottom)* Slow paper speed recording, same patient, showing another seizure. Note temporal discrepancy between EEG discharge (again starting at O₁–T₅) and clinical seizure (Mec. R foot).

The loss of consciousness is related to a wider diffusion of the discharge rather than to a different origin. If the diffusion is restricted, the clinical expression is a simple partial seizure; when the discharge diffuses the simple partial seizure constitutes the *aura* of the complex partial attack. Thus, the classification of partial seizures as simple or complex is of no value to the surgeon and a topographic classification is more useful (Lüders *et al.* 1993).

The most common types of simple partial seizures are somatomotor seizures. These may remain localized to a small cortical area mostly in the primary motor strip or spread from their area of origin to involve progressively the whole motor strip. This slow extension is known as the jacksonian march and may also occur with primary sensory seizures. In most cases, extension of the discharge is irregular, starting in the primary motor or sensory cortex and involving sequentially other, sometimes distant, cortical areas, probably through the activation of long cortico-cortical pathways. Such seizures start with a tonic phase followed by clonic jerking that may remain localized—most commonly in children to the face and mouth, but in some cases also to the hand or foot—or may spread to half the body or even generalize. Postictal paralysis (Todd paralysis) is frequent.

Partial benign epilepsy (rolandic epilepsy, sylvian seizures, benign epilepsy of childhood with centrotemporal (rolandic) spikes)
This is the most common syndrome of idiopathic partial epilepsy in childhood and one of the best-defined epileptic syndromes. Fifteen to 25 per cent of school-age children with epilepsy are affected (Heijbel *et al.* 1975a, Cavazzuti 1980). The syndrome appears to be genetically determined (Lüders *et al.* 1987) but whether a dominant or a multifactorial transmission is responsible remains undecided although the latter seems more likely. The problem is compounded by the fact that only fewer than 10 per cent of children with rolandic spikes have seizures, and the EEG trait seems to be what is inherited. Foci of characteristic rolandic sharp waves are thus frequently encountered in children without epilepsy and their diagnostic value is therefore limited.

The age of onset is almost always between 2 and 13 years, with rare cases recorded as early as 1 year (Heijbel *et al.* 1975b). The typical seizures are simple partial seizures, therefore without impairment of consciousness. They are mainly motor in expression, although buccal or labial paraesthesiae often occur, and they preferentially involve the face and oropharyngeal musculature, with resulting salivation and/or speech arrest (Lerman and Kivity 1986). Individual seizures are brief (30–60s). Sixty to 80 per cent of seizures occur while the patient is asleep or on awakening. Generalized seizures—which are probably secondarily generalized (Dalla Bernardina and Tassinari 1975, Roger *et al.* 1991)—occur in 20 per cent of patients, mainly in the middle part of the night, while focal seizures tend to occur on falling asleep or awakening. Most children have only rare seizures (Lerman and Kivity 1986) and the response to antiepileptic drugs is good, indicatlng a low epileptogenicity of the focus which remains clinically silent in over 90 per cent of cases.

All patients with partial benign epilepsy (and no other disorder) have a normal neurological examination and most make normal neurodevelopmental progress. However, language difficulties of mild to moderate severity have been observed in such cases (Doose *et al.* 1996), and, in a case–control study, Weglage *et al.* (1997) found visuomotor and spatial difficulties in children with centrotemporal spikes.

The typical and necessary EEG abnormality for the diagnosis of benign partial epilepsy is the presence of focal epileptiform discharges. These are usually localized over the midtemporal or lower rolandic area and may diffuse, or occur independently, bilaterally (Fig. 16.13) in 30 per cent of cases. Some patients with similar features and outcome have multiple bilateral foci (Anderson and Kellaway 1994). Multifocal epilepsy with dominant inheritance has been described in an Australian family (Scheffer *et al.* 1995c). Localization over the upper rolandic area is also possible but the middle area is not involved (Legarda *et al.* 1994). However, unusual localizations are not infrequent

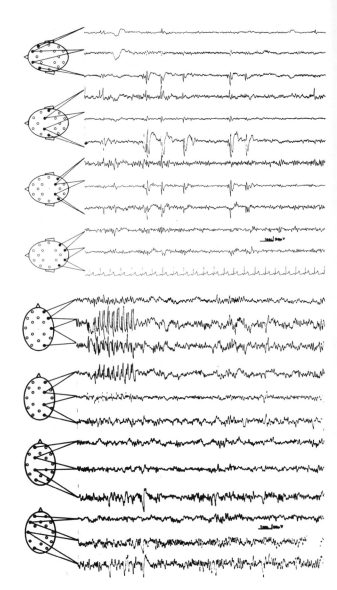

Fig. 16.13. Benign partial epilepsy with centrotemporal spikes. *(Top)* Left-sided focus in an 8-year-old boy. *(Bottom)* Right-sided focus with runs of repetitive rolandic spikes and waves in right centrotemporal region in a 6-year-old boy. In both cases the paroxysmal activity is clearly localized to the lower rolandic, midtemporal electrodes.

(Wirrel *et al.* 1995) and the shape of the spikes (or sharp waves) which are relatively blunted and appear on a normal background tracing, the field distribution with a horizontal dipole (positivity in the frontal area and maximum negativity in the rolandic region), and the activation by sleep are more important for their definition than their precise topography (Lüders *et al.* 1987, Loiseau 1992). Yet, paroxysms quite similar in shape to those found in benign partial epilepsy may rarely exist in epilepsies due to brain injury (Gobbi *et al.* 1989, Santanelli *et al.* 1989, Ambrosetto 1992). Generalized spike–waves are seen in 10–30 per cent of cases (Dravet 1994).

The outcome of benign partial epilepsy is excellent. Recurrences after age 16 years are exceptional (Loiseau *et al.* 1988, 1992) and the prognosis for school and social functioning is good (Loiseau *et al.* 1983, Loiseau 1992). Occasional generalized tonic–clonic seizures have been observed in a few adult patients after the resolution of benign partial epilepsy, and a few cases of status epilepticus of benign partial epilepsy have also been reported. They may feature pseudobulbar symptoms such as drooling and dysarthria (Roulet *et al.* 1989, Boulloche *et al.* 1990, Deonna *et al.* 1993), and some patients require steroids for control (Fejerman and Di Blasi 1987), but this does not affect the overall excellent prognosis of this epileptic syndrome.

However, Scheffer *et al.* (1995b) observed severe and permanent speech dyspraxia and difficulties of orobuccal movements in several members of a family with an autosomal dominant inheritance and possible anticipation, and Guerrini *et al.* (1997) reported the occurrence of paroxysmal dystonia in the form of writer's cramp and ataxia as an autosomal recessive syndrome.

Benign partial epilepsy occasionally occurs under age 2 years (Dulac 1995).

In a few children with rolandic foci and occasional focal nocturnal seizures, atonic and/or myoclonic seizures, often grouped in clusters and repeated many times daily, may occur, so-called *atypical partial benign epilepsy of childhood*. Atonic attacks are particularly prominent and may occur several dozen times daily, often with falls. The clusters may last two to three weeks and be separated by periods of months. The sleep EEG of such children is very much like that of cases of continuous spike–waves during slow sleep (Aicardi and Chevrie 1982, Doose and Baier 1991, Aicardi and Levy Gomes 1992), and the awake EEG shows multiple bilateral discharges of spike–wave complexes. Such patients often receive an erroneous diagnosis of Lennox–Gastaut syndrome (Doose 1989), although the course of this epileptic syndrome is generally favourable, with spontaneous remission before age 10 after two or more clusters. The exact nosological situation of this syndrome is not completely clear (Deonna *et al.* 1986a), especially in relation to the so-called electrical status epilepticus of slow sleep (see pp. 602–604). The atonic episodes seem to represent partial or secondarily generalized negative myoclonus. Such episodes have been reported in patients with benign partial epilepsy treated with carbamazepine (Caraballo *et al.* 1989). However, a number of patients with this syndrome have not received this drug (Aicardi and Levy Gomes 1992).

Occipital epilepsy of childhood

The occipital epilepsies of childhood are a heterogeneous group. The best identified type is an idiopathic and relatively benign epilepsy which is about five times less common than benign partial epilepsy. In fact, in a study of neurologically intact children, Deonna *et al.* (1986b) found no case of occipital epilepsy and only two of 'atypical partial epilepsy', as against 60 of benign partial epilepsy. Genetic factors are probably important in its causation (Kuzniecky and Rosenblatt 1987).

According to Gastaut (1982), the syndrome is characterized by the occurrence of simple partial seizures with predominantly visual symptoms, associated with the presence, over one or both occipital areas, of continuous, more or less rhythmical, spike–

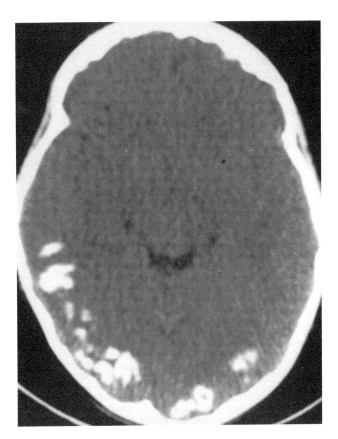

Fig. 16.14. Epilepsy with bilateral occipital calcification in 6-year-old boy with visual seizures. There was no facial naevus, and neither CT nor MRI (with gadolinium enhancement) showed any evidence of pial angioma. This case is similar to those reported by Gobbi *et al.* (1988).

wave activity which is arrested or considerably lessened by eye-opening. Onset is usually between 4 and 9 years (Gobbi and Guerrini 1998). The visual seizures may consist of negative phenomena (transient loss of vision) or of positive symptoms, mainly simple visual hallucinations of colours and/or geometric shapes (Aso *et al.* 1987). Nonvisual seizures may also be the presenting or sole symptom (Panayiotopoulos *et al.* 1989b). Postictal headache, often of a migrainous character, occurs in around one-third of cases of benign occipital epilepsy.

A second syndrome consists of rare nocturnal seizures marked by ictal vomiting, persistent eye deviation and loss of consciousness. Such episodes most often last a few minutes, although in 44 per cent of cases (Ferrie *et al.* 1997) they last for hours with vomiting, unconsciousness and eye deviation. In the latter case they may easily be mistaken for coma of toxic or metabolic origin (Panayiotopoulos 1989a, Kivity and Lerman 1992). This second syndrome is more common than classical benign partial occipital epilepsy in children under 5 years of age (Ferrie *et al.* 1997) and has a regularly benign outcome.

A third group of occipital epilepsies includes idiopathic partial photosensitive epilepsy (Guerrini *et al.* 1995) and a miscellany of nonlesional and lesional cases.

The most characteristic but not constant EEG abnormality in the late-onset syndrome is the presence of unilateral or bilateral spike or spike–wave paroxysms continuously occurring when eyes are closed but disappearing or decreasing markedly on eye opening (fixation-off phenomenon).

The outcome of the syndromes of occipital epilepsy is good. However, 'benign' cases may be difficult to distinguish from cases in brain-damaged children (Newton and Aicardi 1983, Dalla Bernardina et al. 1993).

Other syndromes of occipital epilepsy include seizures characterized by isolated vomiting and partial seizures induced by photic stimulation (Guerrini et al. 1994b).

The syndrome of occipital epilepsy associated with unilateral or bilateral *occipital calcification* (Fig. 16.14) may run a benign course (De Marco and Lorenzin 1990) or a more severe one with secondarily generalized seizures and mental deterioration (Gobbi et al. 1988, 1992; Magaudda et al. 1993; Tiacci et al. 1993). Such cases are closely reminiscent of Sturge–Weber syndrome without cutaneous angioma, and similar vascular abnormalities have been reported (Bye et al. 1993) but are inconstant (Toti et al. 1996). However, there is only minimal or no atrophy of the brain, and enlargement of the choroid plexus and abnormal deep venous drainage is not seen. Most if not all cases of epilepsy with occipital calcification are associated with coeliac disease, although its expression may be reduced to villous atrophy of the intestinal mucosa. The relationship between the coeliac disease and the calcification is not understood.

Frontal lobe epilepsy
Seizures of frontal lobe origin are being increasingly recognized. Multiple seizure types are possible and have been described in great detail by Chauvel et al. (1992). Salanova et al. (1995) found that symptoms and signs clustered into three groups.

In the first group, seizure discharges involved the supplementary motor area and adjacent frontal lobe with preservation of consciousness despite unresponsiveness due to motor phenomena. The seizures may have a sensory aura but consist mainly of motor manifestations with tonic contraction of one or both arms sometimes with a classical 'fencing' attitude, version of the head, bilateral tonic extension of the trunk or neck and vocalization. Such attacks are often mistaken for generalized seizures or for pseudoseizures because of the bizarre manifestations, preservation of awareness and memory, and frequent absence of interictal and sometimes even of ictal EEG anomalies. They may occur in children (Bass et al. 1995, Laskowitz et al. 1995) and are usually symptomatic of a mesial frontal or precentral frontal lesion.

The second group included patients with clonic seizures, speech arrest and head rotation, and appeared to be related to the vicinity of the frontal eye field.

The third group consisted of patients with partial complex seizures. Such children are particularly at risk of misdiagnosis (Fusco et al. 1990, Stores et al. 1991) because of their unusual clinical features and frequent lack of EEG abnormalities. Automatisms do not involve oroalimentary movements but are gestural, complex and often violent with rocking, kicking and dystonic activity. The bizarre appearance of these seizures often suggests a diagnosis of hysteria, the more so as screaming, shout-

ing and the utterance of abusive language are frequent features. Most such attacks seem to originate in the frontobasal area (Chauvel et al. 1992) although this is not fully documented (Williamson et al. 1993b). Like most frontal lobe seizures they are due in most cases to small tumours or dysplasias. In all frontal epilepsies, the seizures tend to be nocturnal, frequently repeated, of brief duration and with only a brief or no postictal manifestation.

Seizures of probable frontal lobe origin can be, in some cases, unrelated to brain lesions and transmitted as an autosomal dominant trait. Such *idiopathic frontal seizures* have been described by Vigevano and Fusco (1993) in 10 children with a syndrome of tonic postural seizures occurring mainly during sleep. These cases had run a favourable course and no lesion could be demonstrated, whereas a family history of epilepsy was prominent. Scheffer et al. (1995a) observed 42 patients, both children and adults, with seizures usually nocturnal and of mainly tonic or dystonic character, often misdiagnosed as parasomnias. The seizures could be either simple or complex (with loss of awareness) even in the same patient, which again underlines the somewhat artificial separation between these two categories. *Familial frontal epilepsy* is dominantly transmitted and can appear at any age. The frontal origin of the seizures was confirmed in a few cases by ictal EEG recording. Linkage to chromosome 20q13 has been shown in one family (Phillips et al. 1995), and a mutation in the gene of a subunit of a nicotinic cholinergic receptor demonstrated (Steinlein et al. 1995). However, no such linkage has been found in several other families.

Temporal lobe epilepsy
Temporal lobe epilepsy is the most common cause of complex partial seizures. A majority of cases are of symptomatic origin, even though demonstration of the lesions may be impossible, short of surgical resection of the epileptogenic area. Recently, however, Berkovic et al. (1996) described idiopathic cases in adults with a dominant transmission and a favourable course, and, in one family, cases of temporal lobe epilepsy with auditory hallucinations have been mapped to chromosome 10q (Ottman et al. 1995). The existence in children of syndromes with complex partial seizures but without pathological damage is suggested by the occurrence of such seizures in children who experience them only for a brief period with a benign outcome (Camfield and Dooley 1987). A benign outcome of some epilepsies with complex partial seizures had been reported by Ounsted et al. (1987). Similarly, a family history of benign partial epilepsy may be present in some children with 'psychomotor' seizures (Dalla Bernardina et al. 1980, Watanabe et al. 1990).

Partial seizures of temporal lobe origin in children are generally similar to those in adults (Kotagal et al. 1987, Devinsky et al. 1988). Onset is often with behavioural arrest and staring. Oro-alimentary automatisms tend to predominate in young children (Duchowny 1987) and include licking, lip-smacking, chewing or swallowing movements while, in older children, gestural automatisms such as fingering or fumbling with clothes are also frequent (Holmes 1986). In children under 2 years of age,

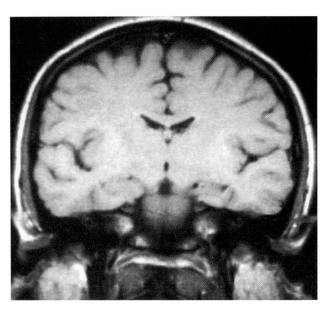

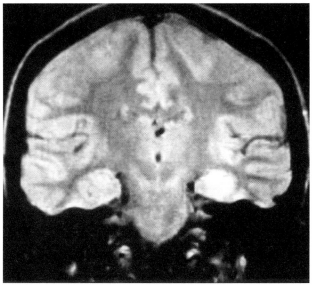

Fig. 16.15. Sclerosis of the left hippocampus in 14-year-old girl who had an episode of right-sided status epilepticus at age 14 months and developed partial complex seizures consistent with a left temporal lobe origin from 4 years of age. *(Top)* T₁-weighted MRI showing global atrophy of left temporal lobe and a markedly shrunken hippocampus. *(Bottom)* T₂-weighted MRI showing intense signal in left hippocampal area.

tonic posturing and head rotation are often the initial and dominant manifestations. The duration of seizures is usually longer than that of absences (60–120 s) and they are followed by a period of confusion and/or of intense tiredness.

Complex seizures of temporal lobe origin are usually preceded by auras with affective or other psychic phenomena such as hallucinations or illusions affecting various sensory modalities (see Aicardi 1994a). In young children, the most common aura is an epigastric sensation often associated with fear. In infants and children under 2 years motor symptoms such as head deviation and posturing may mark the onset of an attack (Jayakar and Duchowny 1990).

In older children and adolescents, the most common syndrome is that of *mesial temporal lobe epilepsy* (Wieser and Kausel 1987, Cendes *et al.* 1993b, French *et al.* 1993, Wieser *et al.* 1993, Williamson *et al.* 1993a). The syndrome is associated with atrophy and gliosis of the hippocampus and often of the amygdala (Fig. 16.15) (see p. 612). A history of febrile seizures, often of long duration and unilateral localization, is found in approximately 40–60 per cent of patients. Partial seizures start in the first 10 years of life and tend to become more severe with increasing age, often after a temporary remission. The seizures are marked by behavioural arrest and staring followed by automatisms involving especially the oroalimentary muscles (lip-smacking, licking, swallowing). A significant proportion of these automatisms are, in fact, conscious (Munari *et al.* 1994, Ebner *et al.* 1995). Dystonic posturing of the arm contralateral to the discharging temporal lobe is often seen (Kotagal *et al.* 1989), while simple automatisms may occur in the ipsilateral arm. The EEG usually shows an interictal anterior temporal spike focus or sometimes a paroxysmal theta rhythm (Gastaut *et al.* 1985), while ictal EEG shows a focal discharge that may diffuse to the contralateral temporal lobe. MRI shows atrophy of the hippocampus, loss of its internal structure and increased T₂ signal (Cendes *et al.* 1993a,b; Cross *et al.* 1993; Jackson *et al.* 1993). PET scan with fluorodeoxyglucose shows local hypometabolism. SPECT with HMPAO shows reduced blood flow to the mesial temporal lobe interictally and increased fixation during the seizure (Harvey *et al.* 1993a, 1995). The outcome of this syndrome following surgery is usually good (Abou-Khalil *et al.* 1993).

A very similar syndrome is produced by small mesial developmental tumours (Wyllie *et al.* 1993, Raymond *et al.* 1994a). Such patients have no antecedent history. Wyllie *et al.* emphasized that, contrary to mesial temporal sclerosis in which the ictal and interictal EEG anomalies are usually localized to the anterior temporal area, the EEG is often diffusely abnormal in small tumours whose diagnosis rests on MRI.

Cortical dysplasias localized to the temporal lobe (Palmini *et al.* 1991) have a less favourable surgical outcome, although Duchowny *et al.* (1992) reported good surgical results in children.

A number of temporal lobe seizures in children may arise from the *basal temporal lobe* rather than from the mesial temporal lobe (Duchowny *et al.* 1994). Such seizures are marked by behavioural arrest followed by automatisms that begin several seconds after seizure onset.

A syndrome of neocortical temporal seizures is also described (Wieser and Muller 1987). According to Blume *et al.* (1993) and to Munari *et al.* (1994), the neocortex is responsible for many features of all temporal lobe seizures.

In general, localization of partial seizures to a particular cortical area is difficult, and distinction between temporal lobe and frontal lobe origin may be clinically impossible (Manford *et al.* 1996a).

Sensory (parietal) epilepsy
Somatosensory seizures can involve any type of sensation, although focal paroxysmal pain (Young *et al.* 1986, Trevathan and

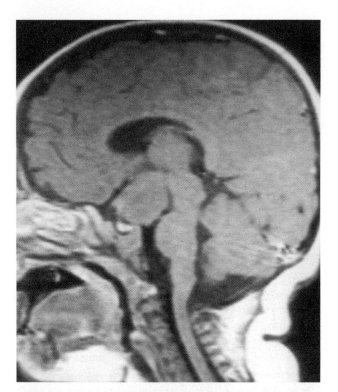

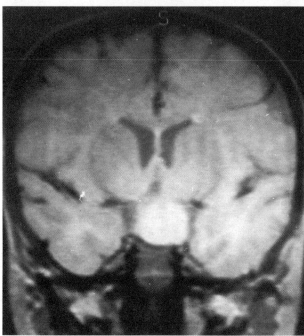

Fig. 16.16. Hamartoma of floor of third ventricle in 8-month-old girl with gelastic seizures from age 2 months. *(Top)* MRI, T₁-weighted sagittal cut showing mass formed within the prepeduncular cistern with same signal as rest of brain. *(Bottom)* MRI, T₂-weighted frontal cut demonstrates more intense signal from hamartoma than from rest of brain.

Cascino 1988, Ho *et al.* 1994) and sensations of heat or cold are rare. Elementary sensations (*e.g.* paraesthesiae, numbness) are most common. Somatosensory seizures may have a jacksonian march (Mauguière and Courjon 1978). They are often associated with motor phenomena.

Some special epilepsy syndromes of lesional origin

A syndrome of *gelastic seizures* (giggling attacks) of early onset (often in the first year and usually before 2 years of age) is associated with the occurrence of a hamartoma of the hypothalamus (Fig. 16.16). The seizures are frequently repeated and highly resistant to treatment (Berkovic *et al.* 1988). Precocious puberty is a frequent feature. Recent work shows that the seizure discharge may arise from the tumour itself, and surgical excision, when possible, may control the seizures (Nishio *et al.* 1994).

Cerebellar hamartomas may produce repeated brief attacks of tonic facial contraction of early onset, similar to the facial hemispasm of adults (Al-Shahwan *et al.* 1994). Harvey *et al.* (1996) showed that these may correspond to a typical epileptic EEG discharge within the lesion.

Cortical dysplasias have also been shown to be the site of epileptic discharges (Palmini *et al.* 1995) and of increased ictal metabolism.

Secondarily generalized seizures are also a frequent manifestation of the *syndrome of bilateral opercular dysgenesis* (Kuzniecky *et al.* 1994). They appear after 3–5 years of age in children with limited voluntary facial motility and severe language disturbances.

Partial and secondarily generalized seizures are also associated with focal dysplasias (Palmini *et al.* 1991) and with diffuse subcortical heterotopias (double cortex). In both cases, they can present with the Lennox–Gastaut syndrome (Ricci *et al.* 1992). A syndrome of *generalized epilepsy and periventricular heterotopias* often with dominant genetic transmission and affecting almost exclusively females has been studied by Huttenlocher *et al.* (1994), Raymond *et al.* (1994b) and Dubeau *et al.* (1995).

Northern epilepsy (Tahvanainen *et al.* 1994, Hirvasniemi *et al.* 1995), a monogenic recessive disease that maps to chromosome 8p, so far reported only from Finland, begins between 2 and 10 years of age with partial seizures, often secondarily generalized, and later features mental deterioration and brain atrophy.

Seizures with purely autonomic manifestations are on record (Zelnik *et al.* 1990). Rare cases of paroxysmal arousal from sleep as the sole clinical manifestation have been recorded by Montagna *et al.* (1990).

STATUS EPILEPTICUS
Status epilepticus is defined as 'an epileptic seizure that is sufficiently prolonged or repeated at sufficiently brief intervals so as to produce an unvarying and enduring epileptic condition' (Gastaut 1973). There are two major categories of status epilepticus: convulsive status that may be generalized or localized, and nonconvulsive status which can be divided in turn into partial complex status and generalized nonconvulsive status, also known as 'petit mal status'.

CONVULSIVE STATUS
Convulsive status may present as a succession of tonic–clonic seizures without recovery of consciousness between individual attacks, or as a single, prolonged, convulsive seizure, most often of a purely clonic type. The duration necessary to diagnose status

epilepticus is variably estimated. Most recent studies accept a duration of 30 minutes or more (Gross-Tsur and Shinnar 1993). Exclusively or predominantly *unilateral* seizures are more common in childhood than bilateral status (Aicardi and Chevrie 1983). In most patients, clonic jerks may wax and wane in intensity and the involved territory may vary from moment to moment as does the rhythm of the jerks, which, generally, are not synchronous in the affected segments.

Convulsive status epilepticus is often preceded by a premonitory stage of serial seizures during which treatment is particularly effective (Shorvon 1994). Established status can be divided into an early or compensated stage during which physiological mechanisms are sufficient to meet the metabolic demands and cerebral tissue is protected from hypoxic or metabolic damage, and a stage of decompensation when compensatory mechanisms break down and brain damage may occur. As the duration of status increases, the clinical seizures tend to become less conspicuous, eventually evolving into coma without visible movements, while autonomic changes become more prominent with resulting respiratory and circulatory impairment often associated with hyperthermia.

The EEG features of convulsive status are variable. Generalized paroxysmal activity as described in adults (Treiman 1993, Shorvon 1994) is less common in children than asymmetrical slow waves irregularly interspersed by spikes and sharp waves. In cases of prolonged status, episodes of 'flattening' of the EEG frequently occur. Periodic generalized or lateralized epileptiform discharges may be seen in very long episodes and indicate a poor prognosis (Garg *et al.* 1995).

The term *partial convulsive status epilepticus* applies only to those cases in which convulsive activity remains localized to a restricted segment on one side of the body without generalization or diffusion to the whole of the affected side. When segmental myoclonic jerks are continuous, the condition is known as *epilepsia partialis continua*. In such instances, intermittent somatomotor seizures may start from the area of the body that is involved by permanent myoclonus; this association defines the Kojewnikow syndrome.

Convulsive status epilepticus is a major complication of epilepsy and remains a dangerous condition even though its prognosis has improved over the past few decades. The pathogenesis of status and of its consequences has been extensively studied (see Brown and Hussain 1991a, Shorvon 1994). It involves multiple factors that include progressive hypoxia, excitotoxicity, substrate failure, ATP depletion and intracellular acidosis. These, in turn, eventually produce a fall in cardiac output, hyperkalaemia, metabolic acidosis and cerebral oedema, all of which participate in the genesis of sequelae, which, however, rarely appear after episodes of status lasting less than 90–120 minutes (Aicardi and Chevrie 1983).

Systemic factors play an important role in the production of sequelae. However, it seems that the epileptic activity itself, in the absence of systemic complications, can generate brain lesions, especially in the temporal lobe (Meldrum 1978, 1983a), possibly by a mechanism of glutamate-induced excitotoxic damage.

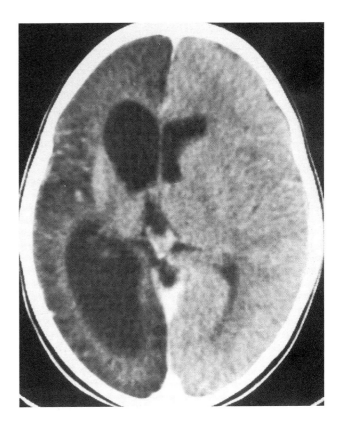

Fig. 16.17. Hemiconvulsion–hemiplegia–epilepsy (HHE) syndrome. CT scan of a 6-year-old girl who had febrile status epilepticus at age 11 months, localized on left side and lasting several hours, followed by permanent hemiplegia. Overall atrophy of right hemisphere and dilatation of whole right ventricle; marked hypodensity of right hemisphere and shift of midline to right. This image is virtually pathognomonic of HHE syndrome and probably corresponds to postconvulsive 'hemiatrophia cerebri'.

In childhood series of epilepsy, the incidence of status epilepticus varies between 3 and 16 per cent. In 77 per cent of infants and children with status epilepticus it is the first epileptic manifestation (Aicardi and Chevrie 1970).

Symptomatic status can be divided into acute symptomatic cases, resulting from an acute brain insult such as trauma, vascular collapse, electrolyte disorders, meningitis or encephalitis; remote symptomatic status, due to chronic nonprogressive brain lesions; and status resulting from progressive encephalopathies (Hauser 1993). Cryptogenic status may occur in the course or at the onset of a recurring seizure disorder. In this case, interruption of treatment is often a precipitating event. It may also represent an occasional seizure, in practice a febrile seizure, that fails to stop for unknown reasons. Such cases do not differ from common febrile seizures in nature but only in duration. Currently, it appears that a large majority of cases of status observed in industrialized countries are of symptomatic origin (Aubourg *et al.* 1985, Dunn 1988, Delorenzo *et al.* 1992). The dramatic decrease in the frequency of cryptogenic status probably results in large part from a better and more prompt treatment of incipient febrile status; the improved outlook for status (Dunn 1988, Maytal *et al.* 1989, Gross-Tsur and Shinnar 1993) should not lead to underestimation of the potential risks (Phillips and Shanahan

TABLE 16.7
Management of status epilepticus

Stage	Procedure
Immediate management	(1) Assessment of vital functions. Establishment of intravenous line, blood sampling (glucose, electrolytes, urea, anticonvulsant levels)
	(2) i.v. diazepam (0.25–0.5 mg/kg, not faster than 2 mg/min). Rectal administration (0.5–0.75 mg/kg) may be used if i.v. line is not established. *Or* i.v. lorazepam (0.05 mg/kg over 2–5 mins)*
Second stage	*Steps 3–4 in all patients:*
	(3) Monitoring of vital functions and correction of disturbances. Tracheal intubation if necessary
	(4) Investigations of the possible cause of status, especially metabolic and infectious (lumbar puncture may be required)
	(5) i.v. administration of 100 mg pyridoxine (under 2 years of age)
	(6) Other treatment of cause if available (meningitis, encephalitis)
	Steps 7–8 if seizures are not controlled within minutes of giving benzodiazepines:
	(7) Repeat dose of diazepam may be given but preferably pass on to step 8
	(8) i.v. phenytoin (loading dose 20 mg/kg to obtain a serum level of 20–25 µg/mL, not faster than 25 mg/min); or i.v. phenobarbitone (loading dose 15–20 mg/kg) (some authors advise larger doses up to 100 mg/kg in intractable cases, if respiratory support available)
	Steps 9–11 for resistant status:
	(9) Close EEG monitoring and supervision by specialized medical and nursing personnel (intensive care unit)
	(10) Available therapeutic agents include paraldehyde (400 mg i.v., 200 mg/kg/h in 5% dextrose), chlormethiazole (0.08 mg/kg/min, i.v.), sodium valproate, lidocaine (lignocaine) (2 mg/kg i.v. as a bolus followed by continuous i.v. infusion of 6 mg/kg/h), i.v. clonazepam (given as bolus, 0.25–0.5 mg repeated up to four times)
Third stage	(11) If above agents fail, general anaesthesia with i.v. barbiturates or halothane may be indicated. Neuromuscular blockade may be necessary for maintaining ventilation. EEG monitoring is imperative

*Lorazepam has a longer half-life than diazepam and no long-life metabolite. It may be less of a respiratory depressant than diazepam, especially in patients who have previously received phenobarbitone (Treiman 1993). Midazolam intramuscularly may be effective in place of diazepam or lorazepam (Jawad *et al.* 1986, Parent and Lowenstein 1994, Appleton *et al.* 1995).

1989) and to neglect of immediate vigorous therapy. A once common syndrome of convulsive status epilepticus is the *hemiconvulsion–hemiplegia or H-H syndrome* (Gastaut *et al.* 1960), characterized by the occurrence, in the course of a febrile disease in a child of less than 4 years of age, of prolonged clonic seizures with a marked unilateral predominance, followed by a long-lasting hemiplegia. After one to several years, partial epilepsy, with seizures originating in the hemisphere contralateral to the hemiplegia, often occurs (*hemiconvulsion–hemiplegia–epilepsy or HHE syndrome*), and affected children are mentally retarded in 85 per cent of cases. CT scan and MRI are characteristic with initial oedematous swelling of one hemisphere followed by a global atrophy independent of any vascular territory (Fig. 16.17) (Labate *et al.* 1991, Aicardi 1994a). Other sequelae of convulsive status include seizures and diffuse neurological signs (Aicardi and Chevrie 1983).

Currently, the mortality of status in children is low, and the sequelae appear to be more often the result of the causal disease rather than that of the status itself. However, neurological sequelae are still observed (Fowler *et al.* 1992) and mesial temporal sclerosis

with late partial epilepsy continues to be an important problem. Recurrent status (Shinnar *et al.* 1992) is frequent in symptomatic cases but occurs rarely in the idiopathic group. The situation is worse in third world countries where cases of HHE syndrome continue to be seen.

The *treatment* of convulsive status in hospital is indicated in Table 16.7 (see also Brown and Hussain 1991b, Shorvon 1994).

Treatment is indicated in all cases after exclusion of pseudo-status epilepticus (Aicardi 1994a, Shorvon 1994). The two objectives of treatment are to quickly stop seizure activity and to maintain adequate respiratory, cardiovascular and metabolic functions. Clearly, the prevention of respiratory and circulatory complications (Table 16.8) has a major place in the prevention of residual damage. There is, however, some experimental and clinical evidence that the convulsive activity itself is probably harmful, so efforts should be made to stop it (see reviews in Meldrum 1978, Aicardi and Chevrie 1983, Brown and Hussain 1991a). The effect of purely EEG discharges is not known so that no firm recommendation is possible regarding the need for drug treatment of residual EEG discharges observed during systematic

TABLE 16.8
Complications of convulsive status epilepticus*

Cardiorespiratory and autonomic
- Hypotension
- Hypertension
- Cardiac failure
- Arrhythmias and cardiac arrest
- Respiratory obstruction
- Pulmonary oedema
- Aspiration pneumonia
- Hyperpyrexia

Metabolic
- Dehydration
- Hypoglycaemia
- Acute renal and liver failure
- Acute pancreatitis

Miscellaneous
- Intravascular coagulopathy
- Rhabdomyolysis
- Infections
- Fractures

Cerebral consequences or complications
- Hypoxic or metabolic damage
- Seizure-induced damage (especially hippocampus)
- Cerebral oedema and raised intracranial pressure
- Cerebral haemorrhage
- Cerebral thrombophlebitis

*Adapted from Shorvon (1994).

EEG monitoring. Prompt intervention is imperative because outcome is related to the duration of status and because therapy becomes progressively more hazardous the longer the seizures continue (Shorvon 1994).

In the premonitory and early phases of serial seizures and incipient status (usually outside the hospital) emergency treatment is based on intravenous or rectal administration of benzodiazepines. Dieckmann et al. (1994) and Alldredge et al. (1995) have adduced evidence that such treatment reduces significantly both the duration of seizures and the likelihood of recurrent seizures in the emergency department, and is reasonably safe. They did not encounter respiratory depression that leads other authors (e.g. Phillips and Shanahan 1989) to advise against emergency benzodiazepine treatment. Intravenous lorazepam has a more prolonged effect and may be equal or superior to phenytoin (Treiman 1993).

The patient should be placed in the lateral prone position and the airways cleared. During transportation the same position should be maintained.

In the hospital, intensive care unit treatment is preferable as adequate surveillance is often difficult to ensure in a regular ward. Maintenance of adequate oxygenation and circulation is clearly essential. Hypoxia is usually more severe than anticipated on clinical grounds and ventilatory support should not be delayed. Pressor therapy (dopamine) is often necessary in protracted status. Any hypoglycaemia, acidosis and electrolyte disorders should be corrected. Regular monitoring, including if necessary oximetry, central venous pressure and, if possible, continuous

EEG, should be established and a rapid search for an underlying cause should be performed following immediate anticonvulsant drug administration. The possibility of pleocytosis due to status epilepticus (Woody et al. 1988) has to be kept in mind when meningitis is suspected. Transient CT and MRI changes (Henry et al. 1994) resulting from convulsive activity can wrongly suggest a lesional cause.

For detailed information on drug treatment, the reader is referred to Shorvon (1994).

Overtreatment is dangerous as anticonvulsant drugs in high doses can induce respiratory depression and hypotension. Maintenance treatment should therefore be substituted for acute therapy as soon as possible.

Because there is some evidence that paroxysmal activity may be deleterious in the absence of complicating systemic factors (Meldrum 1978), there is a tendency to vigorously treat residual EEG discharges observed during systemic monitoring, even though their importance is still in dispute.

In exceptional cases (Gorman et al. 1992) neurosurgical treatment has been used successfully.

Generalized tonic status epilepticus, although it is a form of convulsive status, will be studied with nonconvulsive status with which it is often associated and shares aetiological factors.

Myoclonic status may be observed following hypoxia due to cardiac arrest (Shorvon 1994). A subtle form occurs in children with congenital nonprogressive encephalopathies (Dalla Bernardina et al. 1992) and with Angelman syndrome (Chapter 5). Some myoclonic activity is common in nonconvulsive status epilepticus.

Partial convulsive status epilepticus (epilepsia partialis continua) may be a feature of localized static brain damage involving the motor strip. *Focal dysplasia* (Kuzniecky et al. 1988, 1993) and hemimegalencephaly (Fusco et al. 1992) are common causes but destructive lesions are sometimes encountered (Cockerell et al. 1996). Epilepsia partialis continua may also be a feature of progressive conditions, including indolent tumours, mitochondrial diseases as a result of strokes (Chevrie et al. 1987, Antozzi et al. 1995), subacute measles encephalitis in immunosuppressed children (Chapter 11) and Alpers poliodystrophy (Chapter 10). The most frequent cause is *Rasmussen encephalitis* (Rasmussen and Andermann 1989), a slowly progressive disease that involves exclusively or predominantly one hemisphere, especially the frontotemporal region. Partial seizures are the first symptom and epilepsia partialis continua develops at some stage in over half the patients. Progressive hemiplegia, aphasia, hemianopia and mental deterioration become apparent after months or years of seizure activity. The EEG shows diffuse paroxysmal activity and a slow background tracing over the involved hemisphere. Neuroimaging shows progressive atrophy that begins in the frontemporal area and later spreads to the whole hemisphere and occasionally to the opposite side.

Pathologically, perivascular cuffing and glial nodules are present in areas of neuronal loss and glial proliferation (Vinters and Wasterlain 1996). The disorder is often associated with the presence of antibodies to the R3 glutamate receptors. These have been shown experimentally to be capable of stimulating the receptors and might thus be a cause of the epilepsy.

Antiepileptic drug treatment of the disorder is ineffective and surgery is usually necessary. Only large resections (hemispherectomy) are effective in a majority of cases (Andermann *et al.* 1992; Vining *et al.* 1993, 1997). Corticosteroid and immunoglobulin treatment can be partly effective (Chinchilla *et al.* 1994, Hart *et al.* 1994). Encouraging preliminary results of plasmapheresis have been recently reported (Prasad *et al.* 1996) but they may also be transient. Immunoglobulins are also being tried. The disease seems to run a less severe course in adolescents (Hart *et al.* 1997). A viral infection may be the cause, and both cytomegalovirus and Epstein–Barr virus have been indicted but without definite proof. Herpes simplex virus type 2 has recently been reported as the cause of smouldering encephalitis with temporal lobe epilepsy in two adult patients who presented with many features reminiscent of Rasmussen syndrome (Cornford and McCormick 1997).

Marked hyperglycaemia without ketosis may be responsible in adults for focal status. A similar syndrome of focal spinal myoclonus with extreme hyperglycorrhachia due to accidental dislocation of a venous catheter into a perispinal vein has been reported in a neonate (Bass and Lewis 1995).

GENERALIZED NONCONVULSIVE STATUS EPILEPTICUS
Nonconvulsive status almost always occurs in children with known epilepsy (Porter and Penry 1983, Shorvon 1994). It may belong to several distinct epileptic syndromes. Nonconvulsive status is only seldom a manifestation of typical absence epilepsy. Even when patients have a history of typical absences, many also develop grand mal and/or myoclonic seizures (Porter and Penry 1983).

Generalized nonconvulsive status may occur following an initial convulsive seizure (Cascino 1993) or can culminate in a generalized convulsion.

There are two subgroups of nonconvulsive generalized status (Shorvon 1994). *Typical absence status* occurs in the course of primary generalized epilepsy; *atypical absence status* occurs largely in secondarily generalized epilepsies, specifically in Lennox–Gastaut syndrome, severe myoclonic epilepsy and some of the other myoclonic epilepsies whether of primary (Doose 1992) or of secondarily generalized types. They are difficult to differentiate as the EEG discharge is infrequently of a classical, regular, 3 Hz type reminiscent of typical absences, and in many cases the spike–wave discharge is broken up into frequent bursts, is arrhythmic in frequency or is of less than 3 Hz (Cascino *et al.* 1993).

Consciousness is variably impaired from simple slowing of ideation and expression to profound obtundation or lethargy (Shorvon 1994).

Patients with the Lennox–Gastaut syndrome frequently have prolonged episodes of blurred consciousness, often associated with erratic myoclonus and/or brief head drops due to localized muscle atonia or myoclonic jerks. Such episodes are sometimes accompanied by an increase in the abnormal EEG activity but it may be difficult to fix a limit between ictal and nonictal states

(Erba and Browne 1983). Thus such cases are often excluded from nonconvulsive status. *Repeated tonic seizures* often interrupt such episodes or may replace them, a transition that is sometimes produced by the use of benzodiazepines (Alvarez *et al.* 1981, Di Mario and Clancy 1988).

Episodes of *pure tonic status* are frequent in Lennox–Gastaut syndrome. They may last several days or weeks, the individual seizures becoming shorter and less intense, while autonomic impairment increases with the duration of status. *Atonic status* is characterized by the occurrence of almost continuously repeated brief losses of tone (negative myoclonus) involving the axial and limb musculature (Guerrini *et al.* 1993). Blunting of consciousness is usually associated and erratic myoclonic jerks are often present. Such episodes, lasting hours or days, frequently complicate the course of myoclonic (myoclonic–astatic) epilepsy but may also occur with focal epilepsy, lesional or nonlesional (see below).

PARTIAL NONCONVULSIVE STATUS EPILEPTICUS
This type is rare in children and occurs in the course of temporal lobe or other lesional epilepsies. It may present as frequently recurring complex partial seizures with classical manifestations but without full recovery of mental activity between seizures or as continuous, long-lasting episodes of mental confusion and/or behavioural disturbances with or without automatisms (Aicardi 1994a). An alternation of periods of complete unconsciousness and of partial responsiveness is possible. The diagnosis with generalized nonconvulsive status depends on the EEG which shows permanent or repetitive localized paroxysmal activity, although with variable diffusion (McBride *et al.* 1981, Bauer *et al.* 1989). Partial nonconvulsive status can occur in the course of temporal lobe or of other lesional epilepsies, especially frontal ones. It may produce lasting postictal memory deficits in adults (Aicardi 1994a, Shorvon 1994). Cases of protracted disorder with mental deterioration and variable neurological signs with ultimate recovery have been attributed to partial complex status epilepticus by Mikati *et al.* (1985), although the EEG evidence of epilepsy was rather weak.

Treatment of generalized nonconvulsive status with benzodiazepines (diazepam, clonazepam or lorazepam) usually controls rapidly episodes of nonconvulsive status of the primary generalized type. Atypical absence status, however, is often resistant to drugs. High doses are better avoided, and benzodiazepine administration must be immediately interrupted if tonic components become apparent. Tonic status is highly resistant to therapy (Livingston and Brown 1988). Dexamethasone may be helpful in an emergency situation (Shorvon 1994). Treatment of partial nonconvulsive status epilepticus does not differ from that of status in general.

The outcome of nonconvulsive status is excellent in primary forms but rather poor in secondarily generalized types.

ELECTRICAL STATUS EPILEPTICUS OF SLOW SLEEP (ESESS)
This condition, more correctly termed *continuous slow spike–wave of slow sleep (CSWSS)* is an epilepsy syndrome characterized by

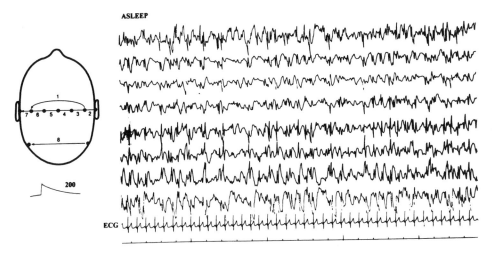

Fig. 16.18. Continuous spike–wave discharges during slow sleep (CSWSS), also termed electrical status epilepticus of slow sleep (ESESS). This 4-year-old girl presented with increasing dysphasia. Isolated seizures had occurred some months before. The EEG taken during non-REM sleep shows practically continuous spikes and spike–wave complexes with left-sided emphasis. (Courtesy Dr Steward Boyd, Great Ormond Street Hospital, London.)

the presence of diffuse bilateral slow (<2.0 Hz) spike–wave complexes (Fig. 16.18) that occupy 85 per cent or more of the slow sleep time (Jayakar and Seshia 1991, Tassinari *et al.* 1992, Bureau 1995). However, cases with a spike–wave index of 50–85 per cent seem not to differ essentially from classical cases in clinical manifestations or outcome (Bureau 1995). Bursts of diffuse spike–wave complexes, sometimes with atypical absences or myoatonic seizures, often occur during wakefulness. Seizures occur in 70 per cent of cases and often include partial nocturnal seizures reminiscent of those of benign partial epilepsy. The electrical abnormalities usually persist for months or years. This syndrome seems to be frequently, although not consistently, associated with behavioural disturbances and/or mental deterioration, the mechanism of which remains unknown. Eventually, the paroxysmal activity disappears, with some recovery of mental function. Morikawa *et al.* (1985) found identifiable brain pathology in 20–30 per cent of cases, and Gaggero *et al.* (1995) demonstrated areas of reduced blood flow by SPECT corresponding to the most actively discharging brain areas in four of their 10 cases. Guerrini *et al.* (1996b) reported seven children with ESESS associated with focal polymicrogyria. These results suggest that the syndrome is heterogeneous and not infrequently caused by multifocal abnormalities. Ethosuximide and corticosteroids may have some efficacy but treatment is often disappointing. Some investigators claim satisfactory results with sulthiame (Gross-Selbeck 1995, Lerman and Lerman-Sagie 1995) or short cycles of high doses of benzodiazepines (De Negri *et al.* 1993). ACTH steroids are, in fact, the most commonly used agents and are considered effective, although only anecdotal evidence is available. Treatment is usually for prolonged periods (months or even years). Recognition of electrical status epilepticus is of great importance as the syndrome is a cause of partially treatable mental deterioration. It is, therefore, essential to obtain a sleep EEG in such cases, even in the absence of clinical seizures.

The same paroxysmal sleep EEG activity may be associated with *acquired aphasia*, a condition also called 'epileptic aphasia' or the *Landau–Kleffner syndrome*. This is defined as acquired aphasia, often but not always predominantly receptive in type, with intense paroxysmal EEG activity, usually more intense in sleep. Awake tracings show uni- or bilateral spike foci often over the temporal lobes (Hirsch *et al.* 1990, Beaumanoir 1992, Maquet *et al.* 1995). There may be a correlation between the intensity of the paroxysmal activity, especially during sleep, and language deterioration. In such cases, there is a rapid or progressive loss of language abilities that often involves mainly verbal auditory discrimination. Approximately 80 per cent of children have convulsive seizures. Most often, these are focal and are not severe. Occasionally, they are atypical absences, frequently repeated. In most cases, the epilepsy and the EEG abnormalities disappear before age 15 years (Dulac *et al.* 1983).

The outlook for language is poor as most patients still have language difficulties as adults, even though the severity is variable from almost no verbal ability to mild or moderate deficits in verbal communication (Bishop 1985, Deonna *et al.* 1989).

A similar EEG activity involving other brain areas may be responsible for disturbance of other functions. Hirsch *et al.* (1995) reported apraxia associated with continuous parietal EEG paroxysms and suggested the mechanism was the same as that of the Landau–Kleffner syndrome. Neville and Boyd (1995) suggested that epilepsy may manifest as a gait disorder that responds to corticosteroid treatment.

In fact, the Landau–Kleffner syndrome is highly heterogeneous (Deonna *et al.* 1977, Hirsch *et al.* 1990, Maquet *et al.* 1995). Some children have predominant disturbances in expressive language or complex patterns of language disturbance. Others do not exhibit the pattern of continuous spike–wave discharges during sleep, and an occasional patient may have severe persisting epilepsy.

The mechanism of the syndrome is unclear. PET studies have given heterogeneous results (Maquet *et al.* 1990, Rintahaka *et al.* 1995). Magnetoencephalographic spikes originated in the left auditory area in one study (Paetau *et al.* 1992), and various techniques also point to this area (Morrell *et al.* 1995). There is evidence to suggest that the paroxysmal EEG abnormality itself may be responsible for the aphasia. Both the Landau–Kleffner syndrome and CSWSS may be examples of the effects of 'sub-clinical' discharges on brain function, and a confirmation that epilepsy is not limited to seizures may have more pervasive effects. Indeed, some cases of Landau–Kleffner syndrome also manifest more diffuse dysfunction, for example in frontal lobe mechanisms (Roulet *et al.* 1991, Hirsch *et al.* 1995), and transient deficits in various localized brain functions such as anterior opercular syndrome (Roulet *et al.* 1989, Boulloche *et al.* 1990) have also been linked to intense, localized, paroxysmal EEG activity.

A definable cause has rarely been found as an explanation of the syndrome.

Pascual-Castroviejo *et al.* (1992) suggested that many cases could be due to unrecognized vasculitis on the basis of angiographic findings and proposed treatment with nicardipine.

The treatment of the condition is disappointing. Anticonvulsant agents usually fail to abolish the paroxysmal activity and to improve language, although some success has been reported with the drugs used in CSWSS. Corticosteroids or ACTH treatment is an accepted practice but has to be continued for one year or more (Lerman *et al.* 1991, Hirsch *et al.* 1995). Only anecdotal reports are available and the relationship between treatment and language improvement has not been proved. The same applies to surgical treatment by multiple temporal transections (Morrell *et al.* 1989, Devinsky *et al.* 1994, Morrell *et al.* 1995).

STIMULUS-SENSITIVE EPILEPSIES
Epileptic seizures are paroxysmal events and it is likely that the majority of them are precipitated by known or unknown factors. Aird (1983) indicated that 40 seizure-precipitating mechanisms are known. These include tension states, alteration of the level of attention or of consciousness, sleep (Baldy-Moulinier 1986), psychological factors and hydration state.

In some epileptic syndromes, there is a regular precipitation of seizures by *specific stimuli*. The same stimuli, in other cases, may be only occasional precipitants of seizures in patients with spontaneous attacks.

PHOTOSENSITIVE EPILEPSIES
These can be observed with various epileptic syndromes and do not constitute a separate syndrome (Harding and Jeavons 1994). Photosensitivity is especially frequent in adolescents with primary generalized epilepsy (Harding and Jeavons 1994), in eyelid myoclonia with absence, and in some types of myoclonic epilepsy (Newmark and Penry 1979). Self-provocation is common in such patients. The role of *television* is emphasized by Harding and Jeavons (1994), although other investigators found it quite limited (Mayr *et al.* 1987). Provocation by *video games* (Maeda *et al.* 1990, Ferrie *et al.* 1994, Graf *et al.* 1994) is also possible, though

computer screens are only rarely a causal factor. This problem as well as that of pattern-sensitive epilepsy is studied in detail by Harding and Jeavons (1994). The treatment of photosensitive epilepsy may be with antiepileptic drugs only, especially sodium valproate. Additional measures may include the use of polarized glasses as well as precautions when watching television: drug therapy may not be necessary if the patient can avoid the stimulus by appropriate measures such as watching TV at a distance of 2–3 m and wearing dark glasses. Self-induced photogenic or pattern-induced seizures (Harding and Jeavons 1994) are difficult to control. Fenfluramine has been used in such cases together with antiepileptic agents, with some measure of success (Aicardi 1994a).

STARTLE EPILEPSY AND MOVEMENT-INDUCED SEIZURES
Startle epilepsy is relatively common in children with congenital brain damage (Aicardi 1994a). Many patients have congenital hemiparesis but others have diffuse brain damage including Down syndrome. Attacks are usually tonic involving one or both sides and follow the startle reaction induced by sudden unexpected stimuli (Chauvel *et al.* 1992). Sound is often particularly effective but proprioceptive or exteroceptive stimuli can also be the cause and some patients may respond electively to particular stimuli. Most cases have their onset in infancy and many patients are mildly to severely retarded. However, recent work (Manford *et al.* 1996b) indicates that about half the patients with the condition have normal intelligence and neurological profile, and these cases may be associated with cortical dysplasia rather than destructive lesions. Treatment is with anticonvulsant drugs but the occurrence of startle seizures usually announces a difficult-to-treat epilepsy. Such seizures should be distinguished from excessive startle disease and from paroxysmal dystonias (Chapter 17). *Touch epilepsy* and movement-induced epilepsy (Ricci *et al.* 1995) are rarer than startle epilepsy.

OTHER 'REFLEX' EPILEPSIES
A host of specific stimuli can induce seizures. These include sound, music, and complex and sometimes specific mental activities (Wilkins and Lindsay 1985). *Eating epilepsy* (Fiol *et al.* 1986) may occur with temporal lobe lesions. *Reading epilepsy* is a well-defined syndrome but is rare in childhood (Wolf 1994). Seizures induced by immersion in hot water (bathing epilepsy) (Roos and Van Dijk 1988) should be distinguished from syncopes (Stephenson 1990) which are probably much more common. Other uncommon precipitating factors are reviewed by Wilkins and Lindsay (1985) and by Aicardi (1994a).

OTHER UNUSUAL EPILEPTIC SEIZURES
Epileptic seizures can disturb all brain functions, and a wide variety of ictal phenomena have been reported. *Abdominal epilepsy* (Mitchell *et al.* 1983) is characterized by attacks of epigastric or periumbilical pain and/or by repeated episodes of unexplained vomiting. However, epilepsy is rarely the cause of the syndrome of recurrent abdominal pain and periodic vomiting, which is probably more often a manifestation of migraine (Aicardi 1994a).

In real cases of abdominal epilepsy, loss of consciousness is a feature. Seizures limited to vomiting rarely occur (Kramer *et al.* 1988). Other autonomic phenomena that can be the sole or main manifestation of a seizure include cardiac arrest (Kiok *et al.* 1986, Smaje *et al.* 1987), ictal arrhythmias (Gilchrist 1985) and apnoea and cyanosis (Southall *et al.* 1987, Donati *et al.* 1995, Hewertson *et al.* 1996). Unusual visual attacks may affect eye movements with ictal gaze deviation or epileptic nystagmus (Thurston *et al.* 1985) and ictal blindness (Barry *et al.* 1985). Pain as a seizure phenomenon is rare (Young *et al.* 1986, Trevathan and Cascino 1988). Shuddering attacks in children have been reported by Holmes and Russman (1986), and isolated disturbances of memory (Gallassi *et al.* 1988) and of sleep with repeated nocturnal awakenings (Peled and Lavie 1986) have also been mentioned.

FEBRILE CONVULSIONS AND OTHER OCCASIONAL SEIZURES

Febrile convulsions are epileptic seizures precipitated by fever that is not due to an intracranial infection or other definable CNS cause and are not preceded by afebrile seizures. Febrile convulsions are the single most common problem in paediatric neurology with a total incidence of 2–5 per cent of children under 5 years of age in Western countries. Excellent reviews of the topic are available (Nelson and Ellenberg 1981, Wallace 1988).

AETIOLOGICAL ASPECTS
Genetic factors are important in the causation of febrile convulsions, and there is a high incidence of a family history of febrile convulsions varying between 17 and 31 per cent in first-degree relatives. Most studies suggest a polygenic mode of transmission (Rich *et al.* 1987). An autosomal dominant pattern, however, may be at play in probands with three or more episodes (Anderson *et al.* 1988), and in some families with multiple affected members and a tendency to long-lasting seizures (Maher and McLachlan 1997).

The genes responsible for febrile convulsions are probably distinct from those that cause afebrile seizures. Only a small proportion of children with febrile convulsions have a first-degree relative with epilepsy (Berg *et al.* 1992). However, febrile seizures not infrequently precede some forms of epilepsy such as absences (Wallace 1991), and the overall risk of later epilepsy remains increased following febrile convulsions into the third decade of life (Hauser 1992). The genetic predisposition to febrile convulsions is age-dependent. Febrile convulsions are rare before age 5–6 months and 85 per cent of children have had their first seizure by 4 years with a median age of 17–23 months.

The fever responsible for febrile seizures is usually high (>38.5°C) and has the same causes as other fever in the same age group including immunizations (Chapter 12). One exception may be exanthema subitum, which is associated with a higher incidence of seizures, varying between 8 (Asano *et al.* 1994) and 13 per cent (Van den Bergh and Yerushalmy 1969). Gastroenteritis, on the contrary, is a relatively rare cause for the degree of temperature (Berg *et al.* 1995). Seizures usually occur early in the course of a fever and are actually the first symptom in 25–42 per cent of cases (Autret *et al.* 1990).

Prenatal and perinatal factors do not play an important role in causation (Nelson and Ellenberg 1990) even though they may influence adversely the prognosis. Some delay in passing early milestones is slightly more frequent than in the general population (Nelson and Ellenberg 1976, Wallace 1988). The only predictors of febrile convulsions are a fever >40.5°C and a family history of febrile seizures (Bethune *et al.* 1993, Berg *et al.* 1995). Febrile convulsions occur mostly between 6 months and 4 years of age: 60 per cent occur under 2 years, 20 per cent between 2 and 3 years, and in only 20 per cent is the first occurrence after age 3 years. An earlier onset is noted in girls and in children with complex seizures (Wallace 1988). *Occurrence of febrile convulsions before age 6 months should suggest the possibility of meningitis.*

CLINICAL FEATURES
The great majority of febrile convulsions are brief, bilateral clonic or tonic–clonic seizures. Unilateral seizures occur in about 4 per cent of patients. These are often prolonged seizures lasting 30 minutes or more (Nelson and Ellenberg 1981). Seizures lasting more than 15 minutes, unilateral seizures, and those followed by a Todd paralysis are termed *complicated febrile convulsions* and have a higher risk (up to 50 per cent) of being followed by epilepsy. Yet most cases of epilepsy subsequent to febrile convulsions occur after brief (so-called simple) febrile convulsions, just because these are overwhelmingly frequent and despite their lower attendant risk of epilepsy (about 1 per cent).

Febrile convulsions lasting 30 minutes or more are one type of status epilepticus and may leave sequelae if allowed to go untreated (Aicardi and Chevrie 1976, Viani *et al.* 1987, Phillips and Shanahan 1989). These include postconvulsive hemiplegia (the HHE syndrome) (Maytal and Shinnar 1990). The role of long-lasting febrile convulsions in the genesis of hippocampal sclerosis and consequent mesial temporal epilepsy remains disputed. A statistical association is well demonstrated (Rocca *et al.* 1987, Kuks *et al.* 1993), and there are strong arguments in favour of an aetiological relationship (Holthausen 1994, Harvey *et al.* 1995; see also p. 597). Thus, vigorous treatment of febrile status is imperative as shown by the persistence of sequelae in areas where emergency treatment is not available and febrile seizures are allowed to go untreated for hours. Such an occurrence is now unusual. Most cases of prolonged febrile convulsions occur during the first 18 months of life and especially before age 12 or 13 months. After 2 years of age, the risk of status epilepticus becomes very small (Aicardi and Chevrie 1976, 1983).

EEG tracings recorded within a week of a febrile convulsion may be abnormally slow for a few days in approximately one-third of patients. Epileptic EEG activitiy is found in about one-third of children with febrile convulsions prospectively followed, whether in the form of rolandic spike foci or of bilateral spike–wave bursts (Kajitani *et al.* 1981, Sofijanov *et al.* 1992). Such abnormalities are poorly correlated with the later occurrence of epilepsy (Sofijanov *et al.* 1992). In particular, they are exceptional in children below 18 months of age who are particularly at risk of recurrences and for the development of afebrile seizures (Viani *et al.* 1987), whereas they occur in up to 50 per cent of 4-year-olds who are at much lower risk. Therefore, the EEG has no place in the management of febrile convulsions.

The differential diagnosis of febrile convulsions includes primarily infections of the CNS (meningitis and encephalitis). In CNS infections, there is almost always an abnormal CSF. Green *et al.* (1993) found that in none of 115 children who had convulsions with meningitis was the disease occult. However, such cases are known to occur (Heijbel *et al.* 1980) so lumbar puncture is advised in children below 18 and especially below 6 months of age. Lumbar puncture is also indicated in children with long-lasting or otherwise atypical convulsions and in those who fail promptly to recover full consciousness. Herpes encephalitis often manifests initially in infants with febrile partial seizures and may pose a real problem. Millner and Puchhammer-Stöckl (1993) found a positive polymerase chain reaction for herpes simplex virus in five cases regarded as complicated febrile convulsions. Two of these patients had no cells in their CSF. In such cases, MRI can be of considerable value by showing signal alterations in a localized or multifocal distribution. Differentiation of acute convulsive encephalopathies from febrile seizures may be difficult when the CSF is normal. Indeed, the distinction is sometimes made only *a posteriori*, cases with sequelae not being regarded as febrile convulsions. However, cases of febrile convulsions with sequelae exist and are important in assessing the prognosis of febrile seizures. Likewise, it is very difficult to separate febrile seizures from 'true' epileptic seizures precipitated by fever as there is a large overlap between these categories.

Nonepileptic paroxysmal events are frequent in febrile children. They include primarily febrile syncopes ('anoxic seizures') (Stephenson 1990). Febrile delirium and rigors can also be mistaken for febrile convulsions.

PROGNOSIS

The prognosis of febrile convulsions is generally extremely favourable. Approximately 60–70 per cent of children have only one episode of febrile convulsions and most of the remaining will have two or three fits. Only 9 per cent of patients experience more than three episodes. Three-quarters of the recurrences take place during the year following the first seizure, and the risk of severe recurrence is quite low (Nelson and Ellenberg 1981, Annegers *et al.* 1990, Van Esch *et al.* 1996).

The risk of recurrences is greater in children who have seizures in the first two hours of fever or with temperature below 40°C, in those with a family history of febrile or afebrile seizures, in children under 1 year of age, and in those who have had already two or more episodes. Complex febrile seizures are also a predictor of a higher risk of recurrence (Berg *et al.* 1990, 1992; Verity *et al.* 1993; Offringa *et al.* 1994).

The risk of developing afebrile seizures is of the order of 2–5 per cent. It is very low in children with simple seizures occurring after age 1 year but increases with a younger age, with the presence of previous delelopmental or neurological abnormality, with a

family history of epilepsy, and in the case of complex febrile convulsions (Verity *et al.* 1993), reaching 50 per cent when all unfavourable factors are present (Annegers *et al.* 1990). A majority of epilepsies following febrile convulsions are primary generalized epilepsies with grand mal attacks, often with only a few seizures (Wallace 1991, Camfield *et al.* 1994). Such cases mainly follow brief, uncomplicated febrile convulsions (Aicardi and Chevrie 1976) and are relatively common. The afebrile seizures are mostly infrequent and generally tend to disappear by 9–10 years of age (Aicardi 1994a). Scheffer and Berkovic (1997) proposed that such 'febrile seizures plus' may be transmitted as an autosomal dominant trait with variable expression including rare cases of myoclonic–atonic seizures. Partial epilepsy (with simple or complex partial seizures) is more common after long-lasting unilateral seizures (Aicardi and Chevrie 1976, 1983). Children with early, often prolonged, febrile convulsions with multiple recurrences in the months following the initial event are suspect of developing polymorphic epilepsy of infants, also called severe myoclonic epilepsy (see p. 588).

The neurodevelopmental prognosis of febrile convulsions is excellent, except in patients who develop epilepsy, some of whom become retarded. This illustrates the tendency of complications to occur in association and is often the case with accidental prolongation of an episode of febrile convulsions. Some such children may have had a previous subclinical brain lesion before the febrile seizure with the result that it was long-lasting and localized. This is in agreement with the relatively high incidence of abnormal pre- and perinatal history found in several studies (Chevrie and Aicardi 1975, Wallace 1988).

TREATMENT

Brief febrile convulsions do not require any treatment except that of the causative febrile illness. Simple measures, such as removal of excess blankets and physical cooling are usually recommended. However, there is no evidence that antipyretic agents are effective in their prevention (Uhari *et al.* 1995). Hospitalization is unnecessary for uncomplicated febrile convulsions if adequate surveillance is possible. In case of doubt, a 12-hour hospitalization is sufficient. Long-lasting episodes should be vigorously treated (see Table 16.7 for the treatment of status epilepticus) as they may be associated with later epilepsy and sequelae, especially when they occur before 1 year of age.

Continuous prophylactic treatment of recurrences is not generally advised (Consensus Developmental Panel 1980) but may be indicated when factors of high risk are present. My own practice is to treat systematically infants under 1 year of age, and treatment for patients with complex partial seizures may be indicated although there is no proof that it prevents the occurrence of later epilepsy (Nelson and Ellenberg 1981, Shinnar and Berg 1996). Although it has been shown that prophylactic treatment with either phenobarbitone or sodium valproate reduces the frequency of recurrences by about two-thirds (Wallace 1988), the balance of risks and advantages of this practice remains to be established. Phenobarbitone (30–40 mg/kg/d) to reach a blood level of around 15 μg is reasonably safe although concern has been

TABLE 16.9
Features of the main types of neonatal seizures

Type of seizures	Clinical features	Ictal paroxysmal EEG discharges
Generalized tonic–clonic	Tonic contraction followed by a few jerks. Seen only with benign familial neonatal convulsions	Present in most cases
Generalized tonic	Sustained symmetrical posturing of neck and trunk sometimes provoked by stimulation	Rarely present
Focal clonic	Rhythmical jerks, focal or multifocal (in this case often asynchronous). Not suppressed by restraint	Almost always present
Focal tonic	Sustained posturing of single limb, sustained eye deviation not suppressed by restraint	Present in some cases
Myoclonic	Arrhythmical, nonrepetitive jerks, generalized, focal or fragmentary	Present in 80% of cases
Subtle or minimal seizures or motor automatisms	Roving eye movements, blinking, grimacing, sucking, chewing, thrusting tongue movements, swimming, boxing or cycling movements, suppressed by restraint and precipitated by stimulation when nonepileptic	Seldom present

expressed about the effects of the drug on IQ levels (Farwell *et al.* 1990). The significance of the small IQ loss observed remains uncertain and various criticisms have been directed at this study. Sodium valproate, although probably effective (Wallace 1988) is not advised because of the risk of hepatic failure.

Intermittent prophylaxis with diazepam orally or rectally is effective provided large enough doses are used (5 mg/kg, t.i.d.) (Autret *et al.* 1990, Rosman *et al.* 1993, Knudsen 1996). However, the efficacy is limited by the early occurrence of seizures, which may be the first symptom of fever—as was the case in 25 per cent of patients in the series reported by Wolf *et al.* (1977). Knudsen *et al.* (1996) followed 289 children up to 14 years of age or for 12 years after their febrile convulsion and found the outcome was excellent both in those receiving preventive treatment of fever before the recurrence of a seizure and in those treated with diazepam for an incipient convulsion. They concluded that it was 'as good to interrupt as to prevent' a seizure and thought that prophylactic treatment at the time of fever should be reserved for special cases. Intermittent treatment of fever with acetaminophen alone (Bethune *et al.* 1993) or combined with low-dose diazepam (Uhari *et al.* 1995) is not effective.

OTHER OCCASIONAL SEIZURES
Occasional seizures may occur with acute febrile diseases in older children. They can also occur in a well child or adolescent without fever (Aicardi 1994a). About half such seizures remain single (Shinnar *et al.* 1990). For that reason, treatment of the first afebrile seizure is not recommended unless specific reasons militate for immediate therapy. Isolated convulsions are especially apt to occur in adolescents during stress and sleep deprivation (Aicardi 1990a). Loiseau and Louiset (1992) have emphasized that generalized tonic–clonic or partial seizures in adolescents often do not recur, especially when the EEG is normal. They describe a *syndrome of partial benign epileptic seizures in teenagers* which, in their experience, accounted for 24 per cent of all partial seizures beginning in adolescence. Simple or complex partial

seizures, often with secondary generalization, occur in isolation or in brief clusters lasting less than 36 hours. Interictal EEGs are normal. The course is benign but distinction from lesional cases is difficult and neuroimaging studies are required.

NEONATAL SEIZURES
Seizures occurring during the first 28 days of life—and in most instances within the first 20 days—are a major problem of neonatal neurology.

CLINICAL FEATURES
The main types of neonatal seizures are shown in Table 16.9.

Only some of the behavioural phenomena classically described as neonatal seizures are regularly associated with rhythmical EEG discharges (Mizrahi and Kellaway 1987, Scher and Painter 1990) similar to those in older patients. These events include *focal clonic seizures* that are always partial with a fixed or shifting location (migratory seizures) and multifocal seizures which often demonstrate asynchronism between the various foci that discharge at different rhythms, either simultaneously or in succession. Generalized tonic–clonic seizures are exceptional in this age group; only familial neonatal convulsions have been associated with an EEG activity reminiscent of that observed at later ages (Hirsch *et al.* 1993, Ronen *et al.* 1993). Myoclonic seizures are also unusual. Tonic seizures and subtle or 'minimal' seizures that comprise such phenomena as oral or ocular movements, grimacing, eye opening, blinking or staring, pedalling or boxing movements, and, rarely, isolated apnoea (Watanabe *et al.* 1982a, Donati *et al.* 1995) are the most common types.

A large group of behavioural phenomena, often regarded as seizures on a clinical basis, are not regularly associated with EEG discharges (Fig. 16.19). These comprise a majority of the tonic (generalized or partial) and 'subtle' seizures. Scher *et al.* (1993a) were able to demonstrate paroxysmal EEG correlates in only 17 per cent of their patients with subtle seizures. Such phenomena can often be elicited by stimulation, the severity varies with

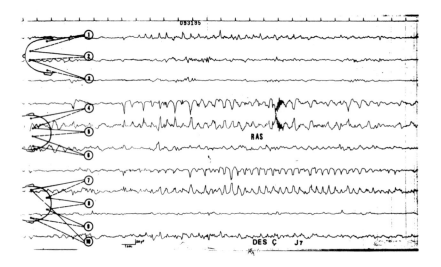

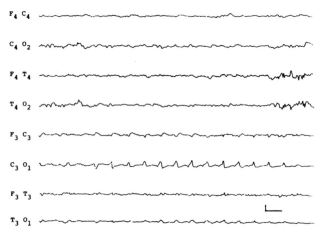

Fig. 16.19. Neonatal seizures. *(Above)* Well-formed EEG discharges occurring independently over two closely spaced areas of right hemisphere in term baby. *(Left)* Rhythmic discharge of low amplitude over posterior left hemisphere in preterm neonate. (Reproduced by permission from Aicardi 1986.)

intensity of stimulation and they may demonstrate temporal or spatial summation (Mizrahi and Kellaway 1987). It has been proposed that they do not represent epileptic seizures but rather 'release' phenomena related to disinhibition of brainstem structures resulting from cortical damage (Camfield and Camfield 1987).

Although this concept seems essentially sound, it should be observed that absence of an EEG discharge on the scalp is no proof of the nonepileptic nature of an event (Volpe 1989, Lombroso 1996). Undoubted epileptic seizures without EEG correlates are known to exist.

The problem is further complicated by the fact that EEG seizure discharges without clinical seizures are very frequent in neonates (Clancy *et al.* 1988, Scher and Painter 1990). Brief discharges lasting less than 10 seconds (brief intermittent rhythmic discharges or BIRDs) (Scher *et al.* 1993a,b) are frequent in the EEG of newborn infants and are not associated with clinical seizure activity. As a result, the definition of neonatal seizures is still imprecise and, consequently, their incidence is poorly known. Figures quoted vary from 0.15 to 1.4 per cent (see Aicardi 1991).

Both term and preterm infants may be affected. Seizures in preterm infants have a limited expression and purely EEG discharges are especially common (Scher *et al.* 1993a,b).

Neonatal seizures rarely occur as isolated events. Most frequently, brief seizures occur repeatedly over a period of a few hours or days (Clancy and Legido 1987a, Scher *et al.* 1993b, Bye and Flanagan 1995) and tend to subside, even without treatment, after 24–96 hours. The mean duration of individual seizures was 14.2 minutes for term infants and 3.1 minutes for preterm babies in the study by Scher *et al.* (1993b), but the difference was the result of the frequency of status in term infants and its rarity in preterm babies.

Ictal EEG discharges may consist of focal rhythmic spikes or sharp wave forms at variable frequencies (from alpha to delta) or of discharges of sharp waves (Tharp 1981, Holmes 1985, Lombroso 1996). Such discharges may be found in both term and preterm infants (Radvanyi-Bouvet *et al.* 1985, Legido *et al.* 1988).

Neonatal seizures should be distinguished from tremors and jitteriness, which are extremely common but are periodic movements at a rhythm of 5–6/s which can be suppressed by restraint or repositioning (Kramer and Harel 1994) and have a favourable outcome; from benign neonatal sleep myoclonus (Chapter 17); and from some vegetative phenomena such as nonepileptic apnoea. The most difficult issue is to decide whether atypical seizures unassociated with EEG paroxysms should be

TABLE 16.10
Main causes of neonatal seizures

Hypoxic–ischaemic encephalopathy (may produce both clearly epileptic attacks and seizures probably nonepileptic in nature)

Intracranial haemorrhage
  Subarachnoid haemorrhage (clonic seizures in term infants 1–5 days of age)
  Intraventricular haemorrhage (mainly tonic seizures and episodes of apnoea without EEG correlates, occasionally typical EEG discharges)
  Intracerebral haematoma (fixed localized clonic seizures)

Intracranial infections
  Bacterial meningitis and/or abcess
  Viral meningoencephalitis

Cerebral malformations
  Myoclonic and focal tonic seizures, infantile spasms, others

Metabolic causes
  Hypocalcaemia (clonic, multifocal seizures)
  Hypoglycaemia
  Hyponatraemia
  Inborn errors of amino acids or organic acids and NH_3 metabolism (often atypical, mostly unassociated with EEG discharges)
  Molybdenum cofactor deficiency
  Bilirubin encephalopathy (atypical, no EEG discharges)
  Pyridoxine dependency
  Biotinidase deficiency
  Folinic-acid-responsive seizures
  Carbohydrate-deficient glycoprotein syndrome

Toxic or withdrawal seizures (probably not true epileptic seizures in most cases)

Familial neonatal convulsions (clonic localized, shifting seizures with EEG correlates)

'Benign' neonatal seizures of unknown origin ('fifth-day fits')
  Clonic and apnoeic seizures with typical EEG correlates

---

regarded as epileptic in nature although the clinical manifestations may be suggestive. The problem remains unsolved in some cases.

CAUSES OF NEONATAL CONVULSIONS

The main causes of neonatal seizures appear in Table 16.10. In fact, many seizures associated with intracranial haemorrhage or with inborn errors of metabolism are probably not epileptic and the same applies to hypoxic–ischaemic encephalopathy even though the latter still represents a common cause of neonatal seizures (Levene and Trounce 1986). It seems likely that many infants with hypoxic–ischaemic encephalopathy have already suffered harm *in utero*, as shown by the frequency of prenatal placental damage (Burke and Tannenberg 1995), and that the perinatal events may not have played the major role. In addition, the definition of hypoxic–ischaemic encephalopathy is difficult and the condition is probably overdiagnosed (Chapter 2).

The seizures of hypoxic–ischaemic encephalopathy occur within the first 48 and often 24 hours of life. They are regularly associated with other manifestations of the disease such as apathy or coma (Chapter 2). The associated EEG in severe cases is of the inactive or discontinuous type (*tracé paroxystique*).

Localized arterial infarction has emerged as an important cause of localized, fixed, clonic seizures (Levy *et al.* 1985). Scher

et al. (1993a) found such infarctions in 58 per cent of their cases of EEG-confirmed neonatal seizures.

The frequency of infections is mainly due to prenatal viral disease. However, the frequency of meningitis and encephalitis is high enough to justify lumbar puncture whenever there is no obvious other cause. On the other hand, hypocalcaemia and hypoglycaemia (Cornblath and Schwartz 1991) are much less common but treatable conditions (Chapter 2). Late hypocalcaemia due to high phosphorus load in artificial milk feeds is now rarely seen, and currently observed cases are often associated with cardiac disease and have a guarded prognosis (Lynch and Rust 1994). Early hypocalcaemia is usually associated with other problems, so another cause for the seizures should be sought in such patients. De Vivo *et al.* (1991) have described a defect of glucose transport across the blood–brain barrier caused by the genetic absence of a specific protein, which results in severe hypoglycorrhachia manifested by isolated seizures without hypoglycaemia. The onset is usually towards the end of the first month of life but truly neonatal cases occur (Chapter 2). Rare metabolic causes include pyridoxine dependency (Chapter 9), spongiform encephalopathy with low activity of Na/K pumps (Renkawek *et al.* 1992), and familial folinic acid-responsive seizures (Hyland *et al.* 1995).

Seizures in infants born to mothers addicted to narcotics or barbiturates are probably often nonepileptic in nature but the EEGs have only rarely been recorded in such cases. Their prognosis appears to be favourable (Doberczak *et al.* 1988). Seizures due to cerebral malformations are often infantile spasms or myoclonic in type.

Neonatal convulsions without detectable cause are not uncommon (Painter *et al.* 1986, Aicardi 1991). *Benign familial convulsions* are dominantly inherited. The most frequent gene is located on chromosome 20q and has been cloned (Leppert *et al.* 1989, Malafosse *et al.* 1994), but rare cases are linked to chromosome 8 (Ryan *et al.* 1991) and no linkage to either locus has been found in still other cases (Plouin 1994). The onset of seizures is within 2–15 days of birth. Seizures recur for a few days then stop. Later relapses have been observed in 14 per cent of cases. The seizures are generalized (Hirsch *et al.* 1993, Ronen *et al.* 1993), although partial attacks have been reported (Aso and Watanabe 1992, Bye 1994). The phenotype is variable, some members of affected families presenting other forms such as febrile convulsions or generalized epilepsies (Berkovic *et al.* 1994). Rare cases of apparently recessively inherited neonatal seizures are on record (Schiffmann *et al.* 1991). The diagnosis rests on a history of similar events in relatives, consistent with an autosomal dominant transmission.

Benign nonfamilial convulsions, also known as 'fifth day seizures', consist of repeated fits mainly clonic or apnoeic in type with onset between 3 and 7 days of age. The interictal neurological state and EEG are normal, although the latter may show peaked theta rhythm (so-called *théta pointu alternant*) (Plouin 1994). In general, seizures of late onset (after 3 days) without known cause tend to have a favourable outcome (Lombroso 1996).

PROGNOSIS AND TREATMENT

The prognosis in neonatal seizures is mainly determined by their cause (Volpe 1989, Lombroso 1996). The possible role of the seizures themselves in generating or increasing brain damage remains disputed (Volpe 1989, Lombroso 1996). Although some aggravating effect of seizures is likely, the occurrence of seizures of long duration without sequelae, such as those of hypocalcaemia or of familial seizures, suggests that the role of paroxysmal activity (Lombroso 1996) is less important than its causes.

The worst outcome is for seizures due to brain dysplasias, followed by hypoxic–ischaemic encephalopathy and neonatal infections with a high mortality rate and a high incidence of later epilepsy, mental retardation and cerebral palsy (Holden *et al.* 1982, Watanabe *et al.* 1982b, Lombroso 1983b, 1996). The prognosis for some metabolic seizures (late hypocalcaemia) is very good and that for seizures of unknown cause with onset after the second day of life is also largely favourable. In a series of patients with electroencephalographically confirmed seizures (Clancy and Legido 1987b), the mortality was 32.5 per cent and sequelae were found in 55.5 per cent of survivors. Late epilepsy occurs in 10–26 per cent of patients but may be as high as 81 per cent when brain malformation is the cause. The prognostic value of the interictal EEG for neurodevelopment has been repeatedly emphasized (Lombroso 1983b, Scher and Beggarly 1989). Whether the occurrence of seizures may augment the original brain damage is controversial (see Aicardi 1991) but active treatment is imperative.

In addition to treatment of the cause of seizures, symptomatic treatment includes maintenance of a free airway and of the vital constants (cardiac rate, blood pressure, etc.). A trial of pyridoxine (a single dose of 100 mg for all neonates) should be made, but too large doses should be avoided as hypotonia and apnoea may result (Kroll 1985). Antiepileptic drug treatment commonly uses phenobarbitone or phenytoin. Large loading doses are usually recommended (phenytoin, a single i.v. dose of 20 mg/kg, not to be repeated—further doses can be administered under control of blood level; phenobarbitone, 20–25 mg/kg/d i.v.—some authors use doses as high as 30–120 mg/kg/d in 10 mg/kg boluses every 30 minutes), provided ventilatory support is available (Crawford *et al.* 1988). However, anticonvulsant agents may have deleterious effects on the neonatal brain (Mikati *et al.* 1994) and their efficacy is not established. Painter *et al.* (1994) found that the apparent effectiveness of phenobarbitone and phenytoin was the same and did not exceed 38 per cent. More importantly, they found that seizure frequency decreased on treatment, mainly when a decreasing trend had been observed previously, and that the drugs failed to prevent the onset of subsequent seizures, to delay the time to onset of recurrent seizures, or to attenuate the severity of recurrence. It has also long been known that antiepileptic agents often eliminate the clinical expression of the seizure but leave unaffected the ictal EEG discharge.

The benzodiazepines, especially lorazepam, may be satisfactory as a first-line or even as the only treatment (Deshmukh *et al.* 1986, Hakeem and Wallace 1990), and are favoured as first-line treatment by Lombroso *et al.* (1983b). My own practice is to use benzodiazepines as first drugs which often avoids the use of other drugs. Lidocaine, primidone and paraldehyde may also be used (Aicardi 1991). Maintenance treatment should be carefully monitored as most antiepileptic drugs are slowly metabolized in the neonatal period with a consequent risk of accumulation (Dodson and Pellock 1993). In fact, prolonged treatment of neonatal seizures is probably not warranted except in the case of major structural brain abnormalities, as neonatal seizures have a strong tendency to be short-lasting (Hellström-Westas *et al.* 1995).

PRENATAL SEIZURES

Prenatal seizures have long been known to occur and have now been demonstrated by ultrasonography (Landy *et al.* 1989, Du Plessis *et al.* 1993). They may occur with pyridoxine dependency (Chapter 9) and with some brain malformations (du Plessis *et al.* 1993).

INVESTIGATIONS IN PATIENTS WITH EPILEPSY

Although history-taking is the cornerstone of diagnosis in epilepsy, and physical examination may give essential clues such as cutaneous and neurological abnormalities (Aicardi and Taylor 1998), technical developments have added considerably to our knowledge in this field and may be of great clinical importance. EEG and neuroimaging are the main investigations performed but functional neuroimaging and biochemical investigations are indicated in selected cases. The EEG is important for diagnosis and differential diagnosis but of little help in the determination of a cause. Neuroimaging is essential for the latter purpose and is therefore of great value in determination of the aetiology. Functional neuroimaging (PET or SPECT scan) seems to be especially useful in conjunction with other methods for research of a focal origin to the seizures when surgery is contemplated.

ELECTROENCEPHALOGRAPHY

An EEG is almost systematically recorded in children with seizure disorders. However, the EEG is of no value in patients with febrile convulsions and in many cases of occasional seizures. In general, an EEG, like any other investigation, should be required only when some sort of hypothesis has been formulated (Stephenson and King 1989). It is essential that the recording technique is correct and that someone with paediatric EEG experience interprets the records, as the EEG profoundly changes with the age of patients, both in terms of background tracing and in the type of abnormalities expected. The reader is referred to the specialized EEG literature (Dreyfus-Brisac and Curzi-Dascalova 1979, Daly and Pedley 1990, Blume and Kalbara 1995) for details. The information obtained must be interpreted in conjunction with the clinical history. A normal EEG, even if repeated, does not exclude the diagnosis of epilepsy nor does an abnormal or even paroxysmal tracing establish it.

ROUTINE EEG

The 'routine' EEG of infants and young children should include a sleep record. A typical tracing, in association with an appropriate history, is extremely useful and often necessary (Blume and Kalbara 1995). For instance, a diagnosis of benign partial epilepsy cannot be made firmly if the characteristic sharp-wave focus has not been demonstrated on at least one tracing. Similarly, a diagnosis of primary generalized epilepsy can only be made when diffuse spike–wave activity is present. The EEG is essential in the establishment of the diagnosis of West syndrome and is indicated in all infants who present with neurodevelopmental deterioration.

The EEG also has a role in the distinction between cryptogenic and symptomatic epilepsies because certain patterns such as bilateral rhythmical spike–waves or rolandic foci are mostly encountered in children with nonlesional epilepsies. In occasional cases, the EEG tracings may suggest an aetiology, *e.g.* the presence of a slow-wave focus may indicate a focal lesion. The lateralizing and localizing value of the EEG has been extensively discussed. Although a consistently focal EEG focus is of considerable value, diffuse paroxysmal EEG abnormalities are not rare in children with focal lesions, especially cortical malformations and developmental tumours (Wyllie *et al.* 1994), and should be kept in mind as not contraindicating the possibility of surgery.

The prognostic significance of the EEG is sometimes clearcut. Such tracings as slow spike–wave complexes or multifocal spikes with abnormally slow background indicate the likelihood of an unfavourable outlook. Likewise, in some studies at least, an abnormal EEG before discontinuation of therapy is associated with a high recurrence rate (Shinnar *et al.* 1990, 1994).

In general, however, the EEG is not an essential guide to therapy. The presence of EEG paroxysms is not an indication to drug treatment nor a necessary contraindication to its discontinuation. In BECRS, for example, the EEG usually normalizes several months or years after cessation of seizures. The greater or lesser paroxysmal EEG activity is rarely, if ever, an indication for stepping up or reducing therapy.

OTHER EEG TECHNIQUES
In addition to hyperventilation, intermittent photic stimulation and brief sleep which are routinely employed, *prolonged sleep studies* are of great interest under certain circumstances (Baldy-Moulinier 1986). All-night sleep records are particularly useful in such epileptic syndromes as the Landau–Kleffner syndrome, atypical partial benign epilepsy, or when continuous spike–waves of slow sleep are suspected. Sleep EEG is essential for recording nocturnal seizures, *e.g.* in frontal lobe epilepsy.

Cassette recordings (ambulatory EEG monitoring) are a useful technique in cases in which the clinical history is not sufficient to establish or rule out the diagnosis of epilepsy and in which seizures are frequent enough to make their occurrence likely during a 24- or 48-hour session. Distinction between true and pseudoseizures is one of the best indications of this technique (Ebersole and Bridgers 1986, Binnie 1991).

Telemetric EEG permits an evaluation of the effect of activity on the occurrence of seizure discharges and assessment of the behavioural status of the child during EEG paroxysms (Binnie *et al.* 1981). Combination of telemetric EEG with video monitoring is particularly useful in this regard. In general, *video–EEG recording* is becoming increasingly important as it permits the study of seizures as a reproducible phenomenon.

Recording of seizures is a necessary requirement when epilepsy surgery is considered as interictal paroxysms may be found at a distance from interictal foci or in patients with bilateral interictal epileptic activity.

Other EEG techniques, beyond the scope of this book to discuss, include semi-invasive electrodes such as sphenoidal or ethmoidal electrodes, foramen ovale electrode, extradural subdural, or intracerebral recordings.

Telemetric EEG monitoring combined with neuropsychological tests has shown that isolated discharges or even single spikes, even rolandic ones, may be associated with transient cognitive dysfunction (Aarts *et al.* 1988). This does not signify that treatment should be used in such cases. Intense paroxysmal EEG abnormalities need not be associated with severe or frequent seizures. Their significance for prognosis is not fully assessed, and whether they indicate treatment is not clear, although it seems reasonable when associated with deterioration or new neurological or developmental abnormalities (Aicardi 1997).

NEUROIMAGING IN EPILEPSY
CT AND MRI
CT scan and MRI play an increasing role in the investigation of children with epilepsy (for details on indications, methods and results, the reader is referred to the admirable review by Duncan 1997). However, CT scan (and even more so MRI) is not routinely indicated for all such patients. Even though the 'yield' of CT scan may be high in focal seizures, a majority of the abnormalities found are not amenable to treatment and are not necessarily of great significance for predicting the prognosis. Only less than 1 per cent of the CT scans performed for epilepsy lead to surgical treatment (see Aicardi 1994a). Conversely, CT scan sometimes leads to the discovery of abnormalities unrelated to the seizures which are best left alone. Such anomalies include lesions such as neurocysticercosis (Chapter 11) and, especially, transient abnormalities following focal seizures (Sammaritano *et al.* 1985), the nature of which is not clearly determined and which appear to be especially frequent in India (Goulatia *et al.* 1987). CT may also be falsely negative by not showing small isointense lesions (Ormason *et al.* 1986).

MRI is clearly the most powerful imaging method and represents an enormous progress in the morphological study of the brain (Kuzniecky and Jackson 1995). It has been especially useful for the demonstration of cortical dysplasias, small indolent tumours and hippocampal sclerosis. When available, MRI is the first imaging technique to be used; CT scan is now a complementary technique when certain types of pathology such as calcification are suspected. Difficulties of interpretation may arise especially when intense convulsive activity is present (Kramer *et al.* 1987, Yaffe *et al.* 1995) and excellent quality imaging is mandatory. When necessary, special techniques such as 3D acquisition and high-resolution MRI should be used (Shorvon 1994, Bergin *et al.* 1995).

The diagnosis of hippocampal sclerosis by MRI rests on a decreased size of the Ammon horn on one side (Jackson *et al.* 1990; Cendes *et al.* 1993a,b), on increased T$_2$ signal (Jackson *et al.* 1993) and on loss of the internal structure of the hippocampus (Fig. 16.20). This lesion is highly correlated with the occurrence of complex partial seizures of temporal lobe origin and is not usually found with frontal lobe lesions (Cascino *et al.* 1993, Raymond *et al.* 1994a, Cendes *et al.* 1995). A careful search for additional anomalies is indicated in cases of hippocampal sclerosis, especially with a view to detection of dual pathology (Raymond *et al.* 1994a, Cendes *et al.* 1995). Both these studies reported the coexistence of cortical dysplasia in 15 per cent of adults with hippocampal sclerosis who were candidates for surgery, and such cases also exist in children even though their actual frequency is not known.

It is my practice *not* to recommend neuroimaging studies for children with classical primary generalized epilepsies (absence epilepsy, juvenile myoclonic epilepsy, grand mal seizures with typical bilateral spike–wave activity) or for children with typical benign rolandic epilepsy. Contrariwise, imaging is in order for children with other types of seizures or for any patient with atypical epilepsy.

OTHER TECHNIQUES OF STRUCTURAL IMAGING
These are only rarely indicated. This applies, in the first place, to plain skull X-rays which should *not* be performed routinely. *Radionuclide studies* have been largely replaced by CT or MRI. *Angiography* is indicated only after an abnormal CT or MRI scan that suggests a vascular lesion.

FUNCTIONAL NEUROIMAGING AND OTHER TECHNIQUES OF INVESTIGATION
FUNCTIONAL NEUROIMAGING
Proton magnetic resonance spectroscopy permits quantification of *N*-acetylaspartate (NAA), a specific neuronal marker in brain tissue in specific regions of interest, most often in the temporal lobe. Low levels of NAA are an indication of neuronal loss. The technique is useful to confirm the results of morphological studies and can demonstrate loss of tissue not detectable by conventional methods (Connelly *et al.* 1994, Cross *et al.* 1996).

Positron emission tomography (Duncan 1997) is used for the detection and localization of metabolic changes associated with seizures. Various positron emitting isotopes and ligands are used; the most commonly employed is ^{18}F-fluorodeoxyglucose which is taken up by actively metabolic cells and not metabolized beyond the stage of deoxyglucose-6-phosphate, so it remains 'trapped' in the metabolically active areas. Epileptogenic lesions have a lower metabolism (so a lower uptake) than the rest of the grey matter, and good correlation has been shown between lesions and hypometabolic areas (Chugani *et al.* 1987, Theodore *et al.* 1992). PET allows quantitation of uptake but its time resolution is limited because of the long duration of the examination. As a result, it does not allow for ictal studies. PET can use other ligands such as flumazenil to study the density of GABA receptors which is decreased in most epileptogenic foci (Burdette *et al.* 1995).

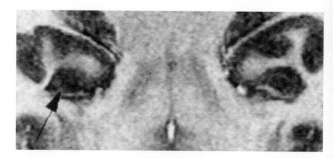
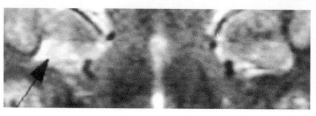

Fig. 16.20. MRI scan of both hippocampi of a patient with mesial temporal sclerosis showing details that can be obtained with high-resolution techniques. *(Top)* Right hippocampus *(arrow)* is of almost normal size but internal structure cannot be made out. *(Bottom)* Increased T$_2$ signal in external part of right hippocampus *(arrow)*. (Courtesy Dr G. Jackson, Melbourne, Australia.)

Single photon emission computed tomography has a somewhat lower spatial resolution than PET, but the use of HMPAO permits study of ictal events as it can be injected during a seizure and is immediately taken up by active cells while actual scanning can be performed for several hours (Harvey *et al.* 1993a,b; Newton *et al.* 1995). Interictal SPECT gives results generally similar to those of PET, *e.g.* decreased localized uptake in the region of origin of seizures, although its accuracy is far from perfect (Cross *et al.* 1997). Ictal SPECT, technically more difficult, is also more precise, and a very good correlation between focal hyperfixation, resulting from increased ictal blood flow and seizure localization, has been found in adults and in children (Harvey *et al.* 1993a,b; Cross *et al.* 1995).

Functional magnetic resonance imaging (Morris *et al.* 1994, Detre *et al.* 1995), still in an early stage of development, is a promising technique for the localization of normal brain such as language or primary motor areas and may eventually replace more invasive methods such as intracarotid injection of amytal to determine language lateralization (the Wada test). The use of functional MRI is limited to presurgical assessment of selected patients for whom convergence of information from several sources is essential but is not useful in the care of the vast majority of children with epilepsy.

OTHER TECHNIQUES
Other techniques that are being investigated include magneto-encephalography (Paetau *et al.* 1992) as well as various computed methods of signal interpretation and EEG topographic studies. Multichannel magnetoencephalography may prove useful in localizing epileptogenic foci (Stefan *et al.* 1990, Paetau *et al.* 1992).

SPECIAL DIAGNOSTIC TECHNIQUES

Biochemical investigations, whether routine (glucose, electrolytes) or more specific (*e.g.* amino acids, organic acids) are indicated in some cases for aetiological investigation. Muscle, skin and, rarely, brain biopsies may be required for specific diagnoses.

Determination of serum prolactin (Molaie *et al.* 1987) has been proposed to distinguish generalized seizures or complex partial seizures from pseudoseizures, as prolactin levels rise in the former within minutes and remain elevated for 60 minutes or more.

SOME AETIOLOGICAL FACTORS OF THE EPILEPSIES

EPILEPSY AND BRAIN TUMOURS

Epileptic seizures in children are due to brain tumours in only 0.2–0.3 per cent of cases (Aicardi 1994a). Nonetheless, brain tumours can be responsible for any type of epilepsy, especially partial seizures. Small astrocytomas, oligodendrogliomas, gangliogliomas and neuroepithelial dysembryoplastic tumours (Chapter 14) can generate epilepsies without any suggestive features, in which association with a tumour is only demontrated by neuroimaging. Small glial tumours were frequent in the large series (39 cases) reported by Morris *et al.* (1993). The commonest tumours are of developmental origin. The so-called *developmental neuroepithelial tumours* (Chapter 14) are frequently found in the temporal lobe, predominantly involve the cortex, and are often associated with adjacent cortical dysplasia. They are very slowly growing or static lesions (Raymond *et al.* 1994a), and their resection, in association with that of neighbouring epileptogenic cortex, gives excellent results. Gangliogliomas and gangliocytomas are less common epileptogenic tumours. It seems that they are not always distinguished from developmental neuroepithelial tumours, which probably explains their variable frequencies in different series. In one mixed series (Hirsch *et al.* 1989), excision of small tumours resulted in disappearance of seizures in 81 per cent of cases. However, resection of the epileptogenic cortex adjacent to the tumour may ensure more stable results (Cascino *et al.* 1992).

POST-TRAUMATIC EPILEPSY

Early seizures have been considered in Chapter 13. Late post-traumatic epilepsy occurs in approximately 5 per cent of patients with a post-traumatic amnesia of 24 hours or more (Jennett 1974). The seizures are secondarily generalized in 60–80 per cent of cases but all types can be seen including a picture similar to the Lennox–Gastaut syndrome (Niedermeyer *et al.* 1970). Seizures disappear after 5 years in about half the cases (Aicardi 1994a). Persistent focal seizures may be very difficult to control (Marks *et al.* 1995).

MIGRATION ABNORMALITIES AND CORTICAL MALFORMATIONS

These have proved to be one of the most common epileptogenic lesions, especially in infants and young children (Wyllie *et al.* 1994, Kuzniecky and Jackson 1995). Both diffuse malformations such as lissencephaly and focal dysplasias (Chapter 3) can cause generalized as well as partial seizures (Hirabayashi *et al.* 1993, Raymond *et al.* 1995). Virtually all types of seizures can occur, including infantile spasms, Lennox–Gastaut syndrome, atonic seizures, atypical absences, simple or complex partial seizures (Guerrini *et al.* 1992, 1996a) and epilepsia partialis continua (Fusco *et al.* 1992). Epilepsy can begin at any age but is usually early in diffuse disorders and can be as late as adolescence or adulthood in focal dysplasias. There is evidence that areas of cortical dysplasia can produce epileptic EEG activity (Palmini *et al.* 1995), justifying efforts to completely remove such lesions.

EPILEPSY AND CHROMOSOMAL ABNORMALITIES

Epilepsy occurs in 6–8 per cent of patients with Down syndrome. Infantile spasms are especially common (Stafstrom and Konkol 1994) and reflex seizures are often observed (Guerrini *et al.* 1998). The fragile X syndrome may be frequently associated with seizures and EEG abnormalities. Angelman syndrome, trisomy 12p and ring chromosomes 14 and 20 are uncommon conditions frequently complicated by epileptic seizures (Guerrini *et al.* 1998, Inoue *et al.* 1997).

EPILEPSY IN BRAIN-INJURED CHILDREN

Seizures in brain-injured children may be of any type and no seizure variety is specific for 'lesional' epilepsy. Some types of fits are highly suggestive of brain damage, *e.g.* startle seizures (Saenz-Lope *et al.* 1984), focal myoclonus (Kuzniecki *et al.* 1988) and gelastic epilepsy associated with hamartoma of the floor of the third ventricle (Berkovic *et al.* 1988). Tonic and atonic seizures and partial seizures evolving into complex seizures are also commonly due to brain damage (Revol 1992).

Seizures in a brain-injured child are usually difficult to control. However, spontaneous remissions can be observed after prolonged periods of seizure activity, even in mentally retarded children (Huttenlocher and Hapke 1990). Seizures may increase any previous brain damage and they are an indication of severe damage since brain lesions associated with seizures tend to be accompanied by more severe symptoms and to have a worse outcome than lesions unassociated with fits (Aicardi 1990a, Vargha-Khadem *et al.* 1992). Such seizures deserve vigorous treatment as they greatly increase the overall disability of affected children.

TREATMENT OF EPILEPSY AND EPILEPTIC SEIZURES

The management of epilepsy is not limited to the prescription of drugs. The impact of epilepsy on the life of the child and the family group is considerable so that education and support of parents, counselling and help with educational problems and management of behavioural difficulties may be even more important than drug therapy of seizures.

EDUCATION AND SUPPORT OF PARENTS

Because the impact of the diagnosis of epilepsy is not only—or not even essentially—concerned with the rational aspects but has also to take into account myths, misunderstandings and prejudices that are traditionally associated with seizure disorders, an adapted yet full explanation should be given to the patient and family. The false idea that epilepsy is a disease in its own right should be dispelled and the fact that epileptic seizures are only a symptom of many types of brain dysfunctions, some of which are quite benign, should be thoroughly explained. False but firmly entrenched ideas, *e.g.* that all epilepsies are life-long conditions or related to psychiatric disorders, should be discussed and dispelled as should the frequently expressed fear that brain tumours or other serious brain disorders are a common cause (Brett 1997). The whole information cannot usually be given in one session and repeated interviews are required.

Full explanation of the aims of therapy, its shortcomings and possible side-effects, is imperative, as is an indication of the probable duration of treatment and of the difficulties that may be encountered when discontinuing it. This is essential for the establishment of a confident relationship between the patient and the physician.

It is extremely important to give the parents precise ideas about what their child can do and what restrictions of activity are warranted. Such restrictions should be limited to a reasonable minimum, with the knowledge that some risks are unavoidable. Swimming is possible with adequate supervision. The use of a bicycle, and especially of a motorbike, is one of the most difficult problems and can be solved only individually and often imperfectly.

EDUCATIONAL, LEARNING AND BEHAVIOUR PROBLEMS

Although a majority of children with epilepsy are not mentally retarded and have no basic behavioural problems, one-fifth to one-third of them are, at least in part as a result of the CNS lesions that are also responsible for their epileptic seizures (Sillanpää 1992). Conversely, 20 per cent of children with mental retardation also have epilepsy and one-third of these also have cerebral palsy (Forsgren *et al.* 1990).

Various educational and behavioural difficulties are present in many children with epilepsy but without mental retardation. The prevalence of psychiatric disorder is several times higher in epileptic children than in the general population (Chapter 30). The reason for this association is not clear as assessment of social and other factors suggests that it is not explained by differences in sex, age, presence of physical disability or low intelligence. Such psychiatric abnormalities are more common in patients with complex partial seizures (Lindsay *et al.* 1979; and Chapter 30).

Underachievement at school is significantly more common in children with epilepsy than in the general population (Seidenberg *et al.* 1986). This is certainly a consequence of the limited intellectual abilities in some children. Bourgeois *et al.* (1983), Rodin *et al.* (1986) and Aldenkamp *et al.* (1990), among others, have shown that some children with epileptic seizures develop intellectual difficulties for which both the disease, the treatment and socioeducational factors may all be partly responsible. However, an undue number of patients with various types of epilepsy, even

well controlled, discontinue educational training prematurely. Over one-third of patients with absence epilepsy in one series were overqualified for their job (Olsson and Campenhausen 1992). This may indicate low self-esteem and/or low parental expectations (Long and Moore 1979, Levin *et al.* 1988, Collings 1990). Sillanpää (1990) showed that professional underachievement was common in adult patients who had had epilepsy starting in childhood, even when the IQ was normal. Loiseau *et al.* (1983) have shown that children with absence epilepsy do less well, in terms of social and professional achievement, than would be expected from their IQ and the relative benignity of their epilepsy, whereas children with benign partial epilepsy have a completely normal outlook from this point of view. The reasons for such differences are obscure. Considerable attention has been given to the interference of infraclinical EEG discharges with learning or other mental processes that may involve attention or concentration but may also interfere specifically with specialized tasks (Aarts *et al.* 1988; Kasteleijn-Nolst Trenité *et al.* 1988, 1990; Aldenkamp *et al.* 1992). However important subclinical discharges may be, they are unlikely to account for all the behavioural and learning difficulties of many epileptic children. Feelings of inadequacy and specialized neuropsychological deficits are clearly correlated with aggressive behaviour, poorer school performance, and having fewer friends and fewer interests (Herman 1982, Viberg *et al.* 1987), but the exact mechanisms need further research. Careful assessment and often remedial help may be needed on an individual basis. In an overwhelming majority of children with isolated epilepsy, regular schooling is possible, and special schools for epileptic patients are rarely—if ever—justified for patients without other neurodevelopmental problems.

DRUG TREATMENT
GENERAL PRINCIPLES
Drug treatment is the major form of therapy for a vast majority of children with seizure disorders. The main drugs currently available are shown in Table 16.11 and the main pharmacokinetic data in Table 16.12. In addition to first-line drugs, favourable results are occasionally obtained with such agents as clorazepate (Naidu *et al.* 1986, Fujii *et al.* 1987), bromides (Steinhof and Kruse 1992) and sulthiame (Lerman and Lerman-Sagie 1995), as well as with other 'minor' agents (Levy *et al.* 1995). In refractory cases, all available agents may deserve a trial (Schmidt 1986a, Aicardi 1988). ACTH and corticosteroids are extremely potent drugs for the treatment not only of infantile spasms but of many types of resistant epilepsy, especially when cognitive and/or major behavioural disturbances appear. They deserve a full trial (two to four weeks or more) in such cases.

New drugs that appear to be promising (Dichter and Brodie 1996) include vigabatrin (gamma-vinyl-GABA), an inhibitor of GABA transaminase that seems to be active in the treatment of partial epilepsies (Ring *et al.* 1990, Richens and Yuen 1991, Nabbout *et al.* 1997). Lamotrigine (Schlumberger *et al.* 1994, Besag *et al.* 1995) acts as an inhibitor of repetitive neuronal firing by stabilizing fast sodium channels and also, probably, as an antagonist of glutamate receptors. This drug seems highly

TABLE 16.11
Main anticonvulsant drugs

Drug	Indication	Total daily dose*	No. of daily doses
Carbamazepine	Partial seizures, generalized convulsive seizures	10–20 mg/kg	2–3[1]
Phenytoin	Generalized convulsive seizures, partial seizures	8–10 mg/kg <3 yrs 4–7 mg/kg >3 yrs	2
Phenobarbitone	Idem	3–5 mg/kg <5 yrs 2–3 mg/kg >5 yrs	2, or 1 at bedtime
Primidone	Idem	10–20 mg/kg	2
Sodium valproate, valproic acid[1]	Primary generalized epilepsies, myoclonic attacks, generalized convulsive and partial seizures	20–50 mg/kg	2–3
Ethosuximide	Absences and myoclonic seizures	20–40 mg/kg	1–2
Clonazepam	All forms	0.05–0.2 mg/kg	2
Clobazam	All forms, development of tolerance frequent	0.25–1.0 mg/kg	2
Diazepam[2]	All forms, mainly status epilepticus	0.25–1.5 mg/kg (0.1–0.3 mg/kg i.v.; 0.25 to 0.5 mg/kg rectally)	—
Nitrazepam	Infantile spasms, myoclonic epilepsies	0.25–1.0 mg/kg	2
Lorazepam[2]	Status epilepticus	0.05 mg/kg i.m. or i.v.	—
Midazolam[2]	Status epilepticus	0.1–0.2 mg/kg i.m.	—
Acetazolamide	Absence seizures, grand mal and partial seizures	10 mg/kg 0–1yr 20–30 mg/kg 1–15yrs	2
Trimethadione[3]	Absence seizures	20–60 mg/kg	2
Lamotrigine[4]	Partial and secondarily generalized seizures, primary generalized and myoclonic seizures, refractory absences, Lennox–Gastaut syndrome	5–20 mg/kg (0.2–5 mg/kg for children receiving sodium valproate)	2
Gabapentin	Partial and secondarily generalized seizures	20–50 mg/kg	2–3
Felbamate[5]	Lennox–Gastaut syndrome (refractory partial seizures)	Up to 45 mg/kg	3–4
Topiramate	Partial and secondarily generalized seizures	Adults 200–800 mg; children 1–5 mg/kg[6]	2
Vigabatrin	Partial seizures, generalized convulsive seizures	40–100 mg/kg	2
ACTH	Infantile spasms, Lennox–Gastaut syndrome, severe myoclonic epilepsy, resistant partial epilepsy	0.1–10 IU/kg	
Corticosteroids	Idem	2 mg/kg (prednisolone) 10–15 mg/kg (hydrocortisone)	

*Oral administration unless otherwise noted (i.v. = intravenously, i.m. = intramuscularly).
[1]Slow release preparation available.
[2]For acute treatment of status.
[3]Largely abandoned because of toxicity.
[4]Progressive increase in dose especially important.
[5]For refractory cases only.
[6]Tentative as little experience with infants, although doses up to 12 mg/kg/d have been used.

active in several types of generalized epilepsy including the Lennox–Gastaut syndrome—especially the astatic attacks, resistant typical absences and myoclonic seizures—and to a lesser extent in partial seizures. Gabapentin, topiramate and tiagabine have been less extensively investigated.

The mode of action of antiepileptic drugs is beyond the scope of this book (see Eadie and Tyrer 1989, Talwar 1990, Macdonald and Kelly 1993, Levy *et al.* 1995) and still imperfectly

known. The main steps in the processing of antiepileptic drugs are shown in Fig. 16.21. Steps from absorption through entry and distribution into the brain constitute the pharmacokinetics of a drug. Considerable knowledge has accumulated over the past two decades about the pharmacokinetics of antiepileptic drugs, especially in children (Dodson and Pellock 1993). Later steps with resulting changes in neuronal excitability constitute the pharmacodynamic phase of drug action. Initial pharmacokinetic steps

TABLE 16.12
Main pharmacokinetic data on anticonvulsant drugs

Drug	Oral availability (%)	T_{max}* (hr)	% protein bound	Apparent volume of distribution (L/kg)	Elim-ination half-life (hr)	Route of elimination	Therapeutic range (mg/L)	Therapeutic range (mmol/L)	Remarks
Phenobarbitone	80–100	2–10	50	0.51–0.57	37–73[1]	Hepatic metabolism	10–30	45–130	Enzyme inducer
Phenytoin	80–95	4–12	90	0.5–0.7	9–40	Saturable hepatic metabolism	10–20	40–80	Zero order kinetics makes small change of dosage result in wide changes of level; numerous interactions
Carbamazepine	70–80	2–10	60–80	0.8–1.6	8–24[2] 24–46[3]	Hepatic metabolism, active metabolite (10,11 epoxide)	4–12	17–50	Autoinduction common;induction of other drug metabolism; multiple interactions
Primidone	90–100	0.5–4	10–20	0.4–0.8	5–10	Hepatic metabolism, active metabolites (PEMA** + phenobarbitone); 40% excreted unchanged	5–12	25–50	Metabolized to PEMA** and phenobarbitone
Ethosuximide	90–100	1–4	0	0.6–0.9	20–40	Hepatic metabolism, 25% excreted unchanged	40–100	300–750	Not an enzyme inducer
Sodium valproate	100	1–3	90	0.10–0.20	7–15	Hepatic metabolism, active metabolites	50–100	345–690	Not an enzyme inducer; mildly inhibits oxidative metabolism; full pharmacological actionmay require weeks
Clonazepam	90	1–3	80–90	2.1–4.3	20–30	Hepatic metabolism	—		

(from absorption to brain entry) are reflected in the *blood levels* of a drug. It has been shown that the blood levels of antiepileptic drugs are more closely related to brain levels than to the dosage ingested, which is the rationale for their determination. However, blood levels are only one link in the chain of processes that take place between ingestion of a drug and its therapeutic and other effects, and their relationship to brain levels and to levels at the receptors is not necessarily close. Such discrepancies are frequent with sodium valproate and can also occur with carbamazepine (Suzuki *et al.* 1991, Scheyer *et al.* 1994). Some children handle anticonvulsant drugs in an atypical manner and in such cases special studies of their metabolism may be indicated (Gilman *et al.* 1994).

PRACTICAL INDICATIONS AND MODALITIES
Institution of treatment
Institution of an antiepileptic treatment is a serious decision that requires a firm diagnosis of epilepsy. Consequently, drug therapy should not be initiated for children with seizures of uncertain origin, for those with a single seizure (unless it is of a type observed only in chronic epilepsies) or for those with epileptic EEG abnormalities without clear-cut clinical manifestation. Likewise, preventive drug treatment for patients with potentially epileptogenic brain lesions is of unproven value and is better avoided as it may result in years of useless drug therapy (Shinnar and Berg 1996).

The problem posed by children with paroxysmal EEG discharges associated with clinical nonparoxysmal manifestations such as behavioural or cognitive difficulties, is delicate. There exist arguments to support a role of EEG paroxysms in such cases, especially when they are intense and prolonged. Treatment is clearly indicated for some syndromes of severe deterioration such as CSWSS or the Landau–Kleffner syndrome, even though there is only anecdotal evidence of efficacy. In fact, these syndromes are often resistant to conventional treatment and the response to any form of therapy is very difficult to assess. Most clinicians are not inclined to treat children with learning difficulties or attention deficit solely because of EEG anomalies.

Children who have had two or more seizures are candidates for drug treatment. Some investigators, however, tend to withhold treatment for patients with infrequent seizures that are of limited

TABLE 16.12
(continued)

Drug	Oral availability (%)	T_{max}* (hr)	% protein bound	Apparent volume of distribution (L/kg)	Elimination half-life	Route of elimination	Therapeutic range (mg/L)	(mmol/L)	Remarks
Clobazam	90	1–3	90	0.7–1.6	10–30	Hepatic metabolism, active metabolites	Not established		Development of tolerance common
Diazepam	75	1–2	95	1.1–1.8	10–20	Hepatic metabolism, active metabolites	0.15–0.25	0.52–0.87	
Vigabatrin	60–80	1–4	0	0.6–1.0	5–7[4]	Excreted largely unchanged	Not established		No drug interaction
Lamotrigine	98	2–3	55	0.9–1.3	12	5% hepatic in enzyme-induced patients, 25% in patients on sodium valproate)	Not established		Elimination inhibited by sodium valproate, increased by enzyme inducers
Gabapentin	51–72	2–3	0	0.57	5–7	>90% renal	Not established		No drug interaction
Felbamate	>90	2–6	22–25	0.7–0.8	2–6	90% renal	Not established		Inhibits elimination of valproate, carbamazepine epoxide, phenytoin and phenobarbitone
Topiramate	80	2	13–17	Not known	21	70% renal, 30% metabolized	Not established		Phenytoin, carbamazepine decrease levels by 40%, sodium valproate by 14%

*T_{max} = time to peak plasma level after administration of single dose.
**PEMA = phenylethylmalonamide.
[1]Half-life may exceed 100 hours in the first two weeks of life.
[2]Half-life in patients receiving the dose chronically, when autoinduction has developed, or receiving other inducing agents.
[3]Half-life in patients receiving the drug as monotherapy, before development of induction.
[4]Not significant as the drug binds irreversibly to glutamate-transaminase thus increasing brain GABA level; therefore the important half-life is that of restoration of enzyme level.

expression and/or occur at socially 'convenient' times, such as benign partial epilepsy (Ambrosetto *et al.* 1987). The decision to start treatment depends heavily on the patient's and parents' preferences when seizures are relatively rare.

Choice of drug(s)
The choice of drug(s) depends, in the first place, on the epileptic syndrome, or at least on the type of seizure experienced by the patient. Table 16.13 indicates the order of preference for the usual antiepileptic drugs in the most frequent types of childhood epilepsy. Any choice is of necessity arbitrary, in part because neither the efficacy nor the unwanted effects of any drug are entirely predictable (Mikati and Browne 1988). Selection of the first drug often depends critically on the toxicity, side-effects and greater or lesser difficulties in handling of any particular drug, as the likely effectiveness of several different drugs is often comparable. Comparative studies both in adults (Mattson *et al.* 1992, Richens *et al.* 1994) and in children (Verity *et al.* 1995, de Silva *et al.* 1996) have failed to show significant differences in the efficacy of the usual drugs (phenobarbitone, phenytoin, carbam-azepine and sodium valproate) used as monotherapy for partial or generalized convulsive seizures. These results do not exclude the possibility of some agents being more effective than others in individual cases or subsets of patients. Clearly they do not apply to absence attacks and many myoclonic seizures for which only sodium valproate, ethosuximide and the benzodiazepines are active, and their applicability to the severe types of childhood epilepsy is doubtful. In many instances the likelihood of side-effects will be a critical factor in the selection of a drug. Major side-effects are rare (see below), but even relatively mild side-effects should be taken into account as their impact on everyday life may be considerable. Thus, given the choice between carbam-azepine, phenobarbitone and phenytoin, the first agent will be preferred because it is much easier to handle than phenytoin and it does not produce the behavioural disturbances, or the 'minor' side-effects such as gingival hyperplasia and hirsutism, that are so common with phenytoin. Such side-effects may indeed be of consequence by making physically obvious the difference that mythically separates patients with epilepsy from the rest of children.

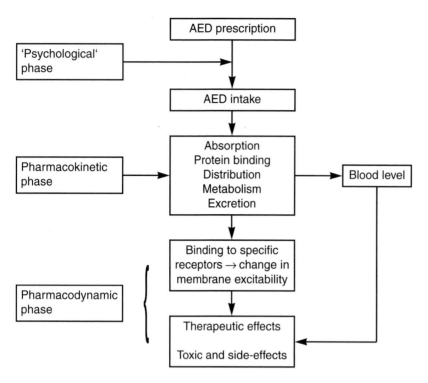

Fig. 16.21. Schematic representation of the successive steps from prescription of antiepileptic drugs (AEDs) to their clinical effects. Note that some toxic or side-effects may be due solely to their presence in blood (*e.g.* skin rashes, liver or kidney toxicity, interference with other drugs) while others (*e.g.* drowsiness, ataxia) necessitate, like their therapeutic effect, their presence at brain sites.

Monotherapy versus polytherapy
Giving only one drug is associated with fewer and less confusing side-effects than polypharmacy and avoids the problem of drug interactions. Therefore treatment should be started with a single agent. Seventy to 90 per cent of newly diagnosed, common forms of epilepsy can be controlled with monotherapy (Forsythe and Sills 1984, Brodie 1990). However, some investigators (*e.g.* Lammers *et al.* 1995) propose that side-effects of polypharmacy are not greater than those of monotherapy when the total dose of multiple drugs therapeutically equivalent to that of the drug given as monotherapy is not larger.

Drug combinations should be used only after single drugs in correct dosages have failed for a period long enough to make an adequate assessment. In case of failure of a drug, progressive substitution by other agents should precede the use of combined therapy. The value of adding a second drug is uncertain. Approximately 10–15 per cent of patients so treated have improved seizure control (Schmidt 1986a, Aicardi 1988, Bourgeois 1992) but a few patients may deteriorate and there is a tendency to increasing side-effects. Some better results with addition of sodium valproate to previous drug regimen are on record (Crawford and Chadwick 1986). Combinations of more than two drugs are rarely indicated (Aicardi and Shorvon 1998). Initial use of two drugs is rarely justified by the occurrence in the same patient of two types of seizure that require different therapy. Associating two drugs with similar side-effects, *e.g.* primidone and

phenobarbitone or phenobarbitone and clonazepam, is to be avoided.

Mode of administration
In principle, the use of more than two doses per day is to be avoided except in cases of very resistant epilepsy treated with drugs of short half-life. Some drugs, *e.g.* phenobarbitone, may be given in a single evening dose (Davis *et al.* 1981). Sodium valproate can also be used as a single dose in adolescents, which improves the compliance and seems to be effective for the control of primary generalized epilepsies (Covanis and Jeavons 1980). In fact, there is indication that the anticonvulsant action of sodium valproate is maintained at very low blood levels (Rowan *et al.* 1979).

A gradual increase or decrease in dosage on initiation or withdrawal of any drug is an essential rule. The first or successive drug should be introduced at low dosage and increased gradually until control is obtained or the limit of tolerance reached. This is especially important with lamotrigine as the frequency of rashes is higher with rapid introduction (Richens and Yuen 1991). Slow withdrawal is especially important for barbiturates, vigabatrin and felbamate whose discontinuation may induce status epilepticus when a first drug has failed. However, in the common epilepsies of childhood, withdrawal over four to eight weeks did not seem to be associated with higher recurrence rate (Dooley *et al.* 1996).

When a first drug has failed and another drug is being introduced, the first agent should be withdrawn progressively. In case

TABLE 16.13
Recommended drugs for the different types of epileptic seizures and syndromes

Type of seizure or epileptic syndrome	Recommended drugs (in order of preference)	
Partial seizures (simple or complex); generalized tonic–clonic seizures (especially secondarily generalized); tonic seizures	1st line:	carbamazepine, phenytoin, phenobarbitone, vigabatrin[1], primidone
	2nd line:	sodium valproate[2], clobazam, acetazolamide, sulthiame[3], lamotrigine
	3rd line:	phenacemide, mephenytoin (mesantoin)[4], bromides, ethotin
Typical absences; myoclonic or atonic seizures; juvenile myoclonic epilepsy	1st line:	sodium valproate, ethosuximide
	2nd line:	clobazam, clonazepam, lamotrigine, acetazolamide, methsuximide, primidone, phenobarbital[1]
	3rd line:	trimethadione[4], paramethadione
Infantile spasms; some cases of Lennox–Gastaut syndrome and some cases of other very resistant epilepsy	1st line:	ACTH, corticosteroids
	2nd line:	sodium valproate, clobazam, clonazepam, nitrazepam
	3rd line:	immunoglobulin i.v.[5]

[1]Some investigators consider it capable of increasing absence frequency.
[2]May be very active for partial seizures especially when secondarily generalized.
[3]May be effective only in association with phenytoin by increasing blood level.
[4]Now abandoned because of toxicity.
[5]Considerable doubt as to efficacy.

of relapse, two-drug therapy is indicated. It should be remembered that achievement of a stable drug level requires approximately four times the plasma half-life. The time to reach stable levels may be much longer as the dose is usually gradually increased and as phenomena of induction progressively modify (usually shorten) the apparent half-life of drugs.

Monitoring of anticonvulsant drug therapy
Regular *clinical supervision* is the only essential measure. Special attention should be given to the search for side-effects such as diplopia or vertigo that some patients come to consider as normal phenomena. In patients receiving sodium valproate, digestive disturbances, drowsiness or a recrudescence of seizures should make one look for incipient hepatic failure and discontinue the drug.

Monitoring of blood cell counts is probably useless except for defensive purposes (Camfield *et al.* 1986), and the same applies to tests of hepatic function as leukopenia and elevation of transaminases are common and do not herald the appearance of hepatic failure or pancytopenia.

In the *evaluation of the efficacy* of any drug regimen, clinical judgement based on seizure recurrences is fundamental. It is relatively easy in patients with frequent seizures regularly repeated (*e.g.* in absence epilepsy) but it becomes long and difficult in patients with rare seizures or in those whose seizures occur irregularly or in clusters, and requires several months or more.

This difficulty must not lead one to forget that the end-point of treatment is the control of seizures, not a normal EEG or a 'therapeutic' blood level however useful these may be.
Monitoring of the blood levels of antiepileptic drugs is *not* routinely indicated. It is useless in children with epilepsies that

are well controlled on regular or low dosage monotherapy. Indeed, many patients are seizure-free with blood levels well below the published ranges, and modification of dosage to obtain 'therapeutic' levels is ineffective (Woo *et al.* 1988) and increases the risk of side-effects. Likewise, discontinuation of a drug because its level is 'subtherapeutic' can result in seizure relapse (Richens 1982). Conversely, in resistant cases, the dose should be pushed to the limit of *clinical* tolerance, regardless of blood levels. Blood level determinations are useful to check the patients' compliance; to confirm suspected toxicity in infants or retarded children for whom it may be difficult to diagnose; and to detect blood interactions in patients on polypharmacy. They are also indicated for patients on phenytoin therapy as the therapeutic ratio (*i.e.* the margin of safety) of this drug is low and, especially, in uncontrolled cases and in the case of 'breakthrough' seizures in previously well-controlled children (Aicardi 1994a). Results of blood level determinations are especially useful when they can be obtained almost immediately (Wallace 1990), allowing immediate adjustment of therapy. Blood levels are useless with some drugs (vigabatrin) and of dubious value with others, *e.g.* sodium valproate whose levels are poorly correlated to clinical effects.

Interpretation of blood levels is not always straightforward, especially in cases of drug interactions (Levy *et al.* 1983, Pippenger 1987) and for drugs whose binding to protein may vary with resultant change in levels of free, unbound, drug and those that have active metabolites, such as carbamazepine, as the rate of formation of the metabolite is not constant and the blood level not measured. Meijer (1991) provides a comprehensive review of the indications, problems and limitations of monitoring of anticonvulsant drugs.

TABLE 16.14
Main side-effects and toxicity of anticonvulsant drugs*

Drug	Side-effects	Severe toxicity
Phenobarbitone	*Drowsiness* *Aggression* *Sleep disturbances* *Hyperactivity* Osteomalacia Rashes	Aplastic anaemia Stevens–Johnson syndrome Rheumatism
Phenytoin	*Ataxia* Anorexia Nausea Acne *Nystagmus* *Gum hypertrophy* *Hirsutism* Megaloblastic anaemia Osteomalacia Reduced IgA Depression Neuropathy	Orofacial dyskinesia Anaemia *Lupus-like syndrome* Pseudolymphoma Stevens–Johnson syndrome Hepatitis Encephalopathy
Primidone	*Drowsiness* Dizziness Nausea Vomiting *Personality change* Diplopia Ataxia Rashes	Agranulocytosis Lupus-like syndrome Thrombocytopenia
Carbamazepine	*Diplopia* *Dizziness* *Ataxia* Nausea Hyponatraemia Rashes (5–10%)	Orofacial dyskinesia Cardiac arrhythmia Hepatotoxicity Lupus-like syndrome Pseudolymphoma
Sodium valproate	*Anorexia* *Nausea* Vomiting *Hair loss* *Weight gain* *Tremor* Drowsiness Thrombocytopoenia *Hyperammonaemia* (usually mild)	*Hepatotoxicity* (especially in retarded infants <3 yrs who may have underlying disorder)[1] Pancreatitis Stupor, encephalopathy
Ethosuximide	Anorexia *Nausea* *Vomiting* Drowsiness *Headache* Hiccups Rashes	*Lupus-like syndrome* Aplastic anaemia Psychosis
Clonazepam/ clobazam	*Fatigue* *Ataxia* *Hyperkinetic syndrome* *Aggression* *Drowsiness* *Hypersalivation*[2] *Bronchorrhoea*[2] *Muscle weakness*	Psychosis Thrombocytopenia
Lamotrigine	Drowsiness Behavioural changes *Rashes*	*Stevens–Johnson syndrome*
Vigabatrin	Drowsiness Hyperactivity Aggression Weight gain	*Psychosis* Depression
Gabapentin	Headache Dizziness	None
Felbamate	Drowsiness Nausea	Aplastic anaemia Hepatic failure (can be lethal)
Topiramate	Loss of appetite Weight loss Slurring of speech Difficulty concentrating	None

*Features in *italics* are frequent or clinically important.
[1]Metabolic diseases can be revealed by administration of sodium valproate (Coulter 1991).
[2]These complications may be responsible for severe aspiration and even sudden death (Murphy *et al.* 1987) in retarded infants and children. This may be due to cricopharyngeal muscle incoordination which has also been reported with nitrazepam (Wyllie *et al.* 1986).

Unwanted Effects of Antiepileptic Drugs

Side-effects of antiepileptic drugs are common (Table 16.14); extensive reviews are available (Schmidt 1986b, Eadie and Tyrer 1989). The most common side-effects are transient and occur at the beginning of treatment. These include mainly digestive disturbances, drowsiness and dizziness. Rashes may occur with certain drugs (*e.g.* carbamazepine, lamotrigine) and are an indication to discontinue the treatment.

Some relatively mild side-effects may be sufficient to necessitate a change of therapy: for example, the behavioural disturbances produced by phenobarbitone or the marked increase in weight in patients receiving sodium valproate. Mental changes may be difficult to assess, and in some cases an attempt at withdrawing the suspect agent(s) may be warranted but requires hospitalization when complete. Mention should be made of the possible induction or aggravation of certain types of seizures with some antiepileptic drugs including phenytoin, carbamazepine, vigabatrin and clonazepam (Lerman 1986, Osorio *et al.* 1989, Lortie *et al.* 1993, Marciani *et al.* 1995). Prevention of hepatic failure by administration of L-carnitine to patients, especially those under 2 years of age, who are receiving sodium valproate is of uncertain value (Coulter *et al.* 1991). Hepatic necrosis is probably due in many cases to latent metabolic disorders (Bicknese *et al.* 1992). Most antiepileptic drugs can adversely affect cognition, drive, performance, mood and behaviour (Kälvinainen *et al.* 1996).

Very long-term side-effects of drugs are poorly known. An example could be the increase in blood levels of both high-density and low-density cholesterol with carbamazepine and phenobarbitone which could theoretically increase the risk of atherosclerosis (Eiris *et al.* 1995).

NONDRUG MEDICAL TREATMENTS
KETOGENIC DIET
The ketogenic diet has long been in use for the treatment of children with severe epilepsies. Although the mechanism of action of the diet is obscure, a high concentration of ketone bodies in the blood is necessary for its effectiveness. Various types of ketogenic diets are available, using either medium-chain triglycerides or conventional 4:1 or 3:1 diet. Although the diet is unpalatable, its taste and appearance can be made acceptable (Freeman *et al.* 1994). Side-effects include diarrhoea, growth failure and, in some children, renal stones and severe episodes of acidosis These may be life-threatening and fatalities have occurred especially when acetazolamide was used concomitantly with the diet (Prasad *et al.* 1996), so this drug should be discontinued two weeks before starting the diet. Elevated levels of cholesterol have occasionally been observed in treated children and the long-term effects of the drug are as yet poorly documented. The short-term beneficial effect of the diet is indisputable for several types of seizures including myoclonic seizures, the Lennox–Gastaut syndrome (Schwartz *et al.* 1989a,b) and some cases of resistant partial or generalized seizures. Kinsman *et al.* (1992) were able to control the seizures completely in 17 of 58 children (29 per cent) and obtained a 50 per cent decrease of frequency in a further 22 (38 per cent). Improvement in awareness may be an additional benefit. The diet has been maintained for two years or more in some children and the effect is said to persist after discontinuation in patients treated for a year or more. However, the drop-out rate is high and in some children the effect of the diet is only transient. Long-term studies are in progress; it now appears that a trial of ketogenic diet is reasonable for at least some refractory epilepsies. Education of parents is all-important and a team approach is essential for optimal results. However, trials have been uncontrolled so the evidence is largely anecdotal and assessment of risks and benefits requires further study.

BEHAVIOURAL METHODS
Behavioural methods of seizure control have been proposed (for review, see Feldman *et al.* 1983).

SURGICAL TREATMENT OF EPILEPSY
It appears increasingly evident that some epilepsies are totally refractory to presently available drugs, and for some such cases surgery deserves to be considered more liberally and earlier than is now customary (Engel 1996).

RESECTIVE SURGERY
Most surgical techniques are intended to remove the epileptogenic tissue which is responsible for initiation and spread of the seizure discharge. Criteria for surgical removal of epileptogenic tissue include refractoriness of seizures, a severity sufficient to interfere seriously with life, clinical and other evidence pointing to a localized brain area, and the possibility of removing such area without producing unacceptable functional sequelae.

The delay before considering surgery is classically three to four years (Schmidt 1986a, Aicardi 1994a). There is a tendency to shorten this delay in children with active epilepsy, especially when an anatomical lesion is detectable (Engel 1993, 1996), and the appearance of neurodevelopmental deterioration may require shorter delays of the order of a few months (Neville *et al.* 1997). Temporal lobe resection is the operation most commonly performed, but more limited resections in the temporal lobe and removal of epileptogenic lesions outside the temporal lobe are also feasible, although the success rate is definitely lower than that of temporal lobe surgery (Polkey 1989, Lüders 1992).

Determination of the epileptogenic area and presurgical evaluation of patients are beyond the scope of this chapter (see Wieser and Elger 1987, Lüders 1992, Engel 1993). Results in children 5–15 years of age are almost identical to those in adults (Guldvog *et al.* 1994). The number of reports of resective surgery in patients under 5 years is now sufficient to indicate that surgery can be effective in this age range and considered even for infants in selected cases (Shields *et al.* 1992). Twenty-two of 33 patients in the study of Gilliam *et al.* (1997) were seizure-free after resective surgery, four had a greater than 90 per cent reduction in seizure frequency, and only four showed no improvement. Six children had an increase in IQ ≥10 points and only one showed a loss >10 IQ points. The association of epilepsy with neurological impairment and/or of mental retardation need not be a contraindication to surgery, as the disturbances resulting from epilepsy tend to multiply the disability rather than simply add to other difficulties. In patients with neurological deficits, some types of surgery such as hemispherectomy may be considered. Hemispherectomy can be performed for large lesions such as some cases of Sturge–Weber syndrome, hemimegalencephaly or other extensive migration disorders, and for widespread destructive lesions, including Rasmussen encephalitis, in patients with hemiplegia (for reviews, see Andermann *et al.* 1992, Vining *et al.* 1997). Various technical modifications appear to limit the risk of secondary complications (Tinuper *et al.* 1987), and the results on epilepsy may be excellent without excessive increase in motor deficit.

Extensive operations are often performed for the 'catastrophic' epilepsies or 'epileptic encephalopathies' of infants in the hope of interrupting or reversing the process of cognitive and/or behavioural deterioration often associated with repeated seizures and severe EEG anomalies. Encouraging results have been reported (Shields *et al.* 1992, Neville *et al.* 1997) but systematic studies with long follow-up and detailed neuropsychological studies are necessary before definitive conclusions can be drawn.

OTHER FORMS OF SURGERY
When resective surgery is not feasible other methods may be applicable. Currently the most widely used is sagittal callosotomy, either partial (anterior two-thirds) or total. Full evaluation of the results of callosotomy is not yet possible. The operation seems to be of some value for epilepsies with generalized tonic and atonic

seizures, especially the Lennox–Gastaut syndrome, and for epilepsies with frontal foci and secondary generalization (Cendes *et al.* 1993c, Reutens *et al.* 1993). Multiple *subpial transections* may be useful in the treatment of focal epilepsy when the focus cannot be removed (Sawhney *et al.* 1995). They may prevent lateral extension of the discharge and favourable results have been reported, especially in the Landau–Kleffner syndrome (Morrell *et al.* 1995).

PROGNOSIS

As already indicated, the prognosis of seizure disorders varies widely with the epileptic syndrome, its aetiology and associated manifestations, and with the age of patients (Sander 1993). Therefore, studies that do not specify the type of children observed are of limited value. They may, however, be an indication of the overall fate of children with epilepsy if the referral of patients is not too selective or biased. Five points will be considered: (1) the risk of recurrence after a first seizure; (2) the risk of relapse after discontinuation of drug therapy; (3) the problem of intractable epilepsy; (4) the social and educational outcome of epilepsy; (5) the risk of sudden death in adolescents and young adults.

RISK OF RECURRENCE AFTER A FIRST UNPROVOKED SEIZURE

Several studies (Annegers *et al.* 1986; Boulloche *et al.* 1989; Shinnar *et al.* 1990, 1996) give figures for generalized tonic–clonic seizures which vary from 25 to 54 per cent. Most recurrences occur within one year of the first seizure. Such studies suggest that treatment of a first seizure, although effective (First Seizure Trial Group 1993), is not indicated as half the children will remain seizure-free. Risk factors for recurrences include an abnormal neurodevelopmental state and, in some studies, a young age (< 4 years) at first seizure, a family history of epilepsy, and an abnormal EEG (Shinnar *et al.* 1994). The recurrence risk in this study was 25 per cent at 24 months with an idiopathic first seizure and a normal EEG, 34 per cent when the EEG was abnormal but nonepileptiform, and 54 per cent with epileptiform abnormalities. An early age of onset (< 2 years) is strongly associated with resistant epilepsies. However, this mainly results from the inclusion of cases of epileptic encephalopathies. When these are excluded, the recurence rate for infants is the same as for older children (Camfield *et al.* 1993).

These figures apply only to cases of isolated seizures or epilepsies. When neurological signs and/or mental retardation are present, the risk of recurrence is much higher. In a longitudinal study of 246 children, Sillanpää (1993) found that the likelihood of a five-year terminal remission after 35 years of follow-up was 79.9 per cent in idiopathic epilepsy, 69.2 per cent in cryptogenic epilepsy, and only 56.3 per cent in symptomatic cases. Whereas 77 per cent of patients with normal neurological and mental status reached a five-year terminal remission, the proportion dropped to 50 per cent for patients with mental retardation, to 46.2 per cent for those with cerebral palsy, and to 29.2 per cent when both mental retardation and cerebral palsy were present. Even minor neurological abnormality significantly decreased the

probability of a remission. However, Cockerell *et al.* (1997) in a large population of both children and adults with newly diagnosed epilepsy found a three-year remission rate of 86 per cent and a five-year remission rate of 68 per cent after a nine-year follow-up.

RISK OF RELAPSE AFTER DISCONTINUATION OF TREATMENT

Several reports have concluded that the risk of relapse is relatively low in children who remain seizure-free for two or three years on therapy (Bouma *et al.* 1987, Aarts *et al.* 1988, Ehrhardt and Forsythe 1989, Aldenkamp *et al.* 1993, Shinnar *et al.* 1994). Figures varied between 12 and 42 per cent, again suggesting that discontinuation of therapy after two years is probably possible in many common types of epilepsy. Dooley *et al.* (1996) found that the recurrence rate was no higher with discontinuation of treatment one year after the last seizure than after two years, and Tennison *et al.* (1994) found no difference in recurrence rate between a six-week and a nine-month weaning period. Similar results were obtained in two prospective studies (Medical Research Council 1991, Peters *et al.* 1995).

INTRACTABLE EPILEPSY

Intractable epilepsy is defined as epilepsy with seizures that have remained uncontrolled, despite 'relevant' therapy (Juul-Jensen 1968). In fact, intractability is a graduated rather than an all-or-none phenomenon. Some cases are indeed inadequately treated epilepsies (Aicardi 1988, Aicardi and Shorvon 1998) and it is therefore essential to look for factors associated with apparent intractibility such as unrecognized progressive causal disease, precipitating factors and treatment irregularities. Misdiagnosis of the type of epilepsy resulting in the use of an inappropriate drug—*e.g.* ethosuximide for partial complex seizures—and failure to recognize that the patient's seizures are not epileptic in nature but rather psychogenic or cardiovascular are other common causes of apparent intractability. About 20 per cent of real epilepsies are resistant to drug therapy. However, some may be controlled after multiple trials and only approximately 10–15 per cent are really intractable. Intractable epilepsies include some of the 'catastrophic syndromes' such as Lennox–Gastaut syndrome or severe myoclonic epilepsy, and cases of partial seizures, mainly those of lesional origin. Even epilepsies associated with brain lesions and mental retardation can remit after variable but often prolonged periods of activity. Huttenlocher and Hapke (1990) found that remission occurred at a rate of 1.4 per cent per year in patients with resistant epilepsy with mental retardation and of 4 per cent per year in those without. In this series of 145 children, 61 per cent of whom were retarded, the remission rate remained unchanged over the years until early adulthood. Children with focal atrophic brain lesions did no worse than those with normal imaging studies.

It is therefore difficult to decide at what point and after how many trials of mono- and polytherapy an epilepsy should be declared intractable (Bourgeois 1992). Clearly when other therapeutic options—especially resective surgery—are available and have a good prospect of success, medical therapy should probably not be prolonged for more than one or two years or even less in case of deterioration. If no alternative to drugs is possible, various drug regimens will be tried for much longer periods.

Intractability is related to the type of epileptic syndrome. Predictors of intractability include infantile spasms, remote symptomatic epilepsy, a history of status epilepticus, neonatal seizures and microcephaly (Berg *et al.* 1996). The poor prognosis of some syndromes, *e.g.* Lennox–Gastaut syndrome and polymorphic epilepsy of infants, has already been emphasized.

SOCIAL AND EDUCATIONAL OUTCOME
The educational level of persons with epilepsy as a group is much lower than that of the general population. In a long-term study of adults with childhood-onset epilepsy, Sillanpää (1992) found that approximately one-third of 176 patients had received less than primary education and 37 per cent only primary education. Only 18 per cent went to secondary school and 9 per cent graduated. Three per cent had a university degree. The proportion of patients having a driving licence (61 per cent), of those married or having a stable relationship (65 per cent), of those having children (49.5 per cent) were all significantly lower than in random matched controls. The proportion who were unemployed (9.1 per cent) was higher. Patients with active epilepsy did signficantly less well than those who had been in remission for five years or more. These figures reflect in part the presence of complicating factors such as neurological impairment, learning difficulties or mental retardation. However, even patients without complicating factors tend to do less well than the general population in terms of professional and social adjustment (Loiseau *et al.* 1983). This is probably due, in part, to school absenteeism, low expectations from parents and teachers, rejection by peers, and practical problems (*e.g.* lack of driving licence). Many such factors reflect prejudice and ill-informedness of the public and patients themselves about their condition and could be improved by a better knowledge.

RISK OF SUDDEN DEATH IN YOUNG PATIENTS WITH EPILEPSY
The mortality of children with uncomplicated epilepsy is probably not significantly different from that of their nonepileptic age peers. The mortality rate of patients with epilepsy associated with mental and/or neurological deficits is considerably greater. Sillanpää (1992) found that between 10 and 20 per cent of such patients were dead by 15 years of age and 20–30 per cent by 25 years. In most cases the primary condition was the cause of death, but a significant proportion of deaths resulted from accidents, suicide or sudden unexpected death.

Sudden unexpected death in patients with epilepsy probably results from seizures associated with apnoea and/or disturbances in cardiac rhythm. Indeed, alarming degrees of oxygen desaturation may occur with apparently regular seizures, not necessarily due to organic lesions. Sudden death mainly occurs in adolescents and young adults and constitutes a significant cause of mortality in this age group. The rate is around 1 per 1000 patients per year (Nashef *et al.* 1995) so the issue clearly warrants continued investigation. The mechanisms of sudden death in epilepsy are obscure. Patients with uncontrolled seizures are at high risk, whereas those with well-controlled attacks have no excess mortality (Sperling *et al.* 1995). Asphyxia and cardiac dysrhythmias are likely factors. However, impressive apnoeic seizures with major cyanosis are not necessarily of bad prognosis. Hewertson *et al.* (1994) reported a benign outcome in four of six infants and children with such events.

REFERENCES

Aarts, W.F.M., Visser, L.H., Loonen, M.C.B., *et al.* (1988) 'Follow-up of 146 children with epilepsy after withdrawal of antiepileptic therapy.' *Epilepsia,* **29,** 244–250.
Abou-Khalil, B., Andermann, E., Andermann, F., *et al.* (1993) 'Temporal lobe epilepsy after prolonged febrile convulsions: excellent outcome after surgical treatment.' *Epilepsia,* **34,** 878–883.
Acharya, J.N., Wyllie, E., Lüders, H.O., *et al.* (1997) 'Seizure symptomatology in infants with localization-related epilepsy.' *Neurology,* **48,** 189–196.
Aicardi, J. (1988) 'Clinical approach to the management of intractable epilepsy.' *Developmental Medicine and Child Neurology,* **30,** 429–440.
—— (1990a) 'Epilepsy in brain-injured children.' *Developmental Medicine and Child Neurology,* **32,** 191–202.
—— (1990b) 'Neonatal myoclonic encephalopathy and early infantile epileptic encephalopathy.' *In:* Wasterlain, C.G., Vert, P. (Eds.) *Neonatal Seizures.* New York: Raven Press, pp. 41–49.
—— (1991) 'Neonatal seizures.' *In:* Dam, M., Gram, L. (Eds.) *Comprehensive Epileptology.* New York: Raven Press, pp. 99–112.
—— (1994a) *Epilepsy in Children, 2nd Edn.* New York: Raven Press.
—— (1994b) 'Syndromic classification in the management of childhood epilepsy.' *Journal of Child Neurology,* **9,** Suppl. 2, 2S14–2S18.
—— (1994c) 'The place of neuronal migration abnormalities in child neurology.' *Canadian Journal of Neurological Sciences,* **21,** 185–193.
—— (1995) 'Typical absences in the first two years of life.' *In:* Duncan, J., Panayiotopoulos, C. (Eds.) *Typical Absences and Related Epileptic Syndromes.* London: Churchill Communication Europe, pp. 284–288.
—— (1996) 'Epileptic syndromes with onset in early childhood.' *In:* Wallace, S.J. (Ed.) *Epilepsy in Children.* London: Chapman & Hall, pp. 247–274.
—— (1997) 'Epilepsy as a nonparoxysmal disorder.' *Acta Neuropediatrica. (In press.)*
—— Chevrie, J.J. (1970) 'Convulsive status epilepticus in infants and children.' *Epilepsia,* **11,** 187–197.
—— —— (1976) 'Febrile convulsions: neurological sequelae and mental retardation.' *In:* Brazier, M.A.B., Coceani, F. (Eds.) *Brain Dysfunction in Infantile Febrile Convulsions.* New York: Raven Press, pp. 247–257.
—— —— (1982) 'Atypical benign partial epilepsy of childhood.' *Developmental Medicine and Child Neurology,* **24,** 281–292.
—— —— (1983) 'Consequences of status epilepticus in infants and children.' *In:* Delgado-Escueta, A.V., Wasterlain, C., Treiman, D.M., Porter, R.J. (Eds.) *Advances in Neurology. Vol. 34. Status Epilepticus.* New York: Raven Press, pp. 115–125.
—— Levy Gomes, A. (1988) 'The Lennox–Gastaut syndrome: clinical and electroencephalographic features.' *In:* Niedermeyer, E., Degen, D. (Eds.) *The Lennox–Gastaut Syndrome.* New York: Alan R. Liss, pp. 25–46.
—— —— (1989) 'The myoclonic epilepsies of childhood.' *Cleveland Clinic Journal of Medicine,* **56** (Suppl., Pt. I), S34–S39.
—— —— (1992) 'Clinical and EEG symptomatology of the "genuine" Lennox–Gastaut syndrome and its differentiation from other forms of epilepsy of early childhood.' *In:* Degen, R. (Ed.) *The Benign Localised and Generalised Epilepsies of Early Childhood, Vol. 6.* Amsterdam: Elsevier, pp. 179–186.
—— Shorvon, S. (1998) 'Intractable epilepsy.' *In:* Engel, J., Pedley, T.A. (Eds.) *Epilepsy: A Comprehensive Textbook. Vol. 2.* New York: Lippincott–Raven, pp. 1325–1331.
—— Taylor, D.C. (1998) 'History and physical examination.' *In:* Engel, J., Pedley, T.A. (Eds.) *Epilepsy: A Comprehensive Textbook. Vol. 1.* New York: Lippincott–Raven, pp. 805–810.
—— Sabril IS Investigator and Peer Review Groups, *et al.* (1996) 'Vigabatrin

as initial therapy for infantile spasms: a European retrospective survey.' *Epilepsia*, **37**, 638–642.

Aird, R.B. (1983) 'The importance of seizure-inducing factors in the control of refractory forms of epilepsy.' *Epilepsia*, **24**, 567–583.

Aldenkamp, A.P., Alpherts, W.C.J., Dekker, M.J.A., Overweg, J. (1990) 'Neuropsychogical aspects of learning disabilities in epilepsy.' *Epilepsia*, **31**, Suppl. 4, S9–S20.

—— Gutter, T., Beun, A.M. (1992) 'The effect of seizure activity and paroxysmal electroencephalographic discharges on cognition.' *Acta Neurologica Scandinavica*, **86**, Suppl. 140, 111–121.

—— Alpherts, W.C.J., Blennow, G., *et al.* (1993) 'Withdrawal of antiepileptic medication in children—effects on cognitive function: the multicenter Holmfrid study.' *Neurology*, **43**, 41–50.

Alldredge, B.K., Wall, D.B., Ferriero, D.M. (1995) 'Effect of prehospital treatment on the outcome of status epilepticus in children.' *Pediatric Neurology*, **12**, 213–216.

Al-Shahwan, S.A., Singh, B., Riela, A.R., Roach, E.S. (1996) 'Hemisomatic spasms in children.' *Neurology*, **44**, 1332–1333.

Alvarez, N., Hartford, E., Doubt, C. (1981) 'Epileptic seizures induced by clonazepam.' *Clinical Electroencephalography*, **12**, 57–65.

—— Shinnar, S., Moshe, S.L. (1987) 'Infantile spasms due to unilateral cerebral infarcts.' *Pediatrics*, **79**, 1024–1026.

Ambrosetto, G. (1992) 'Unilateral opercular macrogyria and benign childhood epilepsy with centrotemporal (rolandic) spikes: report of a case.' *Epilepsia*, **33**, 499–503.

—— Giovanardi Rossi, P., Tassinari, C.A. (1987) 'Predictive factors of seizure frequency and duration of antiepileptic treatment in rolandic epilepsy: a retrospective study.' *Brain and Development*, **9**, 300–304.

Andermann, E. (1982) 'Multifocal inheritance of generalized and focal epilepsy.' *In:* Anderson, V.E., Hauser, W.A., Sing, C.F. (Eds.) *Genetic Basis of the Epilepsies.* New York: Raven Press, pp. 355–374.

—— Straszak, M. (1982) 'Family studies of epileptiform EEG abnormalities and photosensitivity in focal epilepsy.' *In:* Akimoto, H., Kazamatsuri, H. (Eds.) *Advances in Epileptology. XIIIth Epilepsy International Symposium.* New York: Raven Press, pp. 105–112.

Andermann, F., Rasmussen, T.R., Villemure, J.G. (1992) 'Hemispherectomy: results for control of seizures in patients with hemiparesis.' *In:* Lüders, H. (Ed.) *Epilepsy Surgery.* New York: Raven Press, pp. 625–632.

Anderson, A.E., Kellaway, P. (1994) 'Benign epilepsy with multifocal spikes.' *Paper presented at the joint ICNA–CNS Congress, San Francisco, October 1994.*

Anderson, V.E., Hauser, A. (1991) 'Genetics.' *In:* Dam, M., Gram, L. (Eds.) *Comprehensive Epileptology.* New York: Raven Press, pp. 57–76.

—— Wilcox, K.J., Hauser, W.A., Rich, S.S., Jacobs, M.P., Kurland, L.E. (1988) 'A test of autosomal dominant inheritance in febrile convulsions.' *Epilepsia*, **29**, 705–706. *(Abstract.)*

—— Hauser, W.A., Olafsson, E. Rich, S.S. (1990) 'Genetic aspects of the epilepsies.' *In:* Sillanpää, M., Dam, M., Johannessen, S.I., Blennow, G. (Eds.) *Pediatric Epilepsy.* London: Wrightson Biomedical, pp. 37–56.

Annegers, J.F., Shirts, S.B., Hauser, W.A., Kurland, L.T. (1986) 'Risk of recurrence after an initial unprovoked seizure.' *Epilepsia*, **27**, 43–50.

—— Hauser, W.A., Beghi, E., *et al.* (1988) 'The risk of unprovoked seizures after encephalitis and meningitis.' *Neurology*, **38**, 1407–1410.

—— Blakley, S.A., Hauser, W.A., Kurland, L.T. (1990) 'Recurrence of febrile convulsions in a population-based cohort.' *Epilepsy Research*, **5**, 209–216.

Antozzi, C., Franceschetti, S., Filippini, G., *et al.* (1995) 'Epilepsia partialis continua associated with NADH-coenzyme Q reductase deficiency.' *Journal of the Neurological Sciences*, **129**, 152–161.

Ariizumi, M., Baba, K., Hibio, S., *et al.* (1987) 'Immunoglobulin therapy in the West syndrome.' *Brain and Development*, **9**, 422–425.

Appleton, R.E., Panayiotopoulos, C.P., Acomb, B.A., Beirne, M. (1993) 'Eyelid myoclonia with typical absences: an epilepsy syndrome.' *Journal of Neurology, Neurosurgery, and Psychiatry*, **56**, 1312–1316.

—— Sweeney, A., Choonara, I., *et al.* (1995) 'Lorazepam *versus* diazepam in the acute treatment of epileptic seizures and status epilepticus.' *Developmental Medicine and Child Neurology*, **37**, 682–688.

Asano, Y., Yoshikawa, T. Suga, S., *et al.* (1994) 'Clinical features of infants with primary human herpesvirus 6 infection (exanthema subitum, roseola infantum).' *Pediatrics*, **93**, 104–108.

Aso, K., Watanabe, K. (1992) 'Benign familial neonatal convulsions: generalized epilepsy?' *Pediatric Neurology*, **8**, 226–228.

—— —— Negoro, T., *et al.* (1987) 'Visual seizures in children.' *Epilepsy Research*, **1**, 246–253.

Aubourg, P., Dulac, O., Plouin, P., Diebler, C. (1985) 'Infantile status epilepticus as a complication of 'near-miss' sudden infant death.' *Developmental Medicine and Child Neurology*, **27**, 40–48.

Autret, E., Billard, C., Bertrand, P., *et al.* (1990) 'Double-blind randomized trial of diazepam versus placebo for prevention of recurrences of febrile seizures.' *Journal of Pediatrics*, **117**, 490–494.

Babb, T.L., Brown, W.J. (1987) 'Pathological findings in epilepsy.' *In:* Engel, J. (Ed.) *Surgical Treatment of the Epilepsies.* New York: Raven Press, pp. 511–540.

—— Leib, J.P., Brown, W.J., *et al.* (1984) 'Distribution of pyramidal cell density and hyperexcitability in the epileptic human hippocampal formation.' *Epilepsia*, **25**, 721–728.

Baldy-Moulinier, M. (1986) 'Inter-relationships between sleep and epilepsy.' *In:* Pedley, T.A., Meldrum, B.S. (Eds.) *Recent Advances in Epilepsy, Vol. 3.* Edinburgh: Churchill Livingstone, pp. 37–55.

Bancaud, J., Talairach, J. (1975) 'Macro-stereo-electroencephalography in epilepsy.' *In: Handbook of EEG and Clinical Neurophysiology.* Amsterdam: Elsevier, pp. 3–10.

Bankier, A., Turner, M., Hopkins, I.J. (1983) 'Pyridoxine-dependent seizures. A wider clinical spectrum.' *Archives of Disease in Childhood*, **58**, 415–418.

Baram, T.Z., Mitchell, W.G., Tournay, A., *et al.* (1996) 'High-dose corticotropin (ACTH) versus prednisone for infantile spasms: a prospective, randomized, blinded study.' *Pediatrics*, **97**, 375–379.

Barry, E., Sussman, N.M., Bosley, T.M., Harner, R.N. (1985) 'Ictal blindness and status epilepticus amauroticus.' *Epilepsia*, **26**, 577–584.

Bass, N., Wyllie, E., Comair, Y., *et al.* (1995) 'Supplementary sensorimotor area seizures in children and adolescents.' *Journal of Pediatrics*, **126**, 537–544.

Bass, W.T., Lewis, D.W. (1995) 'Neonatal segmental myoclonus associated with hyperglycorrhachia.' *Pediatric Neurology*, **13**, 77–79.

Bauer, J., Stefan, H., Huk, W.J., *et al.* (1989) 'CT, MRI and SPECT neuroimaging in status epilepticus with simple partial and complex partial seizures: case report.' *Journal of Neurology*, **236**, 296–299.

Beaumanoir, A. (1992) 'The Landau–Kleffner syndrome.' *In:* Roger, J., Bureau, M., Dravet, C., *et al.* (Eds.) *Epileptic Syndromes in Infancy, Childhood and Adolescence. 2nd Edn.* London: John Libbey, pp. 231–243.

—— Dravet, C. (1992) 'The Lennox–Gastaut syndrome.' *In:* Roger, J., Bureau, M., Dravet, C., *et al.* (Eds.) *Epileptic Syndromes in Infancy, Childhood and Adolescence. 2nd Edn.* London: John Libbey, pp. 115–132.

—— Foletti, G., Magistris, M., Volanschi, D. (1988) 'Status epilepticus in the Lennox–Gastaut syndrome.' *In:* Niedermeyer, E., Degen, R. (Eds.) *The Lennox–Gastaut Syndrome.* New York: Alan R. Liss, pp. 283–299.

Becker, P.S., Dixon, A.M., Troncoso, S.C. (1989) 'Bilateral opercular microgyria.' *Annals of Neurology*, **25**, 90–92.

Beckung, E., Uvebrant, P. (1997) 'Hidden dysfunction in childhood epilepsy.' *Developmental Medicine and Child Neurology*, **39**, 72–79.

Bellman, M.H., Ross, E.M., Miller, D.L. (1983) 'Infantile spasms and pertussis immunisation.' *Lancet*, **1**, 1031–1034.

Berg, A.T., Shinnar, S., Hauser, W.A., Leventhal, J.M. (1990) 'Predictors of recurrent febrile seizures: a metaanalytic review.' *Journal of Pediatrics*, **116**, 329–337.

—— —— *et al.* (1992) 'A prospective study of recurrent febrile seizures.' *New England Journal of Medicine*, **327**, 1122–1127.

—— Shapiro, E.D., *et al.* (1995) 'Risk factors for a first febrile seizure: a matched case–control study.' *Epilepsia*, **36**, 334–341.

—— Levy, S.R., Novotny, E.J., Shinnar, S. (1996) 'Predictors of intractable epilepsy in childhood: a case–control study.' *Epilepsia*, **37**, 24–30.

Bergin, P.S., Fish, D.R., Shorvon, S.D., *et al.* (1995) 'Magnetic resonance imaging in partial epilepsy: additional abnormalities shown with the fluid attenuated inversion recovery (FLAIR) pulse sequence.' *Journal of Neurology, Neurosurgery, and Psychiatry*, **58**, 439–443.

Berkovic, S.F., Scheffer, I.E. (1997) 'Epilepsies with single gene inheritance.' *Brain and Development*, **19**, 13–18.

—— Andermann, F., Andermann, E., Gloor, P. (1987) 'Concept of absence epilepsies: discrete syndromes or biological continuum?' *Neurology*, **37**, 993–1000.

—— —— Melanson, D., *et al.* (1988) 'Hypothalamic hamartomas and ictal laughter: evolution of a characteristic epileptic syndrome and diagnostic value of magnetic resonance imaging.' *Annals of Neurology*, **23**, 429–439.

—— Kennerson, M.L., Howell, R.A., *et al.* (1994) 'Phenotypic expression of benign familial neonatal convulsions linked to chromosome 20.' *Archives of Neurology*, **51**, 1125–1128.

—— McIntosh, A., Howell, R.A., *et al.* (1996) 'Familial temporal lobe epilepsy: a common disorder identified in twins.' *Annals of Neurology*, **40**, 227–235.

Besag, F.M.C., Wallace, S.J., Dulac, O., *et al.* (1995) 'Lamotrigine for treatment of epilepsy in children.' *Journal of Pediatrics*, **127**, 991–997.

Bethune, P., Gordon, K., Dooley, J., *et al.* (1993) 'Which child will have a febrile seizure?' *American Journal of Diseases of Children*, **147**, 35–39.

Beun, A.M., Beintema, D.J., Binnie, C.D., *et al.* (1984) 'Epileptic nystagmus.' *Epilepsia*, **25**, 609–614.

Bianchi, A., Italian League Against Epilepsy Collaborative Group (1995) 'Study of concordance of symptoms in families with absence epilepsies.' *In:* Duncan, J.S., Panayiotopoulos, C.P. (Eds.) *Typical Absences and Related Epileptic Syndromes.* London: Churchill Communications Europe, pp. 328–337.

Bicknese, A.R., May, W., Hickey, W.F., Dodson, W.E. (1992) 'Early childhood hepatocerebral degeneration misdiagnosed as valproate hepatotoxicity.' *Annals of Neurology*, **32**, 767–775.

Binnie, C.D. (1991) 'Long-term monitoring.' *In:* Dam, M., Gram, L. (Eds.) *Comprehensive Epileptology.* New York: Raven Press, pp. 339–349.

—— Rowan, A.J., Overweg, J., *et al.* (1981) 'Telemetric EEG and video-monitoring in epilepsy.' *Neurology*, **31**, 298–303.

Bird, T.D. (1987) 'Genetic considerations in childhood epilepsy.' *Epilepsia*, **28**, Suppl. 1, S71–S81.

Bishop, D.V.M. (1985) 'Age of onset and outcome in 'acquired aphasia with convulsive disorder' (Landau–Kleffner syndrome).' *Developmental Medicine and Child Neurology*, **27**, 705–712.

Blume, W.T., Kalbara, M. (1995) *Atlas of Adult Electroencephalography.* New York: Raven Press.

—— Borghesi, J., Lemieux, J.F. (1993) 'Interictal indices of temporal seizure origin.' *Annals of Neurology*, **34**, 703–709.

Boniver, C., Dravet, C., Bureau, M., Roger, J. (1987) 'Idiopathic Lennox–Gastaut syndrome.' *In:* Wolf, P., Dam, M., Janz, D., Dreifuss, F. (Eds.) *Advances in Epileptology. XVIth Epilepsy International Symposium.* New York: Raven Press, pp. 195–200.

Boulloche, J., Leloup, P., Mallet, E., *et al.* (1989) 'Risk of recurrence after a single, unprovoked, generalized tonic–clonic seizure.' *Developmental Medicine and Child Neurology*, **31**, 626–632.

—— Husson, A., Le Luyer, B., Le Roux, P. (1990) 'Dysphagie, troubles du langage et pointes-ondes centro-temporales.' *Archives Françaises de Pédiatrie*, **47**, 115–117.

Bouma, P., Peters, A.C.B., Arts, R.J.H.M., *et al.* (1987) 'Discontinuation of antiepileptic therapy: a prospective study in children.' *Journal of Neurology, Neurosurgery, and Psychiatry*, **50**, 1579–1583.

Bourgeois, B. (1992) 'General concepts of medical intractability.' *In:* Lüders, H. (Ed.) *Epilepsy Surgery.* New York: Raven Press, pp. 77–81.

—— Prensky, A.L., Palkes, H.S., *et al.* (1983) 'Intelligence in epilepsy: a prospective study in children.' *Annals of Neurology*, **14**, 438–444.

Brett, E.M. (1997) 'Epilepsy and convulsions.' *In:* Brett, E.M. (Ed.) *Paediatric Neurology, 3rd Edn.* Edinburgh, Churchill Livingstone, pp. 333–395.

Brodie, M.J. (1990) 'Established anticonvulsants and treatment of refractory epilepsy.' *Lancet*, **336**, 350–354.

Brown, J.K., Hussain, I.H.M.I. (1991a) 'Status epilepticus. I: Pathogenesis.' *Developmental Medicine and Child Neurology*, **33**, 3–17.

—— —— (1991b) 'Status epilepticus. II: Treatment.' *Developmental Medicine and Child Neurology*, **33**, 97–109.

Bruton, C.J. (1988) *The Neuropathology of Temporal Lobe Epilepsy. Maudsley Monograph No. 31.* Oxford: Oxford University Press.

Burdette, D.E., Sakurai, S.Y., Henry, T.R., *et al.* (1995) 'Temporal lobe central benzodiazepine binding in unilateral mesial temporal lobe epilepsy.' *Neurology*, **45**, 934–941.

Bureau, M. (1995) 'Continuous spikes and waves during slow sleep (CSWS): definition of the syndrome.' *In:* Beaumanoir, A., Bureau, M., Deonna, T., *et al.* (Eds.) *Continuous Spikes and Waves During Slow Sleep, Electrical Status Epilepticus During Slow Sleep.* London: John Libbey, pp. 17–26.

Burke, C.J., Tannenberg, A.E. (1995) 'Prenatal brain damage and placental infarction—an autopsy study.' *Developmerntal Medicine and Child Neurology*, **37**, 555–562.

Bye, A.M.E., Andermann, F., Robitaille, Y., *et al.* (1993) 'Cortical vascular abnormalities in the syndrome of celiac disease, bilateral occipital calcifications, and folate deficiency.' *Annals of Neurology*, **34**, 399–403.

Bye, A.M.E. (1994) 'Neonate with benign familial neonatal convulsions: recorded generalized and focal seizures.' *Pediatric Neurology*, **10**, 164–165.

—— Flanagan, D. (1995) 'Spatial and temporal characteristics of neonatal seizures.' *Epilepsia*, **36**, 1009–1016.

Camfield, C., Camfield, P., Smith, E., Tibbles, J.A. (1986) 'Asymptomatic children with epilepsy: little benefit from screening for anticonvulsant-induced liver, blood, or renal damage.' *Neurology*, **36**, 838–841.

—— —— Smith, B., *et al.* (1993) 'Outcome of childhood epilepsy: a population-based study with a simple predictive scoring system for those treated with medication.' *Journal of Pediatrics*, **122**, 861–868.

Camfield, P.R., Camfield, C.S. (1987) 'Neonatal seizures: a commentary on selected aspects.' *Journal of Child Neurology*, **2**, 244–251.

—— Dooley, J.M. (1987) 'Multiple brief nontemporal focal seizures in well children: a benign epileptic syndrome with apparent cure in some by very short course of anticonvulsants.' *Annals of Neurology*, **22**, 414A. *(Abstract.)*

—— Camfield, C., Gordon, K., Dooley, J. (1994) 'What types of epilepsy are preceded by febrile seizures? A population-based study of children.' *Developmental Medicine and Child Neurology*, **36**, 887–892.

Caraballo, R., Fontana, E., Michelizza, B., *et al.* (1989) 'Carbamazepina, "assenze atipiche", "crise atoniche", e stato di Po continua del sonno (POCB).' *Bolletino della Lega Italiana Contra l'Epilessia*, **66/67**, 379–381.

Carrazana, E.J., Lombroso, C.T., Mikati, M., *et al.* (1993) 'Facilitation of infantile spasms by partial seizures.' *Epilepsia*, **34**, 97–109.

Cascino, G.D., Kelly, P.J., Sharbrough, F.W., *et al.* (1992) 'Long-term follow-up of stereotactic lesionectomy in partial epilepsy: predictive factors and electroencephalographic results.' *Epilepsia*, **33**, 639–644.

Cascino, G.D. (1993) 'Nonconvulsive status epilepticus in adults and children.' *Epilepsia*, **34**, Suppl. 1, S21–S28.

—— Andermann, F., Berkovic, S.F., *et al.* (1993) 'Gelastic seizures and hypothalamic hamartomas: evaluation of patients undergoing chronic intracranial EEG monitoring and outcome of surgical treatment.' *Neurology*, **43**, 747–750.

Cavazzuti, G.B. (1980) 'Epidemiology of different types of epilepsy in school age children of Modena (Italy).' *Epilepsia*, **21**, 57–63.

—— Ferrari, P., Lalla, M. (1984) 'Follow-up study of 482 cases with convulsive disorders in the first year of life.' *Developmental Medicine and Child Neurology*, **26**, 425–437.

Cendes, F., Andermann, F., Dubeau, F., *et al.* (1993a) 'Early childhood prolonged febrile convulsions, atrophy and sclerosis of mesial structures, and temporal lobe epilepsy: an MRI volumetric study.' *Neurology*, **43**, 1083–1087.

—— —— Gloor, P., *et al.* (1993b) 'Atrophy of mesial structures in patients with temporal lobe epilepsy: cause or consequence of repeated seizures?' *Annals of Neurology*, **34**, 795–801.

—— Ragazzo, P.C., da Costa, V., Martins, L.F. (1993c) 'Corpus callostomy in treatment of medically resistant epilepsy: preliminary results in a pediatric population.' *Epilepsia*, **34**, 910–917.

—— Cook, M.J., Watson, C., *et al.* (1995) 'Frequency and characteristics of dual pathology in patients with lesional epilepsy.' *Neurology*, **45**, 2058–2064.

Chamberlain, M.C. (1996) 'Nitrazepam for refractory infantile spasms and the Lennox–Gastaut syndrome.' *Journal of Child Neurology*, **11**, 31–34.

Chauvel, P., Trottier, S., Vignal, J.P., Bancaud, J. (1992) 'Somatomotor seizures of frontal lobe origin.' *In:* Chauvel, P., Delgado-Escueta, A.V., Halgren, E., Bancaud, J. (Eds.) *Frontal Lobe Seizures and Epilepsies.* New York: Raven Press, pp. 185–232.

Chevrie, J.J., Aicardi, J. (1972) 'Childhood epileptic encephalopathy with slow spike–wave. A statistical study of 80 cases'. *Epilepsia*, **13**, 259–271.

—— —— (1975) 'Duration and lateralization of febrile convulsions. Etiological factors.' *Epilepsia*, **16**, 781–789.

—— —— (1977) 'Convulsive disorders in the first year of life. Etiologic factors.' *Epilepsia*, **18**, 489–498.

—— —— (1978) 'Convulsive disorders in the first year of life. Neurologic and mental outcome and mortality.' *Epilepsia*, **19**, 67–74.

—— —— (1979) 'Convulsive disorders in the first year of life. Persistence of epileptic seizures.' *Epilepsia*, **20**, 643–649.

—— —— Goutières, F. (1987) 'Epilepsy in childhood mitochondrial encephalomyopathies.' *In:* Wolf, P., Dam, M., Janz, D., Dreifuss, F. (Eds.) *Advances in Epileptology. XVIth Epilepsy International Symposium.* New York: Raven Press, pp. 181–184.

Chinchilla, D., Dulac, O., Robain, O., *et al.* (1994) 'Reappraisal of Rasmussen's syndrome with special emphasis on treatment with high doses of steroids.' *Journal of Neurology, Neurosurgery, and Psychiatry*, **57**, 1325–1333.

Chiron, C., Dulac, O., Luna, D., *et al.* (1990) 'Vigabatrin in infantile spasms.' *Lancet*, **335**, 363–364. *(Letter.)*

—— —— Beaumont, D., *et al.* (1991) 'Therapeutic trial of vigabatrin in refractory infantile spasms.' *Journal of Child Neurology*, **6**, Suppl. 2, S52–S59.

625

Chugani, H.T., Conti, J.R. (1996) 'Etiologic classification of infantile spasms in 140 cases: role of positron emission tomography.' *Journal of Child Neurology*, **11**, 44–48.

—— Pinard, J.M. (1994) 'Surgical treatment.' *In:* Dulac, O., Chugani, H.T., Dalla Bernardina, B. (Eds.) *Infantile Spasms and West Syndrome*. Philadelphia: W.B. Saunders, pp. 257–264.

—— Mazziota, J.C., Engel, J., Phelps, M.E. (1987) 'The Lennox–Gastaut syndrome: metabolic subtypes determined by 2-deoxy-2 ^{18}F fluoro-D-glucose positron emission tomography.' *Annals of Neurology*, **21**, 4–13.

—— Shields, W.D., Shewmon, D.A., *et al.* (1990) 'Infantile spasms: I. PET identifies focal cortical dysgenesis in cryptogenic cases for surgical treatment.' *Annals of Neurology*, **27**, 406–413.

—— Da Silva, E., Chugani, D.C. (1996) 'Infantile spasms: III. Prognostic implications of bitemporal hypometabolism on positron emission tomography.' *Annals of Neurology*, **39**, 643–649.

Claes, S., Devriendt, K., Lagae, L., *et al.* (1997) 'The X-linked infantile spasms syndrome (MIM 308350) maps to Xp11.4–Xpter in two pedigrees.' *Annals of Neurology*, **42**, 360–364.

Clancy, R.R., Legido, A. (1987a) 'The exact ictal and interictal duration of electroencephalographic neonatal seizures.' *Epilepsia*, **28**, 537–541.

—— —— (1987b) 'Neurologic outcome after EEG-proven neonatal seizures.' *Pediatric Research*, **21**, 489A. *(Abstract.)*

—— —— Lewis, D. (1988) 'Occult neonatal seizures.' *Epilepsia*, **29**, 256–261.

Cockerell, O.C., Rothwell, J., Thompson, P.D., *et al.* (1996) 'Clinical and physiological features of epilepsia partialis continua. Cases ascertained in the UK.' *Brain*, **119**, 393–407.

—— Johnson, A.L., Sander, J.W.A.S., Shorvon, S.D. (1997) 'Prognosis of epilepsy: a review and further analysis of the first nine years of the British National General Practice Study of Epilepsy, a prospective population-based study.' *Epilepsia*, **38**, 31–46.

Collings, J.A. (1990) 'Psychosocial well-being and epilepsy: an empirical study.' *Epilepsia*, **31**, 418–426.

Commission on Classification and Terminology of the International League against Epilepsy (1981) 'Proposal for revised clinical and electroencephalographic classification of epileptic seizures.' *Epilepsia*, **22**, 489–501.

—— (1989) 'Proposal for revised classification of epilepsies and epileptic syndromes.' *Epilepsia*, **30**, 389–399.

Connelly, A., Jackson, G.D., Duncan, J.S., *et al.* (1994) 'Magnetic resonance spectroscopy in temporal lobe epilepsy.' *Neurology*, **44**, 1411–1417.

Consensus Development Panel (1980) 'Febrile seizures: long-term management of children with fever-associated seizures.' *Pediatrics*, **66**, 1009–1012.

Cornblath, M., Schwartz, R. (1991) *Disorders of Carbohydrate Metabolism in Infancy, 3rd Edn.* Oxford: Blackwell, pp. 225–246.

Cornford, M.E., McCormick, G.F. (1997) 'Adult-onset temporal lobe epilepsy associated with smoldering herpes simplex 2 infection.' *Neurology*, **48**, 425–430.

Coppola, G., Plouin, P., Chiron, C., *et al.* (1995) 'Migrating partial seizures in infancy: a malignant disorder with developmental arrest.' *Epilepsia*, **36**, 1017–1024.

Corsellis, J.A.N., Bruton, C.J. (1983) 'Neuropathology of status epilepticus in humans.' *In:* Delgado-Escueta, A.V., Wasterlain, C., Treiman, D.M., Porter, R.J. (Eds.) *Advances in Neurology. Vol. 34. Status Epilepticus.* New York: Raven Press, pp. 129–139.

Coulter, D.L. (1991) 'Carnitine, valproate and toxicity.' *Journal of Child Neurology*, **6**, 7–14.

Covanis, A., Jeavons, P.M. (1980) 'Once-daily sodium valproate in the treatment of epilepsy.' *Developmental Medicine and Child Neurology*, **22**, 202–204.

Cowan, L.D., Hudson, L.S. (1991) 'The epidemiology and natural history of infantile spasms.' *Journal of Child Neurology*, **6**, 355–364.

Crawford, P., Chadwick, D. (1986) 'A comparative study of progabide, valproate, and placebo as add-on therapy in patients with refractory epilepsy.' *Journal of Neurology, Neurosurgery, and Psychiatry*, **49**, 1251–1257.

Crawford, T.O., Mitchell, W.G., Fishman, L.S., Snodgrass, S.R. (1988) 'Very high-dose phenobarbital for refractory status epilepticus in children.' *Neurology*, **38**, 1035–1040.

Cross, J.H., Jackson, G.D., Neville, B.G.R., *et al.* (1993) 'Early detection of abnormalities in partial epilepsy using magnetic resonance.' *Archives of Disease in Childhood*, **69**, 104–109.

—— Gordon, I., Jackson, G.D., *et al.* (1995) 'Children with intractable focal epilepsy: ictal and interictal [99]Tc[m] HMPAO single photon emission computed tomography.' *Developmental Medicine and Child Neurology*, **37**, 673–681.

—— Connelly, A., Jackson, G.D., *et al.* (1996) 'Proton magnetic resonance spectroscopy in children with temporal lobe epilepsy.' *Annals of Neurology*, **39**, 107–113.

—— Gordon, I., Connelly, A., *et al.* (1997) 'Interictal HMPAO SPECT and H[1] MRS in children with temporal lobe epilepsy.' *Epilepsia*, **38**, 338–345.

Cusmai, R., Dulac, O., Diebler, C. (1988) 'Lésions focales dans les spasmes infantiles'. *Neurophysiologie Clinique*, **18**, 235–241.

Dalla Bernardina, B., Tassinari, C.A. (1975) 'EEG of a nocturnal seizure in a patient with benign epilepsy of childhood with rolandic spikes.' *Epilepsia*, **16**, 497–501.

—— Watanabe, K. (1994) 'Interictal EEG: variations and pitfalls.' *In:* Dulac, O., Chugani, H.T., Dalla Bernardina, B. (Eds). *Infantile Spasms and West Syndrome*. Philadelphia: W.B. Saunders, pp. 63–81.

—— Bureau, M., Dravet, C., *et al.* (1980) 'Epilepsie bénigne de l'enfant avec crises à sémiologie affective.' *Revue d'Electroencéphalographie et de Neurophysiologie Clinique*, **10**, 8–18.

—— Fontana, E., Sgrò, V., *et al.* (1992) 'Myoclonic epilepsy ('myoclonic status') in non-progressive encephalopathies.' *In:* Roger, J., Bureau, M., Dravet, C., *et al.* (Eds.) *Epileptic Syndromes in Infancy, Childhood and Adolescence. 2nd Edn.* London: John Libbey, pp. 89–96.

—— Cappellaro, O., *et al.* (1993) 'The partial occipital epilepsies in childhood.' *In:* Andermann, F., Beaumanoir, H., Mira, L., *et al.* (Eds.) *Occipital Seizures and Epilepsies in Children.* London: John Libbey, pp. 173–181

Daly, D.D., Pedley, T.A. (1990) *Current Practice of Clinical Electro-encephalography, 2nd Edn.* New York: Raven Press.

Davis, A.G., Mutchie, K.D., Thompson, J.A., Myers, G.G. (1981) 'Once-daily dosing with phenobarbital in children with seizure disorders.' *Pediatrics*, **68**, 824–826.

Del Brutto, O.H., Santibañez, R., Noboa, C.A., *et al.* (1992) 'Epilepsy due to neurocysticercosis: analysis of 203 patients.' *Neurology*, **42**, 389–392.

Delgado-Escueta, A.V., Enrile-Bacsal, F. (1984) 'Juvenile myoclonic epilepsy of Janz.' *Neurology*, **34**, 285–294.

—— Greenberg, D.A., Treiman, L., *et al.* (1989) 'Mapping the gene for juvenile myoclonic epilepsy.' *Epilepsia*, **30**, Suppl. 4, S8–S18.

—— Liu, A., Serratosa, J., *et al.* (1994) 'Juvenile myoclonic epilepsy: is there heterogeneity?' *In:* Malafosse, A., Genton, P., Hirsch, E., *et al.* (Eds.) *Idiopathic Generalized Epilepsies.* London: John Libbey, pp. 281–286.

Del Giudice, E., Aicardi, J. (1979) 'Hypertensive encephalopathy in children.' *Neuropädiatrie*, **10**, 150–157.

DeLorenzo, R.J., Towne, A.R., Pellock, J.M., Ko, D. (1992) 'Status epilepticus in children, adults, and the elderly.' *Epilepsia*, **33**, Suppl. 4, S15–S25.

DeMarco, P., Lorenzin, G. (1990) 'Growing bilateral occipital calcifications and epilepsy.' *Brain and Development*, **12**, 342–344.

De Negri, M., Baglietto, M.G., Biancheri, R. (1993) 'Electrical status epilepticus in childhood: treatment with short cycles of high-dosage benzodiazepine (preliminary note).' *Brain and Development*, **15**, 311–312.

Deonna, T., Beaumanoir, A., Gaillard, F., Assal, G. (1977) 'Acquired aphasia in childhood with seizure disorder: a heterogeneous syndrome.' *Neuropädiatrie*, **8**, 263–273.

—— Ziegler, A-L., Despland, P.A. (1986a) 'Combined myoclonic–astatic and "benign" focal epilepsy of childhood ("atypical benign partial epilepsy of childhood"). A separate syndrome?' *Neuropediatrics*, **17**, 144–151.

—— —— —— Van Melle, G. (1986b) 'Partial epilepsy in neurologically normal children: clinical syndromes and prognosis.' *Epilepsia*, **27**, 241–247.

—— Peter, C., Ziegler, A-L. (1989) 'Adult follow-up of the acquired aphasia–epilepsy syndrome in childhood. Report of 7 cases.' *Neuropediatrics*, **20**, 132–138.

—— Roulet, E., Fontan, D., Marcoz, J-P. (1993) 'Speech and oromotor deficits of epileptic origin in benign partial epilepsy of childhood with rolandic spikes (BPERS). Relationship to the acquired aphasia–epilepsy syndrome.' *Neuropediatrics*, **24**, 83–87.

—— Davidoff, V., Maeder-Ingvar, M., *et al.* (1997) 'The spectrum of acquired cognitive disturbances in children with partial epilepsy and continuous spike–waves during sleep. A 4-year follow-up case study with prolonged reversible learning arrest and dysfluency.' *European Journal of Paediatric Neurology*, **1**, 19–29.

Deshmukh, A., Wittert, W., Schnitzler, E., Mangurten, H.H. (1986) 'Lorazepam in the treatment of refractory neonatal seizures: a pilot study.' *American Journal of Diseases of Children*, **140**, 1042–1044.

De Silva, M., McArdle, B., McGowan, M., Hughes, E. (1996) 'Randomized comparative monotherapy trial of phenobarbitone, phenytoin, carbamazepine and sodium valproate for newly diagnosed childhood epilepsy.' *Lancet*, **347**, 709–713.

Detre, J.A., Sirven, J.I., Alsop, D.C., *et al.* (1995) 'Localization of subclinical ictal activity by functional magnetic resonance imaging: correlation with invasive monitoring.' *Annals of Neurology*, **38**, 618–624.

Devinsky, O., Kelley, K., Porter, R.J., Theodore, W.H. (1988) 'Clinical and electro-encephalographic features of simple partial seizures.' *Neurology*, **38**, 1347–1352.

—— Perrine, K., Vazquez, B., *et al.* (1994) 'Multiple subpial transections in the language cortex.' *Brain*, **117**, 255–265.

De Vivo, D.C., Trifiletti, R.R., Jacobson, R.I., *et al.* (1991) 'Defective glucose transport across the blood–brain barrier as a cause of persistent hypoglycorrhachia, seizures and developmental delay.' *New England Journal of Medicine*, **325**, 703–709.

Dichter, M.A., Brodie, M.J. (1996) 'New antiepileptic drugs.' *New England Journal of Medicine*, **334**, 1583–1590.

Dieckmann, R.A. (1994) 'Rectal diazepam for prehospital pediatric status epilepticus.' *Annals of Emergency Medicine*, **23**, 216–224.

Dieterich, E., Doose, H., Baier, W.K., Fichsel, H. (1985) 'Long-term follow-up of childhood epilepsy with absences. II: Absence epilepsy with initial grand mal.' *Neuropediatrics*, **16**, 155–158.

Di Mario, F.J., Clancy, R.R. (1988) 'Paradoxical precipitation of tonic seizures by lorazepam in a child with atypical absence seizures.' *Pediatric Neurology*, **4**, 249–251.

Doberczak, T.M., Shanzer, S., Cutler, R., *et al.* (1988) 'One-year follow-up of infants with abstinence associated seizures.' *Archives of Neurology*, **45**, 649–653.

Dodson, W.E., Pellock, J.M. (Eds.) (1993) *Pediatric Epilepsy: Diagnosis and Therapy*. New York: Demos.

Donat, J.F. (1992) 'The age-dependent epileptic encephalopathies.' *Journal of Child Neurology*, **7**, 7–21.

—— Wright, F.S. (1991a) 'Seizures in series: similarities between seizures of the West and Lennox–Gastaut syndromes.' *Epilepsia*, **32**, 504–509.

—— —— (1991b) 'Simultaneous infantile spasms and partial seizures.' *Journal of Child Neurology*, **6**, 246–250.

—— —— (1991c) 'Unusual variants of infantile spasms.' *Journal of Child Neurology*, **6**, 313–318.

Donati, F., Schäffler, L., Vassella, F. (1995) 'Prolonged epileptic apneas in a newborn: a case report with ictal EEG recording.' *Neuropediatrics*, **26**, 223–225.

Dooley, J., Gordon, K., Camfield, P., *et al.* (1996) 'Discontinuation of anticonvulsant therapy in children free of seizures for 1 year: a prospective study.' *Neurology*, **46**, 969–974.

Doose, H. (1985) 'Myoclonic astatic epilepsy.' *In:* Roger, J., Dravet, C., Bureau, M., *et al.* (Eds.) *Epileptic Syndromes in Infancy, Childhood and Adolescence*. London: John Libbey, pp. 78–88.

—— (1992) 'Myoclonic astatic epilepsy of early childhood.' *In:* Roger, J., Bureau, M., Dravet, C., *et al.* (Eds.) *Epileptic Syndromes in Infancy, Childhood and Adolescence. 2nd Edn.* London: John Libbey, pp. 103–114.

—— Baier, W.K. (1987) 'Genetic factors in epilepsies with primary generalised minor seizures.' *Neuropediatrics*, **18**, Suppl. 1, 1–64.

—— —— (1989) 'Benign partial epilepsy and related conditions: multifactorial pathogenesis with hereditary impairment of brain maturation.' *European Journal of Pediatrics*, **149**, 152–158.

—— —— (1991) 'A genetically determined basic mechanism in benign partial epilepsies and related non-convulsive conditions.' *Epilepsy Research*, **4** (Suppl.), 113–118.

—— Waltz, S. (1993) 'Photosensitivity—genetics and clinical significance.' *Neuropediatrics*, **24**, 249–255.

—— Neubauer, B., Carlsson, G. (1996) 'Children with benign focal sharp waves in the EEG. Developmental disorders and epilepsy.' *Neuropediatrics*, **27**, 227–241.

Dravet, C. (1994) 'Benign epilepsy with centrotemporal spikes: do we know all about it?' *In:* Wolf, P. (Ed.) *Epileptic Seizures and Syndromes*. London: John Libbey, pp. 231–240.

—— Natale, O., Magaudda, A., *et al.* (1985) 'Les états de mal dans le syndrome de Lennox–Gastaut.' *Revue d'Electroencéphalographie et de Neurophysiologie Clinique*, **15**, 361–368.

—— Giraud, N., Bureau, M., *et al.* (1986) 'Benign myoclonus of early infancy or benign non-epileptic infantile spasms.' *Neuropediatrics*, **17**, 33–38.

—— Catani, C., Bureau, M., Roger, J. (1989) 'Partial epilepsies in infancy: a study of 40 cases.' *Epilepsia*, **30**, 807–812.

—— Bureau, M., Roger, J. (1992a) 'Benign myoclonic epilepsy in infants.' *In:* Roger, J., Bureau, M., Dravet, C., *et al.* (Eds.) *Epileptic Syndromes in Infancy, Childhood and Adolescence. 2nd Edn.* London: John Libbey, pp. 67–74.

—— Bureau, M., Guerrini, R. (1992b) 'Severe myoclonic epilepsy in infants.' *In:* Roger, J., Bureau, M., Dravet, C., *et al.* (Eds.) *Epileptic Syndromes in Infancy, Childhood and Adolescence. 2nd Edn.* London: John Libbey, pp. 75–88.

Dreifuss, F., Farwell, J., Holmes, G., *et al.* (1986) 'Infantile spasms: comparative trial of nitrazepam and corticotropin.' *Archives of Neurology*, **43**, 1107–1110.

Dreyfus-Brisac, C., Curzi-Dascalova, L. (1979) 'The EEG during the first year of life.' *In:* Rémond, A. (Ed.) *Handbook of Electroencephalography and Clinical Neurophysiology*. Amsterdam: Elsevier, pp. 24–30.

Duchowny, M.S. (1987) 'Complex partial seizures of infancy.' *Archives of Neurology*, **44**, 911–914.

—— (1992) 'The syndrome of partial seizures in infancy.' *Journal of Child Neurology*, **7**, 66–69.

—— Harvey, A.S. (1996) 'Pediatric epilepsy syndromes: an update and critical review.' *Epilepsia*, **37**, Suppl. 1, S26–S40.

—— Levin, B., Jayakar, P., *et al.* (1992) 'Temporal lobectomy in early childhood.' *Epilepsia*, **33**, 298–303.

—— Jayakar, P., Resnik, T., *et al.* (1994) 'Posterior temporal epilepsy: electro-clinical features.' *Annals of Neurology*, **35**, 427–431.

Dulac, O. (1995) 'Epileptic syndromes in infancy and childhood: recent advances.' *Epilepsia*, **36**, Suppl. 1, S51–S57.

—— N'Guyen, T. (1993) 'The Lennox–Gastaut syndrome.' Epilepsia, **34**, Suppl. 7, S7–S17.

—— Billard, C., Arthuis, M. (1983) 'Aspects électro-cliniques et évolutifs de l'épilepsie dans le syndrome aphasie–épilepsie.' *Archives Françaises de Pédiatrie*, **40**, 299–308.

—— Plouin, P., Jambaqué, I., Motte, J. (1986) 'Spasmes infantiles épileptiques bénins.' *Revue d'Electroencéphalographie et de Neurophysiologie Clinique*, **16**, 371–382.

—— Cusmai, R., de Oliveira, K. (1989) 'Is there a partial benign epilepsy in infancy?' *Epilepsia*, **30**, 798–801.

—— Plouin, P., Chiron, C. (1990) 'Forme "bénigne" d'épilepsie myoclonique chez l'enfant.' *Neurophysiologie Clinique*, **20**, 115–129.

Duncan, J.S. (1997) 'Imaging and epilepsy.' *Brain*, **120**, 339–377.

Dunn, D.W. (1988) 'Status epilepticus in children: etiology, clinical features and outcome.' *Journal of Child Neurology*, **3**, 167–173.

Du Plessis, A.J., Kaufmann, W.E., Kupsky, W.J. (1993) 'Intrauterine-onset myoclonic encephalopathy associated with cerebral cortical dysgenesis.' *Journal of Child Neurology*, **8**, 164–170.

—— Kramer, J., Jonas, R.A., *et al.* (1994) 'West syndrome following deep hypothermic infant cardiac surgery.' *Pediatric Neurology*, **11**, 246–251.

Durner, M. (1994) 'Genetics of juvenile myoclonic epilepsy.' *In:* Wolf, P. (Ed.) *Epileptic Seizures and Syndromes*. London: John Libbey, pp. 169–179.

Eadie, M.J., Tyrer, J.H. (1989) *Anticonvulsant Therapy: Pharmacological Basis and Practice. 3rd Edn.* Edinburgh: Churchill Livingstone.

Ebersole, J.S., Bridgers, S.L. (1986) 'Ambulatory EEG monitoring.' *In:* Pedley, T.A., Meldrum, B.S. (Eds.) *Recent Advances in Epilepsy, Vol. 3*. Edinburgh: Churchill Livingstone, pp. 111–135.

Ebner, A., Dinner, D.S., Noachtar, S., Lüders, H. (1995) 'Automatisms with preserved responsiveness: a lateralizing sign in psychomotor seizures.' *Neurology*, **45**, 61–64.

Echenne, B., Dulac, O., Parayre-Chanez, M.J., *et al.* (1991) 'Treatment of infantile spasms with intravenous gamma-globulins.' *Brain and Development*, **13**, 313–319.

—— Humbertclaude, V., Rivier, F., *et al.* (1994) 'Benign infantile epilepsy with autosomal dominant inheritance.' *Brain and Development*, **16**, 108–111.

Egli, M., Mothersill, I., O'Kane, M., O'Kane, F. (1985) 'The axial spasm—the predominant type of drop seizure in patients with secondary generalised epilepsy.' *Epilepsia*, **26**, 401–415.

Ehrhardt, P., Forsythe, W.I. (1989) 'Prognosis after grand mal seizures: a study of 187 children with three-year remissions.' *Developmental Medicine and Child Neurology*, **31**, 633–639.

Eiris, J.M., Lojo, S., Del Río, M.C., *et al.* (1995) 'Effects of long-term treatment with antiepileptic drugs on serum lipid levels in children with epilepsy.' *Neurology*, **45**, 1155–1157.

Engel, J. (1993) *Surgical Treatment of the Epilepsies, 2nd Edn.* New York: Raven Press.

—— (1996) 'Surgery for seizures.' *New England Journal of Medicine*, **334**, 647–652.

Erba, G., Browne, T.R. (1983) 'Atypical absence, myoclonic, atonic and tonic seizures and the "Lennox–Gastaut syndrome".' *In:* Browne, T.R., Feldman, R.G. (Eds.) *Epilepsy: Diagnosis and Management.* Boston: Little Brown, pp. 75–94.

Farwell, J.R., Lee, Y.J., Hirtz, D.G., *et al.* (1990) 'Phenobarbital for febrile seizures: effects on intelligence and on seizure recurrence.' *New England Journal of Medicine*, **322**, 364–369.

Fejerman, N., Di Blasi, A.M. (1987) 'Status epilepticus of benign partial epilepsies in children: report of two cases.' *Epilepsia*, **28**, 351–358.

Feldman, R.G., Ricks, N.L., Orren, M.M. (1983) 'Behavioral methods of seizure control.' *In:* Browne, T.R., Feldman, K.G. (Eds.) *Epilepsy: Diagnosis and Management.* Boston: Little Brown, pp. 269–279.

Ferrie, C.D., De Marco, P., Grünewald, R.A., *et al.* (1994) 'Video game induced seizures.' *Journal of Neurology, Neurosurgery, and Psychiatry*, **57**, 925–931.

—— Giannakodimos, S., Robinson, R.O., Panayiotopoulos, C.P. (1995) 'Symptomatic typical absence seizures.' *In:* Duncan, J.C., Panayiotopoulos, C.P. (Eds.) *Typical Absences and Related Epileptic Syndromes.* London: Churchill Communications Europe, pp. 241–252.

—— Beaumanoir, A., Guerrini, R., *et al.* (1997) 'Early-onset benign occipital seizure susceptibility syndrome.' *Epilepsia*, **38**, 285–293.

Fiol, M.E., Leppik, I.E., Pretzel, K. (1986) 'Eating epilepsy: EEG and clinical study.' *Epilepsia*, **27**, 441–445.

First Seizure Trial Group (1993) 'Randomized clinical trial on the efficacy of antiepileptic drugs in reducing the risk of relapse after a first unprovoked tonic–clonic seizure.' *Neurology*, **43**, 478–483.

Fisher, R.J., Magistretti, P.J. (Eds.) (1991) 'The role of excitatory aminoacid toxicity in epilepsy.' *Epilepsy Research*, **10**, Suppl. 1, 1–89.

Forsgren, L., Edvinsson, S.O., Blomquist, H.K., *et al.* (1990) 'Epilepsy in a population of mentally retarded children and adults.' *Epilepsy Research*, **6**, 234–248.

Forsythe, W.I., Sills, M.A. (1984) 'One drug for childhood grand mal: medical audit for three-year remissions.' *Developmental Medicine and Child Neurology*, **26**, 742–748.

Fowler, W.E., Kriel, R.L., Krach, L.E. (1992) 'Movement disorders after status epilepticus and other brain injuries.' *Pediatric Neurology*, **8**, 281–284.

Freeman, J.M., Kelly, M.T., Freeman, J. (1994) *The Epilepsy Diet Treatment: an Introduction to the Ketogenic Diet.* New York: Demos Vermande.

French, J.A., Williamson, P.D., Thadani, V.M., *et al.* (1993) 'Characteristics of medial temporal lobe epilepsy. 1. Results of history and physical examination.' *Annals of Neurology*, **34**, 774–780.

Fujii, T., Okuno, T., Go, T., *et al.* (1987) 'Clorazepate therapy for intractable epilepsy.' *Brain and Development*, **9**, 288–291.

Furune, S., Watanabe, K., Negoro, T., *et al.* (1988) 'Long-term prognosis and clinico-electroencephalographic evolution of Lennox–Gastaut syndrome.' *Brain Dysfunction*, **1**, 146–153.

Fusco, L., Iani, C., Faedda, M.T., *et al.* (1990) 'Mesial frontal lobe epilepsy: a clinical entity not sufficiently described.' *Journal of Epilepsy*, **3**, 123–135.

—— Bertini, E., Vigevano, F. (1992) 'Epilepsia partialis continua and neuronal migration anomalies.' *Brain and Development*, **14**, 323–328.

Gabor, A.J. (1974) 'Focal seizures induced by movement without sensory feedback mechanisms.' *Electroencephalography and Clinical Neurophysiology*, **36**, 403–408.

Gaggero, R., Caputo, M., Fiorio, P., *et al.* (1995) 'SPECT and epilepsy with continuous spike waves during slow-wave sleep.' *Child's Nervous System*, **11**, 154–160.

Gaily, E.K., Shewmon, D.A., Chugani, H.T., Curran, J.G. (1995) 'Asymmetric and asynchronous infantile spasms.' *Epilepsia*, **36**, 873–882.

Gallassi, R., Morreale, A., Lorusso, S., *et al.* (1988) 'Epilepsy presenting as memory disturbances.' *Epilepsia*, **29**, 624–629.

Garg, B.P., Patel, H., Markand, O.N. (1995) 'Clinical correlation of periodic lateralized epileptiform discharges in children.' *Pediatric Neurology*, **12**, 225–229.

Gascon, G., Yaqub, B., Waheed, G. (1992) 'Benign myoclonic epilepsy of early childhood.' *Pediatric Neurology*, **8**, 348A. *(Abstract.)*

Gastaut, H. (1973) *Dictionary of Epilepsies. Part I. Definitions.* Geneva: World Health Organization.

—— (1982) 'A new type of epilepsy: benign partial epilepsy of childhood with occipital spike–waves.' *Clinical Electroencephalography*, **13**, 12–22.

—— Zifkin, B.G. (1988) 'Secondary bilateral synchrony and Lennox–Gastaut syndrome.' *In:* Niedermeyer, E., Degen, R. (Eds.) *The Lennox–Gastaut Syndrome.* New York: Alan R. Liss, pp. 221–242.

—— Poirier, F., Payan, H., *et al.* (1960) 'HHE syndrome: hemiconvulsions–hemiplegia–epilepsy.' *Epilepsia*, **1**, 418–447.

—— Gastaut, J.A., Gastaut, L., *et al.* (1973) 'Epilepsie généralisée primaire grand mal.' *In:* Lugaresi, E., Pazzaglia, P., Tassinari, C.A. (Eds.) *Evolution and Prognosis of Epilepsies.* Bologna: Aulo Gaggi, pp. 133–154.

—— Santanelli, P.K., Salinas Jara, M. (1985) 'Une activité EEG intercritique spécifique d'une variété particulière d'épilepsie temporale. Le rythme théta temporal épileptique.' *Revue d'Electroencéphalographie et de Neurophysiologie Clinique*, **15**, 113–120.

—— Aguglia, U., Tinuper, P. (1986) 'Benign versive or circling epilepsy with bilateral 3-cps spike-and-wave discharges in late childhood.' *Annals of Neurology*, **19**, 301–303.

Genton, P., Salas Puig, X., Tunon, A., *et al.* (1994) 'Juvenile myoclonic epilepsy and related syndromes: clinical and neurophysiological aspects.' *In:* Malafosse, A., Genton, P., Hirsch, E., *et al.* (Eds.) *Idiopathic Generalized Epilepsies.* London: John Libbey, pp. 253–265.

Gilchrist, J.M. (1985) 'Arrhythmogenic seizures: diagnosis by simultaneous EEG/ECG recording.' *Neurology*, **35**, 1503–1506.

Gilliam, F., Wyllie, E., Kashden, J., *et al.* (1997) 'Epilepsy surgery outcome: Comprehensive assessment in children.' *Neurology*, **48**, 1368–1374.

Gilman, J.T., Duchowny, M., Jayakar, P., Resnick, T.J. (1994) 'Medical intractability in children evaluated for epilepsy surgery.' *Neurology*, **44**, 1341–1343.

Glaze, D.G., Hrachovy, R.A., Frost, J.D., *et al.* (1986) 'Computed tomography in infantile spasms: effects of hormonal therapy.' *Pediatric Neurology*, **2**, 23–27.

—— —— —— *et al.* (1988) 'Prospective study of outcome of infants with infantile spasms treated during controlled studies of ACTH and prednisone.' *Journal of Pediatrics*, **112**, 389–396.

Gloor, P. (1986) 'Consciousness as a neurological concept in epileptology: a critical review.' *Epilepsia*, **27**, Suppl. 2, S14–S26.

—— Fariello, R.G. (1988) 'Generalized epilepsy: some of its cellular mechanisms differ from those of focal epilepsy.' *Trends in Neurosciences*, **11**, 63–68.

Gobbi, G., Guerrini, R. (1998) 'Childhood epilepsy with occipital spikes and other benign localization-related epilepsies.' *In:* Engel, J., Pedley, T.A. (Eds.) *Epilepsy: A Comprehensive Textbook. Vol. 3.* New York: Lippincott–Raven, pp. 2315–2326.

—— Bruno, L., Pini, A., *et al.* (1987) 'Periodic spasms: an unclassified type of epileptic seizure in childhood.' *Developmental Medicine and Child Neurology*, **29**, 766–775.

—— Sorrenti, G., Santucci, M., *et al.* (1988) 'Epilepsy with bilateral occipital calcifications: a benign onset with progressive severity.' *Neurology*, **38**, 913–920.

—— Tassinari, T.A., Roger, J., *et al.* (1989) 'Particularités électrencéphalographiques des épilepsies partielles symptomatiques sévères de l'enfant.' *Neurophysiologie Clinique*, **19**, 209–218.

—— Ambrosetto, P., Zaniboni, M.G., *et al.* (1992) 'Celiac disease, posterior cerebral calcifications and epilepsy.' *Brain and Development*, **14**, 23–29.

Goodridge, D.M.G., Shorvon, S.D. (1983) 'Epileptic seizures in a population of 6000.' *British Medical Journal*, **287**, 641–647.

Gorman, D.G., Shields, W.D., Shewmon, D.A., *et al.* (1992) 'Neurosurgical treatment of refractory status epilepticus.' *Epilepsia*, **33**, 546–549.

Goulatia, R.K., Verma, A., Mishra, N.K., Ahuja, G.K. (1987) 'Disappearing CT lesions in epilepsy.' *Epilepsia*, **28**, 523–527.

Graf, W.D., Chatrian, G-E., Glass, S.T., Knauss, T.A. (1994) 'Video game-related seizures: a report on 10 patients and a review of the literature.' *Pediatrics*, **93**, 551–556.

Green, S.M., Rothrock, S.G., Clem, K.S., *et al.* (1993) 'Can seizures be the sole manifestation of meningitis in febrile children?' *Pediatrics*, **92**, 527–534.

Greenberg, D.A., Delgado-Escueta, A.V. (1993) 'The chromosome 6p epilepsy locus: exploring mode of inheritance and heterogeneneity through linkage analysis.' *Epilepsia*, **34**, Suppl. 3, S12–S18.

—— Maldonado, H.M., Widelitz, H. (1988) 'Segregation analysis of juvenile myoclonic epilepsy.' *Genetic Epidemiology*, **5**, 81–94.

—— Durner, M., Resor, S., *et al.* (1995) 'The genetics of idiopathic generalized epilepsies of adolescent onset: differences between juvenile myoclonic epilepsy and epilepsy with random grand mal and with awakening grand mal.' *Neurology*, **45**, 942–946.

Greene, S.A., Jefferson, I.G., Baum, J.D. (1990) 'Cerebral oedema complicating diabetic ketoacidosis.' *Developmental Medicine and Child Neurology*, **32**, 633–638.

Gross-Selbeck, G. (1995) 'Treatment of "benign" partial epilepsies of childhood, including atypical forms.' *Neuropediatrics*, **26**, 45–50.

Gross-Tsur, V., Shinnar, S. (1993) 'Convulsive status epilepticus in children.' *Epilepsia*, **34**, Suppl. 1, S12–S20.

Guerrini, R., Dravet, C., Raybaud, C., *et al.* (1992) 'Epilepsy and focal gyral anomalies detected by MRI: electricoclinico-morphological correlations and follow-up.' *Developmental Medicine and Child Neurology*, **34**, 706–718.

—— Genton, P., *et al.* (1993) 'Epileptic negative myoclonus.' *Neurology*, **43**, 1078–1083.

—— —— Gobbi, G., *et al.* (1994a) 'Idiopathic generalized epilepsies with myoclonus in infancy and childhood.' *In:* Malafosse, A., Genton, P., Hirsch, F., *et al.* (Eds.) *Idiopathic Generalized Epilepsies: Clinical, Experimental and Genetic Aspects.* London: John Libbey, pp. 267–280.

—— Ferrari, A.R., Battaglia, A., *et al.* (1994b) 'Occipitotemporal seizures with ictus emeticus induced by intermittent photic stimulation.' *Neurology*, **44**, 253–259.

—— Dravet, C., Genton, P., *et al.* (1995) 'Idiopathic photosensitive occipital lobe epilepsy.' *Epilepsia*, **36**, 883–891.

—— Bureau, M., *et al.* (1996a) 'Diffuse and localized dysplasias of cerebral cortex: clinical presentation, outcome, and proposal for morphologic MRI classification based on a study of 90 patients.' *In:* Guerrini, R., Andermann, F., Canapicchi, R., *et al.* (Eds.) *Dysplasias of Cerebral Cortex and Epilepsy.* New York: Lippincott–Raven, pp. 255–270.

—— Parmeggiani, A., Bureau, M., *et al.* (1996b) 'Localized cortical dysplasia: good seizure outcome after sleep-related electrical status epilepticus.' *In:* Guerrini, R., Andermann, F., Canapicchi, R., *et al.* (Eds.) *Dysplasias of the Cerebral Cortex and Epilepsy.* New York: Lippincott–Raven, pp. 329–335.

—— Bonanni, P., Parmeggiani, L., *et al.* (1997) 'A novel autosomal recessive syndrome with rolandic epilepsy, paroxysmal kinesigenic dystonia (writer's cramp) and ataxia.' *Neurology*, **48**, Suppl. 3, 242. *(Abstract.)*

—— Gobbi, G., Genton, P., *et al.* (1998) 'Chromosomal abnormalities.' *In:* Engel, J., Pedley, T. (Eds.) *Epilepsy: A Comprehensive Textbook. Vol. 3.* New York: Lippincott–Raven, pp. 2533–2546.

Guldvog, B., Løyning, Y., Hauglie-Hanssen, E., *et al.* (1994) 'Surgical treatment for partial epilepsy among Norwegian children and adolescents.' *Epilepsia*, **35**, 554–565.

Guzzetta, F., Crisafulli, A., Crinó, M.I. (1993) 'Cognitive assessment of infants with West syndrome: how useful is it for diagnosis and prognosis?' *Developmental Medicine and Child Neurology*, **35**, 379–387.

Haga, Y., Watanabe, K., Negoro, T., *et al.* (1995) 'Do ictal, clinical, and electroencephalographic features predict outcome in West syndrome?' *Pediatric Neurology*, **13**, 226–229.

Hakeem, V.F., Wallace, S.J. (1990) 'EEG monitoring of therapy for neonatal seizures.' *Developmental Medicine and Child Neurology*, **32**, 858–864.

Hardiman, O., Burke, T., Phillips, J., *et al.* (1988) 'Microdysgenesis in resected temporal neocortex: incidence and clinical significance in focal epilepsy.' *Neurology*, **38**, 1041–1047.

Harding, B.N., Boyd, S.G. (1991) 'Intractable seizures from infancy can be associated with dentato-olivary dysplasia.' *Journal of the Neurological Sciences*, **104**, 157–165.

—— Copp, J.A. (1997) 'Malformations.' *In:* Graham, D.L., Lantos, P.L. (Eds.) *Greenfield's Neuropathology, 6th Edn.* London: Arnold, pp. 397–533.

Harding, G.F.A., Jeavons, P.M. (1994) *Photosensitive Epilepsy. New Edition. Clinics in Developmental Medicine No. 133.* London: Mac Keith Press.

Hart, Y.M., Cortez, M., Andermann, F., *et al.* (1994) 'Medical treatment of Rasmussen's syndrome (chronic encephalitis and epilepsy): effect of high-dose steroids or immunoglobulins in 19 patients.' *Neurology*, **44**, 1030–1036.

—— Andermann, F., Fish, D.N., *et al.* (1997) 'Chronic encephalitis and epilepsy in adults and adolescents.' *Neurology*, **48**, 418–424.

Harvey, A.S., Bowe, J.M., Hopkins, I.J., *et al.* (1993a) 'Ictal ^{99m}Tc-HMPAO single photon emission computed tomography in children with temporal lobe epilepsy.' *Epilepsia*, **34**, 869–877.

—— Hopkins, I.J., Bowe, J.M., *et al.* (1993b) 'Frontal lobe epilepsy: clinical seizure characteristics and localization with ictal ^{99m}Tc-HMPAO SPECT.' *Neurology*, **43**, 1966–1980.

—— Grattan-Smith, J.D., Desmond, P.M., *et al.* (1995) 'Febrile seizures and hippocampal sclerosis: frequent and related findings in intractable temporal lobe epilepsy of childhood.' *Pediatric Neurology*, **12**, 201–206.

—— Jayakar, P., Duchowny, M., *et al.* (1996) 'Hemifacial seizures and cerebellar ganglioglioma: an epilepsy syndrome of infancy with seizures of cerebellar origin.' *Annals of Neurology*, **40**, 91–98.

Hauser, W.A. (1992) 'Seizure disorders: the changes with age.' *Epilepsia*, **33**, Suppl. 4, S6–S14.

—— (1994) 'The prevalence and incidence of convulsive disorders in children.' *Epilepsia*, **35**, Suppl. 2, S1–S6.

Heijbel, J., Blom, S., Bergfors, P.G. (1975a) 'Benign epilepsy of childhood with centrotemporal foci. A study of incidence rate in outpatient care.' *Epilepsia*, **16**, 657–664.

—— —— Rasmuson, M. (1975b) 'Benign epilepsy of childhood with centrotemporal foci: a genetic study.' *Epilepsia*, **16**, 285–293.

—— —— Bergfors, P.G. (1980) 'Simple febrile convulsions. A prospective incidence study and an evaluation of investigations initially needed.' *Neuropediatrics*, **11**, 45–56.

Heiskala, H., Riikonen, R., Santavuori, P., *et al.* (1996) 'West syndrome: individualized ACTH therapy.' *Brain and Development*, **18**, 456–460.

Hellström-Westas, L., Blennow, G., Lindroth, M. (1995) 'Low-risk of seizure recurrence after early withdrawal of anti-epileptic treatment in the neonatal period.' *Archives of Disease in Childhood*, **72**, 97–101.

Henry, T.R., Drury, I., Brunberg, J.A., *et al.* (1994) 'Focal cerebral magnetic resonance changes associated with partial status epilepticus.' *Epilepsia*, **35**, 35–41.

Herman, B.P. (1982) 'Neuropsychological functioning and psychopathology in children with epilepsy.' *Epilepsia*, **23**, 545–554.

Hewertson, J., Poets, C.F., Samuels, M.P., *et al.* (1994) 'Epileptic seizure-induced hypoxemia in infants presenting with apparent life-threatening events.' *Pediatrics*, **94**, 148–156.

—— Boyd, S.G., Samuels, M.P., *et al.* (1996) 'Hypoxaemia and cardiorespiratory changes during epileptic seizures in young children.' *Developmental Medicine and Child Neurology*, **38**, 511–522.

Hirabayashi, S., Binnie, C.D., Janota, I., Polkey, C.E. (1993) 'Surgical treatment of epilepsy due to cortical dysplasia: clinical and EEG findings.' *Journal of Neurology, Neurosurgery, and Psychiatry*, **56**, 765–770.

Hirsch, E., Marescaux, C., Maquet, P., *et al.* (1990) 'Landau–Kleffner syndrome: a clinical and EEG study of five cases.' *Epilepsia*, **31**, 756–767.

—— Velez, A., Sellal, F., *et al.* (1993) 'Electroclinical signs of benign neonatal familial convulsions.' *Annals of Neurology*, **34**, 835–841.

—— Maquet, P., Metz-Lutz, M.N., *et al.* (1995) 'The eponym of "Landau–Kleffner syndrome" should not be restricted to childhood-acquired aphasia with epilepsy.' *In:* Beaumanoir, A., Bureau, M., Deonna, T., *et al.* (Eds.) *Continuous Spikes and Waves During Slow Sleep. Electrical Status Epilepticus During Slow Sleep. Acquired Aphasia and Related Conditions.* London: John Libbey, pp. 161–164.

Hirsch, J.F., Sainte-Rose, C., Pierre-Kahn, A., *et al.* (1989) 'Benign astrocytic and oligodendrocytic tumors of the cerebral hemispheres in children.' *Journal of Neurosurgery*, **70**, 568–572.

Hirvasniemi, A., Herrala, P., Leisti, J. (1995) 'Northern epilepsy syndrome: clinical course and the effect of medication on seizures.' *Epilepsia*, **36**, 792–797.

Ho, S.S., Berkovic, S.F., Newton, M.R., *et al.* (1994) 'Parietal lobe epilepsy: clinical features and seizure localization by ictal SPECT.' *Neurology*, **44**, 2277–2284.

Holmes, G.L. (1985) 'Neonatal seizures.' *In:* Pedley, T.A., Meldrum, B.S. (Eds.) *Recent Advances in Epilepsy, Vol. 1.* Edinburgh: Churchill Livingstone, pp. 207–237.

—— (1986) 'Partial seizures in children.' *Pediatrics*, **77**, 725–731.

—— (1997) 'Epilepsy in the developing brain: lesions from the laboratory and clinic.' *Epilepsia*, **38**, 12–30.

—— Russman, B.S. (1986) 'Shuddering attacks: evaluation using electroencephalographic frequency modulation radiotelemetry and videotape monitoring.' *American Journal of Diseases of Children*, **140**, 72–73.

—— McKeever, M., Adamson, M. (1987) 'Absence seizures in children: clinical and electroencephalographic features.' *Annals of Neurology*, **21**, 268–273.

Holden, K.R., Mellits, E.D., Freeman, J.M. (1982) 'Neonatal seizures. I: Correlation of prenatal and perinatal events with outcomes.' *Pediatrics*, **70**, 165–176.

Holthausen, H. (1994) 'Febrile convulsions, mesial temporal sclerosis and temporal lobe epilepsy.' *In:* Wolf, P. (Ed.) *Epileptic Seizures and Syndromes.* London: John Libbey, pp. 449–467.

Honda, K., Shinomiya, N., Nomura, Y., *et al.* (1985) 'Effects of neurosurgical treatment on diffuse slow spike and wave complex: a case of left frontal mass lesion with diffuse slow spike and wave complex (DSSW).' *Brain and Development*, **7**, 496–499.

Hrachovy, R.A., Frost, J.D. (1989) 'Infantile spasms.' *Pediatric Clinics of North America*, **36**, 311–329.

—— —— Kellaway, P., Zion, T.E. (1983) 'Double-blind study of ACTH vs prednisone therapy in infantile spasms.' *Journal of Pediatrics*, **103**, 641–645.

—— —— Gospe, S.M., Glaze, D.G. (1987) 'Infantile spasms following near-drowning: a report of two cases.' *Epilepsia*, **28**, 45–48.

—— —— Glaze, D.G. (1994) 'High-dose, long-duration versus low-dose, short-duration corticotropin therapy for infantile spasms.' *Journal of Pediatrics*, **124**, 803–806.

Hurst, D.L. (1987) 'Severe myoclonic epilepsy of infancy.' *Pediatric Neurology*, **3**, 269–272.

Huttenlocher, P.R., Hapke, R.J. (1990) 'A follow-up study of intractable seizures in childhood.' *Annals of Neurology*, **28**, 699–705.

—— Taravath, S., Mojtahedi, S. (1994) 'Periventricular heterotopia and epilepsy.' *Neurology*, **44**, 51–55.

Hyland, K., Buist, N.R.M., Powell, S.R. (1995) 'Folinic acid responsive seizures: a new syndrome?' *Journal of Inherited Metabolic Disease*, **18**, 177–181.

Iinuma, K., Yanai, K., Yanagisawa, T., *et al.* (1987) 'Cerebral glucose metabolism in five patients with Lennox–Gastaut syndrome.' *Pediatric Neurology*, **3**, 12–18.

Ikeno, T., Shigematsu, H., Miyakoshi, M., *et al.* (1985) 'An analytic study of epileptic falls.' *Epilepsia*, **26**, 612–621.

Illum, N., Taudorf, K., Heilmann, C., *et al.* (1990) 'Intravenous immunoglobulin: a single-blind trial in children with Lennox–Gastaut syndrome.' *Neuropediatrics*, **21**, 87–90.

Inoue, Y., Fujiwara, T., Matsuda, K., *et al.* (1997) 'Ring chromosome 20 and nonconvulsive status epilepticus. A new epileptic syndrome.' *Brain*, **120**, 939–953.

Jackson, G.D., Berkovic, S.F., Tress, B.M., *et al.* (1990) 'Hippocampal sclerosis can be reliably detected by magnetic resonance imaging.' *Neurology*, **40**, 1869–1875.

—— Connelly, A., Duncan, J.S., *et al.* (1993) 'Detection of hippocampal pathology in intractable partial epilepsy: increased sensitivity with quantitative magnetic resonance T_2 relaxometry.' *Neurology*, **43**, 1793–1799.

Janz, D. (1989) 'Juvenile myoclonic epilepsy—epilepsy with impulsive petit mal.' *Cleveland Clinic Journal of Medicine*, **56** (Suppl.), S23–S33.

—— (1994) 'Pitfalls in the diagnosis of grand mal on awakening.' *In:* Wolf, P. (Ed.) *Epileptic Seizures and Syndromes*. London: John Libbey, pp. 213–220.

—— Beck-Mannagetta, G., Spröder, B., Waltz, S. (1994) 'Childhood absence epilepsy (pyknolepsy) and juvenile absence epilepsy: one or two syndromes?' *In:* Wolf, P. (Ed.) *Epileptic Seizures and Syndromes*. London: John Libbey, pp. 115–126.

Jawad, S., Oxley, J., Wilson, J., Richens, A. (1986) 'A pharmacodynamic evaluation of midazolam as an antiepileptic compound.' *Journal of Neurology, Neurosurgery, and Psychiatry*, **49**, 1050–1054.

Jayakar, P., Duchowny, M.S. (1990) 'Complex partial seizures of temporal lobe origin in early childhood.' *Journal of Epilepsy*, **3**, 41–45.

—— Seshia, S.S. (1991) 'Electrical status epilepticus during slow-wave sleep: a review.' *Journal of Clinical Neurophysiology*, **8**, 299–311.

Jeavons, P.M. (1982) 'Myoclonic epilepsies: therapy and prognosis.' *In:* Akimoto, H., Kazamatsuri, H., Seino, M., Ward, A.A. (Eds.) *Advances in Epileptology. XIIIth Epilepsy International Symposium*. New York: Raven Press, pp. 141–144.

—— (1983) 'Non-epileptic attacks in childhood.' *In:* Rose, F.C. (Ed.) *Research Progress in Epilepsy*. London: Pitman, pp. 224–230.

—— Livet, M.O. (1992) 'West syndrome: infantile spasms.' *In:* Roger, J., Bureau, M., Dravet, C., *et al.* (Eds.) *Epileptic Syndromes in Infancy, Childhood and Adolescence. 2nd Edn.* London: John Libbey, pp. 53–65.

Jellinger, K. (1987) 'Neuropathological aspects of infantile spasms.' *Brain and Development*, **9**, 349–357.

Jennett, B. (1974) 'Post-traumatic epilepsy: incidence and significance after non-missile injuries.' *Archives of Neurology*, **30**, 394–398.

Johnston, M.V. (1996) 'Developmental aspects of epileptogenesis.' *Epilepsia*, **37**, Suppl. 1, S2–S9.

Juul-Jensen, P. (1968) 'Frequency of recurrence after discontinuance of anticonvulsant therapy in patients with epileptic seizures. A new follow-up study after 5 years.' *Epilepsia*, **9**, 11–16.

Kajitani, T., Ueoka, K., Nakamura, M., Kumanomidou, Y. (1981) 'Febrile convulsions and Rolandic discharges.' *Brain and Development*, **3**, 351–359.

Kalayci, Ö., Coskun, T., Tokatli, A., *et al.* (1994) 'Infantile spasms as the initial symptom of biotinidase deficiency.' *Journal of Pediatrics*, **124**, 103–104.

Kälvinainen, R., Aikia, M., Rekkinen, P.J. (1996) 'Cognitive adverse effects of antiepileptic drugs.' *CNS Drugs*, **5**, 358–368.

Kasteleijn-Nolst Trenité, D.G., Bakker, D.J., Binnie, C.D., *et al.* (1988) 'Psychological effects of subclinical epileptiform EEG discharges. I: Scholastic skills.' *Epilepsy Research*, **2**, 111–116.

—— Siebelink, B.M., Berends, S.G.C., *et al.* (1990) 'Lateralized effects of subclinical epileptiform EEG discharges on scholastic performance in children.' *Epilepsia*, **31**, 740–746.

Kinsman, S.L., Vining, E.P.G., Quaskey, S.A., *et al.* (1992) 'Efficacy of the ketogenic diet for intractable seizure disorders: review of 58 cases.' *Epilepsia*, **33**, 1132–1136.

Kiok, M.C., Terrence, C.F., Fromm, G.H., Lavine, S. (1986) 'Sinus arrest in epilepsy.' *Neurology*, **36**, 115–116.

Kivity, S., Lerman, P. (1992) 'Stormy onset prolonged loss of consciousness in benign childhood epilepsy with occipital paroxysms.' *Journal of Neurology, Neurosurgery, and Psychiatry*, **55**, 45–48.

Knudsen, F.U. (1996) 'Febrile seizures: treatment and outcome.' *Brain and Development*, **18**, 438–449.

—— Paerregaard, A., Andersen, R., Andresen, J. (1996) 'Long-term outcome of prophylaxis for febrile convulsions.' *Archives of Disease in Childhood*, **74**, 13–18.

Konishi, Y., Yasujima, M., Kuriyama, M., *et al.* (1992) 'Magnetic resonance imaging in infantile spasms: effects of hormone therapy.' *Epilepsia*, **33**, 304–309.

Koo, B., Hwang, P.A., Logan, W.J. (1993) 'Infantile spasms: outcome and prognostic factors of cryptogenic and symptomatic groups.' *Neurology*, **43**, 2322–2327.

Kotagal, P., Rothner, A.D., Erenberg, G., *et al.* (1987) 'Complex partial seizures of childhood onset.' *Archives of Neurology*, **44**, 1177–1180.

—— Lüders, H., Morris, H.H., *et al.* (1989) 'Dystonic posturing in complex partial seizures of temporal lobe onset: a new lateralizing sign.' *Neurology*, **39**, 196–201.

Kramer, R.E., Lüders, H., Lesser, R.P., *et al.* (1987) 'Transient focal abnormalities of neuroimaging studies during focal status epilepticus.' *Epilepsia*, **28**, 528–532.

—— —— Goldstick, L.P., *et al.* (1988) 'Ictus emeticus: an electroclinical analysis.' *Neurology*, **38**, 1048–1052.

Kroll, J.S. (1985) 'Pyridoxine for neonatal seizures: an unexpected danger.' *Developmental Medicine and Child Neurology*, **27**, 377–379.

Kuks, J.B.M., Cook, M.J., Fish, D.R., *et al.* (1993) 'Hippocampal sclerosis in epilepsy and childhood febrile seizures.' *Lancet*, **342**, 1391–1394.

Kurokawa, T., Sasaki, K., Hanai, T., *et al.* (1981) 'Linear nevus sebaceus syndrome—report of a case with Lennox–Gastaut syndrome following infantile spasms.' *Archives of Neurology*, **38**, 375–377.

Kusse, M.C., van Nieuwenhuizen, O., van Huffelen, A.C., *et al.* (1993) 'The effect of non-depot ACTH$_{(1–24)}$ on infantile spasms.' *Developmental Medicine and Child Neurology*, **35**, 1067–1073.

Kuzniecky, R., Jackson, G. (1995) *Magnetic Resonance in Epilepsy*. New York: Raven Press.

—— Powers, R. (1993) 'Epilepsia partialis continua due to cortical dysplasia.' *Journal of Child Neurology*, **8**, 386–388.

—— Rosenblatt, B. (1987) 'Benign occipital epilepsy: a family study.' *Epilepsia*, **28**, 346–350.

—— Andermann, F., Melanson, D., *et al.* (1988) 'Focal cortical myoclonus and rolandic cortical dysplasia: clarification by magnetic resonance imaging.' *Annals of Neurology*, **23**, 317–325.

—— Garcia, G.H., Faught, E., Morawetz, R.B. (1991) 'Cortical dysplasia in temporal lobe epilepsy: magnetic resonance correlations.' *Annals of Neurology*, **29**, 293–298.

—— Andermann, F., Guerini, R., and the CBPS Multicenter Collaborative Study (1994) 'The epileptic spectrum in the congenital bilateral perisylvian syndrome.' *Neurology*, **44**, 379–385.

Labate, C., Magaudda, A., Fava, C., *et al.* (1991) 'Hemispheric brain atrophy following unilateral status epilepticus.' *Bolletino della Lega Italiana Contro l'Epilessia*, **74**, 103–104.

Lammers, M.W., Hekster, Y.A., Keyser, A., *et al.* (1995) 'Monotherapy or polytherapy for epilepsy revisited.' *Epilepsia*, **36**, Suppl. 3, S59. *(Abstract.)*

Lancman, M.E., Asconapé, J.J., Golimstok, A. (1994) 'Circling seizures in a case of juvenile myoclonic epilepsy.' *Epilepsia*, **35**, 317–318.

Landy, H.J., Khoury, A.N., Heyl, P.S. (1989) 'Antenatal ultrasonographic diagnosis of fetal seizure activity.' *American Journal of Obstetrics and Gynecology*, **161**, 308.

Laskowitz, D.T., Sperling, M.R., French, J.A., O'Connor, M.J. (1995) 'The syndrome of frontal lobe epilepsy: characteristics and surgical management.' *Neurology*, **45**, 780–787.

Lee, W.L., Low, P.S., Rajan, U. (1993) 'Benign familial infantile epilepsy.' *Journal of Pediatrics*, **123**, 588–590.

Legarda, S., Jayakar, P., Duchowny, M., *et al.* (1994) 'Benign rolandic epilepsy: high central and low central subgroups. '*Epilepsia*, **35**, 1125–1129.

Legido, A., Clancy, R.R., Berman, P.H. (1988) 'Recent advances in the diagnosis, treatment and prognosis of neonatal seizures.' *Pediatric Neurology*, **4**, 79–86.

Leppert, M., Anderson, V.E. Quattlebaum, T., *et al.* (1989) 'Benign familial neonatal convulsions linked to genetic markers on chromosome 20.' *Nature*, **337**, 647–648.

Lerman, P. (1986) 'Seizures induced or aggravated by anticonvulsants.' *Epilepsia*, **27**, 706–710.

—— Kivity, S. (1986) 'Benign focal epilepsies of childhood.' *In:* Pedley, T.A., Meldrum, B.S. (Eds.) *Recent Advances in Epilepsy, Vol. 3.* Edinburgh: Churchill Livingstone, pp. 137–156.

—— Lerman-Sagie, T. (1995) 'Sulthiame revisited.' *Journal of Child Neurology*, **10**, 241–242.

—— —— Kivity, S. (1991) 'Effect of early corticosteroid therapy for Landau–Kleffner syndrome.' *Developmental Medicine and Child Neurology*, **33**, 257–260.

Levene, M.I., Trounce, J.Q. (1986) 'Cause of neonatal convulsions: towards a more precise diagnosis.' *Archives of Disease in Childhood*, **61**, 78–87.

Levin, R., Banks, S., Berg, B. (1988) 'Psychosocial dimensions of epilepsy: a review of the literature.' *Epilepsia*, **29**, 805–816.

Levy, R.H., Moreland, T.A., Farwell, J.R. (1983) 'Drug interactions in epileptic children.' *In:* Morselli, P.L., Pippenger, C.E., Penry, J.K. (Eds.) *Antiepileptic Drug Therapy in Pediatrics.* New York: Raven Press, pp. 75–84.

—— Mattson, R.H., Meldrum, B.S (Eds.) (1995) *Antiepileptic Drugs, 4th Edn.* New York: Raven Press.

Levy, S.R., Abrams, I.F., Marshall, P.C., Rosquette, E.E. (1985) 'Seizures and cerebral infarction in the full-term newborn.' *Annals of Neurology*, **17**, 366–370.

Lindsay, J., Ounsted, C., Richards, P. (1979) 'Long-term outcome in children with temporal lobe seizures. III: Psychiatric aspects in childhood and adult life.' *Developmental Medicine and Child Neurology*, **21**, 630–636.

Lipton, S.A., Rosenberg, P.A. (1994) 'Excitatory amino acids as a final common pathway for neurological disorders.' *New England Journal of Medicine*, **330**, 613–622.

Liu, Z., Mikati, M., Holmes, G.L. (1995) 'Mesial temporal sclerosis: pathogenesis and significance.' *Pediatric Neurology*, **12**, 5–16.

Livingston, J.H. (1988) 'The Lennox–Gastaut syndrome.' *Developmental Medicine and Child Neurology*, **30**, 536–540.

Loiseau, P. (1992) 'Childhood absence epilepsy.' *In:* Roger, J., Bureau, M., Dravet, C., *et al.* (Eds.) *Epileptic Syndromes in Infancy, Childhood and Adolescence. 2nd Edn.* London: John Libbey, pp. 135–150.

—— Duché, B. (1995) 'Childhood absence epilepsy.' *In:* Duncan, J.S., Panayiotopoulos, C.P. (Eds.) *Typical Absences and Related Epileptic Syndromes.* London: Churchill Communications Europe, pp. 152–160.

—— Louiset, P. (1992) 'Benign partial seizures of adolescence.' *In:* Roger, J., Bureau, M., Dravet, C., *et al.* (Eds.) *Epileptic Syndromes in Infancy, Childhood and Adolescence. 2nd Edn.* London: John Libbey, pp. 343–345.

—— Pestre, M., Dartigues, J.F., *et al.* (1983) 'Long-term prognosis in two forms of childhood epilepsy: typical absence seizures and epilepsy with rolandic (centrotemporal) EEG foci.' *Annals of Neurology*, **13**, 642–648.

—— Duché, B., Cordova, S., *et al.* (1988) 'Prognosis of benign childhood epilepsy with centrotemporal spikes: a follow-up study of 168 patients.' *Epilepsia*, **29**, 229–235.

—— —— Cohadon, S. (1992) 'The prognosis of benign localized epilepsies in early childhood.' *In:* Degen, R. (Ed.) *The Benign Localized and Generalized Epilepsies of Early Childhood.* Amsterdam: Elsevier, pp. 75–81.

Lombroso, C.T. (1983a) 'A prospective study of infantile spasms: clinical and therapeutic correlations.' *Epilepsia*, **24**, 135–158.

—— (1983b) 'Prognosis in neonatal seizures.' *In:* Delgado-Escueta, A.V., Wasterlain, C.G., Treiman, D.M., Porter, R.J. (Eds.) *Advances in Neurology. Vol. 34. Status Epilepticus.* New York: Raven Press, pp. 101–113.

—— (1990) 'Early myoclonic encephalopathy, early infantile epileptic encephalopathy, and benign and severe infantile myoclonic epilepsies: a critical review and personal contributions.' *Journal of Clinical Neurophysiology*, **7**, 380–408.

—— (1996) 'Neonatal seizures: a clinician's overview.' *Brain and Development*, **18**, 1–28.

—— Fejerman, N. (1977) 'Benign myoclonus in early infancy.' *Annals of Neurology*, **1**, 138–143.

Long, G., Moore, J.R. (1979) 'Parental expectations for their epileptic children.' *Journal of Child Psychology and Psychiatry*, **20**, 299–312.

Lortie, A., Chiron, C., Mumford, J., Dulac, O. (1993) 'The potential for increasing seizure frequency, relapse, and appearance of new seizure types with vigabatrin.' *Neurology*, **43**, Suppl. 5, S24–S27.

Lüders, H. (Ed.) (1992) *Epilepsy Surgery.* New York: Raven Press.

—— Lesser, R.P., Dinner, D.S., Morris, H.H. (1987) 'Benign focal epilepsy of childhood.' *In:* Lüders, H., Lesser, R.P. (Eds.) *Epilepsy: Electroclonical Syndromes.* Berlin: Springer Verlag, pp. 303–346.

—— Burgess, R., Noachtar, S. (1993) 'Expanding the International Classification of Seizures to provide localization information.' *Neurology*, **43**, 1650–1655.

Lynch, B.J., Rust, A.S. (1994) 'Natural history of neonatal hypocalcemic and hypomagnesemic seizures.' *Pediatric Neurology*, **11**, 23–27.

Lyon, G., Gastaut, H. (1985) 'Considerations on the significance attributed to unusual cerebral histological findings recently described in eight patients with primary generalized epilepsy.' *Epilepsia*, **26**, 365–367.

—— Dodge, P.R., Adams, R.D. (1961) 'The acute encephalopathies of obscure origin in infants and children.' *Brain*, 84, 680–708.

Macdonald, R.L., Kelly, K.M. (1993) 'Antiepileptic drug mechanisms of action.' *Epilepsia*, **34**, Suppl. 5, S1–S8.

Maeda, Y., Kurokawa, T., Sakamoto, K., *et al.* (1990) 'Electroclinical study of video-game epilepsy.' *Developmental Medicine and Child Neurology*, **32**, 493–500.

Magaudda, A., Dalla Bernardina, B., De Marco, P., *et al.* (1993) 'Bilateral occipital calcification, epilepsy and coeliac disease: clinical and neuroimaging features.' *Journal of Neurology, Neurosurgery, and Psychiatry*, **56**, 885–889.

Maher, J., McLachlan, R. (1997) 'Febrile convulsions in selected large families: a single-major-locus mode of inheritance?' *Developmental Medicine and Child Neurology*, **39**, 79–84.

Malafosse, A., Leboyer, M., Dulac, O., *et al.* (1992) 'Confirmation of linkage of benign familial neonatal convulsions to D20S19 and D20S20.' *Human Genetics*, **89**, 54–58.

—— Beck, C., Bellet, H., *et al.* (1994) 'Benign infantile familial convulsions are not an allelic form of the benign familial neonatal convulsions gene.' *Annals of Neurology*, **35**, 479–482.

Manford, M., Fish, D.R., Shorvon, S.D. (1996a) 'An analysis of clinical seizure patterns and their localizing value in frontal and temporal lobe epilepsies.' *Brain*, **119**, 17–40.

—— —— —— (1996b) 'Startle provoked epileptic seizures: features in 19 patients.' *Journal of Neurology, Neurosurgery, and Psychiatry*, **61**, 151–156.

Manonmani, V., Wallace, S.J. (1994) 'Epilepsy with myoclonic absences.' *Archives of Disease in Childhood*, **70**, 288–290.

Maquet, P., Hirsch, E., Dive, D., *et al.* (1990) 'Cerebral glucose utilization during sleep in Landau–Kleffner syndrome: a PET study.' *Epilepsia*, **31**, 778–783.

—— —— Metz-Lutz, M.N., *et al.* (1995) 'Regional cerebral glucose metabolism in children with deterioration of one or more cognitive functions and continuous spike-and-wave discharges during sleep.' *Brain*, **118**, 1497–1520.

Marciani, M.G., Maschio, M., Spanedda, F., *et al.* (1995) 'Development of myoclonus in patients with partial epilepsy during treatment with vigabatrin: an electroencephalographic study.' *Acta Neurologica Scandinavica*, **91**, 1–5.

Marks, D.A., Kim, J., Spencer, D.D., Spencer, S.S. (1995) 'Seizure localization and pathology following head injury in patients with uncontrolled epilepsy.' *Neurology*, **45**, 2051–2057.

Mattson, R.H., Cramer, J.A., Collins, J.F., and the Department of Veterans Affairs Epilepsy Cooperative Study No. 264, Group D (1992) 'A comparison of valproate with carbamazepine for the treatment of complex partial seizures and secondarily generalized tonic–clonic seizures in adults.' *New England Journal of Medicine*, **327**, 765–771.

Mathern, G.W., Babb, T.L., Mischel, P.S., *et al.* (1996) 'Childhood generalized and mesial temporal epilepsies demonstrate different amounts and patterns of hippocampal neuron loss and mossy fibre synaptic reorganization.' *Brain*, **119**, 965–987.

Matsuishi, T., Yoshino, M., Tokunaga, O., *et al.* (1985) 'Subacute necrotizing encephalomyelopathy (Leigh disease): report of a case with Lennox–Gastaut syndrome.' *Brain and Development*, **7**, 500–504.

Matsumoto, A., Watanabe, K., Negoro, T., *et al.* (1981) 'Infantile spasms: etiological factors, clinical aspects and long term prognosis in 200 cases.' *European Journal of Pediatrics*, **135**, 239–244.

—— Kumagai, T., Takeuchi, T., *et al.* (1987) 'Clinical effects of thyrotropin-releasing hormone for severe epilepsy in childhood: a comparative study with ACTH therapy.' *Epilepsia*, **28**, 49–55.

Mauguière, F., Courjon, J. (1978) 'Somatosensory epilepsy: a review of 127 cases.' *Brain*, **101**, 307–332.

Mayr, N., Wimberger, D., Pichler, H., *et al.* (1987) 'Influence of television on photosensitive epileptics.' *European Neurology*, **27**, 201–208.

Maytal, J., Shinnar, S. (1990) 'Febrile status epilepticus.' *Pediatrics*, **86**, 611–616.

—— —— Moshé, S.L., Alvarez, L.A. (1989) 'Low morbidity and mortality of status epilepticus in children.' *Pediatrics*, **83**, 323–331.

McBride, M.C., Dooling, E.C., Oppenheimer, E.Y. (1981) 'Complex partial status epilepticus in young children.' *Annals of Neurology*, **9**, 526–530.

McDonald, J.W., Garofalo, E.A., Hood, T., *et al.* (1991) 'Altered excitatory and inhibitory amino acid receptor binding in hippocampus of patients with temporal lobe epilepsy.' *Annals of Neurology*, **29**, 529–541.

McShane, M.A., Finn, J.P., Hall-Craggs, M.A., *et al.* (1990) 'Neonatal hemangiomatosis presenting as infantile spasms.' *Neuropediatrics*, **21**, 211–212.

Medical Research Council Antiepileptic Drug Withdrawal Study Group (1991) 'Randomised study of antiepileptic drug withdrawal in patients in remission.' *Lancet*, **337**, 1175–1180.

Meencke, H.J. (1985) 'Neuronal density in the molecular layer of the frontal cortex in primary generalized epilepsy.' *Epilepsia*, **26**, 450–454.

—— Gerhard, C. (1985) 'Morphological aspects of aetiology and the course of infantile spasms (West-syndrome).' *Neuropediatrics*, 16, 59–66.

—— Janz, D. (1984) 'Neuropathological findings in primary generalized epilepsy: a study of 8 cases.' *Epilepsia*, **25**, 8–21.

—— Veith, G. (1992) 'Migration disturbances in epilepsy.' *In:* Engel, J., Wasterlain, G., Cavalheiro, E.A., *et al.* (Eds.) *Molecular Biology of Epilepsy. Epilepsy Research Supplement No. 9.* Amsterdam: Elsevier, pp. 31–40.

Meijer, J.W.A. (1991) 'Knowledge, attitude and practice in antiepileptic drug monitoring.' *Acta Neurologica Scandinavica*, **83**, Suppl. 134, 1–128.

Meldrum, B.S. (1978) 'Physiological changes during prolonged seizures and epileptic brain damage.' *Neuropädiatrie*, **9**, 203–212.

—— (1983) 'Metabolic factors during prolonged seizures and their relation to nerve cell death.' *In:* Delgado-Escueta, A.V., Wasterlain, C.G., Treiman, D.M., Porter, R.J. (Eds.) *Advances in Neurology. Vol. 34. Status Epilepticus.* New York: Raven Press, 261–275.

—— (1985) 'Possible therapeutic applications of antagonists of excitatory aminoacid-transmitters.' *Clinical Science*, **68**, 113–122.

—— Porter, R.J. (1986) *Curent Problems in Epilepsy. Vol. 4. New Anticonvulsant Drugs.* London: John Libbey.

Metrakos, J.D. Metrakos, K. (1970) 'Genetic factors in epilepsy.' *In:* Niedermeyer, E. (Ed.) *Epilepsy: Modern Problems in Psychopharmacology.* Basel: Karger, pp. 71–86.

Mikati, M.A., Browne, T.R. (1988) 'Comparative efficacy of antiepileptic drugs.' *Clinical Neuropharmacology*, **11**, 130–140.

—— Lee, W.L., De Long, G.R. (1985) 'Protracted epileptiform encephalopathy: an unusual form of partial complex status epilepticus.' *Epilepsia*, **26**, 563–571.

—— Holmes, G.L., Chronopoulos, A., *et al.* (1994) 'Phenobarbital modifies seizure-related brain injury in the developing brain.' *Annals of Neurology*, **36**, 425–433.

Millner, M.M., Puchhammer-Stöckl, E. (1993) 'Herpes simplex virus encephalitis and febrile convulsions: contribution of polymerase chain reaction and magnetic resonance imaging.' *Annals of Neurology*, **34**, 503. *(Abstract.)*

Mitchell, W.G., Greenwood, R.S., Messenheimer, J.A. (1983) 'Abdominal epilepsy: cyclic vomiting as the major symptom of simple partial seizures.' *Archives of Neurology*, **40**, 251–252.

Miyazaki, M., Hashimoto, T., Fujii, E., *et al.* (1994) 'Infantile spasms: localized cerebral lesions on SPECT.' *Epilepsia*, **35**, 988–992.

Mizrahi, E.M., Kellaway, P. (1987) 'Characterization and classification of neonatal seizures.' *Neurology*, **37**, 1837–1844.

Mohnot, D., Snead, O.C., Benton, J.W. (1982) 'Burn encephalopathy in children.' *Annals of Neurology*, **12**, 42–47.

Molaie, M., Culebras, A., Miller, M. (1987) 'Nocturnal plasma prolactin and cortisol levels in epileptics with complex partial seizures and primary generalized seizures.' *Archives of Neurology*, **44**, 699–702.

Montagna, P., Sforza, E., Tinuper, P., *et al.* (1990) 'Paroxysmal arousals during sleep.' *Neurology*, **40**, 1063–1066.

Morikawa, T., Seino, M., Osawa, T., Yagi, K. (1985) 'Five chilldren with continuous spike–wave discharges during sleep.' *In:* Roger, J., Dravet, C.,

Bureau, M., *et al.* (Eds.) *Epileptic Syndromes in Infancy, Childhood and Adolescence.* London: John Libbey, pp. 205–212.

Morrell, F. (1989) 'Variation of human secondary epileptogenesis.' *Journal of Clinical Neurophysiology*, **6**, 227–275.

—— (1995) 'Electrophysiology of CSWS in Landau–Kleffner syndrome.' *In:* Beaumanoir, A., Bureau, M., Deonna, T., *et al.* (Eds.) *Continuous Spikes and Waves During Slow Sleep. Electrical Status Epilepticus During Slow Sleep. Acquired Aphasia and Related Conditions.* London: John Libbey, pp. 77–90.

—— Whisler, W.W., Bleck, T.P. (1989) 'Multiple subpial transection: a new approach to the surgical treatment of focal epilepsy.' *Journal of Neurosurgery*, **70**, 231–239.

—— —— Smith, M.C., *et al.* (1995) 'Landau–Kleffner syndrome. Treatment with subpial intracortical transection.' *Brain*, **118**, 1529–1546.

Morris, G.L., Mueller, W.M., Yetkin, F.Z., *et al.* (1994) 'Functional magnetic resonance imaging in partial epilepsy.' *Epilepsia*, **35**, 1194–1198.

Morris, H.H., Estes, M.L., Gilmore, A., *et al.* (1993) 'Chronic intractable epilepsy as the only symptom of primary brain tumour.' *Epilepsia*, **34**, 1038–1043.

Moshé, S.L. (1987) 'Epileptogenesis and the immature brain.' *Epilepsia*, **28**, Suppl. 1, S3–S15.

—— Ludvig, N. (1988) 'Kindling.' *In:* Pedley, T.A., Meldrum, B.S. (Eds.) *Recent Advances in Epilepsy, Vol. 4.* Edinburgh: Churchill Livingstone, pp. 21–44.

Munari, C., Tassi, L., Kahane, P., *et al.* (1994) 'Analysis of clinical symptomatology during stereo-EEG recorded mesiotemporal lobe seizurres.' *In:* Wolf, P. (Ed.) *Epileptic Seizures and Syndromes.* London: John Libbey, pp. 335–357.

Murphy, J.V., Sawasky, F., Marquardt, K.M., Harris, D.J. (1987) 'Deaths in young children receiving nitrazepam.' *Journal of Pediatrics*, **111**, 145–147.

Murphy, M.J. (1985) 'Long-term follow-up of seizures associated with cerebral arteriovenous malformations. Results of therapy.' *Archives of Neurology*, **42**, 477–479.

Musumeci, S.A., Elia, M., Ferrir, R., *et al.* (1995) 'A further family with epilepsy, dementia and yellow teeth: the Kohlschütter syndrome.' *Brain and Development*, **17**, 133–138.

Nabbout, R.C., Chiron, C., Mumford, J., *et al.* (1997) 'Vigabatrin in partial seizures in children.' *Journal of Child Neurology*, **12**, 172–177.

Naidu, S., Gruener, G., Brazis, D. (1986) 'Excellent results with chlorazepate in recalcitrant childhood epilepsies.' *Pediatric Neurology*, **2**, 18–22.

Nashef, L., Fish, D.R., Garner, S., *et al.* (1995) 'Sudden death in epilepsy: a study of incidence in a young cohort with epilepsy and learing difficulty.' *Epilepsia*, **36**, 1187–1194.

Nelson, K.B., Ellenberg, J.H. (1976) 'Predictors of epilepsy in children who have experienced febrile seizures.' *New England Journal of Medicine*, **295**, 1029–1033.

—— —— (Eds.) (1981) *Febrile Seizures.* New York: Raven Press.

—— —— (1990) 'Prenatal and perinatal antecedents of febrile seizures.' *Annals of Neurology*, **27**, 127–131.

Neville, B.G.R., Boyd, S.G. (1995) 'Selective epileptic gait disorder.' *Journal of Neurology, Neurosurgery, and Psychiatry*, **58**, 371–373.

—— Harkness, W.F.J., Cross, J.H., *et al.* (1997) 'Surgical treatment of autistic regression in childhood epilepsy.' *Pediatric Neurology*, **16**, 137–140.

Newmark, M.E., Penry, J.K. (1979) *Photosensitivity and Epilepsy. A Review.* New York: Raven Press.

Newton, M.R., Berkovic, S.F., Austin, M.C., *et al.* (1995) 'SPECT in the localisation of extratemporal and temporal seizure foci.' *Journal of Neurology, Neurosurgery, and Psychiatry*, **59**, 26–30.

Newton, R., Aicardi, J. (1983) 'Clinical findings in children with occipital spike–wave complexes suppressed by eye-opening.' *Neurology*, **33**, 1526–1529.

Niedermeyer, E., Walker, A.E., Burton, C. (1970) 'The slow spike–wave complex as a correlate of frontal and frontotemporal post-traumatic epilepsy.' *European Neurology*, **3**, 330–346.

Nishio, S., Morioka, T., Fukui, M., Goto, Y. (1994) 'Surgical treatment of intractable seizures due to hypothalamic hamartoma.' *Epilepsia*, **35**, 514–519.

Offringa, M., Bossuyt, P.M.M., Lubsen, J., *et al.* (1994) 'Risk factors for seizure recurrence in children with febrile seizures: a pooled analysis of individual patient data from five studies.' *Journal of Pediatrics*, **124**, 574–584.

Ogino, T., Ohtsuka, Y., Yamatogi, Y., *et al.* (1989) 'The epileptic syndrome sharing common features during early childhood with severe myoclonic epilepsy in infancy.' *Japanese Journal of Psychiatry and Neurology*, **43**, 479–481.

—— Hata, H., Minakuchi, E., *et al.* (1994) 'Neurophysiologic dysfunction in hypomelanosis of Ito: EEG and evoked potential studies.' *Brain and Development*, **16**, 407–412.

Oguni, H., Imaizumi, Y., Uehara, T., *et al.* (1993) 'Electroencephalographic features of epileptic drop attacks and absence seizures: a case study.' *Brain and Development*, **15**, 226–230.

—— Hayashi, K., Oguni, M., *et al.* (1994) 'Treatment of severe myoclonic epilepsy in infants with bromide and its borderline variant.' *Epilepsia*, **35**, 1140–1145.

Ohtahara, S., Ohtsuka, Y., Yamatogi, Y., Oka, E. (1987) 'The early-infantile epileptic encephalopathy with suppression–burst: developmental aspects.' *Brain and Development*, **9**, 371–376.

—— —— —— *et al.* (1993) 'Prenatal etiologies of West syndrome.' *Epilepsia*, **34**, 716–722.

Ohtsuka, Y., Murashima, I., Oka, E., Ohtahara, S. (1994) 'Treatment and prognosis of West syndrome.' *Journal of Epilepsy*, 7, 279–284.

Olsson, I. (1990) 'Absence epilepsy in Swedish children.' (MD thesis.) Göteborg: Vasastadens Bokbinderi AB (ISBN 91-628-0148-1).

—— Campenhausen, G. (1992) 'Social adjustment in young adults with absence epilepsy.' *Epilepsia*, **33**, 325–329.

Ormason, M.J., Kispert, D.B., Sharbrough, F.W., *et al.* (1986) 'Cryptic structural lesions in refractory partial epilepsy: MR imaging and CT studies.' *Radiology*, **160**, 215–219.

Osorio, I., Burnstine, T.H., Remler, B., *et al.* (1989) 'Phenytoin-induced seizures: a paradoxical effect at toxic concentrations in epileptic patients.' *Epilepsia*, **30**, 230–234.

Ottman, R. (1989) 'Genetics of the partial epilepsies: a review.' *Epilepsia*, **30**, 107–111.

—— Annegers, J.F., Kurland, L.T. (1991) 'Familial aggregation and severity of epilepsy.' *Epilepsia*, **32**, 523–529.

—— Risch, N., Hauser, W.A., *et al.* (1995) 'Localization of a gene for partial epilepsy to chromosome 10q.' *Nature Genetics*, **10**, 56–60.

Ounsted, C., Lindsay, J., Richards, P. (1987) *Temporal Lobe Epilepsy. A Biographical Study 1948–1986. Clinics in Developmental Medicine No. 103.* London: Mac Keith Press.

Paetau, R. (1994) 'Sounds trigger spikes in the Landau–Kleffner syndrome.' *Journal of Clinical Neurophysiology*, **11**, 231–241.

—— Kasola, M., Karhu, J., *et al.* (1992) 'Magnetoencephalographic localization of epileptic cortex—impact on surgical treatment.' *Annals of Neurology*, **32**, 106–109.

Painter, M.J., Bergman, I., Crumrine, P. (1986) 'Neonatal seizures.' *Pediatric Clinics of North America*, **33**, 91–109.

—— Scher, M.S., Paneth, N.S., *et al.* (1994) 'Randomized trial of phenobarbital vs phenytoin treatment of neonatal seizures.' *Pediatric Research*, **35**, 384A. *(Abstract.)*

Palm, D.G., Brandt, M., Korithenberg, R. (1988) 'West syndrome and Lennox–Gastaut syndrome in childen with porencephalic cysts.' *In:* Niedermeyer, E., Degen, R. (Eds.) *The Lennox–Gastaut Syndrome.* New York: Alan R. Liss, pp. 419–426.

Palm, L., Blennow, G., Brun, A. (1986) 'Infantile spasms and neuronal heterotopias: a report of six cases.' *Acta Paediatrica Scandinavica*, **75**, 855–859.

Palmini, A., Andermann, F., Olivier, A., *et al.* (1991) 'Neuronal migration disorders: a contribution of modern neuroimaging to the etiologic diagnosis of epilepsy.' *Canadian Journal of Neurological Sciences*, **18**, 580–587.

—— Gambardella, A., Andermann, F., *et al.* (1995) 'Intrinsic epileptogenicity of human dysplastic cortex as suggested by corticography and surgical results.' *Annals of Neurology*, **37**, 476–487.

Panayiotopoulos, C.P. (1989a) 'Benign childhood epilepsy with occipital paroxysms: a 15-year prospective study.' *Annals of Neurology*, **26**, 51–56.

—— (1989b) 'Benign nocturnal childhood occipital epilepsy: a new syndrome with nocturnal seizures, tonic deviation of the eyes and vomiting.' *Journal of Child Neurology*, **4**, 43–48.

—— (1994a) 'Juvenile myoclonic epilepsy: an underdiagnosed syndrome.' *In:* Wolf, P. (Ed.) *Epileptic Seizures and Syndromes.* London: Jonn Libbey, pp. 221–230.

—— (1994b) 'The clinical spectrum of typical absence seizures and absence epilepsies.' *In:* Malafosse, A., Genton, P., Hirsch, E., *et al.* (Eds.) *Idiopathic Generalized Epilepsies: Clinical, Experimental and Genetic Aspects.* London: John Libbey, pp. 75–85.

—— (1998) 'Absence epilepsies.' *In:* Engel, J., Pedley, T.A. (Eds.) *Epilepsy: A Comprehensive Textbook. Vol. 3.* New York: Lippincott–Raven, pp. 2327–2346.

—— Obeid, T., Waheed, G. (1989a) 'Absences in juvenile myoclonic epilepsy: a clinical and video–electroencephalographic study.' *Annals of Neurology*, **25**, 391–397.

—— —— —— (1989b) 'Differentiation of typical absence seizures in epileptic syndromes—a video EEG study of 225 seizures in 20 patients.' *Brain*, **112**, 1039–1056.

Parent, J.M., Lowenstein, D.H. (1994) 'Treatment of refractory generalized status epilepticus with continuous infusion of midazolam.' *Neurology*, **44**, 1837–1840.

Pascual-Castroviejo, I., López-Rodriguez, L., de la Cruz Medina, M., *et al.* (1988) 'Hypomelanosis of Ito. Neurological complications in 34 cases.' *Canadian Journal of Neurological Science*, **15**, 124–129.

—— López Martin, V., Martínez Bermejo, A., Pérez Higueras, A. (1992) 'Is cerebral arteritis the cause of the Landau–Kleffner syndrome? Four cases in childhood with angiographic study.' *Canadian Journal of Neurological Sciences*, **19**, 46–52.

Peled, R., Lavie, P. (1986) 'Paroxysmal awakenings from sleep associated with excessive daytime somnolence: a form of nocturnal epilepsy.' *Neurology*, **36**, 95–98.

Penry, J.K., Porter, R.J., Dreifuss, F.E. (1975) 'Simultaneous recording of absence seizures with video tape and electroencephalography. A study of 374 seizures in 48 patients.' *Brain*, **98**, 427–440.

Peters, A.C.B., Brouwer, O.F., van Donselaar, C.A., *et al.* (1995) 'The Dutch study of epilepsy in childhood: early discontinuation.' *Epilepsia*, **36**, Suppl. 3, 29. *(Abstract.)*

Phillips, H.A., Scheffer, I.E., Berkovic, S.F., *et al.* (1995) 'Localization of a gene for autosomal dominant nocturnal frontal lobe epilepsy to chromosome 20q13.2.' *Nature Genetics*, **10**, 117–118.

Phillipps, S.A., Shanahan, R.J. (1989) 'Etiology and mortality of status epilepticus in children. A recent update.' *Archives of Neurology*, **46**, 74–76.

Pietz, J., Benninger, C., Schäfer, H., *et al.* (1993) 'Treatment of infantile spasms with high-dosage vitamin B_6.' *Epilepsia*, **34**, 757–763.

Pippenger, C.E. (1987) 'Clinically significant carbamazepine drug interactions: an overview.' *Epilepsia*, **28**, Suppl. 3, S71–S76.

Plouin, P. (1994) 'Benign idiopathic neonatal convulsions (familial and non-familial). Open questions about these syndromes.' *In:* Wolf, P. (Ed.) *Epileptic Seizures and Syndromes.* London: John Libbey, pp. 193–202.

—— Dulac, O. (1994) 'Other types of seizures.' *In:* Dulac, O., Chugani, H.T., Dalla Bernardina, B. (Eds.) *Infantile Spasms and West Syndrome.* Philadelphia: W.B. Saunders, pp. 52–62.

Polkey, C.E. (1989) 'Surgery for epilepsy.' *Archives of Disease in Childhood*, **64**, 185–187.

Porter, R.J., Penry, J.K. (1983) 'Petit mal status.' *In:* Delgado-Escueta, A.V., Wasterlain, C.G., Treiman, D.M., Porter, R.J. (Eds.) *Advances in Neurology. Vol. 34. Status Epilepticus.* New York: Raven Press, pp. 61–67.

Prasad, A.N., Stafstrom, C.F., Holmes, G.H. (1996) 'Alternative epilepsy therapies: the ketogenic diet, immunogloblins, and steroids.' *Epilepsia*, **37**, Suppl. 1, S81–S95.

Prats, J.M., Garaizar, C., Rua, M.J., *et al.* (1991) 'Infantile spasms treated with high doses of sodium valproate: initial response and follow-up.' *Developmental Medicine and Child Neurology*, **33**, 617–625.

Radvanyi-Bouvet, M.F., Vallecalle, M.H., Morel-Kahn, F., *et al.* (1985) 'Seizures and electrical discharges in premature infants.' *Neuropediatrics*, **16**, 143–148.

Rasmussen, T., Andermann, F. (1989) 'Update on the syndrome of "chronic encephalitis" and epilepsy.' *Cleveland Clinic Journal of Medicine*, **56** (Suppl.), S181–S184.

Raymond, A.A., Fish, D.R., Stevens, J.M., *et al.* (1994a) 'Association of hippocampal sclerosis with cortical dysgenesis in patients with epilepsy.' *Neurology*, **44**, 1841–1845.

—— —— —— *et al.* (1994b) 'Subependymal heterotopia: a distinct neuronal migration disorder associated with epilepsy.' *Journal of Neurology, Neurosurgery, and Psychiatry*, **57**, 1195–1202.

—— —— Sisokiya, S., Alsanjari, N., *et al.* (1995) 'Abnormalities of gyration, heterotopias, tuberous sclerosis, focal cortical dysplasia, microdysgenesis, dysembryoplastic neuroepithelial tumour and dysgenesis of the archicortex in epilepsy. Clinical, EEG and neuroimaging features in 100 adult patients.' *Brain*, **118**, 629–660.

Renier, W.O. (1988) 'Neuromorphological and biochemical analysis of a brain biopsy in a second case of idiopathic Lennox–Gastaut syndrome.' *In:* Niedermeyer, E., Degen, R. (Eds.) *The Lennox–Gastaut Syndrome.* New York: Alan R. Liss, pp. 427–432.

Renkawek, K., Renier, W.O., De Pont, J.J.H.M., *et al.* (1992) 'Neonatal status convulsions, spongiform encephalopathy and low activity of Na⁺/K⁺ ATPase in the brain.' *Epilepsia*, **33**, 58–64.

Reutens, D.C., Bye, A.M., Hopkins, I.J., *et al.* (1993) 'Corpus callosotomy for intractable epilepsy: seizure outcome and prognostic factors.' *Epilepsia*, **34**, 904–909.

Revol, M. (1992) 'Non idiopathic partial epilepsies and epileptic syndromes in childhood.' *In:* Roger, J., Bureau, M., Dravet, C., *et al.* (Eds.) *Epileptic Syndromes in Infancy, Childhood and Adolescence. 2nd Edn.* London: John Libbey, pp. 347–362.

Ricci, S., Cusmai, R., Fariello, G., *et al.* (1992) 'Double cortex. A neuronal migration anomaly as a possible cause of Lennox–Gastaut syndrome.' *Archives of Neurology*, **49**, 61–64.

—— —— Fusco, L., Vigevano, F. (1995) 'Reflex myoclonic epilepsy in infancy: a new age-dependent idiopathic epileptic syndrome related to startle reaction.' *Epilepsia*, **36**, 342–348.

Rich, S.S., Annegers, J.F., Hauser, W.A., Anderson, V.E. (1987) 'Complex segregation analysis of febrile convulsions.' *American Journal of Human Genetics*, **41**, 249–257.

Richens, A. (1982) 'Clinical pharmacology and medical treatment.' *In:* Laidlaw, J., Richens, A. (Eds.) *A Textbook of Epilepsy, 2nd Edn.* Edinburgh: Churchill Livingstone, pp. 292–348.

—— Yuen, A.W.C. (1991) 'Overview of the clinical efficacy of lamotrigine.' *Epilepsia*, **32**, Suppl. 2, S13–S16.

—— Davidson, D.L.W., Cartlidge, N.E.F., *et al.* (1994) 'A multicentre comparative trial of sodium valproate and carbamazepine in adult onset epilepsy.' *Journal of Neurology, Neurosurgery, and Psychiatry*, **57**, 682–687.

Riela, A.R., Penry, J.K. (1991) 'Magnetic resonance imaging.' *In:* Dam, M., Gram, L. (Eds.) *Comprehensive Epileptology.* New York: Raven Press, pp. 359–374.

Riikonen, R. (1982) 'A long-term follow-up study of 214 children with the syndrome of infantile spasms.' *Neuropediatrics*, **13**, 14–23.

—— (1993) 'Infantile spasms: infectious disorders.' *Neuropediatrics*, **24**, 274–280.

—— Amnell, G. (1981) 'Psychiatric disorders in children with earlier infantile spasms.' *Developmental Medicine and Child Neurology*, **23**, 747–760.

—— Donner, M. (1980) 'ACTH therapy in infantile spasms: side-effects.' *Archives of Disease in Childhood*, **55**, 664–672.

Ring, H.A., Heller, A.J., Farr, I.N., Reynolds, E.H. (1990) 'Vigabatrin: rational treatment for chronic epilepsy.' *Journal of Neurology, Neurosurgery, and Psychiatry*, **53**, 1051–1055.

Rintahaka, P.J., Chugani, H.T., Sankar, R. (1995) 'Landau–Kleffner syndrome with continuous spikes and waves during slow-wave sleep.' *Journal of Child Neurology*, **10**, 127–133.

Ritter, F.J., and the Felbamate Study Group in Lennox–Gastaut Syndrome (1993) 'Efficacy of felbamate in childhood epileptic encephalopathy (Lennox–Gastaut syndrome).' *New England Journal of Medicine*, **328**, 29–33.

Robain, O., Vinters, H.V. (1994) 'Neuropathologic studies.' *In:* Dulac, O., Chugani, H.T., Dalla Bernardina, B. (Eds.) *Infantile Spasms and West Syndrome.* Philadelphia: W.B. Saunders, pp. 99–117.

Rocca, W.A., Sharbrough, F.W., Hauser, W.A., *et al.* (1987) 'Risk factors for complex partial seizures: a population-based case–control study.' *Annals of Neurology*, **21**, 22–31.

Rodin, E.A., Schmaltz, S., Twitty, G. (1986) 'Intellectual functions of patients with childhood-onset epilepsy.' *Developmental Medicine and Child Neurology*, **28**, 25–33.

Roger, J., Gambarelli-Dubois, D. (1988) 'Neuropathological studies of the Lennox–Gastaut syndrome.' *In:* Niedermeyer, E., Degen, R. (Eds.) *The Lennox–Gastaut Syndrome.* New York: Alan R. Liss, pp. 73–93.

—— Bureau, M., Genton, P., Dravet, C. (1991) 'Idiopathic partial epilepsies.' *In:* Dam, M., Gram, L. (Eds.) *Comprehensive Epileptology.* New York: Raven Press, pp. 155–170.

Ronen, G.M., Rosales, T.O., Connolly, M., *et al.* (1993) 'Seizure characteristics in chromosome 20 benign familial neonatal convulsions.' *Neurology*, **43**, 1355–1360.

Rosman, N.P., Colton, T., Labazzo, J., *et al.* (1993) 'A controlled trial of diazepam administered during febrile illnesses to prevent recurrence of febrile seizures.' *New England Journal of Medicine*, **329**, 79–84.

Roos, R.A.C., Van Dijk, J.G. (1988) 'Reflex-epilepsy induced by immersion in hot water: case report and review of the literature.' *European Neurology*, **28**, 6–10.

Ross, E.M., Peckham, C.S. (1983) 'Seizure disorder in the National Child Development Study.' *In:* Rose, F.C. (Ed.) *Research Progress in Epilepsy.* London: Pitman, pp. 46–59.

—— West, P.B., Butler, N.R. (1980) 'Epilepsy in childhood: findings from the National Child Development Study.' *British Medical Journal*, **1**, 207–210.

Roulet, E., Deonna, T., Despland, P.A. (1989) 'Prolonged intermittent drooling and oromotor dyspraxia in benign childhood epilepsy with centrotemporal spikes.' *Epilepsia*, **30**, 564–568.

—— —— Gaillard, F., *et al.* (1991) 'Acquired aphasia, dementia, and behavior disorder with epilepsy and continuous spike and waves during sleep in a child.' *Epilepsia*, **32**, 495–503.

Rowan, A.J., Binnie, C.D., Warfield, C.A., *et al.* (1979) 'The delayed effect of sodium valproate on the photoconvulsive response in man.' *Epilepsia*, **20**, 61–68.

Ruggieri, J., Caraballo, R., Fejerman, N. (1989) 'Intracranial tumors and West syndrome.' *Pediatric Neurology*, **5**, 327–329.

Rugtveit, J. (1986) 'X-linked mental retardation and infantile spasms in two brothers.' *Developmental Medicine and Child Neurology*, **28**, 544–546. *(Letter.)*

Ryan, S.G., Wiznitzer, M., Hollman, C., *et al.* (1991) 'Benign familial neonatal convulsions: evidence for clinical and genetic heterogeneity.' *Annals of Neurology*, **29**, 469–473.

Sagar, H.J., Oxbury, J.M. (1987) 'Hippocampal neuron loss in temporal lobe epilepsy: correlation with early childhood convulsions.' *Annals of Neurology*, **22**, 334–340.

Saenz-Lope, E., Herranz, F.J., Masdeu, J.C. (1984) 'Startle epilepsy: a clinical study.' *Annals of Neurology*, **16**, 78–81.

Salanova, V., Morris, H.H., Van Ness, P., *et al.* (1995) 'Frontal lobe seizures: electroclinical syndromes.' *Epilepsia*, **36**, 16–24.

Salonen, R., Somer, M., Haltia, M., *et al.* (1991) 'Progressive encephalopathy with edema, hypsarrhythmia, and optic atrophy (PEHO syndrome).' *Clinical Genetics*, **39**, 287–293.

Sammaritano, M., Andermann, F., Melanson, D., *et al.* (1985) 'Prolonged focal cerebral edema associated with partial status epilepticus.' *Epilepsia*, **26**, 334–339.

Sander, J.W.A.S. (1993) 'Some aspects of prognosis in the epilepsies: a review.' *Epilepsia*, **34**, 1007–1016.

Santanelli, P., Bureau, M., Magaudda, A., *et al.* (1989) 'Benign partial epilepsy with centrotemporal (or rolandic) spikes and brain lesion.' *Epilepsia*, **30**, 182–188.

Santorelli, F.M., Shanske, S., Macaya, A., *et al.* (1993) 'The mutation at nt 8993 of mitochondrial DNA is a common cause of Leigh's syndrome.' *Annals of Neurology*, **34**, 827–834.

Sawhney, I.M.S., Robertson, I.J.A., Polkey, C.E., *et al.* (1995) 'Multiple subpial transection: a review of 21 cases.' *Journal of Neurology, Neurosurgery, and Psychiatry*, **58**, 344–349.

Scheffer, I.E., Berkovic, S.F. (1997) 'Generalized epilepsy with febrile seizures plus. A genetic disorder with heterogeneous clinical phenotypes.' *Brain*, **120**, 479–501.

—— Bhatia, K.P., Lopes-Cendes, I., *et al.* (1995a) 'Autosomal dominant nocturnal frontal lobe epilepsy. A distinctive clinical disorder.' *Brain*, **118**, 61–73.

—— Jones, L., Pozzebon, M., *et al.* (1995b) 'Autosomal dominant rolandic epilepsy and speech dyspraxia: a new syndrome with anticipation.' *Annals of Neurology*, **38**, 633–642.

—— Phillips, H., Mulley, J., *et al.* (1995c) 'Autosomal dominant partial epilepsy with variable foci is not allelic with autosomal dominant nocturnal frontal lobe epilepsy.' *Epilepsia*, **36**, Suppl. 3, S28. *(Abstract.)*

Scher, M.S., Beggarly, M. (1989) 'Clinical significance of focal periodic discharges in neonates.' *Journal of Child Neurology*, **4**, 175–185.

—— Painter, M.J. (1990) 'Electroencephalographic diagnosis of neonatal seizures: issues of diagnostic accuracy, clinical correlation and survival.' *In:* Wasterlain, C.G., Vert, P. (Eds.) *Neonatal Seizures.* New York: Raven Press, pp. 15–25.

—— Aso, K., Beggarly, M.E., *et al.* (1993a) 'Electrographic seizures in preterm and full-term neonates: clinical correlates, associated brain lesions, and risk for neurologic sequelae.' *Pediatrics*, **91**, 128–134.

—— Hamid, M.Y., Steppe, D.A., *et al.* (1993b) 'Ictal and interictal electrographic seizure durations in preterm and term neonates.' *Epilepsia*, **34**, 284–288.

Scheyer, R.D., During, M.J., Spencer, D.D., *et al.* (1994) 'Measurement of carbamazepine and carbamazepine epoxide in the human brain using in vivo microdialysis.' *Neurology*, **44**, 1469–1472.

Schiffman, R., Shapira, Y., Ryan, S.G. (1991) 'An autosomal recessive form of benign familial neonatal seizures.' *Clinical Genetics*, **40**, 467–470.

Schlumberger, E., Dulac, O. (1994) 'A simple, effective and well-tolerated treatment regime for West syndrome.' *Developmental Medicine and Child Neurology*, **36**, 863–872.

—— Chavez, F., Palacios, L., *et al.* (1994) 'Lamotrigine in treatment of 120 children with epilepsy.' *Epilepsia*, **35**, 359–367.

Schmidt, D. (1986a) 'Diagnostic and therapeutic management of intractable epilepsy.' *In:* Schmidt, D., Morselli, P.L. (Eds.) *Intractable Epilepsy: Experimental and Clinical Aspects.* New York: Raven Press, pp. 237–257.

—— (1986b) 'Toxicity of anti-epileptic drugs.' *In:* Pedley, T.A., Meldrum, B.S. (Eds.) *Recent Advances in Epilepsy, Vol. 3.* Edinburgh: Churchill Livingstone, pp. 211–232.

Schwartz, R.H., Boyes, S., Ainsley-Green, A. (1989a) 'Metabolic effects of three ketogenic diets in the treatment of severe epilepsy.' *Developmental Medicine and Child Neurology*, **31**, 152–160.

—— Eaton, J., Bower, B.D., Aynsley-Green, A. (1989b) 'Ketogenic diets in the treatment of epilepsy: short-term clinical effects.' *Developmental Medicine and Child Neurology*, **31**, 145–151.

Schwartzkroin, P.A. (1994) 'Cellular electrophysiology of human epilepsy.' *Epilepsy Research*, **17**, 185–192.

Seidenberg, M., Beck, N., Geisser, M., *et al.* (1986) 'Academic achievement of children with epilepsy.' *Epilepsia*, **27**, 753–759.

Serratosa, J.M., Delgado-Escueta, A.V., Medina, M.T., *et al.* (1996) 'Clinical and genetic analysis of a large pedigree with juvenile myoclonic epilepsy.' *Annals of Neurology*, **39**, 187–195.

Shewmon, D.A. (1994) 'Ictal aspects with emphasis on unusual variants.' *In:* Dulac, O., Chugani, H.T., Dalla Bernardina, B. (Eds.) *Infantile Spasms and West Syndrome.* Philadelphia: W.B. Saunders, pp. 36–51.

Shields, W.D., Shewmon, D.A., Chugani, H.T., Peacock, W.J. (1992) 'Treatment of infantile spasms: medical or surgical?' *Epilepsia*, **33**, Suppl. 4, S26–S31.

Shinnar, S., Berg, A.T. (1996) 'Does antiepileptic drug therapy prevent the development of "chronic epilepsy"?' *Epilepsia*, **37**, 701–708.

—— —— Moshé, S.L., *et al.* (1990) 'Risk of recurrence following a first unprovoked seizure in childhood: a prospective study.' *Pediatrics*, **85**, 1076–1085.

—— Maytal, J., Krasnoff, L., Moshé, S.L. (1992) 'Recurrent status epilepticus in children.' *Annals of Neurology*, **31**, 598–604.

—— Berg, A.T., Moshé, S.L., *et al.* (1994) 'Discontinuing antiepileptic drugs in children with epilepsy: a prospective study.' *Annals of Neurology*, **35**, 534–545.

—— —— —— *et al.* (1996) 'The risk of seizure recurrence after a first unprovoked afebrile seizure in childhood: an extended follow-up.' *Pediatrics*, **98**, 216–225.

Shorvon, S. (1994) *Status Epilepticus: its Clinical Features and Treatment in Children and Adults.* Cambridge: Cambridge University Press.

Siemes, H., Spohr, H.L., Michael, T., Nau, H. (1988) 'Therapy of infantile spasms with valproate: results of a prospective study.' *Epilepsia*, **29**, 553–560.

Sillanpää, M. (1990) 'Children with epilepsy as adults: outcome after 30 years of follow-up.' *Acta Paediatrica Scandinavica*, Suppl. 368, 1–78.

—— (1992) 'Epilepsy in children: prevalence, disability, and handicap.' *Epilepsia*, **33**, 444–449.

—— (1993) 'Remission of seizures and predictors of intractability in long-term follow-up.' *Epilepsia*, **34**, 930–936.

Sisodiya, S.M., Free, S.L., Stevens, J.M., *et al.* (1995) 'Widespread cerebral structural changes in patients with cortical dysgenesis and epilepsy.' *Brain*, **118**, 1039–1050.

Smaje, J.C., Davidson, C., Teasdale, G.M. (1987) 'Sino-atrial arrest due to temporal lobe epilepsy.' *Journal of Neurology, Neurosurgery, and Psychiatry*, **50**, 112–113.

Snead, O.C. (1995) 'Basic mechanisms of generalized absence seizures.' *Annals of Neurology*, **37**, 146–157.

—— Chiron, C. (1994) 'Medical treatment.' *In:* Dulac, O. Chugani, H.T., Dalla Bernardina, B. (Eds.) *Infantile Spasms and West Syndrome.* London: W.B. Saunders, pp. 244–256.

Sofijanov, N., Emoto, S., Kuturec, M., *et al.* (1992) 'Febrile seizures: clinical characteristics and initial EEG.' *Epilepsia*, **33**, 52–57.

Somer, M., Sainio, K. (1993) 'Epilepsy and the electroencephalogram in progressive encephalopathy with edema, hypsarrhythmia and optic atrophy (the PEHO syndrome).' *Epilepsia*, **34**, 727–731.

Southall, D.P., Stebbens, V., Abraham, N., Abraham, L. (1987) 'Prolonged apnoea with severe arterial hypoxaemia resulting from complex partial seizures.' *Developmental Medicine and Child Neurology*, **29**, 784–789.

Spencer, S.S. (1988) 'Corpus callostomy in the treatment of intractable seizures.' *In:* Pedley, T.A., Meldrum, B.S. (Eds.) *Recent Advances in Epilepsy, No. 4.* Edinburgh: Churchill Livingstone, pp. 181–204.

Sperling, M.R., Liporace, J.D., French, J.A., *et al.* (1995) 'Epilepsy surgery and mortality from epilepsy.' *Epilepsia*, **36**, Suppl. 4, 140. *(Abstract.)*

Stafstrom, C.E., Konkol, R.J. (1994) 'Infantile spasms in children with Down syndrome.' *Developmental Medicine and Child Neurology*, **36**, 576–585.

Stefan, H., Schneider, S., Abraham-Fuchs, K., *et al.* (1990) 'Magnetic source localization in focal epilepsy. Multichannel magnetoencephalography correlated with magnetic resonance brain imaging.' *Brain*, **113**, 1347–1359.

Steinhoff, B.J., Kruse, R. (1992) 'Bromide treatment of pharmaco-resistant epilepsies with general tonic–clonic seizures: a clinical study.' *Brain and Development*, **14**, 144–149.

Steinlein, O.K., Mulley, J.C., Propping, P., *et al.* (1995) 'A missense mutation in the neuronal nicotinic acetylcholine receptor α4 subunit is associated with autosomal dominant nocturnal frontal lobe epilepsy.' *Nature Genetics*, **11**, 201–203.

Stephenson, J.B.P. (1990) *Fits and Faints. Clinics in Developmental Medicine No. 109.* London: Mac Keith Press.

—— King, M.D. (1989) *Handbook of Neurological Investigations in Children.* London: Butterworth.

Stibler, H., Westerberg, B. Hanefeld, F., Hagberg, B. (1993) 'Carbohydrate-deficient glycoprotein (CDG) syndrome—a new variant, type III.' *Neuropediatrics*, **24**, 51–52.

Stores, G., Zaiwalla, Z., Bergel, N. (1991) 'Frontal lobe complex partial seizures in children: a form of epilepsy at particular risk of misdiagnosis.' *Developmental Medicine and Child Neurology*, **33**, 998–1009.

Sutula, T., Cascino, G., Cavazos, J., *et al.* (1989) 'Mossy fiber synaptic re-organization in the epileptic human temporal lobe.' *Annals of Neurology*, **26**, 321–330.

Suzuki, Y., Cox, S., Hayes, J., Walson, P.D. (1991) 'Carbamazepine age–dose ratio relationship in children.' *Therapeutic Drug Monitoring*, **13**, 201–208.

Tahvanainen, E., Ranta, S., Hirvasmiemi, A., *et al.* (1994) 'The gene for a recessively inherited human childhood progressive epilepsy with mental retardation maps to the distal arm of chromosome 8.' *Proceedings of the National Academy of Sciences of the USA*, **91**, 7267–7270.

Talwar, D. (1990) 'Mechanisms of antiepileptic drug action.' *Pediatric Neurology*, **6**, 289–295.

Tassinari, C.A., Bureau, M., Dravet, C., *et al.* (1992) 'Epilepsy with continuous spikes and waves during slow sleep—otherwise described as ESES (epilepsy with electrical status epilepticus during slow sleep).' *In:* Roger, J., Bureau, M., Dravet, C., *et al.* (Eds.) *Epileptic Syndromes in Infancy, Childhood and Adolescence. 2nd Edn.* London: John Libbey, pp. 245–256.

—— Michelucci, R., Rubboli, G., *et al.* (1995) 'Myoclonic absence epilepsy.' *In:* Ducan, J.S., Panayiotopoulos, C.P. (Eds.) *Typical Absences and Related Epileptic Syndromes.* London: Churchill Communications Europe, pp. 187–195.

Tennison, M., Greenwood, R., Lewis, D., Thorn, M. (1994) 'Discontinuing antiepileptic drugs in children with epilepsy. A comparison of a six-week and a nine-month taper period.' *New England Journal of Medicine*, **330**, 1407–1410.

Tharp, B.R. (1981) 'Neonatal and pediatric electroencephalography.' *In:* Aminoff, M.J. (Ed.) *Electrodiagnosis in Clinical Neurology.* Edinburgh: Churchill Livingstone, pp. 67–117.

Theodore, W.H., Rose, D., Patronas, N., *et al.* (1987) 'Cerebral glucose metabolism in the Lennox–Gastaut syndrome.' *Annals of Neurology*, **21**, 14–21.

—— Sato, S., Kufta, C., *et al.* (1992) 'Temporal lobectomy for uncontrolled seizures: the role of positron emission tomography.' *Annals of Neurology*, **32**, 789–794.

—— Porter, R.J., Albert, P., *et al.* (1994) 'The secondarily generalized tonic–clonic seizure: a videotape analysis.' *Neurology*, **44**, 1403–1407.

Thurston, S.E., Leigh, R.J., Osorio, I. (1985) 'Epileptic gaze deviation and nystagmus.' *Neurology*, **35**, 1518–1521.

Tiacci, C., D'Alessandro, P., Cantisani, T.A., *et al.* (1993) 'Epilepsy with bilateral occipital calcifications: Sturge–Weber variant or a different encephalopathy?' *Epilepsia*, **34**, 528–539.

Tinuper, P., Aguglia, V., Laudadio, S., Gastaut, H. (1987) 'Prolonged ictal paralysis: electroencephalographic confirmation of its epileptic nature.' *Clinical Electroencephalography*, **18**, 12–14.

Toti, P., Balestri, P., Cano, M., *et al.* (1996) 'Celiac disease with cerebral calcium and silica deposits.' *Neurology*, **46**, 1088–1092.

Treiman, D.M. (1993) 'Generalized convulsive status epilepticus in the adult.' *Epilepsia*, **34**, Suppl. 1, S2–S11.

Trevathan, E., Cascino, G.D. (1988) 'Partial epilepsy presenting as focal paroxysmal pain.' *Neurology*, **38**, 329–330.

Uhari, M., Rantala, H., Vainionpää, L., Kurttila, R. (1995) 'Effect of acetaminophen and of low intermittent doses of diazepam on prevention of recurrences of febrile seizures.' *Journal of Pediatrics*, **126**, 991–995.

van Bogaert, P., Chiron, C., Adamsbaum, C., *et al.* (1993) 'Value of magnetic resonance imaging in West syndrome of unknown etiology.' *Epilepsia*, **34**, 701–706.

Van den Bergh, B.J., Yerushalmy, J. (1969) 'Studies on convulsive disorders in young children. I. Incidence of febrile and nonfebrile convulsions by age and other factors.' *Pediatric Research*, **3**, 298–304.

Van Esch, A., Ramlal, R.I., van Steesel-Moll, H.A., *et al.* (1996) 'Outcome after febrile status epilepticus.' *Developmental Medicine and Child Neurology*, **38**, 19–24.

Varga-Khadem, F., Isaacs, E., van der Werf, S., *et al.* (1992) 'Development of intelligence and memory in children with hemiplegic cerebral palsy. The deleterious consequences of early seizures.' *Brain*, **115**, 315–329.

Verity, C.M., Ross, E.M., Golding, J. (1993) 'Outcome of childhood status epilepticus and lengthy febrile convulsions: findings of national cohort study.' *British Medical Journal*, **307**, 225–228.

—— Hosking, G., Easter, D.J., on behalf of the Paediatric EPITEG Collaborative Group (1995) 'A multicentre comparative trial of sodium valproate and carbamazepine in paediatric epilepsy.' *Developmental Medicine and Child Neurology*, **37**, 97–108.

Viani, F., Beghi, E., Romeo, A., van Lierde, A. (1987) 'Infantile febrile status epilepticus: risk factors and outcome.' *Developmental Medicine and Child Neurology*, **29**, 495–501.

Viberg, M., Blennow, G., Polski, B. (1987) 'Epilepsy in adolescence: implications for the development of personality.' *Epilepsia*, **28**, 542–546.

Vigevano, F., Cilio, M.R. (1997) 'Vigabatrin versus ACTH as first-line treatment for infantile spasms: a randomized prospective study.' *Epilepsia*, **38**, 270–274.

—— Di Rocco, C. (1990) 'Effectiveness of hemispherectomy in hemimegalencephaly with intractable seizures.' *Neuropediatrics*, **21**, 222–223.

—— Fusco, L. (1993) 'Hypnic tonic postural seizures in healthy children provide evidence for a partial epileptic syndrome of frontal origin.' *Epilepsia*, **34**, 110–119.

—— —— Di Capua, M., *et al.* (1992) 'Benign infantile familial convulsions.' *European Journal of Pediatrics*, **151**, 608–612.

—— —— Cusmai, R., *et al.* (1993) 'The idiopathic form of West syndrome.' *Epilepsia*, **34**, 743–746.

—— —— Ricci, S., *et al.* (1994a) 'Dysplasias.' *In:* Dulac, O., Chugani, H.T., Dalla Bernardina, B. (Eds.) *Infantile Spasms and West Syndrome*. London: W.B. Saunders, pp. 178–191.

—— Santanelli, R., Fusco, L., *et al.* (1994b) 'Benign infantile familial convulsions.' *In:* Malafosse, A., Genton, P., Hirsch, E., *et al.* (Eds.) *Idiopathic Generalized Epilepsies: Clinical, Experimental and Genetic Aspects*. London: John Libbey, pp. 45–49.

Vining, E.P.G., Freeman, J.M., Brandt, J., *et al.* (1993) 'Progressive unilateral encephalopathy of childhood (Rasmussen's syndrome): a reappraisal.' *Epilepsia*, **34**, 639–650.

—— —— Pillas, D.J., *et al.* (1997) 'Why would you remove half a brain? The outcome of 58 children after hemispherectomy. The Johns Hopkins experience: 1968 to 1996.' *Pediatrics*, **100**, 163–171.

Vinters, H.V., Wasterlain, C.G. (1996) 'Pathology of childhood epilepsy.' *In:* Wallace, S.J. (Ed.) *Epilepsy in Children*. London: Chapman & Hall, pp. 87–107.

Volpe, J.J. (1989) 'Neonatal seizures: current concepts and classification.' *Pediatrics*, **84**, 422–428.

Wallace, S.J. (1988) *The Child with Febrile Seizures*. Guildford: Butterworth.

—— (1990) 'Anti-epileptic drug monitoring: an overview.' *Developmental Medicine and Child Neurology*, **32**, 923–926.

—— (1991) 'Epileptic syndromes linked with previous history of febrile seizures.' *In:* Fukuyama, Y., Kamoshita, S., Ohtsuka, C., Suzuki, Y. (Eds.) *Modern Perspectives of Child Neurology*. Tokyo: Japanese Society of Child Neurology, pp. 175–181.

Walther, B., Schmitt, T., Reiter, B. (1987) 'Identification of infants at risk for infantile spasms by neonatal polygraphy.' *Brain and Development*, **9**, 377–390.

Watanabe, K. (1996) 'Recent advances and some problems in the delineation of epileptic syndromes in children.' *Brain and Development*, **18**, 423–437.

—— Hara, K., Miyazaki, S., *et al.* (1982a) 'Apneic seizures in the newborn.' *American Journal of Diseases of Children*, **136**, 980–984.

—— Kuroyanagi, M., Hara, K., Miyazaki, S. (1982b) 'Neonatal seizures and subsequent epilepsy.' *Brain and Development*, **4**, 341–346.

—— Takeuchi, T., Hakamada, S., Hayakawa, F. (1987a) 'Neurophysiological and neuroradiological features preceding infantile spasms.' *Brain and Development*, **9**, 391–398.

—— Yamamoto, N., Negoro, T., *et al.* (1987b) 'Benign complex partial epilepsies in infancy.' *Pediatric Neurology*, **3**, 208–211.

—— Yamamoto, N., Negoro, T., *et al.* (1990) 'Benign infantile epilepsy with complex partial seizures.' *Journal of Clinical Neurophysiology*, **7**, 409–416.

—— Negoro, T., Aso, K. (1993) 'Benign partial epilepsy with secondary generalized seizures in infancy.' *Epilepsia*, **34**, 635–638.

—— —— *et al.* (1994) 'Clinical, EEG and positron emission tomography features of childhood onset epilepsy with localized cortical dysplasia detected by magnetic resonance imaging.' *Journal of Epilepsy*, **7**, 108–116.

Watanabe, M., Fujiwara, T., Terauchi, N., *et al.* (1989) 'Intractable grand mal epilepsy developed in the first year of life.' *In: Advances in Epileptology, Vol. 17. The XVIIth Epilepsy International Symposium*. New York: Raven Press, pp. 327–329.

Weglage, J., Demsky, A., Pietsch, M., Kurlemann, G. (1997) 'Neuropsychological, intellectual, and behavioral findings in patients with centrotemporal spikes with and without seizures.' *Developmental Medicine and Child Neurology*, **39**, 646–651.

Whitehouse, W.P., Rees, M., Curtis, D., *et al.* (1993) 'Linkage analysis of idiopathic generalized epilepsy (IGE) and marker loci on chromosome 6p in families of patients with juvenile myoclonic epilepsy: no evidence for an epilepsy locus in the HLA region.' *American Journal of Human Genetics*, **53**, 652–662.

Wieser, H.G., Elger, C.E. (Eds.) (1987) *Presurgical Evaluation of Epileptics*. Berlin: Springer Verlag.

—— Kausel, W. (1987) 'Limbic seizures.' *In:* Wieser, H.G., Elger, C.E. (Eds.) *Presurgical Evaluation of Epileptics*. Berlin: Springer Verlag, pp. 227–248.

—— Müller, R.V. (1987) 'Neocortical temporal seizures.' *In:* Wieser, H.G., Elger, C.E. (Eds.) *Presurgical Evaluation of Epileptics*. Berlin: Springer Verlag, pp. 252–266.

—— Engel, J., Williamson, P.D., *et al.* (1993) 'Surgically remediable temporal lobe syndromes.' *In:* Engel, J. (Ed.) *Surgical Treatment of the Epilepsies, 2nd Edn.* New York: Raven Press, pp. 49–63.

Wilkins, A., Lindsay, J. (1985) 'Common forms of reflex epilepsy: physiological mechanisms and techniques for treatment.' *In:* Pedley, T.A., Meldrum, B.S. (Eds.) *Recent Advances in Epilepsy, Vol. 2.* Edinburgh: Churchill Livingstone, pp. 239–271.

Williamson, P.D., French, J.A., Thadani, V.M., *et al.* (1993a) 'Characteristics of medial temporal lobe epilepsy: II. Interictal and ictal scalp electroencephalography, neuropsychological testing, neuroimaging, surgical results and pathology.' *Annals of Neurology*, **34**, 781–787.

—— Spencer, D.D., Spencer, S.S., *et al.* (1993b) 'Complex partial seizures of frontal lobe origin.' *Annals of Neurology*, **18**, 497–504.

Wirrel, E.C., Camfield, P.R., Gordon, K.E., *et al.* (1995) 'Benign rolandic epilepsy: atypical features are very common.' *Journal of Child Neurology*, **10**, 455–458.

Wolf, P. (1994) 'Reading epilepsy.' *In:* Wolf, P. (Ed.) *Epileptic Seizures and Syndromes*. London: John Libbey, pp. 67–73.

Wolf, S.M., Carr, A., Davis, D.C., *et al.* (1977) 'The value of phenobarbital in the child who has had a single febrile seizure: a controlled prospective study.' *Pediatrics*, **59**, 378–385.

Woo, E., Chan, Y.M., Yu, Y.L., *et al.* (1988) 'If a well stabilized epileptic patient has a subtherapeutic antiepileptic drug level, should the dose be increased? A randomized prospective study.' *Epilepsia*, **29**, 129–139.

Woody, R.C., Yamauchi, T., Bolyard, K. (1988) 'Cerebrospinal fluid cell counts in childhood idiopathic status epilepticus.' *Pediatric Infectious Disease Journal*, **7**, 298–299.

Wyllie, E. (1992) 'Invasive neurophysiologic techniques in the evaluation for epilepsy surgery in children.' *In:* Lüders, H. (Ed.) *Epilepsy Surgery.* New York: Raven Press, pp. 409–412.

—— Lüders, H., Morris, H.H., *et al.* (1986) 'The lateralizing significance of versive head and eye movements during epileptic seizures.' *Neurology*, **36**, 606–611.

—— Chee, M., Granström, M-L., *et al.* (1993) 'Temporal lobe epilepsy in early childhood.' *Epilepsia*, **34**, 859–868.

—— Baumgartner, C., Prayson, R., *et al.* (1994) 'The clinical spectrum of focal cortical dysplasia and epilepsy.' *Journal of Epilepsy*, **7**, 303–312.

Yaffe, K., Ferriero, D., Barkovich, A.J., Rowley, H. (1995) 'Reversible MRI abnormalities following seizures.' *Neurology*, **45**, 104–108.

Yaqub, B.A. (1993) 'Electroclinical seizures in Lennox–Gastaut syndrome.' *Epilepsia*, **34**, 120–127.

Young, G.B., Barr, H.W.K., Blume, W.T. (1986) 'Painful epileptic seizures involving the second sensory area.' *Annals of Neurology*, **19**, 412. *(Letter.)*

Zelnik, N., Nir, A., Amit, S., Iancu, T.C. (1990) 'Autonomic seizures in an infant: unusual cutaneous and cardiac manifestations.' *Developmental Medicine and Child Neurology*, **32**, 74–78.

17
PAROXYSMAL DISORDERS OTHER THAN EPILEPSY

Epilepsy is the most important of the paroxysmal neurological disorders of childhood but a host of other paroxysmal conditions are observed in children. Indeed, the diagnosis of epilepsy is often made wrongly in the presence of paroxysmal events. An incorrect diagnosis of epilepsy was made in 20–30 per cent of children referred to one epilepsy clinic (Jeavons 1983), in 27 of 124 children (22.1 per cent) reported by Desai and Talwar (1992), and in 10–20 per cent of children according to Metrick *et al.* (1991). Such figures reflect a common experience (Aicardi 1994). Because an incorrect label of epilepsy all too often has profound consequences on a child's life, such misdiagnoses must be avoided. The present chapter reviews the most common nonepileptic paroxysmal conditions that cause faints and other turns.

ANOXIC SEIZURES

So-called 'anoxic' seizures are due to cortical hypoxic failure of energy metabolism as a result of anoxia or hypoxia. They may occur in many circumstances: bradycardia of less than 40 beats per minute, tachycardia of more than 150 beats per minute, asystole of more than four seconds, systolic pressure of less than 50 mmHg or venous O_2 pressure of less than 20 mmHg (Adams and Martin 1983).

Cortical hypoxia results in loss of consciousness and of postural tone. When severe, liberation of tonigenic brainstem centres from corticoreticular inhibition causes decorticate rigidity and/or opisthotonus. Increasing degrees of cortical hypoxia produce slowing of frequency of the dominant cortical rhythms, followed by complete flattening of the EEG tracing, which corresponds to the tonic phase. With correction of hypoxia, slow waves reappear and may be synchronous with a few jerks of the limbs before resumption of normal EEG activity (Gastaut 1974, Stephenson 1990).

Anoxic seizures can be due to several different mechanisms (Table 17.1), several of which may be operative in the same patient or even in the same attack (Stephenson 1990).

REFLEX SYNCOPES AND FAINTS
A syncope is a sudden loss of consciousness and of postural tone associated with a cutting off of energy substrates to the brain usually through a decrease in cerebral perfusion by oxygenated blood, due to reduction in cerebral blood flow or to a drop of the oxygen content, or to a combination of both (Stephenson 1996). Low perfusion is usually the consequence of a cardioinhibitory mechanism mediated through the vagus nerve or of a vasodepressor mechanism with variable vagal accompaniment (vasovagal syncope). Rarely it results from primary cardiac events. In faints, the loss of consciousness is generally preceded by sensations of light-headedness, weakness, or a feeling of things going far away, and the loss of tone is progressive, the patient slowly slumping to the ground. Occasionally, the loss of posture is abrupt with a sudden fall. In such cases the tip of the tongue may be cut, though true tongue-biting with lateral laceration occurs only exceptionally (Stephenson 1990, Lempert *et al.* 1994). Urinary incontinence is not uncommon and does not indicate an epileptic mechanism. The diagnosis of syncope rests essentially on the circumstances of occurrence which include emotional stimuli or stress, a standing posture, especially in a confined atmosphere, or minor pain. In some individuals faints are regularly provoked by the same stimulus such as getting into or out of a bath (Stephenson 1990, Patel *et al.* 1994), combing one's hair (Lewis and Frank 1993) or stretching (Pelekanos *et al.* 1990). During the attack, the patient is pale, the eyes may be deviated vertically and the pulse may be slow. In some cases, a true epileptic attack can be induced by the hypoxia resulting from a syncope (Stephenson 1983, Aicardi *et al.* 1988, Battaglia *et al.* 1989). Such instances are termed anoxic–epileptic seizures by Stephenson (1990). Alternatively, cardiac arrhythmias can occasionally result from an epileptic discharge involving cardioregulatory efferents. Such a phenomenon (epileptic–anoxic seizure) may play a role in sudden death of epileptic patients (Oppenheimer *et al.* 1990, Stephenson 1990). The epileptic nature of such attacks may be difficult to diagnose. Many syncopes have an abrupt onset; clonic movements occur in perhaps 50 per cent of cases and incontinence in 10 per cent (Stephenson 1990). Syncopes can occur in the sitting and even in the supine position, and postictal confusion may be observed. Vasovagal syncopes are often familial in nature (Camfield and Camfield 1990, Cooper *et al.* 1994). Reassurance is usually sufficient therapy, and only for frequently repeated attacks is atropine treatment justified.

Syncopes may occur electively in *febrile children* and such accidents are apt to be mistaken for febrile convulsions. Stephenson (1980) has proposed that the oculocardiac reflex be tested in such cases and that reproduction of a fit identical to the patient's

TABLE 17.1
Possible mechanisms of anoxic seizures

Breath-holding with prolonged expiratory apnoea (Southall *et al.* 1985) and ventilatory/perfusion mismatch or intrapulmonary shunting (Southall *et al.* 1990) responsible for cyanosis

Obstructive apnoea especially awake apnoea associated with gastrointestinal reflux (Spitzer *et al.* 1984)

Suffocation
Self-suffocation or strangulation
Induction of anoxic seizure in an infant by an adult (Munchausen syndrome by proxy or Meadow syndrome)

Valsalva manoeuvre
May play a role in breath-holding
May be exclusive mechanism in some self-induced syncopes (Gastaut 1980)

Cardiac disease
Valvular (aortic stenosis)
Congenital cyanotic heart disease (Daniels *et al.* 1987)
Ventricular tachyarrhythmias
Sick sinus syndrome (Gordon 1994b)

Fainting and reflex anoxic seizures
May alternate with 'true' breath-holding

Other circulatory syncopes
Vagovagal syncope (Woody and Kiel 1986)
'Hypervagism' (Stephenson 1990)
Carotid sinus disorders

Brain compression
Chiari malformation (Stephenson 1990)
Brainstem tumours (Southall *et al.* 1987)

usual attack establishes the diagnosis. This method is not universally accepted as a strong oculocardiac reflex does not exclude the possibility of a febrile convulsion.

One reported cause of fainting and loss of consciousness is the use of niaprazine, an antihistaminic drug. Loss of consciousness is associated with hypotonia and pallor, is of brief duration and occurs within 30 minutes of absorption in most cases (Bodiou and Bavoux 1988). Severe cases are rare (Auduy 1988).

BREATH-HOLDING SPELLS
Breath-holding spells occur in about 4 per cent of all children below the age of 5 years. Two major types of breath-holding spells occur: the cyanotic and the pallid types (Lombroso and Lerman 1967). The mechanisms of the two forms are different and most 'pallid breath-holding attacks', such as occur when a child bumps her/his head and almost immediately loses consciousness, are best regarded as reflex hypoxic syncopes precipitated by painful stimuli or emotion (Stephenson 1980, 1990; Breningstall 1996).

Cyanotic breath-holding attacks are provoked by fright, pain, anger or frustration. The infant cries vigorously, then holds its breath in expiration. This results in cyanosis and eventually culminates in loss of consciousness and limpness. The latter is rarely followed by brief body stiffening before respiration resumes and the attack ends. Polygraphic recordings have shown a sequence of slowing of the EEG tracing with bradycardia such as one would expect in the overshoot phase of a Valsalva

manoeuvre. Despite their frightening appearance breath-holding spasms are harmless (Gordon 1987). The mechanism of cyanotic breath-holding spells is still imperfectly known (DiMario and Burleson 1993). Oxygen desaturation, and reduction of cerebral blood flow because of increased intrathoracic pressure with decreased venous return, play a role. However, cyanosis develops with surprising rapidity and an intrapulmonary right-to-left shunt seems likely as a result of imperfect matching of ventilation to perfusion (Breningstall 1996). Gastaut (1974) made the distinction between breath-holding spells and sobbing spasms or sobbing syncopes in which the child would 'sob intensely and intractably for a long period of time (1–3 minutes)' before losing consciousness.

Exceptional cases of breath-holding attacks resulting in death have been associated with severe underlying conditions (Southall *et al.* 1987, 1990). Such exceptions do not modify the benign prognosis of the condition.

Pallid breath-holding attacks may exist in isolation or alternate with the cyanotic form in the same child. They account for 19 per cent of cases (Lombroso and Lerman 1967). In this type, which is often precipitated by pain, especially from a bump on the head, the children lose consciousness following a minimum of crying or no crying at all. Pallor is marked and stiffening is the rule. In many such patients, the attack is associated with a period of asystole that can also be induced by compression of the eyeballs (Lombroso and Lerman 1967, Stephenson 1980). Urinary incontinence is not rare in this form. The mechanism is reflex cardioinhibition resulting in cardiac standstill with a consequent hypoxic attack. On the EEG tracings, the tonic attack is associated with flattening of the record that follows a run of slow waves. A few clonic jerks are not infrequently observed following the tonic attack (Fig. 17.1). Pallid breath-holding attacks are more frequently mistaken for epilepsy than the cyanotic forms. The diagnosis rests much more on the fact that all attacks are precipitated by an adequate stimulus than on the seizure description which is often indistinguishable by history from an epileptic seizure. Indeed, it is in this form that anoxic–epileptic seizures (Stephenson 1990, 1996) can occur. They are usually brief but prolonged seizures and even status epilepticus have occasionally been reported (Stephenson 1990, Emery 1990, Moorjani *et al.* 1995).

The outlook for this form is also favourable, and explanation and reassurance that the attacks produce no harm and will cease is often followed by a marked diminution of their frequency. Rarely is psychiatric help needed and no drug treatment is necessary or effective (Gordon 1987).

UNUSUAL TYPES OF REFLEX SYNCOPES
Self-induced reflex syncopes are rare but may pose difficult diagnostic problems. Such attacks are seen in retarded psychotic patients (Gastaut 1980, Gastaut *et al.* 1987) and are usually mistaken for absences or drop-attacks. The children stop breathing and inflate their chest or abdomen, producing a Valsalva manoeuvre. After a few seconds, they turn pale with a vacant look and a loss of tone which may be limited to the neck or involve

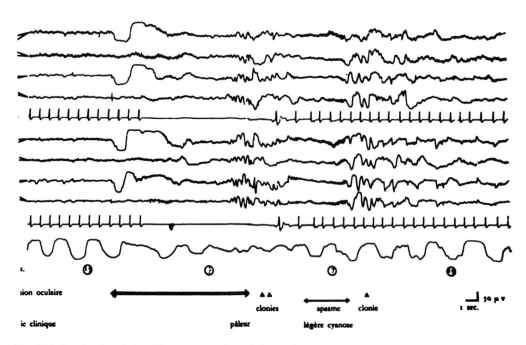

Fig. 17.1. Anoxic seizure induced by pressure on the eyeballs. Ocular pressure was applied at the first horizontal arrow, resulting in cardiac asytole with appearance, after a few seconds, of slow waves on the EEG. The patient turned pale *(pâleur)* and had two clonic jerks *(clonies)*. Later, the EEG flattened while the boy became mildly cyanosed and a tonic spasm occurred (second horizontal arrow). Following resumption of cardiac contractions, slow waves reappeared on the EEG and a further clonic jerk was observed. (Courtesy Prof. H. Gastaut, Hôpital de la Timone, Marseilles.)

also the lower limbs with resultant fall. The same phenomenon may rarely occur in intellectually normal children with behavioural disturbances. The diagnosis rests on a peculiar polygraphic sequence (Aicardi *et al.* 1988). Treatment with fenfluramine may be effective.

ANOXIC SEIZURES DUE TO RESPIRATORY OBSTRUCTION

These are infrequent in children although accidental suffocation or strangulation does occur. Induction of anoxic seizures by an adult, usually the mother, is a relatively common form of the Munchausen syndrome by proxy (Meadow syndrome). The diagnosis may be difficult especially if the mother presses the baby's face into her breast. The constant presence of the mother at the onset of each episode is an essential clue, and a final diagnosis can be established by prolonged polygraphic recording (Stephenson 1990) or by covert EEG–video monitoring.

SYNCOPES OF CARDIAC ORIGIN

Syncopes of cardiac origin are much rarer than reflex vasovagal or cardioinhibitory attacks. It is important to recognize them because they may be due to dangerous conditions which may result in sudden death, so that preventive treatment and monitoring are essential. Cardiac disorders responsible for syncopes include valvular disorders such as aortic stenosis that can produce syncopes on effort, cardiomyopathies, and intrinsic disturbances of cardiac rhythm such as Wolff–Parkinson–White syndrome, congenital atrioventricular block and the *long Q-T syndromes* (Pignata

et al. 1983). The latter include the *Ward–Romano syndrome* which is dominantly transmitted, and the *Jervell–Lange–Nielsen syndrome* that features an associated neurosensory deafness and is recessively inherited. Both syndromes can mimic epilepsy (Gordon 1994b, Pacia *et al.* 1994) and can result in sudden death. Occurrence of episodes during sleep or exercise may be a hint to the correct diagnosis. Attacks can also be precipitated by emotion or stress. Such circumstances as well as a family history of sudden death or 'epilepsy' or a personal history of chest pains, palpitations or of a surgically repaired heart defect require full cardiac investigation. The Q-T_c interval is prolonged in most cases, although occasional cases of cardiac syncope with a normal Q-T have been reported (Bricker *et al.* 1984). Prolonged recording of the electrocardiogram and effort test may be indicated in selected cases (Nousiainen *et al.* 1989), especially when a history of familial syncope or sudden death is present. In some cases, a pacemaker should be inserted as sudden death is possible. Molecular genetic studies (Towbin 1995) have shown that at least five different long Q-T syndromes exist: one is linked to a potassium channel mutation on chromosome 7q35–q36 (*LQT2*), another to a sodium channel protein mutation on chromosome 3 (*LQT3*), and a third to the *ras-1* protein gene on chromosome 11p15.

Acute *attacks of hyperpnoea and cyanosis* are a common feature of congenital cyanotic cardiopathies. They may result in loss of consciousness and may be followed by hemiplegia of vascular origin (Chapter 23). Severe apnoea may also be a feature of the syndrome of alternating hemiplegia (Bourgeois *et al.* 1993).

EPISODES OF APNOEA OR BRADYCARDIA IN YOUNG INFANTS: NEAR-MISS SUDDEN INFANT DEATH SYNDROME/APPARENTLY LIFE-THREATENING EVENTS

Study of the sudden infant death syndrome (SIDS) is beyond the scope of this book. However, some near-miss SIDS cases may be easily mistaken for epileptic events, the more so as they can be followed by neurological sequelae and episodes of status epilepticus (Aubourg *et al.* 1985). Indeed, the true sequence of events may be impossible to establish in some cases. Less severe episodes may manifest as briefer episodes of apnoea, with hypo- or hypertonia and a change of colour which may be wrongly interpreted as epileptic phenomena. Such events may occur in the first few days of life in apparently healthy babies (Grylack and Williams 1996).

Screening for infants at risk of sudden death has been extensively investigated. Most recent studies have found no precise correlation between polygraphic recordings and the later occurrence of sudden death (Krongrad and O'Neill 1986, Kahn *et al.* 1988a, Reerink *et al.* 1995), so that indications for use of electronic monitors in the home remain tentative (Dunne and Matthews 1987). In preterm infants, episodes of marked desaturation can occur without apnoea and remain undetectable by monitoring (Poets *et al.* 1995).

Some apnoeic–bradycardic episodes (the 'awake apnoea syndrome') may be causally related to the presence of gastro-oesophageal reflux (Pedley 1983, Spitzer *et al.* 1984, See *et al.* 1989, Orenstein and Orenstein 1988) or of oesophageal spasm (Fontan *et al.* 1984). The attacks resemble syncope and are often preceded by restlessness and an apprehensive look and accompanied by opisthotonus, so the misdiagnosis of epilepsy is not rare. Such attacks respond to the treatment of gastro-oesophageal reflux.

Other causes of apnoea in neonates and infants appear in Table 17.2.

ACUTE PSYCHIATRIC MANIFESTATIONS

Acute psychiatric manifestations represented the second most common cause of a wrong diagnosis of epilepsy in Jeavons' experience (1983). In most of these cases the resemblance to epileptic seizures is only superficial, and such episodes as attacks of anxiety, acute phobic episodes, attacks of epigastric or laryngeal sensation of pressure, fugues and recurrrent episodes of feelings of derealization do not usually raise major diagnostic problems. However, panic attacks are sometimes mistaken for epilepsy (Genton *et al.* 1995). Hallucinations due to schizophrenia, or to schizophrenia-like states due to substance abuse (Chapter 13), and acute confusional episodes may be difficult to distinguish from some types of nonconvulsive status epilepticus. Recurrent episodes of abnormal paroxysmal behaviour may be due to intermittently manifesting metabolic diseases such as hyperammonaemia or hypoglycaemia, and metabolic screening is in order when such diagnoses are considered. Munchausen syndrome by proxy

may also be regarded as a cause of psychogenic seizures. It can cause great diagnostic difficulties. The mothers may invent a story of seizures and, sometimes, tell it with great sophistication (Meadow 1984, 1991) or even teach the child that s/he has epilepsy, so that the child invents the episodes (Croft and Jervis 1989).

Attacks of rage may occur in adolescents and older children and are sometimes referred to as manifestations of the episodic dyscontrol syndrome (Elliott 1984). Such attacks may be a cause of physical aggression and may be associated with some obscuration of consciousness and postictal sleep. However, at times the attacks are provoked by very slight motives, and the aggression is clearly directed, which differs from what is seen in patients with complex partial seizures fighting against restraint.

PSEUDOSEIZURES

Pseudoepileptic seizures, also known as pseudoseizures, hysterical attacks, psychic or psychogenic seizures, can be very difficult to distinguish from true epileptic attacks (Holmes *et al.* 1980).

They are frequent in adolescents and are not rare in children as early as 4 years of age (Kramer *et al.* 1995). They also occur in children with neurodevelopmental impairment (Neill 1990). Pseudoseizures are commonly observed in children who also have epileptic seizures and are one important cause of apparent 'intractability' of epilepsy (Aicardi 1988). They may also occur in children who have never had epileptic attacks (Holmes *et al.* 1980, Lesser 1996).

Pseudoseizures can mimic any type of seizures, especially generalized ones, but unilateral or focal attacks may be seen. They differ from true seizures by the nature of movements, which are not typical clonias but rather semipurposeful activity, by their violent and theatrical expression and by a nonstereotyped pattern. In one recent series of 21 children (Wyllie *et al.* 1990), 10 had episodes of unresponsiveness, generalized limb jerking and thrashing movements, and six had episodes of staring and unresponsiveness. Most children were responsive immediately after the paroxysm. The average age of 43 patients studied by Lancman *et al.* (1994b) was 12.4 years at onset of seizures and 15 years when the diagnosis was made. Twenty-one of them (49 per cent) received antiepileptic agents. The average duration of attacks was 5.6 minutes, and a majority consisted of violent uncoordinated movements and generalized trembling, although a few patients had only staring seizures. Induction of seizures by suggestion (Lancman *et al.* 1994a) may be helpful. However, the personality of the parents and/or patient and the way they describe the attacks may give rise to serious difficulties. In addition some epileptic seizures—especially frontal ones—may easily suggest hysteria or simulation (Chapter 16). A normal EEG, especially a normal ictal recording, is evidence against epilepsy but certainly does not exclude the diagnosis, and close EEG–video observation of the patients and tests of provocation may be necessary to firmly establish the diagnosis (Wyllie *et al.* 1990).

Contrariwise, recording of typical EEG discharges concomitant to clinical events excludes the diagnosis of pseudoseizures.

TABLE 17.2
Main causes of apnoea in infants and children

Cause	References
Neonates and infants	
Apnoea related to acute neurological disturbances	
Acute hypoxic–ischaemic encephalopathy	Schneider *et al.* (1975)
Brainstem hypoxic injury	Towbin (1969)
Spinal cord birth injury	Towbin (1969)
Mechanical compression of the cord in osteogenesis imperfecta	Pauli and Gilbert (1986)
Neonatal seizures	Watanabe *et al.* (1982)
Apnoea related to chronic neurological disturbances	
CNS malformations	Chapter 3
Joubert syndrome	
Chiari II malformation	
Mohr syndrome	
Dandy–Walker syndrome	
Peripheral malformations	
Vocal cord paralysis	Cohen *et al.* (1982)
Moebius syndrome	Sadarshan and Goldie (1985)
Pierre Robin syndrome	Williams *et al.* (1981)
Degenerative disorders	Parisi *et al.* (1983)
Hyperekplexia	Nigro and Lim (1992)
Neuromuscular diseases	Chapters 20, 21
Congenital myotonic dystrophy	
Congenital myopathies	
Spinal muscular atrophy	
Congenital central alveolar hypoventilation (Ondine's curse)	Commare *et al.* (1993)
Metabolic diseases	Chapter 9
Organic acidurias	
Hypoglycaemia	
Urea cycle disorders	
Nonketotic hyperglycinaemia	
Leigh syndrome	
Cryptogenic apnoeas	
Apnoea of preterm infants due to 'immaturity' of respiratory centres	Takashima and Becker (1986), Poets *et al.* (1995)
Older children	
Rett syndrome	Hagberg *et al.* (1983)
Familial encephalopathy with permanent periodic breathing	Magaudda *et al.* (1988)
Neuromuscular disorders	Ellis *et al.* (1984)
CNS diseases	Southall *et al.* (1987)
Mitochondrial encephalomyopathy with sleep apnoea	Tatsumi *et al.* (1988)
Obstructive apnoea due to hypertrophy of amygdalae and adenoids	Brouillette *et al.* (1982)
Central apnoea of unknown cause	American Academy of Pediatrics Task Force on Infantile Apnea (1985)
Obesity (Pickwickian syndrome)	See text
Leigh disease	Cummiskey *et al.* (1987), Grattan-Smith *et al.* (1990)
Pulmonary diseases	American Academy of Pediatrics Task Force on Infantile Apnea (1985)

Prolonged cassette recording can be especially useful in this regard (Chapter 16).

Pseudoseizures masquerading as absences have been observed in 18 children with hyperventilation syndrome by North *et al.* (1990). The EEG of these patients showed bursts of slow-wave activity without spikes, corresponding to apparently impaired awareness and responsiveness. A similar EEG change associated with altered responsiveness can be observed during hyperventilation in normal children (Epstein *et al.* 1994).

Once the diagnosis is established, previous drug treatment, if any, should be rapidly discontinued. Some form of psychiatric treatment seems beneficial, at least in the short term (Holmes *et al.* 1980). The short-term outcome was favourable in 16 of the 21 children in the series of Wyllie *et al.*, but only 10 of 22 children followed-up for 40 months or more by Lancman *et al.* (1994b) were seizure-free at last visit. A firm diagnosis is critical so that a shift away from antiepileptic medication and toward psychiatric therapy becomes possible.

THE HYPERVENTILATION SYNDROME

Hyperventilation syndrome is relatively common, especially in adolescent girls. The term implies that ventilatory effort is greater than necessitated by metabolic demands. Patients complain variably of chest pain, light-headedness and dyspnoea. Pseudo-absence spells and syncopes may suggest the diagnosis of epilepsy. The diagnosis rests on a high index of suspicion and on the presence of the typical symptoms. Rebreathing in a plastic or paper bag enables control of the symptoms of an impending attack and has both diagnostic and therapeutic value. Underlying family problems should be looked for, but the outlook is somewhat guarded as many children go on to hyperventilate and show chronic anxiety as adults (Herman *et al.* 1981, Oren *et al.* 1987).

SEIZURES OF TOXIC ORIGIN

Attacks of a predominantly motor character are a sequela to an increasing number of drugs. Such seizures are often dystonic in nature, with recurrent episodes of stiffness, hyperextension of the head and opisthotonus. Oculogyric crises are frequent. Any recurrent attack with extrapyramidal manifestation must suggest the diagnosis of drug intoxication, even though any such possibility is denied by the parents or custodians. The drugs most commonly in cause are psychotropic drugs such as phenothiazines and butyrophenones (Pranzatelli 1996) and metoclopramide (Castels-Van Daele 1981), but other agents are being progressively added to the list (Franckx and Noel 1984, Shafrir *et al.* 1986). A familial susceptibility to drugs may exist (Gatrad and Gatrad 1979). There is usually preservation of consciousness, and the diagnosis can be confirmed by urine examination for the commonly responsible drugs.

Most acute drug reactions are self-limited. Treatment with intravenous benztropine or diphenhydramine is useful for controlling rapidly severe dystonic–dyskinetic attacks, although some cases may be resistant to high doses (Leopold 1984).

Rare cases of attacks of endogenous toxic origin (*e.g.* mastocytoma) are on record (Krowchuk *et al.* 1994).

TETANY

Tetany is usually a manifestation of hypocalcaemia or of hypomagnesaemia. The term is sometimes used to designate convulsions due to hypocalcaemia in the newborn infant (Chapters 2, 16). In older infants and children, tetany proper is observed in the same aetiological circumstances but also, occasionally, in normocalcaemic patients. In such cases, tetany appears to be the consequence of a decrease in the level of ionized calcium with a normal level of total calcium. Such a decrease in ionization of calcium can be due to alkalosis as a result of hyperventilation or of repeated vomiting as in pyloric stenosis. Vitamin D deficiency is now a rare cause of tetany. Postoperative hypoparathyroidism and pseudohypoparathyroidism are more frequently the cause.

The clinical manifestations of classical tetany do not appear before 3 months of age. The so-called *carpopedal spasm* is the most striking manifestation. It appears abruptly and affects primarily the fingers, which are flexed at the proximal joint and extended at the distal joints, with the thumbs strongly adducted and opposed. The feet may be similarly involved. Consciousness is clear. *Laryngospasm* often occurs, simultaneously with carpopedal spasm or independently. The vocal cords are adducted so that inspiration becomes noisy, and complete interruption of respiration may rarely occur. Between spasms, signs of latent tetany may be present but the Chvostek sign is not characteristic as it occurs in some normal children. In patients with hypoparathyroidism and pseudohypoparathyroidism, headaches, extrapyramidal signs (Muenter and Whisnant 1968) and calcification of the basal ganglia can be found. Patients with pseudohypoparathyroidism, in addition, are obese, below average height, with a moon-shaped facies and short metacarpals. Mental retardation, cataracts, enamel defect and decreased olfaction and auditory acuity are additional features (Ellie *et al.* 1989).

In all types, epileptic seizures can occur at any age and are, in fact, more commonly observed than the muscle spasms of classical tetany.

The treatment of tetany consists of parenteral administration of calcium salts and vitamin D and occasionally of magnesium salts.

BENIGN PAROXYSMAL VERTIGO AND PAROXYSMAL TORTICOLLIS OF INFANTS

PAROXYSMAL VERTIGO
This condition is characterized by recurrent attacks of vertigo which affect equally boys and girls between 1 and 5 years of age (Koenigsberger *et al.* 1970). The attacks are brief, lasting from one to several minutes and come on suddenly without known precipitant. The child appears in distress, pale but conscious, and may stagger or fall during the attacks. Often, s/he will lie down on the floor, refusing to move. Nystagmus may be noted during attacks. The frequency of attacks is commonly one to a few per month. Many children have fewer than five attacks in total. Affected children otherwise appear normal and in our experience all examinations are negative, although abnormalities in labyrinthine function have been reported by Koenigsberger *et al.* (1970). Most children cease having attacks by 5–6 years of age.

BENIGN PAROXYSMAL TORTICOLLIS OF INFANCY
Benign paroxysmal torticollis of infancy (Deonna and Martin 1981, Cohen *et al.* 1993) is probably closely related to paroxysmal vertigo. The disorder appears before 1 year of age and sometimes from the early weeks of life. The attacks last commonly several hours and up to two or three days. They are marked by repeated

TABLE 17.3
Intermittent and recurrent ataxias in children*

Type	Reference
Vestibular	
Paroxysmal vertigo	Deonna and Martin (1981)
Perilymphatic fistula	Chapter 19
Endolymphatic hydrops	Chapter 19
Vascular	
Basilar migraine	Lapkin and Golden (1978)
Sickle cell disease	Chapter 15
Vasculitis	Chapter 15
Subclavian steal	Kurlan *et al.* (1984)
Emboli of posterior circulation	Chapter 15
Metabolic	
Hypoglycaemia	Chapter 23
Electrolyte disturbances	Chapter 23
Hypoxia	Chapter 23
Urea cycle disorders, esp. ornithine transcarbamylase deficiency	Fowler (1979)
Organic acidaemias including biotinidase and holocarboxylase deficiency	Sander *et al.* (1980b)
Propionic acidaemia	Chapter 9
Leucinosis (intermittent form)	Chapter 9
Leigh disease	Chapter 9
Pyruvate dehydrogenase deficiency	Chapter 9
Hartnup disease	Jepson (1983)
Carnitine acyltransferase deficiency	Di Donato *et al.* (1979)
Acrodermatitis enteropathica	Aguilera-Diaz (1971)
Porphyrias	Chapter 21
Toxic	
Drug ingestion especially antiepileptic agents	Chapter 13
Munchausen syndrome by proxy	Chapter 13
Demyelinating diseases	
Multiple sclerosis	Chapter 12
Tumours (fluctuations due to oedema)	Chapter 14
Recurrent epilepsy	
Epileptic pseudoataxia	Bennett *et al.* (1982)
Recurrent genetic ataxias	
Episodic ataxia type 1 (with continuous myokymia)	Lubbers *et al.* (1995)
Episodic ataxia type 2	Bain *et al.* (1992)
X-linked intermittent**	Livingstone *et al.* (1984)
Dominant with vertigo**	Tibbles *et al.* (1986)
Isolated periodic nystagmuss**	Sogg and Hoyt (1962)
Nystagmus and vertigo**	Farris *et al.* (1986)

*These ataxias may have several different mechanisms (*e.g.* vestibular, cerebellar).
**The nosological situation and autonomy of these forms is uncertain.

vomiting, apparent discomfort and tilting of the head to one side, often with eye movements. The affected side may change with successive attacks. The head can be passively returned to the neutral position but the tilting recurs immediately. In some cases, there may be inclination of the trunk to the same side, sometimes with a degree of ipsilateral stiffness. Ataxia is common, especially in later attacks. If the child can walk, s/he is apt to veer towards the side to which the head is tilted. Although the clinical picture may be impressive, even suggesting a posterior fossa tumour, the abnormalities rapidly subside leaving a completely normal child

free of any neurological anomaly. The diagnosis is greatly helped by a history of previous similar episodes. If these are absent, neuroradiological assessment may be necessary. Familial occurrence has been reported (Lipson and Robertson 1978). A relationship to migraine has been suggested for both paroxysmal vertigo and torticollis, and a family history of migraine is useful for the diagnosis. In some patients, typical migraine will follow the torticollis as the child grows older (Deonna and Martin 1981, Deonna 1988). Other vertiginous episodes may occur in children and are caused by drug intoxication or by acute labyrinthitis of infectious origin (Chapter 19).

RECURRENT FAMILIAL ATAXIA
Benign vertigo of children may be related to recurrent ataxia, a familial condition with dominant (Vighetto *et al.* 1988) or possible X-linked (Livingstone *et al.* 1984) inheritance. Both vertigo and recurrent ataxia have been reported in the same patient (Tibbles *et al.* 1986). Attacks of recurrent ataxia may last from a few hours to a few days. The origin of the ataxia (vestibular or cerebellar) is not clear but the condition is now regarded as belonging in the new category of ionic channel disorders or 'channelopathies' (Griggs and Nutt 1995). At least two distinct forms are known, termed episodic ataxias types 1 and 2 (EA1 and 2). EA1 is characterized by brief episodes lasting seconds to minutes, with onset in early childhood and often induced by startle or exercise, and by the interictal presence of continuous myokymia (Brunt and Van Weerden 1990). The disease maps to chromosome 12p13 (Litt *et al.* 1994) and represents one type of potassium channel disease (KCN A1). EA2 is a calcium channel disorder which is often associated with nystagmus and may have quite variable manifestations; in some patients cerebellar signs are present, and in some families cases of fixed ataxia may coexist with cases of purely episodic disturbances. Linkage of the disease to chromosome 19p13 at the locus for familial hemiplegic migraine has been found in some families (Vahedi *et al.* 1995, Baloh *et al.* 1997) but the mutation is different (Greenberg 1997).

EA2 cases often respond to acetazolamide that interrupts or prevents attacks. Sodium valproate may be a necessary adjunct to acetazolamide (Bain *et al.* 1992). An occasional patient will respond to the calcium-blocking agent flunarizine rather than acetazolamide (Boel and Casaer 1988). EA1 may respond to sulthiame (Brunt and Van Weerden 1990), acetazolamide or phenytoin (Griggs and Nutt 1995).

Autosomal dominant periodic cerebellovestibular ataxia with defective smooth pursuit movements may be genetically distinct from other autosomal dominant ataxias (Damji *et al.* 1996). Nonfamilial cases are on record (Verlooy and Velis 1985). Table 17.3 indicates the main causes of intermittent ataxia in childhood, and Table 17.4 lists the main types of genetically determined cerebellovestibular ataxia.

PAROXYSMAL DYSTONIA, DYSKINESIA AND CHOREOATHETOSIS

The paroxysmal dyskinesias are a complex group of conditions

644

TABLE 17.4

Genetically determined dominantly inherited cerebellar or cerebellovestibular ataxias (progressive or paroxysmal)*

Disorder	Genetic locus	Clinical features	Remarks
Spinocerebellar ataxia type 1 (SCA 1)†	6q22–23	Ataxia, other neurological signs (eye, extrapyramidal)	CAG repeat expansion
Spinocerebellar ataxia type 2 (SCA 2)†	12q23–24	Peripheral nerve involvement, slow saccades	Idem
Spinocerebellar ataxia type 3/Machado–Joseph disease (SCA 3/MJD)†	14q24q32	Extrapyramidal features, ophthalmoplegia	Idem
Spinocerebellar ataxia type 4 (SCA 4)	16q24qter	Ataxia, no ocular involvement, possible axonal neuropathy	
Spinocerebellar ataxia type 5 (SCA 5)	11 centr.	Ataxia	Cerebellar atrophy, no brainstem changes
Spinocerebellar ataxia type 6 (SCA 6)	19p13	Ataxia; migraine in half the cases	CAG repeat expansion, no brainstem atrophy
Autosomal dominant cerebellar ataxia type 2 (ADCA 2)†	3p12–p21	Progressive ataxia, macular degeneration (anticipation)	CAG expansion probable
Episodic ataxia type 1 (EA 1)	12q13	Brief paroxysmal ataxia, permanent myokymias	K-channel disorder, often acetazolamide-sensitive
Episodic ataxia type 2 (EA 2)	19p13	Paroxysmal ataxia (may become fixed), nystagmus	Often sensitive to acetazolamide
Acute paroxysmal cerebellar ataxia (APCA)	19p13	Paroxysmal ataxia	May be allelic to EA 2
Dentatorubropallidoluysian atrophy (DRPLA)†	12p12–12pter	Ataxia, myoclonic epilepsy, movement disorders	CAG repeat expansion
Periodic vestibulocerebellar ataxia	?	Periodic ataxia, defective ocular pursuit	
Acute paroxysmal choreoathetosis/spasticity/ataxia	1p	Abnormal movements, pyramidal tract signs	K channel disorder?

*Modified from Damji *et al.* (1996).
†Occur mostly in adults but sometimes in children.

whose main feature is the occurrence of transient attacks of extrapyramidal movements but whose circumstances of occurrence and aetiology are diverse. Lance (1977) classified the primary paroxysmal dystonias into two subtypes: kinesigenic choreoathetosis and paroxysmal dystonic choreoathetosis. Demirkiran and Jankovic (1995) described, in addition, intermediate cases induced by prolonged exercise, nonkinesigenic dyskinesias and hypnogenic dyskinesia. A majority of their 64 patients had acquired dyskinesia, and a family history was found in only 13 families in contrast to most previous reports.

PAROXYSMAL KINESIGENIC CHOREOATHETOSIS
This disorder is characterized by predominantly unilateral or bilateral attacks of dystonic movements or chorea that are precipitated by sudden movement. Attacks usually last one to a few minutes and may occur up to 100 times daily. Some patients describe an aura of tightness or tingling in the affected segment. Consciousness is preserved but the bizarre, often writhing and sometimes violent ballistic movements may result in falls. About three-quarters of the cases are familial, with a dominant transmission. Other cases probably represent new mutations

or acquired disease. Gay and Ryan (1994) have reviewed the acquired causes of dyskinesia and reported a case induced by methylphenidate. Paroxysmal kinesigenic dyskinesia in many cases responds favourably to anticonvulsant drugs, especially carbamazepine and phenytoin (Lance 1977). The disorder does not affect lifespan but may be socially embarrassing. In some resistant cases, flunarizine has brought about control of the attacks (Lou 1989), but occasional cases are resistant to all known agents.

PAROXYSMAL DYSTONIC CHOREOATHETOSIS OF MOUNT AND REBACK
In this form, attacks are not precipitated by movement but rather by stress, coffee or alcohol (Lance 1977, Bressman *et al.* 1988). Attacks are usually much longer than in kinesigenic forms, lasting from 10 minutes to several hours, and occur less frequently. The condition is rare and appears to be inherited as a dominant mendelian trait. Paroxysmal choreoathetosis generally does not respond to anticonvulsant agents, with the exception of the benzodiazepines, especially clonazepam (Lance 1977) and oxazepam (Kurlan and Shoulson 1983). Acetazolamide has been used

successfully in a patient who also had familial ataxia (Mayeux and Fahn 1982).

OTHER IDIOPATHIC PAROXYSMAL DYSKINESIAS
Intermediate cases do not fall into either of the above groups. Most such cases are induced by continuous exercise with attacks lasting 5–30 minutes (Lance 1977) but cases of dystonias with more variability in expression and response to pharmacological agents have been reported (Bressman *et al.* 1988). Hemidystonia induced by prolonged exercise and cold has been reported by Wali (1992). A rare, distinct type known as autosomal dominant paroxysmal choreoathetosis with spasticity (CSE) maps to chromosome 1p in the vicinity of a potassium gene channels cluster (Auburger *et al.* 1996).

Nocturnal paroxysmal dystonia is discussed below (p. 655).

Paroxysmal dystonia of infancy was reported in nine infants aged between 1 and 5 months (Angelini *et al.* 1988). It consists of brief, frequently repeated episodes of opisthotonus and/or symmetrical or asymmetrical dystonia of the upper limbs. The frequency decreases with age, and the attacks disappear altogether between 8 and 22 months.

The neck–tongue syndrome (Orrell and Marsden 1993) consists of paroxysmal dystonia of the tongue upon rotation of the head.

SYMPTOMATIC PAROXYSMAL DYSTONIA
Paroxysmal dystonia sometimes occurs in patients with fixed, interictal neurological abnormalities such as ataxia, tremor or mental retardation. Attacks are usually focal and have no specific precipitants. Underlying disorders affect mainly the deep grey matter, sometimes with calcification of the basal nuclei with (Kawazawa *et al.* 1985) or without (Micheli *et al.* 1986) hypoparathyroidism. Hart *et al.* (1995) reported a case of paroxysmal dystonia in a patient who also had episodes of hemiplegia, thus representing an intermediary form between dystonias and alternating hemiplegia. Episodes of paroxysmal ballismus precipitated by fever in children with dyskinetic cerebral palsy have been described by Harbord and Kobayashi (1991). In rare adult patients, paroxysmal choreoathetosis has been the presenting manifestation of diabetes mellitus (Haan *et al.* 1989). Paroxysmal dystonia has also been recorded in patients with cystinuria (Cavanagh *et al.* 1974) and with Hartnup disease (Darras *et al.* 1989).

BENIGN MYOCLONUS OF INFANCY
Benign myoclonus of infancy is different from benign neonatal sleep myoclonus (see below). The condition has been described in Chapter 16 as it mimics infantile spasms, although without EEG abnormalities and with an excellent prognosis. Familial recurrence has been reported (Galletti *et al.* 1989).

EXCESSIVE STARTLE DISEASE

HYPEREKPLEXIA
This is a genetically transmitted disease that is characterized by a strikingly excessive response to startle elicited by auditory, visual and other sensory stimuli such as light touch or proprioceptive stimuli that fail to produce a response in normal persons. Nose-tapping is especially effective (Shahar *et al.* 1991). The disorder occurs in two forms: a minor form in which the startle response is excessive but without additional symptoms, and a major form in which other neurological abnormalities are present. In the major form, the startle response is not only quantitatively different from normal but also features momentary generalized stiffness with loss of postural control, producing unprotected falls *'en statue'*. The attacks are different from epileptic seizures as the ictal EEG does not show paroxysmal activity, although some controversy exists regarding the significance of the spikes frequently recorded at the vertex (Matsumoto *et al.* 1992). In addition to abnormal startle, infants with the major form of hyperekplexia may also exhibit marked hypertonia from birth which disappears during sleep and may respond to minor stimuli, such as touching the nose, by episodes of prolonged apnoea that can even be lethal (Pascotto and Coppola 1992). Umbilical and inguinal hernias are frequently present and are probably the consequence of increased abdominal pressure due to permanent muscle contraction. At the time of spontaneous decrease of hypertonia, after the end of the first year of life, violent, often repetitive jerks of the limbs on falling asleep may appear (Andermann and Andermann 1988). The neonatal manifestations of the disease were initially reported as the 'stiff baby syndrome' or congenital stiff-man syndrome (Sander *et al.* 1980a) before the identity of the two conditions was recognized.

The two forms may coexist in the same family. Most cases are dominantly inherited but recessive inheritance has been observed in some pedigrees (Rees *et al.* 1994). Sporadic cases also occur (Nigro and Lim 1992, McAbee *et al.* 1995) with spontaneous resolution and less typical features.

Cases of late onset may occur and may respond to sodium valproate (Dooley and Andermann 1989). A mutation in the alpha 1 subunit of the inhibitory glycine receptor on chromosome 5 (Ryan *et al.* 1992) appears to be responsible for the disease (Shiang *et al.* 1995). Acquired symptomatic causes of hyperekplexia and related excessive startle diseases have been extensively discussed by Brown *et al.* (1991).

The condition is not entirely benign, especially because of repeated falls and episodes of apnoea, and the possibility of death. The attacks can be prevented by sudden flexion of the head and limbs (Vigevano *et al.* 1989). Clonazepam and valproic acid (Dooley and Andermann 1989) are the drugs of choice but do not totally suppress the symptoms.

JUMPING
Jumping has been known for a long time in various populations under picturesque names such as 'jumping Frenchmen of Maine', 'latah' or 'myriachit'. The exact nosological situation of these disorders remains uncertain (Saint-Hilaire *et al.* 1986).

STARTLE EPILEPSY
Startle epilepsy is discussed in Chapter 16.

OTHER PAROXYSMAL ABNORMAL MOVEMENTS

SHUDDERING ATTACKS

Shuddering attacks in infants (Vanasse *et al.* 1976) may be a premonitory symptom of the later development of essential tremor although they may remain isolated (Holmes and Russman 1986).

SANDIFER SYNDROME

Sandifer syndrome is the name given to the contortions of the neck and associated abnormal postures observed in children with hiatus hernia (Sutcliffe 1969). The movements had previously been regarded as involuntary and the mistaken diagnosis of dystonia may be made. The movements primarily consist of sudden extension of the neck in an opisthotonic position, often with continuous twisting of the head from side to side. In some cases, extraordinary positions are assumed (Sutcliffe 1969). Less spectacular manifestations may be more common and often go unrecognized (Werlin *et al.* 1980, Mandel *et al.* 1989). The presence of hiatus hernia or reflux in association with such a dyskinesia allows the correct diagnosis to be made and appropriate therapy to be given. Medical treatment may not be sufficient and fundoplication is often necessary.

HEAD MOVEMENTS AND VISUAL ANOMALIES

A number of abnormal head postures or head movements can be a consequence of visual anomalies. The commonest is head tilt associated with paralysis of the oblique muscles. The head thrusts, characteristic of Cogan ocular motor apraxia, are not infrequently mistaken for myoclonic attacks or tics (Chapter 18).

Benign paroxysmal tonic upgaze of childhood is sometimes associated with forward flexion of the head. Ataxia and repeated falls have been reported (Ouvrier and Billson 1988, Deonna *et al.* 1990). The disorder may respond to L-dopa and be related to dopa-sensitive dystonia (Campistol *et al.* 1993) (Chapter 18).

DYSKINESIAS INDUCED BY TRANSIENT CEREBRAL ISCHAEMIA

Abnormal movements may be seen in patients with vascular disease and are well known in adults (Yanagihara *et al.* 1985). I have seen similar localized rhythmic movements in a child with thrombotic occlusion of the sylvian artery.

ABNORMAL MOVEMENT IN NEONATES

Jitteriness in newborn infants is a common phenomenon (Parker *et al.* 1990, Shuper *et al.* 1991) without pathological significance and is mainly a differential diagnosis of neonatal convulsions (Chapter 16). *Pathological myoclonus* may also be observed in neonates with various disorders (Scher 1985).

RHYTHMIAS, MANNERISMS, GRATIFICATION PHENOMENA, MASTURBATION

Infants and young children often engage in repetitive rhythmic movements such as body-rocking or head-banging. Such movements may occur during the day especially at the time of going to bed or when the child is bored. The movements generally disappear before 3 years of age. Nocturnal head bobbing or lateral movements occurring at night in a rhythmical manner are known as *jactatio capitis nocturna*. Jactatio capitis is a normal phenomenon that occurs in 3–15 per cent of normal children in the first year of life. *Head-banging* is also a normal phenomenon in most cases that usually occurs at the time of going to bed and may last for long periods (Sallustro and Atwell 1978). Excessive head-banging may occur in normal children.

Gratification phenomena (Brett 1997) are stereotyped movements that occur while the child appears withdrawn and from which s/he seems to derive great pleasure. The movements have a ritualistic quality and appear electively when the child is bored. *Masturbation* is commoner in girls in the younger age group. When bored or alone the child will adduct her thighs, stiffen, become flushed and perspire. Such episodes, which are associated with a blank stare, are often mistaken for epileptic seizures (Pranzatelli and Pedley 1991). They are completely benign and do not require any treatment.

MIGRAINE AND RELATED CONDITIONS

Migraine is the most important cause of headache both in children and in adults. The term designates a periodic disorder with symptom-free intervals, characterized by attacks of headache that have several (usually two or three) of the following features: throbbing nature, unilateral location, relief after sleep, presence of an aura, associated abdominal pain or nausea or vomiting, and a family history of similar condition (Prensky 1976, Barlow 1984, Deonna 1988).

The prevalence of migraine in childhood was 3.9 per cent in the classical study of Bille (1962), using restrictive criteria. The incidence of migraine increases with increasing age from 2.7 per cent at age 7, with a slight preponderance of boys, to 6.4 per cent of boys and 14.8 per cent of girls by age 14 years (Sillanpää 1983).

The aetiopathogenesis of migraine is imperfectly understood. Vascular changes clearly play an important role, and some forms of neurovascular instability of genetic origin must exist in migrainous patients. The frequency of a positive family history is very high. Prensky (1976) recorded an average incidence of 72 per cent, and Barlow (1984) found a positive history in 89.7 per cent of his patients. Stewart *et al.* (1997) in a population-based study found the risk of migraine to be 50 per cent higher in patients with a family history than in controls. The mode of inheritance is uncertain although a multifactorial mode seems likely. The syndrome is certainly heterogeneous and some types (*e.g.* familial hemiplegic migraine) clearly follow a dominant pattern of inheritance (Stewart *et al.* 1997). It is possible that the same phenotype is the result of different genotypes, but a definitive answer must await the identification of suitable markers.

A number of hypotheses have incriminated a primary neurogenic origin or a primary vascular involvement with possible humoral factors or platelet abnormalities. The mechanism of the attacks is also uncertain. The pulsating headache is due to the pulsating and presumably dilated arteries. Associated shunting or vasoconstriction of the subcutaneous arterioles accounts for the frequently observable facial pallor, and in an occasional case segmental constrictions of the cerebral arteries have been documented by angiography (Schon and Harrison 1987). However, cerebral blood flow during the headache is highly variable and increased flow cannot account for the pain. The pathophysiology of the aura is classically attributed to cortical ischaemia secondary to either vasospasm or arteriolar shunting. Recent work (Lauritzen 1994, Woods *et al.* 1994) has shown that there is a poor correspondence between regional blood flow, as measured by isotopic methods, and the spread of the aura. In migraine without aura, the blood flow during attacks does not differ from postictal flow (Ferrari *et al.* 1995). A spreading inhibitory phenomenon, akin to Leão spreading depression, might be responsible for the aura but the origin of the inhibition remains unknown. There is still considerable controversy about the primary neurogenic or vascular mechanism of migraine (Olsen *et al.* 1987, Andersen *et al.* 1988).

CLINICAL FEATURES
The age of onset of migraine headaches can be very early in life. Holguin and Fenichel (1967) found that approximately 20 per cent of the patients had their first attack before 5 years of age (Holguin and Fenichel 1967). In many cases, attacks of headache have been preceded by recurrent abdominal pain and/or vomiting (see below) or by motion sickness which is found in 45 per cent of children with migraine, starting from age 2 years (Barabas *et al.* 1983).

The Headache Classification Committee of the International Headache Society (1988) recognize two major forms, migraine with and without aura, otherwise known as classical and common migraine.

The migraine headache is identical in both forms. A major feature of the pain is its throbbing character, and every effort should be made to recognize this feature without inducing the expected answer, by providing the child with several different words—if necessary supplemented by gestures—covering the main types of headache. Throbbing headache is present in 50–60 per cent of the cases of childhood migraine (Barlow 1984), and unilateral location is observed in 25–66 per cent (for review, see Prensky 1976). The duration of headache in children is briefer than in adults, although in most cases it lasts for a few hours.

Nausea and vomiting, photophobia and/or phonophobia, and pallor of the face and 'dark circles' under the eyes are frequent associated features.

The attacks may be precipitated by psychological factors (Leviton *et al.* 1984), by certain foods, by physical exertion (Bille 1962), and by hormonal factors in adolescent girls. Such precipitating factors were present in 25 per cent of the cases reported by Seshia *et al.* (1994).

Sleep is an effective manner of relieving migraine headache—this feature is of diagnostic value so should be asked about when taking the history—although many children resist sleep during the attack.

CLASSICAL MIGRAINE (MIGRAINE WITH AURA)
Classical migraine is defined as an idiopathic recurrent disorder manifesting with attacks of neurological symptoms unequivocally localizable to the cerebral cortex or brainstem, usually developing gradually over 5–20 minutes and lasting less than 60 minutes. The aura may be preceded by symptoms of irritability, pallor or undefinable premonitory feeling. Headache, nausea and/or photophobia normally follow the aura symptoms directly or after a free interval of less than an hour. The headache is generally contralateral to the sensory symptoms, if it is lateralized at all, and usually lasts 4–72 hours although it may be completely absent (migraine aura without headache) (Headache Classification Committee 1988). The most common aura is one of sensory symptoms, mainly visual manifestations. Visual auras include photopsia, fortification spectra, negative scotomata that often consist of a cut-out of a portion of images with smooth, ragged or undulating edges but may also be hemianopic or quadrantic. Total blindness is rare (Bower *et al.* 1994). According to Panayiotopoulos (1994), elementary visual hallucinations in migraine are generally linear and black and white, which might help separate them from those in epilepsy. They may coexist with a scotoma or occur in isolation. More complex visual disturbances consist of illusions of micropsia, macropsia or distortion of objects and may not be described by young children for want of an appropriate vocabulary. Both the positive and the negative scotomata may be of either retinal or cortical origin. When only one eye is involved, a retinal origin (retinal migraine) is likely, whereas hemianopic scotomata are of cortical location.

An aura of light-headedness or vertigo is common, usually in combination with diplopia or blurred vision.

Other sensory auras include sensations of tingling or numbness that may involve both hands and the perioral area or be unilateral, distortions of body image usually associated with visual phenomena to produce the 'Alice in Wonderland syndrome' (Golden 1979), and rarely auditory or olfactory symptoms (Fuller and Guiloff 1987), usually of an unpleasant character.

Neurological signs, especially aphasia and hemiplegia, are included by the current classification in classical migraine. Because of their unusual presentation, they are described here as complicated migraine.

In some children the aura may occur alone without subsequent headaches, nausea or abdominal pain. Such an occurrence is most frequently occasional but, in the rare patient, may be the only manifestation in a given epoch of the migraine (Golden 1979, Barlow 1984, Hockaday 1987, Shevell 1996).

COMMON MIGRAINE (MIGRAINE WITHOUT AURA)
Common migraine accounts for approximately 90 per cent of all cases. Patients with common migraine have no aura before their headache attacks or have an aura only on rare occasions. The international criteria for common migraine include unilateral localization, and a throbbing character of pain which is

moderate or severe and aggravated by physical activity. Such criteria however may not apply to children (Seshia *et al.* 1994), in whom bilateral headache and brief attacks of less than two hours are common.

COMPLICATED MIGRAINE

Neurological signs that develop during the headache phase or persist for hours or days beyond the headache characterize complicated migraine. The term, not used in the International Classification, applies to persistent visual manifestations such as scotoma or hemianopia but is mainly applied to hemiplegic and aphasic migraine, ophthalmoplegic migraine, confusional migraine and basilar artery migraine.

Some authors used the term synonymously with that of 'migraine accompagnée' to include cases with paraesthesiae, often unilateral and with a slow 'march' of several minutes duration, as well as cases with motor deficits (Rossi *et al.* 1980), but it is used here only for cases with prolonged deficits.

The frequency of complicated migraine is between 5 and 10 per cent in series from referral centres, therefore lower in less biased series.

Hemiplegic migraine most frequently occurs as a manifestation of the aura and remains confined to this stage of the attack. It is commonly associated with visual symptoms in the ipsilateral visual field and with ipsilateral sensory phenomena. *Aphasia* of a nonfluent type may also occur as an aura, often in association with other manifestations of left hemisphere affectation such as hemiparesis. In a second type of hemiplegic migraine, hemiparesis with or without aphasia appears after the aura or in its absence and persists for hours or even days. The hemiplegia may be dense and is often associated with confusion and agitation, thus suggesting a diagnosis of meningeal haemorrhage or other vascular accident. CT scan shows the absence of intracranial blood and in some cases a degree of swelling of the involved hemisphere. Prominent slow waves are present in EEG records and may persist up to several weeks. Angiograms are normal and are probably unnecessary when CT scan is fully normal. Angiography may provoke vascular spasms in patients with migraine even though the risk of angiography may have been overestimated (Shuaib and Hachinski 1988). Remarkably, patients with this second type of hemiplegic migraine often have relatives affected with the same form of the disorder, and their recurrences tend to present in a similar manner. Some familial cases have been mapped to chromosome 19q (Joutel *et al.* 1994). Remarkably, some cases of familial hemiplegic migraine can be associated with marked MRI abnormalities of the white matter and have been found in families in which cerebral autosomal dominant arteriopathy with subcortical infarcts and leukoencephalopathy (CADASIL), also mapping to 19q, was present in other adult members (Chabriat *et al.* 1995, Hutchinson *et al.* 1995), suggesting a link between the two disorders. The pattern of recurrence may change, however, sometimes after several years as in one of my patients who had attacks of hemiplegic migraine from 11 months of age and developed visual symptoms at age 10 years. The diagnostic problems posed by such cases can be made even more difficult

by the occasional presence of mild to moderate pleocytosis (Brattström *et al.* 1984, Rossi *et al.* 1985). Bartleson *et al.* (1981) have suggested that some cases of migrainous syndrome with CSF pleocytosis might be symptomatic of a benign underlying inflammatory disorder of the CNS.

Ophthalmoplegic migraine is characterized by the association of a recurrent IIIrd nerve palsy that develops during or following ipsilateral periorbital or temporal headache. The IVth and VIth nerves may be rarely affected (Vijayan 1980). Permanent impairment of the IIIrd nerve may persist after repeated attacks. The syndrome is to be distinguished from other causes of IIIrd nerve palsy, from the painful ophthalmoplegia of Tolosa–Hunt (Chapter 18) and from congenital berry aneurysms. The onset may be as early as the first year of life. In young children, the headache may be absent or overlooked (Durkan *et al.* 1981). Gadolinium enhancement of the cisternal portion of the oculomotor nerve may be a useful sign (Wong and Wong 1997). The occurrence of Raeder type II paratrigeminal syndrome with oculosympathetic paresis as a migraine variant is on record (Shevell *et al.* 1993). Bilateral episodic mydriasis may be a migraine equivalent in childhood (Baziel *et al.* 1991).

Confusional migraine is an uncommon type of migraine that often but not always follows a mild head trauma. An acute confusional state is the presenting feature and headache is often insignificant. Confusion typically lasts for several hours and in some cases may progress to a stuporous state (Barlow 1984). Neurological signs are sometimes associated or alternate with confusion (Feely *et al.* 1982). In a few patients, amnesia dominates the clinical picture so that the term transient global amnesia becomes appropriate (Tirman and Woody 1988, Sheth *et al.* 1995).

Rare cases of coma associated with features of migraine and with frightening symptoms such as autonomic disturbances, apnoea sometimes of long duration, hypotension and cardiac irregularities have been reported (Fitzsimons and Wolfenden 1985). In some of these, ataxia, nystagmus, myokymia and peduncular hallucinosis may be present (Zifkin *et al.* 1995) and cerebellar atrophy may be demonstrated (Elliott *et al.* 1996).

Basilar artery migraine is an established 'complicated' form of migraine (Lapkin and Golden 1978). The main clinical features include variable associations of cranial nerve, cerebellar, cochleovestibular and corticobulbar signs and symptoms, together with visual disturbances attributable to the territory of the posterior cerebral arteries. This form is seen mainly in adolescent girls. Basilar migraine is one cause of intermittent ataxia (see Table 17.3). Visual symptoms are usually first in the sequence and consist of dimming of vision that may amount to almost total blindness. Consciousness may be impaired in some patients and true seizures have been observed (Swanson and Vick 1978). The EEG shows bilateral posterior slow waves, but intense epileptic activity has also been reported (Lapkin *et al.* 1977), so the syndrome may be difficult to distinguish from some forms of occipital epilepsy (Newton and Aicardi 1983). Residual impairment is rare despite an often frightening symptomatology. However, multiple infarcts have been reported in some cases, even in childhood (Caplan 1991). This type of migraine may be related to *amaurosis fugax* which is sometimes observed in adolescents and even in children (Appleton *et al.* 1988) and may occur as a post-traumatic phenomenon (Greenblatt 1973). The prognosis is excellent, and 13 patients followed for 10 years by Bower *et al.* (1994) remained symptom-free.

ATYPICAL MANIFESTATIONS SOMETIMES ASSOCIATED WITH MIGRAINE ATTACKS

Migraine and seizures coexist more often that would be expected by chance alone (Andermann and Lugaresi 1987). The relationship is a complex one: in some cases epilepsy may be the consequence of ischaemia during a severe migraine attack or the sequela thereof; in others it may be the result of a lesion such as an arteriovenous malformation (Barlow 1984). The occurrence of continuous spike–waves over the posterior part of the skull in association with both epileptic phenomena and migraine-like manifestation is of interest (Panayiotopoulos 1989, Newton and Aicardi 1983). Usually the EEG of patients with migraine is normal or shows focal or generalized slow waves, but focal spikes may be far more common than in control subjects (Kinast *et al.* 1982). Postictal slowing may be very marked and persistent (for review, see Barlow 1984).

A further problem may be to differentiate postepileptic headache from migraine (Schon and Blau 1987) and sometimes to distinguish ictal manifestations of partial complex seizures, for example hallucinations or illusions, from those that occur in migraine (Seshia *et al.* 1985).

Syncopes may occur during a migraine attack in around 1 per cent of affected children (Prensky and Sommer 1979). They may be particularly frequent in patients with basilar artery migraine.

Strokes can occur in adults during a migraine attack, especially during complicated attacks. The occurrence of strokes in children with migraine is certainly rare, if it exists at all (Rossi *et al.* 1990, Riikonen and Santavuori 1994, Nezu *et al.* 1997). The occurrence of strokes or stroke-like episodes in childhood migraine should arouse the suspicion of a mitochondrial encephalomyopathy (Chapter 9).

Dvorkin *et al.* (1987) have reported on patients who presented in childhood or adolescence with severe migraine attacks, rapidly associated with epileptic seizures and episodes of *epilepsia partialis continua*. Most patients had a family history of migraine. CT usually showed hypodense lesions. Such cases are probably variants of the mitochondrial encephalopathy with stroke-like episodes and lactic acidosis (MELAS) syndrome and run an unfavourable course.

ATYPICAL FORMS OF MIGRAINE:
THE 'PERIODIC SYNDROME', CYCLIC VOMITING AND ABDOMINAL MIGRAINE

In childhood, and especially in young children, migraine is commonly manifested by atypical features which include cyclic vomiting, recurrent abdominal pain and perhaps other periodic phenomena which have been described as 'the periodic syndrome', such as recurrent fever and paroxysmal limb pains.

CYCLIC VOMITING

Cyclic vomiting presents with repeated episodes of vomiting that may last hours or days and may lead to dehydration and ketosis. Abdominal discomfort is frequent. The onset is commonly in the third or fourth year of life. Two-thirds of patients in one study (Hammond 1974) developed migraine headache in later childhood. The same syndrome has been sometimes attributed to epilepsy, which is certainly exceptional. It may be of psychosomatic origin in some of the cases. The main differential diagnosis is with intestinal malformation or hiatus hernia (Gordon 1994a) and with ketotic or nonketotic hypoglycaemia and other metabolic disorders with periodic manifestations such as disorders of the urea cycle or of oxidation of fatty acids (see Chapter 9).

RECURRENT ABDOMINAL PAIN

Recurrent abdominal pain is much more commonly a psychosomatic disorder than a migrainous manifestation (Hockaday 1987). The incidence of recurrent abdominal pain is between 0.7 and 1.7 per cent of all children, and the condition seems unrelated to migraine (Mortimer *et al.* 1993). In addition. a large number of medical and surgical conditions are manifested in this manner, including brain or spinal tumours. Abdominal migraine is usually associated with vomiting, and the pain is usually periumbilical in location and crampy or more commonly aching in nature (Symon and Russell 1986).

Other manifestations sometimes attributed to migraine include recurrent fever, paroxysmal leg pain (Guiloff and Fruns 1988, Mortimer *et al.* 1993) and paroxysmal chest pain (for review, see Barlow 1984).

THE TREATMENT OF MIGRAINE

Therapy of migraine is empirically based and, at best, only partially successful. Important basic points include reassurance that the condition is benign and general advice about lifestyle, including avoidance of established trigger factors.

Treatment of individual attacks is sufficient for patients with relatively rare episodes. It should be given early at the beginning of headache or at the time of aura if it is present. Antalgic mixtures of aspirin, phenacetin and barbiturates may be valuable. Ibuprofen and acetaminophen often abort attacks in less than two hours (Hämäläinen *et al.* 1997a). Ergot derivatives are probably the drug of choice in combination with antalgic drugs or in isolation. However, they should not be used more than twice weekly and their use in children must be very parsimonious (Silberstein and Young 1995). Antiemetics are useful in children with repeated vomiting and should be given in combination with an analgesic. Metoclopramide has the additional advantage of speeding up gastric emptying thus increasing the absorption of antalgics. Sumatriptan is extremely effective for immediate interruption of an attack but requires injection and is expensive, and has not been fully tested in children, in whom it seems less effective than in adults (Hämäläinen *et al.* 1997b).

Continuous prophylactic treatment (Barlow 1984) is necessary when repeated attacks occur and are considered troublesome enough by the child and family. A vast number of drugs are available (for review, see Welch 1993). *Propanolol* (10–20 mg t.i.d. in children over 7–8 years of age) is highly effective provided the treatment is given for a long enough period in a high enough dosage (Congdon and Forsythe 1979, Rosen 1983). *Pizotifen* was found effective by some authors but had no effect in a recent, relatively large series (Gillies *et al.* 1986). *Clonidine* appeared to be useful in a pilot study of 40 children but this good result was not confirmed in a double-blind study (Sills *et al.* 1982). *Phenytoin and phenobarbitone* are considered drugs of choice by some investigators (Barlow 1984). The side-effects of these drugs are troublesome, however, and propanolol remains probably the drug of choice for severe cases. *Methysergide* is a potent drug but its use in children is made difficult or impossible because of the grave side-effects of retroperitoneal or pulmonary fibrosis. Such side-effects are not observed in patients treated for less than six months. *Calcium channel blocking agents* are vasodilators that prevent the entry of calcium into vascular smooth muscle thus preventing their contraction. Cyproheptadine has been used in children at a dose of 0.2–0.4 mg/kg/d and nifedipine at a dose of 1 mg/kg/d (Barlow 1984). Flunarizine has been also employed in children at a daily dose of 5–7.5 mg. Nimodipine and verapamil have been less extensively tested in young patients. Favourable results have been reported in small groups of patients with uncontrolled studies (Louis 1981). *Sumatriptan*, a selective agonist of serotonin (SHT1) receptors which selectively constricts cranial blood vessels, has been shown to be effective and well-tolerated (Saxena and Den Boer 1991, Visser *et al.* 1996), but is very expensive. Prophylactic treatment is usually given for periods of 6–12 months. If relapse occurs, a further similar course is warranted. Identification of provocative foods or drinks may be helpful but requires a thorough history-taking and may need several trials.

CLUSTER HEADACHES OR MIGRAINOUS NEURALGIA

Cluster headaches appear to be genetically distinct from migraine although they belong to the group of vascular headaches. The fundamental defect is likely to be different from that in migraine, an hypothesis supported by the finding of elevated plasma serotonin and whole blood histamine levels, which is not the case in migraine.

The condition is rare in children and exceptional below 10 years of age. The characteristic periodicity is a basic feature. The headache may occur one or several times in a 24-hour period, during periods that last for several weeks but occur only once or twice a year or even at wider intervals. The headache is unilateral and usually centres about the eye. It is extremely severe but not throbbing and lasts less than 30 minutes in most cases. In approximately one-third of patients pain is located in the lower face (Pearce 1980). Ipsilateral lachrymation and nasal congestion occur in about 50 per cent of attacks. The finding of a Horner syndrome is uncommon in children.

Drugs effective in migraine may be used for cluster headaches

but resistant cases are frequent. Indomethacin or sumatriptan may be useful in some cases (Geaney 1983). Methisergide, ergotamine and ergovonine malleate have been used.

DIFFERENTIAL DIAGNOSIS OF MIGRAINE AND OTHER HEADACHES

Headache is an extremely common complaint in childhood. In most cases it is due to benign causes, including acute infectious disorders, visual difficulties and the like. In some cases such as brain tumours or abscesses headache has a serious significance and the problem is to separate the rare case of headache of severe organic cause from the mass of benign cephalalgias. A list of the main causes of subacute and chronic headache appears in Table 17.5. For all children, a detailed personal and family history, full neurological examination and measurement of blood pressure are in order. Imaging is not indicated for most cases, especially those of common migraine, and only a few basic laboratory investigations should be performed.

Psychogenic headache is comparatively uncommon in childhood but increases significantly in adolescent patients. The term 'tension headache' applies mostly to adults and it is apparently rare in children (Barlow 1984). The diagnosis is based on the characteristics of the headache, which is usually continuous and of an aching or pressing nature, and on some indication of emotional disorder in the child. Tension headache is not associated with nausea, vomiting or transient neurological disturbances. Treatment of tension headache is difficult. Children with moderate to severe depression should be referred to a psychiatrist. Less severe and more common sources of anxiety and concern should be managed by discussing frankly the patient's problem and trying to resolve the conflict. Antidepressant drugs may be useful in rare cases. In children younger than 7 years of age, migraine is by far the most common cause of headache. Chu and Shinnar (1992) found that 75 per cent of such children had migraine (72 of 78 had common migraine) and 12 per cent had post-traumatic headache. None of their 104 patients had a sinister cause to their complaint.

Intracranial hypotension may cause severe headache and commonly follows lumbar puncture. The diagnosis may be difficult when headache lasts for days or even weeks (Kuntz *et al.* 1992).

Other headaches may be due to drugs or toxins such as alcohol that are increasingly used by adolescents in many parts of the world, marijuana which is a peripheral vasodilator, caffeine withdrawal (Greden *et al.* 1980), and certain food additives such as monosodium glutamate which is used in Chinese cooking and produces vasodilation. Sodium glutamate appears to be the cause of the 'Chinese restaurant syndrome' (Schaumburg *et al.* 1969), while nitrites may be responsible, in the United States, for 'hot dog headache' (Henderson and Raskin 1972). *Benign exertional headache* occurs in adolescents following strenuous exercise. The diagnosis is easy as pain begins during or just following exercise and may last minutes to hours (Diamond and Dalessio 1982).

TABLE 17.5
TABLE 17.5
Main causes of persistent headache in childhood outside migraine

Cause	Characters of headache and possible associated symptoms or signs
Organic causes	
Brain tumours	Chronic, progressive, intermittent, often nocturnal, sometimes throbbing, mostly noncharacteristic. Vomiting, neurological signs
Vascular diseases	
Systemic infections	Acute, non-throbbing
Vascular malformations	Throbbing, fixed location. Seizures, neurological signs
Connective tissue diseases	Throbbing
Arterial hypertension	Acute, generalized, sometimes throbbing. Convulsions, transient visual disturbances
Congenital malformations and hydrocephalus	No characteristic quality. Large head and neurological signs
Infectious processes	
Paranasal sinusitis	Focal, acute or chronic, dull pain and pressure, location variable with sinus affected. Tenderness over sinus, nasal discharge
Intracranial suppuration	Neurological or meningeal signs
Chronic meningitis	*Idem*
Cervical osteoarthritis	Chronic, nonprogressive
Pseudotumour cerebri	Nondistinctive. Papilloedema, diplopia
Endocrine and metabolic causes, *e.g.* hypoglycaemia, recurrent metabolic disorders	Nondistinctive. Vomiting, lethargy
Cluster headaches	Characteristic periodicity, extreme pain usually not throbbing, facial pain in 30 per cent. Lachrymation and nasal congestion. Horner syndrome in some cases
Epileptic headache	Acute, non-throbbing
Psychogenic headache and post-traumatic headache	Pressure, aching, tightness, continuous anxiety and/or depression, no aura or visual or neurological symptoms

TABLE 17.6
Alternating hemiplegia in infants: clinical findings in 22 cases

Sex: 10 boys, 12 girls

Age of onset of attacks: 10 days–11 months

Onset with tonic attacks: 11

Paroxysmal symptoms

Onset with bouts of hemiplegia: 4

Hemiplegia: 22 (in 19 cases attacks with bilateral (shifting) involvement were observed)

Tonic seizures: 21 (head turning or tilting with unilateral body stiffening in all cases; bilateral attacks in 5)

Paroxysmal nystagmus: 18 (unilateral in 14 cases)

Paroxysmal strabismus: 9 (may be due to paroxysmal internuclear ophthalmoplegia or 'one and a half' syndrome)

Screaming, apparent pain: 22

Vasomotor disturbances: 17/18 (pallor, flushing, coldness, often limited to one side)

Disappearance with sleep: 22

Paroxysmal respiratory disturbances: 10 (dyspnoea often severe with cyanosis, sometimes life-threatening; may occur without associated tonic seizure)

Nonparoxysmal symptoms

Mental retardation: 20 (some retardation and hypotonia was present before attacks in 4 infants; in remaining cases developed gradually)

Neurological signs: 12 (2 remaining patients under 3 years of age)

  Choreoathetosis: 22

  Ataxia: 22

  Pyramidal tract signs: 5

ALTERNATING HEMIPLEGIA OF CHILDHOOD

Alternating hemiplegia was initially described as a variant of hemiplegic migraine (Verret and Steele 1971). However, the condition is so different from classical migraine that it should be regarded as a specific disorder (Bourgeois *et al.* 1993). Its mechanism remains obscure. Although fewer than 80 cases have been described, the disease is certainly more common as my personal experience is now with 29 patients.

The *onset* of the disorder is always in the first year and usually in the first six months of life. *Paroxysmal manifestations* appear first. They consist of attacks of hemiplegia that are never isolated but variously combined with tonic attacks, ocular motor manifestations and autonomic phenomena. The clinical findings in 22 personal cases are listed in Table 17.6. Localized or generalized tonic and dystonic attacks and episodes of nystagmus often precede the hemiplegias by weeks to months.

The frequency of episodes is usually high, with attacks of hemiplegia occurring several times a month and lasting from a few minutes to several days. A characteristic feature in most cases is the occurrence of episodes when the hemiplegia shifts from one side to the other, with a period of bilateral paralysis associated with mutism, difficulties in swallowing and drooling (Krägeloh and Aicardi 1980). Severe quadriplegic attacks with amimia,

TABLE 17.7

TABLE 17.7
Main causes of recurrent hemiplegia in children

	*Genetics**	*Reference*
Vascular diseases		
Thrombotic		
Homocystinuria	AR	Chapter 15
Dysproteinaemia	AR or AD	Chapter 15
Fabry disease	AR	Chapter 9
Sickle cell disease	AD	
Fibromuscular dysplasia	AD, S	
Hereditary polycythaemia	AD, AR	
Protein C deficiency	AD	Chapter 15
Resistance to activated protein C (factor Leyden)	AR	
Factor XII deficiency	AR	
Cutis marmorata congenita	S	Baxter *et al.* (1993)
Rendu–Osler–Weber disease	AD	Myles *et al.* (1970)
Embolic		
Mitral valve disease	S	
Mitral valve prolapse	AD, S	Riela and Roach (1993)
Auricular myxoma	AD, AR?, S	
Cardiomyopathies	AD, AR, S	Chapter 15
Conduction defects	S or AD	This chapter
Haemorrhagic diseases		
Coagulopathies	XR, AR	
Platelet disorders	XR, AD, AR	Chapter 15
Arteriovenous malformations	S	
Metabolic diseases		
MELAS	AR	Chapter 9
Kearn–Sayre syndrome	Usually S	Chapter 9
Phosphoglycerol kinase deficiency (stroke-like episodes, sometimes myoglobinuria)	AR	DiMauro (1982)
Carbohydrate-deficient glycoprotein syndrome[1]	AR	Jaeken and Carchon (1993)
Sulfite-oxidase deficiency	AR	
Lactic acidosis	XR, AR, AD	Chapter 9
Organic acidaemia (metabolic strokes)	AR	
Pyruvate dehydrogenase deficiency		Silver *et al.* (1995)
Ammonia cycle disorders	AR, XR	Sperl *et al.* (1997)
Miscellaneous genetic diseases		
Hemiplegic migraine	AD	This chapter
Fibromuscular dysplasia	S	Chapter 15
Neurocutaneous diseases (tuberous sclerosis, neurofibromatosis)	AD	Chapter 4
Nongenetic diseases		
Demyelinating diseases		Riikonen and Donner (1987), Kahn *et al.* (1995)
Connective tissue diseases		Chapter 12
Alternating hemiplegia of childhood and variants[2]		Andermann *et al.* (1995)

*AR = autosomal recessive, AD = autosomal dominant, S = sporadic, XR = X-linked recessive.
[1]Stroke-like episodes are on record but their pathological basis is not demonstrated.
[2]Autosomal dominant inheritance has been reported (Mikati *et al.* 1992).

malaise and decreased consciousness are often observed (Fusco and Vigevano 1995). Frightening, possibly life-threatening episodes of apnoea occur in some patients. A very characteristic feature is the disappearance of all symptoms on falling asleep. In prolonged attacks, the child is normal on waking up but all symptoms return within 10–20 minutes. Parents often take advantage of this short period to feed the patient. *Nonparoxysmal manifestations* are present in all patients after a course of a few months or years and run a progressive course. They include mental retardation of variable degree, choreoathetosis and dystonia, ataxia and sometimes pyramidal tract signs. All laboratory investigations and neuroradiological studies including MRI have

TABLE 17.8
Main causes of recurrent obtundation or coma

Disorder	References
Metabolic diseases	Chapters 9, 23
Hypoglycaemia	
Urea cycle disorders	
Mitochondrial disorders	
Organic acidurias	
Diabetes mellitus	
Fructose intolerance	
Glycogenosis type I	
Glutaric aciduria type 2	
Biotinidase deficiency	
Pyruvate dehydrogenase deficiency	
Fatty acid oxidation defects (recurrent Reye-like episodes)	
Addisonian crises	
Methylene-tetrahydrofolate reductase deficiency	Walk *et al.* (1994)
Epilepsy	
Nonconvulsive status epilepticus	Bennett *et al.* (1982)
Benign occipital epilepsy	Panayiotopoulos (1989)
Migraine	
Basilar artery migraine	Lapkin and Golden (1978)
Migraine coma	Zifkin *et al.* (1993)
Hypertensive encephalopathy	Hauser *et al.* (1988)
Recurrent stroke-like episodes	Chapters 9, 15
MELAS, Kearns–Sayre and other mitochondrial diseases	
Carbohydrate-deficient glycoprotein syndromes	
Other vascular disorders	
Intoxication	Chapter 13
Pharmaceutical agents	
Organic solvents	
Street drugs	
Idiopathic recurrent stupor	
Due to accumulation of endozepine-4	Tinuper *et al.* (1992, 1994)
Associated with hypothermia and autonomic disturbances with or without agenesis of the corpus callosum (Shapiro syndrome)	Sheth *et al.* (1994)
Hypersomnias*	This chapter
Narcolepsy	
Idiopathic hypersomnia	
Kleine–Levin syndrome	

*Rarely is the disturbance of consciousness sufficient to suggest coma.

been negative. Transient muscle mitochondrial abnormalities have been reported (Kemp *et al.* 1995) but are inconstant (Kyriakides and Drousiotou 1994). Single photon emission computed tomography (SPECT) has shown variable changes in perfusion, depending probably on the timing of examination (Andermann *et al.* 1995). Ictal EEGs show only a moderate slowing on the affected side. The clinical picture is so characteristic that there are few differential diagnoses. Initially, however, the occurrence of unilateral tonic seizures followed by hemiplegia makes the diagnosis of partial epileptic seizures difficult to avoid for physicians not familiar with the disease. In about half the patients, true seizures may occur with or without temporal relationship to the hemiplegias. The condition occurs mostly sporadically. However, a family with affected members with typical but less severe symptoms and a later onset up to 3 years of age has been reported (Mikati *et al.* 1992), and two pairs of affected monozygotic twins are on record.

The only forms of *treatment* that have brought about partial improvement are the calcium entry blocker flunarizine (Casaer *et al.* 1987, Silver and Andermann 1993, Andermann *et al.* 1995), the NMDA receptor antagonist memantine, which has been found effective in one patient (Korinthenberg 1996), and chloral hydrate or niaprazine, which if given at the onset of an attack may abort it (Veneselli and Biancheri 1997).

A benign form has been reported by Andermann *et al.* (1994). In their two patients, the attacks occurred during sleep. A case associated with paroxysmal dystonia is on record (Kemp *et al.* 1995).

The differential diagnosis is discussed by Andermann *et al.* (1995) and the main causes of paroxysmal hemiplegia are listed in Table 17.7. The cases of cutis marmorata congenita with recurrent alternating hemiplegia described by Baxter *et al.* (1993) can closely simulate the disorder.

PAROXYSMAL DISTURBANCES OF CONSCIOUSNESS

The recurrent occurrence of variable degrees of disturbed consciousness from coma and stupor to lethargy and confusion is a common and difficult diagnostic problem. Most of the conditions that give rise to such problems are described in other chapters. Table 17.8 gives a list of responsible disorders to help diagnostic orientation. In most disorders, the diagnosis is suggested by history of previous similar events and/or by a family history of similar cases. Metabolic disorders are particularly apt to present with recurrent disturbances of consciousness often associated with vomiting and precipitated by infections and fasting. The possibility of drug toxicity should always be considered in such cases. A syndrome of idiopathic recurrent stupor (Tinuper *et al.* 1992, 1994) may be associated with an abnormal level of endogenous benzodiazepine and may respond to flumazenil which blocks benzodiazepine receptors. Associated phenomena may include hypothermia in Shapiro syndrome (Sheth *et al.* 1994) or, rarely, hyperthermia, in the so-called reverse Shapiro syndrome (Hirayama *et al.* 1994).

PAROXYSMAL DISORDERS OF SLEEP

Most disturbances of sleep in children are transient and benign and do not require any treatment. A few common and/or important disorders are discussed in this section.

NIGHT TERRORS AND NIGHTMARES
Night terrors usually occur between the ages of 18 months and 5 years (Guilleminault 1987a) and are associated with partial arousal from deep slow sleep (stages III–IV). They supervene

mainly during the first hours of sleep. The child starts screaming and usually sits up, looking terrified. Although s/he appears to be awake, s/he does not recognize her/his parents and cannot be consoled. An episode lasts a few minutes, the child goes back to sleep and keeps no memory of the event. Night terrors often tend to occur every night for periods, then disappear. They may persist to age 8 in half the children and up to adolescence in one-third (DiMario and Emery 1986).

Nightmares may produce a similar picture but take place during REM sleep.

Both night terrors and nightmares are benign conditions and require only reassurance.

SOMNAMBULISM (SLEEPWALKING), ABNORMAL MOVEMENTS DURING SLEEP, HYPNAGOGIC PHENOMENA

Somnambulism is frequent in older children and adolescents. It is the consequence of incomplete arousal that permits some semi-purposeful activity without clear consciousness or memory of the event. The episodes are usually brief and the activity in which the child engages is usually of simple type such as going to the bathroom. Somnambulism may be associated with somniloquy. It is characterized neurophysiologically by an incomplete arousal from slow sleep (Pedley 1983). Hereditary factors play a role in its genesis (Kales *et al.* 1980).

Night terrors and sleepwalking occur together in more than half the cases and share the same genetic predisposition (DiMario and Emery 1986). They are grouped together under the term 'non-REM parasomnias'.

Involuntary movements occurring during sleep include myoclonic jerks on falling asleep (Oswald 1959), *nocturnal myoclonus* that may be more or less rhythmical (Lugaresi *et al.* 1972), and *jactatio capitis nocturna* (see above). Unconscious violent behaviour may arise from REM sleep in adolescents and adults.

Periodic movements of sleep are more or less regularly repeated rhythmical movements of the limbs. They may be associated with hyperekplexia (see above) or occur in isolation. The *restless legs syndrome* may occur in children. Walters *et al.* (1994) reported dominantly inherited cases in children with the typical features of urge to move, paraesthesiae, motor restlessness and periodic limb movements (nocturnal myoclonus). Affected children may be misdiagnosed as hyperactive or irritable. The syndrome may be one cause of the so-called 'growing pains'.

Benign neonatal sleep myoclonus is a well-defined and easily diagnosed condition, even though it is often mistaken for epileptic seizures or even status epilepticus. Rhythmical jerks of the limbs may be generalized or localized and occur in brief or more prolonged bursts that can be repeated for hours. The trunk and face remain unaffected and the jerks immediately cease on awakening (Resnick *et al.* 1986, Di Capua *et al.* 1993). Induction of the myoclonus by shaking of the crib is a useful diagnostic manoeuvre (Alfonso *et al.* 1995). The myoclonus usually disappears in a few weeks but it can persist up to several months. Physiological myoclonus should be differentiated from pathological newborn myoclonus which is not sleep-related, may involve the face and trunk, and is associated with EEG abnormalities (Scher 1985, Alfonso *et al.* 1993).

Hypnagogic phenomena are brief episodes of auditory or visual hallucinations or distortions of perception, especially auditory or proprioceptive, which occur in the transition between wakefulness and sleep, most commonly on going to sleep. They may be a part of the narcolepsy tetrad (see below) but much more commonly are a normal phenomenon.

The *'exploding head syndrome'*, characterized by an extremely violent and frightening noise that awakens the patient, is probably related to hypnagogic phenomena and may occur in children (Pearce 1989).

Nocturnal paroxysmal dystonia (Lugaresi *et al.* 1986) is characterized by sleep-related seizures with choreoathetoid, dystonic and ballistic movements occurring every night in adult patients. Similar cases occasionally occur in children. The symptomatology is similar to that of some frontal lobe seizures, and the disease often responds well to carbamazepine. Two subtypes are observed: short repeated attacks lasting only seconds to minutes, and long-lasting episodes. It seems likely that at least the short attacks are frontal lobe epileptic seizures that may be familial (Chapter 16).

SLEEP APNOEA SYNDROMES

Several syndromes are characterized by the occurrence of abnormally frequent or prolonged episodes of apnoea during sleep (see Table 17.2, p. 642). Normally, there is an irregular breathing pattern during REM sleep with frequent periods of apnoea lasting less than 10 seconds.

Episodes of apnoea that occur during sleep may be of three types (Thach 1985, Guilleminault 1987b). *Obstructive apnoea* is the unsuccessful maintenance of an airflow in spite of respiratory effort. *Central apnoea* is arrest of respiration because its fails to be initiated by the respiratory centres. *Mixed apnoea* combines both mechanisms.

OBSTRUCTIVE SLEEP APNOEA SYNDROME

This syndrome is defined by the occurrence of at least 30 apnoeic episodes lasting more than 10 seconds in a seven-hour sleep period (Guilleminault 1987b). Associated symptoms and signs may include daytime sleepiness, loud snoring, insomnia, enuresis, behavioural changes and declining school performance. Diagnosis depends on history, and in some cases bursts of increased activity and respiratory pauses during sleep wrongly suggest epilepsy. Polygraphic recording of the EEG, pneumogram and cardiogram are of great use, as is, especially, continuous recording of blood O_2 saturation (Gordon 1988). Severe complications may result including cor pulmonale, failure to thrive and permanent neurological damage (Brouillette *et al.* 1982, Oren *et al.* 1987). Treatment by tonsillectomy and adenoidectomy or, in severe cases, by tracheostomy, or by alternative methods such as nasal continuous positive airway pressure (Guilleminault *et al.* 1986, Marcus *et al.* 1995) can produce spectacular improvement. Rare familial forms of sleep apnoea syndrome with additional features such as anosmia and colour blindness are on record (Manon-Espaillat *et al.*

1988). *Symptomatic cases* of obstructive sleep apnoea are not infrequent in patients with primary neurological conditions, especially abnormalities of the cervicomedullary junction (Chapter 3) or myotonic dystrophy (Chapter 20).

A *syndrome of increased airway resistance* appears to be more frequent than the obstructive sleep apnoea syndrome (Guilleminault *et al.* 1996). In such children, an increased respiratory effort is required to overcome the airway resistance, resulting in disturbed sleep with abnormal brief episodes of rapid shallow respiration, daytime sleepiness and fatigue, although polygraphic recording does not demonstrate obstructive apnoea, thus leading to sleep disturbances being erroneously ruled out. An increased frequency of night terrors and somnambulism may be observed.

CONGENITAL CENTRAL ALVEOLAR HYPOVENTILATION SYNDROME

Congenital central alveolar hypoventilation syndrome, also known as 'Ondine's curse', is characterized by the depression of central ventilatory drive during quiet sleep. Central apnoea is common (Guilleminault *et al.* 1982). Alveolar hypoventilation syndrome is considerably less frequent than the obstructive sleep apnoea syndrome but is difficult to treat and has a high fatality rate (Deonna *et al.* 1974). Ondine's curse may be idiopathic or occur with inflammatory or other disorders of the brainstem (Jensen *et al.* 1988, Miyazaki *et al.* 1991). Swallowing difficulties may be associated, and a history of hydramnios is present in some cases (Alvord and Shaw 1989). Abnormalities of the brainstem auditory evoked potentials have been found in congenital, idiopathic cases (Beckerman *et al.* 1986). Acquired cases also exist. Cases associated with ophthalmoplegia (Dooling and Richardson 1977) and glaucoma (Walsh and Montplaisir 1982) have been reported. Hirschsprung disease (Commare *et al.* 1993) is 10–20 times more common in children with apnoea than in the general population. The association of apnoea with Hirschsprung disease may be genetically determined and due to mutations of the *RET* (receptor tyrosine kinase) gene which is also involved in the determination of multiple endocrine adenomatosis type III and of papillary carcinoma of the thyroid (Leber *et al.* 1995). An association of central apnoea with neuroblastoma seems also unusually common (Commare *et al.* 1993), and the disorder may be associated with neurocristopathies (Poceta *et al.* 1987).

Most cases are unassociated with major organic CNS abnormalities (Brazy *et al.* 1987). Cases may occur in later life as a result of neurological disease (Giangaspero *et al.* 1988, Jensen *et al.* 1988).

OTHER SYNDROMES INCLUDING SLEEP APNOEA

The *Pickwickian syndrome* is a syndrome of hypoventilation with episodes of apnoea observed in some obese children. It is probably due, at least in part, to limitation of diaphragm movements by fat accumulation with resulting oxygen desaturation and hypercapnia. Daytime somnolence is a consequence of the disturbance of night sleep by apnoea.

Other neurological syndromes include, among their major features, apnoea or abnormal respiratory patterns. Rett syndrome

(Chapter 10) is probably the most common syndrome associated with episodes of *awake apnoea*. Boltshauser *et al.* (1987) and Magaudda *et al.* (1987) have reviewed these syndromes, which include Joubert syndrome, Mohr syndrome and Dandy–Walker syndrome (Bordarier and Aicardi 1990). Magaudda *et al.* (1988) have described a syndrome of familial, fixed, congenital encephalopathy with undifferentiated sleep–waking EEG cycle, excessive startles and continuous periodic breathing.

Episodes of 'microsleep' occur especially in patients with nocturnal insomnia (Tassinari 1976), can be mistaken for epileptic absences and may have the same unpleasant or dangerous consequences for the patients.

SYNDROMES OF HYPERSOMNIA

NARCOLEPSY–CATAPLEXY

Narcolepsy consists of attacks of irrepressible sleep occurring during daytime, most often during monotonous activity. In most patients, the attacks appear on a background of more or less continuous sleepiness which may represent the basic disturbance. The diagnosis can be made when sleepiness is associated with one or more of the other elements of the tetrad of symptoms: cataplexy, hypnagogic hallucinations and sleep paralysis. The full tetrad only occurs in 10 per cent of adult patients. Many children present with behaviour problems or learning difficulties, both consequences of sleepiness and efforts to stay awake (Winter *et al.* 1996). Narcolepsy seems to be unusual in children and only short paediatric series are on record (Young *et al.* 1988). However, many adults with narcolepsy retrospectively admit to having had the condition since childhood, and about 80 per cent of cases have their onset before 20 years of age (Kales *et al.* 1982). The earliest recorded onset was in a 2-year-old child (Winter *et al.* 1996). From a neurophysiological point of view, narcolepsy is characterized by a short latency (less than 10 minutes) from sleep onset to the stage of rapid eye movements (REM sleep). However, not every episode of sleep need be associated with early-onset REM which occurs in less than half the episodes (Aldrich 1990). The diagnosis is best assured when a history of cataplexy is present. A positive multiple sleep latency test is confirmatory rather than conclusive. A total REM latency period of less than seven minutes or the occurrence of two sleep-onset REM periods is found in 83 per cent of patients (Moscovich *et al.* 1993). Ninety-eight per cent of the cases of narcolepsy–cataplexy occur in patients who belong to the HLA-DR2 or DQw1 groups (Honda *et al.* 1986, Kramer *et al.* 1987), although exceptional genuine cases exist that do not belong to these HLA groups (Confavreux *et al.* 1988). This relationship is present only in idiopathic cases; it does not always hold for the cases of narcolepsy due to acquired brain injury (Rivera *et al.* 1986, Aldrich and Naylor 1989) that can rarely be observed with hypothalamic or with pontomedullary (D'Cruz *et al.* 1994) lesions. Such lesions most commonly induce coma or excessive permanent hypersomnia or sleepiness. It seems likely that a gene for susceptibility to narcolepsy exists in the vicinity of the DQw1 locus on the short arm of chromosome 6. This gene need not be related to the immune system. Narcolepsy may be genetically related to some instances of idiopathic hypersomnia in which the incidence of HLA-DR2 may be as high as 60 per cent (Parkes and Lock 1989).

The typical tetrad of narcolepsy–cataplexy is rarely complete. *Narcolepsy* proper refers to the brief attacks of sleep that occur three to five times daily on average. Half the patients are easy to awaken during an attack and most feel refreshed afterwards. It occurs by definition in all patients and is usually the sole manifestation before adolescence.

Cataplexy is a sudden loss of muscle tone, precipitated by laughter or excitement. It results in the patient falling to the ground without losing consciousness.

Hypnagogic hallucinations (see p. 655) and *sleep paralysis* are uncommon. The latter consists of generalized hypotonia with inability to move during the transition between sleep and wakefulness. Partial paralysis with inability to move any one body part is more common.

Nocturnal insomnia is also a frequent complaint of narcoleptic patients. In young children, day naps are often long (20–120 minutes) and unrefreshing and the response to stimulants is poor (Kotagal *et al.* 1990).

Episodes of amnesic automatism simulating epilepsy occur in 8 per cent of patients (Aldrich 1990, Schenck and Mahowald 1992).

Sleep paralysis, cataplexy and hypnagogic hallucinations appear to reflect the fact that the motor manifestations of REM sleep, whose immediate or rapid onset after falling asleep characterizes narcolepsy, may also occur in slight chronological dissociation from the behavioural component of sleep in narcoleptic individuals.

The *course* of narcolepsy is lifelong and often psychologically distressing. A good regimen of sleep is an essential component of therapy. This includes a regular schedule of night sleep, the avoidance of long naps and the provision of short periods of day rest. Methylphenidate and the amphetamines may help some patients but their action is often transitory. Imipramine, 50 mg t.i.d., has a beneficial effect on cataplexy. Recently, successful treatment of narcolepsy with modafinil has been reported (Bastuji and Jouvet 1988). Selegiline may also be useful (Hublin *et al.* 1994). Tyrosine seems to produce a subjective improvement in both adults (Elwes *et al.* 1989) and children (Winter *et al.* 1996), perhaps by increasing central catecholamine release. Simple reassurance that the disorder is not a psychiatric one is of great importance to most patients. Isolated cataplexy has been reported with pontomedullary lesions (D'Cruz *et al.* 1994) in patients with Coffin–Lowry syndrome (Stephenson 1996), and in patients with Niemann–Pick C disease and with Norrie syndrome (Chapter 18) in which it may account for the atonic attacks previously reported (Vossler *et al.* 1996).

OTHER SYNDROMES WITH HYPERSOMNIA
Hypersomnia is encountered in patients with *nocturnal insomnia*, especially in children with the obstructive sleep apnoea syndrome or the increased airway resistance syndrome, which are probably the most common causes of diurnal hypersomnia.

Depression and neurotic states are a frequent cause of hypersomnia in adolescent patients.

Occasional cases of *recurrent hypersomnia* are caused by tumours of the third ventricle or appear as sequelae of encephalitis, trauma or vascular accidents (Billiard and Cadilhac 1988).

The *syndrome of Kleine–Levin* occurs in adolescent males (occasional cases are seen in women) and consists of periods of hypersomnia, compulsive megaphagia and behavioural disturbances with sexual disinhibition (Critchley 1962, Billiard and Cadilhac 1988, Fenzi *et al.* 1993). Incomplete forms do not include megaphagia but psychiatric disturbances are often present. These forms are probably more common than the complete syndrome. Involvement of the limbic and diencephalic structures is probable. Endocrinological evidence of episodic hormone secretion during sleep in the Kleine–Levin syndrome has been recently brought forth (Gadoth *et al.* 1987). Rare cases due to brain lesions are on record (Merriam 1986, Fenzi *et al.* 1993). Treatment with clomipramine or lithium has been proposed (Chapter 29).

INSOMNIA

Many young children have periods when they have difficulties going to sleep. This is a physiological event that should be dealt with gently by parents.

The phenomenon occurs less commonly in school-age children, in whom it is often related to anxiety, especially based on school problems or emotional difficulties. Difficulties in getting to sleep are also common in hyperkinetic children (Chapter 27) and in children with learning difficulties (Ferber 1987).

Certain drugs such as phenobarbitone (Camfield *et al.* 1979) are an often unrecognized cause of sleep disturbances in epileptic toddlers or children. Sometimes, a true depressive state is responsible for insomnia.

In a significant proportion of cases no cause is found, and the prognosis is variable, as some cases persist into adolescence and adulthood.

In most cases no drug therapy is indicated. In rare patients the use of hypnotics such as nitrazepam or chloral hydrate may be considered, especially when severe daily fatigue results from insomnia.

Nocturnal awakening in young children, followed by resumption of sleep in the small hours of the morning is a fairly common and benign behaviour that does not require more than reassurance. Seizures are a rare cause of insomnia responsible for excessive daytime somnolence. In some cases, the seizures are limited to awakening associated with paroxysmal EEG bursts (Peled and Lavie 1986).

REFERENCES

Adams, R.D., Martin, J.B. (1983) 'Faintness, syncope and seizures.' *In:* Petersdorf, R.G., Adams, R.D., Braunwald, E., *et al.* (Eds.) *Harrison's Principles of Internal Medicine, 10th Edn.* New York: McGraw Hill, pp. 76–80.
Aguilera-Diaz, M.L.F. (1971) 'Un nouveau symptôme dans l'acro-dermatite entéropathique: la démarche ataxique.' *Bulletin de la Société Française de Dermatologie et Syphiligraphie*, **78**, 259–260.

Aicardi, J. (1988) 'Clinical approach to the management of intractable epilepsy.' *Developmental Medicine and Child Neurology*, **30**, 429–440.

—— (1994) *Epilepsy in Children, 2nd Edn*. New York: Raven Press.

—— Gastaut, H., Mises, J. (1988) 'Syncopal attacks compulsively self-induced by Valsalva's maneuver associated with typical absence seizures: a case report.' *Archives of Neurology*, **45**, 923–925.

Aldrich, M.S. (1990) 'Narcolepsy.' *New England Journal of Medicine*, **323**, 389–394.

—— Naylor, M.W. (1989) 'Narcolepsy associated with lesions of the diencephalon.' *Neurology*, **39**, 1505–1508.

Alfonso, I., Papazian, O., Rodriguez, J.A., Jeffries, H. (1993) 'Benign neonatal sleep myoclonus.' *International Pediatrics*, **8**, 250–252.

—— Papazian, O., Aicardi, J., Jeffries, H.E. (1995) 'A simple maneuver to provoke benign neonatal sleep myoclonus.' *Pediatrics*, **96**, 1161–1163.

Alvord, E.C., Shaw, C-M. (1989) 'Congenital difficulties with swallowing and breathing associated with maternal polyhydramnios: neurocristopathy or medullary infarction?' *Journal of Child Neurology*, **4**, 299–306.

American Academy of Pediatrics Task Force on Infantile Apnea (1985) 'Prolonged infantile apnea: 1985.' *Pediatrics*, **76**, 129–131.

Andermann, E., Andermann, F., Silver, K., *et al.* (1994) 'Benign familial nocturnal alternating hemiplegia of childhood.' *Neurology*, **44**, 1812–1814.

Andermann, F., Andermann, E. (1988) 'Startle disorders of man: hyperekplexia, jumping and startle epilepsy.' *Brain and Development*, **10**, 213–222.

—— Lugaresi, E. (Eds.) (1987) *Migraine and Epilepsy*. London: Butterworths.

—— Aicardi, J., Vigevano, F. (Eds.) (1995) *Alternating Hemiplegia of Childhood*. New York: Raven Press.

Andersen, A.R., Friberg, L., Skyhoj Olsen, T., Olesen, J. (1988) 'Delayed hyperemia following hypoperfusion in classic migraine.' *Archives of Neurology*, **45**, 154–159.

Angelini, L., Rumi, V., Lamperti, E., Nardocci, N. (1988) 'Transient paroxysmal dystonia in infancy.' *Neuropediatrics*, **19**, 171–174.

Appleton, R., Farrell, K., Buncic, J.R., Hill, A. (1988) 'Amaurosis fugax in teenagers: a migraine variant.' *American Journal of Diseases of Children*, **142**, 331–333.

Aubourg, P., Dulac, O., Plouin, P., Diebler, C. (1985) 'Infantile status epilepticus as a complication of "near-miss" sudden infant death.' *Developmental Medicine and Child Neurology*, **27**, 40–48.

Auburger, G., Ratzlaff, T., Lunkes, A., *et al.* (1996) 'A gene for autosomal dominant paroxysmal choreoathetosis/spasticity (CSE) maps to the vicinity of a potassium channel gene cluster on chromosome 1p, probably within 2 cM, between D1S443 and D1S197.' *Genomics*, **31**, 90–94.

Auduy, B. (1988) 'Défaillance cardio-respiratoire aiguë après absorption de Niaprazine.' *Archives Françaises de Pédiatrie*, **45**, 439. *(Letter.)*

Bain, P.G., O'Brien, M.D., Keevil, S.F., Porter, D.A. (1992) 'Familial periodic cerebellar ataxia: a problem of cerebellar intracellular pH homeostasis.' *Annals of Neurology*, **31**, 147–154.

Baloh, R.W., Yue, Q., Furman, J.M., Nelson, S.F. (1997) 'Familial episodic ataxia: clinical heterogeneity in four families linked to chromosome 19p.' *Annals of Neurology*, **41**, 8–16.

Barabas, G., Matthews, W.S., Ferrari, M. (1983) 'Childhood migraine and motion sickness.' *Pediatrics*, **72**, 188–190.

Barlow, C.F. (1984) *Headaches and Migraine in Childhood. Clinics in Developmental Medicine No. 91*. London: Spastics International Medical Publications.

Bartleson, J.D., Swanson, J.W., Whisnant, J.P. (1981) 'A migrainous syndrome with cerebrospinal fluid pleocytosis.' *Neurology*, **31**, 1257–1262.

Bastuji, H., Jouvet, M. (1988) 'Successful treatment of idiopathic hypersomnia and narcolepsy with modafinil.' *Progress in Neuro-psychopharmacology and Biological Psychiatry*, **12**, 695–700.

Battaglia, A., Guerrini, R., Gastaut, H. (1989) 'Epileptic seizures induced by syncopal attacks.' *Journal of Epilepsy*, **2**, 137–146.

Baxter, P., Gardner-Medwin, D., Green, S.H., Moss, C (1993) 'Congenital livedo reticularis and recurrent stroke-like episodes.' *Developmental Medicine and Child Neurology*, **35**, 917–921.

Baziel, G.M., Van Engelen, M.D., Willy, O., *et al.* (1991) 'Bilateral episodic mydriasis as a migraine equivalent in childhood: a case report.' *Headache*, **31**, 375–377.

Beckerman, R., Meltzer, J., Sola, A., *et al.* (1986) 'Brain-stem auditory response in Ondine's syndrome.' *Archives of Neurology*, **43**, 698–701.

Bennett, H.S., Selman, J.E., Rapin, I., Rose, A. (1982) 'Nonconvulsive epileptiform activity appearing as ataxia.' *American Journal of Diseases of Children*, **136**, 30–32.

Bille, B. (1962) 'Migraine in school children.' *Acta Paediatrica Scandinavica*, **51**, Suppl. 136, 1–151.

Billiard, M., Cadilhac, J. (1988) 'Les hypersomnies récurrentes.' *Revue Neurologique*, **144**, 249–258.

Bodiou, C., Bavoux, F. (1988) 'Niaprazine et effets indésirables en pédiatrie. Bilan coopératif des centres français de pharmacovigilance.' *Thérapie*, **43**, 307–311.

Boel, P., Casaer, P. (1988) 'Familial periodic ataxia responsive to flunarizine.' *Neuropediatrics*, **19**, 218–220.

Boltshauser, E., Lange, B., Dumermuth, G. (1987) 'Differential diagnosis of syndromes with abnormal respiration (tachypnea–apnea).' *Brain and Development*, **9**, 462–465.

Bordarier, C., Aicardi, J. (1990) 'Dandy–Walker syndrome and agenesis of the cerebellar vermis: diagnostic problems and genetic counselling.' *Developmental Medicine and Child Neurology*, **32**, 285–294.

Bourgeois, M., Aicardi, J., Goutières, F. (1993) 'Alternating hemiplegia of childhood.' *Journal of Pediatrics*, **122**, 673–679.

Bower, S., Dennis, M., Warlow, C., *et al.* (1994) 'Long term prognosis of transient lone bilateral blindness in adolescents and young adults.' *Journal of Neurology, Neurosurgery, and Psychiatry*, **57**, 734–736.

Brattström, L., Hindfelt, B., Nilsson, O. (1984) 'Transient neurological symptoms associated with mononuclear pleocytosis of the cerebrospinal fluid.' *Acta Neurologica Scandinavica*, **70**, 104–110.

Brazy, J.E., Kinney, H.C., Oakes, W.J. (1987) 'Central nervous system structural lesions causing apnea at birth.' *Journal of Pediatrics*, **111**, 163–175.

Breningstall, G.N. (1996) 'Breath-holding spells.' *Pediatric Neurology*, **14**, 91–97.

Bressman, S.B., Fahn, S., Burke, R.E. (1988) 'Paroxysmal non-kinesigenic dystonia.' *Advances in Neurology*, **50**, 403–413.

Brett, E.M. (Ed.) (1997) *Paediatric Neurology, 3rd Edn*. Edinburgh: Churchill Livingstone.

Bricker, J.T., Garson, A., Gillette, P.C. (1984) 'A family history of seizures associated with sudden cardiac death.' *American Journal of Diseases of Children*, **138**, 866–868.

Brouillette, R.T., Fernbach, S.K., Hunt, C.E. (1982) 'Obstructive sleep apnea in infants and children.' *Journal of Pediatrics*, **100**, 31–40.

Brown, P., Rothwell, J.C., Thompson, P.D., *et al.* (1991) 'The hyperekplexias and their relationship to the normal startle reflex.' *Brain*, **114**, 1903–1928.

Brunt, E.R.P., Van Weerden, T.W. (1990) 'Familial paroxysmal kinesigenic ataxia and continuous myokymia.' *Brain*, **113**, 1361–1382.

Camfield, C.S., Chaplin, S., Doyle, A-B., *et al.* (1979) 'Side-effects of phenobarbital in toddlers: behavioral and cognitive aspects.' *Journal of Pediatrics*, **95**, 361–365.

Camfield, P.R., Camfield, C.S. (1990) 'Syncope in childhood: a case control clinical study of the familial tendency to faint.' *Canadian Journal of Neurological Science*, **17**, 306–308.

Campistol, J., Prats, J.M., Garaizar, C. (1993) 'Benign paroxysmal tonic upgaze of childhood with ataxia. A neuro-ophthalmological syndrome of familial origin?' *Developmental Medicine and Child Neurology*, **35**, 436–439.

Caplan, L.R. (1991) 'Migraine and vertebrobasilar ischemia.' *Neurology*, **41**, 55–61.

Casaer, P., Aicardi, J., Curatolo, P., *et al.* (1987) 'Flunarizine in alternating hemiplegia in childhood. An international study in 12 children.' *Neuropediatrics*, **18**, 191–195.

Castels-Van Daele, M. (1981) 'Metoclopramide poisoning in children.' *Archives of Disease in Childhood*, **56**, 405–406. *(Letter.)*

Cavanagh, N.D.C., Bicknell, J., Howard, F. (1974) 'Cystinuria with mental retardation and paroxysmal dyskinesia in 2 brothers.' *Archives of Disease in Childhood*, **49**, 662–664.

Chabriat, H., Tournier-Lasserve, E., Vahedi, K., *et al.* (1995) 'Autosomal dominant migraine with MRI white-matter abnormalities mapping to the CADASIL locus.' *Neurology*, **45**, 1086–1091.

Chu, M.L., Shinnar, S. (1992) 'Headaches in children younger than 7 years of age.' *Archives of Neurology*, **49**, 79–82.

Cohen, S.R., Geller, K.A., Birns, J.W., Thompson, J.W. (1982) 'Laryngeal paralysis in children: a long-term retrospective study.' *Annals of Otology, Rhinology and Laryngology*, **91**, 417–424.

Cohen, H.A., Nussinovitch, M., Ashkenasi, A., *et al.* (1993) 'Benign paroxysmal torticollis in infancy.' *Pediatric Neurology*, **9**, 488–490.

Commare, M.C., François, B., Estournet, B., Barois, A. (1993) 'Ondine's curse: a discussion of five cases.' *Neuropediatrics*, **24**, 313–318.

Confavreux, C., Gebuhrer, L., Betuel, H., *et al.* (1988) 'HLA et narcolepsie: à propos de 28 cas dont deux HLA-DR2 négatifs.' *Revue Neurologique*, **144**, 327–331.

Congdon, P.J., Forsythe, W.I. (1979) 'Migraine in childhood: a study of 300 children.' *Developmental Medicine and Child Neurology*, **21**, 209–216.

Cooper, C.J., Ridker, P., Shea, J., Creager, M.A. (1994) 'Familial occurrence of neurocardiogenic syncope.' *New England Journal of Medicine*, **331**, 205. (Letter.)

Critchley, M. (1962) 'Periodic hypersomnia and megaphagia in adolescent males.' *Brain*, **85**, 627–656.

Croft, R.D., Jervis, M. (1989) 'Munchausen's syndrome in a 4 year old.' *Archives of Disease in Childhood*, **64**, 740–741.

Cummiskey, J., Guilleminault, C., Davis, R. (1987) 'Automatic respiratory failure, sleep studies and Leigh's disease.' *Neurology*, **37**, 1876–1878.

Damji, K.F., Allingham, R.R., Pollock, S.C., *et al.* (1996) 'Periodic vestibulo-cerebellar ataxia, an autosomal dominant ataxia with defective smooth pursuit, is genetically distinct from other autosomal dominant ataxias.' *Archives of Neurology*, **53**, 338–344.

Daniels, S.R., Bates, S.R., Kaplan, S. (1987) 'EEG monitoring during paroxysmal hyperpnea of tetralogy of Fallot: an epileptic or hypoxic phenomenon?' *Journal of Child Neurology*, **2**, 98–100.

Darras, B.T., Ampola, M.G., Dietz, W.H., Gilmore, H.E. (1989) 'Intermittent dystonia in Hartnup disease.' *Pediatric Neurology*, **5**, 118–120.

D'Cruz, O.F., Vaughn, B.V., Gold, S.H., Greenwood, R.S. (1994) 'Symptomatic cataplexy in pontomedullary lesions.' *Neurology*, **44**, 2189–2191.

Demirkiran, M., Jankovic, J. (1995) 'Paroxysmal dyskinesias: clinical features and classification.' *Annals of Neurology*, **38**, 571–579.

Deonna, T. (1988) 'Paroxysmal disorder which may be migraine or may be confused with it.' *In:* Hockaday, J. (Ed.) *Migraine in Childhood*. London: Butterworths, pp. 75–87.

—— Martin, D. (1981) 'Benign paroxysmal torticollis in infancy.' *Archives of Disease in Childhood*, **56**, 956–959.

—— Arczynska, W., Torrado, A. (1974) 'Congenital failure of automatic ventilation (Ondine's curse).' *Journal of Pediatrics*, **84**, 710–714.

—— Roulet, E., Meyer, H.U. (1990) 'Benign paroxysmal tonic upgaze of childhood—a new syndrome.' *Neuropediatrics*, **21**, 213–214.

Desai, P., Talwar, D. (1992) 'Nonepileptic events in normal and neurologically handicapped children: a video–EEG study.' *Pediatric Neurology*, **8**, 127–129.

Diamond, S., Dalessic, D.J. (1982) *The Practising Physician's Approach to Headache, 3rd Edn.* Baltimore: Williams & Wilkins.

Di Capua, M., Fusco, L., Ricci, S., Vigevano, F. (1993) 'Benign neonatal sleep myoclonus: clinical features and video–polygraphic recordings.' *Movement Disorders*, **8**, 191–194.

DiDonato, S., Rimoldi, M., Moise, A., *et al.* (1979) 'Fatal ataxic encephalopathy and carnitine acetyl-transferase deficiency: a functional defect of pyruvate oxidation?' *Neurology*, **29**, 1578–1583.

DiMario, F.J., Burleson, J.A. (1993) 'Autonomic nervous system function in severe breath-holding spells.' *Pediatric Neurology*, **9**, 268–274.

—— Emery, E.S. (1986) 'The natural history of night terrors.' *Annals of Neurology*, **20**, 440A. (Abstract.)

DiMauro, S. (1982) 'Muscle phosphoglycerate mutase deficiency.' *Neurology*, **32**, 584–591.

Dooley, J.M., Andermann, F. (1989) 'Startle disease or hyperekplexia: adolescent onset and response to valproate.' *Pediatric Neurology*, **5**, 126–127.

Dooling, E.C., Richardson, E.P. (1977) 'Ophthalmoplegia and Ondine's curse.' *Archives of Ophthalmology*, **95**, 1790–1793.

Dunne, K., Matthews, T. (1987) 'Near-miss sudden infant death syndrome: clinical findings and management.' *Pediatrics*, **79**, 889–893.

Durkan, G.P., Troost, B.T., Slamovits, T., *et al.* (1981) 'Recurrent painless oculomotor palsy in children. A variant of ophthalmoplegic migraine.' *Headache*, **21**, 58–62.

Dvorkin, G.S., Andermann, F., Carpenter, S., *et al.* (1987) 'Classical migraine, intractable epilepsy and multiple strokes: a syndrome related to mitochondrial encephalomyopathy.' *In:* Andermann, F., Lugaresi, E. (Eds.) *Migraine and Epilepsy.* London: Butterworths, pp. 203–232.

Ellie, E., Julien, J., Ferrer, X., *et al.* (1989) 'Extensive cerebral calcification and retinal changes in pseudohypoparathyroidism.' *Journal of Neurology*, **236**, 432–434.

Elliott, F.A. (1984) 'The episodic dyscontrol syndrome and aggression.' *Neurologic Clinics*, **2**, 113–125.

Elliott, M.A., Peroutka, S.J., Welch, S., May, E.F. (1996) 'Familial hemiplegic migraine, nystagmus, and cerebellar atrophy.' *Annals of Neurology*, **39**, 100–106.

Ellis, E.R., Bye, P.T.P., Bruderer, J.W., Sullivan, C.E. (1984) 'Treatment of respiratory failure during sleep in patients with neuromuscular disease. Positive-pressure ventilation through a nose mask.' *American Review of Respiratory Disease*, **135**, 148–152.

Elwes, R.D.C., Crewes, H., Chesterman, L.P., *et al.* (1989) 'Treatment of narcolepsy with L-tyrosine: double-blind placebo-controlled trial.' *Lancet*, **2**, 1067–1069.

Emery, E.S. (1990) 'Status epilepticus secondary to breath-holding and pallid syncopal spells.' *Neurology*, **40**, 859.

Epstein, M.A., Duchowny, M., Jayakar, P., *et al.* (1994) 'Altered responsiveness during hyperventilation-induced EEG slowing: a non-epileptic phenomenon in normal children.' *Epilepsia*, **35**, 1204–1207.

Farris, B.K., Smith, J.L., Ayyar, R. (1986) 'Neuro-ophthalmologic findings in vestibulocerebellar ataxia.' *Archives of Neurology*, **43**, 1050–1053.

Feely, M.P., O'Hare, J., Veale, D., Callaghan, N. (1982) 'Episodes of acute confusion or psychosis in familial hemiplegic migraine.' *Acta Neurologica Scandinavica*, **65**, 369–375.

Fenzi, F., Simonati, A., Crosato, F., *et al.* (1993) 'Clinical features of Kleine–Levin syndrome with localized encephalitis.' *Neuropediatrics*, **24**, 292–295.

Ferber, R. (1987) 'The sleepless child.' *In:* Guilleminault, C. (Ed.) *Sleep and its Disorders in Children.* New York: Raven Press, pp. 141–163.

Ferrari, M.D., Haan, J., Blokland, J.A., *et al.* (1995) 'Cerebral blood flow during migraine attacks without aura and effect of sumatriptan.' *Archives of Neurology*, **52**, 135–139.

Fitzsimons, R.B., Wolfenden, W.H. (1985) 'Migraine coma. Meningitic migraine with cerebral oedema associated with a new form of autosomal dominant cerebellar ataxia.' *Brain*, **108**, 555–577.

Fontan, J.P., Heldt, G.P., Heyman, M.B., *et al.* (1984) 'Esophageal spasm associated with apnea and bradycardia in an infant.' *Pediatrics*, **73**, 52–55.

Fowler, G.W. (1979) 'Intermittent ataxia in heterozygote ornithine transcarbamylase deficiency.' *Annals of Neurology*, **6**, 185–186.

Franckx, J., Noel, P. (1984) 'Acute extrapyramidal dysfunction after domperidone administration.' *Helvetica Paediatrica Acta*, **39**, 285–288.

Fuller, G.N., Guiloff, R.J. (1987) 'Migrainous olfactory hallucinations.' *Journal of Neurology, Neurosurgery, and Psychiatry*, **50**, 1688–1690.

Fusco, L., Vigevano, F. (1995) 'Alternating hemiplegia of childhood: clinical findings during attacks.' *In:* Andermann, F., Aicardi, J., Vigevano, F. (Eds.) *Alternating Hemiplegia of Childhood.* New York: Raven Press, pp. 29–41.

Gadoth, N., Dickerman, Z., Bechar, M., *et al.* (1987) 'Episodic hormone secretion during sleep in Kleine–Levin syndrome: evidence for hypothalamic dysfunction.' *Brain and Development*, **9**, 309–315.

Galletti, F., Brinciotti, M., Emanuelli, O. (1989) 'Familial occurrence of benign myoclonus of early infancy.' *Epilepsia*, **30**, 579–581.

Gastaut, H. (1974) 'Syncopes: generalised anoxic seizures.' *In:* Vinken, P.J., Bruyn, G.W. (Eds.) *Handbook of Clinical Neurology, Vol. 15. The Epilepsies.* Amsterdam: North Holland, pp. 815–835.

—— (1980) 'Un syndrome névrotique méconnu de l'enfant oligophrène: les syncopes autoprovoquées de façon compulsive par manoeuvre de Valsalva.' *Bulletin de l'Académie Nationale de Médecine*, **164**, 713–717.

—— Zifkin, B., Rufo, M. (1987) 'Compulsive respiratory stereotypies in children with autistic features: polygraphic recording and treatment with fenfluramine.' *Journal of Autism and Developmental Disorders*, **17**, 391–406.

Gatrad, A.R., Gatrad, A.H. (1979) 'Familial incidence of dystonic reactions to metoclopramide (maloxon).' *British Journal of Clinical Practice*, **33**, 111–115.

Gay, C.T., Ryan, S.G. (1994) 'Paroxysmal kinesigenic dystonia after methylphenidate administration.' *Journal of Child Neurology*, **9**, 45–46.

Geaney, D.P. (1983) 'Indomethacin-responsive episodic cluster headache.' *Journal of Neurology, Neurosurgery, and Psychiatry*, **46**, 860–861.

Genton, P., Bartolomei, F., Guerrini, R. (1995) 'Panic attacks mistaken for relapse of epilepsy.' *Epilepsia*, **36**, 48–51.

Giangaspero, F., Schiavina, M., Sturani, C., *et al.* (1988) 'Failure of automatic control of ventilation (Ondine's curse) associated with viral encephalitis of the brain stem: a clinicopathologic study of one case.' *Clinical Neuropathology*, **7**, 234–237.

Gillies, D., Sills, M., Forsythe, I. (1986) 'Pizotifen (Sanomigran) in childhood migraine. A double-blind controlled trial.' *European Neurology*, **25**, 32–35.

Golden, G.S. (1979) 'The Alice in Wonderland syndrome in juvenile migraine.' *Pediatrics*, **63**, 517–519.

Gordon, N. (1987) 'Breath-holding spells.' *Developmental Medicine and Child Neurology*, **29**, 811–814.

—— (1988) 'Nasal obstruction in childhood: the obstructive sleep apnoea syndrome.' *Developmental Medicine and Child Neurology*, **30**, 261–265.

—— (1994a) 'Recurrent vomiting in childhood, especially of neurological origin.' *Developmental Medicine and Child Neurology*, **36**, 463–467.

—— (1994b) 'The long Q-T syndromes.' *Brain and Development*, **16**, 153–155.

Grattan-Smith, P.J., Shield, L.K., Hopkins, I.J., Collins, K.J. (1990) 'Acute respiratory failure precipitated by general anesthesia in Leigh's syndrome.' *Journal of Child Neurology*, **5**, 137–141.

Greden, J.F., Victor, B.S., Fontaine, P., Lubetsky, M. (1980) 'Caffeine withdrawal headache: a clinical profile.' *Psychosomatics*, 21, 411–413; 417–418.

Greenberg, D.A. (1997) 'Calcium channels in neurological disease.' *Annals of Neurology*, **42**, 275–282.

Greenblatt, S.H. (1973) 'Posttraumatic transient cerebral blindness. Association with migraine and seizure diatheses.' *Journal of the American Medical Association*, 225, 1073–1076.

Griggs, R.C., Nutt, J.G. (1995) 'Episodic ataxias as channelopathies.' *Annals of Neurology*, **37**, 285–287.

Grylack, L.J., Williams, A.D. (1996) 'Apparent life-threatening events in presumed healthy neonates during the first three days of life.' *Pediatrics*, **97**, 349–351.

Guilleminault, C. (1987a) 'Disorders of arousal in children: somnambulism and nignt terrors.' *In:* Guilleminault, C. (Ed.) *Sleep and its Disorders in Children.* New York: Raven Press, pp. 243–252.

—— (1987b) 'Sleep apnea in the full-term infant.' *In:* Guilleminault, C. (Ed.) *Sleep and its Disorders in Children.* New York: Raven Press, pp. 195–211.

—— McQuitty, J., Ariagno, R., *et al.* (1982) 'Congenital central alveolar hypoventilation syndrome in six infants.' *Pediatrics*, **70**, 684–694.

—— Nino-Murcia, G., Heldt, G., *et al.* (1986) 'Alternative treatment to tracheostomy in obstructive sleep apnea syndrome: nasal continuous positive airway pressure in young children.' *Pediatrics*, **78**, 797–802.

—— Pelayo, R., Leger, D., *et al.* (1996) 'Recognition of sleep-disordered breathing in children.' *Pediatrics*, **98**, 871–882.

Guiloff, R.J., Fruns, M. (1988) 'Limb pain in migraine and cluster headache.' *Journal of Neurology, Neurosurgery, and Psychiatry*, **51**, 1022–1031.

Haan, J., Kremer, H.P.H., Padberg, G.W.A.M. (1989) 'Paroxysmal choreoathetosis as presenting symptom of diabetes mellitus.' *Journal of Neurology, Neurosurgery, and Psychiatry*, **52**, 133. *(Letter.)*

Hagberg, B., Aicardi, J., Dias, K., Ramos, O. (1983) 'A progressive syndrome of autism, dementia, ataxia and loss of purposeful use of hands in girls: Rett syndrome: report of 35 cases.' *Annals of Neurology*, **14**, 471–479.

Hämäläinen, M.L., Hoppu, K., Santavuori, P. (1997a) 'Sumatriptan for migraine attacks in children: a randomized placebo-controlled study. Do children with migraine respond to oral sumatriptan differently from adults?' *Neurology*, **48**, 1100–1103.

—— —— Valkeila, E., Santavuori, P. (1997b) 'Ibuprofen or acetaminophen for the acute treatment of migraine in children: A double-blind, randomized, placebo-controlled, crossover study.' *Neurology*, **48**, 103–107.

Hammond, J. (1974) 'The late sequelae of recurrent vomiting of childhood.' *Developmental Medicine and Child Neurology*, **16**, 15–22.

Harbord, M.G., Kobayashi, J.S. (1991) 'Fever producing ballismus in patients with choreoathetosis.' *Journal of Child Neurology*, **6**, 49–52.

Hart, Y.M., Tampieri, D., Andermann, E., *et al.* (1995) 'Alternating paroxysmal dystonia and hemiplegia in childhood as a symptom of basal ganglia disease.' *Journal of Neurology, Neurosurgery, and Psychiatry*, **59**, 453–454. *(Letter.)*

Hauser, R.A., Lacey, M., Knight, M.R. (1988) 'Hypertensive encephalopathy. Magnetic resonance imaging demonstration of reversible cortical and white matter lesions.' *Archives of Neurology*, **45**, 1078–1083.

Headache Classification Committee of the International Headache Society (1988) 'Classification and diagnostic criteria for headache disorders, cranial, neuralgic and facial pain.' *Cephalalgia*, **8**, Suppl. 7, 19–28.

Henderson, W.R., Raskin, N.H. (1972) '"Hot dog headache": individual susceptibility to nitrite.' *Lancet*, **2**, 1162–1163.

Herman, S.P., Stickler, G.B., Lucas, A.R. (1981) 'Hyperventilation syndrome in children and adolescents. Long-term follow-up.' *Pediatrics*, **67**, 183–187.

Hirayama, K., Hoshino, Y., Kamashiro, H., Yamamoto, T. (1994) 'Reverse Shapiro's syndrome. A case of agenesis of the corpus callosum associated with periodic hyperthermia.' *Archives of Neurology*, **51**, 494–496.

Hockaday, J.M. (1987) 'Migraine and its equivalents in childhood.' *Developmental Medicine and Child Neurology*, **29**, 265–270.

Holguin, J., Fenichel, G. (1967) 'Migraine.' *Journal of Pediatrics*, **70**, 290–297.

Holmes, G.L., Russman, B.S. (1986) 'Shuddering attacks.' *American Journal of Diseases of Children*, **140**, 72–74.

—— Sackellares, J.C., McKiernan, J., *et al.* (1980) 'Evaluation of childhood pseudoseizures using EEG telemetry and video tape monitoring.' *Journal of Pediatrics*, **97**, 554–558.

Honda, Y., Juji, T., Matsuki, K., *et al.* (1986) 'HLA-DR2 and Dw2 in narcolepsy and in other disorders of excessive somnolence without cataplexy.' *Sleep*, **9**, 133–142.

Hublin, C., Partinen, M., Heinonen, E.H., *et al.* (1994) 'Selegiline in the treatment of narcolepsy.' *Neurology*, **44**, 2095–2101.

Hutchinson, W., O'Riordan, J., Javed, M., *et al.* (1995) 'Familial hemiplegic migraine and autosomal dominant arteriopathy with leukoencephalopathy (CADASIL).' *Annals of Neurology*, **38**, 817–824.

Jaeken, J., Carchon, H. (1993) 'The carbohydrate-deficient glycoprotein syndromes: an overview.' *Journal of Inherited Metabolic Disease*, **16**, 813–820.

Jeavons, P.M. (1983) 'Non-epileptic attacks in childhood.' *In:* Rose, F.C. (Ed.) *Research Progress in Epilepsy.* London: Pitman, pp. 224–230.

Jensen, T.H., Hansen, P.B., Brodersen, P. (1988) 'Ondine's curse in *Listeria monocytogenes* brain stem encephalitis.' *Acta Neurologica Scandinavica*, **77**, 505–506.

Jepson, J.B. (1983) 'Hartnup disease.' *In:* Stanbury, J.B., Wyngaarden, B.J., Fredrickson, D.S., *et al.* (Eds.) *The Metabolic Basis of Inherited Disease, 5th Edn.* New York: McGraw Hill, pp. 1563–1577.

Joutel, A., Bousser, M.G., Ducros, A., *et al.* (1994) 'Genetic heterogeneity of familial hemiplegic migraine.' *Journal of Neurology*, **241**, Suppl. 1, S85. *(Abstract.)*

Kahn, A., Blum, D., Rebuffat, E., *et al.* (1988a) 'Polysomnographic studies of infants who subsequently died of sudden infant death syndrome.' *Pediatrics*, **82**, 721–727.

—— Rebuffat, E., Sottiaux, M., Blum, D. (1988b) 'Problems in management of infants with an apparent life-threatening event.' *Annals of the New York Academy of Sciences*, **533**, 78–88.

Kahn, S., Yaqub, B.A., Poser, C.M., *et al.* (1995) 'Multiphasic disseminated encephalomyelitis prsenting as alternating hemiplegia.' *Journal of Neurology, Neurosurgery, and Psychiatry*, **58**, 467–470.

Kales, A., Soldatos, C.R., Bixler, E.O., *et al.* (1980) 'Hereditary factors in sleepwalking and night terrors.' *British Journal of Psychiatry*, **137**, 111–118.

—— Cadieux, R.J., Soldatos, C.R., *et al.* (1982) 'Narcolepsy–cataplexy. I. Clinical and electrophysiologic characteristics.' *Archives of Neurology*, **39**, 164–169.

Kawazawa, S., Nogaki, H., Hara, T., *et al.* (1985) 'Paroxysmal dystonic choreoathetosis in a case of pseudoidiopathic hypoparathyroidism.' *Rinsho Shinkeigaku*, **25**, 1152–1158. *(Japanese.)*

Kemp, G.J., Taylor, D.J., Barnes, P.R.J., *et al.* (1995) 'Skeletal muscle mitochondrial dysfunction in alternating hemiplegia of childhood.' *Annals of Neurology*, **38**, 681–684.

Kinast, M., Lenders, H., Rothner, A.D., Erenberg, G. (1982) 'Benign focal epileptiform discharges in childhood migraine.' *Neurology*, **32**, 1309–1311.

Koenigsberger, M.R., Chutorian, A.M., Gold, A.P., Schvey, M.S. (1970) 'Benign paroxysmal vertigo of childhood.' *Neurology*, **20**, 1108–1113.

Korinthenberg, R. (1996) 'Is infantile alternating hemiplegia mediated by glutamate toxicity and can it be treated with memantine?' *Neuropediatrics*, **27**, 277–278.

Kotagal, S., Hartse, K., Walsh, J.K. (1990) 'Characteristics of narcolepsy in preteenaged children.' *Pediatrics*, **85**, 205–209.

Krägeloh, I., Aicardi, J. (1980) 'Alternating hemiplegia in infants: report of five cases.' *Developmental Medicine and Child Neurology*, **22**, 784–791.

Kramer, R.E., Dinner, D.S., Braun, W.E., *et al.* (1987) 'HLA-DR2 and narcolepsy.' *Archives of Neurology*, **44**, 853–855.

Kramer, U., Carmant, L., Riviello, J.J., *et al.* (1995) 'Psychogenic seizures: videotelemetry observations in 27 patients.' *Pediatric Neurology*, **12**, 39–41.

Krongrad, E., O'Neill, L. (1986) 'Near-miss sudden infant death syndrome episodes? A clinical and electroencephalographic correlation.' *Pediatrics*, **77**, 811–815.

Krowchuk, D.P., Williford, P.M., Jorizzo, J.L., Kandt, R.S. (1994) 'Solitary mastocytoma producing symptoms mimicking those of a seizure disorder.' *Journal of Child Neurology*, **9**, 451–453.

Kuntz, K.M., Kokmen, E., Stevens, J.C., *et al.* (1992) 'Post-lumbar puncture headaches: Experience in 501 consecutive procedures.' *Neurology*, **42**, 1884–1887.

Kurlan, R., Shoulson, I. (1983) 'Familial paroxysmal dystonic choreoathetosis and response to alternate day oxazepam therapy.' *Annals of Neurology*, **13**, 456–457.

—— Krall, R.L., Deweese, J.A. (1984) 'Vertebrobasilar ischemia after total repair of tetralogy of Fallot: significance of subclavian steal created by Blalock–Taussig anastomosis. Vertebrobasilar ischemia after correction of tetralogy of Fallot' *Stroke*, **15**, 359–362.

Kyriakides, T., Drousiotou, A. (1994) 'No structural or biochemical evidence for mitochondrial cytopathy in a case of alternating hemiplegia of childhood.' *Annals of Neurology*, **36**, 805–806. *(Letter.)*

Lance, J.W. (1977) 'Familial paroxysmal dystonic choreoathetosis and its differentiation from related syndromes.' *Annals of Neurology*, **2**, 285–293.

Lancman, M.E., Asconapé, J.J., Craven, W.J., et al. (1994a) 'Predictive value of induction of psychogenic seizures by suggestion.' *Annals of Neurology*, **35**, 359–361.

—— —— Graves, S., Gibson, P.A. (1994b) 'Psychogenic seizures in children: long-term analysis of 43 cases.' *Journal of Child Neurology*, **9**, 404–407.

Lapkin, M., French, J., Golden, G., Rowan, J. (1977) 'The electroencephalogram in childhood basilar artery migraine.' *Neurology*, **27**, 580–583.

Lapkin, M., Golden, G. (1978) 'Basilar artery migraine. A review of 30 cases.' *American Journal of Diseases of Children*, **132**, 278–281.

Lauritzen, M. (1994) 'Pathophysiology of the migraine aura. The spreading depression theory.' *Brain*, **117**, 199–210.

Leber, S.M., Carlson, K.M., Barks, J.D.E., Donis-Keller, H. (1995) 'Congenital central alveolar hypoventilation syndrome, Hirschsprung's disease, and ciliary ganglia dysfunction with RET mutation.' *Paper presented at the Child Neurology Society Meeting, Baltimore, October 1995. (Abstract 135.)*

Lempert, T., Bauer, M., Schmidt, D. (1994) 'Syncope: a videometric analysis of 56 episodes of transient cerebral hypoxia.' *Annals of Neurology*, **36**, 233–237.

Leopold, N.A. (1984) 'Prolonged metoclopramide-induced dyskinetic reaction.' *Neurology*, **34**, 238–239.

Lesser, R.P. (1996) 'Psychogenic seizures.' *Neurology*, **46**, 1499–1507.

Leviton, A., Slack, W.V., Moser, B., et al. (1984) 'A computerized behavioral assessment of children with headaches.' *Headache*, **24**, 182–185.

Lewis, D.W., Frank, C.M. (1993) 'Hair-grooming syncope seizures.' *Pediatrics*, **91**, 836–838.

Lipson, E.H., Robertson, W.C. (1978) 'Paroxysmal torticollis of infancy: familial occurrence.' *American Journal of Diseases of Children*, **132**, 422–423.

Litt, M., Kramer, P., Browne, D., et al. (1994) 'A gene for episodic ataxia/myokymia maps to chromosome 12p13.' *American Journal of Human Genetics*, **55**, 702–709.

Livingstone, I.R., Gardner-Medwin, D., Pennington, R.J.T. (1984) 'Familial intermittent ataxia with possible X-linked inheritance.' *Journal of the Neurological Sciences*, **64**, 89–97.

Lombroso, C.T., Lerman, P. (1967) 'Breath-holding spells (cyanotic and pallid infantile syncope).' *Pediatrics*, **39**, 563–581.

Lou, H.C. (1989) 'Flunarizine in paroxysmal choreoathetosis.' *Neuropediatrics*, **20**, 112. *(Letter.)*

Louis, P. (1981) 'A double-blind placebo-controlled prophylactic study of flunarizine (Sibelium) in migraine.' *Headache*, **21**, 235–239.

Lubbers, W.J., Brunt, E.R.P., Scheffer, H., et al. (1995) 'Hereditary myokymia and paroxysmal ataxia linked to chromosome 12 is responsive to acetazolamide.' *Journal of Neurology, Neurosurgery, and Psychiatry*, **59**, 400–405.

Lugaresi, E., Coccagna, G., Mantovani, M., Lebrun, R. (1972) 'Some periodic phenomena arising during drowsiness and sleep in man.' *Electroencephalography and Clinical Neurophysiology*, **32**, 701–705.

—— Cirignotta, F., Montagna, P. (1986) 'Nocturnal paroxysmal dystonia.' *Journal of Neurology, Neurosurgery, and Psychiatry*, **49**, 375–380.

Magaudda, A., Tassinari, C.A., Bureau, M., et al. (1987) 'Awake apnea syndromes: differential diagnosis with epileptic seizures and correlation with Rett syndrome: report of 28 cases.' *In*: Wolf, P., Dam, M., Janz, D., Dreifuss, F.E. (Eds.) *Advances in Epileptology, Vol. 46*. New York: Raven Press, pp. 245–250.

—— Genton, P., Bureau, M., et al. (1988) 'Familial encephalopathy wth permanent periodic breathing: 4 cases in 2 unrelated families.' *Brain and Development*, **10**, 110–119.

Mandel, H., Tirosh, E., Berant, M. (1989) 'Sandifer syndrome reconsidered.' *Acta Paediatrica Scandinavica*, **78**, 797–799.

Manon-Espaillat, R., Gothe, B., Adams, N., et al. (1988) 'Familial "sleep apnea plus" syndrome: report of a family.' *Neurology*, **38**, 190–193.

Marcus, C.L., Davidson Ward, S.L., Mallory, G.B., et al. (1995) 'Use of nasal continuous positive airway pressure as treatment of childhood obstructive sleep apnea.' *Journal of Pediatrics*, **127**, 88–94.

Matsumoto, J., Fuhr, P., Nigro, M., Hallett, M. (1992) 'Physiological abnormalities in hereditary hyperekplexia.' *Annals of Neurology*, **32**, 41–50.

Mayeux, R., Fahn, S. (1982) 'Paroxysmal dystonic choreoathetosis in a patient with familial ataxia.' *Neurology*, **32**, 1184–1186.

McAbee, G.N., Kadakia, S.K., Sisley, K.C., Delfiner, G.S. (1995) 'Complete heart block in nonfamilial hyperekplexia.' *Pediatric Neurology*, **12**, 149–151.

Meadow, R. (1984) 'Fictitious epilepsy.' *Lancet*, **2**, 25–28.

—— (1991) 'Neurological and developmental variants of Munchausen syndrome by proxy.' *Developmental Medicine and Child Neurology*, **33**, 270–272.

Merriam, A.E. (1986) 'Kleine–Levin syndrome following acute viral encephalitis.' *Biological Psychiatry*, **21**, 1301–1304.

Metrick, M.E., Ritter, F.J., Gates, J.R., et al. (1991) 'Nonepileptic events in childhood.' *Epilepsia*, **32**, 322–328.

Micheli, F., Fernandez Pardal, M.M., Casas Parera, I., Giannaula, R. (1986) 'Sporadic paroxysmal dystonic choreoathetosis associated with basal ganglia calcifications.' *Annals of Neurology*, **20**, 750. *(Letter.)*

Mikati, M.A., Maguire, H., Barlow, C.F., et al. (1992) 'A syndrome of autosomal dominant alternating hemiplegia: clinical presentation mimicking intractable epilepsy; chromosomal studies; and physiologic investigations.' *Neurology*, **42**, 2251–2257.

Miyazaki, M., Hashimoto, T., Sakurama, N., et al. (1991) 'Central sleep apnea and arterial compression of the medulla.' *Annals of Neurology*, **29**, 564–565.

Moorjani, B.I., Rothner, A.D., Kotagal, P. (1995) 'Breath-holding spells and prolonged seizures.' *Annals of Neurology*, **38**, 512–513. *(Abstract.)*

Mortimer, M.J., Kay, J., Jaron, A. (1993) 'Clinical epidemiology of childhood abdominal migraine in an urban general practice.' *Developmental Medicine and Child Neurology*, **35**, 243–248.

Moscovitch, A., Partinen, M., Guilleminault, C. (1993) 'The positive diagnosis of narcolepsy and narcolepsy's borderland.' *Neurology*, **43**, 55–60.

Muenter, M.D., Whisnant, J.P. (1968) 'Basal ganglia calcification: hypoparathyroidism and extrapyramidal motor manifestations.' *Neurology*, **18**, 1075–1080.

Myles, S.T., Needham, C.W., LeBlanc, F.E. (1970) 'Alternating hemiparesis associated with hereditary hemorrhagic telangiectasia.' *Canadian Medical Association Journal*, **103**, 509–511.

Neill, J.C. (1990) 'Pseudoseizures in impaired children.' *Neurology*, **40**, 1146. *(Letter.)*

Newton, R., Aicardi, J. (1983) 'Clinical findings in children with occipital spike–wave complexes suppressed by eye-opening.' *Neurology*, **33**, 1526–1529.

Nezu, A., Kimura, S., Ohtsuki, N., et al. (1997) 'Acute confusional migraine and migrainous infarction in childhood.' *Brain and Development*, **19**, 148–151.

Nigro, M.A., Lim, H.C. (1992) 'Hyperekplexia and sudden neonatal death.' *Pediatric Neurology*, **8**, 221–225.

North, K.N., Ouvrier, R.A., Nugent, M. (1990) 'Pseudoseizures caused by hyperventilation resembling absence epilepsy.' *Journal of Child Neurology*, **5**, 288–294.

Nousiainen, U., Mervaala, E., Uusitupa, M., et al. (1989) 'Cardiac arrhythmias in the differential diagnosis of epilepsy.' *Journal of Neurology*, **236**, 93–96.

Olsen, T.S., Friberg, L., Lassen, N.A. (1987) 'Ischemia may be the primary cause of the neurologic deficits in classic migraine.' *Archives of Neurology*, **44**, 156–161.

Oppenheimer, S.M., Cechetto, D.F., Hachinski, V.C. (1990) 'Cerebrogenic cardiac arrhythmias: cerebral electrocardiographic influences and their role in sudden death.' *Archives of Neurology*, **47**, 513–519.

Oren, J., Kelly, D.H., Shannon, D.C. (1987) 'Long-term follow-up of children with congenital central hypoventilation syndrome.' *Pediatrics*, **80**, 375–380.

Orenstein, S.R., Orenstein, D.M. (1988) 'Gastroesophageal reflux and respiratory disease in children.' *Journal of Pediatrics*, **112**, 847–858.

Orrell, R.W., Marsden, C.D. (1993) 'The neck–tongue syndrome.' *Journal of Neurology, Neurosurgery, and Psychiatry*, **57**, 348–352.

Oswald, I. (1959) 'Sudden bodily jerks on falling asleep.' *Brain*, **82**, 92–103.

Ouvrier, R.A., Billson, F. (1988) 'Benign paroxysmal tonic upgaze of childhood.' *Journal of Child Neurology*, **3**, 177–180.

Pacia, S.V., Devinsky, O., Luciano, D.J., Vazquez, B. (1994) 'The prolonged QT syndrome presenting as epilepsy: a report of two cases and literature review.' *Neurology*, **44**, 1408–1410.

Panayiotopoulos, C. (1989) 'Benign nocturnal childhood occipital epilepsy: a new syndrome with nocturnal seizures, tonic deviation of the eyes, and vomiting.' *Journal of Child Neurology*, **4**, 43–48.
—— (1994) 'Elementary visual hallucinations in migraine and epilepsy.' *Journal of Neurology, Neurosurgery, and Psychiatry*, **57**, 1371–1374.
Parisi, J.E., Collins, G.H., Kim, R.C., Crosley, C.J. (1983) 'Prenatal symmetrical thalamic degeneration with flexion spasticity at birth.' *Annals of Neurology*, **13**, 94–97.
Parker, S., Zuckerman, B., Bauchner, H., *et al.* (1990) 'Jitteriness in full-term neonates: prevalence and correlates.' *Pediatrics*, **85**, 17–23.
Parkes, J.D., Lock, C.B. (1989) 'Genetic factors in sleep disorders.' *Journal of Neurology, Neurosurgery, and Psychiatry*, **52** (Suppl.), 101–108.
Pascotto, A., Coppola, G. (1992) 'Neonatal hyperekplexia: a case report.' *Epilepsia*, **33**, 817–820.
Patel, H., Garg, B.P., Markand, O.N. (1994) 'Bathing epilepsy: video/EEG recording and literature review.' *Journal of Epilepsy*, **7**, 290–294.
Pauli, R.M., Gilbert, E.F. (1986) 'Upper cervical cord compression as a cause of death in osteogenesis imperfecta type II.' *Journal of Pediatrics*, **108**, 579–581.
Pearce, J.M.S. (1980) 'Chronic migrainous neuralgia, a variant of cluster headache.' *Brain*, **103**, 149–159.
—— (1989) 'Clinical features of the exploding head syndrome.' *Journal of Neurology, Neurosurgery, and Psychiatry*, **52**, 907–910.
Pedley, T.A. (1983) 'Differential diagnosis of episodic symptoms.' *Epilepsia*, **24**, Suppl. 1, S31–S44.
Peled, R., Lavie, P. (1986) 'Paroxysmal awakenings from sleep associated with excessive daytime somnolence: a form of nocturnal epilepsy.' *Neurology*, **36**, 95–98.
Pelekanos, J.T., Dooley, J.M., Camfield, P.R., Finley, J. (1990) 'Stretch syncope in adolescence.' *Neurology*, **40**, 705–707.
Pignata, C., Farina, V., Andria, G., *et al.* (1983) 'Prolonged Q-T interval syndrome presenting as idiopathic epilepsy.' *Neuropediatrics*, **14**, 235–236.
Poceta, J.S., Strandjord, T.P., Badura, R.J., Milstein, J.M. (1987) 'Ondine curse and neurocristopathy.' *Pediatric Neurology*, **3**, 370–372.
Poets, C.F., Stebbens, V.A., Richard, D., Southall, D.P. (1995) 'Prolonged episodes of hypoxemia in preterm infants undetectable by cardiorespiratory monitors.' *Pediatrics*, **95**, 860–863.
Poole, C.J.M., Russell, R.W.R., Harrison, P., Savidge, G.F. (1987) 'Amaurosis fugax under the age of 40 years.' *Journal of Neurology, Neurosurgery, and Psychiatry*, **50**, 81–84.
Pranzatelli, M.R. (1996) 'Antidyskinetic drug therapy for pediatric movement disorders.' *Journal of Child Neurology*, **11**, 355–359.
—— Pedley, T.A. (1991) 'Differential diagnosis in children.' *In:* Dam, M., Gram, L. (Eds.) *Comprehensive Epileptology.* New York: Raven Press, pp. 423–447.
Prensky, A.L. (1976) 'Migraine and migrainous variants in pediatric patients.' *Pediatric Clinics of North America*, **23**, 461–471.
—— Sommer, D. (1979) 'Diagnosis and treatment of migraine in children.' *Neurology*, **29**, 506–510.
Reerink, J.D., Peters, A.C.B., Verloove-Vanhorick, S.P., *et al.* (1995) 'Paroxysmal phenomena in the first two years of life.' *Developmental Medicine and Child Neurology*, **37**, 1094–1100.
Rees, M.I., Andrew, M., Jawad, S., *et al.* (1994) 'Evidence for recessive as well as dominant forms of startle disease (hyperekplexia) caused by mutations in the alpha-subunit of the inhibitory glycine receptor.' *Human Molecular Genetics*, **3**, 2175–2179.
Resnick, T.J., Moshé, S.L., Perotta, L., Chambers, H.J. (1986) 'Benign neonatal sleep myoclonus: relationship to sleep states.' *Archives of Neurology*, **43**, 266–268.
Riela, A.R., Roach, E.S. (1993) 'Etiology of stroke in children.' *Journal of Child Neurology*, **8**, 201–220.
Riikonen, R., Donner, M. (1987) 'Chronic relapsing course of encephalo-myeloradiculopathy in a 6-year-old boy.' *Neuropediatrics*, **18**, 235–238.
—— Santuavori, P. (1994) 'Hereditary and acquired risk factors for childhood stroke.' *Neuropediatrics*, **25**, 227–233.
Rivera, V.M., Meyer, J.S., Hata, T. , *et al.* (1986) 'Narcolepsy following cerebral hypoxic–ischemia.' *Annals of Neurology*, **19**, 505–508.
Rosen, J.A. (1983) 'Observations on the efficacy of propanolol for the prophylaxis of migraine.' *Annals of Neurology*, **13**, 92–93.
Rossi, L.N., Mumenthaler, M., Vassella, F. (1980) 'Complicated migraine (migraine accompagnée) in children. Clinical characteristics and course in 40 personal cases.' *Neuropädiatrie*, **11**, 27–35.

—— Vassella, F., Bajc, O., *et al.* (1985) 'Benign migraine-like syndrome with CSF pleocytosis in children.' *Developmental Medicine and Child Neurology*, **27**, 192–198.
—— Penzien, J.M., Deonna, T., *et al.* (1990) 'Does migraine-related stroke occur in childhood?' *Developmental Medicine and Child Neurology*, **32**, 1016–1021.
Ryan, S.G., Sherman, S.L., Terry, J.C., *et al.* (1992) 'Startle disease, or hyper-ekplexia: response to clonazepam and assignment of the gene (STHE) to chromosome 5q by linkage analysis.' *Annals of Neurology*, **31**, 663–668.
Sadarshan, A., Goldie, W.D. (1985) 'The spectrum of congenital facial diplegia (Moebius syndrome).' *Pediatric Neurology*, **1**, 180–184.
Saint-Hilaire, M-H., Saint-Hilaire, J-M., Granger, L. (1986) 'Jumping Frenchmen of Maine.' *Neurology*, **36**, 1269–1271.
Sallustro, C., Atwell, C.W. (1978) 'Body rocking, head banging, and head rolling in normal children.' *Journal of Pediatrics*, **93**, 704–708.
Sander, J.E., Layzer, R.B., Goldsobel, A.B. (1980a) 'Congenital stiff-man syndrome.' *Annals of Neurology*, **8**, 195–197.
Sander, J.E., Malamud, N., Cowan, M.J., *et al.* (1980b) 'Intermittent ataxia and immunodeficiency with multiple carboxylase deficiency: a biotin-responsive disorder.' *Annals of Neurology*, **8**, 544–547.
Saxena, P.R., Den Boer, M.O. (1991) 'Pharmacology of anti-migraine drugs.' *Journal of Neurology*, **238**, S28–S35.
Schaumburg, H.H., Byck, R., Gerstl, R. (1969) 'Monosodium L-glutamate. Its pharmacology and role in the Chinese restaurant syndrome.' *Science*, **163**, 826–828.
Schenck, C.H., Mahowald, M.W. (1992) 'Motor dyscontrol in narcolepsy: rapid eye movement (REM) sleep without atonia and REM sleep behavior disorder.' *Annals of Neurology*, **32**, 3–10.
Scher, M.S. (1985) 'Pathologic myoclonus of the newborn: electrographic and clinical correlations.' *Pediatric Neurology*, **1**, 324–328.
Schneider, H., Ballowitz, L., Schachinger, H., *et al.* (1975) 'Anoxic encephalo-pathy with predominant involvement of basal ganglia, brainstem and spinal cord in the perinatal period. Report on seven newborns.' *Acta Neuropatho-logica*, **32**, 287–298.
Schon, F., Blau, J.M. (1987) 'Post-epileptic headache and migraine.' *Journal of Neurology, Neurosurgery, and Psychiatry*, **50**, 1148–1152.
—— Harrison, M.J.H. (1987) 'Can migraine cause multiple segmental cerebral artery constrictions?' *Journal of Neurology, Neurosurgery, and Psychiatry*, **50**, 492–494.
See, C.C., Newman, L.J., Berezin, S., *et al.* (1989) 'Gastroesophageal reflux-induced hypoxia in infants with apparent life-threatening events.' *American Journal of Diseases of Children*, **143**, 951–954.
Seshia, S.S., Reggin, J.D., Stanwick, R.S. (1985) 'Migraine and complex seizures in children.' *Epilepsia*, **26**, 232–236.
—— Wolstein, J.R., Adams, C., Booth, F.A., Reggin, J.D. (1994) 'International Headache Society criteria and childhood headache.' *Developmental Medicine and Child Neurology*, **36**, 419–428.
Shahar, E., Brand, N., Uziel, Y., Barak, Y. (1991) 'Nose tapping test inducing a generalized flexor spasm: a hallmark of hyperekplexia.' *Acta Paediatrica Scandinavica*, **80**, 1073–1077.
Shafrir, Y., Levy, Y. , Beharab, A., *et al.* (1986) 'Acute dystonic reaction to bethanechol—a direct acetylcholine receptor agonist.' *Developmental Medicine and Child Neurology*, **28**, 646–648.
Sheth, R.D., Barron, T.F., Hartlage, P.L. (1994) 'Episodic spontaneous hypothermia with hyperhydrosis: implications for pathogenesis.' *Pediatric Neurology*, **10**, 58–60.
—— Riggs, J.E., Bodensteiner, J.B. (1995) 'Acute confusional migraine: variant of transient global amnesia.' *Pediatric Neurology*, **12**, 129–131.
Shevell, M.I. (1996) 'Acephalgic migraines of childhood.' *Pediatric Neurology*, **14**, 211–215.
—— Silver, K., Watters, G.V., Rosenblatt, B. (1993) 'Transient oculosym-pathetic paresis (Group II Raeder paratrigeminal neuralgia) of childhood: migraine variant.' *Pediatric Neurology*, **9**, 289–292.
Shiang, R., Ryan, S.G., Zhu, Y-Z., *et al.* (1995) 'Mutational analysis of familial and sporadic hyperekplexia.' *Nature Genetics*, **5**, 351–358.
Shuaib, A., Hachinski, V.C. (1988) 'Migraine and the risks from angiography.' *Archives of Neurology*, **45**, 911–912.
Shuper, A., Zalzberg, J., Weitz, R., Mimouni, M. (1991) 'Jitteriness beyond the neonatal period: a benign pattern of movement in infancy.' *Journal of Child Neurology*, **6**, 243–245.
Silberstein, S.D., Young, W.B., for the Working Panel of the Headache and Facial Pain Section of the American Academy of Neurology (1995) 'Safety

and efficacy of ergotamine tartrate and dihydroergotamine in the treatment of migraine and status migrainosus.' *Neurology*, **45**, 577–584.

Sillanpää, M. (1983) 'Changes in the prevalence of migraine and other headache during the first seven school years.' *Headache*, **23**, 15–19.

Sills, M., Congdon, P., Forsythe, I. (1982) 'Clonidine and childhood migraine: a pilot and double-blind study.' *Developmental Medicine and Child Neurology*, **24**, 837–841.

Silver, K., Andermann, F. (1993) 'Alternating hemiplegia of childhood: a study of 10 patients and results of flunarizine treatment.' *Neurology*, **43**, 36–41.

—— Scriver, C., Arnold, D.L., *et al.* (1995) 'Alternating hemiplegia of childhood associated with mitochondrial disease—a deficiency of pyruvate dehydrogenase.' *In:* Andermann, F., Aicardi, J., Vigevano, F. (Eds.) *Alternating Hemiplegia of Childhood.* New York: Raven Press, pp. 165–171.

Sogg, R.L., Hoyt, W.F. (1962) 'Intermittent vertical nystagmus in father and son.' *Archives of Ophthalmology*, **68**, 515–517.

Southall, D.P., Talbert, D.G., Johnson, P., *et al.* (1985) 'Prolonged expiratory apnoea: a disorder resulting in episodes of severe arterial hypoxaemia in infants and young children.' *Lancet*, **2**, 571–577.

—— Lewis, G.M., Buchanan, R., Weller, R.O. (1987) 'Prolonged expiratory apnoea (cyanotic 'breath holding') in association with a medullary tumour.' *Developmental Medicine and Child Neurology*, **29**, 788–793.

—— Samuels, M.P., Talbert, D.G. (1990) 'Recurrent cyanotic episodes with severe arterial hypoxaemia and intrapulmonary shunting: a mechanism for sudden death.' *Archives of Disease in Childhood*, **65**, 953–961.

Sperl, W., Felber, S., Skladal, D., Wermuth, B. (1997) 'Metabolic stroke in carbamyl phosphate synthetase deficiency.' *Neuropediatrics*, **28**, 229–234.

Spitzer, A.R., Boyle, J.T., Tuchman, D.N., Fox, W.W. (1984) 'Awake apnea associated with gastroesophageal reflux: a specific clinical syndrome.' *Journal of Pediatrics*, **104**, 200–205.

Stephenson, J.B.P. (1980) 'Reflex anoxic seizures and ocular compression.' *Developmental Medicine and Child Neurology*, **22**, 380–386.

—— (1983) 'Febrile convulsions and reflex anoxic seizures.' *In:* Rose, F.C. (Ed.) *Research Progress in Epilepsy.* London: Pitman, pp. 244–252.

—— (1990) *Fits and Faints. Clinics in Developmental Medicine No. 109.* London: Mac Keith Press.

—— (1996) 'Nonepileptic seizures: anoxic–epileptic seizures, and epileptic–anoxic seizures.' *In:* Wallace, S. (Ed.) *Epilepsy in Children.* London: Chapman & Hall, pp. 5–26.

Stewart, W.F., Staffa, J., Lipton, R.B., Ottman, R. (1997) 'Familial risk of migraine: a population-based study.' *Annals of Neurology*, **41**, 166–172.

Sutcliffe, J. (1969) 'Torsion spasms and abnormal postures in childen with hiatus hernia: Sandifer's syndrome.' *Progress in Pediatric Neurology*, **2**, 190–197.

Swanson, J.W., Vick, N.A. (1978) 'Basilar artery migraine. 12 patients, with an attack recorded electroencephalographically.' *Neurology*, **28**, 782–786.

Symon, D.N.K., Russell, G. (1986) 'Abdominal migraine: a childhood syndrome defined.' *Cephalalgia*, **6**, 223–228.

Takashima, S., Becker, L.E. (1986) 'Prenatal and postnatal maturation of medullary "respiratory centers".' *Developmental Brain Research*, **26**, 173–177.

Tassinari, C.A. (1976) 'Nosologie et frontières des syndromes avec respiration périodique au cours du sommeil (syndrome de Pickwick, syndrome d'Ondine, obstruction des voies aériennes supérieures, syndrome avec microsommeil, insomnie et narcolepsie).' *Revue d'Electroencéphalographie et de Neurophysiologie Clinique*, **6**, 53–61.

Tatsumi, C., Takahashi, M., Yorifuiji, S., *et al.* (1988) 'Mitochondrial encephalomyopathy with sleep apnea.' *European Neurology*, **28**, 64–69.

Thach, B.T. (1985) 'Sleep apnea in infancy and childhood.' *Medical Clinics of North America*, **69**, 1289–1313.

Tibbles, J.A.R., Camfield, P.R., Cron, C.C. Farrell, K. (1986) 'Dominant recurrent ataxia and vertigo of childhood.' *Pediatric Neurology*, **2**, 35–38.

Tinuper, P., Montagna, P., Cortelli, P., *et al.* (1992) 'Idiopathic recurring stupor: a case with possible involvement of the gamma-aminobutyric acid (GABA)ergic system.' *Annals of Neurology*, **31**, 503–506.

—— —— Plazzi, G., *et al.* (1994) 'Idiopathic recurring stupor.' *Neurology*, **44**, 621–625.

Tirman, P.J., Woody, R.C. (1988) 'Transient global amnesia precipitated by emotion in an adolescent.' *Journal of Child Neurology*, **3**, 185–188.

Towbin, A. (1969) 'Latent spinal cord and brain stem injury in newborn infants.' *Developmental Medicine and Child Neurology*, **11**, 54–68.

Towbin, J.A. (1995) 'New revelations about the long-QT syndrome.' *New England Journal of Medicine*, **333**, 384–385.

Vahedi, K., Joutel, A., van Bogaert, P., *et al.* (1995) 'A gene for hereditary paroxysmal cerebellar ataxia maps to chromosome 19p.' *Annals of Neurology*, **37**, 289–293.

Vanasse, M., Bédard, M., Andermann, F. (1976) 'Shuddering attacks in children: an early clinical manifestation of essential tremor.' *Neurology*, **26**, 1027–1030.

Veneselli, E., Biancheri, R. (1997) 'Alternating hemiplegia of childhood: treatment of attacks with chloral hydrate and niaprazine.' *European Journal of Pediatrics*, **156**, 157–158. *(Letter.)*

Verlooy, P., Velis, D.N. (1985) 'Non-familial periodic ataxia responding to acetazolamide.' *Clinical Neurology and Neurosurgery*, **87**, 35–37.

Verret, S., Steele, J.C. (1971) 'Alternating hemiplegia in childhood: a report of eight patients with complicated migraine beginning in infancy.' *Pediatrics*, **47**, 675–680.

Vigevano, F., Di Capua, M., Dalla Bernardina, B. (1989) 'Startle disease: an avoidable cause of sudden infant death.' *Lancet*, **1**, 216. *(Letter.)*

Vighetto, A., Froment, J.C., Trillet, M., Aimard, J. (1988) 'Magnetic resonance imaging in familial paroxysmal ataxia.' *Archives of Neurology*, **45**, 547–549.

Vijayan, N. (1980) 'Ophthalmoplegic migraine: ischemic or compressive neuropathy?' *Headache*, **20**, 300–304.

Visser, W.H., de Vriend, R.H., Jaspers, N.M.W.H., Ferrari, M.D. (1996) 'Sumatriptan in clinical practice: a 2-year review of 453 migraine patients.' *Neurology*, **47**, 46–51.

Vossler, D.G., Wyler, A.R., Wilkus, R.J., *et al.* (1996) 'Cataplexy and monoamine oxidase deficiency in Norrie disease.' *Neurology*, **46**, 1258–1261.

Wali, G.M. (1992) 'Paroxysmal hemidystonia induced by prolonged exercise and cold.' *Journal of Neurology, Neurosurgery, and Psychiatry*, **55**, 236–237. *(Letter.)*

Walk, D., Kang, S-S., Horwitz, A. (1994) 'Intermittent encephalopathy, reversible nerve conduction slowing, and MRI evidence of cerebral white matter disease in methylene-tetrahydrofolate reductase deficiency.' *Neurology*, **44**, 344–347.

Walsh, J.T., Montplaisir, J. (1982) 'Familial glaucoma with sleep apnea: a new syndrome?' *Thorax*, **37**, 845–849.

Walters, A.S., Picchietti, D.L., Ehrenberg, B.L., Wagner, M.L. (1994) 'Restless legs syndrome in childhood and adolescence.' *Pediatric Neurology*, **11**, 241–245.

Watanabe, K. Hara, K., Miyazaki, S., *et al.* (1982) 'Apneic seizures in the newborn.' *American Journal of Diseases of Children*, **136**, 980–984.

Welch, K.M. (1993) 'Drug therapy of migraine.' *New England Journal of Medicine*, **329**, 1476–1483.

Werlin, S.L., D'Souza, B.J., Hogan, W.J.H., *et al.* (1980) 'Sandifer syndrome: an unappreciated clinical entity.' *Developmental Medicine and Child Neurology*, **22**, 374–378.

Williams, A.J., Williams, M.A., Walker, C.A., Bush, P.G. (1981) 'The Robin anomalad (Pierre Robin syndrome): a follow-up study.' *Archives of Disease in Childhood*, **56**, 663–668.

Winter, E., Prendergast, M., Green, A. (1996) 'Narcolepsy in a 2-year-old boy.' *Developmental Medicine and Child Neurology*, **38**, 356–359.

Wong, V., Wong, W.C. (1997) 'Enhancement of oculomotor nerve: a diagnostic criterion for ophthalmoplegic migraine?' *Pediatric Neurology*, **17**, 70–73.

Woods, R.P., Iacoboni, M., Mazziotta, J.C. (1994) 'Brief report: bilateral spreading cerebral hypoperfusion during spontaneous migraine headache.' *New England Journal of Medicine*, **331**, 1689–1692.

Woody, R.C., Kiel, E.A. (1986) 'Swallowing syncope in a child.' *Pediatrics*, **78**, 507–509.

Wyllie, E., Friedman, D., Rothner, D., *et al.* (1990) 'Psychogenic seizures in children and adolescents: outcome after diagnosis by ictal video and electroencephalographic recording.' *Pediatrics*, **85**, 480–484.

Yanagihara, T., Piepgras, D.G., Klass, D.W. (1985) 'Repetitive involuntary movement associated with episodic cerebral ischemia.' *Annals of Neurology*, **18**, 244–250.

Young, D., Zorick, F., Wittig, R., *et al.* (1988) 'Narcolepsy in a pediatric population.' *American Journal of Diseases of Children*, **142**, 210–213.

Zifkin, B.G., Arnold, D.L., Andermann, F., Andermann, E. (1995) 'Familial hemiplegic migraine with altered consciousness followed by peduncular hallucinosis: migraine coma as a disorder of brain energy metabolism and possible relevance to alternating hemiplegia of childhood.' *In:* Andermann, F., Aicardi, J., Vigevano, F. (Eds.) *Alternating Hemiplegia of Childhood.* New York: Raven Press, pp. 179–187.

PART VIII

DISORDERS OF THE OCULAR, VISUAL, AUDITORY AND VESTIBULAR SYSTEMS

Disorders of the visual, visuomotor, auditory and vestibular systems are of considerable importance in neurology in general and especially in child neurology. The information collected through these major sensory channels plays a decisive role in the development and function of the CNS, and their main dys-functions justify a separate study. Many of these disorders have been described elsewhere in this book, but a number of relatively common conditions do not fit into any of the preceding chapters and warrant a description of their own because of their frequency or therapeutic or diagnostic importance.

18
DISORDERS OF THE OCULAR MOTOR AND VISUAL FUNCTIONS

The visual system plays a primary role in exploration and analysis of the external world. Proper functioning of this system requires the integrity of an extremely complex neuronal network that is easily disturbed by a vast number of CNS disorders. Such disturbances include defects of ocular motility that result not only from peripheral nerve involvement but also from affectation of the highly complex systems that maintain binocular vision, stability of gaze and other mechanisms necessary for adequate collection and interpretation of visual information. Transmission of the visual information received by the retina to the occipital cortex and processing of this information can also be impeded or disturbed by many pathological processes that, in turn, may influence the ocular motor system. Clinical and electrophysiological analysis of the dysfunction of visual system disorders is a sensitive means of exploring CNS function in general, and study of the abnormalities of ocular movements and of visual perception constitute an essential part of the neurological examination.

DISORDERS OF OCULAR MOTOR FUNCTION

INVOLVEMENT OF PERIPHERAL OCULAR MOTOR NERVES OR THEIR NUCLEI

The movements of the eyeballs are controlled by the IIIrd, IVth and VIth cranial nerves and the muscles they innervate. Paralysis of one or several of these muscles results in ophthalmoplegia, which may be acquired or congenital. Such paralysis should be distinguished from nonparalytic strabismus which is a very common condition affecting 3–4 per cent of all children and whose study is beyond the scope of this book (see Taylor 1997).

ACQUIRED OPHTHALMOPLEGIA
Ophthalmoplegia can be due to a large number of causes (Tables 18.1, 18.2), most of which have been described in the preceding chapters.

Acquired IIIrd nerve palsies are common. Their most frequent causes are closed head trauma, infections and tumours. Traumatic palsies result from haemorrhage or oedema into the nerves or muscles or from avulsion or laceration of these structures (Miller 1985). Fourth nerve paralysis is unilateral in more than 60 per cent of cases and resolves spontaneously in two-thirds (Sydnor

et al. 1982). Third and IVth nerve palsies often clear spontaneously, but infrequently they persist or show evidence of aberrant regeneration, the first signs of which may appear by four to six weeks following the causal lesion or infection (Walsh and Hoyt 1969, Miller 1985). The diagnosis of traumatic palsy may be difficult when the trauma has been minimal or not reported, or when the paralysis is delayed, due to secondary orbital oedema, secondary increased intracranial pressure, infections or vascular complications such as carotid–cavernous fistula (Marmor *et al.* 1982). In such cases, neuroimaging investigation is indicated because trauma may be only the precipitating factor of paralysis of a nerve already compromised by a chronic (compressive) lesion. Infection is the next most common cause, especially meningitis (Miller 1985). Tumours may present as an isolated IIIrd nerve palsy, especially craniopharyngiomas. With brainstem tumours other neurological signs become rapidly obvious. Infectious causes include meningitis, encephalitis and abscesses. Partial palsy may be due to frontal sinusitis (Coker and Ros 1996).

Acquired IVth nerve palsies are mainly of traumatic origin (Keane 1993). Avulsion of the superior oblique pulley may explain the relative frequency of paralysis of this muscle (von Noorden *et al.* 1986). The nerve can also be injured by inflammation or compression in its long intracranial course (Sydnor *et al.* 1982).

Paralysis of the VIth nerve is sometimes observed in newborn infants, probably as a result of birth trauma (de Grauw *et al.* 1983), and usually disappears spontaneously in a few weeks. Tumours are the most common cause in older children and the nerve is especially sensitive to any cause of high intracranial pressure including pseudotumour cerebri. Meningitis and postnatal trauma can also produce lateral rectus paralysis (Afifi *et al.* 1992). Acquired paralysis of the VIth nerve may be difficult to distinguish from the sudden appearance of a squint due to decompensation of refractive error or other visual disturbance, often at the time of an acute infectious disorder (Watson and Fielder 1987).

Postinfectious VIth nerve palsy is thought to be secondary to a viral infection on the basis of history but without definite proof. The onset is sudden and the involvement is generally unilateral. The child complains of diplopia, and paralytic strabismus is observed. Full motility is restored within six months to

Site of lesion	Clinical features	Main causes
Oculomotor nuclei	Bilateral involvement frequent, often associated with gaze palsies. Internal ophthalmoplegia indicates midline lesion. Symmetrical ptosis may exist in isolation	Brainstem tumours and other tumours (pineal region, diencephalon). Infections and inflammation, *e.g.* brainstem encephalitis, multiple sclerosis. Vascular disease and vascular malformations. Degenerative diseases (Wernicke, Leigh)
Fascicular portion (between nuclei and emergence from peduncle)	Similar to nuclear involvement but rarely bilateral	Brainstem intrinsic disease
Interpeduncular fossa	May be associated with involvement of pyramidal tract. Pupillary dilatation and accomodative paralysis present	Basilar meningitis. Aneurysms of rostral basilar artery (rare). Dermoid cysts
At or near entrance into dura	Pupillary involvement prominent especially with herniation	Frontal trauma. Aneurysms. Transtentorial herniation from expanding supratentorial masses or haematomas
In cavernous sinus	Associated involvement of other nerves (V, VI, IV, oculosympathetic)	Sinus thrombosis. Aneurysms. Carotid–cavernous fistulas. Pituitary adenomas. Chordomas and other basilar tumours
Orbital apex and/or superior orbital fissure	Involvement may be partial as the nerve divides into two branches. Pupillary involvement only with affectation of lower trunk	Tolosa–Hunt syndrome. Orbital pseudotumour. Orbital cellulitis. Orbital tumours
Diffuse, undetermined or variable	Variable. Associated paralyses in some cases	Ophthalmoplegic migraine. Sarcoidosis, Whipple disease, some toxic causes such as drugs (*e.g.* anticonvulsants, aspirin). Miller Fisher syndrome and related cranial polyneuropathies, postviral palsies. Diabetes mellitus (exceptional)

one year. A recurrent form has been reported (Afifi *et al.* 1990, Cohen 1993).

Involvement of the VIth nerve may be a part of the Gradenigo syndrome which was usually a complication of mastoiditis when infection reached the apex of the petrous, though such cases are now exceptional. Due to the proximity of the cavum trigeminale, the Vth nerve is also affected with pain in the face and eye, and the facial nerve may be involved in its petrous canal. Rarely, Gradenigo syndrome can be the consequence of T-cell lymphoma (Norwood and Haller 1990). The syndrome is now more commonly seen with orbital or retro-orbital disease (Taylor 1997).

The *Tolosa–Hunt syndrome* (Fig. 18.1) is characterized by a dull, persistent pain around the affected eye, ophthalmoplegia and, sometimes, involvement of the optic nerve, the first and/or second branches of the trigeminal nerves and the sympathetic innervation of the affected eye (Rapin and Echenne 1987, Goto *et al.* 1989, Gordon 1994). The IIIrd nerve is usually involved first and more severely than the others but all three ocular motor nerves may be affected. The diagnosis requires exclusion of other known causes of painful ophthalmoplegia such as infection, neoplasm or lymphoma (Spector and Fiandaca 1986). CT scan may show a high-density area in the orbit, and orbital phlebography may show occlusion of the superior ophthalmic vein (Goadsby and Lance 1989). Subtle MRI abnormalities such as thickening

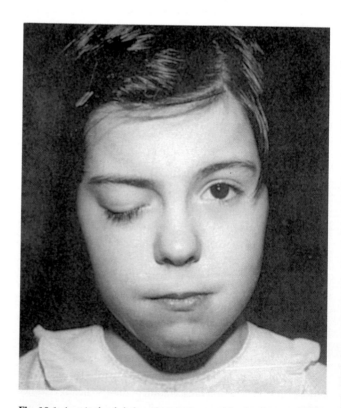

Fig. 18.1. Acquired ophthalmoplegia in 8-year-old girl with Tolosa–Hunt syndrome.

Site of lesion	Clinical features	Causes
Nucleus of IVth nerve	Difficult to determine and to differentiate from IIIrd nerve nuclei involvement and from supranuclear lesions	Brainstem tumours. Inflammatory or demyelinating disease. Vascular obstruction and malformations
Peripheral IVth nerve	Difficult to make a topical diagnosis. Head tilt toward the opposite shoulder	Head trauma
Nucleus of VIth nerve	Conjugate gaze palsy to the ipsilateral side. Does not produce isolated lateral rectus palsy	Same as IVth nerve nucleus involvement
Subarachnoid segment of VIth nerve	Isolated lateral rectus palsy	Aneurysm of basilar artery or its branches. Space-occupying supratentorial lesion (downward movement of neuraxis). Arnold–Chiari malformation. Meningitis and infiltration of the basal meninges
Extradural VIth nerve	Gradenigo syndrome. Involvement of VIIth nerve and gasserian ganglion: pain in the face, reduced corneal sensitivity	Mastoiditis. Rarely bone tumours
Inferior petrosal sinus	May be similar to Gradenigo syndrome	Mastoiditis. Dural arteriovenous malformations of posterior fossa. Fracture of temporal bone. Primitive trigeminal artery
Cavernous sinus and/or superior orbital fissure	Associated involvement of other cranial nerves	Aneurysm, carotid cavernous fistulae, tumours, thrombosis of cavernous sinus
Sphenopalatine fossa	Loss of tearing due to involvement of 2nd division of Vth nerve	Tumours of skull base
Orbit	Indistinguishable from myogenic involvement except by EMG	Tumours, inflammatory lesions
Diffuse, undetermined or variable	Isolated VIth nerve palsy	Postinfectious paralysis, diabetes (rare), migraine (rare), cranial polyneuropathy and Miller Fisher syndrome

of the external wall of the cavernous sinus are being increasingly recognized (Ganesan *et al.* 1996), and detailed imaging of the cavernous sinus is now essential in the investigation of apparently isolated, even painless, cranial nerve palsies. The course usually extends over weeks or, rarely, months. Corticosteroid administration is valuable in the treatment and frequently has a dramatic effect. The condition is related to *orbital pseudotumour* (Grossniklaus *et al.* 1985, Rohr and Gauthier 1988). The latter condition may be either acute or chronic, the so-called sclerosing orbital pseudotumour (Abramovitz *et al.* 1983) which does not respond to steroids. Pseudotumour is rarely seen in children and is usually associated with displacement of the globe downward and outward as well as with oedema and inflammation of the eyelids, both signs that are not present with the Tolosa–Hunt syndrome. Pseudotumours may be very difficult to differentiate from lymphomas and other tumours (Flanders *et al.* 1989).

Acute rectus muscle palsy as a result of orbital myositis (Pollard 1996) is also closely related to orbital pseudotumour and Tolosa–Hunt syndrome. CT or MRI shows swelling of the affected muscle, usually the lateral rectus but occasionally the medial or superior rectus. Muscle involvement has also been observed in Graves ophthalmopathy in infants and adolescents (Uretsky *et al.* 1980).

The painful ophthalmoplegia of Tolosa–Hunt syndrome may be difficult to distinguish from ophthamoplegic migraine,

although involvement of the Vth nerve, increased erythrocyte sedimentation rate and a long duration of pain favour the former diagnosis (Kandt and Goldstein 1985). Enlargement of the optic nerve sheath and of extraocular muscles is also an argument in favour of Tolosa–Hunt syndrome. Treatment with prednisone (1–1.5 mg/d) produces disappearance of pain and of ophthalmoplegia, the latter after several days or weeks. Recurrences may occur on discontinuation of treatment or in spite of it. Involvement of the facial nerve is not rare (Swerdlow 1980). Some authors suggest that the Tolosa–Hunt syndrome may be a form of recurrent cranial nerve neuropathy because of the relative frequency of recurrences that may affect the contralateral side and the involvement of different cranial nerves (Barontini *et al.* 1987).

Cavernous sinus thrombosis may resemble the Tolosa–Hunt syndrome when it produces unilateral (and sometimes bilateral) ophthalmoplegia. However, fever and septic signs are usually marked and there is proptosis and orbital congestion. Vigorous antibiotic treatment is urgently indicated before meningeal involvement sets in (Harbour *et al.* 1984).

CONGENITAL OPHTHALMOPLEGIA
Congenital ophthalmoplegia and ptosis are often not recognized until relatively late or are discounted as representing 'physiological' or pathological strabismus. For this reason, the diagnosis of congenital ophthalmoplegia should not be excluded on the

basis of the child having no ophthalmoplegia at birth by history. Photographs may be extremely useful.

Ocular motor nerve paralysis is relatively common. Victor (1976) reported 16 cases of congenital IIIrd nerve palsy, only one of which was familial. Trauma might have played a role in one child who had a periorbital haematoma and fracture of the zygomatic bone at birth. The paralysis is generally unilateral and complete, although the pupil may be of normal size or even small because of aberrant regeneration. There is exotropia and usually amblyopia of the affected eye. In most cases, evidence of aberrant regeneration is present in the form of lid retraction and/or pupillary constriction on attempted adduction (Prats *et al.* 1993). Cyclic phenomena, with spasm of adduction, pupillary constriction and lid elevation alternating with adductor paresis, ptosis and pupillary constriction may occur.

Treatment is surgical by recession of the lateral rectus or resection of the medial rectus but is of purely cosmetic value.

Congenital trochlear nerve paralysis (Reynolds *et al.* 1984) is sometimes traumatic in origin but most often has no recognized cause. Almost all cases are unilateral (Von Noorden *et al.* 1986). The presenting complaint is frequently a head tilt away from the paralysed side or even scoliosis. When the head is tilted to the paralytic side, hypertropia becomes evident. Surgical therapy is important to avoid torticollis and scoliosis. Congenital IVth nerve palsy has been reported in association with occult cranium bifidum (Bale *et al.* 1988) and as a familial occurrence (Astle and Rosenbaum 1985).

Abducens nerve palsy is unilateral or bilateral and, in the latter case, is easily confused with nonparalytic strabismus. It is often a part of Moebius syndrome (Chapter 21). The *retraction syndrome or Duane syndrome* is characterized by palsy of the lateral rectus, limitation of adduction and narrowing of the palpebral fissure because of globe retraction on attempted adduction (Hotchkiss *et al.* 1980). The syndrome is more often unilateral than bilateral and has been attributed to fibrosis of the lateral rectus, but its pathogenesis is more complex and neural in origin (Huber 1974, Miller 1985, Taylor 1997). Retraction on adduction is due to cocontraction in the superior and inferior as well as the lateral rectus, indicating absence of the VIth nerve, the IIIrd nerve supplying all the extraocular muscles in an abnormal manner. Interestingly, a majority of children with Duane syndrome are able to maintain binocular vision by turning their head toward the side of the lesion. Abnormalities of the brainstem auditory evoked potentials have also been found (Jay and Hoyt 1980). The syndrome is more frequent in girls and may be transmitted as a dominant condition. More complex forms associated with the Marcus Gunn phenomenon (Isenberg and Blechman 1983) (see below) or with the 'crocodile tears' phenomenon (Biedner *et al.* 1979) are on record, indicating that the tendency to abnormal synkineses may be widespread. Crocodile tears are thought to be due to a discrete lesion in the vicinity of the abducens nucleus with innervation of both the lateral rectus and the salivary gland by ocular motor fibres.

Fibrosis of extraocular muscles (congenital familial external ophthalmoplegia) is characterized by the local (Prakash *et al.*

1985) or diffuse (Hiatt and Halle 1983) replacement of muscle fibres by fibrous connective tissue. Most cases are dominantly inherited. The only manifestation is restricted ocular motility in the fields of affected muscles. Ptosis is generally present. Diagnosis requires biopsy of the fibrotic muscles. Recently, the classical type, linked to chromosome 12, has been shown to be associated with absence of the nucleus and nerve fibres normally forming the upper part of the IIIrd nerve complex (Engle *et al.* 1997).

Brown syndrome is caused by shortening of the superior oblique muscle or tendon (Walsh and Hoyt 1969) and is closely related to fibrosis of extraocular muscles. Passive elevation of the globe in adduction is restricted as well as voluntary elevation. Acquired cases may occur as a result of rheumatoid arthritis (Wang *et al.* 1984) or trauma.

Surgical treatment can produce cosmetic benefit in cases of muscle fibrosis.

Congenital ptosis is a common condition caused by absence or fibrosis of the levator palpebrae. Familial cases may occur although the condition is usually sporadic (Walsh and Hoyt 1969). Seventy per cent of cases are unilateral, and in rare cases ptosis is associated with extraocular muscle involvement. Some patients demonstrate a synkinesis between the movements of the jaw and those of the upper lid such that lowering the jaw or moving it sideways produces elevation of the lid which is especially striking in infants when sucking, the so-called jaw-winking or *Marcus Gunn phenomenon* (Pratt *et al.* 1984). An inverted Marcus Gunn phenomenon in which there is drooping of the lid on opening the mouth has been reported as a congenital (Lubkin 1978) or acquired (Rana and Wadia 1985) phenomenon. The mechanism of this phenomenon may be an aberrant regeneration, but a central mechanism is possible and has also been proposed for other synkineses (McLeod and Glaser 1974).

Congenital ptosis should be distinguished from acquired ptosis, especially from myasthenia gravis. Corrective surgery is indicated in severe cases for cosmetic reasons or when vision is impaired by the drooping lid.

GAZE PALSIES
Gaze palsies (Table 18.3) are due to involvement of the supranuclear pathways that control the orientation of the head and eyes (Daroff and Troost 1985). Such control is integrated at several levels including the vestibular nuclei, other brainstem structures, the basal nuclei and the cerebral cortex (Pierrot-Deseilligny *et al.* 1997). The diagnosis of supranuclear ocular palsies rests on the characteristics of abnormal head movements and on the demonstration that the eyes can move normally in response to the doll's head manoeuvre, caloric testing and Bell's phenomenon. The main causes of gaze palsies are listed in Table 18.3 and only some of the manifestations and causes will be discussed.

HORIZONTAL GAZE PALSY
Horizontal gaze palsy can be due to a cortical lesion in the contralateral frontal lobe (area 8), in the anterior occipital lobe or in the ipsilateral para-abducens pontine nucleus. Cortical

TABLE 18.3
Types and causes of gaze palsies in children

Vertical gaze palsy
Tumours (of pineal region and brainstem)
Sylvian aqueduct syndrome in hydrocephalus, especially aqueductal stenosis
Niemann–Pick C disease (DAF syndrome)*
Gaucher disease
Miller Fisher syndrome
Abetalipoproteinaemia (vitamin E deficiency)
Vitamin B$_{12}$ deficiency
Congenital vertical ocular motor apraxia

Horizontal gaze palsy
Frontal lobe destructive lesions (area 8)
Brainstem (pontine) tumours
Central pontine myelinolysis
Familial congenital gaze palsy

Internuclear ophthalmoplegia
Brainstem tumours
Brainstem vascular lesions
Multiple sclerosis
Toxic causes

Convergence palsy
Trauma (may be minor)
Tumour of pineal region

Ocular motor apraxia (paresis or slowing of saccadic eye movements)
Cogan disease (congenital ocular motor apraxia)
Ataxia–telangiectasia
Ataxia–ocular motor apraxia (Chapter 10)
Gaucher disease
Spinocerebellar degenerations

*DAF syndrome: *d*ownward gaze palsy, *a*taxia and *f*oam cells.

lesions are usually associated with hemiplegia or with more complex disturbances such as hemineglect or hemianopia.

Subcortical (pontine) lesions are a common manifestation of brainstem glioma, less commonly of vascular malformations or destructive lesions. They may be a sign of central pontine myelinolysis (Chapter 23). Pontine gaze palsy can be difficult to distinguish from the Moebius syndrome or other causes of bilateral VIth nerve palsy. Familial congenital gaze palsy has been reported (Vetterli and Henn 1981).

VERTICAL GAZE PALSY
Paralysis of vertical gaze, especially upward gaze, may be difficult to distinguish from the simple difficulty in looking upwards which is frequent in patients with mild disturbances of consciousness or even in fatigued patients. Transient disturbances in supranuclear vertical gaze occur in up to 2 per cent of healthy neonates with downward deviation of gaze (Hoyt *et al.* 1980). They can be associated with upbeat nystagmus (Goldblum and Effron 1994). Yokochi (1991) reported episodes of downward gaze deviation in 13 neurologically impaired preterm or term infants with a history of perinatal asphyxia. These episodes lasted several seconds each during wakefulness. All patients had imaging evidence of periventricular leukomalacia, involving predominantly the optic radiations, and half of them had mental retarda-

tion or cerebral palsy at 5 years of age. However, similar episodes with a benign course have also been reported (Kleiman *et al.* 1994). Ouvrier and Billson (1988) reported a syndrome, which they termed *benign paroxysmal tonic upgaze of childhood*, characterized by episodes of sustained tonic conjugate upward deviation of the eyes, lasting from 30 minutes to several hours, with compensatory forward bending of the head. On attempted downward gaze, downbeating ocular saccades would occur. Symptoms were fluctuating, increased by fatigue and intercurrent illnesses and relieved by sleep. The onset was between 6 and 24 months of age. Affected children had no other difficulty except mild ataxia. All symptoms spontaneously disappeared in a few weeks or months. Similar cases have been reported by Deonna *et al.* (1990) who also mentioned the occurrence of occasional atonic falls. Very similar symptoms but with an earlier onset in the first month of life have also been described (Ahn *et al.* 1989).

Familial cases of this syndrome have been reported and the episodes of downward gaze can be abolished by low-dose L-dopa treatment, suggesting a possible link to dopa-sensitive dystonia (Campistol *et al.* 1993). Association with psychomotor retardation has been rarely reported (Sugie *et al.* 1995).

Paralysis of vertical gaze that has been described in intoxication with anticonvulsants, antidepressants and other drugs may be explained in part by disturbance of consciousness, but this does not apply to all cases and true ophthalmoplegia has been repeatedly observed.

The most important cause of vertical gaze palsy is represented by *tumours in the pineal region*. The sylvian aqueduct syndrome can also be seen in patients with hydrocephalus due to aqueductal stenosis. The syndrome features associated eyelid retraction, mydriasis with dilated pupils with better contraction to near objects than to light (light-near dissociation), skew deviation of the eyes, and sometimes convergence–retraction nystagmus (nystagmus retractorius) and disturbances in horizontal gaze. The pretectal syndrome has been reviewed in detail by Keane (1990). Disorders of the basal ganglia such as Huntington disease are frequently associated with vertical supranuclear gaze palsies. Vertical downward gaze palsy is also a feature of Niemann–Pick and Gaucher diseases. In the latter case, paralysis of horizontal gaze is frequently associated (Grosse-Tsur *et al.* 1989) and may be isolated (Patterson *et al.* 1993).

Keane and Finstead (1982) have reported that isolated upward gaze palsy may be the initial manifestation of the Miller Fisher syndrome, and Sandyk (1984) has described the same phenomenon in vitamin B$_{12}$ deficiency.

INTERNUCLEAR OPHTHALMOPLEGIA
Internuclear ophthalmoplegia is characteristic of the involvement of the medial longitudinal fasciculus that connects the abducens nucleus on one side and the opposite ocular motor nucleus to permit conjugate lateral gaze (Fig. 18.2). When these nuclei are disconnected, attempted lateral movements produce abduction of the eye ipsilateral to the fasciculus lesion and absence of the normal adduction of the contralateral eye. The phenomenon may be uni- or bilateral and is mainly due to multiple sclerosis,

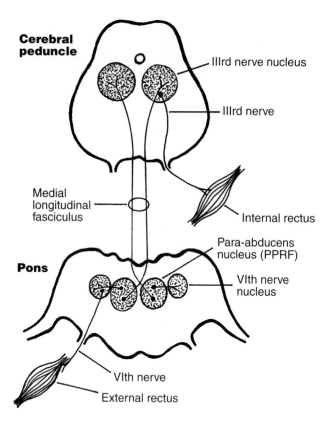

Cerebral peduncle

IIIrd nerve nucleus

IIIrd nerve

Medial longitudinal fasciculus

Internal rectus

Pons

Para-abducens nucleus (PPRF)

VIth nerve nucleus

VIth nerve

External rectus

Fig. 18.2. Internuclear ophthalmoplegia. On attempted gaze to either side, there is no contraction of the internal rectus, due to involvement of the medial longitudinal fasciculus which prevents transmission of influx from the pontine centre for lateral gaze (para-abducens nucleus in the para-median pontine reticular formation: PPRF) to the contralateral IIIrd nerve nucleus, resulting in disconjugate lateral gaze. In unilateral lesions of the medial longitudinal fasciculus, the internuclear ophthalmoplegia is also unilateral. There is usually associated nystagmus of the abducting eye.

although, in children, brainstem tumours and head trauma (Mueller *et al.* 1993) may be a more frequent cause. In mild cases, contraction of the medial rectus may be present but slower than that of the lateral rectus. Nystagmus of the abducting eye is usually present. The *'one-and-a-half syndrome'* is a variant characterized by complete lateral gaze palsy to one side ('one') with contralateral paralysis of adduction ('and a half'). It is caused by a lesion involving the parapontine reticular formation and the longitudinal fasciculus on the same side (Pierrot-Deseilligny *et al.* 1981, Wall and Wray 1983).

CONVERGENCE PALSY

Convergence palsy is an inability to adduct both eyes in the absence of medial rectus paralyses. The commonest cause is probably closed head injury (Krohel *et al.* 1986). Convergence palsy may be encountered even following minor head trauma. It is necessary before accepting the diagnosis of convergence palsy to rule out the presence of a tumour of the quadrigeminal plate or neighbouring structures. Treatment of post-traumatic convergence palsy consists of convergence exercises and/or wearing prisms.

OCULAR MOTOR APRAXIA

Ocular motor apraxia is characterized by abnormal movements of the head and eyes when changes in gaze are being attempted. In its complete form, initiation of a saccade may take up to one second and the movement is slow and hypometric so that several successive hypometric saccades may be necessary to bring the eyes to the desired position. In fact, refixation is commonly performed by head turning rather than by eye deviation. During head rotation, there may be deviation of the eyes in the opposite direction (contraversion) with secondary realignment of the eyes and head when the new objective has been reached (Zee *et al.* 1977). The anomaly is limited to horizontal saccades, whilst vestibular reflex movements, pursuit (slow) movements and vertical saccades are normal.

Most cases are idiopathic. A few cases have been associated with chromosomal abnormalities (Martín Carballo *et al.* 1993) or with immune deficiency (Narbona *et al.* 1980). Shawkat *et al.* (1995) reported that 38 of 62 scans in such children were abnormal, showing delayed myelination, agenesis of the corpus callosum and cerebellar vermian abnormalities, and suggested that lesional causes of delayed saccades may be more common than previously thought. Rare cases of vertical ocular motor apraxia are on record (Hughes *et al.* 1985, Ebner *et al.* 1990). The patient of Ebner *et al.* had a bilateral lesion at the mesencephalic–diencephalic junction demonstrated by CT scan.

Ocular motor apraxia should be distinguished from abnormal eye movements observed in children with very low visual acuity who tend to use head movements rather than saccades for looking at targets (Jan *et al.* 1986) and in children with severe strabismus and low acuity. A syndrome of saccade palsy associated with retinal dystrophy reported by Moore and Taylor (1984) may be simply due to the low visual acuity of affected children.

Ocular motor apraxia is observed as a specific congenital disease also known as Cogan disease, and in various CNS disorders.

Cogan disease or congenital ocular motor apraxia is generally recognized after 6–12 months of age because of the occurrence of head thrusts that may be mistaken for tics or even epileptic seizures. Vertical saccades are normal and mental development is usually preserved. However, many children have clumsiness, difficulties with equilibrium and learning problems. The disease is genetically determined in rare cases, probably transmitted as a recessive trait the expression of which may be very mild, limited for instance to slowness or absence of optokinetic nystagmus. The prognosis is generally favourable with a tendency towards improvement (Zee *et al.* 1977). In addition, older patients tend to use more unobtrusive manoeuvres than head thrusts such as forced blinking for refixation. However, learning problems and clumsiness may be a very significant associated disability (Rappaport *et al.* 1987).

Abnormal eye movements reminiscent of those in Cogan disease may be seen in association with callosal agenesis or vermian aplasia (Bordarier and Aicardi 1990, Leão and Ribeiro-Silva 1995). Slowness of saccades has also been reported with Friedreich disease (Kirkham *et al.* 1979) and other rare spinocerebellar degenerations (Wadia and Swami 1971) including a syndrome of

TABLE 18.4
Various types of nystagmus

Type	Origin	References
Pendular	Congenital; rarely acquired loss of vision	Troost (1989)
	Acquired neurological diseases of brainstem/cerebellum or diffuse degenerations	Harris (1997)
Latent (seen only with monocular vision)	Congenital	Dell'Osso et al. (1979)
Acquired horizontal jerk nystagmus		
Vestibular	Peripheral end-organ (horizontal rotary); central (pure vertical or horizontal)	Troost (1981)
Gaze-evoked/gaze-paretic	Posterior fossa structures; if vertical: brainstem+ cerebellum	Spector and Troost (1981)
Rotary	Vestibular central; medullary lesions; congenital	Troost (1989)
Upbeat	Congenital; acquired brainstem disease; Wernicke encephalopathy	Daroff and Troost (1973)
Downbeat	Chiari I malformation; other lesions of cervicomedullary junction	Pedersen et al. (1980), Baloh and Spooner (1981), Halmagyi et al. (1983)
See-saw (binocular pendular torsional oscillations with superimposed vertical vector moving the eyes in opposite directions)	Lesions of chiasma + floor of 3rd ventricle	Dell'Osso et al. (1974), Daroff et al. (1978)
Retractorius	Quadrigeminal plate; pineal tumours	Walsh and Hoyt (1969)
Periodic alternating (beating successively in one then the opposite direction)	Similar to downbeat nystagmus	Baloh et al. (1976)
Dissociated (major asymmetry between eyes)	Posterior fossa lesions	Cogan (1963)
Voluntary nystagmus	May be a manifestation of hysteria	Walsh and Hoyt (1969)

ataxia–ocular motor apraxia (Aicardi *et al.* 1988; Chapter 10). Abnormal movements are also observed in children with albinism (Collewijn *et al.* 1985).

NYSTAGMUS

Nystagmus is an involuntary, rhythmical, conjugate oscillatory movement of the eyes (Dell'Osso 1984, Hoyt 1987, Troost 1989) which may occur in any plane. It is due to dysfunction of the complex mechanisms that maintain ocular fixation. A time-honoured distinction is between jerk nystagmus in which there is a slow initiating component followed by a fast corrective component, and pendular nystagmus in which the oscillations are of equal speed. However, the distinction between pendular and jerk oscillations may be difficult and even meaningless as the form of eye movements may change with gaze or other factors. In *pendular nystagmus*, the oscillations are slow in each direction, at least in the primary position of gaze, but may change to jerk nystagmus on lateral gaze. The most common form of jerk nystagmus is *gaze-evoked nystagmus* due to a deficit in the mechanisms responsible for holding the eyes in an eccentric position, whose seat is in the

posterior fossa. *Vestibular nystagmus* is also a common type of jerk nystagmus and may result from involvement of the vestibular end organ or central pathways and nuclei (Daroff *et al.* 1978). The direction of the fast jerk conventionally defines the direction of nystagmus. The intensity of jerk nystagmus increases in the horizontal plane when gaze is in the direction of the fast phase (Alexander's law). Other less common types of nystagmus are shown in Table 18.4.

DIFFERENTIAL DIAGNOSIS
The differential diagnosis of nystagmus includes many ophthalmological and neurological conditions. Nystagmus should be differentiated from the roving movements of blind children with pregeniculate lesions. Such movements are indicative of extremely poor vision or complete blindness and may be replaced by nystagmus when some useful vision develops in infants a few months of age (Jan *et al.* 1986, Kömpf and Piper 1987). Monocular vertical oscillations may also occur in amblyopic patients, the so-called Hermann–Bielschowsky phenomenon (Smith *et al.* 1982). Many other types of ocular oscillations are recognized. Some of

TABLE 18.5
Some ocular movements related to or mimicking nystagmus

Type of movement	Clinical features (and common causes)	Reference
Square-wave jerks	Barely visible jerks on steady fixation or smooth pursuit (1–5° saccades) away from fixation point, followed after 200 ms interval by refixation. Only larger jerks clinically visible. (Most common abnormality with cerebellar disease)	Daroff *et al.* (1978)
Ocular dysmetria	Undershooting followed by brief small-amplitude saccadic oscillations or overshooting followed by single or several corrective saccades on refixation. (Cerebellar disease)	Daroff *et al.* (1978)
Ocular flutter and macrosaccadic oscillations	Brief binocular, purely horizontal oscillations occurring spontaneously during straight-ahead fixation. Crescendo amplitude; no intersaccadic latency; whole burst lasts 1–2 s. (Cerebellar disease)	Cogan (1954)
Opsoclonus	Very fast saccadic eye movements in all directions occurring in sudden bursts. (Neuroblastoma, opsomyoclonic syndrome, diffuse cerebellar disease)	Cogan (1954)
Ocular bobbing	Fast downward movement of both eyes followed by slow drift back to mid-position. (Severe brainstem dysfunction, comatose patients)	Mehler (1988)
Ocular dipping	Slow downward and fast upward movement and spontaneous roving horizontal movements. (Same as bobbing)	Ropper (1981)
Superior oblique myokymia	Small-amplitude torsional monocular movement with oscillopsia. (Nonpathological phenomenon. Benign like palpebral myokymia)	Hoyt and Keane (1970)

TABLE 18.6
Main features of congenital nystagmus*

Binocular
Similar amplitude in both eyes
Uniplanar, usually horizontal (may be vertical, rotary)
Increased by attempts at fixation
Inversion of the optokinetic reflex**
Associated head oscillations (in some types)
Abolished in sleep
Distinctive waveforms (require special recording systems)

*Adapted from Troost (1989).
**See Halmagyi *et al.* (1980) for details.

them are listed in Table 18.5, together with their probable or possible anatomical origin and causes.

CAUSES

Congenital nystagmus is usually recognized shortly after birth but may be of the latent type and not detected until visual acuity testing. It may be delayed up to several months of age especially when sensory in type. It persists throughout life and may be ignored by the patient. Congenital nystagmus can be of 'sensory origin', associated with low visual acuity present before 2 years of age (Jan *et al.* 1986, 1990); congenital *motor nystagmus* is caused by a defect in the slow eye movement system. It is not associated with low visual acuity and is usually present from birth. The visual defect may not be causal in all cases although there is controversy

on this point (Dell'Osso *et al.* 1974, Troost 1989, Jan *et al.* 1990).

Congenital nystagmus may be genetically determined. It can be transmitted as an autosomal recessive, autosomal dominant or X-linked character (Dell'Osso *et al.* 1974).

Nystagmus is associated with several types of albinism. This condition is a complex abnormality that includes an excess proportion of nondecussated retinofugal fibres so that only the innermost parts of the nasal fields have a crossed cortical projection. This anomaly can be detected by study of the visual evoked potentials and, in some cases, by MRI showing a sagittally split chiasma (Apkarian *et al.* 1995).

Congenital nystagmus usually oscillates in a constant direction; up to 40 wave forms have been described, most of which are specific for congenital nystagmus but require specialized recordings for their recognition. Such recordings are difficult to calibrate in children (Baker *et al.* 1995) and careful clinical examination is essential. Clinically, congenital nystagmus remains horizontal during vertical gaze rather than converting to gaze-evoked vertical nystagmus (Troost 1989). Additional features of congenital nystagmus are shown in Table 18.6. A unique feature of congenital nystagmus is the so-called inverted optokinetic nystagmus: the fast components are in the direction of rotation of the drum instead of the opposite which is normal (Halmagyi *et al.* 1980).

Head nodding or shaking is present in 6.6–8.0 per cent of children with congenital nystagmus, regardless of the type (motor or sensory) and mode of inheritance (Jan *et al.* 1990). It may be a means of improving foveation time and, therefore, visual acuity.

Latent nystagmus occurs when a single eye is covered. It may be 'manifest–latent' in children with strabismus who are actually viewing with a single eye at a time, even though both eyes are open. The differential diagnosis of congenital nystagmus has been reviewed by Gresty *et al.* (1984).

Acquired nystagmus is usually of the jerk type with a horizontal or horizontal–rotary form. The main causes of acquired nystagmus are indicated in Table 18.4. It is important to keep in mind that drug toxicity is a common cause of jerk nystagmus of horizontal or vertical types, and that certain forms of nystagmus, *e.g.* see-saw nystagmus or downbeat nystagmus, are electively caused by certain conditions such as chiasmatic lesions or the Chiari I malformation.

OCULAR OSCILLATIONS DIFFERENT FROM NYSTAGMUS
(Table 18.5)
Square wave jerks are the most frequent abnormal eye movement associated with cerebellar disease and are often barely visible because of small amplitude.

Opsoclonus is characterized by chaotic, rapid oscillations in all planes of gaze. Opsoclonus is exceptionally observed in newborn infants (Hoyt 1977). It may also be seen in some viral infections and in association with neuroblastoma (Chapter 12).

Ocular flutter and *ocular hypermetria* may be seen in patients with inflammatory or other disorders of the cerebellum (Cogan 1954).

SPASMUS NUTANS
Spasmus nutans consists of a triad of nystagmus, head shaking and head tilt or torticollis. Symptoms appear usually toward the end of the first year of life or during the second year. All three components need not be present at the same time, and head tilt and nodding movements may be transitory or be absent altogether. The nystagmus is constant. It may be binocular but is often predominantly or exclusively monocular. When binocular, it is usually dysconjugate. Vision is normal. The head shaking is horizontal, vertical or gyral, with a rate of 60–120 per minute, while the rate of eye oscillations is around 300 per minute. The nystagmus and head shaking occur in bursts lasting 5–30 seconds in association with fixation. Although infrequent, spasmus nutans is the commonest cause of unilateral nystagmus in infants (Weissman *et al.* 1987) and should be included in the diagnosis of all cases of unilateral nystagmus (Farmer and Hoyt 1984). The cause of the disorder is unknown and the course is benign with resolution in a few months to two years. However, cases of 'sinister' spasmus nutans due to optic gliomas are on record (Albright *et al.* 1984, King *et al.* 1986) so that imaging is indicated in all cases, even when the typical picture is present. Retinal disease can also be a cause (Lambert and Newman 1993), and spasmus nutans has been reported in association with unilateral poor vision due to anterior pathway lesions.

DISORDERS OF VISUAL PERCEPTION

A vast number of CNS disorders include ophthalmological abnormalities which may be their presenting manifestation or represent one of their major diagnostic features.

Assessment of visual acuity is difficult in young children. A full ophthalmological examination is in order and includes fundoscopic examination and evaluation of visual acuity and visual fields. Such examinations are difficult in infants and young children (Hoyt *et al.* 1982) but have been made possible, in many cases, by an adaptation of the preferential looking technique, the acuity card procedure (McDonald *et al.* 1985, Atkinson and van Hof-van Duin 1993). Reflex responses, such as pupillary light reflex, are reliably present after 31 weeks gestation. A blink response to light develops at approximately the same period (dazzle reflex) but the blink response to threat is unreliable and late in appearance. Fixation and following are present from very early in life. Infants turn their head towards a diffuse light from a few days of age. The human face, at a distance of approximately 30 cm, is the best target for fixation. Following in the vertical plane is particularly useful as vertical eye movements are not normally random movements and are therefore more reliable than horizontal ones. Nystagmus induced by rotation about the body axis is present in normal term babies but is inhibited within a few seconds by visual fixation, while, in blind children, it may persist for 15 seconds. The visual evoked response to flashes is an excellent technique to demonstrate the integrity of the visual pathways without patient cooperation (Baker *et al.* 1995). A positive cortical wave with a peak latency of 300 ms is first demonstrable at 30 weeks gestation. The latency then declines by about 10 ms each week through the last 10 weeks of gestation (Taylor *et al.* 1987, Leaf *et al.* 1995). By about 3 months of age, the morphology and latency of the visual evoked responses are relatively mature, but interpretation of the response at earlier periods remains difficult.

Blindness is variably defined. The legal definition in Canada and the USA specifies that distance visual acuity should be no more than 20/200 in the better eye with correction or that the widest diameter of vision should subtend an angle of no more than 20°. In the UK, an acuity of 3/60 or less in the better eye is legally required. Such definitions are not applicable to younger children; these are considered to be blind if there is obviously no vision or if they notice large objects only a few feet away (Jan *et al.* 1977). The main causes of blindness in childhood are listed in Table 18.7.

Amblyopia is defined as defective visual acuity after correction of refractive error. The term is customarily reserved for visual loss associated with strabismus (Friendly 1987).

Cortical blindness is defined as visual loss due to involvement of the retrogeniculate part of the optic pathway. This anomaly is probably more common in children than previously thought (Whiting *et al.* 1985, Roland *et al.* 1986), but some vision is often preserved so that the term *cortical visual impairment* may be more appropriate (Jan *et al.* 1987).

Congenital cataracts or lens opacities are a frequent cause of visual deficits in children and may be a clue to neurological disorders such as the mucopolysaccharidoses, galactosaemia, intrauterine infections, chromosomal aberrations or other syndromes

TABLE 18.7
Main causes of blindness or severe visual impairment in childhood

Diseases of the anterior visual pathway*
Corneal anomalies (scars or metabolic disorders)
Congenital cataracts (hereditary, prenatal infections, metabolic diseases, unknown causes)
Retinopathy of prematurity
Retinitis pigmentosa (several types)
Infectious retinal disease (*e.g.* toxoplasmosis, rubella)
Leber congenital amaurosis
Metabolic and heredodegenerative retinal diseases
Optic nerve hypoplasia
Leber hereditary optic neuropathy
Acquired optic atrophy (see Table 18.8)

Diseases of the posterior visual pathway*
Congenital occipital malformations
Periventricular leukomalacia (due to preterm birth, pre- or postnatal hypoxic–ischaemic events)
Occipital infarcts (thrombosis or compression of posterior cerebral arteries)
Diffuse circulatory failure (vascular collapse, heart failure, status epilepticus, malaria)
Raised intracranial pressure (especially shunt failure)
Heredodegenerative diseases

*Many causes can involve both anterior and posterior pathways.

(Kohn 1976). Further consideration of congenital cataracts is beyond the scope of this book.

Retinopathy of prematurity is still occurring but is now mostly seen in surviving extremely low birthweight (< 1000 g) infants. Up to 30 per cent of preterm infants may suffer from visual problems, most commonly strabismus (Gibson *et al.* 1990). Periventricular leukomalacia and retinopathy of prematurity may coincide in the same patient and share a similar pathogenetic mechanism (Ng *et al.* 1989). Aspects of retinopathy of prematurity have been reviewed by Hoon *et al.* (1988) and the International Committee for Classification of Retinopathy of Prematurity 1988).

CONGENITAL BLINDNESS
Congenital blindness is usually easily detected except in young infants with severe deficit of cognitive and relational functions in whom the distinction between blindness and indifference to surroundings may be difficult to establish.

Visual impairment associated with *lesions of the pregeniculate optic pathways* is most common. In children with involvement of eye media and/or retina, *eye-pressing* with thumb and fingers is common (Jan *et al.* 1983). The mechanism of this digito-ocular phenomenon may be related to the production of phosphenes and other visual sensations by mechanical pressure. The presence of intense eye-pressing should suggest the possibility of retinal disease. It is especially common in blind, mentally retarded children.

Visual impairment due to optic atrophy and other pregeniculate lesions is often accompanied by abnormal eye movements that may be of a 'searching' or roving type, in cases of total blindness, and of congenital nystagmus type when some useful vision is preserved or recovery takes place following an early period of complete visual impairment (Jan *et al.* 1986).

In contrast, *cortical visual impairment* is not associated with abnormal eye movements (Whiting *et al.* 1985) and many patients with this type of deficit seem to be able to spot objects at more than 3 m distance but are unable to identify them without touch. This suggests the probable occurrence in humans of extra-geniculo-calcarine visual pathways (Blythe *et al.* 1987, Braddick *et al.* 1992).

The diagnosis of congenital blindness is essentially clinical. Visual evoked responses may be deceptive, *e.g.* they may be normal despite profound visual loss (Taylor and McCulloch 1991, Wong 1991). An extinguished electroretinogram is helpful but is absent in blindness not due to involvement of the retinal sensory epithelium. The study of the optokinetic nystagmus may be helpful for the diagnosis of malingering if special equipment is available, but in most cases clinical assessment is the best possibility.

Blindness may be responsible for some neurological manifestations such as hypotonia and delayed motor development (Jan and Scott 1974). However, gross retardation is never explained by visual disturbances. Sonksen (1993) followed 600 children with severe visual impairment and carefully assessed the development of their language and social skills. She emphasized the importance of early diagnosis and management to compensate for the increased vulnerability of these children. Visual impairment can also be responsible for EEG abnormalities, particularly the occurrence of occipital spikes that may result from deafferentation of the occipital cortex (Jan and Wong 1988). Such spikes are not indicative of epilepsy, if no clinical seizures are present, and do not require treatment. Neuroimaging techniques may be useful in the assessment of children with visual difficulties (Flodmark *et al.* 1990); they can detect associated cerebral malformations such as absence of the septum pellucidum or agenesis of the corpus callosum and they may also be useful in demonstrating lesions of the optic radiations, especially dilatation of the occipital horns and periventricular leukomalacia (Van Nieuwenhuizen and Willemse 1988, Scher *et al.* 1989).

Congenital blindness may be difficult to distinguish from *delayed visual maturation* (Tresidder *et al.* 1990, Fielder and Mayer 1991). This condition is defined as reduced or absent visual responsiveness with normal ophthalmological examination present from birth but with subsequent improvement at several months of age. Fielder and Mayer (1991) distinguished four types: type I in which there is no ocular or CNS defect; type II where neurological abnormalities are associated; type III in children with albinism and infantile nystagmus: and type IV in which severe structural eye abnormalities are present. A 'roving' nystagmus may be present in some infants when visual recovery begins. Transient strabismus is frequent. Fundoscopic examination is normal but the infantile optic disc is paler than that of older children and the fundus and macula may be somewhat mottled so that an erroneous diagnosis of optic atrophy or retinopathy may be entertained. Delayed maturation of the visual evoked response may be found with abnormal shape, including absence of negative deflections following the first potential (Mellor and Fielder 1980) and increased latency of the evoked response. The

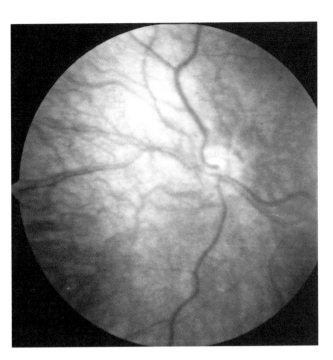

Fig. 18.3. Hypoplasia of the optic papilla. The disc is less than half the normal size. There is a suggestion of a double contour in the nasal region of the disc. (Courtesy Prof. J-L. Dufier, Hôpital des Enfants Malades, Paris.)

ERG is normal. Recovery occurs after the age of 4–6 months, although nystagmus and low acuity may persist in some infants. The cause of this condition is unknown.

OPTIC NERVE HYPOPLASIA

Optic nerve hypoplasia is a developmental defect in the number of optic nerve fibres. The defect may be unilateral or bilateral and it may occur as an isolated defect or be associated with other CNS defects, the most common of which is absence of the septum pellucidum in *septo-optic dysplasia (de Morsier syndrome)*.

In severe bilateral hypoplasia, complete blindness is present. Fundoscopic examination shows a small disc of about half the size of a normal papilla (Fig. 18.3), surrounded by a yellowish, mottled peripapillary halo, bordered on either side by a dark ring of pigment, the 'double-ring' sign. In mild cases, red-free light examination shows various degrees of absence of ganglion cells and axons, which are replaced by a variable number of glial elements (Margalith *et al.* 1984, Ouvrier and Billson 1986, Roberts-Harry *et al.* 1990). Neurological deficits such as quadriplegia or hemiplegia are frequently associated. Endocrinological abnormalities related to defective development of diencephalic derivatives are commonly present. These include dwarfism, often preceded in the neonatal period by manifestations of hypoglycaemia, including seizures. This hypopituitarism of early onset requires emergency treatment, including growth hormone administration, in order to avoid sequelae, especially due to hypoglycaemia. Thus, an early diagnosis of associated cerebral abnormalities is essential. CT scan or MRI permit the diagnosis of septo-optic dysplasia, which may be associated with other congenital abnormalities. The occurrence of bilateral porencephalies

(schizencephalies) is rare (Menezes *et al.* 1988). Optic nerve hypoplasia is observed in infants born to diabetic mothers in an inordinate proportion of the cases (Nelson *et al.* 1986). Therefore, systematic research of maternal diabetes is in order. Fetal alcohol syndrome is another important cause of optic nerve hypoplasia. Strömland and Hellström (1996) found it in 19 of 25 children with the syndrome. The condition is not genetically transmitted.

OTHER DISC ABNORMALITIES

Some disc abnormalities may interfere with vision or may be associated with neurological anomalies of which they may be the presenting manifestation.

Colobomas of the optic nerve may extend to involve the retina, iris, ciliary body and choroid. Colobomas of the optic disc may be isolated, appearing as deep excavations with abnormal emergence of retinal vessels. They may be unilateral or bilateral and are often associated with CNS abnormalities which include, in particular, agenesis of the corpus callosum, in isolation or as a component of the Aicardi syndrome (Chevrie and Aicardi 1986, Aicardi *et al.* 1987). Isolated cases are sometimes transmitted as an autosomal dominant trait (Savell and Cook 1976).

The *'morning glory disc'* is an enlarged papilla with a white excavated centre, surrounded by an annulus of pigmentary change. Retinal vessels emerge at the margins of the disc. Most cases are unilateral (Steinkuller 1980) and some may be associated with CNS abnormalities, especially basal encephalocele.

Drusen of the optic nerve head are cystic formations buried in the head of the optic nerve whose precise mechanism of formation is not known but which may be transmitted as an autosomal dominant trait with variable penetrance. Drusen present in children as a swelling of the optic disc which may mimic papilloedema (Santavuori and Erkkilä 1976, Katz *et al.* 1988). They may occur as an isolated abnormality or be associated with various neurological dysfunctions (Santavuori and Erkkilä 1976). In adult patients they present at fundoscopic examination as polylobulated cystic formations of distinctive appearance, whereas in children they remain buried within the optic nerve head (Fig. 18.4). Therefore, examination of both parents is indicated for any child with pseudopapilloedema as the presence of typical drusen in one of them is of diagnostic importance.

CONGENITAL OPTIC ATROPHY

Congenital optic atrophy is a relatively common finding in children with neurological disorders. In most cases, it occurs as a sporadic phenomenon and does not have a high degree of specificity, as it is observed in a number of apparently heterogeneous congenital nonprogressive encephalopathies as well as in some early progressive encephalopathies.

Congenital optic atrophy is rarely isolated and often represents part of more complex syndromes that also involve the CNS. Many cases are due to infectious fetopathies such as that caused by rubella virus, to brain malformations, to sequelae of hypoxic–ischaemic encephalopathy (probably the most common cause), or to disorders such as osteopetrosis.

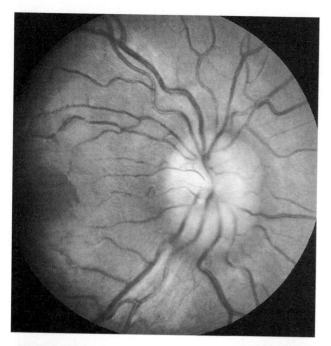

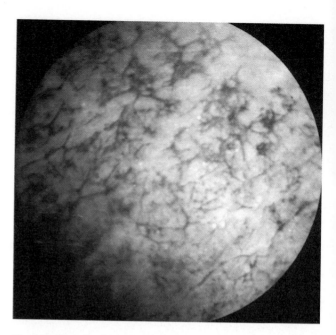

Fig. 18.5. Typical retinitis pigmentosa. Pigment clumps appear as typical bone corpuscles in the retinal periphery. Note considerable attenuation of vessels. (Courtesy Prof. J-L. Dufier, Hôpital des Enfants Malades, Paris.)

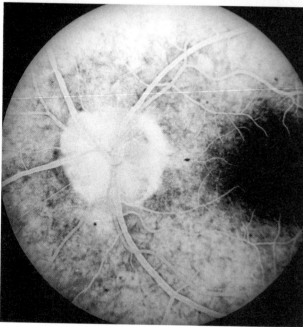

Fig. 18.4. Drusen of the head of the optic disc in a 4-year-old child. *(Top)* Fundus photograph showing protruding papilla with bending of vessels at its margin. *(Bottom)* Following fluorescein injection there is no exudation of substance, contrary to what is observed in papilloedema.

Congenital dominant optic atrophy is a rare variant of the more common type with onset in the first decade of life. *Congenital recessive optic atrophy* is rare and its existence is uncertain (Moeller 1992). The ERG is normal.

Complicated optic atrophy or Behr syndrome (Landrigan *et al.* 1973) includes spastic diplegia and ataxia in association with early-onset optic atrophy. This syndrome is probably heterogeneous. A syndrome of optic atrophy, movement disorder and spastic paraplegia has recently been delineated. It is associated with 3-methylglutaconic aciduria (Costeff *et al.* 1993). Dystonia and pyramidal tract signs in the lower limbs are frequent features (Elpeleg *et al.* 1994). Recessively inherited optic atrophy is a hallmark of the PEHO syndrome (Chapters 10, 16).

LEBER CONGENITAL AMAUROSIS
Leber congenital amaurosis is a generalized rod and cone dystrophy which is present at birth or early in infancy and may be progressive in some cases. The disease may present only with ophthalmological features, but in some cases it is associated with mental retardation or evidence of neurological dysfunction. It is responsible for 10–18 per cent of cases of congenital blindness (Alström and Olson 1957, Schappert-Kimmijser *et al.* 1959). The condition presents as blindness or poor vision with nystagmus from birth or the first months of life. Fundus examination may show pallor of optic discs, thinned retinal vessels, clumps of retinal pigment or white punctate retinopathy (Fig. 18.5) or be altogether normal (Schroeder *et al.* 1987). Extinction of the ERG is an essential diagnostic feature. The finding of a 'flat' ERG in an infant with unexplained neurodevelopmental deficit and/or poor vision indicates the likelihood of the condition being a genetic one with a probable recessive inheritance unless proven otherwise. Some affected infants are hypotonic, mentally retarded or have seizures. Imaging shows hypoplasia of the vermis in 10 per cent of children with Leber amaurosis (Nickel and Hoyt 1982).

Congenital tapetoretinal degeneration with similar characteristics is known to occur in association with structural defects of the CNS such as encephaloceles (Vaizey *et al.* 1977) and, especially, anomalies of the cerebellar vermis (Dekaban 1975, Weinstein *et al.* 1984, Marchal *et al.* 1989, Funakawa *et al.*

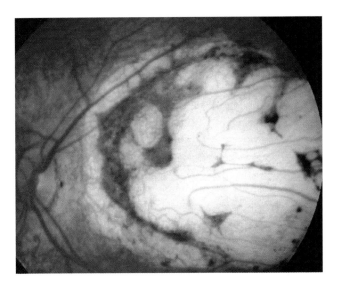

Fig. 18.6. Toxoplasmic choroidoretinitis. Large cicatricial zone involving the macula. Clumps of pigment are haphazardly scattered. (Courtesy Prof. J-L. Dufier, Hôpital des Enfants Malades, Paris.)

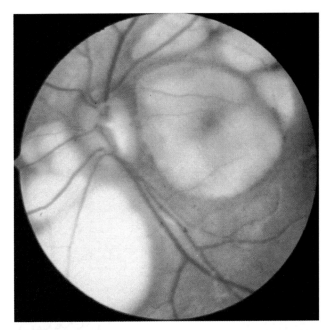

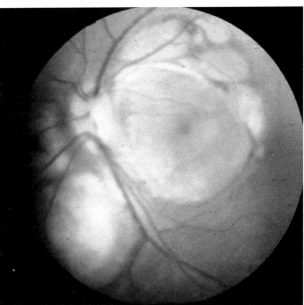

Fig. 18.7. Aicardi syndrome. Typical 'lacunae' in left fundus oculi *(top)* at age 9 months and *(bottom)* at age 4½ years. The size of the 'lacunae' has not changed but the amount of pigment has increased. The peripapillary location of the lesions is usual. (Courtesy Dr I. McCormick, Children's Hospital, Vancouver.)

1995). Retinal degeneration may also be associated with various renal defects (Proesmans *et al.* 1975, Godel *et al.* 1978, Rizzo *et al.* 1986, Warady *et al.* 1994) and with microcephaly (Cantu *et al.* 1977), or be a part of complex syndromes (Mainzer *et al.* 1970, Rizzo *et al.* 1986).

A similar phenotype has been found in patients with peroxisomal disorders such as Zellweger syndrome, as well as in cases with few other abnormalities suggestive of a peroxisomal defect (Ek *et al.* 1986). Such heterogeneity probably accounts for the variable frequency with which neurodevelopmental signs are found in infants with congenital retinal degeneration, with figures as low as 3 per cent of cases (Noble and Carr 1978) or as high as 25–37 per cent (Schappert-Kimmijser *et al.* 1959). Lambert *et al.* (1989) reviewed 75 cases diagnosed with Leber amaurosis and found that 30 had different conditions, including Joubert syndrome, Zellweger syndrome, infantile Refsum disease, congenital stationary night blindness and achromatopsia. Only six of the 45 patients with a diagnosis of Leber amaurosis in their series had mental retardation.

Although some investigators suggested that mental retardation could be a result of visual deprivation (Nickel and Hoyt 1982), this opinion is hardly tenable in view of the pathological findings (Noble and Carr 1978) and the high incidence of severe retardation in some series.

It seems that there is a relatively 'pure' form of Leber amaurosis in which neurodevelopmental abnormalities are rather uncommon. It is transmitted as an autosomal recessive trait (Lambert *et al.* 1993), and a gene has been mapped to chromosome 17p (Camuzat *et al.* 1995). It may be difficult to separate from a group of related conditions, most of which are probably transmitted as mendelian recessive traits (Alstrom and Olson 1957, Baker *et al.* 1995, Casteels *et al.* 1996, Taylor 1997), in which structural CNS defects and neurological and mental dysfunction are more frequent (Vaizey *et al.* 1977).

Miscellaneous retinal diseases are an important cause of impaired vision and may also be a clue to the diagnosis of many neurological disorders. The most common are infectious diseases, especially toxoplasmosis (Fig. 18.6) and cytomegalovirus infection, and congenital anomalies such as the retinal 'lacunae' of Aicardi syndrome (Fig. 18.7). Fundoscopic abnormalities may also be seen in metabolic diseases (see below).

ACQUIRED DISORDERS OF VISUAL PERCEPTION
Acquired disorders of visual perception may be due to a large

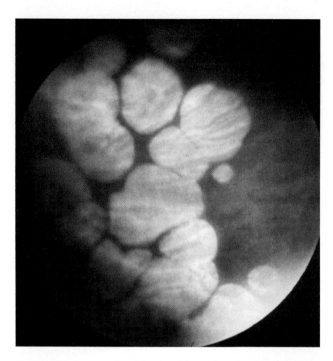

Fig. 18.8. Gyrate atrophy of the choroid. Gyriform areas of atrophy at a distance from the papilla. This aspect may be associated with hyperornithinaemia (see text). (Courtesy Prof. J-L. Dufier, Hôpital des Enfants Malades, Paris.)

number of causes (genetic with late manifestations, or acquired) involving the retina, optic nerve, and retrochiasmatic and retrogeniculate pathways back to the occipital cortex.

RETINAL DISORDERS
Retinal disorders include genetic, traumatic, inflammatory, deficiency and vascular diseases. Several *infectious disorders* can produce retinitis, especially the exanthematous diseases of childhood (Marshall *et al.* 1985; Chapter 12). Choroidoretinitis may be the first manifestation of subacute encephalitis and remain isolated for months or even years. This disease should be included in the differential diagnosis of retinal disorders as early treatment is potentially useful (Tomoda *et al.* 1997).

Gyrate atrophy of the choroid (Fuchs disease)
This is a familial condition, inherited as an autosomal recessive trait. The gene maps to 10q26 and various mutations are known. It is a slowly progressive disease whose initial manifestation is nyctalopia, followed by concentric narrowing of visual field and loss of vision. Fundoscopic examination shows the classical appearance of spider's web retina covered with chocolate dust (Fig. 18.8). Hyperornithinaemia, characteristic of the disease, is due to deficiency of the enzyme ornithine aminotransferase. This is a pyridoxal-dependent enzyme so a small proportion of cases respond to pharmacological doses of pyridoxine (Michaud *et al.* 1995).

Pigmentary retinopathies
A number of other *progressive pigmentary degenerations* of the

retina can be the cause of progressive visual loss in association with neurological dysfunction. Extensive studies of this group are available (Newsome 1988, Taylor 1997). The major initial symptom is hemeralopia, followed after a variable time by concentric narrowing of the visual fields and decrease in visual acuity. The ERG is abnormal early, but fundus examination may remain normal for long periods. There are two main groups of pigmentary retinopathy: in one, only the eyes are involved; in the second, retinal disease is associated with neurodegenerative disorders. These include peroxisomal diseases, mitochondrial disorders including cases of Leigh syndrome, the ceroid–lipofuscinoses, abetalipoproteinaemia, the mucopolysaccharidoses, several types of cerebellar or spinocerebellar degenerations, and genetic syndromes such as the Laurence–Moon, Alström–Hallgren and Usher syndromes. Among the isolated pigmentary retinopathies, multiple types exist with variable inheritance (X-linked, autosomal recessive and dominant), and several DNA mutations have been described (Moore 1997).

Vitamin deficiency
Retinal involvement may be associated with vitamin E deficiency (Chapters 21, 23). Peripheral neuropathy and ocular motor dysfunction are often present.

Vascular disease of the retina
The most common cause of vascular retinal disease is *migraine* that may be responsible for monocular loss of vision ipsilateral to the side of the headache. Visual loss constitutes the aura of a migraine attack and may be partial or total. Rare attacks may be characterized by monocular blindness without headache. Visual loss generally clears in a few minutes but an occasional patient may be left with permanent visual loss. Although patients who develop persistent blindness often have other risk factors for vascular disease, cases have been reported in adolescents without such risk factors (Coppeto *et al.* 1986). Patients with monocular attacks of blindness as a manifestation of migraine ('retinal migraine') should be given vigorous treatment to prevent permanent impairment (Chapter 17). Treatment is that of migraine, sometimes supplemented by antiaggregant drugs (*e.g.* aspirin). Transient bilateral loss of vision is often related to migraine in young patients (Tippin *et al.* 1989) and the same applies to post-traumatic transient blindness (Greenblatt 1973).

Other causes of retinal artery obstruction
These include congenital heart disease causing emboli to the retinal artery (Brown *et al.* 1981), coagulopathies, various types of vasculitis, mitral valve prolapse (Jackson *et al.* 1984), the cardiolipin antibody syndrome (Chapter 15) and cardiac catheterization (Kosmorsky *et al.* 1988).

The onset of symptoms is usually abrupt with a sudden unilateral loss of vision that may be partial or total. Altitudinal defects are present in a majority of cases. Ophthalmological examination shows swelling of the optic disc, oedema of the retina, and narrowing of arteries followed by thickening of the arterial wall. Haemorrhages may be present. Fluorescein angiography can

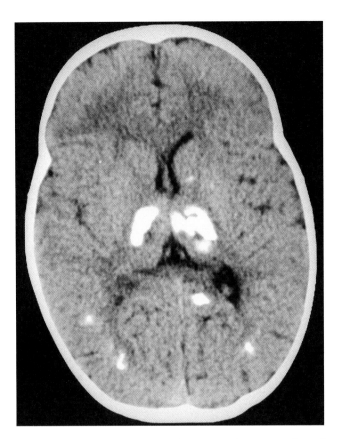

Fig. 18.9. Patient with Coats disease of the retina (telangiectasia of retinal vessel with exudation between retina and choroid), dysplastic nails and extensive intracranial calcification. CT scan. (Courtesy Dr F. Goutières, Hôpital des Enfants Malades, Paris.)

provide objective confirmation of the diagnosis and accurately show the topography and degree of ischaemia.

The outlook for vision depends on the cause of obstruction and on the location of obstructed vessels. The prognosis is better for obliteration of peripheral branches than for that of the central artery itself. Treatment depends on the cause. Anticoagulants may be indicated if a source of emboli is identified. Steroids and immunosuppressors are useful for many vasculitides.

Coats disease
Coats disease, characterized by congenital retinal telangiectasias and exudative retinal detachment, can be part of a rare autosomal recessive syndrome of facioscapulohumeral dystrophy, hearing loss and mental retardation (Taylor *et al.* 1982, Matsuzaka *et al.* 1986). Bilateral Coats disease, facial dysmorphism, abnormal hair and nails, and striking supra- and infratentorial calcification involving the thalami and neighbouring brain areas has been reported as a familial disorder (Tolmie *et al.* 1988) (Fig. 18.9).

Norrie disease
Norrie disease is a sex-linked recessive disorder characterized by bilateral retinal folds, retinal detachment, vitreous haemorrhage and bilateral retrolental masses which may be a cause of congenital or early-onset blindness in boys. About 25 per cent of affected

TABLE 18.8
Main causes of optic neuropathies

Cause	Reference
Developmental lesions	This chapter
Optic nerve hypoplasia	
Septo-optic dysplasia	
Heredodegenerative neuropathies	This chapter
Dominant optic neuropathy	
Leber hereditary optic neuropathy	
Complicated optic neuropathy—Behr syndrome	
Costeff syndrome (3-methylglutaconic aciduria)	
Metabolic diseases	
Diabetes mellitus	Chapter 23
Mitochondrial diseases including Leigh syndrome	Chapter 9
Hyperthyroidism	Chapter 23
Infantile neuroaxonal dystrophy	Chapter 10
Ischaemic neuropathies	
Thrombosis and emboli of retinal arteries	This chapter
Inflammatory arterial diseases (*e.g.* panarteritis nodosa)	Chapter 12
Venous thrombosis	Chapter 15
Compression neuropathies	Chapter 14
Sellar and perisellar tumours	
Meningeal carcinomatosis	
Leukaemia and lymphomas	
Inflammatory demyelinating neuropathies	Chapter 12
Multiple sclerosis	
Neuromyelitis optica	
Schilder disease	
Postviral neuropathies (measles, mumps, chicken pox, infectious mononucleosis, etc.)	
Toxic and nutritional neuropathies	This chapter
Drugs	
Other exogenous toxins	
Protein–caloric malnutrition	
Neighbouring inflammatory lesions	
Sinusitis and ethmoiditis	This chapter
Acute purulent and subacute meningitides	Chapter 11
Intraorbital pseudotumour	This chapter
Cavernous sinus lesions	This chapter

children also develop cochlear hearing loss (Liberfarb *et al.* 1985). Mutations of the responsible gene can be used in genetic diagnosis (Black and Redmond 1994). Cataplectic attacks may be associated (Chapter 17).

DISORDERS OF THE OPTIC NERVE (Table 18.8)
Leber hereditary optic neuropathy (LHON)
This is the most frequent cause of hereditary optic neuropathy with late manifestation. The disease affects men in 85 per cent of cases, and 18 per cent of female carriers are clinically affected. Seventy to 100 per cent of daughters of female carriers are also carriers, and 50–100 per cent of the sons of female carriers are affected. Transmission is always through the female line. Several point mutations of mitochondrial DNA have been shown to be associated with the disease (Wallace *et al.* 1988, Johns *et al.* 1992, Paulus *et al.* 1993, Antozzi *et al.* 1995). Some of these mutations probably act as primary mutations ('major

mutations'), while others may have only a contributory role ('minor mutations').

The mechanism of the disease, however, remains unknown. Onset is usually in adolescence or early adulthood. Occasionally, children as young as 7 years may be affected (Moorman *et al.* 1993). The age of onset may be quite variable even in the same kinship.

Blurred central vision in one eye is the initial complaint. Similar symptoms usually occur in the opposite eye within a few days or weeks but the interval is occasionally of months or years, and in about 20 per cent of cases onset is simultaneous in both eyes (Riordan-Eva *et al.* 1995). Fundoscopic examination at an initial stage shows a peculiar telangiectatic microangiopathy, especially in the peripapillary region (Nikoskelainen *et al.* 1983), although this may be absent in one-third of cases. Such an angiopathy may be present in asymptomatic family members (Nikoskelainen *et al.* 1982). Fluorescein angiography characteristically shows absence of peripapillary retinal staining (Nikoskelainen *et al.* 1984). In symptomatic patients, telangiectasias are accompanied by retinal oedema and haemorrhages. In later stages, atrophy appears first in the maculopapillar bundle, then in the rest of the retina within two months of onset. At that stage, a pale disc with narrow vessels is visible (Lopez and Smith 1986). Visual field loss progresses from an enlarged blind spot to a large centrocaecal scotoma. Loss of visual acuity is usually severe to 6/60 or less. The relationship between individual DNA mutations and phenotype has been studied by Riordan-Eva *et al.* (1995).

In most patients, some useful vision is left or restored after one to several years, and rare patients recover fully. No relapses are observed.

Treatment is limited to avoidance of potential toxins such as alcohol and, especially, tobacco. Hydroxocobalamin and oral cystine have been recommended on the basis of a possible deficit in rhodanese activity in liver and rectal mucosa (Poole and Kind 1986). The efficacy of this regimen remains to be proved.

Hereditary optic atrophy with the characteristics of LHON has been reported in association with neurological symptoms and signs in some kindreds. Associated neurological features have included ataxia and cerebellar manifestations that may suggest multiple sclerosis, dystonia and paraplegia. Some such cases might result from a special susceptibility of patients with specific mitochondrial mutations associated with LHON (*e.g.* 11778 mutation) to demyelinating disease (Flanigan and Johns 1993, Hanefeld *et al.* 1994). Kellar-Wood *et al.* (1994) found both the 11778 and the 3460 mutations in some women with multiple sclerosis with prominent and early optic nerve involvement. In one case, a peripheral neuropathy was also found (Pagès and Pagès 1983). Even classical forms may be associated with abnormalities of auditory evoked potentials (Mondelli *et al.* 1990), suggesting diffusion of lesions to the brainstem in two-thirds of cases.

Cases of *optic atrophy and dystonia* (Novotny *et al.* 1986, Leuzzi *et al.* 1992) are of especial interest as they may also represent a mitochondrial disease. Also of interest is the finding of 'typical' Leber optic atrophy in a patient with a mitochondrial myopathy (Roger 1986). The relationship between pure and complicated forms can now be clarified by DNA studies.

Other hereditary optic atrophies
Dominant hereditary optic atrophy may occur very early in life (see above). However, most cases have an insidious onset between 6 and 10 years of age (Hoyt 1980). The degree of visual loss is variable (Caldwell *et al.* 1971) and may be mild in almost half the patients. Examination shows disc pallor, especially in the temporal sector of the disc, and central or centrocaecal scotomata (Neetens and Martin 1986). There is no angiopathy at any stage of the disorder and this makes it easy to separate dominant optic atrophy from early Leber disease. The outlook is favourable as the condition is stationary in most patients (Elliott *et al.* 1993).

Autosomal recessive optic atrophy is rare and more severe and is usually present at birth (see above) or, in any case, before 3 years of age. An ERG is necessary to exclude Leber congenital amaurosis (Repka and Miller 1988).

Optic atrophy and diabetes mellitus occur together in a progressive syndrome that may also include deafness, diabetes insipidus and other neurological disturbances, known as the DIDMOAD or Wolfram syndrome (Grosse Aldenhövel *et al.* 1991, Barrett *et al.* 1995). This syndrome (Chapter 23) seems to be transmitted as an autosomal recessive trait. The diabetes is usually the first manifestation, followed, in the second decade of life, by visual and hearing loss. Anosmia is also present in some patients. Tremor, ataxia, nystagmus, ptosis, brainstem atrophy and central apnoea have been reported in many cases.

Optic atrophy is also a feature of a vast number of neurological diseases and syndromes (Isler and Boltshauser 1981). It is present in at least 20 per cent of cases of Friedreich ataxia (Pinto *et al.* 1988) but is not a presenting manifestation, whereas this may be the case with other 'spinocerebellar degenerations'.

Compressive optic neuropathies
Compression of the optic nerve on one or both sides is a frequent feature of tumours of the diencephalon and, less commonly, of the hypophysis. In a significant proportion of cases, optic neuropathy is the presenting manifestation, and in such cases it is important to make an early diagnosis and not to accept a wrong diagnosis of demyelinating or vascular optic neuropathy.

Craniopharyngiomas and optic nerve gliomas are the most common causes of compression neuropathy but hypophyseal tumours may rarely be a cause (Reid *et al.* 1985). The onset of visual symptoms may be acute and unilateral, and the classical features of bitemporal hemianopia can be absent as well as any neurological finding. Growth retardation is often present and is an important clue suggesting the possibility of diencephalic disease. Neuroimaging, especially MRI, is essential for a precise diagnosis and should be performed whenever there is doubt about the origin of optic disorder (Eidelberg *et al.* 1988).

Toxic and nutritional optic neuropathies
A large number of chemicals, especially drugs, can be the cause of optic neuropathy (Spiteri and James 1983). Isoniazide, etham-

butol, streptomycin, chloramphenicol, penicillamine, quinine, ergot derivatives and chlorpropamide are among the most important incriminated agents. The halogenated hydroxyquinolines have been responsible, especially in Japan but also, less commonly, in occidental countries, for an optic neuropathy associated with peripheral and spinal involvement (Behrens 1974) This subacute myelo-optic neuropathy has substantially regressed since the dangers of these drugs have been publicized.

Nutritional deficiencies can be responsible for optic neuropathy and visual loss, especially deficiency of vitamin B_{12} and folic acid (Knox *et al.* 1982). This may be especially the case in some of the syndromes of optic atrophy, ataxia and neuropathy which are observed in tropical countries. Not all such diseases are due to HTLV 1 infection (Chapter 11), and nutritional and toxic factors (in particular the use of inadequately prepared cassava) probably play an important role in their genesis. Toxic factors, *e.g.* tobacco, may play an adjunctive role as suggested for a recent epidemic in Cuba (Chapter 21). Indeed, many of the toxic causes of optic neuropathy probably act through interference with the absorption or metabolism of essential nutrients.

Intra-arterial chemotherapy has been implicated as the origin of optic atrophy following therapy of intracranial tumours (Kupersmith *et al.* 1988).

Demyelinating optic neuropathies
Unilateral and bilateral optic neuritis has been studied in Chapter 12. The relationship of optic neuritis to multiple sclerosis is much less close in children than in adults, especially when optic involvement is bilateral, although some controversy exists in this regard (Parkin *et al.* 1984, Kriss *et al.* 1988, Riikonen *et al.* 1988). Optic neuritis following specific infectious diseases has been recorded following measles, rubella, varicella (Selbst *et al.* 1983, Purvin *et al.* 1988b), Epstein–Barr virus infection (Purvin *et al.* 1988a) and coxsackie B5 infection (Spalton *et al.* 1989). Optic neuritis may also occur as a complication of nasal sinus disease (Awerbuch *et al.* 1989) and of sarcoidosis (Graham *et al.* 1986, Chapelon *et al.* 1990).

ACQUIRED CORTICAL BLINDNESS (CORTICAL VISUAL IMPAIRMENT, CVI)
Acquired CVI is frequent in children. The term cortical blindness is confusing as some degree of visual perception is usually preserved. Many children present with puzzling visual behaviour and can be shown to have field and/or agnosic deficits, including difficulties with recognition, orientation and depth, movement and simultaneous perception (Jan *et al.* 1987, Jan 1993). CVI may be transient or lasting. Transient CVI is frequent following head trauma (Eldridge and Punt 1988), and may be a manifestation of epilepsy, migraine or other acute conditions (Barnet *et al.* 1970) such as hypoglycaemia (Garty *et al.* 1987).

Lasting acquired cortical blindness is a complication of infections, especially of purulent meningitis or herpes encephalitis, of acute hypoxia following vascular collapse, of acute dehydration, of status epilepticus, of pernicious attacks of malaria or of severe head trauma. Cortical visual impairment may also result from

shunt dysfunction in hydrocephalus (Arroyo *et al.* 1985, Connolly *et al.* 1991) as a result of infarction in the territory of both posterior cerebral arteries due to their compression while crossing the tentorial edge. Extensive cortical malformations are a less frequent cause (Jan 1993).

Although there may be complete loss of vision lasting weeks or months, most patients recover some degree of vision, even though permanent field defects and low acuity almost always persist (Lambert *et al.* 1987).

The bizarre clinical features of CVI often make its recognition difficult, especially in children with cognitive and/or behavioural manifestations.

It is occasionally difficult to distinguish CVI from *optic ataxia* in which major disturbances in reaching for objects easily suggest blindness (Perenin and Vighetto 1988).

PUPILLARY DISORDERS
HORNER SYNDROME (CLAUDE BERNARD–HORNER SYNDROME)
Horner syndrome is caused by sympathetic denervation which may be congenital or acquired. It may be due to damage to the brachial plexus, especially the lower roots, at birth, or to tumours or other injuries that involve the superior cervical ganglion or the sympathetic trunks around the carotid artery.

Horner syndrome comprises three features (Weinstein *et al.* 1980): miosis, ptosis and anhidrosis of the face. In congenital cases there is also heterochromia of the irides with deficient pigmentation on the affected side. In some cases flushing of the face is present (Saito 1990). Instillation of norepinephrine produces immediate pupillary dilatation while cocaine produces little or no dilatation. In rare cases, the syndrome is transmitted as a dominant trait (Hageman *et al.* 1992).

Horner syndrome should be distinguished from physiological anisocoria which may happen to be associated with mild ptosis of whatever cause, the so-called pseudo-Horner syndrome (Thompson *et al.* 1982). The distinction is important as Horner syndrome may have serious implications. *Raeder syndrome* differs from Horner syndrome by absence of facial anhidrosis and evidence of trigeminal involvement and often of other cranial nerves (Mokri 1982). This syndrome indicates pathology in the region of the cavum of Meckel. Other cases without involvement of other cranial nerves may be a variant of migraine (Shevell *et al.* 1993).

Horner syndrome can be caused by lesions anywhere from the hypothalamus to the eye.

ARGYLL ROBERTSON PUPIL AND OTHER RARE PUPILLARY ANOMALIES
Argyll Robertson pupil is classically associated with tertiary syphilis and is therefore rarely observed in children. However, dissociation of light and near response may occur with pinealomas and other midbrain damage such as encephalitis, diabetes mellitus and some degenerative conditions.

Inverse Argyll Robertson pupil, that is pupils that react to light but not to convergence–accomodation, is rare and difficult to diagnose as one should be certain that there is indeed an attempt at convergence.

The tonic pupil of Adie is rare in children. It may be associated with hyporeflexia or areflexia. The syndrome is thought to result from lesions in the ciliary ganglion with aberrant fibre regeneration. Hemifacial flushing and loss of sweating on exertion may be associated with the tonic pupil, absence of deep tendon reflexes and more widespread sympathetic dysfunction (Ross syndrome), or occur in persons with normal pupils, the 'harlequin syndrome' (Drummond and Lance 1993). Bilateral congenital mydriasis has been observed in association with malformation of the posterior fossa with vermian agenesis (Richardson and Schulenburg 1992).

REFERENCES

Abramovitz, J.N., Kasdon, D.L., Sutula, F., et al. (1983) 'Sclerosing orbital pseudotumor.' Neurosurgery, 12, 463–468.

Afifi, A.K., Bell, W.E., Bale, J.F., Thompson, H.S. (1990) 'Recurrent lateral rectus palsy in childhood.' Pediatric Neurology, 6, 315–318.

—— —— Menezes, A.H. (1992) 'Etiology of lateral rectus palsy in infancy and childhood.' Journal of Child Neurology, 7, 295–299.

Ahn, J.C., Hoyt, W.F., Hoyt, C.S. (1989) 'Tonic upgaze in infancy.' Archives of Ophthalmology, 107, 57–58.

Aicardi, J., Chevrie, J.J., Baraton, J. (1987) 'Agenesis of the corpus callosum.' In: Vinken, P.S., Bruyn, G.W., Klawans, H.L., Myrianthopoulos, N.C. (Eds.) Handbook of Clinical Neurology. Vol. 50. Malformations. Amsterdam: Elsevier, pp. 149–173.

—— Barbosa, C., Andermann, E., et al. (1988) 'Ataxia–ocular motor apraxia: a syndrome mimicking ataxia–telangiectasia.' Annals of Neurology, 24, 497–502.

Albright, A.L., Sclabassi, R.J., Slamovits, T.L., Bergman, I. (1984) 'Spasmus nutans associated with optic gliomas in infants.' Journal of Pediatrics, 105, 778–780.

Alström, C.H., Olson, O. (1957) 'Heredoretinopathia congenitalis monohybrida recessiva autosomalis.' Hereditas, 43, 1–178.

Antozzi, C., Uziel, G., Mariotti, C., et al. (1995) 'Mitochondrial encephalomyopathies.' In: Di Donato, S., Parini, R., Uziel, G. (Eds.) Metabolic Encephalopathies—Therapy and Prognosis. London: John Libbey, pp. 25–36.

Apkarian, P., Bour, L.J., Barth, P.G., et al. (1995) 'Non-decussating retinal–fugal fibre syndrome. An inborn achiasmatic malformation associated with visuotopic misrouting, visual evoked potential ipsilateral asymmetry and nystagmus.' Brain, 118, 1195–1216.

Arroyo, H.A., Jan, J.E., McCormick, A.Q., Farrell, K. (1985) 'Permanent visual loss after shunt malfunction.' Neurology, 35, 25–29.

Astle, W.F., Rosenbaum, A.L. (1985) 'Familial congenital fourth cranial nerve palsies.' Archives of Ophthalmology, 103, 532–535.

Atkinson, J., Van Hof-van Duin, J. (1993) 'Visual assessment during the first years of life.' In: Fielder, A.R., Best, A..B., Bax, M.C.O. (Eds.) The Management of Visual Impairment in Childhood. Clinics in Developmental Medicine No. 128. London: Mac Keith Press, pp. 9–29.

Awerbuch, G., Labadie, E.L., Van Dalen, J.T.W. (1989) 'Reversible optic neuritis secondary to paranasal sinusitis.' European Neurology, 29, 189–193.

Baker, R.S., Schmeisser, E.T., Epstein, A.D. (1995) 'Visual system electrodiagnosis in neurologic disease of childhood.' Pediatric Neurology, 12, 99–110.

Bale, J.F., Scott, W.E., Yuh, W., et al. (1988) 'Congenital fourth nerve palsy and occult cranium bifidum.' Pediatric Neurology, 4, 320–321.

Baloh, R.W., Spooner, J.W. (1981) 'Downbeat nystagmus: a type of central vestibular nystagmus.' Neurology, 31, 304–310.

—— Honrubia, V., Konrad, H.R. (1976) 'Periodic alternating nystagmus.' Brain, 99, 11–26.

Barnet, A.B., Manson, J.I., Wilner, E. (1970) 'Acute cerebral blindness in childhood. Six cases studied clinically and electrophysiologically.' Neurology, 20, 1147–1156.

Barontini, F., Maurri, S., Marrapodi, E. (1987) 'Tolosa–Hunt syndrome versus recurrent cranial neuropathy. Report of two cases with a prolonged follow-up.' Journal of Neurology, 234, 112–115.

Barrett, T.G., Bundey, S.E., Macleod, A.F. (1995) 'Neurodegeneration and diabetes: UK nationwide study of Wolfram (DIDMOAD) syndrome.' Lancet, 346, 1458–1463.

Behrens, M.M. (1974) 'Optic atrophy in children after diiodohydroxyquin therapy.' Journal of the American Medical Association, 228, 693–694. (Letter.)

Biedner, B., Geltman, C., Rothkoff, L. (1979) 'Bilateral Duane's syndrome associated with crocodile tears.' Journal of Pediatric Ophthalmology and Strabismus, 16, 113–114.

Black, G., Redmond, R.M. (1994) 'The molecular biology of Norrie's disease.' Eye, 8, 491–496.

Blythe, I.M., Kennard, C., Ruddock, K.H. (1987) 'Residual vision in patients with retrogeniculate lesions of the visual pathways.' Brain, 110, 887–905.

Bordarier, C., Aicardi, J. (1990) 'Dandy–Walker syndrome and agenesis of the cerebellar vermis: diagnostic problems and genetic counselling.' Developmental Medicine and Child Neurology, 32, 285–294.

Braddick, O., Atkinson, J., Hood, B. (1992) 'Possible blindsight in infants lacking one cerebral hemisphere.' Nature, 360, 461–463.

Brown, G.C., Magargal, L.E., Shields, J.A., et al. (1981) 'Retinal artery obstruction in children and young adults.' Ophthalmology, 88, 18–25.

Caldwell, J.B., Howard, R.O., Riggs, L.A. (1971) 'Dominant juvenile optic atrophy. A study of two families and review of hereditary disease in childhood.' Archives of Ophthalmology, 85, 133–147.

Campistol, J., Prats, J.M., Garaizer, C. (1993) 'Benign paroxysmal upgaze of childhood with ataxia. A neuro-ophthalmological syndrome of familial origin?' Developmental Medicine and Child Neurology, 32, 285–294.

Camuzat, A., Dollfus, H., Rozet, J-M., et al. (1995) 'A gene for Leber's congenital amaurosis maps to chromosome 17p.' Human Molecular Genetics, 4, 1447–1452.

Cantu, J.M., Rojas, J.A., Garcia-Cruz, D., et al. (1977) 'Autosomal recessive microcephaly associated with chorioretinopathy.' Human Genetics, 36, 243–247.

Casteels, I., Spileers, W., Demaerel, P., et al. (1996) 'Leber congenital amaurosis—differential diagnosis, ophthalmological and neuroradiological report of 18 patients.' Neuropediatrics, 27, 189–193.

Chapelon, C., Ziza, J.M., Piette, J.C., et al. (1990) 'Neurosarcoidosis: signs, course and treatment in 35 confirmed cases.' Medicine, 69, 261–276.

Chevrie, J.J., Aicardi, J. (1986) 'Aicardi syndrome.' In: Pedley, T.A., Meldrum, B.S. (Eds.) Recent Advances in Epilepsy, Vol. 3. Edinburgh: Churchill Livingstone, pp. 189–210.

Cogan, D.G. (1954) 'Ocular dysmetria, flutter-like oscillations of the eye and opsoclonus.' Archives of Ophthalmology, 51, 318–335.

—— (1963) 'Dissociated nystagmus with lesions in the posterior fossa.' Archives of Ophthalmology, 70, 361–368.

Cohen, H.A., Nussinovitch, M., Ashkenazi, A., et al. (1993) 'Benign abducens nerve palsy of childhood.' Pediatric Neurology, 9, 394–395.

Coker, S.B., Ros, S.P. (1996) 'Ptosis associated with sinusitis.' Pediatric Neurology, 14, 62–63.

Collewijn, H., Apkarian, P., Spekreijse, H. (1985) 'The oculomotor behaviour of human albinos.' Brain, 108, 1–28.

Connolly, M.B., Jan, J.E., Cochrane, D.D. (1991) 'Rapid recovery from cortical visual impairment following correction of prolonged shunt malfunction in congenital hydrocephalus.' Archives of Neurology, 48, 956–957.

Coppeto, J.R., Lessell, S., Sciarra, R., Bear, L. (1986) 'Vascular retinopathy in migraine.' Neurology, 36, 267–270.

Costeff, H., Elpeleg, O., Apter, N., et al. (1993) '3-methylglutaconic aciduria in "optic atrophy plus".' Annals of Neurology, 33, 103–104.

Daroff, R.B., Troost, B.T. (1973) 'Upbeat nystagmus.' Journal of the American Medical Association, 225, 312. (Letter.)

—— —— (1985) 'Supranuclear disorders of eye movements.' In: Glaser, J.S. (Ed.) Neuroophthalmology. Hagerstown, MD: Harper & Row, pp. 201–218.

—— —— Dell'Osso, L.F. (1978) 'Nystagmus and other ocular oscillations.' In: Glaser, J.S. (Ed.) Neuro-ophthalmology. Hagerstown, MD: Harper & Row, pp. 219–243.

De Grauw, A.J.C., Rotteveel, J.J., Cruysbreg, J.R.M. (1983) 'Transient sixth cranial nerve paralysis in the newborn infant.' Neuropediatrics, 14, 164–165.

Dekaban, A. (1975) 'Neurological disorders associated with congenital retinal blindness.' In: Vinken, P.J., Bruyn, G.W. (Eds.) Handbook of Clinical Neurology. Vol. 22. System Disorders and Atrophies, Part II. Amsterdam: North Holland, pp. 527–543.

Dell'Osso, L.F. (1984) 'Nystagmus and other ocular motor oscillations and intrusions.' In: Lessell, S., Van Dalen, K. (Eds.) Neuro-ophthalmology, Vol. 3. Amsterdam: Elsevier, pp. 157–204.

—— Flynn, J.T., Daroff, R.B. (1974) 'Hereditary congenital nystagmus: an intrafamilial study.' *Archives of Ophthalmology*, **92**, 366–374.

—— Schmidt, D., Daroff, R.B. (1979) 'Latent, manifest–latent and congenital nystagmus.' *Archives of Ophthalmology*, **97**, 1877–1885.

Deonna, T., Roulet, E., Meyer, H.U. (1990) 'Benign paroxysmal tonic upgaze of childhood—a new syndrome.' *Neuropediatrics*, **21**, 213–214.

Drummond, P.D., Lance, J.W. (1993) 'Site of autonomic deficit in harlequin syndrome: local autonomic failure affecting the arm and face.' *Annals of Neurology*, **34**, 814–819.

Ebner, R., Lopez, L., Ochoa, S., Crovetto, L. (1990) 'Vertical ocular motor apraxia.' *Neurology*, **40**, 712–713.

Eidelberg, D., Newton, M.R., Johnson, G., *et al.* (1988) 'Chronic unilateral optic neuropathy: a magnetic resonance study.' *Annals of Neurology*, **24**, 3–11.

Ek, J., Kase, B.F., Reith, A., *et al.* (1986) 'Peroxisomal dysfunction in a boy with neurological symptoms and amaurosis (Leber disease). Clinical and biochemical findings similar to those observed in Zellweger syndrome.' *Journal of Pediatrics*, **108**, 19–24.

Eldridge, P.R., Punt, J.A.G. (1988) 'Transient traumatic cortical blindness in children.' *Lancet*, **1**, 815–816.

Elliott, D., Traboulsi, E.I., Maumenee, I.H. (1993) 'Visual prognosis in autosomal dominant optic atrophy (Kjer type).' *American Journal of Ophthalmology*, **115**, 360–367.

Elpeleg, O.N., Costeff, H., Joseph, A., *et al.* (1994) '3-methylglutaconic aciduria in the Iraqi–Jewish 'optic atrophy plus' (Costeff) syndrome.' *Developmental Medicine and Child Neurology*, **36**, 167–172.

Engle, E.C., Goumnerov, B.C., McKeown, C.A., *et al.* (1997) 'Ocular motor nerve and muscle abnormalities in congenital fibrosis of the extraocular muscles.' *Annals of Neurology*, **41**, 314–325.

Farmer, J., Hoyt, C.S. (1984) 'Monocular nystagmus in infancy and early childhood.' *American Journal of Ophthalmology*, **98**, 504–509.

Fielder, A.R., Mayer, D.L. (1991) 'Delayed visual maturation.' *Seminars in Ophthalmology*, **6**, 182–193.

Flanders, A.E., Mafee, M.F., Rao, J.M., Choi, K.H. (1989) 'CT characteristics of pseudotumors and other orbital inflammatory processes.' *Journal of Computer Assisted Tomography*, **13**, 40–47.

Flanigan, K.M., Johns, D.R. (1993) 'Association of the 11778 mitochondrial DNA mutation and demyelinating disease.' *Neurology*, **43**, 2720–2722.

Flodmark, O., Jan, J.E., Wong, P.K.H. (1990) 'Computed tomography of the brains of children with cortical visual impairment.' *Developmental Medicine and Child Neurology*, **32**, 611–620.

Friendly, D.S. (1987) 'Amblyopia: definition, classification and management considerations for pediatricians, family physicians and general practitioners.' *Pediatric Clinics of North America*, **34**, 1389–1401.

Funakawa, I., Kato, H., Terao, A. *et al.* (1995) 'Cerebellar ataxia in patients with Leber's hereditary optic neuropathy.' *Journal of Neurology*, **242**, 75–77.

Ganesan, V., Lin, J-P., Chong, W.K., *et al.* (1996) 'Painful and painless ophthalmoplegia with cavernous sinus pseudotumour.' *Archives of Disease in Childhood*, **75**, 239–241.

Garty, B.Z., Dinari, G., Nitzan, M. (1987) 'Transient acute cortical blindness associated with hypoglycemia.' *Pediatric Neurology*, **3**, 169–170.

Gibson, N.A., Fielder, A.R., Trounce, J.Q., Levene, M.I. (1990) 'Ophthalmic findings in infants of very low birthweight.' *Developmental Medicine and Child Neurology*, **32**, 7–13.

Goadsby, P.J., Lance, J.W. (1989) 'Clinicopathological correlation in a case of painful ophthalmoplegia: Tolosa–Hunt syndrome.' *Journal of Neurology, Neurosurgery, and Psychiatry*, **52**, 1290–1293.

Godel, V., Blumenthal, M., Iaina, A. (1978) 'Congenital Leber amaurosis, keratoconus, and mental retardation in familial juvenile nephronophthisis.' *Journal of Pediatric Ophthalmology and Strabismus*, **15**, 89–91.

Goldblum, T.A., Effron, L.A. (1994) 'Upbeat nystagmus associated with tonic downward deviation in healthy neonates.' *Journal of Pediatric Ophthalmology and Strabismus*, **31**, 334–335.

Good, W.V., Koch, T.S., Jan, J.E. (1993) 'Monocular nystagmus caused by unilateral anterior visual-pathway disease.' *Developmental Medicine and Child Neurology*, **35**, 1106–1110.

Gordon, N. (1994) 'Ophthalmoplegia in childhood.' *Developmental Medicine and Child Neurology*, **36**, 370–374.

Goto, Y., Goto, I., Hosokawa, S. (1989) 'Neurological and radiological studies in painful ophthalmoplegia: Tolosa–Hunt syndrome and orbital pseudotumour.' *Journal of Neurology*, **236**, 448–451.

Graham, E.M., Ellis, C.J.K., Sanders, M.D., McDonald, W.I. (1986) 'Optic neuropathy in sarcoidosis.' *Journal of Neurology, Neurosurgery, and Psychiatry*, **49**, 756–765.

Greenblatt, S.H. (1973) 'Posttraumatic transient cerebral blindness. Association with migraine and seizure diathesis.' *Journal of the American Medical Association*, **225**, 1073–1076.

Gresty, M.E., Page, N., Barratt, H. (1984) 'The differential diagnosis of congenital nystagmus.' *Journal of Neurology, Neurosurgery, and Psychiatry*, **47**, 936–942.

Grosse Aldenhövel, H.B., Gallenkamp, U., Sulemana, C.A. (1991) 'Juvenile onset diabetes mellitus, central diabetes insipidus and optic atrophy (Wolfram syndrome)—neurological findings and prognostic implications.' *Neuropediatrics*, **22**, 103–106.

Grosse-Tsur, V., Har-Even, Y., Gutman, I., Amir, N. (1989) 'Oculomotor apraxia: the presenting sign of Gaucher disease.' *Pediatric Neurology*, **5**, 128–129.

Grossniklaus, H.E., Lass, J.H., Abramowsky, C.R., Levine, M. (1985) 'Childhood orbital pseudotumor.' *Annals of Ophthalmology*, **17**, 372–377.

Hageman, G., Ippel, P.F., te Nijenhuis, F.C.A.M. (1992) 'Autosomal dominant congenital Horner's syndrome in a Dutch family.' *Journal of Neurology, Neurosurgery, and Psychiatry*, **55**, 28–30.

Halmagyi, G.M., Gresty, M.A., Leech, J. (1980) 'Reversed optokinetic nystagmus (OKN): mechanism and clinical significance.' *Annals of Neurology*, **7**, 429–435.

—— Rudge, P., Gresty, M.A., Sanders, M.D. (1983) 'Downbeating nystagmus. A review of 62 cases.' *Archives of Neurology*, **40**, 777–784.

Hanefeld, F.A., Ernst, B.P., Wilichowski, E., Christen, H-J. (1994) 'Leber's hereditary optic neuropathy mitochondrial DNA mutations in childhood multiple sclerosis.' *Neuropediatrics*, **25**, 331. *(Letter.)*

Harbour, R.C., Trobe, J.D., Ballinger, W.E. (1984) 'Septic cavernous sinus thrombosis associated with gingivitis and parapharyngeal abscess.' *Archives of Ophthalmology*, **102**, 94–97.

Harris, C. (1997) 'Nystagmus and eye movement disorders.' *In:* Taylor, D. (Ed.) *Paediatric Ophthalmology, 2nd Edn.* Oxford: Blackwell, pp. 869–896.

Hiatt, R.L., Halle, A.A. (1983) 'General fibrosis syndrome.' *Annals of Ophthalmology*, **15**, 1103–1109.

Hoon, A.H., Jan, J.E., Whitfield, M.F., *et al.* (1988) 'Changing pattern of retinopathy of prematurity: a 37-year clinic experience.' *Pediatrics*, **82**, 344–349.

Hotchkiss, M.G., Miller, N.R., Clark, A.W., Green, W.R. (1980) 'Bilateral Duane's retraction syndrome: a clinico-pathologic case report.' *Archives of Ophthalmology*, **98**, 870–874.

Hoyt, C.S. (1977) 'Neonatal opsoclonus.' *Journal of Pediatric Ophthalmology*, **14**, 274–277.

—— (1980) 'Autosomal dominant optic atrophy: a spectrum of disability.' *Ophthalmology*, **87**, 245–251.

—— (1987) 'Nystagmus and other abnormal ocular movements in children.' *Pediatric Clinics of North America*, **34**, 1415–1423.

—— Mousel, D.K., Weber, A.A. (1980) 'Transient supranuclear disturbances of gaze in healthy neonates.' *American Journal of Ophthalmology*, **89**, 708–713.

—— Nickel, B.L., Billson, F.A. (1982) 'Ophthalmological examination of the infant. Developmental aspects.' *Survey of Ophthalmology*, **26**, 177–189.

Hoyt, W.F., Keane, J.R. (1970) 'Superior oblique myokymia: report and discussion of five cases of benign, intermittent uniocular microtremor.' *Archives of Ophthalmology*, **84**, 461–466.

Huber, A. (1974) 'Electrophysiology of the retraction syndrome.' *British Journal of Ophthalmology*, **58**, 293–300.

Hughes, J.L., O'Connor, P.S., Larsen, P.D., Mumma, O.V. (1985) 'Congenital vertical ocular motor apraxia.' *Journal of Clinical Neuro-Ophthalmology*, **5**, 153–157.

International Committee for the Classification of the Late Stages of Retinopathy of Prematurity (1988) 'An international classification of retinopathy of prematurity: II. The classification of retinal detachment.' *Pediatrics*, **82**, 37–43.

Isenberg, S., Blechman, B. (1983) 'Marcus Gunn jaw winking and Duane's retraction syndrome.' *Journal of Pediatric Ophthalmology and Strabismus*, **20**, 235–237.

Isler, W., Boltshauser, E. (1981) 'Ocular symptoms in neurodegenerative diseases of childhood.' *In:* Huber, A., Klein, D. (Eds.) *Neurogenetics and Neuro-Ophthalmology.* Amsterdam: Elsevier, pp. 341–346.

Jackson, A.C., Boughner, D.R., Barnett, H.J.M. (1984) 'Mitral valve prolapse and cerebral ischemic events in young patients.' *Neurology*, **34**, 784–787.

Jan, J.E. (1993) 'Neurological causes and investigations.' *In:* Fielder, A.R., Best, A.B., Bax, M.C.O. (Eds.) *The Management of Visual Impairment in Childhood. Clinics in Developmental Medicine No. 128.* London: Mac Keith Press, pp. 48–63.

—— Scott, E. (1974) 'Hypotonia and delayed motor development in congenitally blind children.' *Journal of Pediatrics,* **84,** 929–930.

—— Wong, P.K. (1988) 'Behaviour of the alpha rhythm in electroencephalograms of visually impaired children.' *Developmental Medicine and Child Neurology,* **30,** 444–450.

—— Robinson, G.C., Kinnis, C., MacLeod, P.J.M. (1977) 'Blindness due to optic-nerve atrophy and hypoplasia in children: an epidemiological study (1944–1974).' *Developmental Medicine and Child Neurology,* **19,** 353–363.

—— Freeman, R.D., McCormick, A.Q., *et al.* (1983) 'Eye-pressing by visually impaired children.' *Developmental Medicine and Child Neurology,* **25,** 755–762.

—— Farrell, K., Wong, P.K., McCormick, A.Q. (1986) 'Eye and head movements of visually impaired children.' *Developmental Medicine and Child Neurology,* **28,** 285–293.

—— Groenveld, M., Sykanda, A.M., Hoyt, C.S. (1987) 'Behavioural characteristics of children with permanent cortical visual impairment.' *Developmental Medicine and Child Neurology,* **29,** 571–576.

—— —— Connolly, M.B. (1990) 'Head shaking by visually impaired children: a voluntary neurovisual adaptation which can be confused with spasmus nutans.' *Developmental Medicine and Child Neurology,* **32,** 1061–1066.

Jay, W.M., Hoyt, C.S. (1980) 'Abnormal brain stem auditory-evoked potentials in Stilling–Turk–Duane retraction syndrome.' *American Journal of Ophthalmology,* **89,** 814–818.

Johns, D.R., Smith, K.H., Miller, N.R. (1992) 'Leber's hereditary optic neuropathy. Clinical manifestations of the 3460 mutation.' *Archives of Ophthalmology,* **110,** 1577–1581.

Kandt, R.S., Goldstein, G.W. (1985) 'Steroid responsive ophthalmoplegia in a child. Diagnostic considerations.' *Archives of Neurology,* **42,** 589–591.

Katz, B., Van Patten, P., Rothrock, J.F., Katzman, R. (1988) 'Optic nerve head drusen and pseudotumor cerebri.' *Archives of Neurology,* **45,** 45–47.

Keane, J.R. (1990) 'The pretectal syndrome: 206 patients.' *Neurology,* **40,** 684–695.

—— (1993) 'Fourth nerve palsy: historical review and study of 215 inpatients.' *Neurology,* **43,** 2439–2443.

—— Finstead, B.A. (1982) 'Upward gaze paralysis as the initial sign of Fisher's syndrome.' *Archives of Neurology,* **39,** 781–782.

Kellar-Wood, H., Robertson, N., Govan, G.G., *et al.* (1994) 'Leber's hereditary optic neuropathy mitochondrial DNA mutations in multiple sclerosis.' *Annals of Neurology,* **36,** 109–112.

King, R.A., Nelson, L.B., Wagner, R.S. (1986) 'Spasmus nutans. A benign clinical entity?' *Archives of Ophthalmology,* **104,** 1501–1504.

Kirkham, T.H., Guitton, D., Katsarkas, A., *et al.* (1979) 'Oculomotor abnormalities in Friedreich's ataxia.' *Canadian Journal of Neurological Sciences,* **6,** 167–172.

Kleiman, M.D., DiMario, F.J., Leconche, D.A., Zalneraitis, E.L. (1994) 'Benign transient downward gaze in preterm infants.' *Pediatric Neurology,* **10,** 313–316.

Knox, D.L., Chen, M.F., Guillarte, T.R. (1982) 'Nutritional amblyopia. Folic acid, vitamin B₁₂ and other vitamins.' *Retina,* **2,** 288–291.

Kohn, B.A. (1976) 'The differential diagnosis of cataracts in infancy and childhood.' *American Journal of Diseases of Children,* **130,** 184–192.

Kömpf, D., Piper, H.E. (1987) 'Eye movements and vestibulo-ocular reflex in the blind.' *Journal of Neurology,* **234,** 337–341.

Kosmorsky, G., Hanson, M.R., Tomsak, R.L. (1988) 'Neuro-ophthalmologic complications of cardiac catheterization.' *Neurology,* **38,** 483–485.

Kriss, A., Francis, D.A., Cuendet, F., *et al.* (1988) 'Recovery after optic neuritis in childhood.' *Journal of Neurology, Neurosurgery, and Psychiatry,* **51,** 1253–1258.

Krohel, G.B., Kristan, R.W., Simon, J.W., Barrows, N.A. (1986) 'Posttraumatic convergence insufficiency.' *Annals of Ophthalmology,* **18,** 101–102.

Kupersmith, M.J., Frohman, L.P., Choi, I.S., *et al.* (1988) 'Visual system toxicity following intra-arterial chemotherapy.' *Neurology,* **38,** 284–289.

Lambert, S.R., Newman, N.J. (1993) 'Retinal disease masquerading as spasmus nutans.' *Neurology,* **43,** 1607–1609.

—— Hoyt, C.S., Jan, J.E., *et al.* (1987) 'Visual recovery from hypoxic cortical blindness during childhood. Computed tomographic and magnetic resonance imaging predictors.' *Archives of Ophthalmology,* **105,** 1371–1377.

—— Kriss, A., Taylor, D., *et al.* (1989) 'Follow-up and diagnostic reappraisal of 75 patients with Leber's congenital amaurosis.' *American Journal of Ophthalmology,* **107,** 624–631.

—— Sherman, S., Taylor, D., *et al.* (1993) 'Concordance and recessive inheritance of Leber congenital amaurosis.' *American Journal of Medical Genetics,* **46,** 275–277.

Landrigan, P.J., Berenberg, W., Bresnan, M. (1973) 'Behr's syndrome: familial optic atrophy, spastic diplegia and ataxia.' *Developmental Medicine and Child Neurology,* **15,** 41–47.

Leaf, A.A., Green, C.R., Esack, A., *et al.* (1995) 'Maturation of electroretinograms and visual evoked potentials in preterm infants.' *Developmental Medicine and Child Neurology,* **37,** 814–826.

Leão, M.J., Ribeiro-Silva, M.L. (1995) 'Orofaciodigital syndrome type I in a patient with severe CNS defects.' *Pediatric Neurology,* **13,** 247–251.

Leuzzi, V., Bertini, E., De Negri, A.M., *et al.* (1992) 'Bilateral striatal necrosis, dystonia and optic atrophy in two siblings.' *Journal of Neurology, Neurosurgery, and Psychiatry,* **55,** 16–19.

Liberfarb, R.M., Eavey, R.D., De Long, G.R., *et al.* (1985) 'Norrie's disease: a study of two families.' *Ophthalmology,* **92,** 1445–1451.

Lopez, P.F., Smith, J.L. (1986) 'Leber's optic neuropathy. New observations.' *Journal of Clinical Neuro-Ophthalmology,* **6,** 144–152.

Lubkin, V. (1978) 'The inverse Marcus Gunn phenomenon. An electromyographic contribution.' *Archives of Neurology,* **35,** 249.

Mainzer, F., Saldino, R.F., Ozonoff, M.B., Minaghi, H. (1970) 'Familial nephropathy associated with retinitis pigmentosa, cerebellar ataxia and skeletal abnormaliities.' *American Journal of Medicine,* **49,** 556–562.

Marchal, J.L., Hehunstre, J.P., Deminière, C., *et al.* (1989) 'Nephronophtise, dégénérescence tapétorétinienne, encéphalopathie et agénésie vermienne: une nouvelle association.' *Semaine des Hôpitaux,* **65,** 2186–2191.

Margalith, D., Jan, J.E., McCormick, A.Q., *et al.* (1984) 'Clinical spectrum of congenital optic nerve hypoplasia: review of 51 patients.' *Developmental Medicine and Child Neurology,* **26,** 311–322.

Marmor, M., Wertenbaker, C., Berstien, L. (1982) 'Delayed ophthalmoplegia following head trauma.' *Surveys in Ophthalmology,* **27,** 126–132.

Marshall, G.S., Wright, P.F., Fenichel, G.M., Karzon, D.T. (1985) 'Diffuse retinopathy following measles, mumps, and rubella vaccination.' *Pediatrics,* **76,** 989–991.

Martín Carballo, G., Ramos Lizana, J., García Peñas, J.J., *et al.* (1993) 'Apraxia oculomotora congénita (AOMC) asociada a duplicación de la banda P13 del cromosoma 5 (DUP.5 P13). Revisión de la literatura.' *Anales Españoles de Pediatria,* **38,** 57–60.

Matsuzaka, T., Sakuragawa, M., Terasawa, K., Kuwabara, H. (1986) 'Facioscapulohumeral dystrophy associated with mental retardation, hearing loss, and tortuosity of retinal arteries.' *Journal of Child Neurology,* **1,** 218–223.

McDonald, M.A., Dobson, V., Sebris, S.L., *et al.* (1985) 'The acuity card procedure: a rapid test of infant acuity.' *Investigative Ophthalmology and Visual Science,* **26,** 1158–1162.

McLeod, A.R., Glaser, J.S. (1974) 'Deglutition–trochlear synkinesis.' *Archives of Ophthalmology,* **92,** 171–172.

Mehler, M.F. (1988) 'The clinical spectrum of ocular bobbing and ocular dipping.' *Journal of Neurology, Neurosurgery, and Psychiatry,* **51,** 725–727.

Mellor, J., Fielder, A.R. (1980) 'Dissociated visual development: electrodiagnostic studies in infants who are 'slow to see'.' *Developmental Medicine and Child Neurology,* **22,** 327–335.

Menezes, L., Aicardi, J. , Goutières, F. (1988) 'Absence of the septum pellucidum with porencephalia: a neuroradiologic syndrome with variable clinical expression.' *Archives of Neurology,* **45,** 542–545.

Michaud, J., Thompson, G.N., Brody, L.C., *et al.* (1995) 'Pyridoxine-responsive gyrate atrophy of the choroid and retina: clinical and biochemical correlates of the mutation A226V.' *American Journal of Human Genetics,* **56,** 616–622.

Miller, N.R. (1985) *Walsh and Hoyt Clinical Neuro-ophthalmology, 4th Edn.* Baltimore: Williams & Wilkins.

Moeller, H.V. (1992) 'Recessively inherited simple optic atrophy—does it exist?' *Ophthalmic Paediatrics and Genetics,* **13,** 31–32.

Mokri, B. (1982) 'Raeder's paratrigeminal syndrome: original concept and subsequent deviations.' *Archives of Neurology,* **39,** 395–399.

Mondelli, M., Rossi, A., Scarpini, C., *et al.* (1990) 'BAEP changes in Leber's hereditary optic atrophy: further confirmation of multisystem involvement.' *Acta Neurologica Scandinavica,* **81,** 349–353.

Moore, A. (1997) 'Inherited retinal dystrophies.' *In:* Taylor, D. (Ed.) *Paediatric Ophthalmology.* London: Butterworths, pp. 557–598.

—— Taylor, D.S.I. (1984) 'A syndrome of congenital retinal dystrophy and saccade palsy—a subset of Leber's amaurosis.' *British Journal of Ophthalmology*, **68**, 421–431.

Moorman, C.M., Elston, J.S., Matthews, P. (1993) 'Leber's hereditary optic neuropathy as a cause of severe visual loss in childhood.' *Pediatrics*, **91**, 988–989.

Mueller, C., Koch, S., Toifl, K. (1993) 'Transient bilateral internuclear ophthalmoplegia after minor head-trauma.' *Developmental Medicine and Child Neurology*, **35**, 163–166.

Narbona, J., Crisci, C.D., Villa, I. (1980) 'Familial congenital ocular motor apraxia and immune deficiency.' *Archives of Neurology*, **37**, 325. *(Letter.)*

Neetens, A., Martin, J.J. (1986) 'The hereditary optic atrophies.' *Neuro-ophthalmology*, **6**, 277–285.

Nelson, M., Lessell, S., Sadun, A. (1986) 'Optic nerve hypoplasia and maternal diabetes mellitus.' *Archives of Neurology*, **43**, 20–25.

Newsome, D.A. (Ed.) (1988) *Retinal Dystrophies and Degenerations*. New York: Raven Press.

Ng, Y.K., Fielder, A.R., Levene, M.I., *et al.* (1989) 'Are acute retinopathy of prematurity and severe periventricular leukomalacia both ischaemic insults?' *British Journal of Ophthalmology*, **73**, 111–114.

Nickel, B., Hoyt, C.S. (1982) 'Leber's congenital amaurosis. Is mental retardation a frequent associated defect?' *Archives of Ophthalmology*, **100**, 1089–1092.

Nikoskelainen, E., Hoyt, W.F., Nummelin, K. (1982) 'Ophthalmoscopic findings in Leber's hereditary optic atrophy. I. Fundus findings in asymptomatic family members.' *Archives of Ophthalmology*, **100**, 1597–1602.

—— —— —— (1983) 'Ophthalmoscopic findings in Leber's hereditary optic neuropathy. II. The fundus findings in the affected family members.' *Archives of Ophthalmology*, **101**, 1059–1068.

—— —— Schatz, H. (1984) 'Fundus findings in Leber's hereditary optic neuroretinathy. III. Fluorescein angiographic studies.' *Archives of Ophthalmology*, **102**, 981–989.

Noble, K.G., Carr, R.E. (1978) 'Leber's congenital amaurosis.' *Archives of Ophthalmology*, **96**, 818–821.

Norwood, V.F., Haller, J.S. (1990) 'Gradenigo syndrome as presenting sign of T-cell lymphoma.' *Pediatric Neurology*, **5**, 377–380.

Novotny, E.J., Singh, G., Wallace, D.C., *et al.* (1986) 'Leber's disease and dystonia: a mitochondrial disease.' *Neurology*, **36**, 1053–1060.

Ouvrier, R., Billson, F. (1986) 'Optic nerve hypoplasia: a review.' *Journal of Child Neurology*, **1**, 181–188.

—— (1988) 'Benign paroxysmal tonic upgaze of childhood.' *Journal of Child Neurology*, **3**, 177–180.

Pagès, M., Pagès, A-M. (1983) 'Leber's disease with spastic paraplegia and peripheral neuropathy. Case report with nerve biopsy study.' *European Neurology*, **22**, 181–185.

Parkin, P.J., Hierons, R., McDonald, W.I. (1984) 'Bilateral optic neuritis: a long-term follow-up.' *Brain*, **107**, 951–964.

Patterson, M.C., Horowitz, M., Abel, R.B., *et al.* (1993) 'Isolated horizontal supranuclear gaze palsy as a marker of severe systemic involvement in Gaucher's disease.' *Neurology*, **43**, 1993–1997.

Paulus, W., Straube, A., Bauer, W., Harding, A.E. (1993) 'Central nervous system involvement in Leber's optic neuropathy.' *Journal of Neurology*, **240**, 251–253.

Pedersen, R.A., Troost, B.T., Abel, L.A., Zorub, D. (1980) 'Intermittent downbeat nystagmus and oscillopsia reversed by suboccipital craniectomy.' *Neurology*, **30**, 1239–1242.

Perenin, M.T., Vighetto, A. (1988) 'Optic ataxia: a specific disruption in visuomotor mechanisms. I: Different aspects of the deficit in reaching for objects.' *Brain*, **111**, 643–674.

Pierrot-Deseilligny, C., Chain, F., Serdaru, M., *et al.* (1981) 'The 'one-and-a-half' syndrome. Electro-oculographic analyses of five cases with deductions about the physiological mechanisms of lateral gaze.' *Brain*, **104**, 665–699.

—— Gaymard, B., Müri, R., Rivaud, S. (1997) 'Cerebral ocular motor signs.' *Journal of Neurology*, **244**, 65–70.

Pinto, F., Amantani, A., De Scisciolo, G., *et al.* (1988) 'Visual involvement in Friedreich's ataxia: PERG and VEP study.' *European Neurology*, **28**, 246–251.

Pollard, Z.F. (1996) 'Acute rectus muscle palsy in children as a result of orbital myositis.' *Journal of Pediatrics*, **128**, 230–233.

Poole, C.J., Kind, P.R.N. (1986) 'Deficiency of thiosulphate sulphurtransferase (rhodanese) in Leber's hereditary optic atrophy.' *British Medical Journal*, **292**, 1229–1230.

Prakash, P., Menon, V., Ghosh, G. (1985) 'Congenital fibrosis of superior rectus and superior oblique: a case report.' *British Journal of Ophthalmology*, **69**, 57–59.

Prats, J.M., Monzon, M.J., Zuazo, E., Garaizar, C. (1993) 'Congenital nuclear syndrome of oculomotor nerve.' *Pediatric Neurology*, **9**, 476–478.

Pratt, S.G., Beyer, C.K., Johnson, C.C. (1984) 'The Marcus Gunn phenomenon.' *Ophthalmology*, **90**, 27–30.

Proesmans, W., Van Damme, B., Macken, J. (1975) 'Nephronophthisis and tapetoretinal degeneration associated with liver fibrosis.' *Clinical Nephrology*, **3**, 160–164.

Purvin, V., Herr, J., De Myer, W. (1988a) 'Chiasmal neuritis as a complication of Epstein–Barr virus infection.' *Archives of Neurology*, **45**, 458–460.

—— Hrisolamos, N., Dunn, D. (1988b) 'Varicella optic neuritis.' *Neurology*, **38**, 501–503.

Rana, P.V.S., Wadia, R.S. (1985) 'The Marin–Awat syndrome: an unusual facial synkinesia.' *Journal of Neurology, Neurosurgery, and Psychiatry*, **48**, 939–941.

Rapin, F., Echenne, B. (1987) 'Ophthalmoplégie douloureuse de Tolosa–Hunt: à propos d'une observation chez une fille de 10 ans.' *Archives Françaises de Pédiatrie*, **44**, 299–301.

Rappaport, L., Urion, D., Strand, K., Fulton, A.B. (1987) 'Concurrence of congenital ocular motor apraxia and other motor problems: an expanded syndrome.' *Developmental Medicine and Child Neurology*, **29**, 85–90.

Reid, R.L., Quigley, M.E., Yen, S.S.C. (1985) 'Pituitary apoplexy. A review.' *Archives of Neurology*, **42**, 712–719.

Repka, M.X., Miller, N.R. (1988) 'Optic atrophy in children.' *American Journal of Ophthalmology*, **106**, 191–193.

Reynolds, J.D., Biglan, A.W., Hiles, D.A. (1984) 'Congenital superior oblique palsy in infants.' *Archives of Ophthalmology*, **102**, 1503–1505.

Richardson, P., Schulenburg, W.E. (1992) 'Bilateral congenital mydriasis.' *British Journal of Ophthalmology*, **76**, 632–633.

Riikonen, R., Donner, M., Erkkilä, H. (1988) 'Optic neuritis in children and its relationship to multiple sclerosis: a clinical study of 21 children.' *Developmental Medicine and Child Neurology*, **30**, 349–359.

Riordan-Eva, P., Sanders, M.D., Govan, G.G., *et al.* (1995) 'The clinical features of Leber's hereditary optic neuropathy defined by the presence of a pathogenic mitochondrial DNA mutation.' *Brain*, **118**, 319–337.

Rizzo, J.F., Berson, E.L., Lessell, S. (1986) 'Retinal and neurologic findings in the Laurence–Moon–Bardet–Biedl phenotype.' *Ophthalmology*, **93**, 1452–1456.

Roberts-Harry, J., Green, S.A., Willshaw, H.E. (1990) 'Optic nerve hypoplasia: associations and management.' *Archives of Disease in Childhood*, **65**, 103–106.

Roger, J. (1986) 'Genetic transmission of myoclonus epilepsy with ragged red fibers.' *Annals of Neurology*, **20**, 545. *(Letter.)*

Rohr, J., Gauthier, G. (1988) 'Myosite orbitaire aiguë idiopathique.' *Revue Neurologique*, **144**, 47–48.

Roland, E.H., Jan, J.E., Hill, A., Wong, P.K. (1986) 'Cortical visual impairment following birth asphyxia.' *Pediatric Neurology*, **2**, 133–137.

Ropper, A.H. (1981) 'Ocular dipping in anoxic coma.' *Archives of Neurology*, **38**, 297–299.

Saito, H. (1990) 'Congenital Horner's syndrome with unilateral facial flushing.' *Journal of Neurology, Neurosurgery, and Psychiatry*, **53**, 85–86.

Sandyk, R. (1984) 'Paralysis of upward gaze as a presenting symptom of vitamin B_{12} deficiency.' *European Neurology*, **23**, 198–200.

Santavuori, P., Erkkilä, H. (1976) 'Neurologic and developmental findings in children with optic disc drusen.' *Neuropädiatrie*, **7**, 283–301.

Savell, J., Cook, J.R. (1976) 'Optic nerve colobomas of autosomal-dominant heredity.' *Archives of Ophthalmology*, **94**, 395–400.

Schappert-Kimmijser, J., Henkes, H.E., Van den Borsch, J. (1959) 'Amaurosis congenita (Leber).' *Archives of Ophthalmology*, **61**, 211–218.

Scher, M.S., Dobson, V., Carpenter, N.A., Guthrie, R.D. (1989) 'Visual and neurological outcome of infants with periventricular leukomalacia.' *Developmental Medicine and Child Neurology*, **31**, 353–365.

Schroeder, R., Mets, M.B., Maumenee, I.H. (1987) 'Leber's congenital amaurosis. Retrospective review of 43 cases and new fundus finding in two cases.' *Archives of Ophthalmology*, **105**, 356–359.

Selbst, R.G., Selhorst, J.B., Harbison, J.W., Myer, E.C. (1983) 'Parainfectious optic neuritis. Report and review following varicella.' *Archives of Neurology*, **40**, 347–350.

Shawkat, F.S., Kingsley, D., Kendall, B., *et al.* (1995) 'Neuroradiological and eye movement correlates in children with intermittent saccade failure: "ocular motor apraxia".' *Neuropediatrics*, **26**, 298–305.

Shevell, M., Silver, K., Watters, G., Rosenblatt, B. (1993) 'Transient oculosympathetic paresis (group II Raeder's paratrigeminal neuralgia) of childhood: a migraine variant.' *Pediatric Neurology*, **9**, 289–292.

Smith, J.L., Flynn, J.T., Spiro, H.J. (1982) 'Monocular vertical oscillations of amblyopia: the Hermann–Bielschowsky phenomena.' *Journal of Clinical Neuro-Ophthalmology*, **2**, 85–91.

Sonksen, P.M. (1993) 'Effect of severe visual impairment on development.' *In:* Fielder, A.R., Best, A.B., Bax, M.C.O. (Eds.) *The Management of Visual Impairment in Childhood. Clinics in Developmental Medicine No. 128.* London: Mac Keith Press, pp. 78–90.

Spalton, D.J., Murdoch, I., Holder, G.E. (1989) 'Coxsackie B5 papillitis.' *Journal of Neurology, Neurosurgery, and Psychiatry*, **52**, 1310–1311. *(Letter.)*

Spector, R.H., Fiandaca, M.S. (1986) 'The "sinister" Tolosa–Hunt syndrome.' *Neurology*, **36**, 198–203.

—— Troost, B.T. (1981) 'Neurological review: the ocular motor system.' *Annals of Neurology*, **9**, 517–525.

Spiteri, M.A., James, D.J. (1983) 'Adverse ocular reactions to drugs.' *Postgraduate Medicine*, **59**, 343–349.

Steinkuller, P.G. (1980) 'The morning glory disc anomaly: case report and literature review.' *Journal of Pediatric Ophthalmology and Strabismus*, **17**, 81–87.

Strömland, K., Hellström, A. (1996) 'Fetal alcohol syndrome—an ophthalmological and socioeducational prospective study.' *Pediatrics*, **97**, 845–850.

Sugie, H., Sugie, Y., Ito, M., *et al.* (1995) 'A case of paroxysmal tonic upward gaze associated with psychomotor retardation.' *Developmental Medicine and Child Neurology*, **37**, 362–365.

Swerdlow, B. (1980) 'Tolosa–Hunt syndrome: a case with associated facial nerve palsy.' *Annals of Neurology*, **8**, 542–543.

Sydnor, C.F., Seaber, J.H., Buckley, E.G. (1982) 'Traumatic superior oblique palsies.' *Ophthalmology*, **89**, 134–138.

Taylor, D. (Ed.) (1997) *Pediatric Ophthalmology, 2nd Edn.* Cambridge, MA: Blackwell.

—— Carroll, J.E., Smith, M.E., *et al.* (1982) 'Facioscapulohumeral dystrophy associated with hearing loss and Coats syndrome.' *Annals of Neurology*, **12**, 395–398.

Taylor, M.J., McCulloch, D.L. (1991) 'Prognostic value of VEPs in young children with acute onset of a cortical blindness.' *Pediatric Neurology*, **7**, 111–115.

—— Menzies, R., MacMillan, L.J., Whyte, H.E. (1987) 'VEPs in normal full-term and premature neonates: longitudinal versus cross-sectional data.' *Electroencephalography and Clinical Neurophysiology*, **68**, 20–27.

Thompson, B.M., Corbett, J.J., Kline, L.B., Thompson, S. (1982) 'Pseudo-Horner's syndrome.' *Archives of Neurology*, **39**, 108–111.

Tippin, J., Corbett, J.J., Kerber, R.E., *et al.* (1989) 'Amaurosis fugax and ocular infarction in adolescents and young adults.' *Annals of Neurology*, **26**, 69–77.

Tolmie, J.L., Browne, B.H., McGettrick, P.M., Stephenson, J.B.P. (1988) 'A familial syndrome with Coats' reaction retinal angiomas, hair and nail defects and intracranial calcification.' *Eye*, **2**, 297–303.

Tomoda, A., Miike, T., Miyagawa, S., *et al.* (1997) 'Subacute sclerosing panencephalitis and chorioretinitis.' *Brain and Development*, **198**, 55–57.

Tresidder, J., Fielder, A.R., Nicholson, J. (1990) 'Delayed visual maturation: ophthalmic and neurodevelopmental aspects.' *Developmental Medicine and Child Neurology*, **32**, 872–881.

Troost, B.T. (1981) 'An overview of ocular motor neurophysiology.' *Annals of Otology, Rhinology and Laryngology*, **90**, Suppl. 86, 29–36.

—— (1989) 'Nystagmus: a clinical review.' *Revue Neurologique*, **145**, 417–428.

Uretsky, S.H., Kennerdell, J.S., Gutai, J.P. (1980) 'Graves' ophthalmopathy in childhood and adolescence.' *Archives of Ophthalmology*, **98**, 1963–1964.

Vaizey, M.J., Sanders, M.D., Wybar, K.C., Wilson, J. (1977) 'Neurological abnormalities in congenital amaurosis of Leber. Review of 30 cases.' *Archives of Disease in Childhood*, **52**, 399–402.

Van Nieuwenhuizen, O., Willemse, J. (1988) 'Neuro-imaging of cerebral visual disturbances in children.' *Neuropediatrics*, **19**, 3–6.

Vetterli, A., Henn, V. (1981) 'Congenital horizontal gaze palsy in two brothers.' *In:* Huber, A., Klein, D. (Eds.) *Neurogenetics and Neuro-ophthalmology.* Amsterdam: Elsevier, pp. 81–88.

Victor, D.I. (1976) 'The diagnosis of congenital third-nerve palsy.' *Brain*, **99**, 711–718.

Von Noorden, G.K., Murray, E., Wong, S.Y. (1986) 'Superior oblique paralysis: a review of 270 cases.' *Archives of Ophthalmology*, **104**, 1771–1776.

Wadia, N.H., Swami, R.K. (1971) 'A new form of heredo-familial spinocerebellar degeneration with slow eye movements (nine families).' *Brain*, **94**, 359–374.

Wall, M., Wray, S.H. (1983) 'The one-and-a-half syndrome—a unilateral disorder of the pontine tegmentum: a study of 20 cases and review of the literature.' *Neurology*, **33**, 971–980.

Wallace, D.C., Singh, G., Lott, M.T., *et al.* (1988) 'Mitochondrial DNA mutation associated with Leber's hereditary optic atrophy.' *Science*, **242**, 1427–1430.

Walsh, F.B., Hoyt, W.F. (1969) *Clinical Neuro-Ophthalmology, 3rd Edn.* Baltimore: Williams & Wilkins.

Wang, F.M., Wertenbaker, C., Behrens, M.M., Jacobs, J.C. (1984) 'Acquired Brown's syndrome in children with juvenile rheumatoid arthritis.' *Ophthalmology*, **91**, 23–26.

Warady, B.A., Cibis, G., Alon, V., *et al.* (1994) 'Senior–Loken syndrome: revisited.' *Pediatrics*, **94**, 111–112.

Watson, A.P., Fielder, A.R. (1987) 'Sudden-onset squint.' *Developmental Medicine and Child Neurology*, **29**, 207–211.

Weinstein, J.M., Zweifel, T.J., Thompson, H.S. (1980) 'Congenital Horner's syndrome.' *Archives of Ophthalmology*, **98**, 1074–1078.

—— Gleaton, M., Weidner, W.A., Young, R.S.K. (1984) 'Leber's congenital amaurosis—relationship of structural CNS anomalies to psychomotor retardation.' *Archives of Neurology*, **41**, 204–206.

Weissman, B.M., Dell'Osso, L.F., Abel, L.A., Leigh, R.J. (1987) 'Spasmus nutans. A quantitative prospective study.' *Archives of Ophthalmology*, **105**, 525–528.

Whiting, S., Jan, J.E., Wong, P.K.H., *et al.* (1985) 'Permanent cortical visual impairment in children.' *Developmental Medicine and Child Neurology*, **27**, 730–739.

Wong, V.C.N. (1991) 'Cortical blindness in children: a study of etiology and prognosis.' *Pediatric Neurology*, **7**, 178–185.

Yokochi, K. (1991) 'Paroxysmal ocular downward deviation in neurologically impaired infants.' *Pediatric Neurology*, **7**, 426–428.

Zee, D.S., Yee, R.D., Singer, H.S. (1977) 'Congenital ocular motor apraxia.' *Brain*, **100**, 581–599.

19
DISORDERS OF HEARING AND VESTIBULAR FUNCTION

Hearing and vestibular functions are dependent on the ear, especially the inner ear, on the acoustic nerve (VIIIth nerve), on the central vestibular and cochlear nuclei, and on the respective conduction pathways up to the corresponding cortical areas.

HEARING IMPAIRMENT

GENERAL NOTIONS ON AUDITORY DYSFUNCTION AND ASSESSMENT

The major symptom of auditory dysfunction is hearing impairment. Tinnitus and hyperacusis are accessory symptoms. In infants, hearing impairment, if sufficiently profound, leads to failure to develop speech and to its loss in young children. In less severe hearing loss, speech may be more or less severely impaired with resulting behavioural and learning difficulties.

Hearing impairment is classified according to the part of the system that is affected.

Conduction hearing impairment results from abnormalities or disturbances in the external and/or middle ear. In such cases, sound vibrations are not properly transmitted to the inner ear because of blockade of the external auditory canal or of abnormalities of the tympanic membrane or the chain of ossicles.

Sensorineural hearing impairment results from abnormalities or dysfunction of the cochlea of the inner ear or auditory nerve. In contrast with conductive impairment, sensorineural loss often mainly affects high-frequency sounds.

Central hearing impairment is caused by disturbances of the cochlear nuclei or their cortical projections. With brainstem lesions, hearing impairment is usually bilateral and involves all modalities of auditory perception. With cortical lesions, there may be selective involvement of certain categories of sound perception, while pure tone audiometry is normal. In addition, various distortions in the processing of auditory messages may result in various bizarre impairments.

DIAGNOSIS OF HEARING IMPAIRMENT

The approach to the diagnosis of hearing impairment is dependent on the circumstances.

Screening for hearing impairment may be used for all newborn babies (Parving 1985, Stewart-Brown and Haslum 1987, McCormick 1988). However, many cases of auditory dysfunc-

tion—even congenital—have a delayed postnatal onset, so neonatal screening, in addition to the practical difficulties involved, is no proof of later normal hearing (Brown *et al.* 1989). Some investigators (Bess and Paradise 1994) think that universal screening is not without problems and risks and do not consider it currently justified, despite the contrary advice of the National Institutes of Health (1993). Systematic screening, on the other hand, is probably indicated for newborn babies and infants with intrauterine growth retardation and for those who experienced prenatal or perinatal difficulties such as hyperbilirubinaemia, hypoxia, apnoea, respiratory distress, infections and antibiotic therapy. However, 71 per cent of deaf children in one study (Johnson and Ashurst 1990) did not come from the 'at risk' group. Various techniques are available depending on age (respiratory audiometry, observation audiometry, visual reinforcement audiometry, play audiometry) but none is entirely reliable, so that the examination may have to be repeated, especially if no response to sounds presented is obtained. Later screening during the second semester of life may appear preferable because in many infants onset of deafness is delayed. However, because of technical problems and a high default rate, systematic audiometric testing has been shown to make only a very small contribution to the diagnosis of hearing impairment (Boothman and Ohr 1978).

Clinical examination for hearing impairment should be a part of any neurological examination of infants. Simple methods such as producing an interesting sound behind the child with bells, chimes, rattles or specially designed toys is usually adequate if a clear response is obtained as indicated by an alerting reaction and attemps at localizing the sound. Important clues to a possible hearing deficit may come from listening to abnormal sounds produced by the infant, or from the parents reporting doubts on their infant's hearing, or from the observation that cooing and lallations, initially normal, are disappearing or changing in character.

In older children, hearing examination should be required in all cases of delayed and/or abnormal language development. In such patients, a specialist investigation is often necessary as gross hearing may seem normal and selective loss of high-frequency perception is sufficient to severely disturb language comprehension and production. Indeed, even relatively mild and fluctuating hearing loss associated with otitis media may impair developing language (Gordon 1986, Chalmers *et al.* 1989).

Screening of hearing is performed as a standard procedure for preschool children in certain countries (*e.g.* Sweden) using low intensity levels (15–20 dB).

In all dubious cases, special tests of hearing should be provided. These include *subjective methods* such as pure-tone audiometry, with various techniques of conditioning being used for evaluating the response, and *objective techniques*. Among these, impedance audiometry (Peterson 1978) evaluates the tympanic membrane and ossicles, as does study of the stapedian reflexes that assess the motility of the stapes and the integrity of the reflex arc, which comprises the VIIIth nerve, the cochlear nuclei and the facial nerve. Spontaneous and evoked otoemission (Collet *et al.* 1993) is of value when positive, excluding deafness.

Brainstem auditory evoked responses can be used from an early age, as a response first appears at a conceptional age of 26–27 weeks. Seven different peaks are identified, each corresponding to a particular step in the processing of auditory information. Details on this technique and interpretation of results in neonates, infants and children have been published (Despland and Galambos 1980, Stockard *et al.* 1983, Vies *et al.* 1987).

CAUSES OF HEARING IMPAIRMENT IN CHILDREN

Deafness in childhood can be of acquired or genetic cause. The latter were found to account for approximately 80 per cent of the cases in a study conducted in Göteborg, Sweden (Thiringer *et al.* 1984). In a recent study, Das (1996) found isolated genetic deafness in 23.3 per cent of their cases, chromosomal defects in 6.5 per cent, and syndromes with hearing impairment in 5.3 per cent. Congenital infections accounted for 12.8 per cent of cases, meningitis for 8.5 per cent, and miscellaneous causes for 4.7 per cent. No cause was found in 33.9 per cent of patients. The overall prevalence of bilateral hearing impairment among 8-year-old boys varies between 0.7 and 1.5 per 1000 (Commission of the European Communities 1979).

Hearing Impairment of Prenatal Origin
Many common causes of hearing impairment or deafness have their origin in prenatal life.

Defects and malformations of the ear
Ear defects were the cause of 14 per cent of cases of hearing impairment and deafness in the Göteborg study (Thiringer *et al.* 1984). With involvement of the external and middle ear, impairment is only partial or unilateral and is of the conductive type. Meatal atresia and various auriculofacial syndromes are the usual causes. Minor anomalies such as stenosis of the external canal or abnormalities of the ossicular chain are responsible only for limited deficits (Wildervanck 1982). Auriculofacial syndromes include the Treacher–Collins syndrome (Fazen *et al.* 1967), which is dominantly inherited, Goldenhar oculo-auriculo-vertebral syndrome (Rollnick *et al.* 1987, Cohen *et al.* 1995),

TABLE 19.1
Main types of isolated hereditary deafness in childhood*

Hereditary deafness without associated abnormalities
Dominant congenital severe deafness
(no vestibular involvement in most cases)
Dominant progressive nerve deafness
(childhood-onset of mild high-tone loss)
Dominant unilateral deafness
(common cause of congenital unilateral moderate to severe hearing loss)
Recessive congenital severe deafness
(accounts for 26% of profound congenital deafness. Several genes are probably responsible. Vestibular function normal)
Recessive early-onset deafness
(some hearing at birth; severe neural loss by 5–6 years)
Recessive congenital moderate hearing loss
Sex-linked congenital neural deafness
(rare)
Sex-linked early-onset deafness
(rare)

Hereditary deafness with external ear malformations
Wildervanck syndrome
(deformed auricles, marginal pits, preauricular appendages; dominant transmission; Duane retraction syndrome; Klippel–Feil deformity)
Preauricular pits and neural hearing loss
(preauricular pits, branchial fistulae, dominant transmission)
Dominant thickened ears and incus–stapes abnormality
(conductive hearing loss, hypertrophic earlobes)

*Modified from Konigsmark (1969).

which is usually sporadic, and laterocervical branchial clefts or other anomalies of the first and second branchial arches (Table 19.1). Inner ear involvement may be associated.

Malformations of the inner ear are associated with severe deafnesss. In Mondini defect, there is incomplete development of the bony and membranous labyrinth with dysgenesis of the spiral ganglion. Scheibe (defects in cochlea and sacculus with normal canals and utricle) and Michel (absent or defective labyrinth) defects are rarer. In all cases, abnormalities of the VIIIth nerve are associated with the bony defects. The clinical presentation is usually that of isolated congenital deafness which is frequently detected only by delayed or absent language development. Deafness due to osseous defects is impossible to distinguish from that due to degeneration of the organ of Corti. In some cases, abnormalities of the external or middle ear are associated and always are a definite indication to further testing as they rarely explain major hearing impairment.

Genetic deafness due to VIIIth nerve abnormalities and/or abnormalities of the organ of Corti
Genetic factors are responsible for about 30 per cent of cases of congenital deafness. Most prelingual cases are due to a dominant connexin-26 gene defect, but late cases may have a different transmission (Konigsmark 1969, 1975; Steele 1981). A possible family history of deafness may be an important diagnostic clue. Linkage of syndromic and nonsyndromic deafness to chromosome loci has been found in several conditions (Coucke *et al.* 1994).

TABLE 19.2
Some syndromes of hearing loss of neurological interest*

Usher syndrome	Congenital deafness and atypical pigmentary retinal degeneration
Refsum syndrome	Neuropathy, ataxia, retinitis pigmentosa (Chapters 9, 21)
Alström–Hallgren syndrome	Obesity, atypical retinitis pigmentosa, diabetes mellitus, progressive hearing loss
Small syndrome	Deafness, retinal detachment, muscular dystrophy, mental retardation (Chapter 22)
Norrie syndrome	Vascular and glial retinal proliferation, microphthalmia, mental retardation (Chapter 18)
Recessive optic atrophy	Hearing loss and juvenile diabetes mellitus
Rosenberg–Chutorian syndrome	Familial hearing loss, polyneuropathy, optic atrophy
Richards–Rundle syndrome	Mental retardation, ataxia, muscle wasting, infantilism
May–White syndrome	Photomyoclonus, hearing loss, nephropathy, diabetes mellitus
Cranial osseous disorders (osteopetrosis, metaphyseal dysplasia, etc.)	May produce hearing loss, optic atrophy and involvement of other cranial nerves
Jervell–Lange–Nielsen syndrome	Hearing loss, heart conduction block with syncope (Chapter 17)
Waardenburg syndrome	Laterally displaced inner canthi, heterochromy of irides, white forelock, behavioural disturbances

*Adapted from Konigsmark (1969, 1975).

The main forms of genetic deafness unassociated with involvement of systems other than the ear are shown in Table 19.1.

Genetic deafness associated with other defects
Deafness is a part of a host of degenerative neurological syndromes and occasionally of syndromes with more diffuse systemic involvement (Table 19.2).

Usher syndrome is an autosomal recessive syndrome characterized by the association of congenital deafness with the secondary appearance, usually before 10 years of age, of retinitis pigmentosa slowly leading to blindness. Cataracts and glaucoma may occur. Mental retardation may be present in a quarter of cases and psychotic syndromes may appear. There are at least two subtypes of the syndrome. In type I, deafness is severe to profound with an absent peripheral vestibular response. Many patients have delayed motor development, and difficulties with balance of vestibular origin develop as vision fails. In type II, deafness is milder except at higher frequencies, and vestibular responses are normal (Samuelson and Zahn 1990). Usher syndrome is genetically heterogeneous and at least four different loci can be involved (Kimberling and Smith 1992). Mutations of the gene for myosin VII A have been demonstrated in one form (type 1B) (Weil *et al.* 1995).

Hallgren syndrome shares deafness and retinitis pigmentosa with Usher syndrome but seems genetically distinct. Ataxia due to vestibulocerebellar dysfunction may be prominent (Montandon 1972).

Other deafness syndromes with tapetoretinal degeneration include the *Alström–Hallgren syndrome* which comprises diabetes mellitus and obesity (Alström 1972), the *Bardet–Biedl syndrome* with retinopathy, polydactyly, mental retardation, obesity and hypogenitalism, Cockayne syndrome (Chapter 10) and Refsum disease (Chapter 21). The latter is of special importance as effective treatment is possible in the form of dietary measures and other measures such as exchange transfusion to lower phytanic acid levels (Djupesland *et al.* 1983). In none of these syndromes is deafness present from birth.

Deafness may be *associated with optic atrophy* in several syndromes (Konigsmark 1975). These include the syndrome of dominant optic atrophy, ataxia and progressive hearing loss (Sylvester syndrome), sometimes associated with muscle wasting; the syndrome of recessive optic atrophy, polyneuropathy and hearing loss (Rosenberg–Chutorian syndrome); the syndrome of optico-cochleo-dentate degeneration (Zeman 1975); and an X-linked syndrome of nerve deafness, optic atrophy and dementia (Jensen *et al.* 1987).

Pendred syndrome is a genetic defect in thyroxine synthesis which is transmitted as an autosomal recessive character (Konigsmark and Gorlin 1976). Congenital sensorineural hearing impairment is present at birth and is severe in half the cases. A diffuse, non-nodular goitre becomes apparent in infancy or early childhood but is usually unaccompanied by signs of thyroid insufficiency. Mental development is also normal in most patients.

The diagnosis rests on the perchlorate discharge test which produces a marked decline of the radioiodine content of the thyroid gland to 10 per cent or less of baseline value. Treatment is with exogenous thyroid hormones.

Deafness is a frequent feature of endemic cretinism (Cao *et al.* 1994).

The *Jervell–Lange–Nielsen syndrome* associates deafness and prolonged Q-T transmission which may result in cardiac syncopes and even in sudden death (Chapter 17). Other cardio-auditory syndromes are known, including the lentigines–cardiopathy–deafness syndrome or Leopard syndrome (Chapter 4).

Waardenburg syndrome is characterized by laterally displaced inner canthi, a prominent nasal root, heterochromia iridis, the presence of a white forelock and sometimes behavioural disturbances. It is transmitted as an autosomal dominant character (Preus *et al.* 1983). The defective gene on chromosome 2 is the *Pax3* homeobox gene (Baldwin *et al.* 1992).

Deafness accompanying neurological diseases (Table 19.2) is often associated with a neuropathy and is usually acquired rather than congenital. Special mention should be made of the deafness that not infrequently accompanies facio-scapulo-humeral dystrophy (Korf *et al.* 1985, Voit *et al.* 1986). Deafness is also an essential part of the Vialetto–Van Laere syndrome (Chapter 20) and of the rare ataxia–deafness–retardation syndrome (Koletzko *et al.* 1987).

CONGENITAL DEAFNESS DUE TO FETAL INFECTIONS
Deafness due to viral diseases of the fetus represents approximately

10 per cent of the cases of congenital deafness. The main causes are rubella and cytomegalovirus infection (Chapter 1). In both diseases, deafness may be the sole clinical manifestation. In a study of infants with inapparent congenital cytomegalovirus infection (Brookhouser and Bordley 1973), subsequent hearing loss was demonstrated in 56 per cent of patients referred to otolaryngologists, in contrast to 17 per cent of a control population, and in some cases the hearing impairment was progressive. With rubella, deafness is the only abnormality in 35 per cent of those infected after the 13th gestational week (Miller *et al.* 1982). Deafness has also occurred in infants born to mothers who had received anticoagulation therapy during pregnancy (Hall *et al.* 1980).

ACQUIRED HEARING IMPAIRMENT
Acquired deafness accounts for approximately 12–20 per cent of the cases of hearing impairment in children (Thiringer *et al.* 1984, Das 1996). The main causes of acquired hearing loss are shown in Table 19.2.

Toxic causes of hearing loss
Drugs are by far the most common offenders (Snavely and Hodges 1984). *Antibiotics* of the aminoglycoside group are especially prone to produce hearing impairment. Amikacin and vancomycin are more commonly the cause than kanamycin and neomycin, although neomycin has been implicated even when used as a topical application to infants with extensive burns (Bamford and Jones 1978). Cochlear damage in older patients usually begins as tinnitus and progresses to vertigo and deafness. In infants, however, particularly preterm newborns who are especially at risk (Bergman *et al.* 1985), deafness sets in insidiously. The true incidence of antibiotic-induced hearing impairment in infants is controversial. Some investigators (*e.g.* Thiringer *et al.* 1984) have not found any relationship of deafness to antibiotics use but a connection seems established in many cases (Lynn *et al.* 1985). A genetic factor is operative in at least some cases of antibiotic-induced deafness (Prezant *et al.* 1993).

Other drugs are uncommonly a cause of deafness. Cases have been reported in patients receiving furosemide (Lynn *et al.* 1985), beta-blocking agents (Fäldt *et al.* 1984) and cisplatin, an antineoplastic agent (Rozencweig *et al.* 1977). Salicylates in high doses can produce hearing impairment (Ballantyne 1984).

Bilirubin toxicity has become an uncommon cause of nerve deafness. Deafness in preterm infants with hyperbilirubinaemia may be of multifactorial origin. The classical sequence of kernicterus is no longer seen in industrialized countries.

Risk factors for neonates and especially preterm infants often include hyperbilirubinaemia, together with other factors such as hypothermia, while ototoxic drugs may not be important in all cases (Anagnostakis *et al.* 1982).

Bacterial infections
Acute *bacterial meningitis* is complicated by permanent unilateral or bilateral hearing loss in about 10 per cent of cases (Dodge *et al.* 1984), with the highest frequency of over 30 per cent in pneumococcal meningitis (Bohr *et al.* 1984). Deafness is probably

due to invasion of the labyrinth by the suppurative process and to involvement of the VIIIth nerve as it crosses the subarachnoid space. Checking for deafness should be performed systematically following purulent meningitis (Vienny *et al.* 1984). The use of corticosteroids in conjunction with ceftriaxone may be associated with a lower incidence of postmeningitic deafness (Lebel *et al.* 1988).

Otitis media is only rarely a cause of permanent deafness.

Viral infections
Acquired viral infections are a common cause of hearing loss. Mumps can produce unilateral or, infrequently, bilateral sudden deafness as a result of neuritis or meningitis. The same phenomenon may be observed following measles or chickenpox. Auditory dysfunction has been reported with herpes zoster of the concha in adults (Iragui 1986) and may also occur in cases of sarcoidosis. Exceptionally, hearing loss may be the first manifestation of the opsoclonus–myoclonus syndrome (Rosenberg 1984).

Tumours and compression
Compression by tumours is a rare cause of deafness in children. Unilateral deafness can result from any tumour of the cerebellopontine angle. Acoustic neuroma is the least uncommon of such tumours. It is usually bilateral and belongs to neurofibromatosis type II (Chapter 4). The disorder is observed almost exclusively in adolescents. Sensorineural hearing impairment is associated with facial weakness, paraesthesiae and other neurological signs in one-third of cases. Diagnosis can be confirmed by CT or MRI which demonstrate both the tumour itself and the erosion of the internal auditory canals.

Other causes
Metabolic diseases including the mucopolysaccharidoses and mitochondrial disorders are uncommon but important causes. In rare cases, deafness can be the first and most prominent manifestation of Leigh syndrome or of other mitochondrial diseases. Deafness is a common feature of the MERRF and MELAS syndromes (Chapter 9). The association of deafness and diabetes mellitus may be encountered among members of the maternal lineage of MELAS patients. It may also occur as a specific mitochondrial disease observed mainly in adults (Reardon *et al.* 1992). Recently, familial cases of isolated, nonsyndromic deafness have been shown to result from a mitochondrial DNA mutation involving a mitochondrial RNA gene (Prezant *et al.* 1993, El-Shahazawi *et al.* 1997). Cases of both antibiotic-induced and spontaneous deafness have been reported.

Cases of *auditory neuropathy* in which the integrity of the cochlea could be demonstrated by the presence of a normal otoemission can be observed in cases of genetic (Charcot–Marie–Tooth) or sporadic peripheral neuropathy. Seven such cases with onset in childhood have been reported by Starr *et al.* (1996). In two of these the auditory neuropathy was isolated, although later appearance of more diffuse nerve involvement could not be excluded.

DYSFUNCTION OF THE VESTIBULAR SYSTEM

CLINICAL MANIFESTATIONS OF VESTIBULAR DISORDERS

SYMPTOMS OF VESTIBULAR DYSFUNCTION

Dizziness and vertigo are the major manifestations of vestibular disease. Vertigo is characterized by the illusion of rotation, either of the subject or of her/his environment. True vertigo should be distinguished by careful questioning from sensations of dizziness or lightheadedness which are often reported as vertigo by patients (Tusa *et al.* 1994).

Vertigo may be acute, recurrent or chronic. It may be spontaneous or precipitated, *e.g.* by changes of position. Vomiting and nausea are often associated symptoms.

Less characteristic vestibular symptoms include dizziness and a feeling of instability, especially on changing position in space or on rapid movements of the head.

EXAMINATION OF VESTIBULAR DYSFUNCTION

In addition to the classical tests of vestibular functions that are part of standard neurological examination, special tests are often required for study of a patient with suspected vestibular disease.

The most commonly used procedure is caloric testing, which can be practised at the bedside using small quantities of ice-water for successive irrigation of both ears.

Positional testing can also be used at the bedside. The patient is tilted from the sitting to the supine position with the head hanging down below the level of the examining table. The head is then turned 45° to the left, then several minutes later to the right, and the eyes observed for nystagmus.

Electronystagmography and other elaborate techniques for study of the labyrinth are described in specialized texts (Barber and Stockwell 1976, Oosterveld 1984).

CENTRAL AND PERIPHERAL VESTIBULAR DYSFUNCTION

Peripheral vestibular syndrome is characterized by a concordance of symptoms and signs pointing to one labyrinth. In addition, there are often associated signs such as hearing loss, tinnitus and otalgia. Spontaneous nystagmus is away from the affected labyrinth, past pointing and falling are towards the affected side. Caloric testing indicates ipsilateral vestibular paresis on the same side with absent caloric nystagmus on stimulation of the affected ear, or directional preponderance to the contralateral side.

Central vestibular syndromes are characterized by discordance between the results of various clinical tests of vestibular function. Caloric testing does not indicate vestibular paresis although directional preponderance may be present. Associated neurological signs pointing to the brainstem or cerebellum are often found whereas hearing is intact.

CAUSES OF VESTIBULAR IMPAIRMENT

DRUGS AND OTHER TOXIC CAUSES

Many drugs disturb vestibular function. *Antibiotics* are the major class of drugs affecting the labyrinths, with associated cochlear involvement. Streptomycin is highly toxic for the vestibule but has less effect on cochlear function. Most aminoglycoside drugs have an adverse effect on both vestibular and auditory function.

Anticonvulsant agents, especially phenytoin, produce ataxia, incoordination and vestibular dysfunction when blood levels are high enough (Abu-Arafeh and Wallace 1988). Disturbances of eye movements in patients receiving anticonvulsant therapy may be due in part to toxicity to central vestibular pathways (Remler *et al.* 1990). Vestibular impairment due to drugs and other toxic agents has been reviewed by Ballantyne (1984).

BACTERIAL AND VIRAL INFECTIONS

Acute suppurative labyrinthitis resulting from extension of *middle ear infection* has become rare since widespread use of antibiotics in the therapy of otitis media. A vestibular syndrome is sometimes observed during otitis media which is probably due to serous labyrinthitis resulting from the action of bacterial toxins. The onset of acute labyrinthitis is sudden with vertigo, vomiting or nausea, and unilateral hearing loss. With vigorous antibiotic therapy the course is usually favourable in a few days.

Purulent meningitis can be responsible for bilateral labyrinthine disease which usually becomes evident upon recovery from the acute phase. Labyrinthitis is responsible for most cases of ataxia associated with purulent meningitis (Kaplan *et al.* 1981, Eavey *et al.* 1985). Deafness is associated in most such cases. The ataxia is usually transient but vestibular reflexes often remain abolished.

Mild episodes lasting 24–72 hours are sometimes seen in toddlers and young children who are found to be ataxic and unable to walk, often upon awakening, without any obvious evidence of otitis media. The nature of such episodes is uncertain. In some cases, I have been able to demonstrate transient disturbances in vestibular function, especially on caloric testing.

Such cases may be due to *viral infection* even though in many cases no agent is identifiable. More obvious cases of viral infection may occur during mumps (Thömke and Hopf 1992), measles or infectious mononucleosis. Some such cases may be part of a postinfectious cranial polyneuritis (Adour *et al.* 1981).

Vestibular neuronitis is rare in children. It is characterized by the sudden occurrence of vertigo, instability, nystagmus, nausea and vomiting without hearing loss (Lumio and Aho 1965). The condition is sometimes recurrent. It should be noted that there is no proof of inflammatory phenomena in most such patients. In some cases, vertigo is associated with other neurological manifestations. Such cases may occur in small epidemics and have been reported as 'epidemic vertigo' (Pederson 1959).

TRAUMA

Dizziness occurs in 50 per cent of children following head trauma, even without loss of consciousness (Eviatar *et al.* 1986). Persistent post-traumatic vertigo may result from direct or indirect trauma to the labyrinth (vestibular concussion). Severe vertigo occurs immediately following injury and the child is unstable with deviation toward the affected side. The symptoms usually subside after several days but recurrent episodes of vertigo lasting for a few seconds may continue for several months.

MIGRAINE AND EPILEPSY
Migraine is a common cause of vertigo in adults. Seventeen per cent of patients report vertigo at the time of attacks (Kayan and Hood 1984). In children, it seems likely that paroxysmal vertigo (Chapter 17), and especially benign paroxysmal torticollis of infancy, may be migrainous equivalents (Deonna and Martin 1981).

Vertigo is only rarely an initial manifestation of temporal or parietal lobe *epilepsy* (Deonna *et al.* 1986, Aicardi 1994). Vertigo may also be a feature of vascular disease in the posterior brain circulation, *e.g.* in basilar artery obliteration or with vascular malformations of the brainstem (Chapter 15).

RECURRENT VERTIGO
Benign positional vertigo is an uncommon disorder in childhood. It is characterized by bursts of nystagmus and associated vertigo that can be induced by a rapid position change from the sitting to the head-hanging right or left position (Baloh *et al.* 1987). Positional vertigo of the central type is only rarely associated with intracranial pathology. The peripheral type may be post-traumatic or due to miscellaneous causes. A majority of adult cases are cryptogenic but in young patients symptomatic cases tend to be more frequent. An abnormality of the posterior semicircular canal seems strongly implicated (Baloh *et al.* 1987).

Benign recurrent vertigo, also termed recurrent vestibulopathy (Slater 1979), may be the result of hydrops of the pars superior of the inner ear. It is characterized by attacks of vertigo without cochlear involvement that last from half an hour to four hours. The acute constant vertigo then subsides and may be replaced for a period of hours or days by positional vertigo. This syndrome is mainly seen in adults but may have its onset in childhood. Some cases of recurrent vertigo are associated with eye movement abnormalities and with evidence of cerebellar involvement; they respond remarkably to administration of acetazolamide (Baloh and Winder 1991).

Delayed vertigo is very similar to recurrent vertigo but appears months or years after the onset of severe acute unilateral complete deafness such as occurs following mumps or exanthematous diseases. Attacks of vertigo with nausea and vomiting, lasting from 10 minutes to 24 hours in almost all cases, have their onset several years after the occurrence of juvenile, unilateral total deafness of unknown or known cause. They are not accompanied by cochlear symptoms such as acouphenes, which distinguishes delayed vertigo from Ménière disease (Wolfson and Leiberman 1975, Kamei 1978).

Ménière disease can occur as early as the first decade and even in infants (Sadé and Yaniv 1984), although it is a rare condition in children. The clinical symptoms are hearing impairment, tinnitus and vertigo which occur in attacks lasting one to three hours. Attacks occur at unpredictable intervals. Hearing impairment may be fluctuating and may even return temporarily to normal. Eventually, definitive deafness ensues.

Bilateral impairment may be present in as many as 20 per cent of adult patients. Treatment is only symptomatic.

Benign paroxysmal vertigo has been studied in Chapter 17. Episodic ataxia (Kramer *et al.* 1994) includes a vestibular as well as a cerebellar component.

PROGRESSIVE FAMILIAL VESTIBULOCEREBELLAR DYSFUNCTION
This rare condition is dominantly inherited. Onset is in childhood but not congenital and is often marked by true vertigo (Verhagen and Huygen 1991, Baloh *et al.* 1994, Huygen *et al.* 1994). Tremor and ataxia may be present. Abnormal eye movements include absence of smooth pursuit and gaze, paretic and rebound nystagmus indicating cerebellar involvement, and head and movement-dependent oscillopsia (Harris *et al.* 1993). The disorder does not appear to be progressive after childhood. Lenard *et al.* (1992) have reported four preschool children with acute simultaneous loss of both hearing and vestibular function, muscle weakness and multiple white matter lesions of unknown cause.

PROGRESSIVE FAMILIAL VESTIBULOCOCHLEAR DYSFUNCTION
Head-movement-dependent oscillopsia due to acquired vestibular areflexia in combination with progressive hearing loss has been reported in a few kindreds (Verhagen *et al.* 1987). The pedigrees suggest autosomal dominant inheritance. Head-movement-dependent oscillopsia is a also a very common complaint in patients with total vestibular function loss (Verhagen *et al.* 1987).

MISCELLANEOUS CAUSES
Other causes of vestibular impairment are reviewed by Brandt and Daroff (1980).

Motion sickness is very frequent in children. Antihistamine, diazepam and scopolamine may be effective for prevention. Visual, somatosensory and head-extension vertigo are other types of physiological vertigo. Psychogenic vertigo has been observed in adolescents. Vertigo of central origin may be seen with multiple sclerosis (Chapter 12).

Recurrent ataxia of obscure origin (Chapter 17) may have a vestibular rather than a cerebellar origin and may be associated with vertigo (Tibbles *et al.* 1986) or with other manifestations of vestibular dysfunction such as nystagmus (Sogg and Hoyt 1962, Farris *et al.* 1986).

REFERENCES

Abu-Arafeh, I.A., Wallace, S.J. (1988) 'Unwanted effects of anti-epileptic drugs.' *Developmental Medicine and Child Neurology*, **30**, 117–121.
Adour, K.K., Sprague, M.A., Hilsinger, R.L. (1981) 'Vestibular vertigo. A form of polyneuritis?' *Journal of the American Medical Association*, **246**, 1564–1567.
Aicardi, J. (1994) *Epilepsy in Children, 2nd Edn.* New York: Raven Press.
Alström, C.H. (1972) 'The Lindenov–Hallgren, Alström–Hallgren and Weiss syndromes.' *In:* Vinken, P.J., Bruyn, G.W. (Eds.) *Handbook of Clinical Neurology. Vol. 13. Neuroretinal Degenerations.* Amsterdam: North Holland, pp. 451–467.
Anagnostakis, D., Petmezakis, J., Papazissis, G., *et al.* (1982) 'Hearing loss in low-birthweight infants.' *American Journal of Diseases of Children*, **136**, 602–604.

Baldwin, C.T., Hoth, C.F., Amos, J.A., *et al.* (1992) 'An exonic mutation in the *HuP2* paired domain gene causes Waardenburg's syndrome.' *Nature*, **355**, 637–638.

Ballantyne, J. (1984) 'Ototoxicity.' *In:* Oosterveld, W.J. (Ed.) *Otoneurology.* Chichester: John Wiley, pp. 41–51.

Baloh, R.W., Winder, A. (1991) 'Acetazolamide-responsive vestibulocerebellar syndrome: clinical and oculographic features.' *Neurology*, **41**, 429–433.

—— Honrubia, V., Jacobson, K. (1987) 'Benign positional vertigo—clinical and oculographic features in 240 cases.' *Neurology*, **37**, 371–378.

—— Jacobson, K., Fife, T. (1994) 'Familial vestibulopathy: a new dominantly inherited syndrome.' *Neurology*, **44**, 20–25.

Bamford, M.F.M., Jones, L.F. (1978) 'Deafness and biochemical imbalance after burns treatment with topical antibiotics in young children.' *Archives of Disease in Childhood*, **53**, 326–329.

Barber, H.O., Stockwell, C.W. (1976) *Manual of Electronystagmography.* St Louis: C.V. Mosby.

Bergman, I., Hirsch, R.P., Fria, T.J., *et al.* (1985) 'Cause of hearing loss in the high-risk premature infant.' *Journal of Pediatrics*, **106**, 95–101.

Bess, F.H., Paradise, J.L. (1994) 'Universal screening for infant hearing impairment: not simple, not risk-free, not necessarily beneficial, and not presently justified.' *Pediatrics*, **93**, 330–334.

Bohr, V., Paulson, O.B., Rasmussen, N. (1984) 'Pneumococcal meningitis. Late neurological sequelae and features of prognostic impact.' *Archives of Neurology*, **41**, 1045–1049.

Boothman, R., Orr, N. (1978) 'Value of screening for deafness in the first year of life.' *Archives of Disease in Childhood*, **53**, 570–573.

Brandt, T., Daroff, R.B. (1980) 'The multisensory physiological and pathological vertigo syndromes.' *Annals of Neurology*, **7**, 195–203.

Brookhouser, P.E., Bordley, J.E. (1973) 'Congenital rubella deafness.' *Archives of Otolaryngology*, **98**, 252–257.

Brown, J., Watson, E., Alberman, E. (1989) 'Screening children for hearing loss.' *Archives of Disease in Childhood*, **64**, 1488–1495.

Cao, X-Y., Jiang, X-M., Dou, Z-H., *et al.* (1994) 'Timing of vulnerability of the brain to iodine deficiency in endemic cretinism.' *New England Journal of Medicine*, **331**, 1739–1744.

Chalmers, D., Stewart, I., Silva, P., Mulvena, A. (1989) *Otitis Media with Effusion in Children—the Dunedin Study. Clinics in Developmental Medicine No. 108.* London: Mac Keith Press.

Cohen, M.S., Samango-Sprouse, C.A., Stern, H.J., *et al.* (1995) 'Neurodevelopmental profile of infants and toddlers with oculo-auriculo-vertebral spectrum and the correlation of prognosis with physical findings.' *American Journal of Medical Genetics*, **60**, 535–540.

Collet, L., Gartner, M., Veuillet, E., *et al.* (1993) 'Evoked and spontaneous otoacoustic emissions. A comparison of neonates and adults.' *Brain and Development*, **15**, 249–252.

Commission of the European Communities (1979) *Childhood Deafness in the European Community. EUR Report 6413.* Luxembourg: European Commission.

Coucke, P., Van Camp, G., Djoyodiharjo, B., *et al.* (1994) 'Linkage of autosomal dominant hearing loss to the short arm of chromosome 1 in two families.' *New England Journal of Medicine*, **331**, 425–431.

Das, V.K. (1996) 'Aetiology of bilateral sensorineural hearing impairment in children: a 10 year study.' *Archives of Disease in Childhood*, **74**, 8–12.

Deonna, T., Martin, D. (1981) 'Benign paroxysmal torticollis in infancy.' *Archives of Disease in Childhood*, **56**, 956–959.

—— Ziegler, A.L., Despland, P.A., Van Melle, G. (1986) 'Partial epilepsy in neurologically normal children: clinical syndromes and prognosis.' *Epilepsia*, **27**, 241–247.

Despland, P.A., Galambos, R. (1980) 'Use of the auditory brainstem responses by premature and newborn infants.' *Neuropädiatrie*, **11**, 99–107.

Djupesland, G., Flottorp, G., Refsum, S. (1983) 'Phytanic acid storage disease: hearing maintained after 15 years of dietary treatment.' *Neurology*, **33**, 237–240.

Dodge, P.R., Davis, H., Feigin, R.D., *et al.* (1984) 'Prospective evaluation of hearing impairment as a sequela of acute bacterial meningitis.' *New England Journal of Medicine*, **311**, 869–874.

Eavey, R.D., Gao, Y-Z., Schuknecht, H.F., Gonzalez-Pineda, M. (1985) 'Otologic features of bacterial meningitis of childhood.' *Journal of Pediatrics*, **106**, 402–407.

El-Shahawazi, M., Lopez de Munain, P., Sarrazin, A.M., *et al.* (1997) 'Two large Spanish pedigrees with nonsyndromic sensorineural deafness and the mt DNA mutation at nt 1555 in the 12Sr RNA gene: evidence of heteroplasmy.' *Neurology*, **48**, 453–456.

Eviatar, L., Bergtraum, M., Randel, R.M. (1986) 'Post-traumatic vertigo in children: a diagnostic approach.' *Pediatric Neurology*, **2**, 61–66.

Fäldt, R., Liedholm, H., Aursnes, J. (1984) 'β blockers and loss of hearing.' *British Medical Journal*, **289**, 1490–1492.

Farris, B.K., Smith, J.L., Ayyar, R. (1986) 'Neuro-ophthalmologic findings in vestibulocerebellar ataxia.' *Archives of Neurology*, **43**, 1050–1053.

Fazen, L.E., Elmore, J., Nadler, H.L. (1967) 'Mandibulo-facial dysostosis (Treacher–Collins syndrome).' *American Journal of Diseases of Children*, **113**, 405–410.

Gordon, N. (1986) 'Intermittent deafness and learning.' *Developmental Medicine and Child Neurology*, **28**, 364–369.

Hall, J.G., Pauli, R.M., Wilson, K.M. (1980) 'Maternal and fetal sequelae of anticoagulation during pregnancy.' *American Journal of Medicine*, **68**, 122–140.

Harris, C.M., Walker, J., Shawkat, F., *et al.* (1993) 'Eye movements in a familial vestibulocerebellar disorder.' *Neuropediatrics*, **24**, 117–122.

Huygen, P.L.M., Verhagen, W.I.M., Lenssen, P.P.A., Theunissen, E.J.J.M. (1994) 'Familial vestibulocerebellar disorder.' *Neuropediatrics*, **25**, 277. (*Letter.*)

Iragui, V.J. (1986) 'Auditory dysfunction in Ramsay Hunt syndrome.' *Journal of Neurology, Neurosurgery, and Psychiatry*, **49**, 824–826.

Jensen, P.K.A., Reske-Nielsen, E., Hein-Sørensen, O., Warburg, M. (1987) 'The syndrome of opticoacoustic nerve atrophy with dementia.' *American Journal of Medical Genetics*, **28**, 517–518. (*Letter.*)

Johnson, A., Ashurst, H., for the Steering Committee, Oxford Region Child Development Project (1990) 'Screening for sensorineural deafness by health visitors.' *Archives of Disease in Childhood*, **65**, 841–845.

Kamei, T. (1978) 'Delayed vertigo.' *In:* Hood, J.D. (Ed.) *Vestibular Mechanisms in Health and Disease.* London: Academic Press, pp. 369–374.

Kaplan, S.L., Goddard, J., Van Kleek, M., *et al.* (1981) 'Ataxia and deafness in children due to bacterial meningitis.' *Pediatrics*, **68**, 8–13.

Kayan, A., Hood, J.D. (1984) 'Neuro-otological manifestations of migraine.' *Brain*, **107**, 1123–1142.

Kimberling, W., Smith, R.J.H. (1992) 'Gene mapping of the Usher syndromes.' *Otolaryngologic Clinics of North America*, **25**, 923–934.

Koletzko, S., Koletzko, B., Lamprecht, A., Lenard, H.G. (1987) 'Ataxia–deafness–retardation syndrome in three sisters.' *Neuropediatrics*, **18**, 18–21.

Konigsmark, B.W. (1969) 'Hereditary deafness in man.' *New England Journal of Medicine*, **281**, 713–720; 774–778; 827–832.

—— (1975) 'Hereditary diseases of the nervous system with hearing loss.' *In:* Vinken, P.J., Bruyn, G.W. (Eds.) *Handbook of Clinical Neurology. Vol. 22. System Disorders and Atrophies, Part II.* Amsterdam: North Holland, pp. 499–526.

—— Gorlin, R.J. (1976) *Genetic and Metabolic Deafness.* Philadelphia: W.B. Saunders.

Korf, B.R., Bresnan, M.J., Shapiro, F., *et al.* (1985) 'Facioscapulohumeral dystrophy presenting in infancy with facial diplegia and sensorineural deafness.' *Annals of Neurology*, **17**, 513–516.

Kramer, P., Litt, M., Browne, D., *et al.* (1994) 'Autosomal dominant episodic ataxia represents at least two genetic disorders.' *Annals of Neurology*, **36**, 279. (*Abstract.*)

Lebel, M.H., Freij, B.J., Syrogiannopoulos, G.A., *et al.* (1988) 'Dexamethasone therapy for bacterial meningitis: results of two double-blind, placebo-controlled trials.' *New England Journal of Medicine*, **319**, 964–971.

Lenard, H.G., Voit, T., Lamprecht, A., *et al.* (1992) 'Sudden loss of hearing and vestibular function, muscular weakness, and multiple white matter lesions in preschool children.' *Neuropediatrics*, **23**, 221–224.

Lumio, J.S., Aho, J. (1965) 'Vestibular neuronitis.' *Annals of Otology, Rhinology and Laryngology*, **74**, 264–270.

Lynn, A.M., Redding, G.J., Morray, J.P., Tyler, D.C. (1985) 'Isolated deafness following recovery from neurologic injury and adult respiratory distress syndrome: a sequela of intercurrent aminoglycoside and diuretic use.' *American Journal of Diseases of Children*, **139**, 464–466.

McCormick, B. (1988) *Screening for Hearing Impairment in Young Children.* London: Croom Helm.

Miller, E., Cradock-Watson, J.E., Pollock, T.M. (1982) 'Consequences of confirmed maternal rubella at successive stages of pregnancy.' *Lancet*, **2**, 781–784.

Montandon, A. (1972) 'Usher syndrome.' *In:* Vinken, P.J., Bruyn, G.W. (Eds.) *Handbook of Clinical Neurology. Vol.13. Neuroretinal Degenerations.* Amsterdam: North Holland, pp. 441–450.

National Institutes of Health (1993) *NIH Consensus Statement. Early Identi-*

fication of Hearing Impairment in Infants and Young Children. Baltimore, MD: NIH.

Oosterveld, W.J. (Ed.) (1984) *Otoneurology.* Chichester: John Wiley.

Parving, A. (1985) 'Hearing disorders in childhood, some procedures for detection, identification and diagnostic evaluation.' *International Journal of Pediatric Otorhinolaryngology,* **9,** 31–57.

Pederson, E. (1959) 'Epidemic vertigo. Clinical picture, epidemiology and relation to encephalitis.' *Brain,* **82,** 566–580.

Peterson, M.K. (1978) 'Impedance audiometry and the brain-damaged child.' *Developmental Medicine and Child Neurology,* **20,** 800–802.

Preus, M., Linstrom, C., Polomeno, R.C., Milot, J. (1983) 'Waardenburg syndrome—penetrance of major signs.' *American Journal of Medical Genetics,* **15,** 383–388.

Prezant, T.R., Agapian, J.V., Bohlman, M.C., *et al.* (1993) 'Mitochondrial ribosomal RNA mutation associated with both antibiotic-induced and non-syndromic deafness.' *Nature Genetics,* **4,** 289–294.

Reardon, W., Ross, R.J.M., Sweeney, M.G., *et al.* (1992) 'Diabetes mellitus associated with a pathogenic point mutation in mitochondrial DNA.' *Lancet,* **340,** 1376–1379.

Remler, B.F., Leigh, J., Osorio, I.,Tomsak, R.L. (1990) 'The characteristics and mechanisms of visual disturbance associated with anticonvulsant therapy.' *Neurology,* **40,** 791–796.

Rollnick, B.R., Kaye, C.I., Nagatoshi, K., *et al.* (1987) 'Oculoauriculovertebral dysplasia and variants: phenotypic characteristics of 294 patients.' *American Journal of Medical Genetics,* **26,** 361–375.

Rosenberg, N.L. (1984) 'Hearing loss as an initial symptom of the opso-clonus–myoclonus syndrome.' *Archives of Neurology,* **41,** 998–999.

Rozencweig, M., Von Hoff, D.D., Slavik, M. (1977) 'As-diamine-dichloro-platinum (II). A new anticancer drug.' *Annals of Internal Medicine,* **86,** 803–810.

Sadé, J., Yaniv, E. (1984) 'Ménière's disease in infants.' *Acta Oto-laryngologica,* **97,** 33–37.

Samuelson, S., Zahn, J. (1990) 'Usher's syndrome.' *Ophthalmic Pediatric Genetics,* **11,** 71–76.

Slater, R. (1979) 'Benign recurrent vertigo.' *Journal of Neurology, Neurosurgery, and Psychiatry,* **42,** 363–367.

Snavely, S.R., Hodges, G.R. (1984) 'The neurotoxicity of antibacterial agents.' *Annals of Internal Medicine,* **101,** 92–104.

Sogg, R.L., Hoyt, W.F. (1962) 'Intermittent vertical nystagmus in father and son.' *Archives of Ophthalmology,* **68,** 515–517.

Starr, A., Picton, T.W., Sininger, Y., *et al.* (1996) 'Auditory neuropathy.' *Brain,* **119,** 741–753.

Steele, M.W. (1981) 'Genetics of congenital deafness.' *Pediatric Clinics of North America,* **28,** 973–980.

Stewart-Brown, S., Haslum, M.N. (1987) 'Screening for hearing loss in childhood: a study of national practice.' *British Medical Journal,* **294,** 1386–1388.

Stockard, J.E., Stockard, J.J., Kleinberg, F., Westmoreland, F. (1983) 'Prognostic value of brainstem auditory evoked potentials in neonates.' *Archives of Neurology,* **40,** 360–365.

Thiringer, K., Kankkunen, A., Liden, G., Niklasson, A. (1984) 'Perinatal risk factors in the aetiology of hearing loss in preschool children.' *Developmental Medicine and Child Neurology,* **26,** 799–807.

Thömke, F., Hopf, H.C. (1992) 'Unilateral vestibular paralysis as the sole manifestation of mumps.' *Journal of Neurology, Neurosurgery, and Psychiatry,* **55,** 858–859. *(Letter.)*

Tibbles, J.A.R., Camfield, P.R., Cron, C.C., Farrell, K. (1986) 'Dominant recurrent ataxia and vertigo of childhood.' *Pediatric Neurology,* **2,** 35–38.

Tusa, R.J., Saada, A.A., Niparko, J.K. (1994) 'Dizziness in childhood.' *Journal of Child Neurology,* **9,** 261–274.

Verhagen, W.I.M., Huygen, P.L.M. (1991) 'Familial progressive vestibulo-cochlear dysfunction.' *Archives of Neurology,* **48,** 262. *(Letter.)*

—— —— Horstink, M.W.I.M. (1987) 'Familial congenital vestibular areflexia.' *Journal of Neurology, Neurosurgery, and Psychiatry,* **50,** 933–935.

Vienny, H., Despland, P.A., Lütschg, J., *et al.* (1984) 'Early diagnosis and evolution of deafness in childhood bacterial meningitis: a study using brainstem auditory evoked potentials.' *Pediatrics,* **73,** 579–586.

Vies, J.S.H., Casaer, P., Kingma, H., *et al.* (1987) 'A longitudinal study of brainstem auditory evoked potentials in preterm infants.' *Developmental Medicine and Child Neurology,* **29,** 577–585.

Voit, T., Lamprecht, A., Lenard, H-G., Goebel, H.H. (1986) 'Hearing loss in facioscapulohumeral dystrophy.' *European Journal of Pediatrics,* **145,** 280–285.

Weil, D., Blanchard, S., Kaplan, J., *et al.* (1995) 'Defective myosin VIIA gene responsible for Usher syndrome type 1B.' *Nature,* **374,** 60–61.

Wildervanck, L.S. (1962) 'Hereditary malformations of the ear in three generations. Marginal pits, preauricular appendages, malformations of the auricle and conductive deafness.' *Acta Oto-laryngologica,* **54,** 553–560.

Wolfson, R.J., Leiberman, A. (1975) 'Unilateral deafness with subsequent vertigo.' *Laryngoscope,* **85,** 1762–1766.

Zeman, W. (1975) 'Dégénérescence systématisée optico-cochléo-dentelée.' *In:* Vinken, P.J., Bruyn, G.W. (Eds.) *Handbook of Clinical Neurology. Vol. 21. System Disorders and Atrophies, Part I.* Amsterdam: North Holland, pp. 535–551.

PART IX

NEUROMUSCULAR DISEASES

This part deals with disorders that involve the peripheral nervous and muscular systems from the spinal motor neuron to muscles via the peripheral nerves. The three chapters are devoted to diseases of the motor neuron (Chapter 20), diseases of the axons (or peripheral nerves, whether sensory, motor or sensorimotor) (Chapter 21), and diseases of muscles including motor endplate disorders (Chapter 22). Distinction between the different mechanisms may be difficult, especially in neonates and young infants as they all may result in a 'floppy infant' syndrome.

Moreover, affectation of the peripheral nervous system may be combined with involvement of the CNS in a fairly large number of neurological diseases. The most important are listed in Table 20.3 (p. 707).

Many disorders of childhood feature hypotonia that may be of a marked degree, without actually affecting the motor unit. In addition to CNS disorders such as cerebellar diseases or certain forms of atonic cerebral palsy with diffuse CNS involvement (see Chapter 8), hypotonia may be prominent in acute systemic illnesses, in chromosomal abnormalities such as Down syndrome or the Prader–Willi syndrome (Chapter 5) (Fig. IX.1), in acquired or congenital metabolic diseases, and in connective tissue diseases with musculoligamentous hyperextensibility.

Various types of the Ehlers–Danlos syndrome and congenital laxity of ligaments (arthrochalasis multiplex congenita) (Royce and Steinman 1993) can give rise to abnormalities of gait, which may be broad-based and waddling, and to other motor disturbances such as difficulties in rising unaided from a sitting position, which may suggest a neuromuscular disorder. An excessive range of joint mobility, unusual joint postures, the ability to do various contortions of the limbs and/or hyperelasticity of the skin are important diagnostic clues. Molecular diagnosis is possible for several of these disorders. Patients have normal creatine kinase levels and normal EMGs. Although the cause of these problems is obscure, it is important to be aware of their existence for genetic counselling and to avoid mistaken diagnosis of severe disorders.

Excessive musculoligamentous laxity can, in turn, result in neural damage. Moreira and Wilson (1992) have described non-progressive paraparesis, attributed to possible microtraumas of the spinal cord, and peripheral brachial plexus neuropathy has been reported in Ehlers–Danlos syndrome types 1 and 3 (Galan and Kousseff 1995). Some such children may present with abnormalities of gait, which may be broad-based and waddling, or with other motor disturbances such as difficulties in rising from a sitting position, which may suggest a neuromuscular disorder, especially congenital myopathy (Dubowitz 1995, and personal cases). Other complications of joint hypermobility may include muscle pain and various orthopaedic complications that may sometimes result in a misleading diagnosis of neuromuscular disease.

Muscle hypertrophy is much less common than wasting and hypotonia and may result from various neurological diseases (see below). Physiological hypertrophy may be generalized as a result of training or localized as with masseter hypertrophy. Total or partial lipodystrophy presents with muscular prominence due, at least in part, to loss of subcutaneous fat tissue. Various endocrine, cutaneous, genital and CNS abnormalities are often associated (Senior and Gellis 1964), and insulin-resistant diabetes and kidney disease are severe complications. The condition is probably recessively inherited, although dominant (Lloyd *et al.* 1993) and X-linked inheritance have been suspected.

Investigation of children with neuromuscular disorders often requires special techniques such as electromyography and measurement of motor and sensory conduction velocities, as well as muscle biopsy, which should always be studied by histochemical techniques and sometimes by electron microscopy. A specialized laboratory is increasingly required for full examination of biopsy specimens, and improper study of samples is often worse than no

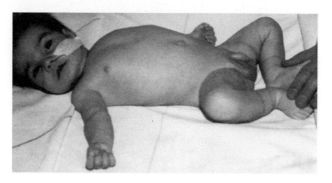

Fig. IX.1. Neonatal hypotonia of 'central' origin: Prader–Willi syndrome in a 5-month-old infant.

biopsy. The reader is referred to specalized texts (Dubowitz and Brooke 1973, Sarnat 1983).

Osteoarticular disorders may simulate neuromuscular disease. Wasting and at times weakness and reflex changes can result from chronic pain and reflex immobilization ('splinting') of adjoining segments. Such 'pseudoparalyses' are observed with slipped epiphyses, minimal fractures, osteomyelitis or congenital syphilis. Osteoid osteoma is a frequent cause in children and adolescents and may be especially difficult to diagnose in patients with gait disturbances, atrophy and diminished or absent reflexes which may affect one segment or a whole lower limb (Kiers *et al.* 1990). Pain, which is usually located over the lesion, may also

be referred or radicular in type and rarely associated with dermatomal sensory loss (Halperin *et al.* 1982).

Other osseous conditions such as polyepiphyseal dysplasia, osteomalacia and osteoporosis may also produce symptoms that simulate neuromuscular disease to the point that in some personally observed patients, muscular biopsy had been required or even performed.

REFERENCES

Dubowitz, V. (1995) *Muscle Disorders in Children.* Philadelphia: W.B. Saunders.
—— Brooke, M.H. (1973) *Muscle Biopsy: a Modern Approach.* Philadelphia: W.B. Saunders.
Galan, E., Kousseff, B.G. (1995) 'Peripheral neuropathy in Ehlers–Danlos syndrome.' *Pediatric Neurology,* **12,** 242–245.
Halperin, N., Gadoth, N., Reif, R., Axer, A. (1982) 'Osteoid osteoma of the proximal femur simulating spinal root compression.' *Clinical Orthopedics,* **162,** 191–194.
Kiers, L., Shield, L.K., Cole, W.G. (1990) 'Neurologic manifestations of osteoid osteoma.' *Archives of Disease in Childhood,* **65,** 851–855.
Lloyd, J., Mansell, P.I., Reckless, J.P.D. (1993) 'Subtotal lipodystrophy with autosomal dominant inheritance.' *Journal of the Royal Society of Medicine,* **86,** 477–478.
Moreira, A., Wilson, J. (1992) 'Non-progressive paraparesis in children with congenital ligamentous laxity.' *Neuropediatrics,* **23,** 49–52.
Royce, P.M., Steinmann, B. (1993) *Connective Tissue and its Heritable Disorders: Molecular, Genetic and Medical Aspects.* New York: Wiley–Liss.
Sarnat, H.B. (1983) *Muscle Pathology and Histochemistry.* Chicago: American Society of Clinical Pathologists.
Senior, B., Gellis, S.S. (1964) 'The syndromes of total lipodystrophy and of partial lipodystrophy.' *Pediatrics,* **33,** 593–612.

20
DISEASES OF THE MOTOR NEURON

Since the almost complete disappearance of acute anterior poliomyelitis in industrialized countries, chronic degenerative diseases account for most cases of anterior horn cell disease. In some developing countries, however, acute poliomyelitis remains a cause of involvement of the motor neurons of the spinal cord.

SPINAL MUSCULAR ATROPHY (SMA)

The spinal muscular atrophies constitute a heterogeneous group of disorders characterized by progressive degeneration of the anterior horn cells in the spinal cord and often of cells of the motor nuclei in the brainstem. Collectively, they represent the commonest degenerative disorder of the CNS and are the second most frequent lethal genetic disorder of childhood after mucoviscidosis. Most are genetic diseases with various modes of inheritance. Onset may be at any age from early infancy, or even the prenatal period, to adulthood. The mechanisms responsible for neuronal degeneration and death are unknown.

Involvement of the motor neurons may be diffuse or restricted to certain muscle groups. Most commonly, muscular weakness and wasting involve the proximal part of the limbs, but distal, scapulohumeral, facioscapulohumeral and segmental forms are known, and both the topography of involvement and mode of inheritance are important for the diagnosis.

Classification of the SMAs (Table 20.1) is difficult and several systems have been proposed, none of which is entirely satisfactory. Agreement has been reached regarding classification of the most common forms into three types. Type I, or Werdnig–Hoffmann disease, designates the easily recognizable early-onset acute form. The chronic forms are divided into type II, in which onset is later in the first year and the topography of weakness is diffuse with resulting deformities and severe disability, and the milder type III, also known as Kugelberg, Kugelberg–Welander or Wohlfart–Kugelberg disease, with mostly proximal involvement (Bundey and Lovelace 1975, Pearn 1980, Emery 1994). This classification has supplanted previous schemes (Hausmanowa-Petrusewicz et al. 1985). The classical SMAs fulfil the following criteria (Munsat and Davies 1992): symmetrical muscle weakness of trunk and limbs more marked proximally than distally and predominating in the lower limbs; presence of tongue fasciculations and/or of tremor of the hands; EMG and biopsy demonstrating neurogenic abnormalities. Conversely, criteria of exclusion are: sensory involvement, evidence of CNS dysfunction, extensive arthrogryposis, elevation of creatine kinase to more than 10 times the

maximum normal level, and reduction of nerve conduction velocity by more than 70 per cent. The three classical types have been shown to be linked to chromosome 5q13 markers (Melki et al. 1990a,b; Brzustowicz et al. 1990), and a gene at this locus, the *SMN* (survival motor neurons) gene, encoding a hitherto unknown protein of 294 amino acids has been identified (Lefebvre et al. 1995). Deletion of exon 7 of this gene is found in 85–95 per cent of all types of SMA (Rodrigues et al. 1996). Homozygous deletion of the *SMN* gene was found in 93 per cent and interruption of the gene in 5.6 per cent of SMA patients by Melki and Munnich (1996). In rare cases, the gene is neither lacking nor truncated, but a point mutation is present in exon 7, supporting the view that the *SMN* gene—and especially exon 7—is responsible for the SMA phenotype. However, the *SMN* gene is present in two copies (central and telomeric) and no function has yet been assigned to any of the normal or mutated copies, and rare normal carriers with homologous deletion of these genes have been identified (Cobben et al. 1995), so some uncertainties persist. DiDonato et al. (1997) have proposed that conversion (i.e. exchange of DNA sequences between central and telomeric *SMN* genes so that the telomeric locus now possesses nucleotides normally associated with the inactive central locus) is frequently the cause of types II and III SMA. Such conversion is indistinguishable from deletion of exon 7 with usual methods, and seems to be commonly associated with chronic, relatively benign SMAs, while true deletion causes type I. Some rarer forms of SMA are not linked to this gene or even to chromosome 5, but cases with associated congenital heart disease and some cases with arthrogryposis show the same deletion as the classical type (Bürglen et al. 1996, Melki and Munnich 1996).

ACUTE INFANTILE SPINAL MUSCULAR ATROPHY, WERDNIG–HOFFMANN DISEASE, SMA TYPE I
The incidence of SMA type I is 1 per 20,000 live births, and the gene carrier frequency is 1 in 60–80 (Pearn et al. 1978b, 1980). It is associated with a deletion of exon 7 of the *SMN* gene in over 95 per cent of cases. A deletion in the *NAIP* (neuronal apoptosis inhibitory protein) gene is also found in 50–60 per cent of cases of SMA type I (Rodrigues et al. 1996), and large deletions of the 5q13 region seem to be correlated with the severe type of SMA. However, 27 per cent of SMA type I cases have only a deletion of the *SMN* gene. Deletions in exon 3 have been found in some patients without exon 7 deletion (Cobben et al. 1995), resulting in a frameshift and a premature stop codon.

TABLE 20.1
Classification of the spinal muscular atrophies (SMAs)

Type	Principal synonyms*	Genetics†
SMA type I	Werdnig–Hoffmann disease; acute infantile SMA; amyotonia congenita	AR
Chronic SMA		
Type II	Arrested Werdnig–Hoffmann disease; chronic generalized SMA; intermediate form of SMA	AR
Type III	Kugelberg disease; Kugelberg–Welander disease; Wohlfart–Kugelberg disease	AR
Others (Pearn 1978b)		AD? Phenocopies?
Distal SMA	Progressive SMA (Charcot–Marie–Tooth type)	AR or AD
Neurogenic scapuloperoneal syndrome		AD, AR, XR
Neurogenic facioscapulohumeral syndrome		AD
Adolescent SMA with hypertrophy of calves (Pearn and Hudgson 1978)		XR AD (rare: d'Alessandro et al. 1982)
Infantile and childhood SMA with cerebellar atrophy	Norman disease; amyotrophic cerebellar hypoplasia	AR?
Adult SMA	SMA type IV	AD or AR
	Kennedy disease	XR

*Some of these terms may not designate the same entity but have been used as synonyms in several studies.
†AR = autosomal recessive, AD = autosomal dominant, XR = X-linked recessive.

PATHOLOGY

Pathologically there is conspicuous loss of anterior horn cells. Residual motor neurons are in the process of degenerating with chromatolysis and eventual phagocytosis by satellite cells. Neurons in the cervical cord may be strikingly preserved (Kuzuhara and Chou 1981). Glial bundles have been observed in the anterior roots (Chou and Nonaka 1978) and in the posterior roots, which are also shrunken (Probst *et al.* 1981). The significance of this finding remains obscure. Evidence of peripheral nerve involvement with loss of large myelinated axons (Chien and Nonaka 1989) is consistent with wallerian degeneration rather than indicating a dying-back process. Supraspinal lesions are regularly present in the motor nuclei of the brainstem, notably in the hypoglossal nucleus, nucleus ambiguus and facial nucleus. Thalamic involvement is also a common feature (Oppenheimer 1976).

CLINICAL FEATURES

The clinical manifestations of the disease are characteristic, permitting an almost immediate diagnosis except at the very onset. In about 30 per cent of cases, the disorder has a prenatal onset and the infant is born with proximal weakness of the limbs and areflexia. The weakness spreads rapidly and, within a few weeks, there is marked quadriplegia with some preservation of distal movements, especially in the upper limbs. The paralysis is symmetrical and also involves axial muscles especially of the neck (Gamstorp 1967).

Paralysis of the intercostal muscle is a key feature of the condition. It produces a characteristic deformity of the thorax that is flattened laterally and remains immobile or paradoxically decreases in circumference during inspiratory movements, whereas the abdomen bulges, in a see-saw manner. Respiratory motions are performed almost exclusively by the diaphragm which is spared until the late stages of the disease. Retrognathism, sometimes associated with fasciculations of the chin muscles, is constant and, together with preserved eye movements and vivid look, completes the characteristic appearance of the patients (Fig. 20.1).

Deep tendon reflexes are abolished. Tongue fasciculations are often present but may be difficult to distinguish from the frequent tremulous tongue movements of normal infants. There is no sensory loss, no pyramidal tract signs and no sphincter disturbances. Intelligence is preserved and the infants are usually described as very attractive.

The disorder in most cases is rapidly progressive, especially in prenatal forms and in acute cases of early onset. Death occurs within the first 18 months of life in 95 per cent of cases and results from respiratory insufficiency, often precipitated and aggravated by intercurrent respiratory infections. Many infants have swallowing difficulties necessitating tube feeding. Patients with disease of neonatal onset often die before 3 months of age. Recent reports (Russman *et al.* 1992, Iannacone *et al.* 1993) indicate a less gloomy outlook with much higher survival rates and better function. However, selection of cases was not excluded and the prognosis of acute infantile SMA remains quite poor.

DIAGNOSIS

The diagnosis of SMA I can be confirmed by EMG examination which shows neurogenic tracings with a reduced pattern of

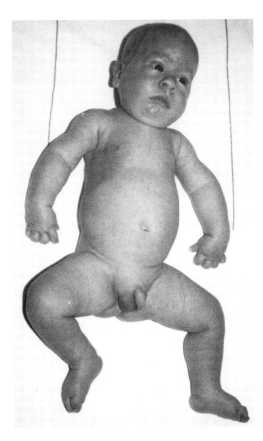

Fig. 20.1. Werdnig–Hoffmann disease (spinal muscular atrophy type I). Note narrow chest due to paralysis of intercostal mucles, flexion position of fingers, retrognathism and alert look.

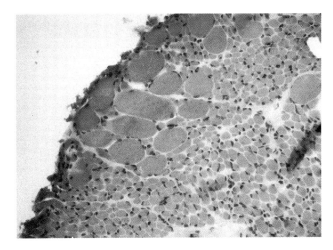

Fig. 20.2. Werdnig–Hoffmann disease. Muscle biopsy specimen showing fascicular atrophy typical of anterior horn cell involvement. Note that atrophic fibres keep a rounded contour which is unusual in spinal muscular atrophy of later onset in which angular atrophic fibres are the rule. (Courtesy Dr M.C. Routon, Hôpital Saint Vincent de Paul, Paris.)

activity during maximal effort, increased duration and amplitude of individual motor unit potentials, and increased incidence of polyphasic potentials. Spontaneous activity, in the form of rhythmical firing of motor units, is present in 69 per cent of cases, and fibrillation and positive sharp waves are found in 35 per cent (Hausmanowa-Petrusewicz and Karwanska 1986), but fasciculations are rarely visible in small infants. Polyphasic potentials are common and probably result from the presence in muscles of numerous groups of small fibres without any sign of reinnervation and of the less tightly packed fibres within the motor unit. Motor nerve conduction velocities are normal or slightly slowed in most patients, but more marked reduction may be observed, especially in severely affected patients (Moosa and Dubowitz 1976, Imai *et al.* 1990).

Serum creatine kinase is usually normal, although it may be mildly elevated in infants with a rapidly progressive form.

Muscle biopsy shows fascicles of small rounded fibres that belong to both types I and II. Hypertrophic fibres are scattered among atrophic fascicles and belong to type I. The normal checkerboard pattern is replaced by type grouping in which large numbers of fibres of the same type are contiguously arranged (Fig. 20.2).

It is this writer's opinion that muscle biopsy is *not* necessary for the diagnosis of SMA when clinical and EMG data are characteristic. Indeed, biopsy may be difficult to interpret in early cases or due to sampling problems, at a time when clinical and EMG diagnosis does not raise any difficulty when interpreted in the light of clinical evidence. Diagnostic tests based on DNA analysis are now available and are discussed below.

The *differential diagnosis* of SMA type I is usually easy even though there are many causes of hypotonia in infancy (Table 20.2). Congenital myopathies and congenital muscular dystrophies may present in a similar manner with absent tendon reflexes. Respiratory involvement is different in such cases, with antero-posterior flattening of the chest as opposed to lateral compression in SMA. Facial affectation is usually present, and a neurogenic EMG pattern is not observed. Creatine kinase levels are raised. Myasthenia gravis should always be considered because it is a treatable condition but the clinical picture is different with predominant facial and ocular involvement in most cases. Transection of the spinal cord and congenital spinal tumours occasionally produce superficially similar features, especially with regard to respiratory muscle involvement and thoracic deformity. Systematic exploration of sensation in the lower part of the body and search for minor pyramidal tract signs are therefore important. Infantile type 2 glycogenosis (Pompe disease) which produces a similar extensive muscle involvement is invariably associated with cardiac affectation and often with CNS signs. Rare cases of congenital or early neuropathy are on record (Goebel *et al.* 1976). Such patients have marked reduction of nerve conduction velocity and may have evidence of sensory impairment. The CSF may contain excess protein (Chapter 21). A rare mitochondrial disease with cytochrome *c* deficiency produces severe hypotonia with respiratory failure in the neonatal period. Renal tubular symptoms and CNS anomalies may be associated (DiMauro *et al.* 1985). An exceptional form of this disease is due to transient deficiency of cytochrome *c* and recovers with delayed maturation of the enzyme (Zeviani *et al.* 1987).

No effective treatment is available. Vigorous treatment of

TABLE 20.2
Main causes of hypotonia in infants and young children*

Hypotonia with paralysis
  Hereditary spinal muscular atrophies
    Werdnig–Hoffmann disease (type I)
    Chronic forms (types II and III)
  Congenital structural myopathies (Chapters 9, 22)
  Metabolic myopathies
    Glycogenosis types II, III, IV
    Mitochondrial myopathies
  Other neuromuscular disorders
    Congenital myotonic dystrophy
    Congenital muscular dystrophy
    Congenital and neonatal myasthenia (may last up to 1 year)
    Congenital neuropathies
    Disorders with combined CNS and PNS involvement
      Carbohydrate-deficient glycoprotein syndrome type 1
      Neuroaxonal dystrophy
      Mitochondrial diseases, Leigh syndrome[1]

Hypotonia without paralysis
  CNS disorders
    Hypotonic cerebral palsy, especially the early stages of dystonic and ataxic cerebral palsy (cerebellar involvement)
  Metabolic disorders
    Aminoacidurias, organic acidurias, lactic acidosis, mitochondrial diseases, Leigh syndrome[1]
    Lowe syndrome[2]
    Degenerative diseases, *e.g.* leukodystrophies[2]
    Glycogen storage disorders
  Chromosomal disorders
    Down syndrome
    Prader–Willi syndrome
  Nutritional and endocrine disorders
    Rickets, hypothyroidism, renal tubular acidosis
    Malnutrition, kwashiorkor[2]
  Connective tissue disorders
    Ehlers–Danlos syndrome
    Congenital laxity of ligaments (arthrochalasis multiplex congenita)
    Marfan syndrome
    Osteogenesis imperfecta
    Mucopolysaccharidoses
  Benign congenital
    Dissociated motor development (hypotonia and delayed walking contrasting with normal fine motor development—Hagberg and Lundberg 1969), with or without 'shuffling'

*Partially adapted from Dubowitz (1995).
[1]Cases with and without paralysis can occur.
[2]In some cases there is involvement of muscles or nerves.

respiratory infections is indicated. The intensity of therapy and especially the indication for long-term mechanical ventilation are extremely difficult to determine (Gilgoff *et al.* 1989, Gordon 1991). In my opinion the latter is not indicated.

ATYPICAL FORMS AND THE LIMITS OF WERDNIG–HOFFMANN DISEASE

Atypical forms of SMA of early onset and unfavourable course are on record.

A few patients have had *initial diaphragmatic involvement* with neonatal onset (Schapira and Swash 1985) or onset before age 5 months (Mellins *et al.* 1974). Weakness and wasting leading to early death developed later. Such cases probably differ from classical type I SMA in which diaphragmatic involvement is a late event despite the typical features of anterior horn cell disease (McWilliam *et al.* 1985) and are not associated with exon 7 deletion in the *SMN* gene (Rudnik-Schöneborn *et al.* 1996).

In a few families, a severe form of congenital SMA, often with arthrogryposis, has occurred *in association with pontocerebellar hypoplasia* (Norman and Kay 1973, Weinberg and Kirkpatrick 1975). Such patients also have mental retardation and evidence of peripheral nerve involvement with markedly slowed motor conduction velocities (Goutières *et al.* 1977, Kamoshita *et al.* 1990). This condition features evidence of both spinocerebellar degeneration and malformation in the form of cerebellar hypoplasia and has also been termed infantile neuronal degeneration (Steinman *et al.* 1980), amyotrophic cerebellar hypoplasia (De Léon *et al.* 1984), Norman disease (Kamoshita 1990) and pontocerebellar hypoplasia type 1 (Barth 1993). It is not linked to chromosome 5.

SMA with arthrogryposis and multiple bone fractures (Lunt *et al.* 1992) is often rapidly lethal and like the previous two disorders is not related to a deletion in the *SMN* gene (Rudnik-Schöneborn *et al.* 1996), although Bürglen *et al.* (1996) demonstrated deletion of exon 7 in six of 12 infants with SMA with arthrogryposis.

Several cases of SMA initially limited to, or clearly *predominating in the cervical muscles* (Fig. 20.3) may also be distinct from classical Werdnig–Hoffmann disease (Goutières *et al.* 1991). Affected children may be able to walk. Secondary diffusion occurs in a descending manner with intercostal muscle paralysis eventually leading to respiratory failure and death. No DNA study is available.

Acute-onset forms following intercurrent infections have been reported (Robb et al 1991).

Progressive SMA with ophthalmoplegia and pyramidal symptoms has been observed in two siblings (Hamano *et al.* 1994). Similar cases with involvement of motor and sensory nerves and a rapidly lethal course have been shown to be associated with large deletions involving the *SMN* gene and several flanking markers (Korinthenberg *et al.* 1997).

Such atypical forms have bred true in several families, indicating that SMA is probably not a homogeneous group.

CHRONIC SMA TYPE II, ARRESTED WERDNIG–HOFFMANN DISEASE

Type II SMA is also inherited as an autosomal recessive character in at least 90 per cent of cases. According to the English SMA study, the gene carrier frequency is 1 in 76–111 for the chronic forms (Pearn 1978b, 1980). The different expression of the acute and chronic forms in which a similar DNA abnormality is present is as yet not understood. However, deletion of the *NAIP* gene has not been found in SMA types II and III, and large-scale deletions of the 5q13 region are suggestive of Werdnig–Hoffmann disease (Burlet *et al.* 1996, Wang *et al.* 1997). Conversion involving centromeric and telomeric *SMN* genes (see above) may be a common mechanism in these cases.

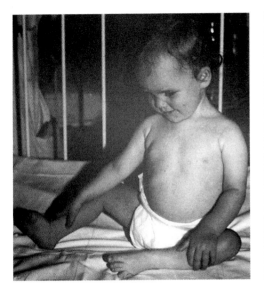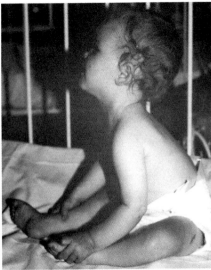

Fig. 20.3. Spinal muscular atrophy with cervical predominance. *(Left)* Head in forward flexion, the patient being unable to keep it erect. *(Right)* After being pulled back, the head cannot be put back to the forward position. (14-month-old girl with complete paralysis of both anterior and posterior cervical muscles with preservation of normal strength in lower limbs but some weakness and wasting of upper limbs.)

Type II SMA has its onset after 3 months of age, although the exact date of the first manifestations is difficult to determine (Pearn and Wilson 1973; Pearn 1978a,b) and may overlap with that of the acute form. Rare cases of occurrence of both type I and type II cases in the same pedigree are on record, but, much more frequently, this is only apparent and results from slow course of a few type I cases. The onset is generally insidious, the infant initially developing normally and attaining the first motor milestones up to the sitting position. Acquisition of standing posture does not develop, and even the sitting position is often abnormal with excessive curvature of the back. In some cases, onset is earlier with failure to reach more than head control. Conversely, in a few patients there is fairly rapid onset of weakness in the legs with loss of previous mobility. Eventually, weakness and atrophy are widespread although some predominance in muscles of the pelvic girdle may persist.

The course is initially one of slowly progressive weakness and wasting. Stabilization is common after one to two years but there is no improvement and late resumption of progression is rare. Deep tendon reflexes are abolished, except occasionally the distal reflexes. Fasciculations are often visible. Swallowing usually remains normal. Involvement of intercostal muscles is present in about half the cases and, in such instances, develops before the age of 3 years. During childhood, contractures tend to develop and major deformities are extremely common (Fig. 20.4). These include hip dislocation and kyphoscoliosis that favours the development of respiratory complications (Merlini *et al.* 1989). Such complications may in turn precipitate neurological decompensation. Even with the best prevention of orthopaedic deformities, ambulation is never achieved when onset is before 2 years. Patients may survive only to age 18 months or live into adulthood; mean age at death is 30 years (Pearn *et al.* 1978).

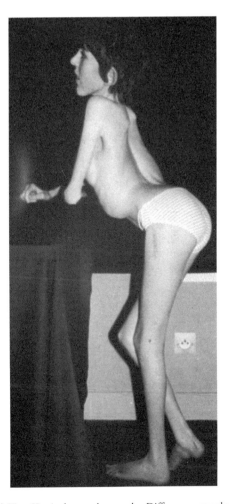

Fig. 20.4. Type II spinal muscular atrophy. Diffuse amyotrophy of limbs and marked kyphoscoliosis in 14-year-old girl. (Courtesy Dr J-P. Padovani, Hôpital des Enfants Malades, Paris.)

703

The pathological and EMG features are similar to those of type I SMA. However, electrical fasciculation is often observed and pseudomyotonic discharges may be seen (Hausmanowa-Petrusewicz and Karwanska 1986). Motor nerve conduction velocities are mildly decreased, especially in the distal portions of nerves (Imai *et al.* 1990).

The *management* of patients with type II SMA poses numerous problems. Physiotherapy, prevention of deformities and attempts at verticalization are of utmost importance. Physiotherapy aims at maintaining articular motility and at preventing muscle retractions and consequent deformities. Orthoses can be used early for the same purpose. Prevention of scoliosis is especially important (Shapiro and Bresnan 1982, Barois *et al.* 1989) whether by orthopaedic or surgical intervention (Aprin *et al.* 1982).

Assisted night-time ventilation by facial mask or buccal canula may be necessary for patients with intercostal muscle involvement. It should be started early enough to promote pulmonary growth and to maintain elasticity of the thorax (Duval-Baupère *et al.* 1985). Long-term mechanical ventilation raises a number of ethical and practical problems (Gilgoff *et al.* 1989).

Integration of affected children into normal schools can be realized through the use of especially adapted school material and electric wheelchairs. Orientation of these normally intelligent patients toward activities that they will be able to perform, such as mathematics and writing, is essential. Active psychological support of the patients and families should be provided.

CHRONIC SMA TYPE III (KUGELBERG DISEASE, KUGELBERG–WELANDER DISEASE, PSEUDOMYOPATHIC SMA, WOHLFART–KUGELBERG DISEASE)

This form is also transmitted as an autosomal recessive trait although sporadic cases are not uncommon. It is also associated, in most cases, with a deletion in the *SMN* gene. The onset of the disease may be at any age between infancy and early childhood and is extremely insidious. The parents may first notice the small volume of the child's thigh muscles or that s/he has difficulty rising from the floor. Weakness and amyotrophy clearly predominate on the proximal segment of the lower limbs and may involve electively the quadriceps. Examination shows a positive Gowers manoeuvre, wasting of proximal muscles and absent knee jerks with preservation of ankle jerks and of reflexes of the upper limbs. The picture thus bears a close clinical resemblance to the muscular dystrophies (Hausmanowa-Petrusewicz *et al.* 1979) with a waddling gait. Calf hypertrophy may be present in some patients, completing the resemblance to Duchenne dystrophy (Pearn and Hudgson 1978, Bouwsma and Van Wijngaarden 1980). The disease progresses very slowly towards either the distal lower limbs or the proximal upper limbs or both. Pes cavus is frequent. Many patients show a coarse tremor of the hands (Moosa and Dubowitz 1973, Dawood and Moosa 1983) that is probably related to imperfect synchronization of a diminished number of large motor units resulting from collateral

reinnervation of fibres by remaining neurons. The ECG shows tremulousness of the baseline, presumably reflecting the same muscular tremor. Most affected individuals can continue to lead normal lives into adulthood but some cases run a faster course; orthopaedic complications can produce severe limitations which should be avoided by appropriate physiotherapy and/or orthopaedic management. In rare cases, congenital (Pachter *et al.* 1976, Oka *et al.* 1995) or progresssive (Alberfeld and Namba 1969) ophthalmoplegia is associated.

Distinguishing type III SMA from muscular dystrophy may be difficult as the clinical picture may be suggestive and the creatine kinase level may be moderately elevated. Muscle biopsy is sometimes difficult to interpret, as 'myopathic' changes such as split or necrotic fibres, central nuclei and some increase in fibrous and fatty tissue may be observed. EMG is the best examination and is sufficient for the diagnosis in this writer's experience. In addition to myogenic diseases, differential diagnosis also includes rare diseases such as 'adult-type' gangliosidosis that may present with isolated anterior horn cell involvement (Navon *et al.* 1995) and exceptional cases of intramedullary tumours presenting as isolated SMA (Aysun *et al.* 1993).

DIAGNOSIS BY MOLECULAR GENETICS OF THE RECESSIVE PROXIMAL SMAs
Diagnosis of the three classical types of SMA by molecular genetics is possible, mostly by demonstration of homozygous deletion of exon 7 in the distal copy of the *SMN* gene (Melki *et al.* 1994). However, a deletion is not present in a variable but small proportion of patients with SMA; rare persons with homozygous deletion may be phenotypically unaffected, and the relationship of the *SMN* gene to SMA has not been fully worked out. Several atypical forms (*e.g.* SMA with olivopontocerebellar atrophy, diaphragmatic form) are not associated with a deletion or linked to chromosome 5 (Lunt *et al.* 1992, Novelli *et al.* 1995, Rudnick-Schöneborn *et al.* 1995). Conversely, a number of cases in which one or several of the accepted exclusion criteria (Munsat and Davies 1992) are present may show a typical deletion, including cases with CNS dysfunction, arthrogryposis or associated malformations (Rudnik-Schöneborn *et al.* 1996). DNA analysis makes prenatal diagnosis of most types of classical SMA possible and reliable (Cobben *et al.* 1993, Wirth *et al.* 1995). A DNA test using polymerase chain reaction is available (Van der Steege *et al.* 1995). The basis of this test is homozygous deletion of exon 7 of the *SMN* gene. It is relatively easy to perform but may be negative in around 2 per cent of affected children who harbour a different DNA defect (Raymond *et al.* 1997).

OTHER TYPES OF SMA
DOMINANT DIFFUSE (OR PROXIMAL) FORMS OF CHRONIC SMA
Dominant forms of chronic SMA are uncommon in childhood (Emery *et al.* 1976a,b; Pearn 1978a,b; Boylan and Cornblath 1992). These forms usually have a slowly progressive course. They represent less than 2 per cent of childhood cases but up to 30 per cent of adult cases (Pearn 1978a) and are also known

in adults as type IV SMA (Dyck 1984). There may be two distinct genes: early-onset forms begin between birth and 8 years of age and do not have a marked selectivity for proximal muscles; late-onset forms are seen in young adults and have a marked proximal selectivity. Some other cases of chronic SMA may represent non-genetic phenocopies or new dominant mutations (Pearn 1980).

SEX-LINKED SMA

Rare cases of sex-linked SMA are on record in adults (Paulson *et al.* 1980) and in children (Skre *et al.* 1978). In the kindred reported by Skre and coworkers, some patients had a pattern of diffuse involvement and others a scapuloperoneal pattern. These X-linked forms may be different from the proximal form of adult proximal neuronopathy, or *Kennedy disease* (Guidetti *et al.* 1986), which features bulbar muscle involvement, gynaecomastia and frequent asymmetry of involvement in addition to proximal SMA. The gene is located on the proximal long arm of chromosome X (Fishbeck *et al.* 1986) and includes a CAG repeat whose expansion is associated with the clinical disease. The gene codes for cell surface androgen receptor (Doyu *et al.* 1992).

DISTAL SMA

This form presents with features similar to those of the peroneal muscle atrophies. In the large series of Harding and Thomas (1980) it accounted for 13 per cent of 262 cases. Several genes are probably implicated but there is no linkage to chromosome 5. Dominant inheritance was predominant, but recessive forms are also known (Meadows and Marsden 1969a, Emery 1971, Harding and Thomas 1980) and sporadic cases are frequent. There is a marked excess of males especially in mild forms, suggesting an X-linked inheritance in some families. The disease is difficult to distinguish from the neural peroneal atrophies, especially as these may not show any sign of sensory impairment at onset. Criteria for diagnosis should therefore include: (1) distal muscular atrophy usually predominant in the lower limbs; (2) absence of sensory anomalies; (3) concordant EMG and pathological evidence of anterior horn cell affectation; (4) a period of at least 18 months free of sensory signs (Harding and Thomas 1980). Pes cavus, often severe, is a common presenting sign. Ankle jerks and upper-limb tendon reflexes are often preserved in contrast to what is seen in Charcot–Marie–Tooth disease. Age of onset varies from infancy to middle life. The course is usually slow but progressive, patients needing calipers or other walking aids by 25–30 years of age, although many are only moderately disabled in adulthood. In rare forms, the upper extremities are affected first and predominantly, with a slow course (Lander *et al.* 1976, O'Sullivan and McLeod 1978). These forms seem to be dominantly inherited or sporadic. An association with optico-acoustic atrophy has been reported (Chalmers and Mitchell 1987). A previously described association of distal SMA with vocal cord paralysis (Young and Harper 1980, Boltshauser *et al.* 1989) has recently been shown to be due to a neuropathy rather than to anterior horn cell disease (Dyck *et al.* 1994). Bertini *et al.* (1989) reported the association of a distal SMA with diaphragmatic paralysis.

SCAPULOPERONEAL SMA

The scapuloperoneal syndrome, characterized by wasting and weakness in the shoulder girdle and anterior muscles of the leg, can be due to myopathic, neural or anterior horn cell involvement (Kaeser 1965). The latter type is the most common (Mercelis *et al.* 1980). It is usually inherited as an autosomal dominant trait (Meadows and Marsden 1969b), but recessive inheritance and X-linked transmission (Thomas *et al.* 1972) may occur. Some investigators (*e.g.* Dubowitz 1995) have expressed doubts about the reality of SMA as a cause of scapuloperoneal syndrome.

Facioscapuloperoneal SMA is a rare type (Fenichel *et al.* 1967) that simulates the more common facioscapulohumeral muscular dystrophy. The genetic transmission is autosomal dominant. Onset is by facial diplegia with progressive downward extension of weakness (Furukawa and Toyokura 1976). In one child, optic atrophy and sensory and autonomic disturbances were associated (Schmitt *et al.* 1994).

BENIGN FAMILIAL SMA WITH HYPERTROPHY OF THE CALVES

Hypertrophy of the calves may be relatively common in chronic SMAs (Bertorini and Igarashi 1985). Bouwsma and Van Wijngaarten (1980) found it in 29 of 100 patients. All were males, suggesting that an X-linked factor might be at play. D'Alessandro *et al.* (1982) described a dominant form in a father and son.

UNCONVENTIONAL PATTERNS OF SMA

MONOMELIC OR ASYMMETRICAL SMA

A monomelic or clearly asymmetrical form of progressive SMA has been reported, originally from Japan where the condition seems to be prevalent (Hirayama *et al.* 1987) but also in other countries (De Visser *et al.* 1988, Peiris *et al.* 1989, Tandan *et al.* 1990, Liu and Specht 1993). The disease predominantly affects males, and clinical features of the condition include a juvenile onset, between 15 and 25 years, of an insidiously progressive muscular atrophy not precipitated by any infection or trauma. The atrophy does not involve the brachioradialis muscle and is associated with weakness exaggerated by cold and with fine irregular tremor. Both sides may be involved, almost always in a very asymmetrical manner. Denervation changes are shown by EMG and muscle biopsy. There is no sensory impairment and conduction velocities are normal. The disorder is usually sporadic but a few familial cases are known (Tandan *et al.* 1990). Pathological lesions (Hirayama *et al.* 1987) include shrinkage and necrosis of large and small motor nerve cells. The aetiology is unknown. A traumatic origin is suspected (Toma and Shiozawa 1995).

COMPLEX PATTERNS OF SMA

Juvenile motor neuron disease is common in southern India. The best defined type is known as Madras type (Jagganathan 1973). The disease predominates in males and its onset is during the second decade of life. The upper limbs are initially and preferentially affected although the lower limbs eventually become involved. Deafness is present in one-third of the patients

(Gourie-Devi and Suresh 1988). The disease is slowly progressive and not uncommonly becomes arrested.

BULBAR AND BULBOPONTINE TYPES OF NEUROGENIC MUSCULAR ATROPHY

CHILDHOOD AND JUVENILE PROGRESSIVE BULBAR PALSY; BULBAR HEREDITARY NEUROPATHY TYPE 2 (BHN2)

Progressive bulbar palsy is a form of motor neuron disease with predominant involvement of bulbar muscles, although muscles innervated by pontine, spinal and, occasionally, midbrain motor neurons may also be involved.

Only those cases with 'pure' involvement of brainstem nuclei are considered here. Some cases that feature both bulbar paralysis and extensive involvement of limb and trunk muscles are difficult to differentiate from the SMAs. Cases with definite involvement of the long tracts, especially the corticospinal tracts, can be regarded as a form of lateral amyotrophic sclerosis and are studied later in this chapter. The mere presence of some pyramidal tract signs may not be sufficient for exclusion from the syndrome. The eponym Fazio–Londe disease is often applied to the childhood form. Age of onset may be variable within the same kindred (Dobkin and Verity 1976, Albers *et al.* 1983). Typically the disease begins between 2 and 12 years by nasal speech, stridor and often repeated respiratory infections. Dysphagia, facial diplegia and sometimes oculomotor paralyses progressively develop and may lead to death in around 18 months to 10 years (Della Giustina *et al.* 1979, Beauvais *et al.* 1988). Involvement of the spinal musculature is variable (Dobkin and Verity 1976). McShane *et al.* (1992) reported five cases and distinguished three different forms: a dominant type is exceptional; recessive forms can present with early onset before 2 years of age, stridor and respiratory difficulties resulting from vocal cord paralysis, involvement of the lower cranial pairs, the facial nerve and, sometimes, the oculomotor nuclei, and are often lethal in two to three years. A more benign and protracted form features dysarthria, dysphagia and facial weakness rather than respiratory symptoms and may be seen even in adults. There is a strong concordance of each pattern within the same family. Pathologically, there is marked degeneration of the cranial motor nuclei with variable involvement of motor neurons in the spinal cord. Cases of childhood and juvenile progressive bulbar palsy are either dominantly or recessively inherited (Dobkin and Verity 1976, Beauvais *et al.* 1988). Recessively inherited forms are not necessarily severe (Beauvais *et al.* 1988). This disorder should be differentiated from other lesions of the brainstem such as myasthenia gravis, tumours or encephalitis, from Miller Fisher syndrome, and from the rare cases of congenital oculobulbar palsy (Jennekens *et al.* 1992) that may be related to congenital myasthenia.

BROWN–VIALETTO–VAN LAERE SYNDROME (BULBAR HEREDITARY NEUROPATHY TYPE 1)

Juvenile-onset bulbospinal muscular atrophy also occurs in association with deafness (Brown–Vialetto–Van Laere syndrome). In this rare syndrome, bilateral neural deafness first appears in late childhood or adolescence. Vestibular areflexia is associated.

Subsequently, involvement of several cranial nerves appears, causing facial diplegia, dysarthria and dysphagia. Optic atrophy is occasionally observed as well as mild cerebellar and pyramidal signs (Brucher *et al.* 1981). The course of the disease is slow and some patients may survive to their fourth decade but respiratory insufficiency and swallowing difficulties develop and lead to death (Gallai *et al.* 1981, Summers *et al.* 1987). Degenerative lesions of the first and second neurons of the auditory and vestibular pathways are evident along with gliosis of the vestibular and cochlear nuclei and superior olives. The condition is apparently inherited as an autosomal recessive trait.

ASSOCIATED OR COMPLICATED SMAs

SMA occurs in association with involvement of CNS structures in several rare multisystem disorders.

JUVENILE AMYOTROPHIC LATERAL SCLEROSIS

Rare cases of typical amyotrophic lateral sclerosis occur before adulthood (Nelson and Prensky 1972, Beauvais *et al.* 1990).

Most of the juvenile cases of associated bilateral pyramidal tract signs with amyotrophy of the limbs and fasciculations that have been reported as juvenile amyotrophic lateral sclerosis are chronic and often familial diseases. Ben Hamida *et al.* (1990) separated three subgroups. One consists of upper-limb and sometimes also bulbar amyotrophy, with bilateral pyramidal tract involvement, and closely resembles adult amyotrophic lateral sclerosis but with a benign, slow course and a common genetic (autosomal recessive) origin. A second group includes spastic paraplegia associated with peroneal atrophy and can be regarded also as a form of spastic paraplegia (Chapter 10). The third group is composed of patients with spastic pseudobulbar syndrome with spastic paraplegia and may also be thought of as a form of spastic paraplegia with pseudobulbar involvement (Chapter 10). In some such cases, intraneuronal inclusions have been found (Nelson and Prensky 1972, Yokochi *et al.* 1989). Linkage to chromosome 2q33–q35 has been reported (Hentati *et al.* 1994).

A familial degenerative disease of the anterior horn cells and pyramidal tracts, often in association with parkinsonism and dementia is seen among the Chamorro tribe on the island of Guam (Mulder 1981).

SMA may also occur in association with familial spastic paraplegia (Ben Hamida *et al.* 1990). Associated involvement of the posterior columns of the spinal cord has also been observed (Engel *et al.* 1959), and more complex cases including pyramidal, spinocerebellar and thalamic involvement are known (Grunnet and Donaldson 1985).

PRIMARY LATERAL SCLEROSIS

This condition is exceptional in children (Grunnett *et al.* 1989). Familial cases associated with a pseudobulbar syndrome and gaze paresis have been reported by Gascon *et al.* (1995).

ANDERMANN SYNDROME

A syndrome featuring agenesis of the corpus callosum, anterior horn cell disease, a mixed sensory and motor neuropathy, and

TABLE 20.3
Disorders with associated peripheral and CNS involvement

Disease	References
With predominant involvement of spinal cord, especially anterior horn cells	
Infantile neuroaxonal dystrophy	Chapter 10
Hexosaminidase A deficiency (chronic and juvenile types)	Chapter 9
Neuronal inclusion disease	Chapter 10
Andermann syndrome (callosal agenesis and neuronopathy)	Chapters 3, 10
Amyotrophic cerebellar hypoplasia (pontocerebellar hypoplasia with anterior horn cell disease, Norman disease)	De Leon *et al.* (1984)
Acute anterior poliomyelitis	Chapter 11
Mycoplasma pneumoniae infection	Francis *et al.* (1988)
Triose-phosphate isomerase deficiency	Poll-Thé *et al.* (1985)
Rett syndrome	Oldfors *et al.* (1988)
Sea-blue histiocytosis	Ashwal *et al.* (1984)
With predominant involvement of nerves	
Leukodystrophies	Chapters 9, 10
Metachromatic	
Krabbe	
Cockayne	
Spinocerebellar degenerations	Chapter 10
Friedreich ataxia	
Behr syndrome	
Ataxia with retained deep tendon reflexes (especially Troyer syndrome, Charlevoix–Saguenay ataxia)	
Azorean disease (Machado–Joseph disease)	
Spastic paraplegia with neuropathy	
Metabolic and degenerative diseases	
Adrenomyeloneuropathy	Chapter 9
Bassen–Korzweig disease (abetalipoproteinaemia)	Chapters 9, 21
Vitamin E malabsorption (isolated or associated with hepatic disease)	Chapter 21
Giant axonal neuropathy	Chapter 21
Leigh disease	Jacobs *et al.* (1990)
Refsum disease	Chapters 9, 21
Carbohydrate-deficient glycoprotein syndrome, type 1	Stibler and Jaeken (1990)
Cerebrotendinous xanthomatosis	Chapter 9
Sialosidosis 1	Steinman *et al.* (1980)
B-mannosidosis	Kleijer *et al.* (1990)
Mitochondrial cytopathy, especially NARP and MELAS	Chapter 9
Lowe syndrome	Charnas *et al.* (1988)
Ataxia–telangectasia	Kwast and Ignatowicz (1990)
Sea-blue histiocytosis	Ashwal *et al.* (1984)
Chronic intestinal obstruction, neuropathy and leukoencephalopathy	Chapter 21
Malnutrition, folate deficiency	Chopra and Sharma (1992)
Short- and long-chain hydroxy acid deficiency (SCHAD and LCHAD)	Dionisi Vici *et al.* (1991), Tein *et al.* (1995)
Malignant diseases (leukaemia, lymphoma)	Chapter 14
Inflammatory diseases	
Inflammatory neuropathy with CNS involvement	Uncini *et al.* (1988)
Collagen disorders (*e.g.* scleroderma, lupus erythematosus)	Chapter 12
Dysimmune disorders	
Chediak–Higashi disease	Van Hale (1987)
Lymphohistiocytosis	Boutin *et al.* (1988)
Toxic disorders	Chapters 13, 21

*Axonal involvement also present.

facial dysmorphism occurs in Quebec and is inherited as an autosomal recessive trait (Andermann 1981). Mild mental retardation is also a feature. The course is slowly progressive but lifespan seems to be normal (Chapter 3).

OTHER COMPLICATED SMAs
The so-called adult form of *hexosaminidase A deficiency* regularly features anterior horn cell involvement with a slowly progressive course, beginning in half the cases before age 10 years. Associated dystonia and pyramidal tract signs are frequent (Specola *et al.* 1990) but pure affectation of the anterior horn cells is occasionally seen (Johnson *et al.* 1982).

SMA WITH RETINITIS PIGMENTOSA
Rare cases of familial progressive atrophy of the arms, shoulders, neck and chest with loss of tendon reflexes and associated deafness, typical bone corpuscle retinopathy and mental retardation have been described (Walsh and Hoyt 1969). A spastic component was probably present. The association of retinitis pigmentosa and muscle weakness is much more commonly due to mitochondrial disease, and the weakness is then usually of myogenic origin (Chapter 9). Several other conditions feature both peripheral and CNS involvement (Table 20.3). In this table, disorders involving the axons rather than the anterior horn are also indicated, as the clinical problems they pose are very similar to those posed by anterior horn involvement.

ACQUIRED MOTOR NEURON DISEASES

Acquired motor neuron diseases are mainly of viral origin; the role of toxic, vascular or other environmental factors has been discussed in the aetiology of lateral amyotrophic sclerosis and other related syndromes.

Most acquired viral diseases of the anterior horn cells run an acute course. They are mainly represented by acute anterior poliomyelitis and similar diseases due to enteroviruses other than the polioviruses.

Acute poliomyelitis is by far the commonest cause of acquired anterior horn cell disease. The disease unfortunately remains prevalent in some developing countries. In industrialized countries only rare cases occur in unvaccinated children. Occasional cases of paralytic poliomyelitis due to attenuated live vaccine virus have been reported in recipients of the vaccine or in contacts, mainly in children with immunodeficiency. Poliomyelitis has been discussed in Chapters 11 and 12. Poliomyelitis-like diseases due to other enteroviruses have been reported.

Hopkins syndrome which consists of acute poliomyelitis-like paralysis following an attack of asthma is also described in Chapter 11.

REFERENCES

Alberfeld, D.C., Namba, T. (1969) 'Progressive ophthalmoplegia in Kugelberg–Welander disease. Report of a case.' *Archives of Neurology,* **20,** 253–256.
Albers, J.W., Zimnowodzki, S., Lowrey, C.M., Miller, B. (1983) 'Juvenile progressive bulbar palsy. Clinical and electrodiagnostic findings.' *Archives of Neurology,* **40,** 351–353.
Andermann, E. (1981) 'Sensorimotor neuropathy with agenesis of the corpus callosum.' *In:* Vinken, P.J., Bruyn, G.W. (Eds.) *Handbook of Clinical Neurology. Vol. 42. Neurogenetic Directory, Part I.* Amsterdam: North Holland, pp. 100–103.
Aprin, H., Bowen, J.R., MacEwen, G.D., Hall, J.E. (1982) 'Spine fusion in patients with spinal muscular atrophy.' *Journal of Bone and Joint Surgery,* **64A,** 1179–1187.
Ashwal, S., Thrasher, T.V., Rice, O.R., Wenger, D.A (1984) 'A new form of sea-blue histiocytosis associated with progressive anterior horn cell and axonal degeneration.' *Annals of Neurology,* **16,** 184–192.
Aysun, S., Cinbis, M., Özcan, O.E. (1993) 'Intramedullary astrocytoma presenting as spinal muscular atrophy.' *Journal of Child Neurology,* **8,** 354–356.
Barois, A., Estournet, B., Duval-Beaupère, G., *et al.* (1989) 'Amyotrophie spinale infantile.' *Revue Neurologique,* **145,** 299–304.
Barth, P.G. (1993) 'Pontocerebellar hypoplasias. An overview of a group of inherited neurodegenerative disorders with fetal onset.' *Brain and Development,* **15,** 411–422.
Beauvais, P., Roubergue, A., Billette de Villemeur, T., Richardet, J.M. (1988) 'Paralysie bulbopontine progressive de l'enfant.' *Archives Françaises de Pédiatrie,* **45,** 653–655.
—— Billette de Villemeur, T., Richardet, J.M. (1990) 'Sclérose latérale amyotrophique probable de l'enfant. Une observation singulière. Revue de la littérature.' *Archives Françaises de Pédiatrie,* **47,** 519–522.
Ben Hamida, M., Hentati, F., Ben Hamida, C. (1990) 'Hereditary motor system diseases (chronic juvenile amyotrophic lateral sclerosis)—conditions combining a bilateral pyramidal syndrome with limb and bulbar amyotrophy.' *Brain,* **113,** 347–363.
Bertini, E., Gadisseux, J.L., Palmieri, G., *et al.* (1989) 'Distal infantile spinal muscular atrophy associated with paralysis of the diaphragm: a variant of infantile spinal muscular atrophy.' *American Journal of Medical Genetics,* **33,** 328–335.
Bertorini, T.E., Igarashi, M. (1985) 'Postpoliomyelitis muscle pseudohypertrophy.' *Muscle and Nerve,* **8,** 644–649.
Boltshauser, E., Lang, W., Spillmann, T., Hof, E. (1989) 'Hereditary distal muscular atrophy with vocal cord paralysis and sensorineural hearing loss: a dominant form of spinal muscular atrophy?' *Journal of Medical Genetics,* **26,** 105–108.
Boutin, B., Routon, M.C., Rocchiccioli, F., *et al.* (1988) 'Peripheral neuropathy associated with erythrophagocytic lymphohistiocytosis.' *Journal of Neurology, Neurosurgery, and Psychiatry,* **51,** 291–294.
Bouwsma, G., Van Wijngaarden, G.K. (1980) 'Spinal muscular atrophy and hypertrophy of the calves.' *Journal of the Neurological Sciences,* **44,** 275–279.
Boylan, K.B., Cornblath, D.R. (1992) 'Werdnig–Hoffmann disease and chronic distal spinal muscular atrophy with apparent autosomal dominant inheritance.' *Annals of Neurology,* **32,** 404–407.
Brucher, J.M., Dom, R., Lombaert, A., Carton, H. (1981) 'Progressive pontobulbar palsy with deafness: clinical and pathological study of two cases.' *Archives of Neurology,* **38,** 186–190.
Brzustowicz, L.M., Lehner, T., Castilla, L.A., *et al.* (1990) 'Genetic mapping of childhood-onset spinal muscular atrophy to chromosome 5q11.2–13.3.' *Nature,* **344,** 540–541.
Bundey, S., Lovelace, R.E. (1975) 'A clinical and genetic study of chronic proximal spinal muscular atrophy.' *Brain,* **98,** 455–472.
Bürglen, L., Amiel, J., Viollet, L., *et al.* (1996) 'Survival motor neuron deletion in the arthrogryposis multiplex congenita–spinal muscular atrophy association.' *Journal of Clinical Investigation,* **98,** 1130–1132.
Burlet, P., Bürglen, L., Clermont, O., *et al.* (1996) 'Large scale deletions of the 5q13 region are specific to Werdnig–Hoffmann disease.' *Journal of Medical Genetics,* **33,** 281–283.
Cavanagh, N.P.C., Eames, R.A., Galvin, R.J., *et al.* (1979) 'Hereditary sensory neuropathy with spastic paraplegia.' *Brain,* **102,** 79–94.
Chalmers, N., Mitchell, J.D. (1987) 'Optico-acoustic atrophy in the distal spinal muscular atrophy.' *Journal of Neurology, Neurosurgery, and Psychiatry,* **50,** 238–239.
Charnas, L., Bernar, J., Pezeshkpour, G.H., *et al.* (1988) 'MRI findings and peripheral neuropathy in Lowe's syndrome.' *Neuropediatrics,* **19,** 7–9.
Chien, Y.Y., Nonaka, I. (1989) 'Peripheral nerve involvement in Werdnig–Hoffmann disease.' *Brain and Development,* **11,** 221–229.
Chopra, J.S., Sharma, A. (1992) 'Protein energy malnutrition and the nervous system.' *Journal of the Neurological Sciences,* **110,** 8–20.

Chou, S.M., Nonaka, I. (1978) 'Werdnig–Hoffmann disease: proposal of a pathogenetic mechanism.' *Acta Neuropathologica*, **41**, 45–54.

Cobben, J.M., de Visser, M., Scheffer, H., *et al.* (1993) 'Confirmation of clinical diagnosis in requests for prenatal prediction of SMA type 1.' *Journal of Neurology, Neurosurgery, and Psychiatry*, **56**, 319–321.

—— van der Steege, G., Grootscholten, P.M., *et al.* (1995) 'Deletions of the survival motor neuron gene in unaffected siblings of patients with spinal muscular atrophy.' *American Journal of Human Genetics*, **57**, 805–808.

D'Alessandro, R., Montagna, P., Govoni, E., Pazzaglia, P. (1982) 'Benign familial spinal muscular atrophy with hypertrophy of the calves.' *Archives of Neurology*, **39**, 657–660.

Dawood, A.A., Moosa, A. (1983) 'Hand and ECG tremor in spinal muscular atrophy.' *Archives of Disease in Childhood*, **58**, 376–378.

De Leon, G.A., Grover, W.D., D'Cruz, C.A. (1984) 'Amyotrophic cerebellar hypoplasia: a specific form of infantile spinal atrophy.' *Acta Neuropathologica*, **63**, 282–286.

Della Giustina, E., Ferrière, G., Evrard, P., Lyon, G. (1979) 'Progressive bulbar paralysis in childhood.' *Acta Paediatrica Belgica*, **32**, 129–133.

De Visser, M., Ongerboer de Visser, B.W., Verbeeten, B. (1988) 'Electromyographic and computed tomographic findings in five patients with monomelic spinal muscular atrophy.' *European Neurology*, **28**, 135–138.

DiDonato, C.J., Ingraham, S.E., Mendell, J.R., *et al.* (1997) 'Deletion and conversion in spinal muscular atrophy patients: is there a relationship with severity?' *Annals of Neurology*, **41**, 230–237.

DiMauro, S., Bonilla, E., Zeviani, M., *et al.* (1985) 'Mitochondrial myopathies.' *Annals of Neurology*, **17**, 521–538.

Dionisi Vici, C., Burlina, A.B., Bertini, E., *et al.* (1991) 'Progressive neuropathy and recurrent myoglobinuria in a child with long-chain 3-hydroxyacyl-coenzyme A dehydrogenase deficiency.' *Journal of Pediatrics*, **118**, 744–746.

Dobkin, B.H., Verity, A. (1976) 'Familial progressive bulbar and spinal muscular atrophy. Juvenile onset and late morbidity with ragged-red fibers.' *Neurology*, **26**, 754–763.

Doyu, M., Sobue, G., Mukai, E., *et al.* (1992) 'Severity of X-linked recessive bulbospinal neuronopathy correlates with size of the tandem CAG repeat in androgen receptor gene.' *Annals of Neurology*, **32**, 707–710.

Dubowitz, V. (1995) *Muscle Disorders in Children, 2nd Edn.* Philadelphia: W.B. Saunders.

Duval-Baupère, G., Barois, A., Quinet, I., Estournet, B. (1985) 'Les problèmes thoraciques, rachidiens et respiratoires de l'enfant atteint d'amyotrophie spinale à évolution prolongée.' *Archives Françaises de Pédiatrie*, **42**, 625–634.

Dyck, P.J. (1984) 'Inherited neuronal degeneration and atrophy.' *In:* Dyck, P.J., Thomas, P.K., Lambert, E.M. (Eds.) *Peripheral Neuropathy. Vol. 2. 2nd Edn.* Philadelphia: W.B. Saunders, pp. 1600–1655.

—— Litchy, W.J., Minnerath, S., *et al.* (1994) 'Hereditary motor and sensory neuropathy with diaphragm and vocal cord paresis.' *Annals of Neurology*, **35**, 608–615.

Emery, A.E.H. (1971) 'The neurology of spinal muscular atrophies.' *Journal of Medical Genetics*, **8**, 481–495.

—— (1994) *Diagnostic Criteria for Neuromuscular Disorders.* Barn, The Netherlands: ENMC.

—— Davie, A.M., Holloway, D., Skinner, R. (1976a) 'International collaborative study of the spinal muscular atrophies. Part II: Analysis of genetic data.' *Journal of the Neurological Sciences*, **30**, 375–384.

—— Hausmanowa-Petrusewicz, I., Davie, M.H., *et al.* (1976b) 'International collaborative study of the spinal muscular atrophies. Part I: Analysis of clinical and laboratory data.' *Journal of the Neurological Sciences*, **29**, 83–94.

Engel, K., Kurland, L.T., Klatzo, I. (1959) 'An inherited disease similar to amyotrophic lateral sclerosis with a pattern of posterior column involvement: an intermediate form?' *Brain*, **82**, 203–220.

Fenichel, G.M., Emery, E.S., Hunt, P. (1967) 'Neurogenic atrophy simulating facioscapulohumeral dystrophy.' *Archives of Neurology*, **17**, 257–260.

Fishbeck, K.H., Ionasescu, V., Ritter, A.W., *et al.* (1986) 'Localization of the gene for X-linked spinal muscular atrophy.' *Neurology*, **36**, 1595–1598.

Francis, D.A., Brown, A., Miller, D.H., *et al.* (1988) 'MRI appearances of the CNS manifestations of *Mycoplasma pneumoniae*: a report of two cases.' *Journal of Neurology*, **235**, 441–443.

Furukawa, T., Toyokura, Y. (1976) 'Chronic spinal muscular atrophy of facioscapulohumeral type.' *Journal of Medical Genetics*, **13**, 285–289.

Galan, E., Kousseff, B.G. (1995) 'Peripheral neuropathy in Ehlers–Danlos syndrome.' *Pediatric Neurology*, **12**, 242–245.

Gallai, V., Hockaday, J.M., Hughes, J.T., *et al.* (1981) 'Ponto-bulbar palsy with deafness (Brown–Vialetto–Van Laere syndrome): a report of three cases.' *Journal of the Neurological Sciences*, **50**, 259–275.

Gamstorp, I. (1967) 'Progressive spinal muscular atrophy in infancy or early childhood.' *Acta Paediatrica Scandinavica*, **56**, 408–423.

Gascon, G.G., Chavis, P., Yaghmour, A., *et al.* (1995) 'Familial childhood primary lateral sclerosis with associated gaze paresis.' *Neuropediatrics*, **26**, 313–319.

Gilgoff, I.S., Kahlstrom, E., McLaughlin, E., Keens, T.G. (1989) 'Long-term ventilatory support in spinal muscular atrophy.' *Journal of Pediatrics*, **115**, 904–909.

Goebel, H.H., Zeman, W., De Myer, W. (1976) 'Peripheral motor and sensory neuropathy of early childhood simulating Werdnig–Hoffmann disease.' *Neuropädiatrie*, **7**, 182–195.

Gordon, N. (1991) 'The spinal muscular atrophies.' *Developmental Medicine and Child Neurology*, **33**, 934–938.

Gourie-Devi, M., Suresh, T.G. (1988) 'Madras pattern of motor neuron disease in South India.' *Journal of Neurology, Neurosurgery, and Psychiatry*, **51**, 773–777.

Goutières, F., Aicardi, J., Farkas, A. (1977) 'Anterior horn cell disease associated with ponto-cerebellar hypoplasia in infants.' *Journal of Neurology, Neurosurgery, and Psychiatry*, **40**, 370–378.

—— Bogicevic, D., Aicardi, J. (1991) 'A predominantly cervical form of spinal muscular atrophy.' *Journal of Neurology, Neurosurgery, and Psychiatry*, **54**, 223–225.

Grunnet, M.L., Donaldson, J.O. (1985) 'Juvenile multisystem degeneration with motor neuron involvement and eosinophilic intracytoplasmic inclusions.' *Archives of Neurology*, **42**, 1114–1116.

—— Leicher, C., Zimmerman, A., *et al.* (1989) 'Primary lateral sclerosis in a child.' *Neurology*, **39**, 1530–1532.

Guidetti, D., Motti, L., Marcello, N., *et al.* (1986) 'Kennedy disease in an Italian kindred.' *European Neurology*, **25**, 188–196.

Hagberg, B., Lundberg, K. (1969) 'Dissociated motor development simulating cerebral palsy.' *Neuropädiatrie*, **1**, 187–199.

Hamano, K., Tsukamoto, H., Yazawa, T., *et al.* (1994) 'Infantile progressive spinal muscular atrophy with ophthalmoplegia and pyramidal symptoms.' *Pediatric Neurology*, **10**, 320–324.

Harding, A.E., Thomas, P.K. (1980) 'Hereditary distal spinal muscular atrophy. A report of 34 cases and a review of the literature.' *Journal of the Neurological Sciences*, **45**, 337–348.

Hausmanowa-Petrusewicz, I., Karwanska, A. (1986) 'Electromyographic findings in different forms of infantile and juvenile proximal spinal muscular atrophy.' *Muscle and Nerve*, **9**, 37–46.

—— Zaremba, J., Borkowska, J. (1979) 'Chronic form of childhood spinal muscular atrophy. Are the problems of genetics really solved?' *Journal of the Neurological Sciences*, **43**, 317–326.

—— —— —— (1985) 'Chronic spinal muscular atrophy of childhood and adolescence: problems of classification and genetic counselling.' *Journal of Medical Genetics*, **22**, 350–353.

Hentati, A., Bejaoui, K., Pericak-Vance, M.A., *et al.* (1994) 'Linkage of recessive familial amyotrophic lateral sclerosis to chromosome 2q33–q35.' *Nature Genetics*, **7**, 425–428.

Hirayama, K., Tomonaga, M., Kitano, K., *et al.* (1987) 'Focal cervical poliopathy causing juvenile muscular atrophy of distal upper extremity: a pathological study.' *Journal of Neurology, Neurosurgery, and Psychiatry*, **50**, 285–290.

Iannaccone, S.T., Browne, R.H., Samaha, F.J., Buncher, C.R. (1993) 'Prospective study of spinal muscular atrophy before age 6 years. DCN/SMA group.' *Pediatric Neurology*, **9**, 187–193.

Imai, T., Minami, R., Nagaoka, M., *et al.* (1990) 'Proximal and distal motor nerve conduction velocities in Werdnig–Hoffmann disease.' *Pediatric Neurology*, **6**, 82–86.

Jacobs, J.M., Harding, B.N., Lake, B.D., *et al.* (1990) 'Peripheral neuropathy in Leigh's disease.' *Brain*, **113**, 447–462.

Jagganathan, K. (1973) 'Juvenile motor neuron disease.' *In:* Spillane, J.D. (Ed.) *Tropical Neurology.* Oxford: Oxford University Press, pp. 127–130.

Jennekens, F.G.I., Veldman, H., Vroegindeweij-Claessens, L.J.H.M., *et al.* (1992) 'Congenital oculo-bulbar palsy.' *Journal of Neurology, Neurosurgery, and Psychiatry*, **55**, 404–406.

Johnson, W.G., Wigger, H.J., Karp, H.R., *et al.* (1982) 'Juvenile spinal muscular atrophy: a new hexosaminidase deficiency phenotype.' *Annals of Neurology*, **11**, 11–16.

Kaeser, H.E. (1965) 'Scapuloperoneal muscular atrophy.' *Brain*, **88**, 407–418.

709

Kamoshita, S., Takei, Y., Miyao, M., *et al.* (1990) 'Pontocerebellar hypoplasia associated with infantile motor neuron disease (Norman's disease).' *Pediatric Pathology*, **10**, 133–142.

Kleijer, W.J., Hu, P., Thoomes, R., *et al.* (1990) 'β-mannosidase deficiency: heterogenous manifestation in the first female patient and her brother.' *Journal of Inherited Metabolic Disease*, **13**, 867–872.

Korinthenberg, R., Sauer, M., Ketelsen, U-P., *et al.* (1997) 'Congenital axonal neuropathy caused by deletion in the spinal muscular atrophy region.' *Annals of Neurology*, **42**, 364–368.

Kuzuhara, S., Chou, S.M. (1981) 'Preservation of the phrenic motoneurons in Werdnig–Hoffmann disease.' *Annals of Neurology*, **9**, 506–510.

Kwast, O., Ignatowicz, R. (1990) 'Progressive peripheral neuron degeneration in ataxia–telangiectasia: an electrophysiological study in children.' *Developmental Medicine and Child Neurology*, **32**, 800–807.

Lander, C.M., Eadie, M.J., Tyrer, J.H. (1976) 'Hereditary motor peripheral neuropathy predominantly affecting the arms.' *Journal of the Neurological Sciences*, **28**, 389–393.

Lefebvre, S., Bürglen, L., Reboullet, S., *et al.* (1995) 'Identification and characterization of a spinal muscular atrophy-determining gene.' *Cell*, **80**, 155–165.

Liu, G.T., Specht, L.A. (1993) 'Progressive juvenile segmental spinal muscular atrophy.' *Pediatric Neurology*, **9**, 54–56.

Lunt, P.W., Mathew, C., Clark, S., *et al.* (1992) 'Can prenatal diagnosis be offered in neonatally lethal spinal muscular atrophy (SMA) with arthrogryposis and fractures?' *Journal of Medical Genetics*, **29**, 282. *(Abstract.)*

McShane, M.A., Boyd, S., Harding, B., *et al.* (1992) 'Progressive bulbar paralysis of childhood. A reappraisal of Fazio–Londe disease.' *Brain*, **115**, 1889–1900.

McWilliam, R.C., Gardner-Medwin, D., Doyle, D., Stephenson, J.B.P. (1985) 'Diaphragmatic paralysis due to spinal cord atrophy.' *Archives of Disease in Childhood*, **60**, 145–149.

Meadows, J.C., Marsden, C.D. (1969a) 'A distal form of chronic spinal muscular atrophy.' *Neurology*, **19**, 53–58.

—— —— (1969b) 'Scapuloperoneal amyotrophy.' *Archives of Neurology*, **20**, 9–12.

Melki, J., Munnich, A. (1996) 'Molecular genetics of spinal muscular atrophy.' *In:* Arzimanoglou, A., Goutières, F. (Eds.) *Trends in Child Neurology.* Paris: John Libbey, pp. 137–141.

—— Abdelhak, S., Sheth, M.F., *et al.* (1990a) 'The gene responsible for chronic proximal spinal muscular atrophies of childhood maps to chromosome 5q.' *Nature*, **344**, 767–768.

—— Sheth, P., Abdelhak, S., *et al.* (1990b) 'Mapping of acute (type I) spinal muscular atrophy to chromosome 5q12–q14.' *Lancet*, **336**, 271–273.

—— Lefebvre, S., Bürglen, P., *et al.* (1994) 'De novo and inherited deletions of the 5q13 region in spinal muscular atrophies.' *Science*, **264**, 1474–1477.

Mellins, R.B., Hays, A.P., Gold, A.P., *et al.* (1974) 'Respiratory distress as the initial manifestation of Werdnig–Hoffmann disease.' *Pediatrics*, **53**, 33–40.

Mercelis, R., Demeester, J., Martin, J.J. (1980) 'Neurogenic scapuloperoneal syndrome in childhood.' *Journal of Neurology, Neurosurgery, and Psychiatry*, **43**, 888–896.

Merlini, L., Granata, C., Bonfiglioli, S., *et al.* (1989) 'Scoliosis in spinal muscular atrophy: natural history and management.' *Developmental Medicine and Child Neurology*, **31**, 501–508.

Moosa, A., Dubowitz, V. (1973) 'Spinal muscular atrophy in childhood: two clues to clinical diagnosis.' *Archives of Disease in Childhood*, **48**, 386–388.

—— —— (1976) 'Motor nerve conduction velocity in spinal muscular atrophy of childhood.' *Archives of Disease in Childhood*, **51**, 974–977.

Mulder, D.W. (1981) 'Amyotrophic lateral sclerosis and Parkinson-dementia in Guam.' *In:* Vinken, P.J., Bruyn, G.W. (Eds.) *Handbook of Clinical Neurology. Vol. 42. Neurogenetics Directory, Part I.* Amsterdam: North Holland, pp. 70–71.

Munsat, T.L., Davies, K.E. (1992) 'International SMA consortium meeting (26–28 June 1992, Bonn, Germany).' *Neuromuscular Disorders*, **2**, 423–428.

Navon, R., Khosravi, R., Korczyn, T., *et al.* (1995) ' A new mutation in the HEXA gene associated with a spinal muscular atrophy phenotype.' *Neurology*, **45**, 539–543.

Nelson, J.S., Prensky, A.L. (1972) 'Sporadic juvenile amyotrophic lateral sclerosis: a clinicopathological study of a case with neuronal cytoplasmic inclusions containing RNA.' *Archives of Neurology*, **27**, 300–306.

Norman, R.M., Kay, J.M. (1965) 'Cerebello-thalamo-spinal degeneration in infancy: an unusual variant of Werdnig–Hoffmann disease.' *Archives of Disease in Childhood*, **40**, 302–308.

Novelli, G., Capon, F., Tamisari, L., *et al.* (1995) 'Neonatal spinal muscular atrophy with diaphragmatic paralysis is unlinked to 5q11.2–q13.' *Journal of Medical Genetics*, **32**, 216–219.

Oka, A., Matsushita, Y., Sakakihara, Y., *et al.* (1995) 'Spinal muscular atrophy with oculomotor palsy, epilepsy, and cerebellar hypoperfusion.' *Pediatric Neurology*, **12**, 365–369.

Oldfors, A., Hagberg, B., Nordgren, H., *et al.* (1988) 'Rett syndrome: spinal cord neuropathology.' *Pediatric Neurology*, **4**, 172–174.

Oppenheimer, D.R. (1976) 'Diseases of the basal ganglia, cerebellum and motor neurons.' *In:* Blackwood, W., Corsellis, J.A.N. (Eds.) *Greenfield's Neuropathology, 3rd Edn.* London: Edward Arnold, pp. 608–651.

O'Sullivan, D.G., McLeod, J.G. (1978) 'Distal chronic spinal muscular atrophy involving the hands.' *Journal of Neurology, Neurosurgery, and Psychiatry*, **41**, 653–658.

Pachter, B.R., Pearson, J., Davidowitz, J., *et al.* (1976) 'Congenital total external ophthalmoplegia associated with infantile spinal muscular atrophy. Fine structure of extraocular muscle.' *Investigative Ophthalmology*, **15**, 320–324.

Paulson, G.W., Liss, L., Sweeney, P.J. (1980) 'Late-onset spinal muscle atrophy. A sex-linked variant of Kugelberg–Welander.' *Acta Neurologica Scandinavica*, **61**, 49–55.

Pearn, J. (1978a) 'Incidence, prevalence and gene-frequency studies of chronic childhood spinal muscular atrophy.' *Journal of Medical Genetics*, **15**, 409–413.

—— (1978b) 'Autosomal dominant spinal muscular atrophy. A clinical and genetic study.' *Journal of the Neurological Sciences*, **38**, 263–275.

—— (1980) 'Classification of spinal muscular atrophies.' *Lancet*, **1**, 919–922.

—— Hudgson, P. (1978) 'Anterior-horn cell degeneration and gross calf hypertrophy with adolescent onset. A new spinal muscular atrophy syndrome.' *Lancet*, **1**, 1059–1061.

—— Wilson, J. (1973) 'Chronic generalised spinal muscular atrophy of infancy and childhood: arrested Werdnig–Hoffmann disease.' *Archives of Disease in Childhood*, **48**, 768–774.

—— Gardner-Medwin, D., Wilson, J. (1978) 'A clinical study of chronic childhood muscular atrophy. A review of 141 cases.' *Journal of the Neurological Sciences*, **38**, 23–37.

Peiris, J.B., Seneviratne, K.N., Wickremasinghe, H.R., *et al.* (1989) 'Non familial juvenile distal spinal muscular atrophy of upper extremity.' *Journal of Neurology, Neurosurgery, and Psychiatry*, **52**, 314–319.

Poll-Thé, B.T., Aicardi, J., Girot, R., Rosa, R. (1985) 'Neurological findings in triosephosphate isomerase deficiency.' *Annals of Neurology*, **17**, 439–443.

Probst, A., Ulrich, J., Bischoff, A., Boltshauser, E. (1981) 'Sensory ganglioneuropathy in infantile spinal muscular atrophy. Light and electronmicroscopic findings in two cases.' *Neuropediatrics*, **12**, 215–231.

Raymond, F.L. (1997) 'Spinal muscular atrophy of childhood: genetics.' *Developmental Medicine and Child Neurology*, **39**, 419–420.

Robb, S.A., McShane, M.A., Wilson, J., Payan, J. (1991) 'Acute onset spinal muscular atrophy in siblings.' *Neuropediatrics*, **22**, 45–46.

Rodrigues, N.R., Owen, N., Talbot, K., *et al.* (1995) 'Deletions in the survival motor neuron gene on 5q13 in autosomal recessive spinal muscular atrophy.' *Human Molecular Genetics*, **4**, 631–634.

—— —— —— *et al.* (1996) 'Gene deletions in spinal muscular atrophy.' *Journal of Medical Genetics*, **33**, 93–96.

Rudnik-Schöneborn, S., Wirth, B., Röhrig, D., *et al.* (1995) 'Exclusion of the gene locus for spinal muscular atrophy on chromosome 5q in a family with infantile olivopontocerebellar atrophy (OPCA) and anterior horn cell degeneration.' *Neuromuscular Disorders*, **5**, 19–23.

—— Forkert, R., Hahnen, E., *et al.* (1996) 'Clinical spectrum and diagnostic criteria of infantile spinal muscular atrophy: further delineation on the basis of SMN gene deletion findings.' *Neuropediatrics*, **27**, 8–15.

Russman, B.S., Iannacone, S.T., Buncher C.R., *et al.* (1992) 'Spinal muscular atrophy: new thoughts on the pathogenesis and classification schema.' *Journal of Child Neurology*, **7**, 347–353.

Schapira, D., Swash, M. (1985) 'Neonatal spinal muscular atrophy presenting as respiratory distress: a clinical variant.' *Muscle and Nerve*, **8**, 661–663.

Schmitt, H.P., Härle, M., Koelfen, W., Nissen, K-H. (1994) 'Childhood progressive spinal muscular atrophy with facioscapulo-humeral predominance, sensory and autonomic involvement and optic atrophy.' *Brain and Development*, **16**, 386–392.

Shapiro, F., Bresnan, M.J. (1982) 'Orthopaedic management of childhood neuromuscular disease. Part I: Spinal muscular atrophy.' *Journal of Bone and Joint Surgery*, **64A**, 785–789.

Skre, H., Mellgren, S.I., Bergsholm, P., Slagsvold, J.E. (1978) 'Unusual type of neural muscular atrophy with a possible X-chromosomal inheritance pattern.' *Acta Neuropathologica Scandinavica*, **58**, 249–260.

Specola, N., Vanier, M., Goutières, F., *et al.* (1990) 'The juvenile and chronic forms of GM2 gangliosidosis. Clinical and enzymatic heterogeneity.' *Neurology*, **40**, 145–150.

Steinman, G.S., Rorke, L.B., Brown, M.J. (1980) 'Infantile neuronal degeneration masquerading as Werdnig–Hoffmann disease.' *Annals of Neurology*, **8**, 317–324.

Stibler, H., Jaeken, J. (1990) 'Carbohydrate deficient serum transferrin in a new systemic hereditary syndrome.' *Archives of Disease in Childhood*, **65**, 107–111.

Summers, B.A., Swash, M., Schwartz, M.S., Ingram, D.A. (1987) 'Juvenile-onset bulbospinal muscular atrophy with deafness: Vialetto–Van Laere syndrome or Madras-type motor neuron disease?' *Journal of Neurology*, **234**, 440–442.

Tandan, R., Sharma, K.R., Bradley, W.G., *et al.* (1990) 'Chronic segmental spinal muscular atrophy of upper extremities in identical twins.' *Neurology*, **40**, 236–239.

Tein, I., Donner, E.J., Hale, D.E., Murphy, E.G. (1995) 'Clinical and neurophysiologic response of myopathy and neuropathy in long-chain L-3-hydroxyacyl-CoA dehydrogenase deficiency to oral prednisone.' *Pediatric Neurology*, **12**, 68–76.

Thomas, P.K., Calne, D.B., Elliott, C.F. (1972) 'X-linked scapuloperoneal syndrome.' *Journal of Neurology, Neurosurgery, and Psychiatry*, **35**, 208–215.

Toma, S., Shiozawa, Z. (1995) 'Amyotrophic cervical myelopathy in adolescence.' *Journal of Neurology, Neurosurgery, and Psychiatry*, **58**, 56–64.

Uncini, A., Treviso, M., Basciani, M., *et al.* (1988) 'Associated central and peripheral demyelination: an electrophysiological study.' *Journal of Neurology*, **235**, 238–240.

Van der Steege, G., Grootscholten, P.M., Van der Vlies, P., *et al.* (1995) 'PCR-based DNA test to confirm clinical diagnosis of autosomal recessive spinal muscular atrophy.' *Lancet*, **345**, 985–986. *(Letter.)*

Van Hale, P. (1987) 'Chediak–Higashi syndrome.' *In:* Gomez, M.R. (Ed.) *Neurocutaneous Diseases: a Practical Approach.* London: Butterworths, pp. 209–213.

Walsh, F.B., Hoyt, W.F. (1969) *Clinical Neuro-ophthalmology, 3rd Edn.* Baltimore: Williams & Wilkins.

Wang, C.H., Carter, J.A., Das, K., *et al.* (1997) 'Extensive DNA deletion associated with severe disease alleles on spinal muscular atrophy homologues.' *Annals of Neurology*, **42**, 41–49.

Weinberg, A.G., Kirkpatrick, J.B. (1975) 'Cerebellar hypoplasia in Werdnig–Hoffmann disease.' *Developmental Medicine and Child Neurology*, **17**, 511–516.

Wirth, B., Rudnick-Schöneborn, S., Hahnen, E., *et al.* (1995) 'Prenatal prediction in families with autosomal recessive proximal spinal muscular atrophy (5q11.2–q13.3): molecular genetics and clinical experience in 109 cases.' *Prenatal Diagnosis*, **15**, 407–417.

Yokochi, K., Oda, M., Satoh, J., Morimatsu, Y. (1989) 'An autopsy case of atypical infantile motor neuron disease with hyaline intraneuronal inclusions.' *Archives of Neurology*, **46**, 103–107.

Young, I.D., Harper, P.S. (1980) 'Hereditary distal spinal muscular atrophy with vocal chord paralysis.' *Journal of Neurology, Neurosurgery, and Psychiatry*, **43**, 413–418.

Zeviani, M., Peterson, P., Servidei, E., *et al.* (1987) 'Benign reversible muscle cytochrome c oxidase deficiency: a second case.' *Neurology*, **37**, 64–67.

21
DISORDERS OF THE PERIPHERAL NERVES

This chapter considers only those disorders in which the primary pathological process affects the axons of motor or sensory cells or both, or their myelin sheath and associated Schwann cells. Diseases in which axonal damage results in primary lesions of the neuronal perikarya have been described in Chapter 20.

Hereditary neuropathies may be purely sensory in type. More often they involve both sensory and motor fibres (Hagberg 1990). Nerve fibre function can be disturbed in several manners (Fig. 21.1). *Wallerian degeneration* occurs when an axon is separated from the cell perikaryon or when the cell dies. *Axonal neuropathies* are characterized primarily by involvement of the axon which may be the result of toxins, genetic disease, vascular disturbances and so on. In many cases, axonal neuropathies begin and remain more severe distally than proximally, perhaps because the enormous length of axons makes the metabolic needs of their most distal parts difficult to meet. This may also be due to disturbances in the axonal transport systems. In axonal neuropathies, nerve conduction velocities are normal or only slightly slowed despite evidence of denervation. *Diseases of the Schwann cell and the myelin sheath* are also of multiple (genetic or acquired) causes, especially inflammatory diseases. The lesions are diffuse or segmental, limited to the length of nerve depending on one Schwann cell (internode). Such a process may produce a *conduction block* in some fibres or only a slowing of nerve conduction velocities. Slowing may be diffuse and uniform as in metabolic neuropathies (Miller *et al.* 1985). Conduction block and temporal dispersion are indicative of multifocal segmental demyelination. With conduction block, defined as failure of an action potential to propagate throughout the length of an axon, both the amplitude and the area under the curve of the evoked muscle action potential are reduced when proximal stimulation is compared to distal stimulation of the motor nerve. With pure temporal dispersion, increased duration occurs together with reduced amplitude but the area under the curve is preserved. Demyelination and axonal disease are not independent processes, but the exact nature of their relationship remains unclear.

HEREDITARY MOTOR AND SENSORY NEUROPATHIES (HMSNs)

HMSNs are the most common degenerative disorders of the peripheral nervous system, accounting for approximately 40 per cent of childhood chronic neuropathies (Ouvrier 1992). Degeneration of myelin sheaths and/or axons produces a predominantly distal paralytic amyotrophy involving preferentially the lower limbs and associated with areflexia. Sensory disturbances are overshadowed by motor involvement.

The current classification of the HMSNs remains based in part on their pathology (axonal or myelinic), their electroclinical manifestations, especially the motor and sensory conduction velocities, and their mode of inheritance. Progress in molecular genetics is rapidly changing the criteria for classification. A composite classification is given in Table 21.1.

HEREDITARY MOTOR AND SENSORY NEUROPATHY TYPE I (HMSN I)

HMSN I is characterized pathologically by extensive segmental demyelination and remyelination with the development of 'onion bulbs' around nerve fibres, by slow motor and sensory nerve conduction velocities and by a dominant inheritance (Dyck 1984). However, autosomal recessive forms have been reported (Harding and Thomas 1980a, Gabreëls-Festen *et al.* 1992) and X-linked inheritance has been demonstrated (Hahn 1990, Ionasescu *et al.* 1991). The prevalence of HMSN I is 3.8 per 100,000 population, accounting for 51 per cent of pooled paediatric cases of hereditary neuropathies (Hagberg and Lyon 1981). Although the penetrance of the disease is high (83 per cent) there is a broad variability in clinical and pathological expression (Harding and Thomas 1980b, Van Weerden *et al.* 1982). In some cases, even nerve biopsy findings can be minimal (Dyck *et al.* 1983a). Mild and even asymptomatic cases occur, and systematic examination of parents and relatives therefore improves the diagnostic yield in propositi. Most cases are of paternal origin (Harding 1995).

HMSN I is genetically heterogeneous. It is usually referred to as Charcot–Marie–Tooth disease type I (CMT 1) in the gene mapping literature. Most cases are linked to chromosome 17 (CMT 1A). The defect in such cases is usually a submicroscopic duplication, approximately 1.5 megabases in length, within band 17p11.2 (Raeymaekers *et al.* 1991, Hallam *et al.* 1992). The duplication includes the gene encoding peripheral myelin protein 22 (PMP-22) (Patel *et al.* 1992) so that the gene is present in three

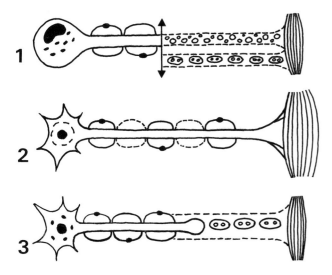

Fig. 21.1. Different types of peripheral nerve involvement.

1. Wallerian degeneration. Following interruption of axon, there is chromatolysis of the cell body. In distal axon, myelin initially disintegrates (upper part of schema). Later, Schwann cells divide and line up inside basement membrane to regenerate an axon (lower part of schema). Axonal sprouting is also observed. Nerve conduction is normal in proximal axon and absent distally. Muscle atrophy is present.

2. Segmental demyelination. Patchy damage to Schwann cells with secondary paranodal, axonal degeneration. Secondary remyelination generates short internodes with thin myelin sheath. Repeated episodes of demyelination and remyelination may produce 'onion bulb' formations. Conduction block or slowing of conduction in demyelinated segments. Increased mechanical irritability.

3. 'Dying back' neuropathy. Degeneration begins in terminal axon. Secondary demyelination often occurs. Conduction is normal proximally and absent distally in affected fibres. Preferential involvement of large fibres explains the mild/moderate reduction in nerve conduction velocity, as the measured velocity is that of small fibres.

TABLE 21.1
Classification of the hereditary motor and sensory neuropathies (HMSNs)*

Type	Genetics†
Type I (hypertrophic, demyelinating, remyelinating, low conduction velocity)	
CMT 1A (duplication of chromosome 17p11.2, including *PMP22* gene or mutation of gene)	AD
CMT 1B (linkage to chromosome 1q21–q23 with defect in P_o gene)	AD
CMT 1C (no linkage to chromosomes 1 or 17)	AD
Autosomal recessive types (CMT 4)	AR
With basal lamina onion bulbs	
With focally folded myelin	
Linked to chromosome 8q (CMT 4A)	
Type II (neuronal, low-normal conduction velocities)	
Classical-type linkage to chromosome 1p36 in some families (CMT 2A)	AD
Autosomal recessive type (CMT 2B)	AR
Severe childhood form	Usually AR, Rare cases AD
Type III (hypertrophic with hypomyelination)	AR or S
With basal lamina onion bulbs	
Amyelinic type	
With classical onion bulbs (may be associated with mutations of *PMP22* or of P_o; highly heterogeneous)	
X-linked forms (CMT X)	
Linked to Xq13.1: mutations, deletions or insertions in connexin 32 gene (responsible for most so-called intermediate forms as behaves like hypertrophic type in males and more as axonal type in females) (CMT X1)	XD
Linked to Xq26 (often with mental retardation and deafness; rare)	XR
Linked to Xp22.2 (axonal form, rare)	XR
Complex forms[1]	
With spasticity (type V)[2]	AD
With optic atrophy (type VI) (genetically heterogeneous)	AR
With deafness (type VII)	AR?
With pigmentary retinopathy (type VIII)	AR?

*Data from Dyck (1984), Gabreëls-Festen *et al.* (1993), Harding (1995).
†AD = autosomal dominant, AR = autosomal recessivec, XD = X-linked dominant, XR = X-linked recessive, S = sporadic.
[1]Rare, classification still uncertain.
[2]The nosological situation vis-à-vis the spastic paraplegias is unclear. Refsum syndrome, sometimes termed HMSN type IV, is usually not included among the HMSNs.

copies. In a few cases without duplication, a point mutation of the *PMP22* gene has been found (Roa *et al.* 1993), thus indicating that this gene is the disease gene in HMSN I. The duplication is thought to result from unequal crossing-over during meiosis. The mechanism by which overexpression of PMP-22 produces the clinical manifestations is not understood.

In a few families, the disease is caused by mutations of the P_o gene (CMT 1B) which maps to chromosome 1q21–q23 (Hayasaka *et al.* 1993, Harding 1995).

Some cases do not map to either of these loci. In some dominantly transmitted cases the gene is not known (CMT 1C) (Chance *et al.* 1992). A fourth type mapping to chromosome 8q has been described with an autosomal recessive inheritance (Ben Othmane *et al.* 1993a).

In approximately 10 per cent of cases, the disorder is linked to the X chromosome. At least two different loci have been found (Ionasescu *et al.* 1991, 1992), the most frequent one on the long arm of the chromosome (Xq13.1). Several mutations at this locus are known to involve the gene for connexin 32 (Bergoffen *et al.* 1993, Bone *et al.* 1995), which are membrane-spanning proteins localized adjacent to the nodes of Ranvier. The neurophysiological features of the X-linked type in males may resemble those of HMSN I, whereas in females they are more axonal in type (Harding 1995). It seems likely that 'intermediate' types of HMSN I with mildly slowed conduction velocities are mainly X-linked. A rare X-linked axonal form maps to Xp22.2, and another axonal form with associated deafness and mental retardation maps to Xq24–q26 (Priest *et al.* 1995).

PATHOLOGY
The pathology of HMSN I has been mainly studied by muscle and nerve biopsy. Only a few post-mortem examinations have been reported: these cases showed degeneration of the posterior columns, some loss of anterior horn cells and degeneration of the

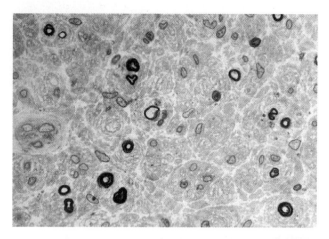

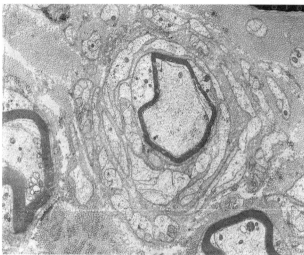

Fig. 21.2. Hereditary motor and sensory neuropathy type I. *(Top)* Proliferation of Schwann cells with 'onion bulb' formations. Note also the small number of myelinated fibres. *(Bottom)* 'Onion bulb' formation as seen with electron microscope. The axon is thinly myelinated in comparison with two normal axons. (Courtesy Dr M.C. Routon, Hôpital Saint Vincent de Paul, Paris.)

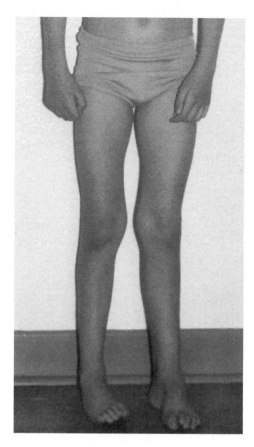

Fig. 21.3. Hereditary motor and sensory neuropathy type I in an 8-year-old girl. Note wasting of lower limbs below the lower third of thigh and deformed feet.

anterior and posterior spinal roots (De Recondo 1975). There is a reduction in the numbers of myelinated fibres with the greatest loss among those of large calibre. The distribution of fibre diameters is thus unimodal. Unmyelinated fibres are not affected. Proliferation of the sheath of Schwann produces the classical 'onion bulb' formations (Fig. 21.2) that can be shown by electron microscopy to contain only Schwann cells and their processes (Behse and Buchtal 1977). Nerve-fibre teasing shows numerous images of segmental and paranodal demyelination and remyelination predominating on the distal part of nerves. Pathological lesions, in particular onion bulbs, are nonspecific and indicate only the succession of demyelinating and remyelinating episodes that can also be observed in many other neuropathies. When marked, the process leads to hypertrophy of nerve roots and plexi. Degenerative changes in muscle are secondary to neural damage. The mechanism of the malady is not understood. Nukuda and Dyck (1984) have suggested that demyelination–remyelination might be secondary to alterations of the axons.

CLINICAL MANIFESTATIONS

Onset of the disease is usually within the first decade although cases of later onset are known. A very early onset during the neonatal period or the first year is not as rare as once thought (Hagberg and Lyon 1981, Vanasse and Dubowitz 1981). Foot deformity or gait disturbances are the usual presenting manifestations. Pes cavus is typical and is often associated with hammer toes. Some children present with pes planus and marked valgus deviation of the feet. Pes planus was more common than pes cavus in a series of 17 children diagnosed early because of a positive family history; seven had areflexia and the ankle jerk was absent in only three of them (Feasby *et al.* 1992). Gait disturbances include poor stability or stepping gait, difficulties running and frequent falls. Such symptoms develop insidiously so that most patients are seen only after several years. The contrast between marked neurological signs and good preservation of function is then striking.

Examination reveals symmetrical atrophy of the peroneal muscles (hence the term peroneal amyotrophy classically applied to HMSN), later involving the calves and eventually the lower third of the thigh (Fig. 21.3). In the upper extremity, atrophy of the small muscles of the hand may occur, although it is usually a late manifestation. Asymmetrical and even unilateral involvement has been rarely reported (Ouvrier 1992). In many cases, muscle bulk remains normal for prolonged periods, and in my experience approximately half of affected children and adolescents do not have any wasting. Hypertrophy of the calves occurs in some families (Sakashita *et al.* 1992, Uncini *et al.* 1994).

Deep tendon reflexes, especially the ankle jerks, are often lost early, and this may be a useful sign for the clinical diagnosis of the condition in young children with affected relatives or in parents of children with the disease.

Sensory abnormalities are mild and may be difficult to evidence when they are limited to subtle deficits of epicritic or deep sensation. Pain and touch sensation is not impaired, and dysaesthesia or pain are not a feature, except for pain due to foot deformities or calluses which may be severe in some patients.

Vasomotor disturbances are common, with frequent cyanosis and marbling of the skin. Palpable nerve enlargement is rare in children and difficult to assess objectively. Scoliosis, lordosis and recurrent patellar dislocation may occur (Harding and Thomas 1980c). The CSF protein level is elevated in over half the cases, but lumbar puncture is not indicated.

Progression of HMSN I is slow, and arrests are common and often prolonged. Most patients remain active indefinitely but some severe cases exist. In an occasional patient, intercurrent infections or rapid growth may be associated with acceleration of the disease process. Rare cases of proven HMSN I with rapid deterioration and response to steroid treatment are on record (Mitchell *et al.* 1987, Dyck *et al.* 1993). The interpretation of such cases of prednisone-responsive HMSN I is difficult. They resemble chronic inflammatory polyneuropathy but a coincidence of two different nerve disorders seems unlikely. In practice a trial of steroid is indicated in cases with sudden deterioration.

RECESSIVE TYPES OF HMSN I
A few patients with a clinical picture indistinguishable from that of classical HMSN I but with an autosomal recessive transmission are on record (Gabreëls-Festen *et al.* 1992, 1993). Pathologically, they are of two different types: one features onion bulbs made only of basal lamina, the other focally folded myelin sheaths. The latter type may present with relatively severe symptoms and signs (Gabreëls-Festen *et al.* 1990, 1993; Quattrone *et al.* 1996).

DIAGNOSIS
The diagnosis of HMSN I is easy in typical forms. The presence of sensory deficit is important to distinguish the condition from distal forms of myopathy or spinal amyotrophy.

Marked slowing of motor and sensory nerve conduction velocities to less than 50 per cent of normal values and increased distal latencies separate HMSN I from type II. There is no correlation between slowing of conduction velocities and clinical severity. EMG abnormalities appear early and, in the study by Ouvrier (1992), were present in most secondary cases by 3 years of age. Conduction velocities are also abnormal in one of the parents, whether or not clinically affected. Neurogenic EMG changes are usually moderate.

Nerve biopsy is not specific and is not necessary for diagnosis, especially when there is a clear family history of the disease.

Cases of HMSN I are not uncommonly associated with tremor of the upper limbs and sometimes with some degree of ataxia. Such cases are probably identical with the Roussy–Levy syndrome (Lapresle and Salisachs 1973) and do not deserve individualization. HMSN I is clearly different clinically and genetically from Friedreich ataxia with which it is all too often confused but whose prognosis is completely different (Chapter 10), even though asymptomatic anomalies of visual and auditory evoked potentials have been reported in some cases (Carroll *et al.* 1983). Molecular genetic techniques can be used for the diagnosis of HMSN I, especially when a duplication is present. The main indication would be differentiation from chronic inflammatory neuropathy. In other cases, nerve biopsy and/or trial of steroid treatment may be warranted. Prenatal diagnosis is possible in principle, but the presence of a duplication does not enable one to predict the severity of the disorder. Approximately 20 per cent of cases have a significant disability but a similar proportion remain asymptomatic (Harding 1995).

HEREDITARY MOTOR AND SENSORY NEUROPATHY TYPE II (HMSN II)
HMSN II also produces a clinical picture consistent with the description of Charcot–Marie–Tooth disease. Its frequency in children is classically much lower than that of type I (Ouvrier *et al.* 1990, Ouvrier 1992). The high prevalence of the disease in Swedish children (Hagberg and Westerberg 1983) may be due to ethnic factors; however, the frequency of an asymptomatic or very mild form in young children makes the diagnosis difficult and may partly explain the discrepant figures.

PATHOLOGY
The pathology is characterized by the presence of signs of old axonal affectation without involvement of the myelin sheath or Schwann cell. Large-calibre fibres are reduced in number, and the internodes are shortened and of irregular length on teasing. Acute axonal lesions are rare and the pathological abnormalities may be inconspicuous. No onion bulbs are present.

CLINICAL FEATURES
The clinical manifestations are similar to those of HMSN I but with a later onset, during the second or third decade, and a slower course. Atrophy of posterior tibial and calf muscles is commonly as marked as in the anterolateral compartment (Harding 1995). Absent reflexes and foot deformity are less frequent than in type I, but foot ulcers may occur making these cases difficult to distinguish from hereditary sensory and autonomic neuropathy type I (see below) (Elliott *et al.* 1997). Sensory manifestations are difficult to demonstrate. There is no nerve hypertrophy and raised CSF protein is rare. Upper limb tremor is uncommon (Salisachs *et al.* 1979, Harding and Thomas 1980c, Westerberg *et al.* 1983).

Differentiation from type I is by electrophysiological investigation. Motor and sensory conduction velocities are normal or only mildly decreased to 60 per cent or more of normal values (Berciano *et al.* 1986). In patients over 2 years of age, a motor conduction velocity of greater than 38 m/s in the median nerve is compatible with the diagnosis of HMSN II, whereas values below 38 m/s are more in favour of HMSN I (Harding and Thomas 1980c).

HETEROGENEITY OF HMSN II

HMSN II is a heterogeneous group. In most kindreds, the disease is inherited as an autosomal dominant trait, mapping in some families to chromosome 1p35–p36 (Ben Othmane *et al.* 1993b) (CMT 2A) with a large number (60 per cent) of very mild or asymptomatic forms (Westerberg *et al.* 1983), and runs a mild course, only rarely leading to marked disability. Cases not mapping to 1p36—especially those that map to 3q—are termed CMT 2B, and a form with vocal cord paralysis (Dyck *et al.* 1994), in which no linkage has been found, is known as CMT 2C. Autosomal recessive forms are known. One of them maps to chromosome 8q (Ben Othmane *et al.* 1993b), although in other families this linkage has not been found. X-linked cases mapping to Xp22.2 are also on record. Ouvrier *et al.* (1981) have described 11 children with onset within the first five years of life and significant impairment with loss of ambulation before 12 years or age. In two kindreds, the disease was inherited as an autosomal recessive trait and in one as an autosomal dominant trait. Clinical features included rapid progression of weakness, usually to almost complete paralysis below the elbows and knees by the teens, and moderate sensory changes. Motor conduction velocities were unmeasurable in five patients because of absent motor response, but were over 35 m/s in all other patients. Gabreëls-Festen *et al.* (1991) reported 18 further cases, only one being dominantly transmitted. The association of glomerular nephropathy with HMSN type II seems to be a nonfortuitous association with a dominant inheritance (Deniau *et al.* 1986). Accumulation of neurofilaments has been found in one typical case (Vogel *et al.* 1985).

HEREDITARY MOTOR AND SENSORY NEUROPATHY TYPE III (HMSN III)

The terms HMSN III and Déjerine–Sottas disease are applied to a heterogeneous group of inherited or sporadic neuropathies (Ouvrier *et al.* 1987, 1990; Ouvrier 1992, Harding 1995) with various ages of onset and severity. There is no universal agreement as to the limits of this group especially with respect to the congenital types, and considerable genetic heterogeneity is being recognized in this group (Harding 1995). Mutations and deletions of the P_o and of the *PMP22* genes, homozygosity for the HMSN IA genotype with or without duplication, and homozygosity for the HMSN II abnormality have all been reported (Sghirlanzoni *et al.* 1992, Tyson *et al.* 1997), and the inheritance pattern is variable even for the same genetic defect (Ionasescu *et al.* 1997).

Pathologically, nerve alterations are reminiscent of those in type I but they are more intense. Onion bulbs are well formed and the ratio of the axon diameter over the onion bulb diameter is lower than in HMSN I (Ouvrier *et al.* 1987). These structures also include collagen fibres and there is massive interstitial collagen hypertrophy.

CLASSICAL PHENOTYPE

The most typical form (Ouvrier *et al.* 1987) has an early onset, and slow motor development and hypotonia are commonly present during the first year of life. Ambulation is delayed in 30–50 per cent of patients. Weakness is more profound and more diffuse than in type I cases and frequently involves severely the proximal muscles. Ataxia is consistently present and the weakness may be asymmetrical. Thickening and eversion of the upper limb is a common feature (Dyck 1984, Ouvrier *et al.* 1987). Pupillary abnormalities and even an Argyll Robertson pupil are occasionally observed. Tendon reflexes are abolished and nerve hypertrophy is frequent.

The course is often more severe than in the other forms, and loss of independent walking before adolescence may occur. However, some variability in expression may be present and the age of onset was widely different in the two patients originally reported by Déjerine and Sottas.

Nerve conduction velocities are severely diminished to below 10 m/s or even cannot be measured as no evoked muscle response can be obtained. Parents have no clinical signs or slowing of nerve conduction velocities, thus ruling out the possibility of a type I neuropathy, but EMG may reveal signs of mild neurogenic muscular involvement in some.

CONGENITAL NEUROPATHIES

The congenital hereditary neuropathies are usually considered as a form of HMSN III, although an early onset may also be observed in some type I cases (Hagberg and Lyon 1981, Vanasse and Dubowitz 1981, Harati and Butler 1985). They are also a heterogeneous group and no agreement has been reached regarding their nosological situation. Guzzetta *et al.* (1982) distinguished two groups of congenital cases. A severe form may resemble acute Werdnig–Hoffmann disease with congenital hypotonia and paralysis, wasting and respiratory impairment that may be lethal in a few months or years (Goebel *et al.* 1976) and is aggravated by swallowing difficulties. A raised CSF protein level is constant, and nerve conduction velocities are unmeasurable or extremely low. Less severe cases exist that permit survival for many years but with severe motor impairment. Some sensory impairment may be observed in the course of such cases.

The pathological picture in most cases is that of complete absence of myelin (amyelinic form) or *hypomyelination neuropathy* (Kennedy *et al.* 1977, Guzzetta *et al.* 1982) with formation of onion bulbs containing mainly layers of Schwann cells with little or no myelin. The pathological findings have been interpreted as indicating that the pathological process is one of deficient myelin deposition rather than one of demyelination–remyelination. In some cases, there is proliferation of neurofilaments in Schwann cells, along with demyelination (Ulrich *et al.* 1981). In others, unstable myelin with infolding of myelin lamellae has been described (Peudenier *et al.* 1993). Cases with congenital arthrogryposis have been reported (Boylan *et al.* 1992, Balestrini *et al.* 1991).

A special form of congenital neuropathy, with associated osseous fragility, mental retardation and CNS involvement has been reported in one family by Neimann *et al.* (1973). A second family with two affected siblings has been observed in our institution. Agenesis of the corpus callosum was present together with severe degenerative CNS lesions and an apparently axonal neuropathy. A case with brain dysfunction and opsoclonus is on record (Rust and Hichey 1990).

Johnson *et al.* (1989) have described central hypomyelination in association with hypomyelination polyneuropathy. The cases of relapsing axonal neuropathy reported in siblings by Quinlivan *et al.* (1994) are difficult to classify. Such cases may be difficult to distinguish from the rare infantile forms of Guillain–Barré syndrome.

UNCOMMON NEUROPATHIES WITH MOTOR AND SENSORY INVOLVEMENT

HEREDITARY NEUROPATHY WITH LIABILITY TO PRESSURE PALSIES (HNPP)

This is a rare, dominantly inherited disease, characterized by an abnormal susceptibility to pressure palsies (Behse *et al.* 1972), usually with evidence of an underlying generalized neuropathy with moderate slowing of nerve conduction velocities and prolonged distal motor and sensory latencies. In most cases the disease is due to a deletion of the region of chromosome 17 that is duplicated in cases of HMSN I (Mariman *et al.* 1994, Silander *et al.* 1994, Verhalle *et al.* 1994). This is probably the reciprocal of HMSN I duplication as a result of unequal crossing-over during meiosis.

Affected subjects may develop symptoms during the first decade, although a later onset is more usual. The paralyses usually involve a single nerve trunk, especially the popliteal nerve, following prolonged maintenance of attitudes such as squatting or sitting cross-legged, or the cubital nerve following pressure on the elbow. Paralysis also occurs following a brief, unusual effort such as intense physical activity, especially sport. Many patients develop a carpal tunnel syndrome of early onset, which may be clinically manifested but is present on electrophysiological examination in most cases.

Recovery from palsies is usually complete over a period of days to weeks, but in some cases permanent generalized motor and sensory neuropathy eventually develops. Dunn *et al.* (1978) noted brachial plexus involvement in some patients. Although this suggested a relationship to hereditary brachial plexopathy, the two conditions are genetically distinct (Chance *et al.* 1994, Gouider *et al.* 1994).

The diagnosis is suggested by the disproportion between minor trauma and the occurrence of paralysis. The frequent presence of a similar history in relatives is virtually diagnostic. Electrophysiological examination confirms the suspicion of an underlying neuropathy by showing slowed conduction velocities outside the affected territory. Examination of family members may demonstrate a neuropathy even in the absence of attacks. Nerve biopsy, which is not necessary in most cases, can show segmental thickenings of myelin sheaths known as tomaculas (Verhagen *et al.* 1993). Such findings have been found in definite cases of familial brachial plexus palsy (Martinelli *et al.* 1989) and

in one patient with a clinical picture of recurrent polyneuropathy (Joy and Oh 1989). HNPP is due to a deletion of the same area of chromosome 17p11.2 as is duplicated in CMT 1 cases (Mandich *et al.* 1995). Recent data (Tyson *et al.* 1996) indicate that the same DNA abnormalities may occasionally be found in cases of multifocal paralysis without pressure liability, thus widening the spectrum of the disease.

No treatment is known, but avoidance of repeated episodes that may leave sequelae may require changes in lifestyle.

HEREDITARY NEURALGIC AMYOTROPHY (BRACHIAL PLEXOPATHY)

This is also a dominantly transmitted condition. The onset is usually in the second decade but earlier onset can occur and brachial plexus paralyses at birth may be the first manifestation. Attacks closely resemble those observed in the nonhereditary type of plexopathy. Pain may be intense and precedes weakness usually by a few days. Weakness persists for variable periods. It is mainly proximal. Recovery takes place over a few weeks to months and is usually complete. The frequency of recurrences is extremely variable (Geiger *et al.* 1974, Arts *et al.* 1983, Airaksinen *et al.* 1985). Occasional patients may experience episodes of lumbar plexopathy (Awerbuch *et al.* 1989, Thomson 1993). In several families a particular kind of mild dysmorphism with a long face and hypotelorism is present in affected members (Dunn *et al.* 1978). In some cases, involvement may be limited to a single branch of the brachial plexus, *e.g.* the long thoracic nerve with isolated palsy of the serratus anterior (Philips 1986). The disease maps to chromosome 17q (Pellegrino *et al.* 1996).

Diagnosis with a sporadic brachial plexopathy is not possible at the first episode unless affected relatives are known and/or dysmorphism is present.

Treatment is purely symptomatic.

MISCELLANEOUS TYPES OF HEREDITARY DEGENERATIVE MOTOR AND SENSORY NEUROPATHIES

SCAPULOPERONEAL AMYOTROPHY OF NEURAL ORIGIN (DAWIDENKOW SYNDROME)

This is a rare cause of the scapuloperoneal syndrome (Chapter 22). Evidence of neural involvement and nerve hypertrophy enable linkage of such cases to the hereditary motor and sensory neuropathies, Both axonal and demyelinating forms exist (Hyser *et al.* 1988). Such cases are to be distinguished from those of spinal cord origin (De Long and Siddique 1992).

HMSN type IV, better known as Refsum disease, and other metabolic neuropathies are described below. For a more complete description of the rare types, see Ouvrier *et al.* (1990).

THERMOSENSITIVE NEUROPATHY

Magy *et al.* (1997) reported on a remarkable family with intermittent episodes of extensive paralysis precipitated by body temperature elevations above 38.5°C with onset in childhood or adolescence and not allelic to CMT 1 or hereditary pressure-sensitive neuropathy.

TABLE 21.2
The various types of hereditary sensory neuropathy (HSN)

	HSN I	HSN II	HSN III	HSN IV	HSN V	Congenital sensory neuropathy with skeletal dysplasia (Axelrod et al. 1983b)	Progressive pan-neuropathy with hypotonia (Orbeck and Ofedal 1977)	Congenital autonomic dysfunction with universal pain loss (Axelrod et al. 1983a)	Sensory + autonomic neuropathy X-linked (Jestico et al. 1985)	Hereditary sensory neuropathy with spastic paraplegia (Cavanagh et al. 1979)
Inheritance*	AD	AR	AR	AR	?	?	?	AR?	XR	AR?
Insensitivity to pain	++ Localized	++ Diffuse	+ Diffuse	++ ± Diffuse	++ Localized	+	++ (Self-mutilation)	++ Localized	++	
Deep tendon reflexes	Absent	Absent	Often absent	N		Absent	N	+		
Objective sensory loss	+	++	+	++	++				+	
Muscle hypotonia	Absent	Absent	+	Absent	Absent	+	++	++		
Fungiform papillae of tongue	Present	Present	Absent	Present		Absent				
Hypohidrosis/anhidrosis	Absent	Absent		++		Hyperhidrosis	Hyperhidrosis	Absent		
Histamine flare	Present	May be present	Absent	Absent		Absent		Absent		
Mecholyl-induced miosis	Absent	Absent	Present	Present			Present		?	Absent
Overflow tears	Present	Present	Absent	Present		Sparse	Present	+	Absent	
Blood pressure		N	Low[1]	N						
Blotching	Absent		Present	+					Absent	Absent
Oesophageal + gastrointestinal involvement	Absent	Sometimes	++	Absent				+		
Mental retardation	Absent	±	±	++	±				+	Absent
Motor nerve conduction velocity	N	N	N	N or decreased	N					Absent
Sensory nerve conduction velocity	Low/absent	Low/absent	Low/absent	Low/absent	N					N
Skeletal dysplasia	Absent	Absent	Absent			+			Frontal bone prominence	Absent

Key to symbols: + mild; ++ moderate/severe; ± some cases only; N = normal.
*AD = autosomal dominant; AR = autosomal recessive; XR = X-linked recessive.
[1]Orthostatic hypotension.

HEREDITARY SENSORY AND AUTONOMIC NEUROPATHIES

Inherited peripheral sensory neuropathies are rare and their definitive diagnosis is difficult. Controversy over terminology confuses their classification (Axelrod and Pearson 1984), and some diagnostic tests may not be easily available outside specialized centres. Dyck (1984) has proposed a classification into four types to which rare forms have been added by other investigators (Table 21.2).

HEREDITARY SENSORY AND AUTONOMIC NEUROPATHY TYPE I (HSAN I), SENSORY RADICULAR NEUROPATHY, *ACROPATHIE ULCEROMUTILANTE*

HSAN I differs from all other HSANs in that the symptoms appear late rather than congenitally. The transmission is autosomal dominant, the gene mapping to 9q22.1–q22.3 (Nicholson *et al.* 1996). Pathological examination shows a marked reduction in the number of unmyelinated fibres. Small myelinated fibres are decreased to a smaller extent and large myelinated fibres are hardly or not affected (Dyck 1984). The dorsal root ganglia and the spinal dorsal roots supplying the lower limbs are degenerated. Symptoms appear in late childhood or adolescence with a progressive loss of sensation in the lower extremities, rapidly complicated by episodes of cellulitis and trophic ulcerations of the feet. Spontaneous stabbing pain may occur. There is loss of pain and temperature sensation with preservation of tactile sensation. Later, all sensation may disappear and the distal upper limbs may become involved. Neural deafness is frequently present (Horoupian 1989). Nerve conduction velocity and EMG are not changed. The course is slowly progressive. HSAN I may be heterogeneous. A form with early-onset dementia is on record (Wright and Dyck 1995).

HEREDITARY SENSORY AND AUTONOMIC NEUROPATHY TYPE II (HSAN II), CONGENITAL SENSORY NEUROPATHY

This is an autosomal recessive condition with a congenital or early onset. Nerve biopsy often shows grossly atrophic nerves. Myelinated axons are severely reduced in number but unmyelinated fibres are usually normal or at least not greatly diminished. Clinically, most patients have a universal absence of pain sensation resulting in burns and mutilations of the lips or fingertips and in painless fractures, especially of the metatarsals. Areas of normal sensation are preserved in some patients in whom the limbs and face are predominantly affected (Dyck 1984). Bladder sensation may be impaired with vesical distension (Verity *et al.* 1982). Deafness has been described in some patients (Verity *et al.* 1982). In most patients, the disease does not seem progressive or is only very slowly evolving (Ferrière *et al.* 1992). Some cases may run a faster course with clinical evidence of progression (Johnson and Spalding 1964) which is in agreement with nerve biopsy findings of fibre degeneration and regeneration. Motor conduction velocities are preserved but sensory velocities are unobtainable.

Cortical evoked somatosensory potentials were lacking in the lower limbs in some patients.

HEREDITARY SENSORY AND AUTONOMIC NEUROPATHY TYPE III (HSAN III), FAMILIAL DYSAUTONOMIA, RILEY–DAY SYNDROME

HSAN III is the most common of the sensory and autonomic neuropathies. The disorder is prevalent among Ashkenazi Jews in whom the disease frequency is between 0.5 and 1 per 10,000 live births with an estimated carrier frequency of 1 in 50. Scattered case reports on non-Jewish patients can be found (*e.g.* Guzzetta *et al.* 1986). The disorder is transmitted as an autosomal recessive trait and maps to chromosome 9q31–q33.

Histopathological findings include loss of neurons in the posterior root, Lissauer tract and intermediolateral grey columns (Pearson and Pytel 1978) and loss of unmyelinated and myelinated fibres in peripheral nerves where catecholamine endings are lacking (Pearson *et al.* 1974). Substance P-immune reactivity in the substantia gelatinosa of the spinal cord and in the medulla is consistently depleted (Pearson *et al.* 1982). Sympathetic ganglia are hypoplastic.

Clinical manifestations are mainly referable to the autonomic nervous system. Onset is congenital, and hypotonia, sucking difficulties, a poor cry and vomiting are present from birth. Growth retardation becomes evident later in life. Patients do not have overflow tears. Skin blotching, motor incoordination, unstable temperature and blood pressure, cyclic vomiting and drooling are variably present. Relative indifference to pain is usual (Axelrod *et al.* 1981). Bouts of apnoea and pneumonia are common and are a usual cause of death in infancy and childhood. Oesophageal dilatation and impaired gastric motility are frequent findings. Postural hypotension is almost always present. Scoliosis is a major problem.

Diagnostic criteria include the absence of fungiform papillae on the tongue, diminished or absent deep tendon reflexes, lack of overflow tears, miosis following instillation of 2.5% metacholine chloride in the eyes, and lack of an axon flare after intradermal histamine injection (Axelrod *et al.* 1974). None of these criteria is individually characteristic, and any of them can be found in other sensory neuropathies. Prenatal diagnosis is possible by studying closely located markers (Blumenfeld *et al.* 1993, Eng *et al.* 1995).

The *course* of familial dysautonomia is severe; in the early studies in the 1960s only 20 per cent of patients survived to adulthood, although by the 1980s due to improvements in management this proportion had risen to 50 per cent (Axelrod and Abularrage 1982). Digestive and respiratory complications are common and may be aggravated by the frequent occurrence of kyphoscoliosis. Emotional lability with repeated severe breath-holding spells is common. Intelligence remains normal.

Treatment is symptomatic. The risk of aspiration pneumonia should be minimized by attention to posture and by meticulous precautions during feeding that may necessitate gavage or even gastrostomy or fundoplication. Diazepam is effective in association with chlorpromazine for the treatment of acute crises and

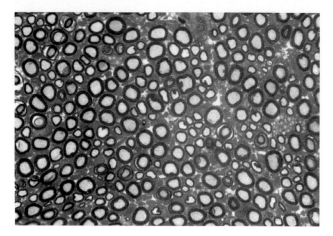

Fig. 21.4. Hereditary sensory neuropathy type IV. There is almost complete absence of small unmyelinated fibres.

of hypertension. Families of affected children need considerable psychological support.

HEREDITARY SENSORY AND AUTONOMIC NEUROPATHY TYPE IV (HSAN IV), CONGENITAL INSENSITIVITY TO PAIN AND ANHIDROSIS

In this rare disorder, there is virtual absence of unmyelinated nerve fibres in peripheral nerves (Goebel *et al.* 1980) (Fig. 21.4). The Lissauer tract and dorsal spinal roots are also affected.

The onset of the disease is congenital with episodes of unexplained fever often related to environmental temperature. Absence of sweating (anhidrosis) is an essential feature. Insensitivity to pain is universal and leads to injuries, self-mutilation and osteomyelitis, especially of the lower extremities. Tongue-biting is frequent. Blotching of the skin and pupillary hypersensitivity to metacholine chloride occur (Axelrod and Pearson 1984). Mental retardation is the rule. Motor nerve conduction velocity may be slowed. A mild form without anhidrosis has been reported by Pavone *et al.* (1992).

OTHER FORMS OF HEREDITARY SENSORY AND AUTONOMIC NEUROPATHY AND INSENSITIVITY OR INDIFFERENCE TO PAIN

Several rare and/or controversial types of HSAN have been described and are shown in Table 21.3.

Hereditary sensory and autonomic neuropathy type V presents as a congenital indifference to pain (Dyck 1984) and is characterized pathologically by an almost complete disappearance of small fibres and a moderate decrease of unmyelinated fibres.

Additional types include HSAN with growth hormone deficiency (Liberfarb *et al.* 1993), progressive panneuropathy with hypotension (Axelrod and Pearson 1984), HSAN type II without trophic changes (Bye *et al.* 1990), HSAN with neurotrophic keratitis (Donaghy *et al.* 1987), and HSAN with cataracts, mental retardation and skin lesions (Heckmann *et al.* 1995). HSAN associated with spastic paraplegia includes two distinct types, one affecting mainly the small sensory fibres (Cavanagh *et*

TABLE 21.3
Metabolic and degenerative CNS disorders in which a peripheral neuropathy may occur

Disease	References
Sulfatidosis (metachromatic leukodystrophy)	Bardosi *et al.* (1987)
Krabbe leukodystrophy	Tada *et al.* (1992)
Adrenomyeloneuropathy	Powers (1985)
Cockayne syndrome	Grunnet *et al.* (1983)
Leigh disease	Jacobs *et al.* (1990), Chabrol *et al.* (1994)
Mitochondrial diseases, especially NARP	Rusanen *et al.* (1995)
Carbohydrate-deficient glycoprotein (CDG) syndrome	Jaeken and Carchon (1993)
Bassen–Korzweig disease (abetalipoproteinaemia)	Wichman *et al.* (1985), Brin *et al.* (1986)
Hypobetalipoproteinaemia	Brown *et al.* (1974), Matsuo *et al.* (1994)
Tangier disease	Pollock *et al.* (1983)
Niemann–Pick A disease	Gumbinas *et al.* (1975)
Cerebrotendinous xanthomatosis	Donaghy *et al.* (1990), Tokimura *et al.* (1992)
Refsum disease (adult and infantile forms)	Skjeldal *et al.* (1987), Dickson *et al.* (1989)
GM2 gangliosidosis	Specola *et al.* (1990)
Farber disease	Vital *et al.* (1976)
Chediak–Higashi disease	Lockman *et al.* (1967)
Peroxisomal diseases	MacCollin *et al.* (1990)
Adrenal insufficiency, achalasia and alachrymia	Tsao *et al.* (1994)
Ataxia–telangiectasia	Kwast and Ignatowicz (1990)
Xeroderma pigmentosum	Mimaki *et al.* (1986), Tachi *et al.* (1988)
Lowe syndrome	Charnas *et al.* (1988)
Polyneuropathy, ophthalmoplegia, chronic intestinal pseudo-obstruction and leukoencephalopathy	Simon *et al.* (1990)
Trichothiodystrophy	Personal cases
Vitamin E deficiency or abnormal metabolism	Burck *et al.* (1981), Harding *et al.* (1985), Stumpf *et al.* (1987)
Vitamin B$_1$, B$_6$, B$_{12}$ and folate deficiency	Chapter 23
Vitamin B$_{12}$ deficiency or abnormal metabolism	Steiner *et al.* (1988)
Amyloidosis	Benson (1995)
Porphyria	Becker and Kramer (1977)
Mitochondrial diseases	Yiannikas *et al.* (1986)

al. 1979), the other involving the large fibres with few neuropathic symptoms (Schady and Smith 1994).

Cases of sensory polyneuropathy associated with CNS involvement are on record (Cilio *et al.* 1997), with autonomic dysfunction, microcephaly and agenesis of the corpus callosum in one case.

Some cases of sensory neuropathy can simulate child abuse (Makari *et al.* 1994).

The term *insensitivity to pain* in principle applies to patients in whom analgesia is the result of abnormalities of peripheral nerves, cutaneous nerve endings or central sensory pathways, whereas indifference to pain applies to those who have normal sensory pathways but fail to appreciate the painful nature of stimuli (Manfredi *et al.* 1981). Such a distinction may well be artificial, and Dyck *et al.* have emphasized the fact that precise analysis of cases of indifference to pain shows abnormalities of the peripheral sensory system when sophisticated methods are used (Dyck *et al.* 1983b). However, a case with normal morphometric nerve study has been reported (Landrieu *et al.* 1990). The differential diagnosis of such cases is discussed by Gorke (1981).

MISCELLANEOUS SENSORY AND AUTONOMIC NEUROPATHIES
Rare cases of *involvement of the autonomic nervous system* are marked by pain. A familial syndrome of paroxysmal rectal pain of early onset, associated with unilateral or bilateral vasodilatation of the lower limbs and abdomen and often precipitated by defaecation has been described (Hayden and Grossman 1959). Later, ocular and submaxillary pain may appear. Although Schubert and Gracco (1992) proposed considering it as a form of epilepsy, a peripheral origin seems indisputable (Singman *et al.* 1990). I have seen a similar sporadic case in which rectal pain induced repeated syncopes, severe submaxillary pain developing later. Treatment with carbamazepine is effective.

A polyneuropathy of variable severity with demyelination and interstitial fibrosis has been reported in association with chronic intestinal pseudo-obstruction and often ophthalmoplegia. The condition appears to be familial (Steiner *et al.* 1987). A leukoencephalopathy has been shown by MRI in similar cases for which the acronym 'POLIP' (*p*olyneuropathy, *o*phthalmoplegia, *l*eukoencephalopathy and *i*ntestinal *p*seudo-obstruction) has been proposed (Simon *et al.* 1990). Some such cases were recently shown to be associated with cytochrome *c* oxidase deficit in muscle biopsy samples (Lerman-Sagie *et al.* 1997).

The *restless legs syndrome*, which is a special type of sensory neuropathy frequent in adults, also exists in children. Walters *et al.* (1994) reported five cases. The related syndrome of periodic limb movements in sleep has its onset before 10 years in 20 per cent of cases.

COMPLEX NEUROPATHIES ASSOCIATED WITH CNS INVOLVEMENT AND METABOLIC NEUROPATHIES

Hereditary neuropathies may constitute a part of more complex neurological diseases (see Table 21.3) involving the CNS. Friedreich ataxia, a common cause of neuropathy with CNS involvement, is reviewed in Chapter 10.

HEREDITARY MOTOR AND SENSORY NEUROPATHIES WITH CNS INVOLVEMENT
Rare types of HMSN include affectation of the optic pathways and retina and, sometimes, more widespread disturbances. HMSN type V features pyramidal tract signs associated with a motor and sensory neuropathy. There is no clinical spasticity (Harding and Thomas 1984, Frith *et al.* 1994). Dyck (1984) recognizes type VI HMSN associated with optic atrophy, type VII

with deafness (Satya-Murti *et al.* 1979), and type VIII with pigmentary retinopathy. The neuropathy in type VI is mainly sensory and the condition is heterogeneous (Ippel *et al.* 1995, Chalmers *et al.* 1996). Some cases of HMSN VI also feature mental retardation and pyramidal signs (McDermot and Walker 1987). The latter have been reported also by Pagès and Pagès (1983) in association with Leber optic atrophy. Sommer and Schröder (1989) indicate that in such cases the neuropathy is axonal in type and represents a distinct form. HMSN VII has been described in association with protanopia (Khoubesserian *et al.* 1979). Polyneuropathy can also be associated with opticoacoustic degeneration (Rosenberg and Chutorian 1967) and with neural deafness (Pinhas-Hamiel *et al.* 1993) and palmar–plantar keratosis (Ouvrier 1992). Wright and Dyck (1995) described early-onset dementia and deafness in association with HMSN I. Axonal neuropathy associated with juvenile parkinsonism and ophthalmoplegia is on record (van der Wiel and Staal 1981).

GIANT AXONAL NEUROPATHY
This condition is characterized pathologically by the presence of massive axonal enlargements filled with neurofilaments. Normal sized axons may be demyelinated and show 'onion bulb' structures. The disease probably represents a disorder of cytoplasmic microfilament formation affecting both the peripheral and central nervous system (Treiber-Held *et al.* 1994). It is transmitted as an autosomal recessive trait.

The onset is in the first year of life with motor deficit and areflexia. Orthopaedic deformities include scoliosis and deformed feet. Sensory abnormalities are sometimes present (Maia *et al.* 1988, Ouvrier 1989). Cranial nerves may be involved, and variable mental retardation is the rule. System degenerations may be associated (Ben Hamida *et al.* 1990), and diffuse involvement with endocrinological abnormalities has been reported (Takebe *et al.* 1981). Nerve conduction velocities are sometimes slowed. The EEG is often disorganized with spike discharges, and brainstem auditory evoked potentials are altered. A high signal from white matter on T_2 sequences may be present. One remarkable feature is the presence of 'frizzy' hair, although this is inconstant (seven of 37 reviewed cases) (Treiber-Held *et al.* 1994). The course is progressive with increasing disability, and no treatment is known.

REFSUM DISEASE, HEREDITARY MOTOR AND SENSORY NEUROPATHY TYPE IV (HMSN IV), HEREDOPATHIA ATACTICA POLYNEURITIFORMIS
Classical Refsum disease is rare in childhood, although some manifestations of the condition may appear early or even be congenital, *e.g.* bone deformities, especially short metatarsals (Skjeldal *et al.* 1987). Although Dyck classified Refsum disease as type IV of the hereditary motor and sensory neuropathies, the condition deserves a special place because of its well-established metabolic disturbance, its remarkable symptomatology and its partially treatable nature. The disease is caused by an abnormal accumulation of phytanic acid (a C16 branched-chain fatty acid)

whose beta-oxidation is blocked due to phytanic oxidase deficiency. Most phytanic acid is of exogenous origin so that reduction of intake, sometimes in association with plasma exchanges (Gibberd *et al.* 1985, Dickson *et al.* 1989), results in lowering of abnormally high plasma levels when patients are placed on a phytol-free diet (Chapter 9). This change is accompanied by increased nerve conduction velocity, return of reflexes and sensory and motor improvement. Plasmapheresis is often used at onset of treatment to deplete the accumulated phytanic acid.

The clinical manifestations of Refsum disease usually begin after 4–7 years of age but are often recognized much later as the progression of the disorder is slow. A few patients have presented in infancy with neurological features (Herbert and Clayton 1994). The picture is one of partial and intermittent peripheral neuropathy but the clinical expression is very variable (Skjeldal *et al.* 1987). Ataxia is often marked. Atypical retinitis pigmentosa is present and hemeralopia may be the first symptom. Anosmia, deafness, ichthyosis and disorders of cardiac function are common. The CSF protein level is >1 g/L but there is no excess of cells. The diagnosis can be confirmed by measurement of plasma level of phytanic acid which is considerably increased (300–1600 µmol/L instead of <10 µmol/L; 10–50 mg/dL vs <0.3 mg/dL).

OTHER NEUROPATHIES WITH KNOWN METABOLIC ABNORMALITY

A number of metabolic diseases feature a neuropathy which may be overshadowed by other neurological or systemic manifestations but may occasionally be the predominant or presenting feature. The main disorders in this group are shown in Table 21.3 and studied in Chapter 9.

In some cases of *metachromatic leukodystrophy*, involvement of the peripheral nerves may be the only manifestation for periods of up to several months. Neuropathy with absence of deep tendon reflexes is common in Krabbe disease and has been reported in sialidosis type 1 (Steinman *et al.* 1980).

Neuropathy due to *inherited disorders of porphyrin metabolism* is rare in childhood. It can be observed with four diseases: variegate porphyria due to deficiency of protoporphyrinogen oxidase, acute intermittent porphyria due to deficiency of porphobilinogen deaminase (mapping on chromosome 11q23–11qter), hereditary coproporphyrinuria due to deficient coproporphyrin oxidase and delta-aminolaevulinic aciduria. These diseases are transmitted as autosomal dominant traits with variable penetrance. Prepubertal cases may occur. The symptoms and signs are similar to those in adult patients and are similar in the three types, except for the presence of photosensitivity in variegate porphyria and coproporphyria. The polyneuropathy can involve both the lower and the upper limbs. The weakness is both proximal and distal and may involve the respiratory muscles. Sensory involvement is minimal. Acute attacks of colicky abdominal pain, dysautonomic signs such as hypertension, and psychiatric disturbances may be observed. Bouts of paralysis are often precipitated by administration of drugs, especially barbiturates but also several antibiotics, oral contraceptives, oestrogens, imipramine and methyldopa among others (Crimlisk 1997). Convulsions

may be more frequent in children than in adults (Houston *et al.* 1977) and this is of considerable importance as antiepileptic agents including phenytoin, carbamazepine, ethosuximide and sodium valproate can trigger attacks. Paraldehyde and chloral hydrate can be safely used, and so far no toxicity has been reported with diazepam, clonazepam (Suzuki *et al.* 1992), gabapentin (Tatum and Zachariah 1995) and magnesium sulfate (Sadeh *et al.* 1991).

The diagnosis is confirmed by the finding of an increased urinary excretion of porphobilinogen and delta-aminolaevulinic acid. Between attacks, excretion of these compounds may be absent. Assay of erythrocyte porphobilinogen deaminase is the most accurate way of detecting acute intermittent porphyria, often resulting in a red discoloration of urine.

Treatment includes prevention of attacks by avoidance of precipitating drugs. During attacks, intravenous administration of glucose up to 100 g/d is indicated. If there is no improvement in 48 hours, intravenous haematin (2 mg/kg/d) should be given (Lamon *et al.* 1979). Side-effects (thrombophlebitis, coagulopathy) are frequent. Haem arginate (Crimlisk 1997) seems both effective and well tolerated. Avoidance of skin trauma and light is important only in variegate porphyria in which transient polyneuritis is accompanied by increased skin sensitivity.

Abetalipoproteinaemia (Bassen–Kornzweig disease) is an autosomal recessive disorder of the synthesis of the beta-apoprotein. As a consequence, fat absorption is deficient. Apparently, lipids are not transported from the intestinal mucosal cells into the lymphatic system, because beta-lipoproteins are necessary for the formation of chylomicrons. Fat-soluble vitamins are also poorly absorbed, and levels of vitamins A and E in the serum are quite low (Wichman *et al.* 1985, Kane and Havel 1995).

Neurological symptoms are the result of the deficit in vitamin E, resulting in peroxidation of the unsaturated myelin phospholipids.

Pathologically, there is extensive demyelination of the posterior columns and spinocerebellar tracts with severe depletion and segmental demyelination of large myelinated fibres in peripheral nerves and posterior roots. Involvement of the anterior horn cells and cerebellar cortex has been reported (Kane and Havel 1995).

The neurological picture is one of spinocerebellar degeneration with progressive ataxia, loss of tendon reflexes, disturbances of deep sensation and pes cavus in association with pigmentary retinal degeneration that gives rise to decreased visual acuity and night blindness. Paralysis of vertical gaze is a frequent feature. Muscle weakness and atrophy may supervene. Indeed, the picture is highly suggestive of a primary spinocerebellar degeneration and it is likely that many cases reported as Friedreich ataxia with retinitis pigmentosa were in fact cases of abetalipoproteinaemia.

Neurological manifestations may appear as early as 2 years of age, and one-third of patients are symptomatic by 10 years. About the same proportion of patients have mental retardation. A history of coeliac syndrome during the first year of life with foul, bulky stools and abdominal distension is usually obtained, and most children exhibit growth retardation.

The diagnosis rests on the presence of retinal lesion with an extinguished ERG, on the finding of a low serum cholesterol level, on the presence of acanthocytosis on blood smears, and ultimately on the absence of beta-lipoproteins. Electromyography shows denervation, and conduction velocities are diminished.

Abetalipoproteinaemia is a treatable condition, and supplementation of the diet with high-dose vitamin E (100 mg/kg/d orally) prevents the development or progression of eye and nervous disease (Kane and Havel 1995). Intramuscular vitamin E is not superior. Administration of vitamin A (200–400 IU/kg/d) and vitamin K₁ (5 mg every two weeks) is also advised.

Acanthocytosis is also observed in another dominantly inherited condition, known as *amyotrophic choreoacanthocytosis*, which includes symptoms of basal ganglia dysfunction, peripheral nerve involvement and other neurological features but is observed mostly in adults (Spencer *et al.* 1987), and in Hallervorden–Spatz disease (Chapter 10).

Hypobetalipoproteinaemia is a condition distinct from abetalipoproteinaemia (Mawatari *et al.* 1972) which may produce acanthocytosis and neurological manifestations. These are usually limited to loss of deep tendon reflexes. Occasional cases may feature ataxia, hearing loss and retinitis pigmentosa (Matsuo *et al.* 1994).

Vitamin E deficiency may be due, in addition to absence of betalipoproteins, to biliary insufficiency that prevents normal emulsion of fat in the bowel lumen and results in poor absorption, in association with steatorrhoea (Guggenheim *et al.* 1982, Harding *et al.* 1982). A similar result has been observed in a case of intestinal lymphangiectasia (Gutmann *et al.* 1986). The clinical picture, indistinguishable from that observed with abetalipoproteinaemia, is observed in children with chronic liver disease, especially ductular hypoplasia (Sokol *et al.* 1985). The condition is amenable to the same therapy as abetalipoproteinaemia.

Rare cases of a similar syndrome mimicking spinocerebellar degeneration have been described in children without liver disease or apparent fat malabsorption (Burck *et al.* 1981, Harding *et al.* 1985, Stumpf *et al.* 1987). This disorder is relatively frequent in Tunisia and has been shown to map to chromosome 8 (Ben Hamida *et al.* 1993). For unknown reasons, these patients had a normal retina, as did the one patient I have seen with this condition. The disorder results from genetically determined absence of the alpha-tocopherol transfer protein (Gotada *et al.* 1995, Hentati *et al.* 1996).

Tangier disease is a rare condition characterized by a decrease of high-density lipoproteins and a low cholesterol level. Accumulation of cholesterol esters in Schwann cells produces a sensorimotor neuropathy that often remains subclinical.

Neuropathies are a major manifestation of the various types of amyloidosis but this condition is exceptional before adulthood (Scelsi *et al.* 1989, Benson 1995).

Several *mitochondrial disorders* can cause a neuropathy. These include the MELAS (*m*itochondrial *e*ncephalomyopathy, *l*actic *a*cidosis and *s*troke-like episodes) and NARP (*n*europathy, *a*taxia, *r*etinitis *p*igmentosa) syndromes as well as cases of Leigh syndrome (Goebel *et al.* 1986, Jacobs *et al.* 1990, Chabrol *et al.*

1994) and other rare mitochondrial diseases (Hagberg 1990, Rusanen *et al.* 1995).

A neuropathy is also a frequent feature of the carbohydrate-deficient glycoprotein syndrome (Jaeken and Carchon 1993).

Vitamin deficiencies in association with poorly defined other nutritional factors is a major cause of endemic neuropathy in several developing countries (Chapter 23).

COMPLEX NEUROPATHIES OF OBSCURE ORIGIN
Large series of polyneuropathies in children include a variable proportion of unclassifiable cases that usually feature both peripheral and CNS involvement. This was the case in 16 of 61 patients of Evans (1979) who received a diagnosis of undefined 'degenerative disorder' or of 'spinocerebellar degeneration'.

ACQUIRED DIFFUSE NEUROPATHIES

Acquired neuropathies are most often inflammatory in origin but various toxins and undetermined processes may also cause them.

Inflammatory disorders of the peripheral nervous system include two groups of diffuse diseases: the acute polyneuropathies, also termed polyradiculoneuritis, and the much less common chronic progressive polyneuropathies. Localized inflammatory neuropathies are relatively common although their mechanisms are poorly known.

ACUTE INFLAMMATORY NEUROPATHY, ACUTE POLYRADICULONEURITIS, GUILLAIN–BARRÉ SYNDROME AND RELATED DISORDERS
The Guillain–Barré syndrome (GBS) is an acute demyelinating disease of peripheral nerves characterized clinically by progressive weakness that usually appears a few days after a viral illness or immunization. The nature of the relationship between nerve dysfunction and infection is not well understood but an immunological mechanism apparently plays an important role.

PATHOLOGY
GBS is characterized by the presence of inflammatory lesions scattered throughout the peripheral nervous system from the anterior and posterior roots to distal twigs (Prineas 1981). The lesions consist of circumscribed areas of myelin loss associated with the presence of lymphocytes and macrophages. The initial site of lesions is at the Ranvier node. Myelin damage is produced mainly by macrophages that penetrate the basement membrane around nerve fibres and strip myelin away from the axon and the body of Schwann cells. Interruption of the axons with subsequent wallerian degeneration is present only in the most severe cases with intense inflammation. In a minority of cases, macrophage-associated demyelination occurs despite a paucity of lymphocytes. These cases may be due to the action of an antibody rather than a T-cell autoimmune process (Honavar *et al.* 1991). Proliferation of Schwann cells occurs later in the disease, probably as a first step in the remyelination process. However, the concept of GBS as a primarily demyelinating neuropathy has been recently challenged

by the discovery of clinically similar cases with severe and probably primary axonal damage (Feasby et al. 1986, McKhann et al. 1993), suggesting the likelihood of two different mechanisms (Thomas 1992, Feasby et al. 1993).

PATHOGENESIS
The pathological changes seen in GBS resemble those of acute allergic neuritis produced in experimental animals by immunization with homogenates of peripheral nerves or, more specifically, with a peptide of the myelin basic protein (peptide P2). In humans, the immunological mechanisms are still unclear and the respective roles of humoural and cellular factors are still in debate. Although lymphocytes from GBS patients may be sensitized to peripheral nerve proteins, several studies have failed to confirm an elevation of anti-P2 antimyelin antibody titres (Iqbal et al. 1981), suggesting that this may not be the actual antigen.

Humoral factors are probably important. Intraneural injection of sera from GBS patients produces demyelination in animals (Feasby et al. 1982). Antimyelin antibodies have been demonstrated in GBS patients by fixation of the C1 component of complement and are especially high at onset of the disease (Koski et al. 1986). However, attempts at fractionation and characterization of the active components have so far failed. Similarly, no antibodies have been regularly found in nerve biopsies and no circulating immune complexes have been detected (Pollard et al. 1987). Activated complement components C3a and C5a have been found in CSF (Hartung et al. 1987). High titres of antibodies against gangliosides GM1 and GD1b are found in a high proportion of cases, especially those associated with *Campylobacter* infection (Gregson et al. 1993, Kuroki et al. 1993, Vriesendarp et al. 1993). The antibodies are of various serotypes, probably indicating heterogeneity in the aetiology of GBS. The most attractive hypothesis remains that a pathogenic agent may damage the Schwann cell with release of Schwann cell antigens triggering a cascade of events leading to segmental demyelination which, in turn, is responsible for *multiple conduction blocks* (Sumner 1981) which are the elecrophysiological basis of the clinical manifestations of GBS.

EPIDEMIOLOGY
GBS occurs usually in children over 3–4 years of age but cases of early and even neonatal onset (Al-Qudah et al. 1988) are on record. The overall frequency of GBS is 1.9 cases per 100,000 population (Larsen et al. 1985). The disease usually follows infection or immunization by two to four weeks (Jones 1996). Among the identified viral agents, herpes viruses (cytomegalovirus, Epstein–Barr virus) have been frequently indicted (Dowling and Cook 1981), and immunization against rabies (Hemachuda et al. 1988) and against influenza (Poser and Behan 1982) have received considerable attention. Other viral agents such as that of non-A, non-B hepatitis (MacLeod 1987, De Klippel et al. 1993) and varicella-zoster virus (Sanders et al. 1987) are less frequently found, and a firm connection has been established only with CMV and EB viruses (Jones 1996). Poliovirus infection is not a cause (Rantala et al. 1994). *Campylobacter jejuni* infection,

often with diarrhoea, is the most common infection preceding GBS and, even more so, the Miller Fisher variant (Kohler et al. 1988, Ropper 1988, Kinnunen et al. 1989, Kuroki et al. 1993, Vriesendorp et al. 1993, Rees et al. 1995, Jones 1996). In 100 patients studied by Winer et al. (1988), 38 per cent had had respiratory symptoms and 17 per cent gastrointestinal symptoms. Serological evidence of *C. jejuni* (14 per cent) and CMV (11 per cent) infection was significantly more frequent in patients than in controls.

CLINICAL FEATURES
The onset of GBS is usually fairly sudden with weakness generally affecting the lower limbs. The paralyses then follow an ascending course. Paralysis is generalized in half the cases, predominates in the distal parts of the limbs in 30 per cent, and is symmetrical, although minor differences are not uncommon and gross asymmetry has been reported in rare patients (Jones 1996). Predominantly proximal involvement is present in 20 per cent of the patients. The facial nerve is involved in 50 per cent of cases, often bilaterally (Hung et al. 1994). Ophthalmoplegia occurs in 3 per cent of cases (Dehaene et al. 1986). Optic neuritis is uncommon (Nikoskelainen and Riekkinen 1972, Behan et al. 1976). Papilloedema may also be associated with increased intracranial pressure (Morley and Reynolds 1966), but although altered consciousness is not rare, objective evidence of CNS involvement is highly unusual (Willis and van den Bergh 1988). Sensory symptoms are present in about half the cases. Pain is often a prominent feature at onset, while paraesthesiae are inconspicuous and hypoaesthesiae present only in a minority of older children. Deep tendon reflexes are abolished early in 83 per cent of cases, even in nonparalytic territories (Winer et al. 1988) Plantar responses are flexor. Loss of deep sensation is frequently found at examination.

Paralysis of the respiratory muscles is a common complication of GBS and often requires respirator treatment (Ropper 1992). Mild respiratory impairment is even more frequent with resulting hypercarbia. Autonomic involvement is present in many patients and may be responsible for hypotension, hypertension, cardiac arrhythmia and even cardiac arrest (Winer et al. 1988). CNS manifestations were found in five of 24 patients of Bradshaw and Jones (1992). Urinary retention or overflow incontinence may be present in up to 10 per cent of cases. Ataxia of probable sensory mechanism is not uncommon and a Babinski response may be seen (Jones 1996).

The CSF is most often normal during the first days of the illness. Elevation of CSF protein appears between two and 15 days and reaches a peak by four to five weeks after clinical onset. The CSF total protein concentration and the IgG percentage seem to depend mainly on the degree of blood–brain barrier damage, which in turn correlates with the clinical course. Oligoclonal IgGs are frequently present in the CSF but come essentially from serum. Oligoclonal IgG banding in GBS is transitory and correlates with the development of blood–brain barrier damage, the presence of cranial nerve involvement and the severity of the disease (Segurado et al. 1986). In occasional cases, the CSF protein may remain normal (Sullivan and Reeves 1977). In contrast to protein, cell content of CSF remains normal in GBS, the classical albuminocytological dissociation with fewer than 10 cells/mm³. The presence of more than 50 mononuclear leukocytes/mm³ should cast doubt on the diagnosis (Asbury *et al.* 1978, Asbury and Cornblath 1990), but a lesser number of cells is acceptable and has no prognostic value.

ELECTROPHYSIOLOGY

Electrophysiological studies (McLeod 1981, Cornblath *et al.* 1988, Ropper *et al.* 1990) show marked slowing of motor conduction velocities, along with prolonged distal latencies consistent with demyelination in about 50 per cent of the patients. Some abnormalities of motor or sensory conduction velocities are present in 90 per cent of patients but, because of the patchy distribution of lesions, the probability of finding abnormalities increases with the number of nerves studied, and the degree of involvement can vary with the nerve studied. In 20 per cent of cases abnormalities are found in only one or two but not all nerves studied. The amplitude of the sensory action potentials and of the motor action potential is diminished. A conduction block could be demonstrated in at least one nerve in 74 per cent of the cases of Bradshaw and Jones (1992). Measurement of F-wave latency may detect abnormalities of proximal nerves or roots that escape routine examination. The amplitude of the mean compound muscle action potential bears a significant relationship to the prognosis (Cornblath *et al.* 1988). Signs of denervation and fibrillations indicate greater axonal involvement and may be of poor prognostic significance (Triggs *et al.* 1992).

Evoked potential studies have shown anomalies of both brainstem auditory evoked potentials and somatosensory evoked potentials (Ropper and Chiappa 1986).

COURSE

The initial phase of gradually increasing involvement lasts 10–30 days. Prolongation beyond four weeks excludes the diagnosis of GBS (Asbury 1981) and suggests a diagnosis of chronic inflammatory polyneuropathy. In some forms (Ropper 1986a) paralysis progresses very rapidly with complete quadriplegia in two to five days. Such patients often have severe respiratory involvement and sequelae are more likely than in average cases.

A plateau phase then follows. A long plateau phase was found by some investigators (Billard *et al.* 1979) but not by others (Winer *et al.* 1988) to be associated with a relatively poor prognosis and the persistence of motor sequelae.

Death occurs in 2–3 per cent of childhood cases, although in some adult series (Winer *et al.* 1988) mortality was as high as 15 per cent, mostly in older adult patients.

Recovery is usually complete. Motor sequelae, often mild, occur in 5–25 per cent of patients. Relapses and late recurrences occur in about 3 per cent of patients (Thomas *et al.* 1969, Wijdicks and Ropper 1990). Late recurrences that supervene several years after the first episode probably have a different mechanism to those seen after discontinuation of plasma exchange or corticosteroid therapy and are usually only partial (Ropper *et al.* 1988).

Factors giving an unfavourable prognosis include a rapid development of the paralyses, possibly a long duration of the plateau phase, a marked distal deficit, the presence of fibrillation potentials and of a low amplitude of the mean compound motor unit potentials (Ropper 1986a). The prevalent impression that the disease has a better prognosis in children than in adults has been questioned by Kleyweg *et al.* (1989) and by Jansen *et al.* (1993) who found no difference in severity between 18 children and 50 adults and therefore recommended that the same treatments should be used in both groups. However, recent findings of a large collaborative study (Korinthenberg and Mönting 1996) confirm the lesser severity of the disease in children. Rantala *et al.* (1997) found three major risk factors for more severe cases: onset of symptoms within eight days of the preceding infection, cranial nerve involvement, and a CSF protein level > 800 mg/L during the first week of the disease.

TREATMENT

Symptomatic treatment is an essential part of the management of GBS. Careful monitoring of vital functions, avoidance of aspiration pneumonia, and tube feeding and respiratory assistance when needed have considerably lessened the mortality rate.

Treatments that aim at correcting the immunological abnormalities described earlier are not yet fully assessed. Corticosteroid treatment has been shown in controlled studies to have no beneficial effects and even to prolong hospitalization (Hughes 1991). Plasmapheresis is clearly effective in adults (French Cooperative Group 1987, McKhann *et al.* 1988) when performed during the first week of the disease and repeated over a period of 7–14 days. This treatment has been shown to reduce the duration of hospitalization, to avoid respiratory insufficiency and to limit the extension of the paralyses. Such a treatment is probably indicated for severe cases when rapid extension is evident early. However, the exact indications are not yet firmly established. Plasmaphereses are difficult to use in children of less than 15 kg, although Khatri *et al.* (1990) and Jansen *et al.* (1993) have reported favourable results with the use of a specially adapted technique. Epstein and Sladky (1990) found that plasmapheresis diminishes morbidity in childhood Guillain–Barré syndrome by shortening the interval until recovery of independent walking. Results similar to those in adult patients have also been reported by Jansen *et al.* (1993).

The demonstration that high-dose (2 g/kg) intravenous gammaglobulins (Kleyweg *et al.* 1988, Van der Meché *et al.* 1992, Azulay *et al.* 1994, Thornton and Griggs 1994, Hartung *et al.* 1995) are also an effective therapy opens a new avenue for therapy. Doses of 0.4 g/kg/d for five days given during the first days of the disease seem to give results similar to those of plasmapheresis (Van der Meché *et al.* 1992). Administration of the total dose in two days may be more effective than conventional fractionated therapy (Kanra *et al.* 1997). This technique will probably replace plasmapheresis in children. Recent reports have questioned the efficacy of immunoglobulin therapy. Castro and Ropper (1993) reported worsening in seven of 15 adults, and relapses following initially good results have been reported (Irani

TABLE 21.4
Causes of acute flaccid paralysis

Cause	References
Peripheral neuropathy	
Guillain–Barré syndrome (acute demyelinating neuropathy)	This chapter
Acute axonal neuropathy	This chapter
Neuropathies of infectious diseases (diphtheria, neuroborreliosis)	This chapter, Chapter 11
Acute toxic neuropathies	
Heavy metals	This chapter
Snake (elapid) toxins	This chapter
Wild berries, buckthorn	Villalobos and Santos (1996)
Arthropod bites	Créange *et al.* (1993)
Anterior horn cell disease	
Acute anterior poliomyelitis	Chapters 11, 20
Vaccinal poliomyelitis	Chapters 11, 20
Other neurotropic viruses (coxsackie, echoviruses, enteroviruses 70 and 71	Melnik (1984)
Acute myelopathy	
Cord compression (tumours, trauma, paraspinal abscess)	Chapter 14
Vascular malformation with thrombosis or bleeding	Chapter 15
Demyelinating diseases (multiple sclerosis, Devic syndrome, acute disseminated encephalomyelitis)	Chapters 11, 12
Systemic disease	
Acute porphyrias	This chapter
Critical illness neuropathy	This chapter
Acute myopathy in intensive care patients	Zochodne *et al.* (1993)
Disorders of neuromuscular transmission	
Myasthenia gravis	Chapter 22
Botulism	Chapters 2, 11
Insecticide (organophosphate) poisoning	Zwiener and Ginsberg (1988)
Tick paralysis	Smith (1992)
Snake bites	Saini *et al.* (1986)
Muscle disorders	
Polymyositis, dermatomyositis	Chapter 22
Trichinosis	Fourestié *et al.* (1993)
Periodic paralyses	Chapter 22
Corticosteroid and blocking agents	Hirano *et al.* (1992)
Mitochondrial diseases (infantile type)	Chapters 9, 22

et al. 1993). However, immunoglobulins appear to be an effective and safe treatment (van der Meché *et al.* 1992, Jones 1996, Korinthenberg and Mönting 1996, Shahar *et al.* 1997). The exact indications are yet to be established; cases with rapid extension or impending respiratory insufficiency are obvious candidates but whether all incipient cases should be treated is not known. Rantala *et al.* (1995) suggested early administration at time of diagnosis when risk factors are present. Combined therapy with high-dose immunoglobulins and methylprednisolone may be more effective than globulins alone with a 73 per cent success rate as compared with 50 per cent (Dutch Guillain–Barré Group 1994).

DIAGNOSIS
GBS is a major cause of acute flaccid paralysis (Table 21.4). The diagnosis of GBS is easy in typical cases. Diagnostic criteria (Asbury 1981, Asbury and Cornblath 1990) include symmetrical weakness and areflexia, the presence of mild sensory symptoms and signs, progression of the symptoms lasting no more than four weeks after onset, absence of fever, sphincter dysfunction and evidence of CNS involvement. The last two criteria may not apply to all childhood cases (see above). Typical CSF and electrophysiological findings confirm the clinical diagnosis.

The conditions that may simulate GBS are common in children (Table 21.4) but only a few raise difficult problems. It is imperative to exclude conditions that require immediate specific treatment, especially spinal cord compression. Transverse myelitis can be distinguished because of sensory and sphincter involvement. Rare cases of metabolic disease such as Leigh syndrome (Coker 1993) can closely simulate GBS. Poliomyelitis is now exceptional but some toxic neuropathies may be confused with acute polyneuritis. In adolescents the possibility of volatile solvent abuse neuropathy should be kept in mind. Diphtheritic neuropathy closely mimics GBS but is rare. Botulism and diphtheria can be excluded by the intrinsic eye involvement which is never present in GBS.

CLINICAL VARIANTS OF THE GUILLAIN–BARRÉ SYNDROME AND RELATED DISORDERS
Miller Fisher syndrome is characterized by the triad of ophthalmoplegia, ataxia and areflexia (Fig. 21.5), which comes on rapidly and follows the same illnesses as classical GBS (Kohler *et al.* 1988). However, a history or serological evidence of *C. jejuni* infection is particularly common in this syndrome (Gregson *et al.* 1993, Rees *et al.* 1995, Jones 1996) and antiganglioside GQ1b antibodies are almost always present. CSF protein becomes elevated in most patients with few or no cells, and electrodiagnostic features indicate peripheral nerve involvement in some cases (Asbury 1981). Abnormalities of brainstem evoked potentials have been reported (Unishi *et al.* 1988), and some investigators have regarded the syndrome as a form of brainstem encephalitis (Al-Din *et al.* 1982, Petty *et al.* 1993) because of MRI anomalies. Similar anomalies of evoked potentials may occur in classical GBS and Miller Fisher syndrome (Ropper and Chiappa 1986), and the bulk of evidence indicates that Miller Fisher syndrome is a form of acute polyneuritis. The ataxia may be due to involvement of large sensory fibres (Weiss and White 1986). Transitional cases with variable peripheral motor weakness also link the Miller Fisher syndrome to GBS (Gibberd 1970). The course is similar to that of GBS although recurrences are quite rare (Vincent and Vincent 1986).

An *acute axonal form of GBS* has been described in adults (Feasby *et al.* 1986, Azouvi *et al.* 1989, van der Meché *et al.* 1991) and tends to run a severe course with motor sequelae. Recent reports from China (McKhann *et al.* 1993; Griffin *et al.* 1995, 1996) have underlined the frequency of an acute inflammatory neuropathy in children that predominantly involves axons rather than myelin sheaths. The clinical picture is one of severe

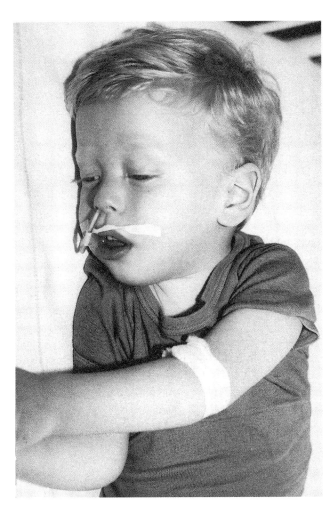

Fig. 21.5. Miller Fisher syndrome in a 20-month-old boy. Note ptosis of eyelids, unexpressive facies, open mouth and tube feeding (due to swallowing difficulties).

neuropathy with features of denervation but with an overall good recovery. Sensory manifestations may be marked, and the role of *C. jejuni* appears prominent (Yuki *et al.* 1990) with a clear peak of incidence in summer. Similar cases have been reported from other Asian countries and from Mexico.

Cases of GBS without sensory loss (acute motor neuropathy) have also been reported in adult patients with features suggestive of axonal involvement (Visser *et al.* 1995) and also seem to be commonly associated with *C. jejuni* infection.

Cases of sensory loss and areflexia without motor deficit probably represent GBS if the onset is rapid, the distribution widespread and symmetrical, and recovery complete with elevated CSF protein (Dawson *et al.* 1988). In rare instances, GBS may present mainly with painful manifestations (Mikati and DeLong 1985). Sensory neuropathy as described in adults is a different condition (Sterman *et al.* 1980).

The nosological situation of the case of childhood peripheral neuropathy with antibodies to P_o myelin glycoprotein (Ben Jelloun-Dellagi *et al.* 1992) is unclear.

Some cases of *acute polyneuritis cranialis* are probably variants of GBS provided that cranial nerves I and II are uninvolved

and other features of GBS are present (Asbury 1981, Polo *et al.* 1992).

Rare instances of *acute pure pandysautonomia (acute acquired dysautonomia)* (Young *et al.* 1975, Pavesi et al. 1992) may be atypical aspects of acute polyneuritis. The clinical picture of such cases is highly polymorphic with various combinations of hypotension, disorders of sweating and lachrymation, diarrhoea or intestinal obstruction, pupillary abnormalities and vasomotor disturbances (McLeod and Tuck 1987, Takayama *et al.* 1987). Acute or subacute cholinergic dysautonomia is characterized by failure of postganglionic cholinergic fibres (including sympathetic efferents to sweat glands), sometimes preceded by a transient increase in function resulting in hypersalivation, increased sweating and more frequent bowel movements. Symptoms include blurred vision, alachrymia, dry mouth, dysphagia, abdominal distension, urinary retention and anhidrosis. Pupils are fixed and dilated, and heart rate is invariable. Paralytic ileus may occur. Pure pandysautonomia features in addition symptoms and signs of sympathetic failure with resulting postural hypotension, depressed pressor responses and a syncopal tendency. The course is variable, with substantial recovery in some cases. Treatment is symptomatic. Sensory dysfunction may be associated (Nass and Chutorian 1982, Kanda *et al.* 1990). In some cases, vasomotor dysfunction occurs in isolation, *e.g.* with unilateral flushing (Lance *et al.* 1988). Dopamine beta-hydroxylase deficiency is a rare cause of similar sympathetic failure (Mathias and Bannister 1992).

In some patients (mostly adults) the course of diffuse inflammatory polyneuropathy is longer than in classical GBS. In particular, the period of progression of the paralyses exceeds four weeks and may last up to eight weeks (Hughes *et al.* 1992). These patients represent intermediate cases between GBS and the chronic inflammatory neuropathies.

CHRONIC INFLAMMATORY DEMYELINATING POLYNEUROPATHY
Chronic inflammatory polyneuropathies (CIDPs) are much rarer than GBS. The diagnostic criteria for CIDP include: (1) a clinical course of either a monophasic illness with an initial progressive phase lasting more than eight weeks, or a relapsing–remitting course: (2) electrophysiological and pathological evidence of demyelination; and (3) the absence of systemic disease that may cause demyelinating neuropathy (Ouvrier 1992). An immunological origin to the condition is likely (Dalakas and Engel 1981). Contrary to what is observed in GBS, there is an increased frequency of certain HLA groups (A1, B8, DRw3) in patients with chronic inflammatory neuropathy (Stewart *et al.* 1978, Adams *et al.* 1979) and the disease has been seen in siblings (Gabreëls-Festen *et al.* 1986).

CLINICAL FEATURES
The disease occurs predominantly in children 5–15 years of age but cases with infantile or early childhood onset are on record (Pasternak *et al.* 1982, Sladky *et al.* 1986). Clinical characteristics include the slow subacute onset over several weeks of a sensory motor neuropathy involving the distal and proximal

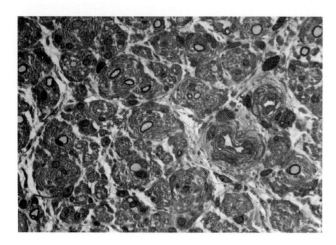

Fig. 21.6. Chronic inflammatory neuropathy. Note well-developed 'onion bulb' formation and paucity of myelinated fibres.

limbs but respecting the respiratory muscles and cranial nerves (Colan *et al.* 1980, Sladky *et al.* 1986). However, an acute onset as in GBS is possible, cranial nerve involvement occurs in 10–40 per cent of patients, and weakness of bulbar or respiratory muscles severe enough to necessitate assisted ventilation is present in about 10 per cent of cases (Ouvrier 1992). Due to the usual predominance of weakness in the lower limbs, difficulties with ambulation are usually the first manifestation and in early cases may be responsible for delayed motor milestones. The weakness is not infrequently asymmetrical. It is associated with amyotrophy and sensory disturbances although these are generally inconspicuous (McCombe *et al.* 1987b, Barohn *et al.* 1989). Action or postural tremor is present in some patients.

Two different courses are possible. In about one-third of cases, the disease is monophasic although lasting several months. In the remaining cases there is a relapsing course with a variable number of exacerbations and remissions, often incomplete, which may extend over several years (Barohn *et al.* 1989).

The CSF shows a protein/cell dissociation as in GBS in 90 per cent of patients. The presence of a monoclonal or of oligoclonal bands is frequent but the oligoclonal proteins seem to be plasma-derived (Segurado *et al.* 1986).

There is consistently electrophysiological evidence of demyelination with slowed motor and sensory conduction velocities, often varying in different segments of the same nerve, increased distal latencies and a neurogenic EMG.

Nerve biopsy (Fig. 21.6) shows endoneural and subperineural inflammatory exudates and mononuclear cell infiltration. In some cases, hypertrophic changes with marked enlargement of the roots may be present and can be demonstrated by MRI of the cauda equina (Crino *et al.* 1993). Onion bulbs are present in about 50 per cent of cases. The condition is aetiologically related to chronic dysimmune neuropathy as observed mostly in adults (Maisonobe *et al.* 1996).

DIAGNOSIS
The main diagnostic difficulty is to distinguish CIDP from some

types of hereditary motor and sensory neuropathy (types I and III). It is indeed not clear whether steroid-responsive HMSN is actually a distinct condition (Baba *et al.* 1995), and so a course of steroids is worth trying in dubious cases (Gabreëls-Festen *et al.* 1986). Metabolic neuropathies, such as in metachromatic leukodystrophy, may exhibit similar features with increased CSF protein.

CNS involvement in association with chronic demyelinating neuropathy has been described in some adult patients (Thomas *et al.* 1987, Ohtake *et al.* 1990). Such cases raise the question of a relationship with multiple sclerosis. Systematic MRI in adult patients with chronic neuropathy has shown the occasional presence of areas of abnormal white matter signal (Feasby *et al.* 1990). The significance of this finding is unclear.

PROGNOSIS AND TREATMENT
The disorder does not usually threaten life, but its protracted course and the possible motor sequelae make it a disabling condition.

Therapy with corticosteroids is effective both in childen and in adults (Dyck *et al.* 1982) but the modalities of treatment are not fully codified. Relapses following minimal decreases in dosage are extremely common so that prolonged treatment with careful monitoring is necessary (Wertman *et al.* 1988).

The development of steroid resistance is possible. In such cases, the addition of immunosuppressors and/or the use of a bolus of methylprednisolone should be tried. *Plasma exchange* is effective and has less side-effects than protracted steroid therapy (Hahn *et al.* 1996). In my experience, plasmapheresis has been associated with remarkable, although transitory, improvement. Many patients may be maintained adequately with one exchange every two to three weeks. High-dose intravenous immunoglobulins (Faed *et al.* 1989, Van Doorn *et al.* 1990, Hughes *et al.* 1992, Hahn *et al.* 1996) may prove to be an effective therapy. However, Vermeulen *et al.* (1993) in a comparative study of seven adults did not confirm the efficacy of the treatment. Recent reviews (Azulay *et al.* 1994, Otten *et al.* 1996) of immunoglobulin treatment in neuropathies are available.

LEPROSY
Leprosy is still a major health problem in several developing countries and together with vitamin deficiency is the main cause of neuropathy in many regions. The disease is due to infection with *Mycobacterium leprae* and is transmitted by intimate person to person contact. HLA-linked genes control the susceptibility to the organism and the course of the illness. Leprosy is a systemic disease with a marked predilection for nerves and skin. Hosts with a low resistance to the organism develop lepromatous or nodular infection. Hosts with high resistance develop tuberculoid infection. In lepromatous leprosy, most infiltrates consist of macrophages heavily infected by *M. leprae*. In tuberculoid leprosy, the lesions contain only remnants of bacteria surrounded by well-organized granulomas with epithelioid and giant cells. Borderline cases intermediate between lepromatous and tuberculoid leprosy occur frequently, and unstable cases can oscillate between the two forms.

In lepromatous leprosy neural damage may produce a purely sensory polyneuritis with loss of touch, pain and temperature sensation in a glove and stocking distribution while deep sensitivity is preserved. Sensory loss first appears in cool areas of the body (ears, dorsal surface of the hands, forearms, feet and lateral aspect of the legs). Sensory motor neuropathy is less common (Sabin *et al.* 1993). Pure mononeuritis is rare. In most patients the onset is insidious but an abrupt onset is possible. Shooting pains are uncommon. Enlargement of peripheral nerves may be present. The diagnosis may be difficult in nonendemic areas. A serological test is available (Young and Buchanan 1983). Nerve biopsy is useful for both diagnosis and detection of persistent infection (Chimelli *et al.* 1997). Treatment uses sulfone derivatives, rifampicin and clofazimine (Sabin *et al.* 1993).

ENDOGENOUS AND EXOGENOUS TOXIC NEUROPATHIES

Toxic neuropathies of both endogenous and exogenous origin are uncommon in childhood at least in symptomatic form (Gamstorp 1968, Evans 1979).

ENDOGENOUS TOXIC NEUROPATHIES

Subclinical neuropathy may not be rare in patients with *juvenile diabetes* as judged by electrophysiological findings. Gamstorp (1968) found mildly slowed conduction velocities and increased distal latencies in 11 of 42 children with polyneuropathy, whereas only one of the 61 patients of Evans (1979) had diabetes mellitus.

More recently, Gallai *et al.* (1988) found decreased motor conduction velocity in the median nerve in 10 per cent, in the posterior tibial nerve in 32 per cent, and in the sural nerve in 44 per cent of 50 juvenile diabetics with a mean age of 13 years. The neuropathy appeared to be more marked in poorly controlled diabetes.

Clinically manifest diabetic neuropathy is rare (Bastron and Thomas 1981, Fiçicioglu *et al.* 1994), even though the study of spinal sensory evoked potentials confirms that subclinical involvement of neural transmission in young diabetic patients is common (Cracco *et al.* 1984). Cranial nerve palsies are exceptional in juvenile diabetes. Autonomic involvement with gastrointestinal features is sometimes apparent. A neurogenic bladder may be relatively common but usually remains asymptomatic (Faerman *et al.* 1971).

Uraemic neuropathy is also subclinical in a large majority of cases. Seventy-six per cent of uraemic children had a significant slowing of peroneal nerve conduction velocity without other evidence of neuropathy in the study by Mentser *et al.* (1978). Symptomatic patients may experience sensory abnormalities in the lower extremities that may evolve into a sensory motor polyneuropathy with flaccid paraplegia or quadriplegia. Any type of neuropathy (purely axonal, axonomyelinic or predominantly demyelinating) may be observed (Saïd *et al.* 1983). A purely motor type of uraemic neuropathy (McGonigle *et al.* 1985) may occur. The neuropathy of uraemia is usually reversed by successful renal transplant. A case of Miller Fisher syndrome with a relapsing course and fluctuations temporally related to uraemia and

TABLE 21.5
Some exogenous toxic causes of polyneuropathy

Agent	Reference
Drugs	
Isoniazid	Evans (1979)
Ethionamide	Argov and Mastaglia (1979)
Ethambutol	
Nitrofurantoin	Toole and Parrish (1973)
Chlorambucil	Argov and Mastaglia (1979)
Vincristine	Casey *et al.* (1973)
Cisplatin	Gastaut and Pellissier (1985), Riggs *et al.* (1988)
Phenytoin	Lovelace and Horwitz (1968)
Lithium	Chang *et al.* (1988)
Thalidomide	Hess *et al.* (1986)
Metronidazole	
Amphotericin	Argov and Mastaglia (1979)
Amitriptylin	
Amiodarone	Bono *et al.* (1993)
Complication of bone marrow and solid transplants	Amato *et al.* (1993), Patchell (1994)
Heavy metals	
Mercury	Swaiman and Flager (1971)
Lead	Browder *et al.* (1973)
Arsenic	Evans (1979)
Thallium	Bank *et al.* (1972)
Organic chemicals	
N-hexane	Korobkin *et al.* (1975)
Triorthocresylphosphate	Evans (1979)
Carbon monoxide	Hopkins (1975)
Cyanate	Peterson *et al.* (1974)
Hydroxyquinolines	Baumgartner *et al.* (1970)
Pyridoxine abuse	Schaumburg *et al.* (1983)
Organophosphates	Zwiener and Ginsberg (1988)
Biological toxins	
Immunizations	Evans (1979)
Serum sickness	Chapter 12
Arthropod bites	Haller and Fabara (1972), Créange *et al.* (1993)

haemodialysis session has been observed (Galassi *et al.* 1990).

Polyneuropathy may also occur in *hypothyroidism* (Nemni *et al.* 1987).

EXOGENOUS TOXIC NEUROPATHIES

A vast number of chemicals can induce polyneuropathy (Table 21.5). Only the most important ones, especially drugs, are mentioned here. *Isoniazid* can cause a distal mixed sensory and motor neuropathy through interference with the metabolism of pyridoxine. Supplementation with pyridoxine is therefore indicated in patients treated for tuberculosis. *Vincristine* is a relatively common cause of neuropathy in children with malignancies. The drug interferes with the formation of neurotubules. Abolition of reflexes starting with the ankle jerk is virtually constant following vincristine therapy. In more severe cases paraesthesiae develop, followed by sensory loss then by weakness which may be initially focal and may remain asymmetrical (Casey *et al.* 1973). Severe pain, in the parotid region, is frequent during vincristine treatment, and oculomotor palsies have been observed. *Nitrofurantoin* causes neuropathy mainly in children with renal insufficiency. Axonal involvement is the rule, and distal sensory symptoms are usually predominant. Differential diagnosis with uraemic neuropathy may be difficult.

Most drug-induced neuropathies are reversible after discontinuation of treatment but recovery may be slow especially when intoxication was prolonged. *Phenytoin* toxicity is almost always subclinical.

Accidental neuropathies due to heavy metals are rare. *Insecticides* should be suspected in rural communities along with arsenic. N-*hexane neuropathy* may result from glue-sniffing, a practice that has become popular among adolescents and even children (Korobkin *et al.* 1975). A history of glue-sniffing should be routinely searched for in this age group.

Biological toxins are rarely a cause. Tick paralysis is seen in America and in Australia. It results in a flaccid, rapidly extensive paralysis, involving the respiratory muscles and may be lethal if the tick is not removed. Careful search is clearly imperative and removal leads to cure in a few hours to several days (Grattan-Smith *et al.* 1997). In Western Europe, paralysis following tick bite is due to *Borrelia* disease (Chapter 11).

NEUROPATHIES OF SYSTEMIC AND VASCULAR DISEASES

A neuropathy may be a manifestation of most vasculitides (Chapter 12) including lupus erythematosus (McCombe *et al.* 1987a), rheumatoid arthritis, polyarteritis nodosa, anaphylactoid purpura (Ritter *et al.* 1983) and other, less well-defined collagen disorders and vasculitides (Harati and Niakan 1986, Dyck *et al.* 1987). Such complications are rare in children. They may present either as mononeuritis multiplex or as diffuse polyneuropathy.

Neuropathy may occur in gravely ill patients with multiple visceral deficiency (Zochodne *et al.* 1987) or following major surgery (Gross *et al.* 1988). The nature of these 'critically ill neuropathies' is obscure. They may entail compression, hypoxia (Pfeiffer *et al.* 1990) and other mechanisms. Similar cases have been observed in childhood (Heckmatt *et al.* 1993, Tsao *et al.* 1995). A neuropathy can occur in burn patients; it most frequently presents as mononeuritis multiplex, less often as a mononeuropathy (Marquez *et al.* 1993). A neuropathy with optic atrophy has been associated with malnutrition combined with tobacco toxicity in Cuba (Cuba Neuropathy Field Investigation Team 1995, Thomas *et al.* 1995).

LOCALIZED DISORDERS OF THE PERIPHERAL NERVES (EXCEPT CRANIAL NERVES)

INFLAMMATORY LOCALIZED NEUROPATHIES
These may involve a single nerve or branch or several nerves as in plexopathies. Transitional forms with the generalized neuropathies exist, *e.g.* neuropathy with liability to pressure palsies or cases of familial brachial plexopathy that may also affect the lumbar plexus and presumably are the result of a more or less diffuse process.

PAINFUL BRACHIAL NEUROPATHY OR PLEXOPATHY, PARSONAGE–TURNER SYNDROME, NEURALGIC AMYOTROPHY
Brachial plexopathy occurs from infancy although paediatric cases are much rarer than in adults (Charles and Jayam-Trouth 1980). It may follow a nonspecific respiratory infection, a specific viral disease such as infectious mononucleosis (Watson and Ashby 1976, Dussaix *et al.* 1986) or parvovirus infection (Denning *et al.* 1987), or an immunization (Petrera and Trojaborg 1984, Hamati-Haddad and Fenichel 1997).

The disorder usually begins with pain localized to the shoulder or involving the whole upper limb. Pain may last from hours to weeks and is often intense. It is followed by weakness that may be the first manifestation in 5 per cent of the cases. Paralysis affects the upper brachial roots in over half the patients, the whole plexus in one-third, but may be limited to the hand and fingers in a small proportion. Amyotrophy sets in rapidly and objective sensory signs may be present (England and Sumner 1987).

Recovery is virtually constant but it may take months or years and some residua may rarely persist (Zeharia *et al.* 1990).

The diagnosis requires exclusion of spinal cord compression which often demands an imaging study of the cervical cord. The CSF is usually normal although a mild inflammatory reaction may be present at onset. EMG and nerve conduction studies are useful for determining the extent of involvement of the ipsilateral and, occasionally, the contralateral plexus.

Treatment is based on antalgics and physiotherapy. Steroids are not indicated.

Involvement of only one nerve from the brachial plexus may be seen. The long thoracic nerve is commonly affected with consequent paralysis of the serratus anterior, producing a unilateral winged scapula (Petrera and Trojaborg 1984)

OTHER LOCALIZED INFLAMMATORY NERVE DISORDERS
Lumbosacral plexopathy is the counterpart in the lower limb of neuralgic amyotrophy but is even rarer in children. Occasional cases are on record in adolescents (Evans *et al.* 1981) and even in 2- to 3-year-old children (Sander and Sharp 1981, Thomson 1993). Pain is located in a femoral or sciatic distribution and children will limp or refuse to walk. Weakness of the leg follows in about a week. Recovery is almost universal although mild residual weakness may persist. When the lower plexus is involved it may be confused with sciatica due to disc or vertebral disease. In some countries, schistosomiasis is an important cause (Marra 1983).

Sacral radiculomyelitis (Elsberg syndrome) is observed mainly in young adults and presents with a tetrad of acute urinary retention, sensory deficit in sacral dermatomes, paraesthesiae in the same terriroty and pleocytosis of the CSF (Herbaut *et al.* 1987). Most cases are due to genital herpes simplex virus but other viral agents, *e.g.* echovirus and cytomegalovirus, may be the cause (Vanneste *et al.* 1980, Michaelson *et al.* 1983). One case in a 6-year-old boy has been diagnosed at our institution and a similar patient has been reported (Gerber and Cromie 1996).

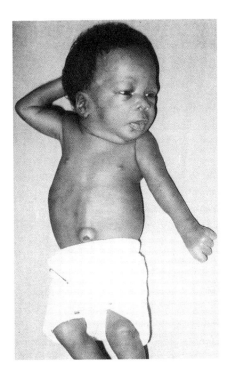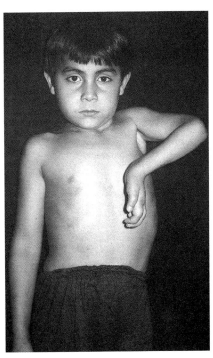

Fig. 21.7. Obstetric paralysis of the brachial plexus. *(Far left)* 1-month-old boy with proximal (Duchenne–Erb) palsy. The left arm is internally rotated, the forearm is extended and pronated. The intrinsic hand muscles are normal. *(Left)* 6-year-old boy with severe sequelae of total plexus involvement. Synkinetic contraction of proximal muscles is evident. The left hand is paralysed and atrophic. There is ipsilateral Horner syndrome. (Courtesy Dr J-P. Padovani, Hôpital des Enfants Malades, Paris.)

TRAUMATIC NERVE INJURIES
BRACHIAL PLEXUS INJURY
The incidence of brachial plexus injury in neonates has decreased in recent years probably because of improved obstetric techniques. Since 1980, the incidence has varied from 0.37 to 0.87 per 1000 live births (Painter 1988). Women over 35 years of age, those with preeclampsia or diabetes mellitus, and those who had previously delivered children with brachial plexus injuries are more likely to have affected babies. In one series (Rossi *et al.* 1982) up to 50 per cent of affected children weighed more than 4000g at birth. Abnormal birth presentations are also a factor but the frequency of breech delivery varies with the series (Rossi *et al.* 1982, Painter 1988). Occasional cases of prenatal plexus injury due to deformation from uterine constraint, such as that of bicornuate uterus, are on record and are a possible cause of paralysis in siblings (Dunn and Engle 1985).

Pathology
Lesions affect the upper plexus (C5 and C6 roots)—the Duchenne–Erb type of plexus paralysis—in 55–72 per cent of cases. Lesions of the entire plexus occur on an average in 10 per cent of patients; those of C5, C6 and C7 in 10–20 per cent; and those of C8–T1 (Déjerine–Klumpke type) in less than 10 per cent. Bilateral, but often asymmetrical, involvement is not rare. In most instances there is stretching of the upper cord of the plexus due to traction on the shoulder during delivery of the aftercoming head or to turning the head away from the shoulder in difficult cephalic presentation. Injury to the lower cord seems to result from traction on the abducted forearm during vertex delivery or from traction on the trunk with breech presentation. The most common lesions are haemorrhages and oedema within the nerve sheath of primary plexus cords. Actual avulsion of the roots from the spinal cord with segmental damage of the grey matter or tearing of the nerves is uncommon but occurs when the degree of traction is severe enough.

Clinical manifestations
In a large majority of patients, the paralysis is recognized from the first days of life. The affected arm hangs limply adducted and internally rotated, the elbow extended, the forearm pronated and the wrist variably flexed (Fig. 21.7). The grasp remains normal. The biceps and brachioradialis reflexes are absent. Weakness of the triceps and extensors of forearm and digits may complicate the picture when there is significant C7 involvement. In lower plexus lesions, intrinsic hand muscles are paralysed, the grasp is absent and a Horner syndrome with ptosis and miosis is frequently present. If the Horner syndrome does not resolve, the iris fails to pigment and heterochromia iridum develops. Winging of the scapula and Horner syndrome generally herald a poor outcome. In some cases, there is significant sensory involvement with the possible appearance of whitlows on the fingers. Involvement of the diaphragm, due to lesion of the fourth cervical root, is present in approximately 5 per cent of cases and may produce symptoms of respiratory distress. This occurs most often in association with upper plexus palsy but may be present in isolation (Schifrin 1952).

Diagnosis
The diagnosis of plexus paralysis is readily apparent. Study of the somatosensory evoked potentials may help distinguish between an avulsed root or a more distal lesion of better prognosis (Jones 1979) in older patients. MRI of the spinal cord and roots may

also be used for the same purpose. EMG may be helpful in determining the extent of paralysis.

Prognosis and management
A majority of neonates with brachial plexus injury recover. Gordon *et al.* (1973) studied 59 such infants: examination showed recovery in 46/52 at 4 months of age, in 48/52 at 12 months, and in 53/56 at 4 years, with only three patients lost to follow-up. Similarly, Greenwald *et al.* (1984) found that 23 of their 38 patients had recovered by 1 week, 35 by 3 months, and 36 at several years. Children with residual deficits may continue to improve even during preschool years. Sequelae may affect various muscles depending on the lesions but tend to predominate on the proximal limb (Rossi *et al.* 1982). Sequelae include weakness, amyotrophy and sensory deficits. Contractures are often more marked than weakness. They are due to faulty re-innervation and result in paradoxical synkinesias. In particular, attempts at any movement of the upper limb tend to provoke contraction of the deltoid and biceps with abduction of the flexed limb. In virtually all cases there is internal rotation of the arm and pronation of the forearm.

The average case of plexus palsy in the newborn infant does not require more than range of motion exercises starting no sooner than 7–10 days after birth. Splinting is contraindicated as it may promote the development of contracture. For infants who have not significantly improved by age 6 months, the question of surgical therapy, including neural lysis, nerve anastomosis or grafting, arises (Gilbert and Tassin 1987, Gilbert *et al.* 1991). Laurent and Lee (1994) reported satisfactory results in 50 of 70 operated infants but controversy persists in the absence of a prospective controlled study and no firm statement seems currently possible (Bodensteiner *et al.* 1994). Surgical intervention after 6 months to 1 year of age is recommended by some groups but the precise indications are not agreed upon (Hunt 1988).

Surgical procedures on joints and tendon transfers have variable results but may become indicated in older children to improve specific functions.

Postnatal injuries to the brachial plexus are mainly due to motor vehicle (especially motorcycle) and sports accidents and consequently affect principally adolescents. The prognosis of these injuries is often guarded. Traumatic lesions of the lumbosacral plexus are rare. Both neonatal (Hope *et al.* 1985) and childhood (Egel *et al.* 1995) cases have been reported with a favourable outcome.

SCIATIC NERVE INJURIES
Injury to the sciatic nerve is often the result of injections into the nerve or in its vicinity. Such accidents are particularly prone to occur in small preterm infants because of the small volume of the buttock allowing substances to diffuse right up to the nerve with resulting injury and dysfunction (Gilles and French 1961). Therefore, intramuscular injections into the buttocks of such infants are prohibited. The sciatic nerve can also be injured following injection of drugs into the umbilical artery. This is caused by thrombosis of the inferior gluteal artery and is accompanied by circulatory changes in the buttock (San Agustin *et al.* 1962, Wynne *et al.* 1978) or gangrenous skin areas in the leg. Similar changes may occur following injection of viscid substances into the buttocks.

Paralysis may affect the whole territory of the sciatic nerve or only one of its two main divisions, most commonly the peroneal nerve. Foot-drop and amyotrophy and growth disturbances of the leg are the most frequent manifestations. Surgical exploration of the nerve should be considered when no improvement occurs after a few weeks and/or when a granuloma is palpable at the site of injection. The prognosis is poor in severe cases especially as a result of trophic and growth disturbances.

Breech delivery is a rare cause of neonatal sciatic palsy (Jones *et al.* 1988).

Sciatic neuralgia due to disc herniation is rare in childhood, and pain in the territory of the lower lumbar and upper sciatic roots is more commonly due to tumours than to disc pathology.

In children above 10 years of age typical sciatica is occasionally observed. Spine rigidity and scoliosis or kyphosis may be prominent manifestations (Kurihara and Kataoka 1980, Epstein *et al.* 1984).

Other causes of sciatic neuropathy in childhood include compression by tumour or lymphoma, stretch injury after closed reduction of hip dislocation, hypersensitivity vasculitis and prolonged posture. In rare cases no cause is found (Jones *et al.* 1988).

CARPAL TUNNEL SYNDROME AND OTHER ENTRAPMENT SYNDROMES
Carpal tunnel syndrome is rare in childhood: Sainio *et al.* (1987) collected only 32 published cases and added three of their own. As in adults, the syndrome occurs most commonly in females. Motor symptoms tend to dominate the clinical picture in children with typical affectation of the thenar muscles. Pain and paraesthesiae are often less marked than in adults. Sensory and motor distal latencies are prolonged.

Mucopolysaccharidoses types IS, II and IV may cause the carpal tunnel syndrome through hypertrophy of the flexor retinaculum and related structures. Other rare causes include neuropathy with liability to pressure palsies (see p. 717) and the Schwartz–Jampel syndrome (Cruz Martínez *et al.* 1984). Occasional familial idiopathic cases are on record (Danta 1975). Other entrapment neuropathies of the upper extremities have been reviewed by Dawson (1993).

Other entrapment syndromes are exceptional in childhood. A more complete description is given by Ouvrier and Shield (1990). Entrapment of the sciatic nerve due to a congenital iliac bony abnormality has been reported (Lester and McAlister 1970). Hypertrophy of the piriformis muscle can also compress the nerve when it emerges from the greater sciatic foramen (Boespflug-Tanguy *et al.* 1994). Section of the muscle relieves compression. Occasional adolescent cases of the thoracic outlet syndrome with cervical rib or fibrous band are known (Smith and Trojaborg 1987). Radial neuropathies in childhood have been reviewed by Escobar and Jones 1996).

MRI helps to diagnose the causes of such cases (Panegyres et al. 1993). The neck–tongue syndrome (Lance and Anthony 1980) consists of numbness of one side of the tongue with abnormal proprioception and sometimes twisting, on head turning. It may occur with degenerative or malformative abnormalities of the upper spine, although in many cases the cervical spine appears normal.

OTHER TRAUMATIC NERVE INJURIES

Neonatal *injuries to the radial nerve* as a result of subcutaneous fat necrosis of the upper arm (Eng *et al.* 1996) and of the median nerve as a result of attempts at catheterization of the radial or humeral artery have been reported (Chapter 2). I have seen two infants with transient paralysis of the femoral nerve after difficult puncture of the femoral vein and two similar cases following herniorrhaphy and appendectomy. In the latter procedure (for retrocaecal appendicitis), nerve injury was probably due to trauma of the nerve along the psoas muscle. Similar cases are reported in the literature (Stultz and Pfeiffer 1982).

Traumatic palsy of the peroneal nerve may be due to orthopaedic appliance to the region (Jones 1986) and has been reported following infiltration of intravenous fluid (Kreusser and Volpe 1984). Radial paralysis following constraint of the forearm for intravenous infusion is relatively common and always transient.

Lumbar plexus injuries are rare and occur only following major trauma to the pelvis, especially as a result of motor vehicle accidents. Rare cases have been seen following difficult breech delivery (Hope *et al.* 1985).

Glossopharyngeal neuralgia following amygdalectomy or tonsillectomy has been exceptionally recorded (Ekbom and Westerberg 1966). Occipital neuralgia is not rare especially in adolescents (Dugan *et al.* 1962).

Nerve tumours are quite rare in children excepting the benign tumours of neurofibromatosis I which require no treatment. Detection of malignant nerve tumours is important, however, as effective treatment should not be delayed.

REFLEX SYMPATHETIC DYSTROPHY (REFLEX NEUROVASCULAR DYSTROPHY)

Reflex sympathetic dystrophy is a syndrome of unknown cause characterized by pain, tenderness, swelling, vasomotor disturbances and dystrophic skin changes typically affecting a single extremity (Schwartzman and McLellan 1987). Three diagnostic criteria have been suggested: (1) diffuse pain often not localized to anatomical nerve territories and out of proportion to the cause; (2) loss of function or impaired movements; (3) some objective evidence of autonomic dysfunction such as skin changes, oedema or osteoporosis. The disorder follows trauma, usually minor, in 40 per cent of cases and typically occurs in young adolescent girls (Ashwal *et al.* 1988, Silber and Majd 1988, Dietz *et al.* 1990, Gordon 1996). Pain may be so severe as to produce pseudoparalysis. In children, symptoms tend to be self-limited but a significant minority have protracted and disabling illness. Affected children may have a special psychological profile (Sherry and Weisman 1988). Bone scan may help in diagnosing the condition

by showing localized hypofixation rather than the hyperfixation seen in adults. Study by cutaneous thermography of local vasomotor reflex or by monitoring of near-surface blood flow may be of diagnostic value (Gordon 1996). Numerous forms of treatment have been used (Schwartzman and McLellan 1987, Kesler *et al.* 1988, Dietz *et al.* 1990) with variable results, including steroids, betablockers, calcitonin, vasodilators and physiotherapy (Gordon 1996). Infiltration of the regional sympathetic ganglia may be hepful although involvement of the sympathetic system in the disorder has been contested. Sympathectomy may be used when infiltration proves helpful. Trophic changes may persist in long-standing cases.

Other rare autonomic disturbances of neural origin include Harlequin syndrome (Lance *et al.* 1988) and Ross syndrome (anhydrosis, Adie's pupil, syncope and other autonomic symptoms) (Drummond and Lance 1993) which have been occasionally reported in children.

LOCALIZED DISORDERS OF CRANIAL NERVES (EXCEPT OPTIC AND AUDITORY NERVES)

The cranial nerves are affected together with the rest of the peripheral nerves in many diffuse nerve disorders. Certain conditions more specific to the cranial nerves, whether congenital or acquired, are described in this section.

FACIAL NERVE PARALYSES

Facial paralysis can be due to lesions located anywhere between the motor nucleus of the nerve and its terminal ramifications. Depending on the site of the lesion, variable symptoms and signs may accompany the facial weakness (Table 21.6, Fig. 21.8).

CONGENITAL FACIAL PARALYSES
Birth injury to the facial nerve
The facial nerve is the most commonly involved in birth trauma or prenatal compression. Congenital unilateral facial nerve palsy is observed in approximately 0.3 per 1000 live births (McHugh *et al.* 1969) but is more common in large infants with an incidence of up to 6.5–7.5 per 1000 (Levine *et al.* 1984). In a majority of cases injury to the nerve is probably the result of pressure on the facial nerve distal to its emergence from the stylomastoid foramen against the sacral prominence of the maternal pelvis. This is suggested by the consistent relationship between fetal position and side of palsy, with left and right palsies observed subsequent to, respectively, left and right occipital positions. Paralysis resulting from application of forceps is comparatively rare.

The clinical expression of unilateral facial palsy even when it is complete is not always evident at birth, and partial involvement is not uncommon. In such cases, the orbicularis oculi is most often spared. This is because fibres that course upward just after leaving the foramen are not involved by compression over the parotid gland. The palpebral fissure is wider on the affected side and the eye fails to close completely (Fig. 21.9). Finding a

TABLE 21.6
Facial nerve paralysis: features associated with weakness as a function of localization of the lesion

Localization	Taste	Hyperacousis	Lachrymation	Salivation
Motor nucleus	Normal	Present[2]	Normal	Normal
Facial nerve trunk between pons and internal auditory meatus	Normal	Present[2]	Impaired[3]	Impaired[1]
Geniculate ganglion	Impaired[1]	Present[2]	Impaired[3]	Impaired[1]
Facial nerve trunk between geniculate ganglion and emergence of stapedius nerve	Impaired[1]	Present[2]	Normal	Impaired[1]
Facial nerve trunk between stapedius nerve and chorda tympani	Impaired[1]	Absent	Normal	Impaired[1]
Lower facial nerve below chorda tympani	Normal	Absent	Normal	Normal

[1]Function subserved by the chorda tympani (fibres orginating from the solitary tract nucleus and joining the facial nerve through its anastomosis with the IXth cranial nerve).
[2]Function subserved by the stapedius nerve.
[3]Function subserved by the greater superficial petrosal nerve (fibres originating from the solitary tract nucleus, coursing through the ganglion).

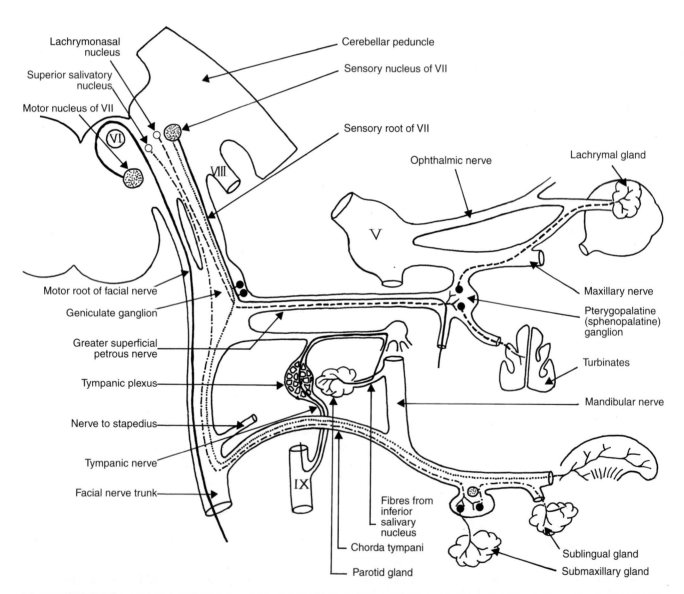

Fig. 21.8. Schematic representation of the facial nerve, indicating the distribution of sensory fibres and of autonomic fibres to lacrimal and salivary glands. (This schema helps explain the consequences to taste and hearing sensation, lacrimation and salivation of lesions at various levels—see also Table 21.6.)

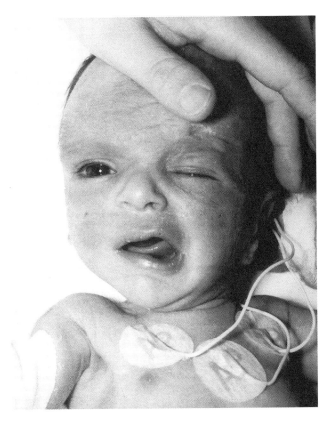

Fig. 21.9. Congenital facial palsy. 2-day-old infant born by forceps extraction. Note involvement of whole of right side of face, with failure of right eye to close.

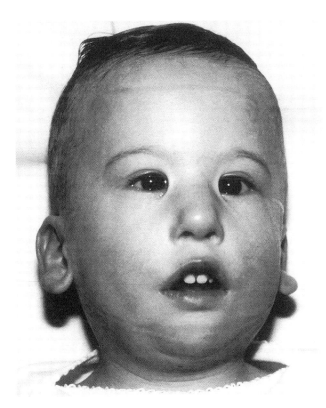

Fig. 21.10. Moebius syndrome. Mask-like facies due to bilateral facial paralysis. Note also bilateral internal strabismus due to involvement of both abducens nerves.

periauricular ecchymosis or a haemotympanum helps diagnose traumatic palsy with a likely recovery (Shapiro *et al.* 1996).

In most cases, resolution of the paralysis is observed in a few weeks. Severe injuries with extensive disruption of the nerve seem to be rare. Surgical exploration of the nerve may be considered when no recovery is apparent after three to six months.

Congenital nontraumatic facial palsy
Congenital facial palsy can result from various anomalies of the nerve or its nucleus. Lesions of the inner ear may be associated with visible anomalies of the auricle and may be demonstrated by CT scan studies showing osseous abnormalities. More often, the nucleus or the nerve itself is abnormal or interrupted (Zucker 1990). Such patients present with unilateral complete paralysis and have no tendency to spontanous recovery. Electrical stimulation at the stylomastoid foramen shows no muscle contraction, in contrast to what obtains in traumatic palsy, and is of great value (Shapiro *et al.* 1996). Surgical exploration of the nerve may be indicated. Cleidocranial dysostosis and other bony dysplasias of the base of the skull are an unusual cause.

Moebius syndrome
Moebius syndrome is characterized by facial diplegia typically associated with bilateral abducens palsy (Fig. 21.10) and, occasionally, with involvement of several cranial nerves, especially the lower cranial pairs with frequent tongue involvement (Sudarshan and Goldie 1985). Affectation of the IIIrd nerves is uncommon. The syndrome often results in speech and sometimes feeding difficulties. Mental deficiency is present in about 10–27 per cent of affected children, although the immobile facies, drooling and speech difficulties often wrongly suggest subnormality. Unilateral Moebius syndrome has been reported (Towfighi *et al.* 1979).

The mechanism of the Moebius syndrome is probably multiple. Some cases may be due to congenital muscle aplasia or to other muscle disorders (Hanson and Rowland 1971). Others may be due to absence of the brainstem nucleus (Towfighi *et al.* 1979). It seems more likely that many cases result from prenatal brainstem ischaemia with necrosis and sometimes calcification of the facial nuclei (Thakkar *et al.* 1977, Govaert *et al.* 1989, Fujita *et al.* 1991). Bavinck and Weaver (1986) have speculated that the Moebius syndrome and other regional malformations such as the Poland anomaly and the Klippel–Feil syndrome might all be consequences of disrupted blood supply in the territory of the subclavian artery. Hamaguchi *et al.* (1993) separate three subgroups: children with only cranial nerve involvement, primarily of the VIth and VIIth pairs; patients with associated arthrogryposis; and those with absence or structural deformities of the extremities. The last type were found in 48 per cent of 106 cases collected by Engler *et al.* (1979) who also encountered absence of the pectoralis major in 9 per cent and micrognathia in 6 per cent of their cases. Rare cases of familial Moebius syndrome are on record (Garcia-Erro *et al.* 1989). In some familial cases, other abnormalities such as Poland anomaly or arthrogryposis may be associated (Gadoth *et al.* 1979, Sudarshan and Goldie 1985).

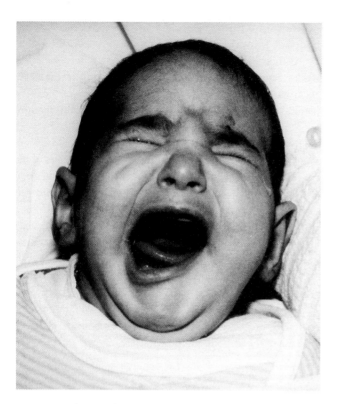

Fig. 21.11. Absence of depressor anguli muscle. Upper part of face is normal. Left corner of mouth fails to be lowered on crying.

Hypoplasia (or paralysis) of the depressor anguli oris muscle
This is a common minor anomaly (Nelson and Eng 1972). The corner of the mouth on the involved side fails to move downward on crying (Fig. 21.11). The lower lip may be slighlty everted on the same side. This anomaly has been thought to be associated with other manifestations, especially congenital heart disease (Levin *et al.* 1982, Raymond and Holmes 1993), the so-called cardiofacial syndrome. A vast majority of children with this anomaly do not have other problems and a referral bias cannot be excluded. Beck *et al.* (1989) reported cases of *isolated auriculo-temporal syndrome* in children, characterized by localized flushing of the face when eating.

Diagnosis of congenital facial palsies
The major causes of facial weakness are shown in Table 21.7. Congenital palsies represent about 8 per cent of cases of child-hood facial paralysis (Manning and Adour 1972), but it is not always easy to distinguish acquired from congenital cases and to separate nerve involvement from weakness due to muscle diseases.

For all cases with paralysis lasting more than a few weeks without improvement, imaging studies of the base of the brain are indicated. In cases of Moebius syndrome, brain CT or MRI should be performed.

ACQUIRED FACIAL PARALYSES
Paralysis of unknown cause—Bell palsy
Bell palsy is an acute idiopathic paralysis involving the territory of one facial nerve. The *pathological changes* include considerable

TABLE 21.7
Main causes of facial weakness in childhood*

Congenital
Congenital facial palsy due to birth injury
Congenital absence of depressor anguli oris muscle
Abnormalities of inner ear and/or facial nerve
Moebius syndrome of peripheral or central (nuclear) origin
Congenital or neonatal myasthenic syndromes
Congenital myotonic dystrophy
Other congenital myopathies or muscular dystrophies
Acquired
Diffuse neuromuscular diseases
   Muscular dystrophy (facioscapulohumeral type) and myopathies (*e.g.* nemaline myopathy)
   Acquired myasthenia and myasthenic syndromes
   Juvenile bulbar palsy (Fazio Londe and Van Laere types)
Involvement of facial nerve
   Inflammatory
      Bell palsy
      Idiopathic cranial neuropathy
      Miller Fisher syndrome and atypical forms of Guillain–Barré syndrome (Ropper 1986b)
      Herpes zoster (Ramsay Hunt syndrome)
      Lyme disease
      Otitis media and mastoiditis
      Infectious mononucleosis and other herpes viruses (Dowling and Cook 1981)
      Tuberculosis (tuberculoma or meningitis)
      Trichinosis (Lopez-Lozano *et al.* 1988)
      Sarcoidosis (Heerfordt syndrome)
      Multiple sclerosis
   Trauma and compression
      Fracture of petrous bone and other traumas
      Parotid gland tumours
      Osseous dysplasia of the base of the skull (*e.g.* cleidocranial dysostosis, osteopetrosis, hyperostosis cranialis interna) (Manni *et al.* 1990)
      Brainstem glioma and other intracranial tumours
      Langerhans histiocytosis (histiocytosis X)
      Intracranial hypertension
   Malformations
      Chiari malformation
      Syringobulbia
   Unknown mechanism
      Hyperparathyroidism
      Hypothyroidism
   Genetic
      Melkersson–Rosenthal syndrome
      Recurrent familial cranial neuropathy
   Vascular
      Arterial hypertension
      Vascular syndromes of the cranial nerve

*References are given only for conditions not discussed in text.

oedema but there are few inflammatory signs. The pathogenesis is still uncertain but autoimmune demyelination probably plays a major role. The incidence of Bell palsy is 2.7 per 100,000 in the first decade of life and 10.1 per 100,000 in the second decade (Katusik *et al.* 1986). Both sides of the face are equally involved. Approximately 1.4 per cent of patients have a family history of the disorder. A history of prior viral infection is frequently recorded but its significance is undecided. Multiple viral infections have been suspected. CSF studies in many cases have demonstrated pleocytosis, disordered blood–brain barrier and intrathecal immunoglobulin synthesis (Roberg *et al.* 1991). There is evidence that Bell palsy may be only the most striking manifestation of an autoimmune disorder affecting other cranial nerves, particularly the sensory trigeminal nerve which may be involved in up to 50 per cent of cases (Adour *et al.* 1978, Lapresle *et al.* 1980).

The first *clinical manifestations* may be pain or paraesthesiae in the ear or the face unilaterally but these are usually mild or absent. The paralysis reaches its maximum in a few hours and involves all muscles on one side of the face. The face is pulled to the side opposite the paralysis with efforts to use muscles of expression. The eye cannot be fully closed, and drinking may become difficult. Lachrymation is preserved in many cases but taste sensation is lost in about half the patients (see Table 21.6, p. 734).

Weakness remains maximal for two to four weeks and then begins to lessen spontaneously (Adour 1982). Complete recovery is the rule in children especially when palsy is partial. Wong (1995) found complete recovery in 21 of 24 children. When de-nervation is complete, the onset of improvement may be delayed and recovery may not be total, reaching its maximum within six months (Adour 1982). Aberrant regeneration with 'crocodile tears' or auriculotemporal syndrome (Levin 1987) is exceptional in children. Recurrent paralysis is observed in around 6 per cent of cases (Katusik *et al.* 1986). Electrical stimulation studies may be useful: incomplete denervation predicts complete recovery whereas complete denervation may herald the persistence of some weakness. The CSF is abnormal in 10 per cent (Weber *et al.* 1987) to 75 per cent (Sandstedt *et al.* 1985) of patients, with increased protein and mononuclear cells, but lumbar puncture is rarely indicated.

The treatment of Bell palsy is purely symptomatic. Protection of an exposed cornea (by lubrication and patching) is essential. Corticosteroids are often advocated for adult patients but they are not indicated for children and there is indeed no proof of their efficacy (Burgess *et al.* 1984). It is important to exclude the possibility of otitis or mastoiditis and of any other lesional cause and to rule out Lyme disease (Clark *et al.* 1985) which may be the sole manifestation of the disease although involvement of the chorda tympani is less frequent in Lyme disease.

Paralyses of known cause
Facial palsy is frequently the only manifestation of *Lyme disease*, especially in summer and autumn (Harkby 1989, Grundfast *et al.* 1990). Christen *et al.* (1993) found that 32.9 per cent of their cases were due to Lyme disease whereas viruses were apparently responsible for 18.4 per cent. Facial palsy in neuroborreliosis may be unilateral; the occurrence of bilateral palsy a few days after in-volvement of one side is highly suggestive of borreliosis (Keane 1994, Kindstrand 1995). Stiff neck may be found in a quarter of cases. The CSF in such cases consistently shows pleocytosis and increased protein and may contain antibodies against *Borrelia burgdorferi* (Chapter 11).

Herpes zoster of the geniculate ganglion (Ramsay Hunt syndrome) is an uncommon cause of facial palsy in children. It may occur without any vesicular rash in the concha (Manning and Adour 1972). Other viruses may cause facial paralysis including Epstein–Barr, chicken pox and mumps viruses.

Otitis media and mastoiditis, although now uncommon causes, should always be thought of, as antibiotic and/or surgical treatment may be required and as local signs may be extremely subtle. X-rays or CT of the temporal bone are indicated if there is any doubt about the possibility of a local otogenic process.

Tumours, especially rhabdomyosarcomas, may compress the nerve and should always be considered.

Hypertension is a frequent cause of facial palsy (Lloyd *et al.* 1966) and should be systematically looked for (Chapter 15).

Traumatic paralysis is easy to suspect but demonstration may also require X-ray investigations (May *et al.* 1981). It may lead to aberrant regeneration and contractures.

Facial palsy is also the most common manifestation of *neurosarcoidosis*, a rare disorder in childen (Scott 1993).

Melkersson–Rosenthal syndrome is characterized by recurrent facial palsy, associated with swelling of the lips, face or eyelids and furrowing of the tongue (Wadlington *et al.* 1984). Facial swelling and palsy may occur in isolation or simultaneously. Often swelling is the initial manifestation. Lingual involvement is inconstant. With repeated attacks, residual paralysis may appear and increase, leading to severe impairment.

Recurrent facial palsy may also be due to hypertension and to familial Bell palsy (Hageman *et al.* 1990).

Bilateral facial palsy is most commonly due to neuroborreli-osis. Other causes in a mixed series of 43 children and adults (Keane 1994) included Guillain–Barré syndrome (six cases), tumours of brainstem or meninges (nine cases), brainstem encephalitis and other miscellaneous causes. Ten cases were idiopathic (bilateral Bell palsy).

Hemifacial spasm has been reported in a few infants and children (Al Shahwan *et al.* 1994, Arzimanoglou *et al.* 1996). The onset is usually in the first days of life with repeated attacks of unilateral tonic facial contracture lasting a minute or less and repeated many times daily. The syndrome is regularly associated with a small mass lesion in the region of the nucleus of the ipsi-lateral VIIth nerve probably hamartomatous in nature (Al Shah-wan *et al.* 1994, Arzimanoglou *et al.* 1996, Harvey *et al.* 1996). Harvey *et al.* have recorded the mass paroxysmal discharges syn-chronous with the attack that may thus be regarded as a form of subcortical epilepsy. Their patient remained free of attacks following resection of the lesion. Such attacks differ from true peripheral hemifacial spasm, a rare condition in childhood, which is usually attributed to compression of the VIIth nerve trunk (Ronen *et al.* 1986). A case presenting in a newborn infant has been reported with a benign course (Zefeiriou *et al.* 1997).

LOWER CRANIAL NERVE PALSIES
CONGENITAL LOWER CRANIAL NERVE PALSIES
Impairment of function of lower cranial nerves VII to XII is present in cases of Chiari I and II malformation (Chapter 3).

Involvement of the abductors of the vocal cords is particularly important as it often gives rise to severe respiratory insufficiency. Some cases are improved by treatment of the accompanying hydrocephalus.

Congenital traumatic laryngeal paralyses are probably related to intrauterine posture with rotation and lateral flexion of the head causing compression of the superior branch of the laryngeal nerve against the thyroid bone and that of the recurrent nerve against the cricoid cartilage. This produces a dual syndrome of the laryngeal nerve with both disturbances of swallowing due to sensory dysfunction of the superior laryngeal nerve and dysphonia due to involvement of the recurrent nerve (Chapple 1956). The prognosis of such cases is usually good (Narcy *et al.* 1978).

Hoarseness due to paralysis of the left recurrent nerve is in rare cases a presenting or accompanying symptom of congestive heart failure in infancy or a manifestation of congenital anomaly of the great vessels of the base of the heart, the cardiovocal syndrome (Condon *et al.* 1985).

Congenital dysfunction of the vocal cords may occur in isolation and may be genetically transmitted. The posterior cricoarytenoid muscle, which is the sole abductor of the vocal cords and the only laryngeal muscle innervated solely by neurons of the ventral division of the ipsilateral nucleus ambiguus, is affected resulting in stridor and respiratory impairment. The condition may be familial (Cunningham *et al.* 1985). The course is towards spontaneous recovery in some cases, while other patients require a tracheostomy to maintain a free airway (Cohen *et al.* 1982).

Neurogenic stridor may also be of traumatic origin following forceps delivery or accidental trauma at birth (Maze and Bloch 1979). It may also be a feature of CNS involvement and occurs in association with nystagmus in connatal Pelizaeus–Merzbacher disease (Chapter 10).

Congenital dysphagia is rarely due to peripheral nerve involvement and is more often a part of pseudobulbar palsy that may be due to brain malformations or vascular and degenerative disorders. Severe dysarthria is often present in such cases (Van Dongen *et al.* 1987). Prolonged congenital dysphagia was reported by Mbonda *et al.* (1995). One of their four patients had associated paralysis of the adductors of the vocal cords. Cineradiographic study of swallowing showed major difficulties with the pharyngeal stage with only minimal involvement of the first oral stage. Two of the patients died; the others recovered in 20 and 40 months respectively. This syndrome is to be distinguished from benign transient pharyngeal dysfunction observed usually in preterm infants with recovery in a few weeks. EMG of the tongue and pharyngeal muscle confirms the peripheral involvement and helps predict the outcome.

ACQUIRED LESIONS OF LOWER CRANIAL NERVES
Traumatic neonatal paralyses of the lower cranial pairs are uncommon. A few cases of glossopharyngeal paralysis variably associated with involvement of the IXth, Xth and XIth pairs are on record (Greenberg *et al.* 1987), and hypoglossal palsy accompanied by brachial plexus injury has also been reported (Haenggeli and Lacourt 1989).

Intracranial disorders that produce raised intracranial pressure can be responsible for unilateral or, more commonly, bilateral vocal cord palsy often requiring tracheostomy. Spontaneous regression occurred in four of seven cases reported by Chaten *et al.* (1991).

Isolated neuropathies probably related to viral or postviral diseases may raise serious diagnostic problems in children. Some may affect only one nerve, *e.g.* the hypoglossal nerve (Edin *et al.* 1976, Wright and Lee 1980), the recurrent nerve (Blau and Kapadia 1972) or the vagus nerve (Berry and Blair 1980). Others may involve both the IXth and Xth pairs usually on one side and produce an isolated temporary paralysis of the pharynx that may raise the suspicion of brainstem disease (Aubergé *et al.* 1979, Roberton and Mellor 1982, Suarez-Zeledon and Brian-Gago 1995). The onset is sudden, often following an upper respiratory infection, more rarely after a specific viral infection such as infectious mononucleosis (Wright and Lee 1980, Sugama *et al.* 1992, Connelly and De Witt 1994), with nasal reflux and/or dysphagia. Examination shows unilateral paresis of the soft palate and of the posterior pharyngeal wall. Spontaneous recovery occurs in a few days or weeks. Such cases are probably related to postinfectious abducens palsy (Chapter 18). XIIth nerve palsy is rare in children (Keane 1996).

Glossopharyngeal neuralgia is exceptional in children. Kandt and Daniel (1986) reported a case relieved by section of the glossopharyngeal nerve.

ANOSMIA AND KALLMANN SYNDROME
Cranial trauma affecting the first cranial nerve may result in anosmia, which is often definitive. Anosmia also occurs in boys with cleft palate (Richman *et al.* 1988).

Congenital anosmia is a part of a usually but not exclusively X-linked syndrome of anosmia and eunuchoidism, sometimes associated with mild mental retardation, known as Kallmann syndrome, mapping to Xp22.3 (Chapter 3). It results from an arrest of migration of axons from the olfactory placode that fail to reach the olfactory bulbs. Neurological defects are often present including mirror movements, cerebellar signs, hearing loss and abnormal eye movements (Schwankhaus *et al.* 1989). The syndrome is rarely associated with ichthyosis, short stature, chondrodystrophia punctata and ocular albinism, representing a contiguous gene syndrome associated with deletion of the entire short arm of the X chromosome (Gomez 1994).

MULTIPLE CRANIAL NERVE PARALYSES
As indicated above, multiple involvement of cranial nerves may be more frequent than suspected, and Bell palsy is often the visible part of a subclinical multiple neuropathy. Such multiple nerve involvement in adults may be of vascular origin (Lapresle and Lasjaunias 1986). Affected nerves are few in such cases and belong to a localized arterial territory. In children, multiple cranial neuropathy is more often a manifestation of acute polyneuritis akin to the Guillain–Barré syndrome (Ropper 1986a, Waddy *et al.* 1989). In occasional cases, a known virus is implicated, *e.g.* the varicella-zoster virus (Mayo and Booss 1989).

Idiopathic cranial polyneuropathy is observed mainly in adults (Hokkanen *et al.* 1978, Juncos and Beal 1987, Uldry and Regli 1988) but may also affect children. Various patterns of multiple cranial nerve involvement can obtain. The most commonly involved nerves are the facial nerves, the ocular motor nerves and the lower cranial nerves, but optic nerve involvement has been reported. The course of multiple cranial neuropathies is often recurrent and such cases pose difficult diagnostic problems with myasthenia gravis, recurrent facial plasy, the syndrome of Tolosa–Hunt (Sorensen 1988), and some mitochondrial diseases. A migrating course is sometimes oberved (Takahashi 1978). The condition may be familial (Sorensen 1988) but little is known about its mechanism.

A similar picture may be produced by tumours invading the base of the skull or basal meninges, hence the necessity of a careful radiological examination of such patients. Brainstem gliomas and encephalitis may also pose a diagnostic problem although they commonly produce signs of long tract affectation. Osseous diseases (hyperostosis cranialis interna) (Manni *et al.* 1990) may be a rare cause of multiple cranial nerve entrapment.

REFERENCES

Adams, D., Festenstein, H., Gibson, J.D., *et al.* (1979) 'HLA antigens in chronic relapsing idiopathic inflammatory polyneuropathy.' *Journal of Neurology, Neurosurgery, and Psychiatry*, **42**, 184–186.

Adour, K.K. (1982) 'Diagnosis and management of facial paralysis.' *New England Journal of Medicine*, **307**, 348–351.

—— Byl, F.M., Hilsinger, R.L., *et al.* (1978) 'The true nature of Bell's palsy: analysis of 1000 consecutive patients.' *Laryngoscope*, **88**, 787–801.

Airaksinen, E.M., Iivanainen, M., Karli, P., *et al.* (1985) 'Hereditary recurrent brachial plexus neuropathy with dysmorphic features.' *Acta Neurologica Scandinavica*, **71**, 309–316.

Al-Din, A.N., Anderson, M., Bickestaff, E.R., Harvey, I. (1982) 'Brainstem encephalitis and the syndrome of Miller Fisher.' *Brain*, **105**, 481–495.

Al-Qudah, A.A., Shahar, E., Logan, W.J., Murphy, E.G. (1988) 'Neonatal Guillain–Barré syndrome.' *Pediatric Neurology*, **4**, 255–256.

Al-Shahwan, S.A., Singh, B., Riela, A.R., Roach, E.S. (1994) 'Hemisomatic spasms in children.' *Neurology*, **44**, 1332–1333.

Amato, A.A., Barohn, R.J., Sahenk, Z., *et al.* (1993) 'Polyneuropathy complicating bone marrow and solid organ transplantation.' *Neurology*, **43**, 1513–1518.

Argov, Z., Mastaglia, F.L. (1979) 'Drug-induced peripheral neuropathies.' *British Medical Journal*, **1**, 663–666.

Arts, W.F.M., Busch, H.F.M., Van der Brand, H.D., *et al.* (1983) 'Hereditary neuralgic amyotrophy.' *Journal of Neurological Sciences*, **62**, 261–279.

Arzimanoglou, A. (1996) 'Hemifacial spasm or subcortical (infratentorial) epilepsy: a case report of a child with Goldenhar syndrome and a postmedullary junction lesion.' *In:* Arzimanoglou, A., Goutières, F. (Eds.) *Trends in Child Neurology.* Paris: John Libbey, pp. 43–51.

Asbury, A.K. (1981) 'Diagnostic considerations in Guillain–Barré syndrome.' *Annals of Neurology*, **9** (Suppl.), 1–5.

—— Cornblath, D.R. (1990) 'Assessment of current diagnostic criteria for Guillain–Barré syndrome.' *Annals of Neurology*, **27** (Suppl.), S21–S24.

—— Arnason, B.G., Karp, H.R., McFarlin, D.E. (1978) 'Criteria for diagnosis of Guillain–Barré syndrome.' *Annals of Neurology*, **3**, 565–566.

Ashwal, S., Tomasi, L., Neumann, M., Schreider, S. (1988) 'Reflex sympathetic dystrophy syndrome in children.' *Pediatric Neurology*, **4**, 38–42.

Aubergé, C., Ponsot, G., Gayraud, P., *et al.* (1979) 'Les hémiparésies vélopalatines isolées et acquises chez l'enfant.' *Archives Françaises de Pédiatrie*, **36**, 283–286.

Awerbuch, G.I., Nigro, M.A., Dabrowski, E., Levin, J.R. (1989) 'Childhood lumbosacral plexus neuropathy.' *Pediatric Neurology*, **5**, 314–316.

Axelrod, F.B., Abularrage, J.J. (1982) 'Familial dysautonomia: a prospective study of survival.' *Journal of Pediatrics*, **101**, 234–236.

—— Pearson, J. (1984) 'Congenital sensory neuropathies: diagnostic distinction from familial dysautonomia.' *American Journal of Diseases of Children*, **138**, 947–954.

—— Nachtigall, R., Dancis, J. (1974) 'Familial dysautonomia: diagnosis, pathogenesis and management.' *Advances in Pediatrics*, **21**, 75–96.

—— Iyer, K., Fish, I., *et al.* (1981) 'Progressive sensory loss in familial dysautonomia.' *Pediatrics*, **67**, 517–522.

—— Cash, R., Pearson, J. (1983a) 'Congenital autonomic dysfunction with universal pain loss.' *Journal of Pediatrics*, **103**, 60–64.

—— Pearson, J., Tepperberg, J., Ackerman, B.D. (1983b) 'Congenital sensory neuropathy with skeletal dysplasia.' *Journal of Pediatrics*, **102**, 727–730.

Azouvi, P., Hostachy, T., Desi, M., Saïd, G. (1989) 'Polyneuropathie axonale aiguë et réversible dans les suites d'une leptospirose.' *Revue Neurologique*, **145**, 805–807.

Azulay, J-P., Blin, O., Pouget, J., *et al.* (1994) 'Intravenous immunoglobulin treatment in patients with motor neuron syndromes associated with anti-GM₁ antibodies: a double-blind, placebo-controlled study.' *Neurology*, **44**, 429–432.

Baba, M., Takada, H., Miura, H., *et al.* (1995) '"Pseudo" hypertrophic neuropathy of childhood.' *Journal of Neurology, Neurosurgery, and Psychiatry*, **58**, 236–237.

Balestrini, M.R., Cavaletti, G., D'Angelo, A., Tredici, G. (1991) 'Infantile hereditary neuropathy with hypomyelination: report of two siblings with different expressivity.' *Neuropediatrics*, **22**, 65–70.

Bank, W.J., Pleasure, D.E., Suzuki, K., *et al.* (1972) 'Thallium poisoning.' *Archives of Neurology*, **26**, 456–464.

Bardosi, A., Creutzfeldt, W., DiMauro, S., *et al.* (1987) 'Myo-, neuro-, gastrointestinal encephalopathy (MNGIE syndrome) due to partial deficiency of cytochrome-c-oxidase. A new mitochondrial multisystem disorder.' *Acta Neuropathologica*, **74**, 248–258.

Bardosi, R., Friede, R., Ropte, S., Goebel, H.H. (1987) 'A morphometric study on sural nerves in metachromatic leukodystrophy.' *Brain*, **110**, 683–694.

Barohn, R.J., Kissel, J.T., Warmolts, J.R., Mendell, J.R. (1989) 'Chronic inflammatory demyelinating polyradiculoneuropathy: clinical characteristics, course and recommendation for diagnostic criteria.' *Archives of Neurology*, **46**, 878–884.

Bastron, J.A., Thomas, J.E. (1981) 'Diabetic polyneuropathy: clinical and electromyographic findings in 105 patients.' *Mayo Clinic Proceedings*, **56**, 725–732.

Baumgartner, G., Gawel, M.J., Kaeser, H.E., *et al.* (1970) 'Neurotoxicity of halogenated hydroxyquinolines: clinical analysis of cases reported outside Japan.' *Journal of Neurology, Neurosurgery, and Psychiatry*, **42**, 1073–1083.

Bavinck, J.N.B., Weaver, D.D. (1986) 'Subclavian artery supply disruption sequence: hypothesis of a vascular etiology for Poland, Klippel–Feil and Möbius anomalies.' *American Journal of Medical Genetics*, **23**, 903–918.

Beck, S.A., Burks, A.W., Woody, R.C. (1989) 'Auriculotemporal syndrome seen clinically as food allergy.' *Pediatrics*, **83**, 601–603.

Becker, D.M., Kramer, S. (1977) 'The neurological manifestations of porphyria: a review.' *Medicine*, **56**, 411–423.

Behan, P.O., Lessell, S., Roche, M. (1976) 'Optic neuritis in the Landry–Guillain–Barré–Strohl syndrome.' *British Journal of Ophthalmology*, **60**, 58–59.

Behse, F., Buchtal, F. (1977) 'Peroneal muscular atrophy (PMA) and related disorders. II. Histological findings in sural nerves.' *Brain*, **100**, 67–86.

—— —— Carlsen, F., Knappeis, G.G. (1972) 'Hereditary neuropathy with liability to pressure palsies.' *Brain*, **95**, 777–794.

Ben Hamida, M., Hentati, F., Ben Hamida, C. (1990) 'Giant axonal neuropathy with inherited multisystem degeneration in a Tunisian kindred.' *Neurology*, **40**, 245–250.

—— Belal, S., Svingo, G., *et al.* (1993) 'Friedreich's ataxia phenotype not linked to chromosome 9 and associated with selective autosomal recessive vitamin E deficiency in two inbred Tunisian families.' *Neurology*, **43**, 2179–2183.

Ben Jelloun-Dellagi, S., Dellagi, K., Burger, D., *et al.* (1992) 'Childhood peripheral neuropathy with antibodies to myelin glycoprotein Po.' *Annals of Neurology*, **32**, 700–702.

Ben Othmane, K., Hentati, F., Lennon, F., *et al.* (1993a) 'Linkage of a locus (CMT4A) for autosomal recessive Charcot–Marie–Tooth disease to chromosome 8q.' *Human Molecular Genetics*, **2**, 1625–1628.

—— Middleton, L.T., Loprest, L.J., *et al.* (1993b) 'Localization of a gene (CMT2A) for autosomal dominant Charcot–Marie–Tooth disease type 2 to chromosome 1p and evidence of genetic heterogeneity.' *Genomics*, **17**, 370–375.

Benson, M.D. (1995) 'Amyloidosis.' *In:* Scriver, C.R., Beaudet, A.L., Sly, W.S., Valle, D. (Eds.) *The Metabolic Basis of Inherited Disease, 6th Edn.* New York: McGraw Hill, 2439–2460.

Berciano, J., Combarros, O., Figols, J., *et al.* (1986) 'Hereditary motor and sensory neuropathy type II. Clinicopathological study of a family.' *Brain*, 109, 897–914.

Bergoffen, J., Scherer, S.S., Wang, S., *et al.* (1993) 'Connexin mutations in X-linked Charcot–Marie–Tooth disease.' *Science*, 262, 2039–2042.

Berry, H., Blair, R.L. (1980) 'Isolated vagus nerve palsy and vagal mononeuritis.' *Archives of Otolaryngology*, 106, 333–338.

Billard, C., Ponsot, G., Lyon, G., Arthuis, M. (1979) 'Polyradiculonévrites aiguës de l'enfant. Aspects cliniques et évolutifs. Facteurs pronostiques à propos de 100 observations.' *Archives Françaises de Pédiatrie*, 36, 149–161.

Blau, J.N., Kapadia, R. (1972) 'Idiopathic palsy of the recurrent laryngeal nerve: a transient cranial mononeuropathy.' *British Medical Journal*, 4, 259–261.

Blumenfeld, A., Slaugenhaupt, S.A., Axelrod, F.B., *et al.* (1993) 'Localization of the gene for familial dysautonomia on chromosome 9 and definition of DNA markers for genetic diagnosis.' *Nature Genetics*, 4, 160–164.

Bodensteiner, J.B., Rich, K.M., Landau, W.M. (1994) 'Early infantile surgery for birth-related brachial plexus injuries: justification requires a prospective controlled study.' *Journal of Child Neurology*, 9, 109–110.

Boespflug-Tanguy, O., Gimbergues, P., Campagne, D., *et al.* (1994) 'The piriformis muscle syndrome: a rare cause of acquired sciatic paralysis in children.' *Journal of Neurology*, 241, Suppl. 1, S141. *(Abstract.)*

Bone, L.J., Dahl, N., Lensch, M.W., *et al.* (1995) 'New connexin 32 mutations associated with X-linked Charcot–Marie–Tooth disease.' *Neurology*, 45, 1863–1866.

Bono, A., Beghi, E., Bogliun, G., *et al.* (1993) 'Antiepileptic drugs and peripheral nerve function: a multicenter screening investigation of 141 patients with chronic treatment. Collaborative Group for the Study of Epilepsy.' *Epilepsia*, 34, 323–331.

Boylan, K.B., Ferriero, D.M., Greco, C.M., *et al.* (1992) 'Congenital hypomyelination neuropathy with arthrogryposis multiplex congenita.' *Annals of Neurology*, 31, 337–340.

Bradshaw, D.Y., Jones, H.R. (1992) 'Guillain–Barré syndrome in children: clinical course, electrodiagnosis, and prognosis.' *Muscle and Nerve*, 15, 500–506.

Brin, M.F., Pedley, T.A., Lovelace, R.E., *et al.* (1986) 'Electrophysiologic features of abetalipoproteinemia: functional consequences of vitamin E deficiency.' *Neurology*, 36, 669–673.

Browder, A.A., Joselow, M.M., Louria, D.B. (1973) 'The problem of lead poisoning.' *Medicine*, 52, 121–139.

Brown, B.J., Lewis, L.A., Mercer, R.D. (1974) 'Familial hypobetalipoproteinemia: report of a case with psychomotor retardation.' *Pediatrics*, 54, 111–113.

Burck, U., Goebel, H.H., Kuhlendahl, H.D., *et al.* (1981) 'Neuromyopathy and vitamin E deficiency in man.' *Neuropediatrics*, 12, 267–278.

Burgess, L.P.A., Yim, D.W.S., Lepore, L.M. (1984) 'Bell's palsy: the steroid controversy revisited.' *Laryngoscope*, 94, 1472–1476.

Bye, A.M., Baker, W.deC., Pollard, J., Wise, G. (1990) 'Hereditary sensory neuropathy type II, without trophic changes.' *Developmental Medicine and Child Neurology*, 32, 164–167.

Carroll, J.E., Jedziniak, M., Guggenheim, M.A. (1977) 'Guillain–Barré syndrome. Another cause of the "floppy infant".' *American Journal of Diseases of Children*, 131, 699–700.

Carroll, W.M., Jones, S.J., Halliday, A.M. (1983) 'Visual evoked potential abnormalities in Charcot–Marie–Tooth disease and comparison with Friedreich's ataxia.' *Journal of the Neurological Sciences*, 61, 123–133.

Casey, E.B., Jellife, A.M., Le Quesne, P.M., Millett, Y. (1973) 'Vincristine neuropathy. Clinical and electrophysiological observations.' *Brain*, 96, 69–86.

Castro, L.H.M., Ropper, A.H. (1993) 'Human immunoglobulin infusion in Guillain–Barré syndrome: worsening during and after treatment.' *Neurology*, 43, 1034–1036.

Cavanagh, N.P.C., Eames, R.A., Galvin, R.J., *et al.* (1979) 'Hereditary sensory neuropathy with spastic paraplegia.' *Brain*, 102, 79–94.

Chabrol, B., Mancini, J., Benelli, C., *et al.* (1994) 'Leigh syndrome: pyruvate dehydrogenase defect. A case with peripheral neuropathy.' *Journal of Child Neurology*, 9, 52–55.

Chalmers, R.M., Bird, A.C., Harding, A.E. (1996) 'Autosomal dominant optic atrophy with asymptomatic peripheral neuropathy.' *Journal of Neurology, Neurosurgery, and Psychiatry*, 60, 195–196.

Chance, P.F., Matsunami, N., Lensch, M.W., *et al.* (1992) 'Analysis of the DNA duplication 17p11.2 in Charcot–Marie–Tooth neuropathy type I pedigrees: additional evidence for a third autosomal CMT1 locus.' *Neurology*, 42, 2037–2041.

—— Lensch, M.W., Lipe, H., *et al.* (1994) 'Hereditary neurologic amyotrophy and hereditary neuropathy with liability to pressure palsies: two distinct genetic disorders.' *Neurology*, 44, 2253–2257.

Chang, Y.C., Yip, P.K., Chiu, Y.N., Lin, H.N. (1988) 'Severe generalised polyneuropathy in lithium intoxication.' *European Neurology*, 28, 39–41.

Chapple, C.C. (1956) 'A duosyndrome of the laryngeal nerve.' *American Journal of Diseases of Children*, 91, 14–18.

Charles, L.M., Jayam-Trouth, A. (1980) 'Brachial plexus neuropathy. Three cases in children.' *American Journal of Diseases of Children*, 134, 299–300.

Charnas, L., Bernar, J., Pezeshkpour, G.H., *et al.* (1988) 'MRI findings and peripheral neuropathy in Lowe's syndrome.' *Neuropediatrics*, 19, 7–9.

Chaten, F.C., Lucking, S.E., Young, E.S., Mickell, J.J. (1991) 'Stridor: intracranial pathology causing postextubation vocal cord paralysis.' *Pediatrics*, 87, 39–43.

Chimelli, L., Freitas, M., Nascimento, O. (1997) 'Value of nerve biopsy in the diagnosis and follow-up of leprosy: the role of vascular lesions and usefulness of nerve studies in the detection of persistent bacilli.' *Journal of Neurology*, 244, 318–323.

Christen, H-J., Hanefeld, F., Eiffert, H., Thomssen, R. (1993) 'Epidemiology and clinical manifestations of Lyme borreliosis in childhood. A prospective multicentre study with special regard to neuroborreliosis.' *Acta Paediatrica*, 83, Suppl. 386, 1–76.

Cilio, M.R., Bertini, E., Sabatelli, M., *et al.* (1997) 'Congenital panneuropathy with central nervous system involvement.' *Annals of Neurology*, 42, 531. *(Abstract.)*

Clark, J.R., Carlson, R.D., Sasaki, C.T., *et al.* (1985) 'Facial paralysis in Lyme disease.' *Laryngoscope*, 95, 1341–1345.

Cohen, S.R., Geller, K.A., Birns, J.W., Thompson, J.W. (1982) 'Laryngeal paralysis in children: a long-term retrospective study.' *Annals of Otology, Rhinology and Laryngology*, 91, 417–424.

Coker, S.B. (1993) 'Leigh disease presenting as Guillain–Barré syndrome.' *Pediatric Neurology*, 9, 61–63.

Colan, R.V., Snead, O.C., Oh, S.J., Benton, J.W. (1980) 'Steroid responsive polyneuropathy with subacute onset in childhood.' *Journal of Pediatrics*, 97, 374–377.

Condon, L.M., Katkov, H., Singh, A., Helseth, H.K. (1985) 'Cardiovocal syndrome in infancy.' *Pediatrics*, 76, 22–25.

Connelly, K.P., De Witt, L.D. (1994) 'Neurologic complications of infectious mononucleosis.' *Pediatric Neurology*, 10, 181–184.

Cornblath, D.R., Mellits, E.D., Griffin, J.W., *et al.* (1988) 'Motor conduction studies in Guillain–Barré syndrome: description and prognostic value.' *Annals of Neurology*, 23, 354–359.

Cracco, J., Castells, S., Mark, E. (1984) 'Spinal somatosensory evoked potentials in juvenile diabetics.' *Annals of Neurology*, 15, 55–58.

Créange, A., Saint-Val, C., Guillevin, L., *et al.* (1993) 'Peripheral neuropathies after arthropod stings not due to Lyme disease: a report of five cases and review of the literature.' *Neurology*, 43, 1483–1488.

Crimlisk, H.L. (1997) 'The little imitator—porphyria: a neuropsychiatric disorder.' *Journal of Neurology, Neurosurgery, and Psychiatry*, 62, 319–328.

Crino, P.B., Grossman, R.I., Rostami, A. (1993) 'Magnetic resonance imaging of the cauda equina in chronic inflammatory demyelinating polyneuropathy.' *Annals of Neurology*, 33, 311–313.

Cruz Martínez, A., Arpa, J., Pérez Conde, M.C., Ferrer, M.T. (1984) 'Bilateral carpal tunnel in childhood associated with Schwartz–Jampel syndrome.' *Muscle and Nerve*, 7, 66–72.

Cuba Neuropathy Field Investigation Team (1995) 'Epidemic optic neuropathy in Cuba—clinical characterization and risk factors.' *New England Journal of Medicine*, 333, 1176–1182.

Cunningham, M.J., Eavey, R.D., Shannon, D.C. (1985) 'Familial vocal cord dysfunction.' *Pediatrics*, 76, 750–753.

Dalakas, M.C., Engel, W.K. (1981) 'Chronic relapsing (dysimmune) polyneuropathy: pathogenesis and treatment.' *Annals of Neurology*, 9 (Suppl.), 134–145.

Danta, G. (1975) 'Familial carpal tunnel syndrome with onset in childhood.' *Journal of Neurology, Neurosurgery, and Psychiatry*, 38, 350–355.

Dawson, D.M. (1993) 'Entrapment neuropathies of the upper extremities.' *New England Journal of Medicine*, 329, 2013–2018.

—— Samuels, M.A., Morris, J. (1988) 'Sensory form of acute polyneuritis.' *Neurology*, 38, 1728–1731.

740

Dehaene, I., Martin, J.J., Geens, K., Cras, P. (1986) 'Guillain–Barré syndrome with ophthalmoplegia: clinicopathologic study of the central and peripheral nervous systems including the oculomotor nerves.' *Neurology*, **36**, 851–854.

De Klippel, N., Hautekeete, M.L., De Keyser, J., Ebinger, G. (1993) 'Guillain–Barré syndrome as the presenting manifestation of hepatitis C infection.' *Neurology*, **43**, 2143.

De Long, R., Siddique, T. (1992) 'A large New England kindred with autosomal dominant neurogenic scapuloperoneal amyotrophy with unique features.' *Archives of Neurology*, **49**, 905–908.

Deniau, F., Guillot, M., Plus, A., *et al.* (1986) 'Maladie de Charcot–Marie–Tooth et néphropathie glomérulaire.' *Archives Françaises de Pédiatrie*, **43**, 791–793.

Denning, D.W., Amos, A., Rudge, P., Cohen, B.J. (1987) 'Neuralgic amyotrophy due to parvovirus infection.' *Journal of Neurology, Neurosurgery, and Psychiatry*, **50**, 641–642.

De Recondo, J. (1975) 'Hereditary neurogenic muscular atrophies.' *In:* Vinken, P.J., Bruyn, G.W. (Eds.) *Handbook of Clinical Neurology, Vol. 21.* Amsterdam: North Holland, pp. 271–317.

Dickson, N., Mortimer, J.G., Faed, J.M., *et al.* (1989) 'A child with Refsum's disease: successful treatment with diet and plasma exchange.' *Developmental Medicine and Child Neurology*, **31**, 92–97.

Dietz, F.R., Mathews, K.D., Montgomery, W.J. (1990) 'Reflex sympathetic dystrophy in children.' *Clinical Orthopaedics*, **258**, 225–231.

Donaghy, M., Hakin, R.N., Bamford, J.M., *et al.* (1987) 'Hereditary sensory neuropathy with neurotrophic keratitis. Description of an autosomal recessive disorder with selective reduction of small myelinated nerve fibres and a discussion of the classification of the hereditary sensory neuropathies.' *Brain*, **110**, 563–583.

—— King, R.H.M., McKeran, R.O., *et al.* (1990) 'Cerebrotendinous xanthomatosis: clinical, electrophysiological and nerve biopsy findings and response to treatment with chenodeoxycholic acid.' *Journal of Neurology*, **237**, 216–219.

Dowling, P.C., Cook, S.D. (1981) 'Role of infection in Guillain–Barré syndrome: laboratory confirmation of herpes viruses in 41 cases.' *Annals of Neurology*, **9** (Suppl.), 44–55.

Drummond, P.D., Lance, J.W. (1993) 'Site of autonomic deficit in harlequin syndrome: local autonomic failure affecting the arm and the face.' *Annals of Neurology*, **34**, 814–819.

Dugan, M.D., Locke, S., Gallagher, R.J. (1962) 'Occipital neuralgia in adolescents and young adults.' *New England Journal of Medicine*, **267**, 1166–1172.

Dunn, D., Engle, W.A. (1985) 'Brachial plexus palsy: intrauterine onset.' *Pediatric Neurology*, **1**, 367–369.

Dunn, H.G., Daube, J.R., Gomez, M.R. (1978) 'Heredofamilial brachial plexus neuropathy (hereditary neuralgic amyotrophy with brachial predilection) in childhood.' *Developmental Medicine and Child Neurology*, **20**, 28–46.

Dussaix, E., Le Touzé, P., Tardieu, M. (1986) 'Neuropathie du plexus brachial compliquant une mononuclérose infectieuse chez un enfant de 18 mois.' *Archives Françaises de Pédiatrie*, **43**, 129–130.

Dutch Guillain–Barré Group (1994) 'Treatment of Guillain–Barré syndrome with high-dose immune globulins combined with methylprednisolone.' *Annals of Neurology*, **35**, 749–752.

Dyck, P.J. (1984) 'Inherited neuronal degeneration and atrophy affecting peripheral motor sensory and autonomic neurons.' *In:* Dyck, P.J., Thomas, P.K., Lambert, E.M. (Eds.) *Peripheral Neuropathy. Vol. 2. 2nd Edn.* Philadelphia: W.B. Saunders, pp. 1600–1655.

—— Swanson, C.J., Low, P.A., *et al.* (1982) 'Prednisone responsive hereditary motor and sensory neuropathy.' *Mayo Clinic Proceedings*, **57**, 239–246.

—— Karnes, J.L., Windebank, A.J., *et al.* (1983a) 'Minimal pathologic expression of a mutant gene for hereditary motor and sensory neuropathy.' *Mayo Clinic Proceedings*, **58**, 419–425.

—— Mellinger, J.F., Reagan, T.J., *et al.* (1983b) 'Not "indifference to pain" but varieties of hereditary sensory and autonomic neuropathy.' *Brain*, **106**, 373–390.

—— Benstead, T.J., Conn, D.L., Stevens, J.C., *et al.* (1987) 'Nonsystemic vasculitic neuropathy.' *Brain*, **110**, 843–854.

—— Chance, P., Lebo, R., Carney, J.A. (1993) 'Hereditary motor and sensory neuropathies.' *In:* Dyck, P.J., Thomas, P.K., Griffin, J.W., *et al.* (Eds.) *Peripheral Neuropathy, 3rd Edn.* Philadelphia: W.B. Saunders, pp. 1094–1136.

—— Litchy, W.J., Minnerath, S., *et al.* (1994) 'Hereditary motor and sensory neuropathy with diaphragm and vocal cord paresis.' *Annals of Neurology*, **35**, 608–615.

Edin, M., Sveger, T., Tegner, H., Tjernström, U. (1976) 'Isolated temporary pharyngeal paralysis in childhood.' *Lancet*, **1**, 1047–1049.

Egel, R.T., Cueva, J.P., Adair, R.L. (1995) 'Posttraumatic childhood lumbosacral plexus neuropathy.' *Pediatric Neurology*, **12**, 62–64.

Ekbom, K.A., Westerberg, C.E. (1966) 'Carbamazepine in glossopharyngeal neuralgia.' *Archives of Neurology*, **14**, 595–596.

Elliott, J.L., Kwon, J.M., Goodfellow, P.J., Yee, W-C. (1997) 'Hereditary motor and sensory neuropathy IIB: Clinical and electrodiagnostic characteristics.' *Neurology*, **48**, 23–28.

Eng, C.M., Slaugenhaupt, S.A., Blumenfeld, A., *et al.* (1995) 'Prenatal diagnosis of familial dysautonomia by analysis of linked CA-repeat polymorphisms on chromosome 9q31–q33.' *American Journal of Medical Genetics*, **59**, 349–355.

Eng, G.D., Binder, H., Getson, P., O'Donnell, R. (1996) 'Obstetrical brachial plexus palsy (OBPP) outcome with conservative management.' *Muscle and Nerve*, **19**, 884–891.

England, J.D., Sumner, A.J. (1987) 'Neuralgic amyotrophy: an increasingly diverse entity.' *Muscle and Nerve*, **10**, 60–68.

Engler, R.J.M., Oetgen, W.J., Hyman, L.R. (1979) 'Congenital facial diplegia (Mobius syndrome) and diabetes insipidus: case report.' *Military Medicine*, **144**, 117–120.

Epstein, J.A., Epstein, N.E., Marc, J., *et al.* (1984) 'Lumbar intervertebral disk herniation in teenage children: recognition and management of associated abnormalities.' *Spine*, **9**, 427–432.

Epstein, M.A., Sladky, J.T. (1990) 'The role of plasmapheresis in childhood Guillain–Barré syndrome.' *Annals of Neurology*, **28**, 65–69.

Escobar, D.M., Jones, H.R. (1996) 'Pediatric radial mononeuropathies: a clinical and electromyographic study of sixteen children with review of the literature.' *Muscle and Nerve*, **19**, 876–883.

Evans, B.A., Stevens, J.C., Dyck, P.J. (1981) 'Lumbosacral plexus neuropathy.' *Neurology*, **31**, 1327–1330.

Evans, O.B. (1979) 'Polyneuropathy in childhood.' *Pediatrics*, **64**, 96–105.

Faed, J.M., Pollock, M., Taylor, P.K., *et al.* (1989) 'High-dose intravenous human immunoglobulin in chronic inflammatory demyelinating polyneuropathy.' *Neurology*, **39**, 422–425.

Faerman, I., Maler, M., Jadzinsky, M., *et al.* (1971) 'Asymptomatic neurogenic bladder in juvenile diabetes.' *Diabetologia*, **7**, 168–172.

Feasby, T.E., Hahn, A.F., Gilbert, J.J. (1982) 'Passive transfer studies in Guillain–Barré polyneuropathy.' *Neurology*, **32**, 1159–1167.

—— Gilbert, J.J., Brown, W.F., *et al.* (1986) 'An acute axonal form of Guillain–Barré polyneuropathy.' *Brain*, **109**, 1115–1126.

—— Hahn, A.F., Koopman, W.J., Lee, D.H. (1990) 'Central lesions in chronic inflammatory demyelinating polyneuropathy: an MRI study.' *Neurology*, **40**, 476–478.

—— —— Bolton, C.F., *et al.* (1992) 'Detection of hereditary motor sensory neuropathy type I in childhood.' *Journal of Neurology, Neurosurgery, and Psychiatry*, **55**, 895–897.

—— —— Brown, W.F., *et al.* (1993) 'Severe axonal degeneration in acute Guillain–Barré syndrome: evidence of two different mechanisms?' *Journal of the Neurological Sciences*, **116**, 185–192.

Ferrière, G., Guzzetta, F., Kulakowski, S., Evrard, P. (1992) 'Nonprogressive type II hereditary sensory autonomic neuropathy: a homogeneous clinicopathologic entity.' *Journal of Child Neurology*, **7**, 364–370.

Fiçicioglu, C., Aydin, A., Haktan, M., Kiziltan, M. (1994) 'Peripheral neuropathy in children with insulin-dependent diabetes mellitus.' *Turkish Journal of Pediatrics*, **36**, 97–104.

Fourestié, V., Douceron, H., Brugières, P., *et al.* (1993) 'Neurotrichinosis. A cerebrovascular disease associated with myocardial injury and hypereosinophilia.' *Brain*, **116**, 603–616.

French Cooperative Group on Plasma Exchange in Guillain–Barré Syndrome (1987) 'Efficency of plasma exchange in Guillain–Barré syndrome: role of replacement fluids.' *Annals of Neurology*, **22**, 753–761.

Frith, J.A., McLeod, J.G., Nicholson, G.A., Yang, F. (1994) 'Peroneal muscular atrophy with pyramidal tract features (hereditary motor and sensory neuropathy type V): a clinical, neurophysiological, and pathological study of a large kindred.' *Journal of Neurology, Neurosurgery, and Psychiatry*, **57**, 1343–1346.

Fujita, I., Koyanagi, T., Kukita, J., *et al.* (1991) 'Moebius syndrome with central hypoventilation and brainstem calcification: a case report.' *European Journal of Pediatrics*, **150**, 582–583.

Gabreëls-Festen, A.A.W.M., Hageman, A.T.M., Gabreëls, F.J.M., *et al.* (1986) 'Chronic inflammatory demyelinating polyneuropathy in two siblings.' *Journal of Neurology, Neurosurgery, and Psychiatry*, **49**, 152–156.

—— Joosten, E.M.G., Gabreëls, F.J.M., *et al.* (1990) 'Congenital demyelinating motor and sensory neuropathy with focally folded myelin sheaths.' *Brain*, **113**, 1629–1643.

—— —— *et al.* (1991) 'Hereditary motor and sensory neuropathy of neuronal type with onset in early childhood.' *Brain*, **114**, 1855–1870.

—— Gabreëls, F.J.M., Jennekens, F.G.I., *et al.* (1992) 'Autosomal recessive form of hereditary motor and sensory neuropathy type I.' *Neurology*, **42**, 1755–1761.

—— —— —— (1993) 'Hereditary motor and sensory neuropathies. Present status of types I, II and III.' *Clinical Neurology and Neurosurgery*, **95**, 93–107.

Gadoth, N., Biedner, B., Torok, G. (1979) 'Mobius syndrome and Poland anomaly: Case report and review of the literature.' *Journal of Pediatric Ophthalmology and Strabismus*, **16**, 374–376.

Galassi, G., Cappelli, G., Trevisan, G. (1990) 'Acute Fisher's syndrome during the course of chronic uremia: is the hemodialysis implicated in relapses?' *European Neurology*, **30**, 84–86.

Gallai, V., Firenze, C., Mazzotta, G., Del Gatto, F. (1988) 'Neuropathy in childen and adolescents with diabetes mellitus.' *Acta Neurologica Scandinavica*, **78**, 136–140.

Gamstorp, I. (1968) 'Polyneuropathy in childhood.' *Acta Pediatrica Scandinavica*, **57**, 230–238.

Garcia-Erro, M.I., Correale, J., Arberas, C., *et al.* (1989) 'Familial congenital facial diplegia: electrophysiologic and genetic studies.' *Pediatric Neurology*, **5**, 262–264.

Gastaut, J.L., Pellissier, J.F. (1985) 'Neuropathie au cisplatine. Étude clinique, électrophysiologique et morphologique.' *Revue Neurologique*, **141**, 614–626.

Geiger, L.R., Mancall, E.L., Penn, A.S., Tucker, S.H. (1974) 'Familial neuralgic amyotrophy: report of three families with review of the literature.' *Brain*, **27**, 87–102.

Gerber, S.I., Cromie, W.J. (1996) 'Herpes simplex virus type 2 infection associated with urinary retention in the absence of genital lesions.' *Journal of Pediatrics*, **128**, 250–251.

Gibberd, F.B. (1970) 'Ophthalmoplegia in acute polyneuritis.' *Archives of Neurology*, **23**, 161–164.

—— Billimoria, J.D., Goldman, J.M., *et al.* (1985) 'Heredopathia atactica polyneuritiformis: Refsum's disease.' *Acta Neurologica Scandinavica*, **72**, 1–17.

Gilbert, A., Tassin, J.L. (1987) 'Obstetrical palsy. A clinical, pathological and surgical overview.' *In:* Terzis, J. (Ed.) *Microreconstruction of Nerve Injuries.* Philadelphia: W.B. Saunders, pp. 529–553.

—— Brockman, R., Carlioz, H. (1991) 'Surgical treatment of brachial plexus birth palsy.' *Clinical Orthopaedics and Related Research*, **264**, 39–47.

Gilles, F.H., French, J.H. (1961) 'Postinjection sciatic nerve palsies in infants and children.' *Journal of Pediatrics*, **58**, 193–204.

Goebel, H.H., Zeman, W., DeMyer, W. (1976) 'Peripheral motor and sensory neuropathy in early childhood, simulating Werdnig–Hoffmann disease.' *Neuropädiatrie*, **7**, 182–195.

—— Veit, S., Dyck, P.J. (1980) 'Confirmation of virtual unmyelinated fiber absence in hereditary sensory neuropathy type IV.' *Journal of Neuropathology and Experimental Neurology*, **39**, 670–675.

—— Bardosi, A., Friede, R.L., *et al.* (1986) 'Sural nerve biopsy studies in Leigh's subacute necrotizing encephalomyelopathy.' *Muscle and Nerve*, **9**, 165–173.

Gomez, M.R. (1994) 'New observations in neurocutaneous angiomatosis.' *Acta Neuropediatrica*, **1**, 81–95.

Gordon, M., Rich, H., Deutschberger, J., Green, M. (1973) 'The immediate and long-term outcome of obstetric birth trauma. I. Brachial plexus paralysis.' *American Journal of Obstetrics and Gynecology*, **117**, 51–56.

Gordon, N. (1996) 'Reflex sympathetic dystrophy.' *Brain and Development*, **18**, 257–262.

Gorke, W. (1981) 'The differential diagnosis of congenital analgesia and other diseases with diminished pain perception in childhood.' *Neuropediatrics*, **12**, 33–43.

Gotoda, T., Arita, M., Arai, H., *et al.* (1995) 'Adult-onset spinocerebellar dysfunction caused by a mutation in the gene for the α-tocopherol-transfer protein.' *New England Journal of Medicine*, **333**, 1313–1318.

Gouider, R., Le Guern, E., Emile, J., *et al.* (1994) 'Hereditary neuralgic amyotrophy and hereditary neuropathy with liability to pressure palsies: two distinct clinical, electrophysiologic, and genetic entities.' *Neurology*, **44**, 2250–2252.

Govaert, P., Vanhaesebrouck, P., De Praeter, C., *et al.* (1989) 'Moebius sequence and prenatal brainstem ischemia.' *Pediatrics*, **84**, 570–573.

Grattan-Smith, P.J., Morris, J.G., Johnston, H.M., *et al.* (1997) 'Clinical and neurophysiological features of tick paralysis.' *Brain*, **120**, 1975–1987.

Greenberg, S.J., Kandt, R.S., D'Souza, B.J. (1987) 'Birth injury-induced glossolaryngeal paresis.' *Neurology*, **37**, 533–535.

Greenwald, A.G., Schute, P.C., Shiveley, J.L. (1984) 'Brachial plexus birth palsy: a 10-year report on the incidence and prognosis.' *Journal of Pediatric Orthopedics*, **4**, 689–692.

Gregson, N.A., Koblar, S., Hughes, R.A. (1993) 'Antibodies to gangliosides in Guillain–Barré syndrome: specificity and relationship to clinical features.' *Quarterly Journal of Medicine*, **86**, 111–117.

Griffin, J.W., Li, C.Y., Ho, T.W., *et al.* (1995) 'Guillain–Barré syndrome in northern China. The spectrum of neuropathological changes in clinically defined cases.' *Brain*, **118**, 577–595.

—— —— —— *et al.* (1996) 'Pathology of the motor-sensory axonal Guillain–Barré syndrome.' *Annals of Neurology*, **39**, 17–28.

Gross, M.L.P., Fowler, C.J., Ho, R., *et al.* (1988) 'Peripheral neuropathy complicating pancreatitis and major pancreatic surgery.' *Journal of Neurology, Neurosurgery, and Psychiatry*, **51**, 1341–1344.

Grundfast, K.M., Guarisco, J.L., Thomsen, J.R., Koch, B. (1990) 'Diverse etiologies of facial paralysis in children.' *International Journal of Pediatric Otorhinolaryngology*, **19**, 223–239.

Grunnet, M.L., Zimmerman, A.W., Lewis, R.A. (1983) 'Ultrastructure and electrodiagnosis of peripheral neuropathy in Cockayne's syndrome.' *Neurology*, **33**, 1606–1609.

Guggenheim, M.A., Ringel, S.P., Silverman, A., Grabert, B.E. (1982) 'Progressive neuromuscular disease in children with chronic cholestasis and vitamin E deficiency: diagnosis and treatment with alpha tocopherol.' *Journal of Pediatrics*, **100**, 51–58.

Gumbinas, M., Larsen, M., Liu, H.M. (1975) 'Peripheral neuropathy in classic Niemann–Pick disease: ultrastruture of nerves and skeletal muscles.' *Neurology*, **25**, 107–113.

Gutmann, L., Shockcor, W., Gutmann, L., Kien, C.L. (1986) 'Vitamin E-deficient spinocerebellar syndrome due to intestinal lymphangiectasia.' *Neurology*, **36**, 554–556.

Guzzetta, F., Ferrière, G., Lyon, G. (1982) 'Congenital hypomyelination polyneuropathy. Pathological fndings compared with neuropathies starting later in life.' *Brain*, **105**, 395–416.

—— Tortorella, G., Cardia, E., Ferrière, G. (1986) 'Familial dysautonomia in a non-Jewish girl with histological evidence of progression in the sural nerve.' *Developmental Medicine and Child Neurology*, **28**, 62–68.

Haenggeli, C.A., Lacourt, G. (1989) 'Brachial plexus injury and hypoglossal paralysis.' *Pediatric Neurology*, **5**, 197–198.

Hagberg, B. (1990) 'Polyneuropathies in paediatrics.' *European Journal of Pediatrics*, **149**, 296–305.

—— Lyon, G. (1981) 'Pooled European series of hereditary peripheral neuropathies in infancy and childhood.' *Neuropediatrics*, **12**, 9–17.

—— Westerberg, B. (1983) 'The nosology of genetic peripheral neuropathies in Swedish children.' *Developmental Medicine and Child Neurology*, **25**, 3–18.

Hageman, G., Ippel, P.F., Jansen, E.N.H., Rozeboom, A.R. (1990) 'Familial, alternating Bell's palsy with dominant inheritance.' *European Neurology*, **30**, 310–313.

Hahn, A.F., Brown, W.F., Koopman, W.J., Feasby, T.E. (1990) 'X-linked dominant hereditary motor and sensory neuropathy.' *Brain*, **113**, 1511–1525.

—— Bolton, C.F., Pillay, N., *et al.* (1996) 'Plasma exchange therapy in chronic demyelinating polyneuropathy. A double-blind, sham-controlled, cross-over study.' *Brain*, **119**, 1055–1066.

—— —— Zochodne, D., Feasby, T.E. (1996) 'Intravenous immunoglobulin treatment in chronic inflammatory demyelinating polyneuropathy. A double-blind, placebo-controlled, cross-over study.' *Brain*, **119**, 1067–1077.

Hallam, P.J., Harding, A.E., Berciano, J., *et al.* (1992) 'Duplication of part of chromosome 17 is commonly associated with hereditary motor and sensory neuropathy type I (Charcot–Marie–Tooth disease type 1).' *Annals of Neurology*, **31**, 570–572.

Haller, J.S., Fabara, J.A. (1972) 'Tick paralysis: case report with emphasis on neurologic toxicity.' *American Journal of Diseases of Children*, **124**, 915–917.

Hamaguchi, H., Hashimoto, T., Mori, K., *et al.* (1993) 'Moebius syndrome:

continuous tachypnea verified by a polygraphic study.' *Neuropediatrics*, **24**, 319–323.

Hamati-Haddad, A., Fenichel, G.M. (1997) 'Brachial neuritis following routine childhood immunization for diphtheria, tetanus, and pertussis (DTP): report of two cases and review of the literature.' *Pediatrics*, **99**, 602–603.

Hanson, P.A., Rowland, L.P. (1971) 'Möbius syndrome and facioscapulo-humeral muscular dystrophy.' *Archives of Neurology*, **24**, 31–39.

Harati, Y., Butler, I.J. (1985) 'Congenital hypomyelinating neuropathy.' *Journal of Neurology, Neurosurgery, and Psychiatry*, **48**, 1269–1276.

—— Niakan, E. (1986) 'The clinical spectrum of inflammatory–angiopathic neuropathy.' *Journal of Neurology, Neurosurgery, and Psychiatry*, **49**, 1313–1316.

Harding, A.E. (1995) 'From the syndrome of Charcot, Marie and Tooth to disorders of peripheral myelin proteins.' *Brain*, **118**, 809–818.

—— Thomas, P.K. (1980a) 'Autosomal recessive forms of hereditary motor and sensory neuropathy.' *Journal of Neurology, Neurosurgery, and Psychiatry*, **43**, 669–678.

—— —— (1980b) 'Genetic aspects of hereditary motor and sensory neuropathy (types I and II).' *Journal of Medical Genetics*, **17**, 329–336.

—— —— (1980c) 'The clinical features of hereditary motor and sensory neuropathy types I and II.' *Brain*, **103**, 259–280.

—— —— (1984) 'Peroneal muscular atrophy with pyramidal features.' *Journal of Neurology, Neurosurgery, and Psychiatry*, **47**, 168–172.

—— Muller, D.P.R., Thomas, P.K., Willison, H.J. (1982) 'Spinocerebellar degeneration secondary to chronic intestinal malabsorption: a vitamin E deficiency syndrome.' *Annals of Neurology*, **12**, 419–424.

—— Matthews, S., Jones, S., *et al.* (1985) 'Spinocerebellar degeneration associated with a selective defect of vitamin E absorption.' *New England Journal of Medicine*, **313**, 32–35.

Hartung, H-P., Schwenke, C., Bitter-Suermann, D., Toyka, K.Y. (1987) 'Guillain–Barré syndrome: activated complement components C3a and C5a in CSF.' *Neurology*, **37**, 1006–1009.

—— Pollard, J.D., Harvey, G.K., Toyka, K.V. (1995) 'Immunopathogenesis and treatment of the Guillain–Barré syndrome—Part II.' *Muscle and Nerve*, **18**, 154–164.

Harvey, A.S., Jayakar, P., Duchowny, M., *et al.* (1996) 'Hemifacial seizures and cerebellar ganglioglioma: an epilepsy syndrome of infancy with seizures of cerebellar origin.' *Annals of Neurology*, **40**, 91–98.

Hayasaka, K., Himoro, M., Sato, W., *et al.* (1993) 'Charcot–Marie Tooth neuropathy type 1B is associated with mutations of the myelin P₀ gene.' *Nature Genetics*, **5**, 31–34.

Hayden, R., Grossman, M. (1959) 'Rectal, ocular, and submaxillary pain. A familial autonomic disorder related to proctalgia fugax: report of a family.' *American Journal of Diseases of Children*, **97**, 479–482.

Heckmann, J.M., Carr, J.A., Bell, N. (1995) 'Hereditary sensory and autonomic neuropathy with cataracts, mental retardation, and skin lesions: five cases.' *Neurology*, **45**, 1405–1408.

Heckmatt, J.Z., Pitt, M.C., Kirkham, F. (1993) 'Peripheral neuropathy and neuromuscular blockade presenting as prolonged respiratory paralysis following critical illness.' *Neuropediatrics*, **24**, 123–125.

Hemachudha, P., Griffin, D., Chen, W.W., Johnson, R.T. (1988) 'Immunologic studies of rabies vaccination-induced Guillain–Barré syndrome.' *Neurology*, **38**, 375–378.

Hentati, A., Deng, H-X., Hung, W-Y., *et al.* (1996) 'Human α-tocopherol transfer protein: gene structure and mutations in familial vitamin E deficiency.' *Annals of Neurology*, **39**, 295–300.

Herbaut, A.G., Voordecker, P., Monseu, G., Germeau, F. (1987) 'Benign transient urinary retention.' *Journal of Neurology, Neurosurgery, and Psychiatry*, **50**, 354–355.

Herbert, M.A., Clayton, P.T. (1994) 'Phytanic acid a-oxidase deficiency (Refsum disease) presenting in infancy.' *Journal of Inherited Metabolic Disease*, **17**, 211–214.

Hess, C.W., Hunziker, T., Küpfer, A., Ludin, H.P. (1986) 'Thalidomide-induced peripheral neuropathy—a prospective clinical, neurophysiological and pharmacogenetic evaluation.' *Journal of Neurology*, **233**, 83–89.

Hirano, M., Ott, B.R., Raps, E.C., *et al.* (1992) 'Acute quadriplegic myopathy: a complication of treatment with steroids, nondepolarizing blocking agents, or both.' *Neurology*, **42**, 2082–2087.

Hokkanen, E. Haltia, T., Myllyä, V.V. (1978) 'Recurrent multiple cranial neuropathies.' *European Neurology*, **17**, 32–37.

Honavar, M., Tharakan, J.K., Hughes, R.A., *et al.* (1991) 'A clinicopathological study of the Guillain–Barré syndrome. Nine cases and literature review.' *Brain*, **114**, 1245–1269.

Hope, E.E., Bodensteiner, J.B., Thong, N. (1985) 'Neonatal lumbar plexus injury.' *Archives of Neurology*, **42**, 94–95.

Hopkins, A. (1975) 'Toxic neuropathy due to industrial agents.' *In:* Dyck, P.J., Thomas, P.K., Lambert, E.H. (Eds.) *Peripheral Neuropathy.* Philadelphia: W.B. Saunders, pp. 1207–1226.

Horoupian, D.S. (1989) 'Hereditary sensory neuropathy with deafness: a familial multisystem atrophy.' *Neurology*, **39**, 244–248.

Houston, A.B., Brodie, M.J., Moore, M.R., Stephenson, J.B.P. (1977) 'Hereditary coproporphyria and epilepsy.' *Archives of Disease in Childhood*, **52**, 646–650.

Hughes, R.A.C. (1991) 'Ineffectiveness of high-dose intravenous methyl-prednisolone in Guillain–Barré syndrome.' *Lancet*, **338**, 1142. *(Letter.)*

—— Sanders, E., Hall, S., *et al.* (1992) 'Subacute idiopathic demyelinating polyradiculoneuropathy.' *Archives of Neurology*, **49**, 612–616.

Hung, K-L., Wang, H-S., Liou, W-Y., *et al.* (1994) 'Guillain–Barré syndrome in children: a cooperative study in Taiwan.' *Brain and Development*, **16**, 204–208.

Hunt, D. (1988) 'Surgical management of brachial plexus birth injuries.' *Developmental Medicine and Child Neurology*, **30**, 824–828.

Hyser, C.L., Kissel, J.T., Warmolts, J.R., Mendell, J.R. (1988) 'Scapuloperoneal neuropathy: a distinct clinicopathologic entity.' *Journal of the Neurological Sciences*, **87**, 91–102.

Ionasescu, V.V., Trofatter, J., Haines, J.L., *et al.* (1991) 'Heterogeneity in X-linked recessive Charcot–Marie–Tooth neuropathy.' *American Journal of Human Genetics*, **48**, 1075–1083.

—— —— —— *et al.* (1992) 'Mapping of the gene for the X-linked dominant Charcot–Marie–Tooth neuropathy.' *Neurology*, **42**, 903–908.

—— Searby, C.C., Ionasescu, R., *et al.* (1997) 'Déjerine–Sottas neuropathy in mother and son with same point mutation of PMP 22 gene.' *Muscle and Nerve*, **20**, 97–99.

Ippel, P.F., Wittebol-Post, D., Jennekens, F.G., Bijlsma, J.B. (1995) 'Genetic heterogeneity of hereditary motor and sensory neuropathy type VI.' *Journal of Child Neurology*, **10**, 459–463.

Iqbal, A., Oger, J.J.F., Arnason, B.W.G. (1981) 'Cell-mediated immunity in idiopathic polyneuritis.' *Annals of Neurology*, **9** (Suppl.), 65–69.

Irani, D.N., Cornblath, D.R., Chaudry, V., *et al.* (1993) 'Relapse in Guillain–Barré syndrome after treatment with human immune globulin.' *Neurology*, **43**, 872–875.

Jacobs, J.M., Harding, B.N., Lake, B.D. *et al.* (1990) 'Peripheral neuropathy in Leigh's disease.' *Brain*, **113**, 447–462.

Jaeken, J., Carchon, H. (1993) 'The carbohydrate-deficient glycoprotein syndromes: an overview.' *Journal of Inherited Metabolic Disease*, **16**, 813–820.

Jansen, P.W., Perkin, R.M., Ashwal, S. (1993) 'Guillian–Barré syndrome in childhood: natural course and efficacy of plasmapheresis.' *Pediatric Neurology*, **9**, 16–20.

Jestico, J.V., Urry, P.A., Efphimiou, J. (1985) 'An hereditary sensory and autonomic neuropathy transmitted as an X-linked recessive trait.' *Journal of Neurology, Neurosurgery, and Psychiatry*, **48**, 1259–1264.

Johnson, M.D., Glick, A.D., Whetsell, W.O. (1989) 'Central hypomyelination associated with congenital hypomyelinating polyneuropathy: report of an autopsied case.' *Clinical Neuropathology*, **8**, 28–34.

Johnson, R.H., Spalding, J.M.K. (1964) 'Progressive sensory neuropathy in children.' *Journal of Neurology, Neurosurgery, and Psychiatry*, **27**, 125–130.

Jones, H.R. (1986) 'Compressive neuropathy in childhood: a report of 14 cases.' *Muscle and Nerve*, **9**, 720–723.

—— (1996) 'Childhood Guillain–Barré syndrome: clinical presentation, diagnosis, and therapy.' *Journal of Child Neurology*, **11**, 4–12.

—— Gianturco, L.E., Gross, P.T., Buchhalter, J. (1988) 'Sciatic neuropathies in childhood: a report of ten cases and review of the literature.' *Journal of Child Neurology*, **3**, 193–199.

Jones, S.J. (1979) 'Investigations of brachial plexus traction lesions by peripheral and spinal somatosensory evoked potentials.' *Journal of Neurology, Neurosurgery, and Psychiatry*, **42**, 107–116.

Joy, J.L., Oh, S.J. (1989) 'Tomaculous neuropathy presenting as acute recurrent polyneuropathy.' *Annals of Neurology*, **26**, 98–100.

Juncos, J.L., Beal, M.F. (1987) 'Idiopathic cranial polyneuropathy: a fifteen-year experience.' *Brain*, **110**, 197–211.

Kanda, F., Uchida, T., Jinnai, K., *et al.* (1990) 'Acute autonomic and sensory neuropathy: a case report.' *Journal of Neurology*, **237**, 42–44.

743

Kandt, R.S., Daniel, F.L. (1986) 'Glossopharyngeal neuralgia in a child: a diagnostic and therapeutic dilemma.' *Archives of Neurology*, **43**, 301–302.

Kane, J.P., Havel, R.J. (1995) 'Disorders of the biogenesis and secretion of lipoproteins containing the b-apolipoproteins.' *In:* Scriver, C.R., Beaudet, A.L., Sly, W.S., Valle, D. (Eds.) *The Metabolic Basis of Inherited Disease, 7th Edn. Vol. 2.* New York: McGraw Hill, pp. 1853–1885.

Kanra, G., Ozon, A., Vajsur, J., et al. (1997) 'Intravenous immunoglobulin treatment in children with Guillain–Barré syndrome.' *European Journal of Paediatric Neurology*, **1**, 7–12.

Katusik, S., Beard, C.M., Wiederholt, W.C., et al. (1986) 'Incidence, clinical features and prognosis in Bell's palsy, Rochester, Minnesota 1968–1982.' *Annals of Neurology*, **20**, 622–627.

Keane, J.R. (1994) 'Bilateral seventh nerve palsy. Analysis of 43 cases and review of the literature.' *Neurology*, **44**, 1198–1202.

—— (1996) 'Twelfth nerve palsy: analysis of 100 cases.' *Archives of Neurology*, **53**, 561–566.

Kennedy, W.R., Sung, J.H., Berry, J.F. (1977) 'A case of congenital hypomyelination neuropathy. Clinical, morphological and chemical studies.' *Archives of Neurology*, **34**, 337–345.

Kesler, R.W., Saulsbury, F.T., Miller, L.T., Rowlingson, J.C. (1988) 'Reflex sympathetic dystrophy in children: treatment with transcutaneous electric nerve stimulation.' *Pediatrics*, **82**, 728–732.

Khatri, B.O., Flamini, J.R., Baruah, J.K., et al. (1990) 'Plasmapheresis with acute inflammatory polyneuropathy.' *Pediatric Neurology*, **6**, 17–19.

Khoubesserian, P., Van Regemorter, N., Ohrn-Degueldre, O., et al. (1979) 'Charcot–Marie–Tooth disease associated with retinal pigment dystrophy and protanopia.' *Journal of Neurology*, **222**, 1–10.

Kinnunen, E., Färkkilaä, M., Juntunen, J., Weckström, P. (1989) 'Incidence of Guillain–Barré syndrome during a nationwide oral poliovirus vaccine campaign.' *Neurology*, **39**, 1034–1036.

Kindstrand, E. (1995) 'Lyme borreliosis and cranial neuropathy.' *Journal of Neurology*, **242**, 658–663.

Kleyweg, R.P., van der Meché, F.G.A., Meulstee, J. (1988) 'Treatment of Guillain–Barré syndrome with high-dose gammaglobulin.' *Neurology*, **38**, 1639–1641.

—— —— Loonen, M.C.B., et al. (1989) 'The natural history of the Guillain–Barré syndrome in 18 children and 50 adults.' *Journal of Neurology, Neurosurgery, and Psychiatry*, **52**, 853–856.

Kohler, A., Torrenté, A., Inderwildi, B. (1988) 'Fisher's syndrome associated with *Campylobacter jejuni* infection.' *European Neurology*, **28**, 150–151.

Korinthenberg, R., Mönting, J.S. (1996) 'Natural history and treatment effects in Guillain–Barré syndrome: a multicentre study.' *Archives of Disease in Childhood*, **74**, 281–287.

Korobkin, R., Asbury, A.K., Sumner, A.J., Nielsen, S.L. (1975) 'Glue sniffing neuropathy.' *Archives of Neurology*, **32**, 158–162.

Koski, C.L., Gratz, E., Sutherland, J., Mayer, R.F. (1986) 'Clinical correlation with anti-peripheral-nerve myelin antibodies in Guillain–Barré syndrome.' *Annals of Neurology*, **19**, 573–577.

Kreusser, K.L., Volpe, J.J. (1984) 'Peroneal palsy produced by intravenous fluid infiltration in a newborn.' *Developmental Medicine and Child Neurology*, **26**, 522–524.

Kurihara, A., Kataoka, O. (1980) 'Lumbar disc herniation in children and adolescents. A review of 70 operated cases and their minimum 5-year follow-up studies.' *Spine*, **5**, 443–451.

Kuroki, S., Saida, T., Nukina, M., et al. (1993) '*Campylobacter jejuni* strains from patients with Guillain–Barré syndrome belong mostly to Penner serogroup 19 and contain beta-N-acetylglucosamine residues.' *Annals of Neurology*, **33**, 243–247.

Kwast, O., Ignatowicz, R. (1990) 'Progressive peripheral neuron degeneration in ataxia–telangiectasia: an electrophysiological study in children.' *Developmental Medicine and Child Neurology*, **32**, 800–807.

Lamon, J.M., Frykholm, B.C., Hess, R.A., Tschudy, D.P. (1979) 'Hematin therapy for acute porphyria.' *Medicine*, **58**, 252–269.

Lance, J.W., Anthony, M. (1980) 'Neck–tongue syndrome on sudden turning of the head.' *Journal of Neurology, Neurosurgery, and Psychiatry*, **43**, 97–101.

—— Drummond, P.D., Gandevia, J.C., Morris, J.G.L. (1988) 'Harlequin syndrome: the sudden onset of unilateral flushing and sweating.' *Journal of Neurology, Neurosurgery, and Psychiatry*, **51**, 635–642.

Landrieu, P., Saïd, G., Allaire, C. (1990) 'Dominantly transmitted congenital indifference to pain.' *Annals of Neurology*, **24**, 574–578.

Lapresle, J., Lasjaunias, P. (1986) 'Cranial nerve ischaemic arterial syndromes. A review.' *Brain*, **109**, 207–215.

—— Salisachs, P. (1973) 'Onion bulbs in a nerve biopsy in an original case of Roussy–Lévy disease.' *Archives of Neurology*, **29**, 346–348.

—— Fernandez Manchola, I., Lasjaunias, P. (1980) 'L'atteinte trigéminale sensitive au cours de la paralysie faciale périphérique essentielle.' *Nouvelle Presse Médicale*, **9**, 291–293.

Larsen, J.P., Kvåle, G., Nyland, H. (1985) 'Epidemiology of the Guillain–Barré syndrome in the county of Hordaland, Western Norway.' *Acta Neurologica Scandinavica*, **71**, 43–47.

Laurent, J.P., Lee, R.T. (1994) 'Birth-related upper brachial plexus injuries in infants: operative and nonoperative approaches.' *Journal of Child Neurology*, **9**, 111–117.

Lee, E.L., Oh, G.C., Lam, K.L., Parameswaran, N. (1976) 'Congenital sensory neuropathy with anhidrosis: a case report.' *Pediatrics*, **57**, 259–262.

Lerman-Sagie, T., Lev, D., Barash, V., et al. (1997) 'Familial neurogenic bladder and intestinal pseudoobstruction: a new mitochondrial syndrome with cytochrome c oxidase deficiency.' *European Journal of Paediatric Neurology*, **1**, A27. *(Abstract.)*

Lester, P.D., McAlister, W.H. (1970) 'Congenital iliac anomaly with sciatic palsy.' *Radiology*, **96**, 397–399.

Levin, S.E., Silverman, N.H., Milner, S. (1982) 'Hypoplasia or absence of the depressor anguli oris muscle and congenital abnormalities with special reference to the cardiofacial syndrome.' *South African Medical Journal*, **61**, 227–233.

Levin, S.L. (1987) 'Syndromes of a complex lesion of greater and lesser superficial petrosal nerves.' *Journal of Neurology*, **234**, 31–35.

Levine, M.G., Holroyde, J., Woods, J.R. (1984) 'Birth trauma: incidence and predisposing factors.' *Obstetrics and Gynecology*, **63**, 792–797.

Liberfarb, R.M., Jackson, A.H., Eavey, R.D., Robb, R.M. (1993) 'Unique hereditary sensory and autonomic neuropathy with growth hormone deficiency.' *Journal of Child Neurology*, **8**, 271–276.

Lloyd, A.V.C., Jewitte, D.E., Still, J.D.L. (1966) 'Facial paralysis in children with hypertension.' *Archives of Diseases in Childhood*, **41**, 292–294.

Lockman, L.A., Kennedy, W.R., White, J.G. (1967) 'The Chediak–Higashi sydrome: electrophysiologic and electron microscopic observations on the peripheral neuropathy.' *Journal of Pediatrics*, **70**, 942–981.

Lopez-Lozano, J.J., Garcia Merino, J.A., Liano, H. (1988) 'Bilateral facial paralysis secondary to trichinosis.' *Acta Neurologica Scandinavica*, **78**, 194–197.

Lovelace, R.E., Horwitz, S.J. (1968) 'Peripheral neuropathy in long-term diphenylhydantoin therapy.' *Archives of Neurology*, **18**, 69–77.

MacCollin, M., De Vivo, D.C., Moser, A.B., Beard, M. (1990) 'Ataxia and peripheral neuropathy: a benign variant of peroxisome dysgenesis.' *Annals of Neurology*, **28**, 833–836.

MacLeod, W.N. (1987) 'Sporadic non-A, non-B hepatitis and Epstein–Barr hepatitis associated with the Guillain–Barré syndrome.' *Archives of Neurology*, **44**, 438–442.

Magy, L., Birouk, N., Vallat, J.M., et al. (1997) 'Hereditary thermosensitive neuropathy: An autosomal dominant disorder of the peripheral nervous system.' *Neurology*, **48**, 1684–1690.

Maisonobe, T., Chassande, B., Vérin, M., Jouni, M., et al. (1996) 'Chronic dysimmune demyelinating polyneuropathy: a clinical and electrophysiological study of 93 patients.' *Journal of Neurology, Neurosurgery, and Psychiatry*, **61**, 36–42.

Maia, M., Pires, M.M., Guimaraes, A. (1988) 'Giant axonal disease: report of three cases and review of the literature.' *Neuropediatrics*, **19**, 10–15.

Makari, G.S.H., Carroll, J.E., Burton, E.M. (1994) 'Hereditary sensory neuropathy manifesting as possible child abuse.' *Pediatrics*, **93**, 842–844.

Mandich, P., James, R., Nassani, R., et al. (1995) 'Molecular diagnosis of hereditary neuropathy with liability to pressure palsies (HNPP) by detection of 17p11.2 deletion in Italian patients.' *Journal of Neurology*, **242**, 295–298.

Manfredi, M., Bini, G., Cruccu, G., et al. (1981) 'Congenital absence of pain.' *Archives of Neurology*, **38**, 507–511.

Manni, J.J., Scaf, J.J., Huygen, P.L.M., et al. (1990) 'Hyperostosis cranialis interna. A new hereditary syndrome with cranial-nerve entrapment.' *New England Journal of Medicine*, **322**, 450–454.

Manning, J.J., Adour, K.K. (1972) 'Facial paralysis in children.' *Pediatrics*, **49**, 102–109.

Mariman, E.C., Gabreëls-Festen, A.A.W.M., Van Beersum, S.E.C., et al. (1994) 'Prevalence of the 1.5-Mb 17p deletion in families with hereditary neuropathy with liability to pressure palsies.' *Annals of Neurology*, **36**, 650–655.

Markby, D.P. (1989) 'Lyme disease facial palsy: differentiation from Bell's palsy.' *British Medical Journal*, **299**, 605–606.

Marquez, S., Turley, J.J.E., Peters, W.J. (1993) 'Neuropathy in burn patients.' *Brain*, **116**, 471–483.

Marra, T.A. (1983) 'Recurrent lumbosacral and brachial plexopathy associated with schistosomiasis.' *Archives of Neurology*, **40**, 586–588.

Martinelli, P., Fabbri, R., Moretto, G., *et al.* (1989) 'Recurrent familial brachial plexus palsies as the only clinical expression of 'tomaculous' neuropathy.' *European Neurology*, **29**, 61–66.

Mathias, C.J., Bannister, E.R. (1992) 'Dopamine beta-hydroxylase deficiency and other genetically determined autonomic disorders.' *In:* Bannister, E.R., Mathias, C.J. (Eds.) *Autonomic Failure. A Textbook of Clinical Disorders of the Autonomic Nervous System. 3rd Edn.* Oxford: Oxford University Press, pp. 719–746.

Matsuo, H., Nomura, S., Hara, T., *et al.* (1994) 'A variant form of hypobetalipo-proteinaemia associated with ataxia, hearing loss and retinitis pigmentosa.' *Developmental Medicine and Child Neurology*, **36**, 1015–1020.

Mawatari, S., Iwashita, H., Kuroiwa, Y. (1972) 'Familial hypo-β-lipoproteinaemia.' *Journal of the Neurological Sciences*, **16**, 93–101.

May, M., Fria, T.J., Blumenthal, F., Curtin, H. (1981) 'Facial paralysis in children: differential diagnosis.' *Otolaryngology—Head and Neck Surgery*, **89**, 841–848.

Mayo, D.R., Booss, J. (1989) 'Varicella-zoster-associated neurologic disease without skin lesions.' *Archives of Neurology*, **46**, 313–315.

Maze, A., Bloch, E. (1979) 'Stridor in pediatric patients.' *Anesthesiology*, **50**, 132–135.

Mbonda, E., Claus, D., Bonnier, C., *et al.* (1995) 'Prolonged dysphagia caused by congenital pharyngeal dysfunction.' *Journal of Pediatrics*, **126**, 923–927.

McCombe, P.A., McLeod, J.G., Pollard, J.D., *et al.* (1987a) 'Peripheral sensorimotor and autonomic neuropathy associated with systemic lupus erythematosus. Clinical, pathological and immunological features.' *Brain*, **110**, 533–549.

—— Pollard, J.D., McLeod, J.G. (1987b) 'Chronic inflammatory demyelinating polyradiculoneuropathy: a clinical and eletrophysiological study of 92 cases.' *Brain*, **110**, 1617–1630.

McDermot, K.D., Walker, R.W.H. (1987) 'Autosomal recessive hereditary motor and sensory neuropathy with mental retardation, optic atrophy and pyramidal signs.' *Journal of Neurology, Neurosurgery, and Psychiatry*, **50**, 1342–1347.

McGonigle, R.J.S., Bewick, M., Weston, M.J., Parsons, V. (1985) 'Progressive, predominantly motor, uraemic neuropathy.' *Acta Neurologica Scandinavica*, **71**, 379–384.

McHugh, H.E., Sowden, K.A., Levitt, M.N. (1969) 'Facial paralysis and muscle agenesis in the newborn.' *Archives of Otolaryngology*, **89**, 131–143.

McKhann, G.M., Griffin, J.W., Cornblath, D.R., *et al.* (1988) 'Plasmapheresis and Guillain–Barré syndrome: analysis of prognostic factors and the effect of plasmapheresis.' *Annals of Neurology*, **23**, 347–353.

—— Cornblath, D.R., Griffin, J.W., *et al.* (1993) 'Acute motor axonal neuropathy: a frequent cause of acute flaccid paralysis in China.' *Annals of Neurology*, **33**, 332–342.

McLeod, J.G. (1981) 'Electrophysiological studies in the Guillain–Barré syndrome.' *Annals of Neurology*, **9** (Suppl.), 20–27.

—— Tuck, R.R. (1987) 'Disorders of the autonomic nervous system: Part I: Pathophysiology and clinical features.' *Annals of Neurology*, **21**, 419–430.

Melnick, J.L. (1984) 'Enterovirus type 71 infections: a varied clinical pattern sometimes mimicking paralytic poliomyelitis.' *Reviews of Infectious Diseases*, **6**, S387–S390.

Mentser, M.I., Clay, S., Malekzadeh, M.H., *et al.* (1978) 'Peripheral motor nerve conduction velocities in children undergoing chronic hemodialysis.' *Nephron*, **22**, 337–341.

Michaelson, R.A., Benson, G.S., Friedman, H.M. (1983) 'Urinary retention as the presenting symptom of acquired cytomegalovirus infection.' *American Journal of Medicine*, **74**, 526–528.

Mikati, M.A., DeLong, J.R. (1985) 'Childhood Guillain–Barré syndrome masquerading as a protracted pain syndrome.' *Archives of Neurology*, **42**, 839. *(Letter.)*

Miller, R.G., Gutmann, L., Lewis, R.A., Sumner, A.J. (1985) 'Acquired versus familial demyelinative neuropathies in children.' *Muscle and Nerve*, **8**, 205–210.

Mimaki, T., Itoh, N., Abe, J., *et al.* (1986) 'Neurological manifestations in xeroderma pigmentosum.' *Annals of Neurology*, **20**, 70–75.

Mitchell, G.W., Bosch, E.P., Hart, M.N. (1987) 'Response to immunosuppressive therapy in patients with hereditary motor and sensory neuropathy

and associated dysimmune neuromuscular disorders.' *European Neurology*, **27**, 188–196.

Morley, J.B., Reynolds, E.H. (1966) 'Papilloedema and Landry–Guillain–Barré syndrome. Case reports and review.' *Brain*, **89**, 205–222.

Narcy, P., Manac'h, Y., Sitbon, G., Pons, G. (1978) 'Paralysies laryngées néonatales. Evolution et traitement. A propos de 56 observations.' *Annales d'Otolaryngologie et de Chirurgie Cervico-Faciale*, **95**, 461–468.

Nass, R., Chutorian, A. (1982) 'Dysaesthesias and dysautonomia: a self-limited syndrome of painful dysaesthesias and autonomic dysfunction in childhood.' *Journal of Neurology, Neurosurgery, and Psychiatry*, **45**, 162–165.

Neimann, N., Vidailhet, M., Martin, J-J., *et al.* (1973) 'Fragilité osseuse, amyotrophie, arriération et lésions dégénératives du système nerveux central. Une nouvelle affection familiale.' *Archives Françaises de Pédiatrie*, **30**, 899–913.

Nelson, K.B., Eng, C.D. (1972) 'Congenital hypoplasia of the depressor anguli oris muscle: differentiation from congenital facial palsy.' *Journal of Pediatrics*, **81**, 16–20.

Nemni, R., Bottacchi, E., Fazio, R., *et al.* (1987) 'Polyneuropathy in hypothyroidism: clinical, electrophysiological and morphological findings in four cases.' *Journal of Neurology, Neurosurgery, and Psychiatry*, **50**, 1454–1460.

Nicholson, G.A., Dawkins, J.L., Blair, I.P., *et al.* (1996) ''The gene for hereditary sensory neuropathy type I (HSN-I) maps to chromosome 9p22.1–q22.3.' *Nature Genetics*, **13**, 101–104. *(Letter.)*

Nikoskelainen, E., Riekkinen, P. (1972) 'Retrobulbar neuritis as an early symptom of Guillain–Barré syndrome: report of a case.' *Acta Ophthalmologica*, **50**, 111–115.

Nukuda, H., Dyck, P.J. (1984) 'Decreased axon caliber and neurofilaments in hereditary motor and sensory neuropathy, type I.' *Annals of Neurology*, **16**, 238–241.

Ohtake, T., Komori, T., Hirose, K., Tanabe, H. (1990) 'CNS involvement in Japanese patients with chronic inflammatory demyelinating polyradiculoneuropathy.' *Acta Neurologica Scandinavica*, **81**, 108–112.

Orbeck, H., Oftedal, G. (1977) 'Familial dysautonomia in a non-Jewish child.' *Acta Paediatrica Scandinavica*, **66**, 774–781.

Otten, A., Vermeulen, M., Bossuyt, P.M.M., Otten, A. (1996) 'Intravenous immunoglobulin treatment in neurological diseases.' *Journal of Neurology, Neurosurgery, and Psychiatry*, **60**, 359–361.

Ouvrier, R.A. (1989) 'Giant axonal neuropathy—a review.' *Brain and Development*, **11**, 207–214.

—— (1992) 'Peripheral neuropathies in childhood.' *In:* Fukuyama, Y., Suzuki, Y., Kamoshita, S., Casaer, P. (Eds.) *Fetal and Perinatal Neurology.* Basel: Karger, pp. 60–78.

—— Shield, L. (1990) 'Focal lesions of peripheral nerves.' *In:* Ouvrier, R., McLeod, J.G., Pollard, J. (Eds.) *Peripheral Neuropathy in Childhood.* New York: Raven Press, pp. 219–233.

—— McLeod, J.G., Morgan, G.J., *et al.* (1981) 'Hereditary motor and sensory neuropathy of neuronal type with onset in early childhood.' *Journal of the Neurological Sciences*, **51**, 181–197.

—— —— Conchin, T.E. (1987) 'The hypertrophic forms of hereditary motor and sensory neuropathy: a study of hypertrophic Charcot–Marie–Tooth disease (HMSN type I) and Dejerine–Sottas disease (HMSN type III) in childhood.' *Brain*, **110**, 121–148.

—— —— Pollard, J. (1990) *Peripheral Neuropathy in Childhood. International Review of Child Neurology Series.* New York: Raven Press.

Pagès, M., Pagès, A-M. (1983) 'Leber's disease with spastic paraplegia and peripheral neuropathy. Case report with nerve biopsy study.' *EuropeanNeurology*, **22**, 181–185.

Painter, M.J. (1988) 'Brachial plexus injuries in neonates.' *International Pediatrics*, **3**, 120–124.

Panegyres, P.K., Moore, N., Gibson, R., *et al.* (1993) 'Thoracic outlet syndromes and magnetic resonance imaging.' *Brain*, **116**, 823–841.

Pasternak, J.F., Fulling, K., Nelson, J., Prensky, A.L. (1982) 'An infant with chronic, relapsing polyneuropathy responsive to steroids.' *Developmental Medicine and Child Neurology*, **24**, 504–510.

Patchell, R.A. (1994) 'Neurological complications of organ transplantation.' *Annals of Neurology*, **36**, 688–703.

Patel, P.I., Roa, B.B., Welcher, A.A., *et al.* (1992) 'The gene for the peripheral myelin protein PMP-22 is a candidate for Charcot–Marie–Tooth disease type 1A.' *Nature Genetics*, **1**, 159–165.

Pavesi, G., Gemignani, F., Macaluso, G.M., *et al.* (1992) 'Acute sensory and autonomic neuropathy: possible association with Coxsackie B virus infection.' *Journal of Neurology, Neurosurgery, and Psychiatry*, **55**, 613–615.

Pavone, L., Huttenlocher, P., Siciliano, L., *et al.* (1992) 'Two brothers with a variant of hereditary sensory neuropathy.' *Neuropediatrics*, **23**, 92–95.

Pearson, J., Pytel, B. (1978) 'Quantitative studies of sympathetic ganglia and spinal cord intermediolateral gray columns in familial dysautonomia.' *Journal of the Neurological Sciences*, **39**, 47–59.

—— Dancis, J., Axelrod, F. (1974) 'The sural nerve in familial dysautonomia.' *Journal of Neuropathology and Experimental Neurology*, **34**, 413–424.

—— Brandeis, L., Cuello, A.C. (1982) 'Depletion of substance P-containing axons in substantia gelatinosa of patients with diminished pain sensitivity.' *Nature*, **295**, 61–63.

Pellegrino, J.E., Rebbeck, T.R., Brown, M.J., *et al.* (1996) 'Mapping of hereditary neuralgic amyotrophy (familial brachial plexus neuropathy) to distal chromosome 17q.' *Neurology*, **46**, 1128–1132.

Peterson, C.M., Tsairis, P., Ohnishi, A., *et al.* (1974) 'Sodium cyanate induced polyneuropathy in patients with sickle-cell disease.' *Annals of Internal Medicine*, **81**, 152–158.

Petrera, J.E., Trojaborg, W. (1984) 'Conduction studies of the long thoracic nerve in serratus anterior palsy of different etiology.' *Neurology*, **34**, 1033–1037.

Petty, R.K.H., Duncan, R., Jamal, G.A., *et al.* (1993) 'Brainstem encephalitis and the Miller Fisher syndrome.' *Journal of Neurology, Neurosurgery, and Psychiatry*, **56**, 201–203.

Peudenier, S., Deleuze, J-F., Pham-Dinh, D., *et al.* (1993) 'Infantile neuropathy with unstable myelin: study of the Po protein.' *Journal of Neurology*, **240**, 291–294.

Pfeiffer, G., Künze, K., Brüch, M., *et al.* (1990) 'Polyneuropathy associated with chronic hypoxaemia: prevelance in patients with chronic obstructive pulmonary disease.' *Journal of Neurology*, **237**, 230–233.

Philipps, L.H. (1986) 'Familial long thoracic nerve palsy: a manifestation of brachial plexus neuropathy.' *Neurology*, **36**, 1251–1253.

Pinhas Hamiel, O., Raas-Rothschild, A., Upadhyaya, M., *et al.* (1993) 'Hereditary motor–sensory neuropathy (Charcot–Marie–Tooth disease) with nerve deafness: a new variant.' *Journal of Pediatrics*, **123**, 431–434.

Pollard, J.D., Beverstock, J., McLeod, J.G. (1987) 'Class II antigen expression and inflammatory cells in the Guillain–Barré syndrome.' *Annals of Neurology*, **21**, 337–341.

Pollock, M., Nukuda, H., Frith, R.W., *et al.* (1983) 'Peripheral neuropathy in Tangier disease.' *Brain*, **106**, 911–928.

Polo, A., Manganotti, P., Zanette, G., De Grandis, D. (1992) 'Polyneuritis cranialis: clinical and electrophysiological findings.' *Journal of Neurology, Neurosurgery, and Psychiatry*, **55**, 398–400.

Poser, C.M., Behan, P.O. (1982) 'Late onset of Guillain–Barré syndrome.' *Journal of Neuroimmunology*, **3**, 27–41.

Powers, J.M. (1985) 'Adrenoleukodystrophy (adreno-testiculo-leuko-myelo-neuropathic complex). A review.' *Clinical Neuropathology*, **4**, 181–199.

Priest, J.M., Fischbeck, K.H., Nouri, N., Keats, B.J.B. (1995) 'A locus for axonal motor–sensory neuropathy with deafness and mental retardation maps to Xq24–q26.' *Genomics*, **29**, 409–412.

Prineas, J.W. (1981) 'Pathology of the Guillain–Barré syndrome.' *Annals of Neurology*, **9** (Suppl.), 6–19.

Quattrone, A., Gambardella, A., Bono, F., *et al.* (1996) 'Autosomal recessive hereditary motor and sensory neuropathy with focally folded myelin sheaths: clinical, electrophysiologic, and genetic aspects of a large family.' *Neurology*, **46**, 1318–1324.

Quinlivan, R.M., Robb, S.A., Hall, M.A., *et al.* (1994) 'Infantile axonal neuropathy in two siblings.' *Neuromuscular Disorders*, **4**, 227–232.

Raeymaekers, P., Timmerman, V., Nelis, E., *et al.* (1991) 'Duplication in chromosome 17p11.2 in Charcot–Marie–Tooth neuropathy type 1a (CMT 1a). The HMSN Collaborative Research Group.' *Neuromuscular Disorders*, **1**, 93–97.

Rantala, H., Cherry, J.D., Shields, W.D., Uhari, M. (1994) 'Epidemiology of Guillain–Barré syndrome in children: relationship of oral polio vaccine administration to occurrence.' *Journal of Pediatrics*, **124**, 220–223.

—— Uhari, M., Cherry, J.D., Shields, D. (1995) 'Risk factors of respiratory failure in children with Guillain–Barré syndrome.' *Pediatric Neurology*, **13**, 289–292.

Raymond, G., Holmes, G.B. (1993) 'Cardio-facio-cutaneous (CFC) syndrome: neurological features in two children.' *Developmental Medicine and Child Neurology*, **35**, 727–732.

Rees, J.H., Soudain, S.E., Gregson, N.A., Hughes, R.A.C. (1995) '*Campylobacter jejuni* infection and Guillain–Barré syndrome.' *New England Journal of Medicine*, **333**, 1374–1379.

Richman, R.A., Sheehe, P.R., McCanty, S., *et al.* (1988) 'Olfactory deficits in boys with cleft palate.' *Pediatrics*, **82**, 840–844.

Riggs, J.E., Ashraf, M., Snyder, R.D., Gutmann, L. (1988) 'Prospective nerve conduction studies in cisplatin therapy.' *Annals of Neurology*, **23**, 92–94.

Ritter, F.J., Seay, A.R., Lahey, M.E. (1983) 'Peripheral mononeuropathy complicating anaphylactoid purpura.' *Journal of Pediatrics*, **103**, 77–78.

Roa, B.B., Garcia, C.A., Suter, U., *et al.* (1993) 'Charcot–Marie–Tooth disease type 1A. Association with a spontaneous point mutation in the PMP22 gene.' *New England Journal of Medicine*, **329**, 96–101.

Roberg, M., Ernerudh, J., Forsberg, P., *et al.* (1991) 'Acute peripheral facial palsy: CSF findings and etiology.' *Acta Neurologica Scandinavica*, **83**, 55–60.

Roberton, D.M., Mellor, D.H. (1982) 'Asymmetrical palatal paresis in childhood: a transient cranial mononeuropathy?' *Developmental Medicine and Child Neurology*, **24**, 842–849.

Ronen, G.M., Donat, J.R., Hill, A. (1986) 'Hemifacial spasm in childhood.' *Canadian Journal of Neurological Sciences*, **13**, 342–343.

Ropper, A.H. (1986a) 'Severe acute Guillain–Barré syndrome.' *Neurology*, **36**, 429–432.

—— (1986b) 'Unusual clinical variants and signs in Guillain–Barré syndrome.' *Archives of Neurology*, **43**, 1150–1152.

—— (1988) '*Campylobacter* diarrhea and Guillain–Barré syndrome.' *Archives of Neurology*, **45**, 655–656.

—— (1992) 'The Guillain–Barré syndrome.' *New England Journal of Medicine*, **326**, 1130–1136.

—— Chiappa, K.H. (1986) 'Evoked potential in Guillain–Barré syndrome.' *Neurology*, **36**, 587–590.

—— Albers, J.W., Addison, R. (1988) 'Limited relapse in Guillain–Barré syndrome after plasma exchange.' *Archives of Neurology*, **45**, 314–315.

—— Wijdicks, E.F.M., Shahani, B.T. (1990) 'Electrodiagnostic abnormalities in 113 consecutive patients with Guillain–Barré syndrome.' *Archives of Neurology*, **47**, 881–887.

Rosenberg, R.N., Chutorian, A., (1967) 'Familial opticoacoustic nerve degeneration and polyneuropathy.' *Neurology*, **17**, 827–832.

Rossi, L.N., Vassella, F., Mumenthaler, M. (1982) 'Obstetrical lesions of the brachial plexus. Natural history in 34 personal cases.' *European Neurology*, **21**, 1–7.

Rusanen, H., Majamaa, K., Tolonen, U., *et al.* (1995) 'Demyelinating polyneuropathy in a patient with the tRNA$^{Leu (UUR)}$ mutation at base pair 3243 of the mitochondrial DNA.' *Neurology*, **45**, 1188–1192.

Rust, R.S., Hickey, W. (1990) 'Congenital hypomyelination neuropathy (CHMN) with CSF findings: report of a case.' *In: Proceedings of the 5th International Child Neurology Congress, Tokyo*, p. 646.

Sabin, T.D., Swift, T.R., Jacobsen, R.R. (1993) 'Leprosy.' *In:* Dyck, P., Thomas, P.K., Griffin, J.W., *et al.* (Eds.) *Peripheral Neuropathy, Vol. 2.* Philadelphia: W.B. Saunders, pp. 1354–1372.

Sadeh, M., Blatt, I., Martonovits, G., *et al.* (1991) 'Treatment of porphyric convulsions with magnesium sulfate.' *Epilepsia*, **32**, 712–715.

Saïd, G., Boudier, L., Selva, J., *et al.* (1983) 'Different patterns of uremic polyneuropathy: clinicopathologic study.' *Neurology*, **33**, 567–574.

Saini, R.K., Singh, S., Sharma, S., *et al.* (1986) 'Snake bite poisoning presenting as early morning neuroparalytic syndrome in jhuggi dwellers.' *Journal of the Association of Physicians of India*, **34**, 415–417.

Sainio, K., Merikanto, J., Larsen, T.A. (1987) 'Carpal tunnel syndrome in childhood.' *Developmental Medicine and Child Neurology*, **29**, 794–797.

Sakashita, Y., Sakato, S., Komai, K., Takamori, M. (1992) 'Hereditary motor and sensory neuropathy with calf muscle enlargement.' *Journal of the Neurological Sciences*, **113**, 118–122.

Salisachs, P., Codina, A., Gimenez-Roldan, S., Zarranz, J.J. (1979) 'Charcot–Marie–Tooth disease associated with 'essential tremor' and normal or slightly diminished conduction velocity: report of 7 cases.' *European Neurology*, **18**, 49–58.

San Agustin, M., Nitowsky, H.M., Borden, J.N. (1962) 'Neonatal sciatic palsy after umbilical vessel injection.' *Journal of Pediatrics*, **60**, 408–413

Sander, J.E., Sharp, F.R. (1981) 'Lumbosacral plexus neuritis.' *Neurology*, **31**, 470–473.

Sanders, E.A.C.M., Peters, A.C.B., Gratana, J.W., Hughes, R.A.C. (1987) 'Guillain–Barré syndrome after varicella-zoster infection. Report of two cases.' *Journal of Neurology*, **234**, 437–439.

Sandstedt, P., Hyden, D., Odkvist, L.M., Kostulas, V. (1985) 'Peripheral facial palsy in children. A cerebrospinal fluid study.' *Acta Paediatrica Scandinavica*, **74**, 281–285.

Satya-Murti, S., Cacace, A., Hanson, P.A. (1979) 'Abnormal auditory evoked potentials in hereditary motor–sensory neuropathy.' *Annals of Neurology*, **5**, 445–448.

Scelsi, R., Verri, A.P., Bono, G., Marbini, A. (1989) 'Familial amyloid polyneuropathy: report of an autopsy case with neuropathy, vitreous opacities and polycystic kidney.' *European Neurology*, **29**, 27–32.

Schady, W., Smith, C.M.L. (1994) 'Sensory neuropathy in hereditary spastic paraplegia.' *Journal of Neurology, Neurosurgery, and Psychiatry*, **57**, 693–698.

Schaumburg, H., Kaplan, J., Windebank, A., *et al.* (1983) 'Sensory neuropathy from pyridoxine abuse. A new megavitamin syndrome.' *New England Journal of Medicine*, **309**, 445–448.

—— Berger, A.R., Thomas, P.K. (Eds.) (1992) 'Part VI. Toxic neuropathy.' *In: Disorders of Peripheral Nerves.* Philadelphia: F.A. Davis, pp. 257–302.

Schifrin, N. (1952) 'Unilateral paralysis of the diaphragm in the newborn infant due to phrenic injury with and without associated brachial palsy.' *Pediatrics*, **9**, 69–76.

Schubert, R., Cracco, J.B. (1992) 'Familial rectal pain: a type of reflex epilepsy?' *Annals of Neurology*, **32**, 824–826.

Schwankhaus, J.D., Currie, J., Jaffe, M.J., *et al.* (1989) 'Neurologic findings in men with isolated hypogonadotrophic hypogonadism.' *Neurology*, **39**, 223–226.

Schwartzman, R.J., McLellan, T.L. (1987) 'Reflex sympathetic dystrophy: a review.' *Archives of Neurology*, **44**, 555–561.

Scott, T.F. (1993) 'Neurosarcoidosis: progress and clinical aspects.' *Neurology*, **43**, 8–12.

Segurado, O.G., Krüger, H., Mertens, H.G., (1986) 'Clinical significance of serum and CSF findings in the Guillain–Barré syndrome and related disorders.' *Journal of Neurology*, **233**, 202–208.

Sghirlanzoni, A., Pareyson, D., Balestrini, M.R., *et al.* (1992) 'HMSN III phenotype due to homozygous expression of a dominant HMSN II gene.' *Neurology*, **42**, 2201–2203.

Shahar, E., Shorer, E., Roifman, C.M., *et al.* (1997) 'Immune globulins are effective in severe pediatric Guillain–Barré syndrome.' *Pediatric Neurology*, **16**, 32–36.

Shapiro, N.L., Cunningham, M.J., Parikh, S.R., *et al.* (1996) 'Congenital unilateral facial paralysis.' *Pediatrics*, **97**, 261–265.

Sherry, D.D., Weisman, R. (1988) 'Psychologic aspects of childhood reflex neurovascular dystrophy.' *Pediatrics*, **81**, 572–578.

Silander, K., Halonen, P., Sara, R., *et al.* (1994) 'DNA analysis in Finnish patients with hereditary neuropathy with liability to pressure palsies (HNPP).' *Journal of Neurology, Neurosurgery, and Psychiatry*, **57**, 1260–1262.

Silber, T.J., Majd, M. (1988) 'Reflex sympathetic dystrophy in children and adolescents. Report of 18 cases and review of the literature.' *American Journal of Diseases of Children*, **142**, 1325–1330.

Simon, L.T., Horoupian, D.S., Dorfman, L.J., *et al.* (1990) 'Polyneuropathy, ophthalmoplegia, leukoencephalopathy and intestinal pseudo-obstruction: POLIP syndrome.' *Annals of Neurology*, **28**, 349–360.

Singman, R., Segan, S., Gracco, J. (1990) 'Is "familial rectal pain" a form of reflex epilepsy?' *Annals of Neurology*, **28**, 432. (Abstract.)

Skjeldal, O.H., Stokke, O., Refsum, S., *et al.* (1987) 'Clinical and biochemical heterogeneity in conditions with phytanic acid accumulation.' *Journal of the Neurological Sciences*, **77**, 87–96.

Sladky, J.T., Brown, H.J., Berman, P.H. (1986) 'Chronic inflammatory demyelinating polyneuropathy of infancy. A corticosteroid responsive disorder.' *Annals of Neurology*, **20**, 76–81.

Smith, T., Trojaborg, W. (1987) 'Diagnosis of thoracic outlet syndrome. Value of sensory and motor conduction studies and quantitative electromyography.' *Archives of Neurology*, **44**, 1161–1163.

Sokol, R.J., Guhggenheim, M.A., Heubi, J.E., *et al.* (1985) 'Frequency and clinical progression of the vitamin E deficiency neurologic disorder in children with prolonged neonatal cholestasis.' *American Journal of Diseases of Children*, **139**, 1211–1215.

Sommer, C., Schröder, J.M. (1989) 'Hereditary motor and sensory neuropathy with optic atrophy. Ultrastructural and morphometric observations on nerve fibers, mitochondria and dense-cored vesicles.' *Archives of Neurology*, **46**, 973–977.

Sorensen, T.T. (1988) 'Familial recurrent cranial nerve palsies.' *Acta Neurologica Scandinavica*, **78**, 542–543.

Specola, N., Vanier, M.T., Goutières, F., *et al.* (1990) 'The juvenile and chronic forms of GM2 gangliosidosis. Clinical and enzymatic heterogeneity.' *Neurology*, **40**, 145–150.

Spencer, S.E., Walker, F.O., Moore, S.A. (1987) 'Chorea-amyotrophy with chronic hemolytic anemia: a variant of chorea–amyotrophy with acanthocytosis.' *Neurology*, **37**, 645–649.

Steiner, I., Kidron, D., Soffer, D., *et al.* (1988) 'Sensory peripheral neuropathy of vitamin B$_{12}$ deficiency: a primary demyelinating disease?' *Journal of Neurology*, **235**, 163–164.

Steiner, I., Steinberg, A., Argov, Z., *et al.* (1987) 'Familial progressive neuronal disease and chronic idiopathic intestinal pseudo-obstruction.' *Neurology*, **37**, 1046–1050.

Steinman, L., Tharp, B.R., Dorfman, L.J., *et al.* (1980) 'Peripheral neuropathy in the cherry-red-spot–myoclonus syndrome (sialidosis type 1).' *Annals of Neurology*, **7**, 450–456.

Sterman, A.B., Schaumburg, H.H., Asbury, A.K. (1980) 'The acute sensory neuropathy syndrome: a distinct clinical entity.' *Annals of Neurology*, **7**, 354–358.

Stewart, G.J., Pollard, J.D., McLeod, J.G., Wolnizer, C.M. (1978) 'HLA antigens in the Landry–Guillain–Barré syndrome and chronic relapsing polyneuritis.' *Annals of Neurology*, **4**, 285–289.

Stultz, P., Pfeiffer, K.M. (1982) 'Peripheral nerve injuries resulting from common surgical procedures in the lower portion of the abdomen.' *Archives of Surgery*, **117**, 324–327.

Stumpf, D.A., Sokol, R., Bettis, D., *et al.* (1987) 'Friedreich's disease. V. Variant form with vitamin E deficiency and normal fat absorption.' *Neurology*, **37**, 68–74.

Suarez-Zeledon, A., Brian-Gago, R. (1995) 'Acute pharyngeal paralysis in childhood: report of three cases.' *Acta Neuropediatrica*, **1**, 130–133.

Sudarshan, A., Goldie, W.D. (1985) 'The spectrum of congenital facial diplegia (Moebius syndrome).' *Pediatric Neurology*, **1**, 180–184.

Sugama, S., Matsunaga, T., Ito, F., *et al.* (1992) 'Transient unilateral, isolated hypoglossal nerve palsy.' *Brain and Development*, **14**, 122–123.

Sullivan, R.L., Reeves, A.G. (1977) 'Normal cerebrospinal fluid protein, increased intracranial pressure and the Guillain–Barré syndrome.' *Annals of Neurology*, **1**, 108–109.

Sumner, A.J. (1981) 'The physiological basis for symptoms in Guillain–Barré syndrome.' *Annals of Neurology*, **9** (Suppl.), 28–30.

Suzuki, A., Aso, K., Ariyoshi, C., Ishimaru, M. (1992) 'Acute intermittent porphyria and epilepsy: safety of clonazepam.' *Epilepsia*, **33**, 108–111.

Swaiman, K.F., Flagler, D.G. (1971) 'Mercury poisoning with central and peripheral nervous system involvement treated with penicillamine.' *Pediatrics*, **48**, 639–642.

Tachi, N., Sasaki, K., Kusano, T., *et al.* (1988) 'Peripheral neuropathy in four cases of group A xeroderma pigmentosum.' *Journal of Child Neurology*, **3**, 114–119.

Tada, K., Taniike, M., Ono, J., *et al.* (1992) 'Serial magnetic resonance imaging studies in a case of late-onset globoid leukodystrophy.' *Neuropediatrics*, **23**, 306–309.

Takahashi, A. (1978) 'Migrating disseminated multiple cranial neuropathy.' *Clinical Neurology*, **14**, 843–853.

Takayama, H., Kazahaya, Y., Kashihara, N., *et al.* (1987) 'A case of post-ganglionic cholinergic dysautonomia.' *Journal of Neurology, Neurosurgery, and Psychiatry*, **50**, 915–918.

Takebe, Y., Koide, N., Takahashi, G. (1981) 'Giant axonal neuropathy: report of two siblings with endocrinological and histological studies.' *Neuropediatrics*, **12**, 392–404.

Tatum, W.O., Zachariah, S.B. (1995) 'Gabapentin treatment of seizures in intermittent porphyria.' *Neurology*, **45**, 1216–1217.

Thakkar, N., O'Neil, W., Duvally, J., *et al.* (1977) 'Möbius syndrome due to brain stem segmental necrosis.' *Archives of Neurology*, **34**, 124–126.

Thomas, P.K. (1992) 'The Guillain–Barré syndrome: no longer a simple concept.' *Journal of Neurology*, **239**, 361–362.

—— Lascelles, R.G., Hallpike, J.F., Hewer, R.L. (1969) 'Recurrent and chronic relapsing Guillain–Barré polyneuritis.' *Brain*, **92**, 589–606.

—— Walker, R.W.H., Rudge, P., *et al.* (1987) 'Chronic demyelinating peripheral neuropathy associated with mulifocal central nervous system demyelination.' *Brain*, **110**, 53–76.

—— Plant, G.T., Baxter, P., *et al.* (1995) 'An epidemic of optic neuropathy and painful sensory neuropathy in Cuba: clinical aspects.' *Journal of Neurology*, **242**, 629–638.

Thomson, A.J.G. (1993) 'Idiopathic lumbosacral plexus neuropathy in two children.' *Developmental Medicine and Child Neurology*, **35**, 258–261.

Thornton, C.A., Griggs, R.C. (1994) 'Plasma exchange and intravenous immunoglobulin treatment of neuromuscular disease.' *Annals of Neurology*, **35**, 260–268.

Tokimura, Y., Kuriyama, M., Arimura, K., *et al.* (1992) 'Electrophysiological studies in cerebrotendinous xanthomatosis.' *Journal of Neurology, Neurosurgery, and Psychiatry*, **55**, 52–55.

Toole, J.F., Parrish, M.L. (1973) 'Nitrofurantoin polyneuropathy.' *Neurology*, **23**, 554–559.

Towfighi, J., Marks, K., Palmer, E., Vannucci, K. (1979) 'Möbius syndrome. Neuropathologic observations.' *Acta Neuropathologica*, **48**, 11–17.

Treiber-Held, S., Budjarjo-Welim, H., Riemann, D., *et al.* (1994) 'Giant axonal neuropathy: a generalized disorder of intermediate filaments with longitudinal grooves in the hair.' *Neuropediatrics*, **25**, 89–93.

Triggs, W.J., Cros, D., Gominak, S.C., *et al.* (1992) 'Motor nerve inexcitability in Guillain–Barré syndrome. The spectrum of distal conduction block and axonal degeneration.' *Brain*, **115**, 1291–1302.

Tsao, C.Y., Romshe, C.A., Lo, W.D., *et al.* (1994) 'Familial adrenal insufficiency, achalasia, alacrimia, peripheral neuropathy, microcephaly, normal plasma very long chain fatty acids, and normal muscle mitochondrial respiratory chain enzymes.' *Journal of Child Neurology*, **9**, 135–138.

—— Lo, W.D., Mendell, J.R., Batley, R.J. (1995) 'Critical illness polyneuropathy in a 2-year-old girl with hemorrhagic shock encephalopathy syndrome.' *Journal of Child Neurology*, **10**, 486–488.

Tyson, J., Malcolm, S., Thomas, P.K., Harding, A.E. (1996) 'Deletions of chromosome 17p11.2 in multifocal neuropathies.' *Annals of Neurology*, **39**, 180–186.

—— Ellis, D., Fairbrother, U., *et al.* (1997) 'Hereditary demyelinating neuropathy of infancy. A genetically complex syndrome.' *Brain*, **120**, 47–63.

Uldry, P.A., Regli, F. (1988) 'Multinévrite des nerfs crâniens et syndrome d'immunodéficience acquise (SIDA): 5 cas.' *Revue Neurologique*, **144**, 586–589.

Ulrich, J., Hirt, H.R., Kleihues, P., Oberholzer, M. (1981) 'Connatal polyneuropathy—a case with proliferated microfilaments in Schwann cells.' *Acta Neuropathologica*, **55**, 39–46.

Uncini, A., Di Muzio, A., Chiavaroli, F., *et al.* (1994) 'Hereditary motor and sensory neuropathy with calf hypertrophy is associated with 17p11.2 duplication.' *Annals of Neurology*, **35**, 552–558.

Unishi, G., Yasuhara, A., Hori, A., *et al.* (1988) 'Electrophysiologic study of Fisher syndrome.' *Pediatric Neurology*, **4**, 296–300.

Vanasse, M., Dubowitz, V. (1981) 'Dominantly inherited peroneal muscular atrophy (hereditary motor and sensory neuropathy type I) in infancy and childhood.' *Muscle and Nerve*, **4**, 26–30.

Van der Meché, F.G.A., Meulstee, J., Kleyweg, R.P. (1991) 'Axonal damage in Guillain–Barré syndrome.' *Muscle and Nerve*, **14**, 997–1002.

—— Schmitz, P.I.M., and the Dutch Guillain–Barré Study Group (1992) 'A randomized trial comparing intravenous immune globulin and plasma exchange in Guillain–Barré syndrome.' *New England Journal of Medicine*, **326**, 1123–1129.

Van der Wiel, H.L., Staal, A. (1981) 'External ophthalmoplegia, juvenile parkinsonism and axonal neuropathy in two siblings.' *Clinical Neurology and Neurosurgery*, **83**, 247–252.

Van Dongen, H.R., Arts, W.F.M., Yousef-Bak, E. (1987) 'Acquired dysarthria in childhood: an analysis of dysarthric features in relation to neurologic deficits.' *Neurology*, **37**, 296–299.

Van Doorn, P.A., Brand, A., Strengers, P.F.W., *et al.* (1990) 'High-dose intravenous immunoglobulin treatment in chronic inflammatory demyelinating polyneuropathy: a double-blind, placebo-controlled crossover study.' *Neurology*, **40**, 209–212.

Vanneste, J.A., Karthaus, P.P.M., Davies, G. (1980) 'Acute urinary retention due to sacral myeloradiculitis.' *Journal of Neurology, Neurosurgery, and Psychiatry*, **43**, 954–956.

Van Weerden, T.W., Houthoff, H.J., Sie, O., Minderhoud, J.M. (1982) 'Variability in nerve biopsy findings in a kinship with dominantly inherited Charcot–Marie–Tooth disease.' *Muscle and Nerve*, **5**, 185–196.

Verhagen, W.I.M., Gabreëls-Festen, A.A.W.M., Van Wensen, P.J.M., *et al.* (1993) 'Hereditary neuropathy with liability to pressure palsies: a clinical, electrophysiological and morphological study.' *Journal of the Neurological Sciences*, **116**, 176–184.

Verhalle, D., Löfgren, A., Nelis, E., *et al.* (1994) 'Deletion in the CMT1A locus on chromosome 17p11.2 in hereditary neuropathy with liability to pressure palsies.' *Annals of Neurology*, **35**, 704–708.

Verity, C.M., Dunn, H.G., Berry, K. (1982) 'Children with reduced sensitivity to pain: assessment of hereditary sensory neuropathy types II and IV.' *Developmental Medicine and Child Neurology*, **24**, 785–797.

Vermeulen, M., Van Doorn, P.A., Brand, A., *et al.* (1993) 'Intravenous immunoglobulin treatment in patients with chronic inflammatory demyelinating polyneuropathy: a double blind, placebo controlled study.' *Journal of Neurology, Neurosurgery, and Psychiatry*, **56**, 36–39.

Villalobos, R., Santos, M.A. (1996) 'Karwinskia palsy in children.' *Acta Neuropediatrica*, **2**, 155–159.

Vincent, F.M., Vincent, T. (1986) 'Relapsing Fisher's syndrome.' *Journal of Neurology, Neurosurgery, and Psychiatry*, **49**, 604–606.

Visser, L.H., Van der Meché, F.G.A., Van Doorn, P.A., *et al.* (1995) 'Guillain–Barré syndrome without sensory loss (acute motor neuropathy). A subgroup with specific clinical, electrodiagnostic and laboratory features.' *Brain*, **118**, 841–847.

Vital, C., Battin, J., Rivel, J., Heheunstre, J.P. (1976) 'Aspects ultrastructuraux des lésions du nerf périphérique dans un cas de maladie de Farber.' *Revue Neurologique*, **132**, 419–423.

Vogel, P., Gabriel, M.M., Goebel, H.H., Dyck, P.J. (1985) 'Hereditary motor sensory neuropathy type II with neurofilament accumulation: new finding or new disorder?' *Annals of Neurology*, **17**, 455–461.

Vriesendorp, F.J., Mishu, B., Blaser, M.J., Koski, C.L. (1993) 'Serum antibodies to GM1, GD1b, peripheral nerve myelin, and *Campylobacter jejuni* in patients with Guillain–Barré syndrome and controls: correlation and prognosis.' *Annals of Neurology*, **34**, 130–135.

Waddy, H.M., Misra, V.P., King, R.H.M., *et al.* (1989) 'Facial cranial involvement in chronic inflammatory demyelinating polyneuropathy: clinical and MRI evidence of peripheral and central lesions.' *Journal of Neurology*, **236**, 400–405.

Wadlington, W.B., Riley, H.D., Lowbeer, L. (1984) 'The Melkersson–Rosenthal syndrome.' *Pediatrics*, **73**, 502–506.

Walters, A.S., Picchietti, D.L., Ehrenberg, B.L., Wagner, M.L. (1994) 'Restless legs syndrome in childhood and adolescence.' *Pediatric Neurology*, **11**, 241–245.

Watson, P., Ashby, P. (1976) 'Brachial plexus neuropathy associated with infectious mononucleosis.' *Canadian Medical Association Journal*, **114**, 766–767.

Weber, T., Jürgens, S., Lüer, W. (1987) 'Cerebrospinal fluid immunoglobulins and virus-specific antibodies in disorders affecting the facial nerve.' *Journal of Neurology*, **234**, 308–314.

Weiss, J.A., White, J.C. (1986) 'Correlation of 1A afferent conduction with the ataxia of Fisher syndrome.' *Muscle and Nerve*, **9**, 327–332.

Wertman, E., Argov, Z., Abrmasky, O. (1988) 'Chronic inflammatory demyelinating polyradiculoneuropathy: features and prognostic factors with corticosteroid therapy.' *European Neurology*, **28**, 199–204.

Westerberg, B., Hagne, I., Sellden, U. (1983) 'Hereditary motor and sensory neuropathies in Swedish children. Neuronal–axonal types.' *Acta Paediatrica Scandinavica*, **72**, 685–693.

Wichman, A., Buchthal, F., Pezeshkpour, G.H., Gregg, R.E. (1985) 'Peripheral neuropathy in abetalipoproteinemia.' *Neurology*, **35**, 1279–1289.

Wijdicks, E.F.M., Ropper, A.H. (1990) 'Acute relapsing Guillain–Barré syndrome after long asymptomatic intervals.' *Archives of Neurology*, **47**, 82–84.

Willis, J., Van den Bergh, P. (1988) 'Cerebral involvement in children with acute and relapsing inflammatory polyneuropathy.' *Journal of Child Neurology*, **3**, 200–204.

Winer, J.B., Hughes, R.A.C., Osmond, C. (1988) 'A prospective study of acute idiopathic neuropathy. I: Clinical features and their prognostic value.' *Journal of Neurology, Neurosurgery, and Psychiatry*, **51**, 605–612.

Wong, V. (1995) 'Outcome of facial nerve palsy in 24 children.' *Brain and Development*, **17**, 294–296.

Wright, A., Dyck, P.J. (1995) 'Hereditary sensory neuropathy with sensorineural deafness and early-onset dementia.' *Neurology*, **45**, 560–562.

Wright, G.D.S., Lee, K.D. (1980) 'An isolated right hypoglossal nerve palsy in association with infectious mononucleosis.' *Postgraduate Medical Journal*, **56**, 185–186.

Wynne, J.M., Williams, G.L., Ellman, B.A.H. (1978) 'Accidental intraarterial injection.' *Archives of Disease in Childhood*, **53**, 396–400.

Yiannikas, C., McLeod, J.G., Pollard, J.D., Baverstock, J. (1986) 'Peripheral neuropathy associated with mitochondrial myopathy.' *Annals of Neurology*, **20**, 249–257.

Young, D.B., Buchanan, T.M. (1983) 'A serological test for leprosy with a glycolipid specific for *Mycobacterium leprae*.' *Science*, **221**, 1057–1059.

Young, R.R., Asbury, A.K., Corbett, J.L., Adams, R.D. (1975) 'Pure pandysautonomia with recovery: description and discussion of diagnostic criteria.' *Brain*, **98**, 613–636.

Yuki, N., Yoshino, H., Sato, S., Miyatake, T. (1990) 'Acute axonal polyneuropathy associated with anti-GM1 antibodies following *Campylobacter* enteritis.' *Neurology*, **40**, 1900–1902.

Zefeiriou, D.I., Mauromatis, I.V., Hatjisevastou, H.K., *et al.* (1997) 'Benign congenital hemifacial spasm.' *Pediatric Neurology*, **17**, 174–176.

Zeharia, A., Mukamel, M., Frishberg, Y., *et al.* (1990) 'Benign plexus neuropathy in children.' *Journal of Pediatrics*, **116**, 276–278.

Zochodne, D.W., Bolton, C.F., Wells, G.A., *et al.* (1987) 'Critical illness polyneuropathy. A complication of sepsis and multiple organ failure.' *Brain*, **110**, 819–841.

—— Ramsay, D.A., Saly, V., Semmler, R. (1993) 'Acute myopathy of intensive care unit patients: serial electrophysiological studies.' *Canadian Journal of Neurological Sciences*, **20**, Suppl. 2, S27. *(Abstract.)*

Zucker, R.M. (1990) 'Facial paralysis in children.' *Clinics in Plastic Surgery*, **17**, 95–99.

Zwiener, R.J., Ginsberg, C.M. (1988) 'Organophosphate and carbamate poisoning in infants and children.' *Pediatrics*, **81**, 121–126.

22
PRIMARY MUSCLE DISEASE

The primary muscle diseases include a large number of conditions of multiple causes, the majority of which are genetically determined. The most common diseases in this group are the progressive muscular dystrophies and other degenerative muscle diseases known as congenital myopathies, and the myotonic dystrophies. An increasing number of metabolic myopathies is being recognized.

THE PROGRESSIVE MUSCULAR DYSTROPHIES

The progressive muscular dystrophies are a group of heredo-familial diseases with onset in early life, involvement of proximal more than distal muscle and often pseudohypertrophy of muscles (Walton and Gardner-Medwin 1981). All muscular dystrophies share common pathological features. These include necrosis of fibres with signs of regeneration such as 'splitting' of fibres, forked, hyalinized fibres, and a mixture of atrophic and hypertrophic fibres. These fibres are randomly distributed without any grouping of abnormally small fibres, nor elective involvement of a specific histoenzymological fibre type. Proliferation of collagen and fat is marked, especially in late stages, and collagen and fat cells accumulate between remaining muscle fibres. This is largely responsible for the pseudohypertrophy which is characteristic of some major types of muscular dystrophy. In some types, there is also involvement of cardiac muscle with myocardial degeneration and fibrosis (Fig. 22.1).

These histological features seem to be the result of repeated episodes of necrosis and regeneration of muscle cell which are probably initiated by a breakdown of the muscle cell membrane. Recent discoveries in the biochemistry and molecular genetics of Duchenne muscular dystrophy seem to substantiate the membrane origin of muscular dystrophies. Likewise, observations with the electron microscope have shown breaks in the membrane and changes in intramembranous particles in freeze–fracture studies.

DUCHENNE MUSCULAR DYSTROPHY (DMD)

AETIOLOGY, GENETICS, INCIDENCE AND MECHANISMS
DMD is inherited as an X-linked recessive condition with an incidence of 1 in 3500 male births. Approximately one-third of cases appear to be due to new mutations. Female carriers are usually asymptomatic although in some women the disease is

clinically manifest, either in a subtle or in a more patent manner (Moser 1984). Girls with a complete Duchenne phenotype are on record. Some of these girls had a negative X-chromatin pattern, and XO/XX mosaicism or a structurally abnormal X chromosome. DMD in females has been reported in several patients with X autosome translocations and these have been helpful in identifying the location of the *DMD* gene (Emanuel *et al.* 1983). Rare cases of typical DMD in girls with an XX genotype are on record (Meola *et al.* 1986), probably due to unequal lyonization. However, formal proof now requires demonstration of absent dystrophin and/or deletion in the *DMD* gene. *DMD* carriers may have a mosaic expression of dystrophin with more or less numerous abnormal fibres correlating with the degree of clinical involvement (Witkowski 1989, Wessel 1990).

Approximately 60–70 per cent of asymptomatic carriers of DMD have mildly increased levels of creatine kinase and pyruvate kinase in their serum (Hyser *et al.* 1987). Affected males (hemizygotes) have very high creatine kinase levels detectable from birth. In practice, the persistence of elevated creatine kinase levels beyond the fourth day of life is suggestive, making neonatal screening feasible, as practical methods for determining the amounts of creatine kinase in dried filter paper blood specimens are available (Scheuerbrandt *et al.* 1986). Improved methods using dystrophin testing (Witkowski 1989, Wessel 1990) or DNA analysis (Rowland 1988) are available.

A tremendous impetus to the study and understanding of DMD has been given by the discovery of the gene localization and the cloning of the gene and its product, dystrophin, by reverse genetics (reviewed in Rowland 1988, Witkowski 1989, Wessel 1990, Dubowitz 1995).

The gene is located on the short arm of the X chromosome in the band Xp21. It is extremely large, encompassing at least 2000 kilobases or 0.05 per cent of the total human genome (Kunkel 1986). However, Duchenne RNA encompasses only 14kb, implying that less than 1 per cent of the total genomic DNA is eventually transcribed into protein. The complex splicing procedure needed to remove the noncoding introns provides ample opportunity for errors in the processing of the gene and manufacture of gene product.

DMD is due to a deletion of parts of the gene detectable in 60–70 per cent of cases when studied by cDNA probes, compared to about 10 per cent by genomic probes. This finding considerably increased the potential for carrier detection, antenatal diagnosis and diagnosis of isolated cases (Gutmann and Fischbeck

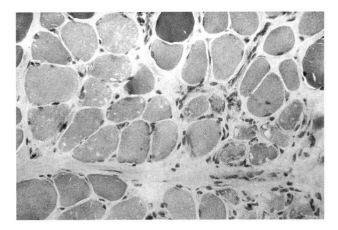

Fig. 22.1. Duchenne dystrophy. Haematoxylin–eosin stained histological section of muscle. Note necrotic fibres, irregular calibre of fibres, and intramuscular fibrosis. (Courtesy Dr F. Renault, Hôpital Trousseau, Paris.)

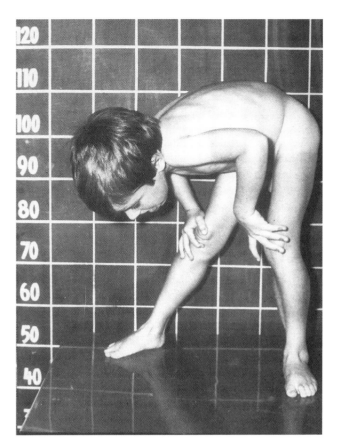

Fig. 22.2. Duchenne dystrophy. Gower's manoeuvre. (Courtesy Dr F. Renault, Hôpital Trousseau, Paris.)

1989). Both DMD and Becker dystrophy are caused by defects in the same gene (Monaco and Kunkel 1987) but DMD patients produce no functional protein, while patients with Becker dystrophy express abnormal but partially functional mRNA and protein.

Dystrophin is localized to the membrane of cell muscles and is absent in virtually all patients with DMD but almost never in controls (Hoffman *et al.* 1988, Wessel 1990). Dystrophin is also present in brain cells and other tissues but the significance of this finding in relation to mental retardation in DMD patients is unclear. In general, the role of dystrophin is poorly understood although it seems to be concerned with the maintenance of the membrane in muscular contractions and/or in transmembrane ion fluxes. The discovery of animal models in which dystrophin is also absent has made it probable that other factors are involved. For example, the mdx mouse (without dystrophin) develops only a transient disorder, whereas dogs without dystrophin have a severe DMD-like disorder.

CLINICAL FEATURES

DMD has its onset in early childhood. The disease is slowly progressive and the first manifestations are often overlooked. Delay in passing milestones and difficulties with climbing stairs, arising from the floor or other signs of pelvic muscle weakness are usually the initial symptoms. When fully developed, pelvic weakness produces the classical Gowers' sign in which the patient arises by climbing up the thighs (Fig. 22.2). Lordosis and a waddling gait progressively develop and some degre of muscle atrophy may become apparent, although hypertrophy of the calves and less frequently of the vastus lateralis and deltoids is much more striking in most cases. Echography and radiological examination by CT or MRI have confirmed the pathological finding that this is indeed a pseudohypertrophy related to fat and collagen proliferation (Fischer *et al.* 1988, Heckmatt *et al.* 1988). Such examinations are not normally needed in DMD.

Muscle weakness and atrophy are symmetrical and relentlessly progressive. However, immobilization in bed and surgical opera-

tion may be associated with rapid progress of the disease. Patients with typical DMD become wheelchair-dependent by 12 years of age; deep tendon reflexes progressively decrease, and severe deformations, especially scoliosis, often develop and may be rapidly progressive (Rodillo *et al.* 1988). Respiratory failure occurs, in part related to scoliosis and in part to involvement of respiratory muscles.

Cardiac involvement is consistently present. In the early stages this is reflected only in the ECG changes but later overt signs of cardiac decompensation may develop.

The involvement of smooth muscle is rare if it occurs at all. Barohn *et al.* (1988) observed acute gastric dilatation, bladder paralysis or megacolon in a few of their patients, often as a late event, although gastric hypomotility was relatively common.

Intellectual impairment is a remarkable feature of many cases of DMD. Psychometric assessment in several large series showed a mean IQ of about 85 with a range from about 40–130. Approximately 20–30 per cent of patients fall in the subnormal range with IQs <70 (Dubowitz 1995). Moreover, there is a high concordance between the intelligence levels of affected siblings. Early verbal disability is characteristic of DMD (Dorman *et al.* 1988), although other skills may also be impaired. The distribution of intelligence levels is gaussian and unimodal, therefore consistent with a general shift in IQ to lower values rather than selective involvement in only some cases, with a different genetic basis. No pathological basis for the intellectual impairment has been consistently found (Dubowitz and Crome 1969, Jagadha and Becker 1988), although abnormal dendritic arborization has been reported (Jagadha and Becker 1988). MRI scans have been reportedly normal in a few patients. Contrary to previous opinions, intellectual impairment in DMD does not seem to be due to the effects of physical disability but rather is a part of the spectrum of the disease. There is no correlation between the severity and duration of weakness and mental impairment.

The total duration of the disease is variable. Some patients lose the ability to walk by 6–7 years of age, the median age is 10 years, and in the more slowly progressive cases patients may walk till 12 or 13 years. Some patients with apparently typical DMD continue to walk beyond age 13. It is difficult to know whether these are mild cases of DMD or severe cases of Becker dystrophy. Such 'outliers' were found in one study (Hoffman *et al.* 1989) to have detectable levels of dystrophin in muscle biopsy samples and, therefore, were regarded as cases of severe Becker dystrophy. Death from cardiorespiratory problems occurs in most cases during the second or early third decade of life. DMD is rarely if ever responsible for malignant hyperthermia (Wedel 1992), but less severe anaesthetic reactions with tachycardia, fever and elevation of creatine kinase may occur (Sethna *et al.* 1988). Patients whose muscles are stronger are more likely to die of cardiomyopathy, whereas weaker patients die from respiratory failure (Brooke *et al.* 1989).

The *diagnosis* of DMD is generally easy as the clinical features of the disease are sterotyped. However, the disorder is often recognized late, which is especially regrettable for genetic counselling. Confirmation of the diagnosis rests on determination of the creatine kinase level which is extremely high (> 5000 UI) early in the course and slowly decreases in older patients while remaining far above normal values. Due to the difficulty in early recognition, systematic determination of the creatine kinase level should always be obtained in children who do not walk by 18 months of age. These represent about a half of the cases of DMD. Rare atypical presentations may occur such as neonatal rhabdomyolysis revealing an X-linked severe dystrophy (Breningstall *et al.* 1988). Screening for DMD based on systematic creatine kinase determination at the same time as the Guthrie test for phenylketonuria has been proposed but not generally accepted. The conditions required for such testing have been reviewed recently by van Ommen and Scheuerbrandt (1993).

Electromyography shows a typical myogenic pattern, and the conjunction of this with elevated creatine kinase and clinical signs is sufficient evidence for the diagnosis in most cases. Muscle biopsy confirms the dystrophic nature of the disorder and excludes other causes. It may not be necessary when a deletion is demonstrated in blood samples but remains necessary for dystrophin studies.

Dystrophin testing now appears to be the best way of confirming the diagnosis of DMD and of separating DMD from Becker dystrophy (see below) (Witkowski 1989, Wessel 1990). However, rare patients with different disorders (<5 per cent) may lack normal dystrophin (Hoffman *et al.* 1988), and other

dystrophin-related phenotypes may exist such as the cases of X-linked nonprogressive disorder with muscle cramps and myalgia reported by Gospe *et al.* (1989), the case of X-linked myoglobinuria described by Fischbeck *et al.* (1988), and the cases of myalgia and cramps with abnormal dystrophin reported by Samaha and Quinlan (1996b), which has obvious consequences for genetic counselling. Absence of dystrophin has also been demonstrated in rare cases of neonatal muscular dystrophy (Mendell *et al.* 1990, 1995).

The opinion that all myopathic disorders related to the *DMD* gene constitute a single entity (Rowland 1988) is no longer tenable, as a disease cannot be defined without reference to its phenomenology and as variable mutations or deletions with different phenotypes and courses exist (Samaha and Quinlan 1996a), *e.g.* McLeod syndrome, characterized by the absence of Kell antigen, acanthocytosis and elevated creatine kinase, usually in asymptomatic individuals (Witt *et al.* 1992) but occasionally in persons with neuromuscular involvement (Danek *et al.* 1994). In McLeod syndrome, however, Danek *et al.* (1990) have shown the presence of normal dystrophin, suggesting that the *DMD* gene, albeit close to the McLeod locus, is not involved in McLeod myopathy. The diagnosis of DMD can now be made in some girls with a suggestive clinical picture by demonstrating abnormalities in the dystrophin gene or dystrophin. A chromosomal abnormality, especially an X autosomal translocation, is usually present but not in every case (Medori *et al.* 1989).

A *prenatal diagnosis* of DMD through dystrophin testing of fetal muscle appears impractical given sampling problems and fetal risks. Prenatal diagnosis is possible from about 10 weeks gestational age using chorionic villus sampling with almost 100 per cent accuracy for cases in which a DNA deletion is present (Gutmann and Fischbeck 1989), especially using cDNA probes. In cases without deletion, study of linkage with DNA markers can be used in informative kinships. Genetic counselling is possible with a greater or lesser precision, depending on the characteristics of a kinship and numbers of testable members, by DNA analysis or by traditional genetics if the kinship is not informative. Recent techniques utilize polymerase chain reaction analysis of dystrophin following activation of myogenesis in amniocytes or chorionic villus cells (Sancho *et al.* 1993) or even single fetal nucleated erythrocytes from maternal blood (Sekizawa *et al.* 1996). Carrier detection by histochemical staining of dystrophin has been performed (Bonilla *et al.* 1988). Carriers demonstrate two populations of fibres, one with normal dystrophin staining, the other with irregular and weak staining. Even in the most favourable cases, however, the possibility of intragenic recombination and germline mosaicism, although rare, makes certainty unattainable in isolated cases (Gutmann and Fischbeck 1989).

No satisfactory treatment is currently available for DMD or other muscular dystrophies. However, management of DMD patients is essential for the prevention of deformities, especially scoliosis (Rideau *et al.* 1984). The use of orthoses (Rodillo *et al.* 1988) remains controversial but may prolong walking. Orthopaedic interventions should be used conservatively due to the risk of immobilization and should be combined with early mobilization and in many cases with the use of lightweight orthoses. In late stages, respiratory problems become prominent. The use of nocturnal oral intermittent positive pressure may be helpful (Bach *et al.* 1987).

Trials of corticosteroid administration have shown that prednisone produces a small but significant increase in muscle strength—greater with a dose of 0.75 mg/kg than with one of 0.3 mg/kg—reaching a maximum after three months and persisting thereafter (Griggs *et al.* 1993a). More importantly this therapy was associated with absence of further deterioration over the 18-month period of treatment, whereas deterioration was observed in the control group. Whether a long-term treatment with attendant side-effects is justified remains to be explored (Dubowitz 1991). Deflazocort has been claimed to produce similar benefits with fewer side-effects (Mesa *et al.* 1991). Cyclosporine may also be effective (Sharma *et al.* 1993). *Gene therapy* is being intensively studied but has not yet reached the stage of practical use (for a review, see Dubowitz 1995).

BECKER MUSCULAR DYSTROPHY (BMD)
GENETICS AND NOSOLOGY
The birth incidence of BMD is one-third that of DMD (5.4 *vs* 17.8 per 100,000) but the prevalence is about equal because of longer survival (Bushby and Gardner-Medwin 1993). This disorder is allelic to DMD and results from a deletion or other anomaly in the dystrophin gene which is responsible for the production of dystrophin of lower than normal molecular weight and/or of low amounts of dystrophin (Hoffman *et al.* 1988, 1989). DNA studies have indicated that deletions in the DMD gene are detectable in 90 per cent of cases and there is no good correlation between the size of the deletion when present and the severity of the disease, as some large deletions are compatible with a mild disease and the presence of dystrophin, while smaller deletions may be associated with DMD (Bushby and Gardner-Medwin 1993, Bushby *et al.* 1993, Comi *et al.* 1994). However, deletions of exons 45 to 52 are preferentially associated with a regular or benign course whereas heterogeneous DNA deletions are found in severe cases (Bushby *et al.* 1993). A tandem duplication has been found in association with severe disease (Gold *et al.* 1994). Deletions resulting in a BMD phenotype have been found to start within the same 1.5 kb region at the 5′ end of the gene and include a different number of exons (Medori *et al.* 1989). Deletions that result in a BMD phenotype may maintain an open reading frame but this is still conjectural (Gold *et al.* 1994).

In most cases, BMD is clearly distinct from DMD as to age of onset, severity and course. Whereas DMD patients are wheelchair-dependent by 13 years of age, BMD patients remain ambulatory beyond 13 years of age and often much later. Onset is between 5 and 10 years. However, intermediate forms are observed, in which patients become wheelchair-dependent between 13 and 16 years.

The nosological situation of these 'outliers' is uncertain (Dubowitz 1995). Most of them seem to have a deletion similar to that of BMD patients (Medori *et al.* 1989). Their dystrophin

level ranges between 3 and 10 per cent, while that of typical BMD is usually above 20 per cent (Hoffman *et al.* 1989).

CLINICAL FEATURES AND DIAGNOSIS
The onset of BMD is after 5 years of age and up to adolescence. Patients can walk at least to age 16 and often well into adulthood. Pseudohypertrophy is often present although less commonly than in DMD. Pes cavus is present in 60 per cent of cases. Tendon reflexes are usually retained but the ankle reflexes are often lost. Creatine kinase levels are as high as in DMD. Mental retardation is not present in definite cases, although it may exist in the 'outliers'. Cramps are a common symptom. The course is very variable. Atypical manifestations may include myalgia, myoglobinuria and, rarely, malignant hyperthermia, Achilles tendon contracture (Hoffman *et al.* 1989) and cardiomyopathy (Yazawa *et al.* 1987). Most patients are intellectually normal, although some cases—in particular those with deletions involving exons 48 and 49 (Bushby *et al.* 1993)—may show a relatively low IQ.

The diagnosis of classical types rests on clinical and EMG examination and on muscle biopsy. CT scanning of muscles may help distinguish BMD from unusual forms of benign spinal muscular atrophy (De Visser and Verbeeten 1985). Currently, dystrophin analysis is required for accurately distinguishing between severe BMD, DMD and some autosomal recessive myopathies (Gardner-Medwin and Sharples 1989).

The expression of BMD may be extremely variable. Mild forms include cases with only cramps on exercise (Mastaglia and Laing 1996), cases of exercise intolerance with myoglobinuria (Doriguzzi *et al.* 1993), and focal forms, especially limited to the quadriceps muscles (Sunohara *et al.* 1990). Cardiomyopathy is not rare (de Visser *et al.* 1992), and at least some cases of familial hypercreatine-kinasaemia are probably variants of BMD.

EMERY–DREIFUSS MUSCULAR DYSTROPHY
This is a rare X-linked muscle dystrophy characterized clinically by muscle weakness with humeroperoneal preponderance, joint contractures and cardiac involvement. However, these features tend to develop independently from one another so that the diagnosis can be difficult in young patients (Voit *et al.* 1988). Weakness predominates in the biceps, triceps and peroneal muscles. Flexion contractures at the elbows, Achilles tendon, neck and spine are a prominent early sign. Cardiac involvement is characterized by sinoatrial and atrioventricular conduction defects, impairment of impulse generation, increased atrial and ventricular heterotopia and functional impairment of the ventricular myocardium. As many as 40 per cent of Emery–Dreifuss patients die suddenly, often without preceding cardiac symptoms (Merlini *et al.* 1986). Early detection of arrhythmia with 24-hour Holter ECG is important as the provision of a cardiac pacemaker may be life-saving and considerably improve the prognosis. Carriers may also develop cardiac arrhythmias and may need a pacemaker. The earliest changes consist of first-degree block while complete heart block often develops later. Some patients may show evidence of nocturnal hypoventilation and may benefit from night-time ventilatory support.

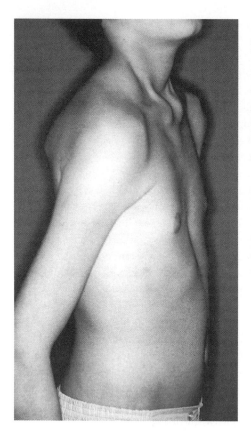

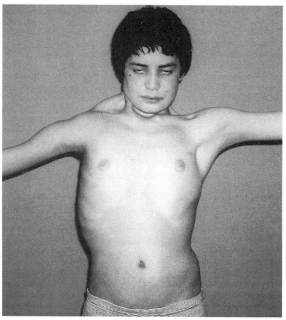

Fig. 22.3. Facioscapulohumeral dystrophy in a 13-year-old boy. *(Above)* Marked involvement of the scapular girdle, predominantly on right side. The eyes cannot be completely closed. *(Left)* Same patient, demonstrating atrophy of cervical muscles and amyotrophy of proximal arm with winged scapula. (Courtesy Dr F. Renault, Hôpital Trousseau, Paris.)

Creatine kinase levels are mildly elevated but may be in the normal range in patients with isolated initial cardiac involvement (Voit *et al.* 1988). Histological findings at muscle biopsy are nonspecific features.

Despite the homogeneity of the clinical picture, the genetic transmission of Emery–Dreifuss dystrophy indicates genetic heterogeneity (Petty *et al.* 1986). Most cases are transmitted as an X-linked character. The gene has been mapped to Xq28 and the gene product is a protein termed emerin. This is a nuclear membrane protein whose absence can be demonstrated in lymphocytes or by skin biopsy (Mora *et al.* 1997). Dominant transmission has been demonstrated in a few families (Fenichel *et al.* 1982, Miller *et al.* 1985). A few cases in girls are on record (Voit *et al.* 1988), and autosomal recessive inheritance has been postulated in one such case on the basis of parental consanguinity (Takamoto *et al.* 1984). However, the manifestation rate in heterozygotes may be as high as 50 per cent, so virtually any mode of transmission could be responsible for sporadic female cases. In *scapulohumeral syndrome with dementia*, also transmitted as an X-linked recessive disease, affected children, who are normal until age 5 years, develop first learning disability, then mental retardation, weakness, contractures and cardiomyopathy (Bergia *et al.* 1986).

The *rigid spine syndrome* shares several features with Emery–Dreifuss dystrophy. It occurs predominantly in boys, and muscle weakness is noticed at between a few months to 13 years of age (average 4 years). Spine rigidity in forward flexion is constant, and elbow and ankle contractures may also be present. A mild increase

of creatine kinase is usual and electromyography shows a myopathic pattern. Most cases are sporadic although rare cases in siblings are on record (Vanneste *et al.* 1988). Merlini *et al.* (1989) propose distinguishing the rigid spine sign which may be present in several types of myopathy, in particular Emery–Dreifuss myopathy, and the rigid spine syndrome which is an axial myopathy with a characteristic natural history leading to progressive scoliosis and often respiratory difficulties. There is no cardiac involvement (Van Munster *et al.* 1986).

FACIO-SCAPULO-HUMERAL DYSTROPHY (LANDOUZY–DÉJERINE) AND FACIO-SCAPULO-HUMERAL SYNDROMES

Progressive weakness and wasting with a facio-scapulo-humeral distribution is often due to a muscular dystrophy with autosomal dominant inheritance. New mutations are common, especially in early-onset forms (Jardine *et al.* 1994). However, similar involvement has also been reported in polymyositis, congenital myopathies and spinal muscular atrophy (Rothstein *et al.* 1971). From a clinical point of view, facio-scapulo-humeral dystrophy is not homogeneous. Many cases have their onset in late childhood and adolescence, and usually lead to disability only late in the course. Clinical presentation often varies within a single family, and minimally affected parents may have severely affected offspring.

In the usual, late-onset form, the initial symptoms are wasting of the shoulder girdle, winging of the scapulae, and facial affectation with inability to purse the lips and to close the eyes tightly, and weakness of the zygomatic muscle with a transverse smile. Involvement tends to be symmetrical (Fig. 22.3). Depending on the families and individuals, there may be more or less severe involvement of the biceps and triceps in the upper limbs and of the quadriceps and/or peroneal muscles in the lower extremities. Progression of the weakness is insidious and may be interrupted by periods of apparent arrest. Some patients are only mildly affected and may not be recognized as affected. In such forms, the life span is often normal (Gardner-Medwin 1980, Tawil *et al.* 1993). Onset may be early within some families (Bailey *et al.* 1986), and onset in infancy or early childhood with facial weakness has been observed. Bulbar dysfunction hypotonia, progressive proximal weakness and subsequent respiratory insufficiency may develop in some cases, thus precluding a favourable prognosis. Infantile forms are not genetically distinct from late-onset types, and the histological and EMG findings do not differ from classical cases. A definitive diagnosis may be difficult as the pathology is inconspicuous and atypical for a dystrophy and creatine kinase levels are normal in a substantial proportion of patients.

Facio-scapulo-humeral dystrophy has been described in association with hearing loss (Voit *et al.* 1986, Jardine *et al.* 1994), and with retinal Coats disease, sensorineural hearing loss and mental retardation (Taylor *et al.* 1982, Wulff *et al.* 1982, Matsuzaka *et al.* 1986). Such cases often have an early onset and a rapid progression (Yasukohchi *et al.* 1988).

Most cases appear to be linked to a locus on chromosome 4q35-ter. A number of closely linked markers enable accurate diagnosis in familial and sporadic cases (Upadhyaya *et al.* 1992, Griggs *et al.* 1993b, Lunt 1994) and open the way to prenatal diagnosis. However, genetic heterogeneity has been demonstrated in some pedigrees (Speer *et al.* 1992, Gilbert *et al.* 1993).

The *scapulohumeral muscular dystrophy* (or Erb dystrophy) is rare and probably related to Landouzy–Déjerine form. The *scapuloperoneal syndrome* includes cases of muscular dystrophy and neuropathies, and several modes of transmission are known to occur. Both X-linked and autosomal dominant transmission are possible (Thomas *et al.* 1972, Chakrabarti and Pearce 1981, Bergia *et al.* 1986). A cardiomyopathy is frequently associated. No linkage to 4q35 has been found (Tawill *et al.* 1995). A dominant form has recently been shown to be linked to chromosome 12 (Wilhelmsen *et al.* 1996).

LIMB–GIRDLE MUSCULAR DYSTROPHIES (LGMDs)
THE CONCEPT OF LIMB–GIRDLE MUSCULAR DYSTROPHY
The concept of LGMD originally applied to cases of muscle weakness mainly affecting the proximal muscles of limbs either in a pelvifemoral or in a scapulofemoral distribution (Gardner-Medwin 1980). The group in fact includes several unrelated muscle diseases, in particular manifesting carriers of DMD and BMD, benign cases of congenital muscular dystrophy, inflammatory disorders of muscle, and mild types of spinal atrophy. There are, however, authentic cases of autosomal muscular dystrophies with such presentation, and recent progress in molecular genetics has now helped establish several distinct conditions

within this group (Table 22.1). A complete investigation including EMG, muscular biopsy and specialized genetic techniques is necessary in such cases especially for genetic counselling purposes.

THE VARIOUS TYPES OF LGMD
Several types have been reported (Table 22.1). The discovery of dystrophin and of dystrophin-associated glycoproteins (sarcoglycans) has enabled a clear separation of such cases from the much more common X-linked muscular dystrophy (Gardner-Medwin and Sharples 1989).

Severe autosomal recessive muscular dystrophy of childhood (SCARD or LGMD type 2C)
This a well-defined type that appears to be prevalent in North Africa (Ben Hamida *et al.* 1983) but is also observed elsewhere. Onset is between 3 and 12 years of age. In the most severe cases children lose ambulation by 10–15 years of age, whereas less severe forms allow walking to be preserved to age 15–20 years. The disease is due to a selective loss of the 50 kDa dystrophin-associated glycoprotein adhalin (Fardeau *et al.* 1993) and maps to chromosome 13q12 (Azibi *et al.* 1993). However, adhalin is coded for by a different gene located on chromosome 17, so its deficiency in SCARD is a secondary phenomenon (Romero *et al.* 1994). In fact, some cases showed no linkage to 13q12 and showed mutations on the adhalin gene itself mapping at 17q12–q21.33. This latter type is termed LGMD type 2D (Roberds *et al.* 1994) and may vary considerably in severity (Eymard *et al.* 1997).

Other types of LGMD
Other autosomal recessive dystrophies have less severe manifestations. Affected patients of both sexes may have prominent toe-walking before difficulty in ambulation appears. The intelligence is normal as is the EEG (Gardner-Medwin and Sharples 1989). Molecular biology has enabled separation of subtypes (LGMD types 2A to 2E). Type 2A maps to 15q15–q21.1 (Beckmann *et al.* 1991, Fardeau *et al.* 1996), coding for the enzyme calpain 3; type 2B maps to 2q13–p16. These forms also involve the manufacture of dystrophin-associated glycoproteins or sarcoglycans that form a complex with dystrophin whose role seems to be to link the subsarcolemmal skeleton to the extracellular protein laminin (Matsumura and Campbell 1994). Still other types responsible for deficiency of sarcoglycans have not yet been mapped (Duggan *et al.* 1997).

Autosomal dominant limb–girdle dystrophies are usually of mild to moderate severity (Tohyama *et al.* 1994). A gene locus on chromosome 5q22–q24 has been identified (Yamaoka *et al.* 1994) and defines LGMD type 1A, but in other families with type 1B no gene has yet been localized. The condition is characterized by proximal weakness, greater in the legs than in the arms, and has usually a late onset in adulthood.

An early-onset form starting around 5 years of age, with slow progression and early flexion contractures of elbows, ankles and interphalangeal joints and without cardiac involvement and preservation of walking, has been described by Bethlem and van

TABLE 22.1
Main muscular dystrophies: genetic and molecular data*

Name (acronym)	Gene location	Gene product
X-linked dystrophies		
Dystrophinopathies	Xq21.2	Dystrophin
Duchenne muscular dystrophy (DMD)		
Becker muscular dystrophy (BMD)		
Quadriceps myopathy		
Myalgia and cramps		
Hypercreatine kinasaemia		
Emery–Dreiffus dystrophy (EMD)	Xq28	Emerin
Centronuclear myopathy	Xq28	?
Autosomal dominant dystrophies		
Facioscapulohumeral dystrophy (FSH)	4q3.5 (second type possible)	?
Limb–girdle dystrophies (LGMD)		
Dominant type 1A (LGMD 1A)	5q22–q34	?
Dominant type 1B (LGMD 1B)	?	?
Bethlem myopathy	?	?
Distal dominant dystrophies		
Welander type	14q	?
Autosomal recessive dystrophies		
Limb–girdle dystrophies (LGMD)		
Type 2A (LGMD 2A)	15q15–q21	Calpain 3
Type 2B (LGMD 2B)	2p13–p16	?
Type 2C (LGMD 2C) (severe childhood autosomal recessive dystrophy, SCARD)	13q12	γ-sarcoglycan
Type 2D (LGMD 2D)	17q12–q21.33	α-sarcoglycan (adhalin)
Type 2E (Amish)	4q12	β-sarcoglycan
Type 2F	5q33–q34	δ-sarcoglycan
Distal (Miyoshi) type	2p12–p14	?
Congenital dystrophies		
Fukuyama type	9q31–q33	?
Walker–Warburg syndrome (WW)	?	?
Muscle–eye–brain disease	?	?
Merosin-negative dystrophy (heterogeneous)	6q2	Merosin
Merosin-positive dystrophy	?	?

*Modified from Mastaglia and Laing (1996).

Wijngaarden and is known as 'Bethlem myopathy' (Merlini *et al.* 1994, Dubowitz 1995). Another type with cardiac involvement has been recently reported (van der Kooi *et al.* 1996).

Cole *et al.* (1988) have described an apparently recessive muscular dystrophy with onset in early childhood, slowly progressive course, filamentous bodies similar to those in inclusion body myositis, and a leukoencephalopathy demonstrated by markedly abnormal appearance of the white matter on CT scan and MRI. These patients had no evidence of CNS dysfunction.

The differential diagnosis of LGMD includes atypical forms of DMD, symptomatic DMD carriers, congenital myopathies, metabolic myopathies and spinal muscular atrophy, all of which can present with similarly distributed weakness. Muscle biopsy and dystrophin studies will settle the issue. Rare cases of myositis can also produce a limb–girdle syndrome. Dalakas and Engel (1987) reported a child with apparent LGMD who responded dramatically to steroids despite the absence of inflammatory signs at biopsy. A trial of prednisone might be worth conducting in some atypical cases.

DISTAL MUSCULAR DYSTROPHIES

These disorders are quite rare and are mainly encountered in adults. Cases of distal dystrophy with onset in late adolescence or early childhood have been reported.

A *dominant type* linked to chromosome 14q is observed in adults. Rare cases in children (Bautista *et al.* 1978, Kinoshita *et al.* 1995) may belong to a different entity.

Recessive distal muscular dystrophy (Miyoshi type) has its onset in adolescence or early adulthood and runs a progressive course (Miyoshi *et al.* 1986). Creatine kinase levels are grossly elevated, and muscle biopsy shows clear evidence of dystrophy. Linkage to 2p12–14 has been established.

Another recessive form (Nonaka *et al.* 1981a) is characterized pathologically by fibre atrophy and rimmed vacuoles, and a form with filamentous inclusions (Matsubara and Tanabe 1982) is on record.

OCULAR MUSCULAR DYSTROPHY

Involvement of the eye muscles is a manifestation of various types of dystrophy. It is especially common with mitochondrial myopathies, although cases without morphological abnormalities of the mitochondria are not uncommon. Even in such cases, however, abnormalities of mitochondrial DNA have often been found.

Ophthalmoplegia may rarely be a feature of congenital myopathy (Riggs *et al.* 1989a).

CONGENITAL MUSCULAR DYSTROPHY

The term congenital muscular dystrophy is used to describe a group of disorders in infants characterized by muscle weakness, usually associated with hypotonia from birth, with muscle showing pathological changes reminiscent of those of muscular dystrophy in older patients (Dubowitz 1995). The condition is clearly heterogeneous, varying with regard to severity, associated manifestations and outcome. Some cases are associated with brain abnormalities. In a few cases, the absence of dystrophin in muscle has been demonstrated, indicating that congenital onset can occur with DMD (Mendell *et al.* 1990).

In typical cases, weakness is predominantly proximal and slowly progressive. A great variability is evident in most reports (Donner *et al.* 1975, McMenamin *et al.* 1982, Echenne *et al.* 1986, Leyten *et al.* 1989), and some authors have separated severe and benign forms of congenital dystrophy (Zellweger *et al.* 1967a,b). In most cases the inheritance seems to be autosomal recessive. Dominant inheritance has also been rarely reported. The extraocular muscles are spared. Tendon reflexes are usually abolished and fixed joint deformities are frequent.

The course is usually static or slowly progressive, and contractures tend to become more extensive. Involvement of respiratory muscles, especially the diaphragm, is not rare and may be responsible for respiratory complications and death.

The diagnosis rests on clinical findings, creatine kinase determinations that usually indicate a moderate increase, and muscle biopsy that shows a variable picture from severe muscle destruction with fat replacement to minimal changes (Dubowitz 1995).

The congenital dystrophies can be classified into two major groups: those with obvious involvement of the CNS and those without, usually termed 'classical forms'.

CONGENITAL DYSTROPHIES WITH CNS INVOLVEMENT

Fukuyama-Type Congenital Muscular Dystrophy

Fukuyama-type congenital muscular dystrophy was the first clearly individualized entity in this group. It is transmitted as an autosomal recessive trait (Fukuyama and Osawa 1984) and the gene has been mapped to chromosome 9q31–33 (Toda *et al.* 1993). Pathologically, there is extensive muscle necrosis. The brain demonstrates abnormalities of gyration such as pachygyria or microgyria and severe cortical disorganization (Takada *et al.* 1984, Takashima *et al.* 1987). Clinical features include severe neonatal hypotonia, marked facial involvement, the presence of contractures and severe mental retardation often associated with epilepsy. CT and MRI scans show extensive lucencies of the white matter and migration abnormalities with a thick, poorly sulcated cortex (Yoshioka *et al.* 1986). Creatine kinase levels are high. The outcome is poor, death usually occurring in the second decade. Prenatal diagnosis is possible by linkage analysis in informative families.

Other Congenital Dystrophies with CNS Involvement

The *Walker–Warburg syndrome*, described in Chapter 3, features a severe muscle dystrophy in virtually all cases. The disorder may be genetically identical to Fukuyama-type congenital dystrophy (Toda et el 1995).

Muscle–eye–brain disease, originally reported from Finland, features major eye abnormalities (visual failure, glaucoma, myopia of > 6 dioptres) and a grossly abnormal brain with hydrocephalus and abnormal gyration. Its nosological situation vis-à-vis Fukuyama-type congenital dystrophy and mucle–eye–brain disease is unclear. Ranta *et al.* (1995) adduced evidence that it is not allelic to Fukuyama dystrophy. The disease is present at birth but is apparently progressive as shown by the flattening of the EEG after infancy. Flash-evoked potentials are of high amplitude in three-quarters of patients (Santavuori *et al.* 1989).

Marinesco–Sjögren syndrome (Chapter 10) is usually marked in its later stages by a peculiar muscle disease (Zimmer *et al.* 1992).

'CLASSICAL' CONGENITAL MUSCULAR DYSTROPHIES

In this group, there are no specific brain malformations and no characteristic neurological symptoms or signs. However, it has been apparent for some time that neurodevelopmental abnormalities are present in some of these cases and that abnormal lucencies in the white matter are not uncommon. The nosological situation has been considerably clarified by the discovery that the phenotype is correlated with the expression of merosin (or laminin-M) in skeletal muscles. Merosin is an extrasarcolemmal protein which links with dystrophin through glycoproteins (Matsumura and Campbell 1994) and is probably essential in the stabilization of cell membrane.

Merosin-Negative Congenital Dystrophy

This form is characterized by the absence of merosin expression in muscle. The clinical features are fairly homogeneous with hypotonia, severe weakness and early development of contractures. Weakness frequently involves facial muscles. Creatine kinase levels are markedly elevated in the first year of life. Mental retardation is usually severe and epilepsy is common. MR imaging shows extensive areas of low T_1 and high T_2 signal from hemispheral white matter (Topaloglu *et al.* 1995, North *et al.* 1996,

TABLE 22.2
Main congenital myopathies

Myopathy	Suggestive clinical features	Histology	References
Central core	Skeletal deformities	Type 1 preponderance cores (see text)	See text
Nemaline	Several types (see text)	Type 1 preponderance rod-like structures	See text
Congenital fibre type disproportion	Variable	Type 1 preponderance Type 1 hypotrophy	See text
Centronuclear	Variable (see text)	Type 1 preponderance Central nuclei	See text
Multicore (minicore)	Nonprogressive weakness, neck weakness	Multiple areas devoid of enzyme activity	Paljärvi et al. (1987)
Zebra-body	None	Zebra bodies on electron microscopy	Reyes et al. (1987)
Fingerprint	Tremor, weakness, mental retardation	Sarcolemmic inclusions	Fardeau et al. (1976)
Reducing body	None	Inclusion rich in sulfhydril groups and RNA	Kiyomoto et al. (1995)
Cytoplasmic body (spheroid body)	Heterogeneous; severe infantile forms; severe late cases	Type 1 predominance Subsarcolemmal inclusions	Mizuno et al. (1989), Chapon et al. (1989)
Sarcotubular	None	Dilated and fragmented tubules in type II fibres	
Tubular aggregates	Cramps, muscle pain, weakness	Tubular arrays in subsarcolemmic region	Pierobon-Bormioli et al. (1985), Orimo et al. (1987)
Trilaminar	Neonatal rigidity; decreasing with age	3-zone fibres	Ringel et al. (1978)
Specific type 1 hypertrophy	Ptosis, myopathic facies	Elective type 1 hypertrophy	Young and Anderson (1987)
Cylindrical spiral	Cramp, myotonia	Cylindrical spiral formations	Bove et al. (1980)
Uniform type 1 fibres	Nonprogressive	No fibre type differentiation	Pellegrini et al. (1985)
Autophagic vacuoles	X-linked; cardiomyopathy + mental retardation	Increased number of autophagic vacuoles	Kalimo et al. (1988), Hart et al. (1987)
Minimal change	Variable	Limited abnormalities, nonspecific	Dubowitz (1995)

Reed et al. 1996). Evoked potentials are delayed and decreased (Mercuri et al. 1995). The presence of cortical migration abnormalites has been recently reported in three European patients (Pini et al. 1996).

MEROSIN-POSITIVE CONGENITAL DYSTROPHY
This form is also known as 'occidental' type congenital dystrophy. It is usually of lesser severity than merosin-negative type and not associated with clinical evidence of CNS involvement. Of 50 patients studied by Kobayashi et al. (1996), 46 were able to walk and all but two had a normal IQ. This group is probably heterogeneous with some severe cases (Topaloglu et al. 1994). Areas of white matter lucency are present in some cases. Occasional patients suffer severe CNS abnormalties (De Stefano et al. 1996). The cases of 'occidental' congenital muscular dystrophy with lucency of the white matter on MRI (Echenne et al. 1986) or various CNS brain malformations (Krijgsman et al. 1980, Korithenberg et al. 1984, Peters et al. 1984) are difficult to classify and probably represent a heterogeneous group. MRI studies show that cortical dysplasia is associated with abnormal signal from white matter (low in T_1- and high in T_2-weighted sequences) in cases of Walker–Warburg syndrome and muscle–eye–brain disease but not in merosin-negative congenital dystrophy (van der Knaap et al. 1997). Abnormal white matter signal is rarely present in merosin-positive cases. In some children, abnormal signal from the white matter is associated with occipital agyria and hypoplasia of the pons and vermis, and these may constitute a new syndrome.

RARE TYPES OF CONGENITAL DYSTROPHY
ULLRICH CONGENITAL MUSCULAR DYSTROPHY
This rare autosomal recessive disorder is characterized by proximal joint contractures, distal hyperextensibility, normal intelligence, normal deep tendon reflexes, hyperhidrosis and minor dysmorphism (Nonaka et al. 1981b, de Paillette et al. 1989). Death due to respiratory failure may occur.

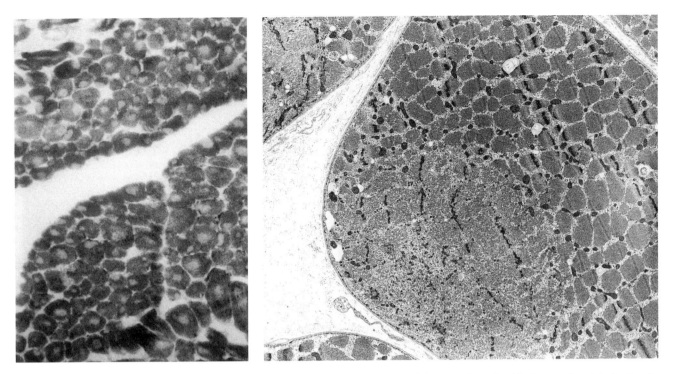

Fig. 22.4. Central core myopathy. *(Left)* Note uniformity of fibre type (type 1) and presence of clear central area devoid of enzymatic activity in virtually all fibres (NADH ×150). *(Right)* Electron microscopy shows that the 'core' region (which is lateral rather than central in this particular fibre) is devoid of normal muscle fibrils and of mitochondria and shows disorganization of myofilaments (×23,000). (Courtesy Drs M-C. Routon and O. Robain, Hôpital Saint Vincent de Paul, Paris.)

CONGENITAL MYOPATHIES

Congenital myopathies are disorders characterized clinically by hypotonia and weakness from birth and by morphological changes on histological and/or electron microscopic examination. Signs of muscle dystrophy are not present and creatine kinase levels are normal or only mildly elevated. The morphological changes are not specific for any congenital myopathy and type identification may sometimes remain tentative. Although congenital myopathies of all grades of severity exist, they are often relatively mild and responsible for a significant proportion of the cases of otherwise unexplained *benign congenital hypotonia* (Brooke *et al.* 1979) The congenital myopathies, in general, should be distinguished from the Prader–Willi syndrome (Chapter 5) which presents in the neonatal period with marked hypotonia and features suggestive of a myopathy, and from hereditary diseases of the collagen that may present with massive hypotonia and hyperextensibility (Wenstrup *et al.* 1989) in early infancy or later childhood. There is also an overlap clinically between the congenital myopathies and some metabolic myopathies (mitochondrial or lipid storage myopathies) which may also present as a 'floppy infant' syndrome or as neuromuscular diseases. A list of the congenital myopathies appears in Table 22.2.

CENTRAL CORE DISEASE
Central core disease was the first congenital myopathy to be described. It is a rare disease with autosomal dominantly inherited

and sporadic cases (Byrne *et al.* 1982). It is linked to chromosome 19q13.1, as is malignant hyperthermia, and it is likely that the two conditions may be different expressions of the same gene. The gene appears to be allelic with the ryanodine receptors gene which has also been implicated in malignant hyperthermia (Mulley *et al.* 1993). However, discrepant families have been reported. The disorder is characterized pathologically by central areas within fibres which are devoid of the normal histochemical reactions for oxidative enzymes, myophosphorylase and glycogen. Ultrastructurally, the cores consist of closely packed myofibrils with loss of the intermyofibrillary spaces and of mitochondria, cytoplasmic reticulum and glycogen; almost all fibres are type I (Fig. 22.4).

The clinical features are hypotonia from birth or early infancy, proximal weakness, mild facial weakness in some cases, and depressed or absent deep tendon reflexes. Congenital hip dislocation, pes cavus and kyphoscoliosis are frequently present. Although the condition is usually nonprogressive and compatible with a normal lifespan, some children become progressively weaker with marked deformities and involvement of the respiratory muscles which can lead to early death. Central core disease is one of the myopathies associated with susceptibility to malignant hyperthermia so that extreme care is in order when surgery is contemplated for such patients and for patients directly related to known cases. The diagnosis rests on muscle biopsy. The creatine kinase level is usually normal. No treatment is available.

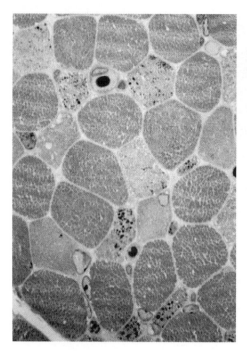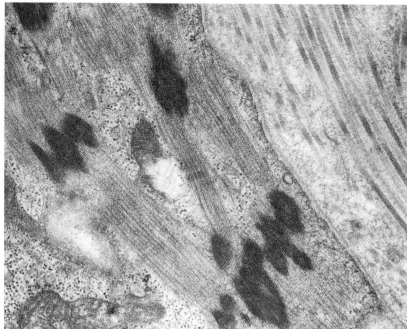

Fig. 22.5. Nemaline myopathy. *(Left)* Severe neonatal form. Semi-thin section stained with toluidine blue. Rod-like structures are visible in numerous, generally atrophic, angular fibres. *(Right)* Childhood form, electron microscopy (×47,000). Eosinophilic structures are made of Z-band protein irregularly organized. (Courtesy Dr M-C. Routon, Hôpital Saint Vincent de Paul, Paris.)

NEMALINE MYOPATHY

Nemaline myopathy is transmitted as an autosomal dominant trait in rare cases and, more commonly, as a recessive trait. Many cases appear sporadic (Dubowitz 1995). In dominant cases penetrance is variable as is expressivity, and some affected individuals are almost normal with only poorly developed muscles. A gene for the dominant form (*NEM1*) has been mapped to chromosome 1q21–q23, but the locus for the recessive type has not yet been located.

Histologically, multiple small rod-like particles, thought to represent Z-band proteins, are present within most if not all muscle fibres (Fig. 22.5). Even though such structures are non-specific as they can be oberved in cases of myositis, they are rarely of similar abundance, and type I fibre predominance is present in cases of nemaline myopathy but not in the other conditions. Type 2B fibre deficiency is also found (Shimomura and Nonaka 1989).

There are three main clinical presentations (Martinez and Lake 1987, Shimomura and Nonaka 1989). In the *severe neonatal form*, severe hypotonia and weakness, breathing difficulties, myopathic facies, high-arched palate and depressed deep reflexes are present from birth, with early death of almost all affected infants (Schmalbruch *et al.* 1987a).

In the *moderate congenital form*, there is mild to moderate hypotonia and weakness in the neonatal period. Motor delay, swallowing and feeding problems, neck hypotonia and frequent respiratory infections may occur later, and contractures often develop. These children are usually able to walk although with variable difficulties and easy fatiguability. The outlook for survival is usually favourable although respiratory problems may arise and sudden death occur. It is important to detect nocturnal hypoventilation as nasal mask ventilation is then indicated. Cardiac involvement is possible (Ishibashi-Ueda *et al.* 1990).

In the *mild form*, muscle function is relatively preserved but muscle bulk is poor.

The diagnosis is by muscle biopsy.

CONGENITAL FIBRE-TYPE DISPROPORTION MYOPATHY

This term applies to congenital myopathies in which biopsies demonstrate an excessive disparity of size between type 1 and type 2 fibres in the absence of other obvious histological abnormalities. In some cases, type 2 hypertrophy is associated, but type 1 hypotrophy and type 1 predominance are the main anomalies. This condition may be a common type of congenital myopathy. The inheritance may be autosomal dominant but there may be marked variation in clinical expression and age of onset, some cases presenting only in childhood or even in adulthood, but recessive heredity has also been reported. Many sporadic cases are on record.

The clinical features are similar to those in other congenital myopathies with proximal weakness and diffuse hypotonia. Facial weakness and ptosis may be present. Skeletal deformities frequently develop. A high degree of clinical variability is encountered with some patients having only mild hypotonia, while others may be severely affected (Clancy *et al.* 1980). In most cases, the course is stationary and some improvement is frequent after the end of infancy.

The diagnosis requires muscle biopsy. Cases of fibre disproportion should not be confused with simple type 2 fibre hypertrophy or hypotrophy which can be observed in many situations. Both type 1 predominance and type 1 fibre hypotrophy are necessary criteria. In some cases neurogenic EMG features and some grouping of atrophic fibres may pose problems in the differential diagnosis with neurogenic conditions (Sulaiman *et al.* 1983). The disease may not be totally distinct from other forms of congenital myopathy.

MYOTUBULAR MYOPATHY (CENTRONUCLEAR MYOPATHY)

Several disorders produce a histological picture of type 1 fibre predominance and centrally located nuclei with or without fibre hypotrophy (Heckmatt *et al.* 1985). The term 'myotubular' probably applies only to the X-linked neonatal form. In other cases, the term is inaccurate because muscle fibres in centronuclear myopathy show differentiation into two types and are different from immature myotubes.

The *X-linked neonatal form* is characterized by marked diffuse hypotonia with rapid respiratory failure which usually leads to death in early infancy (Barth *et al.* 1975). The onset is intrauterine with decreased fetal movements and polyhydramnios; sucking difficulties are present, and ptosis and ophthalmoplegia are frequently found. Creatine kinase levels are normal, and the EMG is uncharacteristic as both myogenic and neurogenic features may be found. This form is linked to Xq28, and prenatal diagnosis using DNA markers is possible (Liechti-Gallati *et al.* 1993). Some carriers may demonstrate muscle histological abnormalities.

The chronic types of *centronuclear myopathy* may be sporadic or transmitted by autosomal dominant or autosomal recessive inheritance, and their clinical presentation is also variable (De Angelis *et al.* 1991). The onset may be at any age from birth to adulthood. Ophthalmoplegia is often a feature but usually is not present at birth. Facial involvement is frequent, and mental retardation and convulsions are sometimes observed in recessive and sporadic forms. The course is highly variable (Reske-Nielsen *et al.* 1987).

The diagnosis is by muscle biopsy. In most cases, creatine kinase levels are normal or mildly elevated. The EMG is myogenic or nonspecific. There is often deficiency of type 2B fibres (Sasaki *et al.* 1989). The heterogeneity of centronuclear myopathy is further confirmed by the presence of different types of myosin in different forms (Sawchak *et al.* 1991).

OTHER CONGENITAL MYOPATHIES

A large number of congenital myopathies have been reported. Most of them are rare diseases. They are shown in Table 22.2.

The clinical features of these diseases include mostly hypotonia with variable degrees of weakness. In some cases, suggestive features are present. Trilaminar myopathy and myopathy with tubular aggregates are mainly manifested by muscle rigidity, myalgia or cramps. They are considered in the next section.

MYOTONIC DISEASES AND RELATED CONDITIONS

Myotonia designates a disturbance in muscle relaxation following contraction of voluntary muscles (decontraction myotonia) and a slow, tonic response to mechanical and electrical stimulation. Myotonia is characterized, electromyographically, by repetitive response of motor units producing the classical 'dive bomber' aspect (crescendo–decrescendo). Myotonia is related to instability of the muscle cell membrane and is purely of muscular origin.

Myotonia is a nonspecific abnormality that belongs to several genetic diseases and syndromes.

Many of the diseases that feature myotonia have been recently recognized to be caused by mutations in the genes that clone for ion channels. However, the same phenomena can occur without ion channel anomalies as in myotonic dystrophy, the most common myotonic disorder.

I shall include in this section disorders characterized by other forms of abnormal muscle contractions even though their mechanism may be completely different from that of 'channelopathies' (ion channel disorders) because of clinical resemblances.

MYOTONIC DYSTROPHY (DYSTROPHIA MYOTONICA, STEINERT DISEASE)

Myotonic dystrophy is a relatively common disease with an incidence of 13.5 per 100,000 live births. It is transmitted as an autosomal dominant trait and is characterized by the association of myotonia with a dystrophic process of muscles and with various endocrine and other systemic abnormalities. The onset of symptoms is usually in adolescence or adulthood, and in such cases the disease is transmitted slightly more often by fathers than by mothers. In contrast, in neonatal forms the inheritance is virtually always from the mother (Harper 1975b), although an occasional paternal transmission can occur (Nakagawa *et al.* 1994, Ohya *et al.* 1994), and the disease is of great severity and often lethal in infancy. Neonatal forms occur in kindreds in which a regular transmission through either parent had occurred in preceding generations (Aicardi *et al.* 1974). The basic molecular abnormality is the presence of an expansion of a CTG triplet repeat, associated with the gene for myotonin protein kinase. As is usual with disorders associated with DNA expansion, anticipation and sex bias in genetic transmission are observed in this disease. The length of the repeat usually increases in successive generations, especially when maternally transmitted. There is a good correlation between the length of the expansion and the clinical severity and age of onset, the longer repeats being associated with congenital forms (Jaspert *et al.* 1995, Takahashi *et al.* 1996).

CLINICAL FEATURES OF THE CLASSICAL FORM
The clinical presentation of myotonic dystrophy is variable. Some patients have severe generalized myotonia with few dystrophic features that develop late in life, while in others atrophy and weakness are prominent. Both varieties may occur in the same kindred (Aicardi *et al.* 1974). Myotonia is demonstrated by

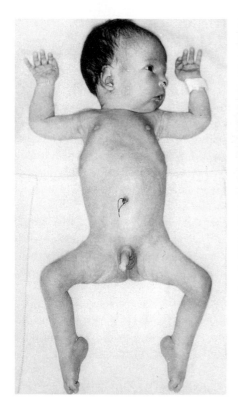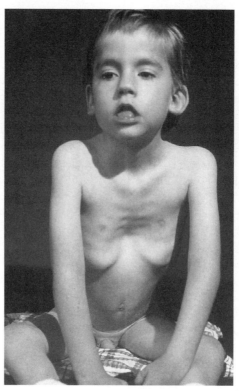

Fig. 22.6. Dystrophia myotonica (Steinert disease). *(Left)* Neonatal form. Note equinovarus feet. *(Right)* Child with neonatal onset of mild form. Note tent-shaped upper lip, open mouth, mild ptosis and pectus excavatum. (Courtesy Dr F. Renault, Hôpital Trousseau, Paris.)

percussion of muscle, *e.g.* the thenar eminence or tongue, the thumb remaining opposed, the tongue being dimpled for several seconds after percussion of its side. Relaxation myotonia is demonstrated by shaking hands with the patient: release of grip is performed by forcing the flexors of the fingers open by flexion of the wrist.

The distribution of muscular atrophy and weakness is characteristic. Atrophy begins in the face—especially the masseters and temporal muscles, giving all the patients a similar appearance with a long, thin face and hollowed temporal fossae—and in the sternomastoid muscles. The shoulder girdle is then involved and, characteristically, the brachioradialis and the muscles of the anterior compartment of the leg are also wasted. In some patients, there is only minimal weakness, even in the presence of visible atrophy, but when it is present before 20 years of age it is likely to be relentlessly progressive, severe distal weakness being present by middle adult life. Smooth muscle involvement may be present with decreased gastrointestinal motility, and constipation is a well-recognized feature. In adult patients baldness, testicular atrophy, hyperinsulinism and disturbances in growth hormone secretion may occur. Peripheral nerve involvement has been reported in several cases and an occasional patient may have an association of motor and sensory conduction neuropathy with myotonic dystrophy (Spaans *et al.* 1986). About half the patients have abnormal ECG, arrhythmias or other cardiac disturbances (Morgenlander *et al.* 1993).

Posterior cataracts are not seen before 8–10 years of age, even by slit-lamp examination, but occur later and may be the first and occasionally the presenting feature of the disease.

Intellectual impairment is rare in patients with the adult form of myotonic dystrophy and seems to be correlated to the presence of morphological CNS abnormalities (Glantz *et al.* 1988, Huber *et al.* 1989, Hashimoto *et al.* 1995).

CLINICAL FEATURES OF THE CONGENITAL FORM
The congenital form of the disease has a completely different presentation (Harper 1975a,b; A.T.M. Hageman *et al.* 1993; Roig *et al.* 1994). The onset is prenatal; hydramnios is present in about half the cases. Birth is often by breech delivery and the infant may be small for gestational age. Arthrogryposis is common (Harper 1975a,b). Hypotonia, weakness and facial diplegia are the most striking features (Fig. 22.6). Respiratory insufficiency due to diaphragmatic and intercostal muscle involvement occurs in about half the patients and usually leads to an early death. Myotonia is never observed even by EMG before 3–4 years of age, often much later. In less severely affected patients who survive the neonatal period, mental impairment is present in almost all cases. Ventricular dilatation may be a common correlate of mental retardation and of the macrocephaly which is sometimes found (Regev *et al.* 1987). Severe and relatively mild forms of congenital myotonic dystrophy may occur in the same sibship (Aicardi *et al.* 1974).

DIAGNOSIS AND TREATMENT

The diagnosis of the classical form of myotonic dystrophy is usually easy, and EMG examination helps to confirm the diagnosis (Jamal *et al.* 1986). In infants, the differential diagnosis is more difficult although the overall appearance of the infant, especially the facial involvement and the presence of pes equinus, is suggestive. Patients with congenital myopathies and congenital dystrophies may look very similar to those with myotonic dystrophy. Examination of the mothers, especially for myotonia, is the best diagnostic clue, although an occasional mother may have no myotonia, even by EMG, until months or years after the birth of an affected infant (personal cases). Of 20 or so congenital cases I have seen, the disease in the mother was undiagnosed at the time of birth of the infant in over half of the cases.

Presymptomatic and prenatal diagnosis is based on detection of an increase in repeat length (Harley *et al.* 1992, Shelbourne *et al.* 1993) and can be performed on chorionic villus samples thus enabling an early diagnosis to be made. The risk of a congenital form for women with known disease is at least 10 per cent and increases with multisystem maternal involvement. It reaches 20–40 per cent after birth of an affected child (Koch *et al.* 1991).

Rare cases of apparent myotonic dystrophy without trinucleotide repeat expansion have been reported in adults (Thornton *et al.* 1994). Such cases have been shown not to be linked to the gene of myotonic dystrophy or to those of Na and K channels associated with other myotonic disorders. They tend to be relatively benign (Moxley 1997) and are currently termed proximal myotonic dystrophy. The clinical presentation is also unusual with exclusively proximal weakness, muscle pain and hypertrophy (Ricker *et al.* 1995).

Treatment is of limited indication as myotonia is rarely severe enough to justify the use of procaine amide, quinine or steroids. Nifedipine may be useful in some patients (Grant *et al.* 1987).

ION CHANNEL DISORDERS

These are listed in Table 22.3. Although myasthenia gravis and related diseases are part of this group, they are described later as their clinical features are very different.

CHLORIDE CHANNEL DISEASE: MYOTONIA CONGENITA

Myotonia congenita is a genetic disorder, transmitted as either a dominant or autosomal recessive trait and also often occurring sporadically (Kuhn *et al.* 1979). It is characterized by myotonia and muscle hypertrophy. Both the dominant and the recessive forms are caused by mutations in the same chloride channel gene (*CLCN1*) on chromosome 7q, although the mutations are different (Koch *et al.* 1992; Ptácek *et al.* 1993, 1994b).

The *clinical presentation* varies from case to case from mild myotonia, which may not be known to the patient even in adulthood, to severe stiffness that severely interferes with everyday life. In general the *autosomal dominant form* (Thomsen disease) is more benign than the recessive type. The disorder is often present from birth or infancy. After rest, muscles are stiff and movement is difficult to initiate. The stiffness disappears with activity, and movement may become normal. Many patients have generalized

TABLE 22.3
Ion channel disorders involving muscle function

Disorder	Genetics
Chloride channel disorders	
Thomson myotonia congenita	AD[1]
Becker myotonia congenita	AR[1]
Sodium channel disorders[2]	
Hyperkalaemic periodic paralysis	AD
Paramyotonia congenita	AD
Myotonia fluctuans (K-sensitive)	AD
Calcium channel disorders	
Hypokalaemic periodic paralysis	AD
Acetylcholine receptor	
Myasthenia gravis	S, AR[3]
Imperfectly characterized disorders	
Malignant hyperthermia (some cases involve the ryanodine receptor)	AD?[4]
Lambert–Eaton syndrome (probably involves Ca channel)	S
Neuromyotonia[5]	—

[1]Different mutations in same channel.
[2]Multiple mutations known.
[3]Congenital cases usually genetically transmitted.
[4]Heterogeneous group.
[5]Acquired K channel disorder.

muscle hypertrophy as a consequence of continuous muscle contraction. Stiffness is painless and increased by exposure to cold.

The *recessive form* (Becker disease) (Sun and Streib 1983) begins between 3 and 12 years of age. Muscle stiffness is prominent and always associated with weakness, and distal atrophy may coexist with hypertrophy. The disease is often progressive to age 30.

The *diagnosis* is established clinically and confirmed by EMG, which records repetitive discharges when the needle is inserted in the muscle and on voluntary contraction. Muscle biopsy is rarely necessary. It shows the absence of type 2B fibres (Heine 1986).

Malignant hyperthermia may occur in patients with myotonia congenita (Heiman-Patterson *et al.* 1988).

Unusual forms with mental retardation (Richieri-Costa *et al.* 1981) or with painful stiffness precipitated by fasting or potassium administration (Trudell *et al.* 1987) have been reported in single families.

Treatment, when justified, may be with carbamazepine or phenytoin in usual anticonvulsant dosage. In the family reported by Trudell *et al.*, a dramatic response was obtained with acetazolamide.

SODIUM CHANNEL DISEASES

Three disorders are due to various mutations in the sodium channel gene (*SCN4A* gene on chromosome 17q) and variably produce myotonia, weakness or a mixture of both (Hudson *et al.* 1995).

Paramyotonia congenita (Eulenburg disease)

In this disease, which is dominantly inherited, myotonia is present from infancy and involves especially the eyelids, facial muscles and hand muscles, and sometimes the pharyngeal muscles. The myotonia may paradoxically be augmented by exercise and is very sensitive to cold (Johnsen and Friis 1980). Many patients also experience episodes of weakness and may develop muscular atrophy. Weakness is of two types: generalized attacks of weakness that can be brought on by cold; and localized weakness that is also precipitated by cold but may also occur in hot surroundings, provoked by exercise alone. This second type, when brought on by cold, may persist for hours after rewarming (Haas *et al.* 1981). The condition is also associated pathologically with absence of type 2B fibres (Heine 1986). The responsible mutation has been studied in great detail (Lerche *et al.* 1996).

Hyperkalaemic periodic paralysis (adynamia episodica hereditaria)

This disorder may occur at an early age, even in infancy. Attacks are often triggered by moderate exercise and are often brief and frequently repeated, sometimes several times daily. Severe attacks, however, resemble those in the hypokalaemic form and may last several hours. Some patients can delay the paralysis by walking or moving about. Myotonia of a mild degree is often associated with the weakness and may not be increased by exposure to cold (Subramony *et al.* 1986). It is especially well shown in the eyelids. Cardiac dysrhythmia has been reported (Baquero *et al.* 1995) and may be due to a different sodium channel mutation.

The diagnosis may be confirmed by demonstration of ECG changes such as peaked T waves and the finding of elevated potassium concentration, although many children have concentrations still within the normal range, and by direct DNA study (Feero *et al.* 1993). Oral administration of 2–5 g potassium chloride after exercise may provoke an attack.

Treatment of attacks is required only in severe cases and includes administration of 2 g/kg glucose and 10–20 units of insulin subcutaneously. Prevention is by avoidance of cold and by administration of acetazolamide if the attacks are frequent.

Myotonia fluctuans (potassium-aggravated myotonia)

This rare condition resembles Thomson disease but the myotonia is aggravated by potassium intake. Muscle weakness is not a significant feature (Heine *et al.* 1993, Ricker *et al.* 1994).

Sodium channel myotonia

This fourth sodium channel disorder has been recently reported (Moxley 1997). It may respond to acetazolamide and/or mexiletin.

CALCIUM CHANNEL DISEASE: HYPOKALAEMIC PERIODIC PARALYSIS

This dominant disorder is caused by a mutation in the dihydro-pyridine receptor, a subunit of the DHP-sensitive calcium channel, whose gene maps to 1q31–32 (Ptácek *et al.* 1994a).

It has its onset between 5 and 16 years of age in 60 per cent of the cases. Attacks of paralysis are at first infrequent and are often precipitated by meals rich in carbohydrate or by exercise following rest and thus commonly occur in the early morning.

Exposure to cold may also be a trigger. The intensity and extent of weakness are very variable. In some patients, only the proximal limb muscles are affected while others have diffuse paralysis. However, facial muscles are rarely affected and extraocular and respiratory muscles are not involved. Most attacks last from four to six hours and some for a whole day or more. In severe cases, tendon reflexes are absent and muscles can be swollen. Frequent repetition of the attacks may leave permanent residual weakness which is not observed in the paediatric age range. In such cases vacuolization of muscle fibres is present histologically, together with centralization of nuclei and unequal fibre diameter.

The attacks tend initially to increase in frequency, then decrease after 25–30 years and may even disappear.

The diagnosis rests on the characteristics of paralysis and the family history. Potassium concentration during attacks may be as low as 1.5 mmol/L but is often only slightly lowered. ECG changes are present, including bradycardia, prolonged P-R and Q-T intervals and flattening of T waves. Attacks can be provoked by oral administration of 2 g/kg of glucose with 10–20 units of insulin subcutaneously. Hypokalaemia and weakness usually results within two or three hours. A negative test does not exclude the diagnosis. The adrenalin test (2 μg/min by intraarterial route for five minutes) is positive if the action potential simultaneously recorded in a hand muscle is decreased by more than 30 per cent 10 minutes after injection.

Treatment of acute attacks in patients with normal renal function is by oral potassium chloride administration, 5–10 g per dose, which may be repeated. Prevention of attacks may be achieved by a low sodium regimen and supplementation in potassium. Acetazolamide is beneficial in many families (Links *et al.* 1988).

OTHER PRIMARY PERIODIC PARALYSES

Normokalaemic periodic paralysis has been observed in several families. The features are not different from those in other forms. During attacks, there is an increase in natriuresis and a decrease in kaliuresis but no detectable change in potassium concentration in blood. The nosological situation of these rare cases is unclear.

Periodic paralysis with disturbances in cardiac rhythm and dysmorphism (Andersen syndrome) has been reported in a few cases (Tawill *et al.* 1994, Sansone *et al.* 1997). Variable neurological signs may also be present, and hyperkalaemic and hypokalaemic cases are on record. The Q-T interval is lengthened and arrhythmias may be the first manifestation. The disease is not linked to the gene of hyperkalaemic periodic paralysis (Sansone et al. 1997).

SECONDARY PERIODIC PARALYSES

These are mainly caused by urinary or gastrointestinal losses of potassium, as occurs with primary hyperaldosteronism, renal tubular defects, thiazide treatment, amphotericin B therapy, gastrointestinal fluid loss due to vomiting, draining of intestinal fistulae or liquorice intoxication and prolonged diarrhoea (Comi *et al.* 1985).

In Oriental patients, hypokalaemic periodic paralysis is often associated with hyperthyroidism (Oh *et al.* 1990), which occurs only rarely in Western countries. Hyperkalaemic paralysis may result from renal or adrenal insufficiency or spironolactone therapy. It has been reported in an adolescent with Gordon syndrome (hypertension, tubular acidosis and hyperkalaemia possibly related to a lack of sensitivity to atrial natriuretic peptide) (Pasman *et al.* 1989).

Patients with secondary dyskalaemic paralysis should receive treatment of their primary disease. Administration of potassium is indicated for hypokalaemia, while hyperkalaemia should be treated with intravenous glucose and insulin and occasionally with peritoneal dialysis. Hypermagnesaemia due to disturbances in the renal tubular system may be a rare cause of periodic paralysis (Emser 1982).

Periodic attacks of paralysis have been reported in one patient with multiple deletions of mitochondrial DNA (Prelle *et al.* 1993).

MALIGNANT HYPERTHERMIA
Although the mechanisms of this condition are not yet completely clear, it seems likely that it belongs to the group of ion channel disorders and involves a channel for calcium release in muscle sarcoplasmic reticulum (Moroni *et al.* 1995).

It is characterized by the occurrence of muscular rigidity and necrosis associated with a rapid rise in body temperature, triggered by the administration of anaesthetics or myorelaxants. Malignant hyperthermia occurs in 1 in 15,000 children submitted to anaesthesia but there is a spectrum of severity from lethal to less severe cases (Nelson and Flewellen 1983). The inhalation anaesthetics, especially fluothane, and succinylcholine are most often implicated, but malignant hyperthermia has also rarely been reported with other inhalation anaesthetics, including nitrous oxide (Ellis *et al.* 1975), although it does not follow the use of local anaesthetics (Berkowitz and Rosenberg 1985). A less severe syndrome of acidosis, fever and elevated creatine kinase levels has been observed in patients receiving ketamine (Roervik and Stovner 1974), and some cases may be revealed only by rhabdomyolysis and consequent renal failure (Burns 1993). Malignant hyperthermia may occur exceptionally without exposure to exogenous agents as a result of intense stress (Wingard and Gatz 1978).

The disorder is inherited as an autosomal dominant trait, so a family history of accidents during anaesthesia is of extreme diagnostic importance. Creatine kinase levels in relatives are often elevated but not all patients at risk have increased levels.

The syndrome may occur in two different settings: in patients with a specific inherited predisposition, and in those with certain muscular diseases. Cases have been documented in patients with central core disease (Frank *et al.* 1980), the Schwartz–Jampel syndrome (Seay and Ziter 1978), Thomsen disease (Heiman-Patterson *et al.* 1988), myoadenylate deaminase deficiency (Fishbein *et al.* 1985) and other classical forms of muscular disorder, though it seems rare in Duchenne dystrophy. Several cases of hyperthermia have occurred in boys with multiple minor dysmorphisms such as pectus carinatum, kyphoscoliosis, cryptorchidism, small mandible and short size (King and Denborough 1973, Stewart *et al.* 1988). Such children often have mildly elevated levels of creatine kinase which may also be found in siblings without dysmorphism. It also seems that some patients with muscular hypertrophy associated with myo-oedema and raised creatine kinase may be prone to anaesthetic hyperthermia (personal observations).

The genetic predisposition to malignant hyperthermia appears to be heterogeneous. Linkage to the ryanodin receptor gene on chromosome 19q12–q13.2 is found in some cases but not in all (Moroni *et al.* 1995). Another locus on chromosome 17q11–q24 has been found that may be related to the *SCN4A* gene (Levitt *et al.* 1992), and linkage to 7q21–q22, possibly in association with another calcium channel, is also on record (Greenberg 1997).

The *clinical features* of malignant hyperthermia include tachycardia, tachypnoea, muscle fasciculation and increasing muscle tone which usually first appears in the masseters and pterygoid muscles. The rise in body temperature is extremely fast, and severe acidosis develops rapidly. Death occurs if vigorous treatment is not promptly given.

Treatment includes termination of anaesthesia, body cooling, treatment of acidosis, and intravenous injection of dantrolene at a dose of 1–2 mg/kg which may be repeated every 5–10 minutes up to a total dose of 10 mg/kg (Gronert 1980).

Siblings and relatives of patients with hyperthermia should be screened for high creatine kinase levels, and this also should be done in patients with suggestive dysmorphisms or recognized muscular disorders, and in patients who have experienced hyperthermia and/or tachycardia during anaesthesia. In such cases, an *in vitro* caffeine provocation test on a muscle biopsy sample may be indicated (European Malignant Hyperpyrexia Group 1984, Krivosic-Horber *et al.* 1990, Ellis 1992). Pretreatment with dantrolene prior to the use of anaesthetics should be given in children who might be at risk of hyperthermia.

NEUROLEPTIC MALIGNANT SYNDROME
Although its mechanism is unknown, the neuroleptic malignant syndrome shares several features with malignant hyperthermia induced by anaesthetics (Levenson 1985, Moore *et al.* 1986). The syndrome has been observed following the use of phenothiazines, butyrophenones, thioxanthenes and sulpiride (Kashihara and Ishida 1988).

Rigidity, high fever, sweating and hypertension develop over a few hours or days and the outcome may be fatal in up to 20 per cent of patients.

Bromocriptine should be promptly administered as it is capable of completely reversing the syndrome.

CRAMPS AND ABNORMAL MUSCLE CONTRACTIONS
DEFINITIONS AND CLINICAL FEATURES
Cramps are involuntary painful contractions of a muscle or part of a muscle. When cramps occur in normal individuals they are

characterized on EMG by the repetitive firing of normal motor unit potentials. Such 'normal' cramps are often precipitated by vigorous exercise or by excessive loss of fluids and electrolytes. Stretching the involved muscle usually relieves the cramp. Night cramps are also physiological events, although they occur much more frequently in partially denervated muscles.

Cramps induced by exercise occur in patients with disorders of muscle energy metabolism. These cramps are electrically silent (Rowland 1985).

Muscle spasms are also involuntary and often painful muscle contractions that are more prolonged in duration and less explosive in onset than cramps and can result in the assumption of unusual postures.

Myokymias are rippling fascicular contractions that occur spontaneously in healthy children and adults, especially about the eyes but also in other muscles. They are a physiological phenomenon unless they are excessively diffuse and intense.

Cramps associated with metabolic diseases are studied below. Severe cramps can be observed in patients on peritoneal dialysis and these may be reversed by the administration of hypertonic dextrose (Neal *et al.* 1981). Cramps are also a common feature of many muscle disorders including muscular dytrophy, especially Becker dystrophy, the neuromyotonic syndromes and neuromuscular or endocrinological diseases.

NONPHYSIOLOGICAL CRAMPS
Certain conditions are characterized exclusively or predominantly by an abnormal intensity or frequency of cramps.

Some patients develop excessive cramps in their second or third decade. The cramps may occur at rest or be induced by exercise and involve mainly the lower limbs. Cramps are often made worse by cold, and myalgia is commonly present in addition. Some patients may have brief episodes, reminiscent of myotonia, that affect the mouth and tongue and may interfere with speech. Neurological examination is normal and there is no weakness. This syndrome of myalgia and cramps is often associated with the presence in muscles of *tubular aggregates* that consist of densely packed, double-walled tubules originating from the sarcoplasmic reticulum (Rosenberg *et al.* 1985). Such aggregates are nonspecific and can be found in several muscle disorders, but their association with myalgia and cramps appears to be greater than expected (Niakan *et al.* 1985). The condition predominates, or occurs exclusively, in males. Autosomal dominant transmission is possible, although most cases are sporadic.

A nonprogressive X-linked myopathy, associated with a deletion in the dystrophin gene (Gospe *et al.* 1989), features cramps, calf hypertrophy and a high creatine kinase level. Other genetic cramp disorders include hereditary persistent distal cramps (Jusic *et al.* 1972).

OTHER ABNORMAL MUSCLE CONTRACTIONS
Hereditary myokymia (Sheaff 1952) is characterized by the diffusion and intensity of myokymia and is dominantly transmitted. In the curious condition of *rippling muscle disease* (Ricker *et al.* 1989, Burns *et al.* 1994, Stephan *et al.* 1994), 'mounding'

is produced by percussion of muscles and rolling movements occur after contraction followed by stretching. Muscle pain and stiffness after exercise may occur but the condition is benign. Linkage to chromosome 1q41 has been found in one family (Stephan *et al.* 1994). This condition may be related to the cases of familial myo-oedema, muscular hypertrophy and stiffness (Sadeh *et al.* 1990). In one personally observed family the disorder was associated with mildly elevated creatine kinase levels in three generations, with late development of weakness and mild atrophy in some patients and anaesthetic hyperthermia with massive elevation of enzyme levels in one.

Rare cases of hereditary permanent myokymia associated with periodic ataxia and sometimes with truncal jerks or carpopedal spasm are on record (Brunt and van Weerden 1990; see Chapter 17).

SARCOPLASMIC RETICULUM ADENOSINE TRIPHOSPHATASE (ATP) DEFICIENCY (BRODY DISEASE)
This is a rare genetic myopathy caused by deficiency of calcium-activated ATPase in sarcoplasmic reticulum (Karpati *et al.* 1986, Danon *et al.* 1988, Taylor *et al.* 1988) whose mode of inheritance is still debated (Danon *et al.* 1988).

The disorder presents as atypical myotonia: the main clinical manifestation is difficulty in muscle relaxation, which is different from myotonia in being electrically silent and increasing with continued exercise.

The diagnosis can be confirmed only by demonstration of the biochemical defect, as conventional histological examination shows only atrophy of type 2 fibres.

CONTINUOUS MUSCLE FIBRE ACTIVITY (NEUROMYOTONIA), STIFF MAN SYNDROME AND RELATED DISORDERS
The term neuromyotonia designates a clinical syndrome of abnormal, continuous muscle fibre activity which is of primary *neural origin*. Characteristic features are muscle cramps or stiffness and pseudomyotonic discharges, differing from true myotonia by the absence of electrical silence on EMG at rest and by the absence of crescendo–decrescendo muscle discharges. Neuromyotonia is a feature of several rare diseases and syndromes.

ISAACS SYNDROME
This syndrome (De Grandis *et al.* 1988, Oda *et al.* 1989, Ono *et al.* 1989) features mainly stiffness, while cramps and myokymia are less prominent. The legs are most affected, often with an asymmetrical distribution at onset. Deep tendon reflexes are usually abolished. The EMG shows continuous fibre activity which appears to originate in the distal part of axons as it is not abolished by proximal nerve blocks. Sensory involvement in the form of paraesthesiae is present in 30 per cent of cases. The condition is mainly sporadic and probably acquired (Newsom-Davis and Mills 1993), and antibodies directed against potassium ion channels have been detected (Shillito *et al.* 1995). Hart *et al.* (1997) found such antibodies in all of 12 patients with neuromyotonia but in none of the controls; they consider the disorder to be an

acquired antibody-mediated channelopathy. A few hereditary cases are on record (McGuire *et al.* 1984).

Treatment by carbamazepine or phenytoin suppresses totally the abnormal activity in some but not all cases.

SCHWARTZ–JAMPEL SYNDROME (DYSTONIC CHONDRODYSTROPHY)

This is an hereditary (autosomal recessive) condition that features a neuromyotonic muscle abnormality, a chondrodysplasia and short stature.

The skeletal abnormalities are present in infancy and include coxa vara or valga, vertebral flattening, pectus carinatum and dwarfism, reminiscent of the Morquio syndrome. Continuous activity is most prominent in the face and results in blepharophimosis, pursing of the mouth and puckering of the chin. The limbs are stiff, and contracture of the pharyngeal muscles can produce an abnormally high-pitched voice. Creatine kinase is normal or only mildly increased. EMG demonstrates the abnormal muscle fibre activity. Muscle histology is usually normal. Treatment with phenytoin or carbamazepine is rarely completely effective (Cao *et al.* 1978, Spaans *et al.* 1990).

OTHER FORMS OF NEUROMYOTONIA

The nosology and terminology of this group of disorders are confusing. The term Isaacs syndrome should be reserved for cases in which the ectopic nerve impulses are of distal origin, probably in the terminal axonal arborizations. Forms with a more proximal impulse generation exist. They are associated in some cases with evidence of neuropathy as indicated by EMG. In such cases, myokymias and cramps are often prominent and muscular atrophy of the limbs may be present (Hahn *et al.* 1991). Most cases are sporadic and occur in adults. In rare cases, the disorder is genetically determined (Auger *et al.* 1984) and transmitted as an autosomal dominant trait (Ashizawa *et al.* 1983). A neonatal onset has been reported (Black *et al.* 1972).

Continuous muscle fibre activity may also be due to peripheral nerve injury (Medina *et al.* 1976) or to toxic substances such as gold salts.

STIFF MAN SYNDROME

This is ordinarily a sporadic disease of adults with rare cases in adolescents (Daras and Spiro 1981). Rigidity is permanently present except in sleep and is intermittently reinforced by painful spasms. The EMG shows a continuous motor unit activity of normal configuration, distinct from the fibre activity of the conditions mentioned above. However, some cases demonstrate the existence of an overlap between continuous muscle fibre activity and the stiff man syndrome (Valli *et al.* 1983).

The cause of the disorder is unknown. Antibodies against GABA-ergic neurons are present in two-thirds of cases (Solimena *et al.* 1990, Grimaldi *et al.* 1993). A similar condition may occasionally result from progressive encephalomyelitis (Whiteley *et al.* 1976, Meinck and Ricker 1987).

An *early genetic type* of stiff man syndrome has been described. This condition is in fact quite different from the adult stiff man syndrome and appears to be an early manifestation of the startle disease or hyperekplexia (Sander *et al.* 1980; see Chapter 17). The infants are rigid and are often misdiagnosed as cases of diplegia. They may have, in addition, inguinal and umbilical hernias and attacks of apnoea. A family with a recessively inherited syndrome of rapidly progressive rigidity of skeletal muscles and early respiratory deficiency and death reported by Lacson *et al.* (1995) may be related to both the stiff man syndrome and neuromyotonia.

METABOLIC MYOPATHIES

Several metabolic disturbances interfere with muscle function and can be responsible for muscular symptoms that may be intermittent, occur on muscular effort, or be permanent. The metabolic myopathies are infrequent diseases caused by enzyme deficiencies affecting three main metabolic pathways: the glycogenolytic and glycolytic pathway; the transport and oxidation of lipids; and oxidative phosphorylation.

DISORDERS OF GLYCOGENOLYSIS AND GLYCOLYSIS—THE GLYCOGENOSES

Disorders of glycogenolysis and glycolysis can present in two distinct manners. Some feature permanent and progressive weakness: these include glycogenoses types II, III and IV and occasional other rare types such as muscle phosphoglucomutase deficiency (DiMauro *et al.* 1982, Sugie *et al.* 1988) and muscle fructose diphosphatase deficiency (Kar *et al.* 1980). Others present with intermittent attacks of weakness, muscle pain and/or myoglobinuria including glycogenosis types V (McArdle disease), deficits in phosphofructokinase, phosphoglycerate kinase, phosphoglycerate mutase, lactate dehydrogenase and glucose-6-phosphate dehydrogenase (Bresolin *et al.* 1989), and abnormal hexosaminidase (Poulton and Nightingale 1988).

Some cases are difficult to classify into either clinical presentation. These include the fatal infantile forms of phosphofructokinase deficiency (Danon *et al.* 1981, Servidei *et al.* 1986).

ACID MALTASE DEFICIENCY (TYPE II GLYCOGENOSIS)

Acid maltase is a lysosomal enzyme present in all tissues, which hydrolyses maltose to yield glucose. Three distinct forms of maltase deficiency are recognized (infantile, childhood and adult types) all transmitted as autosomal recessive diseases due to various mutations in the same gene, localized to 17q23–q25.

The *infantile form* of acid maltase deficiency, known as *Pompe disease* or type IIa glycogenosis, is characterized by the onset at birth, or during the first weeks of life, of profound hypotonia accompanied by macroglossia, cardiomegaly and cardiac failure. Deep tendon reflexes are often abolished as a result of involvement of the anterior horn cells. Death from cardiac failure occurs before 1 year of age. Giant QRS complexes and a very short P-R interval are suggestive features.

In the *childhood form*, only skeletal muscle is involved and the patients present with slowly progressive proximal limb weakness. Mild hypertrophy of the calves has been documented.

The illness is progressive, leading to increasing disability and respiratory insufficiency by the end of the second or the third decade (Danon *et al.* 1986).

The *adult form*, also known as type IIb glycogenosis, has features similar to those of the juvenile form with which it overlaps.

In all types, the diagnosis depends on the demonstration of glycogen storage by muscle biopsy, with a classical vacuolar appearance, and on the absence of acid maltase in muscle, leukocytes or fibroblasts. Attempts at therapy with enzyme replacement have been unsuccessful. Prenatal diagnosis is possible on trophoblasts or amniotic cells. A condition clinically resembling glycogenosis type IIa, with vacuolization of fibres, glycogen storage but no acid maltase deficiency, has been reported in children and adults (Danon *et al.* 1981, Tachi *et al.* 1989) as an X-linked condition. A similar case with dominant inheritance has been described (Byrne *et al.* 1986). Cardiac involvement may be prominent (Muntoni *et al.* 1994). The nosological situation of such cases is unclear and they may not belong to the glycogenoses, glycogen accumulation being a secondary phenomenon (Dubowitz 1995).

GLYCOGENOSES TYPES III AND IV
These forms are usually characterized by predominant hepatic involvement. In occasional patients and families, muscle involvement may be the major clinical feature with weakness and pseudohypertrophy (Marbini *et al.* 1989), and myocardiopathy may be associated. Dietary treatment may be helpful.

McARDLE DISEASE (GLYCOGENOSIS TYPE V).
McArdle disease (myophosphorylase deficiency) is the prototype of those glycogenoses that manifest with intermittent symptoms. The disease is usually transmitted by autosomal recessive inheritance, although occasional dominant transmission has been reported (Chui and Munsat 1976). Myophosphorylase is coded for by a gene mapping to chromosome 11q13 (Tsujino *et al.* 1993). The incidence of the disease is 1 per 50,000 births (DiMauro and Tsujino 1994). The severity of symptoms depends on the proportion of residual activity.

Onset is usually after 5 years of age. Symptoms occur only on effort, with muscle aching from the first minutes of exercise, severe cramps and, sometimes, myoglobinuria. In children, however, easy fatiguability can be the only symptom. Most children reduce their overall level of physical activity as a result of pain. Some patients experience the so-called 'second wind phenomenon' (Braakhekke *et al.* 1986) whereby exercise may be pursued normally. This phenomenon largely results from a switch from glucose to free fatty acid as a substrate of muscle metabolism. Permanent weakness may be observed many years after the first manifestations of the disease.

Rare patients have a different phenotype characterized by slowly progressive proximal weakness with onset in childhood, without any cramp, myalgia or myoglobinuria (Abarbanel *et al.* 1987).

The diagnosis of McArdle disease is confirmed by the ischaemic exercise test and by muscle biopsy. Lactate increase,

which is normally more than 2 mmol/L, fails to develop and cramps may appear during the test. Muscle biopsy shows moderate increase in subsarcolemmic glycogen. Absence of phosphorylase can be demonstrated histochemically. Muscle fibre degeneration may be seen following a recent episode. About 90 per cent of patients have increased levels of creatine kinase, and about half show EMG abnormalities of myogenic type at rest. Definitive diagnosis requires the biochemical demonstration of decreased myophosphorylase activity (Servidei *et al.* 1988).

Treatment with a high-protein diet has been advised (Slonim and Goans 1985).

A fatal infantile type has been described (Milstein *et al.* 1989).

PHOSPHOFRUCTOKINASE DEFICIENCY (TARUI DISEASE)
Phosphofructokinase deficiency, which impairs glycolysis, is rare. It usually presents with cramps on exercise and myoglobinuria (Di Mauro and Tsujino 1994). Phosphofructokinase consists of several isoenzymes. In muscle, only M subunits are present, while M and L subunits are found in erythrocytes and all three subunits in most other tissues. In addition to muscle symptoms, deficit in M subunit may present with bouts of haemolysis. A neonatal form has been reported (Servidei *et al.* 1986). It is marked by hypotonia, weakness, respiratory insufficiency and joint deformities. Cerebral involvement is present and death supervenes during the first year.

PHOSPHORYLASE B KINASE (PBK) DEFICIENCY
PBK deficiency is an uncommon disease that almost always begins in infancy or childhood. The spectrum of reported cases includes a benign autosomal recessive form with weakness and hepatomegaly, similar X-linked cases, and muscle disease usually presenting as exercise intolerance in childhood sometimes with weakness in infancy and cardiac disease (van den Berg and Berger 1990, DiMauro and Tsujino 1994). Similar cases have been reported in adults (Wilkinson *et al.* 1994).

OTHER GLYCOGENOSES
Muscle disorder presenting with intolerance to exercise and associated myoglobinuria has been reported in glycogenosis type IX (phosphoglycerate kinase deficiency) (DiMauro *et al.* 1981, Sugie *et al.* 1989), type X (phosphoglycerate mutase deficiency) (Vita *et al.* 1994) and type XI (lactate dehydrogenase deficiency) (Bryan *et al.* 1990, DiMauro and Tsujino 1994). Type IV glycogenosis can also generate muscle symptoms (Marbini *et al.* 1989).

MYOADENYLATE DEAMINASE DEFICIENCY
Myoadenylate deaminase deficiency is a familial trait that has been found in muscle samples of patients with infantile hypotonia and with progressive myopathies of childhood onset and in asymptomatic individuals. Although the significance of the deficit is still unclear (Mercelis *et al.* 1987), there is increasing evidence that it may be responsible for symptoms of exercise intolerance (Kelemen *et al.* 1982). Sabina (1993) found that 85 of 187 documented cases (45 per cent) had no other identifiable muscle

abnormality, and in 77 of these there was exertional myalgia and fatigue, thus supporting a causal role of the deficit.

Children may present with intermittent pain and weakness. Cramps may be associated with muscle swelling or tenderness (Ashwal and Peckham 1985). The condition does not appear to be progressive. Muscles of the face and eyes are consistently spared. The diagnosis can be suspected by ischaemic exercise test showing normal lactate production but failure of the blood ammonia level to rise. Confirmation requires demonstration of the enzyme deficit in muscle biopsy samples. A mutation in the gene on chromosome 1p13–p21 identifies primary deficiency and distinguishes it from secondary cases (Sabina 1993). The condition is transmitted by autosomal recessive inheritance.

DISORDERS OF LIPID UTILIZATION AND METABOLISM (see also Chapter 9)
Fatty acids are very important fuels for striate muscle. They are especially important for sustained exercise and under fasting conditions. Carnitine is an essential cofactor in the transfer of long-chain fatty acids into the mitochondrion where fatty acids of long, medium and short chain are metabolized by beta-oxidation.

CARNITINE DEFICIENCY
Carnitine deficiency is mainly secondary to other metabolic disorders (Chapter 9).

PRIMARY MUSCLE CARNITINE DEFICIENCY
Primary *muscle* carnitine deficiency is an autosomal recessive disease which is characterized by progressive proximal limb weakness. A cardiomyopathy is often associated. Muscle biopsy shows lipid storage and a reduced carnitine content. Dietary treatment with L-carnitine is effective in some cases. Corticosteroids may be helpful in occasional children. Primary *systemic* carnitine deficit can produce muscle symptoms (Chapter 9).

DEFICITS IN CARNITINE–PALMITOYL TRANSFERASE
Deficits in carnitine–palmitoyl transferase (CPT) are mostly associated with intermittent manifestations which appear in the course of prolonged effort or in fasting conditions. There is no 'second wind' phenomenon. In such cases, entry of long-chain fatty acid into mitochondria is limited because of the absence of the specific transfer enzyme system. This system consists of two enzymes (Meola *et al.* 1987, Zierz 1994). CPT I deficiency is rare and has been identified in a few patients who presented with episodes of severe hypoglycaemia without ketonaemia triggered by fasting or intercurrent illnesses. CPT II deficiency can also present in infants with liver disease (infantile hepatomuscular phenotype) or as a lethal neonatal form (Uziel *et al.* 1995). The clinical features are myalgia and fatiguability but severe cramps are not observed. Myoglobinuria is common. The onset of the disease is usually in late childhood or adolescence. The severity of the disease is variable and partial deficiencies may be observed (Kieval *et al.* 1989). Respiratory muscles may be involved. Fatal rhabdomyolysis has been exceptionally observed (Kelly *et al.*

1989). Permanent weakness is rarely observed (Gieron and Korthals 1987, Kieval *et al.* 1989). Biochemical estimation shows marked reduction or complete absence of the enzyme in muscle and also in leukocytes, platelets and cultured fibroblasts.

The disease is genetically determined and transmitted as an autosomal recessive trait. A similar clinical picture may obtain with mitochondrial trifunctional protein deficiency (Schaefer *et al.* 1996).

Treatment consists mainly of avoidance of fasting. A high-carbohydrate low-fat diet seems to reduce the frequency of attacks.

OTHER DEFECTS OF LIPIDIC METABOLISM
Other causes of lipid disorders, often associated with cardiac, neurological or ocular manifestations, include deficit in acyl-CoA-dehydrogenase activities, either specific for long-chain fatty acids or global, resulting from multiple acyl-CoA-dehydrogenase defect (Jackson and Turnbull 1993), from lack of electron transfer flavoprotein ubiquinone reductase (glutaric aciduria type II) (Turnbull *et al.* 1988a,b) or from long-chain 3-hydroxyacyl-CoA dehydrogenase deficiency (Jackson *et al.* 1991). In some cases treatment with riboflavine may be effective (DiDonato *et al.* 1989; see Chapter 9).

Rare cases of *multisystem triglyceride storage disease* with ichthyosis, steatorrhoea and Jordans anomaly of leukocytes are on record (Angelini *et al.* 1980).

MITOCHONDRIAL MYOPATHIES
Abnormal mitochondria are a feature of a wide range of diseases involving especially the CNS and muscular systems. The field of mitochondrial diseases has become extremely vast over the past few years and considerable progress has been made in the understanding of their genetic, biochemical, pathological and clinical features (DiMauro 1993). Mitochondrial dysfunction may occur at various steps in the mitochondrial metabolism of lipids and other metabolites (Jackson *et al.* 1995). These aspects have been reviewed in Chapter 9. The present section deals only with the muscular aspects of mitochondrial diseases limited to dysfunction of the electron transfer system (respiratory chain). Many of these are characterized morphologically by the so-called ragged red fibres. This appearance (Fig. 22.7) is due to the accumulation of mitochondria which are seen to have an abnormal structure and often contain paracrystalline inclusions of proteinic nature (Fig. 22.8). However, ragged red fibres may be permanently or temporarily absent in proven mitochondrial diseases. Knowledge of the specific biochemical and enzymatic defects associated with mitochondrial diseases has recently rapidly increased but much remains to be learnt about multiple aspects of these disorders. Many mitochondrial diseases are complex illnesses that involve other systems in addition to muscles: these are described in Chapter 9. In fact, the distinction between purely muscular and more complex forms is to some extent artificial as the ubiquitous presence of mitochondria in all cells is likely to be responsible for various dysfunctions; on the other hand, the proportion of abnormal mitochondria can vary

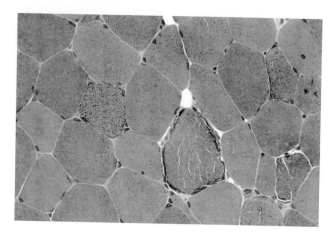

Fig. 22.7. Ragged red fibres in a case of Kearns–Sayre syndrome. Note subsarcolemmal deposits of red material representing mitochondria in most affected fibres, while similar but less marked changes are beginning to appear in other fibres. (Courtesy Prof. B. Lake, Great Ormond Street Hospital, London.)

enormously from tissue to tissue thus accounting for different presentations of the same defect.

CLINICAL FEATURES

Mitochondrial myopathies may be extremely variable in their age of presentation, severity and outcome (Harding *et al.* 1988, DiMauro 1993, Morgan-Hughes 1994). Some are part of complex encephalomyopathies (Chapter 9), while others are purely or essentially limited to striated muscle involvement. One frequent and highly suggestive presentation is *progressive external ophthalmoplegia* with more or less severe involvement of other muscles (Moraes *et al.* 1989). Another type presents as a proximal myopathy, sometimes associated with cardiomyopathy and other symptoms (Holt *et al.* 1989). Some features are suggestive of a mitochondrial disease, such as a history of exercise intolerance, general body underdevelopment and hearing loss. Associated symptoms and signs, such as CNS disease, retinitis pigmentosa and cardiac or multisystem involvement, and/or a family history of neuromuscular diseases, diabetes mellitus or retinal disease are of great diagnostic value, and lactic acidosis may be found in the blood and/or CSF (Zeviani *et al.* 1991).

One remarkable form presents with severe congenital hypotonia that can be isolated or be associated with tubular and/or cardiac involvement. Such infants become symptomatic by a few weeks to 3 months of age and usually run a rapidly downward course with respiratory insufficiency (Zeviani *et al.* 1985). This type is caused in most cases by cytochrome *c* oxidase deficiency. A reversible form of cytochrome *c* oxidase deficiency with an identical clinical presentation but a favourable course is exceptional (Zeviani *et al.* 1987). Cytochrome *c* oxidase deficiency manifesting acutely at 7 years of age by ptosis, ophthalmoplegia and respiratory arrest with recovery following coenzyme Q10 administration has been reported (Nozaki *et al.* 1990). This patient was the sister of an infant with the congenital form of the disorder who died at age 3 months. Atypical presentations include

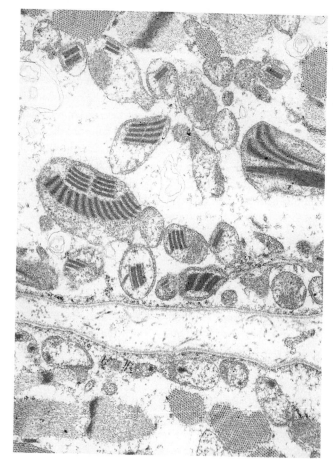

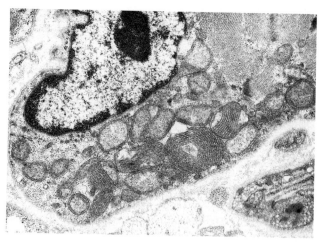

Fig. 22.8. Mitochondrial myopathy (electron microscopy, ×28,500). *(Top)* 13-year-old patient with typical history. Note classical 'parking lot' inclusions within mitochondria. *(Bottom)* 5-year-old patient. Note proliferation of the cristae within mitochondria. 'Parking lots' and paracrystalline arrays do not generally become apparent before 7–8 years of age. (Courtesy Prof. B. Lake, Great Ormond Street Hospital, London.)

predominent hypokinesia and rigidity (van Erven *et al.* 1989), although suggestive signs were present in the three patients reported.

Many patients with mitochondrial myopathy have elevated lactate levels which may appear only on effort or glucose loading.

PATHOLOGICAL FEATURES

Ragged red fibres are evident in most cases on Gomori trichrome staining. Other features include intensely reactive fibres with oxidative enzymes and ultrastructural alterations on biopsy specimens. Staining with succinate dehydrogenase clearly shows mitochondrial proliferation. Staining for cytochrome c oxidase (cox) usually shows that ragged red fibres are cox-negative (Byrne et al. 1985). However, in patients with MELAS syndrome, ragged red fibres are usually cox-positive. An excess of lipids or of glycogen is seen in some cases.

As indicated in Chapter 9, there is some specificity in the metabolic defect associated with some syndromes. Myopathies, however, can be associated with a wide spectrum of metabolic abnormalities including deficiency in complexes I and IV.

A large number of biochemical defects have been found, most commonly involving complexes I and IV (Roodhoft et al. 1986, Shimoizumi et al. 1989). Such defects may be partial (Turnbull et al. 1985) and may be evidenced only in some fibres (Reichmann 1988). Defects in complex III have been less commonly reported (Reichmann et al. 1986).

Myopathies are also frequently observed with deletions or duplications of mitochondrial DNA, and are a common feature of the recently described syndromes of multiple DNA deletions and of mtDNA depletion (Tritschler et al. 1992, Mariotti et al. 1995, Bohlega et al. 1996, Suomalainen et al. 1997).

Progressive extraocular ophthalmoplegia is associated with the mitochondrial DNA mutation mt 3243 in 80 per cent of cases (Hirano and Pavlakis 1994). Atypical presentations, e.g. forms simulating spinal muscular atrophy, are on record (Pons et al. 1996).

The treatment of mitochondrial diseases is reviewed in Chapter 9. In some cases, the muscle disease may respond to riboflavine, nicotinamide and carnitine (Bernsen et al. 1991, Bakker et al. 1994). The value of coenzyme Q10 remains disputed.

Secondary mitochondrial myopathy induced by long-term zidovudine therapy (Dalakas et al. 1990) or associated with chronic renal magnesium loss (Riggs et al. 1992) has been reported in adults.

MYOGLOBINURIA

Myoglobinuria is a syndrome with multiple causes (Table 22.4). Many of these are metabolic. However, the cause remains undetermined in about half the cases (Tonin et al. 1990) even though an underlying metabolic abnormality is likely in many. The clinical syndrome may feature, in addition to pigmenturia, muscle pain and swelling, sometimes disturbances of consciousness, renal failure and cardiac arrhythmias largely due to hyperkalaemia. Respiratory failure may occur. Tein et al. (1991a,b) recognized two groups in 40 children, exertional myoglobinuria, in which a metabolic cause was often found; and 'toxic' myoglobinuria, precipitated by fever and infection, and with a more severe outcome, the frequent presence of bulbar signs and no recognized metabolic defect. Fasting may also be a triggering factor in patients with cartinine palmitoyl deficiency but not in the glycogenoses. A careful search for a metabolic defect

TABLE 22.4
Main causes of myoglobinuria*

Genetic, usually recurrent myoglobinuria (Tein et al. 1991a)
With known biochemical anomaly:
  Of glycolysis/glycogenolysis (see text)
    Phosphorylase kinase
    Phosphofructokinase
    Phosphoglycerate mutase
    Lactic dehydrogenase
    Aldolase A (Kreuder et al. 1996)
  Of fatty acid oxidation
    Carnitine palmitoyl transferase
    Long-chain acyl-CoA dehydrogenase
    Very-long-chain acyl-CoA dehydrogenase (Ogilvie et al. 1994)
    Short-chain hydroxyacyl-CoA dehydrogenase (Tein et al. 1991b)
  Of pentose-phosphate pathway
    Glucose-6-phosphate dehydrogenase
  Of purine nucleotide cycle
    Myoadenylate deaminase (see text)
  Of respiratory chain
    Complex II deficiency (Haller et al. 1991)
    Multiple mitochondrial deletions (Ohno et al. 1991)
With incompletely characterized anomaly (see text)
  Excess lactate production
  Impaired long-chain fatty acid oxidation
  Impaired sarcoplasmic reticulum function in malignant hyperthermia
With unknown metabolic abnormality (see text)
  Duchenne and Becker muscular dystrophy
  Familial recurrent myoglobinuria
  Reported attacks in individual patients
  X-linked myoglobinuria (Fischbeck et al. 1988)
Nongenetic, usually not recurrent myoglobinuria (Chamberlain 1991)
Mechanical trauma (Bywater syndrome)
Myotoxic agents (animal poisons, numerous drugs, alcohol)
Salt/water imbalance
Extreme hyperthermia
Hypothermia
Infections, especially viral

*Modified from Tein et al. (1991b).

is in order in all cases, once haematuria and other causes of pigmenturia have been ruled out.

INFLAMMATORY MYOPATHIES

The inflammatory myopathies are a heterogeneous group of acquired muscle disorders. Some are due to known specific agents whilst in most cases no agent is recognized and a dysimmune mechanism appears likely. In childhood or adolescence, dermatomyositis has a distinctive clinical presentation and is relatively common, whereas polymyositis is much less common and has a more variable presentation. Localized myositis is much less frequent than generalized forms (Whitaker 1982).

DERMATOMYOSITIS

Dermatomyositis is a systemic angiopathy mainly affecting small vessels, capillaries, arterioles and venules (Silver and Maricq 1989). The angiopathy accounts for all pathological changes in muscle, small nerves, gastrointestinal tract, connective tissue and skin.

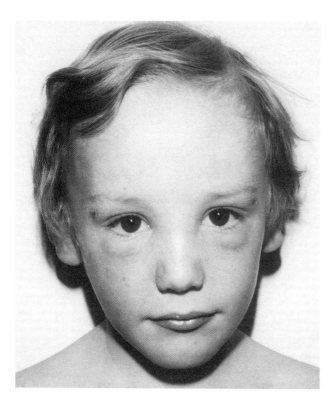

Fig. 22.9. Dermatomyositis in 11-year-old boy. Eyelid oedema is evident and was associated with heliotrope discoloration.

Immunological abnormalities are found in some cases (Mastaglia and Ojeda 1985). Contrary to what is seen in adults, dermatomyositis in children is never associated with malignancy. Dermatomyositis may occur in patients with X-linked agammaglobulinaemia, usually in association with involvement of the CNS (Chapter 12), and as a result of graft-versus-host reaction (Urbano-Márquez *et al.* 1986). A dermatomyositis-like syndrome due to *Toxoplasma gondii* infestation has been reported (Topi *et al.* 1979).

CLINICAL FEATURES AND DIAGNOSIS
The main clinical features of dermatomyositis have been reported in detail by Dubowitz (1995). Onset is commonly between 5 and 10 years of age but infantile cases are known. The illness presents acutely in one-third of cases with fever, muscle pain or arthralgia. In the remaining patients, the onset is insidious with fatigue, anorexia and mild fever. Cutaneous manifestations and weakness may become manifest only after weeks or even months. The rash is constant, involves the upper eyelids and spreads to the periorbital and malar regions. The heliotrope discolouration is suggestive. Periorbital oedema is associated (Fig. 22.9). A similar rash may appear on the extensor surfaces overlying the knuckles, elbows and knee. The skin manifestations are very variable. They are occasionally widespread involving the trunk as well as the face and extremities. In other patients, they may appear only late in the course and be transient, so the borderline with polymyositis may be difficult to trace.

Muscle weakness affects mainly the proximal muscles, is accompanied in most cases by muscle pain and stiffness, and sometimes involves the pharyngeal muscles with swallowing difficulties. Periarticular contractures tend to develop early and to produce joint deformities.

Gastrointestinal symptoms are present in about 20 per cent of patients. Ulcerations may extend over the whole length of the bowel and are an important cause of death (Bowyer *et al.* 1983). In a few children, retinal exudates are present. Respiratory distress as a result of parenchymal involvement is possible and ECG abnormalities are common. Calcinosis of subcutaneous tissue and muscle itself occurs in 25–50 per cent of the children. It may be located under the discoloured areas of skin or be extensive (*calcinosis universalis*) with occasional extrusion of calcium through the skin. Chronic cases feature generalized muscle wasting and severe contractures. The skin over the knuckles becomes thickened and discoloured and calcinosis is frequent. Such cases may be slowly progressive or burnt out and are often the result of late diagnosis and inadequate treatment. Some such cases may overlap with childhood scleromyositis (Blazsczyk *et al.* 1991).

The *diagnosis* of dermatomyositis is difficult before a rash or definite weakness appears and is often delayed for several months. The diagnosis can be made if four of the five following criteria are present: cutaneous rash; symmetrical muscle weakness; elevated creatine kinase levels; fibrillation potentials at EMG; perifascicular atrophy and mononuclear perivascular infiltrates (Bohan and Peter 1975). It should always be suspected in a child with weakness and misery (Dubowitz 1995) even in the absence of skin lesions.

Creatine kinase may be normal, especially late in the course. The EMG usually shows insertional activity, fibrillation and positive waves at rest and is of the 'myogenic' type with polyphasic small-amplitude potentials on contraction. Muscle ultrasound and MRI have been found useful in adults (Reimers *et al.* 1994), although results may be normal. Perifascicular atrophy on muscle biopsy is the usual finding. Perivascular infiltrates are commonly found but they may be missed because they are focally distributed.

TREATMENT
Corticosteroids are the standard treatment for dermatomyositis; since their introduction, the mortality has been reduced from 30 per cent to around 5–10 per cent (Bowyer *et al.* 1983). Many authors use doses of 2–2.5 mg/kg initially and maintain treatment at smaller doses for 18 months or two years which corresponds to the average duration of the active phase of the disorder, which is suppressed rather than cured by steroids. Other investigators (Miller *et al.* 1983, Dubowitz 1995) advise smaller doses (1.0–1.5 mg/kg) that can induce satisfactory remission of the active disease for shorter periods, gradually tapering the dosage once response begins without waiting for a full remission. The total duration may be as short as three to six months. The dose of steroids is progressively tapered at a rate of 5–10 mg per month. Some advise the continuance of a maintenance dose, sufficient to suppress symptoms. Relapses occur if treatment is discontinued too early, requiring stepping up the dose temporarily. Intravenous pulses of high-dose methylprednisolone can be tried in resistant cases (Laxer *et al.* 1987).

Some 10–20 per cent of affected children do not respond to steroids. For such patients immunosuppressant drugs are indicated. Methotrexate, in doses of 10–20 mg/m² given twice weekly by intravenous or oral route, is effective in 75 per cent of patients (Hanissian *et al.* 1982, Miller *et al.* 1983). Cyclosporin is a valuable agent for resistant cases (Heckmatt *et al.* 1989).

Other therapies include intravenous pulse methylprednisolone (Laxer *et al.* 1987), intravenous immunoglobulins which appeared to be effective in a controlled study (Dalakas *et al.* 1993), and plasmapheresis (Miller *et al.* 1992). Their value, however, is not proved (Mancias *et al.* 1994).

Prevention of the development of contractures by active and passive mobilization and the use of night splints is an essential part of therapy.

Early treatment is important to prevent sequelae, especially contracture and calcinosis whose treatment is disappointing.

POLYMYOSITIS

The clinical picture and course of polymyositis in children is similar to the adult disorder (Mastaglia and Ojeda 1985). It is characterized variably by insidious muscular weakness without cutaneous manifestations, sometimes with muscle pain, or by general ill-being and mild fever associated with the weakness. Usually creatine kinase levels are elevated and biopsy shows necrosis and inflammatory infiltrates, but in some cases all laboratory examinations may be normal. The diagnosis should be suspected in any child with misery and weakness (Dubowitz 1995) until proved otherwise, as steroids are effective although in a less predictable manner than in dermatomyositis. Muscle biopsy shows fibre necrosis and inflammatory infiltrates but not the perivascular atrophy characteristic of dermatomyositis.

The course of polymyositis can be extremely slow with spontaneous arrest or periods of remission, and such cases may be mistaken for limb–girdle muscular dystrophy.

INCLUSION BODY MYOSITIS

This disorder is exceptional in childhood (Riggs *et al.* 1989b, Griggs *et al.* 1995). It presents like a chronic myositis simulating muscular dystrophy. Muscle biopsy shows necrosed and regenerating fibres, mononuclear cell infiltration and sarcoplasmic vacuoles containing basophilic and eosinophilic inclusions. On electron microscopy, the vacuoles are shown to include membranous bodies and intranuclear and cytoplasmic filamentous inclusions. The cause of this special form of 'myositis' is unknown and anti-inflammatory treatment is ineffective.

INFANTILE AND CONGENITAL MYOSITIS

This is a rare condition that presents in the neonatal period or between 1 and 12 months of age (Shevell *et al.* 1990, Nagai *et al.* 1992). Hypotonia may be extreme, and breathing difficulties may necessitate resuscitation and assisted ventilation. Weakness and hypotonia can suggest a diagnosis of spinal amyotrophy (Thompson 1982, Roddy *et al.* 1986). Muscle biopsy, however, shows diffuse inflammation and proliferation of connective tissue.

Some cases respond to corticosteroid therapy at usual doses. These should be rapidly tapered in young patients.

TRANSIENT ACUTE MYOSITIS OF VIRAL, BACTERIAL, PARASITIC OR PROTOZOAN ORIGIN

VIRAL MYOSITIS

Epidemic pleurodynia (Bornholm disease) due to coxsackievirus B infection is a well-recognized disease involving the intercostal muscles. Myalgias are a regular feature of some other viral diseases, especially of influenza. In some epidemics of influenza A or B, muscular involvement may be prominent, and in rare cases influenza virus has been isolated from muscle (Gamboa *et al.* 1979).

The characteristic picture is one of intense pain, mainly in the calves and thighs, with tightness, swelling and tenderness of muscles. Some children can walk only on tip-toe as result of gastrocnemius–soleus involvement (Dietzman *et al.* 1976, Buchta 1977) or cannot walk at all.

A picture of acute diffuse polymyositis is uncommon, and severe cases with myoglobinuria are rare (DiBona and Morens 1977, Gamboa *et al.* 1979). A possible role of viral infections as triggers of myositis has been suggested, as raised antibody titres to coxsackievirus B have been found in some patients (Dubowitz 1995).

Other viruses (adenoviruses, parainfluenza viruses) rarely produce myositis. Association with rotavirus gastroenteritis has been reported (Hattori *et al.* 1992).

BACTERIAL MYOSITIS (PYOMYOSITIS)

Bacterial myositis is rare in industrialized countries. In tropical countries, purulent myositis is common. It is mainly due to staphylococcal infections. Abscess formation occurs following a first phase of muscle induration and often raises diagnostic problems, as the condition may be difficult to distinguish from rhabdomyosarcoma or haematoma. Surgical drainage may be necessary, in addition to antibiotic treatment. The course is usually favourable (Mastaglia and Ojeda 1985). Pyomyositis has been reported in an infant with AIDS (Raphael *et al.* 1989). Nonsuppurative myositis is also observed in cases of *Borrelia burgdorferi* infection (Reimers *et al.* 1993).

PARASITIC MYOSITIS

Trichinosis is the commonest cause of parasitic myositis (Chapter 11). In cysticercosis, muscle involvement is frequent in heavy infection, and radiological examination of muscles in search of calcified cysts may be useful for diagnosis. Toxoplasmosis is an unusual cause of polymyositis (Karasawa *et al.* 1981).

FOCAL MYOSITIS

Focal myositis of unknown origin is rare (Lederman *et al.* 1984) especially in children. It is marked by a painful swelling of a muscle or group of muscles which may suggest the diagnosis of rhabdomyosarcoma. The diagnosis can be made only by biopsy.

Fascial inflammations are also a rare condition in children. One form is associated with eosinophilia (eosinophilic fasciitis). The condition has been reviewed by Simon *et al.* (1982).

OSSIFYING MYOSITIS

This is a rare condition characterized by the successive appearance of localized swellings over the neck, spine and limbs with an inflammatory character. These lesions subside spontaneously, leaving behind ossification of underlying ligaments and soft tissues. Congenital abnormality of the first metatarsal is often a cue to the diagnosis. This is a dominantly transmitted disease with irregular penetrance. No effective treatment is known, although corticosteroids or other inflammatory agents and nifedipine have been tried (Smith *et al.* 1996).

EFFECTS OF ENDOCRINE AND SYSTEMIC DISEASE ON MUSCLE

Myopathic diseases are frequent in endocrinological disorders in adults but are uncommon in children. Disorders of calcium, phosphate or magnesium metabolism and drugs can also produce muscle weakness.

MYOPATHY AND THYROID DISEASE

Hypothyroidism is often associated with muscular symptoms or signs. In fact, a special form of pseudomyotonia is extremely common in congenital hypothyroidism as shown by the increased latency of the ankle jerk reflex. Clinical manifestations such as cramp or myo-oedema are relatively common (Kaminsky and Ruff 1994). In children with congenital hypothyroidism, muscle hypertrophy producing a pseudoathletic appearance and pseudomyotonia constitute the Debré–Sémelaigne syndrome (Kaminsky and Ruff 1994).

Muscular manifestations can be corrected by treatment of the hypothyroidism.

Hyperthyroidism produces involvement of ocular muscles. Hyperthyroid myopathies are observed in adulthood. The incidence of myasthenia is increased in patients with hyperthyroidism. In Orientals, a form of periodic paralysis with hypokalaemia is the commonest type of periodic paralysis (see p. 765).

MYOPATHY AND STEROIDS

Cushing disease and steroid treatment give rise to a similar myopathy. This disorder may occur at any age and following variable doses and durations of steroid treatment. The onset is insidious with progressive weakness, chiefly affecting the pelvic girdle with associated wasting and sometimes pain. The diagnosis may be difficult in patients receiving steroids as a treatment of inflammatory muscle diseases or if the administration of steroids escapes notice (*e.g.* cutaneous treatment with steroid unguents under occlusive dressing). Treatment is by diminution of dose or alternate-day therapy if complete discontinuation of steroids is not possible (Kaminsky and Ruff 1994). An acute form of steroid myopathy has been observed in children following treatment of status asthmaticus (Kaplan *et al.* 1986) and in patients receiving high-dose steroid therapy with or without associated nondepolarizing blocking agents for the treatment of various disorders (Hirano *et al.* 1992, Panegyres *et al.* 1993, Lacomis *et al.* 1996). Such cases present as an acute quadriplegia that may be life-threatening and require assisted ventilation, and muscle has been found to be completely inexcitable (Rich *et al.* 1996).

MYOPATHIES ASSOCIATED WITH OTHER SYSTEMIC DISEASES AND DRUGS

Muscle weakness and hypotonia are a common feature of *rickets and osteomalacia*. In some children, weakness may be the presenting manifestation and raise diagnostic problems if bone X-rays are not obtained (Torres *et al.* 1986).

Phosphate depletion (Goodman *et al.* 1978), magnesium deficiency (Riggs *et al.* 1992) and hypermagnesaemia (Emser 1982) are rare causes of myopathy. Muscle disease may also be seen in malnourished children (Donley and Evans 1989), although the respective roles of neural and muscular involvement in this case are unclear, and following administration of drugs like procainamide (Lewis *et al.* 1985). A syndrome of eosinophilia and myalgia has been reported in persons taking tryptophan preparations (Medsger 1990). Acute type II fibre atrophy may be seen in acute critical illnesses (Gutmann *et al.* 1996).

ARTHROGRYPOSIS MULTIPLEX CONGENITA

The term arthrogryposis multiplex congenita applies to a heterogeneous group of cases whose common feature is congenital immobilization of several joints. It can be due to multiple causes all involving fetal immobilization whether due to lesions of the neuromuscular system or CNS, to a functional disturbance such as congenital myasthenia or the use of curarizing agents during pregnancy (Hageman and Willemse 1983, Hageman *et al.* 1987b), or to external mechanical factors in the presence of an anatomically and functionally intact neuromuscular apparatus. Such is the case, for example, with uterine constraint associated with Potter syndrome and other causes of oligohydramnios. A number of complex syndromes of chromosomal or genetic origin feature arthrogryposis in association with dysmorphism and multisystem abnormalities. The most common is Pena–Shokeir syndrome (Pena and Shokeir 1974, Hageman *et al.* 1987a) that is recessively inherited and features pulmonary hypoplasia, facial dysmorphism and a variety of cerebral malformations. Other rare progressive syndromes can also be the cause (Hageman *et al.* 1988a,b; Di Rocco *et al.* 1995), including a syndrome of multiple pterygia (Hall *et al.* 1982b) and the syndrome of congenital contractural arachnodactyly (Wong 1997).

A majority of cases are caused by neuromuscular or CNS disorders. *Anterior horn cell disease* of prenatal origin is the most common neuromuscular cause (Fedrizzi *et al.* 1993). These cases differ from Werdnig–Hoffmann disease in which major contractures are unusual. The EMG may show signs of denervation, although in many cases these are rather minor or undetectable, suggesting a stable condition in which muscles or fascicles have either become fibrotic and electrically silent or remained normal. Pathologically, the smaller anterior horn neurons are present or increased, whereas in spinal muscular atrophy both large and

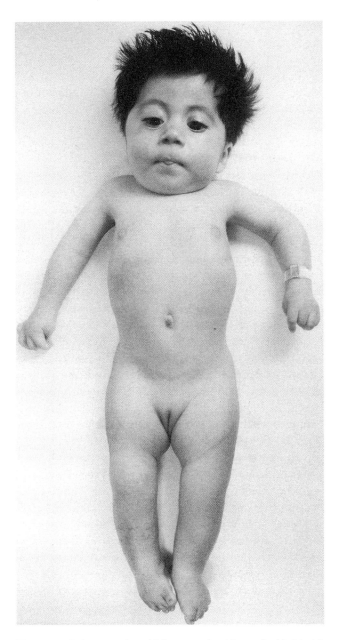

Fig. 22.10. Arthrogryposis multiplex congenita. 18-month-old girl with classical form (sometimes termed amyoplasia congenita) illustrating attitude in extension of the limbs, flexion contractures of the fingers, absence of skin creases and tube-shaped limbs.

small neurons are absent. A variant of anterior horn cell disease, frequent in Finland and lethal prenatally, is termed congenital contracture syndrome and is probably a recessive disease (Vuopala *et al.* 1994). *Muscle disease*, mainly congenital dystrophies but occasionally other disorders including congenital myasthenia (Vajsar *et al.* 1995), is a less common cause of arthrogryposis (Banker 1994). Cases have been reported in which antibodies inhibiting fetal acetylcholine receptors were found (Vincent *et al.* 1994). Neural causes are rare (Charnas *et al.* 1988). *CNS abnormalities* are frequent, either in isolation or associated with anterior horn cell disease (Fedrizzi *et al.* 1993). Both destructive (Perlman *et al.* 1995) and malformative lesions (Hageman *et al.* 1985, 1987b,

1988b; Massa *et al.* 1988; Baker *et al.* 1996) can be responsible. Intracranial calcification may be seen (Illum *et al.* 1988).

Familial lesions of the anterior horn spinal roots and non-progressive congenital neuropathies (Yuill and Lynch 1974, Boylan *et al.* 1992) are rare causes. A case of arthrogryposis with ragged red muscle fibres and complex I deficiency (Laubscher *et al.* 1997) suggests that mitochondrial cytopathy should be looked for in some cases.

Most cases of arthrogryposis are sporadic. However, some forms are genetically transmitted. These include distal arthrogryposis, the lethal congenital contracture syndrome, and several complex malformation syndromes (Lebenthal *et al.* 1970).

The *clinical presentation* is very variable depending on the cause, the number and location of immobilized joints, and the presence or absence of brain abnormalities and other signs.

The most common form, sometimes termed *amyoplasia congenita*, occurs in 1 in 3000 live births (Hall *et al.* 1983, Sells *et al.* 1996) and has a suggestive presentation. In most cases, there is symmetrical involvement of all four limbs with reduced muscle mass, internal rotation of the arms, sloping of the shoulders, equinovarus feet, flexion of the wrists, clenched hands, extension of elbows and flexion of the hips and knees (Fig. 22.10). Some passive mobility may be preserved, and in such cases paralysis of the muscles normally moving the involved joint is evident. Flexion creases are usually absent or abnormal, an indication of early intrauterine onset, and abnormal dimples are frequently present. Sensorium is normal. Retrognathism is common and about one-quarter of affected patients have contracture of the temporomandibular joint. A midline facial flat capillary angioma is visible in 80–90 per cent of cases.

Major feeding difficulties in infancy were present in 51 of 87 patients reported by Robinson (1990). Subsequent language problems and poor growth were commonly associated, and such patients require continuing therapy from many disciplines.

Other forms of neurogenic arthrogryposis include localized forms such as observed in spina bifida or sacral agenesis, and a rare type affecting only the neck and upper limb that seems to be due to segmental spinal cord involvement (Darwish *et al.* 1981, G. Hageman *et al.* 1993).

The *distal types of arthrogryposis* are much more benign than the diffuse forms. Depending on associated abnormalities, they have been classified by Hall and Reed (1982b) into five subgroups, some of them with a dominant inheritance.

X-linked forms of arthrogryposis have also been described (Hall *et al.* 1982a). One rapidly lethal type maps to Xp11.3–q11.2 (Kobayashi *et al.* 1995).

The course of arthrogryposis is obviously variable with the cause. In the common amyoplasia congenita type, the outcome is relatively good despite the extension of deformities. Of 68 children studied by Sells *et al.* (1996), two-thirds were fully ambulatory by 5 years of age, most were completely or relatively independent, and a majority went to normal schools in the appropriate grade. Most of them had undergone around five to seven orthopaedic procedures, including castings. Clearly, appropriate surgical and orthopaedic treatment, physiotherapy and rehabilitation, and careful follow-up are essential.

CONGENITAL ABSENCE OF MUSCLES

Local absence of muscles is common and may involve a number of muscles or parts of muscle, including, in decreasing order of frequency, the pectoralis, trapezius, sternocleidomastoid, serratus anterior and quadriceps femori. One common condition is the *Poland syndrome* in which absence of the sternal head of the pectoralis major is associated with ipsilateral brachysyndactyly of fingers and hypoplasia of the upper limb. Focal agenesis of muscles is usually asymptomatic. Vascular abnormalities may be a cause in some cases (Lee *et al.* 1995). The *prune belly syndrome* is characterized by absence or hypoplasia of abdominal wall muscles that may be primary or secondary (Moerman *et al.* 1984).

TRAUMATIC LESIONS OF MUSCLES

Trauma to muscle may result from excessive strain (Cameron 1983) or overuse as in *compartmental syndromes.* The rectus abdominis syndrome (Rutgers 1986) and the anterior compartment syndrome of the leg (Sloane *et al.* 1994) are of clinical importance for diagnosis and treatment.

Deltoid, gluteal or vastus lateralis *fibrotic contracture* results from repeated intramuscular injections usually in the neonatal period or in infancy (Chen *et al.* 1988). Fibrotic retractions produce, after a variable latent period, limitation of joint movements and abnormal gait or postures and may require surgical lengthening of affected muscle. The best treatment is preventive by avoidance of intramuscular injections in children.

Congenital torticollis due to fibrosis of the sternomastoid muscle is probably traumatic in origin. It should be distinguished from neurological, vertebral or ocular causes of torticollis which include, *inter alia*, superior oblique palsy, posterior fossa tumours and osteoarticular lesions of the cervical column (Sarnat and Morrissy 1981, Morrison and MacEwen 1982). Spontaneous disappearance is frequent toward the end of the first year of life. Surgical treatment is reserved for the most severe cases.

Muscle hypertrophy may be caused by several myopathic or neurogenic disorders. It may also be due to intensive exercise. Familial hypertrophy of masticatory muscles has been reported (Martinelli *et al.* 1987). Muscle hypertrophy may also be seen in a syndrome of rigidity, muscle hypertrophy and extensive brain damage involving especially the basal ganglia, described by Cornelia de Lange (1934).

MYASTHENIA AND DISORDERS OF THE NEUROMUSCULAR JUNCTION

Diseases of the neuromuscular junction are characterized clinically by weakness and increased fatiguability on muscular exercise. The group includes two autoimmune diseases, myasthenia gravis and the Eaton–Lambert syndrome, several congenital myasthenic syndromes, and various types of neuromuscular blockade due to drugs, toxins or other exogenous factors.

AUTOIMMUNE MYASTHENIA GRAVIS
Myasthenia gravis is the most common cause of neuromuscular block in children and adolescents. Approximately 10 per cent of all cases of myasthenia gravis occur in this age range.

MECHANISMS, PATHOLOGY, PATHOGENESIS
The functional lesion is located at the postsynaptic site of the neuromuscular junction and is the consequence of binding of antibodies directed against acetylcholine receptors to the postsynaptic membrane. The receptors have been located on the postsynaptic folds, and their number is considerably reduced in myasthenic patients. This reduction has been shown to result from the action of autoantibodies whose presence has been demonstrated in serum and at the neuromuscular junction of human patients (Andrews *et al.* 1993, Drachman 1994), and a myasthenia-like disease has been produced in animals by repeated injection of antibody-containing sera. The antibody response is polyclonal in type and only one fraction of the antibodies can prevent the binding of alpha-bungarotoxin to the receptors. Further investigations have demonstrated the nature of the epitopes recognized by the antibodies and have shown that they bind at a site distinct from that of the acetylcholine binding-site (Penn *et al.* 1993).

The mechanism responsible for the production of autoantibodies is unknown. A role of the thymus is suggested by the association of myasthenia with thymus tumours, by the presence of thymus hyperplasia and by the effects of thymectomy, but the pathogenesis remains obscure. A genetic susceptibility is suggested by the relative frequency of clinical or EMG manifestations in relatives of myasthenic patients and by increased frequency of some HLA groups (Kerzin-Storrar *et al.* 1988).

Other autoimmune disorders including thyroid disease (Ichiki *et al.* 1992), diabetes, rheumatoid arthritis and lupus erythematosus may be associated. Malignant disease was present in 5 per cent of children in one series (Rodriguez *et al.* 1983).

The microscopical changes are limited in most cases, although denervation atrophy may be present in cases of longstanding. Focal collections of small lymphocytes (lymphorrhages) have been found repeatedly around necrotic fibres but are often lacking. Lymphoid hyperplasia of the thymus is frequently found.

CLINICAL FEATURES OF THE JUVENILE FORM
The onset of symptoms is always after 1 year of age and adolescent girls are most often affected (Oosterhuis 1989). The onset may be insidious or sudden, often following an acute febrile illness. In the *generalized form*, onset is usually marked by involvement of the extraocular muscles, with unilateral or asymmetrical ophthalmoplegia and ptosis (Afifi and Bell 1993). Involvement rapidly extends to proximal limbs and bulbar muscles which may cause difficulty in swallowing. Involvement of the lower limbs is less common but may cause diagnostic

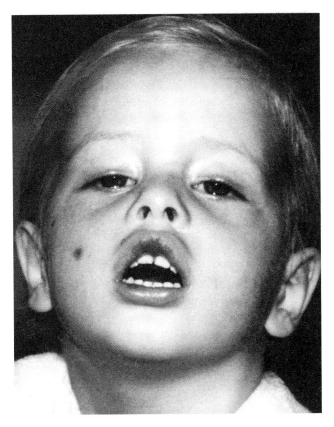

difficulties in the rare cases in which it represents the first manifestation of the disease (Drachman 1994).

In other cases, the spread from ocular muscles to the body muscles is clearly secondary after several weeks, months or years. In 20–40 per cent of patients weakness remains limited to the extraocular mucles without involvement of bulbar or limb muscles.

In all cases, myasthenic weakness is characterized by its variability, at least during the initial phase of the disease. This is an essential diagnostic clue that should be carefully enquired about as it may not be obvious. Many patients may only complain of increasing fatigue. The patients feel normal on awakening but fatigue and weakness appear following muscular exercise and are more marked towards the end of the day. By the evening the children may have difficulty chewing and choke on food.

The natural course of juvenile myasthenia gravis is variable. The course tends to be slowly progressive with marked fluctuation. About half the patients experience one or more remissions. In others, the symptoms initially progress, later becoming stationary. In some untreated patients, weakness becomes fixed with some degree of muscle wasting. In 20–40 per cent of patients, involvement remains limited to the extraocular muscles (Afifi and Bell 1993, Sommer *et al.* 1997). Myasthenic crises with increased weakness and especially with involvement of respiratory muscles may occur spontaneously or following febrile illnesses. They may require assisted ventilation and intubation or even lead to death.

Rodriguez *et al.* (1983) observed spontaneous remissions in 30 per cent of patients after a 15-year follow-up, but in patients with extremity weakness the remission rate was significantly lower.

A more benign type of early onset (mainly in the first two years of life) and limited in 80 per cent of cases to the extraocular muscles is frequently observed in Oriental children (Wong *et al.* 1992).

DIAGNOSIS
The diagnosis of the juvenile form can be confirmed by three main types of investigation.

(1) The edrophonium chloride (Tensilon) test consists in observing the response to intravenous administration of this short-acting anticholinesterase agent. The dose varies with age from 1mg in infants to up to 8mg in older children. A test dose of 1 or 2mg is given first, the rest being injected after 30 seconds if there is no response. This should be evident within one minute and does not last more than 5–10 minutes. Taking photographs of the child before and one minute after injection allows objective documentation of any change (Fig. 22.11). Subcutaneous atropine before injection neutralizes the muscarinic effects of the drug. Serious side-effects may occur in rare cases so the test should always be performed with resuscitation equipment available. Intramuscular neostigmine may also be used (0.04 mg/kg). The effect is obtained more slowly, starting after 10–15 minutes and reaching a maximum at 30 minutes. Tests using anticholinesterase agents can be negative in confirmed cases of myasthenia,

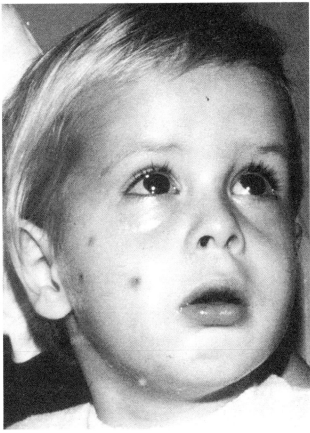

Fig. 22.11. Myasthenia gravis in 3-year-old boy. *(Top)* Note asymmetrical ptosis, open mouth and lack of expression. *(Bottom)* Three minutes after i.v. administration of 8mg of edrophonium chloride (Tensilon): complete disappearance of all previous abnormalities.

especially in ocular forms (Seybold 1986); conversely, a positive test is nonspecific and should not be the only basis of diagnosis (Drachman 1994, Sommer *et al.* 1997).

(2) Electromyography is another manner of confirming the diagnosis by evidencing the presence of a neuromuscular block (Oh *et al.* 1992). Repetitive stimulation at 3–20 Hz induces a decrement in amplitude of more than 20 per cent from the third to the fifth response. Faster stimulation (50 Hz) produces the same decrement instead of the normal potentiation and an increase in the latency of the responses. Repetition of the EMG following injection of edrophonium shows correction of the abnormalities. EMG is also important to determine the extension of the disorder. In many cases apparently limited to eye muscles, EMG abnormalities are present in limb muscles (especially the extensor digitorum brevis), indicating that the disease is in fact generalized. Single-fibre EMG to demonstrate increased 'jitter' in contraction of pairs of fibres is more sensitive than classical EMG but difficult to perform in children.

(3) Demonstration of the presence of antibodies directed against acetylcholine receptors by radioimmunoassay can be made in 60–80 per cent of juvenile cases (Tindall 1981). Seronegative cases of myasthenia do not appear to be clinically distinct from seropositive ones (Soliven *et al.* 1988), although seronegativity is more frequent in ocular myasthenia. Some seronegative patients have evidence of impaired neuromuscular transmission mediated by immunoglobulins directed against other antigenic determinants than the acetylcholine receptor (Mossman *et al.* 1986). The antibody titre declines in successfully treated patients.

The choice of a diagnostic test largely depends on the experience of each institution. Tensilon test is regarded as the best test by some (Affi and Bell 1993), while others found electrical stimulation more useful in different cases (Oh *et al.* 1992).

Differential diagnosis includes other neuromuscular disorders in which fatiguability can sometimes be marked, and rare cases of myasthenic syndromes, especially resulting from the use of agents such as penicillamine, carnitine and aminoglycosides. Structural lesions of the midbrain such as tumours may be responsible for fatiguable ptosis and ophthalmoplegia and thus mimic myasthenia, but complete neurological examination shows additional defects (Ragge and Hoyt 1992).

TREATMENT
The aims of treatment are to improve neuromuscular transmission through the use of anticholinesterase agents and to prevent continuing immunological interference with synthesis, maintenance and catabolism of acetylcholine receptors by immunosuppressive therapy, plasma exchange or thymectomy.

The treatment of immunologically determined myasthenia gravis is usually started by the use of *anticholinesterase agents*. These drugs increase the half-life of acetylcholine released into the synaptic cleft by inhibiting its hydrolysis by acetylcholinesterase, thus increasing the probability of acetylcholine molecules reaching the reduced number of receptors (Drachman 1994). Commonly used anticholinergic drugs include neostigmine,

pyridostigmine and ambenomium. The initial dose of neostigmine is 0.5 mg/kg every four hours in children younger than 5 years and 0.25 mg/kg in older children, not to exceed 15 mg per dose. The equivalent doses of pyridostigmine and ambenomium are four times the dose of neostigmine. The dose should be slowly increased as a function of the response and needs. Overdose may result in diaphoresis, nausea, vomiting and abdominal cramps, bradycardia and miosis. It may also produce an increased muscle weakness (cholinergic crises). Theoretically, administration of edrophonium can separate cholinergic from myasthenic crises, but the evaluation may be impossible, and in severe cases assisted ventilation and weaning from drugs may be necessary.

The long-term use of anticholinergic drugs may damage the endplate region of the neuromuscular junction in animals and produce a state not unlike myasthenia itself (Hudson *et al.* 1978).

There is currently a trend toward the use of immunosuppression or thymectomy rather than anticholinesterase drugs which rarely produce complete normality and have undesirable long-term effects. Most of the experience is in adults (Newsom-Davis 1994), and extrapolation to children may be hazardous as no controlled comparative studies are available in this age group (Dubowitz 1995).

Corticosteroid treatment is usually with oral prednisone in doses of 1–2 mg/kg/d (daily or on an alternate-day schedule) until a good response is sustained, followed by progressive tapering. Cholinesterase inhibitors are used as needed during steroid administration. Exacerbation of myasthenic symptoms is not rare at the beginning of steroid therapy. In order to avoid this, some investigators prefer to use gradually incremented doses on an alternate-day therapy regime until an effect is obtained, then maintaining the effective dose for a three month period before tapering (Newsom-Davis 1994). High-dose pulses of methylprednisolone is an alternative method (Sakano *et al.* 1989) which has been used successfully in children with refractory disease.

For cases that do not respond to steroids, azathioprine may be used in conjunction with steroids or in isolation, with satisfactory results (Myasthenia Gravis Study Group 1993). There is some evidence in adults that long-term immunosuppressive treatment and thymectomy may prevent generalization of localized disease (Sommer *et al.* 1997). Intravenous immunoglobulin has given promising results in a few children (Sakano *et al.* 1989). Cyclosporine seems to be effective in adults (Tindall *et al.* 1987). Plasma exchange can produce rapid but short-lived improvement and has been used for the treatment of myasthenic crises, and for pre- and postoperative support (Snead *et al.* 1987, Stricker *et al.* 1993). Recent work (Gajdos *et al.* 1997) suggests that administration of immunoglobulins may be as effective as plasma exchange and is easier to perform especially in children.

Thymectomy is usually considered when stabilization has been obtained but may also be performed once a diagnosis of severe or moderate disease has been made. It frequently results in significant and lasting improvement, although long-term therapy remains necessary in many cases. It may be the treatment

TABLE 22.5
Myasthenic syndromes in childhood

Disorder*	Neurophysiological type*	Clinical features	Genetics	References
Defect in ACh resynthesis and packaging (familial infantile myasthenia)	Presynaptic defect Decremental response, normal AChR	Ptosis, apnoea, sudden death, no extraocular involvement, neonatal onset	AR	Engel (1994)
Paucity of synaptic vesicles and reduced ACh release	Presynaptic defect Decremental response	Respiratory difficulties from birth, no extraocular involvement	AR	Walls et al. (1993)
Endplate AChE deficiency	Pre- and postsynaptic defect Repetitive potentials on single-nerve stimulation	Neonatal onset, ptosis, ophthalmoparesis and diffuse weakness, negative Tensilon test	AR	Hutchinson et al. (1993)
Reduced number of AChRs	Postsynaptic defect Decremental response at slow-speed stimulation, single response to stimulation	Respiratory distress, ptosis, feeding difficulties, positive Tensilon test	AR	Smit et al. (1988), Wokke et al. (1989)
Slow channel syndrome (+ variant with epsilon subunit mutation)	Postsynaptic defect Repetitive potentials on single-nerve stimulation, decremental response	Onset <2y, limb weakness with slow progressive ptosis, variable Tensilon reponse	AD	Engel (1988) Engel (1994)
High-conductance fast channel syndrome	Postsynaptic defect Single response to nerve stimulation	Neonatal onset, extraocular weakness	?	Engel et al. (1993)
Abnormal ACh–AChR interaction	Postsynaptic defect Single response to nerve stimulation	Neonatal or childhood onset, ocular weakness absent	?	Uchitel et al. (1993)
AChR deficiency with paucity of secondary synaptic clefts	Postsynaptic? Partially characterized, single response to nerve stimulation	Onset <2y, extraocular involvement	AR	Engel (1994)
Other AChR deficiencies	Postsynaptic? Partially characterized	Onset <2y	?	Shillito et al. (1993)

*ACh = acetylcholine; AChE = acetylcholine esterase; AChR = acetylcholine receptor.

of choice for children because of the possible side-effects of long-term treatment with anticholinesterasic agents or immunosuppressants. For children, it increases significantly the remission rate up to 67 per cent (Adams et al. 1990). Most remissions occur during the first postoperative year. In a recent study (Lindner et al. 1997) of 79 patients with juvenile-onset myasthenia (onset 12–18 years), 65 received thymectomy, usually in association with immunosuppressive treatment. Thirty-nine (60 per cent) of these went into remission, as against only four of 14 nonoperated patients, thus suggesting the value of thymectomy in such cases.

TRANSIENT NEONATAL MYASTHENIA
Approximately 10–15 per cent of infants born to myasthenic mothers are affected by transient neonatal myasthenia gravis. The disorder is due to the transfer of antibodies directed against acetylcholine receptors from the maternal to the fetal circulation. It is not clear why only some infants are clinically affected whereas all have high antibody titres, and there is no relation between the severity of maternal disease and involvement of the infant. However, mothers with a high titre of antibodies specifically directed against the fetal type of acetylcholine receptors are more likely to give birth to further affected infants following a first affected baby, and the ratio of antibodies against fetal vs adult type receptors in maternal serum is a reliable predictor of neonatal disease (Gardnerova et al. 1997).

The clinical features of transient myasthenia are usually distinctive (Papazian 1992). The onset is delayed to a few hours after birth, sometimes as long as three days and is marked by hypotonia, feeding difficulties due to poor sucking and/or swallowing, poor crying and facial diplegia. Ptosis is present in only a minority of cases. Respiratory distress requiring mechanical ventilation may be present in some infants. These features permit an easy diagnosis when myasthenia is known in the mother, but maternal disease can be latent in some cases. The diagnosis can be confirmed by intramuscular or subcutaneous injection of Tensilon (1 mg), which can also be given intravenously with initial administration of a test dose of 0.03 mg/kg followed by repeated fractional doses to a maximum of 0.15 mg/kg, or by electrical stimulation.

Treatment with neostigmine: 0.1 mg prior to feeding is often sufficient to permit adequate nutrition. In severe forms with respiratory distress and/or profound hypotonia, exchange transfusion may be indicated (Pasternak et al. 1981).

In some atypical cases marked hypotonia and weakness may persist well beyond the first three or four weeks, up to several months (Morel et al. 1988).

Neonatal myasthenic arthrogryposis with respiratory distress, hydramnios during pregnancy, and a high rate of stillbirth and neonatal death has been observed often as a recurrent condition even when there were initially no obvious signs of maternal disease (Barnes et al. 1995). Such cases can be associated with the presence of antibodies directed against fetal acetylcholine receptors (Vincent *et al.* 1994).

CONGENITAL AND FAMILIAL MYASTHENIA GRAVIS

These genetic forms of myasthenia are not antibody-mediated (Misulis and Fenichel 1989). They are the expression of several different defects in neuromuscular transmission. Their classification is still tentative (Engel 1994) and their exact diagnosis often requires sophisticated techniques that are only available in very few laboratories. The main types are listed in Table 22.5. All these syndromes, with the exception of the dominantly inherited slow channel syndrome, are probably recessively transmitted.

It is convenient to classify these disorders according to the site and mechanism of the transmission defect (Misulis and Fenichel 1989, Engel 1994) into presynaptic and postsynaptic defects, but some cases may share both mechanisms and several are only partially characterized.

The clinical picture is also heterogeneous. In about half the cases, symptoms are present at birth or appear within the first two years of life. In some of these, there is a history of reduced fetal movements. In general, presynaptic defects tend to present in a relatively homogeneous manner with the features of the familial infantile form, while postsynaptic defects exhibit considerable phenotypic variability and usually produce milder symptoms. Some cases may be associated with facial dysmorphism and be limited to certain ethnic groups (Goldhammer *et al.* 1990).

Familial infantile myasthenia is characterized by hypotonia from birth with variable but sometimes severe weakness, so that assisted ventilation may be required. In contrast, extraocular motility is usually normal although facial muscles may be involved. The course is fluctuating. Hypotonia and weakness often improve within a few weeks of birth, but repeated episodes of weakness, at times with life-threatening apnoeic episodes, may supervene. Apnoea may occur in isolation without premonitory weakness. The disease lasts throughout infancy and childhood (Albers *et al.* 1984) and may even sometimes persist up to adult life. Although this phenotype is characteristically associated with a presynaptic defect and especially with deficient acetylcholine resynthesis and packaging, clinical manifestations are quite variable and different phenotypes may be observed even within the same sibship (Vincent *et al.* 1981). In most patients with congenital myasthenias no antibodies are present in blood and the response to Tensilon is variable. The response to treatment depends on the defect. It is usually good in familial infantile myasthenia in which treatment may have to be continued throughout childhood to prevent sudden apnoeic episodes.

LAMBERT–EATON SYNDROME AND OTHER DEFECTS IN NEUROMUSCULAR TRANSMISSION
THE LAMBERT–EATON SYNDROME
This syndrome that is mainly due to visceral malignancies in adult patients (O'Neill *et al.* 1988) is extremely rare in children. It is due to a presynaptic block. The major characteristic of this myasthenic syndrome is the marked increase in the amplitude

of evoked muscle potentials on 50 Hz stimulation of the motor nerve, which contrasts with the occurrence of a decrement at slow (3–10 Hz) stimulation. A congenital form has been reported (Bady *et al.* 1987).

A few cases of muscular disorders affecting the proximal muscles with weakness and wasting in a limb–girdle distribution, associated with myasthenic features, are on record (Husain *et al.* 1989). Limb weakness in such cases of limb–girdle myasthenia responds to injection of edrophonium. The EMG indicates a combination of myopathic features and decremental response to repetitive stimulation. Some cases are familial with apparently autosomal recessive inheritance. Tubular aggregates have been described in some patients.

OTHER NEUROMUSCULAR BLOCKS
These have been reviewed in detail by Swift (1981). Agents that impair neuromuscular transmission at a presynaptic level include immunosuppressants, arthropod venoms, and some insect bites. Such agents may reveal a latent myasthenia. At a postsynaptic level several snake venoms and several drugs including phenytoin, trimethadione and many antibiotics can produce a neuromuscular block. This applies especially to polymyxins B and E, and to aminoglycosides, in particular neomycin and clindamycin, and possibly to ampicillin (Argov *et al.* 1986). D,L-carnitine has been reported to induce a myasthenia-like syndrome (Bazzato *et al.* 1981). Such drugs may be the cause of postoperative apnoeic episodes, especially when used in combinations with muscle relaxants. Calcium infusions and anticholinesterase drugs may be an effective treatment in some but not all cases. Magnesium intoxication acts antagonistically to calcium at the neuromuscular junction.

A prolonged myasthenic syndrome has been reported in patients treated with muscle relaxants (Benzing *et al.* 1990).

REFERENCES

Abarbanel, J.M., Potashnik, R., Frisher, S., *et al.* (1987) 'Myophosphorylase deficiency: the course of an unusual congenital myopathy.' *Neurology*, **37**, 316–318.

Adams, C., Theodorescu, D., Murphy, G., Shandling, B. (1990) 'Thymectomy in juvenile myasthenia gravis.' *Journal of Child Neurology*, **5**, 216–218.

Afifi, A.K., Bell, W.E. (1993) 'Tests for juvenile myasthenia gravis: comparative diagnostic yield and prediction of outcome.' *Journal of Child Neurology*, **8**, 404–411.

Aicardi, J., Conti, D., Goutières, F. (1974) 'Les formes néonatales de la dystrophie myotonique de Steinert.' *Journal of the Neurological Sciences*, **22**, 149–164.

Albers, J.W., Faulkner, J.A., Dorovini-Zis, K., *et al.* (1984) 'Abnormal neuromuscular transmission in an infantile myasthenic syndrome.' *Annals of Neurology*, **16**, 28–34.

Andrews, P.I., Massey, J.M., Sanders, D.B. (1993) 'Acetylcholine receptor antibodies in juvenile myasthenia gravis.' *Neurology*, **43**, 977–982.

Angelini, C., Philippart, M., Borrone, C., *et al.* (1980) 'Multisystem triglyceride storage disorder with impaired long-chain fatty acid oxidation.' *Annals of Neurology*, **7**, 5–10.

Argov, Z., Brenner, T., Abramsky, O. (1986) 'Ampicillin may aggravate clinical and experimental myasthenia gravis.' *Archives of Neurology*, **43**, 255–256.

Ashizawa, T., Butler, I.J., Harati, Y., Roongta, S.M. (1983) 'A dominantly inherited syndrome with continuous motor neuron discharges.' *Annals of Neurology*, **13**, 285–290.

Ashwal, S., Peckham, N. (1985) 'Myoadenylate deaminase deficiency in children.' *Pediatric Neurology*, **1**, 185–188.

Auger, R.G., Daube, J.R., Gomez, M.R., Lambert, E.H. (1984) 'Hereditary form of sustained muscle activity of peripheral nerve origin causing generalised myokymia and muscle weakness.' *Annals of Neurology*, **15**, 13–21.

Azibi, K., Bachner, L., Beckmann, J.S., *et al.* (1993) 'Severe childhood autosomal recessive muscular dystrophy with the deficiency of the 50 kDa dystrophin-associated glycoprotein maps to chromosome 13q12.' *Human Molecular Genetics*, **2**, 1423–1428.

Bach, J.R., O'Brien, J., Krotenberg, R., Alba, A.S. (1987) 'Management of end stage respiratory failure in Duchenne muscular dystrophy.' *Muscle and Nerve*, **10**, 177–182.

Bady, B., Chauplannaz, G., Carrier, H. (1987) 'Congenital Lambert–Eaton myasthenic syndrome.' *Journal of Neurology, Neurosurgery, and Psychiatry*, **50**, 476–478.

Bailey, R.O., Marzulo, D.C., Harris, M.B. (1986) 'Infantile facioscapulohumeral muscular dystrophy: new observations.' *Acta Neurologica Scandinavica*, **74**, 51–58.

Baker, E.M., Khorasgani, G., Gardner-Medwin, D., *et al.* (1996) 'Arthrogryposis multiplex congenita and bilateral parietal polymicrogyria in association with intrauterine death of a twin.' *Neuropediatrics*, **27**, 54–56.

Bakker, H.D., Scholte, H.R., Jeneson, J.A.L., *et al.* (1994) 'Vitamin-responsive complex I deficiency in a myopathic patient with increased activity of the terminal respiratory chain and lactic acidosis.' *Journal of Inherited Metabolic Disease*, **17**, 196–204.

Banker, B.Q. (1994) 'Congenital deformities.' *In*: Engel, A.G., Franzini-Armstrong, C. (Eds.) *Myology, Basic and Clinical. 2nd Edn.* New York: McGraw Hill, pp. 1905–1937.

Baquero, J.L., Ayala, R.A., Wang, J., *et al.* (1995) 'Hyperkalemic periodic paralysis with cardiac dysrhythmia: a novel sodium channel mutation?' *Annals of Neurology*, **37**, 408–411.

Barnes, P.R., Kanabar, D.J., Brueton, L., *et al.* (1995) 'Recurrent congenital arthrogryposis leading to a diagnosis of myasthenia gravis in an initially asymptomatic mother.' *Neuromuscular Disorders*, **5**, 59–65.

Barohn, R.J., Levine, E.J., Olson, J.O., Mendell, J.R. (1988) 'Gastric hypomotility in Duchenne's muscular dystrophy.' *New England Journal of Medicine*, **319**, 15–18.

Barth, P.G., van Wijngaarden, G.K., Bethlem, J. (1975) 'X-linked myotubular myopathy with fatal neonatal asphyxia.' *Neurology*, **25**, 531–536..

Bautista, J., Rafael, E., Castilla, J.M., Alberca, R. (1978) 'Hereditary distal myopathy with onset in early infancy: observation of a family.' *Journal of the Neurological Sciences*, **37**, 149–158.

Bazzato, C., Coli, U., Landini, S., *et al.* (1981) 'Myasthenia-like syndrome after D,L- but not L-carnitine.' *Lancet*, **1**, 1209. *(Letter.)*

Beckmann, J.S., Richard, I., Hillaire, D., *et al.* (1991) 'A gene for limb–girdle muscular dystrophy maps to chromosome 15 by linkage.' *Comptes Rendus de l'Académie des Sciences*, **312**, 141–148.

Ben Hamida, M., Fardeau, M., Attia, N. (1983) 'Severe childhood muscular dystrophy affecting both sexes and frequent in Tunisia.' *Muscle and Nerve*, **6**, 469–480.

Benzing, G., Iannacone, S.T., Bove, K.E., *et al.* (1990) 'Prolonged myasthenic syndrome after one week of muscle relaxants.' *Pediatric Neurology*, **6**, 190–196.

Bergia, B., Sybers, H.D., Butler, I.J. (1986) 'Familial lethal cardiomyopathy with mental retardation and scapuloperoneal muscular atrophy.' *Journal of Neurology, Neurosurgery, and Psychiatry*, **49**, 1423–1426.

Berkowitz, A., Rosenberg, H. (1985) 'Femoral block with mepivacaine for muscle biopsy in malignant hyperthermia patients.' *Anaesthesiology*, **62**, 651–652.

Bernsen, P.L.J.A., Gabreëls, F.J.M., Ruitenbeek, W., *et al.* (1991) 'Successful treatment of pure myopathy, associated with complex I deficiency, with riboflavin and carnitine.' *Archives of Neurology*, **48**, 334–338.

Black, J.T., Garcia-Mullin, R., Good, E., Brown, S. (1972) 'Muscle rigidity in a newborn due to continuous peripheral nerve hyperactivity.' *Annals of Neurology*, **27**, 413–425.

Blaszczyk, M., Jablonska, S., Szymanska-Jagiello, W., *et al.* (1991) 'Childhood scleromyositis: an overlap syndrome associated with PM-Scl antibody.' *Pediatric Dermatology*, **8**, 1–8.

Bohan, A., Peter, J.B. (1975) 'Polymyositis and dermatomyositis.' *New England Journal of Medicine*, **292**, 344–347; 403–407.

Bohlega, S., Tanji, K., Santorelli, F.M., *et al.* (1996) 'Multiple mitochondrial DNA deletions associated with autosomal recessive ophthalmoplegia and severe cardiomyopathy.' *Neurology*, **46**, 1329–1334.

Bonilla, E., Samitt, C.E., Miranda, A.F., *et al.* (1988) 'Duchenne muscular dystrophy: deficiency of dystrophin at the muscle cell surface.' *Cell*, **54**, 447–452.

Bove, K.E., Iannaccone, S.T., Hilton, P.K., Samaha, F. (1980) 'Cylindrical spirals in a familial neuromuscular disorder.' *Annals of Neurology*, **7**, 550–556.

Bowyer, S.L., Blane, C.E., Sullivan, D.B., Cassidy, J.T. (1983) 'Childhood dermatomyositis: factors predicting functional outcome and development of dystrophic calcification.' *Journal of Pediatrics*, **103**, 882–888.

Boylan, K.B., Ferriero, D.M., Greco, C.M., *et al.* (1992) 'Congenital hypomyelination neuropathy with arthrogryposis multiplex congenita.' *Annals of Neurology*, **31**, 337–340.

Braakhekke, J.P., De Bruin, M.I., Stegeman, D.F., *et al.* (1986) 'The second wind phenomenon in McArdle's disease.' *Brain*, **109**, 1087–1101.

Breningstall, G.N., Grover, W.D., Barbera, S., Marks, H.G. (1988) 'Neonatal rhabdomyolysis as a presentation of muscular dystrophy.' *Neurology*, **38**, 1271–1272.

Bresolin, N., Bet, L., Moggio, M., *et al.* (1989) 'Muscle glucose-6-phosphate dehydrogenase deficiency.' *Journal of Neurology*, **236**, 193–198.

Brooke, M.H., Carroll, J.E., Ringel, S.P. (1979) 'Congenital hypotonia revisited.' *Muscle and Nerve*, **2**, 84–100.

—— Fenichel, G.M., Griggs, R.C., *et al.* (1989) 'Duchenne muscular dystrophy: patterns of clinical progression and effects of supportive therapy.' *Neurology*, **39**, 475–481.

Brunt, E.R.P., van Weerden, T.W. (1990) 'Familial paroxysmal kinesigenic ataxia and continuous myokymia.' *Brain*, **113**, 1361–1382.

Bryan, W., Lewis, S.F., Bertocci, I., *et al.* (1990) 'Muscle lactate dehydrogenase deficiency: a disorder of anaerobic glycogenolysis associated with exertional myoglobinuria.' *Neurology*, **40**, Suppl. 1, 203. *(Abstract.)*

Buchta, R.M., (1977) 'Myositis and influenza.' *Pediatrics*, **60**, 761–762.

Burns, A.P. (1993) 'Rhabdomyolysis and acute renal failure in unsuspected malignant hyperthermia.' *Quarterly Journal of Medicine*, **86**, 431–434.

Burns, R.J., Bretag, A.H., Blumbergs, P.C., Harbord, M.G. (1994) 'Benign familial disease with muscle mounding and rippling.' *Journal of Neurology, Neurosurgery, and Psychiatry*, **57**, 344–347.

Bushby, K.M.D., Gardner-Medwin, D. (1993) 'The clinical, genetic and dystrophin characteristics of Becker muscular dystrophy. I. Natural history.' *Journal of Neurology*, **240**, 98–104.

—— —— Nicholson, L.V.B., *et al.* (1993) 'The clinical, genetic and dystrophin characteristics of Becker muscular dystrophy. II. Correlation of phenotype with genetic and protein abnormalities.' *Journal of Neurology*, **240**, 105–112.

Byrne, E., Blumbergs, P.C., Hallpike, J.F. (1982) 'Central core disease. Study of a family with five affected generations.' *Journal of the Neurological Sciences*, **53**, 77–83.

—— Dennett, X., Trounce, I., Henderson, R. (1985) 'Partial cytochrome oxidase (aa3) deficiency in chronic progressive external ophthalmoplegia. Histochemical and biochemical studies.' *Journal of the Neurological Sciences*, **71**, 257–271.

—— —— Crotty, B., *et al.* (1986) 'Dominantly inherited cardioskeletal myopathy with lysosomal glycogen storage and normal acid maltase levels.' *Brain*, **109**, 523–536.

Cameron, P.F. (1983) 'Strained abdominal muscles as a cause of acute abdominal pain in children and young adults and its treatment with Paramax.' *British Journal of Clinical Practice*, **37**, 178–180.

Cao, A., Cianchetti, C., Calisti, L., *et al.* (1978) 'Schwartz–Jampel syndrome: clinical, electrophysiological and histopathological study of a severe variant.' *Journal of the Neurological Sciences*, **35**, 175–187.

Chakrabarti, A., Pearce, J.M.S. (1981) 'Scapuloperoneal syndrome with cardiomyopathy: report of a family with autosomal dominant inheritance and unusual features.' *Journal of Neurology, Neurosurgery, and Psychiatry*, **44**, 1146–1152.

Chamberlain, M.C. (1991) 'Rhabdomyolysis in children: a 3-year retrospective study.' *Pediatric Neurology*, **7**, 226–228.

Chapon, F., Viader, F., Fardeau, M., *et al.* (1989) 'Myopathie familiale avec inclusions de type "corps cytoplasmiques" (ou "sphéroïdes") révélée par une insuffisance respiratoire.' *Revue Neurologique*, **145**, 460–465.

Charnas, L., Trapp, B., Griffin, J. (1988) 'Congenital absence of peripheral myelin: abnormal Schwann cell development causes lethal arthrogryposis mutiplex congenita.' *Neurology*, **38**, 966–974.

Chen, S.S., Chien, C.H., Yu, H.S. (1988) 'Syndrome of deltoid and/or gluteal fibrotic contracture: an injection myopathy.' *Acta Neurologica Scandinavica*, **78**, 167–176.

Chui, L.A., Munsat, T.L. (1976) 'Dominant inheritance of McArdle syndrome.' *Archives of Neurology*, **33**, 636–641.

Clancy, R.R., Kelts, K.A., Oehlert, J.W. (1980) 'Clinical variability in congenital fiber type disproportion.' *Journal of the Neurological Sciences*, **46**, 257–266.

Cole, A.J., Kuzniecky, R., Karpati, G., *et al.* (1988) 'Familial myopathy with changes resembling inclusion body myositis and periventricular leuco-encephalopathy. A new syndrome.' *Brain*, **111**, 1025–1037.

Comi, G., Testa, D., Cornelio, F., Comola, M., Canal, N. (1985) 'Potassium depletion myopathy: a clinical and morphological study of 6 cases.' *Muscle and Nerve*, **8**, 17–21.

—— Prelle, A., Bresolin, N., *et al.* (1994) 'Clinical variability in Becker muscular dystrophy. Genetic, biochemical and immunohistochemical correlates.' *Brain*, **117**, 1–14.

Dalakas, M.C., Engel, W.K. (1987) 'Prednisone-responsive limb–girdle syndrome: a special disorder?' *Neuropediatrics*, **18**, 88–90.

—— Illa, I., Pezeshkpour, G.H., *et al.* (1990) 'Mitochondrial myopathy caused by long-term zidovudine therapy.' *New England Journal of Medicine*, **322**, 1098–1105.

—— —— Damibrosia, J.M., *et al.* (1993) 'A controlled trial of high-dose in-travenous immune globulin infusions as treatment for dermatomyositis.' *New England Journal of Medicine*, **329**, 1993–2000.

Danek, A., Witt, T.N., Stockmann, H.B.A.C., *et al.* (1990) 'Normal dystrophin in McLeod myopathy.' *Annals of Neurology*, **28**, 720–722.

—— Uttner, I., Vogl, T., *et al.* (1994) 'Cerebral involvement in McLeod syndrome.' *Neurology*, **44**, 117–120.

Danon, M.J., Oh, S.J., DiMauro, S. (1981) 'Lysosomal glycogen storage disease with normal acid maltase.' *Neurology*, **31**, 51–57.

—— DiMauro, S., Shanske, S., *et al.* (1986) 'Juvenile-onset acid maltase deficiency with unusual familial features.' *Neurology*, **36**, 818–822.

—— Karpati, G., Charuk, J., Holland, P. (1988) 'Sarcoplasmic reticulum adenosine triphosphatase deficiency with probable autosomal dominant inheritance.' *Neurology*, **38**, 812–815.

Daras, M., Spiro, A.J. (1981) ''Stiff-man syndrome' in an adolescent.' *Pediatrics*, **67**, 725–726.

Darwish, H., Sarnat, H., Archer, C., *et al.* (1981) 'Congenital cervical spinal atrophy.' *Muscle and Nerve*, **4**, 106–110.

De Angelis, M.S., Palmucci, L., Leone, M., Doriguzzi, C. (1991) 'Centro-nuclear myopathy: clinical, morphological and genetic characters. A review of 288 cases.' *Journal of the Neurological Sciences*, **103**, 2–9.

De Grandis, D., Bertolasi, L., Polo, A. (1988) 'Activité musculaire continue: aspects cliniques et neurophysiologiques différents du syndrome d'Isaacs.' *Revue Neurologique*, **144**, 447–451.

De Lange, C. (1934) 'Congenital hypertrophy of the muscles, extrapyramidal motor disturbances and mental deficiency. A clinical entity.' *American Journal of Diseases of Children*, **48**, 243–268.

De Paillette, L., Aicardi, J., Goutières, F. (1989) 'Ullrich's congenital atonic sclerotic muscular dystrophy: a case report.' *Journal of Neurology*, **236**, 108–110.

De Stefano, N., Dotti, M.T., Villanova, M., *et al.* (1996) 'Merosin positive congenital muscular dystrophy with severe involvement of the central nervous system.' *Brain and Development*, **18**, 323–326.

De Visser, M., Verbeeten, B. (1985) 'Computed tomography of the skeletal musculature in Becker-type muscular dystrophy and benign infantile spinal muscular atrophy.' *Muscle and Nerve*, **8**, 435–444.

—— de Voogt, W.G., La Rivière, G.V. (1992) 'The heart in Becker muscular dystrophy, facioscapulohumeral dystrophy and Bethlem myopathy.' *Muscle and Nerve*, **15**, 591–596.

DiBona, F.J., Morens, D.M. (1977) 'Rhabdomyolysis associated with influenza A. Report of a case with unusual fluid and electrolyte abnormalities.' *Journal of Pediatrics*, **91**, 943–945.

DiDonato, S., Gellera, C., Peluchetti, D., *et al.* (1989) 'Normalization of short-chain acylcoenzyme A dehydrogenase after riboflavin treatment in a girl with multiple acylcoenzyme A dehydrogenase-deficient myopathy.' *Annals of Neurology*, **25**, 479–484.

Dietzman, D.E., Schaller, J.G., Ray, C.G., Reed, M.E. (1976) 'Acute myositis associated with influenza B infection.' *Pediatrics*, **57**, 255–258.

DiMauro, S. (1993) 'Mitochondrial encephalomyopathies.' *In:* Rosenberg, R.N., Prusiner, S.B., DiMauro, S. (Eds.) *The Molecular and Genetic Basis of Neurological Disease*. Boston: Butterworth-Heinemann, pp. 665–694.

—— Tsujino, S. (1994) 'Phosphorylase deficiency.' *In:* Engel, A.G., Franzini-Armstrong, C. (Eds.) *Myology, Basic and Clinical. 2nd Edn*. New York: McGraw Hill, pp. 1557–1561.

—— Dalakas, M., Miranda, A.F. (1981) 'Phosphoglycerate kinase deficiency: a new cause of recurrent myoglobinuria.' *Annals of Neurology*, **10**, 90. *(Abstract.)*

—— Miranda, A.F., Olarte, M., Friedman, R. Hays, A.P. (1982) 'Muscle phos-phoglycerate mutase deficiency.' *Neurology*, **32**, 584–591.

Di Rocco, M., Callea, F., Pollice, B., *et al.* (1995) 'Arthrogryposis, renal dysfunction and cholestasis syndrome: report of five patients from three Italian families.' *European Journal of Pediatrics*, **154**, 835–839.

Donley, D.K., Evans, B.K. (1989) 'Reversible neuromuscular syndrome in malnourished children.' *Developmental Medicine and Child Neurology*, **31**, 797–803.

Donner, M., Rapola, J., Somer, H. (1975) 'Congenital muscular dystrophy: a clinico-pathological and follow-up study of 15 patients.' *Neuropädiatrie*, **6**, 239–258.

Doriguzzi, C., Palmucci, L., Mongini, T., *et al.* (1993) 'Exercise intolerance and recurrent myoglobinuria as the only expression of Xp21 Becker type muscular dystrophy.' *Journal of Neurology*, **240**, 269–271.

Dorman, C., DesNoyers Hurley, A., D'Avignon, J. (1988) 'Language and learning disorders of older boys with Duchenne muscular dystrophy.' *Developmental Medicine and Child Neurology*, **30**, 316–327.

Drachman, D.B. (1994) 'Myasthenia gravis.' *New England Journal of Medicine*, **330**, 1797–1810.

Dubowitz, V. (1991) 'Prednisone in Duchenne dystrophy.' *Neuromuscular Disorders*, **1**, 161–163.

—— (1995) *Muscle Disorders in Childhood, 2nd Edn*. London: W.B. Saunders.

—— Crome, L. (1969) 'The central nervous system in Duchenne muscular dystrophy.' *Brain*, **92**, 505–508.

Duggan, D.J., Gorospe, J.R., Fanin, M., *et al.* (1997) 'Mutations in the sarco-glycan genes in patients with myopathy.' *New England Journal of Medicine*, **336**, 618–624.

Echenne, B., Arthuis, M., Billard, C., *et al.* (1986) 'Congenital muscular dystrophy and cerebral CT anomalies. Results of a collaborative study of the Société de Neurologie Infantile.' *Journal of the Neurological Sciences*, **75**, 7–22.

Ellis, F.R. (1992) 'Detecting susceptibility to malignant hyperthermia.' *British Medical Journal*, **304**, 791–792.

—— Clarke, I.M.C., Appleyard, T.N., Dinsdale, R.C.W. (1975) 'Malignant hyperpyrexia induced by nitrous oxide successfully treated by steroids.' *British Journal of Anaesthesia*, **47**, 632. *(Abstract.)*

Emanuel, B.S., Zackai, E.H., Tucker, S.H. (1983) 'Further evidence for Xp21 location of Duchenne muscular (DMD) locus: X;9 translocation in a female with DMD.' *Journal of Medical Genetics*, **20**, 461–463.

Emser, W. (1982) 'Hypermagnesemic periodic paralysis: treatment with digitalis and lithium carbonate.' *Archives of Neurology*, **39**, 727–730.

Engel, A.G. (1988) 'Congenital myasthenic syndromes.' *Journal of Child Neurology*, **3**, 233–246.

—— (1994) 'Myasthenic syndromes.' *In:* Engel, A.G., Franzini-Armstrong, C. (Eds.) *Myology, Basic and Clinical. 2nd Edn*. New York: McGraw Hill, pp. 1798–1835.

—— Uchitel, O.D., Walls, T.J., *et al.* (1993) 'Newly recognized congenital myasthenic syndrome associated with high conductance and fast closure of the acetylcholine receptor channel.' *Annals of Neurology*, **34**, 38–47.

European Malignant Hyperpyrexia Group (1984) 'A protocol for the investi-gation of malignant hyperpyrexia (MH) susceptibility.' *British Journal of Anaesthesia*, **56**, 1267–1269.

Eymard, B., Romero, N.B., Leturcq, F., *et al.* (1997) 'Primary adhalinopathy (α-sarcoglycanopathy): clinical, pathologic and genetic correlation in 20 patients with autosomal recessive muscular dystrophy.' *Neurology*, **48**, 1227–1234.

Fardeau, M., Tomé, F.M.S., Derambure, S. (1976) 'Familial fingerprint body myopathy.' *Archives of Neurology*, **33**, 724–725.

—— Matsumura, K., Tomé, F.M.S., *et al.* (1993) 'Deficiency of the 50kDa dystrophin associated glycoprotein (adhalin) in severe autosomal recessive muscular dystrophies in children native from European countries.' *Comptes Rendus de l'Académie des Sciences*, **316**, 799–804.

—— Hillaire, D., Mignard, C., *et al.* (1996) 'Juvenile limb–girdle muscular dystrophy. Clinical, histopathological and genetic data from a small community living in the Reunion Island.' *Brain*, **119**, 295–308.

Fedrizzi, E., Botteon, G., Inverno, M., *et al.* (1993) 'Neurogenic arthrogryposis multiplex congenita: clinical and MRI findings.' *Pediatric Neurology*, **9**, 343–348.

Feero, W.G., Wang, J., Barany, F., *et al.* (1993) 'Hyperkalemic periodic paralysis: rapid molecular diagnosis and relationship of genotype to phenotype in 12 families.' *Neurology*, **43**, 668–673.

Fenichel, G.M., Sul, Y.C., Kilroy, A.W., Blovin, R. (1982) 'An autosomal dominant dystrophy with humeropelvic distribution and cardiomyopathy.' *Neurology*, **32**, 1399–1401.

Fischbeck, K.H., Kamholz, J., Shi, Y.J., *et al.* (1988) 'X-linked myoglobinuria.' *Neurology*, **39**, Suppl. 1, 174. *(Abstract.)*

Fischer, A.Q., Carpenter, D.W., Hartlage, P.L., *et al.* (1988) 'Muscle imaging in neuromuscular disease using computerized real-time sonography.' *Muscle and Nerve*, **11**, 270–275.

Fishbein, W.N., Muldoon, S.M., Deuster, P.A., Armbrustmacher, V.W. (1985) 'Myoadenylate deaminase deficiency and malignant hyperthermia susceptibility: is there a relationship?' *Biochemical Medicine*, **34**, 344–354.

Frank, J.P., Harati, Y., Butler, I.J., *et al.* (1980) 'Central core disease and malignant hyperthermia syndrome.' *Annals of Neurology*, **7**, 11–17.

Fukuyama, Y., Osawa, M. (1984) 'A genetic study of the Fukuyama type congenital muscular dystrophy.' *Brain and Development*, **6**, 373–390.

Gajdos, P., Chevret, S., Clair, B., *et al.* (1997) 'Clinical trial of plasma exchange and high-dose intravenous immunoglobulin in myasthenia gravis.' *Annals of Neurology*, **41**, 789–796.

Gamboa, E.T., Eastwood, A.B., Hays, A.P., *et al.* (1979) 'Isolation of influenza virus from muscle in myoglobinuric polymyositis.' *Neurology*, **29**, 1323–1335.

Gardner-Medwin, D. (1980) 'Clinical features and classification of the muscular dystrophies.' *British Medical Bulletin*, **36**, 109–116.

—— Sharples, P. (1989) 'Some studies of the Duchenne and autosomal recessive types of muscular dystrophy.' *Brain and Development*, **11**, 91–97.

Gardnerova, M., Eymard, B., Morel, E., *et al.* (1997) 'The fetal/adult acetylcholine receptor antibody ratio in mothers with myasthenia gravis as a marker for transfer of the disease to the newborn.' *Neurology*, **48**, 50–54.

Gieron, M.A., Korthals, J.K. (1987) 'Carnitine palmityltransferase deficiency with permanent weakness.' *Pediatric Neurology*, **3**, 51–53.

Gilbert, J.R., Stajich, J.M., Wall, S., *et al.* (1993) 'Evidence for heterogeneity in facioscapulohumeral muscular dystrophy (FSHD).' *American Journal of Human Genetics*, **53**, 401–408.

Glantz, R.H., Wright, R.B., Huckman, M.S., *et al.* (1988) 'Central nervous system magnetic resonance imaging findings in myotonic dystrophy.' *Archives of Neurology*, **45**, 36–37.

Gold, R., Kreß, W., Bettecken, T., *et al.* (1994) 'A 400-kb tandem duplication within the dystrophin gene leads to severe Becker muscular dystrophy.' *Journal of Neurology*, **241**, 331–334.

Goldhammer, Y., Blatt, I., Sadeh, M., Goodman, R.M. (1990) 'Congenital myasthenia associated with facial malformations in Iraqi and Iranian Jews. A new genetic syndrome.' *Brain*, **113**, 1291–1306.

Goodman, M., Solomons, C.L., Miller, P.D. (1978) 'Distinction between the common symptoms of the phosphate-depletion syndrome and glucocorticoid-induced disease.' *American Journal of Medicine*, **65**, 868–872.

Gospe, S., Lazaro, R.P., Lava, N.S., *et al.* (1989) 'Familial X-linked myalgia and cramps: a nonprogressive myopathy associated with a deletion in the dystrophin gene.' *Neurology*, **39**, 1277–1280.

Grant, R., Sutton, D.L., Behan, P.O., Ballantyne, J.P. (1987) 'Nifedipine in the treatment of myotonia in myotonic dystrophy.' *Journal of Neurology, Neurosurgery, and Psychiatry*, **50**, 199–206.

Greenberg, D.A.. (1997) 'Calcium channels in neurological disease.' *Annals of Neurology*, **42**, 275–282.

Griggs, R.C., Moxley, R.T., Mendell, J.R., *et al.* (1993a) 'Duchenne dystrophy: randomized, controlled trial of prednisone (18 months) and azathioprine (12 months).' *Neurology*, **43**, 520–527.

—— Tawil, R., Storvick, D., *et al.* (1993b) 'Genetics of facioscapulohumeral muscular dystrophy: new mutations in sporadic cases.' *Neurology*, **43**, 2369–2372.

—— Askanas, V., DiMauro, S., *et al.* (1995) 'Inclusion body myositis and myopathies.' *Annals of Neurology*, **38**, 705–713.

Grimaldi, L.M., Martino, G., Braghi, S., *et al.* (1993) 'Heterogeneity of autoantibodies in stiff-man syndrome.' *Annals of Neurology*, **34**, 57–64.

Gronert, G.A. (1980) 'Malignant hyperthermia.' *Anesthesiology*, **53**, 395–423.

Gutmann, D.H., Fischbeck, K.H. (1989) 'Molecular biology of Duchenne and Becker's muscular dystrophy: clinical applications.' *Annals of Neurology*, **26**, 189–194.

Gutmann, L., Blumenthal, D., Gutmann, L., Schochet, S.S. (1996) 'Acute type II myofiber atrophy in critical illness.' *Neurology*, **46**, 819–821.

Haas, A., Ricker, K., Rüdel, R., *et al.* (1981) 'Clinical study of paramyotonia congenita with and without myotonia in a warm environment.' *Muscle and Nerve*, **4**, 388–395.

Hageman, A.T.M., Gabreëls, F.J.M., Liem, K.D., *et al.* (1993) 'Congenital myotonic dystrophy: a report on thirteen cases and a review of the literature.' *Journal of the Neurological Sciences*, **115**, 95–101.

Hageman, G., Willemse, J. (1983) 'Arthrogryposis multiplex congenita. Review and comment.' *Neuropediatrics*, **14**, 6–11.

—— Gooskens, R.H.M.J., Willemse, J. (1985) 'A cerebral cause of arthrogryposis: unilateral cerebral hypoplasia.' *Clinical Neurology and Neurosurgery*, **87**, 119–122.

—— Willemse, J., van Ketel, B.A., *et al.* (1987a) 'The heterogeneity of the Pena–Shokeir syndrome.' *Neuropediatrics*, **18**, 45–50.

—— —— Verdonck, A.F.M.M. (1987b) 'The pathogenesis of fetal hypokinesia. A neurological study of 75 cases of congenital contractures with emphasis on fetal lesions.' *Neuropediatrics*, **18**, 22–33.

—— Ippel, E.P.F., Beemer, F.A., *et al.* (1988a) 'The diagnostic management of newborns with congenital contractures: a nosologic study of 75 cases.' *American Journal of Medical Genetics*, **30**, 883–904.

—— Jennekens, F.G.I., Vete, U.K., Willemse, J. (1988b) 'The heterogeneity of distal arthrogryposis.' *Brain and Development*, **6**, 273–283.

—— Ramaekers, V.T., Hilhorst, B.G.J., Rozeboom, A.R. (1993) 'Congenital cervical spinal muscular atrophy: a non-familial, non-progressive condition of the upper limbs.' *Journal of Neurology, Neurosurgery, and Psychiatry*, **56**, 365–368.

Hahn, A.F., Parkes, A.W., Bolton, C.F., Stewart, S.A. (1991) 'Neuromyotonia in hereditary motor neuropathy.' *Journal of Neurology, Neurosurgery, and Psychiatry*, **54**, 230–235.

Hall, J.G., Reed, S.D., Greene, G. (1982a) 'The distal arthrogryposes: delineation of new entities—review and nosologic discussion.' *American Journal of Medical Genetics*, **11**, 185–239.

—— —— Rosenbaum, K.N., *et al.* (1982b) 'Limb pterygium syndromes: a review and report of eleven patients.' *American Journal of Medical Genetics*, **12**, 377–409.

—— —— Scott, C.I., *et al.* (1982c) 'Three distinct types of X-linked arthrogryposis seen in 6 families.' *Clinical Genetics*, **21**, 81–97.

—— —— Driscoll, E.P. (1983) 'The syndromes of arthrogryposis congenita. Part I. Amyoplasia: a common, sporadic condition with congenital contractures.' *American Journal of Medical Genetics*, **15**, 571–590.

Haller, R.G., Henriksson, K.G., Jorfeldt, L., *et al.* (1991) 'Deficiency of skeletal muscle succinate dehydrogenase and aconitase: pathophysiology of exercise in a novel human muscle oxidative defect.' *Journal of Clinical Investigation*, **88**, 1197–1206.

Hanissian, A.S., Masi, A.T., Pitner, G., *et al.* (1983) 'Polymyositis and dermatomyositis in children: an epidemiologic and clinical comparative analysis.' *Journal of Rheumatology*, **9**, 390–394.

Harding, A.E., Petty, R.K.H., Morgan-Hughes, J.A. (1988) 'Mitochondrial myopathy: a genetic study of 71 cases.' *Journal of Medical Genetics*, **25**, 528–535.

Harley, H.G., Rundle, S.A., Reardon, W., *et al.* (1992) 'Unstable DNA sequence in myotonic dystrophy.' *Lancet*, **339**, 1125–1128.

Harper, P.S. (1975a) 'Congenital myotonic dystrophy in Britain. I. Clinical aspects.' *Archives of Disease in Childhood*, **50**, 505–513.

—— (1975b) 'Congenital myotonic dystrophy in Britain. II. Genetic basis.' *Archives of Disease in Childhood*, **50**, 514–521.

Hart, I.K., Waters, C., Vincent, A., *et al.* (1997) 'Antibodies detected to expressed K⁺ channels are implicated in neuromyotonia.' *Annals of Neurology*, **41**, 238–246.

Hart, Z.H., Servidei, S., Peterson, P.L., *et al.* (1987) 'Cardiomyopathy, mental retardation and autophagic vacuolar myopathy.' *Neurology*, **37**, 1065–1068.

Hashimoto, T., Tayama, M., Miyazaki, M., *et al.* (1995) 'Neuroimaging study of myotonic dystrophy. I. Magnetic resonance imaging of the brain.' *Brain and Development*, **17**, 24–27.

Hattori, H., Torii, S., Nagafuji, H., *et al.* (1992) 'Benign acute myositis associated with rotavirus gastroenteritis.' *Journal of Pediatrics*, **121**, 748–749.

Heckmatt, J.Z., Sewry, C.A., Hodes, D., Dubowitz, V. (1985) 'Congenital centronuclear (myotubular) myopathy. A clinical, pathological and genetic study of eight children.' *Brain*, **198**, 941–964.

—— Pier, N., Dubowitz, V. (1988) 'Real-time ultrasound imaging of muscles.' *Muscle and Nerve*, **11**, 56–65.

—— Hasson, N., Saunders, C., *et al.* (1989) 'Cyclosporin in juvenile dermatomyositis.' *Lancet*, **1**, 1063–1066.

Heiman-Patterson, T., Martino, C., Rosenberg, H., *et al.* (1988) 'Malignant hyperthermia in myotonia congenita.' *Neurology*, **38**, 810–812.

Heine, R. (1986) 'Evidence of myotonic origin of type 2B muscle fibre deficiency in myotonia and paramyotonia congenita.' *Journal of the Neurological Sciences*, **76**, 357–359.

—— Pika, U., Lehmann-Horn, F. (1993) 'A novel SCN4A mutation causing myotonia aggravated by cold and potassium.' *Human Molecular Genetics*, **2**, 1349–1353.

Hirano, M., Pavlakis, S.G. (1994) 'Mitochondrial myopathy, encephalopathy, lactic acidosis, and stroke-like episodes (MELAS): current concepts.' *Journal of Child Neurology*, **9**, 4–13.

—— Ott, B.R., Raps, E.C., *et al.* (1992) 'Acute quadriplegic myopathy: a complication of treatment with steroids, nondepolarizing blocking agents, or both.' *Neurology*, **42**, 2082–2087.

Hoffman, E.P., Fischbeck, K.H., Brown, R.H., *et al.* (1988) 'Characterization of dystrophin in muscle-biopsy specimens from patients with Duchenne's or Becker's muscular dystrophy.' *New England Journal of Medicine*, **318**, 1363–1368.

—— Kunkel, L.M., Angelini, C., *et al.* (1989) 'Improved diagnosis of Becker muscular dystrophy by dystrophin testing.' *Neurology*, **39**, 1011–1017.

Holt, I.J., Harding, A.E., Cooper, J.M., *et al.* (1989) 'Mitochondrial myopathies: clinical and biochemical features of 30 patients with major deletions of muscle mitochondrial DNA.' *Annals of Neurology*, **26**, 699–708.

Huber, S.J., Kissel, J.T., Shuttleworth, E.C., *et al.* (1989) 'Magnetic resonance imaging and clinical correlates of intellectual impairment in myotonic dystrophy.' *Archives of Neurology*, **46**, 536–540.

Hudson, A.J., Ebers, G.C., Bulman, D.E. (1995) 'The skeletal muscle sodium and chloride channel diseases.' *Brain*, **118**, 547–563.

Hudson, C.S., Rash, J.E., Tiedt, T.N., Albuquerque, E.X. (1978) 'Neostigmine-induced alterations at the mammalian neuromuscular junction. II. Ultrastructure.' *Journal of Pharmacology and Experimental Therapeutics*, **205**, 340–355.

Husain, F., Ryan, N.J., Hogan, G.R. (1989) 'Concurrence of limb–girdle muscular dystrophy and myasthenia gravis.' *Archives of Neurology*, **46**, 101–102.

Hutchinson, D.O., Walls, T.J., Nakano, S., *et al.* (1993) 'Congenital endplate acetylcholinesterase deficiency.' *Brain*, **116**, 633–653.

Hyser, C.L., Griggs, R.C., Mendell, J.R., *et al.* (1987) 'Use of serum creatine kinase, pyruvate kinase and genetic linkage for carrier detection in Duchenne and Becker dystrophy.' *Neurology*, **37**, 4–10.

Ichiki, S., Komatsu, C., Ogata, H., Mitsudome, A. (1992) 'A case of myasthenia gravis complicated with hyperthyroidism and thymic hyperplasia in childhood.' *Brain and Development*, **14**, 164–166.

Illum, N., Reske-Nielsen, E., Skovby, F., *et al.* (1988) 'Lethal autosomal recessive arthrogryposis multiplex congenita with whistling face and calcifications of the nervous system.' *Neuropediatrics*, **19**, 186–192.

Ishibashi-Ueda, H., Imakita, M., Yutani, C., *et al.* (1990) 'Congenital nemaline myopathy with dilated cardiomyopathy: an autopsy study.' *Human Pathology*, **21**, 77–82.

Jackson, M.J., Schaefer, J.A., Johnson, M.A., *et al.* (1995) 'Presentation and clinical investigation of mitochondrial respiratory chain disease. A study of 51 patients.' *Brain*, **118**, 339–357.

Jackson, S., Turnbull, D.M. (1993) 'Lipid disorders of muscle.' *In:* Rosenberg, R.N., Prusiner, S.B., DiMauro, S. (Eds.) *The Molecular and Genetic Basis of Neurological Disease.* Boston: Butterworth-Heinemann, pp. 651–661.

—— Bartlett, K., Land, J., *et al.* (1991) 'Long-chain 3-hydroxyacyl CoA dehydrogenase deficiency.' *Pediatric Research*, **29**, 406–411.

Jagadha, V., Becker, L.E. (1988) 'Brain morphology in Duchenne muscular dystrophy: a Golgi study.' *Pediatric Neurology*, **4**, 87–92.

Jamal, G.M., Weir, A.I., Hansen, S., Ballantyne, J.P. (1986) 'Myotonic dystrophy—a reassessment by conventional and more recently introduced neurophysiological techniques.' *Brain*, **109**, 1279–1296.

Jardine, P.E., Koch, M.C., Lunt, P.W., *et al.* (1994) 'De novo facioscapulohumeral muscular dystrophy defined by DNA probe p 13E-11 (D4F104S1).' *Archives of Disease in Childhood*, **71**, 221–227.

Jaspert, A., Fahsold, R., Grehl, H., Claus, D. (1995) 'Myotonic dystrophy: correlation of clinical symptoms with the size of the CTG trinucleotide repeat.' *Journal of Neurology*, **242**, 99–104.

Johnsen, T., Friis, M.L. (1980) 'Paramyotonia congenita (von Eulenburg) in Denmark.' *Acta Neurologica Scandinavica*, **62**, 78–87.

Jong, Y.J., Shishikura, K., Aoyama, M., *et al.* (1987) 'Nonspecific congenital myopathy (minimal change myopathy): a case report.' *Brain and Development*, **9**, 61–64.

Jusic, A., Dogan, S., Stojanovic, V. (1972) 'Hereditary persistent distal cramps.' *Journal of Neurology, Neurosurgery, and Psychiatry*, **35**, 379–384.

Kalimo, H., Savontaus, M.L., Lang, H., *et al.* (1988) 'X-linked myopathy with excessive autophagy: a new hereditary muscle disease.' *Annals of Neurology*, **23**, 258–265.

Kaminsky, H.J., Ruff, R.L. (1994) 'Endocrine myopathies (hyper- and hypofunction of adrenal, thyroid, pituitary, and parathyroid glands and iatrogenic corticosteroid myopathy.' *In:* Engels, A.G., Franzini-Armstrong, C. (Eds.) *Myology, Basic and Clinical. 2nd Edn.* New York: McGraw Hill, pp. 1726–1752.

Kaplan, P.W., Rocha, W., Sanders, D.B., *et al.* (1986) 'Acute steroid-induced tetraplegia following status asthmaticus.' *Pediatrics*, **78**, 121–123.

Kar, N.C., Pearson, C.M., Verity, M.A. (1980) 'Muscle fructose 1,6-diphosphatase deficiency associated with an atypical central core disease.' *Journal of the Neurological Sciences*, **48**, 243–256.

Karasawa, T., Takizawa, I., Morita, K., *et al.* (1981) 'Polymyositis and toxoplasmosis.' *Acta Pathologica Japonica*, **31**, 675–680.

Karpati, G., Charuk, J., Carpenter, S., *et al.* (1986) 'Myopathy caused by a deficiency of Ca^{2+}-adenosine triphosphatase in sarcoplasmic reticulum (Brody's disease).' *Annals of Neurology*, **20**, 38–49.

Kashihara, K., Ishida, K. (1988) 'Neuroleptic malignant syndrome due to sulpiride.' *Journal of Neurology, Neurosurgery, and Psychiatry*, **51**, 1109–1110.

Kelemen, J., Rice, D.R., Bradley, W.G., *et al.* (1982) 'Familial myoadenylate deaminase deficiency and exertional myalgia.' *Neurology*, **32**, 857–863.

Kelly, K.J., Garland, J.S., Tang, T.T., *et al.* (1989) 'Fatal rhabdomyolysis following influenza infection in a girl with familial carnitine palmityl transferase deficiency.' *Pediatrics*, **84**, 312–316.

Kerzin-Storrar, L., Metcalfe, R.A., Dyer, P.A., *et al.* (1988) 'Genetic factors in myasthenia gravis: a family study.' *Neurology*, **38**, 38–42.

Kieval, R.I., Sotrel, A., Weinblatt, M.E. (1989) 'Chronic myopathy with a partial deficiency of the carnitine palmityltransferase enzyme.' *Archives of Neurology*, **46**, 575–576.

King, J.O., Denborough, M. (1973) 'Anesthetic-induced malignant hyperpyrexia in children.' *Journal of Pediatrics*, **83**, 37–40.

Kinoshita, H., Sugai, K., Goto, Y-i., Nonaka, I. (1995) 'Early onset distal muscular dystrophy.' *Brain and Development*, **17**, 206–209.

Kiyomoto, B.H., Murakami, N., Kobayashi, Y., *et al.* (1995) 'Fatal reducing body myopathy. Ultrastructural and immunohistochemical observations.' *Journal of the Neurological Sciences*, **128**, 58–65.

Kobayashi, H., Baumbach, L., Matise, T.C., *et al.* (1995) 'A gene for a severe lethal form of X-linked arthrogryposis (X-linked infantile spinal muscular atrophy) maps to human chromosome Xp11.3–q11.2.' *Human Molecular Genetics*, **4**, 1213–1216.

Kobayashi, O., Hayashi, Y., Arahata, K., *et al.* (1996) 'Congenital muscular dystrophy: clinical and pathologic study of 50 patients with the classical (Occidental) merosin-positive form.' *Neurology*, **46**, 815–818.

Koch, M.C., Grimm, T., Harley, H.G., Harper, P.S. (1991) 'Genetic risks for children of women with myotonic dystrophy.' *American Journal of Human Genetics*, **48**, 1084–1091.

—— Steinmeyer, K., Lorenz, C., *et al.* (1992) 'The skeletal muscle chloride channel in dominant and recessive human myotonia.' *Science*, **257**, 797–800.

Korithenberg, R., Palm, D., Klein, J. (1984) 'Congenital muscular dystrophy, brain malformation and ocular problems (muscle, eye and brain disease) in two German families.' *European Journal of Pediatrics*, **142**, 64–68.

Kreuder, J., Borkhardt, A., Repp, R., *et al.* (1996) 'Inherited metabolic myopathy and hemolysis due to a mutation of aldolase A.' *New England Journal of Medicine*, **334**, 1100–1104.

Krijgsman, J.B., Barth, P.G., Stam, F.C., *et al.* (1980) 'Congenital muscular dystrophy and cerebral dysgenesis in a Dutch family.' *Neuropediatrics*, **11**, 108–120.

Krivosic-Horber, R., Adnet, P., Krivosic, I., Reyford, H. (1990) 'Diagnostic de la sensibilité à l'hyperthermie maligne chez l'enfant.' *Archives Françaises de Pédiatrie*, **47**, 421–424.

Kuhn, E., Fiehn, W., Seiler, D., Schröder, J.M. (1979) 'The autosomal recessive (Becker) form of myotonia congenita.' *Muscle and Nerve*, **2**, 109–117.

Kunkel, L.M., Mejmancik, J.F., Caskey, C.T. (1986) 'Analysis of deletions in DNA from patients with Becker and Duchenne muscular dystrophy.' *Nature*, **322**, 73–77.

Lacomis, D., Giuliani, M.J., van Cort, A., Kramer, D.J. (1996) 'Acute myopathy of intensive care: clinical, electromyographic, and pathological aspects.' *Annals of Neurology*, **40**, 645–650.

Lacson, A.G., Seshia, S.S., Sarnat, H.B., *et al.* (1995) 'Autosomal recessive, fatal infantile hypertonic muscular dystrophy among Canadian natives.' *Canadian Journal of Neurological Sciences*, **21**, 203–212.

Laubscher, B., Janzer, R.C., Krühenbühl, S., Deonna, T. (1997) 'Ragged-red fibers and complex I deficiency in a neonate with arthrogryposis congenita.' *Pediatric Neurology*, **17**, 249–251.

Laxer, R.M., Stein, L.D., Petty, R.E. (1987) 'Intravenous pulse methyl-prednisolone treatment of juvenile dermatomyositis.' *Arthritis and Rheumatism*, **30**, 328–334.

Lebenthal, E., Schochet, S.R., Adam, A., *et al.* (1970) 'Arthrogryposis multiplex congenita—23 cases in an Arab kindred.' *Pediatrics*, **46**, 891–899.

Lederman, R.J., Salanga, V.D., Wilbourn, A.J., *et al.* (1984) 'Focal inflammatory myopathy.' *Muscle and Nerve*, **7**, 142–146.

Lee, W.T., Wang, P.J., Young, C., *et al.* (1995) 'Thenar hypoplasia in Klippel–Feil syndrome due to aberrant radial artery.' *Pediatric Neurology*, **13**, 343–345.

Lerche, H., Mitrovic, N., Dubowitz, V., Lehmann-Horn, F. (1996) 'Paramyotonia congenita: the R1448P Na+ channel mutation in adult human skeletal muscle.' *Annals of Neurology*, **39**, 599–608.

Levenson, J.L. (1985) 'Neuroleptic malignant syndrome.' *American Journal of Psychiatry*, **142**, 1137–1145.

Levitt, R.C., Olckers, A., Meyers, S., *et al.* (1992) 'Evidence for the localization of a malignant hyperthermia susceptibility locus (MHS2) to human chromosome 17q.' *Genomics*, **14**, 562–566.

Lewis, C.A., Boheimer, N., Rose, P., Jackson, G. (1985) 'Myopathy after short term administration of procainamide.' *British Medical Journal*, **292**, 593–594.

Leyten, Q.H., Fons, J.M., Gabreëls, J.M., *et al.* (1989) 'Congenital muscular dystrophy.' *Journal of Pediatrics*, **115**, 214–221.

Liechti-Gallati, S., Wolff, G., Ketelsen, U-P., Braga, S. (1993) 'Prenatal diagnosis of X-linked centronuclear myopathy by linkage analysis.' *Pediatric Research*, **33**, 201–204.

Lindner, A., Schalke, B., Toyka, K.V. (1997) 'Outcome in juvenile-onset myasthenia gravis: a retrospective study with long-term follow-up of 79 patients.' *Journal of Neurology*, **244**, 515–520.

Links, T.R., Zwarts, M.J., Oosterhuis, H.J.G.H. (1988) 'Improvement of muscle strength in familial hypokalaemic periodic paralysis with azetazolamide.' *Journal of Neurology, Neurosurgery, and Psychiatry*, **51**, 1142–1145.

Lunt, P.W. (1994) 'Report of the Sixth International Workshop on Facioscapulohumeral Muscular Dystrophy: San Francisco, 11 November 1992; and current guidelines for clinical application of DNA rearrangements at locus D4S810.' *Neuromuscular Disorders*, **4**, 83–86.

Mancias, P., Bohan, T.P., Butler, I.J., Bhattacharjee, M.B. (1994) 'Treatment-resistant eosinophilic polymyositis in a child.' *Journal of Child Neurology*, **9**, 446–448.

Marbini, A., Gemignani, F., Saccardi, F., Rimoldi, M. (1989) 'Debrancher deficiency neuromuscular disorder with pseudohypertrophy in two brothers.' *Journal of Neurology*, **236**, 418–420.

Mariotti, C., Uziel, G., Carrara, F., *et al.* (1995) 'Early-onset encephalomyopathy associated with tissue-specific mitochondrial DNA depletion: a morphological, biochemical and molecular–genetic study.' *Journal of Neurology*, **242**, 547–556.

Martinelli, P., Fabbri, R., Gabellini, A.S., *et al.* (1987) 'Familial hypertrophy of masticatory muscles.' *Journal of Neurology*, **234**, 251–253.

Martinez, B.A., Lake, B.D. (1987) 'Childhood nemaline myopathy: a review of clinical presentation in relation to prognosis.' *Developmental Medicine and Child Neurology*, **29**, 815–820.

Massa, G., Casaer, P., Ceulemans, B., Van Eldere, S. (1988) 'Arthrogryposis multiplex congenita associated with lissencephaly: a case report.' *Neuropediatrics*, **19**, 24–26.

Mastaglia, F.L., Laing, N.G. (1996) 'Investigation of muscle disease.' *Journal of Neurology, Neurosurgery, and Psychiatry*, **60**, 256–274.

—— Ojeda, V.J. (1985) 'Inflammatory myopathies.' *Annals of Neurology*, **17**, 215–227; 317–323.

Matsubara, S., Tanabe, H. (1982) 'Hereditary distal myopathy with filamentous inclusions.' *Acta Neurologica Scandinavica*, **65**, 363–368.

Matsumura, K., Campbell, K.P. (1994) 'Dystrophin–glycoprotein complex: its role in the molecular pathogenesis of muscular dystrophies.' *Muscle and Nerve*, **17**, 2–15.

Matsuzaka, T., Sakuragana, N., Terasawa, K., Kuwabara, H. (1986) 'Facioscapulohumeral dystrophy associated with mental retardation, hearing loss and tortuosity of retinal arterioles.' *Journal of Child Neurology*, **1**, 218–233.

McGuire, S.A., Tomosovic, J.J., Ackerman, N. (1984) 'Hereditary continuous muscle fiber activity.' *Archives of Neurology*, **41**, 395–396.

McMenamin, J.B., Becker, L.E., Murphy, E.G. (1982) 'Congenital muscular dystrophy: a clinicopathological report of 24 cases.' *Journal of Pediatrics*, **100**, 692–697.

Medina, J.L., Chokroverty, S., Reyes, M. (1976) 'Localised myokymia caused by peripheral nerve injury.' *Archives of Neurology*, **33**, 587–588.

Medori, R., Brooke, M.H., Waterston, R.H. (1989) 'Genetic abnormalities in Duchenne and Becker dystrophies: clinical correlations.' *Neurology*, **39**, 461–465.

Medsger, T.A. (1990) 'Tryptophan-induced eosinophilia–myalgia syndrome.' *New England Journal of Medicine*, **322**, 926–928.

Meinck, H.M., Ricker, K. (1987) 'Long-standing "stiff-man" syndrome: a particular form of disseminated inflammatory CNS disease.' *Journal of Neurology, Neurosurgery, and Psychiatry*, **50**, 1556–1557.

Mendell, J.R., Iannaccone, S.T., Burrow, K.L. (1990) 'Dystrophin analysis in a congenital myopathy.' *Annals of Neurology*, **28**, 270.

—— Sahenk, Z., Prior, T.W. (1995) 'The childhood muscular dystrophies: diseases sharing a common pathogenesis of membrane instability.' *Journal of Child Neurology*, **10**, 150–159.

Meola, G., Scarpini, E., Velicogna, M., *et al.* (1986) 'Cytogenetic analysis and muscle differentiation in a girl with severe muscular dystrophy.' *Journal of Neurology*, **233**, 168–170.

—— Bresolin, N., Rimoldi, M., *et al.* (1987) 'Recessive carnitine palmityl transferase deficiency: biochemical studies in tissue cultures and platelets.' *Journal of Neurology*, **235**, 74–79.

Mercelis, R., Martin, J.J., De Barsy, T., Van den Berghe, G. (1987) 'Myoadenylate deaminase deficiency: absence of correlation with exercise intolerance in 452 muscle biopsies.' *Journal of Neurology*, **234**, 385–389.

Mercuri, E., Muntoni, F., Berardinelli, A., *et al.* (1995) 'Somatosensory and visual evoked potentials in congenital muscular dystrophy: correlations with MRI changes and muscle merosin status.' *Neuropediatrics*, **26**, 3–7.

Merlini, L., Granata, C., Dominici, P., Bonfiglioni, S. (1986) 'Emery–Dreifuss muscular dystrophy: report of five cases in a family and review of the literature.' *Muscle and Nerve*, **9**, 481–485.

—— —— Ballestrazzi, A., Marini, M.L. (1989) 'Rigid spine syndrome and rigid spine sign in myopathies.' *Journal of Child Neurology*, **4**, 273–282.

—— Morandi, L., Granata, C., Ballestrazzi, A. (1994) 'Bethlem myopathy: early-onset benign autosomal dominant myopathy with contractures. Description of two new families.' *Neuromuscular Disorders*, **4**, 503–511.

Mesa, L.E., Dubrowsky, A.L., Corderi, J. (1991) 'Steroids in Duchenne muscular dystrophy—deflazacort trial.' *Neuromuscular Disorders*, **1**, 261–266.

Miller, F.W., Leitman, S.F., Cronin, M.E., *et al.* (1992) 'Controlled trial of plasma exchange and leukapheresis in polymyositis and dermatomyositis.' *New England Journal of Medicine*, **326**, 1380–1384.

Miller, G., Heckmatt, J.Z., Dubowitz, V. (1983) 'Drug treatment of juvenile dermatomyositis.' *Archives of Disease in Childhood*, **58**, 445–450.

Miller, R.G., Layzer, R.B., Mellenthin, M.A., *et al.* (1985) 'Emery–Dreifuss muscular dystrophy with humeropelvic distribution and cardiomyopathy.' *Neurology*, **35**, 1230–1233.

Milstein, J.M., Herron, T.M., Haas, J.E. (1989) 'Fatal infantile muscle phosphorylase deficiency.' *Journal of Child Neurology*, **4**, 186–188.

Misulis, K.E., Fenichel, G.M. (1989) 'Genetic forms of myasthenia gravis.' *Pediatric Neurology*, **5**, 205–210.

Miyoshi, K., Kawai, H., Iwasa, M., *et al.* (1986) 'Autosomal recessive distal muscular dystrophy as a new type of progressive muscular dystrophy—seventeen cases in eight families including an autopsied case.' *Brain*, **109**, 31–54.

Mizuno, Y., Nakamura, Y., Komiya, K. (1989) 'The spectrum of cytoplasmic body myopathy: report of a congenital severe case.' *Brain and Development*, **11**, 20–25.

Moerman, P., Fryns, J-P., Goddeeris, P., Lauweryns, J.M. (1984) 'Pathogenesis of the prune-belly syndrome: a functional urethral obstruction caused by prostatic hypoplasia.' *Pediatrics*, **73**, 470–475.

Monaco, A.P., Kunkel, L.M. (1987) 'A giant locus for the Duchenne and Becker muscular dystrophy gene.' *Trends in Genetics*, **3**, 33–37.

Moore, A., O'Donohoe, N.V., Monaghan, H. (1986) 'Neuroleptic malignant syndrome.' *Archives of Disease in Childhood*, **61**, 793–795.

Mora, M., Cartegni, L., Di Blasi, C., *et al.* (1997) 'X-linked Emery–Dreifuss muscular dystrophy can be diagnosed from skin biopsy or blood sample.' *Annals of Neurology*, **42**, 249–253.

Moraes, C.T., DiMauro, S., Zeviani, M., *et al.* (1989) 'Mitochondrial DNA deletions in progressive external ophthalmoplegia and Kearns–Sayre syndrome.' *New England Journal of Medicine*, **320**, 1293–1299.

Morel, E., Eymard, B., Vernet-der Garabedian, B., *et al.* (1988) 'Neonatal myasthenia gravis: A new clinical and immunologic appraisal on 30 cases.' *Neurology*, **38**, 138–142.

Morgan-Hughes, J.A. (1994) 'Mitochondrial myopathy.' *In:* Engel, A.G., Franzini-Armstrong, C. (Eds.) *Myology, Basic and Clinical. 2nd Edn.* New York: McGraw Hill, pp. 1610–1660.

Morgenlander, J.C., Nohria, V., Saba, Z. (1993) 'EKG abnormalities in pediatric patients with myotonic dystrophy.' *Pediatric Neurology*, **9**, 124–126.

Moroni, I., Gonano, E.F., Comi, G.P., *et al.* (1995) 'Ryanodine receptor gene point mutation and malignant hyperthermia susceptibility.' *Journal of Neurology*, **242**, 127–133.

Morrison, D.L., MacEwen, G.D. (1982) 'Congenital muscular torticollis: observations regarding clinical findings, associated conditions and results of treatment.' *Journal of Pediatric Orthopedics*, **2**, 500–505.

Moser, H. (1984) 'Duchenne muscular dystrophy: pathogenetic aspects and genetic prevention.' *Human Genetics*, **66**, 17–40.

Mossman, S., Vincent, A., Newsom-Davis, J. (1986) 'Myasthenia gravis without acetylcholine-receptor antibody: a distinct clinical entity.' *Lancet*, **1**, 116–119.

Moxley, R.T. (1997) 'Myotonic disorders in childhood: diagnosis and treatment.' *Journal of Child Neurology*, **12**, 116–129.

Mulley, J.C., Kozman, H.M., Phillips, H.A., *et al.* (1993) 'Refined genetic localization for central core disease.' *American Journal of Human Genetics*, **52**, 398–405.

Muntoni, F., Catani, G., Mateddu, A., *et al.* (1994) 'Familial cardiomyopathy, mental retardation and myopathy associated with desmin-type intermediate filaments.' *Neuromuscular Disorders*, **4**, 233–241.

Myasthenia Gravis Clinical Study Group (1993) 'A randomized clinical trial comparing prednisone and azathioprine in myasthenia gravis. Results of the second interim analysis.' *Journal of Neurology, Neurosurgery, and Psychiatry*, **56**, 1157–1163.

Nagai, T., Hasegawa, T., Saito, M., *et al.* (1992) 'Infantile polymyositis: a case report.' *Brain and Development*, **14**, 167–169.

Nakagawa, M., Yamada, H., Higuchi, I., *et al.* (1994) 'A case of paternally inherited congenital myotonic dystrophy.' *Journal of Medical Genetics*, **31**, 397–400.

Neal, C.R., Resnikoff, E., Unger, A.M. (1981) 'Treatment of dialysis-related muscle cramps with hypertonic dextrose.' *Archives of Internal Medicine*, **141**, 171–173.

Nelson, T.E., Flewellen, E.H. (1983) 'The malignant hyperthermia syndrome.' *New England Journal of Medicine*, **309**, 416–418.

Newsom-Davis, J. (1994) 'Myasthenia gravis and related syndromes.' *In:* Walton, J., Karpati, G., Hilton-Jones, D. (Eds.) *Disorders of Voluntary Muscles.* Edinburgh: Churchill Livingstone, pp. 761–780.

—— Mills, K.R. (1993) 'Immunological associations of acquired neuromyotonia (Isaacs's syndrome). Report of five cases and literature review.' *Brain*, **116**, 453–469.

Niakan, E., Harati, Y., Danon, M.J. (1985) 'Tubular aggregates: their association with myalgia.' *Journal of Neurology, Neurosurgery, and Psychiatry*, **48**, 882–886.

Nonaka, I., Sunohara, N., Ishiura, S., Satoyoshi, E. (1981a) 'Familial distal myopathy with rimmed vacuole and lamellar (myeloid) body formation.' *Journal of the Neurological Sciences*, **51**, 141–155.

—— Une, Y., Ishihara, T., *et al.* (1981b) 'A clinical and histological study of Ullrich's disease (congenital atonic–sclerotic muscular dystrophy).' *Neuropediatrics*, **12**, 197–208.

North, K.N., Specht, L.A., Sethi, R.K., *et al.* (1996) 'Congenital muscular dystrophy associated with merosin deficiency.' *Journal of Child Neurology*, **11**, 291–295.

Nozaki, H., Hamano, S.I., Jeoka, Y., *et al.* (1990) 'Cytochrome c oxidase deficiency with acute onset and rapid recovery.' *Pediatric Neurology*, **6**, 330–332.

Oda, K., Fukushima, N., Shibasaki, H., Ohnishi, A. (1989) 'Hypoxia-sensitive hyperexcitability of the intramuscular nerve axons in Isaacs' syndrome.' *Annals of Neurology*, **25**, 140–145.

Ogilvie, I., Pourfarzam, M., Jackson, S., *et al.* (1994) 'Very long-chain acyl coenzyme A dehydrogenase deficiency presenting with exercise-induced myoglobinuria.' *Neurology*, **44**, 467–473.

Oh, S.J., Kim, D.E., Kuruoglu, R., *et al.* (1992) 'Diagnostic sensitivity of the laboratory tests in myasthenia gravis.' *Muscle and Nerve*, **15**, 720–724.

Oh, V.M.S., Taylor, E.A., Yeo, S.H., Lee, K.D. (1990) 'Cation transport across lymphocyte plasma membranes in euthyroid and thyrotoxic men with and without hypokalaemic periodic paralysis.' *Clinical Science*, **78**, 199–206.

Ohno, K., Tanaka, M., Sahashi, K., *et al.* (1991) 'Mitochondrial DNA deletions in inherited recurrent myoglobinuria.' *Annals of Neurology*, **29**, 364–369.

Ohya, K., Tachi, N., Chiba, S., *et al.* (1994) 'Congenital myotonic dystrophy transmitted from an asymptomatic father with a DM-specific gene.' *Neurology*, **44**, 1958–1960.

O'Neill, J.H., Murray, N.M.F., Newsom-Davis, J. (1988) 'The Lambert–Eaton myasthenic syndrome: a review of 50 cases.' *Brain*, **111**, 577–596.

Ono, S., Munakata, S., Nagao, K., *et al.* (1989) 'The syndrome of continuous muscle fibre activity: light and electron microscopic studies in muscle and nerve biopsies.' *Journal of Neurology*, **236**, 377–381.

Oosterhuis, H.J.G.H. (1989) 'The natural course of myasthenia gravis: a long term follow up study.' *Journal of Neurology, Neurosurgery, and Psychiatry*, **52**, 1121–1127.

Orimo, S., Araki, M., Ishii, H., *et al.* (1987) 'A case of "myopathy with tubular aggregates" with increased muscle fibre sensitivity to caffeine.' *Journal of Neurology*, **234**, 424–426.

Paljärvi, L., Kalimo, H., Lang, H., *et al.* (1987) 'Minicore myopathy with dominant inheritance.' *Journal of the Neurological Sciences*, **77**, 11–22.

Panegyres, P.K., Squier, M., Mills, K.R., Newsom-Davis, J. (1993) 'Acute myopathy associated with large parenteral dose of corticosteroid in myasthenia gravis.' *Journal of Neurology, Neurosurgery, and Psychiatry*, **56**, 702–704.

Papazian, O. (1992) 'Transient neonatal myasthenia gravis.' *Journal of Child Neurology*, **7**, 135–141.

Pasman, J.W., Gabreëls, F.J., Semmekrot, B., *et al.* (1989) 'Hyperkalemic periodic paralysis in Gordon's syndrome: a possible defect in atrial natriuretic peptide function.' *Annals of Neurology*, **26**, 392–395.

Pasternak, J.F., Hageman, J., Adams, A., *et al.* (1981) 'Exchange transfusion in neonatal myasthenia.' *Journal of Pediatrics*, **99**, 644–646.

Pellegrini, G., Barbieri, S., Moggio, M., *et al.* (1985) 'A case of congenital neuromuscular disease with uniform type I fibres, abnormal mitochondrial network and jagged Z-line.' *Neuropediatrics*, **16**, 162–166.

Pena, S.D.J., Shokeir, M.H.K. (1974) 'Syndrome of camptodactyly, mutiple ankyloses, facial anomalies and pulmonary hypoplasia: a lethal condition.' *Journal of Pediatrics*, **85**, 373–375.

Penn, A.S., Richman, D.P., Ruff, R.L., Lennon, V.A. (1993) 'Myasthenia gravis and related disorders: experimental and clinical aspects.' *Annals of the New York Academy of Sciences*, **681**, 425–514.

Perlman, J.M., Burns, D.K., Twickler, D.M., Weinberg, A.G. (1995) 'Fetal hypokinesia syndrome in the monochorionic pair of a triplet pregnancy secondary to severe disruptive cerebral injury.' *Pediatrics*, **96**, 521–523.

Peters, A.C.B., Bots, G.T.A., Roos, R.A.C., Van Gelderen, H.H. (1984) 'Fukuyama type congenital muscular dystrophy: two Dutch siblings.' *Brain and Development*, **6**, 406–416.

Petty, R.K.H., Thomas, P.K., Landon, D.N. (1986) 'Emery–Dreifuss syndrome.' *Journal of Neurology*, **233**, 108–114.

Pierobon-Bormioli, S., Armani, M., Ringel, P., *et al.* (1985) 'Familial neuromuscular disease with tubular aggregates.' *Muscle and Nerve*, **8**, 291–298.

Pini, A., Merlini, L., Tomé, F.M.S., *et al.* (1996) 'Merosin-negative congenital muscular dystrophy, occipital epilepsy with periodic spasms and focal cortical dysplasia. Report of three Italian cases in two families.' *Brain and Development*, **18**, 316–322.

Pons, R., Andreeta, P., Wang, C.H., *et al.* (1996) 'Mitochondrial myopathy simulating spinal muscular atrophy.' *Pediatric Neurology*, **15**, 153–158.

Poulton, K.R., Nightingale, S. (1988) 'A new metabolic muscle disease due to abnormal hexokinase activity.' *Journal of Neurology, Neurosurgery, and Psychiatry*, **51**, 250–255.

Prelle, A., Moggio, M., Checcarelli, N., *et al.* (1993) 'Multiple deletions of mitochondrial DNA in a patient with periodic attacks of paralysis.' *Journal of the Neurological Sciences*, **117**, 24–27.

Ptácek, L.J., Johnson, K.J., Griggs, R.C. (1993) 'Genetics and physiology of the myotonic muscle disorders.' *New England Journal of Medicine*, **328**, 482–489.

—— Tawil, R., Griggs, R.C., *et al.* (1994a) 'Dihydropyridine receptor mutations cause hypokalemic periodic paralysis.' *Cell*, **77**, 863–868.

786

—— —— —— *et al.* (1994b) 'Sodium channel mutations in acetazolamide-responsive myotonia congenita, paramyotonia congenita, and hyperkalemic periodic paralysis.' *Neurology*, **44**, 1500–1503.

Ragge, N.K., Hoyt, W.F. (1992) 'Midbrain myasthenia: fatigable ptosis, 'lid twitch' sign, and ophthalmoparesis from a dorsal midbrain glioma.' *Neurology*, **42**, 917–919.

Ranta, S., Pihko, H., Santavuori, P., *et al.* (1995) 'Muscle–eye–brain disease and Fukuyama type congenital muscular dystrophy are not allelic.' *Neuromuscular Disorders*, **5**, 221–225.

Raphael, S.A., Wolfson, B.J., Parker, P., *et al.* (1989) 'Pyomyositis in a child with acquired immunodeficiency syndrome.' *American Journal of Diseases of Children*, **143**, 779–781.

Reed, U.C., Marie, S.K., Vainzof, M., *et al.* (1996) 'Congenital muscular dystrophy with cerebral white matter hypodensity. Correlation of clinical features and merosin deficiency.' *Brain and Development*, **18**, 53–58.

Regev, R., De Vries, L.S., Heckmatt, J.Z., Dubowitz, V. (1987) 'Cerebral ventricular dilatation in congenital myotonic dystrophy.' *Journal of Pediatrics*, **111**, 372–376.

Reichmann, H. (1988) 'Enzyme activity measured in single muscle fibers in partial cytochrome c oxidase deficiency.' *Neurology*, **38**, 244–249.

—— Rohkamm, R., Zeviani, M., *et al.* (1986) 'Mitochondrial myopathy due to complex III deficiency with normal reducible cytochrome b concentration.' *Archives of Neurology*, **43**, 957–961.

Reimers, C.D., de Koning, J., Neubert, U., *et al.* (1993) '*Borrelia burgdorferi* myositis: report of eight patients.' *Journal of Neurology*, **240**, 278–283.

—— Schedel, H., Fleckenstein, J.L., *et al.* (1994) 'Magnetic resonance imaging of skeletal muscles in idiopathic inflammatory myopathies of adults.' *Journal of Neurology*, **241**, 306–314.

Reske-Nielsen, E., Hein-Sorensen, O., Vorre, P. (1987) 'Familial centronuclear myopathy: a clinical and pathological study.' *Acta Neurologica Scandinavica*, **76**, 115–122.

Reyes, M.G., Goldbarg, H., Fresco, K., Bouffard, A. (1987) 'Zebra body myopathy: A second case of ultrastructurally distinct congenital myopathy.' *Journal of Child Neurology*, **2**, 307–310.

Rich, M.M., Teener, J.W., Raps, E.C., *et al.* (1996) 'Muscle is electrically inexcitable in acute quadriplegic myopathy.' *Neurology*, **46**, 731–736.

Richieri-Costa, A., Leonel José, J., Silva, S.M.G., Frota-Pessoa, O. (1981) 'Late infantile autosomal recessive myotonia, mental retardation, and skeletal abnormalities.' *In:* Huber, A., Klein, D. (Eds.) *Neurogenetics and Neuro-ophthalmology.* Amsterdam: Elsevier, pp. 59–60.

Ricker, K., Moxley, R.T., Rohkamm, R. (1989) 'Rippling muscle disease.' *Archives of Neurology*, **46**, 405–408.

—— Heine, R., Lehmann-Horn, F. (1994) 'Myotonia fluctuans: a third type of muscle sodium channel disease.' *Archives of Neurology*, **51**, 1095–1102.

—— Koch, M.C., Lehmann-Horn, F., *et al.* (1995) 'Proximal myotonic myopathy: clinical features of a multisystem disorder similar to myotonic dystrophy.' *Archives of Neurology*, **52**, 25–31.

Rideau, Y., Glorion, B., Delaubier, A., *et al.* (1984) 'The treatment of scoliosis in Duchenne muscular dystrophy.' *Muscle and Nerve*, **7**, 281–286.

Riggs, J.E., Schochet, S.S., Goldfarb, G.R., Price, R.A. (1989) 'Congenital myopathy with progressive external ophthalmoplegia.' *Journal of Child Neurology*, **4**, 194–196.

—— —— Gutmann, L., Lerfald, S.C. (1989) 'Childhood onset inclusion body myositis mimicking limb–girdle muscular dystrophy.' *Journal of Child Neurology*, **4**, 283–285.

—— Klingberg, W.G., Flink, E.B., *et al.* (1992) 'Cardioskeletal mitochondrial myopathy associated with chronic magnesium deficiency.' *Neurology*, **42**, 128–130.

Ringel, S.P., Neville, H.E., Duster, M.C., Carroll, J.E. (1978) 'A new congenital neuromuscular diease with trilaminar muscle fibers.' *Neurology*, **28**, 282–289.

Roberds, S.L., Leturcq, F., Allamand, V., *et al.* (1994) 'Missense mutations in the adhalin gene linked to autosomal recessive muscular dystrophy.' *Cell*, **78**, 625–633.

Robinson, R.O. (1990) 'Arthrogryposis multiplex congenita: feeding, language and other health problems.' *Neuropediatrics*, **21**, 177–188.

Roddy, S.M., Ashwal, S., Peckham, N. (1986) 'Infantile myositis: a case diagnosed in the neonatal period.' *Pediatric Neurology*, **2**, 241–243.

Rodillo, E.B., Fernandez-Bermejo, E., Heckmatt, J.Z., Dubowitz, V. (1988) 'Prevention of rapidly progressive scoliosis in Duchenne muscular dystrophy by prolongation of walking with orthoses.' *Journal of Child Neurology*, **3**, 269–274.

Rodriguez, M., Gomez, M.R., Howard, F.M., Taylor, W.F. (1983) 'Myasthenia gravis in children: long-term follow-up.' *Annals of Neurology*, **13**, 504–510.

Roervik, S., Stovner, J. (1974) 'Ketamine-induced acidosis, fever, and creatine-kinase rise.' *Lancet*, **2**, 1384–1385.

Roig, M., Balliu, P.R., Navarro, C., *et al.* (1994) 'Presentation, clinical course, and outcome of the congenital form of myotonic dystrophy.' *Pediatric Neurology*, **11**, 208–213.

Romero, N.B., Tomé, F.M.S., Leturcq, F., *et al.* (1994) 'Genetic heterogeneity of severe childhood autosomal recessive muscular dystrophy with adhalin (50kDa dystrophin-associated glycoprotein) deficiency.' *Comptes Rendus de l'Académie des Sciences*, **317**, 70–76.

Roodhoft, A.M., Van Acker, K.J., Martin, J.J., *et al.* (1986) 'Benign mitochondrial myopathy with deficiency of NADH-CoQ reductase and cytochrome c oxidase.' *Neuropediatrics*, **17**, 221–226.

Rosenberg, N.L., Neville, H.E., Ringel, S.P. (1985) 'Tubular aggregates: their association with neuromuscular diseases including the syndrome of myalgias/cramps.' *Archives of Neurology*, **42**, 973–976.

Rothstein, T.L., Carlson, C.B., Sumi, S.M. (1971) 'Polymyositis with facio-scapulohumeral distribution.' *Archives of Neurology*, **25**, 313–319.

Rowland, L.P. (1985) 'Cramps, spasms and muscle stiffness.' *Revue de Neurologique*, **141**, 261–273.

—— (1988) 'Clinical concepts of Duchenne muscular dystrophy. The impact of molecular genetics.' *Brain*, **111**, 479–495.

Rutgers, M.J. (1986) 'The rectus abdominis syndrome: a case report.' *Journal of Neurology*, **233**, 180–181.

Sabina, R. (1993) 'Myoadenylate deaminase deficiency.' *In:* Rosenberg, R.N., Prusiner, S.B., DiMauro, S. (Eds.) *The Molecular and Genetic Basis of Neurological Disease.* Boston: Butterworth-Heinemann, pp. 261–275.

Sadeh, M., Berg, M., Sandbank, U. (1990) 'Familial myoedema, muscular hypertrophy and stiffness.' *Acta Neurologica Scandinavica*, **81**, 201–204.

Sakano, T., Hamasaki, T., Kinoshita, Y., *et al.* (1989) 'Treatment for refractory myasthenia gravis.' *Archives of Disease in Childhood*, **64**, 1191–1193.

Samaha, F.J., Quinlan, J.G. (1996a) 'Dystrophinopathies: clarification and complication.' *Journal of Child Neurology*, **11**, 13–20.

—— —— (1996b) 'Myalgia and cramps: dystrophinopathy with wide-ranging laboratory findings.' *Journal of Child Neurology*, **11**, 21–24.

Sancho, S., Mongini, T., Tanji, K., *et al.* (1993) 'Analysis of dystrophin expression after activation of myogenesis in amniocytes, chorionic-villus cells, and fibroblasts. A new method for diagnosing Duchenne's muscular dystrophy.' *New England Journal of Medicine*, **329**, 915–920.

Sander, J.E., Layzer, R.B., Goldsobel, A.B. (1980) 'Congenital stiffman syndrome.' *Annals of Neurology*, **8**, 195–197.

Sansone, V., Griggs, R.C., Meola, G., *et al.* (1997) 'Andersen's syndrome: a distinct periodic paralysis.' *Annals of Neurology*, **42**, 305–312.

Santavuori, P., Somer, H., Sainio, K., *et al.* (1989) 'Muscle–eye–brain disease (MEB).' *Brain and Development*, **11**, 147–153.

Sarnat, H.B., Morrissy, R.T. (1981) 'Idiopathic torticollis: sternocleidomastoid myopathy and accessory neuropathy.' *Muscle and Nerve*, **4**, 374–380.

Sasaki, T., Shikura, K., Sugai, K., *et al.* (1989) 'Muscle histochemistry in myotubular (centronuclear) myopathy.' *Brain and Development*, **11**, 26–32.

Sawchak, J.A., Sher, J.H., Norman, M.G., *et al.* (1991) 'Centronuclear myopathy heterogeneity: distinction of clinical types by myosin isoform patterns.' *Neurology*, **41**, 135–140.

Schaefer, J., Jackson, S., Dick, D.J., Turnbull, D.M. (1996) 'Trifunctional enzyme deficiency: adult presentation of a usually fatal β-oxidation defect.' *Annals of Neurology*, **40**, 597–602.

Scheuerbrandt, G., Lundin, A., Lövgren, T. Mortier, W. (1986) 'Screening for Duchenne muscular dystrophy: an improved screening test for creatine kinase and its application in an infant screening program.' *Muscle and Nerve*, **9**, 11–23.

Schmalbruch, H., Kamienlecka, Z., Arrøe, M. (1987) 'Early fatal nemaline myopathy: case report and review.' *Developmental Medicine and Child Neurology*, **29**, 800–804.

Seay, A.R., Ziter, F.A. (1978) 'Malignant hyperpyrexia in a patient with Schwartz–Jampel syndrome.' *Journal of Pediatrics*, **93**, 83–84.

Sekizawa, A., Kimura, T., Sasaki, M., *et al.* (1996) 'Prenatal diagnosis of Duchenne muscular dystrophy using a single fetal nucleated erythrocyte in maternal blood.' *Neurology*, **46**, 1350–1353.

Sells, J.M., Jaffe, K.M., Hall, J.G. (1996) 'Amyoplasia, the most common type of arthrogryposis: the potential for good outcome.' *Pediatrics*, **97**, 225–231.

Servidei, S., Bonilla, E., Diedrich, R.G., *et al.* (1986) 'Fatal infantile form of muscle phosphofructokinase deficiency.' *Neurology*, **36**, 1465–1470.

—— Shanske, S., Zeviani, M., *et al.* (1988) 'McArdle's disease: biochemical and molecular genetic studies.' *Annals of Neurology*, **24**, 774–781.

Sethna, N.F., Rockoff, M.A., Worthen, H.M., Rosnow, J.M. (1988) 'Anesthesia-related complications in children with Duchenne muscular dystrophy.' *Anesthesiology*, **68**, 462–465.

Seybold, M.E. (1986) 'The office Tensilon test for ocular myasthenia gravis.' *Archives of Neurology*, **43**, 842–844.

Sharma, K.R., Mynhier, M.A., Miller, R.G. (1993) 'Cyclosporine increases muscular force generation in Duchenne muscular dystrophy.' *Neurology*, **43**, 527–532.

Sheaff, H.M. (1952) 'Hereditary myokymia.' *Archives of Neurology and Psychiatry*, **68**, 236–247.

Shelbourne, P., Davies, J., Buxton, J., *et al.* (1993) 'Direct diagnosis of myotonic dystrophy with a disease-specific DNA marker.' *New England Journal of Medicine*, **328**, 471–475.

Shevell, M., Rosenblatt, B., Silver, K., *et al.* (1990) 'Congenital inflammatory myopathy.' *Neurology*, **40**, 1111–1114.

Shillito, P., Vincent, A., Newsom-Davis, J. (1993) 'Congenital myasthenic syndromes.' *Neuromuscular Disorders*, **3**, 183–190.

—— Molenaar, P.C., Vincent, A., *et al.* (1995) 'Acquired neuromyotonia: evidence for autoantibodies directed against K+ channels of peripheral nerves.' *Annals of Neurology*, **38**, 714–722.

Shimoizumi, H., Momoi, M.Y., Ohta, S., *et al.* (1989) 'Cytochrome c oxidase-deficient myogenic cell lines in mitochondrial myopathy.' *Annals of Neurology*, **25**, 615–621.

Shimomura, C., Nonaka, I. (1989) 'Nemaline myopathy: comparative muscle histochemistry in the severe neonatal, moderate congenital, and adult-onset forms.' *Pediatric Neurology*, **5**, 25–31.

Silver, R.M., Maricq, H.R. (1989) 'Childhood dermatomyositis: serial microvascular studies.' *Pediatrics*, **83**, 278–283.

Simon, D.B., Ringel, S.P., Sufit, R.L. (1982) 'Clinical spectrum of fascial inflammation.' *Muscle and Nerve*, **5**, 525–537.

Sloane, A.E., Vajsar, J., Laxer, R.M., *et al.* (1994) 'Spontaneous non-traumatic anterior compartment syndrome with peroneal neuropathy and favorable outcome.' *Neuropediatrics*, **25**, 268–270.

Slonim, A.E., Goans, P.J. (1985) 'Myopathy in McArdle's syndrome. Improvement with a high-protein diet.' *New England Journal of Medicine*, **312**, 355–359.

Smit, L.M., Hageman, G., Veldman, H., *et al.* (1988) 'A myasthenic syndrome with congenital paucity of secondary synaptic clefts: CPSC syndrome.' *Muscle and Nerve*, **11**, 337–348.

Smith, R., Athanasou, N.A., Vipond, S.E. (1996) 'Fibrodysplasia (myositis) ossificans progressiva: clinicopathological features and natural history.' *Quarterly Journal of Medicine*, **89**, 445–456.

Snead, O.C., Kohaut, E.C., Oh, S.J., Bradley, R.J. (1987) 'Plasmapheresis for myasthenic crisis in a young child.' *Journal of Pediatrics*, **110**, 740–742.

Solimena, M., Folli, F., Aparasi, R., *et al.* (1990) 'Antibodies to GABA-ergic neurons and pancreatic beta-cells in stiff-man syndrome.' *New England Journal of Medicine*, **322**, 1555–1560.

Soliven, B.C., Lange, D.J., Penn, A.S., *et al.* (1988) 'Seronegative myasthenia gravis.' *Neurology*, **38**, 514–517.

Sommer, N., Sigg, B., Melms, A., *et al.* (1997) 'Ocular myasthenia gravis: response to long term immunosuppressive treatment.' *Journal of Neurology, Neurosurgery, and Psychiatry*, **62**, 156–162.

Spaans, F., Jennekens, F.G.I., Mirandolle, J.F., *et al.* (1986) 'Myotonic dystrophy associated with hereditary motor and sensory neuropathy.' *Brain*, **109**, 1149–1168.

—— Theunissen, P., Reekers, A.D., *et al.* (1990) 'Schwartz–Jampel syndrome: I. Clinical, electromyographic and histologic studies.' *Muscle and Nerve*, **13**, 516–527.

Speer, M.C., Yamaoka, L.H., Gilchrist, J.H., *et al.* (1992) 'Confirmation of genetic heterogeneity in limb–girdle muscular dystrophy: linkage of an autosomal dominant form to chromosome 5q.' *American Journal of Human Genetics*, **50**, 1211–1217.

Stephan, D.A., Buist, N.R.M., Chittenden, A.B., *et al.* (1994) 'A rippling muscle disease gene is localized to 1q41: evidence for multiple genes.' *Neurology*, **44**, 1915–1920.

Stewart, C.R., Kahler, S.O., Gilchrist, J.M. (1988) 'Congenital myopathy with cleft palate and increased susceptibility to malignant hyperthermia: King syndrome?' *Pediatric Neurology*, **4**, 371–374.

Stricker, R.B., Kwiatkowska, B.J., Habis, J.A, Kiprov, D.D. (1993) 'Myasthenic crisis. Response to plasmapheresis following failure of intravenous γ-globulin.' *Archives of Neurology*, **50**, 837–840.

Subramony, S.H., Wee, A.S., Mishra, S.K. (1986) 'Lack of cold sensitivity in hyperkalemic periodic paralysis.' *Muscle and Nerve*, **9**, 700–703.

Sugie, H., Kobayashi, J., Sugie, Y., *et al.* (1988) 'Infantile muscle glycogen storage disease: phosphoglucomutase deficiency with decreased muscle and serum carnitine levels.' *Neurology*, **38**, 602–605.

—— Sugie, Y., Nishida, M., *et al.* (1989) 'Recurrent myoglobinuria in a child with mental retardation: phospoglycerate kinase deficiency.' *Journal of Child Neurology*, **4**, 95–99.

Sulaiman, A.R., Swick, H.M., Kinder, D.S. (1983) 'Congenital fibre type disproportion with unusual clinico-pathologic manifestations.' *Journal of Neurology, Neurosurgery, and Psychiatry*, **46**, 175–182.

Sun, S.F., Streib, E.W. (1983) 'Autosomal recessive generalized myotonia.' *Muscle and Nerve*, **6**, 143–148.

Sunohara, N., Arahata, K., Hoffman, E.P., *et al.* (1990) 'Quadriceps myopathy: forme fruste of Becker muscular dystrophy.' *Annals of Neurology*, **28**, 634–639.

Suomalainen, A., Majander, A., Wallin, M., *et al.* (1997) 'Autosomal dominant progressive external ophthalmoplegia with multiple deletions of DNA: clinical, biochemical and molecular genetic features of the 10q-linked disease.' *Neurology*, **48**, 1244–1253.

Swift, T.R. (1981) 'Disorders of neuromuscular transmission other than myasthenia gravis.' *Muscle and Nerve*, **4**, 334–353.

Tachi, N., Tachi, M., Sasaki, K., *et al.* (1989) 'Glycogen storage disease with normal acid maltase: skeletal and cardiac muscles.' *Pediatric Neurology*, **5**, 60–63.

Takada, K., Nakamura, H., Tanaka, J. (1984) 'Cortical dysplasia in congenital muscular dystrophy with central nervous system involvement (Fukuyama type).' *Journal of Neuropathology and Experimental Neurology*, **43**, 395–407.

Takahashi, S., Miyamoto, A., Oki, J., Okuno, A. (1996) 'CTG trinucleotide repeat length and clinical expression in a family with myotonic dystrophy.' *Brain and Development*, **18**, 127–130.

Takamoto, K., Hirose, K., Uono, M., Nonaka, I. (1984) 'A genetic variant of Emery–Dreifuss disease. Muscular dystrophy with humeropelvic distribution, early joint contracture, and permanent atrial paralysis.' *Archives of Neurology*, **41**, 1292–1293.

Takashima, S., Becker, L.E., Chan, F., Takada, K. (1987) 'A Golgi study of the cerebral cortex in Fukuyama-type congenital muscular dystrophy, Walker type "lissencephaly" and classical lissencephaly.' *Brain and Development*, **9**, 621–626.

Tawil, R., Storvick, D., Feasby, T.E., *et al.* (1993) 'Extreme variability of expression in monozygotic twins with FSH muscular dystrophy.' *Neurology*, **43**, 345–348.

—— Ptácek, L.J., Pavlakis, S.G., *et al.* (1994) 'Andersen's syndrome: potassium-sensitive periodic paralysis, ventricular ectopy, and dysmorphic features.' *Annals of Neurology*, **35**, 326–330.

—— Myers, G.J., Weiffenbach, B., Griggs, R.C. (1995) 'Scapuloperoneal syndrome. Absence of linkage to the 4q35 FSHD locus.' *Archives of Neurology*, **52**, 1069–1072.

Taylor, D.A., Carroll, J.E., Smith, M.E., *et al.* (1982) 'Facioscapulohumeral dystrophy associated with hearing loss and Coats syndrome.' *Annals of Neurology*, **12**, 395–398.

Taylor, D.J., Brosnan, M.J., Arnold, D.L., *et al.* (1988) 'Ca2+-ATPase deficiency in a patient with an exertional muscle pain syndrome.' *Journal of Neurology, Neurosurgery, and Psychiatry*, **51**, 1425–1433.

Tein, I., De Vivo, D.C., Hale, D.E., *et al.* (1991a) 'Short-chain L-3-hydroxy-acyl-CoA dehydrogenase deficiency in muscle: a new cause for recurrent myoglobinuria and encephalopathy.' *Annals of Neurology*, **30**, 415–419.

—— DiMauro, S., De Vivo, D.C. (1991b) 'Recurrent childhood myoglobinuria.' *Advances in Pediatrics*, **37**, 77–117.

Thomas, P.K., Calne, D.B., Elliott, C.F. (1972) 'X-linked scapuloperoneal syndrome.' *Journal of Neurology, Neurosurgery, and Psychiatry*, **35**, 208–215.

Thompson, C.E. (1982) 'Infantile myositis.' *Developmental Medicine and Child Neurology*, **24**, 307–313.

Thornton, C.A., Griggs, R.C., Moxley, R.T. (1994) 'Myotonic dystrophy with no trinucleotide repeat expansion.' *Annals of Neurology*, **35**, 269–272.

Tindall, R.S.A. (1981) 'Humoral immunity in myasthenia gravis: biochemical characterization of acquired antireceptor antibodies and clinical correlations.' *Annals of Neurology*, **10**, 437–447.

—— Rollins, J.A, Phillips, J.T., *et al.* (1987) 'Preliminary results of a double-blind, randomized, placebo-controlled trial of cyclosporine in myasthenia gravis.' *New England Journal of Medicine*, **316**, 719–724.

Toda, T., Segawa, M., Nomura, Y., *et al.* (1993) 'Localization of a gene for Fukuyama type congenital muscular dystrophy to chromosome 9q31–33.' *Nature Genetics*, **5**, 283–286.

—— Yoshioka, M., Nakahori, Y., *et al.* (1995) 'Genetic identity of Fukuyama-type congenital muscular dystrophy and Walker–Warburg syndrome.' *Annals of Neurology*, **37**, 99–101.

Tohyama, J., Inagaki, M., Nonaka, I. (1994) 'Early onset muscular dystrophy with autosomal dominant heredity. Report of a family and CT findings of skeletal muscle.' *Brain and Development*, **16**, 402–406.

Tonin, P., Lewis, P., Servidei, S., DiMauro, S. (1990) 'Metabolic causes of myoglobinuria.' *Annals of Neurology*, **27**, 181–185.

Topaloglu, H., Kale, G., Yalnizoglu, D., *et al.* (1994) 'Analysis of "pure" congenital muscular dystrophies in thirty-eight cases. How different is the classical type 1 from the occidental type cerebromuscular dystrophy?' *Neuropediatrics*, **25**, 94–100.

—— Cila, A., Tasdemir, A.H., Saatçi, I. (1995) 'Congenital muscular dystrophy with eye and brain involvement. The Turkish experience in two cases.' *Brain and Development*, **17**, 271–275.

Topi, G.C., D'Alessandro, L., Catricala, C., Zardi, O. (1979) 'Dermatomyositis-like syndrome due to *Toxoplasma*.' *British Journal of Dermatology*, **101**, 589–591.

Torres, C.F., Forbes, G.B., Decancq, G.H. (1986) 'Muscle weakness in infants with rickets: distribution, course and recovery.' *Pediatric Neurology*, **2**, 95–98.

Tritschler, H-J., Andreetta, F., Moraes, C.T., *et al.* (1992) 'Mitochondrial myopathy of childhood associated with depletion of mitochondrial DNA.' *Neurology*, **42**, 209–217.

Trudell, R.G., Kaiser, K.K., Griggs, R.C. (1987) 'Acetazolamide-responsive myotonia congenita.' *Neurology*, **37**, 488–491.

Tsujino, S., Shanske, S., DiMauro, S. (1993) 'Molecular basis of myophosphorylase deficiency (McArdle's disease).' *Neurology*, **43**, Suppl. 2, A279. *(Abstract.)*

Turnbull, D.M., Johnson, M.A., Dick, D.J., *et al.* (1985) 'Partial cytochrome oxidase deficiency without subsarcolemmal accumulation of mitochondria in chronic progressive ophthalmoplegia.' *Journal of the Neurological Sciences*, **70**, 93–100.

—— Bartlett, K., Eyre, J.A., *et al.* (1988a) 'Lipid storage myopathy due to glutaric aciduria type II: treatment of a potentially fatal myopathy.' *Developmental Medicine and Child Neurology*, **30**, 667–672.

—— Shepherd, I.M., Ashworth, B., *et al.* (1988b) 'Lipid storage myopathy associated with low acyl-CoA dehydrogenase activities.' *Brain*, **111**, 815–828.

Uchitel, O., Engel, A.G., Walls, T.J., *et al.* (1993) 'Congenital myasthenic syndrome attributed to an abnormal interaction of acetylcholine with its receptor.' *Annals of the New York Academy of Sciences*, **681**, 487–495.

Upadhyaya, M., Lunt, P.W., Sarfarazi, M., *et al.* (1992) 'The mapping of chromosome 4q markers in relation to facioscapulohumeral muscular dystrophy (FSHD).' *American Journal of Human Genetics*, **51**, 404–410.

Urbano-Márquez, A., Estruch, R., Grau, J.M., *et al.* (1986) 'Inflammatory myopathy associated with chronic graft-versus-host disease.' *Neurology*, **36**, 1091–1093.

Uziel, G., Taroni, F., DiDonato, S. (1995) 'Fatty acid oxidation disorders.' *In:* DiDonato, S., Parini, R., Uziel, G. (Eds.) *Metabolic Encephalopathies. Therapy and Prognosis.* London: John Libbey, pp. 11–24.

Vajsar, J., Sloane, A., MacGregor, D.L., *et al.* (1995) 'Arthrogryposis multiplex congenita due to congenital myasthenic syndrome.' *Pediatric Neurology*, **12**, 237–241.

Valli, G., Barbieri, S., Cappa, S., *et al.* (1983) 'Syndromes of abnormal muscular activity: overlap between continuous muscle fiber activity and the stiff man syndrome.' *Journal of Neurology, Neurosurgery, and Psychiatry*, **46**, 241–247.

van den Berg, I.E.T., Berger, R. (1990) 'Phosphorylase b kinase deficiency in man: a review.' *Journal of Inherited Metabolic Diseases*, **13**, 442–451.

van der Knaap, M.S., Smit, L.M.E., Bart, P.G., *et al.* (1997) 'Magnetic resonance imaging in classification of congenital muscular dystrophies with brain abnormalities.' *Annals of Neurology*, **42**, 50–59.

van der Kooi, A.J., Ledderhof, T.M., de Voogt, W.G., *et al.* (1996) 'A newly recognized autosomal dominant limb girdle muscular dystrophy with cardiac involvement.' *Annals of Neurology*, **39**, 636–642.

Van Erven, P.M.M., Renier, W.O., Gabreëls, F.J.M., *et al.* (1989) 'Hypokinesia and rigidity as clinical manifestations of mitochondrial encephalomyopathy: report of three cases.' *Developmental Medicine and Child Neurology*, **31**, 81–91.

Van Munster, E.T.L., Joosten, E.M.G., Van Munster-Uijtdehaage, M.A.M., *et al.* (1986) 'The rigid spine syndrome.' *Journal of Neurology, Neurosurgery, and Psychiatry*, **49**, 1292–1297.

Vanneste, J.A.L., Augustijn, P.B., Stam, F.C. (1988) 'The rigid spine syndrome in two sisters.' *Journal of Neurology, Neurosurgery, and Psychiatry*, **51**, 131–135.

van Ommen, G.J.B., Scheuerbrandt, G. (1993) 'Neonatal screening for muscular dystrophy. Consensus recommendation of the 14th Workshop sponsored by the European Neuromuscular Center (ENMC).' *Neuromuscular Disorders*, **3**, 231–239.

Vincent, A., Cull-Candy, S.G., Newsom-Davis, J., *et al.* (1981) 'Congenital myasthenia: end-plate acetylcholine receptors and electrophysiology in five cases.' *Muscle and Nerve*, **4**, 306–318.

—— Riemersma, S., Hawke, S., *et al.* (1994) 'Arthrogryposis associated with antibodies inhibiting fetal acetylcholine receptor function.' *Annals of Neurology*, **36**, 325. *(Abstract.)*

Vita, G., Toscano, A., Bresolin, N., *et al.* (1994) 'Muscle phosphoglycerate mutase (PGAM) deficiency in the first caucasian patient: biochemistry, muscle culture and ^{31}P-MR spectroscopy.' *Journal of Neurology*, **241**, 289–294.

Voit, T., Lamprecht, A., Goebel, H.H. (1986) 'Hearing loss in facioscapulohumeral dystrophy.' *European Journal of Pediatrics*, **145**, 280–285.

—— Krogmann, O., Lenard, H.G., *et al.* (1988) 'Emery–Dreifuss muscular dystrophy: disease spectrum and differential diagnosis.' *Neuropediatrics*, **19**, 62–71.

Vuopala, K., Leisti, J., Herva, R. (1994) 'Lethal arthrogryposis in Finland—a clinico-pathological study of 83 cases during thirteen years.' *Neuropediatrics*, **25**, 308–315.

Walls, T.J., Engel, A.G., Nagel, A.S., *et al.* (1993) 'Congenital myasthenic syndrome associated with paucity of synaptic vesicles and reduced quantal release.' *Annals of the New York Academy of Sciences*, **681**, 461–468.

Walton, J.N., Gardner-Medwin, D. (1981) 'Progressive muscular dystrophy and the myotonic disorders.' *In:* Walton, J.N. (Ed.) *Disorders of Voluntary Muscle, 4th Edn.* Edinburgh: Churchill Livingstone, pp. 481–524.

Wedel, D.J. (1992) 'Malignant hyperthermia and neuromuscular disease.' *Neuromuscular Disorders*, **2**, 157–164.

Wenstrup, R.J., Murad, S., Pinnell, S.R. (1989) 'Ehlers–Danlos syndrome type VI. Clinical manifestations of collagen and lysil hydroxylase deficiency.' *Journal of Pediatrics*, **115**, 405–409.

Wessel, H.B. (1990) 'Dystrophin: a clinical perspective.' *Pediatric Neurology*, **6**, 3–12.

Whitaker, J.N. (1982) 'Inflammatory myopathy: a review of etiologic and pathogenetic factors.' *Muscle and Nerve*, **5**, 573–592.

Whiteley, A.M., Swash, M., Urich, H. (1976) 'Progressive encephalomyelitis with rigidity.' *Brain*, **99**, 27–42.

Wilhelmsen, K.C., Blake, D.M., Lynch, T., *et al.* (1996) 'Chromosome 12-linked autosomal dominant scapuloperoneal muscular dystrophy.' *Annals of Neurology*, **39**, 507–520.

Wilkinson, D.A., Tonin, P., Shanske, S., *et al.* (1994) 'Clinical and biochemical features of 10 adult patients with muscle phosphorylase kinase deficiency.' *Neurology*, **44**, 461–466.

Wingard, D.W., Gatz, E.E. (1978) 'Some observations in stress susceptible patients.' *In:* Aldrete, J.A., Britt, B.A. (Eds.) *Second International Symposium on Malignant Hyperthermia.* New York: Grune & Stratton, pp. 363–372.

Witkowski, J.A. (1989) 'Dystrophin-related muscular dystrophies.' *Journal of Child Neurology*, **4**, 251–271.

Witt, T.N., Danek, A., Reiter, M., *et al.* (1992) 'McLeod syndrome: a distinct form of neuroacanthocytosis. Report of two cases and literature review with emphasis on neuromuscular manifestations.' *Journal of Neurology*, **239**, 302–306.

Wokke, J.H.J., Jennekens, F.G.I., Molenaar, P.C., *et al.* (1989) 'Congenital paucity of secondary synaptic clefts (CPSC) syndrome in 2 adult sibs.' *Neurology*, **39**, 648–654.

Wong, V. (1997) 'The spectrum of arthrogryposis in 33 Chinese children.' *Brain and Development*, **19**, 187–196.

—— Hawkins, B.R., Yu, Y.L. (1992) 'Myasthenia gravis in Hong Kong Chinese. 2. Paediatric disease.' *Acta Neurologica Scandinavica*, **86**, 68–72.

Wulff, J.D., Lin, J.T., Kepes, J.J. (1982) 'Inflammatory facioscapulohumeral muscular dystrophy and Coats syndrome.' *Annals of Neurology*, **12**, 398–401.

Yamaoka, L.H., Westbrook, C.A., Speer, M.C., *et al.* (1994) 'Development of a microsatellite genetic map spanning 5q31–q33 and subsequent placement of the LGMD1A locus between D5S178 and IL9.' *Neuromuscular Disorders*, **4**, 471–475.

Yasukohchi, S., Yagi, Y., Akabane, T., *et al.* (1988) 'Facioscapulohumeral dystrophy associated with sensorineural hearing loss, tortuosity of retinal arterioles, and an early onset and rapid progression of respiratory failure.' *Brain and Development*, **10**, 319–324.

Yazawa, M., Ikeda, S.I., Owa, M., *et al.* (1987) 'A family of Becker's progressive muscular dystrophy with severe cardiomyopathy.' *European Neurology*, **27**, 13–19.

Yoshioka, M., Saiwai, S. (1988) 'Congenital muscular dystrophy (Fukuyama type). Changes in the white matter low density on CT.' *Brain and Development*, **10**, 41–44.

Young, J.A., Anderson, J.M. (1987) 'Infantile myopathy with type I fibre specific hypertrophy.' *Developmental Medicine and Child Neurology*, **29**, 680–685.

Yuill, G.M., Lynch, P.G. (1974) 'Congenital non-progressive peripheral neuropathy with arthrogryposis multiplex.' *Journal of Neurology, Neurosurgery, and Psychiatry*, **37**, 316–323.

Zellweger, H., Afifi, A., McCormick, W.F., Mergner, W. (1967a) 'Benign congenital muscular dystrophy: a special form of congenital hypotonia.' *Clinical Pediatrics*, **6**, 655–663.

—— —— —— —— (1967b) 'Severe congenital muscular dystrophy.' *American Journal of Diseases of Children*, **114**, 591–612.

Zeviani, M., Nonaka, I., Bonilla, E., *et al.* (1985) 'Fatal infantile myopathy and renal dysfunction caused by cytochrome c oxidase deficiency: immunological studies in a new patient.' *Annals of Neurology*, **17**, 414–417.

—— Peterson, P., Servidei, S., *et al.* (1987) 'Benign reversible muscle cytochrome c oxidase deficiency: a second case.' *Neurology*, **37**, 64–67.

—— Gellera, C., Antozzi, C., *et al.* (1991) 'Maternally inherited myopathy and cardiomyopathy: association with mutation in mitochondrial DNA tRNA[leu (UUR)].' *Lancet*, **338**, 143–147.

Zierz, S. (1994) 'Carnitine palmitoyl transferase deficiency.' *In:* Engel, A.G., Franzini-Armstrong, C. (Eds.) *Myology, Basic and Clinical. 2nd Edn.* New York: McGraw Hill, pp. 1577–1585.

Zimmer, C., Gosztonyi, G., Cervos-Navarro, J., *et al.* (1992) 'Neuropathy with lysosomal changes in Marinesco–Sjögren syndrome: fine structural findings in skeletal muscle and conjunctiva.' *Neuropediatrics*, **23**, 329–335.

PART X

NEUROLOGICAL MANIFESTATIONS
OF SYSTEMIC DISEASES

Some degree of neurological involvement is common in many systemic diseases, some of which have already been discussed or alluded to in several chapters of this book. A complete coverage of this vast field is not the aim of this part, which is limited to the most important disorders that can produce major neurological disturbances and have not been previously dealt with. These include neurological syndromes due to disturbances of the electrolyte and acid-base metabolism to which the nervous system is extremely sensitive, nutritional diseases involving the CNS which represent a major cause of neurological disease in developing countries, and CNS involvement in endocrine and visceral diseases. Both the peripheral and the central nervous system can be affected in several of these conditions.

23

ELECTROLYTE AND ACID-BASE METABOLISM DISTURBANCES, NUTRITIONAL DISORDERS AND OTHER SYSTEMIC DISEASES

DISORDERS OF WATER AND ELECTROLYTE METABOLISM

COMPLICATIONS OF ACUTE DEHYDRATION

Acute dehydration can be seen at all ages, although it is more common in infancy because of the frequency of gastroenteritis, especially in developing countries. Other causes include renal and adrenal disease, heat exhaustion, limited water intake and diabetes insipidus. Acute dehydration can act on the CNS by at least two different mechanisms which are not mutually exclusive. One is volume loss that may lead to circulatory insufficiency and vascular collapse with resulting hypoxic brain damage. The second mechanism is electrolyte imbalance with hypernatraemia or hyponatraemia.

Hypovolaemia and Vascular Collapse as a Cause of Neurological Complications of Dehydration

There is evidence that in most cases of diarrhoeal disorders of infants, hypovolaemia and resulting circulatory insufficiency play a major role in the genesis of neurological complications (Aicardi and Goutières 1973). Such disturbances can result in vascular collapse that is observed in infants with either hyper- or hyponatraemic dehydration. The resulting *acute hypoxic encephalopathy* involves diffuse areas of the brain involving predominantly the territory fed by the carotid arteries and relatively sparing that fed by the posterior circulation (Fig. 23.1). The neurological features include coma and convulsive seizures which occur usually after a few hours, even though they are not necessarily related to the correction of hypernatraemia. Indeed, the occurrence of convulsive seizures is better correlated to indices of volume loss such as a high urea level (Stephenson 1971, Aicardi and Goutières 1973, Andrew 1991) than to sodium level or to the more or less rapid fall of natraemia. Sequelae of acute hypoxic encephalopathy include diplegia, microcephaly, mental retardation and seizures. Cortical blindness is not uncommon following the acute phase but useful recovery is usually observed.

Hypovolaemia with slowed venous circulation is one of the major factors of the *venous and sinus thromboses* that often occur with acute dehydration. These are probably responsible for the subarachnoid haemorrhage not uncommonly present in such cases and can also produce focal neurological symptoms and signs (Aicardi and Goutières 1973, Barron *et al.* 1992).

Hypernatraemia and the Intracranial Complications of Dehydration

Hypernatraemia is usually present in cases of severe dehydration and has been held responsible for the neurological complications observed in such cases.

An increased concentration of sodium in body fluids results in shrinkage of the brain as fluid is drawn from the cells into the hyperosmolar vascular compartment which becomes engorged and overdistended. Subdural haemorrhage has been experimentally produced in this way (Luttrell *et al.* 1959) but the clinical relevance in children remains uncertain (Luttrell and Finberg 1959, Elton *et al.* 1963, Aicardi and Goutières 1973, Andrew 1991). Small haemorrhages in the choroid plexus have been found by CT scan (Larsen 1989), and haemorrhage (of whatever source) is probably the cause of elevated CSF protein in dehydration.

Other consequences of hypernatraemia may occur in the absence of structural alteration of the CNS. Clinical manifestations include varying degrees of impaired consciousness, fever and spasticity. About one-third of infants experience convulsions which usually do not start until 24–48 hours following onset of rehydration. These have been attributed to oedema resulting from rapid return of fluid into the brain on lowering plasma osmolality. Fluid is attracted into the cells because of increased intracellular chloride level and the release by the brain tissue of as yet unidentified intracellular osmotically active particles called 'idiogenic osmoles' during the hypertonic phase of dehydration, which produces intracellular hypertonicity and consequently limits the degree of cellular dehydration (Arieff

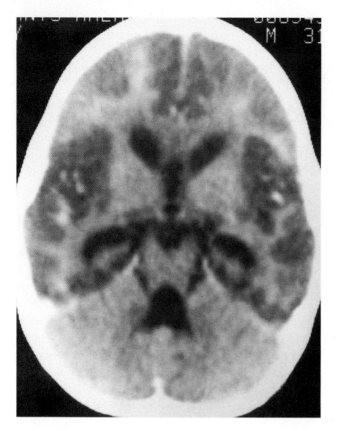

Fig. 23.1. Extensive ischaemic cortical necrosis in 18-month-old boy who suffered acute dehydration with vascular collapse and cardiac arrest at age 13 months.

1985, Lee *et al.* 1994). Seizures may well be due also to the return to basal value, during rehydration, of the convulsive threshold which had been maintained during the initial phase at supranormal level as a result of hypertonicity of body fluids. This may result in 'unmasking' the convulsive effects of vascular or hypoxic brain damage.

HYPONATRAEMIA

Hyponatraemia is uncommon in acute dehydration, unless it results from therapeutic errors or the occurrence of intense vomiting. Severe alkalosis is usually associated in such cases. Vascular collapse and hypoxic encephalopathy may supervene if dehydration is severe enough.

ELECTROLYTE DISTURBANCES IN OTHER CONDITIONS

Severe electrolyte disturbances may occur in conditions other than acute dehydration resulting from diarrhoeal disease.

HYPERNATRAEMIA

Hypernatraemia may be due to excessive evaporative losses of pure water or excess of salt caused by heat or hyperpnoea, salt poisoning or sodium retention as observed in hyperaldosteronism or Cushing disease. Hypernatraemia is virtually always associated with dehydration and it is difficult to determine which neuro-

logical features are due to the various factors. Rare cases of hypernatraemia are attributed to 'central' neurological causes (a disordered function of the hypothalamus). Hypernatraemia may be part of the syndrome of idiopathic hypothalamic dysfunction, in association with obesity, poor thermoregulation and disturbances of pituitary functions (North *et al.* 1994). A similar syndrome is more often caused by hypothalamic lesions including neoplasms. True central hypernatraemia without chronic dehydration is rare and most such cases are due to abnormal thirst resulting in adipsic hypernatraemia (Radetti *et al.* 1991), or to hyperosmolar alimentation in patients on tube feeding receiving concentrated formulas, or occur in unconscious patients unable to have proper access to water. In all three cases there is associated latent dehydration (Hammond *et al.* 1986, Diringer *et al.* 1989). The condition of central diabetes insipidus (Greger *et al.* 1986) is a primary failure of antidiuretic hormone secretion that may lead to hypernatraemia. It is most often due to brain tumours, especially craniopharyngioma, to malformations of the midline of the brain such as septo-optic dysplasia and to CNS infections; no cause was found in five of the 35 cases studied by Wang *et al.* (1994). The persistently increased diuresis in the face of marked hyperosmolality distinguishes diabetes insipidus from primary 'central' hypernatraemia.

HYPONATRAEMIA

Hyponatraemia occurs in patients with inappropriate secretion of antidiuretic hormone, due to CNS disorders, or as a side-effect of some drugs such as vincristine or carbamazepine (Van Amelsvoort *et al.* 1994), or occurring during the postoperative period. It is also observed in children with water retention due to heart or liver failure, in patients who receive excessive amounts of solute-poor fluids in the face of impaired renal function, and in cases of excess salt depletion as occurs with adrenal insufficiency, malnutrition or the use of diuretics. Oral water intoxication as a result of compulsive water drinking may occur in psychotic patients. A change of the solute content in formulas used for oral rehydration and the more widespread use of hypotonic solutes by parents for children with diarrhoea has resulted in an 'epidemic' increase of cases of hyponatraemia in infants (Keating *et al.* 1991, *Lancet* 1992). Ingestion of 3-4-methylenedioxymethamphetamine (MDMA, 'ecstasy') may be associated with severe hyponatraemia (Parr *et al.* 1997) and should be thought of in unexplained coma or abnormal behaviour in adolescents.

Neurological manifestations are headache, incoordination, disturbances of consciousness and, especially, convulsive seizures (Finberg 1991). These are usually brief and are often associated with low body temperature, apnoea, and an opisthotonic posture (Finberg 1991). Any neurological symptom in patients dependent on a third party for their fluid requirements should lead to the suspicion of abnormal electrolyte concentrations.

CHLORIDE DEFICIENCY

Deficiency in chloride obtains with profuse vomiting such as occurs in infants with pyloric stenosis and results in metabolic alkalosis. The latter decreases ionization of calcium and can result in *normocalcaemic tetany*.

Chloride deficiency rarely results from intestinal losses in children with chloride diarrhoea and in children who have ingested a chloride-deficient formula for periods of one month or more. Clinical features include lethargy, failure to thrive, weakness and delayed milestones, reversible on chloride administration. Head growth is slowed or arrested (Grossman *et al.* 1980). Although chloride supplementation rapidly reverses the symptoms, cognitive sequelae may persist (Willoughby *et al.* 1987). In rare cases chloride deprivation may occur as a result of a maternal chloride deficiency in breast-fed infants (Hill and Bowie 1983).

CENTRAL PONTINE MYELINOLYSIS AND RELATED CONDITIONS

Central pontine myelinolysis is characterized pathologically by symmetrical demyelination of the central basis pontis (Cadman and Rorke 1969, Valsalmis *et al.* 1971). The clinical picture is marked by confusion and quadriplegia, sometimes with cranial nerve dysfunction. The disease used to be considered fatal in most cases. More recently, neuroimaging techniques, especially MRI, have enabled *in vivo* diagnosis in patients who went on to recover (Brunner *et al.* 1990). The condition seems to be associated with rapid correction of hyponatraemia (Weissman and Weissman 1989, Brunner *et al.* 1990), but the safe rates for correction of hyponatraemia have not been determined (Harris *et al.* 1993). Some investigators emphasize the role of hyperosmolality rather than that of hyponatraemia (McKee *et al.* 1988). The disease is more common in adults with alcoholism but it also occurs in children with debilitating conditions (Kotagal *et al.* 1984), kernicterus (Ho *et al.* 1980), or following liver transplantation (Estol *et al.* 1989) or viral gastroenteritis (Gregorio *et al.* 1997).

Under similar circumstances to those responsible for the classic form of the disease, it may also involve extrapontine structures (Dickoff *et al.* 1988, Laureno and Karp 1988) such as the basal nuclei and/or central white matter.

OTHER ELECTROLYTE DISTURBANCES

Calcium and phosphorus disturbances occur preferentially in the neonatal period (Chapter 2) or as a complication of parathyroid disease.

Hypercalcaemia may occur with hyperparathyroidism, either acquired or congenital. Neonatal severe hyperparathyroidism features marked muscular hypotonia in association with failure to thrive and vomiting (Cooper *et al.* 1986).

Primary hypomagnesaemia with secondary hypocalcaemia has been considered in Chapter 2. This condition occurs mainly in males, but study of large pedigrees does not support an X-linked disease but rather sex-limitation of an autosomal recessive disorder (Teebi 1983). It can produce focal neurological deficits (Leicher *et al.* 1991). Chronic magnesium deficiency was described in a child with nephropathy in association with carpo-pedal spasm, convulsions and mitochondrial myopathy (Riggs *et al.* 1992).

NUTRITIONAL DISORDERS OF THE NERVOUS SYSTEM

The nervous system may be affected by nutritional deficiencies whether they involve a globally deficient nutrition as a result of grossly reduced quantities of food, poor protein intake, dietary imbalances, or lack of specific necessary nutriments. In many cases, intercurrent parasitic or bacterial infections, poor hygiene, and educational and emotional deprivation combine to produce a complex clinical picture. The growing nervous system is particularly at risk under such circumstances.

The total complement of neurons in the cerebrum is virtually complete at birth, but the growth of dendritic and axonal trees and of glial cells and the process of myelination are all very active during the first two years of life (Fox *et al.* 1972). In fact, the weight of the infant brain almost trebles during the first year of life. In the cerebellum, proliferation of the granule cells continues postnatally for at least the first year. The cerebellum may thus be especially vulnerable and this might be a factor in the origin of the clumsiness frequently observed in individuals submitted to early malnutrition. The first two or three years of life thus constitute, together with the prenatal period, a 'critical period' as the brain growth spurt begins about midgestation and ends between the second and third year of life (Dobbing 1980, 1981; Ballabriga 1989). Dendritic development has been shown to be subnormal in malnourished infants (Cordero *et al.* 1993). During this period both brain insults and neglect are especially apt to result in brain growth disturbances and dysfunction. The effects of prenatal deprivation have been discussed in Chapter 1. This section is devoted to the neurological consequences of postnatal nutritional deficiencies.

PROTEIN–CALORIE MALNUTRITION (PCM)
Winick (1969) estimated that 300 million children in the world suffer varying degrees of malnutrition and the figure may have increased since. The sequelae of this problem may represent a large proportion of cases of mental retardation, learning difficulties and abnormal behaviour in many parts of the world.

CLINICAL FEATURES
PCM may present as one of two main syndromes. *Marasmus* is primarily due to caloric insufficiency and is observed in infants weaned before 1 year of age or when the amount of breast milk becomes markedly reduced. The major clinical manifestations are emaciation, loss of muscle mass and growth failure.

Kwashiorkor results from a diet containing sufficient calories but deficient in proteins. Other factors such as infections, specific vitamin deficiencies and lack of appropriate stimulation also play a role (Jelliffe and Jelliffe 1992). Kwashiorkor is most common in children weaned between 2 and 3 years of age. The clinical features include oedema, growth failure, muscle wasting and behavioural disturbances. Abnormal pigmentation of the hair and skin, anaemia and hepatomegaly may be associated.

The neurological features of marasmus and kwashiorkor are similar. Indeed, the two conditions are often associated, as symptoms of kwashiorkor may develop in children already suffering from PCM. They include apathy which may be of such degree that children may manifest little interest in food despite severe wasting (Chavez and Martinez 1979). Muscle wasting and hypotonia are common and tendon reflexes may be decreased. This reflects involvement of peripheral nerves with reduction of nerve conduction velocities and segmental demyelination (Kumar *et al.* 1977, Chopra *et al.* 1986, Chopra and Sharma 1992). Soft neurological signs are significantly more frequent in malnourished than in well-fed children (Agarwal *et al.* 1989). CT scan may show brain atrophy, and MRI confirms the possibility of reversible atrophy but shows appropriate-for-age myelination (Gunston *et al.* 1992). Nonspecific EEG abnormalities have been reported (Agarwal *et al.* 1989).

NEUROLOGICAL COMPLICATIONS OF THE TREATMENT OF PCM

Up to 20 per cent of children with PCM experience neurological problems within three to seven days after being started on a normal diet. In most cases this is limited to drowsiness but rare cases of coma and even of fatality are on record (Balmer *et al.* 1968). This syndrome may result from hepatic failure when a large protein load is presented to an atrophic liver.

In some patients with PCM, coarse tremor, myoclonus, bradykinesia and rigidity are observed one to several weeks after protein refeeding (Kahn and Falcke 1956, Woodd-Walker 1971). The syndrome usually resolves in a few days or weeks. The tremor is usually generalized but localized jerking is occasionally seen and may be difficult to distinguish from epileptic jerking, especially from partial continuous epilepsy, as in two of my patients. The mechanism of this syndrome is unknown. A role of magnesium deficiency has been proposed and magnesium therapy was said to accelerate recovery. The syndrome may also be observed in cases of renutrition following protracted diarrhoea (unpublished data). Megaloblastic anaemia may be associated (Priolisi 1969). A relationship between this syndrome and that of infantile tremor syndrome as observed in India (Garewal *et al.* 1988) remains to be explored; the latter is associated with vitamin B_{12} deficiency in 87 per cent of cases and occurs in malnourished children in 82 per cent. It usually leaves behind a significant degree of mental retardation despite control with vitamin B_{12} therapy.

Other complications of treatment include thrombosis of the superior vena cava following prolonged catheterization responsible for increased intracranial pressure (Newman *et al.* 1980). In some cases, increased T_1 signal from the basal ganglia has been found on MRI in patients receiving total parenteral nutrition (Mirowitz *et al.* 1991). This may be related to manganese toxicity (Barron *et al.* 1994).

LONG-TERM NEURODEVELOPMENTAL EFFECTS OF PCM

Extreme PCM has been shown to result in reduced brain growth and behavioural abnormalities, both in experimental animals and in man (Winick 1969). In human beings, however, the role of malnutrition is more difficult to assess because malnourished infants also suffer several other adverse conditions such as crowd-

ing, poor hygiene, infections, deficient education and care, and such factors have a cumulative effect (Werner *et al.* 1967). However, there is little doubt that head growth—which reflects brain growth in humans—is slowed in severely malnourished infants (Stoch *et al.* 1982) and that the younger the infant at the time of deprivation the greater the effect on head circumference. 'Catch-up' growth of the brain can occur if renutrition is provided during the first one or two years of life but not later, even though catch-up of size and weight occurs (Stoch *et al.* 1982). CT scans have confirmed the presence of atrophy in the temporoparietal region bilaterally in patients with kwashiorkor followed up to early adulthood (Househam 1991). However, this is largely reversible (Gunston *et al.* 1992). Even though a small head does not necessarily mean a reduction in neuronal number, as neurons represent only a small fraction of human brain (Dobbing 1981), experience has shown that microcephaly is correlated with low IQ and learning difficulties (Smith 1981a, Gillberg and Rasmussen 1982) and that brain growth in low-birthweight infants is the best predictor of later IQ (Hack *et al.* 1984, Hack and Breslau 1986). There is also evidence that intellectual attainments in patients with PCM are inferior to those of normally fed children (Evans *et al.* 1980, Moodie *et al.* 1980), even though other factors such as sex, education and home environment may play a role as great or greater than nutrition proper. It is of note that malnutrition occurring in children older than 1–2 years of age has much less effect on the eventual IQ than earlier PCM. Disentangling the multiple factors responsible for developmental delay in malnourished children is difficult as lack of stimulation has been shown to be a possible cause. A recent study comparing four groups (supplemented, stimulated, supplemented and stimulated, and controls) showed a significantly greater benefit when both supplementation and stimulation were offered than when each was offered alone (Grantham-McGregor *et al.* 1991), and Colombo *et al.* (1992) found that neurodevelopment of adopted children who had had PCM reverted to normal levels thus indicating both the reversibility of the condition and the value of environmental stimulation.

NONORGANIC FAILURE TO THRIVE

The complexity of the relationships between malnutrition and somatic and mental development is illustrated by the common problem of 'nonorganic failure to thrive' (Casey *et al.* 1984). Growth retardation is commonly found in children from underprivileged homes even in industrialized countries. Such infants may also be the victims of abuse (King and Taitz 1985). Their failure to thrive is poorly understood and does not simply result from food deprivation, as shown by the rapid growth gain on changing the environment. The parents of children with 'deprivation dwarfism' differ in several respects from control parents. They have less emotional responsivity, the level of maternal acceptance of the child is lower and they are less able to organize the physical home environment (Casey *et al.* 1984). Such parents fail to 'read' the child's needs and respond to them. Poor feeding-skills can be an important cause of nonorganic growth failure, particularly in infants with early feeding difficulties

(Ramsay *et al.* 1993), and children with neurological problems often have feeding difficulties that may be responsible for poor nutrition and growth (Morton *et al.* 1993).

The syndrome of psychosocial or psychosomatic dwarfism appears to result from reversible inhibition of somatotropin secretion (Green *et al.* 1984). Affected children may have behaviour problems, bizarre eating habits, self-mutilation and poor response to pain (Fehrolt *et al.* 1985). All symptoms are reversible when the child's domicile is changed to a more benign environment. Such behavioural disturbances may be the presenting manifestation of nonorganic failure to thrive (Mouridsen and Nielson 1990), and this syndrome should be considered in the differential diagnosis of every child with short stature, low IQ, learning disabilities or bizarre behaviour in various combinations.

VITAMIN DEFICIENCIES
In addition to dietary deficiency, the action of vitamins in intermediary metabolism can be disturbed by abnormally high requirements—which may be of dietary origin, *e.g.* an excess of carbohydrates increases the need for B group vitamins—or by the action of inhibitory substances, or by an alteration of configuration of apoenzymes protein which also results in a considerable increase in vitamin requirements. Some inborn errors of metabolism can be corrected by large doses of certain vitamins (Chapter 9).

THIAMINE (VITAMIN B₁) DEFICIENCY
Thiamine plays an important role in the decarboxylation of pyruvate and alpha-ketoglutarate, two steps of the Krebs cycle, and the conversion of 5-carbon to 6-carbon sugars by means of the enzyme transketolase. Therefore, thiamine deficiency decreases energy available to the brain and increases the concentration of the two keto acids.

The clinical features of thiamine deficiency are variable. *Classical beriberi*, as seen in Asia and Africa, is marked by the sudden onset of weakness due to acute peripheral neuropathy, neck stiffness, aphonia and cardiac failure. In industralized countries, cases of *Wernicke encephalopathy* are sometimes seen in patients receiving parenteral nutrition (Barrett *et al.* 1993), in those on dialysis (Jagadha *et al.* 1987), and in children with malignant or debilitating diseases especially when they are taking a high-carbohydrate diet (Seear and Norman 1988, Pihko *et al.* 1989). The clinical picture is highly variable from sudden collapse and death to chronic cognitive impairment, through the classic picture of acute ataxia, global confusion and ocular abnormalities. The diagnosis is often missed and it should be thought of in all appropriate settings as Wernicke encephalopathy is a preventable cause of death (Pihko *et al.* 1989, Barrett *et al.* 1993). CT scan may be of considerable help if it shows hypodense areas with contrast enhancement in the paraventricular region of both thalami and along the cerebral aqueduct (Mensing *et al.* 1984). MRI better shows a low-intensity signal from the same regions. Abnormal MR images from the thalamic areas have also been described (Donnal *et al.* 1990). In patients on parenteral nutrition, unusual location of haemorrhagic lesions in the superior vermis

and lower brainstem without involvement of the mamillary bodies has been observed (Vortmeyer *et al.* 1992). The condition may occur even in children receiving conventional doses of vitamin B₁ if the requirements are increased by the carbohydrate intake (Seear and Norman 1988). Treatment is with large amounts of intravenous thiamine. The condition should be differentiated from Leigh disease (Chapter 9) which does not affect the mamillary bodies in most cases, contrary to their almost constant involvement in thiamine deficiency. Vitamin B₁ deficiency may favour the occurrence of epileptic seizures in patients with a latent predisposition (Keyser and DeBruijn 1991).

PYRIDOXINE (VITAMIN B₆) DEFICIENCY AND PYRIDOXINE DEPENDENCY
Vitamin B₆ in the form of its aldehyde derivative pyridoxal-5-phosphate is essential for correct functioning of the CNS. It is, in particular, necessary for the decarboxylation of glutamic acid to GABA, an essential inhibitory neurotransmitter in cerebral cortex.

Pyridoxine deficiency is responsible for heightened brain excitability and seizures. It appears during the first year of life in infants on a diet providing less than 0.1 mg/d such as powdered goat's milk (Johnson 1982). Less rarely, pyridoxine deficiency may occur in patients who have a jejunal bypass or in those who receive treatment with hydrazide drugs such as isoniazid or penicillamine. In such cases, however, peripheral neuropathy (Chapter 21) is more common than convulsions.

Pyridoxine dependency (Chapter 9) is an uncommon familial disease transmitted as an autosomal recessive trait, characterized by seizures, usually severe and repeated, which occurs soon after birth or even *in utero* (Haenggeli *et al.* 1991). Recently, several investigators have pointed out that seizures manifesting pyridoxine dependency may occur relatively late, up to 16 months, respond to anticonvulsants and remain controlled for periods of several weeks or even months after receiving pyridoxine (Bankier *et al.* 1983). Such seizures are apt to occur repeatedly in bouts of status epilepticus but may also present as infantile spasms or myoclonic attacks (Goutières and Aicardi 1985). Treatment of pyridoxine dependency requires large doses of vitamin B₆. In case of status, intravenous administration of 50–100 mg should stop the seizures in less than 10 minutes. In the case of brief seizures oral administration of 50 mg/d as a single dose produces immediate discontinuation of attacks. Intravenous doses of more than 200 mg may produce hypotonia and apnoea (Kroll 1985). Megadoses of pyridoxine (over 1 g) can produce a chronic neuropathy (Schaumburg *et al.* 1983).

CYANOCOBALAMIN (VITAMIN B₁₂) DEFICIENCY
Deficiency of cyanocobalamin in adults is responsible for the classical picture of subacute combined degeneration of the posterior and lateral columns of the spinal cord. This condition is exceptional in children in whom it may accompany congenital pernicious anaemia or be associated with intestinal disease. The clinical features of such cases are ataxia, weakness and spasticity of the lower extremities, loss of vibratory sensation and

intellectual deficit (Pearson *et al.* 1964, Chanarin *et al.* 1985).

Dietary vitamin B_{12} deficiency is relatively common in India (Jadhav *et al.* 1962). In Western countries, cases of vitamin B_{12} deficiency are being observed in breast-fed infants of mothers deficient in B_{12} as a result of pernicious anaemia or a strict vegetarian (vegan) diet lacking in the vitamin (Sadowitz *et al.* 1986, Grattan-Smith *et al.* 1997). In such cases, excretion of homocystine and methylmalonic acid is present, although not constantly (Stollhoff and Schulte 1987). The clinical picture is one of normal development during the first months of life, followed by developmental regression, pyramidal tract signs and CT evidence of brain atrophy. In some patients, choreomyoclonic movements are present (Grattan-Smith *et al.* 1997; and personal case) or develop at the time of starting vitamin B_{12}. With therapy, there is rapid improvement and the atrophy can disappear. Sequelae may persist (Graham *et al.* 1992). Neurological disease may be present in the absence of anaemia or macrocytosis (Lindenbaum *et al.* 1988).

A similar picture but with an earlier onset from the first months of life may occur in rare infants with *inborn errors of vitamin B_{12} metabolism* (Chapter 9).

Cobalamin deficiency usually responds favourably to therapy with vitamin B_{12}. Administration of folate is to be avoided as it may increase the neurological anomalies (Pearson *et al.* 1964). There is some suggestion that the spectrum of neurological manifestations of vitamin B_{12} deficiency may be wide in adult patients and include psychiatric disorders (Nijst *et al.* 1990) but no data are available in children.

FOLATE DISORDERS

Errors in folate metabolism are studied in Chapter 9.

Congenital folate malabsorption is a rare metabolic error with selective inability to absorb folates from the intestine and across the blood–brain barrier. The disease presents in early infancy with diarrhoea, poor weight gain and megaloblastic anaemia. Neurological manifestations may include mental retardation, seizures, ataxia, extrapyramidal disease and peripheral neuropathy (Steinschneider *et al.* 1990). The diagnosis is confirmed by low serum and CSF folate concentration. Treatment with folinic acid may be more effective than folic acid and the condition may be reversible if recognized early. Similar manifestations may occur in patients with deficiency of folate-binding protein in the CNS (Wevers *et al.* 1994).

NICOTINIC ACID DEFICIENCY

This is a rare condition which was commonly observed in areas where corn is the staple food. Mildly affected children are apathetic or irritable. In severe cases there is polyneuropathy, and degeneration of Betz cells in the motor cortex and of the pyramidal and spinocerebellar tract in the spinal cord. The clinical disease known as *pellagra* is probably the result of multivitamin deficiency but responds to nicotinic acid. Skin rash is a prominent feature. In addition to peripheral involvement, there may be obtundation or delirium, optic atrophy and coarse tremors (Still 1977).

LIPOSOLUBLE VITAMIN DEFICIENCY

Deficiency of vitamin A can produce increased intracranial pressure, reversible by dietary treatment (Keating and Feigin 1970). The same effect is more frequently the result of excess vitamin A intoxication (Feldman and Schlezinger 1970).

Deficiency of vitamin E is encountered in cases of mucoviscidosis (Willison *et al.* 1985), biliary disease and other malabsorptive conditions including the blind-loop syndrome (surgically diverted intestinal loop), and, rarely, as an isolated deficiency (Krendel *et al.* 1987). The resulting neuropathy is described in Chapter 21. Muscular involvement with accumulation of electron-dense material in muscle fibres is frequent (Werlin *et al.* 1983), and elevation of creatine kinase may occur (Kohlschütter 1993).

The neuropathy of abetalipoproteinaemia probably has a similar mechanism (Brin *et al.* 1986).

TROPICAL PARAPLEGIAS AND TROPICAL ATAXIC NEUROPATHY

These disorders are observed in several developing countries, and in southern Japan where a similar disorder is known as HTLV1-associated myelopathy (HAM). Patients with tropical paraplegia slowly develop bilateral spasticity of the lower limbs with few or no sensory defects. In ataxic neuropathy, paraesthesiae and loss of deep sensation and reflexes are associated.

The role of HTLV1 infection seems predominant in the genesis of tropical paraplegia in some parts of the world (Chapter 11). Some cases, however, are not associated with HTLV1 infection and may be of multifactorial origin: malnutrition, deficiency in B_{12} and other vitamins, and chronic malabsorption due to persistent parasitic infestation may all play a role. Improperly prepared cassava is a major factor in some epidemics (Roman *et al.* 1985, Carton *et al.* 1986) and may be a major causal factor of the so-called konzo observed in Tanzania (Howlett *et al.* 1990). A good review of the tropical neuropathies, especially those due to rare biological toxins and nutritional deficiencies, is available (Thomas 1997).

In other parts of the world, a similar disease known as lathyrism is caused by consumption of the chick pea *Lathyrus sativus* (Ludolph *et al.* 1987).

The possible role of *deficiency in oligoelements* remains unsettled. Ramaekers *et al.* (1994) have suggested that selenium deficiency could play a role in triggering seizures.

NEUROLOGICAL COMPLICATIONS OF DIABETES MELLITUS

DIABETIC KETOACIDOSIS AND OTHER COMAS IN DIABETIC CHILDREN

Ketoacidosis is a frequent cause of unconsciousness in young diabetic patients. Although the pathogenesis of CNS involvement in diabetic ketoacidosis is still unclear, a drastic reduction in cerebral blood flow and oxygen uptake by the brain is well-established. There is no good correlation between the degree of obtundation and blood or CSF glucose or osmolality levels, pH,

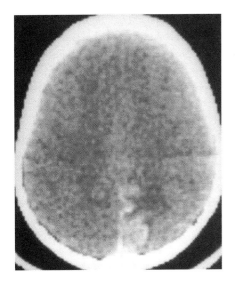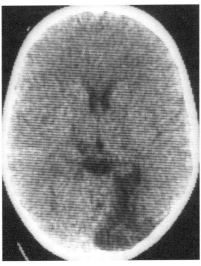

Fig. 23.2. Cerebrovascular accident during an episode of diabetic ketoacidosis. 7-year-old girl who, following an episode of ketoacidotic coma, developed acute psychosis with delirium and hallucinations and was left with right hemianopia. *(Far left)* First CT scan shows an infarct in the territory of the left posterior artery (note cortical take-up of contrast). *(Left)* Seven months later an area of cavitation is present.

or concentrations of ketone bodies, hydroxybutyrate and aceto-acetate.

Diabetic ketoacidosis may be complicated by the occurrence of *cerebral oedema* that can be lethal or leave severe sequelae (Rosenbloom *et al.* 1980, Greene *et al.* 1990). A rapid reduction of blood hyperosmolality in the face of a more slowly decreasing cerebral osmolality is thought to account for the entrance of water into the brain, but oedema may occur even with cautiously conducted rehydration (Greene *et al.* 1990). The diagnosis of brain oedema is difficult as there is no specific clinical feature and papilloedema has no time to develop. Oedema should be suspected when the child fails to regain consciousness despite adequate treatment. CT scan may show small cerebral ventricles and hypodensity of the white matter. Krane *et al.* (1985) found that subclinical oedema was frequently present on systematic CT scanning as shown by decreased parenchymal density. Treatment is based on cautious rehydration to prevent the occurrence of this complication. Mannitol therapy (Chapter 14) may be effective when given early (Franklin *et al.* 1982).

Nonketotic hyperosmolar diabetic coma is rare in children (Vernon and Postellon 1986). Clinical features may include generalized or focal seizures, ophthalmoplegia and hemiparesis.

Hypoglycaemic coma is frequent in treated diabetic patients. Hypoglycaemic attacks are marked by sudden or progressive impairment of neurological function (Koh *et al.* 1988). During the initial stages, cortical dysfunction is the main feature, with somnolence, slowed intellectual activity or bizarre behaviour. Focal neurological signs, especially hemiplegia, may be transiently present (Shintani *et al.* 1993). At a late stage unconsciousness occurs, and in many cases generalized or partial seizures supervene. Response to intravenous glucose is immediate. Severe hypoglycaemic attacks may leave neurological residua.

ACUTE HEMIPLEGIA
Transient hemiparesis may acutely develop in some patients with insulin-dependent diabetes mellitus in the absence of hypoglycaemia or of any disorder of consciousness (McDonald and Brown 1979, Korobkin 1980).

Hemiplegia frequently appears during sleep and may be precipitated by a febrile illness. Headache is a constant feature and a migrainous mechanism has been proposed but is entirely conjectural (Korobkin 1980). The hemiplegia remits after a few hours and recovery is complete. Recurrences can occur. CT scan in such cases does not show any abnormality. The EEG usually shows slowing contralateral to the hemiplegia.

The condition should be distinguished from strokes, which do not occur in juvenile diabetes except during episodes of keto-acidotic coma (Fig. 23.2). Spontaneous intracerebral haematomas have been rarely reported, possibly as a result of venous thrombosis (Atluru 1986). There is no established form of treatment.

PERIPHERAL NEUROPATHY
Clinically manifest polyneuropathy is exceptional in diabetic children. Subclinical involvement of the peripheral nerves, however, is frequent. There is some evidence from electrophysiological studies that both a long duration and poor control of the diabetes are correlated with the development of polyneuropathy (Eeg-Olofsson and Petersen 1966, Hoffman *et al.* 1983).

Polyradiculopathy, which is common in adults, may be seen in rare cases of juvenile diabetes (Bastron and Thomas 1981). It is marked by pain, dysaesthesiae and weakness, and electrical studies point to involvement of several nerve roots or proximal segments of nerves. Cranial nerve involvement is exceptional before adulthood. I have seen one 14-year-old patient with typical acute IIIrd nerve paralysis.

OPTIC NERVE INVOLVEMENT
A syndrome of *d*iabetes *i*nsipidus, *d*iabetes *m*ellitus, *o*ptic *a*trophy, *d*eafness and other neurological abnormalities (DIDMOAD or Wolfram syndrome) has been reported in several kindreds (Rando *et al.* 1992). The syndrome is probably genetically determined and transmitted as an autosomal recessive trait (Chapter 18).

The diabetes has its onset in the first decade and is insulin-dependent. Optic atrophy occurs later in the first decade. Central diabetes insipidus and deafness usually appear in the second decade followed by dilatation of the lower urinary tract. Other manifestations such as vestibulo-ocular central disturbances, anosmia or tremor are on record. This is a progressive degenerative condition, and, in adult life, cerebellar ataxia, nystagmus, dysarthria and episodes of apnoea develop. Atrophy of the CNS, especially the cerebellum and brainstem, becomes evident after 30 years (Grosse Aldenhövel *et al.* 1991, Barrett *et al.* 1995, Scolding *et al.* 1996). The optic neuropathy is considered not to be the result of diabetes but to represent an independent feature of a genetic syndrome.

HYPOGLYCAEMIA

Cerebral function requires glucose even though the brain of infants and young children can utilize ketone bodies more efficiently and has a greater glycolytic ability than that of adults (Altman *et al.* 1993). Neonates tolerate levels of < 1.1 mmol/L (< 20 mg/dL) without clinical manifestations, and, in general, there is no constant relationship between blood glucose levels and the severity of neurological manifestations. Nevertheless, hypoglycaemia lasting 10–20 minutes or more can produce selective neuronal necrosis of the superficial cortical laminae, the CA1 sector of Ammon's horn and the caudate nuclei (Banker 1967). The most common causes of symptomatic hypoglycaemia outside the neonatal period include nonketotic hypoglycaemia, which usually occurs in infants with low birthweight for gestational age; congenital hypopituitarism; various metabolic disorders such as mitochondrial defects in fatty acid metabolism; and pancreatic tumours or nesidioblastosis (Cornblath and Schwartz 1991).

The clinical manifestations in older children are due to the adrenaline response to low glucose levels and the deficiency of available energy delivery to the brain. The adrenalin response is responsible for autonomic manifestations such as pallor, sweating, palpitations and anxiety. It tends to disappear in patients with frequently repeated hypoglycaemic attacks, whereas increasing impairment of brain function produces headache, dizziness, blurred vision, somnolence and eventually coma and epileptic seizures. These manifestations respond immediately to intravenous administration of glucose (Cornblath and Schwartz 1991). Focal seizures or deficits are not rare (Wayne *et al.* 1990). The diagnosis rests on the circumstances of occurrence, type of symptoms, history of previous similar symptoms and, in case of doubt, response to therapy. The outcome is favourable for brief episodes, but prolonged unconsciousness is of poor prognostic significance.

NEUROLOGICAL COMPLICATIONS OF CARDIAC DISEASES

CONGENITAL HEART DISEASE
Congenital heart disease, especially cyanotic heart disease, is an important cause of neurological problems.

COGNITIVE DEVELOPMENT AND HEART MALFORMATIONS
The cognitive development of children with congenital heart disease is usually normal. However, cognitive functions in children with cyanotic heart disease may be abnormal more often than in noncyanotic disease (Silbert *et al.* 1969), and especially in children with left-heart hypoplasia. Rogers *et al.* (1995) found that seven of 11 survivors with this condition had major mental disabilities. Many mechanisms for such cognitive difficulties are possible, including associated malformations, the consequences of infarcts or of hypoxic attacks, and chronic hypoxia. The role of hypoxia is suggested by the finding that the age at which surgery is performed for great vessel transposition is inversely correlated to the cognitive level attained (Newburger *et al.* 1984), indicating that postponement of surgical repair may be associated with impairment of higher brain functions. Chronic hypoxia in cyanotic children was found to be associated with impaired motor function, inability to sustain attention and low academic achievement (O'Dougherty *et al.* 1985, Wright and Nolan 1994).

Brain malformations are more frequent in children with congenital heart disease than in the general population. In studies of cyanotic heart disease, CNS abnormalities have been found in 2–5 per cent of cases of great vessel transposition, 5–10 per cent of those of tetralogy of Fallot, 4–10 per cent of those of truncus arteriosus, and up to 29 per cent of those of hypoplasia of the left heart (Fyler *et al.* 1980, Glauser *et al.* 1990a). Brain malformations may include both major and minor abnormalities, and micrencephaly is common. In noncyanotic disease brain anomalies are especially frequent, with endocardial cushion defects because of their association with Down syndrome, but are sometimes found with coarctation of the aorta or aortic stenosis. Coarctation of the aorta is commonly associated with cerebral aneurysms and may also produce cerebral haemorrhage in their absence (Freedom 1989).

NEUROLOGICAL COMPLICATIONS OF NONOPERATED CONGENITAL HEART DISEASE
Paroxysmal episodes of syncope can occur in patients with valvular aortic stenosis. *Cyanotic attacks* constitute a major complication of cyanotic heart disease. The episodes are precipitated by exertion, feeding or bowel movement and are marked by hyperpnoea and a sudden increase in previous cyanosis. Consciousness may be decreased and a generalized convulsion may occur in severe cases. EEG monitoring indicates that such seizures are of hypoxic rather than epileptic nature (Daniels *et al.* 1987). In some cases, cyanotic attacks are followed by the acute appearance of a cerebrovascular accident.

Cerebrovascular accidents occur during the first 20 months of life in 75 per cent of the cases, and tetralogy of Fallot and transposition of the great vessels account for 90 per cent of cases (Cottrill and Kaplan 1973, Phornphutkul *et al.* 1973). Their incidence has considerably decreased as most children undergo early surgical treatment. However, cerebrovascular accidents also occur following complete repair. Du Plessis *et al.* (1995a) observed stroke in 17 (2.6 per cent) of 645 children undergoing the Fontan operation. These occurred from the first postoperative day

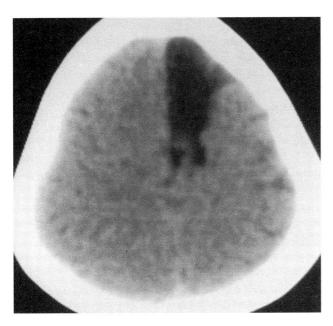

Fig. 23.3. Infarct in territory of anterior cerebral artery in 3-year-old patient with transposition of the great vessels. There was sudden onset of hemiplegia with crural predominance following corrective surgery.

to 30 months after surgery. The infarcts are mainly located in the territory of the middle cerebral artery but other large vessels may be involved (Fig. 23.3). Venous thrombosis also occurs and is particularly correlated to dehydration and a high haematocrit, whereas arterial infarcts are often observed in patients with iron-deficiency anaemia (Tyler and Clark 1957). The latter is often associated with increased blood viscosity (Linderkamp *et al.* 1979). Hemiplegia of sudden onset is the usual clinical presentation but other focal deficits such as hemianopia or aphasia may be seen. CT scan shows the usual images of arterial infarction of large vessels but lacunar infarcts are unusual (Dusser *et al.* 1986). Mental retardation and residual epilepsy are seen in a quarter of cases.

Brain abscesses have been studied in Chapter 11. About 80 per cent of them occur in cases of tetralogy of Fallot and transposition of the great vessels. They are rare before 2 years of age, perhaps because they develop on previous small infarcts. Systematic administration of antibiotics in patients with suspected stroke has been suggested (Kurlan and Griggs 1983). Papilloedema is of little value in the diagnosis of brain abscess in patients with cyanotic heart disease, because retinal vessels are frequently engorged and tortuous with blurring of the disc margins (Peterson and Rosenthal 1972).

Neurological complications of acquired heart disease are much less common than those of congenital disease. They include chorea (Chapter 12) and cerebral embolization that may be due to cardiac arrhythmias or bacterial endocarditis.

NEUROLOGICAL COMPLICATIONS OF SURGERY FOR HEART DISEASE
Surgical complications of cardiac surgery in children are common as a result of the increasing number of severe malformations now amenable to operation. They represent a significant cause

of neurodevelopmental sequelae of congenital heart disease (Ferry 1987).

Acute complications that occur during or immediately following operation include coma or lesser alterations of consciousness, seizures (generalized, partial or multifocal), hemiparesis, changes in muscle tone, organic mental syndromes, gaze palsies, dyskinesia and personality changes. Seizures in particular are frequent (occurring in 4–26 per cent of patients following heart surgery with deep hypothermia) and usually subside without sequelae (Du Plessis *et al.* 1994). However, they may be prolonged and severe, and neuroimaging shows that some of them are associated with evidence of focal ischaemia. Ehyai *et al.* (1984) observed seizures in 15 of 166 operated infants, associated in two cases with hypocalcaemia and hypomagnesaemia. CT and MR imaging studies (Ferry 1990, McConnell *et al.* 1990) have shown that the incidence of ischaemic accidents, unsuspected cerebral atrophy and subdural haemorrhages was greater than suspected. A majority of these complications are due to impaired perfusion and embolic phenomena (Du Plessis *et al.* 1995b) and are associated with marked EEG abnormalities (Olson and Shewmon 1989). Pathologically, they consist of periventricular leukomalacias, cerebral necrosis and occasionally brainstem necrosis (Glauser *et al.* 1990b): these are common during and after cardiopulmonary bypass and consist of microthrombi, fat emboli and especially air emboli (Malone *et al.* 1981, Furlan and Breuer 1984). The mechanisms responsible for cerebral extradural or subdural haemorrhages remain poorly understood although reperfusion probably plays a role (Humphreys *et al.* 1975). Choreoathetotic dyskinesias (Robinson *et al.* 1988, Wical and Tomasi 1990, Huntley *et al.* 1993, Curless *et al.* 1994), especially involving the orofacial muscles, are particularly observed following induced profound hypothermia (Newburger *et al.* 1993). Abnormal movements usually appear a few days after operation. Medlock *et al.* (1993) observed this complication in eight (1.2 per cent) of 668 children undergoing cardiopulmonary bypass surgery. In three of them the abnormal movements were transient, disappearing in a few days or weeks, but in the other five they were persistent. None of these eight children had normal development 22–130 months after surgery.

Ischaemic spinal cord injury may occur not only following repair of coarctation of the aorta but also in open heart surgery, following vascular collapse (Puntis and Green 1985).

Late sequelae of cardiac surgery include mental retardation, cerebral palsy, gait disorders, seizures sometimes in the form of West syndrome (Du Plessis *et al.* 1994), and learning disorders. Abnormal MRI scans are found in a high proportion of operated children. Such changes include ventriculomegaly, atrophy and white matter infarcts (McConnell *et al.* 1990) and are not necessarily associated with neurological or developmental sequelae (Miller *et al.* 1994). There is an unexplained frequency of hearing loss but impairment of communication is of multifactorial origin. Hydrocephalus due to increased intracranial venous pressure may occur following Mustard operation (Ferry 1990). Vertebrobasilar ischaemia after a Blalock–Taussig anastomosis can be the result of a significant subclavian steal but is rare (Kurlan *et al.* 1984).

Complications of cardiac transplantation include those of cardiopulmonary bypass surgery and those of immunosuppressant therapy (Adair *et al.* 1992).

INFECTIVE ENDOCARDITIS
Bacterial endocarditis can complicate a known cardiac disease but it may also occur in an apparently normal heart (Jones and Siekert 1989). The commonest manifestations are emboli, purulent meningitis, brain abcess and mycotic aneurysm with possible meningeal or parenchymal haemorrhage.

In children, seizures are not uncommon and were observed in 14 of 141 patients of Johnson *et al.* (1975).

The CSF is abnormal in 70 per cent of cases either with a purulent appearance or with a lymphocytic pleocytosis. The CSF is haemorrhagic in 13 per cent of cases (Pruitt *et al.* 1978).

PULMONARY DISEASES

Pulmonary diseases can affect the CNS through chronic hypoxia or chronic retention of carbon dioxide or both.

PROGRESSIVE CNS DISEASE IN PRETERM INFANTS WITH BRONCHOPULMONARY DYSPLASIA
This condition is encountered in preterm infants with severe respiratory failure followed by CNS symptoms including increasing hypotonia and loss of developmental milestones with eventual EEG deterioration and death. In other cases, the clinical features consist of progressive apnoea, bradycardia and sudden death (Ellison and Farina 1980). Under similar circumstances, a peculiar movement disorder has been reported (Perlman and Volpe 1989, Hadders-Algra *et al.* 1994; see Chapter 2). Chronic hypoventilation has also been implicated as a cause of brainstem gliosis which, in turn, might be responsible for sudden death (Becker and Takashima 1985).

CHRONIC CARBON DIOXIDE RETENTION
CO_2 retention is usually associated with at least some degree of hypoxia and with respiratory acidosis. It is primarily observed in chronic lung disease in older children, such as mucoviscidosis. The main clinical feature is progressively deepening lethargy which may evolve into coma often as a result of pulmonary infection. Cognitive impairment as a result of chronic lung disease is usually mild in adults (Manni *et al.* 1987). CO_2 retention can produce intracranial hypertension as a consequence of dilatation of the cerebral vasculature with the possible development of papilloedema.

A subclinical neuropathy has been reported in adults (Faden *et al.* 1981) but no case is known in childhood.

COMPLICATIONS OF EXTRACORPOREAL MEMBRANE OXYGENATION (ECMO)
ECMO is currently used in many centres for the treatment of neonatal respiratory distress. The technique necessitates ligation of the right common carotid artery and anticoagulation. Neurological complications are frequently associated with this method. In children dying during or following ECMO both ischaemic and haemorrhagic lesions are found at post-mortem examination (Mendoza *et al.* 1991, Jarjour and Ahdab-Barmada 1994). Clinical manifestations include hemiplegia and seizures (Schumacher *et al.* 1991, Korinthenberg *et al.* 1993). Seizures predominantly involve the right cerebral hemisphere (Campbell *et al.* 1991, Hahn *et al.* 1993). The EEG is essential for the diagnosis as children are ventilated and paralysed (Streletz *et al.* 1992). Electrical status epilepticus and periodic or repetitive discharges are common (Hahn *et al.* 1993). Seizures indicate a greatly increased risk of permanent sequelae, which usually present as quadriparesis, residual epilepsy and cognitive difficulties. They are present in 20–50 per cent of survivors (Graziani *et al.* 1994, Glass *et al.* 1995, Lago *et al.* 1995). Neuroimaging may show both ischaemic and haemorrhagic lesions. The former were said to be mainly right-sided and the latter left-sided (Mendoza *et al.* 1991) but this has not been substantiated by later studies (Lago *et al.* 1995). The mechanism of damage in ECMO is poorly understood. Reversed flow in the right vertebral artery is observed in 30 per cent of cases but is not correlated with a greater frequency of sequelae (Graziani *et al.* 1994). Deafness is not rare in survivors, but no more frequently than in infants with similar problems not undergoing ECMO.

RENAL DISEASES

Cerebral symptoms and signs frequently accompany uraemia, although the mechanisms of neurological impairment are poorly understood. Some procedures, *e.g.* dialysis, may have complications mainly due to one specific factor; in most cases the aetiology is probably multifactorial and includes such factors as electrolyte disorders, hypertension or entrance into the brain of toxic substances such as organic acids.

Peripheral uraemic neuropathy may occur in a subclinical form in as many as 76 per cent of uraemic children (Mentser *et al.* 1978). This complication has been considered in Chapter 21 and only CNS abnormalities are mentioned here. A primary myopathy has been rarely encountered (Berretta *et al.* 1986).

URAEMIC ENCEPHALOPATHY
The main neurological complication of renal insufficiency is uraemic encephalopathy which is marked by alteration in mental status, hypotonia, seizures, athetoid movements, nystagmus and ataxia (Tyler 1968, Foley *et al.* 1981, Rotundo *et al.* 1982). Myoclonus is a suggestive symptom as are peripheral cramps. Transient focal cerebral symptoms, including hemiparesis and cortical blindness, may be more closely related to hypertensive encephalopathy.

In children with moderate to severe chronic renal failure, a small head and developmental delay are commonly encountered (McGraw and Haka-Ikse 1985). Bock *et al.* (1989) found that children with the most severe renal insufficiency had a small head circumference early in life, motor developmental delay and progressive decrease in IQ in the absence of neurological signs.

Uraemic encephalopathy is reversible upon correction of renal insufficiency by haemodialysis or kidney transplantation. The latter is highly efficacious for uraemic polyneuropathy, whereas haemodialysis does not correct sensory symptoms. Treatment of seizures is with standard anticonvulsant therapy, taking into account the changes in metabolism and excretion of the drugs. Benzodiazepines are effective against the myoclonus.

Cognitive deficits, cortical atrophy and disseminated brain calcification are often associated with nephropathic cystinosis (Nichols *et al.* 1990). The effect of kidney transplant in such cases is not yet known.

COMPLICATIONS OF TREATMENT OF CHRONIC RENAL FAILURE

Dialysis may be associated with aggravation of neurological manifestations as a result of the *dialysis dysequilibrium syndrome*. This syndrome is due to failure of the urea to equilibrate rapidly between brain and blood, thus resulting in a shift of extracellular water into the brain. This complication can be avoided by gradual changes in blood electrolytes and earlier dialysis (Tyler 1965).

Repeated dialysis may be associated with a variety of symptoms probably related to deficiency of vitamins, other nutritional factors or electrolyte dysequilibrium. These include the 'burning feet syndrome', a form of sensorimotor neuropathy that may respond to supplementation with group B vitamins (Tyler 1965), central pontine myelinolysis and Wernicke encephalopathy.

Dialysis encephalopathy is characterized by personality changes, dysarthria, apraxia of speech, myoclonus and seizures. The EEG shows slowing of background tracings and multiple paroxysms (Hughes and Schreeder 1980, Foley *et al.* 1981). The disorder is fatal in a few years. Aluminium toxicity is probably the cause of such cases as a result of a high content of this metal in the dialysis bath, and the incidence of the syndrome has decreased sharply with the use of aluminium-free water. Moreover, reversal of dialysis dementia has been achieved by discontinuation of the use of aluminium gels and by aluminium chelation (Ackrill *et al.* 1980). Cases of dialysis encephalopathy have been seen in patients not on dialysis (Griswold *et al.* 1983, Andreoli *et al.* 1984, Sedman *et al.* 1984). These patients were receiving large quantities of aluminium salts and had levels of serum and bone aluminium considerably in excess of the average figures.

Acute hypercalcaemia in haemodialysis patients may mimic dialysis dementia (Rivera-Vásquez *et al.* 1980) and has an excellent prognosis on correction of serum calcium.

Symptomatic hypoglycaemia has been observed months to years following renal transplantation (Wells *et al.* 1988). It occurred in children receiving propanolol and responded to discontinuation of the drug.

Patients with *renal transplants* run the risks attendant to immunosuppression, especially opportunistic infections. Aspergillosis of the CNS with multiple brain abcesses is a particularly common infection in immunocompromised children. In addition, they can be contaminated by the donated kidney, especially with cytomegalovirus (Schneck 1965). The development of reticulum cell neoplasms may also be a result of immunodeficiency (Penn 1979). Toxicity of immunosuppressant agents, especially cyclosporin, is dealt with below.

An acute neurological syndrome, termed *rejection encephalopathy*, occurs in some renal transplant recipients (Gross *et al.* 1982). It is important to recognize that this syndrome is not due to disturbances in electrolytes, hypertension, fever or steroids, so steroid treatment may be continued.

It is also important to keep in mind that drugs such as most anticonvulsants accelerate the catabolism of steroids resulting in possible reduction of allograft survival (Wassner *et al.* 1976). Treatment of seizures should be with non-enzyme-inducing drugs such as valproate or benzodiazepines.

HEPATIC DISEASE

HEPATIC ENCEPHALOPATHY

Hepatic encephalopathy constitutes the end stage of acute or chronic liver disease and culminates in hepatic coma. This complication has been attributed to hyperammonaemia (Cooper *et al.* 1984). However, the mechanism of ammonia toxicity is obscure and occasional patients with hepatic encephalopathy have normal or mildly elevated levels of ammonia in the blood and CSF. The toxicity of ammonia is well shown by the possible occurrence of encephalopathy in patients receiving essential amino acid hyperalimentation (Grazer *et al.* 1984) but does not account for all features of the encephalopathy of liver failure. Its role as a cause of the stuporous episodes sometimes observed during valproate therapy (Marescaux *et al.* 1982) remains unclear.

Neuropathological changes are limited. Gross examination of the brain shows no abnormalities. Microscopically, the main alteration is enlargement and increase in the number of protoplasmic astrocytes, the so-called Alzheimer type II astrocytes. These are seen throughout the cerebral cortex, basal ganglia and brainstem nuclei.

The *clinical features* of hepatic encephalopathy are observed in children with liver failure due to acute hepatitis, drug toxicity, Wilson disease or metabolic diseases, less commonly with chronic hepatitis or various terminal liver illnesses, including cystic fibrosis of the pancreas and deficiency in alpha 1 antitrypsin. Acute hepatic failure has been observed repeatedly in epileptic patients receiving valproic acid or sodium valproate (Schmidt 1984, Fenichel and Greene 1985, Scheffner *et al.* 1988). This rare complication occurs mainly in infants and young children, usually mentally retarded and receiving valproate as part of a multidrug treatment (Dreifuss *et al.* 1989). In the USA the incidence has been estimated to be as high as 1 in 500 treated infants under 2 years, which seems vastly in excess of what is observed in Western Europe. However, a dramatic decrease in fatal hepatotoxicity has been recently reported from the USA (Dreifuss *et al.* 1989). It is doubtful in this writer's opinion that this decrease is due to preventive measures. It is more likely that stricter criteria are now required for hepatic failure to be attributed to valproate. Valproate toxicity closely resembles Reye syndrome (Chapter 11) or cases of impaired fatty acid beta-oxidation (Chapter 9). It is possible that metabolites of the drug interfere with fatty acid or other metabolisms in patients with some latent enzyme defect. This has been observed in patients with deficiencies of enzymes of the urea cycle (Christmann *et al.* 1990, Coulter 1991) and of the respiratory chain, especially cytochrome *c* oxidase (Chabrol *et al.* 1994; and personal case) and medium-chain acyl-CoA dehydrogenase (Njølstad *et al.* 1997).

A proportion of the cases may in fact be due to liver failure, which accompanies naturally some cases of poliodystrophy (Alpers disease, Chapter 10) and may be precipitated by administration of the drug (Bicknese *et al.* 1992). Cases of liver failure induced by valproate cannot be prevented by determination of the blood levels of transaminases, which remain normal up to the onset of failure in most cases but may be moderately increased in patients with a normal course (Dreifuss *et al.* 1989). The preventive value of carnitine is not demonstrated (Coulter 1991). Parents should be warned that they should report any vomiting, lethargy or increase in seizure frequency. Other drugs, notably anticonvulsants such as phenytoin and carbamazepine may occasionally produce fatal hepatitis (Pellock 1987).

The onset of hepatic encephalopathy is sometimes fulminating but it is often heralded by malaise, anorexia and vomiting. Disorders of consciousness are the principal symptoms. Disorientation, anxiety, depression and slurred speech appear first. They are rapidly followed by drowsiness, lethargy, disorientation and inappropriate behaviour. Delirium, lethargy and disorentiation precede coma. Asterixis or 'flapping tremor' may be an early feature. Extrapyramidal rigidity and choreic movements are frequent in children (Danks 1990). Ataxia, seizures, myoclonus and hyperventilation with resulting alkalosis frequently develop in advanced stages. Decerebrate posturing may occur in the terminal phase. Cerebral oedema is a major cause of death (Lidofsky *et al.* 1992). The EEG often shows diffuse bursts of high-voltage, slow-wave activity and sometimes triphasic spikes (Tasker *et al.* 1988).

The course may be rapidly lethal or fluctuate considerably, and symptoms may be rapidly reversible if the course of the liver disease is favourable.

In cases of chronic liver failure, hyperintensity of the globus pallidus on T_1-weighted MRI is associated with the severity of liver failure (Pujol *et al.* 1993). Manganese toxicity, which is reversible by discontinuation of parenteral manganese in parenteral nutrition (Ejima *et al.* 1992, Barron *et al.* 1994), may be an important factor in such cases.

Treatment of hepatic encephalopathy is beyond the scope of this book (see Devictor *et al.* 1993, Riordan and Williams 1997). Liver transplantation is being increasingly used. It should be performed before there is evidence of cerebral oedema as the results are exceedingly poor in its presence. It is customary to stop protein intake and to sterilize the intestinal tract with antibiotics, although the relationship between diet and hepatic encephalopathy is complex.

OTHER COMPLICATIONS OF HEPATIC FAILURE AND ITS TREATMENT
Mental development and somatic growth in children with chronic

liver disease are frequently impaired (Stewart *et al.* 1988), especially in liver disease of early onset. Part of the impairment is perhaps due to vitamin E deficiency which is frequent in disorders of biliary secretion.

CNS complications of liver transplantation (Stein *et al.* 1992, Garg *et al.* 1993, Patchell 1994) include immunological problems related to increased sensitivity to certain types of infection as well as toxic complications. *Listeria monocytogenes, Cryptococcus neoformans* and *Aspergillus fumigatus* are responsible for 80 per cent of infections in immunosuppressed children (Patchell 1994). *Cyclosporin toxicity* occurs in 15–40 per cent of treated children and manifests with tremor, ataxia, seizures and neuropathy. In about 5 per cent of cases it presents as an acute encephalopathy with hallucination, confusion, cortical blindness, quadriparesis, seizures, intracranial haemorrhage, white matter changes and coma (Stein *et al.* 1992, Patchell 1994). CT scan shows hypodensity of the white matter and MRI an abnormally intense signal on T_2-weighted sequences. Other agents used with liver transplantation such as FK506 (Wijdicks *et al.* 1994), azathioprine and corticosteroids may contribute to the occurrence of neurological complications. The presence of infection, haemorrhage and noncholestatic liver disease are predictive factors of CNS complications following transplantation (Pujol *et al.* 1994).

ENDOCRINE DISEASE

THYROID DISEASES
Thyroid hormones are crucial to normal neural maturation and function. In the human fetus, thyroxine (T4) is synthesized from 10 to 14 weeks gestation.

Therefore, early in gestation, neurological maturation, dependent on thyroid hormone, relies on T4 from the mother. The view that the placenta is impermeable to thyroid hormones, even in late gestation, is now being revised. Work with animals has shown that substantial amounts of T4 and T3 are present in all fetal tissues and that iodothyronines are transferred in significant quantity from mother to fetus early in gestation (Pharoah and Connolly 1995). In humans, T4 levels of 35–70 nmol/L have been found in cord blood of infants with complete failure of T4 synthesis (Vulsma *et al.* 1989). T4 but not T3 has been shown to be associated with measures of fetal neurological development, and the availability of circulating T4 is crucial to the normal maturation of neuronal cells (Pharoah and Connolly 1995). In this view, the timing of any T4 deficiency will determine the clinical picture. Early deficiency of exclusively maternal origin will be responsible for endemic cretinism. Later deficiency due to more or less severe failure of fetal thyroid hormone synthesis, with only partial maternal compensation, will result in congenital hypothyroidism of variable severity.

Absent or insufficient thyroxine results in impaired RNA and protein synthesis, reduced size and number of cortical neurons, hypoplasia of dendrites and axons and retarded myelination (Smith 1981b).

In *neonatal nongoitrous hypothyroidism* the thyroid gland is absent or too small to produce adequate amounts of hormones. The diagnosis is difficult at birth and many countries have introduced systematic screening at birth for its detection. Untreated infants are placid or hypotonic with a grunting cry. They have a protuberant abdomen and may have prolonged jaundice. They are pale and have coarse, lustreless hair and widely open fontanelles and sutures. One-third of affected infants have neurological abnormalities including spasticity, incoordination and cerebellar ataxia (Smith *et al.* 1975). Sensorineural hearing loss is present in 10 per cent of infants (Vanderschueren-Lodeweyckx *et al.* 1983) as a result of developmental cochlear abnormalities.

Neonatal goitrous hypothyroidism is due to at least five different defects in the synthesis of thyroid hormones. Impairment of intelligence varies with the responsible defect. Pendred syndrome (Chapter 19), transmitted as an autosomal recessive anomaly, includes goitre, deafness and hypothyroidism.

Treatment of neonatal hypothyroidism with synthetic laevo-thyroxine is essential to avoid developmental retardation. The outcome depends on the date of onset and the dose used. Infants with prenatal onset of thyroid insufficiency as shown by low T4 levels and retarded bone age at birth tend to have lower than normal scores on visuospatial, perceptual, motor and language subtests despite a normal global IQ (Rovet and Ehrlich 1995). Most children treated within the first four weeks of life do well, although subtle developmental difficulties may be present in later life (Gottschalk *et al.* 1994) even in infants detected by neonatal screening and immediately treated, although there are divergent opinions in this regard (Iliki and Larsson 1988, Mitchell 1994, Kooistra *et al.* 1994, Simons *et al.* 1994). An increased incidence of cerebral palsy in preterm infants with transient hypothyroxinaemia has been reported by Reuss *et al.* (1996).

In infants treated after 3 months of age, developmental delay and a cerebellar ataxic syndrome (Wiebel 1976) are common.

The prognosis for hypothyroidism that develops during childhood is clearly better. In such patients, in addition to mental slowing and slow movements, there is sometimes muscle hypertrophy which is often associated with a degree of myotonia or, at least, of reduced speed of contraction and relaxation, constituting the Kocher–Debré–Sémelaigne syndrome (Spiro *et al.* 1971).

Endemic cretinism is a worldwide problem with an estimated 800 million people at risk in many developing countries (Hetzel 1994). There are two forms of the condition, myxoedematous and nervous cretinism, but neurological signs are common to both types (Halpern *et al.* 1991) and include mental retardation and a nonprogressive neurological syndrome of bilateral spasticity, extrapyramidal features, notably dystonia, and parkinsonian gait. Deafness is usually associated. Calcification of the basal ganglia is present in 30 per cent of patients (Ma *et al.* 1993).

Endemic cretinism is a consequence of iodine deficiency in the mothers of affected children (Cao *et al.* 1994, Hetzel 1994, Pharoah and Connolly 1995), with consequent deficit of maternal T4 during pregnancy. The exact timing of deficiency, however, is still unclear. Pharoah and Connolly (1995) consider

that the first trimester is critical. Cao *et al.* (1994) believe that iodine supplementation begun before the end of the second trimester prevents neurological consequences. It is likely that there is a wide spectrum of manifestations from fetal wastage to mild mental or neurological deficits and/or deafness, depending on the degree of maternal iodine deficiency, so preventive administration of iodine could significantly improve the heath of at-risk populations (Pharoah and Connolly 1995).

An acute encephalopathy featuring quadriparesis, ataxia and seizures followed by progressive brain atrophy may be related to immunological abnormalities in Hashimoto thyroiditis and respond partially to corticosteroids (Takahashi *et al.* 1994).

Hyperthyroidism is much less common than hypothyroidism. CNS involvement may be marked by irritability and nervousness, abnormal movements, especially chorea in the adult patient, that may be permanent or paroxysmal (Swanson *et al.* 1981, Pozzon *et al.* 1992), and rarely seizures as a manifestation of thyrotoxic crisis (Radetti *et al.* 1993). Exophthalmos may be accompanied by ocular motor nerve palsies. Several reports of papilloedema, sometimes associated with other neurological symptoms and signs, are on record (Ono *et al.* 1987). Myasthenia gravis may be more common in patients with thyrotoxicosis, and one type of periodic paralysis is associated with thyrotoxicosis in Oriental populations (Chapter 22).

OTHER ENDOCRINE DISORDERS

The neurological symptoms of *parathyroid disease* are directly related to calcium and phosphorus metabolism and have been described elsewhere (Chapters 2, 10). CNS manifestations have been reviewed by Cogan *et al.* (1978).

Pituitary diseases have been considered in Chapter 14. Neonatal hypopituitarism is often missed, with the risk of death or cerebral damage because of growth hormone deficiency and hypoglycaemia. Costello and Gluckman (1988) studied 12 patients. Six had septo-optic dysplasia (Chapter 3), one agenesis of the corpus callosum, one an empty fossa on CT scan, and one pituitary hypoplasia. Two had idiopathic hypopituitarism and one dominant growth hormone deficiency. These infants were not small at birth and most had early seizures. Hyperbilirubinaemia was common and hypoglycaemia was documented in 11 patients. A microphallus was noted in seven males. Immediate treatment with growth hormone is imperative to prevent neurodevelopmental sequelae.

Isolated hypogonadotrophic hypogonadism is found in adult patients but is associated with developmental abnormalities that permit an early diagnosis (Schwankhaus *et al.* 1989). These include anosmia, hyposmia, mirror movements, ocular motor abnormalities, cerebellar dysfunction and pes cavus deformity. Delayed sexual maturation becomes apparent at adolescence. The mechanism of associated abnormalities is poorly known.

ADRENAL INSUFFICIENCY

This can produce neurological disturbances by disrupting water and electrolyte metabolism or by inducing hypoglycaemia. Papilloedema and pseudotumour cerebri may occur and this may be likened to pseudotumour following withdrawal of corticosteroids (Donaldson 1981).

HAEMATOLOGICAL DISORDERS

HEREDITARY HAEMOGLOBINOPATHIES

SICKLE-CELL DISEASE (DREPANOCYTOSIS)

Sickle-cell disease is a genetic disorder affecting Black populations, transmitted as an autosomal recessive trait that may manifest mildly in heterozygotes. Neurological complications occur in up to 25 per cent of cases and constitute a major cause of disability in this disorder. Neurological complications usually appear before 5 years of age. They are, at least in part, the consequence of vascular disease.

The mechanism of neurological accidents is probably twofold (Huttenlocher *et al.* 1984). Occlusive disease of large vessels at the base of the brain is common (13–17 per cent) and may be one cause of increased collateral circulation or moyamoya syndrome (Seeler *et al.* 1978). The second mechanism involves reduction in capillary flow which may be a direct consequence of the sickling phenomenon and produces diffuse signs such as stupor or coma.

From a pathological viewpoint, there is intimal proliferation and sometimes thrombosis of vessels. Microinfarcts are frequently present and are usually disseminated. Large vessels are more involved than small ones.

Neurological symptoms often appear at the time of sickle-cell crises that may be precipitated by dehydration, hypoxia or intercurrent disease including operations. Their description, diagnosis and therapy are discussed in Chapter 15. Hyperventilation should be avoided in patients with sickle-cell disease as it may result in neurological impairment precipitated by the reduction of blood flow which occurs during the test (Allen *et al.* 1976). Other neurological complications of sickle-cell disease include an increased risk of pneumococcal meningitis that may be due to decreased phagocytic potential of the reticuloendothelial system. Children with sickle-cell trait have a low incidence of neurological accidents, of the order of 6 per cent.

OTHER HAEMOGLOBINOPATHIES

Neurological symptoms are uncommon in other haemoglobinopathies. They have been observed, however, in haemoglobin SC disease (Fabian and Peters 1984).

Thalassaemia rarely gives rise to overt neurological disorder. About 20 per cent of patients have myalgia, proximal weakness and a myopathic EEG pattern (Logothetis *et al.* 1972). Spinal compression due to bone marrow hyperplasia as a result of extramedullary haematopoiesis has been occasionally observed (Issaragrisil *et al.* 1981). A syndrome of mental retardation associated with alpha-thalassaemia has been reported in children with a deletion of chromosome 16 (Wilkie *et al.* 1990). Another alpha-thalassaemia mental retardation syndrome featuring specific dysmorphic features has been recognized (Wilkie *et al.* 1991). It is not associated with a chromosomal deletion and seems to be transmitted as an X-linked character (Gibbons and Higgs 1996).

HAEMOLYTIC ANAEMIAS DUE TO DEFICIENCY OF GLYCOLYTIC ENZYMES

Pyruvate kinase deficiency can produce neurological complications only as a result of kernicterus.

Erythrocyte *phosphoglycerate kinase deficiency* is a sex-linked recessive disorder which may give rise to a slowly progressive extrapyramidal disorder that features dystonia, hyperlordosis, resting tremor and other extrapyramidal signs (Konrad *et al.* 1973). More recently, it has been recognized that neuromuscular manifestations associated with glycerol kinase deficiency are not directly due to the enzymatic deficit but rather are the consequence of a contiguous gene syndrome due to a microdeletion affecting the glycerol kinase locus as well as neighbouring loci, so the clinical picture may include sex-linked muscular dystrophy and/or congenital adrenogenital hypoplasia (Wise *et al.* 1987, Darras and Francke 1988).

Triose phosphate isomerase deficiency is regularly associated with a progressive neurological disease that features extrapyramidal manifestations of a dystonic type, tremor, cerebellar symptoms, pyramidal tract signs and involvement of the anterior horn cell (Poll-Thé *et al.* 1985). Cortical function is preserved. Spinal cord disease has also been reported in *hereditary spherocytosis* (McCann and Jacob 1976) which is a disorder related to erythrocyte membrane abnormality rather than to glycolysis.

OTHER ANAEMIAS

All anaemias may be accompanied by minor neurological symptoms such as irritability, listlessness and fatigue. A bruit can be heard over the head in some patients. Headache, and papilloedema due to increased intracranial pressure may be encountered in severe cases (Shahidi and Diamond 1961). Superior sagittal sinus thrombosis has been reported in patients receiving androgen therapy for the treatment of aplastic anaemia (Shiozawa *et al.* 1982). Symptoms subsided slowly upon withdrawal of treatment. Subacute combined degeneration of the posterior and lateral columns of the spinal cord is a classical complication of pernicious anaemia. In children, the most likely cause is a congenital defect of vitamin B_{12} absorption which is also associated with mental deficiency and abnormalities of brain myelination (Salameh *et al.* 1991). Congenital deficiency of intrinsic factor is rare (Chanarin *et al.* 1985). Deficiency of B_{12} due to an unbalanced vegetarian diet has been described above. Iron-deficiency anaemia may have a bearing on the neurological development of affected infants and children (Lozoff *et al.* 1991).

POLYCYTHAEMIA

Polycythaemia can be associated with neurological symptoms whether it is primary or secondary. The latter type is much more common in infants and especially in neonates (Chapter 2). Vertigo, headaches, tinnitus and seizures may be encountered in older patients. Cerebrovascular accidents are possible and may not always be transient especially in newborn infants. Neurological sequelae were present in 38 per cent of newborn infants with polycythaemia in one series (Black *et al.* 1982), but the genesis of neurological involvement is probably multifactorial as infants with polycythaemia are often born post-term and also suffer from hypoglycaemia and hypoxia. Seizures, visual disturbances and, rarely, intracranial haemorrhage have been reported (Wiswell *et al.* 1986).

Peripheral neuropathy has been reported in adults with polycythaemia vera (Yiannikas *et al.* 1983). It has not been recognized in children.

DISORDERS OF COAGULATION AND PLATELETS

Haemophilia is a major cause of intracranial haemorrhage that may occur at any age. Bleeding may be extradural, subdural or intraparenchymal. CT scan indicates the extent and origin of the haemorrhage, which is best treated by medical means (coagulation factors) whenever possible. Surgery, when indicated, should be deferred until factor VIII replacement therapy has been completed.

Other causes of bleeding include factor IX deficiency and Von Willebrand disease (Davies-Jones *et al.* 1980).

In infants, factor XIII deficiency is an important cause of idiopathic intracranial bleeding (Larsen *et al.* 1990).

Thrombocytopenic purpura, whether acute or chronic, is a relatively uncommon cause of intracranial haemorrhage (Davies-Jones *et al.* 1980). Intracranial bleeding can occur, however, and is one of the indications for splenectomy in this disease.

Alloimmunization against platelet antigens (usually PA1 antigen) produces prenatal (Chapter 1) or neonatal thrombocytopenia that may be responsible for intracranial haemorrhage (Muller *et al.* 1985, Matsui *et al.* 1995). Treatment with maternal platelets and immunoglobulins (Massey *et al.* 1987) is indicated. Effective prevention by immunoglobulin administration during pregnancy (1 g/kg/w) and delivery by caesarian section is possible (Menell and Bussel 1994).

NEUROLOGICAL COMPLICATIONS OF BONE MARROW TRANSPLANTATION

These are becoming increasingly common as the indications for the procedure are widening. CNS complications were observed in 46 per cent of patients in one childhood series (Wiznitzer *et al.* 1984). Infection, cerebrovascular accidents and metabolic encephalopathy were the main causes (Grams *et al.* 1996). Peripheral nervous system involvement was present in 24 per cent of children (Amato *et al.* 1993). Metabolic encephalopathy was the most frequent complication in a large series including adults and children (Patchell 1994). Myasthenia gravis has been reported in isolation (Bolger *et al.* 1986) and in association with myositis and peripheral neuropathy (Adams *et al.* 1995). A syndrome of acute parkinsonism with white matter demyelination has been observed (Lockman *et al.* 1991), especially in patients receiving amphotericin for the treatment of aspergillosis (Mott *et al.* 1995). Polymyositis in association with other features of graft-versus-host syndrome is on record (Schmidley and Galloway 1990).

GASTROINTESTINAL DISEASES

Gluten enteropathy is a disorder of intestinal malabsorption characterized by villous atrophy, absence of surface mucosa and crypt hyperplasia. Neurological complications reported in adults include peripheral neuropathy, cerebellar dysfunction, myelopathy and disordered mentation (Kinney *et al.* 1982), and a syndrome of ataxia and myoclonus similar to the Ramsay–Hunt syndrome (Lu *et al.* 1986, Bhatia *et al.* 1995), but these have not been reported in children. The possibility of neurological complications should be kept in mind, however, as it may represent a disorder treatable with gluten restriction (Kaplan *et al.* 1988).

The role played by vitamins B$_6$, B$_{12}$ and E in this disorder is not determined.

Multiple cases of gluten enteropathy associated with epilepsy and cerebral calcification have been reported, especially from Italy (Gobbi *et al.* 1988, 1992; Magaudda *et al.* 1993; Tortorella *et al.* 1993). The enteropathy may be overt or latent, revealed only by villous atrophy on intestinal biopsy, and is usually, but not always, accompanied by low folate levels in plasma. Brain calcification is often bilateral, predominating in the parieto-occiptal regions and reminiscent of that seen in Sturge–Weber syndrome and in methotrexate encephalopathy. However, there is usually no atrophy, contrary to what obtains in Sturge–Weber cases, and hypodensities underlie the calcified areas (Toti *et al.* 1996). The epilepsy was initially reported as severe (Gobbi *et al.* 1988) but cases with a favourable course are not rare. Exclusion of gluten may result in control or reduction of seizures (Gobbi *et al.* 1992). Whether it can prevent the development of epilepsy and calcification is not known (Bardella *et al.* 1994). The histopathological basis of the syndrome is imperfectly known. Bye *et al.* (1993) found vascular abnormalities reminiscent of, but not similar to those in Sturge–Weber in one biopsy sample, but this does not seem to be a common finding.

Other causes of malabsorption can produce neurological disease, in particular optic neuropathy associated with peripheral neuropathy, sometimes observed in patients with resection or exclusion of significant lengths of intestine (Pallis and Lewis 1980).

Whipple disease is very unusual in childhood (Barakat *et al.* 1973). In older patients, neurological involvement most commonly consists of myoclonus, ataxia and ophthalmoplegia (Louis *et al.* 1996). Oculomasticatory and oculofacioskeletal myorhythmias are pathognomonic. Dementia may develop. Diagnosis can be made by the discovery of bacilli-like structures in biopsy samples of the jejunal mucosa, although these may be absent in rare instances.

In some infants, *intussusception* may present initially with disturbances of consciousness (obtundation or even coma) that may suggest a primary neurological disease. This condition may be due to electrolytic disturbances, shock or release of enterotoxins, gut hormones or peptides. In such unexplained *intussusception encephalopathy*, one should enquire for abdominal symptoms and vomiting, and abdominal film or ultrasound should be obtained (Goetting *et al.* 1990).

BONE DISORDERS

Several bone disorders may be associated with neurological symptoms and signs, through various mechanisms that include compression of nerves at the skull base, venous compression with resulting hydrocephalus, narrowing of the foramen magnum or of the vertebral canal with resulting compression of the medulla, spinal cord or nerve roots, and craniosynostosis. Several of these disorders are mentioned elsewhere in this book.

Fibrous dysplasia of bone is characterized by proliferation of fibrous tissue in osseous tissue. Onset is in childhood or adolescence in over half the cases. Up to 34 per cent of cases may exhibit the association of skin pigmentation (Derome *et al.* 1983).

Osteopetrosis, especially in its severe infantile form, is often associated with neurological problems (Lehman *et al.* 1977). Compression of the optic nerves in their bony canal is most common and frequently leads to visual impairment and blindness. Nystagmus and strabismus may occur. Compression of the facial nerve with facial paralysis is not uncommon, and anosmia and trigeminal nerve involvement have been reported. Not uncommonly, patients with infantile osteopetrosis are mentally retarded and brain atrophy is apparent on their CT scans. The reasons for mental involvement, sometimes associated with signs of upper neuron affectation, are not understood, but neurological assessment is essential before considering medullary transplant. Ceroid–lipofuscin storage was found in several cases (Chapter 10) but the mechanism remains unclear.

REFERENCES

Ackrill, P., Ralston, A.J., Day, J.P., Hodge, K.C. (1980) 'Successful removal of aluminium from a patient with dialysis encephalopathy.' *Lancet*, **2**, 692–693.

Adair, J.C., Call, G.K., O'Connell, J.B., Baringer, J.R. (1992) 'Cerebrovascular syndromes following cardiac transplantation.' *Neurology*, **42**, 819–823.

Adams, C., August, C.S., Maguire, H., Sladky, J.T. (1995) 'Neuromuscular complications of bone marrow transplantation.' *Pediatric Neurology*, **12**, 58–61.

Agarwal, K.N., Das, D., Agarwal, D.K., *et al.* (1989) 'Soft neurological signs and EEG pattern in rural malnourished children.' *Acta Paediatrica Scandinavica*, **78**, 873–878.

Aicardi, J., Goutières, F. (1973) 'Les thromboses veineuses intracrâniennes. Complications des déshydratations aiguës du nourrisson.' *Archives Françaises de Pédiatrie*, **30**, 809–830.

Allen, J.P., Imbus, C.E., Powars, D.R., Harwood, L.J. (1976) 'Neurologic impairment induced by hyperventilation in children with sickle cell anemia.' *Pediatrics*, **58**, 124–126.

Altman, D.I., Perlman, J.M., Volpe, J.J., Powers, N.J. (1993) 'Cerebral oxygen metabolism in newborns.' *Pediatrics*, **92**, 99–104.

Amato, A.A., Barohn, R.J., Sahenk, Z., *et al.* (1993) 'Polyneuropathy complicating bone marrow and solid organ transplantation.' *Neurology*, **43**, 1513–1518.

Andreoli, J.P., Bergstein, J.M., Sherrard, D.J. (1984) 'Aluminium intoxication from aluminium-containing phosphate binders in children with azotemia not undergoing dialysis.' *New England Journal of Medicine*, **310**, 1079–1084.

Andrew, R.D. (1991) 'Seizure and acute osmotic change: clinical and neurophysiological aspects.' *Journal of the Neurological Sciences*, **101**, 7–18.

Arieff, A.I. (1985) 'Effects of water, acid-base and electrolyte disorders on the central nervous system.' *In:* Arieff, A.I., De Fronzo, R.A. (Eds.) *Fluid, Electrolyte and Acid-base Disorders.* New York: Churchill Livingstone, pp. 969–1040.

Atluru, V.L. (1986) 'Spontaneous intracerebral hematomas in juvenile diabetic ketoacidosis.' *Pediatric Neurology*, **2**, 167–169.

Ballabriga, A. (1989) 'Some aspects of clinical and biochemical changes related to nutrition during brain development in humans.' *In:* Evrard, P., Minkowski, A. (Eds.) *Developmental Neurobiology. Nestlé Nutrition Workshop Series No. 12.* New York: Raven Press, pp. 271–286.

Balmer, S., Howells, G., Wharton, B. (1968) 'The acute encephalopathy of kwashiorkor.' *Developmental Medicine and Child Neurology*, **10**, 766–771.

Banker, B.Q. (1967) 'The neuropathological effects of anoxia and hypoglycaemia in the newborn.' *Developmental Medicine and Child Neurology*, **9**, 544–550.

Bankier, B., Turner, M., Hopkins, I.J. (1983) 'Pyridoxine dependent seizures: a wider clinical spectrum.' *Archives of Disease in Childhood*, **58**, 415–418.

Barakat, A.V., Bitar, J., Nassar, V.H. (1973) 'Whipple's disease in a seven-year-old child: report of a case.' *American Journal of Proctology*, **24**, 312–314.

Bardella, M.T., Molteni, N., Prampolini, L., *et al.* (1994) 'Need for follow-up in coeliac disease.' *Archives of Disease in Childhood*, **70**, 211–213.

Barrett, T.G., Forsyth, J.M., Nathavitharana, K.A., Booth, I.W. (1993) 'Potentially lethal thiamine deficiency complicating parenteral nutrition in children.' *Lancet*, **341**, 901.

—— Bundey, S.E., McLeod, A.F. (1995) 'Neurodegeneration and diabetes: UK nationwide study of Wolfram (DIDMOAD) syndrome.' *Lancet*, **316**, 1458–1463.

Barron, T.F., Gusnard, D.A., Zimmerman, R.A., Clancy, R.R. (1992) 'Cerebral venous thrombosis in neonates and children.' *Pediatric Neurology*, **8**, 112–116.

—— Devenyi, A.G., Mamourian, A.C. (1994) 'Symptomatic manganese neurotoxicity in a patient with chronic liver disease: correlation of clinical symptoms with MRI findings.' *Pediatric Neurology*, **10**, 145–148.

Bastron, J.A., Thomas, J.E. (1981) 'Diabetic polyradiculopathy: clinical and electromyographic findings in 105 patients.' *Mayo Clinic Proceedings*, **56**, 725–732.

Becker, L.E., Takashima, S. (1985) 'Chronic hypoventilation and development of brain stem gliosis.' *Neuropediatrics*, **16**, 19–23.

Berretta, J.S., Holbrook, C.T., Haller, J.S. (1986) 'Chronic renal failure presenting as proximal muscle weakness in a child.' *Journal of Child Neurology*, **1**, 50–52.

Bhatia, K.P., Brown, P., Gregory, R., *et al.* (1995) 'Progressive myoclonic ataxia associated with coeliac disease. The myoclonus is of cortical origin but the pathology is in the cerebellum.' *Brain*, **118**, 1087–1093.

Bicknese, A.R., May, W., Hickey, W.F., Dodson, W.E. (1992) 'Early childhood hepatocerebral degeneration misdiagnosed as valproate hepatotoxicity.' *Annals of Neurology*, **32**, 767–775.

Black, V.D., Lubchenco, L.O., Luckey, D.W., *et al.* (1982) 'Developmental and neurologic sequelae of neonatal hyperviscosity syndrome.' *Pediatrics*, **69**, 426–431.

Bock, G.H., Conners, C.K., Ruley, J., *et al.* (1989) 'Disturbances of brain maturation and neurodevelopment during chronic renal failure.' *Journal of Pediatrics*, **114**, 231–238.

Bolger, G.B., Sullivan, K.M., Spence, A.M., *et al.* (1986) 'Myasthenia gravis after allogeneic bone marrow transplantation: relationship to chronic graft-versus-host disease.' *Neurology*, **36**, 1087–1091.

Brin, M.F., Pedley, T.A., Lovelace, R.E., *et al.* (1986) 'Electrophysiologic features of abetalipoproteinemia: functional consequences of vitamin E deficiency.' *Neurology*, **36**, 669–673.

Brunner, J.E., Redmond, J.M., Haggar, A.M., *et al.* (1990) 'Central pontine myelinosis and pontine lesions after rapid correction of hyponatremia: a prospective magnetic resonance study.' *Annals of Neurology*, **27**, 61–66.

Bye, A.M.E., Andermann, F., Robitaille, Y., *et al.* (1993) 'Cortical vascular abnormalities in the syndrome of celiac disease, epilepsy, bilateral occipital calcifications, and folate deficiency.' *Annals of Neurology*, **34**, 399–403.

Cadman, T.E., Rorke, L.B. (1969) 'Central pontine myelinolysis in childhood and adolescence.' *Archives of Disease in Childhood*, **44**, 342–350.

Campbell, L.R., Bunyapen, C., Gangarosa, M.E., *et al.* (1991) 'Significance of seizures associated with extracorporeal membrane oxygenation.' *Journal of Pediatrics*, **119**, 789–792.

Cao, X-Y., Jiang, X-M., Dou, Z-H., *et al.* (1994) 'Timing of vulnerability of the brain to iodine deficiency in endemic cretinism.' *New England Journal of Medicine*, **331**, 1739–1744.

Carton, H., Kayembe, K., Kabeya, M., *et al.* (1986) 'Epidemic of spastic paraparesis in Bandudu (Zaïre).' *Journal of Neurology, Neurosurgery, and Psychiatry*, **49**, 620–627.

Casey, P.H., Bradley, R., Wortham, B. (1984) 'Social and nonsocial home environments of infants with nonorganic failure-to-thrive.' *Pediatrics*, **73**, 348–353.

Chabrol, B., Mancini, J., Chretien, D., *et al.* (1994) 'Valproate-induced hepatic failure in a case of cytochrome *c* oxidase deficiency,' *European Journal of Pediatrics*, **153**, 133–135.

Chanarin, I., Deacon, R., Lumb, M., *et al.* (1985) 'Cobalamin–folate interrelations: a critical review.' *Blood*, **66**, 479–489.

Chavez, A., Martinez, C. (1979) 'Behavioral effects of under-nutrition and food supplementation.' *In: Proceedings of the International Nutrition Conference: Behavioral Effects of Energy and Protein Deficits.* Washington, DC: US Dept of Education and Welfare, p. 216.

Chopra, J.S., Sharma, A. (1992) 'Protein energy malnutrition and the nervous system.' *Journal of the Neurological Sciences*, **110**, 8–20.

—— Dhand, U.K., Mehta, S., *et al.* (1986) 'Effect of protein calorie malnutrition on peripheral nerves. A clinical, electrophysiological and histopathological study.' *Brain*, **109**, 307–323.

Christmann, D., Hirsch, E., Mutschler, V., *et al.* (1990) 'Argininémie congénitale diagnostiquée tardivement à l'occasion de la prescription de valproate de sodium.' *Revue Neurologique*, **146**, 764–766.

Cogan, M.G., Covey, C.M., Arieff, A.I., *et al.* (1978) 'Central nervous system manifestations of hyperparathyroidism.' *American Journal of Medicine*, **65**, 963–970.

Colombo, M., de la Perra, A., López, I. (1992) 'Intellectual and physical outcome of children undernourished in early life is influenced by later environmental conditions.' *Developmental Medicine and Child Neurology*, **36**, 611–622.

Cooper, A.J.L., Ehrlich, M.E., Plum, F. (1984) 'Hepatic encephalopathy: GABA or ammonia?' *Lancet*, **2**, 158–159.

Cooper, L., Wertheimer, J., Levey, R., *et al.* (1986) 'Severe primary hyperparathyroidism in a neonate with two hypercalcemic parents: management with parathyroidectomy and heterotopic autotransplantation.' *Pediatrics*, **78**, 263–268.

Cordero, M.E., D'Acuña, E., Benveniste, S., *et al.* (1993) 'Dendritic development in neocortex of infants with early postnatal life undernutrition.' *Pediatric Neurology*, **9**, 457–464.

Cornblath, M., Schwartz, R. (1991) *Disorders of Carbohydrate Metabolism in Infancy, 3rd Edn.* Oxford: Blackwell.

Costello, J.M., Gluckman, P.D. (1988) 'Neonatal hypopituitarism: a neurological perspective.' *Developmental Medicine and Child Neurology*, **30**, 190–199.

Cottrill, C.M., Kaplan, S. (1973) 'Cerebral vascular accidents in cyanotic congenital heart disease.' *American Journal of Diseases of Children*, **125**, 484–487.

Coulter, D.L. (1991) 'Carnitine, valproate, and toxicity.' *Journal of Child Neurology*, **6**, 7–14.

Curless, R.G., Katz, D.A., Perryman, R.A., *et al.* (1994) 'Choreoathetosis after surgery for congenital heart disease.' *Journal of Pediatrics*, **124**, 737–739.

Daniels, S.R., Bates, S.R., Kaplan, S. (1987) 'EEG monitoring during paroxysmal hyperpnea of Fallot: an epileptic or hypoxic phenomenon?' *Journal of Child Neurology*, **2**, 98–100.

Danks, D.M. (1990) 'Copper-induced dystonia secondary to cholestatic liver disease.' *Lancet*, **335**, 410. *(Letter.)*

Darras, B.T., Francke, U. (1988) 'Myopathy in complex glycerol kinase deficiency patients is due to 3′ deletions of the dystrophin gene.' *American Journal of Human Genetics*, **43**, 126–130.

Davies-Jones, G.A.B., Preston, F.E., Timperly, W.R. (1980) *Neurological Complications in Clinical Haematology.* Oxford: Blackwell.

Derome, P.J., Visot, A., Akerman, M., *et al.* (1983) 'La dysplasie fibreuse cranienne.' *Neurochirurgie*, **21**, Suppl. 1, 1–117.

Devictor, D., Tahiri, C., Rousset, A., *et al.* (1993) 'Management of fulminant hepatic failure in children—analysis of 56 cases.' *Critical Care Medicine*, **21**, Suppl. 9, S348–S349.

Dickoff, D.J., Raps, M., Yahr, M.D. (1988) 'Striatal syndrome following hyponatremia and its rapid correction: a manifestation of extrapontine myelinolysis confirmed by magnetic resonance imaging.' *Archives of Neurology*, **45**, 112–114.

Diringer, M., Ladenson, P.W., Borel, C., *et al.* (1989) 'Sodium and water regulation in a patient with cerebral salt wasting.' *Archives of Neurology*, **46**, 928–930.

Dobbing, J. (1980) 'Nutrition and brain development.' *In:* Harel, S. (Ed.) *The At-risk Infant.* Amsterdam: Excerpta Medica, pp. 124–128.

—— (1981) *Scientific Foundation of Pediatrics, 2nd Edn.* London: Heinemann.

Donaldson, J.O. (1981) 'Pathogenesis of pseudotumor cerebri syndrome.' *Neurology*, **31**, 877–880.

Donnal, J.F., Heinz, E.R., Burger, P.C. (1990) 'MR of reversible thalamic lesions in Wernicke syndrome.' *American Journal of Neuroradiology*, **11**, 893–894.

Dreifuss, F.E., Langer, D.H., Moline, K.A., Maxwell, J.E. (1989) 'Valproic acid hepatic fatalities. II. US experience since 1984.' *Neurology*, **39**, 201–207.

Du Plessis, A.J., Kramer, U., Jonas, R.A., *et al.* (1994) 'West syndrome following deep hypothermic infant cardiac surgery.' *Pediatric Neurology*, **11**, 246–251.

—— Chang, A.C., Wessel, D.L., *et al.* (1995a) 'Cerebrovascular accidents following the Fontan operation.' *Pediatric Neurology*, **12**, 230–236.

—— Newburger, J., Jonas, R.A., *et al.* (1995b) 'Cerebral oxygen supply and utilization during infant cardiac surgery.' *Annals of Neurology*, **37**, 488–497.

Dusser, A., Goutières, F., Aicardi, J. (1986) 'Ischemic strokes in children.' *Journal of Child Neurology*, **1**, 131–136.

Eeg-Olofsson, O., Petersen, I. (1966) 'Childhood diabetic neuropathy.' *Acta Paediatrica Scandinavica*, **55**, 165–176.

Ehyai, A., Fenichel, G.M., Bender, H.W. (1984) 'Incidence and prognosis of seizures in infants following cardiac surgery with profound hypothermia and circulatory arrest.' *Journal of the American Medical Association*, **252**, 3165–3167.

Ejima, A., Imamura, T., Nakamura, S., *et al.* (1992) 'Manganese intoxication during total parenteral nutrition.' *Lancet*, **339**, 426. (Letter.)

Ellison, P.H., Farina, M.A. (1980) 'Progressive central nervous system deterioration: a complication of advanced chronic lung disease of prematurity.' *Annals of Neurology*, **8**, 43–46.

Elton, N.W., Elton, W.J., Nazareno, J.P. (1963) 'Pathology of acute salt poisoning in infants.' *American Journal of Clinical Pathology*, **39**, 252–264.

Estol, C.J., Faris, A.A., Martinez, J., Ahdab-Barmada, M. (1989) 'Central pontine myelinolysis after liver transplantation.' *Neurology*, **39**, 493–498.

Evans, D.E., Bowie, M.D., Hansen, J.D.L., *et al.* (1980) 'Intellectual development and nutrition.' *Journal of Pediatrics*, **97**, 358–363.

Fabian, R.H., Peters, B.H. (1984) 'Neurological complications of hemoglobin SC disease.' *Archives of Neurology*, **41**, 289–292.

Faden, A., Mendoza, E., Flynn, F. (1981) 'Subclinical neuropathy associated with chronic obstructive pulmonary disease. Possible pathophysiologic role of smoking.' *Archives of Neurology*, **38**, 639–642.

Feldman, M.H., Schlezinger, N.S. (1970) 'Benign intracranial hypertension associated with hypervitaminosis A.' *Archives of Neurology*, **22**, 1–7.

Fenichel, G.M., Greene, H.L. (1985) 'Valproate hepatotoxicity: two new cases, a summary of others and recommendations.' *Pediatric Neurology*, **1**, 109–113.

Fehrolt, J.B., Rotnen, D.L., Genel, M., *et al.* (1985) 'A psychodynamic study of psychosomatic dwarfism: a syndrome of depression, personality disorder and impaired growth.' *Journal of the American Academy of Child Psychiatry*, **24**, 49–57.

Ferry, P.C. (1987) 'Neurologic sequelae of cardiac surgery in children.' *American Journal of Diseases of Children*, **141**, 309–312.

—— (1990) 'Neurologic sequelae of open heart surgery in children: an 'irritating question'.' *American Journal of Diseases of Children*, **144**, 369–373.

Finberg, L. (1991) 'Water intoxication. A prevalent problem in the inner city.' *American Journal of Diseases of Children*, **145**, 981–982.

Foley, C.M., Polinsky, M.S., Gruskin, A.B., *et al.* (1981) 'Encephalopathy in infants and children with chronic renal disease.' *Archives of Neurology*, **38**, 656–658.

Fox, J.H., Fishman, M.A., Dodge, P.R., Prensky, A.L. (1972) 'The effect of malnutrition on human central nervous system myelin.' *Neurology*, **22**, 1213–1216.

Franklin, B., Liu, J., Ginsberg-Fellner, F. (1982) 'Cerebral edema and ophthalmoplegia reversed by mannitol in a new case of insulin-dependent diabetes mellitus.' *Pediatrics*, **69**, 87–90.

Freedom, R.M. (1989) 'Cerebral vascular disorders of cardiovascular origin in infants and children.' *In:* Edwards, B.S., Hoffman, H.J. (Eds.) *Cerebral Vascular Disease in Children and Adolescents.* Baltimore: Williams & Wilkins, pp. 423–428.

Furlan, A.J., Breuer, A.C. (1984) 'Central nervous system complications of open heart surgery.' *Stroke*, **15**, 912–915.

Fyler, D.C., Buckey, L.A., Hellenbrand, W.E., Cohn, H.E. (1980) 'Report of the New England Regional Infant Program.' *Pediatrics*, **85** (Suppl.), 375–468.

Garewal, G., Narang, A., Das, K.C. (1988) 'Infantile tremor syndrome: a vitamin B_{12} deficiency syndrome in infants.' *Journal of Tropical Medicine*, **34**, 174–178.

Garg, B.P., Walsh, L.E., Pescovitz, M.D., *et al.* (1993) 'Neurologic complications of pediatric liver transplantation.' *Pediatric Neurology*, **9**, 444–448.

Gibbons, R.J., Higgs, D.R. (1996) 'The alpha-thalassemia/mental retardation syndromes.' *Médecine*, **75**, 45–52.

Gillberg, C., Rasmussen, P. (1982) 'Abnormal head circumference and learning disability.' *Developmental Medicine and Child Neurology*, **24**, 198–199. *(Letter.)*

Glass, P., Wagner, A.E., Papero, P.H., *et al.* (1995) 'Neurodevelopmental status at age five years of neonates treated with extracorporal membrane oxygenation.' *Journal of Pediatrics*, **127**, 447–457.

Glauser, T.A., Rorke, L.B., Weinberg, P.M., Clancy, R.R. (1990a) 'Congenital brain anomalies associated with the hypoplastic left heart syndrome.' *Pediatrics*, **85**, 984–990.

—— —— —— (1990b) 'Acquired neuropathologic lesions associated with the hypoplastic left heart syndrome.' *Pediatrics*, **85**, 991–1000.

Gobbi, G., Bouquet, F., Greco, L., *et al.* (1988) 'Coeliac disease, epilepsy, and cerebral calcifications.' *Lancet*, **340**, 439–443.

—— Ambrosetto, P., Zaniboni, M.G., *et al.* (1992) 'Celiac disease, posterior cerebral calcifications and epilepsy.' *Brain and Development*, **14**, 23–29.

Goetting, M.G., Tiznado-Garcia, E., Bakdash, T.F. (1990) 'Intussusception encephalopathy: an underrecognized cause of coma in children.' *Pediatric Neurology*, **6**, 419–421.

Gottschalk, B., Richman, R., Lewandowski, L. (1994) 'Subtle speech and motor deficits of children with congenital hypothyroid treated early.' *Developmental Medicine and Child Neurology*, **36**, 216–220.

Goutières, F., Aicardi, J. (1985) 'Atypical presentations of pyridoxine-dependent seizures: a treatable cause of intractable epilepsy in infants.' *Annals of Neurology*, **17**, 117–124.

Graham, S.M., Arvela, O.M., Wise, G.A. (1992) 'Long-term neurologic consequences of nutritional vitamin B$_{12}$ deficiency in infants.' *Journal of Pediatrics*, **121**, 710–714.

Grantham-McGregor, S.M., Powell, C.A., Walker, S.P., Himes, J.H. (1991) 'Nutritional supplementation, psychosocial stimulation, and mental development of stunted children: the Jamaican Study.' *Lancet*, **338**, 1–5.

Grattan-Smith, P.J., Wilcken, B., Procopis, P.G., Wise, G.A. (1997) 'The neurological syndrome of infantile cobalamin deficiency: developmental regression and involuntary movements.' *Movement Disorders*, **12**, 39–46.

Graus, F., Saiz, A., Sierra, J., *et al.* (1996) 'Neurologic complications of autologous and allogeneic bone marrow transplantation in patients with leukemia. A comparative study.' *Neurology*, **46**, 1004–1009.

Grazer, R.E., Sutton, J.M., Friedstrom, S., McBarron, F.D. (1984) 'Hyperammonemic encephalopathy due to essential amino acid hyperalimentation.' *Archives of Internal Medicine*, **144**, 2278–2279.

Graziani, L.J., Streletz, L.J., Mitchell, D.G., *et al.* (1994) 'Electroencephalographic, neuroradiologic, and neurodevelopmental studies in infants with subclavian steal during ECMO.' *Pediatric Neurology*, **10**, 97–103.

Green, W.H., Campbell, M., David, R. (1984) 'Psychosocial dwarfism: a critical review of the evidence.' *Journal of the American Academy of Child Psychiatry*, **23**, 39–48.

Greene, S.A., Jefferson, I.G., Baum, J.D. (1990) 'Cerebral oedema complicating diabetic ketoacidosis.' *Developmental Medicine and Child Neurology*, **32**, 633–638.

Greger, N.G., Kirkland, R.T., Clayton, R.W., Kirkland, J.L. (1986) 'Central diabetes insipidus: 22 years' experience.' *American Journal of Diseases of Children*, **140**, 551–554.

Gregorio, L., Sutton, C.L., Lee, D.A. (1997) 'Central pontine myelinolysis in a previously healthy 4-year-old child with acute rotavirus gastroenteritis.' *Pediatrics*, **99**, 738–743.

Griswold, W.R., Reznik, V., Mendoza, S.A., *et al.* (1983) 'Accumulation of aluminum in a nondialyzed uremic child receiving aluminum hydroxide.' *Pediatrics*, **71**, 56–58.

Gross, M.L.P., Sweny, P., Pearson, R.M., *et al.* (1982) 'Rejection encephalopathy: an acute neurological syndrome complicating renal transplantation.' *Journal of the Neurological Sciences*, **56**, 23–34.

Grosse Aldenhövel, H.B., Gallenkamp, U., Sulemana, C.A. (1991) 'Juvenile onset diabetes mellitus, central diabetes insipidus and optic atrophy (Wolfram syndrome)—neurological findings and prognostic implications.' *Neuropediatrics*, **22**, 103–106.

Grossman, H., Duggan, E., McCamman, S., *et al.* (1980) 'The dietary chloride deficiency syndrome.' *Pediatrics*, **66**, 366–374.

Gunston, G.D., Burkimsher, D., Malan, H., Sive, A.A. (1992) 'Reversible cerebral shrinkage in kwashiorkor: an MRI study.' *Archives of Disease in Childhood*, **67**, 1030–1032.

Hack, M., Breslau, N. (1986) 'Very low birth weight infants: effects of brain growth during infancy on intelligence quotient at 3 years of age.' *Pediatrics*, **77**, 196–202.

—— Merkatz, I.R., McGrath, S.K., *et al.* (1984) 'Catch-up growth in very-low-birth-weight infants. Clinical correlates.' *American Journal of Diseases of Children*, **138**, 370–375.

Hadders-Algra, M., Bos, A.F., Martijn, A., Prechtl, H.F.R. (1994) 'Infantile chorea in an infant with severe bronchopulmonary dysplasia: an EMG study.' *Developmental Medicine and Child Neurology*, **36**, 177–182.

Haenggeli, C-A., Girardin, E., Paunier, L. (1991) 'Pyridoxine-dependent seizures, clinical and therapeutic aspects.' *European Journal of Pediatrics*, **150**, 452–455.

Hahn, J.S., Vaucher, Y., Bejar, R., Coen, R.W. (1993) 'Electroencephalographic and neuroimaging findings in neonates undergoing extracorporeal membrane oxygenation.' *Neuropediatrics*, **24**, 19–24.

Halpern, J.P., Boyages, S.C., Maberly, G.F., *et al.* (1991) 'The neurology of endemic cretinism. A study of two endemias.' *Brain*, **114**, 825–841.

Hamano, S-i., Nakanishi, Y., Nara, T., *et al.* (1993) 'Neurologic manifestations of hemorrhagic colitis in the outbreak of *Escherichia coli* O157:H7 infection in Japan.' *Acta Paediatrica*, **82**, 454–458.

Hammond, D.N., Moll, G.W., Robertson, G.L., Chelmicka-Schorr, E. (1986) 'Hypodipsic hypernatremia with normal osmoregulation of vasopressin.' *New England Journal of Medicine*, **315**, 433–436.

Harris, C.P., Townsend, J.J., Baringer, J.R. (1993) 'Symptomatic hyponatremia: can myelinolysis be prevented by treatment?' *Journal of Neurology, Neurosurgery, and Psychiatry*, **56**, 626–632.

Hetzel, B.S. (1994) 'Iodine deficiency and fetal brain damage.' *New England Journal of Medicine*, **331**, 1770–1771.

Hill, I.D., Bowie, M.D. (1983) 'Chloride deficiency syndrome due to chloride-deficient breast milk.' *Archives of Disease in Childhood*, **58**, 224–226.

Ho, K-C., Hodach, R., Varma, R., *et al.* (1980) 'Kernicterus and central pontine myelinolysis in a 14-year-old boy with fulminating viral hepatitis.' *Annals of Neurology*, **8**, 633–636.

Hoffman, W.H., Hart, Z.H., Franck, R.N. (1983) 'Correlates of delayed motor nerve conduction velocity and retinopathy in juvenile-onset diabetes mellitus.' *Journal of Pediatrics*, **102**, 351–356.

Househam, K.C. (1991) 'Computed tomography of the brain in kwashiarkor: a follow up study.' *Archives of Disease in Childhood*, **66**, 623–626.

Howlett, W.P., Brubaker, G.R., Mlingi, N., Rosling, H. (1990) 'Konzo, an epidemic upper motor neuron disease studied in Tanzania.' *Brain*, **113**, 223–235.

Hughes, J.R., Schreeder, M.T. (1980) 'EEG in dialysis encephalopathy.' *Neurology*, **30**, 1148–1154.

Humphreys, R.P., Hoffman, H.J., Mustard, W.T. (1975) 'Cerebral hemorrhage following heart surgery.' *Journal of Neurosurgery*, **43**, 671–675.

Huntley, D.T., Al-Mateen, M., Menkes, J.H. (1993) 'Unusual dyskinesia complicating cardiopulmonary bypass surgery.' *Developmental Medicine and Child Neurology*, **35**, 631–636.

Huttenlocher, P.R., Moohr, J.W., Johns, L., Brown, F.D. (1984) 'Cerebral blood flow in sickle cell cerebrovascular disease.' *Pediatrics*, **73**, 615–621.

Iliki, A., Larsson, A. (1988) 'Psychomotor development of children with congenital hypothyroidism diagnosed by neonatal screening.' *Acta Paediatrica Scandinavica*, **77**, 142–147.

Issaragrisil, S., Piankigagum, A., Wasi, P. (1981) 'Spinal cord compression in thalassemia: report of 12 cases and recommendations for treatment.' *Archives of Internal Medicine*, **141**, 1033–1036.

Jadhav, M., Webb, J.K.G., Vaishnava, S., Baker, S.J. (1962) 'Vitamin B$_{12}$ deficiency in Indian infants.' *Lancet*, **2**, 903–907.

Jagadha, V., Deck, J.H.N., Halliday, W.C., Smyth, H.S. (1987) 'Wernicke's encephalopathy in patients on peritoneal dialysis or hemodialysis.' *Annals of Neurology*, **21**, 78–84.

Jarjour, I.T., Ahdab-Barmada, M. (1994) 'Cerebrovascular lesions in infants and children dying after extracorporeal membrane oxygenation.' *Pediatric Neurology*, **10**, 13–19.

Jelliffe, D.B., Jelliffe, E.F.P. (1992) 'Causation of kwashiorkor: toward a multifactorial consensus.' *Pediatrics*, **90**, 110–113.

Johnson, D.H., Rosenthal, A., Nadas, A.S. (1975) 'A forty-year review of bacterial endocarditis in infancy and childhood.' *Circulation*, **51**, 581–588.

Johnson, G.M. (1982) 'Powdered goat's milk: pyridoxine deficiency and status epilepticus.' *Clinical Pediatrics*, **21**, 494–495.

Jones, H.R., Siekert, R.G. (1989) 'Neurological manifestations of infective endocarditis. Review of clinical and therapeutic challenges.' *Brain*, **112**, 1295–1315.

Kahn, E., Falcke, H.C. (1956) 'A syndrome simulating encephalitis affecting children recovering from malnutrition (kwashiorkor).' *Journal of Pediatrics*, **49**, 37–45.

Kaplan, J.G., Pack, D., Horoupian, D., *et al.* (1988) 'Distal axonopathy associated with chronic gluten enteropathy: a treatable disorder.' *Neurology*, **38**, 642–645.

810

Keating, J.P., Feigin, R.D. (1970) 'Increased intracranial pressure associated with probable vitamin A deficiency in cystic fibrosis.' *Pediatrics*, **46**, 41–46.

—— Schears, G.J., Dodge, P.R. (1991) 'Oral water intoxication in infants. An American epidemic.' *American Journal of Diseases of Children*, **145**, 985–990.

Keyser, A., De Bruijn, S.F.T.M. (1991) 'Epileptic manifestations and vitamin B_1 deficiency.' *European Neurology*, **31**, 121–125.

King, J.M., Taitz, L.S. (1985) 'Catch up growth following abuse.' *Archives of Disease in Childhood*, **60**, 1152–1154.

Kinney, H.C., Burger, P.C., Hurwitz, P.J., et al. (1982) 'Degeneration of the central nervous system associated with celiac disease.' *Journal of the Neurological Sciences*, **53**, 9–22.

Koh, T.H.H.G., Aynsley-Green, A., Tarbit, M., Eyre, J.A. (1988) 'Neural dysfunction during hypoglycaemia.' *Archives of Disease in Childhood*, **63**, 1353–1358.

Kohlschütter, A. (1993) 'Vitamin E and neurological problems in childhood: a curable neurodegenerative process.' *Developmental Medicine and Child Neurology*, **35**, 642–646.

Konrad, P.N., McCarthy, D.J., Mauer, A.M., et al. (1973) 'Erythrocyte and leukocyte phosphoglycerate kinase deficiency with neurologic disease.' *Journal of Pediatrics*, **82**, 456–460.

Kooistra, L., Laane, C., Vulsma, T., et al. (1994) 'Motor and cognitive development in children with congenital hypothyroidism: a long-term evaluation of the effects of neonatal treatment.' *Journal of Pediatrics*, **124**, 903–909.

Korinthenberg, R., Kachel, W., Koelfen, W., et al. (1993) 'Neurological findings in newborn infants after extracorporeal membrane oxygenation, with special reference to the EEG.' *Developmental Medicine and Child Neurology*, **35**, 249–257.

Korobkin, R. (1980) 'Acute hemiparesis in juvenile insulin-dependent diabetes mellitus (JIDDM).' *Neurology*, **30**, 220–221 *(Letter.)*

Kotagal, S., Rolfe, U., Schwarz, K.B., Escober, W. (1984) '"Locked-in" state following Reye's syndrome.' *Annals of Neurology*, **15**, 599–601.

Krane, E.J., Rockoff, M.A., Wallman, J.K., Wolfsdorf, J.I. (1985) 'Subclinical brain swelling in children during treatment of diabetic ketoacidosis.' *New England Journal of Medicine*, **312**, 1147–1151.

Krendel, D.A., Gilchrist, J.M., Johnson, A.O., Bossen, E.H. (1987) 'Isolated deficiency of vitamin E with progressive neurologic deterioration.' *Neurology*, **37**, 538–540.

Kroll, J.S. (1985) 'Pyridoxine for neonatal seizures: an unexpected danger.' *Developmental Medicine and Child Neurology*, **27**, 377–379.

Kumar, A., Ghai, O.P., Singh, N., Singh, R. (1977) 'Delayed nerve conduction velocities in children with protein–calorie malnutrition.' *Journal of Pediatrics*, **90**, 149–153.

Kurlan, R., Griggs, R.C. (1983) 'Cyanotic congenital heart disease with suspected stroke: should all patients receive antibiotics?' *Archives of Neurology*, **40**, 209–212.

—— Krall, R.L., Deweese, J.A. (1984) 'Vertebrobasilar ischemia after total repair of tetralogy of Fallot. Significance of subclavian steal created by Blalock–Taussig anastomosis.' *Stroke*, **15**, 359–362.

Lago, P., Rebsamen, S., Clancy, R.R., et al. (1995) 'MRI, MRA, and neurodevelopmental outcome following neonatal ECMO.' *Pediatric Neurology*, **12**, 294–304.

Lancet (1992) 'Excess water administration and hyponatraemic convulsions in infancy.' *Lancet*, **339**, 153–155. *(Editorial.)*

Larsen, P.D. (1989) 'Hypernatremic dehydration with hemorrhage into the choroid plexus.' *Pediatric Neurology*, **5**, 114–117.

—— Wallace, J.W., Frankel, L.S., Crisp, B. (1990) 'Factor XIII deficiency and intracranial hemorrhages in infancy.' *Pediatric Neurology*, **6**, 277–278.

Laureno, R., Karp, B.I. (1988) 'Pontine and extrapontine myelinolysis following rapid correction of hyponatraemia.' *Lancet*, **1**, 1439–1440.

Lee, J.H., Arcinue, E., Ross, B.D. (1994) 'Brief report: organic osmolytes in the brain of an infant with hypernatremia.' *New England Journal of Medicine*, **331**, 439–442.

Lehman, R.A.W., Reeves, J.D., Wilson, W.B., Wesenberg, R.I. (1977) 'Neurological complications of infantile osteopetrosis.' *Annals of Neurology*, **2**, 378–384.

Leicher, C.R., Mezoff, A.G., Hyams, J.S. (1991) 'Focal cerebral deficits in severe hypomagnesemia.' *Pediatric Neurology*, **7**, 380–381.

Lidofsky, S.D., Bass, N.M., Prager, M.C., et al. (1992) 'Intracranial pressure monitoring and live transplantation for fulminant hepatic failure.' *Hepatology*, **16**, 1–7.

Lindenbaum, J., Healton, E.B., Savage, D.G., et al. (1988) 'Neuropsychiatric disorders caused by cobalamin deficiency in the absence of anemia or macrocytosis.' *New England Journal of Medicine*, **318**, 1720–1728.

Linderkamp, O., Klose, H.J., Betke, K., et al. (1979) 'Increased blood viscosity in patients with cyanotic congenital heart disease and iron deficiency.' *Journal of Pediatrics*, **95**, 567–569.

Lockman, L.A., Sung, J.H., Krivit, W. (1991) 'Acute parkinsonian syndrome with demyelinating leukoencephalopathy in bone marrow transplant recipients.' *Pediatric Neurology*, **7**, 457–463.

Logothetis, J., Constantoulakis, M., Economidou, J., et al. (1972) 'Thalassemia major (homozygous beta thalassemia): a survey of 138 cases with emphasis on neurologic and muscular aspects.' *Neurology*, **22**, 294–304.

Louis, E.D., Lynch, T., Kaufmann, P., et al. (1996) 'Diagnostic guidelines in central nervous system Whipple's disease.' *Annals of Neurology*, **40**, 561–568.

Lozoff, B., Jimenez, E., Wolf, A.W. (1991) 'Long-term developmental outcome of infants with iron deficiency.' *New England Journal of Medicine*, **325**, 687–694.

Lu, C-S., Thompson, P.D., Quinn, N.P., et al. (1986) 'Ramsay Hunt syndrome and coeliac disease: a new association?' *Movement Disorders*, **1**, 209–219.

Ludolph, A.C., Hugon, J., Dwivedi, M.P., et al. (1987) 'Studies on the aetiology and pathogenesis of motor neuron diseases. 1. Lathyrism: clinical findings in established cases.' *Brain*, **110**, 149–165.

Luttrell, C.N., Finberg, L. (1959) 'Hemorrhagic encephalopathy induced by hypernatremia. I: Clinical, laboratory and pathological observations.' *Archives of Neurology and Psychiatry*, **81**, 424–432.

—— Drawdy, L.P. (1959) 'Hemorrhagic encephalopathy induced by hypernatremia. II: Experimental observations on hyperosmolarity in cats.' *Archives of Neurology*, **1**, 153–160.

Ma, T., Lian, Z.C., Qi, S.P., et al. (1993) 'Magnetic resonance imaging of brain and the neuromotor disorder in endemic cretinism.' *Annals of Neurology*, **34**, 91–94.

Magaudda, A., Dalla Bernardina, B., De Marco, P., et al. (1993) 'Bilateral occipital calcification, epilepsy and coeliac disease: clinical and neuroimaging features.' *Journal of Neurology, Neurosurgery, and Psychiatry*, **56**, 885–889.

Malone, M., Prior, P., Scholz, C.L. (1981) 'Brain damage after cardiopulmonary by-pass: correlations between neurophysiological and neuropathological findings.' *Journal of Neurology, Neurosurgery, and Psychiatry*, **44**, 924–931.

Manni, R., Tartara, A., Marchioni, E., et al. (1987) 'A clinical, EEG and CT study in 21 cases of chronic respiratory failure.' *Journal of Neurology*, **234**, 83–85.

Marescaux, C., Warter, J.M., Micheletti, G., et al. (1982) 'Stuporous episodes during treatment with sodium valproate: report of seven cases.' *Epilepsia*, **23**, 297–305.

Massey, G.V., McWilliams, N.B., Mueller, D.G., et al. (1987) 'Intravenous immunoglobulin in treatment of neonatal isoimmune thrombocytopenia.' *Journal of Pediatrics*, **111**, 133–135.

Matsui, K., Ohsaki, E., Koresawa, M., et al. (1995) 'Perinatal intracranial hemorrhage due to severe neonatal alloimmune thrombocytopenic purpura (NAITP) associated with anti-Yuk[b] (HPA-4a) antibodies.' *Brain and Development*, **17**, 352–355.

McCann, S.R., Jacob, H.S. (1976) 'Spinal cord disease in hereditary spherocytosis: report of two cases with a hypothesized common mechanism for neurologic and red cell abnormalities.' *Blood*, **48**, 259–263.

McConnell, J.R., Fleming, W.H., Chu, W-K., et al. (1990) 'Magnetic resonance imaging of the brain in infants and children before and after cardiac surgery. A prospective study.' *American Journal of Diseases of Children*, **144**, 374–378.

McDonald, J.T., Brown, D.R. (1979) 'Acute hemiparesis in juvenile insulin-dependent diabetes mellitus (JIDDM).' *Neurology*, **29**, 893–896.

McGraw, M.E., Haka-Ikse, K. (1985) 'Neurologic–developmental sequelae of chronic renal insufficiency.' *Journal of Pediatrics*, **106**, 579–583.

McKee, A.C., Winkelman, M.D., Banker, B.Q. (1988) 'Central pontine myelinolysis in severely burned patients: relationship to serum hyperosmolarity.' *Neurology*, **38**, 1211–1217.

Medlock, M.D., Cruse, R.S., Winek, S.J., et al. (1993) 'A 10-year experience with postpump chorea.' *Annals of Neurology*, **34**, 820–826.

Mendoza, J.C., Shearer, L.L., Cook, L.N. (1991) 'Lateralization of brain lesions following extracorporeal membrane oxygenation.' *Pediatrics*, **88**, 1004–1009.

Menell, J.S., Bussel, J.B. (1994) 'Antenatal management of the thrombocytopenias.' *Clinics in Perinatology*, **21**, 591–614.

Mensing, J.W.A., Hoogland, P.H., Sloof, J.L. (1984) 'Computed tomography in the diagnosis of Wernicke's encephalopathy: a radiological–neuropathological correlation.' *Annals of Neurology*, **16**, 363–365.

Mentser, M.I., Clay, S., Malekzadeh, H., *et al.* (1978) 'Peripheral motor nerve conduction velocities in children undergoing chronic hemodialysis.' *Nephron*, **22**, 337–341.

Meyers, C.C., Schochet, S.S., McCormick, W.F. (1978) 'Wernicke's encephalopathy in infancy: development during parenteral nutrition.' *Acta Neuropathologica*, **43**, 267–271.

Miller, G., Mamourian, A.C., Tesman, J.R., *et al.* (1994) 'Long-term MRI changes in brain after pediatric open heart surgery.' *Journal of Child Neurology*, **9**, 390–397.

Mirowitz, S.A., Westrich, T.J., Hirsch, J.D. (1991) 'Hyperintense basal ganglia on T1-weighted MR images in patients receiving parenteral nutrition.' *Radiology*, **181**, 117–120.

Moodie, A.D., Bowie, M.D., Mann, M.D., Hansen, J.D. (1980) 'A prospective 15-year follow-up study of kwashiorkor patients. Part II. Social circumstances, educational attainment and social adjustment.' *South African Medical Journal*, **58**, 677–681.

Morton, R.E., Bonas, R., Fourie, B., Minford, J. (1993) 'Videofluoroscopy in the assessment of feeding disorders of children with neurological problems.' *Developmental Medicine and Child Neurology*, **35**, 388–395.

Mott, S.H., Packer, R.J., Vezina, L.G., *et al.* (1995) 'Encephalopathy with parkinsonian features in children following bone marrow transplantations and high-dose amphotericin B.' *Annals of Neurology*, **37**, 810–814.

Mouridsen, S.E., Nielsen, S. (1990) 'Reversible somatotropin deficiency (psychosocial dwarfism) presenting as conduct disorder and growth hormone deficiency.' *Developmental Medicine and Child Neurology*, **32**, 1093–1098.

Muller, J.Y., Reznikoff-Etievant, M.F., Patereau, C., *et al.* (1985) 'Thrombopénies néonatales allo-immunes: étude clinique et biologique de 84 cas.' *Presse Médicale*, **14**, 83–86.

Newburger, J.W., Silbert, A.R., Buckley, L.P., Fyler, D.C. (1984) 'Cognitive functions and age at repair of transposition of the great arteries in children.' *New England Journal of Medicine*, **310**, 1495–1499.

—— Jonas, R.A., Wernovsky, G., *et al.* (1993) 'A comparison of the perioperative neurologic effects of hypothermic circulatory arrest versus low-flow cardiopulmonary bypass in infant heart surgery.' *New England Journal of Medicine*, **329**, 1057–1064.

Newman, L.J., Heitlinger, L., Hiesiger, E., *et al.* (1980) 'Comunicating hydrocephalus following total parenteral nutrition.' *Journal of Pediatric Surgery*, **15**, 215–217.

Nichols, S.L., Press, G.A., Schneider, J.A., Trauner, D.A. (1990) 'Cortical atrophy and cognitive performance in infantile nephropathic cystinosis.' *Pediatric Neurology*, **6**, 379–381.

Nijst, T.Q., Wevers, R.A., Schoonder-Waldt, H.C., *et al.* (1990) 'Vitamin B$_{12}$ and folate concentrations in serum and cerebrospinal fluid of neurological patients with special reference to multiple sclerosis and dementia.' *Journal of Neurology, Neurosurgery, and Psychiatry*, **53**, 951–954.

Njølstad, P.R., Skjeldal, O.H., Agsterribe, E., *et al.* (1997) 'Medium-chain acyl-CoA dehydrogenase deficiency and fatal valproate toxicity.' *Pediatric Neurology*, **16**, 160–162.

North, K.N., Ouvrier, R.A., McLean, C.A., Hopkins, I.J. (1994) 'Idiopathic hypothalamic dysfunction with dilated unresponsive pupils: report of two cases.' *Journal of Child Neurology*, **9**, 320–325.

O'Dougherty, M., Wright, F.S., Loewenson, R.B., Torres, F. (1985) 'Cerebral dysfunction after chronic hypoxia in children.' *Neurology*, **35**, 42–46.

Olson, D.M., Shewmon, D.A. (1989) 'Electroencephalographic abnormalities in infants with hypoplastic left heart syndrome.' *Pediatric Neurology*, **5**, 93–98.

Ono, S., Morooka, S., Shimizu, N., Saimizu, N. (1987) 'Hyperthyroidism associated with papilloedema and pyramidal tract involvement.' *Journal of Neurology*, **235**, 62–63.

Pallis, C.A., Lewis, P.D. (1980) 'Neurology of gastrointestinal disease.' *In:* Vinken, P.J., Bruyn, G.W. (Eds.) *Handbook of Clinical Neurology. Vol. 39. Neurologic Manifestations of Systemic Disorders, Part II.* Amsterdam: North Holland, pp. 449–468.

Parr, M.J.A., Low, H.M., Botterill, P. (1997) 'Hyponatraemia and death after "ecstasy" ingestion.' *Medical Journal of Australia*, **166**, 136–137.

Patchell, R.A. (1994) 'Neurological complications of organ transplantation.' *Annals of Neurology*, **36**, 688–703.

Pearson, H.A., Vinson, R., Smith, R.T. (1964) 'Pernicious anemia with neurologic involvement in childhood. Report of a case with emphasis on dangers of folic acid therapy.' *Journal of Pediatrics*, **65**, 334–339.

Pellock, J.M. (1987) 'Carbamazepine side-effects in children and adults.' *Epilepsia*, **28**, Suppl. 3, S64–S70.

Penn, I. (1979) 'Tumor incidence in human allograft recipients.' *Transplantation Proceedings*, **11**, 1047-1051.

Perlman, J.M., Volpe, J.J. (1989) 'Movement disorder of premature infants with severe bronchopulmonary dysplasia: a new syndrome.' *Pediatrics*, **84**, 215–218.

Peterson, R.A., Rosenthal, A. (1972) 'Retinopathy and papilledema in cyanotic congenital heart disease.' *Pediatrics*, **49**, 243–249.

Pharoah, P.O.D., Connolly, K.J. (1995) 'Iodine and brain development.' *Developmental Medicine and Child Neurology*, **37**, 744–747.

Phornphutkul, C., Rosenthal, R., Nadas, A.S., Berenberg, W. (1973) 'Cerebrovascular accidents in infants and children with cyanotic congenital heart disease.' *American Journal of Cardiology*, **32**, 329–334.

Pihko, H., Saarinen, U., Paetau, A. (1989) 'Wernicke encephalopathy. A preventable cause of death. Report of 2 children with malignant disease.' *Pediatric Neurology*, **5**, 237–242.

Poll-Thé, B.T., Aicardi, J., Girot, R., Rosa, R. (1985) 'Neurological findings in triose phosphate isomerase deficiency.' *Annals of Neurology*, **17**, 439–443.

Pozzon, G.B., Battistella, P.A., Rigon, F., *et al.* (1992) 'Hyperthyroid-induced chorea in an adolescent girl.' *Brain and Development*, **14**, 126–127.

Priolisi, A. (1969) 'Treatment of kwashiorkor in Sicily.' *Journal of Pediatrics*, **75**, 1080–1081.

Pruitt, A.A., Rubin, R.H., Karchmer, A.W., Duncan, G.W. (1978) 'Neurologic complications of bacterial endocarditis.' *Medicine*, **57**, 329–343.

Pujol, A., Pujol, J., Graus, F., *et al.* (1993) 'Hyperintense globus pallidus on T1-weighted MRI in cirrhotic patients is associated with severity of liver failure.' *Neurology*, **43**, 65–69.

—— Graus, F., Rimola, A., *et al.* (1994) 'Predictive factors of in-hospital CNS complications following liver transplantation.' *Neurology*, **44**, 1226–1230.

Puntis, J.W., Green, S.H. (1985) 'Ischaemic spinal cord injury after cardiac surgery.' *Archives of Disease in Childhood*, **60**, 517–520.

Radetti, G., Rizza, F., Mengarda, G., Pittschieler, K. (1991) 'Adipisic hypernatremia in two sisters.' *American Journal of Diseases of Children*, **145**, 321–325.

—— Dordi, B., Mengarda, G., *et al.* (1993) 'Thyrotoxicosis presenting with seizures and coma in two children.' *American Journal of Diseases of Children*, **147**, 925–927.

Ramaekers, V.T., Calomme, M., Vanden Berghe, D., Makropoulos, W. (1994) 'Selenium deficiency triggering intractable seizures.' *Neuropediatrics*, **25**, 217–223.

Ramsay, M., Gisel, E.G., Boutary, M. (1993) 'Non-organic failure to thrive: growth failure secondary to feeding-skills disorders.' *Developmental Medicine and Child Neurology*, **35**, 285–297.

Rando, T.A., Horton, J.C., Layzer, R.B. (1992) 'Wolfram syndrome: evidence of a diffuse neurodegenerative disease by magnetic resonance imaging.' *Neurology*, **42**, 1220–1224.

Reuss, M.L., Paneth, N., Pinto-Martin, J.A., *et al.* (1996) 'The relation of transient hypothyroxinemia in preterm infants to neurologic development of two years of age.' *New England Journal of Medicine*, **334**, 821–827.

Riggs, J.E., Klingberg, W.G., Flink, E.B., *et al.* (1992) 'Cardioskeletal mitochondrial myopathy associated with chronic magnesium deficiency.' *Neurology*, **42**, 128–130.

Riordan, S.M., Williams, R. (1997) 'Treatment of hepatic encephalopathy.' *New England Journal of Medicine*, **337**, 473–479.

Rivera-Vásquez, A.B., Noriega-Sánchez, A., Ramírez-González, R., Martinez-Maldonado, M. (1980) 'Acute hypercalcemia in hemodialysis patients: distinction from 'dialysis dementia'.' *Nephron*, **25**, 243–246.

Robinson, R.O., Samuels, M., Pohl, K.R.E., (1988) 'Choreic syndrome after cardiac surgery.' *Archives of Disease in Childhood*, **63**, 1466–1469.

Rogers, B.T., Msall, M.E., Buck, G.M., *et al.* (1995) 'Neurodevelopmental outcome of infants with hypoplastic left heart syndrome.' *Journal of Pediatrics*, **126**, 496–498.

Roman, G.C., Spencer, P.S., Schoenberg, B.S. (1985) 'Tropical myeloneuropathies. The hidden endemias.' *Neurology*, **35**, 1158–1170.

Rosenbloom, A.L., Riley, W.J., Weber, F.T., *et al.* (1980) 'Cerebral edema complicating diabetic ketoacidosis in childhood.' *Journal of Pediatrics*, **96**, 357–361.

Rotundo, A., Nevins, T.E., Lipton, M., *et al.* (1982) 'Progressive encephalopathy in children with chronic renal failure.' *Kidney International*, **21**, 486–491.

Rovet, J.F., Ehrlich, R.M. (1995) 'Long-term effects of L-thyroxine therapy for congenital hypothyroidism.' *Journal of Pediatrics*, **126**, 380–386.

Sadowitz, P.D., Livingston, A., Cavanaugh, R.M. (1986) 'Developmental regression as an early manifestation of vitamin B$_{12}$ deficiency.' *Clinical Pediatrics*, **25**, 369–371.

Salameh, M.M., Banda, R.W., Mohdi, A.A. (1991) 'Reversal of severe neurological abnormalities after vitamin B$_{12}$ replacement in the Imerslund–Grasbeck syndrome.' *Journal of Neurology*, **238**, 349–350.

Schaumburg, H., Kaplan, J., Windebank, A., *et al.* (1983) 'Sensory neuropathy from pyridoxine abuse: a new megavitamin syndrome.' *New England Journal of Medicine*, **309**, 445–448.

Scheffner, D., König, S., Rauterberg-Ruland, I., *et al.* (1988) 'Fatal liver failure in 16 children with valproate therapy.' *Epilepsia*, **29**, 530–542.

Schmidley, J.W., Galloway, P. (1990) 'Polymyositis following autologous bone marrow transplantation in Hodgkin's disease.' *Neurology*, **40**, 1003–1004.

Schmidt, D. (1984) 'Adverse effects of valproate.' *Epilepsia*, **25** (Suppl.), S44–S49.

Schneck, S.A. (1965) 'Neuropathological features of human organ transplantation. I. Probable cytomegalovirus infection.' *Journal of Neuropathology and Experimental Neurology*, **24**, 415–429.

Schumacher, R.E., Palmer, T.W., Roloff, T.W., *et al.* (1991) 'Follow-up of infants treated with extracorporeal membrane oxygenation for newborn respiratory failure.' *Pediatrics*, **87**, 451–457.

Schwankhaus, J.D., Currie, J., Jaffe, M.J., *et al.* (1989) 'Neurologic findings in men with isolated hypogonadotrophic hypogonadism.' *Neurology*, **39**, 223–226.

Scolding, N.J., Kellar-Wood, H.F., Shaw, C., *et al.* (1996) 'Wolfram syndrome: hereditary diabetes mellitus with brainstem and optic atrophy.' *Annals of Neurology*, **39**, 352–360.

Sedman, A.B., Wilkening, G.M., Warady, B.M., *et al.* (1984) 'Encephalopathy in childhood secondary to aluminium toxicity.' *Journal of Pediatrics*, **105**, 836–838.

Seear, M.D., Norman, M.G. (1988) 'Two cases of Wernicke's encephalopathy in children: an underdiagnosed complication of poor nutrition.' *Annals of Neurology*, **24**, 85–87.

Seeler, R.A., Royal, J.E., Powe, L., Goldbarg, H.R. (1978) 'Moyamoya in children with sickle cell anemia and cerebrovascular occlusion.' *Journal of Pediatrics*, **93**, 808–810.

Shahidi, N.T., Diamond, L.K. (1961) 'Testosterone-induced remission in aplastic anemia of both acquired and congenital types. Further observations in 24 cases.' *New England Journal of Medicine*, **264**, 953–957.

Shintani, S., Tsuruoka, S., Shiigai, T. (1993) 'Hypoglycaemic hemiplegia: a repeat SPECT study.' *Journal of Neurology, Neurosurgery, and Psychiatry*, **56**, 700–701.

Shiozawa, Z., Yamada, H., Mabuchi, C., *et al.* (1982) 'Superior sagittal sinus thrombosis associated with androgen therapy for hypoplastic anemia.' *Annals of Neurology*, **12**, 578–580.

Silbert, A., Wolff, P.H., Mayer, B., *et al.* (1969) 'Cyanotic heart disease and psychological development.' *Pediatrics*, **43**, 192–200.

Simons, W.F., Fuggle, P.W., Grant, D.B., Smith, I. (1994) 'Intellectual development at 10 years in early treated congenital hypothyroidism.' *Archives of Disease in Childhood*, **71**, 232–234.

Smith, D.W., Klein, A.M., Henderson, J.R., Myrianthopoulos, N.C. (1975) 'Congenital hypothyroidism: signs and symptoms in newborn period.' *Journal of Pediatrics*, **87**, 958–962.

Smith, R. (1981a) 'Abnormal head circumference in learning-disabled children.' *Developmental Medicine and Child Neurology*, **23**, 626–632.

—— (1981b) 'Thyroid hormones and brain development in children.' *In:* Hetzel, B.S., Smith, R.M. (Eds.) *Fetal Brain Disorders—Recent Approaches to the Problem of Mental Deficiency.* Amsterdam: Elsevier, pp. 149–185.

Spiro, A.J., Hirano, A., Beilin, R.L., Finkelstein, J.W. (1970) 'Cretinism with muscular hypertrophy (Kocher–Debré–Sémelaigne syndrome): histochemical and ultrastructural study of skeletal muscle.' *Archives of Neurology*, **23**, 340–349.

Stein, D.P., Lederman, R.J., Vogt, D.P., *et al.* (1992) 'Neurological complications following liver transplantation.' *Annals of Neurology*, **31**, 644–649.

Steinschneider, M., Sherbany, A., Pavlakis, S., *et al.* (1990) 'Congenital folate malabsorption: reversible clinical and neurophysiologic abnormalities.' *Neurology*, **40**, 1315.

Stephenson, J.B.P. (1971) 'Uraemia as a determinant of convulsions in acute infantile hypernatraemia.' *Archives of Disease in Childhood*, **46**, 676–679.

Stewart, S.M., Uauy, R., Kennard, B.D., *et al.* (1988) 'Mental development and growth in children with chronic liver disease of early and late onset.' *Pediatrics*, **82**, 167–172.

Still, C.N. (1977) 'Nicotinic acid and nicotinamide deficiency: pellagra and related disorders of the nervous system.' *In:* Vinken, P.J., Bruyn, G.W. (Eds.) *Handbook of Clinical Neurology. Vol. 28. Metabolic and Deficiency Diseases of the Nervous System, Part II.* Amsterdam: North Holland, pp. 59–104.

Stoch, M.B., Smythe, P.M., Moodie, A.D., Bradshaw, D. (1982) 'Psychosocial outcome and CT findings after gross undernourishment during infancy: a 20-year developmental study.' *Developmental Medicine and Child Neurology*, **24**, 419–436.

Stollhoff, K., Schulte, F.J. (1987) 'Vitamin B$_{12}$ and brain development.' *European Journal of Pediatrics*, **146**, 201–205.

Streletz, L.J., Bej, M.D., Graziani, L.J., *et al.* (1992) 'Utility of serial EEGs in neonates during extracorporeal membrane oxygenation.' *Pediatric Neurology*, **8**, 190–196.

Swanson, J.W., Kelley, J.J., McConahey, W.M. (1981) 'Neurologic aspects of thyroid dysfunction.' *Mayo Clinic Proceedings*, **56**, 504–512.

Takahashi, S., Mitamura, R., Itoh, Y., *et al.* (1994) 'Hashimoto encephalopathy: etiologic considerations.' *Pediatric Neurology*, **11**, 328–331.

Tasker, R.C., Boyd, S., Harden, A., Matthew, D.J. (1988) 'Monitoring in non-traumatic coma. Part II: Electroencephalography.' *Archives of Disease in Childhood*, **63**, 895–899.

Teebi, A.S. (1983) 'Primary hypomagnesaemia, an X-borne allele?' *Lancet*, **1**, 701.

Thomas, P.K. (1997) 'Tropical neuropathies.' *Journal of Neurology*, **244**, 475–482.

Tortorella, G., Magaudda, A., Mercuri, E., *et al.* (1993) 'Familial unilateral and bilateral occipital calcifications and epilepsy.' *Neuropediatrics*, **24**, 341–342.

Toti, P., Balestri, P., Cano, M., *et al.* (1996) 'Celiac disease with cerebral calcium and silica deposits: X-ray spectroscopic findings, an autopsy study.' *Neurology*, **46**, 1088–1092.

Tyler, H.R. (1965) 'Neurological complications of dialysis, transplantation and other forms of treatment in chronic uremia.' *Neurology*, **15**, 1081–1088.

—— (1968) 'Neurologic disorders in renal failure.' *American Journal of Medicine*, **44**, 734–748.

—— Clark, D.B. (1957) 'Cerebrovascular accidents in patients with congenital heart disease.' *Archives of Neurology and Psychiatry*, **77**, 483–497.

Valsalmis, M.P., Peress, N.S., Wright, L.D. (1971) 'Central pontine myelinolysis in childhood.' *Archives of Neurology*, **25**, 307–312.

Van Amelsvoort, T., Bakshi, R., Devaux, C.B., Schwabe, S. (1994) 'Hyponatremia associated with carbamazepine and oxcarbazepine therapy: a review.' *Epilepsia*, **35**, 181–188.

Vanderschueren-Lodeweyckx, M., Debruyne, F., Dooms, L., *et al.* (1983) 'Sensorineural hearing loss in sporadic congenital hypothyroidism.' *Archives of Disease in Childhood*, **58**, 419–422.

Vernon, D.D., Postellon, D.C. (1986) 'Nonketotic hyperosmolal diabetic coma in a child: management with low-dose insulin infusion and intracranial pressure monitoring.' *Pediatrics*, **77**, 770–772.

Vortmeyer, A.O., Hagel, C., Laas, R. (1992) 'Haemorrhagic thiamine deficient encephalopathy following prolonged parenteral nutrition.' *Journal of Neurology, Neurosurgery, and Psychiatry*, **55**, 826–829.

Vulsma, T., Gons, M.H., De Vijlder, J.J.M. (1989) 'Maternal–fetal transfer of thyronine in congenital hypothyroidism due to a total organification defect or thyroid agenesis.' *New England Journal of Medicine*, **321**, 13–16.

Wang, L.C., Cohen, M.E., Duffner, P.K. (1994) 'Etiologies of central diabetes insipidus in children.' *Pediatric Neurology*, **11**, 273–277.

Wassner, S.J., Pennisi, M.H., Malekzadeh, M.H., Fine, R.N. (1976) 'The adverse effect of anticonvulsant therapy on renal allograft survival: a preliminary report.' *Journal of Pediatrics*, **88**, 134–137.

Wayne, E.A., Dean, H.J., Booth, F., Tenenbein, M. (1990) 'Focal neurologic deficits associated with hypoglycemia in children with diabetes.' *Journal of Pediatrics*, **117**, 575–577.

Weissman, J.D., Weissman, B.M. (1989) 'Pontine myelinolysis and delayed encephalopathy following the rapid correction of acute hyponatremia.' *Archives of Neurology*, **46**, 926–927.

Wells, T.G., Ulstrom, R.A., Nevins, T.E. (1988) 'Hypoglycemia in pediatric renal allograft recipients.' *Journal of Pediatrics*, **113**, 1002–1007.

Werlin, S.L., D'Souza, B.J., Hogan, W.J.H., *et al.* (1980) 'Sandifer syndrome: an unappreciated clinical entity.' *Developmental Medicine and Child Neurology*, **22**, 374–378.

Werner, E., Simonian, K., Bierman, J.M., French, F.E. (1967) 'Cumulative effects of prenatal complications and deprived environment on physical, intellectual and social development of preschool children.' *Pediatrics*, **39**, 490–505.

Wevers, R.A., Ingemann Hansen, S., Van Hellenberg Hubar, J.L.M., *et al.* (1994) 'Folate deficiency in cerebrospinal fluid associated with a defect in folate binding protein in the central nervous system.' *Journal of Neurology, Neurosurgery, and Psychiatry*, **57**, 223–226.

Wical, B.S., Tomasi, L.G. (1990) 'A distinctive syndrome after induced profound hypothermia.' *Pediatric Neurology*, **6**, 202–205.

Wiebel, J. (1976) 'Cerebellar–ataxic syndrome in children and adolescents with hypothyroidism under treatment.' *Acta Paediatrica Scandinavica*, **65**, 201–205.

Wijdicks, E.F., Wiesner, R.H., Dahlke, L.J., Krom, R.A. (1994) 'FK506-induced neurotoxicity in liver transplantation.' *Annals of Neurology*, **35**, 498–501.

Wilkie, A.O.M., Zeitlin, H.C., Lindenbaum, R.H., *et al.* (1990) 'Clinical features and molecular analysis of the α thalassemia mental retardation syndromes. II. Cases without detectable abnormality of the α globulin complex.' *American Journal of Human Genetics*, **46**, 1127–1140.

—— Gibbons, R.J., Higgs, D.R., Pembrey, M.E. (1991) 'X linked α thalassemia/mental retardation: spectrum of clinical features in three related males.' *Journal of Medical Genetics*, **28**, 738–741.

Willison, H.J., Muller, D.P.R., Matthews, S., *et al.* (1985) 'A study of the relationship between neurological function and serum vitamin E concentrations in patients with cystic fibrosis.' *Journal of Neurology, Neurosurgery, and Psychiatry*, **48**, 1097–1102.

Willoughby, A., Moss, H.A., Hubbard, V.S., *et al.* (1987) 'Developmental outcome in children exposed to chloride-deficient formula.' *Pediatrics*, **79**, 851–857.

Winick, M. (1969) 'Malnutrition and brain development.' *Journal of Pediatrics*, **74**, 667–679.

Wise, J.E., Matalon, R., Morgan, A.M., McCabe, E.R.B. (1987) 'Phenotypic features of patients with congenital adrenal hypoplasia and glycerol kinase deficiency.' *American Journal of Diseases of Children*, **141**, 744–747.

Wiznitzer, M., Packer, R.J., August, C.S., Burkey, E. (1984) 'Neurological complications of bone marrow transplantation in childhood.' *Annals of Neurology*, **16**, 569–576.

Wiswell, T.E., Cornish, J.D., Northam, R.S. (1986) 'Neonatal polycythemia: frequency of clinical manifestations and other associated findings.' *Pediatrics*, **78**, 26–30.

Woodd-Walker, R.B. (1970) 'Kwashi shakes.' *Lancet*, **1**, 299. *(Letter.)*

Wright, M., Nolan, T. (1994) 'Impact of cyanotic heart disease on school performance.' *Archives of Disease in Childhood*, **71**, 64–70.

Yiannikas, C., McLeod, J.G., Walsh, J.C. (1983) 'Peripheral neuropathy associated with polycythemia vera.' *Neurology*, **33**, 139–143.

PART XI

DEVELOPMENTAL AND NEUROPSYCHIATRIC DISORDERS OF CHILDHOOD

Christopher Gillberg

Neuropsychiatric disorders of childhood include those conditions presenting mainly with emotional and/or behavioural symptoms, but for which an exclusive or partial biological basis has been documented or presumed to exist.

Many of the mental retardation syndromes present initially only with psychiatric or developmental problems or with a combination of both. Among these are the so-called 'behavioural phenotype syndromes' (*i.e.* syndromes with a known or presumed genetic cause—such as Prader–Willi syndrome and Williams syndrome—in which behaviour in some key respects is similar from one case to another). In mental retardation of unknown origin, it is perhaps even more common to encounter developmental, emotional and behavioural presenting problems rather than major neurological or other physical deficits.

Autism and the different autistic-like conditions (including Asperger syndrome) have gradually come to be accepted as mainly biologically determined syndromes. Unfortunately, the term 'pervasive developmental disorders' has come into use in some quarters to cover autism and autistic-like conditions. Autism, however, need not be pervasive (and Asperger syndrome usually is not). It is conceptually confusing to use such a term but not to include severe or profound mental retardation under this label.

Tourette syndrome and other severe tic disorders are now conceptualized more and more as a biologically determined spectrum of problems. Genetic and other family studies plus the partially successful pharmacological treatment of some of these cases have combined to produce a picture of an inherited liability to decreased motor and impulse control, sometimes with

far-reaching consequences for psychological development.

Obsessions and compulsions are phenomena which are now believed to be biological in nature. They are part and parcel of Tourette syndrome and obsessive–compulsive disorders and are common in several of the other neuropsychiatric disorders referred to in these chapters.

Most of the various symptom constellations comprising attentional, motor control and perceptual deficits (*e.g.* attention deficit–hyperactivity disorders and specific developmental disorders, including dyslexia) have a clear or surmised biological basis (and a very strong correlation with emotional and behavioural disorders). They are therefore an important part of child neuropsychiatry. These are common problems, affecting 5–10 per cent of the general population of school-age children.

A number of 'minor' developmental problems presenting as sleep disorders, speech disorders and disorders of bladder and bowel control also often cause or are in other ways associated with psychiatric problems.

Finally, child neuropsychiatry encompasses a number of 'borderline' problems, such as behavioural and emotional problems associated with known neurological disorders (epilepsy, hydrocephalus, cerebral palsy, etc.) and a number of psychiatric disorders not yet documented to have a biological basis but in which biological factors play an essential role (anorexia nervosa, schizophrenia, etc.).

In the following chapters, all of the above-mentioned problems and syndromes will be briefly surveyed or at least referred to in more general terms. Before that, however, some comments on normal mental and behavioural development will be made.

24
NORMAL MENTAL AND BEHAVIOURAL DEVELOPMENT

This brief chapter is not a comprehensive summary of all aspects of normal development; rather, it is intended as a background for better understanding of the degree to which symptoms seen in abnormal states deviate qualitatively or quantitatively from the norm. The reader wanting a more detailed description and fuller theoretical background of normal development is referred to specific textbooks on this topic (*e.g.* Illingworth 1979, Lewis 1982) or to comprehensive appraisals of the 'state of the art' as regards research findings (Cicchetti and Cohen 1995; Gillberg 1995; Harris 1995a,b).

However, recent developments in social/cognitive psychology (*e.g.* Astington *et al.* 1988; Frith 1989; Baron-Cohen 1990, 1995)—and in particular in the fields of 'shared attention' and 'theory of mind'—have changed some of the conceptual framework for understanding normal social, communicative and cognitive development, and as yet there is no good comprehensive text on normal development that adequately takes these changes into account. Because of this dearth of good reviews, the current section will focus mostly on the recent expansion of knowledge in the fields of social interaction and communication.

DEVELOPMENTAL MILESTONES

Before discussing the important new insights gained with reference to the child's 'inner world', Table 24.1, outlining some of the outwardly obvious developmental milestones, is presented as a crude point of reference. The table shows the approximate dates at which these milestones are usually attained.

NORMAL VARIABILITY
These are just rough guidelines. Normal interindividual variation is wide for many variables. For instance, it is stated that unsupported walking is achieved at age 10–16 months, but in fact a child starting to walk at age 10 months may well be abnormal—perhaps having so-called attention deficit–hyperactivity disorder (ADHD, see below)—whereas another starting to walk at age 20 months may turn out to be a highly intelligent child with familial late-onset walking.

SEX DIFFERENCES
Girls are, on the whole, earlier in their development than boys (Rutter 1980) and demonstrate a more rapid rate of maturation. This does not hold for certain gross motor skills (such as onset of walking) and visuospatial skills (boys are, for instance, generally earlier and better than girls at jigsaw puzzles). Girls, as a group, seem to be particularly early in the development of some social and communication skills (Maccoby and Jacklin 1980). Most girls have a 'peak' spurt of speech and language development around age $1^1/_2$–2 years. Some boys show a similar spurt even before this age, but for most it occurs considerably later, between the ages of 2 and 3 years. The normal range of variation in the development of speech and language skills appears to be considerably greater in boys than in girls. Limited evidence from studies of CSF levels of homovanillic acid (the end-product of brain dopamine) indicates that girls may have significantly lower levels than boys (Gillberg *et al.* 1983, Shaywitz *et al.* 1984), a finding that could be taken to reflect a higher degree of maturation in CNS functioning, given the well-established negative correlation between homovanillic acid and age.

The systematic scientific study of sex differences in development is relatively scanty. Studies of development and of developmental disability should always subdivide according to sex, but so far not enough attention has been paid to this need.

SHARED ATTENTION AND SOCIAL REFERENCING

Around the age of 9–14 months, normal children of both sexes begin to show clear signs that they want to share other people's attention, indicating joint points of reference (such as the lamp above the kitchen table). Not only do they indicate the objects as such; in doing this, they also look at people as if to check whether they too are interested and perhaps looking at the same thing. It is possible that this drive for shared attention (Mundy and Sigman 1989) is present in even younger infants, but no clear examples of shared attention *behaviours* have yet been documented before the end of the second half of the first year of life. It is also possible that mentalizing abilities—equivalent to having a 'theory of mind' (see below)—might be necessary for the appearance of signs of shared attention and that shared attention is the first outward reflection of the presence of this mind theory.

Parallel to the emergence of shared attention behaviours, there is usually also the typical interest in 'peek-a-boo' games and objects that disappear out of sight. This is not necessarily connected with shared attention, and the child may participate in peek-a-boo games in an imitative fashion, without really sharing a joint external reference point with the other person.

Similar to the notion of shared attention is the concept of social referencing (Walden and Ogan 1988). Social referencing is a process of emotional communication in which one's perception of other individuals' interpretations is used to form one's own understanding of that event (Feinman 1982). A four-level sequence of development leading to the ability to participate in social referencing has been proposed (Plutschik and Kellerman 1983). First emerges the ability to discriminate among emotional expressions, for instance on mother's or father's face. Then follows the gradual recognition of the meaning of these various expressions. After that comes emotional responsiveness. Finally, the ability to refer to another person and interactive regulation of behaviour appear. It is this final stage that is usually referred to as social referencing. The first links in this chain of development are already observable at age 6–9 months (Walden and Ogan 1988).

THE 'EYE-DIRECTION DETECTOR' CONSTRUCT

A recently developed hypothesis (Baron-Cohen 1995) postulates an 'eye-direction detector' developing early in normal child development. We can infer an eye-direction detector in 2-month-old human babies (Maurer and Barrera 1981). The eye-direction detector discerns the presence of eyes or eye-like stimuli, computes whether eyes are directed toward it or toward something else, and infers—from its own case—that the other organism's eyes see what they are looking at. Unless a child has a well-functioning eye-direction detector, s/he will not automatically notice and register the same things and actions that are seen by other people. If the eye-direction detector is defective, conceptions of the real world will be different from those of others, dependent more on internal and proximal stimuli than on external and distant events. Shared attention will not develop in a smooth and automatic fashion. Children with autism, very likely, are deficient in their development of an eye-direction detector.

EXECUTIVE FUNCTIONS

The abilities to plan, to sequentially arrange events in an orderly way, and to postpone to a later time the need for gratification are often referred to as 'executive abilities' or 'executive functions'. They are believed to be specific functions of the frontal lobes, or of the frontal lobes in interaction with other areas of the brain (Ozonoff *et al.* 1991). It is obvious that such functions are necessary for the development of time concepts, motivation and 'common sense'. It is unclear what the earliest 'markers' of executive functions might be, but school-age children usually have remarkable skills in this area. It is well known that executive

TABLE 24.1
Some developmental milestones

Developmental milestone	Approx. age first noted
Gaze contact	1–2 hrs
Smile	0–4 wks
Vocalizing other than crying	2–8 wks
Social smile	2–3 mths
Begins to lift head in prone position	2–3 mths
Laughs aloud	2–4 mths
Bimanual (visually guided) coordination in reaching for objects	4–6 mths
Pulls to stand holding onto furniture	5–10 mths
Sits steadily unsupported	7–10 mths
Responds to own name	7–10 mths
Sits up on floor	8–10 mths
Pincer grip	9–12 mths
Waves goodbye	9–12 mths
Holds out object to adult but will not release it	9–12 mths
One word with meaning	9–14 mths
Simple pretend play (*e.g.* 'peek-a-boo')	10–14 mths
Walks unsupported	10–16 mths
Holds out object to adult and will release it	11–14 mths
Shakes head for 'No'	12–16 mths
Complex pretend play (with toys)	18–24 mths
Goes up and down stairs alone, both feet on each step	20–26 mths
Uses 'I', 'me', 'you'	2–2½ yrs
Mutual play with other children	2–2½ yrs
Five-word sentences comprehensible to strangers	2–3 yrs
Mainly dry by day	2–5 yrs
Mainly dry by night	2½–6 yrs
Speech generally intelligible to strangers	2½–5 yrs
(Imaginary companion)	(3–4 yrs)*
Skips on one foot	3½–4½ yrs
Tells stories	3½–4½ yrs
Draws a person	3½–4½ yrs
Emerging time concepts: distinguishes morning/evening	4½–6 yrs

*Not a universal phenomenon.

functions are deficient in many of the syndromes on the autism spectrum (Happé 1994). They are also often dysfunctional in syndromes comprising attention deficits and motor control problems.

CENTRAL COHERENCE

It now seems that one of the most basic 'instincts' of young human beings is the drive to seek out meaning, pattern and coherence from details presented to them (Frith 1989, Happé 1994). Again, it is unclear which might be the earliest signs of this 'drive for central coherence', but it is present in preschool children, who, for instance, will see a 'cat' when being presented with images of various cat body-parts. Children with neuropsychiatric disorder, particularly those on the autism spectrum, have a low drive for central coherence, and tend to be fixated on details rather than on wholes.

MORE COMPLEX FORMS OF SOCIAL INTERACTION AND EMPATHY: THE EMERGENCE OF MENTALIZING ABILITIES ('THEORY OF MIND')

The normal infant is already socially responsive and ready to interact immediately after birth. Newborn infants have been demonstrated to fixate, give gaze contact and even to imitate slightly after intensive coaxing. This should not be taken to mean that the newborn baby has good social interaction skills typical of older children. It does imply that the old notion of a 'normal autistic phase' in early development was mistaken.

The necessary basic skills for developing a superficially acceptable 'social competence' are, in a sense, there from the beginning. Gaze contact, imitation, detection of eye-direction and turntaking are all necessary if the kinds of behaviours associated with gossiping, interaction at cocktail parties or small talk at the bus station—best termed 'superficial social competence skills'—are ever to develop. It is likely that such skills can be strengthened through training and practice. This is evidenced by the observation that girls tend to be better at such things than boys (girls often get more training in these areas than boys when they are young). On the other hand, there could already be qualitative biological differences between boys and girls in this respect from infancy.

Possibly separate from superficial social competence skills, there appear towards the end of the child's first year obvious signs that s/he is developing mentalizing skills (or a 'theory of mind'), that is, an ability to impute mental states such as knowing and believing to other people and to oneself. For instance, if a 12-month-old baby, turning the pages of a picture book, is stopped in this activity by another person firmly putting her/his hand over the child's, the child will often look the other person in the eye rather than just try to get rid of the hand. It seems reasonable to assume that underlying this kind of gaze contact would be the presumption on the part of the child that the other person has an intention in doing what s/he is doing. In other words, the child has a mentalizing ability, or a theory of mind. As s/he grows older s/he will become aware that there are a variety of mental states in other people and that there is not necessarily a correspondence between superficial social competence skills and these states of mind. The child even begins to be able to think: 'He thinks she thinks'. S/he will then also be able gradually to develop a more sophisticated understanding of complex social cues and interactions and of other people's many-faceted feelings. A theory of mind would also be necessary for the development of a generally good 'human' intelligence. Without a theory of mind the child will not be able to ask meaningful questions of other people (either verbally or non-verbally) and her/his use of language and 'communication' will not be appropriate for acquiring new skills. Rote memory skills need not be affected at all, however, and some children who appear to lack a theory of mind may be thought of as '*idiots savants*' (see Frith 1989) and show remarkable skill in one or a few areas.

Mentalizing ability is a prerequisite for developing empathy (the ability to reflect intuitively and correctly about other people's thoughts and feelings). Empathy, in turn, is necessary for the development of sympathy and compassion (terms often semantically confused with empathy). However, empathy is not all that is necessary to develop these 'talents'. For instance, sociopaths/psychopaths may basically have good empathic skills (necessary when deliberately trying to deceive people) yet generally show little compassion or sympathy with anybody but themselves.

Many children show signs of compassion and sympathy before age 2 years, for instance in approaching and wanting to hug, kiss and comfort somebody who has been hurt or is crying.

Executive functions and the drive for central coherence probably need to be relatively well developed in order for empathy skills to emerge in a smooth and harmonious fashion. When deficient, even with a relatively well developed theory of mind, empathy would tend to be 'unfocused', 'piecemeal', flimsy and shallow.

It is common knowledge that we are all different in our superficial social competence skills and in respect of empathy skills and compassion. Perhaps all these three variables are to a considerable extent biologically determined, discrete or only partly overlapping functions which are distributed in much the same way as IQ along a spectrum from superior skills to severe dysfunction. Maybe, in the lowermost portion of each spectrum there exists a small group affected by environmentally caused dysfunction (such as in the case of brain damage in individuals with very low IQ). If this were the case, there would be similar types of social dysfunction caused either by brain damage/dysfunction or by simply being at the lowermost end of the normal distribution.

SOCIAL DYSFUNCTION SYNDROMES SEEN IN THE LIGHT OF NEW DEVELOPMENTS IN NORMAL SOCIAL/COGNITIVE PSYCHOLOGY

Social dysfunctions of various kinds are the hallmarks of many of the neuropsychiatric disorders of childhood. Autism and Asperger syndrome are now the best known of such conditions. Both seem to share severe problems of empathy. People with autism are generally deficient in superficial social competence skills, empathy and, to some extent, compassion. IQ is often low as well. People with Asperger syndrome are, invariably, deficient in empathy and, to some extent, compassion. IQ is often normal or high. Such people are likely to be diagnosed as Asperger syndrome cases if superficial social competence skills are also impaired. However, there could be Asperger cases with relatively well developed superficial skills of this kind who would then be accepted as belonging in a normal group in spite of severe empathy deficits. Girls in particular might have relatively good social competence skills and yet be severely deficient in the development of empathy skills. A diagnosis of Asperger syndrome in such girls will probably not be thought of, much less made. Children with deficits in attention, motor control and perception often have slight dysfunction in all three areas (and sometimes in overall intelligence as well). Psychopaths need only be deficient in compassion, and must—almost by definition—have some, or even good, empathy skills. It appears that an analysis in terms of superficial social competence skills, empathy, compassion and IQ in patients showing social dysfunction might be useful and have far-reaching practical implications. So far, most psychiatric/neuropsychiatric evaluations do not make use of this model for analysis. The following presentation of neuropsychiatric problems in childhood will also rely on a more conservative phenotypical structure, and various syndromes will be described mainly as they show in outward symptoms and signs. Nevertheless, an awareness of the briefly surveyed expansion of our knowledge as regards children's social and cognitive development is likely to be helpful when trying to understand children affected with neuropsychiatric problems in more depth.

INTELLECTUAL DEVELOPMENT

Intellectual development and the development of intelligence are often considered synonymous. Intelligence is 'the broadest and most pervasive cognitive trait, and is conceived of as being involved in virtually every kind of cognitive skill' and 'it is a quintessentially high-level skill at the summit of a hierarchy of intellectual skills' (Butcher 1970). Intelligence is also 'what intelligence tests measure—a sample of current intellectual performance' (Madge and Tizard 1980). Tested IQ is a *relatively* stable variable: more than 90 per cent of all children show less than 30 points IQ variation from age 2 to 18 years if several tests are performed during this period (Honzik *et al.* 1948), and more than 80 per cent show less than 15 points variation if only one retest is undertaken (Vernon 1976). Stability over time is further increased if the first IQ test is undertaken after age 6 years. Before age 2 years, developmental tests have strong predictive validity only in the case of severely and profoundly mentally retarded children.

The remarkable stability of IQ over time was demonstrated in the long-term follow-up study from Dunedin (Moffitt *et al.* 1993). Almost 800 children were followed with IQ tests at ages 7, 9, 11 and 13 years. Only 13 per cent showed IQ changes that exceeded what was expected from sources of measurement errors. However, even in this rather small subgroup, IQ changes tended not to be major and to return to previous levels at continued follow-up.

Cognitive development is rapid during the first few years of life and continues at a fast rate throughout childhood to adolescence. Thereafter the rate is much slower and most people reach a point (perhaps in early adult life) beyond which they do not increase their intelligence capacities. In adults, IQ is defined by tests which yield normally distributed results in the general population and have a mean of 100. In children, IQ can be conceptualized in similar terms, but also as the equivalent of a developmental quotient (DQ) in which mental age is divided by chronological age and multiplied by 100. When used in this way, a child with an IQ of 50 around age 8 years can be seen as having roughly 50 per cent of normal development for chronological age and therefore as performing similarly to a normal 4-year-old.

Spearman (1927) found that people who did well on one cognitive task usually also did well on most of the other cognitive tasks. He hypothesized that a 'general' (g) factor, or 'mental energy', was in operation. Children with emotional and behavioural problems, as we shall see, very often have cognitive profiles which are extremely uneven and which cannot be predicted by a specific g-factor level.

Both genetic and environmental factors play a part in determining individual differences in IQ, but their relative contribution is not clearly established. That there are strong genetic determinants for IQ is now widely accepted. The overall effects of environment on the development of intelligence in individuals falling within the normal range of intelligence are probably less significant except in grossly abnormal situations such as extreme psychosocial deprivation and long-term near-starvation (Madge and Tizard 1980).

REFERENCES

Astington, J., Harris, P., Olson, D.R. (Eds.) (1988) *Developing Theories of Mind.* Cambridge: Cambridge University Press.
Baron-Cohen, S. (1990) 'Autism: a specific cognitive disorder of "mind-blindness".' *International Review of Psychiatry,* **2**, 81–90.
—— (1995) *Mind Blindness. An Essay on Autism and Theory of Mind.* Cambridge: MIT Press.
Butcher, H.J. (1970) *Human Intelligence: Its Nature and Assessment.* London: Methuen.
Cicchetti, D., Cohen, D.J. (1995) *Developmental Psychopathology. Vol. 1. Theory and Methods.* New York: John Wiley.
Feinman, S. (1982) 'Social referencing in infancy.' *Merrill-Palmer Quarterly,* **29**, 83–87.
Frith, U. (1989) *Autism: Explaining the Enigma.* Oxford: Basil Blackwell.
Gillberg, C. (1995) *Clinical Child Neuropsychiatry.* Cambridge: Cambridge University Press.
—— Svenson, B., Carlström, G., *et al.* (1983) 'Mental retardation in Swedish urban children: some epidemiological considerations.' *Applied Research in Mental Retardation,* **4**, 207–218.
Happé, F.G.E. (1994) 'Current psychological theories of autism: the "theory of mind" account and rival theories.' *Journal of Child Psychology and Psychiatry,* **35**, 215–229.
Harris, J.C. (1995a) *Developmental Neuropsychiatry. Vol. I. The Fundamentals.* Oxford: Oxford University Press.
—— (1995b) *Developmental Neuropsychiatry. Vol. II. Assessment, Diagnosis and Treatment of Developmental Disorders.* Oxford: Oxford University Press.
Honzik, M.P., MacFarlane, J.W., Allen, L. (1948) 'The stability of mental test performance between two and eighteen years.' *Journal of Experimental Education,* **17**, 309–324.
Illingworth, R.S. (1979) *The Normal Child, 7th Edn.* Edinburgh: Churchill Livingstone.
Lewis, M. (1982) *Clinical Aspects of Child Development.* Philadelphia: Lea & Febiger.
Maccoby, E.E., Jacklin, C.N. (1980) 'Sex differences in aggression: a rejoinder and reprise.' *Child Development,* **51**, 964–980.
Madge, N., Tizard, J. (1980) 'Intelligence.' *In:* Rutter, M. (Ed.) *Developmental Psychiatry.* London: Heinemann Medical, pp. 245–265.
Maurer, D., Barrera, M. (1981) 'Infants' perception of natural and distorted arrangements of a schematic face.' *Child Development,* **52**, 196–202.
Moffitt, T.E., Caspi, A., Harkness, A.R., Silva, P.A. (1993) 'The natural history of change in intellectual performance: Who changes? How much? Is it meaningful?' *Journal of Child Psychology and Psychiatry,* **34**, 455–506.
Mundy, P., Sigman, M. (1989) 'Specifying the nature of the social impairment in autism.' *In:* Dawson, G. (Ed.) *Autism: New Perspectives on Nature, Diagnosis and Treatment.* New York: Guilford, pp. 3–31.

Ozonoff, S., Pennington, B.F., Rogers, S.J. (1991) 'Executive function deficits in high-functioning autistic individuals: relationship to theory of mind.' *Journal of Child Psychology and Psychiatry*, **32**, 1081–1105.

Plutschik, R., Kellerman, H. (Eds.) (1983) *Emotion: Theory, Research and Experience. Vol. 2. Emotions in Early Development*. Orlando, FL: Academic Press.

Rutter, M. (Ed.) (1980) *Developmental Psychiatry*. London: Churchill Livingstone.

Shaywitz, S.E., Shaywitz, B.A., Cohen, D.J., Young, J.G. (1984) 'Monoaminergic mechanisms in hyperactivity.' *In:* Rutter, M. (Ed.) *Developmental Neuropsychiatry*. London: Churchill Livingstone, pp. 330–347.

Spearman, C. (1927) 'The doctrine of two factors.' *Reprinted in:* Wiseman, S. (Ed.) (1967) *Intelligence and Ability: Selected Readings*. Harmondsworth: Penguin, pp. 58–68.

Vernon, P.E. (1976) 'Development of intelligence.' *In:* Hamilton, V., Vernon, M.D. (Eds.) *The Development of Cognitive Processes*. London and New York: Academic Press, pp. 507–547.

Walden, T.A., Ogan, T.A. (1988) 'The development of social referencing.' *Child Development*, **59**, 1230–1240.

25
MENTAL RETARDATION

Mental retardation is not a disease, disorder, syndrome or specific disability. It is an administrative blanket term for a wide variety of different genetic, social and specific medical conditions sharing the one common feature that affected individuals score consistently below 70 (or below a range of 67–73) on specific IQ tests (see below).

Mental retardation is subgrouped according to the level of tested IQ. It is becoming increasingly common to include only two levels: *severe mental retardation*, for IQs < 50; and *mild mental retardation*, for IQs in the 50–70 range. *Borderline intellectual functioning* is the term applied when IQ is in the 71–84 range. This subgrouping system will be used in this chapter.

The category of severe mental retardation as defined above is sometimes subdivided further into moderate mental retardation (IQ 36–49), severe mental retardation (IQ 20–35) and profound mental retardation (IQ < 20).

PREVALENCE

Mild mental retardation is more common than severe mental retardation, but claims that it is as much as six times more common—such as in the DSM-IV (American Psychiatric Association 1994)—seem to have relatively weak support in the modern literature.

Recent Swedish studies have suggested that clear mental retardation occurs in less than 1 per cent of school-age children. Hagberg *et al.* (1981) found that 0.7 per cent of 10- to 13-year-olds in one Swedish urban area had IQ scores < 70 and were in need of extra educational support. Slightly less than half of these children had severe mental retardation (IQ < 50) and the rest had mild mental retardation (IQ 50–70). Hagberg's group acknowledged that a number of borderline cases might have been missed and that tested IQ in the Swedish population of children tended toward a higher mean than 100. On follow-up during the teenage period, almost 1 per cent of the population were classified as mentally retarded. Mild mental retardation was about twice as common as severe mental retardation. Gillberg *et al.* (1983) found that 1 per cent of the whole 7- to 8-year-old population had tested IQ < 73 and needed special education. They also found that a further 1 per cent of children in this age-group had tested IQs close to 73 without clearly and constantly falling below this level, and also required special education.

These prevalence figures are considerably lower than reported in earlier studies from Sweden and from other Western countries.

One possible explanation is that the IQ tests used were standardized long ago and that for some reason they now yield a 'falsely high' IQ score. Another contributory factor could be the early stimulation in nurseries, day-care centres and similar settings which could lead to a 'transiently higher' IQ score in early childhood. This is supported by the finding of Hagberg *et al.* that 'new' mental retardation cases continue to be diagnosed even in adolescence, after the impact of the early stimulation has to some extent subsided.

Interestingly, a recent study from a rural Swedish county (Landgren *et al.* 1996) suggested that mild mental retardation may occur in as many as 1.5 per cent of all 7-year-old children, a finding which is in fair accord both with the older studies and with the results of a newer Swedish urban study by Fernell (1996).

The rate of diagnosed severe mental retardation is already 0.3–0.4 per cent at age 3 years, because it is usually recognized in the first few years of life. The rate is then relatively stable for a number of years, and eventually begins to drop a little because of the increased mortality rate. Diagnosed mild mental retardation is at a very low rate during the first years of life, because milder degrees of retardation become progressively more difficult to recognize. Most cases of mild mental retardation are diagnosed from age 3 to 7 years, but the prevalence will continue to increase throughout the school years, at least if screening tests are not performed at a young age.

The rate of mental retardation will also depend upon cultural factors, such as early stimulation, social deprivation, tolerance (in both the positive and negative senses of the word) and access to and provision of special education services.

Boys are affected by mental retardation more often than girls. The boy/girl ratio is in the range of 1.3:1 to 1.9:1. Some mental retardation conditions are much more common in boys than in girls (*e.g.* the fragile X syndrome and autism), but in a few instances the reverse is true (*e.g.* Rett syndrome).

BACKGROUND FACTORS

Having a low tested IQ can be dependent on a wide variety of factors. Several hundred different medical conditions can lead to mental retardation. Genetic and social factors of various kinds can also contribute to cause mental retardation. The panorama of aetiologies varies with the degree of mental retardation and, to a considerable extent, with a number of geographical/cultural factors and factors associated with ante- and perinatal care.

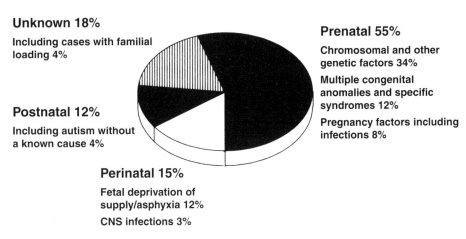

Unknown 18%

Including cases with familial
loading 4%

Prenatal 55%

Chromosomal and other
genetic factors 34%

Multiple congenital
anomalies and specific
syndromes 12%

Pregnancy factors including
infections 8%

Postnatal 12%

Including autism without
a known cause 4%

Perinatal 15%

Fetal deprivation of
supply/asphyxia 12%

CNS infections 3%

Fig. 25.1. Aetiological panorama of severe mental retardation. (Adapted from Hagberg and Kyllerman 1983.)

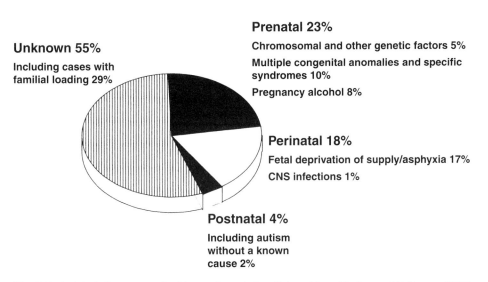

Prenatal 23%

Chromosomal and other genetic factors 5%

Multiple congenital anomalies and specific
syndromes 10%

Pregnancy alcohol 8%

Unknown 55%

Including cases with
familial loading 29%

Perinatal 18%

Fetal deprivation of supply/asphyxia 17%

CNS infections 1%

Postnatal 4%

Including autism
without a known
cause 2%

Fig. 25.2. Aetiological panorama of mild mental retardation. (Adapted from Hagberg and Kyllerman 1983.)

BACKGROUND FACTORS IN SEVERE MENTAL RETARDATION

The aetiology of severe mental retardation can often be established with accuracy. Several chromosomal abnormalities are associated with severe mental retardation (Chapter 5). Enzyme deficiencies due to single or (in some cases) multiple gene defects can sometimes be demonstrated. Certain disorders carrying a high risk of severe mental retardation have an autosomal recessive mode of inheritance. In such disorders, carrier status in clinically unaffected (or very mildly affected) relatives can sometimes be identified. In other cases, physical or behavioural features cluster together in such a typical way that the diagnosis of a specific syndrome can be made even without the identification of a biological marker. However, there are 'borderline' variants for which a case can be made both for inclusion and exclusion. In some cases aetiology cannot be established with certainty but a plausible cause can be inferred. This applies to many cases of perinatal asphyxia, infections and disorders due to environmental toxins (such as intrauterine alcohol poisoning), in which there may be demonstrable brain damage but for which there is no proven cause–effect relationship in the individual case. Finally, there are cases of unknown aetiology, including some with familial clustering and some with great reduction of pre-, peri- and neonatal optimality (see below).

In a study of the aetiology of severe mental retardation in Sweden, Hagberg and Kyllerman (1983) found a definite or highly probable cause in just over 80 per cent of cases (Fig. 25.1). Two-thirds of these were of prenatal origin and about one-sixth each were of peri- and postnatal origin. The *prenatal factors* were chromosomal in more than half the cases (trisomy 21 being much the most common type). In a further 20 per cent, multiple anomalies were present in the absence of chromosomal abnormalities. Prenatal infections accounted for 13 per cent of cases, while clear genetic disorders without demonstrable chromosomal abnormality constituted less than 10 per cent. The *perinatal factors* were fetal deprivation and asphyxia in most cases and perinatal CNS infections in a minority. The *postnatal factors* were very variable and could not be easily grouped. Of the 18 per cent of severe mental retardation cases of unknown aetiology, slightly less than one in four had a familial clustering.

BACKGROUND FACTORS IN MILD MENTAL RETARDATION

In mild mental retardation it is more difficult to arrive at a correct aetiological diagnosis. In the study by Hagberg and Kyllerman (1983), a definite or highly probable cause was found in just under 45 per cent of cases (Fig. 25.2).

More than half of the known or probable causes were of *pre-natal origin*. However, the pattern was very different from that seen in severe mental retardation. Fetal alcohol exposure was the single most common factor, accounting for one-third of the pre-natal cases. Identifiable chromosomal abnormalities were much less common than in the severely retarded group, but syndromes with multiple congenital anomalies were relatively common. *Perinatal factors* were relatively common, and almost all of these were associated with fetal deprivation and asphyxia. Only one out of 91 cases of mild mental retardation appeared to have been caused by perinatal CNS infection. *Postnatal factors* were a rare cause for mild mental retardation. Of the 55 per cent of mild mental retardation cases without a known or probable cause, more than half showed familial clustering.

BACKGROUND FACTORS IN BORDERLINE INTELLECTUAL FUNCTIONING

In borderline intellectual functioning it becomes very difficult to establish the cause. A number of these cases can be accounted for by their being on the lower portion of the normal distribution for intellectual capacity, and the same probably applies to some of the mild mental retardation cases. Indirect evidence from studies of children with deficits in attention, motor control and perception (Gillberg and Rasmussen 1982) suggests that pre-, peri- and postnatal brain-damaging factors play a role in about one-third of the cases. *Reduced optimality* in pregnancy and in the peri- and postnatal periods might be more important than the occurrence of single major events. Reduced optimality is defined as any departure from the defined optimal state for any specified factor/condition during the pre-, peri- and neonatal periods. A high score for reduced optimality would indicate a low level of optimality. The level of reduced optimality seems to be greater in borderline intellectual functioning than in severe mental retardation (Gillberg *et al.* 1990, Gillberg and Gillberg 1991). The reduced optimality could reflect both constitutional defects in the fetus and events that could lead to brain dysfunction. Important interactions between genetic and environmental factors might be associated with the reduced optimality. Many studies also suggest that *psychosocial factors* (including understimulation) are of considerable importance in this group (see Craft 1985).

SUMMARY OF BACKGROUND FACTORS

Known genetic disorders (including Down syndrome) accounted for 47 per cent of severe mental retardation cases but for only 5 per cent of mild mental retardation cases in the Hagberg and Kyllerman (1983) study. With recent developments in molecular genetics, it is likely that the fractions with a specific genetic disorder would be bigger had the study been performed in the late 1990s. Intrauterine infections were responsible for 10 per cent of severe retardation cases, but were not encountered at all in the mildly retarded group. Fetal alcohol exposure was not a contributory factor in the severely retarded group, but accounted for 9 per cent of the mild mental retardation cases. Fetal deprivation with or without asphyxia contributed about 20 per cent of cases in both groups. Aetiology was uncertain in 18 per cent of the severely retarded group and in 55 per cent of the mildly retarded group, but the tendency to familial clustering was much greater in the latter group, indicating the possible presence of one or several genetic factors. In the group with borderline intellectual functioning, genetic factors, psychosocial factors and reduced optimality in the pre-, peri- and neonatal periods appear to interact in a complex pattern to cause mild (but often clinically important) reductions of IQ.

A number of environmental factors, such as fetal exposure to drugs and postnatal exposure to lead, benzene and other toxins, could theoretically contribute to cause mental retardation in certain individuals. There is ample evidence that lead can lower IQ (Needleman and Gatsonis 1990), but the extent to which it may be involved in the causation of mental retardation has not been analysed. More research is warranted in this field.

Depending on the part of the world under view, the aetiological panorama of mental retardation will differ. For instance, if there is widespread starvation, intrauterine malnourishment will be a major cause of mental retardation. Certain genetic conditions are more common in some countries than in others. These and other factors account for the wide variation as regards both prevalence and background factors in mental retardation.

THE CLINICAL PICTURE IN THE MENTAL RETARDATION SYNDROMES

Mental retardation is not a single syndrome and there is no clinical picture common to all people with mental retardation. Depending on underlying aetiology, the clinical presentation varies enormously from one syndrome to another. Within syndromes, it may vary considerably as a consequence of such factors as personality ('temperament') and psychosocial environment. Moreover, it is rare for the 'cognitive profile' to be smooth and even. It is the rule rather than the exception that there is some degree of irregularity in the test profile. For example, if a person has an overall tested IQ of about 60, it would not be surprising if in one area s/he would score a subscale IQ of 80 and in another area one of 45. Unfortunately, even though this insight is acknowledged by most clinicians, in clinical practice it is still common to encounter the notion of 'simple' or 'uncomplicated' mental retardation, with generally (and evenly) low IQ. The term 'uncomplicated mental retardation' is also, usually inadvertently, used to infer that there is nothing else the matter besides the generally low IQ level. Such 'uncomplicated' cases are extremely rare. In fact, 'anonymous' (Hagberg 1995) or 'undefined' would constitute more reasonable terms than 'uncomplicated' in this

TABLE 25.1
Associated disorders in severe (SMR) and mild (MMR) mental retardation*

Associated disorder	SMR (%)	MMR (%)
Cerebral palsy	21	9
Epilepsy	37	12
Severe hearing impairment/deafness	8	7
Severe visual impairment/blindness	15	1
Hydrocephalus	5	2
One or more of above disorders	40	24
Infantile autism	8	4
Other severe psychiatric abnormality	56	53

*Adapted from Rasmussen (1990), based on data from Hagberg and Kyllerman (1983) and Gillberg *et al.* (1986).

context, given that what is usually inferred is a mental retardation syndrome without a known cause.

Finally, there are people with Down syndrome who have low-normal or normal tested IQs. The same applies in Prader–Willi syndrome, Williams syndrome and other disorders originally conceptualized as consistently associated with mental retardation. In fact, mental retardation may not be the most typical symptom in many of these syndromes. Prader–Willi syndrome, for instance, appears to be more clearly defined by the presence of a certain set of behavioural psychiatric problems than by the degree of the learning disorder (which seems to be universal). Thus, the mental retardation syndromes are better grouped in an overall class of 'neuropsychiatric disorders', in which mental retardation is a common but certainly not invariable feature.

For these reasons, the clinical picture of mental retardation is not detailed here, but will instead be presented in connection with a number of named syndromes both in the chapter dealing with autism and autistic-like conditions (Chapter 26) and in that describing other neuropsychiatric syndromes (Chapter 28).

ASSOCIATED DISABILITIES IN MENTAL RETARDATION

The fact that mental retardation is often associated with localized or widespread brain damage accounts for its common association with other types of CNS disorders. Thus, cerebral palsy, epilepsy, autism, and visual and hearing impairments are much more common in people with mental retardation than in the general population. Table 25.1 shows the prevalence of associated neurological and psychiatric disorders in severe and mild mental retardation.

PSYCHIATRIC/BEHAVIOURAL PROBLEMS IN MENTAL RETARDATION

Children with mental retardation show much higher rates of moderate and severe psychiatric abnormality than do children of normal intelligence (Rutter *et al.* 1970, Corbett 1979). A recent Swedish study revealed that more than half of school-age children with mild mental retardation and almost two-thirds of those with severe mental retardation had major psychiatric/behavioural problems (Gillberg *et al.* 1986).

Some behavioural problems are particularly common in the population of children with mental retardation. *Autism and other severe social impairments* appear to be more than one hundred times more common in children with mental retardation than in those of normal intelligence. Classical autism affects about 5 per cent of all children with mental retardation but less than 0.05 per cent of normally intelligent children. Autistic-like conditions—including Lorna Wing's triad (Wing and Gould 1979, see Chapter 26)—are even more common. One in three to one in four children with severe mental retardation are affected by such conditions (Gillberg *et al.* 1986).

Other behavioural features commonly associated with mental retardation include *motor stereotypies* (regardless of associated autistic-like symptoms) (Corbett 1985) and extremes of hyperactive behaviour (see below). Strange eating habits (or rather mouthing habits) are very common in severe mental retardation. Pica is overrepresented in mentally retarded populations. It consists of extremely odd and potentially self-injurious mouthing behaviours such as putting flowers, newspaper, razor-blades, soil or sand into the mouth and then swallowing. Pica can lead to gastrointestinal obstruction, diarrhoea and stomach ache, sometimes requiring immediate surgical intervention.

The symptoms mentioned so far are especially prevalent in the severely retarded population. In children with mild mental retardation, these problems are relatively common also, but, in general, the behavioural/psychiatric problems encountered in mildly retarded subjects are more like those of children (particularly young children) with normal intelligence.

MEDICAL WORK-UP

An adequate medical work-up must include a thorough history taking, concentrating on hereditary/familial and psychosocial circumstances on the one hand and on psychomotor development and associated impairments on the other. The clinical examination of the child must include a full paediatric and neuromotor assessment (including a meticulous search for skin changes and examination of hand function), evaluation of the child's growth chart and assessment of minor physical anomalies and other signs which might help suggest a specific medical syndrome. A brief evaluation of neuropsychiatric/behavioural traits, which might help in differential diagnosis, should also be included. This should focus on symptoms suggestive of autism, Tourette syndrome and other specific neuropsychiatric syndromes.

Hearing and vision must always be examined as comprehensively as possible. This may have to involve auditory brainstem response examination and neuro-ophthalmological assessment under general anaesthesia in certain cases.

Laboratory investigations should always be considered only after some sort of preliminary diagnostic evaluation has been undertaken. However, chromosomal analysis is often indicated, particularly if there are several minor physical anomalies, congenital malformations or autism. The same holds for neuro-radiological examinations, particularly if there is a suspicion of cerebral malformation; for EEG, which is mandatory in all syndromes suspected of having a convulsive or episodic character; and for certain biochemical blood and urine screens (*e.g.* amino acids, organic acids and mucopolysaccharides).

NEUROPSYCHOLOGICAL WORK-UP

No child should be said to suffer from mental retardation until at least two IQ tests (or Vineland interviews or clinical assessments), three months apart, have shown an IQ level < 70.

One cannot expect to make accurate 'IQ diagnoses' in children under 3 years of age, other than to separate out those with severe and profound levels of mental retardation from the rest. From around age 7–8 years more reliable IQ estimates can be made, using well-standardized tests such as the WISC-R (Wechsler 1974). Because of the well-known difficulties associated with testing children with social and language impairments, some more details of various tests used with children are provided in Chapter 26.

TREATMENT, MANAGEMENT AND EDUCATION

For most mental retardation conditions, no cure is currently available. Nevertheless, some forms of mental retardation are preventable through immunization programmes (*e.g.* rubella embryopathy) and screening followed by diet (*e.g.* phenylketonuria) or substitution therapy (*e.g.* hypothyroidism).

Early diagnosis, education of the family and special education measures for the affected child are crucial elements in most treatment/management programmes for children with mental retardation. In individual mental retardation syndromes, more or less specific interventions may be available. These and other aspects of treatment, as well as the need for special services, are illuminated in more detail in Chapters 26 and 27.

OUTCOME

No general prognosis can be given for all children with mental retardation. Outcome is heavily dependent on underlying aetiology. Children with progressive brain disorders have a worse prognosis than those with nonprogressive brain damage. Even in disorders that have traditionally been regarded as 'nonprogressive', empirical study has revealed that the picture is more complicated. For instance, Down syndrome is very often associated with Alzheimer-type dementia, and the type of familial mental retardation associated with the fragile X chromosome abnormality may become worse at puberty. However, it is possible to make the general statement that most children diagnosed in the preschool period as having an IQ < 50 will still be mentally retarded in adult life. Those having an IQ < 70 in the early school years are also likely to have significant intellectual impairment in adulthood.

REFERENCES

American Psychiatric Association (1994) *Diagnostic and Statistical Manual of Mental Disorders, 4th Edn.* Washington, DC: APA.
Corbett, J.A. (1979) 'Psychiatric morbidity and mental retardation.' *In:* James, F.E., Snaith, R.P. (Eds.) *Psychiatric Illness and Mental Handicap.* London: Gaskell Press, pp. 28–45.
—— (1985) 'Mental retardation: psychiatric aspects.' *In:* Rutter, M., Hersov, L. (Eds.) *Child and Adolescent Psychiatry: Modern Approaches. 2nd Edn.* Oxford: Blackwell Scientific, pp. 661–678.
Craft, M. (1985) 'Classification, criteria, epidemiology and causation.' *In:* Craft, M., Bicknell, D.J., Hollins, S. (Eds.) *Mental Handicap: a Multidisciplinary Approach.* London: Baillière Tindall, pp. 75–88.
Fernell, E. (1996) 'Mild mental retardation in schoolchildren in a Swedish suburban municipality: prevalence and diagnostic aspects.' *Acta Paediatrica*, **85**, 584–588.
Gillberg, C., Gillberg, I.C. (1991) 'Note on the relationship between population-based and clinical studies: the question of reduced optimality in autism.' *Journal of Autism and Developmental Disorders*, **21**, 251–253. *(Letter.)*
—— Rasmussen, P. (1982) 'Perceptual, motor and attentional deficits in seven-year-old children: background factors.' *Developmental Medicine and Child Neurology*, **24**, 752–770.
—— Svenson, B., Carlström, G., *et al.* (1983) 'Mental retardation in Swedish urban children: some epidemiological considerations.' *Applied Research in Mental Retardation*, 4, 207–218.
—— Persson, E., Grufman, M., Themnér, U. (1986) 'Psychiatric disorders in mildly and severely mentally retarded urban children and adolescents: epidemiological aspects.' *British Journal of Psychiatry*, **149**, 68–74.
—— Gillberg, I.C., Steffenburg, S. (1990) 'Reduced optimality in the pre-, peri-, and neonatal periods is not equivalent to severe peri- or neonatal risk: a rejoinder to Goodman's technical note [comment]. Comment on: J Child Psychol Psychiatry 1990, Jul 31, 5, 809–12.' *Journal of Child Psychology and Psychiatry*, **31**, 813–815.
Hagberg, B. (1995) 'Rett syndrome: clinical peculiarities and biological mysteries.' *Acta Paediatrica*, **84**, 971–976.
—— Kyllerman, M. (1983) 'Epidemiology of mental retardation—a Swedish survey.' *Brain and Development*, **5**, 441–449.
—— Hagberg, G., Lewerth, A., Lindberg, U. (1981) 'Mild mental retardation in Swedish school children. I. Prevalence.' *Acta Paediatrica Scandinavica*, **70**, 441–444.
Landgren, M., Pettersson, B., Kjellman, B., Gillberg, C. (1996) 'ADHD, DAMP and other neurodevelopmental/psychiatric disorders in 6-year-old children: epidemiology and co-morbidity.' *Developmental Medicine and Child Neurology*, **38**, 891–906.
Needleman, H.L., Gatsonis, C.A. (1990) 'Low-level lead exposure and the IQ of children. A meta-analysis of modern studies.' *Journal of the American Medical Association*, **263**, 673–678.
Rasmussen, P. (1990) 'Psykisk utvecklingsstörning.' *In:* Gillberg, C., Hellgren, L. (Eds.) *Barn- och ungdomspsykiatri.* Stockholm: Natur & Kultur, pp. 269–285.
Rutter, M., Graham, P., Yule, W. (1970) *A Neuropsychiatric Study in Childhood. Clinics in Developmental Medicine No. 35/36.* London: Spastics International Medical Publications.
Wechsler, D. (1974) *Manual of the Wechsler Intelligence Scale for Children—Revised.* New York: Psychological Corporation.
Wing, L., Gould, J. (1979) 'Severe impairments of social interaction and associated abnormalities in children: epidemiology and classification.' *Journal of Autism and Developmental Disorders*, **9**, 11–29.

26
AUTISM AND AUTISTIC-LIKE CONDITIONS

There are descriptions in the literature (*e.g.* Haslam 1809, Malson 1964, Frith 1989) of people living several hundred years ago, who, according to our present-day terminology, would have fulfilled criteria for infantile autism (Rutter 1978a,b; American Psychiatric Association 1980) or autistic disorder (American Psychiatric Association 1987). Obviously autistic syndromes are not 'new' conditions typical of Western societies of the 20th century (as has been proposed by Tinbergen and Tinbergen 1983), even though current concepts and definitions are less than 50 years old.

AUTISM

PREVIOUS DEFINITIONS AND CONCEPTS
The US child psychiatrist Leo Kanner (1943) and the Austrian paediatrician Hans Asperger (1944) were possibly the first to describe the type of empathy disorders encompassed in the 'autistic continuum' (Wing 1989), highlighting the specificity of the social interaction deficit which has, ever since, been regarded as the core symptom of autism. Before them, however, Ssucharewa (1926), a Russian clinical assistant working in a 'psychoneurological clinic', described 'schizoid personality disorder' in children in a way which makes it clear that she was referring to the disorder now known as Asperger syndrome.

Whether to regard Kanner's 'early infantile autism' and Asperger's 'autistic psychopathy' as synonymous, as different sections on an autism spectrum, as partly biologically and psychologically overlapping disabilities or as clearly different conditions has been the subject of considerable debate. Here they will be described separately, even though they can probably—at least regarding some key features—be conceptualized as existing on a continuum.

A number of labelled conditions and syndromes, some of which can be regarded as synonymous and others that can be seen as partly overlapping entities, are shown in Table 26.1.

The word autism does not only refer to the syndrome of autism, but is also used in its original Bleulerian sense to describe the particular quality of thought encountered as a first-rank symptom in schizophrenia (Bleuler 1911). In the following, unless otherwise specified, 'autism' will be used throughout when referring to the syndrome of autism (outlined below).

CURRENT DEFINITIONS OF AUTISM
All currently accepted definitions of autism include three main criteria which have to be met for a diagnosis to be made. These are: (1) disturbance of reciprocal social interaction; (2) disturbance of communication (including language comprehension and spoken language); (3) disturbance of normal variation in behaviour and imaginative activities, leading to extreme restriction in the behavioural repertoire. The various specific symptoms associated with each criterion tend to be slightly differently emphasized by different authors, but the basic symptom categories are the same throughout. Some authors also require an onset before age 30–36 months to make the diagnosis of autism.

The criteria currently most used in the field are those of the DSM-III (American Psychiatric Association 1980), DSM-III-R (American Psychiatric Association 1987), and DSM-IV (American Psychiatric Association 1994). These three sets of criteria are outlined in Table 26.2. The ICD-10 criteria for childhood autism (WHO 1993) are also in use. They are almost identical to those of the DSM-IV. It is believed that DSM-III identifies a more narrow subtype of autism. The DSM-IV criteria are actually rather vague and, if used by clinicians unfamiliar with autism, would probably tend towards overinclusion of cases.

Lorna Wing (1989) has argued that the specificity of infantile autism or 'Kanner autism' is in doubt. She has shown that a number of mentally handicapping conditions and brain damage syndromes show the same triad of social, communicative and behavioural impairments, and that a case for separating out a diagnosis of 'pure' Kanner autism sometimes cannot be made. Even when the phenomenology is concordant with Kanner's description, background factors and outcome tend to vary considerably (Wing and Gould 1979, Gillberg and Steffenburg 1987, Gillberg *et al.* 1987). Wing has also shown that, in mentally impaired individuals, the presence of one of the problems included in the triad dramatically increases the risk that one or both of the other two types of problems will be present as well. Gillberg and Coleman (1992) have advocated a similar line of reasoning when referring to the 'autistic syndromes'. It has gradually become accepted that autism is a behavioural symptom constellation signalling underlying nervous system dysfunction. The evidence for a specific 'nuclear autism' disease entity is largely lacking.

TABLE 26.1
Synonyms and partly overlapping labels in the spectrum of autism disorders

Label	References
Infantile autism	Rutter (1978a,b), American Psychiatric Association (1980)
Autistic disorder	American Psychiatric Association (1987, 1994)
Early infantile autism	Kanner (1943)
Childhood autism	Wing (1981b)
Autistic syndrome	Gillberg and Coleman (1992)
Triad of social impairments	Wing and Gould (1979)
Pervasive developmental disorder	American Psychiatric Association (1987)
Childhood schizophrenia	Bender (1947)
Autistic psychopathy	Asperger (1944)
Asperger syndrome	Wing (1981b)
Atypical child syndrome	Rank (1949)
Symbiotic psychosis	Mahler (1952)

PREVALENCE

Recent studies suggest that in industrialized countries the prevalence of autism—defined according to DSM-III, DSM-III-R or Rutter criteria—is at least in the range of 1–1.2 per 1000, not including Asperger syndrome cases (for overviews see Gillberg *et al.* 1991c, Wing 1993). Older reports suggested a lower prevalence rate (around 0.2–0.5 per 1000). One study (Arvidsson *et al.* 1997) has shown a rate as high as 1 in 1000 for the classical 'Kanner variant' of autism (characterized by aloofness and elaborate repetitive routines). Hertzig *et al.* (1990) proposed that the increased prevalence could be accounted for by the use of more inclusive criteria in later diagnostic manuals such as the DSM-III-R. However, there is no good evidence from population studies to support this notion. To the contrary, there is limited evidence that the reasons for the relatively high recent figures are an increasing awareness of the existence of autism generally and particularly in severely and profoundly mentally retarded people, and the fact that a higher incidence of autism has been observed in recent years among children of immigrants from remote countries (Akinsola and Fryers 1986, Gillberg *et al.* 1987).

SEX RATIOS

In classic autism cases, boys tend to outnumber girls by at least 3:1 (Wing 1981b). Among cases with severe and profound mental retardation, the ratio tends to be lower, and in those with higher IQ it tends to be considerably higher.

ASSOCIATED DISABILITIES

Mental retardation is present in 65–88 per cent of autism cases.

Epilepsy occurs in 30–40 per cent of autism cases before 30 years of age (Gillberg 1991c). Slightly less than half this proportion comprises various epilepsy types (including infantile spasms) with onset in early childhood. The other half is mostly adolescent-onset epilepsy. Partial complex seizures and generalized tonic–clonic seizures are the most common types of epilepsy.

Hearing problems are relatively common. A hearing deficit of 25 dB or more is present in about 20 per cent of children with typical autism (Steffenburg 1991).

Visual problems are also common (but also difficult to diagnose). On the basis of results from one Swedish study (Steffenburg 1991), about half of those children with autism who function at a level sufficient to permit a comprehensive ophthalmological assessment have refraction errors or squints or both. Recent studies (Hobson 1993, Jacobsson *et al.* 1998) suggest that children who are blind may have a high rate of autistic disorder, particularly if the blindness is associated with so-called retinopathy of prematurity.

A considerable proportion of people with autism have expressive dysphasia 'superimposed' on their autistic-type speech and language abnormalities.

Major motor control abnormalities are uncommon in classical autism in childhood. However, follow-up into adulthood (von Knorring 1991) reveals that many patients develop disturbances of gait, ataxic movements and overall motor clumsiness with increasing age. Hypotonia and mild ataxia sometimes occur in early childhood autism cases (Gillberg and Coleman 1992). Also, children with spastic tetraplegia exhibit social interaction and communication deficits in a relatively large proportion of cases, even when the effects of concomitant severe mental retardation are taken into account.

ASSOCIATED SPECIFIC MEDICAL CONDITIONS

A large number of specific medical conditions have been found to be associated with autism or autistic symptoms at a rate higher than that found in the general population. Conversely, in autism there is a high rate of associated medical conditions such as fragile X syndrome, other chromosomal abnormalities, tuberous sclerosis, neurofibromatosis, Moebius syndrome and Rett syndrome. In a population-based study of autism in western Sweden, Steffenburg (1991) found that 37 per cent had an associated medical condition of this type. Table 26.3 shows some of the correlations between autism and specific medical conditions that have been reported in the literature to date.

SOCIAL COGNITION IN AUTISM

Three basic sets of psychological functions are often impaired in autism: (1) mentalizing (also referred to as 'theory of mind' and 'empathy'); (2) executive functions; and (3) drive for central coherence (Happé 1994). Of these, (1) and (3) appear to be more 'autism-specific', and (2) less so. Attachment behaviours, originally believed to be severely abnormal in autism, are usually not primarily affected (Sigman and Mundy 1989, Dissanayake and Crossley 1996).

Mentalizing is the ability to attribute mental states (such as knowing, believing, etc.) to other people. It has been clearly demonstrated that young children with autism have severe problems in this domain as compared to normal and mentally retarded children who do not have autistic features.

Executive functions comprise initiation of responses to the environment, maintaining the response, and shifting to a new set

TABLE 26.2
Diagnostic criteria for autism

Label	Diagnostic criteria
Infantile autism (DSM-III: American Psychiatric Association 1980)	Onset before age 30 months Pervasive lack of responsiveness to other people Gross deficits in language development and, if speech is present, peculiar patterns such as echolalia, metaphorical language and pronominal reversals Bizarre responses to environment, *e.g.* resistance to change, peculiar interests (+ Absence of clear signs suggestive of schizophrenia)
Autistic disorder (DSM-III-R: American Psychiatric Association 1987)	Onset during infancy or childhood Qualitative impairment in reciprocal social interaction as manifested by at least two of the following: • marked lack of awareness of the existence of feelings of others • no or abnormal seeking of comfort at times of distress • no or impaired imitation • no or abnormal social play • gross impairment in ability to make peer friendships Qualitative impairment in verbal and nonverbal communication, and in imaginative activity, as manifested by at least one of the following: • no mode of communication, such as communicative babbling, facial expression, gesture, mime or spoken language • markedly abnormal nonverbal communication, as in the use of eye-to-eye gaze, facial expression, body posture or gestures to initiate or modulate social interaction • absence of imaginative activity, *e.g.* play-acting of adult roles, fantasy characters or animals; lack of interest in stories about imaginary events • marked abnormalities in speech production, including volume, pitch, stress, rate, rhythm and intonation • marked abnormalities in the use of speech, including stereotyped and repetitive speech • marked impairment in the ability to initiate or sustain a conversation with others, despite adequate speech Markedly restricted repertoire of activities and interests, as manifested by at least one of the following: • stereotyped body movements, *e.g.* hand flicking, twisting, spinning, head banging or complex whole-body movements • persistent preoccupation with parts of objects • marked distress over changes in trivial aspects of environment, *e.g.* when a vase is moved from its usual position • unreasonable insistence on following routines in precise detail, *e.g.* insisting that exactly the same route always be followed when shopping • markedly restricted range of interest and a preoccupation with one narrow interest, *e.g.* lining up objects, amassing facts about meteorology, or pretending to be a fantasy character At least 8 of the 16 specified items above must be fulfilled

Autistic disorder DSM-IV: (American Psychiatric Association 1994)	A. A total of six (or more) items from (1), (2), and (3) with at least two from (1), and one each from (2) and (3):
	(1) qualitative impairment in social interaction, as manifested by at least two of the following:
	  (a) marked impairment in the use of multiple nonverbal behaviours such as eye-to-eye gaze, facial expression, body postures and gestures to regulate social interaction
	  (b) failure to develop peer relationships appropriate to developmental level
	  (c) a lack of spontaneous seeking to share enjoyment, interests or achievements with other people (*e.g.* by a lack of showing, bringing or pointing out objects of interest)
	  (d) lack of social or emotional reciprocity
	(2) qualitative impairments in communication as manifested by at least one of the following:
	  (a) delay in, or total lack of, the development of spoken language (not accompanied by an attempt to compensate through alternative modes of communication such as gesture or mime)
	  (b) in individuals with adequate speech, marked impairment in the ability to initiate or sustain a conversation with others
	  (c) stereotyped and repetitive use of language or idiosyncratic language
	  (d) lack of varied, spontaneous make-believe play or social imitative play appropriate to developmental level
	(3) restricted repetitive and stereotyped patterns of behaviour, interests and activities, as manifested by at least it one of the following:
	  (a) encompassing preoccupation with one or more stereotyped and restricted patterns of interest that is abnormal either in intensity or focus
	  (b) apparently inflexible adherence to specific, nonfunctional routines or rituals
	  (c) stereotyped and repetitive motor mannerisms (*e.g.* hand or finger flapping or twisting, or complex whole-body movements)
	  (d) persistent preoccupation with parts of objects
	B. Delays or abnormal functioning in at least one of the following areas, with onset prior to age 3 years:
	(1) social interaction,
	(2) language as used in social communication,
	(3) symbolic or imaginative play
	C. The disturbance is not better accounted for by Rett syndrome or Childhood Disintegrative Disorder

Childhood autism (WHO 1993)	Qualitative impairments in reciprocal social interaction Qualitative impairments in communication Restricted, repetitive and stereotyped patterns of behaviour, interests and activities Developmental abnormalities must have been present in the first 3 years for the diagnosis to be made
Autism (Denckla 1986)	Social impairment Delayed and deviant language Repetitive, stereotypic or ritualistic behaviour

TABLE 26.3
Associated medical conditions in autism documented in at least two studies

Medical condition	Important reference
Fragile X syndrome	Hagerman (1989)
Other sex chromosome anomalies	Hagerman (1989)
Marker chromosome syndrome	Gillberg *et al.* (1991b)
Other chromosome anomalies	Hagerman (1989)
Tuberous sclerosis	Hunt and Dennis (1987)
Neurofibromatosis	Gillberg and Forsell (1984)
Hypomelanosis of Ito	Åkefeldt and Gillberg (1991)
Rett syndrome	Gillberg and Coleman (1992)
Angelman syndrome	Steffenburg *et al.* (1996)
Moebius syndrome	Ornitz *et al.* (1977)
Phenylketonuria	Friedman (1969)
Lactic acidosis	Coleman and Blass (1985)
Rubella embryopathy	Chess *et al.* (1971)
Herpes encephalitis	Gillberg (1986)
Cytomegalovirus infection	Stubbs (1978)
Williams syndrome	Reiss *et al.* (1985)
Duchenne muscular dystrophy	Komoto *et al.* (1984)

of responses. Attentional ability, planning, sequencing, impulse control and time conceptualization are all examples of such executive functions, which are usually impaired in autism. However, they are also commonly impaired in other disorders, such as attention deficit–hyperactivity disorder.

The *drive for central coherence*—i.e. the seeking to find a coherent theme or 'picture' behind a set of details—is usually weak in autism.

It is not clear 'where in the brain' these cognitive psychological abilities are located. However, it is generally assumed that executive functions involve the frontal lobes (Harris 1995a,b). One PET scan study of mentalizing abilities in normal and Asperger syndrome males suggested that such functions may be located in the medial portion of the left frontal lobe (Happé *et al.* 1996).

PATHOGENETIC CHAIN OF EVENTS IN AUTISM

Reduced optimality in the pre-, peri- and neonatal periods has been found to be considerably more 'pathological' in autism than in a number of other developmental disorders such as mental retardation without autistic traits, syndromes associated with deficits in attention, motor control and perception and teenage psychosis (Gillberg and Gillberg 1991). These disorders are in turn associated with reductions of optimality greater than those to be expected in normal children. Bleeding in pregnancy, high maternal age, pre- and post-term birth, clinical dysmaturity and hyperbilirubinaemia are among the factors which contribute to a high prevalence of reduced optimality scores in autism (Gillberg and Gillberg 1983, Bryson *et al.* 1988). The added negative effects of several factors that deviate from the optimal state in pregnancy and the newborn period could lead to a suboptimal environment for the developing nervous system which could cause brain dysfunction showing later as autistic symptomatology. However, the interpretation of reduced optimality is not straightforward.

Clear brain-damage risks (such as haemolytic anaemia caused by blood-group incompatibility, severe and protracted asphyxia, etc.) are also associated with some cases of autism (*e.g.* Folstein and Rutter 1977). Such findings imply that typical autism can arise on the basis of nonspecific brain damage.

There is increasing evidence that, in many cases, genetic factors are in operation in autism. Three well-designed twin studies have all shown a strong concordance for autism in monozygotic twins and no concordance in dizygotic twins (Bolton and Rutter 1990). Family studies of population-based series of autism cases have demonstrated a 50- to 100-fold autism risk increase for siblings of children with autism as compared with children in the general population. Family studies (*e.g.* Bowman 1988, Bolton *et al.* 1994) show that in certain families Asperger syndrome, autistic-like conditions (including a 'condition' which is sometimes referred to as a 'lesser variant of autism') and autism 'proper' cluster in such a way as to suggest the presence of a strong heritability for some kind of autism-associated traits. Folstein and Rutter (1977) have suggested that it is not autism as such which is inherited, rather that some kind of cognitive disorder is transmitted which will in certain cases turn into autism if environmental insults are added. Other authors (*e.g.* Gillberg *et al.* 1992) have argued that a genetically transmitted social or 'social cognitive' deficit factor might be present in some families of children with autism. The family studies favour the notion of an 'Asperger trait' running in some kinships. If combined with brain damage, such as in the case of intrauterine rubella infection, this trait might produce autism (Gillberg 1991a). Most family studies show support for the notion of a language-associated cognitive deficit running in certain families, but a few have not found any evidence for this (*e.g.* Steffenburg 1990). Several different hereditary factors, interacting with other factors, could produce the same end result. Thus, there might be Asperger-associated heredity in some families and dyslexia-associated heredity in others.

In an overview of all studies providing detailed information about associated medical disorders (Gillberg and Coleman 1996), the rate of such conditions in typical autism cases was estimated at about one in four individuals. In a study by Steffenburg (1991) of a total population cohort of children with autism, about one-third had a clear associated medical condition, less than 10 per cent had a 'pure' hereditary form, and the majority of the remainder had major signs of brain dysfunction revealed by comprehensive neurobiological work-up. The aetiology of the disorder was unknown in more than half of all affected individuals. Genetic factors alone or interacting with pre-, peri- or postnatal brain damaging factors may account for much or all of the variance in this 'idiopathic' group.

Several theories regarding the aetiology of autism have been proposed over the last 20 years. It is clear that autism can be the end result of a number of different conditions, ranging from tuberous sclerosis and the fragile X chromosome abnormality to metabolic disorders. Do these aetiologies share a common feature, namely that they impinge on the same brain structures or functional systems? In recent years, the brainstem, the temporal lobes and the prefrontal areas of the frontal lobes of the brain have been most often implicated in studies of neurophysiology/neuro-radiology in autism. A few studies have drawn attention to the possible role of the cerebellum and the basal ganglia. The target areas for the brain's dopaminergic nerve fibres arising in the brainstem are the mesolimbic structures in the temporal lobes and prefrontal areas and in the basal ganglia. The dopamine system has been reported to be abnormal in autism (Gillberg and Svennerholm 1987, Barthélémy *et al.* 1988, Nordin *et al.* 1998). One theory proposes that the diverse aetiologies all affect this functional dopamine system in the brain and that when dopamine systems become dysfunctional, many of the typical autism symptoms ensue (Gillberg and Coleman 1992). Support for this theory is also provided by recent observations that babies born to mothers addicted to the cocaine derivative 'crack' show many of the characteristic features of autism from the first few months of life (Gillberg and Coleman 1992). Crack affects the brain's dopamine systems. However, alternative theories, such as hyperserotoninaemia problems, locus ceruleus dysfunction and endorphin imbalance, have been advanced (Cook 1990). The various theories need not be exclusive. It does not seem likely that one pathogenetic chain of events will ever be discovered to account for all autism cases.

In summary, autism is best conceptualized as a behavioural disorder—not so specific as previously believed—with multiple aetiologies. Autism is a sign that there is something wrong in the nervous system. It is best regarded as belonging with the other major neurodisabling conditions such as mental retardation, cerebral palsy and epilepsy. It often occurs in conjunction with other disorders and there should no longer be a need to discuss whether a child has, for example, 'autism or a hearing deficit', in a case where it is clear that both diagnoses apply.

MEDICAL WORK-UP IN AUTISM

Studies by Steffenburg (1991) and others have demonstrated that a comprehensive medical work-up should be performed in all cases of autism. Steffenburg found a clear aetiology in about one-third of cases (and signs of major nonspecific brain dysfunction in another 50 per cent). More than half of the clear aetiologies would not have been disclosed without an exhaustive work-up of the kind suggested in Tables 26.4 and 26.5. These tables list the essentials in any work-up of a child under 10 years of age who receives a diagnosis of autism for the first time. In older children, and in children for whom a clear aetiology is suspected, the work-up may be differently tailored.

If there is a nearby laboratory testing CSF amino acids (phenylalanine in particular), CSF monoamines and CSF endorphins, these tests should be considered if the child has a lumbar puncture anyway (to exclude progressive encephalitis/encephalopathy).

Even in those many cases for which a clear aetiology cannot be established, the medical work-up may be important for psychological reasons. The parents need to know that their doctor has done what is currently the best possible work-up in the field of autism. The fact that so many cases turn out to have

TABLE 26.4
Neuropsychiatric assessment in autism

(1) History

Detailed, structured assessment in relation to autism using standard questionnaire (including handedness)

Review of optimality in pre-, peri- and neonatal periods (medical records required)

Review of postnatal, potentially brain-damaging events (medical records usually needed)

Review of previous medical illness, growth patterns, etc.

Detailed psychiatric history:
- family factors and psychosocial milieu
- temperament and attention span of child
- heredity (especially autism, Asperger syndrome, 'autistic-like conditions' (including so-called 'lesser variants of autism'), learning disorders, mental retardation, 'childhood psychosis', childhood schizophrenia, affective disorders, obsessive–compulsive disorders, psychiatric disorders generally including anorexia nervosa and elective mutism, tuberous sclerosis, neurofibromatosis, geniuses, kinship)

(2) General physical examination

Measurement of cranial circumference, height, weight, auricle length and interpupillary distance

Assessment with respect to minor physical anomalies: meticulous physical examination (often needs repeating), including search for diagnostic skin changes (tuberous sclerosis, neurofibromatosis, hypomelanosis of Ito)

Assessment of heartbeat variation

In boys, inspection of external genitalia (prepuce, penile and testicular size and volume)

(3) Age-appropriate neurodevelopmental neurological examination

(4) Psychological evaluation

Has to be performed by an experienced clinical psychologist who knows how to do cognitive testing in children with autism and knows which test is appropriate according to child's age, developmental level, language and degree of cooperation

(5) Laboratory examinations (see Table 26.5)

demonstrable signs of brain dysfunction—even when no exact cause can be established—is often helpful rather than, as some seem to fear, contributing to pessimistic attitudes in parents and others working to help the affected child. The disorder becomes less mysterious, and some of the child's problems take on a less baffling, less threatening character.

NEUROPSYCHOLOGICAL WORK-UP

All children with autism also need a neuropsychological work-up. This must include some kind of cognitive/intellectual testing or evaluation. No single measure in childhood will be able to predict outcome in autism better than an IQ test: IQ < 50 around age 5–8 years almost invariably means a relatively poor outcome, whereas IQ > 70 at this age predicts that outcome may be relatively good (see below).

The test used will vary from one culture to another. It should be performed by a psychologist both clinically and theoretically experienced with testing and evaluating children with autism.

At least four different cognitive/developmental scales seem to be useful in autism: the WISC-R (Wechsler 1974), the Leiter International Scale (Leiter 1980), the Vineland Social Maturity Scale (Doll 1965) and the Griffiths Developmental Scale II (Griffiths 1970). For language evaluation, the Reynell

TABLE 26.5
Relevant laboratory analyses in all medium- and low-functioning, and certain high-functioning cases with autism and autistic-like conditions

Analysis	Finding	Reference
Chromosomal (including folic acid-depleted medium)	Fragile Xq27.3	Hagerman (1989)
	XYY	Gillberg *et al.* (1984)
	Deletions, *e.g.* 15q12	Kerbeshian *et al.* (1990)
	Marker chromosome (15q)	Gillberg *et al.* (1991b)
	Other	Hagerman (1989)
CT/MRI	Tuberous sclerosis	Gillberg *et al.* (1987)
	Intrauterine infections	Chess *et al.* (1971)
	Neurofibromatosis	Gillberg and Forsell (1984)
	Hypomelanosis of Ito	Åkefeldt and Gillberg (1991)
	Other	Tsai (1989)
CSF protein*	Progressive encephalopathy	Wing and Gould (1979)
EEG	Tuberous sclerosis	Steffenburg (1990)
	Subclinical epilepsy	Gillberg and Schaumann (1983)
	Epileptic discharges	Gillberg and Schaumann (1983)
Auditory brainstem response	Brainstem dysfunction	Gillberg and Coleman (1992)
Ophthalmology	Poor vision, fundus signs	Steffenburg (1990)
Otolaryngology (including hearing test)	Poor hearing, anatomical defects	Smith *et al.* (1988)
Blood:		
Phenylalanine	High	Friedman (1969)
Uric acid	High	Gillberg and Coleman (1992)
Lactic acid	High	Coleman and Blass (1985)
Pyruvic acid	High	Gillberg and Coleman (1992)
Herpes titre	Seroconversion	Gillberg (1986)
24-hour urine:		
Metabolic screening including mucopolysaccharidosis	Abnormal	Gillberg and Coleman (1992)
Uric acid	High	Gillberg and Coleman (1992)
Calcium	Low	Coleman (1989)

*If there is a nearby laboratory testing CSF amino acids (phenylalanine in particular), CSF monoamines and CSF endorphins, these tests should be considered since the child has to have a lumbar puncture anyway (to exclude progressive encephalitis/encephalopathy).

Developmental Language Scales (Reynell 1969) and the Peabody Picture Vocabulary Test (Dunn 1970) can be useful. A recently developed neuropsychological test battery, the NEPSY (Korkman *et al.* 1997) may prove worthwhile in the evaluation of childhood autism, but so far no systematic studies exist.

The WISC-R can be used only for children aged 6 years or over but is particularly useful in cases with moderate or high-functioning autism (those with IQ levels >50). The 'typical' profile is one in which Verbal scores are lower than Performance scores. Also, scores tend to be exceptionally low (relative to the child's other scores) for Picture Arrangement and Comprehension (tests which, to a considerable degree, require 'common sense' and the ability to reflect on other people's inner thoughts and to take account of context), and exceptionally high for Block Design (a test which does not require the child to take account of context other than that provided by the visible patterns on the cubes).

The Leiter is a nonverbal test that is easy to administer (for a skilled psychologist) even to nonspeaking children with autism. Many of the subtests of the Leiter reflect underlying abilities akin to those tested in the Block Design test of the WISC-R. Therefore, some children with autism will receive a high Leiter IQ even when overall IQ (verbal and nonverbal) is below normal.

Nevertheless, the Leiter has been shown to have relatively good correlation with other IQ tests in many cases of autism and is widely used in the field.

The Vineland Social Maturity Scale is not an ordinary test but rather a structured interview with the closest carer. The examiner comes up with a social quotient, which, in autism, fairly well indicates the intelligence level also. The Vineland scale is therefore especially useful in patients considered 'untestable'.

The Griffiths scale seems to be relatively useful in young children with autism (aged 2–7 years) for discriminating between those with IQ <50 and those >50 (Dahlgren Sandberg *et al.* 1993). For a more detailed evaluation, the Griffiths scale appears inadequate and usually has to be followed up with a WISC-R test during the early school years.

In making the diagnosis of autism, various questionnaires and other evaluation tools are available. Currently the two most used manuals are the CARS (Childhood Autism Rating Scale—Schopler *et al.* 1988) and the ABC (Autism Behavior Checklist—Krug *et al.* 1980). The CARS has good reliability and validity, at least in cases with clear-cut and obvious autism. The ABC comprises an interview containing 57 statements which can be used to elicit information about the child in about 30 minutes; it

TABLE 26.6
**Important components of management/treatment regimes in autism
and autistic-like conditions**

Early diagnosis
Specific treatments such as diets
Rehabilitation team well acquainted with basic problems of autism
Home-based treatment programme
Structured environment, including 'ritualizing' of everyday routines
Continuity as regards people, place and approach
Graded change
Physical exercise
Education focusing on activities of daily life and interest patterns which can
form the basis for future work
Pharmacotherapy
Psychotherapy
Long-term (lifetime) perspective

should not be used as the sole instrument for making a diagnosis of autism. The suggested cut-off point (above 67 for autism) leads to many false-negative cases (Nordin *et al.* 1998).

For the educational evaluation, which is an important part of the neuropsychological work-up, the PEP (Psycho-Educational Profile—Schopler *et al.* 1980) is useful. It provides a concise picture of the child's current educational status in a number of areas and forms the basis for goal-directed educational interventions in the individual case. The PEP is intended to be used at regular intervals in an educational treatment programme in order to promote and evaluate intervention effects.

TREATMENT, MANAGEMENT AND EDUCATION
There can be no clear dividing line between education, management and treatment in autism. A few cases can be rationally treated (*e.g.* by diet in phenylketonuric autism, and by neurosurgery in tuberous sclerosis–autism–epilepsy syndrome), others may be helped by way of classic treatment, such as pharmacotherapy or psychotherapy or both. However, in the majority of cases, such measures do not produce significant change. On the other hand, education and 'management', in a broad sense of that word, can lead to worthwhile improvements. The crucial elements in any management/treatment programme for autism (or autistic-like conditions) are outlined in Table 26.6.

SPECIFIC TREATMENTS (INCLUDING PREVENTION)
Diet-based treatments
Phenylketonuria, if untreated, can cause autism. If it is appropriately treated with a diet from the first few days of life, autistic symptoms never develop. In fact, one is here dealing with prevention rather than cure, since the autistic symptoms are never allowed to appear before treatment is started.

Other diet-based treatments are possible for autism. Coleman and Blass (1985) described lactic acidosis associated with autism and showed that in such cases dietary treatment could lead to disappearance of autistic symptoms.

Pharmacotherapy
Pharmacotherapy plays a minor, but important, role in the treatment of autism. No medication is available for which benefits outweigh side-effects in a majority of cases of autism. Nevertheless, some drugs, adequately tested in controlled studies, have positive effects in a sufficient number of cases to warrant recommendation for treatment trials if there is a clinically felt need for pharmacological intervention. This is sometimes the case when thorough educational measures have not led to expected gains; when overactivity, destructiveness and/or self-injurious behaviour cause such turmoil that other interventions cannot be used at all; or when adolescent aggravation of symptoms (see below) prevents developmental progress. Drugs should never be used as the sole kind of intervention but should always be accompanied by educational and psychosocial approaches. Anti-epileptic pharmacotherapy is quite often indicated in autism with epilepsy.

The nonspecific drugs most often used are vitamin B_6, neuroleptics and sedating drugs. Lithium, naltrexone and clomipramine may become alternatives in the near future but are still being investigated. In the treatment of epilepsy, carbamazepine and valproic acid are drugs of first choice in many cases.

Vitamin B_6 has been shown to have at least some positive effects in relatively well-designed studies (*e.g.* Lelord *et al.* 1981). It is given in doses of 300–900 mg/d, supplemented with magnesium in cases with severe nonspecific behaviour problems (including restlessness, aggressiveness, sleep problems and self-injurious behaviour).

Neuroleptics (particularly haloperidol and pimozide) have been examined in a number of double-blind placebo-controlled studies (see Campbell 1989). They seem to exert some positive effects on the basic problems associated with autism (social withdrawal, communication, learning and rigid behaviour patterns). However, it is difficult to recommend their use in the long term because of the high incidence of severe or moderate extrapyramidal side-effects (25–30 per cent in most series). Neuroleptics can be of some value in breaking up 'vicious circles', particularly in adolescent symptom aggravation.

Sedative drugs are not indicated for more than short-term use (days/weeks). They are most often considered in the treatment of sleep problems. They often have paradoxical effects, the child reacting with even more hyperactivity and difficulty settling down in the evening. Benzodiazepines usually have extremely negative effects on behaviour and cognition in autism (Gillberg 1991c) and should, if possible, be avoided.

In the treatment of epilepsy in autism, many drugs have detrimental side-effects on behaviour and learning (Gillberg 1991c). There are no well-controlled double-blind studies in the field, but a systematic survey of the literature and clinical experience suggest that valproic acid and carbamazepine may be less negative than other drugs with respect to behavioural side-effects. The side-effects of phenobarbitone (irritability, hyperactivity, aggressive outbursts and decreased learning) are well known, but the benzodiazepines (clonazepam in particular) are often even worse. It is not uncommon for a child with complex partial seizures to appear autistic while on clonazepam but nonautistic as soon as s/he is taken off the drug.

Folic acid has been tried in the treatment of autism associated with fragile X syndrome (in doses ranging from 0.5 to 1.5 mg/kg/d). The findings so far are equivocal, but there appears to be a mild stimulant effect which can be useful in alleviating some of the nonspecific symptoms such as concentration difficulties and hyperactivity.

Stimulant medication (methylphenidate and amphetamine in particular) has—by and large—been avoided in the treatment of autism. However, recently a new trend has emerged in this field, so that some mildly retarded children with autism who also have severe attention deficits are indeed treated with central stimulants, usually with few side-effects.

The new serotonin reuptake inhibitors (such as fluvoxamine, fluoxetine and sertraline) are currently being evaluated, and although some promising results have been reported, it is as yet too early to determine their possible role in the treatment of autism.

Lithium may be an adjunct in controlling mood swings (and perhaps aggressiveness) occurring particularly during the adolescent period. Serum concentration should be kept at the lowest possible level (0.4–0.7 mmol/L).

Naltrexone and other opiate blockers have recently been tried in autism after the report of associated endogenous opioid dysfunction (Gillberg 1995). Naltrexone seems to be a relatively safe drug and might become more used in future in autism, perhaps particularly if there is concomitant hyperactivity. Self-injurious behaviours in autism have been reported to be associated with particularly high levels of CSF endorphins (Gillberg *et al.* 1985), but evidence that naltrexone reduces self-injury is lacking.

Fenfluramine, an anorexogenic drug with serotonin-lowering properties, appears, despite early enthusiastic reports, to have little place in the treatment of most cases of autism (Gualtieri 1987). However, if autism is associated with severe attention deficits/hyperactivity, and treatment with stimulants has been unsuccessful, fenfluramine might be worth a trial.

For a good overview of drug treatment in autism, the reader is referred to Campbell (1989).

Non-drug medical/biological treatments
Physical exercise is effective in reducing major behaviour problems (self-injury, aggressiveness, hyperactivity and sleep problems) in autism (McGimsey and Favell 1988, Haracopos 1989) and should be used much more than is currently the case. Jogging programmes (two half-hour sessions a day for instance) can be very helpful.

Psychotherapy
In a wide sense of the word, there can be no treatment for autism without psychotherapeutic elements. However, classical analytically oriented psychotherapy for children with autism has never been shown to have lasting or even positive effects and should not be used, unless as part of a systematic research trial, since there have been reports of negative effects both on the child and on the family (Gillberg 1989). If analytically oriented techniques are employed by somebody very experienced who also knows about the basic disabilities involved in autism (Tustin 1981, Hobson 1990), it is possible that in some cases such therapy can have some positive effects. Certainly, some people with autism who have high-functioning verbal ability benefit from individual talks with somebody well acquainted with the various aspects of autism, from around the time of puberty, when many of them begin to realize the extent to which they differ from other people.

Family therapy usually has no place in autism. However, regular contact with the family and teaching the family to become the child's best advocate (see below) should be essential parts of any good treatment/management programme.

EARLY DIAGNOSIS
To give autism a name as soon as possible can have far-reaching positive consequences. An early diagnosis can mean (1) the discovery of treatable underlying conditions, (2) the identification of genetic disorders requiring genetic counselling, (3) getting the family out of a vicious circle including elements of self-blame, practical problems, loss of sleep and inappropriate behaviour management techniques, and (4) appropriate treatments and education for the child. Also, siblings can be better informed so that they may better understand the deviant child's strange behaviour (Bågenholm and Gillberg 1992).

HOME-BASED APPROACHES
Howlin and Rutter (1987) and Schopler (1989) have shown that home-based approaches to autism can have beneficial effects for both child and family. Parents should be regarded as co-therapists. All parents need to receive as much education as possible about autism, including symptoms, aetiology and available treatments. Seminars for groups of parents are often useful. The family should be informed about the existence of available autism support groups. An integrated education/behaviour modification programme for the child, including elements of 'graded change' (Howlin and Yates 1989), should be planned in collaboration with the parents. Activities of daily life (such as feeding, hygiene and sleeping) should be the focus of home-based interventions. 'Institutional handling' of problems in this field usually does not generalize to the home situation without proper training at home.

EDUCATION
For at least 200 years it has been recognized that education has particular merit in relation to autism. Education in autism is a vast and growing area (Schopler 1989), beyond the scope of this volume. However, some brief comments are warranted.

Children with autism need a structured environment with as much predictability as possible. Their own need to insist on routine and 'sameness' should be met by adults introducing useful routines that can be accepted by child and adult alike. Once routines have been established by adults, the child with autism is more likely to stop introducing new, bizarre routines, and even to abandon some of the old ones. Whereas normal children —and indeed most mentally retarded children without autism— learn 'automatically' as they seek new experiences and interact with other people, children with autism do not get anything for free and need to learn through training. Training needs to be planned, and this requires an evaluation tool. The PEP (see above) is a useful instrument for pinpointing individual skills and deficits in autism. The PEP can then also be used in the follow-up of management to document that the child has actually developed 'according to plan'.

Some principles of education in autism are essential. First, there is a need to individualize: in spite of similarities, people with autism are, first and foremost, individuals with different personalities, different IQs and different social backgrounds. Second, there is a need for structure and continuity in relation to time, place and teacher. In other words, the same thing should be trained at the same time in the same room by the same person. This style of structure might have to be applied with some rigour in the early stages of education, whereas the long-term goal is, wherever possible, to be able gradually to introduce a little more flexibility. Third, children with autism can usually harbour only one thought at a time, which means that instruction about several things cannot be given at once. Fourth, and interconnected with the third point, is their deficient sense of time in most cases. This should be met, for instance, by ensuring that one task is finished before the next task is introduced. Last, but not least, education has to take account of the fact that children with autism—even those labelled high-functioning—usually have extremely deficient comprehension of spoken language and poor understanding of abstract symbols, but often relatively good visual or visuospatial skills. Spoken language has to be reduced to a minimum in interactions with people with autism, and one must find ways of ensuring that they actually understand any communication used. Long sentences must be avoided in most cases, as must use of metaphorical language. Token and sign language can often be as difficult to cope with as spoken language. Instead, pictures containing photos of concrete situations which the child knows well are often very helpful.

Some of the higher functioning individuals with autism may need specific help in training mentalizing abilities (Ozonoff and Miller 1995, Howlin 1997).

Special education and treatment facilities for people with autism
There is a need for special preschools, special classrooms. special job facilities and services planning work, and special group homes for people with autism and autistic-like conditions. Such facilities are also needed for people with other kinds of social and communicative impairments, most of whom are likely to have some kind of minor or major intellectual impairment. For some children with autism the best option would be placement in a class specifically for children with autism, for others it would be better to attend a class for the communication-impaired with or without autism, while for some a class for the mentally retarded would be more suitable. Many children with autism do not need any special services, but they and their families might need the help of an expert autism team to guide them through childhood, adolescence and adult life.

The most important thing is that true options should exist for the child and family and that no extreme philosophy of segregation or integration should govern the kind of help and service that can be provided.

OUTCOME IN AUTISM
Most follow-up studies of autism agree that psychosocial outcome is variable but often quite poor. According to one recent survey of the literature (Gillberg 1991b), the mortality rate seems to be slightly increased. Almost 2 per cent of people with autism surviving the first two years of life die before age 25 years. Of those who survive much longer, about 60 per cent become totally dependent on other people for their everyday lives. Only a small number of these can hold even half-sheltered jobs. Another 25 per cent show considerable progress, but still remain dependent on other people for many things. About 10 per cent (recruited almost exclusively from the group with tested IQ >60 in childhood) function independently and hold ordinary jobs, but may still be perceived as somewhat odd in their style of social interaction. At most, about 5 per cent in different follow-up studies have been considered 'cured', or rather as having grown out of symptoms associated with autism.

About 10–20 per cent of all children with autism deteriorate in adolescence and, as it appears, never return to their preadolescent level of functioning. Another 30 per cent show symptom aggravation in adolescence. This aggravation may run a periodic course, but will usually become less of a problem by 25–30 years of age. The symptoms encountered in these pubertal change cases are often similar to those seen in the same child in the preschool period, *i.e.* overactivity, aggressiveness, self-injurious behaviour, sleep problems, incoherent language, and bladder and bowel incontinence. A trial of lithium can be indicated in some such cases (see above), and may occasionally be helpful. Epilepsy is sometimes the first sign that deterioration may follow, although some cases with the combination of epilepsy and symptom aggravation do not later develop deterioration. The reason for deterioration is not known (even though in some instances progressive neurological/neurometabolic disorders are suspected), and usually there is no treatment available. Neuroleptics are often tried but sometimes with little effect. Physical exercise frequently yields positive results.

There is also a subgroup of children with autism who deteriorate during the first few years of life (Rapin 1996). Although previously a matter of considerable debate, it is now clear that a relatively small group of children with classic autism symptoms have a period of deterioration around 16–24 months of age. Some of these are normal before deterioration, others show mild autism symptoms before the onset of regression. It is possible that this group constitutes a separate clinical entity or one which is more closely linked to childhood disintegrative disorder (see below) than to Kanner's variant of autism. Deterioration may be temporally linked with the appearance of seizure activity on EEG (or clinical seizures), but in many cases no such association is found.

In adulthood, three broad groups of people with autism can be discerned (Wing 1989): those who remain autistic in many respects; those who are passive and friendly; and those who appear active and odd. The second (passive) group quite often is not recognized as having autism unless a clear diagnosis of autism had been made in early childhood. The third group too is often not recognized as suffering from autism, but, because of the conspicuous problems they show (*e.g.* undressing or masturbating in public, touching other people in unexpected ways), they more often are brought to a psychiatrist who might be able to discern the original nature of the disorder.

The natural history in the individual case will also depend on the natural history of the particular associated medical condition (*e.g.* tuberous sclerosis, fragile X syndrome).

Finally, symptomatology in autism changes over the years, even in the subgroup that remains 'autistic'. Many clinicians are surprised when faced with a 10-year-old child given a diagnosis of autism at age 4 years. The child may no longer be gaze-avoidant (in fact s/he might never have been clearly gaze-avoidant, but perhaps only 'gaze-odd'), and may accept the company of other people and even try to interact with them in a number of different ways. In these circumstances it is common for clinicians to confront the parents with the self-assured remark, 'This child does not have autism', sometimes followed by, 'and I do not think s/he ever had autism!' Autism symptomatology is not a 'once and for all' thing.

ATYPICAL AUTISM/AUTISTIC-LIKE CONDITIONS

In clinical practice cases with most but not all of the symptoms typical of autism are not unusual. Also, some people with profound mental retardation show all the three clusters of symptoms considered necessary and sufficient to diagnose autism (Lorna Wing's triad, see above), but are difficult to classify as autism cases because it is difficult to decide whether the social, language and behavioural 'symptoms' are out of keeping with the degree of overall mental development. Finally, there is a group of children with deficits in attention, motor control and perception (see Chapter 27) who show varying degrees of social, communication and behavioural problems, but who do not fit the full clinical picture of autism or Asperger syndrome.

At present no adequate diagnostic category is available for all these cases. 'Pervasive developmental disorder not otherwise specified (including atypical autism)' is used for some of these cases by the DSM-IV. This term is often seriously misleading, particularly when one is dealing with children of normal intelligence. 'Autistic-like conditions' (Nordin and Gillberg 1996a) has been proposed by others to cover the group of 'autism-like' problems which do not fit readily into the classification systems. Some clinicians use the term 'autistic traits'.

Many children with so-called autistic traits fulfil currently accepted criteria for the full syndrome of autism but for some reason do not receive the correct diagnosis of autism. This appears to be particularly common in cases where obvious brain dysfunction has been diagnosed at an early stage in the development of the child's problems, for instance when there is hydrocephalus, infantile spasms, tuberous sclerosis or some other well-known neurological disorder.

The prevalence of autistic traits is possibly much higher than that of autism proper. Wing's studies of mentally retarded individuals under 15 years of age in London and my own studies in the general 7-year-old population in Göteborg suggest that at least 2–6 per 1000 children exhibit severe autistic traits.

Some children do not show overt evidence of autism until after age 3 years. These cases can be classified as 'autistic disorder' according to the DSM-III-R, but doubt remains whether they represent the same type of condition as autism with early onset. In some, a case can be made for diagnosing childhood disintegrative disorder (Heller dementia).

CHILDHOOD DISINTEGRATIVE DISORDER—HELLER DEMENTIA INFANTILIS

Heller (1930) described children who appeared to develop normally up until about the age of 2–4 years but who then dramatically regressed, became confused and hyperactive, and were left, months later, in a more or less aloof and demented state (Burd *et al.* 1989). Many of these children are clinically indistinguishable from those with autism once the regression period is over after 2–20 months. Others follow a gradually more downhill course. Some have neurodegenerative conditions, but less is known about the aetiology of childhood disintegrative disorder than about that of autism. Long-term outcome appears to be even worse than in autism.

ASPERGER SYNDROME

In 1944, the Austrian paediatrician Hans Asperger described what he considered to be an unusual personality variant in young children, most of whom were boys. He alluded to 'autistic psychopathy' but, after an influential paper by Wing (1981a), the particular combination of problems that Asperger described is now generally referred to as Asperger syndrome. Asperger syndrome is believed by many to be on a continuum with autism and autistic-like conditions, but it is not yet clear whether it represents autism in people of generally good intelligence or a specific cognitive profile involving at least some areas of superior functioning.

DIAGNOSIS
Diagnostic criteria have been proposed (Table 26.7) but have not yet been validated. These should not be taken to imply that Asperger syndrome is clearly distinct from autism (the criteria for Asperger syndrome obviously overlap with those for autism). The symptom criteria of the ICD-10 (WHO 1993) and DSM-IV (APA 1994) are virtually identical. These diagnostic manuals regard normal early language development and intellectual functioning and normal curiosity about the environment in the first three years of life as prerequisites for a diagnosis of Asperger's disorder/Asperger syndrome. However, Asperger himself included cases with abnormal language development and mild mental retardation in his series of cases. The DSM-IV and ICD-10 further

TABLE 26.7
Diagnostic criteria for Asperger syndrome/disorder

Asperger syndrome (Gillberg and Gillberg 1989)

1. Severe impairment in reciprocal social interaction (at least two of the following):
   - inability to interact with peers
   - lack of desire to interact with peers
   - lack of appreciation of social cues
   - socially and emotionally inappropriate
2. All-absorbing narrow interests (at least one of the following):
   - exclusion of other activities
   - repetitive adherence
   - more rote than meaning
3. Imposition of routines and interests (at least one of the following):
   - on self, in aspects of life
   - on others
4. Speech and language problems (at least three of the following):
   - delayed development
   - superficially perfect expressive language
   - formal, pedantic language
   - odd prosody, peculiar voice characteristics
   - impairment of comprehension including misinterpretations of literal/implied meanings
5. Nonverbal communication problems (at least one of the following):
   - limited use of gestures
   - clumsy/gauche body language
   - limited facial expression
   - inappropriate expression
   - peculiar, stiff gaze
6. Motor clumsiness, poor performance on neurodevelopmental examination

Asperger's disorder (ICD-10: WHO 1993)

A. There is no clinically significant general delay in spoken or receptive language or cognitive development. Diagnosis requires that single words should have developed by 2 years of age or earlier and that communicative phrases be used by 3 years of age or earlier. Self-help skills, adaptive behaviour, and curiosity about the environment during the first 3 years should be at a level consistent with normal intellectual development. However, motor milestones may be somewhat delayed and motor clumsiness is usual (although not a necessary diagnostic feature). Isolated special skills, often related to abnormal preoccupations, are common, but are not required for diagnosis
B. There are qualitative abnormalities in reciprocal social interaction (criteria as for autism)
C. The individual exhibits an unusually intense, circumscribed interest or restricted, repetitive, and stereotyped patterns of behaviour, interests, and activities (criteria as for autism; however, it would be less usual for these to include either motor mannerisms or preoccupations with part-objects or nonfunctional elements of play materials)
D. The disorder is not attributable to the other varieties of pervasive developmental disorder: simple schizophrenia; schizotypal disorder; obsessive–compulsive disorder; anancastic personality disorder; reactive and disinhibited attachment disorders of childhood

Asperger syndrome (DSM-IV: American Psychiatric Association 1994)

A. Qualitative impairment in social interaction, as manifested by at least two of the following:
   (1) marked impairment in the use of multiple nonverbal behaviours such as eye-to-eye gaze, facial expression, body postures, and gestures to regulate social interaction
   (2) failure to develop peer relationships appropriate to developmental level
   (3) a lack of spontaneous seeking to share enjoyment, interests, or achievements with other people (*e.g.* by lack of showing, bringing, or pointing out objects of interest to other people)
   (4) lack of social or emotional reciprocity
B. Restricted repetitive and stereotyped patterns of behaviour, interests, and activities, as manifested by at least one of the following:
   (1) encompassing preoccupation with one or more stereotyped and restricted patterns of interest that is abnormal either in intensity or focus
   (2) apparently inflexible adherence to specific, nonfunctional routines or rituals
   (3) stereotyped and repetitive motor mannerisms (*e.g.* hand or finger flapping or twisting, or complex whole-body movements)
   (4) persistent preoccupation with parts of objects
C. The disturbance causes clinically significant impairments in social, occupational or other important areas of functioning
D. There is no clinically significant general delay in language (*e.g.* single words used by age 2 years, communicative phrases used by age 3 years)
E. There is no clinically significant delay in cognitive development or in the development of age-appropriate self-help skills, adaptive behaviour (other than in social interaction), and curiosity about the environment in childhood
F. Criteria are not met for another specific pervasive developmental disorder or for schizophrenia

draw a distinct line between autistic disorder and Asperger's, and this is out of keeping with clinical experience suggesting that some individuals meet criteria for autistic disorder early on and later fit the clinical picture of Asperger syndrome much better (and vice versa).

The most distinctive feature of Asperger syndrome in very young children may be a decreased ability of subjects to conceptualize the mental states of other people, similar to that seen in autism. This inability is nowhere near as pronounced as in autism, and some reflection on other people's 'inner' needs can usually be prompted by reminding the subject of their existence, but the degree of empathy to be expected is generally low. A partial lack of a 'theory of mind' in Asperger syndrome has been supported by studies in experimental psychology (for a review, see Frith 1991). However, in later childhood most individuals with the syndrome pass simple theory of mind tests, but show clear deficits in executive functions.

Asperger syndrome is sometimes evident in the first year of life as a restricted interest in social interaction, but usually it is not until the second to fourth year that parents become concerned. Often there is worry about the apparent lack of need for playmates and the relatively late language development, often superseded by the development of formally impeccable, pedantic and prematurely adult-type language. Some cases do not attract attention until well into school age and then only because of extremely limited interests, motor clumsiness and lack of empathy. There is usually an odd prosody with a flat or staccato intonation or a shrill, monotonous quality. In certain cases there is an exceptional tendency to cluttering. Speech therapists often refer to the speech and language problems as 'semantic–pragmatic disorder' (Bishop 1989).

Because of their socially abnormal behaviour, peculiar, restricted interest patterns and unusual language characteristics, children with Asperger syndrome are variously perceived as odd, original, eccentric, 'the little professor', hilarious, cold, naive, lacking in common sense or immature. Some become the subject of teasing or bullying at school, but most manage fairly well in this respect, possibly as a result of their 'untouchability'.

Asperger syndrome is usually associated with normal or above-normal intelligence, but occasional typical cases in children with subnormal intelligence have been described. Associated impairments/medical conditions are much less common than in autism, but the available evidence suggests that the rate of epilepsy may be slightly higher than in the general population, and associated chromosomal abnormalities (*e.g.* fragile X, XYY) may not be altogether uncommon. Cases of Asperger syndrome in children with mild cerebral palsy have also been described (Gillberg 1989).

EPIDEMIOLOGY
Asperger syndrome is about 10 times more frequent in boys than in girls. It is possible that a similar core condition might be present in girls but with a slightly different phenotype.

The overall prevalence has been estimated to be at least 3 per 1000 children born (Ehlers and Gillberg 1993), but could be higher.

BACKGROUND FACTORS
Most cases are thought to be caused by genetic factors. In many instances there is a close relative with similar problems or sometimes clear-cut autism. Brain damage without a genetic predisposition can probably also cause Asperger syndrome (Wing 1981a). Perinatal brain insults, postnatal brain infections and congenital hypothyroidism have been reported as causing brain damage in children who later received a diagnosis of Asperger syndrome.

In a recent study (Happé *et al.* 1996), it appeared that portions of the left medial frontal lobe may be specifically dysfunctional in Asperger syndrome and that this impairment might underlie the difficulties individuals with the syndrome have when solving mentalizing tasks.

DIFFERENTIAL DIAGNOSIS
The distinction of Asperger syndrome from sociopathy, severe antisocial behaviour ('psychopathy'), borderline conditions and various types of manipulating personality disorders is based on the fact that because of their limitations in conceiving of other people's minds, Asperger subjects do not have a well-developed capacity for lying, luring or manipulating other people. 'Borderline conditions' (a dubious notion anyway) are supposed to be characterized by intense swings in relationships with other people (love–hate: 'cannot live with you, cannot live without you'). This is the opposite of Asperger syndrome, in which stability of relationship and behaviour over time is usually highly characteristic.

MEDICAL AND PSYCHOLOGICAL WORK-UP
The work-up in a child or adolescent suspected of having Asperger syndrome is similar to that in high-functioning autism (see above). A screen for visual and hearing problems should also be made in all cases. If there is academic failure, the WISC-R (with typically relatively lower results on Comprehension and Picture Arrangement) and a more exhaustive neuropsychological work-up might be appropriate.

TREATMENT
Specific treatment for Asperger syndrome is not available. The best approach is to make a proper diagnosis, to give oral and written information to those concerned, to offer educational and other measures intended to improve school adjustment, and to follow up (yearly if appropriate, more often if necessary). Attempts should be made to find areas of interest that might eventually provide a basis for a good education and adult hobbies, and to actively avoid areas that may hold potential danger (*e.g.* 'violent' sports). Medication makes little difference in most cases and may have harmful side-effects. The new serotonin reuptake inhibitors (*e.g.* sertraline and fluoxetine) may be effective in reducing ritualistic behaviours and may improve mood. Psychotherapy is usually not indicated, but supportive talks on a regular basis with somebody knowledgeable in the field can be helpful, particularly in the teenage period when some insight into the situation is often gained and the experience of being different from one's peers can become overwhelming. For younger children

with Asperger syndrome, group sessions can also be of value (Mesibov and Stephens 1990).

Parents often ask about the genetic risk for themselves, for the affected child and for his/her siblings. There is a risk that more cases of Asperger syndrome will occur in the family (Bowman 1988). At least half of all children with Asperger syndrome have a parent with the same (or very similar) condition. This should be acknowledged truthfully, while at the same time emphasizing the relatively benign character of the problems. However, the possibility that Asperger syndrome might be genetically linked to classic autism makes counselling in this respect somewhat difficult. Recent estimates for siblings are not available. In a study of 23 children with Asperger syndrome (Gillberg 1989), one boy had a brother with autism (and another brother with mild Asperger syndrome) and one girl had a sister with elective mutism (and Asperger traits).

Adult psychiatrists need to be aware of the existence of Asperger syndrome. In stressful situations, young adults with the syndrome are often referred to psychiatrists because of obsessiveness, feelings of helplessness and chaotic reactions. Because of limited facial expression, mimicry and gestures they may be diagnosed as depressed or paranoid and accordingly treated with antidepressants or neuroleptic drugs which usually do little to alter the cause of the disorder. Quite often, stress relief combined with the appreciation that this is only part of a life-long condition will go a long way in reducing acute symptoms.

OUTCOME

Only a fraction of all children with Asperger syndrome apply for paediatric or psychiatric help specifically as a consequence of their 'Asperger problems'. Therefore, follow-up of cases seen in clinics will not necessarily yield a true picture of outcome. So far, the only studies of outcome available refer either to such populations or to groups assessed in adult psychiatric clinics and diagnosed retrospectively as possibly having suffered from Asperger syndrome from early childhood (Tantam 1988). The overall impression is that many children with Asperger syndrome diagnosed in childhood, although not outgrowing the basic problems, manage fairly well in adult life, at least with respect to education, employment and marriage. Equally obvious, however, is the tendency for some to have severe psychiatric problems (often diagnosed as depression, paranoia, pseudoneurotic schizophrenia or 'borderline'), to attempt suicide or develop alcoholism (Wing 1981a), and for others to commit criminal offences (usually directly associated with one or other extreme interest, *e.g.* gunpowder, poisonous chemicals, fire) (Baron-Cohen 1988, Everall and Le Couteur 1990, Scragg and Shah 1994).

ELECTIVE MUTISM

Some children do not speak to more than a very limited number of people from early childhood, throughout the early school years and often into adolescence and adult life. It is not that they cannot speak, indeed some of them can be verbally demanding and talkative when in their home environment. They do, however, refuse to say a word to most people outside of the immediate family (perhaps excluding even one or more members of the family). A few have one or two friends with whom they will communicate verbally. Some are mute most of the time but will occasionally give up their complete silence to whisper a few words. This group of children who can speak but who do so only with a very limited number of people are referred to as having '(s)elective mutism' (Kolvin and Fundudis 1981). Many 'shy' children are temporarily silent on entering preschool or school. If their silence is of a transient nature, they should not be considered for a diagnosis of elective mutism.

The child with elective mutism probably can have normal language development but often shows delay and deviance; there are frequently minor associated developmental disorders such as enuresis and slight motor delay; it appears that there may be a markedly increased rate of epilepsy; IQ tends to be lower than in the general population of children; typical symptoms usually appear before the child's fourth birthday; there is often a family history of psychiatric disorder, 'shyness' and elective mutism; and the outcome is variable but probably restricted, although it may be excellent in individual cases. Many features of elective mutism are similar to those encountered in relatively high-functioning autistic-like conditions.

Children with elective mutism are usually shy, avoidant and sometimes clearly withdrawn. Also, many are described as being strong-willed and have outbursts of rage if demands or changes of routine are made. A recent report has mentioned the association of elective mutism and Asperger straits (see above).

Elective mutism is rare, occurring in severe forms (with a duration of more than one year) in 0.6–2 in 1000 children (Kolvin and Fundudis 1981, Kopp and Gillberg 1997). The boy/girl ratio appears to be equal, or with a slight preponderance in females.

The psychological and medical work-up should include a cognitive test and a thorough clinical examination aimed at detecting hearing deficits and symptoms and signs suggestive of autistic disorder. The possibility of associated medical conditions should be entertained. I know of two cases with the combination of elective mutism and neurofibromatosis.

Treatment in elective mutism has to focus on training of basic social skills and activities of daily life, to enable the child/ adolescent to accept the company of others and to express—at least in writing—her/his academic skills. Psychotherapeutic or psychopharmacological approaches have not been successful according to clinical experience.

CHILDHOOD SCHIZOPHRENIA

Autism and autistic-like conditions were long considered synonymous with childhood schizophrenia. Since about 1970, however, childhood schizophrenia has been regarded as a clearly separate condition, implying a severe disorder of affect and thought, showing before 10 years of age with typical schizophrenic thought disorder, hallucinations and emotional bluntness. It appears to be very rare, maybe occurring in no more than 2–3 per 100,000 children. Some authors have even questioned the existence of typical schizophrenia in early childhood. In recent years, however, US authors have reintroduced the term when referring to early-onset conditions on the autism spectrum (*e.g.* Asarnow *et al.* 1988). Others regard it as a more distinct syndrome with symptom onset at any age between 5 and 12 years (Caplan *et al.* 1989, Werry *et al.* 1991, Murray 1994, Remschmidt *et al.* 1994). The male:female ratio in this very early onset variant of schizophrenia is reported to be in the range of 2–3:1. From the age of 13 years and up, authors in the USA and elsewhere agree that schizophrenia is more common and that the male:female ratio is closer to equality as seen in adulthood (Harris 1995a,b).

Neuroleptics are likely to be more effective than in autism, and outcome is supposedly better. However, no good population-based follow-up studies exist, and the matter cannot be regarded as settled.

REFERENCES

Åkefeldt, A., Gillberg, C. (1991) 'Hypomelanosis of Ito in three cases with autism and autistic-like conditions.' *Developmental Medicine and Child Neurology*, **33**, 737–743.

Akinsola, H.A., Fryers, T. (1986) 'A comparison of patterns of disability in severely mentally handicapped children of different ethnic origins.' *Psychological Medicine*, **16**, 127–133.

American Psychiatric Association (1980) *Diagnostic and Statistical Manual of Mental Disorders, 3rd Edn (DSM-III)*. Washington, DC: APA.

—— (1987) *Diagnostic and Statistical Manual of Mental Disorders, 3rd Edn—Revised (DSM-III-R)*. Washington, DC: APA.

—— (1994) *Diagnostic and Statistical Manual of Mental Disorders, 4th Edn (DSM-IV)*. Washington, DC: APA.

Arvidsson, T., Danielsson, B., Forssberg, P., *et al.* (1997) 'Autism in 3–6-year-old children in a suburb of Göteborg, Sweden.' *Autism*, **1**, 163–173.

Asarnow, J.W., Goldstein, M.J., Ben-Meir, S. (1988) 'Parental communication deviance in childhood onset schizophrenia spectrum and depressive disorders.' *Journal of Child Psychology and Psychiatry*, **29**, 825–838.

Asperger, H. (1944) 'Die autistischen Psychopathen im Kindesalter.' *Archiv für Psychiatrie und Nervenkrankheiten*, **117**, 76–136.

Bågenholm, A., Gillberg, C. (1992) 'Autism och mental retardation. Vid hjälp till familjer med svårt handikappade barn bör syskonrelationer beaktas mer än idag.' *Läkartidningen*, **89**, 555–560.

Baron-Cohen, S. (1988) 'An assessment of violence in a young man with Asperger's syndrome.' *Journal of Child Psychology and Psychiatry*, **29**, 351–360.

Barthélémy, C., Bruneau, N., Cottet-Eymard, J.M., *et al.* (1988) 'Urinary free and conjugated catecholamines and metabolites in autistic children.' *Journal of Autism and Developmental Disorders*, **18**, 583–591.

Bender, L. (1947) 'Childhood schizophrenia. Clinical study of one hundred schizophrenic children.' *American Journal of Orthopsychiatry*, **17**, 40–56.

Bishop, D.V.M. (1989) 'Autism, Asperger's syndrome and semantic–pragmatic disorders. Where are the boundaries?' *British Journal of Disorders of Communication*, **24**, 107–121.

Bleuler, E. (1911) *Dementia Praecox or the Group of Schizophrenias*. Vienna: F. Deuticke. (Translated by J. Zinkin, 1950. New York: International Universities Press.)

Bolton, P., Rutter, M. (1990) 'Genetic influences in autism.' *International Review of Psychiatry*, **2**, 67–80.

—— Macdonald, H., Pickles, A., *et al.* (1994) 'A case–control family history study of autism.' *Journal of Child Psychology and Psychiatry*, **35**, 877–900.

Bowman, E.P. (1988) 'Asperger's syndrome and autism: the case for a connection.' *British Journal of Psychiatry*, **152**, 377–382.

Bryson, S.E., Clark, B.S., Smith, I.M. (1988) 'First report of a Canadian epidemiological study of autistic syndromes.' *Journal of Child Psychology and Psychiatry*, **29**, 433–445.

Burd, L., Fisher, W., Kerbeshian, J. (1989) 'Pervasive disintegrative disorder: are Rett syndrome and Heller dementia infantilis subtypes?' *Developmental Medicine and Child Neurology*, **31**, 609–616.

Campbell, M. (1989) 'Pharmacotherapy in autism: an overview.' *In:* Gillberg, C. (Ed.) *Diagnosis and Treatment of Autism*. New York: Plenum, pp. 203–218.

Caplan, R., Guthrie, D., Fish, B., *et al.* (1989) 'The Kiddie Formal Thought Disorder Rating Scale: clinical assessment, reliability, and validity.' *Journal of the American Academy of Child and Adolescent Psychiatry*, **28**, 408–416.

Chess, S., Korn, S.J., Fernandez, P.B. (1971) *Psychiatric Disorders of Children with Congenital Rubella*. New York: Brunner/Mazel.

Coleman, M., Blass, J.P. (1985) 'Autism and lactic acidosis.' *Journal of Autism and Developmental Disorders*, **15**, 1–8.

Cook, E.H. (1990) 'Autism: review of neurochemical investigation.' *Synapse*, **6**, 292–308.

Dahlgren Sandberg, A., Nydén, A., Gillberg, C., Hjelmquist, E. (1993) 'The cognitive profile in infantile autism—a study of 70 children and adolescents using the Griffiths Mental Development Scale.' *British Journal of Psychology*, **84**, 365–373.

Denckla, M.B. (1986) 'New diagnostic criteria for autism and related behavioural disorders—guidelines for research protocols.' *Journal of the American Academy of Child and Adolescent Psychiatry*, **25**, 221–224. *(Editorial.)*

Dissanayake, C., Crossley, S.A. (1996) 'Proximity and sociable behaviours in autism: evidence for attachment.' *Journal of Child Psychology and Psychiatry*, **37**, 149–156.

Doll, E.A. (1965) *Vineland Social Maturity Scale*. Circle Pines, MN: American Guidance Service.

Dunn, L.M. (1970) *Peabody Picture Vocabulary Test*. Circle Pines, MN: American Guidance Service.

Ehlers, S., Gillberg, C. (1993) 'The epidemiology of Asperger syndrome. A total population study.' *Journal of Child Psychology and Psychiatry*, **34**, 1327–1350.

Everall, I.P., LeCouteur, A. (1990) 'Firesetting in an adolescent boy with Asperger's syndrome.' *British Journal of Psychiatry*, **157**, 284–287.

Folstein, S., Rutter, M. (1977) 'Infantile autism: a genetic study of 21 twin pairs.' *Journal of Child Psychology and Psychiatry*, **18**, 297–321.

Friedman, E. (1969) 'The autistic syndrome and phenylketonuria.' *Schizophrenia*, **1**, 249–261.

Frith, U. (1989) *Autism: Explaining the Enigma*. Oxford: Basil Blackwell.

—— (Ed.) (1991) *Autism and Asperger Syndrome*. Cambridge: Cambridge University Press.

Gillberg, C. (1986) 'Onset at age 14 of a typical autistic syndrome. A case report of a girl with herpes simplex encephalitis.' *Journal of Autism and Developmental Disorders*, **16**, 369–375.

—— (1989) 'Asperger syndrome in 23 Swedish children.' *Developmental Medicine and Child Neurology*, **31**, 520–531.

—— (1991a) 'Clinical and neurobiological aspects of Asperger syndrome in six family studies.' *In:* Frith, U. (Ed.) *Autism and Asperger Syndrome*. Cambridge: Cambridge University Press, pp. 122–146.

—— (1991b) 'Outcome in autism and autistic-like conditions.' *Journal of the American Academy of Child and Adolescent Psychiatry*, **30**, 375–382.

—— (1991c) 'The treatment of epilepsy in autism.' *Journal of Autism and Developmental Disorders*, **21**, 61–77.

—— (1995) 'Endogenous opioids and opiate antagonists in autism: brief review of empirical findings and implications for clinicians.' *Developmental Medicine and Child Neurology*, **37**, 239–245.

—— Coleman, M. (1992) *The Biology of the Autistic Syndromes, 2nd Edn. Clinics in Developmental Medicine No. 126*. London: Mac Keith Press.

—— —— (1996) 'Autism and medical disorders: a review of the literature.' *Developmental Medicine and Child Neurology*, **38**, 191–202.

—— Forsell, C. (1984) 'Childhood psychosis and neurofibromatosis—more than a coincidence?' *Journal of Autism and Developmental Disorders*, **14**, 1–8.

—— Gillberg, I.C. (1983) 'Infantile autism: a total population study of reduced optimality in the pre-, peri-, and neonatal period.' *Journal of Autism and Developmental Disorders*, **13**, 153–166.

—— —— (1991) 'Note on the relationship between population-based and clinical studies: the question of reduced optimality in autism.' *Journal of Autism and Developmental Disorders*, **21**, 251–254. *(Letter.)*

—— Schaumann, H. (1983) 'Epilepsy presenting as infantile autism? Two case studies.' *Neuropediatrics*, **14**, 206–212.

—— Steffenburg, S. (1987) 'Outcome and prognostic factors in infantile autism and similar conditions: a population-based study of 46 cases followed through puberty.' *Journal of Autism and Developmental Disorders*, **17**, 273–287.

—— Svennerholm, L. (1987) 'CSF-monoamines in autistic syndromes and other pervasive developmental disorders of early childhood.' *British Journal of Psychiatry*, **151**, 89–94.

—— Winnergård, I., Wahlström, J. (1984) 'The sex chromosomes—one key to autism? An XYY case of infantile autism.' *Applied Research in Mental Retardation*, **5**, 353–360.

—— Terenius, L., Lönnerholm, G. (1985) 'Endorphin activity in childhood psychosis. Spinal fluid levels in 24 cases.' *Archives of General Psychiatry*, **42**, 780–783.

—— Steffenburg, S., Jakobsson, G. (1987) 'Neurobiological findings in 20 relatively gifted children with Kanner-type autism or Asperger syndrome.' *Developmental Medicine and Child Neurology*, **29**, 641–649.

—— —— Schaumann, H. (1991a) 'Is autism more common now than 10 years ago?' *British Journal of Psychiatry*, **158**, 403–409.

—— Steffenburg, S., Wahlström, J., *et al.* (1991b) 'Autism associated with marker chromosome.' *Journal of the American Academy of Child and Adolescent Psychiatry*, **30**, 489–494.

—— Gillberg, I.C., Steffenburg, S. (1992) 'Siblings and parents of children with autism: a controlled population-based study.' *Developmental Medicine and Child Neurology*, **34**, 389–398.

Gillberg, I.C., Gillberg, C. (1989) 'Asperger syndrome—some epidemiological considerations: a research note.' *Journal of Child Psychology and Psychiatry*, **30**, 631–638.

Griffiths, R.G. (1970) *The Abilities of Young Children. A Comprehensive System of Mental Measurement for the First Eight Years of Life.* High Wycombe, Bucks: The Test Agency.

Gualtieri, C.T. (1987) 'Reappraisal of "Fenfluramine and autism: careful reappraisal is in order." Reply.' *Journal of Pediatrics*, **110**, 159–160. *(Letter.)*

Hagerman, R.J. (1989) 'Chromosomes, genes and autism.' *In:* Gillberg, C. (Ed.) *Diagnosis and Treatment of Autism.* New York: Plenum Press, pp. 105–132.

Happé, F.G.E. (1994) 'Current psychological theories of autism: the "theory of mind" account and rival theories.' *Journal of Child Psychology and Psychiatry*, **35**, 215–229.

—— Ehlers, S., Fletcher, P., *et al.* (1996) '"Theory of mind" in the brain. Evidence from a PET scan study of Asperger syndrome.' *NeuroReport*, **8**, 197–201.

Haracopos, D. (1989) 'Comprehensive treatment program for autistic children and adults in Denmark.' *In:* Gillberg, C. (Ed.) *Diagnosis and Treatment of Autism.* New York: Plenum Press, pp. 251–261.

Harris, J.C. (1995a) *Developmental Neuropsychiatry. I. The Fundamentals.* Oxford: Oxford University Press.

—— (1995b) *Developmental Neuropsychiatry. II. Assessment, Diagnosis and Treatment of Developmental Disorders.* Oxford: Oxford University Press.

Haslam, J. (1809) *Observations on Madness and Melancholy.* London: Hayden.

Heller, T. (1930) 'Über Dementia infantilis.' *Zeitschrift für Kinderforschung*, **37**, 661–667.

Hertzig, M.E., Snow, M.E., New, E., Shapiro, T. (1990) 'DSM-III and DSM-III-R diagnosis of autism and pervasive developmental disorder in nursery school children.' *Journal of the American Academy of Child and Adolescent Psychiatry*, **29**, 123–126.

Hobson, R.P. (1990) 'On psychoanalytic approaches to autism.' *American Journal of Orthopsychiatry*, **60**, 324–336.

—— (1993) *Autism and the Development of Mind.* London: Lawrence Erlbaum.

Howlin, P. (1997) 'Prognosis in autism: do specialist treatments affect long-term outcome?' *European Child and Adolescent Psychiatry*, **6**, 55–72.

—— Rutter, M. (1987) *Treatment of Autistic Children. Wiley Series on Studies in Child Psychiatry.* London: John Wiley.

—— Yates, P. (1989) 'Treating autistic children at home. A London based programme.' *In:* Gillberg, C. (Ed.) *Diagnosis and Treatment of Autism.* New York: Plenum, pp. 307–322.

Hunt, A., Dennis, J. (1987) 'Psychiatric disorder among children with tuberous sclerosis.' *Developmental Medicine and Child Neurology*, **29**, 190–198.

Jacobsson, L., Broberger, U., Fernell, E., *et al.* (1998) 'Children with blindness due to retinopathy of prematurity: a population-based study. I. Perinatal data, ophthalmological aspects and neurological outcome.' *Developmental Medicine and Child Neurology. (In press.)*

Kanner, L. (1943) 'Autistic disturbances of affective contact.' *Nervous Child*, **2**, 217–250.

Kerbeshian, J., Burd, L., Randall, T., *et al.* (1990) 'Autism, profound mental retardation and atypical bipolar disorder in a 33-year-old female with a deletion of 15q12.' *Journal of Mental Deficiency Research*, **34**, 205–210.

Kolvin, I., Fundudis, T. (1981) 'Elective mute children: psychological development and background factors.' *Journal of Child Psychology and Psychiatry*, **22**, 219–232.

Komoto, J., Udsui, S., Otsuki, S., Terao, A. (1984) 'Infantile autism and Duchenne muscular dystrophy.' *Journal of Autism and Developmental Disorders*, **14**, 191–195.

Kopp, S., Gillberg, C. (1997) 'Selective mutism: a population-based study: a research note.' *Journal of Child Psychology and Psychiatry*, **38**, 257–262.

Korkman, M., Kirk, V., Kemp, S.L. (1997) *A Developmental Neuropsychological Assessment.* San Antonio, TX: The Psychological Corporation.

Krug, D.A., Arick, J., Almond, P. (1980) 'Behavior checklist for identifying severely handicapped individuals with high levels of autistic behavior.' *Journal of Child Psychology and Psychiatry*, **21**, 221–229.

Leiter, R.G. (1980) *Leiter International Performance Scale: Instruction Manual.* Chicago: Stoelting.

Lelord, G., Muh, J.P., Barthélémy, C., *et al.* (1981) 'Effects of pyridoxine and magnesium on autistic symptoms—initial observations.' *Journal of Autism and Developmental Disorders*, **11**, 219–230.

Mahler, M.S. (1952) 'On child psychoses and schizophrenia: autistic and symbiotic infantile psychoses.' *Psychoanalytic Study of the Child*, 7, 286–305.

Malson, L. (Ed.) (1964) *Les Enfants Sauvages—Mythe et Realité.* Paris: Union Generale d'Editions.

McGimsey, J.F., Favell, J.E. (1988) 'The effects of increased physical exercise on disruptive behavior in retarded persons.' *Journal of Autism and Developmental Disorders*, **18**, 167–169.

Mesibov, G.B., Stephens, J. (1990) 'Perception of popularity among a group of high-functioning adults with autism.' *Journal of Autism and Developmental Disorders*, **20**, 33–43.

Murray, R.M. (1994) 'Neurodevelopmental schizophrenia: the rediscovery of dementia praecox.' *British Journal of Psychiatry*, **25** (Suppl.), 6–12.

Nordin, V., Gillberg, C. (1996a) 'Autism spectrum disorders in children with physical or mental disability or both. Part I: Clinical and epidemiological aspects.' *Developmental Medicine and Child Neurology*, **38**, 297–313.

—— —— (1996b) 'Autism spectrum disorders in children with physical or mental disability or both. II: Screening aspects.' *Developmental Medicine and Child Neurology*, **38**, 314–324.

—— Lekman, A., Johansson, M., *et al.* (1998) 'Gangliosides in cerebrospinal fluid in children with autism spectrum disorders.' *Developmental Medicine and Child Neurology. (In press.)*

Ornitz, E.M., Guthrie, D., Farley, A.J. (1977) 'The early development of autistic children.' *Journal of Autism and Childhood Schizophrenia*, 7, 207–229.

Ozonoff, S., Miller, J.N. (1995) 'Teaching theory of mind. A new approach to social skills training for individuals with autism.' *Journal of Autism and Developmental Disorders*, **25**, 415–433.

Rank, B. (1949) 'Adaptation of the psycho-analytic technique for the treatment of young children with atypical development.' *American Journal of Orthopsychiatry*, **19**, 130–139.

Rapin, I. (Ed.) (1996) *Preschool Children with Inadequate Communication. Developmental Language Disorder, Autism, Low IQ. Clinics in Developmental Medicine No. 139.* London: Mac Keith Press.

Remschmidt, H.E., Schulz, E., Martin, M., *et al.* (1994) 'Childhood-onset schizophrenia: history of the concept and recent studies.' *Schizophrenia Bulletin*, **20**, 727–745.

Reynell, J. (1969) *Reynell Developmental Language Scales.* Windsor, Berks: NFER.

Rutter, M. (1978a) 'Diagnosis and definition.' *In:* Rutter, M., Schopler, E. (Eds.) *Autism. A Reappraisal of Concepts and Treatment.* New York: Plenum Press, pp. 1–25.

—— (1978b) 'Diagnosis and definition of childhood autism.' *Journal of Autism and Childhood Schizophrenia*, **8**, 139–161.

Schopler, E. (1989) 'Principles for directing both educational treatment and research.' *In:* Gillberg, C. (Ed.) *Diagnosis and Treatment of Autism.* New York: Plenum Press, pp. 167–183.

—— Reichler, R.J., DeVellis, R.F., Daly, K. (1980) 'Towards objective classification of childhood autism: Childhood Autism Rating Scale (CARS).' *Journal of Autism and Developmental Disorders*, **10**, 91–103.

—— —— Renner, B.R. (1988) *The Childhood Autism Rating Scale (CARS). Revised.* Los Angeles: Western Psychological Services.

Scragg, P., Shah, A. (1994) 'Prevalence of Asperger's syndrome in a secure hospital.' *British Journal of Psychiatry*, **165**, 679–682.

Sigman, M., Mundy, P. (1989) 'Social attachments in autistic children.' *Journal of the American Academy of Child and Adolescent Psychiatry*, **28**, 74–81.

Ssucharewa, G.E. (1926) 'Die schizoiden Psychopathien im Kindesalter.' *Monatsschrift für Psychiatrie und Neurologie*, **60**, 235–261.

Steffenburg, S. (1990) 'Neurobiological correlates of autism.' MD thesis, University of Göteborg.

—— (1991) 'Neuropsychiatric assessment of children with autism: a population-based study.' *Developmental Medicine and Child Neurology*, **33**, 495–511.

—— Gillberg, C., Steffenburg, U., Kyllerman, M. (1996) 'Autism in Angelman syndrome. A population-based study.' *Pediatric Neurology*, **14**, 131–136.

Stubbs, E.G. (1978) 'Autistic symptoms in a child with congenital cytomegalovirus infection.' *Journal of Autism and Childhood Schizophrenia*, **8**, 37–43.

Tantam, D. (1988) 'Asperger's syndrome.' *Journal of Child Psychology and Psychiatry*, **29**, 245–255.

Tinbergen, N., Tinbergen, E.A. (1983) *Autistic Children. New Hope for a Cure.* London: Allen & Unwin.

Tsai, L.Y. (1989) 'Recent neurobiological findings in autism.' *In:* Gillberg, C. (Ed.) *Diagnosis and Treatment of Autism.* New York: Plenum Press, pp. 83–104.

Tustin, F. (1981) *Autistic State in Children.* London: Routledge & Kegan Paul.

von Knorring, A-L. (1991) 'Outcome in autism.' *Svensk Medicin*, **23**, 34–36.

Wechsler, D. (1974) *Manual of the Wechsler Intelligence Scale for Children—Revised.* New York: Psychological Corporation.

Werry, J.S., McClellan, J.M., Chard, L. (1991) 'Childhood and adolescent schizophrenic, bipolar, and schizoaffective disorders: a clinical and outcome study.' *Journal of the American Academy of Child and Adolescent Psychiatry*, **30**, 457–465.

Wing, L. (1981a) 'Asperger's syndrome: a clinical account.' *Psychological Medicine*, **11**, 115–129.

—— (1981b) 'Sex ratios in early childhood autism and related conditions.' *Psychiatry Research*, **5**, 129–137.

—— (1989) 'Autistic adults.' *In:* Gillberg, C. (Ed.) *Diagnosis and Treatment of Autism.* New York: Plenum Press, pp. 419–432.

—— (1993) 'The definition and prevalence of autism: a review.' *European Child and Adolescent Psychiatry*, **2**, 61–74.

—— Gould, J. (1979) 'Severe impairments of social interaction and associated abnormalities in children: epidemiology and classification.' *Journal of Autism and Developmental Disorders*, **9**, 11–29.

WHO (1993) *The ICD-10 Classification of Mental and Behavioural Disorders. Clinical Descriptions and Guidelines.* Geneva: World Health Organization.

27
ATTENTION DEFICITS AND SPECIFIC LEARNING DISORDERS

Over the past 60 years, a number of behavioural and learning disorders have been lumped together under the uninformative label of 'minimal brain dysfunction' (MBD). The roots of this unfortunate diagnostic etiquette are to be found at the beginning of this century, when, on the basis of studies of children with encephalitis, it was surmised that a characteristic syndrome of overactivity often developed as a consequence of brain damage sustained *in utero* or in early childhood. Reciprocally, the notion gradually emerged that overactivity was in itself a sign that the child was brain-damaged. Subsequent empirical study has shown that (a) overactivity is not *usually* a sign of brain damage, and (b) brain damage does not usually lead to overactivity (Rutter 1982).

SYNONYMS

A comprehensive survey of all the many synonyms and partly overlapping concepts used in this field is beyond the scope of this book. However, a list of some of the most common diagnostic labels (Table 27.1) is appropriate, as an introduction to a description of the symptom profiles encountered in children who have been given the (often inappropriate) label of MBD over the last 30 years.

The array of labels testifies to the confusion in this field. Unfortunately, it does not appear that it is yet time for consensus. In North America, inflectional versions of the attention deficit disorder/attention deficit–hyperactivity disorder spectrum are mostly used. In the British Isles, the 'hyperkinetic disorders' and 'clumsy child' concepts seem to be more popular. In Scandinavia and Central Europe yet other concepts are emerging.

Not in the table, but certainly on the map of confusion in the field, is the concept of dyslexia and 'specific developmental disorders' which show considerable overlap with all the previously named 'syndromes'. Reading and writing difficulties and developmental motor coordination disorders are almost part and parcel of many of the so-called MBD syndromes. Dyslexia is also problematic in itself, in that most currently used definitions are conceptually unsound.

Further complication stems from the fact that many other neuropsychiatric syndromes (*e.g.* autism, many of the mental retardation syndromes and Tourette syndrome) often comprise elements of the MBD disorders. At present, the most common practice seems to be to diagnose only one syndrome. For instance, if a boy of 10 years suffers from the combination of multiple motor and vocal tics, pervasive attention deficit problems and dyslexia, it is quite common to diagnose only Tourette syndrome, although a case could be made for diagnosing attention deficit–hyperactivity disorder and dyslexia as well. This should become less of a problem once it becomes generally accepted that 'comorbidity' is common in child neuropsychiatry.

ATTENTION DEFICIT–HYPERACTIVITY DISORDER

DEFINITION
Some children show a persistent pattern of inattention, often associated with hyperactivity and impulsivity, from the first years of life. The terms 'attention deficit disorder' (ADD) (American Psychiatric Association 1980) and 'attention deficit–hyperactivity disorder' (ADHD) (American Psychiatric Association 1994) to cover this group of problems have been widely accepted in North America, and criteria for diagnosis have become increasingly operationalized. In the latest version of the DSM, three subtypes of AD-HD are recognized: (1) mainly inattentive, (2) mainly hyperactive–impulsive, and (3) mixed, plus a residual category of ADHD not otherwise specified (Table 27.1).

EPIDEMIOLOGY
ADHD occurs at a rate of 3–9 per cent of all school-age children (Landgren *et al.* 1996). It is several times more common in boys than in girls. IQ tends to be skewed downwards, even though the majority of children receiving this diagnosis are of normal intelligence.

THE VALIDITY OF THE ADHD CONCEPT
ADHD is valid from the behavioural point of view, although there is considerable symptom overlap with 'conduct disorder' and 'oppositional defiant disorder' (ODD) (Gillberg 1995). It tends to signal a poor psychosocial outcome (Hechtman 1996), but it is possible that prognosis is better predicted by some of the often associated problems (such as specific learning disorders and conduct problems) rather than by the attention deficit symptoms *per se* (Hellgren *et al.* 1994). This is one of the major reasons why

TABLE 27.1
Syndromes attributed to so-called 'minimal brain dysfunction' (MBD): synonyms and partly overlapping concepts

Diagnostic label	Comments
MBD (minimal brain dysfunction)	Once referred to as minimal brain *damage* (before *c.*1960). Almost universally used until *c.*1980. Still in *clinical* use in many countries. Usually refers to various combinations of attention and motor/learning problems. Inappropriate in that it infers brain dysfunction on phenotypical grounds and in its use of the word 'minimal'
ADD (attention deficit disorder)	DSM-III label (American Psychiatric Association 1980). Widespread use in USA. Semantically confusing (should be either 'deficit' or 'disorder'). Diagnostic criteria very loose and subjective. Pervasiveness not required. With or without motor/learning problems
ADHD (attention deficit–hyperactivity disorder)	DSM-III-R label (American Psychiatric Association 1987). Does not account for cases without clear hyperactivity. If categorized as 'severe', then pervasiveness required. With or without motor/learning problems
DAMP (deficits in attention, motor control and perception)	Accepted term in Nordic countries. Umbrella term to cover the various combinations of motor control, perceptual and attentional problems encountered in children without mental retardation or cerebral palsy
Hyperkinetic syndrome/disorder	Mostly used in the UK. Usually refers to a syndrome of pervasive hyperactivity. In the past, this diagnosis was often made only if there were no major associated conduct problems. The syndrome was then regarded as exceedingly rare. As used in the late 1980s, it has become obvious that it is not quite so rare, that conduct disorders often coincide, and that motor/speech/learning problems are the rule
MND (minor neurological dysfunction)	Sometimes used to describe summary score for minimal motor/neurological problems or 'soft neurological signs'
MCD (minimal cerebral dysfunction)	Rarely used. Refers mostly to overriding concept of cerebral dysfunction rather than to any specific clinical syndrome
Clumsy child syndrome	UK concept. Highlights only one aspect of what is usually a multifaceted syndrome
Motor/perceptual impairment	Common Scandinavian concept. Attention problems are common in this group
Organic brain syndrome	Central European concept. Highlights certain behavioural features, but essentially similar to MBD
OBD (organic brain dysfunction)	Used particularly by groups who stress the importance of neonatal reflexes in the genesis of learning and attention problems

the term DAMP ('deficits in attention, motor control and perception') has come to be the preferred diagnostic label in the Scandinavian countries. Children with DAMP also meet many, indeed often full, criteria for ADHD. The clinical profile and background factors in ADHD will therefore be presented in the following section on DAMP.

HYPERKINETIC DISORDERS

DEFINITION
The term hyperkinetic disorder has gradually come to refer to a constellation of childhood symptoms that closely resemble those described under the ADHD label. However, only 30 years ago it was usually thought of as a rare 'disorder' characterized by extremes of hyperactivity. The definition of hyperkinetic disorders in the ICD-10 (WHO 1993a,b) is very similar to that of ADHD in the DSM-IV.

EPIDEMIOLOGY
In the Isle of Wight population study in the 1960s, the 'pure' hyperkinetic syndrome was encountered in less than 1 in 2000

10- to 11-year-olds without 'neuroepileptic' disorders who attended normal schools (Rutter *et al.* 1970). In marked contrast, 7 per cent of all children with neuroepileptic disorders and children excluded from school because of severe mental subnormality were considered to suffer from a hyperkinetic syndrome.

THE VALIDITY OF THE HYPERKINESIS CONCEPT
The notion that hyperkinesis is extremely uncommon has lingered in Europe, despite the fact that reports from the USA have described 4–15 or even 30 per cent of all schoolchildren as hyperactive/hyperkinetic (see Wender 1971). It was not until the early 1980s, when a reanalysis of the Isle of Wight material (Schachar *et al.* 1981) revealed that about 2 per cent of the population showed hyperactive behaviour both at home and at school, that it became accepted that hyperactivity—even pervasive forms—is a common problem in school-age children. Up until then, European children tended to be diagnosed as hyperactive/ hyperkinetic only if this was their only (or at least main) problem. It is now becoming more common to make dual and triple diagnoses in child psychiatry. As a consequence, rates of hyperkinetic syndromes reported from Europe and the USA are no longer so

discrepant. Nevertheless, there is still some difference, which is difficult to account for. The most recent British study (Taylor *et al.* 1991) yielded a prevalence of 1.7 per cent for 'hyperkinetic disorder' among 6- to 7-year-old boys in London. No similar recent study from the USA is available for comparison; however, this prevalence is very similar to that for 7-year-old boys with severe DAMP in Göteborg (2.1 per cent).

The concept of hyperactivity has become linked with that of attention deficit. It is not clear, however, whether attention deficit underlies hyperactivity in the majority of cases: recent findings suggest that it may not (Taylor *et al.* 1991). Attention deficits are quite often associated with normoactive behaviour, hypoactivity and fluctuating degrees of activity. It is possible that in the next 10 years pervasive hyperkinesis may emerge as a distinct clinical entity. However, it does not appear to be the umbrella term needed to cover all disorders involving deficits in attention, motor control and perception (DAMP).

Stimulant treatment (see below) is often recommended for the hyperkinetic syndromes. Such treatment should be reserved for very specific cases with severe DAMP who also meet other criteria, and should never be seen as the sole solution to the 'problem of hyperactivity in childhood'.

DEFICITS IN ATTENTION, MOTOR CONTROL AND PERCEPTION (DAMP)

DEFINITION

Surveying the literature on MBD it became apparent that the problems inferred were perceptual, motor and attention deficits in various combinations in children without mental retardation or cerebral palsy. The concept of DAMP was therefore launched in the mid-1980s to cover most of the syndromes previously referred to as 'MBD' but without any implicit aetiological meaning (Gillberg *et al.* 1989). This label has now been accepted in the Nordic countries (Airaksinen *et al.* 1990). Diagnostic criteria have been proposed by Landgren *et al.* (1996) and are shown in Table 27.2. In brief, DAMP is defined as the combination of pervasive attention deficit and motor coordination/perception dysfunction in any child of normal or low-normal intelligence who does not meet criteria for cerebral palsy.

According to a recent Swedish study (Landgren *et al.* 1996), about three-quarters of 6- and 7-year-old children diagnosed as suffering from DAMP also meet many criteria for ADHD, even though only about one in four have the full DSM-III-R syndrome of ADHD (with eight or more of a possible 14 symptoms). However, it has been argued (Barkley 1990) that the threshold for diagnosing ADHD according to the DSM-III-R (and the DSM-IV) might be too high: with a slightly lower level, the majority of children with DAMP would also be diagnosed as having ADHD (Fig. 27.1).

Attention deficits have to be present in several observational settings such as at home, in school and in the peer group. Reliable rating scales are available. The most used is that of Conners (1969), which exists in 39-item and 10-item versions designed for use either by parents or by teachers. The minimum require-

TABLE 27.2
Diagnostic criteria for DAMP*

A. ADD (attention deficit disorder) as manifested by:
  (a) severe problems in at least one or moderate problems in at least two of the following areas: attention span, activity level, vigilance and ability to sit still; and
  (b) cross-situational problems in the areas mentioned under (a), documented at two or more of the following: psychiatric, neurological, psychological evaluation and maternal report
B. MPD (motor perception dysfunction) as manifested by marked
  (a) gross motor dysfunction according to detailed neurological examination (see Gillberg *et al.* 1983a), or
  (b) fine motor dysfunction according to detailed neurological examination (see Rasmussen *et al.* 1983), or
  (c) perceptual dysfunction according to testing with the Block Design and Object Assembly subtests of the WISC-R (a discrepancy of 15 IQ points or more on any of these, relative overall IQ) (Wechsler 1974) or visuomotor dyscoordination test outlined in Rasmussen *et al.* (1983)
C. Problems not accounted for or associated with mental retardation or cerebral palsy

*From Landgren *et al.* (1996).

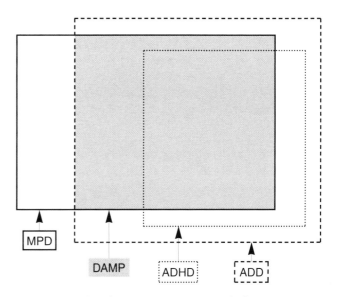

Fig. 27.1. Overlap of MPD (motor perception dysfunction), DAMP (deficits in attention, motor control and perception), ADHD (attention deficit–hyperactivity disorder) and ADD (attention deficit disorder).

ment for diagnosing attention deficit is that the child is rated as abnormal on a rating scale of this kind by at least two independent observers (*e.g.* parent and teacher). Not all children with attention deficit are hyperactive. Some are rather hypoactive, and many fluctuate between hyper- and hypoactivity. Many are best described as disorganized in their activity. This is one of the reasons why the hyperactivity label is inadequate. The DSM-IV acknowledges three different types of attention disorders: one with predominantly attentional problems, one with predominant problems in the field of impulsivity–hyperactivity, and one combined type.

The motor coordination problems are usually best described as immature performance on various neurological/motor tests

845

such as diadochokinesis, finger tapping, alternating movements, standing and skipping on one leg, walking on the lateral sides of the feet, and various fine motor performance tests such as tracing in a maze, cutting out paper, etc. These problems are evident in everyday settings as overall clumsiness, poor table manners, difficulties in dressing and tying shoe-laces, and difficulties learning to draw, write, ride a bicycle, swim, ski and skate. Many such children are poor at games, particularly ball games, and especially if such games involve small balls. The Touwen manual for examination of the child with minor neurological dysfunction (Touwen 1979) is helpful to the clinician wanting to acquire the skills necessary to perform an age-appropriate neuromotor evaluation in this field. A number of other such manuals are available (Denckla 1985, Whitmore and Bax 1986, Gillberg 1987, Michelsson and Ylinen 1989).

The perceptual problems appear on formal tests—such as the Performance part of the WISC-R (Block Design, Picture Completion and Object Assembly are often problematic) and the Southern California Sensory Integration Tests (Ayres 1974)—and on specific tests of perception that may vary from one country to another. There are often perceptual problems in several domains (visual, auditory, tactile, etc.), but most tests focus on visual–perceptual tasks and it is sometimes difficult to determine whether one is dealing with a pure visual–perceptual problem, a fine motor problem, a dysfunction of eye–hand coordination or a combination of these. Perceptual problems often show in impaired perception of form, space and shape, in drawing and writing immaturities, and in severe problems in acquiring automatic reading skills. Disturbance of body image is also a common consequence of various perceptual difficulties.

Attentional problems are often reflected in poor results on the Coding and Digit Span subtests of the WISC-R. As the child grows older the Information and Arithmetic subtests may yield gradually poorer results. In some cases this can be seen as a reflection of the gradually more important DAMP-associated problem of dyslexia, which leads to a relative decline in skills for which good reading is essential.

Children with DAMP often show various types of speech and language difficulties, some of which may be a consequence of motor problems or reflect auditory perceptual problems, while others are related to some basic and specific language deficit.

DAMP can be subdivided into *severe cases*, showing all five of (1) attention, (2) gross motor, (3) fine motor, (4) perceptual and (5) speech/language dysfunction, and *mild cases* showing some but not all of these dysfunctions.

An adequate working diagnosis in severe cases (*i.e.* a formulation in diagnostic terms which can serve as a basis for intervention suggestions) requires the collaboration of the paediatrician (or a child psychiatrist), a clinical neuropsychologist and, optimally, a speech therapist, all of whom should make independent evaluations and then combine their data. In mild cases, the paediatrician (or school doctor) will have to do most of the diagnostic work alone, considering the high prevalence of the disorder and the lack of diagnostic resources.

EPIDEMIOLOGY
DAMP in severe form is present in about 1.2 per cent of all 7-year-old children, and mild variants are present in another 3–6 per cent according to various Nordic studies. Social class and IQ are generally a little lower in DAMP subjects than in the general population, but children with DAMP come from all social classes and some have very high IQs.

BACKGROUND FACTORS
According to Swedish studies, DAMP is 'idiopathic' in about 10 per cent of cases, mainly hereditary in slightly more than one-third of cases, mainly due to pre-, peri- or postnatal brain damage in slightly less than one-third of cases, and in the remaining 20 per cent of cases is caused by a combination of hereditary and potentially brain-damaging factors (Gillberg and Rasmussen 1982). Some of the variance attributed to brain damage could be due to hereditary factors (Chapter 25). Findings from a twin study of hyperactivity (Stevenson *et al.* 1987) are compatible with a model for the development of DAMP in which hereditary factors are of dominating importance.

CLINICAL PICTURE AND COURSE
The diagnosis of DAMP requires the presence of both attention and motor/perception dysfunction. According to two Swedish studies (Gillberg *et al.* 1989, Landgren *et al.* 1996) there are about as many children with attention problems only as there are children with DAMP, who, in turn, are about twice as prevalent as those with motor/perception dysfunction only. Follow-up studies suggest that children with the combination of problems require treatment and interventions of various kinds but that outcome in the other two groups, in broad terms, is often relatively good. The identification of 'pervasively hyperkinetic' (as opposed to 'situationally hyperkinetic') children (Sandberg *et al.* 1978) has revealed that motor/perception and speech/language problems are almost universal in this group. This argues for the clinical separation of a diagnostic category with the combination of attention and motor/perception dysfunctions from groups with only one of the two types of dysfunction.

Situational attention deficit or hyperactivity can be a sign of psychological problems specific to a particular situation. Follow-up at age 13 years of children who had situational as compared to pervasive hyperkinesis at age 6–7 years (Gillberg and Gillberg 1988) has shown that outcome is much better in the former group and not very different to that of children without attention deficits of any kind.

Isolated motor/perception difficulties sometimes cause considerable academic problems, particularly during the early school years. Nevertheless, limited systematic follow-up and clinical experience suggest that, in this group also, outcome is usually considerably better than for those with the combination of attention problems and motor/perception difficulties (Hellgren *et al.* 1994).

In the following, reference will often be made to the longitudinal study of more than 100 children with DAMP (and comparison children without DAMP) examined from early childhood through age 20 years in the city of Göteborg, Sweden

TABLE 27.3
Children with DAMP: outcome from age 7 to 16 years*

Area of dysfunction	% of children with dysfunction			
	7 yrs	10 yrs	13 yrs	16 yrs
Attention	100	55	49	40
Motor control	100	55	30	25
Perception/reading–writing	69	76	67	55
Psychiatric/behavioural	69	81	64	55
DAMP problem requiring specialist treatment	40	50	52	70
Accidents requiring hospital treatment	12	—	24	—

*Gillberg (1987) and unpublished results.

(*e.g.* Gillberg 1987), though the considerable data bank that exists in neighbouring fields (*e.g.* Taylor 1986, Barkley 1990, Taylor *et al.* 1991) is also taken into consideration.

THE INFANTILE PERIOD
Retrospective analysis of case histories of children suffering from DAMP at age 4–6 years provides important clues to the clinical picture of DAMP in infancy. It seems that there may be at least two clinically distinct subgroups with respect to infant development: (1) the hyperactive group; and (2) the hypo- or normoactive group.

Infants in the hyperactive group usually show sleep problems, feeding difficulties, 'colicky' stomach pains and a generally high level of motor activity even from the first months of life. They often start walking before 10 months of age. From that time on (and sometimes even before), parents often have to change their domestic habits dramatically: anything moveable will have to be removed, not only from the level of the child's reach, but completely out of sight.

Children in the hypoactive/normoactive group were often thought to have low IQ. These infants are regarded by parents as 'good' (*i.e.* well-behaved), sometimes even 'exceptionally good'. Some of them show repetitive behaviours from a very early age (head rolling, even head banging, and repetitive sounds).

THE PRESCHOOL YEARS
From about the age of starting to walk, the two subgroups, for a number of years, often appear to be indistinguishable from each other. Children of both groups appear hyperactive, or at least inattentive. Parents may worry because their child does not seem to listen, shouting being the only way of attracting their attention. Motor coordination problems may surface already around age 2–4 years, but are often obscured by the high activity level and lack of appropriate fear, which is also very common. Speech is delayed in about two-thirds of cases, but only in about half of these is the delay severe enough to warrant consultation. Toward the end of the preschool years the child's 'unwillingness' to draw and paint, and the constant clashes in games with age-peers, become a major source of concern and of increasing scolding.

THE EARLY SCHOOL YEARS
Some children with DAMP can manage fairly well through

infancy and the preschool years but their behavioural and academic performance almost invariably deteriorates during the first few years at school. They have difficulties in concentrating, sitting still and listening, problems with impulse control, and major difficulties interacting in an age-appropriate fashion with peers. They may find it very problematic to participate in physical education and games, and sometimes they have almost insurmountable difficulties acquiring basic automatic reading and writing skills. All these problems peak around age 7–10 years in the vast majority of DAMP cases and cause emotional upset in the child, parents and teachers. Problems will be especially difficult to cope with if the diagnosis and its implications are not explained to those involved with the child (see below).

At age 6 years, children with DAMP, by definition, will have motor control problems and pervasive attention deficits. Around age 10 years, only about half of these children will have persistent obvious motor difficulties, and attentional problems will also have subsided to a considerable degree. Unfortunately, however, the prevalence of psychiatric/behavioural problems will have increased from just over 60 to 80 per cent, and dyslexia/dysgraphia will also be present in 80 per cent of cases (Table 27.3). In age-peers without DAMP, such problems will be found at a very much lower level.

PREADOLESCENCE AND ADOLESCENCE
Many preadolescent and adolescent children with DAMP experience persistent difficulties in concentrating. Some are described by their teachers or parents as daydreaming. Dyslexia is a very common complaint. The motor clumsiness is often less conspicuous than it used to be. There is a considerable risk for various types of psychiatric problems. If a child with DAMP attends a clinic for the first time in the teenage years, the psychiatric disorder is often seen as primary and a 'new' problem, not specifically associated with DAMP. The child's problems then run the risk of not being put into perspective, and suggestions for intervention might be inappropriate.

COMORBID PSYCHIATRIC PROBLEMS IN DAMP AND ADHD
There are four main groups of comorbid psychiatric problems in DAMP/ADHD: (1) depression; (2) conduct and oppositional defiant disorders; (3) tics and Tourette syndrome; (4) autistic traits.

Depression and feelings of low self-esteem are already common during the early school years but appear to peak around age 10 years, when they frequently coincide with various kinds of behaviour problems. The child with DAMP often becomes increasingly aware of her/his 'otherness' during the school years. Feeling that 'there is nobody to help', the child often becomes depressed and even contemplates suicide (which is uncommon in groups without DAMP). In the midst of depression there is also often much anger and resentment that may show outwardly as some kind of behaviour disorder. The child's predicament may be mistaken for 'antisocial problems with an outlook to psychopathy'. Personal interview with the child will soon reveal, however, that this is (usually) not a hardened criminal-to-be, but rather an immature and sad child who needs to have certain basic learning problems recognized.

The behaviour problems encountered in DAMP can be of any kind: a general oppositional defiant attitude to adults, stealing, firesetting, lying, bullying, running away from home, or drug/alcohol abuse. In the preschool years there is often aggression towards other children in connection with inadvertent disruption of play and games. About 10 per cent of children with DAMP already show severe conduct problems on school entry. This figure increases to about 50 per cent around age 10 years, but seems to decline to around 30 per cent during the teenage years.

Children with DAMP often have tics and some meet full criteria for Tourette syndrome. The association of DAMP and Tourette syndrome appears to be stronger if looked at from the perspective of the tic disorder: about half of all children with Tourette syndrome have major attention problems. It is not uncommon for children and adolescents with Tourette syndrome to have an early childhood history compatible with a diagnosis of DAMP or ADHD.

At least half of all children with severe DAMP show autistic traits. These comprise motor stereotypies, preoccupations with certain topics, objects or parts of objects, peculiarities of language (pronoun reversal, repetitive questioning and immaturities of grammar) and similar, but milder, social interaction problems as in autism. Occasionally, the differentiation of severe DAMP from Asperger syndrome may be very difficult. Children with mild DAMP usually do not exhibit autistic-type features.

TREATMENT

No single treatment is applicable for a group of disorders as heterogeneous as DAMP.

A recent study of a representative group of children receiving various kinds of intervention at age 6–7 years (Gillberg *et al.* 1993) suggested a positive effect of making the diagnosis and informing child, parents and teachers. Outcome in the three-year perspective for school adjustment and achievement and for behaviour both at school and at home was much better than for children who had not received information about the diagnosis.

The most important part of any treatment plan for a child with DAMP is the physical, psychiatric and neuromotor/neuropsychological examination, followed by oral and written information to parents, child, siblings and teachers, about the type of problems the child exhibits and their possible aetiology. This usually takes away much of the feeling of self-blame which has been strongly felt by both parents and children. Secondary behavioural/emotional problems tend to be minimized if information is given in this way.

Many children with DAMP need special educational measures. Most need individualized (*i.e.* one-on-one) education for some hours every day in order to be able to acquire new academic skills. A minority need special physical education or the help of a physiotherapist. Most importantly, the physical education teacher has to be informed about the child's disability, so that s/he will not treat the child as one who is simply badly behaved.

A limited number of children with DAMP/ADHD should be tried on stimulants (Taylor 1986). Both D-amphetamine (10–40 mg/d given in two to three doses with three-hour intervals in order to last through the school day) and methylphenidate (40–200 mg/d given in the same fashion) have been shown to be effective in the amelioration of hyperactivity, concentration difficulties, some learning problems, feelings of low self-esteem and family interaction problems. Both drugs have also been shown to be relatively free of major side-effects. Relatively common side-effects are loss of appetite, a tendency to increase the likelihood of tics (questioned by many and seen by some authorities to be the 'unmasking' of Tourette syndrome rather than a side-effect provoked in a child not genetically liable to tics) and stereotypies, reduced mimicry, and hallucination—all of which cease promptly upon drug discontinuation. A recent placebo-controlled long-term study (over a period of 15 months) demonstrated remaining beneficial effects of amphetamine throughout the study period (Gillberg *et al.* 1997). Ultimate height may be decreased by 1 cm if the treatment is continued throughout puberty. The risk for increasing doses and developing drug dependence and abuse appears to be nonexistent. Side-effects are much less pronounced than with the commonly used tricyclic antidepressants. The risk of provoking epileptic seizures is small. Nevertheless, prescribing stimulants to children is a delicate matter. Therefore, and also because the possible long-term benefits of using stimulants have been poorly examined, stimulant treatment should be selected only for children with very severe DAMP problems and no major psychosocial problems. Stimulants should never be given as the only mode of treatment. Stimulants may also be a helpful adjunct in the treatment of attention deficit problems and autism spectrum problems. Contrary to old notions in the field, children on the autism spectrum who have mild mental retardation and severe ADHD often benefit from stimulant treatment. Side-effects appear to be mild in most such cases.

Various motor training programmes have not been documented to have a lasting effect on the overall clinical problems associated with DAMP. For most children with DAMP, the motor coordination problems are those with the best prognosis, even without treatment. Therefore, it seems unwise to focus too much energy on this domain. In the long term (see below), problems associated with reading and writing are the most handicapping, and every effort should therefore be made in this field.

LONG-TERM OUTCOME

Many people who had DAMP in childhood and adolescence have overcome most or all of the severe problems by early adult life. However, about half have severe persisting problems. Criminal activity (*e.g.* arson, poisoning and bizarre violent behaviour—motivated by curiosity rather than malevolence) seems to be common, as do major psychiatric problems requiring in- or outpatient psychiatric treatment. Even among the many who outwardly appear to be doing relatively well, low self-esteem is common. Severe dyslexia, quite uncommon in adulthood in those who never had DAMP, is possibly present in 30–50 per cent of cases. Even though the motor control problems appear to have the best prognosis of all, a substantial minority (probably about one in five) continue to have important problems with motor clumsiness well into adulthood.

DYSLEXIA, DYSGRAPHIA AND DYSCALCULIA

Dyslexia constitutes one of the most challenging problems in child neuropsychiatry in that it is an invisible disabling condition with possible consequences for the emotional well-being of the individual affected. Dyslexia is often referred to as 'reading disorder' (the DSM-IV terminology).

At least 5–10 per cent of a school-age population of children are affected by dyslexia/dysgraphia. The figures are likely to be somewhat (though not much) lower in the adult population. The male:female ratio is similar to that in most neuropsychiatric disorders of childhood, at around 2:1 to 4:1 in different studies. However, there is a clear possibility that the male:female ratio in dyslexia *per se* may not be as high as suggested by clinical studies. In studies of children with 'pure' dyslexia, *i.e.* reading disorder without comorbidity, girls have been reported to have problems at least as often as boys. Boys tend to have much more associated disruptive behaviour problems, and it may be these, not the reading disorder, that get them referred to clinical specialists (Sanson *et al.* 1996).

Dyslexia and dysgraphia are often collectively referred to as dyslexia, which is quite inadequate, considering that spelling and other writing problems do not necessarily overlap with reading problems and vice versa. The twin study of Stevenson *et al.* (1987) suggests that spelling problems may have a considerably stronger genetic load than reading backwardness, which would support the separation of these two problems. Nevertheless, the two are usually treated as one, and it is indeed very common for the two to occur together. Dyscalculia is less frequently associated with dyslexia. Dyscalculia and dyslexia often seem to reflect separate conditions. One study demonstrated the strong correlation of DAMP problems with dyscalculia but not with dyslexia (Rosenberg 1989).

Dyslexia (and dysgraphia) often develop during the school years in children with DAMP. Extrapolating the results of the Göteborg studies, it would appear that almost half of all children with severe dyslexia have a DAMP background. The majority of children still showing severe dyslexic/dysgraphic problems in the

early teenage years had been diagnosed in the preschool period to have DAMP. Clinical experience indicates that the true number of children with dyslexia/dysgraphia/dyscalculia who also have attention/motor/perception problems may be even greater, and that it is uncommon for a child to have isolated dyslexia/dysgraphia/dyscalculia without associated attention/motor or major behaviour problems (Sanson *et al.* 1996).

Dyslexia is often defined as a reading level two years below grade (or below the level expected on the basis of IQ results). It is extraordinary that this illogical definition has managed to survive almost uncriticized. It goes without saying that being two years behind at age 7 is very different (minus 29 per cent) from being two years behind at age 13 (minus 15 per cent) years. The only sound way of defining dyslexia would be on the basis of some sort of quotient conceptually similar to that used in defining overall intelligence. Another important diagnostic issue is whether to relate the reading problems to full scale IQ or to performance IQ only. It is self-evident that if verbal IQ measures are included, the determining overall IQ level for a child with dyslexia is likely to be lower than if only nonverbal subtests are included.

Dyslexia has a tendency to become chronic. Even though with appropriate remediation there is usually a gradual amelioration of some of the most severe reading and writing problems, many dyslexic children become slow readers and poor spellers in adult life. In a review of the best follow-up studies in the field, Schonaut and Satz (1983) concluded that outcome in dyslexia is variable but poor with respect to reading skills and psychosocial adjustment. However, it is still open to debate whether it is the dyslexia, the often associated behaviour problems or both that tend to predict poor psychosocial adjustment. There is some evidence that reading disorder without behaviour problems or DAMP has a relatively good outcome (Sanson *et al.* 1996), at least as regards psychosocial adjustment.

Most recent authors in the field regard dyslexia as a biological/developmental problem. Nevertheless, a number of studies have demonstrated a relationship between dyslexia on the one hand and low socioeconomic status and being later-born in a large sibship on the other. These associations most likely reflect both genetic and environmental influences (Rutter and Madge 1976). Dyslexia, like DAMP, tends to cluster in families, and this has been taken as evidence for a genetic model. However, some of this familial tendency could be accounted for by social factors (Stevenson *et al.* 1984) such as low availability of books and low interest in reading in the parents and siblings. There is growing evidence for a quantitative trait locus for dyslexia on chromosome 6p21.3 (Cardon *et al.* 1994). Recent studies (of brain autopsies and magnetic resonance *in vivo* imaging) have suggested that abnormalities of corticogenesis in the planum temporale of the brain might be specifically associated with dyslexia (Galaburda *et al.* 1987, Hynd *et al.* 1990).

Various approaches to the remediation of dyslexia and dysgraphia, and to a lesser extent dyscalculia, have been suggested. An almost unbelievable array of claims regarding the efficacy of various programmes has been made, but the fact remains that in order to achieve better reading and writing skills, reading and writing have to be trained. Several studies have demonstrated that if parents of preschool children can be encouraged to listen to their children reading on a regular basis, this has some preventive effect on the development of reading problems.

Increasing the speed of reading nonsense phonemes also appears to increase reading skills. Computer-based reading and spelling programmes are valuable aids for some children with dyslexia/dysgraphia. Computers have the added advantage of allowing the dysgraphic child to have as 'beautiful' a written output (on the screen or on the print-out) as the child without dysgraphia. Also, computers do not take offence (as teachers and parents can) when the child makes mistakes, which makes 'interactions' less emotionally stressful.

The interest in pharmacological approaches to the treatment of dyslexia has recently increased with the advent of studies of piracetam (derived from GABA) in children with dyslexia (Wilsher 1986). Even before, limited benefits of stimulant medication (in combination with reading remediation) had been reported (Gittelman *et al.* 1983), but the effects appeared to be more on attention problems than on reading. Piracetam seems to have a modest, positive effect on reading skills in many children with dyslexia, regardless of associated attention problems. The drug is well tolerated in most cases. So far, in many countries, piracetam has not been registered for the treatment of dyslexia, but it appears to hold promise and may eventually come to be included as an adjunct in management of severe dyslexia.

Hyperlexia, superficially the opposite of dyslexia, is a condition in which single-word reading occurs in the absence of intensive instruction in children. The recognition of written words is much better than would be expected in view of a child's age and general intellectual level. However, there is usually a pervasive deficit in semantics and pragmatics. In normal reading acquisition it appears that the semantic system is more developed than the decoding system; in hyperlexia, the opposite appears to be the case. Reading appears to be mechanical and perfect without a corresponding level of comprehension. Hyperlexia is relatively common in high-functioning autism and Asperger syndrome, and may occur in moderately mentally retarded individuals

SPEECH AND LANGUAGE DISORDERS

Disorders of speech and language are part of all severe DAMP syndromes and are very common generally in children with perceptual/motor/attention deficits. In fact, delayed language development and other disorders of speech are among the most common early signs that the child might be at risk for the development of neuropsychiatric or psychological problems (Richman 1985). There is also a very strong correlation between speech/language problems in early childhood and dyslexia/dysgraphia in school-age. Thus, the trajectory is often one of DAMP showing in early life as language delay (with or without significant behaviour problems), later as abnormalities of speech production, motor clumsiness and attention problems, and in school-age as behaviour problems, dyslexia and other learning problems.

Abnormalities of speech and language development are very common in the age range of 3–6 years, the prevalence varying as a consequence of the definition used. Boys, again, are much more frequently affected than girls. However, it is difficult to say whether this reflects higher rates of pathology in boys than in girls, or whether our standards for normal language development tend to be based on the norm for girls (or girls and boys combined).

This presentation will briefly survey a few problem areas, namely developmental language delay (isolated), stuttering, abnormalities of pitch, semantic–pragmatic disorder and Landau–Kleffner syndrome.

DEVELOPMENTAL LANGUAGE DISORDER
Developmental language disorder is often treated as a separate diagnostic category (or rather, two different categories: (i) expressive language disorder, and (ii) receptive language disorder, also referred to as mixed receptive/expressive disorder), clearly different from autistic-like conditions, DAMP and behaviour problems. It is said to occur in about 1 in 2000 children and to affect expressive more than receptive language. However, the available evidence runs counter to this notion of an isolated syndrome of specific expressive language delay. Almost all studies which have included behavioural/psychiatric measures have shown that there is a very strong correlation between 'isolated' language delay and all sorts of rather severe behavioural problems, including autistic traits, elective mutism and aggression (Cantwell and Baker 1985). Also, the receptive language problems of children diagnosed as suffering from expressive delay have often been sadly neglected. Finally, the language delay is usually associated with other developmental delays and DAMP problems as well.

STUTTERING
Stuttering consists of outbursts of repetitions of consonants and word-blocking. It usually starts around 3–4 years of age. Most children show some degree of sound/word production reminiscent of stuttering, but only about 3 per cent (4 per cent of boys and 2 per cent of girls) have problems which take a clinical dimension (Barker 1979, Graham 1986). The course is often chronic, even though the problems for most affected children tend to diminish with age. Stuttering is thought to be genetic in origin. It is not specifically associated with psychiatric problems, either in the individual or in the family, but, in severe forms, it does lead to great anxiety and distress.

Stuttering is managed differently from one clinic to another. Most children who stutter do not need any kind of treatment other than encouragement to ignore it as far as possible. Parents and siblings need to be informed of the devastating emotional effects than can come from being teased mercilessly for many years. In severe cases it is often helpful to advise the child to tell other people about the stuttering before they have started to tease or otherwise react negatively.

Various psychological techniques (including biofeedback) have been used, but their effectiveness has yet to be demonstrated.

Occasionally, Tourette syndrome can present as stuttering. The diagnosis will be evident if gradually more severe motor and vocal tics emerge. However, one must keep in mind the possibility that someone who stutters and wants to control the stuttering can develop facial movements that can be misinterpreted as grimaces or tics.

ABNORMALITIES OF PITCH

The reason for including a special section on abnormalities of pitch is that they are a very common symptom in child neuropsychiatry and one that is usually overlooked. Abnormalities of pitch do not constitute a special subclass of disorders, but may be a pointer to other syndromes.

Inability to adjust the tone or volume of voice to varying circumstances is typical of many children with DAMP, autism. autistic-like conditions (including Asperger syndrome) and semantic–pragmatic disorder (see below). Many children with DAMP have a monotonous, loud voice, which can cause considerable irritation at the dinner table or in classroom settings. Verbal children with autism and those with Asperger syndrome almost invariably exhibit abnormalities of pitch, such as exaggerated shrillness, half-whispering huskiness, etc., usually in the context of monotonous speech production.

Some of these abnormalities may reflect motor coordination problems in the larynx, whereas others are possibly caused by auditory feedback difficulties leading to problems in timing adjustment of voice level to the prevailing situation. In still other cases, more fundamental deficits in understanding the meaning of spoken language could underlie the problems in regulating pitch.

SEMANTIC–PRAGMATIC DISORDER

Disorders of semantics and pragmatics have only recently come to the attention of doctors and speech therapists (Allen and Rapin 1980). Their boundaries are not yet clear, and there are currently no good tests available for establishing a clear diagnosis. Clinical experience has not yet reached a sufficient level of sophistication to allow even the suggestion of operational diagnostic criteria. In spite of this, it is already clear that semantic–pragmatic disorder(s) will be an important sub-branch of child neuropsychiatric research and clinical activity in the coming decade.

Children with 'semantic problems' have specific difficulties applying the rules of grammar and conveying meaning when interacting with other people. They may rely too heavily on certain grammatical rules. Others may seem to ignore such rules to the extent that their language becomes self-centred. They may have mild, moderate or severe problems in producing readily comprehensible spoken sentences.

Children with 'pragmatic problems' have specific difficulties in applying their sometimes excellent language skills in situations of social interaction. They may sound 'more like a book than a human being' as one teacher put it. They may ask endless questions and sometimes upset the persons being asked by giving evidence that they already know all the answers. One of the reasons for this is that they cannot divine that other people may know things that they themselves do not know. Because of this they will not be able to formulate questions suitable for unknown answers.

Many children have both semantic and pragmatic problems. On closer inspection, such children will often demonstrate severe problems comprehending spoken language. These same children may have less (or indeed no) problems comprehending a written text.

Recently, there has been increasing concern with the distinction of semantic–pragmatic disorder from Asperger syndrome (Bishop 1989). The two often overlap. The main uncertainties are: (1) Are there persons with Asperger syndrome without semantic–pragmatic disorder? and (2) Are there persons with semantic–pragmatic disorders without other symptoms of Asperger syndrome? Given the kinds of definition for Asperger syndrome currently in use, it seems unlikely that Asperger syndrome could exist without severe pragmatic problems. However, the second issue has not been resolved. Given the enormous importance in social interaction of being able to use language for smooth communication, it would seem likely that most children with semantic–pragmatic disorder would show at least some signs of social interaction problems even if not meeting all the criteria for Asperger syndrome.

Treatment of semantic–pragmatic disorder has to take into account the full clinical picture of associated behavioural difficulties and social oddities. Role play and videotaped sessions with 'playback feedback' are currently used in some centres, but it is too early to decide their efficacy.

LANDAU–KLEFFNER SYNDROME

The onset of Landau–Kleffner syndrome is usually between the ages of 3 and 9 years and relatively abrupt. It is characterized by aphasia occurring after normal or almost normal language development and usually ushered in by receptive problems ('verbal auditory agnosia'), quickly followed by expressive difficulties in association with typical EEG abnormalities (Chapter 16). It has a variable prognosis even though after the first several weeks to months it usually becomes 'quiet' and does not lead to further regression.

Emotional and behavioural symptoms are the rule. Some of these can be seen as anxiety reactions in a child suddenly bereft of the understanding of spoken language. In other instances, some of the symptoms are reminiscent of those seen in typical autism cases. Some children fit the diagnostic criteria both for childhood disintegrative disorder (Heller dementia) and for Landau–Kleffner syndrome.

Anticonvulsant treatment may not have any effect on language; it has not even been demonstrated that the effect on seizures is very good, and the paroxysmal EEG changes usually do not disappear. Some clinicians maintain that antiepileptic drugs (in particular carbamazepine) may have a beneficial effect on emotional and behavioural problems. Corticosteroids and surgical treatment may also be indicated (see Chapter 16).

Many children with Landau–Kleffner syndrome are suspected of being deaf. It is essential that a clear diagnosis be established early so that they can benefit from special education in classrooms for children with aphasia or high-functioning autism/learning disorders.

REFERENCES

Airaksinen, E., Bille, B., Carlström, G., *et al.* (1990) 'Barn och ungdomar med DAMP/MBD.' *Läkartidningen*, **88**, 714.

Allen, D.A., Rapin, I. (1980) 'Language disorders in preschool children: predictors of outcome—a preliminary report.' *Brain and Development*, **2**, 73–80.

American Psychiatric Association (1980) *Diagnostic and Statistical Manual of Mental Disorders, 3rd Edn (DSM-III)*. Washington, DC: APA.

—— (1987) *Diagnostic and Statistical Manual of Mental Disorders, 3rd Edn—Revised (DSM-III-R)*. Washington, DC: APA.

—— (1994) *Diagnostic and Statistical Manual of Mental Disorders, 4th Edn (DSM-IV)*. Washington, DC: APA.

Ayres, A.J. (1974) *Southern California Sensory Integration Test*. Los Angeles: Western Psychological Services.

Barker, P. (1979) *Basic Child Psychiatry*. London: Granada.

Barkley, R.A. (1990) *Attention Deficit Hyperactivity Disorder*. New York: Guilford Press.

Bishop, D.V.M. (1989) 'Autism, Asperger's syndrome and semantic–pragmatic disorders. Where are the boundaries?' *British Journal of Disorders of Communication*, **24**, 107–121.

Cantwell, D.P., Baker, L. (1985) 'Speech and language: development and disorders.' *In:* Rutter, M., Hersov, L. (Eds.) *Child and Adolescent Psychiatry. Modern Approaches. 2nd Edn*. Oxford: Blackwell Scientific, pp. 526–544.

Cardon, L.R., Smith, S.D., Fulker, D.W., *et al.* (1994) 'Quantitative trait locus for reading disability on chromosome 6.' *Science*, **266**, 276–279.

Conners, C.K. (1969) 'A teacher rating scale for use in drug studies with children.' *American Journal of Psychiatry*, **126**, 884–888.

Denckla, M.B. (1985) 'Neurological examination for subtle signs (PANESS).' *Psychopharmacology Bulletin*, **21**, 773–800.

Galaburda, A.M., Corsiglia, J., Rosen, G.D., Sherman, G.F. (1987) 'Planum temporale assymmetry, reappraisal since Geschwind and Levitsky.' *Neuropsychologia*, **25**, 853–868.

Gillberg, C. (1995) *Clinical Child Neuropsychiatry*. Cambridge: Cambridge University Press.

—— Rasmussen, P. (1982) 'Perceptual, motor and attentional deficits in seven-year-old children: background factors.' *Developmental Medicine and Child Neurology*, **24**, 752–770.

—— Carlström, G., Rasmussen, P., Waldenström, E. (1983) 'Perceptual, motor and attentional deficits in seven-year-old children. Neurological screening aspects.' *Acta Paediatrica Scandinavica*, **72**, 119–124.

—— Melander, H., von Knorring, A-L., *et al.* (1997) 'Long-term stimulant treatment of children with attention-deficit hyperactivity disorder symptoms. A randomized, double-blind, placebo-controlled trial.' *Archives of General Psychiatry*, **54**, 857–864.

Gillberg, I.C. (1987) 'Deficits in attention, motor control and perception: follow-up from pre-school to early teens.' MD thesis, University of Uppsala.

—— Gillberg, C. (1988) 'Generalized hyperkinesis: follow-up study from age 7 to 13 years.' *Journal of the American Academy of Child and Adolescent Psychiatry*, **27**, 55–59.

—— —— Groth, J. (1989) 'Children with preschool minor neurodevelopmental disorders. V: Neurodevelopmental profiles at age 13.' *Developmental Medicine and Child Neurology*, **31**, 14–24.

—— Winnergård, I., Gillberg, C. (1993) 'Screening methods, epidemiology and evaluation of intervention in DAMP in preschool children.' *European Child and Adolescent Psychiatry*, **2**, 121–135.

Gittelman, R., Klein, D.F., Feingold, I. (1983) 'Children with reading disorders. II. Effects of methylphenidate in combination with reading remediation.' *Journal of Child Psychology and Psychiatry*, **24**, 193–212.

Graham, P. (1986) *Child Psychiatry. A Developmental Approach*. Oxford: Oxford Medical.

Hechtman, L. (1993) 'Aims and methodological problems in multimodal treatment studies.' *Canadian Journal of Psychiatry*, **38**, 458–464.

—— (Ed.) (1996) *Do They Grow Out Of It? Long-term Outcomes of Childhood Disorders*. Washington, DC: American Psychiatric Press.

Hellgren, L., Gillberg, I.C., Bågenholm, A., Gillberg, C. (1994) 'Children with Deficits in Attention, Motor control and Perception (DAMP) almost grown up: psychiatric and personality disorders at age 16 years.' *Journal of Child Psychology and Psychiatry*, **35**, 1255–1271.

Hynd, G.W., Semrud-Clikeman, M., Lorys, A.R., *et al.* (1990) 'Brain morphology in developmental dyslexia and attention deficit disorder/hyperactivity.' *Archives of Neurology*, **47**, 919–926.

Landgren, M., Pettersson, R., Kjellman, B., Gillberg, C. (1996) 'ADHD, DAMP and other neurodevelopmental/neuropsychiatric disorders in 6-year-old children: epidemiology and co-morbidity.' *Developmental Medicine and Child Neurology*, **38**, 891–906.

Michelsson, K., Ylinen, A. (1989) 'A neurodevelopmental screening examination for five-year-old children.' *Early Child Development and Care*, **29**, 9–22.

Rasmussen, P., Gillberg, C., Waldenström, E., Svenson, B. (1983) 'Perceptual, motor and attentional deficits in seven-year-old children: neurological and neurodevelopmental aspects.' *Developmental Medicine and Child Neurology*, **25**, 315–333.

Richman, N. (1985) 'Disorders in pre-school children.' *In:* Rutter, M., Hersov, L. (Eds.) *Child and Adolscent Psychiatry. Modern Approaches. 2nd Edn*. Oxford: Blackwell Scientific, pp. 336–350.

Rosenberg, P.B. (1989) 'Perceptual–motor and attentional correlates of developmental dyscalculia.' *Annals of Neurology*, **26**, 216–220.

Rutter, M. (1982) 'Syndromes attributed to "minimal brain dysfunction" in childhood.' *American Journal of Psychiatry*, **139**, 21–33.

—— Madge, N. (1976) *Cycles of Disadvantage: a Review of Research*. London: Heinemann Educational.

—— Graham, P., Yule, W. (1970) *A Neuropsychiatric Study in Childhood. Clinics in Developmental Medicine No. 35/36*. London: Spastics International Medical Publications.

Sandberg, S.T., Rutter, M., Taylor, E. (1978) 'Hyperkinetic disorder in psychiatric clinic attenders.' *Developmental Medicine and Child Neurology*, **20**, 279–299.

Sanson, A., Prior, M., Smart, D. (1996) 'Reading disabilities with and without behaviour problems at 7–8 years: prediction from longitudinal data from infancy to 6 years.' *Journal of Child Psychology and Psychiatry*, **37**, 529–541.

Schachar, R., Rutter, M., Smith, A. (1981) 'The characteristics of situationally and pervasively hyperactive children: implications for syndrome definition.' *Journal of Child Psychology and Psychiatry*, **22**, 375–392.

Schonhaut, S., Satz, P. (1983) 'Prognosis for children with learning disabilities: a review of follow-up studies.' *In:* Rutter, M. (Ed.) *Developmental Neuropsychiatry*. New York: Guilford Press, pp. 542–563.

Stevenson, J., Graham, P., Fredman, G., McLoughlin, V. (1984) 'The genetics of reading ability.' *In:* Turner, C. (Ed.) *The Biology of Human Intelligence*. London: Eugenics Society.

—— —— —— —— (1987) 'A twin study of genetic influences on reading and spelling ability and disability.' *Journal of Child Psychology and Psychiatry*, **28**, 229–247.

Taylor, E.A. (Ed.) (1986) *The Overactive Child. Clinics in Developmental Medicine No. 97*. London: Mac Keith Press.

—— Sandberg, S., Thorley, G., Giles, S. (1991) *The Epidemiology of Childhood Hyperactivity. Maudsley Monographs No 33*. Oxford: Oxford University Press.

Touwen, B.C.L. (1979) *Examination of the Child with Minor Neurological Dysfunction, 2nd Edn. Clinics in Developmental Medicine No. 71*. London: Spastics International Medical Publications.

Wechsler, D. (1974) *Manual of the Wechsler Intelligence Scale for Children—Revised*. New York: Psychological Corporation.

Wender, P.H. (1971) *Minimal Brain Dysfunction in Children*. New York: Wiley.

Whitmore, K., Bax, M. (1986) 'The school entry medical examination.' *Archives of Disease in Childhood*, **61**, 807–817.

WHO (1993a) *The ICD-10 Classification of Mental and Behavioural Disorders. Clinical Descriptions and Guidelines*. Geneva: World Health Organization.

—— (1993b) *The ICD-10 Classification of Mental and Behavioural Disorders. Diagnostic Criteria for Research*. Geneva: World Health Organization.

Wilsher, C.R. (1986) 'The nootropic concept and dyslexia.' *Annals of Dyslexia*, **36**, 118–137.

28
TICS, TOURETTE SYNDROME AND OBSESSIVE–COMPULSIVE DISORDERS

TOURETTE SYNDROME

In 1885 the French neurologist Georges Gilles de la Tourette described a syndrome of multiple motor tics and coprolalia and concluded that this was a neuropsychiatric disorder with a chronic course and a variable, but often gloomy, outcome. It now appears that Tourette described only part of a continuum of tic disorders involving the combination of multiple motor and vocal tics. Exactly where on the continuum to draw the line in differential diagnosis of 'Tourette syndrome' is the subject of considerable controversy. This is one reason why reliable population prevalence rates for Tourette syndrome are not available.

DIAGNOSIS
The criteria for diagnosing Tourette syndrome according to the DSM-IV (American Psychiatric Association 1994) are outlined in Table 28.1. The combination of multiple motor and one or more vocal tics is required, but other symptoms, such as coprolalia (the urgent need to say out loud 'dirty words'), echolalia (the often 'meaningless' repetition of phrases or parts of phrases), attention problems, fidgetiness, obsessiveness, compulsions and self-injurious behaviours may or may not be present. ADHD (Chapter 27) is often a concomitant of Tourette syndrome, but there are cases with few or no attention deficit symptoms. Obsessively recurrent thoughts or compulsions (*e.g.* to touch things in passing) seem to be extremely common. Some individuals with Tourette syndrome are more handicapped by their attentional and obsessional/compulsive symptoms than by the tics themselves. Some surveys (Shapiro *et al.* 1988, Comings 1990) have indicated that a number of other problems are commonly associated with Tourette syndrome, *e.g.* difficulties with mathematics (>50 per cent of cases), severe conduct problems, and compulsive public exposure of genitals (<10 per cent of cases). A few studies have suggested a connection between Tourette syndrome on the one hand and autism, Asperger syndrome and anorexia nervosa on the other (*e.g.* Råstam *et al.* 1991).

EPIDEMIOLOGY
Simple motor tics are extremely common phenomena, occurring at some time during the late preschool and early school years in at least 10 per cent of all children (Comings 1990). Full-blown

Tourette syndrome is relatively rare, but mild/moderate degrees of the combination of motor tics (*e.g.* in the upper parts of the body: blinking, nodding or shaking the head, shrugging the shoulders) and vocal tics (ranging from repetitive throat-clearing and snorting to convulsive-like sounds variously described as barking, roaring or shouting) may exist in some patients. and most such cases may nowadays be diagnosed as Tourette syndrome. Onset of Tourette syndrome is usually between 5 and 8 years of age (Corbett *et al.* 1969). Tics usually affect facial muscle groups first, then tend to spread downwards to affect muscles of the neck, trunk, arms and, rarely, legs. Prevalence rates vary widely. To date, only one study has been based on a nonreferred sample. In that study Tourette syndrome was present in 1 per cent of school-age boys and 0.1 per cent of school-age girls (Comings 1990).

PATHOGENESIS
The aetiology of tics and Tourette syndrome remains obscure, but genetic factors play an essential part in the pathogenetic chain of events (Harris 1995a,b). The study of large family trees has implicated a genetic link between Tourette syndrome, tics and obsessive–compulsive disorders. One possible model is that obsessive–compulsive disorders without tics and tics with or without obsessive–compulsive problems are outward manifestations of the same underlying genetically determined trait. Most authorities believe that Tourette syndrome is inherited as an autosomal single dominant gene with incomplete penetrance (van de Wetering and Heutink 1993). Possible nongenetic factors in symptom expression include prenatal factors that stress the mother during pregnancy or other events which might increase sensitivity in the fetal nervous system (Leckman *et al.* 1990). It is not clear which neural networks in the brain are involved in Tourette syndrome. Dopamine dysfunction is believed to be involved, based mainly on the beneficial effect of dopamine antagonists. Post-mortem analyses have revealed a decrease of 5-hydroxytryptamine and glutamate in many areas of the basal ganglia, a reduction also in cyclic AMP, and an increased number of dopamine uptake carrier sites in the striatum (Singer *et al.* 1991, Anderson *et al.* 1992). Nevertheless, it seems unlikely that only one monoamine in one circumscribed brain area will be implicated.

TABLE 28.1
Diagnostic criteria for Tourette syndrome*

A. Both multiple motor and one or more vocal tics have been present at some time during the illness, although not necessarily concurrently (a *tic* is a sudden, rapid, recurrent, nonrhythmic, stereotypic motor movement or vocalization)

B. The tics occur many times a day (usually in bouts), nearly every day or intermittently throughout a period of more than 1 year, and during this period there was never a tic-free period of more than 3 consecutive months

C. The disturbance causes marked distress or significant impairment in social, occupational or other important areas of functioning

D. The onset is before age 18 years

E. The disturbance is not due to the direct physiological effects of a substance (*e.g.* stimulants) or a general medical condition (*e.g.* Huntington disease or postviral encephalitis)

*DSM-IV: American Psychiatric Association (1994).

DIFFERENTIAL DIAGNOSIS

Tourette syndrome should be considered in any child who shows even mild tics at physical examination. Tourette syndrome or multiple tics are sometimes the underlying problem and even occasionally the cause of symptoms such as conduct problems and obsessions, and physicians have to be aware of the syndrome and systematically enquire about it. Tourette originally surmised that outcome was often poor, with intellectual deterioration in many cases. This now seems to be the exception rather than the rule. Nevertheless, it is important to exclude the possibility of underlying neurological disorder, and occasionally it can be difficult to decide whether tic-like movements are really tics or myoclonic jerks.

WORK-UP

Medical and psychological work-up in a child with clear or suspected Tourette syndrome must include a detailed medical, neurobiological, psychological and developmental history, sometimes an EEG, and neuropsychological examination with the WISC-R (which often yields a characteristic profile with low results on Arithmetic and Block Design against an overall background of normal or above-normal results, particularly on Verbal subtests) and with some more specific neuropsychological battery in cases where there is associated academic failure.

TREATMENT

Dopamine blockers—particularly dopamine 2 antagonists such as pimozide—have been shown to reduce tics (Comings 1990) and should be tried in cases where specific treatment for severe tics is sought. Dosage is often much lower than when 'antipsychotic' action is requested. Pimozide, for instance, can often be effective in school-age children in doses of 1–4 mg/d (usually divided into morning and afternoon medication). Certain other drugs, such as clonidine, may also be effective, particularly if there is associated severe attention deficits (this beneficial clonidine effect suggests that the dopamine hypothesis in relation to tics should be seen as an intriguing possibility rather than a scientific fact). It is quite common for the associated neuropsychiatric

problems to be more burdensome to the affected individual than the tics *per se*. Attention deficits and/or obsessive–compulsive symptoms may be severe and cause considerable suffering. In such cases, stimulants may be as effective in reducing attentional and behavioural problems as they are in ADHD/DAMP without tics. Tics do not usually exacerbate during stimulant treatment (Gillberg *et al.* 1997). A selective serotonin reuptake inhibitor (SSRI) can be effective in reducing obsessive and compulsive symptoms. Rarely an individual patient may benefit from a combined treatment with two or all three of neuroleptic, stimulant and SSRI drugs.

The majority of patients with multiple tics and Tourette syndrome do not require 'specific treatment'. Usually, the best approach is to make a correct diagnosis and to inform parents and child that this is not primarily a psychological problem and that, in most cases, the tics do not indicate an underlying severe psychiatric or neurological disorder. Supportive psychotherapeutic techniques are often useful in the management of Tourette patients. Long-term outcome has received little study, but available evidence supports the notion of a chronic disorder with a rather stable course, only rarely remitting altogether and only rarely carrying a clearly negative prognosis. Tics without associated neuropsychiatric symptomatology usually require no other intervention than diagnosis and often have a self-limiting course.

OUTCOME

The outcome is usually relatively good in Tourette syndrome and in tics generally. This does not mean that all 'tiqueurs cease to tic' at a certain age, even though quite a large proportion stop having severe tics before adolescence, but rather that most of them can learn to live with the problem without too much embarrassment. Characteristically there may be waxing and waning of symptoms with periods of exacerbation, often associated with either stress or relaxation, and other, sometimes long periods when few or no tics occur.

OBSESSIVE–COMPULSIVE DISORDER

Obsessive and compulsive problems are common in people with tics and particularly in Tourette syndrome. Many authorities consider Tourette syndrome and so-called 'obsessive–compulsive disorder' (OCD) to be part of the same spectrum of disorders. Nevertheless, there are many children and adolescents who have OCD without tics. The available evidence suggests that Tourette syndrome and OCD belong to the same 'family' of neuropsychiatric disorders.

DIAGNOSIS

The diagnosis of OCD is usually made according to criteria set out in the DSM-IV. There are either obsessions or compulsions, that cause marked distress, consume more than one hour per day, or interfere with the person's life in significant ways. Adults have had a period during which they recognized that the obsessions or compulsions are excessive or unrealistic. This does not apply to children. The most common obsessions are fear of being contaminated, of death, disease and disaster. Obsessions about symmetry and sex and religion are also common, but tend to vary more according to culture (Thomsen 1996). The most common compulsions are rituals involving washing (mostly hand-washing), checking and repeating.

EPIDEMIOLOGY

There have been very few studies of the epidemiology of OCD in the general population of children. Only one study—from Germany—of young children has been published: the rate of severe obsessive–compulsive problems was about 3 per cent among 8-year-olds (Esser *et al.* 1990). Flament *et al.* (1988) reported that strictly defined OCD occurred in 0.35 per cent of 15- to 18-year-olds in the USA. In Israel, the rate of OCD was as high as 3.6 per cent among male and female military conscripts (Zohar *et al.* 1992). In summary, it seems that OCD in childhood is not an uncommon problem and that, at least in some countries, it may be a frequent phenomenon.

OCD appears to be about twice as common in boys as in girls, but in the late adolescent period the male:female ratio equalizes.

PATHOGENESIS

The pathogenesis of OCD is unknown. However, it is no longer assumed that psychogenesis plays an important role in the aetiology of the disorder, although it may be involved in the development of symptoms and contribute to outcome. Most authors believe that OCD results from basal ganglia dysfunction (*e.g.* Rapoport 1989), a hypothesis gaining support from the association of Huntington and Sydenham chorea on the one hand and severe obsessive–compulsive symptoms on the other. Direct evidence for a causal link is scant. There is clear familial clustering of cases, and it is now generally agreed that there is a strong genetic liability to OCD traits, although, in the individual case, the exact type of obsession or compulsion cannot be predicted by the family history of symptomatology.

DIFFERENTIAL DIAGNOSIS AND COMORBIDITY

The most important differential diagnoses are tics, Tourette syndrome, Asperger syndrome and other autism spectrum disorders. All of these disorders can also occur in conjuction with OCD and represent a considerable proportion of the comorbidity spectrum. The distinction of tics and compulsions is sometimes a matter of words: some of the complex motor tics seen in Tourette syndrome might equally be described as compulsive acts or 'compulsions'. Some authors consider OCD and Tourette syndrome to be on the same spectrum of disorders involving obsessions, compulsions and spasmodic compulsive motor activities (= tics).

Depressive symptoms and socially avoidant behaviours often develop in the course of OCD. These may be seen to represent reactions to the underlying OCD or, sometimes, be regarded as biologically associated neuropsychiatric symptoms.

'Obsessive–compulsive personality disorder' (OCPD) is seen in only a small proportion of individuals with OCD. It represents a long-standing disabling condition hallmarked by rigidity, social interaction problems and a lack of generosity. It overlaps with Asperger syndrome much more than with OCD.

OUTCOME

OCD has a variable outcome. About one-third of children affected by severe symptoms are symptom-free at follow-up several years later. Another one-third have persisting problems that tend to wax and wane and to be handicapping only at times and in certain situations. The final third of young people with OCD are severely incapacitated by obsessions and compulsions for many, many years, possibly well into adult age and maybe for life (Thomsen 1996). However, outcome studies in the literature were performed before the advent of effective pharmacological and psychotherapeutic interventions, and it is probably realistic to assume that with modern treatment, outcome may be considerably better.

WORK-UP

There is usually no need for further work-up once the clinical diagnosis has been established; the clinical picture is so striking, and underlying disorders so rare, that OCD is not often a candidate for in-depth medical work-up. However, very rarely OCD can be the only symptomatology in the early stages of childhood-onset Huntington chorea (or other rare disorders involving basal ganglia dysfunction). This has to be borne in mind so that appropriate diagnostic examinations can be made whenever there is a suspicion of deterioration or clear neurological signs. A careful history and a meticulous neurological examination of all children presenting with OCD will usually be sufficient to rule out such underlying neurological disorders.

TREATMENT

Cognitive behavioural therapy and pharmacological treatment, alone or in combination, are now the mainstay of treatment in OCD (Thomsen 1996). The new serotonin reputake inhibitors (such as fluoxetine, sertraline and fluvoxamine in doses ranging from 10 to 60 mg/d depending on child's age/weight and severity of symptoms) are often effective in reducing obsessions and compulsions and also have an ameliorating effect on the often concomitant depressed mood. They should be used in all severe cases in order to reduce suffering and to open up the possibility of cogntive psychotherapy.

REFERENCES

American Psychiatric Association (1994) *Diagnostic and Statistical Manual of Mental Disorders, 4th Edn (DSM-IV).* Washington, DC: APA.
Anderson, G.M., Pollak, E.S., Chatterjee, D., *et al.* (1992) 'Postmortem analysis of subcortical monoamines and amino acids in Tourette syndrome.' *Advances in Neurology,* **58,** 123–133.
Comings, D.E. (1990) *Tourette Syndrome and Human Behaviour.* Duarte, CA: Hope Press.
Corbett, J.A., Mathews, A.M., Connell, P.H., Shapiro, D.A. (1969) 'Tics and Gilles de la Tourette's syndrome: a follow-up study and critical review.' *British Journal of Psychiatry,* **115,** 1229–1241.
de la Tourette, G. (1885) 'Étude sur une affection nerveuse caractérisée par de

l'incordination motrice accompagnée d'écholalie et de coprolalie (jumping, latah, myriachit).' *Archives de Neurologie*, **9**, 19–52, 158–200.

Esser, G., Schmidt, M.H., Woerner, W. (1990) 'Epidemiology and course of psychiatric disorders in school-age children—results of a longitudinal study.' *Journal of Child Psychology and Psychiatry*, **31**, 243–263.

Flament, M.F., Whitaker, A., Rapoport, J.L., *et al.* (1988) 'Obsessive compulsive disorder in adolescence: an epidemiological study.' *Journal of the American Academy of Child and Adolescent Psychiatry*, **27**, 764–771.

Gillberg, C., Melander, H., von Knorring, A-L., *et al.* (1997) 'Long-term central stimulant treatment of children with attention-deficit hyperactivity disorder. A randomized double blind placebo-controlled trial.' *Archives of General Psychiatry*, **54**, 857–864.

Harris, J.C. (1995a) *Developmental Neuropsychiatry. I. The Fundamentals.* Oxford: Oxford University Press.

—— (1995b) *Developmental Neuropsychiatry. II. Assessment, Diagnosis and Treatment of Developmental Disorders.* Oxford: Oxford University Press.

Leckman, J.F., Dolnansky, E.S., Hardin, M.T., *et al.* (1990) 'Perinatal factors in the expression of Tourette's syndrome: an exploratory study.' *Journal of the American Academy of Child and Adolescent Psychiatry*, **29**, 220–226.

Rapoport, J.L. (1989) 'The biology of obsessions and compulsions.' *Scientific American*, **260**, 82–89.

Råstam, M., Gillberg, C., Wahlström, J. (1991) 'Chromosomes in anorexia nervosa. A study of 47 cases including a population-based group: a research note.' *Journal of Child Psychology and Psychiatry*, **32**, 695–701.

Shapiro, A.K., Shapiro, E.S., Young, J.G., Feinberg, T.E. (1988) *Gilles de la Tourette Syndrome, 2nd Edn.* New York: Raven Press.

Singer, H.S., Hahn, I.H., Moran, T.H. (1991) 'Abnormal dopamine uptake sites in postmortem striatum from patients with Tourette's syndrome.' *Annals of Neurology*, **30**, 558–562.

Thomsen, P.H. (1996) 'Treatment of obsessive–compulsive disorder in children and adolescents.' *European Child and Adolscent Psychiatry*, **5**, 55–66.

van de Wetering, B.J.M., Heutink, P. (1993) 'The genetics of the Gilles de la Tourette syndrome: a review.' *Journal of Laboratory and Clinical Medicine*, **121**, 638–645.

Zohar, A.H., Ratzoni, G., Pauls, D.L., *et al.* (1992) 'An epidemiological study of obsessive–compulsive disorder and related disorders in Israeli adolescents.' *Journal of the American Academy of Child and Adolescent Psychiatry*, **31**, 1057–1061.

29

OTHER NEUROPSYCHIATRIC SYNDROMES

In the past decade it has become widely recognized that a number of disorders, usually of genetic origin, have a distinctive behavioural phenotype (O'Brien and Yule 1995). In some of these, such as Angelman syndrome, fragile X syndrome, Prader–Willi syndrome and Williams syndrome, the behaviours in themselves are often so characteristic as to arouse suspicion that the child might be suffering from a specific chromosomal abnormality. Oftentimes, the behaviours are more 'pathognomonic' than any of the physical symptoms or stigmata. Many of these disorders are named after the clinician who first described the characteristic syndrome. Some of the most well-known of these behavioural phenotype syndromes are briefly described in this chapter. For convenience, they are listed in alphabetical order.

ANGELMAN SYNDROME
(see also Chapter 5)

Angelman syndrome encompasses jerky movements, unprovoked laughter and varying degrees of mental retardation, mostly severe or profound (Angelman 1965). Studies supporting the notion of a particular behavioural phenotype in this syndrome are only just being published, and it is too early to suggest details in this respect. One study of adolescents and young adults with Angelman syndrome (Clayton-Smith 1993) indicated that hyperactivity, often prominent in early childhood, usually gives way to more controllable behaviour in late childhood. Most studies to date suggest that muteness may be a constant feature, but that sign language may be acquired by some individuals. In my own centre we have seen one young boy with Angelman syndrome and autism. Many children with Angelman syndrome have marked autistic features in spite of seeming happy and sociable in the sense that they may like the proximity of other people. However, contact is only accepted if it is on their own terms. Stubbornness, insistence on sameness and fascination with water are all highly suggestive of the behavioural phenotype of the classical syndrome of autism (Steffenburg et al. 1996).

DOWN SYNDROME
(see also Chapter 5)

Down syndrome (trisomy 21), unlike other mental retardation syndromes, seems to be associated with a relatively low incidence of psychiatric disorder (Gillberg et al. 1986). Even though the stereotype of the happy, amiable and tractable personality is unsupported in many cases, and temper tantrums, irritability and stubbornness may be relatively common features in childhood, it seems clear that the majority of adolescents and young adults with Down syndrome do not have major psychiatric problems. However, severe problems can occur in Down syndrome, and even autism has been described in some cases. It seems that additional brain damage—or specific genetic influences on constitution—might be a prerequisite for the development of autism in Down syndrome and that the autistic symptoms are unassociated with the chromosomal abnormality as such.

Most children with Down syndrome have IQs <50, and of the 10–20 per cent who test higher, many are cases of mosaicism. Such cases comprise around 2–3 per cent of all cases of Down syndrome. The cognitive profile in Down syndrome, in spite of a generally low level, shows considerable interindividual variation.

In recent years, several studies have indicated that with early intervention programmes, mainly focusing on physiotherapy and educating parents to train affected children (Spiker 1990), IQ can be pushed up by 10–20 points and motor problems associated with hypotonia can be substantially reduced. Because in almost all cases the diagnosis of Down syndrome is made in the first few days of life, intensive intervention should start at once. For a detailed description of the training programme—which includes a language stimulation programme—the reader is referred to Rogers and Coleman (1992). In addition to the education programme, children with Down syndrome always require a medical work-up because major medical problems are frequently associated.

FRAGILE X SYNDROME
(see also Chapter 5)

The fragile X syndrome constitutes a combination of physical and behavioural characteristics associated with a fragile site (and a gene locus) on the long arm of the X chromosome at Xq27.3. It is second only to Down syndrome as a cause of mental retardation, with IQ levels <50. It is the most common known cause of familial mental retardation and it underlies a variety of behavioural problems including autism and hyperactivity syndromes (Percy *et al.* 1990, Reiss and Freund 1990).

PREVALENCE

The fragile X syndrome is present in around 1 per 1000 males as measured by total screen of retarded individuals in one area (Hagerman 1989). In females, the prevalence may be as high as 1 per 500 (Reiss and Freund 1990). Considering that not all persons with fragile X syndrome have IQ < 70 and that there are carrier males and females with only slight or no learning problems, the true prevalence is likely to be considerably higher. Most affected males appear to have moderate or severe problems, though there are healthy men with the confirmed chromosomal abnormality, whereas most females are less severely affected, although about one-third have IQ < 70.

BEHAVIOURAL PHENOTYPE

Most males test below IQ 70 (the most common level of cognitive functioning seems to be 35–40) on standard IQ tests, but a proportion have IQs in the normal or low-normal range. Verbal abilities are usually superior to performance and visuospatial skills.

There is clear evidence of social dysfunction in a vast majority of male cases. Almost all males exhibit 'autistic' features, but only a minority exhibit the full syndrome of autism, with or without mental retardation. The fragile X abnormality is the most common of the known causes of autism. Hyperkinetic syndromes, with and without autism, usually with many autistic features, are common. The cognitive test profile in the fragile X syndrome is different from that ordinarily seen in low-functioning autism, but is quite commonly encountered in high-functioning autism cases and Asperger syndrome. Several authors have described the concurrence of Asperger syndrome and the fragile X chromosome abnormality (see Hagerman 1989).

Some of the behaviours most often encountered in males with fragile X syndrome are: gaze avoidance, tactile defensiveness and social withdrawal (age 0–2 years); gaze avoidance, avoidant greeting behaviour (turning away with head and body on greeting other people), shyness, motor stereotypies of various kinds and hyperactivity (3–4 years); echolalia, cluttering, 'nervous fidgetiness', hand flapping, stereotypic waving of things, wrist or knuckle biting, and gaze avoidance and avoidant greeting behaviour in spite of signs that there is a drive for social 'proximity' and interest in other humans (5–8 years); continuing shyness, gaze avoidance and 'nervousness', and often also a preoccupation with certain objects or human beings in the general setting of moderate mental retardation, with fast, cluttering echolalic speech (very often used in a half whispering, half 'nervously' laughing manner) (9–12 years); continuing difficulties of the same type, often aggravated by various problems associated with onset of puberty, including cross-dressing, self-injurious behaviours and clothing problems (because of large genital size) (13–20 years). Often there is cognitive stagnation, or even setback, around the time of puberty.

The same picture is occasionally seen in affected females, but the majority of girls have less severe problems. A small proportion

have full-blown autism, and shyness and gaze avoidance appear to be rather common phenomena even in the relatively large group with no major difficulties. Various kinds of learning problems appear to affect one-third to one-half of all fragile-X-positive females. These range from dyslexia to mild/moderate mental retardation. There have been occasional reports of the development of schizoaffective psychosis in some young women with the fragile X chromosome abnormality (see Hagerman 1989). Some of these have had relatively minor learning problems before the onset of psychosis, but have otherwise, at least outwardly, appeared to be doing well.

TREATMENT

As yet, there is no specific treatment for fragile X syndrome (see Hagerman 1989). Folic acid (0.5–1.5 mg/kg b.i.d.) has been used by several authors. It appears to have a mild stimulant effect, which could lead to better ability to concentrate and perhaps an amelioration of hyperkinetic problems. Some reports have suggested a beneficial effect of folic acid on autistic symptoms, at least if given from the preschool period, but no or even a slightly negative effect if given after puberty. A few authors have used stimulants to counter excessive hyperactivity (in doses recommended for children with severe hyperkinetic syndromes regardless of aetiology) and reported fair or good results.

Genetic counselling has to be provided in all families with the syndrome.

GOLDENHAR SYNDROME
(see also Chapter 6)

Goldenhar syndrome, which commonly involves the eyes (*e.g.* conjunctival dermoid tumours), the external ears and the vertebrae, shows occasional association with mild/moderate mental retardation. It is too early to decide whether there might be a more specific behavioural phenotype in this syndrome, but I have seen two female patients with smiling face, generally happy predisposition, slightly subnormal intelligence and many features of an autistic-like condition.

HYPOMELANOSIS OF ITO
(see also Chapter 4)

Hypomelanosis of Ito features diagnostic skin changes and a variable degree of involvement of other organs including the brain. Recently, many cases of hypomelanosis of Ito associated with psychiatric disorder including symptoms compatible with the diagnoses of autism, atypical autism and Asperger syndrome have been described (Åkefeldt and Gillberg 1991, Zappella 1992).

KLEINE–LEVIN SYNDROME

Originally described in the 1930s, the Kleine–Levin syndrome has received attention in paediatrics and child psychiatry only in recent years (see Gillberg 1987).

DIAGNOSIS

The Kleine–Levin syndrome occurs mostly in adolescent boys (population prevalence unknown), and presents with the combination of intense hunger or specific craving for certain foods, increased need for sleep (somnolence and withdrawal or fugue-like states may be difficult to distinguish from each other) and a variety of emotional/behavioural/neuropsychiatric problems. This symptom constellation appears abruptly and is present for a few days to a few weeks, whereafter symptoms subside. Weeks to months later a new episode occurs and follows a similar pattern, albeit quite often of more limited duration. New episodes can occur for a period of one to several years. Gradually, however, relapses tend to occur less often and the episodes become shorter and shorter.

PATHOGENESIS

Hypothalamic dysfunction may account for the symptomatology because: (a) the appetite and sleep symptoms implicate hypothalamic systems; (b) the syndrome occurs mostly in the teenage period; (c) it affects mostly boys and its episodic nature could be seen as a counterpart to variable behaviour in connection with onset of menarche in girls; and (d) some EEG findings are compatible with hypothalamic dysfunction.

WORK-UP

The work-up should include a neuropsychiatric assessment. If the history and symptoms are typical there is no need for further work-up, but in case of doubt, neurological and laboratory work-up to exclude other neurological disorders and metabolic problems may be essential. A urine and/or blood screen for narcotics and other drugs might also be appropriate in some cases. The EEG sometimes shows mild to moderate increase of low-frequency activity and there may be subtle signs of damage to the CSF blood–brain barrier.

TREATMENT

Management need often consist only of assessment and a proper diagnosis. In severe cases affecting school attendance over long periods, a trial of stimulants (*e.g.* D-amphetamine, two or three doses of 5–15 mg given at three- to four-hour intervals) might be indicated (Lishman 1978). In most cases, however, information given to the affected child/teenager and to his/her parents and teachers will suffice.

OUTCOME

Long-term outcome is good, although a year or two of school work may be wasted and there is quite often the need to repeat a form (grade), and most cases do well by early adult life.

The behaviour problems encountered are extremely variable and are often associated with some degree of somnolence and clouded consciousness. All sorts of psychiatric diagnoses may be discussed before a correct diagnosis is established. These may range from depression or manic depression to schizophrenia and drug abuse. Encephalitis is commonly suspected if the family seeks help during the first episode. The episodic nature of the disorder might not be evident until three or more episodes have occurred. There is also commonly partial or total amnesia for the episodes.

PARTIAL TETRASOMY 15

This syndrome comprises mental retardation (often severe), autistic and hyperkinetic behaviours and, often, skeletal abnormalities (a characteristic facies, high arched palate, kyphosis and short stature) and epilepsy (Gillberg *et al.* 1991). It is associated with two extra copies of the q11–13 portion of chromosome 15. These copies are usually maternally derived and are located in an extra 'marker' chromosome, visible at ordinary karyotyping. There is delayed development early on and a spectrum of behaviour and communication problems that usually fits the diagnosis of autistic disorder or atypical autism. Hand stereotypies in the midline are common, as is a characteristic 'high-strung' oversensitivity to environmental stimuli. Management should be geared to alleviating, if possible, the behavioural problems and to the treatment of epilepsy (often of the minor motor type).

PRADER–WILLI SYNDROME
(see also Chapter 5)

The Prader–Willi syndrome is caused by an absence of paternal DNA at the chromosome 15q11 locus. The paternally derived gene may be deleted or there may be maternal disomy. Preconception exposure to benzene in the fathers has been documented in one study (Åkefeldt *et al.* 1995).

EPIDEMIOLOGY

Prader–Willi syndrome occurs at a rate of about 1 in 7000 children surviving the first year of life (Åkefeldt *et al.* 1991). The male to female ratio is about equal.

CLINICAL PICTURE

Common symptoms are neonatal hypotonia, early feeding problems, overeating, obesity, short stature, small hands and feet, scoliosis, learning problems and a peculiar behavioural phenotype. There is often a characteristic facies with a small, 'round' head and almond-shaped eyes.

Recent studies have shown that mental retardation is not an invariable feature (Clarke *et al.* 1989) and that there are cases with microdeletions at 15q11 with all the characteristics of the syndrome except for mental retardation, short stature and small hands and feet (Åkefeldt *et al.* 1991). It now seems that Prader–Willi syndrome as originally described may be part of a wider phenotype involving a particular behavioural profile with onset in the first year of life.

As the child in the second or third year of life begins to grow fat, many parents often apply for help. By this time the child may be unusually docile and placid but have occasional episodes of irritability and exceptionally severe and destructive temper tantrums. The tantrums are usually immediately followed by the 'baseline' hypoactivity and remorse.

The majority of children with Prader–Willi syndrome exhibit the strange habit of picking their skin and inflicting wounds, bruises and scratches.

Most children with the syndrome are bulimic during exacerbations. They will go to any ends to gain access to food in the fridge, freezer or pantry. Almost all parents have had to install lock mechanisms to limit the amount of food otherwise bolted by the child. Even in scientific investigations, their inability to stop eating (in an experimental setting) has been amply demonstrated.

DIFFERENTIAL DIAGNOSIS

It now appears that there may be relatively wide clinical variation across cases, including milder forms. Many children may not have a severe learning disorder. This means that the diagnosis of Prader–Willi syndrome should be considered for all 'extremely fat and hungry' children who show features of the behavioural phenotype. All children with severe neonatal hypotonia should be screened for the disorder.

MANAGEMENT

Parents need to be informed about the nature of their child's condition. Oral and written information is essential in all cases. The parents have frequently been blamed by doctors, dietitians and psychologists (and by themselves) for the child's extreme obesity. The associated behavioural problems often lead to referral to a child psychiatric service. Without a proper diagnosis, there is a great risk that counselling may focus on child-rearing practices with the underlying implication that they might be at the root of the child's problems. Informing the parents about the almost identical behaviour problems encountered in other children with Prader–Willi syndrome often has very positive psychological consequences. For the family to belong to a national or local Prader–Willi support group is almost always valuable.

The parents may need to be advised (although most will have already found out for themselves) about locking fridges, cupboards, etc. With a very strict attitude on the part of parents and staff at school, it is sometimes feasible to make the child lose weight and even to achieve normal weight. However, maintaining this strict regime is by no means easy and the family who cannot cope with all the restrictions is not to be blamed. Various diets and drug treatments including fenfluramine have been tried in Prader–Willi syndrome in attempts to reduce weight (and the unusually high level of cerebrospinal fluid serotonin), but the long-term effects, if any, remain to be demonstrated.

So far, no effective treatment has been found for the other symptoms involved in the syndrome.

RETT SYNDROME

The neurological hallmarks of Rett syndrome have been described in Chapter 10. This section will provide a brief survey of the associated behavioural/psychiatric problems.

DIAGNOSIS

The diagnostic criteria of Rett syndrome are detailed in Table

TABLE 29.1
Diagnostic[1] and exclusion[2] criteria for Rett syndrome (RS) variant cases

Inclusion criteria

A girl of at least 10 years of age with mental retardation of unexplained origin and with at least three of the six following primary criteria:

A1   Loss of (partial or subtotal) acquired fine finger skill in late infancy/early childhood

A2   Loss of acquired single words/phrases/modulated babble

A3   RS hand stereotypies, hands together or apart

A4   Early deviant communicative ability

A5   Deceleration of head growth of 2 SD (even when still within normal limits)

A6   The RS disease profile: a regression period (stage II) followed by a certain recovery of contact and communication (stage III) in contrast to slow neuromotor regression through school age and adolescence

and, in addition, at least 5 of the following 11 supportive manifestations:

B1   Breathing irregularities (hyperventilation and/or breath-holding)

B2   Bloating/marked air swallowing

B3   Characteristic RS teeth grinding

B4   Gait dyspraxia

B5   Neurogenic scoliosis or high kyphosis (ambulant girls)

B6   Development of abnormal lower limb neurology

B7   Small blue/cold impaired feet, autonomic/trophic dysfunction

B8   Characteristic RS EEG development

B9   Unprompted sudden laughing/screaming spells

B10 Impaired/delayed nociception

B11 Intensive eye communication, 'eye pointing'

Exclusion criteria

Evidence of intrauterine growth retardation

Organomegaly or other signs of storage disease

Retinopathy or optic atrophy

Microcephaly at birth

Evidence of perinatally acquired brain damage

Existence of identifiable metabolic or other progressive neurological disorder

Acquired neurological disorders resulting from severe infections or head trauma

[1]Hagberg and Skjeldal (1994).
[2]Rett Syndrome Diagnostic Criteria Work Group (1988).

10.15 (p. 356). Many girls with Rett syndrome in the early stages of the disorder show many autistic features without clear-cut neurological signs. Therefore, the diagnosis of autism is commonly made in patients under 3 years of age. The diagnosis of Rett syndrome should be considered in all very young girls presenting with autistic symptoms. In one study, 80 per cent of girls with Rett syndrome had initially been suspected of suffering from autism or autistic features (Witt-Engerström and Gillberg 1987), and on the basis of available prevalence estimates for Rett syndrome and autism it was estimated that of all girls presenting in the first few years of life with autistic symptoms, one-third to one-half will eventually turn out to have Rett syndrome. An occasional child with Rett syndrome runs an unusually slow course. In such cases, the diagnosis of 'pure autism' with severe/moderate mental retardation can be retained for many years.

In recent years, it has become apparent that there are many variants of clinical presentation in Rett syndrome. Hagberg and Skjeldal (1994) have presented tentative diagnostic criteria for such Rett syndrome variant cases (Table 29.1).

PSYCHIATRIC/BEHAVIOURAL ASPECTS

Most girls with Rett syndrome show normal or almost normal development up to the age of 6–16 months. Many then stagnate or rapidly begin to lose skills (social smile, interaction and some language skills might be lost). Some, but not all, become aloof, emotionally detached and are described as 'autistic'. Others slowly develop an emotionally stunted style of social interaction which may eventually also be described as autistic. A few are affected with attacks of rage, anxiety, confusion and chaotic hyperactivity. If there is an autistic or autistic-like phase, this may last from one month to several years. Usually by school age—or at least by puberty—the autistic symptoms begin to subside. The available evidence shows that the same type of development applies in most people with autism almost regardless of underlying cause.

Girls with Rett syndrome show a variety of hand stereotypies, most of which involve 'midline procedures', *i.e.* both hands are 'washed' or clapped in the midline or used to slap the forehead or neck in the midline. At an early stage some patients may show more typical 'autism-type' hand-flapping stereotypies.

Some affected girls are reported to laugh in the middle of the night. This occurs in a number of neurometabolic/neurological disorders affecting the brain (*e.g.* the Sanfilippo variant of mucopoly-saccharidosis) and in many autism cases without Rett syndrome.

Bruxism and hyperventilation are common features in Rett syndrome and are sometimes interpreted as signs of extreme anxiety, a notion for which there is generally no empirical support.

DIFFERENTIAL DIAGNOSIS

A number of children show symptoms in the borderland of Rett syndrome and autism (Gillberg 1989). These include the so-called 'forme fruste' and 'preserved speech' variants (Hagberg and Rasmussen 1986, Zappella *et al.* 1998). These borderline cases show many of the features of classical Rett syndrome but do not fulfil all the criteria; they usually also meet most, or all, of the criteria for autistic disorder (or infantile autism). The girls with preserved speech may have a vocabulary of from 20 to several hundred words, and some speak in long—usually echolalic—sentences. Some girls show the classical symptoms of autism only after a prolonged premorbid (or stage I) period of the disorder. A few boys with these borderline conditions have been described in the literature (*e.g.* Gillberg 1989). Rett-like symptoms also occur in conjunction with other neurological disorders such as polyunsaturated fatty acid lipidosis (Hagberg 1989), Moebius syndrome (Gillberg and Steffenburg 1989) and mucopolysaccharidosis.

TREATMENT AND MANAGEMENT

Management of the behavioural/psychiatric problems encountered in Rett syndrome requires knowledge of the natural course of the disorder so that symptoms such as autism and night laughter are not inappropriately interpreted as signalling specific psychological or interactional problems. The degree of language comprehension is extremely low in Rett syndrome. Communication should be achieved by other means such as through eye gaze and manual prompting. Some degree of hand function can often

be maintained if both hands are trained separately for long periods of time every day.

Pharmacologically, some worthwhile results with bromocriptine (20 mg/kg/d) have been reported (Zappella *et al.* 1990), but confirmatory double-blind placebo-controlled studies are needed. Naloxone has also been tried, with conflicting results.

OUTCOME

The ultimate course of Rett syndrome is only partially known. It is clear that the vast majority of patients—possibly all—become extremely mentally and/or neurologically impaired and remain dependent on other people for virtually all matters in everyday life. Epilepsy, constipation, scoliosis, progressive motor (and vasomotor) control problems complicate the clinical picture in a majority of cases. The psychiatric/behavioural problems can be frustrating through childhood and, sometimes, adolescence, but usually cause less concern in the adult age group.

SEX CHROMOSOME ANEUPLOIDIES

Most cases of sex chromosome aneuploidies (which occur in about 0.3 per cent of all live births) have an increased risk of psychiatric disorders. Conversely, sex chromosome aneuploidies are relatively common in child psychiatric clinic attenders. In one study (Crandall *et al.* 1972), 1.6 per cent of children referred to a child psychiatry clinic had sex chromosome aneuploidies.

XYY SYNDROME

Boys with an extra Y chromosome (about 0.1 per cent in the general male population) are at much increased risk of delay and other problems in language development and of temper tantrums and aggressiveness. They also often show hypotonia, and early-onset attention deficits and hyperactivity. Temper tantrums are frequent in early childhood. Poor sociability is a common feature, and the risk of autism appears to be increased (Hagerman 1989). IQ is usually in the normal range, but learning disorders are very common and the incidence of mental retardation is possibly increased as compared with the general male population. A slightly increased tendency to aggressiveness and features of sadism in sexual orientation in adult life is suggested by at least one unbiased prospective study (Schiavi *et al.* 1988). The majority are tall and proportionate with regard to leg and head size. Affected individuals are usually at least 13 cm taller than their fathers. There is a need to consider XYY in all tall boys with behaviour and learning disorders.

XXY SYNDROME (KLINEFELTER SYNDROME)

Boys with one or more extra X chromosomes (around 0.1–0.2 per cent of all live-born males) are collectively referred to as having Klinefelter syndrome. About two-thirds of all cases are 47,XXY. Height, weight and head circumference are small at birth. From about 2–4 years of age there is increased growth velocity, particularly with regard to leg length. Mean adult height is on average 13 cm more than paternal height. Head size does not show catch-up. It appears that the extra X chromosome inhibits brain growth *in utero*. Boys with Klinefelter syndrome usually have a relatively low verbal IQ even though full-scale IQ is often in the normal (or slightly subnormal) range (IQs are usually reported to be in the 60–130 range). Speech and language is delayed, and the vast majority receive speech and language therapy long before a chromosomal diagnosis has been made. Affected boys are often described as clumsy and show many of the problems typical of children with DAMP, sometimes with a tendency towards hypoactivity. These problems may be enhanced by abnormal body build and neuromotor performance. Reading and writing disorders are often severe and out of keeping with the general IQ level. From middle childhood their legs tend to be long and arm span exceeds height. The penis may or may not be small and the testicles are almost always small with failed sperm production. Many develop breast enlargement, and the incidence of breast cancer is increased as compared with normal males. They are often described as timid and with poor self-confidence. Most have mild/moderate social interaction problems, and tend to withdraw from group activities. A small number have autism. One prospective study suggests that in adult life they may be less sexually active and more submissive in sexual orientation than other men (Schiavi *et al.* 1988).

XO SYNDROME (TURNER SYNDROME)
The majority of 45,X individuals may be recognized at birth because of the characteristic oedema of the dorsum of their hands and feet and the webbing of the neck. In addition, they are often born preterm with low birthweight and short stature. Girls with this syndrome have a low rate of psychiatric disorder. IQ is usually normal, but performance IQ shows a downward shift. About 10 per cent are mentally retarded. Visuospatial skills are often particularly poor and this tends to affect mathematical skills. On the WISC-R, the results on the Block Design and Object Assembly subtests are usually poor. Many individuals with XO syndrome are hyperactive in early childhood but tend to be hypoactive from adolescence (Swillen *et al.* 1993). An association of X0 syndrome with anorexia nervosa (particularly in X0 mosaicism) has been suggested, but a recent systematic chromosome study including a population sample did not support this (Råstam *et al.* 1991). After adolescence, subjects are of short stature and have infantile external and internal genitalia. Replacement therapy with oestrogen is essential but there is, as yet, no consensus as to the optimal age to initiate such treatment. Many women with Turner syndrome marry and lead well-adjusted lives in adulthood.

Individuals with Turner syndrome who have inherited their X chromosome from their mother tend to have more social interaction problems than those whose X chromosome is paternally derived (Skuse *et al.* 1997).

XXX SYNDROME
Girls with triple X syndrome constitute 0.1 per cent of all live-born females. They are at much increased risk of language disorder, learning disorder (with a need for special education in most cases, and IQs in the low-normal range; however, reading and writing disorders tend to correspond to the general level of

IQ), shyness, immaturity and conduct problems of various kinds (Linden *et al.* 1988). They are tall and have poorly coordinated movements. This, in connection with their odd behaviour and conduct problems, leads to a high rate of referral for institutional treatment.

SMITH–MAGENIS SYNDROME

This rare syndrome presents with a highly characteristic behavioural phenotype. It is caused by an interstitial deletion of chromosome 17p11.2. Affected individuals are delayed in overall development and usually test in the moderately mentally retarded range (although some are only mildly mentally retarded). The majority have brachycephaly, midface hypoplasia, ear malformations and brachydactyly. There are major behaviour problems in most cases with aggressive and self-mutilatory symptoms (including onychotillomania and insertion of foreign objects into various body orifices). Head banging, hand biting and another stereotypic behaviour, unusual in other conditions, of hand or arm clasping, now sometimes referred to as 'spasmodic upper body squeeze' or 'self-hugging' (Finucane *et al.* 1994), are all characteristic of the syndrome. This behaviour, a major clinical clue to the diagnosis, and one which should prompt chromosomal analysis, is often elicited in a familiar setting when the patient is relaxed and in a good mood. The history is important in that it is quite uncommon for this type of behaviour to be readily observable in a clinic setting. Most affected individuals are affectionate and have a positive affective tone in spite of the outbursts of aggression and self-mutilation.

SOTOS SYNDROME

This disorder, of unknown etiology, is characterized by cerebral gigantism and rapid body growth. The vast majority of patients have behaviour and learning disorders. It is uncommon, but there have been no reliable estimates of incidence so far. It may not be very rare in children who present with behaviour and learning problems who, in addition, have large body size.

Cole and Hughes (1991) have presented the following diagnostic criteria: (a) a distinctive facies with macrocephalus, a prominent jaw, antimongoloid slant and hypertelorism; (b) a period of accelerated growth in early childhood; (c) advanced bone age during development; and (d) early developmental delay. At adolescence growth rate may be normal.

Low frustration tolerance, irritability, aggressiveness, destructiveness and poor peer relationships are common problems. ADHD is present in about one-third of all young children (Finegan *et al.* 1994), and autistic disorder appears to be over-represented (Morrow *et al.* 1990, Zappella 1990).

TUBEROUS SCLEROSIS
(see also Chapter 4)

The triad of mental retardation, epilepsy and adenoma sebaceum (the typical skin rash that appears in many severely affected cases, at least before adolescence) is diagnostic. In recent years it has been discovered that most patients with tuberous sclerosis presenting with major symptoms before age 2 years have autism or autistic features with severe hyperactivity (Hunt and Dennis 1987). The triad of mental retardation, epilepsy and autism—rather than the classic triad—is a clinical warning that the underlying cause might be tuberous sclerosis.

At least half of all children with tuberous sclerosis diagnosed before age 3 years have autism. In the remaining cases, autistic features and hyperactivity are common. The reason for the link between tuberous sclerosis and autism/hyperactivity remains obscure. It appears that there may be two or more forms of tuberous sclerosis: two definite loci have been identified on chromosomes 9 and 16. The possibility of a gene defect close to loci for enzymes which are important in dopamine metabolism has led to increased interest in the hypothesis that the connection between autism and tuberous sclerosis may be a genomic change involving both the 'pure' tuberous sclerosis gene and neighbouring dopamine genes (which might be involved in the pathogenesis of autism).

Autism and hyperactivity in tuberous sclerosis are almost invariably connected with epilepsy, which is often hard to treat. Unfortunately, both the autism and hyperactivity may also be difficult to treat.

WILLIAMS SYNDROME

Williams syndrome consists of feeding problems, transient hypercalciuria, a specific abnormality of the face, facial skeleton and skull ('elfin facies'), and variable stenosis of large blood vessels (particularly the aorta). The pathogenesis and the neurological and other physical features of this syndrome have been briefly described in Chapter 5. The disorder, in typical cases, is associated with a defective elastine gene, located on chromosome 7.

EMOTIONAL AND BEHAVIOURAL FEATURES
In studies by Udwin *et al.* (1987) and Udwin (1990), a possibly specific behavioural phenotype has been identified in Williams syndrome. In the first two years of life there is often a considerable feeding problem, and the child may seem fussy and could have a sleep problem. Subsequently, overall development is slow. Some children with Williams syndrome show autistic-type behaviour up to about age 5 years. A few of these fulfil criteria for autistic disorder/infantile autism, but most later show more normal social and communication abilities. By age 6 years the typical Williams syndrome behavioural/emotional profile is usually present. Intellectual level is usually in the mildly to moderately retarded range, but a few patients have severe/profound mental retardation and even fewer have low-normal levels of intelligence. Superficial language capacities are usually relatively good, and the most typical feature is the way the affected individual will approach other people to make superficial conversation in a seemingly happy-go-lucky manner. Questions may be asked in a highly repetitive manner, but with a social amiability such that most people will not, at first, feel pestered by their monotony. Usually

TABLE 29.2
Behavioural and emotional problems in Williams syndrome*

Feature	% children	% adults
Solitary	84	71
Worried	71	88
Irritable	68	67
Over-friendly with strangers	64	73
Fearful	64	73
Temper tantrums	61	47
Disobedient	59	34
Eating difficulties	57	45
Obsessive/preoccupations	52	82
Incessant chatter	48	58
Destructive	48	25
Fights	48	20
Excessive use of social phrases/clichés	46	51
Sleeping difficulties	46	40
Complains of aches and pains	39	67
Fussy	39	40
Fear of heights and uneven surfaces	25	33
Cannot manage money	—	94
Cannot settle	—	77
Restless	—	71

*Adapted from Udwin (1990).

underlying this superficial sociability is an anxious obsession and preoccupation with certain ideas and also an emotional problem bordering on a chronic anxiety state. There are generally severe problems with visual perception, but these may be effectively obscured by the talkativeness. Eventually, however, the learning problem becomes increasingly obvious.

COURSE AND OUTCOME OF BEHAVIOUR PROBLEMS
Udwin's studies of adults with Williams syndrome have demonstrated that many of the behavioural and emotional problems persist throughout childhood and adolescence into adult life. Table 29.2 outlines the frequency of various problems shown by children and adults with Williams syndrome.

TREATMENT
It is essential to provide parents with up-to-date information concerning the typical psychological problems shown by most (if not all) children with the syndrome. This will go a long way toward alleviating feelings parents may have of guilt and concern that they might have contributed to the development of a particular behavioural style.

Sleep and anxiety problems in affected children may sometimes require at least short-term pharmacological treatment. Benzodiazepines, which can cause aggressive behaviour and (rarely) addiction problems, should be used sparingly. A trial of clomipramine (10–75 mg/d at 12 years or younger, 25–150 mg/d in the teenage period) is sometimes helpful.

Educational measures of various kinds (including instructing the child/teenager that you cannot approach strangers in the street and immediately ask them a lot of questions) are in order. Placement in a class for the mentally retarded is often required. Teachers should be informed about all the behavioural/emotional aspects of Williams syndrome: this will often make life for the child, family and teacher much easier to cope with.

REFERENCES

Åkefeldt, A., Gillberg, C. (1991) 'Hypomelanosis of Ito in three cases with autism and autistic-like conditions.' *Developmental Medicine and Child Neurology*, **33**, 737–743.

—— —— Larsson, C. (1991) 'Prader–Willi syndrome in a Swedish rural county: epidemiological aspects.' *Developmental Medicine and Child Neurology*, **33**, 715–721.

—— Anvret, M., Grandell, U., *et al.* (1995) 'Parental exposure to hydrocarbons in Prader–Willi syndrome.' *Developmental Medicine and Child Neurology*, **37**, 1101–1109.

Angelman, H. (1965) '"Puppet children." A report on three cases.' *Developmental Medicine and Child Neurology*, **7**, 681–688.

Clarke, D.J., Waters, J., Corbett, J.A. (1989) 'Adults with Prader–Willi syndrome: abnormalities of sleep and behaviour.' *Journal of the Royal Society of Medicine*, **82**, 21–24.

Clayton-Smith, J. (1993) 'Clinical research on Angelman syndrome in the United Kingdom: observations on 82 affected individuals.' *American Journal of Medical Genetics*, **46**, 12–15.

Cole, T.R.P., Hughes, H.E. (1991) 'Autosomal dominant macrocephaly: benign familial macrocephaly or a new syndrome?' *American Journal of Medical Genetics*, **41**, 115–124.

Crandall, B.F., Carrel, R.E., Sparkes, R.S. (1972) 'Chromosome findings in 700 children referred to a psychiatric clinic.' *Journal of Pediatrics*, **80**, 62–68.

Finegan, J-A.K., Cole, T.R.P., Kingwell, E., *et al.* (1994) 'Language and behavior in children with Sotos syndrome.' *Journal of the American Academy of Child and Adolescent Psychiatry*, **33**, 1307–1315.

Finucane, B.M., Konar, D., Haas-Givler, B., *et al.* (1994) 'The spasmodic upper-body squeeze: a characteristic behavior in Smith–Magenis syndrome.' *Developmental Medicine and Child Neurology*, **36**, 78–83.

Gillberg, C. (1987) 'Kleine–Levin syndrome: unrecognized diagnosis in adolescent psychiatry.' *Journal of the American Academy of Child and Adolescent Psychiatry*, **26**, 793–794.

—— (1989) 'The borderland of autism and Rett syndrome: five case histories to highlight diagnostic difficulties.' *Journal of Autism and Developmental Disorders*, **19**, 545–559.

—— Steffenburg, S. (1989) 'Autistic behaviour in Moebius syndrome.' *Acta Paediatrica Scandinavica*, **78**, 314–316.

—— Persson, E., Grufman, M., Themnér, U. (1986) 'Psychiatric disorders in mildly and severely mentally retarded urban children and adolescents: epidemiological aspects.' *British Journal of Psychiatry*, **149**, 68–74.

—— Steffenburg, S., Wahlström, J., *et al.* (1991) 'Autism associated with marker chromosome.' *Journal of the American Academy of Child and Adolescent Psychiatry*, **30**, 489–494.

Hagberg, B. (1989) 'Rett syndrome: clinical peculiarities, diagnostic approach and possible cause.' *Pediatric Neurology*, **5**, 75–83.

—— Rasmussen, P. (1986) '"Forme fruste" of Rett syndrome—a case report.' *American Journal of Medical Genetics*, **24**, Suppl. 1, 175–181.

—— Skjeldal, O.H. (1994) 'Rett variants: a suggested model for inclusion criteria.' *Pediatric Neurology*, **11**, 5–11.

Hagerman, R.J. (1989) 'Chromosomes, genes and autism.' *In:* Gillberg, C. (Ed.) *Diagnosis and Treatment of Autism.* New York: Plenum Press, pp. 105–131.

Hunt, A., Dennis, J. (1987) 'Psychiatric disorder among children with tuberous sclerosis.' *Developmental Medicine and Child Neurology*, **29**, 190–198.

Linden, M.G., Bender, G.G., Harmon, R.J., *et al.* (1988) '47XXX: what is the prognosis?' *Pediatrics*, **82**, 619–630.

Lishman, W.A. (1978) *Organic Psychiatry. The Psychological Consequenses of Cerebral Disorder.* Oxford: Blackwell Scientific.

Morrow, J.D., Whitman, B.Y., Accardo, P.J. (1990) 'Autistic disorder in Sotos syndrome: a case report.' *European Journal of Pediatrics*, **149**, 567–569.

O'Brien, G., Yule, W. (Eds.) (1995) *Behavioural Phenotypes. Clinics in Developmental Medicine No. 138.* London: Mac Keith Press.

Percy, A., Gillberg, C., Hagberg, B., Witt-Engerström, I. (1990) 'Rett syndrome and the autistic disorders.' *Neurologic Clinics*, **8**, 659–676.

Reiss, A.L., Freund, L. (1990) 'Fragile X syndrome.' *Biological Psychiatry*, **27**, 223–240.

Råstam, M., Gillberg, C., Wahlström, J. (1991) 'Chromosomes in anorexia nervosa. A study of 47 cases including a population-based group: a research note.' *Journal of Child Psychology and Psychiatry*, **32**, 695–701.

Rett Syndrome Diagnostic Criteria Work Group (1988) 'Diagnostic criteria for Rett syndrome.' *Annals of Neurology*, **23**, 425–428.

Rogers, P.T., Coleman, M. (1992) *Medical Care in Down Syndrome.* New York: Marcel Dekker.

Schiavi, R.C., Theilgaard, A., Owen, D.R., White, D. (1988) 'Sex chromosome anomalies, hormones, and sexuality.' *Archives of General Psychiatry*, **45**, 19–24.

Skuse, D., James, R.S., Bishop, D.V., *et al.* (1997) 'Evidence from Turner syndrome of an imprinted X-linked locus affecting cognitive function.' *Nature*, **387**, 705–708.

Spiker, D. (1990) 'Early intervention from a developmental perspective.' *In:* Cicchetti, D., Beeghly, M. (Eds.) *Children with Down's Syndrome: a Developmental Perspective.* Cambridge: Cambridge University Press, pp. 424–448.

Steffenburg, S., Gillberg, C.L., Steffenburg, U., Kyllerman, M. (1996) 'Autism in Angelman syndrome: a population-based study.' *Pediatric Neurology*, **14**, 131–136.

Swillen, A., Fryns, J.P., Kleczkowska, A., *et al.* (1993) 'Intelligence, behaviour and psychosocial development in Turner syndrome. A cross-sectional study of 50 pre-adolescent and adolescent girls (4–20 years).' *Genetic Counseling*, **4**, 7–18.

Udwin, O. (1990) 'A survey of adults with Williams syndrome and idiopathic infantile hypercalcaemia.' *Developmental Medicine and Child Neurology*, **32**, 129–141.

—— Yule, W., Martin, N. (1987) 'Cognitive abilities and behavioural characteristics of children with idiophathic hypercalcaemia.' *Journal of Child Psychology and Psychiatry*, **2**, 297–309.

Witt-Engerström, I., Gillberg, C. (1987) 'Rett syndrome in Sweden.' *Journal of Autism and Developmental Disorders*, **17**, 149–150. *(Letter.)*

Zappella, M. (1990) 'Autistic features in children affected by cerebral gigantism.' *Brain Dysfunction*, **3**, 241–244.

—— (1992) 'Hypomelanosis of Ito is common in autistic syndromes.' *European Child and Adolescent Psychiatry*, **1**, 170–177.

—— Genazzani, A., Facchinetti, F., Hayek, G. (1990) 'Bromocriptine in the Rett syndrome.' *Brain and Development*, **12**, 221–225.

—— Gillberg, C., Ehlers, S. (1998) 'The preserved speech variant: a subgroup of the Rett complex. A clinical report of 30 cases.' *Journal of Autism and Developmental Disorders. (In press.)*

30

PSYCHIATRIC AND BEHAVIOURAL PROBLEMS IN EPILEPSY, HYDROCEPHALUS AND CEREBRAL PALSY

Psychiatric, behavioural and emotional problems in children with various neurological disorders constitute a neglected area from the point of view of systematic scientific study. In spite of the fact that behavioural and emotional problems are often extremely frustrating for families of children with neurological disorder, very little is in fact known about epidemiology or transactional chains of events in pathogenesis and intervention.

EPILEPSY

According to the Isle of Wight study, uncomplicated epilepsy carries a four-fold increase in the risk that the child will also have psychiatric problems: almost 30 per cent of 10- and 11-year-old children with uncomplicated epilepsy and 60 per cent with epilepsy accompanying other neurological disorders had psychiatric problems (Rutter *et al.* 1970). The latter represented a prevalence rate almost 10 times that found in the general population of the Isle of Wight. Only children with DAMP (see Chapter 27) have severe psychiatric problems at an equally high rate (Gillberg 1983).

The reasons for psychiatric disorder in epilepsy are manifold and include abnormal brain activity, the influence of various drugs, and environmental and social factors. The location of the brain dysfunction causing epilepsy is important in determining the type and degree of problems encountered. Temporal lobe dysfunction (as in complex partial seizures) tends to carry a particularly high risk for certain types of severe psychiatric problems (Taylor 1975, Lindsay *et al.* 1979). Many antiepileptic drugs can contribute to behavioural problems (Gillberg 1991). Social factors, especially stigmatization associated with prejudice and ignorance, contribute most to the development of emotional problems in epilepsy (Herrington 1969).

PSYCHIATRIC DISORDER ASSOCIATED WITH EPILEPSY

Any kind of psychiatric problem can coexist with epilepsy and

be either related (most likely) or unrelated to it. Hyperkinetic syndromes, rage and 'psychosis' are relatively common complications of temporal lobe seizures. Autistic-type behaviours are very frequent in epilepsy associated with mental retardation.

In one large British series, hyperkinetic syndrome was present in 30 per cent of complex partial seizure patients followed through childhood to adult age (Lindsay *et al.* 1979). It was particularly common in males whose medical history showed a clear insult to the brain and a very early onset of seizures. Hyperkinetic syndromes tended to be associated with relatively low IQ (median 70), and the social outcome in adult life was relatively poor. Hyperkinetic syndromes may now be less common among children with complex partial seizures, partly because of the less widespread use of drugs that can induce it (particularly phenobarbitone, primidone and some of the benzodiazepines).

Rage was also a common phenomenon in the British follow-up study, affecting about 40 per cent of the whole group, with a poor prognosis with regard to social adjustment and development of adult psychiatric disorder. Girls with rage had very low IQ levels, whereas most boys functioned in the normal IQ range.

About 10 per cent of the group with complex partial seizures had developed psychosis (often of a schizophrenic character) in early adult life. Almost all these patients were male, had not shown early remission and were still on anticonvulsants. In no case did the EEG show a right-sided focus, and there was a tendency for left-sided foci to be very common.

There may be two further psychiatric subgroups of people with temporal lobe seizures (most likely overlapping with some of the subgroups already described). Children with autism seem to show a very high risk of developing complex partial seizures (Gillberg 1991). Whether or not there is also a high rate of autism or autistic-like problems in complex partial seizures generally remains to be investigated. A study of all children in one geographical area who had the combination of epilepsy and mental retardation revealed a strong relationship between complex partial seizures and autistic disorder/atypical autism (Steffenburg *et al.*

1996). Obsessive–compulsive features in relation to such seizures have not been systematically examined, but clinical experience suggests that they may be relatively more common than in the general population (D. Taylor, personal communication 1996).

In other types of seizures, the evidence for a connection with specific emotional and behavioural problems is very limited. Autistic symptoms may accompany childhood absence epilepsy (Gillberg and Schaumann 1983), juvenile myoclonic epilepsy and infantile spasms (Gillberg and Coleman 1992). Childhood absence epilepsy is a rare but important underlying problem in certain cases of DAMP. Because of the strong association of certain seizure types with mental retardation, there is also an especially strong correlation between such seizures and psychiatric disorder.

ANTICONVULSANT DRUGS

Anticonvulsants constitute a major psychiatric risk for some children with epilepsy. Phenobarbitone and phenytoin both very often cause somnolence, irritability, restlessness, hyperactivity, rage and decreased learning. Similar symptoms, sometimes even more dramatic, have been noted with the benzodiazepines. Clonazepam appears to have a particularly deleterious effect in the treatment of early childhood epilepsies in which behaviour problems are already associated at the time of commencing treatment, and major psychotic/autistic symptoms may develop (Gillberg 1991). Withdrawal of the drug can occasionally lead to complete remission of such symptoms without increasing the seizure rate. Carbamazepine and valproic acid can also cause psychic reactions (including increased compulsiveness and, in exceptional cases, psychosis), but probably at much lower rates (Gualtieri *et al.* 1987). However, both these drugs have also been reported to have some genuinely positive effects on psychic functions (Gualtieri *et al.* 1987).

PSYCHOSOCIAL FACTORS IN EPILEPSY

The dramatic psychological effects that seeing a child have a major seizure might have on parents, siblings, friends, peers, teachers and others can generate transactional effects which may lead to stigmatization of the child. Most parents seeing their child have a first major convulsion feel convinced that the child is going to die. These almost inevitable psychological consequences need to be dealt with in a tactful and neutral way by the child's doctor. Lack of education about the condition is one reason for the stigmatization so often associated with epilepsy, and educative measures aimed at decreasing such ignorance are important in any treatment plan for childhood epilepsy. In the eyes of uneducated observers, the child with seizures often appears to have 'gone mad'. The mechanisms underlying this 'madness' should be explained to those involved in interactions with the child, so that the strange behaviour does not take on mythical implications.

TREATMENT OF PSYCHIATRIC PROBLEMS IN EPILEPSY

Planning treatment of psychiatric problems in epilepsy involves (1) analysing the various factors that contribute to the psychiatric disorder (the epilepsy itself, the type of associated brain damage/dysfunction, the effects of drug treatment, constitutional factors related or unrelated to the epilepsy and various psychosocial factors), and (2) determining which type of problem (the epilepsy or the psychiatric disorder) is currently having the most negative impact on the child and family. The doctor in charge will then have to discuss the various treatment options at some length with the parents, and sometimes with the patient, depending on developmental level.

No detailed guidelines have yet been published. The management of psychiatric problems in childhood epilepsy constitutes a very delicate balance between environmental measures, education, drugs, and, in treatment-resistant epilepsy, surgery. A neuropsychiatrist well acquainted with epilepsy must be an integral part of the team in charge of treatment of children with epilepsy. In the past, too many children with epilepsy received only drug treatment and diets, and their seizure frequency was used as the only measure of outcome without due attention being paid to behaviour and emotion. Behavioural problems, once the seizure disorder has become less psychologically dramatic to people in the child's environment, are often considered by the parents and teachers as more difficult to cope with than the epilepsy itself. Alleviating some of the psychiatric problems may reduce the frequency and severity of fits.

Finally it should be stressed that children with treatment-resistant epilepsy elected for surgical treatment should receive neuropsychiatric (and not only neuropsychological) assessments before and a year after surgery at the very least. Outcome after surgical interventions can never be comprehensively evaluated unless there is a full appreciation of the neuropsychiatric problems associated with the epilepsy.

HYDROCEPHALUS

In the presurgical treatment days of infantile hydrocephalus, major neurological impairment was often so debilitating as to preclude the study of psychiatric problems.

In a Swedish study of a population-based group of subjects with surgically treated infantile hydrocephalus, behavioural problems and autistic symptoms were found to be common (Fernell *et al.* 1991a,b). About a quarter of all children with hydrocephalus had developed many autistic features by the time they reached school age. Hyperactivity problems and restlessness, often associated with DAMP problems, were also frequent. Autistic features, or full-blown autism, which was present in 5 per cent of all children with infantile hydrocephalus, were associated with severe mental retardation and severe brain damage. Other behavioural problems were associated generally with low IQ scores. Children with hydrocephalus who did not have a learning disorder did not appear to be at increased risk of psychiatric disturbance. Self-esteem was somewhat lower than in children in general.

CEREBRAL PALSY

Cerebral palsy (CP) is accompanied by an increased rate of

psychiatric problems at about the same level as or slightly higher than that seen in uncomplicated epilepsy. Psychiatric disorders in CP fall into several categories. Some of the conditions encountered are secondary to the physical disability, *i.e.* adjustment disorder. In addition, major psychiatric disorder may occur as a comorbid problem in CP.

In severe forms of CP, such as spastic tetraplegia, indirect evidence suggests that the triad of autistic impairments (Chapter 26) may be frequent (Wing and Gould 1979, Edebol-Tysk 1989, Nordin *et al.* 1998). If upheld in other systematic studies, this could be taken to reflect the underlying severe widespread damage not only to high cortical brain areas but to lower centres also.

In milder forms of CP, clinical experience suggests that more common types of psychiatric problems may be prevalent. Emotional disorders, including anxiety states, are not uncommon in CP but since such problems are also common in the general population of children, it is difficult to decide whether they are more (or less) common in CP.

Individuals with CP are sometimes emotionally labile, irritable, have attention deficits, are often impulsive and may have limited social problem-solving skills (Breslau 1990). Depressive symptoms and inattention tend to be particularly common (Breslau 1990, Goodman and Alberman 1996).

There are some case reports in the literature (*e.g.* Gillberg 1989) of Asperger syndrome associated with mild CP (hemiplegia, diplegia and ataxia). In the author's experience, Asperger syndrome and other autism spectrum problems tend to be more often associated with left-sided hemiplegia (which in turn may be associated with right hemisphere damage and a 'nonverbal learning disability'). This association could represent clues to the underlying brain dysfunction in Asperger syndrome. Treatment in such cases should be along lines suggested both for the CP problems and for the Asperger-related problems.

Psychosis (affective disorders and schizophrenia) occurs in CP and should be managed along the same lines as psychosis in the non-cerebral-palsied population.

REFERENCES

Breslau, N. (1990) 'Does brain dysfunction increase children's vulnerability to environmental stress?' *Archives of General Psychiatry*, **47**, 15–20.

Edebol-Tysk, K. (1989) 'Spastic tetraplegic cerebral palsy.' MD thesis, University of Göteborg.

Fernell, E., Gillberg, C., von Wendt, L. (1991a) 'Autistic symptoms in children with infantile hydrocephalus.' *Acta Paediatrica Scandinavica*, **80**, 451–457.

—— —— —— (1991b) 'Behavioural problems in children with infantile hydrocephalus.' *Developmental Medicine and Child Neurology*, **33**, 388–395.

Gillberg, C. (1983) 'Perceptual, motor and attentional deficits in Swedish primary school children. Some child psychiatric aspects.' *Journal of Child Psychology and Psychiatry*, **24**, 377–403.

—— (1989) 'Asperger syndrome in 23 Swedish children.' *Developmental Medicine and Child Neurology*, **31**, 520–531.

—— (1991) 'The treatment of epilepsy in autism.' *Journal of Autism and Developmental Disorders*, **21**, 61–77.

—— Coleman, M. (1992) *The Biology of the Autistic Syndromes, 2nd Edn. Clinics in Developmental Medicine No. 126.* London: Mac Keith Press.

—— Schaumann, H. (1983) 'Epilepsy presenting as infantile autism? Two case studies.' *Neuropediatrics*, **14**, 206–212.

Goodman, R., Alberman, E. (1996) 'A twin study of congenital hemiplegia.' *Developmental Medicine and Child Neurology*, **38**, 3–12.

Gualtieri, T., Evans, R.W., Patterson, D.R. (1987) 'The medical treatment of autistic people: problems and side-effects.' *In:* Schopler, E., Mesibov, G.B. (Eds.) *Neurobiological Issues in Autism.* New York: Plenum Press, pp. 374–388.

Herrington, C.R. (Ed.) (1969) *Current Problems in Neuropsychiatry. British Journal of Psychiatry, Special Publication No. 4.* Ashford, Kent: Hedley, for the Royal Medico-Psychological Association.

Lindsay, J., Ounsted, C., Richards, P. (1979) 'Long-term outcome in children with temporal lobe seizures. III: Psychiatrics aspects in childhood and adult life.' *Developmental Medicine and Child Neurology*, **21**, 630–636.

Nordin, V., Nydén, A., Gillberg, C. (1998) 'The Swedish Childhood Autism Rating Scale in a clinical setting.' *Journal of Autism and Developmental Disorders. (In press.)*

Rutter, M., Graham, P., Yule, W. (1970) *A Neuropsychiatric Study in Childhood. Clinics in Developmental Medicine No. 35/36.* London: Spastics International Medical Publications.

Steffenburg, S., Gillberg, C., Steffenburg, U. (1996) 'Psychiatric disorders in children and adolescents with mental retardation and active epilepsy.' *Archives of Neurology*, **53**, 904–912.

Taylor, D. (1975) 'Factors influencing the occurrence of schizophrenia-like psychosis in patients with temporal lobe epilepsy.' *Psychological Medicine*, **5**, 249–254.

Wing, L., Gould, J. (1979) 'Severe impairments of social interaction and associated abnormalities in children: epidemiology and classification.' *Journal of Autism and Developmental Disorders*, **9**, 11–29.

INDEX

Antiepileptic drugs, *see* Epilepsy, drug treatment
Antiphospholipid antibodies, 439, 440, 554
   cerebral vein thrombosis, 559
Antiphospholipid syndrome, primary, 554
Antituberculous chemotherapy, 390
Anxiety, chronic, 643
Apert syndrome, 176, 177 *(fig.)*
Apgar score
   cerebral palsy, 211–212
   hypoxic–ischaemic encephalopathy, 43, 44, 47
Aphasia, acquired, 603
Apnoea
   alternating hemiplegia, 653
   awake, 641, 656
   causes, 642 *(table)*
   central, 655
   mixed, 655
   obstructive, 655–656
   sleep, 655–656
Apnoeic–bradycardic episodes, 641
Apoptosis
   cortical microdysgenesis, 107
   focal cortical dysplasia, 105
Aprosencephaly, 74
Aqueductal stenosis
   infantile hydrocephalus, 193–194
   X-linked, 165
Arachnia spp., 390
Arachnoid cysts, 516–517
   of cerebellopontine angle, 499
   of incisura, 518
   infratentorial, 518
   neurofibromatosis type 1, 136
   spinal, 525
Arbovirus, encephalitis, 403–404
Arena virus, 398
Arginase deficiency, 284
Argininosuccinic aciduria, 284
Argyll Robertson pupil, 683–684
Arhinencephaly without holoprosencephaly, 89
Arsenic poisoning, 481
Arterial hypertension, neurological complications, 560
Arterial infarction, clonic seizures, 609
Arterial occlusive disorders, 547–549, 550 *(fig.)*, 551–559
   angiography, 551
   cardiac disorders, 556
   causes, 552–553 *(table)*, 554–558
   clinical features, 548–549, 550 *(fig.)*, 551
   differential diagnosis, 551–552
   fibromuscular dysplasia, 556
   imaging, 549, 550 *(fig.)*, 551
   lacunar infarcts, 549, 551
   mechanisms, 547–548
   moyamoya disease, 554–556
   outcome, 552–553
   pathology, 547–548
   posterior circulation, 549
   prognosis, 552–553
   radiological features, 548–549, 551
   syndromes, 548 *(table)*
   therapy, 552–553
   traumatic hemiplegia, 558
   vertebrobasilar, 549
   see also Sickle-cell disease; Vasculitides; Vasculitis
Arterial wall dissection, 554

Arteriovenous malformations, 534–538
   aneurysm of vein of Galen, 537–538
   arteriovenous fistula, 534
   clinical signs, 535
   dural, 537
   embolization, 536
   epilepsy, 536
   haemorrhage, 534, 536
   imaging, 535–536
   internal carotid–cavernous, 537
   pial, 534–536
   rebleeding risk, 536
   of the vein of Galen causing hydrocephalus, 196–197
Arthritis, chronic, 394
Arthrochalasis multiplex congenita, 697
Arthrogryposis, 735
   multiplex congenita, 774–776
   neonatal myasthenic, 779–780
Arylsulfatase deficiency, 251, 324
Aspartylglucosaminidase deficiency, 255–256
Aspartylglucosaminuria, 255–256
Asperger syndrome, 819–820, 836, 837 *(table)*, 838–839
   cerebral palsy, 867
   diagnosis, 836, 837 *(table)*, 838
   epidemiology, 838
   language, 838
   outcome, 839
   pitch abnormalities of speech, 851
   social interaction, 838
   theory of mind, 838
   treatment, 838–839
Asperger trait, 830
Aspergillosis, 419
Aspergillus flavus toxin in Reye syndrome, 408
Aspergillus fumigatus, 804
Asphyxia
   acute total, 40–41
   hypoxic–ischaemic encephalopathy, 39
   peri-intraventricular haemorrhage, 36
   prolonged partial, 41
Ataxia
   autosomal dominant cerebellar (ADCA), 352–353
   autosomal dominant periodic cerebello-vestibular, 644, 645 *(table)*
   cerebellovestibular, 644, 645 *(table)*
   congenital and cerebellar atrophies, 353 *(table)*
   familial
      recurrent, 644
      spastic, 351
   intermittent, 644 *(table)*
   recurrent, 644, 694
   spastic, 351 *(table)*
   see also Spinocerebellar ataxia
Ataxia–deafness–retardation syndrome, 691
Ataxia–ocular motor apraxia, 142, 350, 352, 673
Ataxia–telangiectasia, 140–143, 491
   atypical forms, 142
   clinical features, 141
   course, 141–142
   diagnosis, 142
   gene, 140–141
   infection sensitivity, 141
   laboratory markers, 142
   management, 142–143

   mechanisms, 141
   neurological findings, 141
   pathology, 141
   prognosis, 141–142
   telangiectasias, 141
   variant forms, 142
Ataxic diplegia, 210, 212
Atelencephaly, 74
Atlantoaxial dislocation, 180, 181
Atlantoaxial instability in Down syndrome, 474
ATP-synthase subunit c, 330
ATPase 6 gene, 417
Attention deficit disorder, 345, 843, 845 *(fig.)*
Attention deficit–hyperactivity disorder (ADHD), 817, 843–844, 845 *(fig.)*
   comorbid problems with DAMP, 847–848
   concept validity, 843–844
   epidemiology, 843
   Sotos syndrome, 862
Attention deficits, 843
Auditory brainstem potentials, hydrocephalus, 198
Auditory dysfunction, 689
Auriculofacial syndromes, 690
Auriculotemporal syndrome, 737
   isolated, 736
Austin disease, *see* Mucosulfatidosis
Autism, 819–820, 827–828, 829 *(table)*, 830–836
   adults, 835–836
   aetiology, 830–831
   atypical, 836
   behavioural phenotype, 857
   central coherence, 818, 828, 830
   definitions, 827
   deterioration, 835
   diagnosis, 834
   diagnostic criteria, 829 *(table)*
   diet-based treatment, 833
   dopamine system, 831
   Down syndrome, 857
   education, 833, 834–835
   epilepsy, 865
   evaluation questionnaires, 832–833
   executive function, 828, 830
   eye-direction detector, 818
   family support, 834
   fragile X syndrome, 828
   genetic factors, 830
   hearing deficit, 828
   home-based treatment, 834
   hydrocephalus, 866
   infantile, 827
      with presence of succinylpurines in body fluids, 308
   IQ, 819
   Kanner, 827
   laboratory studies, 832 *(table)*
   language, 828, 835
   medical work-up, 831
   mental retardation, 825, 828
   mentalizing, 828
   minimal brain dysfunction syndromes, 843
   Moebius syndrome, 828
   neurofibromatosis, 828
   neuropsychiatric work-up, 831–833
   outcome, 835–836
   pathogenic chain of events, 830–831
   pharmacotherapy, 833–834

phenylketonuria, 833
physical exercise, 834
pitch abnormalities of speech, 851
prevalence, 828
psychotherapy, 834
retinopathy of prematurity, 828
Rett syndrome, 828
seizures, 828
sex ratio, 828
social cognism, 828, 830
speech, 828
symptom changes, 836
theory of mind, 828
treatment facilities, 835
tuberous sclerosis, 828, 863
visual defects, 828
Autistic features
hydrocephalus, 866
Rett syndrome, 860
Autistic impairment triad, cerebral palsy, 867
Autistic syndromes, 827
Autistic traits, 836
ADHD and DAMP, 847, 848
Autistic-like conditions, 836
Autosomal dominant cerebellar ataxia (ADCA),
352–353
Awake apnoea syndrome, 641, 656
Axonal development, 72
disorders, 356
Axonal neuropathy, 712

B
Babinski sign, congenital hemiplegia, 215
Bacillus spp., 385
Baclofen, cerebral palsy, 232
Bacterial endocarditis, 802
Bacterial infection
deafness, 692
hydrocephalus, 196
neonatal, 56
nonsuppurative, 393–395
vestibular system dysfunction, 693
Bacterial myositis, 773
Bacteroides, cerebral abscess, 391
Ballismus, paroxysmal, 646
Baló concentric sclerosis, 446
Barbiturates, 478
Basal ganglia
calcification, 340, 342, 343 *(table)*, 344, 514
haemorrhage, 468
haemorrhagic necrosis, 34
lesions in hypoxic–ischaemic encephalo-
pathy, 42–43, 47
lucencies, 341 *(table)*
tumours, 511–512
Basilar impression, 179, 180
Basket brain, 110
Bassen–Kornzweig disease, *see* Abetalipoprotein-
aemia
Batten disease, *see* Ceroid–lipofuscinosis
BCG vaccination, 387
Becker disease, 763
Behaviour in autism, 827
Behavioural problems
cerebral palsy, 233
epilepsy, 614
Behçet disease, midbrain mass, 500
Behçet syndrome, 416
Behr syndrome, 352, 678

Bell palsy, 736–737, 738
facial nerve paralysis, 737
Benzodiazepines, teratogenicity, 20
Beriberi, 797
Beta-galactocerebrosidase, 251
Beta-galactosidase deficiency, 248, 255
Beta-glucocerebrosidase deficiency, 247 *(fig.)*,
248
Bethlem myopathy, 756
Bickers–Adams syndrome, 193, 194
Bifrontal dysgenesis, 103
Biliary disease, 798
Bilirubin
kernicterus, 49, 50 *(fig.)*, 51
staining, 49
Biochemical abnormality diagnosis, 5
Biopterin synthesis, 278
Biotin metabolism, 285–286
Biotinidase deficiency, 285
Bladder, neuropathic, 233
Blalock–Taussig type anastomoses, 542
Blastopathies, 72–87, 88 *(fig.)*, 89
Blind-loop syndrome, 798
Blindness, 675
acquired cortical, 683
acute bacterial meningitis, 378–379
causes, 676 *(table)*
congenital, 676–679
cortical, 675
neurological manifestations, 676
post-traumatic, 463
see also Visual impairment; Visual loss; Visual
perception disorders
Blink response, 675
Bloch–Schulzberger syndrome, 145
Blood disease, fetal, 23
Blood flow
head injury, 461
uterine, 13
Blood flow velocity
hydrocephalus, 198
peri-intraventricular haemorrhage, 36
Blood transfusion, fetal, 14
Blood–brain barrier disturbance, 561
Bobble-head doll syndrome, 191, 518
Bonding, impaired, 471
Bone disorders, 807–808
Bone marrow transplantation, 807
Bordetella pertussis, 422
encephalitis, 398
Bornholm disease, 397, 773
Borrelia burgdorferi, 12, 393, 394, 737
Borreliosis, 393–394, 737
paralysis following tick bite, 730
Botulinum toxin
cerebral palsy, 232
dystonia, 339
Botulism, 421–422
Bovine spongiform encephalopathy, 413
Brachial neuropathy, painful, 730
Brachial plexopathy, 717, 730
Brachial plexus injury, 58, 731–732
Brachman–de Lange syndrome, 161
Brain
abscess
acute bacterial meningitis, 378, 384
congenital heart disease, 801
see also Cerebral abscess
atrophy in hydrocephalus, 199

basket, 110
blood supply in fetus, 13
death, 475
dysgenesis and infantile spasms, 583
dysplasia and neonatal seizures, 610
malformations
cerebral palsy, 211
tetraplegia, 220
microabscesses with *Candida* infection, 418
swelling in head injury, 463
weight of infant, 795
Brain damage
contusion, 461
acute subdural haematoma, 467
epilepsy, 613
fetal, 6
head trauma, 460, 461
hypoxic–ischaemic, 48
ischaemic, 461
laceration, 461
shearing injury, 461
Brain oedema
cytotoxic, 520
hydrostatic, 520–521
hypoosmotic, 520
interstitial, 521
intramyelinic, 521
vasogenic, 520
Brainstem
auditory evoked potentials, 690
Leigh syndrome, 295
demyelination, 514
displacement, 494
dysfunction, 494
encephalitis, 409
glioma, 499, 500
haemorrhage, 34
hypoxic–ischaemic encephalopathy, 47
primary injury, 461
signs, 464
tetraplegia, 220
tumours, 499–500
diagnosis, 500
neurofibromatosis type 1, 134
Brain tumours
aetiology, 491–492
base of brain, 500–507
brain movement, 494
cerebellar, 498, 499
cerebral hemisphere, 507–512
chemotherapy, 496
classification, 493
clinical manifestations, 493–495
diagnosis, 495
epilepsy, 613
focal features, 495
fourth ventricle, 499
frequency, 491–492
histology, 494 *(table)*
imaging, 495
immunotherapy, 496
infants, 512
infratentorial, 491
intracranial hypertension, 493–495
location, 494 *(table)*
lumbar puncture, 495
metastases, 493
extracranial tumours, 510
midline, 500–507

Diphtheria–tetanus–pertussis (DTP) vaccine, 452–453
Diplegia
  ataxic, 217, 220
  spastic, 217–220
    aetiology, 217
    clinical features, 218–219
    differential diagnosis, 219–220
    imaging, 218
    pathology, 217–218
    prenatal factors, 217
    preterm infants, 219
Diplomyelia, 83
Disc herniation, sciatic neuralgia, 732
Disc space infection/inflammation, 393
Discitis, 393
Disialotransferrin developmental deficiency, 256
Distal axial palmar triradius, 166
DMD gene, 750, 752
DNA
  analysis, 5
  repair disorders, 309
Dolicocephaly, 93
Dopamine dysfunction, Tourette syndrome, 853
Dopamine system, autism, 831
Dorsal dermal sinus, 81, 82
Dorsal rhizotomy, cerebral palsy, 231–232
Double-ring sign, 677
Down syndrome, 154–156
  Alzheimer-type dementia, 826
  atlantoaxial dislocation, 181
  atlantoaxial instability, 474
  autism, 857
  basal ganglia calcification, 344
  circle of Willis obstruction, 555
  clinical features, 155
  diagnosis, 155–156
  distal axial palmar triradius, 166
  dysmorphisms, 155
  facies, 155 (fig.)
  hypotonia, 697
  ligamentous hyperlaxity, 180
  management, 155–156
  mental retardation, 824, 825
  neuropsychiatric syndromes, 857
  odontoid process hypoplasia, 179–180
  pathology, 154–155
  prenatal screening, 155–156
  recurrence rate, 154
  translocations, 154
Drepanocytosis, see Sickle-cell disease
Dromoic acid, 479
Drowning, prevention, 476
Drugs, prescription, 478
Duane syndrome, 670
Duchenne muscular dystrophy, 750–753
  carriers, 750
  clinical features, 751–753
  diagnosis, 752
  disease duration, 752
  gene deletion, 750–751
  gene therapy, 753
  inheritance, 750
  intellectual impairment, 751–752
  muscle weakness, 751
  patient management, 752–753
  prenatal diagnosis, 752
Duchenne–Erb palsy, 731
Dural sinus thrombosis, 559

Dwarfism
  deprivation, 796
  thanatophoric, 102
Dying back neuropathy, 713 (fig.)
Dysautonomia, familial, 719–720
Dyscalculia, 849–850
Dysequilibrium syndrome, 223, 225
  dialysis, 803
  hypoosmotic oedema, 520
Dysequilibrium–diplegia syndrome, 142, 308, 415
Dysgammaglobulinaemia, 142
Dysgraphia, 849–850
Dyskinesia
  choreoathetotic, 801
  hypnogenic, 645
  nonkinesigenic, 645
  paroxysmal
    intermediate, 646
    kinesigenic, 645
  transient cerebral ischaemia, 647
  volitional, 469
Dyslexia, 843, 849–850
Dysmorphic syndromes
  Angelman syndrome, 158–160
  with CNS involvement, 159 (table), 161–163
  minor morphological anomalies, 165–166
Dysphagia, congenital, 738
Dysraphism, 73
  cranial, 74–76
  spinal, 76–85
    developmental abnormalities, 85–87
    occult, 85
    spina bifida occulta, 81–85
Dystonia, 337–340
  atypical, 340
  classical torsion, 337–339
    differential diagnosis, 338
    late-onset, 338
    therapy, 339
    variants, 338
  dopa-responsive/sensitive, 339–340
  drug-induced, 338
  dyskinetic cerebral palsy, 221, 223
  hereditary progressive with marked diurnal fluctuations, 339–340
  musculorum deformans, 337–339
  myoclonic, 340
    alcohol-sensitive, 340
  optic atrophy, 682
  parkinsonism, 340
  paroxysmal, 654
    of infancy, 646
    nocturnal, 646, 655
    symptomatic, 646
  progressive with bilateral putaminal hypo-densities, 340
  secondary, 338 (table)
  transient, 212, 219, 338
Dystonic chondrodystrophy, see Schwartz–Jampel syndrome
Dystonic lipidosis, juvenile, 303
Dystrophia myotonica, 761–763
Dystrophin, 751
  deletion in nonprogressive X-linked myopathy, 766
  testing, 752
DYT-1 gene, 340

E
Ear defects, 690
Early infantile epileptic encephalopathy, 584, 585
Echinococcosis, 420
Echovirus, 57, 397
  acute focal encephalitis, 416
Ecstasy (MDMA), 794
Edrophonium chloride (Tensilon) test, 777
Education
  autism, 833, 834–835
  cerebral palsy, 228
  DAMP, 848
  epilepsy, 613–614
  mental retardation, 826
  Williams syndrome, 863–864
Edwards syndrome, 156
Ehlers–Danlos syndrome, 697
Ekbom syndrome, 347
Elastin gene disruption, 160
Electrical injuries, 477
Electroencephalography (EEG) in epilepsy, 610–611
Electrolyte metabolism
  disorders, 793–798
  neonatal disturbance, 52–53
Elsberg syndrome, 730
Embolism, 548
Embryo
  circulatory disorders, 12
  infectious diseases, 6–12
Empathy, 819
Empty sella syndrome, 518–519
Encephalitis, 398–409
  acute, 398–409
    focal, 416
  adenovirus subacute focal, 414
  aetiology, 398–399
  arbovirus, 403–404
  atypical, 401
  brain biopsy, 402, 403
  brainstem, 409
  cerebellar, 409
  chickenpox, 406
  chronic, 409–413
    with CSF pleocytosis, 411
    protracted of unknown origin, 411
  clinical signs, 399, 400–401
  CSF, 399, 402
  differential diagnosis, 399–400
  EEG, 401–402
  enterovirus, 403
  Epstein–Barr virus, 407
  herpes simplex virus, 57, 399, 400, 401, 402
    neuroimaging, 402 (fig.)
    treatment, 403
  imaging, 399, 402
  immunoallergic mechanism, 451
  influenza, 407
  lethargic, 417
  management, 400, 401 (table)
  measles, 404, 406
    delayed type acute, 413–414
  mumps, 409
  Mycoplasma pneumoniae, 394, 404
  paraneoplastic limbic, 402
  periaxialis diffusa, 445
  postinfectious, 399, 404–407
    clinical manifestations, 404, 405

Lymphomatoid granulomatosis, 448
Lymphoproliferative syndrome, X-linked, 414
Lymphoreticular malignancies, ataxia–telangi-
    ectasia, 142
Lysinuric protein intolerance, 282, 283, 284
Lysosomal acid lipase (LAL) deficiency, 303
Lysosomal diseases, 246–251, 252 (fig.), 253–
    254

M
Machado–Joseph disease, 353, 355
Macrocephaly, 91–92
    achondroplasia, 180
    causes, 92 (table)
    glutaric aciduria type I, 270
    hydrocephalus, 191
    hypomelanosis of Ito, 145
    infratentorial arachnoid cysts, 518
    neurofibromatosis type 1, 133
Macrocrania, facial naevi and anomalous venous
    return, 545–547
Magnesium
    deficiency and protein–calorie malnutrition,
        796
    malabsorption, 53
Major malformations, diagnosis, 5
Malaria, 419–420
    congenital, 12
Maleylacetoacetate, 266
Malignant hyperthermia, 765
    central core disease, 759
    chloride channel disease, 763
Mamillary bodies, subacute necrotizing enceph-
    alopathy, 293
Manganese poisoning, 481
Mannerisms, 647
Mannosidosis, 254
Maple syrup urine disease, 267, 268
    clinical features, 269
    diagnosis, 270
    pathogenesis, 269
Marasmus, 795–796
Marble bones–marble brain disease, 344
Marcus Gunn phenomenon, 670
Marfan syndrome, 540
Marijuana intoxication, 479
Marinesco–Sjögren syndrome, 226, 354, 757
Maroteaux–Lamy disease, 254
Martin–Bell syndrome, see Fragile X syndrome
MASA syndrome, 165, 194, 354
Mastoiditis, facial nerve paralysis, 737
Masturbation, 647
Maternal disorders, 3
May–White syndrome, 347
MCAD gene, 299
McArdle disease, 768
McCune–Albright syndrome, 178
McLeod syndrome, 752
Meadow syndrome, see Munchausen syndrome
    by proxy
Measles
    deafness, 692
    encephalitis, 404, 406
        delayed type, acute, 413–414
    immunization, 451
    leukaemia, opportunistic infections, 516
    optic neuritis, 446, 683
Meckel–Gruber syndrome, 76, 87, 190
Median cleft face syndromes, 89

Median nerve injury, 58
Medulloblastoma, 496–497
    outcome, 512
Megalencephalic leukodystrophies, 329
Megalencephaly, 92
    cryptogenic pericerebral collections, 205
    mechanisms, 92
Megaloblastic anaemia, 796
    folate metabolism defects, 288
Melanotic neuroectodermal tumour, 499
MELAS syndrome, 290, 291, 295–296, 650
    deafness, 692
    encephalitis, 402
Melioidosis, 385
Melkersson–Rosenthal syndrome, 737
Ménière disease, 694
Meningeal cyst
    infantile hydrocephalus, 194–195
    spinal, 525
Meningioma
    cerebellopontine angle, 499
    neurofibromatosis type 2, 136
Meningitis
    acute bacterial, 373–387
        adjuvant treatment, 381–382
        antibacterial chemotherapy, 379–381
        antibiotics, 385 (table)
        bacterial penetration, 374
        blindness, 378–379
        brain abscess, 378, 384
        brain swelling, 374
        clinical signs, 374
        complications, 376–378
        congenital dermal sinus, 385, 387
        convulsions, 382
        corticosteroid therapy, 381–382
        CSF examination, 374–375
        cytokines, 373, 374
        dermoid cyst, 386 (fig.)
        diagnosis, 375
        endotoxin, 373, 374
        epidemiology, 373
        fever, 378
        hydrocephalus, 374, 379, 381 (fig.)
        infants/children, 374–376
        intracranial hypertension, 377–378
        laboratory diagnosis, 374–376
        latex particle agglutination, 375
        lumbar puncture, 374, 375, 381, 383–
            384
        management, 379–383
        meningococcal infection, 382–383
        mental deficit, 379
        neuroimaging, 376
        neurological sequelae, 379
        newborn infants, 383–385
            clinical manifestations, 384
            diagnosis, 383
            lumbar puncture, 383–384
            outcome, 384
        onset, 374
        pathology, 373–374
        patients with shunt, 385
        pneumococcal, 377 (fig.), 380, 383
        puncture porencephaly, 381 (fig.)
        rare causes, 385
        recurrent, 385, 386 (table), 387
        seizures, 376
        sensorineural hearing loss, 378

        sequelae, 378–379
        spinal cord infarction, 376–377
        stages, 373
        staphylococcal, 383
        subdural effusion, 377, 382
        subdural empyema, 378
        supportive treatment, 381–382
        traumatic leaks, 385
        treatment monitoring, 381
        vasculitis, 376
        ventriculitis, 378, 381
        vessel involvement, 374
    aseptic, 393, 395, 396–398, 441–442
        chronic in HIV infection, 412
        immunization-induced, 453
        syndrome, 375, 376 (table)
    caseous, 387–388
    chemical, 196
    chronic, 390
        basilar, 555
        lymphocytic, 414
    coxsackie, 397
    Cryptococcus neoformans, 390
    deafness, 692
    echovirus, 397
    enteroviral, 397
    eosinophilic, 420, 516
    Epstein–Barr virus, 397–398
    granulomatous, 387–390
    herpes virus infection, 397
    hydrocephalus, 204
    Mollaret, 416–417
    pneumococcal, 383, 806
    poliovirus, 397
    purulent, 373, 693
    recurrent, 75
    shunt procedures, 201
    staphylococcal, 383
    streptococcal, 383, 384, 385
    subacute/chronic, 387–390
    subdural empyema, 392
    syphilitic, 12
    transient aseptic, 390
    tuberculous, 387–390
        clinical manifestations, 387–388
        CSF culture, 388
        diagnosis, 388–390
        imaging, 388, 389
        pathology, 387
        prognosis, 390
        spinal, 388
        treatment, 390
        vasculitis, 388
    varicella-zoster virus, 397
    viral, 395, 396–398
Meningoangiomatosis, 136
Meningocele, 77 (fig.), 81
    antenatal diagnosis, 74
    cranial, 75
Meningocerebral angiodysplasia, diffuse, 540
Meningoencephalitis, 57, 398–409
    immunodepressed children, 413–415
    postinfectious, 398
    viral, 390
Meningoencephalocele, 75
Menkes disease, 306, 307 (fig.), 308
Mental deficit, acute bacterial meningitis, 379
Mentalizing ability, 819
    autism, 828

congenital form, 762–763
diagnosis, 763
muscular atrophy, 762
neonatal, 55
treatment, 763

N

N-acetylaspartic acid, 272
N-acetylaspartic aciduria, *see* Canavan disease
N-acetylglutamate synthetase deficiency, 284
N-acetylaspartate (NAA), 612
NAD, 264
Naevoid basal cell carcinoma syndrome, 131, 147
Naevus
angiomatous, 542
linear, 143
verrucous, 143
NAIP gene deletion, 702
Narcolepsy, 656–657
Narcotic substances, 22
Near-drowning, 474, 476
Neck hyperextension, 57
Neck–tongue syndrome, 733
Necrotizing fasciitis, 557
Negri bodies, 403
Neisseria meningitidis, 373, 379, 380
meningococcal meningitis, 382–383
NEM1 gene, 760
Nemaline myopathy, 760
Nerve injuries, traumatic, 731–733
Nerve tumours, 733
Neural crest cells, developmental abnormality, 131
Neural plate formation, 70, 71 *(fig.)*
Neural tube closure, abnormal, 70
Neural tube defects, 4, 70, 73
viral infection, 6
Neural tube formation, caudal, disorders, 72–87, 88 *(fig.)*, 89
Neuralgia
migrainous, 651
occipital, 181, 733
Neuralgic amyotrophy, hereditary, 717
Neuraminidase deficiency, 255
Neurinoma of VIIIth cranial nerve, 499
Neuritis, optic, 444
Neuroaxonal dystrophy, 241, 333–334
Neuroblastoma
brain metastases, 510
cerebellar ataxia, 449
opsoclonus–myoclonus syndrome, 450
Neurobrucellosis, 390
Neurocutaneous melanosis, 146
Neurocutaneous syndromes, 131–147
abnormal pigmentation, 145–146
ataxia–telangiectasia, 140–143, 491
linear naevus syndrome, 93, 143, 145
neuroichthyosis syndromes, 146–147
with prominent vascular anomalies, 542–547
Sturge–Weber syndrome, 542–545
rare, 144 *(table)*
von Hippel–Lindau disease, 131, 140, 524, 547
Neurocysticercosis, 420
Neurodegenerative disorders, inherited with fetal onset, 19
Neurofibrin, 492

Neurofibromas
multiple, 132
neurofibromatosis type 5, 136
plexiform, 132–133
Neurofibromatosis, 93, 131, 131–137
autism, 828
diagnosis, 137
diagnostic criteria, 131, 132 *(table)*
management, 137
moyamoya disease, 555
predisposition to malignant tumours, 491
segmental (NF5), 136
type 1 (NF1), 131–136
brainstem tumours, 499
cutaneous manifestations, 132–133
hydrocephalus, 197
inheritance, 131
neurological manifestations, 133–136
prevalence, 131
visual pathway glioma, 502, 503 *(fig.)*
type 2 (NF2), 131, 136
acoustic neuroma, 692
cerebellar calcification, 344
Neurofibromatosis–Noonan syndrome, 137
Neurogenic muscular atrophy, bulbar/bulbo-pontine types, 706
Neurogenic stridor, 738
Neuroichthyosis syndromes, 146–147
Neuroleptic malignant syndrome, 765
Neuromuscular diseases, 697–698
investigations, 697–698
Neuromuscular junction disorders, 776–780
Neuromyelitis optica, 445
Neuromyotonia, 766–767
Neuron migration, 72
Neuronal ceroid–lipofuscinoses, 330
adult, 332
congenital, 332
fingerprint inclusions, 332
infantile, 330–331
late, 331
juvenile, 331
treatment, 332–333
see also Ceroid–lipofuscinosis
Neuronal degeneration, progressive of childhood (PNDC) with hepatic involvement, 329
Neuronal intranuclear inclusion disease, 334
Neuronal necrosis
parasagittal pattern, 42, 43 *(fig.)*
selective, 42
Neurons, energy metabolism defect, 348
Neuropathy with liability to pressure palsies, 732
Neurosarcoidosis, 737
Neurosyphilis, 12
Neurotic states, hypersomnia, 657
Neurotoxins, 421–422
Neurotransmitter metabolism disorders, 277–282
Neurotrichosis, 147
Neurulation disorders, 72–87, 88 *(fig.)*, 89
NF1 gene, 131, 137, 492
NF2 gene, 131, 492
N-hexane neuropathy, 730
Niaprazine, fainting induction, 639
Nicotinic acid deficiency, 798
Niemann–Pick disease, 249–241, 671
cherry-red spot, 247
type C, 302–303, 657

type D, 303
Night blindness, congenital stationary, 679
Night terrors, 654–655
Nightmares, 654–655
Nitric oxide, hypoxic–ischaemic encephalopathy, 40
Nitrites, 651
Nitrofurantoin, toxic neuropathy, 729–730
NMDA receptors, 576
Nocardia, 390
cerebral abscess, 391
Nocturnal awakening, 657
Nonaccidental injury, subdural haematoma, 466
Non-Hodgkin lymphoma, 516
ataxia–telangiectasia, 142
Noncalcifying meningeal angiomatosis of Divry and van Bogaert, 327
Nonketotic hyperglycinaemia, 278–280
atypical cases, 279
clinical features, 279–280
diagnosis, 280
early-onset, 279
inheritance, 278
neuropathology, 279
pathogenesis, 279
treatment, 280
Noonan phenomenon, 137
Norrie disease, 681
Notochord, 70
Nutritional disorders, 795–798
Nystagmus, 673–675
acquired, 675
albinism, 674
causes, 674–675
cerebellar ataxia, 450
congenital motor, 674
congenital sensory, 674
connatal Pelizaeus–Merzbacher disease, 738
convergence retraction, 671
differential diagnosis, 673–674
gaze-evoked, 673
head nodding, 674
head shaking, 674–675
internuclear ophthalmoplegia, 672
jerk, 673
latent, 675
osteopetrosis, 808
paroxysmal vertigo, 643
Pelizaeus–Merzbacher disease, 325–326
pendular, 673
retractorius, 197
vestibular, 673

O

O-HAHA syndrome, 356
Obsessive–compulsive disorder, 854–855
Obsessive–compulsive traits, 345
Occipital neuralgia, 181, 733
OCT gene, 283
Ocular abnormalities, hydrocephalus, 191, 197
Ocular flutter, 675
Ocular hypermetria, 675
Ocular motor apraxia, 672–673
Ocular motor function disorders
gaze palsies, 670–673
ocular motor apraxia, 672–673
peripheral ocular motor nerve involvement, 667–670
see also Nystagmus

Ocular motor nerve palsy/paralysis, 499, 670
  acquired, 667, 668 (table)
    IVth nerve, 667
    postinfectious VIth nerve, 667–668
Ocular oscillations, 673
  different from nystagmus, 675
Oculocardiac reflex, 638–639
Oculocerebrorenal syndrome, 246
Oculogyric crises, 643
Odontoid process, abnormal, 179–180
Ohtahara syndrome, 93, 584
Oligosaccharidoses, 256
Olivopontocerebellar atrophy, 274
  neonatal onset, 256
Ollier disease, 506
Ondine's curse, 656
One-and-a-half syndrome, 672
Opercular dysgenesis, syndrome of bilateral, 598
Opercular dysplasia, unilateral, 103
Ophthalmoplegia
  acquired, 667–669
  congenital, 669–670
    myopathy, 757
  internuclear, 671–672
  progressive
    external, 770
    extraocular, 771
  spinal muscular atrophy type III, 704
Oppositional defiant disorder, 843
  ADHD and DAMP, 847, 848
Opsoclonus, 675
Opsoclonus–myoclonus syndrome, 449,
    450–451
  deafness, 692
Optic atrophy, 676
  autosomal recessive, 682
  complicated, 678
  congenital, 677–678
  deafness, 691
  diabetes mellitus, 682
  dominant hereditary, 682
  dystonia, 682
  head injury, 469
  neuropathy, 730
Optic chiasm, visual pathway glioma, 502
Optic glioma, 502–504
  diagnosis, 133–134
  neurofibromatosis type 1, 133–134, 135
    (fig.)
  treatment, 134
Optic nerve
  coloboma, 677
  compression, 177
  disorders, 681–682
  glioma, 682
  hypoplasia, 677
  involvement in diabetic children, 799–800
Optic nerve head drusen, 677, 678 (fig.)
Optic neuritis, 446, 683
Optic neuropathy
  compressive, 682
  demyelinating, 683
  nutritional, 682–683
  toxic, 682–683
Optic tract hamartoma, neurofibromatosis
    type 1, 134, 135 (fig.)
Optico-cochleo-dentate degeneration, 691
Oral contraceptives, cerebral vein thrombosis,
    559

Orbital pseudotumour, 669
Organ of Corti
  abnormalities, 690–691
  degeneration, 690
Organic acid catabolism disorders, 264–277
Organic acidaemia, 54
Organic aciduria, 33
  neurological signs, 273 (fig.)
Organophosphates, 479
Ornithine carbamoyltransferase (ornithine trans-
    carbamylase)deficiency, 283, 284, 357
Oro-facial-digital syndrome type I, 109
Oscillopsia, 694
Osmoles, idiogenic, 793
Osseous dysplasia, neurofibromatosis type 1,
    136
Ossifying myositis, 774
Osteoarticular disorders, 698
Osteogenesis imperfecta, 178, 179, 472
Osteoid osteoma, 698
Osteomalacia, 698
  myotonia, 774
Osteomyelitis, vertebral, 393
Osteopetrosis, 177, 808
  congenital optic atrophy, 677
  with renal acidosis and cerebral calcification,
    344
Osteoporosis, 698
Osteosarcoma, brain metastases, 510
Otitis media
  deafness, 692
  facial nerve paralysis, 737
Oxycephaly, 174 (fig.)

P
P_0 gene mutations, 713, 716
$P21^{ras}$ oncogene, 492
$P53$ tumour suppressor gene, 492
Pachygyria, 94, 96–100, 101
  and leukodystrophy, 327
Pachygyria-like cortex with extracerebral abnor-
    malities, 103
Pain, indifference to, 720–721
  insensitivity, 720
Palatal myoclonus and progressive ataxia syn-
    drome, 334
Pallister–Hall syndrome, 506
Panarteritis nodosa, inflammatory vasculitides,
    558
Pandysautonomia, acute pure, 727
Panhypopituitarism, empty sella syndrome, 518
Panic attacks, 641
Papilloedema
  brain tumours, 395 (fig.), 493
  Guillain–Barré syndrome, 724
  visual pathway glioma, 502
Paragonimus spp., 420
Paralysis
  flaccid, 726 (table), 730
  postictal, 594
  see also Hemiplegia; Paraplegia; Spastic para-
    plegia; Tetraplegia
Paramyotonia congenita, 763–764
Paranasal sinus mucocele, 507
Paraneoplastic cerebellar syndrome, 516
Paraneoplastic limbic encephalitis, 402
Paraplegia
  spinal cord injury, 57–58
  tropical, 798

X-linked type 2, 355
  see also Hemiplegia; Paralysis; Spastic para-
    plegia; Tetraplegia
Parasitic infestation, 419, 420
Parasitic myositis, 773
Paraspinal neuroblastoma, 523 (fig.), 524
Parathyroid disease, 805
Parinaud syndrome, 197, 505
  aneurysm of vein of Galen, 537
Parkinsonism, infantile/juvenile, 340
Paroxysmal depolarization shift, 575
Paroxysmal disorders, 573
  breath-holding attacks, 573
  of consciousness, 654
  faints, 573
  febrile convulsions, 573
  of sleep, 654–655
  see also Epilepsy
Paroxysmal dyskinesias, 644–646
Paroxysmal dystonia, 646
  nocturnal, 655
Paroxysmal EEG discharge, 616
Paroxysmal events, nonepileptic, 606
Paroxysmal pain syndrome of early onset, 721
Paroxysmal tonic upgaze of childhood, benign,
    647, 671
Paroxysmal torticollis of infancy, benign, 643–
    644
Parry–Romberg disease, 147
Parsonage–Turner syndrome, 730
Parvovirus B19, 12, 23
Pasteurella spp., 385
Patau syndrome, 156
Pearson syndrome, 290
Pectus carinatum, malignant hyperthermia, 765
PEHO syndrome, 254
  optic atrophy, 678
Pelizaeus–Merzbacher disease, 222, 226, 325–
    326, 354, 355, 738
  diagnosis, 326
  types, 325
Pellagra, 798
Pena–Shokeir syndrome, 774
Pencil glioma, 506
Pendred syndrome, 691
Peri-intraventricular haemorrhage, see Periven-
    tricular–intraventricular haemorrhage
Pericerebral collections
  cryptogenic, 204–205
  nontraumatic, 204–205
Perinatal disease, prenatal factors, 32
Periodic hypothermia and diaphoresis, 109
Periodic paralysis
  with disturbances in cardiac rhythm and dys-
    morphism, 764
  dyskalaemic secondary, 765
  hyperkalaemic, 764
  hypokalaemic, 764, 765, 774
  normokalaemic, 764
  secondary, 764–765
  thyrotoxicosis, 805
Periodic syndrome, 650
Peripheral malformations, 70
Peripheral nerve disorders, 712
  localized, 730–733
  neurofibromatosis type 2, 136
  radiation-induced lesions, 515
Peripheral nerve tumours in neurofibromatosis
    type 1, 135

polyarteritis nodosa, 440, 730
Schönlein–Henoch purpura, 441, 558
Sydenham chorea, 438–439
Rheumatoid arthritis, 440–441
neuropathy, 730
Rhizomelic chondrodysplasia punctata, 259, 260, 262
Rhizopus, 418
Rhomboencephalosynapsis, 115
Rhythmias, 647
Rickets, myotonia, 774
Rickettsial infection, 395
Kawasaki disease, 441
Rigid spine syndrome, 754
Riley–Day syndrome, 719–720
Ring chromosomes 14 and 20 in epilepsy, 613
Rippling muscle disease, 766
Rochalimaea henselae, 395
Rosenberg–Chutorian syndrome, 691
Rosenthal fibres, 328
Ross syndrome, 733
Rossolimo sign, 524
congenital hemiplegia, 215
Rotavirus infection
encephalopathy, 409
transient acute myositis, 773
Roussy–Lévy syndrome, 350–351
Rubella, 3, 6
congenital, 8–9
deafness, 692
optic atrophy, 677
encephalitis, 406
optic neuritis, 683
progressive panencephalitis, 9, 411
vaccination, 452
Rubinstein–Taybi syndrome, 162
Russell–Silver syndrome, 23

S
Saccade palsy syndrome, 672
Saccades slowness, 672–673
Sacral agenesis, 73, 86
Saethre–Chotzen syndrome, 176–177
Sagittal callosotomy, 621–622
St Vitus dance, *see* Sydenham chorea
Salicylate toxicity, Reye syndrome, 408
Salla disease, 246, 255
Salmonella spp., 385
Salt excess, 794
Sandhoff disease, 247–248
Sandifer syndrome, 647
Sanfilippo disease, 254
Santavuori–Haltia–Hagberg disease, 330–331
Saponin, 246
Sarcoidosis, 448
deafness, 692
Sarcoplasmic reticulum, adenosine triphosphate deficiency, 766
Scalp, congenital defects, 86–87
Scaphocephaly, 174 *(fig.)*
Scapulohumeral muscular dystrophy, 755
Scapulohumeral syndrome with dementia, 754
Scapuloperoneal amyotrophy of neural origin, 717
Scapuloperoneal syndrome, 705, 755
Scheibe defect, 690
Scheie disease, 254
Schilder myelinoclastic diffuse sclerosis, 445–446

Schistosomiasis, 730
Schizencephaly, 69, 110
clinical features, 110
congenital hemiplegia, 214
diagnosis, 110, 111
see also Porencephaly
Schizophrenia, 641
childhood, 839–840
Schönlein–Henoch purpura, 441
inflammatory vasculitides, 558
Schwann cell diseases, 712
Schwannoma, neurofibromatosis type 2, 136
Schwartz–Jampel syndrome, 732, 767
malignant hyperthermia, 765
Sciatic nerve injuries, 732
Sciatic neuralgia, disc herniation, 732
Sclerosing panencephalitis, subacute, *see* Subacute sclerosing panencephalitis
SCN4A gene, 763, 765
Scoliosis
diastematomyelia, 84
Duchenne muscular dystrophy, 752
Friedreich ataxia, 350
glutaric aciduria type I, 271 *(fig.)*
hydrocephalus due to myelomeningocele, 80
hypomelanosis of Ito, 145
neurofibromatosis type 1, 136
syringomyelia, 86
Sebaceous naevus of Jadassohn, 143
Segawa disease, 339–340
Segmental demyelination, 712, 713 *(fig.)*
Seitelberger disease, *see* Neuroaxonal dystrophy
Seizures
acute bacterial meningitis, 376
aetiology of disorders, 577–579
Alpers disease, 296
Angelman syndrome, 159
anoxic, 606, 638–641
respiratory obstruction, 640
arterial occlusive disorders, 553
ataxic cerebral palsy, 224
atypical tonic–clonic, 592
autism, 828
behavioural control, 621
cavernous angioma, 538
cerebral hemisphere
glioma, 507
meningioma, 509
complex of temporal lobe origin, 597
congenital heart disease surgery, 801
Crouzon syndrome, 176
diabetic ketoacidosis, 799
diphtheria–tetanus–pertussis (DTP) vaccine, 452
Down syndrome, 155
drug treatment, 614–621
ECMO, 802
epileptic, 575
epileptic–anoxic, 638
febrile, 575
focal clonic, 607
focal cortical dysplasia, 105
gelastic, 598
generalized, 575, 579
generalized tonic–clonic syndromes, 591–592
head injury, 464
hemimegalencephaly, 93, 94
hydrocephalus, 191

hypernatraemia, 794
hypomelanosis of Ito, 145
idiopathic frontal, 596
incontinentia pigmenti, 145
inherited neonatal metabolic disorders, 54
late hypocalcaemia, 52–53
Lennox–Gastaut syndrome, 585–587
maternal narcotic addiction, 609
measles immunization, 451
MELAS syndrome, 296
migraine, 650
mild/minor head injuries, 463
movement-induced, 604
multicarboxylase deficiency, 285
multiple sclerosis, 444
mumps–measles–rubella vaccine, 452
myoclonic, 587
ketogenic diet, 621
myoclonic–atonic, 606
neonatal, 607–610
causes, 609–610
clinical features, 607–609
prognosis, 610
treatment, 610
neurocutaneous melanosis, 146
neurofibromatosis type 1, 133, 135 *(fig.)*
nocturnal, 595
nodular heterotopia, 96
nonconvulsive, 575
occasional, 607
partial, 579, 589
complex, 593
epileptic syndromes of childhood, 593–598
migratory, 589
simple, 593
temporal lobe origin, 596–597
post-traumatic, 469
prenatal, 610
preterm infants, 608
psychiatric disorders, 865–866
psychic/psychogenic, 641
pyridoxine dependency, 797
selenium deficiency, 798
self-induced photomyoclonic, 593
serial, 599
somatomotor, 593–594
somatosensory, 597–598
Sturge–Weber syndrome, 543
sylvian, 594
symptomatic, 578
thrombosis, 559–560
tonic repeated, 602
toxic origin, 643
tricyclic antidepressants, 478
tuberous sclerosis, 137–138
tyrosinaemia type I, 267
see also Pseudoseizures
Selenium deficiency, 798
Sellar region tumours, 506–507
Semantic–pragmatic disorder, 838, 851
Sensory neuropathy, congenital/radicular, 719
Septo-optic dysplasia, 111, 117, 677
Serratia marcescens, 56, 385
cerebral abscess, 392
Serum sickness, 453
Setting sun sign, 191, 466
Severe autosomal recessive muscular dystrophy of childhood (SCARD), 755

893

Systemic lupus erythematosus, 439–440, 558, 730

T
T-cell leukaemia virus type 1, *see* HTLV-1 infection
Taenia solium, 420
Takayasu arteritis, 557 *(fig.)*, 558
Tangier disease, 723
Tapetoretinal degeneration
    congenital, 678–679
    deafness syndromes, 691
Tardive dyskinesia, 344–345
Tarui disease, 768
Tay disease, *see* Trichothiodystrophy
Tay–Sachs disease, 246–247
Tectocerebellar dysraphia, 115
Telangiectasia, 141, 539
    hereditary haemorrhagic, 547
Telemetric EEG, 611
Telencephalic pseudo-monoventricle, 89
Telencephalic vesicles, 70
Temporal horn entrapment, 192
Tendon reflex, congenital hemiplegia, 215
Tensilon test, 777
Tentorial haemorrhage, 33
Terry bodies, 246
Tetanus, 421
    antitoxin, 453
Tetany, 643
    neonatal, 52
    normocalcaemic, 795
Tethered cord syndrome, *see* Diastematomyelia
Tetrad of Perlstein, 222
Tetradihydrobiopterin, 264
Tetrahydrobiopterin deficiency, 277–278
    clinical manifestations, 278
    diagnosis, 278
    genetic background, 277
    treatment, 278
Tetrahydrofolate, 288
Tetrahydrofolate reductase, 73
Tetraplegia, 212, 217, 220
    autosomal recessive, 220
    brain malformations, 220
Tetrasomy 15, partial, 859
Thalamic haemorrhage, 34
Thalamic necrosis, acute symmetrical, 417
Thalamic reticular system excitation, 575–576
Thalamus tumours, 511–512
Thalassaemia, 23, 806
Thallium poisoning, 481
Thanatophoric dwarfism, 178
Theophylline, 479
Theory of mind, 817, 819
    Asperger syndrome, 838
    autism, 828
Thermosensitive neuropathy, 717
Thiamine deficiency, 797
Third ventricle tumours, 506–507
Thomsen disease, 763
    malignant hyperthermia, 765
Thrombocytopenia
    immune, 34
    intrauterine, 23
Thrombocytopenic purpura, 807
Thrombocytosis, cerebral vein thrombosis, 559
Thrombosis, 548
    cerebral vein, 559–560

hypovolaemia, 793
    sinus, 560, 669
    venous
        intracranial haemorrhage, 35
        neonatal, 55
Thrombotic occlusion, sylvian artery, 647
Thyroid disease, 804–805
    Hashimoto thyroiditis, 441
    myopathy, 774
Thyrotoxicosis, 805
Thyrotropin, 502
Thyroxine synthesis, genetic defect, 691
Tibial pseudoarthrosis, neurofibromatosis type 1, 136
Tick paralysis, 730
Tick-borne encephalitides, 403–404
Tics, 345, 439
    ADHD and DAMP, 847, 848
    management, 854
    Tourette syndrome, 853
Tight filum terminale syndrome, 83
Tobacco smoking, 22
    Leber hereditary optic neuropathy, 682
Tocolytic drugs, 21
Todd paralysis, 594, 605
Tolosa–Hunt syndrome, 668–669
    idiopathic cranial polyneuropathy, 739
    ophthalmoplegia, 669
Toluene, 22
Tonic pupil of Adie, 684
Torticollis
    benign paroxysmal of infancy, 643–644
    congenital, 776
    paroxysmal, 338
Tourette syndrome, 345, 853–854
    ADHD and DAMP, 847, 848
    diagnosis, 853, 854
    epidemiology, 853
    minimal brain dysfunction syndromes, 843
    obsessive–compulsive disorder, 855
    outcome, 854
    pathogenesis, 853
    stuttering, 850–851
    tics, 439
    treatment, 854
    work-up, 854
Toxi-infections, 421–422
Toxic neuropathies
    endogenous, 729
    exogenous, 729–730
Toxic shock syndrome, influenza virus, 409
Toxoplasma, 3
    fetal infection, 6
Toxoplasma gondii, 9, 10, 420
    cerebral abscess, 391
    dermatomyositis-like syndrome, 772
Toxoplasmosis
    acquired, 420
    choroidoretinitis, 679
    congenital, 9–11
    clinical manifestations, 9–10
    diagnosis, 10, 11
    prevention, 10–11
    hydrocephalus, 196, 204
    severe neonatal, 9
Transferrin deficiency, 258
Transient cerebral ischaemia, dyskinesia, 647
Transient ischaemic attacks, 551
Translocase deficiency, 298

Transverse myelitis, 446–447
    acute, 522
    immunization-induced, 453
Trauma
    head injuries, 460–462
    intracerebellar haematoma, 467
Traumatic nerve injuries, 731–733
Traumatic paralysis with facial nerve paralysis, 737
Treacher–Collins syndrome, 690
Tremor
    dyskinetic cerebral palsy, 221
    essential, 345–346
    hereditary, 345–346
    protein–calorie malnutrition, 796
Treponema pallidum
    DNA, 12
    fetal infection, 6
    immobilization test, 12
Trichinosis, parasitic myositis, 773
Trichopoliodystrophy, *see* Menkes disease
Trichothiodystrophy, 147
Tricyclic antidepressants, 478
Triglyceride storage disease, multisystem, 769
Trigonocephaly, 89
Trihydroxycholestanaemia, 263
Trihydroxycholestanoic acid, 259, 262, 263
Triose phosphate isomerase deficiency, 806
Triplegia, 220
Trisomy 8, 156
Trisomy 12p, 613
Trisomy 13, 156
Trisomy 18, 156
    minor morphological anomalies, 166
Trisomy 21, 4
    see also Down syndrome
Trochlear nerve paralysis, 669
    congenital, 670
Tropheryma whippleii, 395
Troyer syndrome, 351
Tuberculoma, 387, 389
Tuberculosis, cerebral abscess, 391
Tuberculous encephalopathy, 387, 388
Tuberous sclerosis, 89, 131, 137–140, 862–863
    autism, 828, 863
    clinical manifestations, 137–138
    cutaneous manifestations, 138–139
    diagnosis, 140, 242
    formes frustes, 577
    genetic counselling, 140
    infantile spasms, 583
    inheritance, 137
    management, 140
    neurodevelopmental difficulties, 138
    pathology, 137
    prevalence, 137
Tuberous sclerosis–autism–epilepsy syndrome, 833
Turcot syndrome of colonic polyposis and brain tumours, 491
Turner syndrome, 163, 862
Twin pregnancy
    cerebral palsy, 211
    singleton birth, 3
Twins
    craniosynostoses, 171
    hydranencephaly–porencephaly, 14
Typus degenerativus amstelodamensis, 161
Tyrosinaemia type I, 266–267

NOTES

NOTES

NOTES